Kuntz / Kuntz † · Hepatology, Textbook and Atlas

Erwin Kuntz · Hans-Dieter Kuntz †

HEPATOLOGY

TEXTBOOK AND ATLAS

History · Morphology
Biochemistry · Diagnostics
Clinic · Therapy

With 530 Coloured Illustrations and 321 Coloured Tables

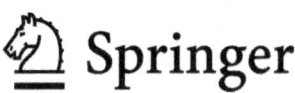

Professor Dr. med. Dr. med. h.c. Erwin Kuntz
Auf dem Kronberg 6

35582 Wetzlar
Germany

ISBN 978-3-662-49970-2   ISBN 978-3-540-76839-5 (eBook)
DOI 10.1007/978-3-540-76839-5

Springer Medizin Verlag Heidelberg

This work is subject to copyright. All rights are reserved, whether the whole or part of the material is concerned, specifically the rights of translation, reprinting, reuse of illustrations, recitation, broadcasting, reproduction on microfilm or in any other way, and storage in data banks. Duplication of this publication or parts thereof is permitted only under the provisions of the German Copyright Law of September 9, 1965, in its current version, and permission for use must always be obtained from Springer-Verlag. Violations are liable for prosection under the German Copyright Law.

Springer Medizin Verlag

springer.de

© Springer Medizin Verlag Heidelberg 2002, 2006, 2008
Printed in Germany

Softcover reprint of the hardcover 3rd edition 2008

The use of general descriptive names, registered names, trademarks, etc. in this publication does not imply, even in the absence of a specific statement, that such names are exempt from the relevant protective laws and regulations and therefore free for general use.
Product liability: The publishers cannot guarantee the accuracy of any information about the application of operative techniques and medications contained in this book. In every individual case the user must check such information by consulting the relevant literature.

Cover design: deblik Berlin
Typesetting: paginamedia GmbH, Hemsbach/Bergstraße
Printing and Binding: Stürtz GmbH, Würzburg

Printed on acid-free paper   SPIN 11979746   2126/SM   5 4 3 2 1 0

Dedication

In 1978, my son and I began with the planning and preparation of a joint textbook on hepatology. In 1997, one year before completion of this work, Hans-Dieter died of a malignant disease. It was his wish that I should realize our mutual aim.

I have dedicated the **German edition** of the book "Praktische Hepatologie" (1998) to:

my unforgettable son *Hans-Dieter*

whose knowledge and manual skill I have always admired,

whose critical as well as creative ideas for our joint book were
so valuable,

who did not live to see the completion of this work as a
co-author

dedicated in love and gratitude

Dedications

The 1st **English edition** of the book "Hepatology · Principles and Practice" (2002) is dedicated — also at my son's request — to:

Dr. med. Dr. rer. nat. *Herbert Falk* (Freiburg)

the most generous patron of hepatological research and further education,

the initiator of worldwide, international hepatology

dedicated in admiration and friendship

The 2nd **English edition** of the book "Hepatology · Principles and Practice" (2006) is dedicated to:

Prof. Dr. med. *Heribert Thaler* (Vienna)

who has united the histopathologic and clinical aspects of hepatology in such an excellent manner,

from whom I have learned so much in many years of friendship

dedicated in esteem and cordiality

The 3rd **English edition** of the book "Hepatology · Textbook and Atlas" (2008) is dedicated to:

Prof. Dr. med. Dr. h.c. mult. *Hubert E. Blum* (Freiburg)

who has enriched hepatology as a scientist, teacher and clinician in such an exemplary manner,

he remains a physician with a strong sense of vocation

dedicated in appreciation and respect

Authors

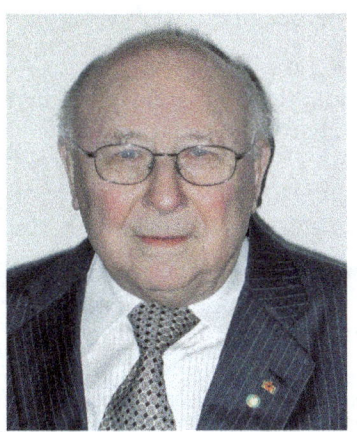

Prof. Dr. med. Dr. med. h. c. Erwin Kuntz
The author spent the first 16 years of his clinical career at the Medical University Hospital in Giessen (6 years as senior physician). Then followed 20 years as head physician at the Internal Department of the Academic Hospital in Schwäbisch Hall and at the Internal Department of the Academic Hospital in Wetzlar. For 45 years, he has taken an active part in the postgraduate education of physicians; he has been an organizer of numerous scientific congresses. Erwin Kuntz has received more than 25 national and international awards and honorary memberships. He has been presented the Honorary Doctorate of the University of Debrecen (Hungary) and is an Honorary Citizen of the region of Waldsolms. He is holder of the "Great Merit Cross of the Federal Republic of Germany", the "Great Merit Cross of the Republic of Italy" and the "Paracelsus Medal", which is the highest award given by the medical profession in Germany.

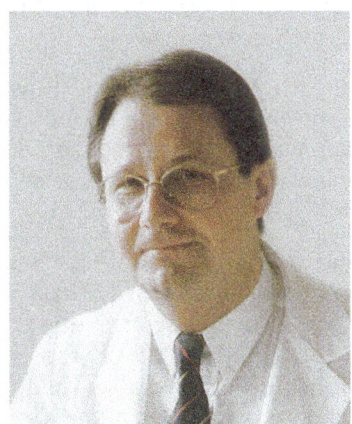

Prof. Dr. med. Hans-Dieter Kuntz
The co-author was certified as a specialist in internal medicine at the Academic Hospital in Duisburg. In 1980, he obtained his qualification as a gastroenterologist and became senior physician at the Department of Gastroenterology/Hepatology of the University Hospital in Bochum. As from 1989, he was head physician at the Department of Internal Medicine and Gastroenterology at Augusta Academic Hospital in Bochum. His many activities included the postgraduate education of physicians for 17 years. He was granted honorary membership of the Society of Gastroenterology of Uruguay (1993) and became a Fellow of the European Board of Gastroenterology (EUMS) (1996). Before the introduction of the German textbook "Praktische Hepatologie" (1998) together with his father he died due to a malignant disease at the age of 48.

Preface to the third Edition

Like the first edition, the second edition was sold out within one year, as was a special reprint available exclusively in the Far East. The extremely positive response from different countries around the world made it easy for both publisher and author to consider a third edition in the near future. We wished to create a textbook with an integrated hepatological atlas based on a form, colour design and scope that had not existed before. Nevertheless, we decided to keep the tried and tested concept of the original version: to serve as a teaching manual, textbook and reference work. Like its predecessor, the new edition has 40 self-contained chapters, each with its own detailed list of contents (using up to three decimal points). Once again, a big black dot is inserted whenever the following sentence represents a semantic leap from the preceding statement. The same fonts and letter sizes have been used. Each chapter finishes with an extensive bibliography. All authors are listed in full in semi-bold type and ordered alphabetically. About 7,000 references have been cited. I have retained historical papers which appeared to me to be in some way remarkable, but literature up to 2008 has also been included.

Due to the updating of the individual chapters, a revised index was required with about 3,000 terms and 12,000 page references. Using this index and the detailed table of contents at the beginning of each chapter, the reader is able to find everything easily and quickly. Furthermore, in the text itself, there are numerous cross-references to related descriptions, figures and tables in other chapters. This makes it possible to interconnect the extensive information contained in the 935-page textbook like a network.

There are more citations of first-time authors (with year) regarding syndromes, diagnostic methods, therapeutic measures, medicotechnical developments, surgical procedures, etc. Some 1,500 initial descriptions are mentioned (whereby numerous corrections had to be made in this respect). Such creative or innovative ideas have often led directly to significant progress or served as a new starting point for subsequent path-breaking developments. The notable achievements of earlier physicians or clinicians deserve great respect! Regrettably, such important scientists of the past tend to be forgotten in our fast-moving times. In this context, we would do well to remember the 2,000-year-old tradition of hepatology.

For that reason, I took great care in revising the chapter on "History of Hepatology". With its 20 historical figures, which have never before been published together, this chapter represents a special feature for all interested readers.

The comprehensive selection of colour illustrations has been extended to 530, so that the textbook has become a real atlas of hepatology. The 320 tables have been designed in different shades and colours. All figures and tables have been integrated in the textflow, making this edition especially attractive. So the book itself is designed to lead from "seeing" to "understanding" and, ultimately, to diagnostic and therapeutic "doing".

I should like to express my special gratitude for all the friendly assistance and helpful advice to the pathologist Prof. Dr. H. P. Fischer (Bonn), the radiologist Prof. Dr. K. Rauber (Wetzlar) as well as the gastroenterologists Prof. Dr. R. Jakobs (Wetzlar) and Dr. G. Schmidt (Kreuztal). In addition, I wish to thank the numerous colleagues who offered their support in preparing the first and second editions and whose names appear in the respective prefaces (see pp X and XII). The abbreviations or symbols frequently used are listed in the preface to the first edition together with all other information regarding dictionary and technical terms.

All my personal thoughts and emotions, which are written down in the first and second edition, have constantly been with my beloved son Hans-Dieter. This comprehensive volume must be seen as our joint life's work.

My special thanks go to the company Pagina Media (Hemsbach) for their excellent setting of all three editions and for their most friendly collaboration over many years. Finally, I thank the employees at Springer Publishing House (Heidelberg) for completing this book, with special mention of Hinrich Küster, senior editor, and Meike Seeker, project manager, for their encouragement and kind support at all times.

Wetzlar, May 2008   Erwin Kuntz

Foreword to the third edition

"...because the liver is a source of many diseases, and is a noble organ that serves many organs, almost all of them: so it suffers, it is not a small suffering, but a great and manifold one" (Paracelsus, 1493–1541). • This quotation already appears as a motto for the German edition "Praktische Hepatologie" (1998) written by Erwin Kuntz and his deceased son Hans-Dieter (1997 †). Even with our present-day level of knowledge, it is not possible to give a better definition of the key role played by the liver and of the various clinical pictures involved, which require a holistic approach.

Despite the fact that "empirical liver research" can boast of a long and cult-related tradition dating back to Babylonian and ancient Egyptian times and although the liver and/or its components have always been an important subject of basic research, clinical hepatology is a relatively recent discipline. A large number of biochemical, cell-biological and metabolic respondent mechanisms were studied and developed in connection with the liver; however, it took time for the results to be applied to clinical practice. Clinical hepatology became more widespread mainly due to the social relevance of liver diseases, which resulted from the significance of the liver as the central metabolic organ and the fact that the liver is the principal target and modulator of environmental influences on the human organism (e. g. toxic substances, alcohol, infections, diet), including drug therapy. The need for experts in clinical hepatology has evolved due to recent developments, such as discovery and characterization of hepatitis viruses, more specific treatment of viral liver diseases, liver transplantation, adverse effects of obesity with associated nonalcoholic fatty liver disease and frequency of complications in chronic liver diseases rising with age of the affected patients. Drug-induced liver damage is the price for medical progress in today's world. In spite of modern concepts used in the design of medicines, the liver remains particularly sensitive to side effects due to its biotransformational function and the pharmacogenetic characteristics of each individual person.

In his foreword to the first English edition of "Hepatology. Principles and Practice", Charles S. Lieber praises it as an international landmark in the field of clinical hepatology. And rightly so! The concept was, and still is, innovative in many respects. This is confirmed by the worldwide success of the book and the fact that the first two editions were completely sold out. The third edition entitled "Hepatology. Textbook and Atlas" with its numerous figures and coloured tables is a further extension of the original concept. In order to understand liver diseases in more depth, it is essential to have a basic knowledge of morphology, pathology, physiology and molecular biology in a clinical context. This book does justice to present-day liver research (also known as "biomolecular hepatology") without losing sight of the patient as the main focus of all efforts.

The new edition comprises 40 chapters, each with its own detailed table of contents for easy reference. The individual chapters deal in a lucid manner with historical aspects, modern diagnostic methods (not forgetting the classical form of bedside examination: "One good feel of the liver is worth any two liver function tests" – F. M. Hanger jr., 1971), symptomatology and general as well as specific effects of liver disease. The fluent and uniform style of presentation underlines the special value of a "one-author" book as opposed to "collective-author" books, which are more common today! Clearly structured information about aetiology, pathogenesis, clinical-pathological correlations, therapy and prognostic assessment helps the reader to gain a complete understanding of the material. A total of more than 500 figures turn the book into a true "atlas". All figures are excellently integrated into the textflow and literally illustrate the content. With the help of the high-quality laparoscopy- and histology-related figures, reading becomes a real pleasure, even for the pathologist. But it is not only the figures which give the book its "completeness". Another special feature are the historical aspects, which describe the development of hepatology up to the present day, and the general evolution of knowledge concerning the liver. This is achieved by stating the first-time authors of the respective clinical pictures, syndromes and advances in diagnostics, technology or therapy. The originators of relevant scientific theories are also mentioned.

The didactic approach which runs through the whole book is a clear indication of the author's immense practical experience in the field of hepatology as well as his understanding of the results of basic research, including the biological and pathological aspects which determine the given disease. Like Paracelsus, the author also looks beyond the liver in his deliberations. The reader also senses the long-term engagement of the author (and his son) in postgraduate education and the lessons learned from this. According to Papyrus Ebers (ca. 1550 BC), the liver is the "seat of emotions". And indeed, it is the emotions with which father and son began their undertaking that are clearly palpable and, at the same time, the key to success. It is only possible to impart knowledge and to convey enthusiasm if one has great personal involvement. This certainly applies to the authors, Erwin and Hans-Dieter Kuntz.

The current edition contains up-to-date information, but also stands for tradition and progress in hepatology. The reader is carefully introduced into the subject matter and learns to experience and understand everything to the full extent. Consequently, the book is not only a source of knowledge for the relatively small circle of hepatologists; due to the chosen form in which the material is presented, the book will surely arouse the interest of less specialized readers, including those involved in research. Thus this work serves as a starting point for new "liver enthusiasts". It is food for thought and a trigger for continued research. Our thirst for knowledge is unquenchable. This book lays out in an admirable fashion what is state of the art, but it makes no dogmatic statements. Therefore we have every reason to look forward to the next edition.

O. Univ. Prof. Dr. Helmut Denk, FRCPath
Director of the Institute of Pathology
University of Graz
Auenbruggerplatz 25
A-8036 Graz (Austria)

Preface to the second edition

Originally, it was the intention of both my son and me that the German edition of "Praktische Hepatologie" should be followed by an English translation. After Hans-Dieter's premature death due to a serious illness, I made it my aim to complete an English-language version of the textbook by myself, knowing that this would have been his great wish. The memory of my dear son was an inspiration to me in my efforts at all times.

It was a great sense of achievement for both author and publisher that the first edition (2002) was sold out within such a short period and that a reprint was necessary. This fact, supported by the positive response shown directly by readers and reviewers, was the main motivation to prepare a second edition.

A decision was made to keep the well-established division of hepatology into six specialist areas; once again, forty chapters were used. Each chapter has been revised and updated with regard to content and language. At the beginning, there is a detailed table of contents and, at the end, a list of references. Like its predecessor, the second edition contains a visually comprehensive arrangement of the text into sections, incorporating various script sizes and types as well as 306 tables in half-tone colouring; significant conclusions are set in coloured boxes. A big, black dot is inserted whenever the following sentence represents a semantic leap from the preceding statement. (For further details regarding the structural concept of the chapters, see preface to 1st edition, page VII, paragraph 2.)

Altogether, about 7,000 references have been cited, of which some 1,500 have been replaced by more recent papers, including many from 2005. The Vancouver-style layout has been used again, since it proved to be clear and easy to read. (For further details regarding the extensive bibliography, see preface to 1st edition, page VII, paragraph 3.)

Every effort has been made to maintain and improve the concept of citing, whenever possible, the first-time authors of syndromes, clinical entities, morphological or clinical findings, imaging or endoscopic techniques and conservative or surgical measures. (For further details, see preface to 1st edition, page VII, paragraph 4.)

The number of coloured figures has been increased by 97 to a total of 477; developments in printing techniques make possible an even more colourful presentation with brilliant reproduction. All the figures are integrated in the text-flow. In this way, a hepatological atlas has been created, leading from "seeing" to "understanding", thereby facilitating diagnostic and therapeutic "acting".

My special thanks for their friendly assistance and helpful advice go to the pathologists Prof. Dr. H.-P. Fischer (Bonn) and Prof. Dr. G. Korb (Weiden), the radiologist Prof. Dr. K. Rauber (Wetzlar), the hepatologist Prof. Dr. J. Eisenburg (Munich), the virologist Prof. Dr. G. Berencsi (Budapest), the immunologist Prof. Dr. W. Storch (Weinheim) and the gastroenterologist Dr. G. Schmidt (Kreuztal). (In addition, numerous colleagues offered their support in preparing the first edition; they are named in the preface to 1st edition – see page VII, paragraphs 5 and 6.)

The abbreviations or symbols frequently used in the text are listed in the preface to the first edition (see page VIII).

All my personal thoughts and emotional feelings, which were written down in the first edition, are unchanged. This applies also to the two quotations from **PARACELSUS** at the beginning and end of the book. But, above all, how extremely happy and proud I would have been if my son Hans-Dieter could have joined me as co-author in achieving our common aim.

It is my sincere wish that this textbook will not only promote interest in the field of hepatology, but also deepen understanding of pathophysiological and morphological changes regarding liver as well as supporting successful application of the various diagnostic and therapeutic possibilities.

Finally, I should like to express my gratitude to the employees at Springer Publishing House (Heidelberg) for their professional help in completing this book, especially to Hinrich Küster, senior editor, and Meike Seeker, project manager, who gave their encouragement and kind support at all times.

Wetzlar, October 2005   Erwin Kuntz

Foreword to the second edition

The first edition of "Hepatology: Principles and Practice" by Erwin Kuntz, which appeared in 2002, was rapidly sold out. This was not astonishing since the textbook offered a comprehensive, lucid and scholarly presentation of liver disease. Informative figures and tables made reading a pleasure. The second edition has now been revised and updated to 2005 by Erwin Kuntz. Once again, the author, a distinguished hepatologist, has produced an encyclopedic masterpiece of hepatology. The book combines a complete scientific and historical discussion of the many aspects of hepatology together with the wise insight of a physician who has enormous practical experience in caring for patients with liver disease.

The second edition has been enlarged to more than 900 pages, a change necessitated by the enormous increase in our understanding of liver disease. The number of references that are cited now stands at 7,000; references are given in full and in alphabetical order, a feature that will prove most helpful to physicians engaged in teaching and research. The judicious use of color for figures and tables made the first edition extremely attractive to the reader. This practice is continued in the second edition which contains a further 97 figures and 30 tables, making a total of 477 figures and 306 tables. A special feature is the quality of the superb laparoscopic and histological pictures. Indeed, the colored figures are of such superior quality that they can be scanned directly for computer-based presentations. The histological illustrations are especially valuable as the number of autopsies and liver biopsies continues to decline worldwide. Moreover, these illustrations have been integrated perfectly into the text. The publishers, true to their long tradition, have done justice to the quality of this work in every way. The book is not only a true handbook of liver disease, but also a hepatological atlas.

Like its predecessor, the second edition also comprises 40 chapters. At the beginning of each chapter, there is a complete table of contents, which, together with the general index, makes it possible for the reader to find specific topics easily. The first chapter "History of Hepatology" is an indication of the depth and breadth of the knowledge which the author brings to the current edition. This chapter contains a richness of historical illustrations depicting the birth of knowledge of this multifaceted organ. The following chapters of the book show the profound knowledge and interest of Erwin Kuntz in the multiple spectra of hepatology. Each topic shows the evolution of our knowledge and acknowledges by name the individuals who contributed to our present knowledge. In this way, hepatology is not only discussed as a contemporary branch of internal medicine, but also related to the pioneering achievements of our ancestors, who deserve our full respect and recognition. The historical emphasis is global, rather than European. Throughout the book, detailed histological depictions of hepatic pathology have been fused with scientific aspects and clinical procedures. All forms of treatment have been updated, so that this work can be used as a manual of therapy which will be highly useful to both practitioners and teachers.

As Charles S. Lieber, New York, wrote three years ago in his foreword to the first edition, such a textbook could not have appeared at a better time. This statement applies to the second edition in the year 2005. Great progress has been made in hepatology with regard to diagnostics and therapy, and consequently, the number of publications dealing with, for example, the treatment of viral hepatitis has grown immensely. Likewise, there is much new information on the pathogenesis of autoimmune liver diseases and so-called overlap syndromes. Thus it is essential that the current body of knowledge is presented in an intensive and accurate form.

It is a pleasure to know Prof. Dr. Erwin Kuntz personally. His enthusiasm for hepatology is contagious and can be sensed in every chapter. To be shown his enormous private library and pictorial archive is a moving experience. This impressive collection contains important papers and original monographs of authors from past and present and provides the data base for this fascinating textbook.

We would like to wish this new edition from Erwin Kuntz the same resounding success which was enjoyed by the first edition. We are convinced that the book will not only find its place in every medical library, but also be consulted repeatedly by scientists and physicians who seek to understand how we can use its contents to improve the care of our patients with liver disease.

Ulrich F. Leuschner, M. D.
Professor of Medicine,
Johann Wolfgang Goethe University
Frankfurt/M., Germany

Alan F. Hofmann, M. D.
Professor Emeritus of Medicine
University of California, San Diego
La Jolla, USA

Preface to the first edition

It is a wonderful experience for a father to work with his son on an enormous number of lectures, seminars, courses, congresses and publications over a period of many years. For a total of 35 (overlapping) years we were both active as clinicians in the field of hepatology. From this experience arose our wish to co-author a book on this fascinating subject. We were greatly encouraged in this project by friends and colleagues. • The joint work, supported by an extensive personal archive, a large number of clinical, endoscopic and morphological illustrations, and documentation of imaging technique findings, is intended to serve as a *teaching manual*, a *textbook*, and a *reference book* — for use in the doctor's surgery, in daily clinical practice, and in the specialist fields associated with hepatology.

After weighing up the various approaches and objectives of the book, the *concept* of subdividing the subject matter into 40 self-contained chapters presented itself. We set value on: — a systematic structure of the chapters, — a coherent presentation of facts and evidence, — a visually comprehensible arrangement of the text into sections, incorporating various script sizes and types, — half-tone colouring of tables and conclusions considered to be of exceptional importance, — consistent cross-referencing of figures, tables and text between different chapters, and the incorporation within the text of 276 tables, 380 figures, and numerous boxed texts (all in colour). • A big, black dot is inserted whenever the following sentence represents a mental leap from the preceding statement, which enables a more structured approach. • Our constant aim was to improve the readability and clarity of the book.

Each chapter has an extensive *bibliography*. We used a modified Vancouver-style layout, which we consider clear and easy to read. Authors' names (all authors are listed in full in the chapter bibliography) appear in semi-bold type and are ordered alphabetically for easy reference. As far as possible, we subdivided more extensive chapter bibliographies thematically. A total of 7,300 *publications* up to 2001 are cited. This detailed bibliography is intended to assist the interested reader in exploring specific areas in more depth. • We have therefore included both historical references and those older publications which we consider of particular significance or interest — there is always the danger, in hepatology as well as in other fields, that such works might regrettably become victims of our fast-moving times. There is certainly a subjective influence in this selection, and in this context any additions or corrections to the bibliography will be gratefully received.

A further conceptual concern was to cite, whenever possible, the *first authors* of publications on syndromes, clinical research, laboratory parameters, imaging or endoscopic techniques, morphological findings of special interest, and conservative, invasive and surgical procedures (and to correct previous information given in the literature). In the past, the creative or innovative ideas of these inaugurators have often led directly to significant progress or have served as a new starting point for subsequent, ground-breaking developments. Despite arduous research, it has not always been possible to attribute work correctly to the first author(s). Yet, the notable achievements of earlier physicians, clinicians and scientists deserve to be remembered with respect! In this connection, further information or corrections will be welcomed.

The extensive selection of *colour illustrations* incorporated into the text covers a wide range of clinical and morphological findings in hepatology: it is designed to lead from *"seeing"* to *"understanding"*, thereby facilitating diagnostic and therapeutic *"acting"*. Although we had collected an extensive picture archive of our own over a period of more than 30 years of clinical practice, we were nevertheless able to complement this and close any gaps thanks to numerous illustrations and impressive findings generously made available to us by colleagues. My special thanks for their friendly assistance go to the pathologists Prof. Dr. H.-P. Fischer (Bonn) and Prof. Dr. O. Klinge (Kassel), and to the radiologists Prof. Dr. K. Rauber (Wetzlar) and Prof. Dr. R. Heckemann (Bochum). Some very valuable documentations of findings could be used by courtesy of Prof. Dr. J. Eisenburg (Munich), Prof. Dr. K.-M. Müller (Bochum), Prof. Dr. G. Piekarski (Bonn), Prof. Dr. H. Thaler (Vienna), Prof. Dr. G. Volkheimer (Berlin), Prof. Dr. O. Vorländer (Berlin), and Prof. Dr. W. Wermke (Berlin).

We repeatedly enlisted the *helpful advice* of friends and colleagues to supplement or confirm our own interpretations. Our opinions not infrequently diverged (and in the field of hepatology, this can only be an advantage) and personal opinions were modified or confirmed. The contacts arising from these discussions have been immensely rewarding to me. Here I should like to express my special thanks to: Prof. Dr. G. Berencsi (Budapest), Prof. Dr. R. Klein (Tuebingen), Prof. Dr. H. K. Seitz (Heidelberg) and Prof. Dr. W. Storch (Weinheim). • Very many thanks for advisory support also go to: Prof. Dr. H.-R. Duncker (Institute of Anatomy, Univ. of Giessen), Priv. Doz. Dr. Marietta Horster (Institute of Classics and Ancient History, Univ. of Cologne) and Prof. Dr.

Preface

N. Katz (Institute of Biochemistry, Univ. of Giessen). • Receiving such varied and kind assistance and advice has filled me with gratitude and encouragement during the years spent compiling this book.

In preparing the book my thoughts and my loving gratitude have constantly been with *my son, Hans-Dieter*, whose death was so sudden and incomprehensible to us all. I have tried to represent his inspirations and detailed ideas as well as incorporating his particular clinical insights. This volume is thus our joint life's work. He will always be remembered as an example to us all.

At the beginning and end of the book I have purposely cited two quotations from PARACELSUS which have always made a deep impression on me. • In the course of such intensive engagement with the history of hepatology, one is repeatedly filled with respect and admiration for how our forebears, solely through sight, hearing and touch, and an ingenuity of methods − and through logical deduction − drew medical conclusions, recognized correlations and established an astounding body of theoretical and practical knowledge. Many of these empirical findings were subsequently confirmed − some (still) remain "empirical", without, however, having been disproved. *"Empiricism, Intuition and Logic"* (R. Gross, Cologne, 1988) will always be the leitmotif of the physician! • The considerable and fascinating developments in hepatology, especially those of the last ten years, remain a central theme. • The current stage of this development may well become known as the 4th (biomolecular) epoch of hepatology, as I have proposed in the first chapter of our book.

Finally, my thanks to the employees at *Springer* for the speedy completion of this book and especially to Jörg Engelbrecht and Dr. Dorothee Guth for their encouragement and kind support at all times.

Wetzlar, July 2001   Erwin Kuntz

Frequently used *abbreviations* and *symbols* in the textbook are listed in alphabetical order below:

s. fig.	see figure	ca.	circa	a.-v.	arterio-venous
s. figs.	see figures	e.g.	exempli gratia, for example	N.B.	nota bene, important
s. p.	see page	etc.	et cetera, and so on	i.m.	intramuscular
s. pp	see pages	i.e.	id est, that is	i.v.	intravenous
s. tab.	see table	quot.	quoted, quotation	s.c.	subcutaneous
s. tabs.	see tables	vs	versus	v.v.	vice versa, conversely

As regards the *half-tone colouring* and colour intensity, blue is used − as far as possible − for normal findings, classification, causes, indications, therapy regimen, etc., red applies to pathological findings, contraindications, complications, side effects, etc., yellow to methods, test procedures, etc., and grey to historical details.

Medical and technical terms, orthography and hyphenation in this textbook are based on: (*1.*) P. PROCTER (editor): Cambridge International Dictionary of English (Cambridge Univ. Press) 1999, 3rd edition; (*2.*) J. CROWTHER (editor): Oxford Advanced Learner's Dictionary (Oxford Univ. Press), 1999, 5th edition; (*3.*) J. DORLAND, W.A. NEWMAN (editors): Illustrated Medical Dictionary (W.B. Saunders, Philadelphia, et al.), 2000, 29th edition; (*4.*) F.J. NÖHRING (editor): Langenscheidt's Fachwörterbuch Medizin (Langenscheidt, Berlin, et al.), 1996, 3rd edition; (*5.*) W.E. BUNJES (editor): Medical and Pharmaceutical Dictionary (Thieme, Stuttgart, et al.), 1985, 4th edition; (*6.*) S. DRESSLER (editor): Dictionary of Clinical Medicine (Chapman & Hall, London, et al.), 1996.

Foreword to the first edition

The textbook "Hepatology. Principles and Practice" by Erwin Kuntz and Hans-Dieter Kuntz will undoubtedly become an international landmark. It reflects the scholarship, encyclopedic knowledge of the authors and the outstanding craftsmanship of the publishers. Professor Erwin Kuntz's stature was not only well established in Germany and the rest of Europe but his fame had crossed the Atlantic and I have known of him for many years. I also had the privilege of getting acquainted with him personally at an international meeting on phospholipids in Cologne in 1989 where I had the pleasure of enjoying both his intellectual and his broad humanistic qualities.

The book is not only an unusual combination of an extremely thorough textbook of all aspects of hepatology, including important pathogenic mechanisms and their clinical application, but it also has a very didactic approach which effectively highlights most points while not neglecting those details the academician or practitioner may want to find for needed clarification. It synthesizes more than 30 years of practical experience in clinical hepatology. Accordingly, it can be used as a teaching manual for students, postgraduate clinicians and practitioners, as a textbook for internists, gastroenterologists and hepatologists, as well as a reference book for teachers, scientists and authors. The original text has been revised and updated to 2000/2001. The bibliography now consists of about 7,300 papers and the number of colored figures has been increased to 380. It is a distillate of hundreds of personal publications and presentations and thousands of literature references of classic and contemporary scholars. The information is presented in such a way that it makes the facts very accessible and the chore of retrieval becomes a pleasure. The very vivid display of information gives unique insights providing a very rational approach to the practice of hepatology. This volume brilliantly achieves the basic aim of its authors, which is to guide the user from "seeing" to "understanding" and finally to "acting".

The book could have come at no better time. There is real blossoming of hepatology worldwide and its importance has increased logarithmically with the availability of transplantation and the pandemic of hepatitis C, with effective treatments finally evolving. Diagnostic procedures have also gained much greater sophistication and "interventional" hepatology is now finally on the rise. Being familiar with German, I had the pleasure of enjoying the original textbook but felt envious that this opus was limited to those fluent in that language. I am delighted to see that this work will now be shared worldwide in an English edition which has been thoroughly updated, with the most recent concepts and therapies reported and carefully assessed. Its comprehensive yet crisp and clear presentation will open the gates of hepatology to all health professionals. Last but not least, this work represents the highly humanistic qualities of its authors and is obviously an act of life time love, with abundant citations not only to our modern masters, but also giving proper credit to those who preceded them. Hippocrates already stated that the liver was the site of the soul; it is obvious that both Erwin Kuntz and his son, Hans-Dieter, have put their souls in this opus.

Charles S. Lieber M.D., M.A.C.P.
Professor of Medicine and Pathology
Mount Sinai School of Medicine
Director, Alcohol Research Center &
Section of Liver Disease & Nutrition
Bronx VA Medical Center
New York, USA

Abbreviations

Abbreviation:	Meaning:
A	
AA	Amino acid
AAA	Acitiactin antibody
AAA	Aromatic amino acid
AAT	α_1-antitrypsin
ABT	Aminopyrine breath test
AcCoA	Acetyl coenzyme A
ACE	Angiotensin-converting enzyme
ACTH	Adrenocorticotropic hormone
ADF	Adenofir
ADH	Antidiuretic hormone
ADH	Alcohol dehydrogenase
ADP	Adenosine diphosphate
ADR	Adverse drug reaction
ADT	Placebo (**a**ny – what you **d**esire – **t**hing)
AE	Anion exchanger
AFP	α_1-foetoprotein
Ag	Antigen
AHA	Antibody histone (2B)-A
AIC	Autoimmune cholangitis
AIH	Autoimmune hepatitis
AIP	Acute intermittent porphyria
ALA	δ-aminolaevulinic acid
ALAD	δ-aminolaevulinic acid-dehydratase
ALD	Aldolase
ALD	Alcohol liver disease
ALDH	Aldehyde dehydrogenase
ALF	Acute liver failure
ALG	Antilymphocytic globulin
ALL	Acute lymphatic leukaemia
ALT	Alanine aminotransferase (= GPT)
AMA	Antimitochondrial antibody
AML	Acute myelogenous leukaemia
AMP	Adenosine monophosphate
ANA	Antinuclear antibody
ANCA	Antineutrophil cytoplasmic antibody
ANF	Atrial natiuretic factor
AP	Alkaline phosphatase
APOLT	Auxiliary partial orthotopic liver transplantation
APTT	Activated partial thromboplastin time
APUD	Amine precursor uptake and decarboxylation
ARA-AMP	Adenine arabinoside monophosphate
ARP	Anti-ribosomal P antibody
ASA	Acetylsalicylic acid
ASGPR	Asialoglycoprotein receptor
ASH	Alcoholic steatohepatitis
AST	Aspartate aminotransferase (= GOT)
AT III	Antithrombin III
ATP	Adenosine triphosphate
ATPase	Adenosine triphosphatase
AVP	Arteriovenous pressure
AWS	Alcohol withdrawal syndrome
B	
BAC	Blood alcohol concentration
BAL	Bioartificial liver device
BBB	Blood-brain barrier
BCAA	Branched-chain amino acid
BCS	Budd-Chiari syndrome
BELS	Berlin extracorporeal liver support
BICAP	Bipolar circumactive probe

Abbreviation:	Meaning:
BLSS	Bioartificial liver support system
BMI	Body mass index
BMP	Bone morphogenetiv factor
BRIC	Benign recurrent intrahepatic cholestasis
BSEP	Bile salt export pump
BSR	Blood sedimentation rate (= ESR)
BUN	Blood urea nitrogen
BW	Body weight
C	
CAGE	Alcoholism test
CAH	Chronic active hepatitis
CAM	Cell adhesion molecule
cAMP	Cyclic adenosine monophosphate
CBAT	Canalicular bile acid transporter
CBG	Corticosteroid-binding globulin
CC	Cystadenocarcinoma
CCC	Cholangiocellular carcinoma
CDCA	Chenodeoxycholic acid
CDK	Cyclin-dependent kinase
CDT	Carbohydrate-deficient transferrin
CEA	Carcinoembryonic antigen
CEDS	Colour-encoded Doppler sonography
CEP	Congenital erythropoietic porphyria
CESD	Cholesterolester storage disease
CET	Caffeine elimination test
CETP	Cholesterolester transfer protein
CEUS	Contrast-enhanced ultrasonography
CF	Cystic fibrosis
CFR	Complement fixation reaction
CFT	Complement fixation test
CFTR	Cystic fibrosis transmembrane regulator
cGMP	Cyclic guanosine-3', 5'-monophosphate
CH	Cavernous haemangioma
ChE	Cholinesterase
CHBV	Crane hepatitis B virus
CHP	Chronic hepatic porphyria
CIBD	Chronic inflammatory bowel disease
CLH	Chronic lobular hepatitis
CLL	Chronic lymphatic leukaemia
CM	Contrast medium
CML	Chronic myeloid leukaemia
CMV	Cytomegalovirus
CNDC	Chronic non-suppurative destructive cholangitis
CNS	Central nervous system
CO	Cardiac output (vol./min)
CPH	Chronic persistent hepatitis
CREST	Calcinosis-Raynaud-esophagus-sclerodactyly-telangiectasia syndrome
CRP	C-reactive protein
CSF	Cerebrospinal fluid
CSH	Chronic septal hepatitis
CSI	Cholesterol saturation index
CT	Computer tomography
CTAP	CT arterioportography
CTL	Cytotoxic T lymphocyte
CVP	Central venous pressure
CYP	Cytochrome P-450
D	
DBP	Vitamin D-binding protein

XV

Abbreviations

DCP	Des-gamma-carboxy prothrombin
DCP	Divalent cation transporter
DDT	Dichlorodiphenyltrichloroethane
DHBV	Duck hepatitis virus
DIC	Disseminated intravascular coagulation
DLPC	Dilinoleoylphosphadidylcholine
DNA	Deoxyribonucleic acid
DOD	Degree of disability
DRQ	DeRitis quotient
DSA	Digital subtraction angiography

E

EBV	Epstein-Barr virus
EC	Elimination capacity
ECLP	Extracorporeal liver perfusion
ECM	Extracellular matrix
ECP	Erythropoietic coproporphyria
ECS	Extracellular space
EDRF	Endothelium-derived relaxing factor
EDTA	Ethylenediaminetetraacetic acid
EEG	Electroencephalography
EEP	Endogenous evoked potentials
EGF	Epidermal growth factor
EHP	Erythrohepatic porphyria
EHT	Electrohydrothermic probe
EIA	Enzyme immunoassay
ELAD	Extracorporeal liver assist device
ELISA	Enzyme-linked immunosorbent assay
EPL	Essential phospholipids
EPP	Erythropoietic protoporphyria
ER	Endoplasmic reticulum
ERC	Endoscopic retrograde cholangiography
ET	Endothelin
EUS	Endoscopic ultrasound
EvG	Elastica van Gieson
EVR	Early viral response

F

FA	Fatty acid
FBP	Folate-binding protein
FENa	Fractional sodium excretion
FFA	Free fatty acid
FFP	Fresh frozen plasma
FGF	Fibroblast growth factor
FHCC	Fibrolamellar hepatocellular carcinoma
FHF	Fulminant hepatic failure (= ALF)
FHVP	Free hepatic venous pressure
FIA	Fluorescence immunoassay
FM	Fibrin monomer
FNB	Fine needle biopsy
FNH	Focal nodular hyperplasia

G

GABA	Gamma-aminobutyric acid
GBV	GB-Virus
GDH	Glutamate dehydrogenase
GEC	Galactose elimination capacity
GFR	Glomerular filtration rate
GGT	Gamma-glutamyl transpeptitase
GHRF	Growth hormone-releasing factor
GMCSF	Granulocyte macrophage colonic stimul. factor
GOT	Glutamic oxaloacetic transaminase (= AST)
GPT	Glutamic pyruvic transaminase (= ALT)
GSH	Reduced glutathione
GSHV	Ground squirrel hepatitis virus
GSSG	Oxidized glutathione
GST	Glutathione-S-transferase
GVHD	Graft-versus-host disease

H

HAI	Hepatitis activity index
HAV	Hepatitis-A virus
HBDH	α-Hydroxybutyrate dehydrogenase
HBIG	Hepatitis-B immunoglobulin
HBP	Hepatic binding protein
HBSS	Hepatobiliary sequence scintigraphy
HBV	Hepatitis-B virus
HCC	Hepatocellular carcinoma
HCP	Hereditary coproporphyria
HCV	Hepatitis-C virus
HDL	High-density lipoprotein
HDV	Hepatitis-D virus
HE	Haemotoxylin eosin
HE	Hepatic encephalopathy
HEP	Hepatoerythropoietic porphyria
HES	Hydroethyl starch
HEV	Hepatitis-E virus
hFABP	Hepatic fatty acid-binding protein
HGBV	Hepatitis-GB virus
HGF	Hepatocyte growth factor
HGV	Hepatitis-G virus
HHBV	Heron hepatitis B virus
HHC	Hereditary haemochromatosis
HHT	Hereditary hepatic telangiectasia
HHV	Human herpes virus
HIDA	Hepatic iminodiacetic acid
HIV	Human immunodeficiency virus
HL	Half-life
HLA	Human leucocyte antigen
HLT	Heterotopic liver transplantation
HMG-CoA	Hydroxymethylglutaryl-CoA
HMV	Heart minute volume
HNF	Hepatocyte nuclear factor
HPI	Hepatic proliferation inhibitor
HPLC	High-pressure liquid chromatography
HPS	Hepatopulmonary syndrome
HRGP	Histidine-rich glycoprotein
HRQL	Health-related quality of live
HRS	Hepatorenal syndrome
HSS	Hepatic stimulatory substance
HSV	Herpes simplex virus
HTL	Hepatic triglyceride lipase
HVF	Hepatocyte volume fraction
HVPG	Hepatic vein pressure gradient

I

IBC	Iron-binding capacity
IBP	Iron-binding protein
ICAM	Intercellular adhesion molecule
ICDH	Isocitrate dehydrogenase
ICG	Indocyanine green
ICP	Intracranial pressure
ICS	Intracellular space
ICU	Intensive care unit
IDL	Intermediate density lipoprotein
IDUS	Intraductal ultrasound
IFN	Interferon
IFT	Immunofluorescence test
IGF	Insulin-like growth factor
IHAT	Indirect haemagglutination test
IL	Interleukin
INR	International normalization ratio
IOUS	Intraoperative ultrasound
IRF	Iron regulation factor
ISAGA	Immunosorbent agglutination assay
ISC	Iron saturation capacity
IU	International unit

K

KB	Ketone bodies
kDa	Kilo-Dalton
KKS	Kallikrein-kinin system

L

LAM	Lamivudine
LAP	Laparoscopy
LAP	Liver active protein
LAP	Leucine aminopeptidase
LASER	Light amplification by stimulated emission of radiation
LB	Liver biopsy
LC1	Liver cytosol typ 1 antibody
LCAT	Lecithin-cholesterol acyl transferase
LCT	Lipiodol-computer tomography
LD	Lethal dose
LDH	Lactate dehydrogenase
LDL	Low-density lipoprotein
LDLT	Living donor liver transplantation
LE	Lupus erythematosus
LFA	Lymphocyte function antigen
LFT	Liver function test
LIP	Liver inhibitor protein
LITT	Laser-induced thermotherapy
LKM	Liver-kidney microsomal antigen
LMA	Liver membrane autoantibody
LPA	Liver-pancreas antibody
LPL	Lipoprotein lipase
LP X	Lipoprotein-X
LR	Liver resection
LSP	Liver-specific protein
LT	Liver transplantation
LTC	Laparoscopic transhepatic cholangiography
LTT	Line-tracing test
LTT	Lymphocyte transformation test
LWW	Liver wet weight

M

MALT	Munich alcoholism test
MALT	Mucous membrane associated lymphoid tissue
MAO	Monoamine oxidase
MARS	Molecular adsorbend recirculatory system
MAST	Michigan alcoholism screening test
mAST	Mitochondrial aspartate aminotransferase
MBq	Megabecquerel
MCL	Midclavicular line
MCT	Medium-chain triglyceride
MCV	Mean corpuscular volume
MEGX	Monoethylglycinexylidide test
MELD	Model for endstage liver disease
MELS	Modular extracorporeal liver support
MEOS	Microsomal ethanol-oxidizing system
MFH	Malignant fibrous histiocytoma
mGOT	Mitochondrial glutamic-oxalacetic transaminase
MHC	Major histocompatibility complex
MIGET	Multiple inert gas elimination technique
MMF	Mycophenolate mofetil
MMP	Matrix metalloproteinase
MOAT	Multi-organic anion transporter
MPS	Mononuclear phagocyte system
MRC	Magnetic resonance cholangiography
MRI	Magnetic resonance imaging (= MRT)
mRNA	Messenger RNA
MRP	Multi-drug resistance protein
MT	Metallothionein
MTP	Microsomal triglyceride transfer protein

N

NAD	Nicotinamide adenine dinucleotide
NADP	Nicotinamide adenine dinucleotide phosphate
NAFLD	Non-alcoholic fatty liver disease
NALD	Non-alcoholic liver disease
NASH	Non-alcoholic steatohepatitis
NCT	Number-connection test
nDNA	Nuclear DNA
NHL	Non-Hodgkin lymphoma
NLCT	Number-letter combination test
NO	Nitrous oxide
NRH	Nodular regenerative hyperplasia
NSAR	Non-steroidal antirheumatics
NU	5'-Nucleotidase

O

OA	Ornithine aspartate
OATP	Natrium-independent transport system for organic anions
OCT	Ornithine carbamoyltransferase
OGTT	Oral glucose tolerance test
OLS	Overlap syndrome
OLT	Orthotopic liver transplantation
ORF	Open reading frame

P

PAF	Platelet-activating factor
PAH	Para-aminohippuric acid
PAI	Percutaneous acetic acid injection
PAI	Plasminogen activator inhibitor
PAIR	Punction/Aspiration/Injection/Re-Aspiration
pANCA	Perinuclear antineutrophilic cytoplasmic antibody
PAP	Pulmonary artery pressure
PAS	Para-aminosalicylic acid
PAS	Periodic acid-Schiff reaction
PBC	Primary biliary cholangitis/cirrhosis
PBG	Porphobilinogen
PCB	Polychlorinated biphenyl
PCNA	Proliferating cell nuclear antigen
PCO_2	Partial pressure carbon dioxide
PCP	Pentachlorophenol
PCR	Polymerase chain reaction
PCT	Porphyria cutanea tarda
PCWP	Pulmonary capillary wedge pressure
PDGF	Platelet-derived growth factor
PDR	Plasma disappearance rate
PEEP	Positive end-expiratory pressure
PELAM	Platelet endothelial cell adhesion molecule
PEI	Percutaneous ethanol injection
PEM	Protein-energy malnutrition
PET	Positron emission tomography
PG	Prostaglandin
PHI	Phosphohexose isomerase
Pi	Protease inhibitor
P III-P	Procollagen-III-peptide
PMN	Polymorphonuclear neutrophilic leucocytes
PPC	Polyenylphosphatidylcholine
PPH	Primary pulmonary hypertension
PPSB	Prothrombin complex (prothrombin, proconvertin, Stuart factor, antihaemophilic factor B)
PSC	Primary sclerosing cholangitis
PSE	Portosystemic encephalopathy
PT	Prothrombin time (= Quick)
PTC	Percutaneous transhepatic cholangiography
PTH	Parathormone
PTP	Percutaneous transhepatic portography
PTT	Partial thromboplastin time

XVII

Abbreviations

PVC	Polyvinyl chloride		TACE	Transarterial chemoembolization
PVS	Peritoneovenous shunt		TAE	Transarterial embolization
			TBG	Thyroxine-binding globulin
			TCDD	Dioxin
Q			TGF	Transforming growth factor
QOL	Quality of life		TIBC	Total iron-binding capacity
			TIMP	Tissue inhibitor metalloproteinase
R			TIPS	Transjugular intrahepatic portosystemic shunt
RAAS	Renin-angiotensin-aldosterone system		TNF	Tumour necrosis factor
RAST	Radio-allergo-sorbent test		TNM	Malignant tumour classification system (tumour, node, metastasis)
RBP	Retinol-binding protein		tPA	Tissue plasminogen activator
RCE	Reduction in earning capacity		TPT	Thromboplastin time
REE	Resting energy expenditure		TRH	Thyreotropin-releasing hormone
RER	Rough endoplasmic reticulum		tRNA	Transfer RNA
RES	Reticuloendothelial system		TSH	Thyroid-stimulating hormone
RFA	Radio frequency ablation		TT	Thrombin time
RFTA	Radiofrequency thermal ablation		TTR	Transthyretin
RHS	Reticulohisticytic system		TUDCA	Tauro-ursodeoxycholic acid
RIA	Radioimmunoassay		TVC	Transvenous cholangiography
RIBA	Recombinant immunoblot assay			
RNA	Ribonucleic acid		**U**	
RNF	Renal natriuretic factor		UDCA	Ursodeoxycholic acid
ROI	Reactive oxygen intermediates		UDP	Uridine diphosphate
rRNA	Ribosomal RNA		UES	Undifferentiated embryonal sarcoma
RT-PCR	Reverse transcription-polymerase chain reaction		uPA	Urokinase plasminogen activator
			US	Ultrasound
S			UTP	Uridine triphosphate
SAMe	S-adenosylmethionine		UV	Ultraviolet
SBP	Spontaneous bacterial peritonitis		UW	University of Wisconsin solution
SDH	Sorbitol dehydrogenase			
SeHCAT	Selenohomotaurocholic acid test		**V**	
SEP	Somatosensory evoked potentials		VBDS	Vanishing bile duct syndrome
SER	Smooth endoplasmic reticulum		VC	Vinyl chloride
SLA	Soluble liver antigen		VCAM	Vascular cell adhesion molecule
SLT	Split liver transplantation		VEGF	Vascular endothelial growth factor
SMA	Smooth muscle antibody		VEP	Visually evoked potentials
SOD	Superoxide dismutase		VIP	Vasoactive intestinal polypeptide
SOL	Space-occupying lesion		VLDL	Very low-density lipoprotein
SPECT	Single-photon emission computer tomography		VOD	Veno-occlusive disease
SPIO	Superparamagnetic particles of iron oxide		VZV	Varicella-zoster virus
SQUID	Superconducting quantum-interference device			
SSC	Secondary sclerosing cholangitis		**W**	
STD	Sexually transmitted disease		WAIS	Wechsler adult intelligence scale
STH	Somatotropic hormone		WHV	Woodchuck hepatitis virus
STP	Standard temperature (0 °C) and pressure (760 mg Hg)		WHVP	Wedged hepatic venous pressure
SVR	Sustained viral response		WNV	West Nile virus
T			**Y**	
TAC	Transarterial chemotherapy		YF	Yellow fever

> "... because the liver is a source of many diseases, and is a noble organ that serves many organs, almost all of them: so it suffers, it is not a small suffering, but a great and manifold one"

Theophrastus Bombastus von Hohenheim, known as Paracelsus (1493−1541)

(Liber tertius paramiri, de morbis ex Tartaro. St. Gallen, 1531)

The first and the last page of this book on hepatology (1st German edition 1998; 1st, 2nd and 3rd English edition 2002, 2004, 2008) are devoted to *Theophrastus Bombastus von Hohenheim,* called **Paracelsus**. The life and work of this great man have fascinated me since my youth.

Therefore, it was an indescribable feeling for me when, in 2006, I was awarded the **Paracelsus Medal** as the greatest distinction of the German Medical Profession It bears the inscription (see last page in all editions!) *"the highest ground is love"*, which is part of a well-known quotation of Paracelsus himself concerning the benefit of remedies.

Contents

- *Dedications*
- *Authors*
- *Prefaces*
- *Forewords*
- *Abbreviations*
- *Contents*

Introduction to hepatology

1. History of hepatology
2. Morphology of the liver
3. Biochemistry and functions of the liver

Diagnostics in liver diseases

4. Clinical findings
5. Laboratory diagnostics
6. Sonography
7. Liver biopsy and laparoscopy
8. Radiological diagnostics
9. Scintigraphic diagnostics
10. Neurological and psychological diagnostics

Symptoms and syndromes

11. Hepatomegaly and splenomegaly
12. Jaundice
13. Cholestasis
14. Portal hypertension
15. Hepatic encephalopathy
16. Oedema and ascites
17. Hepatorenal syndrome
18. Hepatopulmonary syndrome
19. Coagulopathy and haemorrhage
20. Acute and chronic liver insufficiency

Clinical aspects of liver diseases

21. Clinical and morphological principles
22. Acute viral hepatitis (A−SEN)
23. Acute concomitant viral hepatitis
24. Bacterial infections and the liver
25. Parasitic infections and the liver
26. Mycotic infections and the liver
27. Liver abscess
28. Alcohol-induced liver damage
29. Drug-induced liver damage
30. Liver damage due to toxic substances
31. Metabolic disorders and storage diseases
32. Autoimmune hepatitis
33. Cholangitis and cholangiodysplasia
34. Chronic hepatitis
35. Liver cirrhosis
36. Benign hepatic lesions and tumours
37. Malignant liver tumours
38. Systemic diseases and the liver
39. Cardiovascular diseases and the liver
40. Therapy of liver diseases

- *Subject index*

1 History of Hepatology

		Page:
1	*Liver research in antiquity*	2
1.1	Hepatoscopy	2
1.2	Mythological-speculative medicine	5
1.2.1	Liver as the seat of inner emotions	5
1.2.2	Liver and mythology	5
1.3	Natural-philosophical medicine	6
1.4	Corpus Hippocraticum	6
1.5	Platon of Athens	6
1.6	Aristoteles of Stagira	6
1.7	Alexandrian School of Medicine	7
1.8	Roman Medicine	7
1.9	Aretaios of Cappadocia	7
1.10	Galenos of Pergamon	7
2	*Liver research in the Middle Ages*	8
3	*Liver research up to modern times*	11
	• References (1–26)	13
	(Figures 1.1–1.20)	

1 History of Hepatology

Hepatology from ancient to modern times

Over the millennia, the conception of the liver has been subject to more remarkable change than that of almost any other organ. • In antiquity, mantic, religious and speculative thinking combined with anatomical and physiological observations resulted in a most imposing body of knowledge concerning the liver. • The features and disease processes of the liver were described more accurately than in the case of any other organ, and modern medicine has repeatedly afforded resounding confirmation of those ancient observations.

> It may therefore be both interesting and instructive to trace the roots of our present knowledge of hepatology back to antiquity and to commemorate with admiration and respect the tireless spirit of medical and scientific research in this area.

1 Liver research in antiquity

> Even in primeval times, the liver must have been well-known as the most powerful and most blood-rich organ of the animal body. Varied and important processes were attributed to this impressive part of the entrails — it was even regarded as the "seat of life". • The Indo-Germanic word "lîp" meant both liver and life, and there are obvious similarities between the English "liver-live/life" (Old English: "lifer-līf") and the German "Leber-Leben". In Old High German, the liver was termed "leb(a)ra". The Hebrew "kábe(r), kábe(d)" (or "cheber") is the probable root of the Greek word "hepar".

1.1 Hepatoscopy

Evidently, priests and fortune-tellers at that time became interested primarily in the liver and thus great mantic-religious significance was attributed to this organ. *For the Babylonians and Assyrians, the* **inspection of entrails,** *in reality* **inspection of the liver,** *was the most important method of foretelling events.* This "hepatoscopy" was based on the premise that the god to whom the sacrifice was offered would show his pleasure by revealing the future through variations in the appearance of the sacrificial animal's liver.

The sacrificial priests of Mesopotamia had acquired a precise knowledge of the size, colour and external structure of animal liver, especially that of the sheep — the most common sacrificial animal. They assigned specific names to the individual parts of the liver and gall bladder and to their different variations in form and appearance, reflecting similarities to everyday objects e.g. mountains, rivers, roads, nose, ear, tooth, hand, finger. Hepatoscopy was carried out in accordance with stipulated ceremonial rites and in the face of an image of a god. It was strictly limited to assessing the outer appearance of the liver; the organ itself was not dissected.

The Babylonian sacrificial priests taught the art of hepatoscopy systematically, using specially devised **models of the liver.** These models also served as topographical aids for the mantic interpretation of variations in the appearance of the animal liver. The no doubt oldest clay model of a sheep's liver is from a Babylonian temple and dates from ca. 2000 BC. (s. fig. 1.1) Clearly recognizable on the concave surface are 2 lobes: the coniform gall bladder with the cystic duct and the caudate lobe (= pyramidal process) and the smaller papillary process (→). Carved lines divide the lower surface into approximately 40 small, rectangular fields, which contain cuneiform inscriptions of sacral symbols and mantic readings, one of the recurrent themes being ***"May your liver be smooth"***. • Many of the rectangles show small holes, presumably used to insert tiny wooden pins according to the variations in form observed in the animal liver. Such a topographical fixation of findings facilitated a more accurate prophecy. (5, 22, 23)

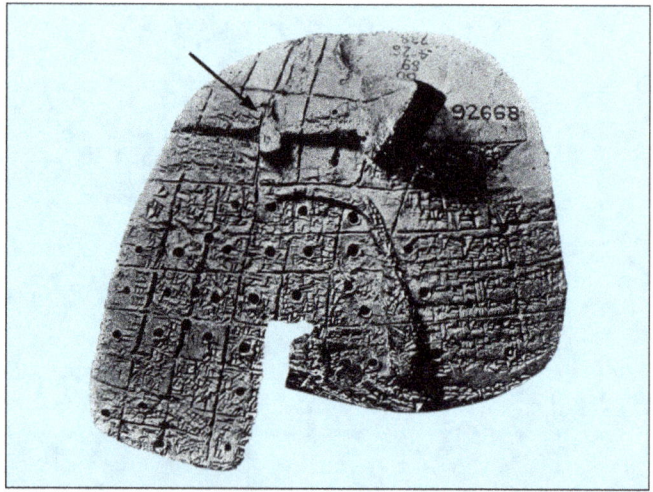

Fig. 1.1: Babylonian terracotta model of a sheep's liver with papillary process (↓), ca. 2000 BC (British Museum, London) (13)

Sumerian culture has also yielded artefacts concerned with hepatoscopy. More than 30 such clay models of the liver with cuneiform inscriptions dating from the 17th century BC were found during the excavations of Mari. (21) (s. fig. 1.2) • Further clay models with cuneiform inscriptions dating from the 13th–12th century BC were also unearthed during the excavations of Bogazköy (1933/34). (10) (s. fig. 1.3)

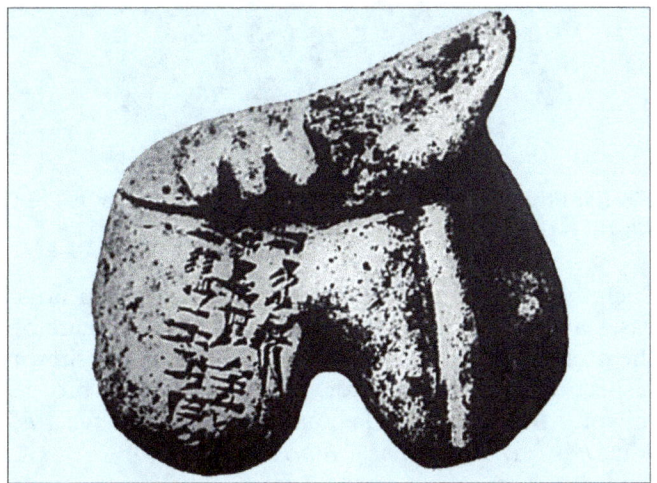

Fig. 1.2: Sumerian clay model of the liver, 1700–1600 BC (excavations of Mari) (21)

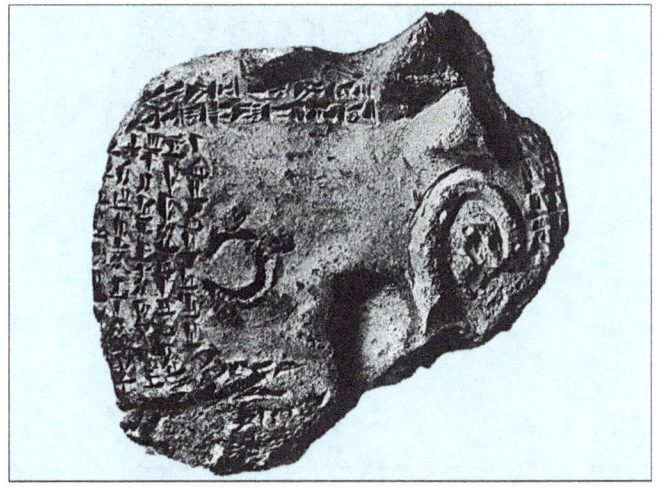

Fig. 1.3: Sumerian clay model of the liver, ca. 1260 BC (excavations of Bogazköy) (10)

The art of hepatoscopy spread from Mesopotamia to Greece, where it received widespread acceptance, as evidenced by various illustrations and accounts of the inspection of entrails. EURIPIDES (Elektra, 826–829) described hepatoscopy as follows: *"Aigisthos took the entrails in his hands and inspected them. Now the liver had no head, while the portal vein and nearby gall bladder revealed threatening events to the one who was observing it."* • Hepatoscopy was applied not only in political decision-making, but also in foretelling the medical prognoses and life events of prominent persons. Babylonian hepatoscopy was also referred to in the Old Testament (EZEKIEL 21, v. 21): *"For the king of Babylon stood at the parting of the way, at the head of the two ways, to use divination: he made his arrows bright, he consulted with images and he looked at the liver."*

A red-figured illustration on a Greek bellied amphora by EUTHYMIDES shows an animal liver being presented to a Greek hoplite before his departure to do battle in the Theban War. (17) (s. fig. 1.4) • The same motif of liver inspection with soldiers departing for battle appears in black on an Attic neck amphora (2) (s. fig. 1.5) as well as on an amphora of pan-Athenian form. (24) (s. fig. 1.6)

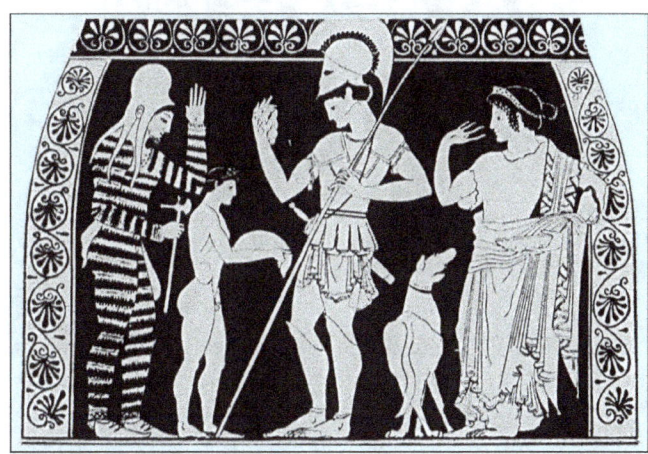

Fig. 1.4: Red-figured illustration of inspection of the liver on a Greek bellied amphora (17)

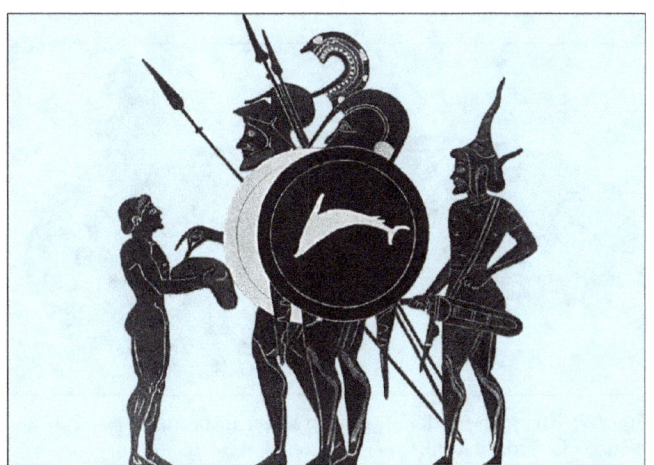

Fig. 1.5: Black-figured illustration of inspection of the liver on an Attic neck amphora (2)

The **Etruscans** also appear to have adopted hepatoscopy from the Babylonians and Assyrians. Etruscan fortune-tellers (= hostiae consultatoriae) were particularly renowned and served so to speak as teachers of the Romans both in augury and in religious rites. Thus the Etruscans virtually held sole rights to carry out the inspection of the liver (LIVIUS 1, 56, 5). M. T. CICERO (106–43 BC) always referred to the haruspices as "etrusci". Liver models such as that of a sheep's liver cast in bronze (3rd–2nd century BC) and a clay liver model (2nd century BC) (7) have survived from the Etruscan civilization. Cir-

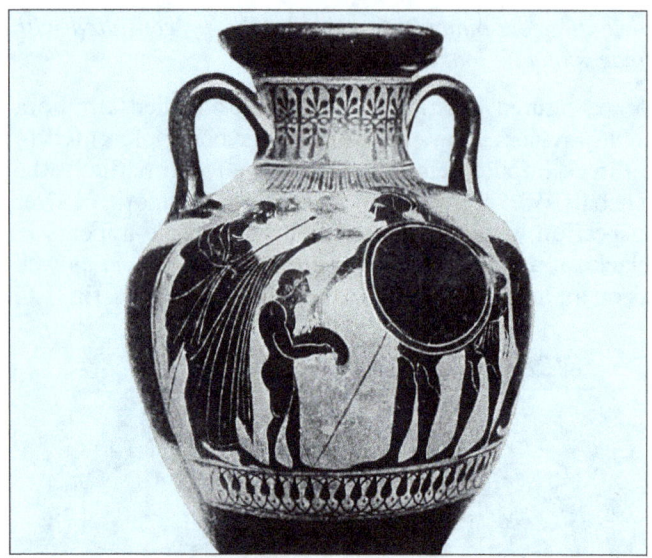

Fig. 1.6: Black-figured illustration of inspection of the liver on an Attic amphora of pan-Athenian form (24)

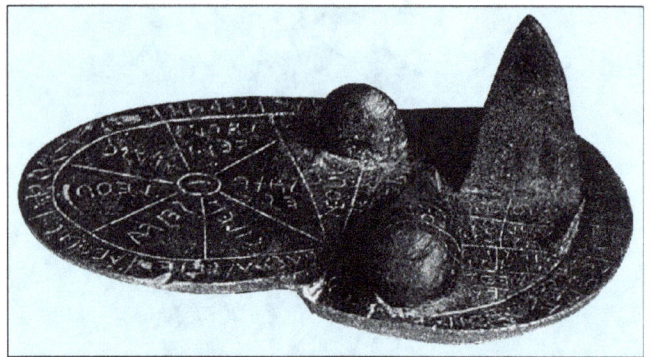

Fig. 1.7: Etruscan model of a sheep's liver in bronze, 300–200 BC (Museo Civico, Piacenza) (7)

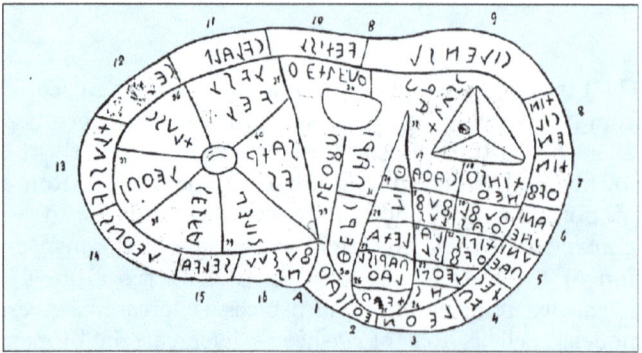

Fig. 1.8: Etruscan model of a sheep's liver in bronze, 300–200 BC, showing inscriptions (Museo Civico, Piacenza) (7)

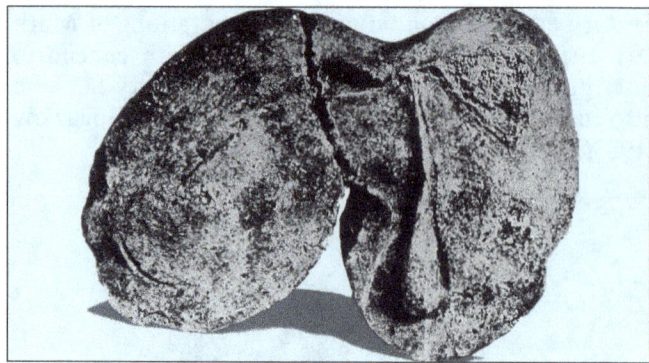

Fig. 1.9: Etruscan clay model of a liver, ca. 200 BC (excavations of Falerii) (7)

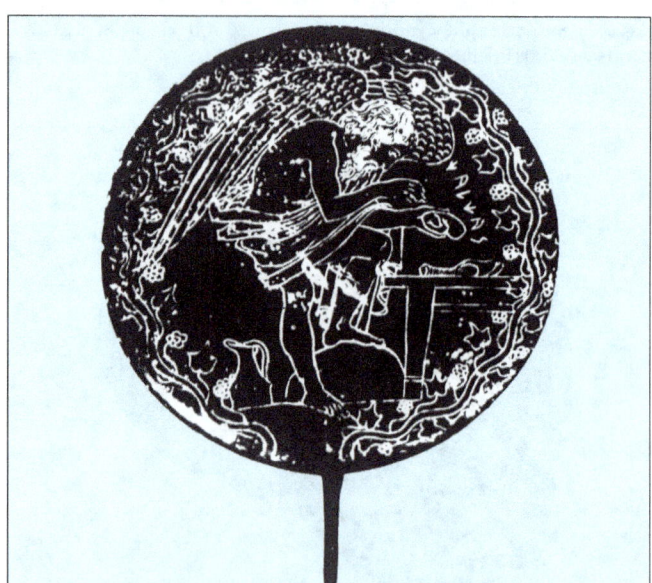

Fig. 1.10: Etruscan hand mirror in bronze, 500–400 BC: KALCHAS (son of Thestor of Mykene), the most famous of the sacrificial priests, inspects the animal liver with large caudate process; on the table are the trachea and lungs of the sacrificial animal (7)

cular and radial carved lines can be seen on the former model, forming approximately 40 small subdivisions containing Etruscan symbols and names of gods. In addition, a pear-shaped gall bladder, the pyramidal process and the papillary process are mounted on the flat, stylized depiction of the visceral face of the animal liver. (s. figs. 1.7, 1.8, 1.9)

Such liver inspections are also depicted on burial urns, vases and hand mirrors. The bearded, winged figure of the sacrificial priest KALCHAS, son of Thestor, is shown inspecting an animal liver on an Etruscan bronze mirror. • HOMER once said about him: "He knew what *is*, what *has been*, and what *will be*." (s. fig. 1.10)

In addition to the *pyramidal process*, the left and right lobes of the liver (pars hostilis and pars familiaris, respectively) were differentiated. Predictions pertaining to the questioner were derived largely from the appearance of the *pars familiaris*, whereas those concerning his opponent were derived from the *pars hostilis*. Based on the presence or absence of specific features in the sacrificial liver, favourable and unfavourable influences were defined and weighed up, thereby allowing the final prediction to be made. If the edge of the liver fell towards the right, the imminent recovery of the sick person was assured; furthermore, the questioner would live or survive if the gall bladder was long.

Numerous predictions based on hepatoscopy have proved to be of **historical interest**: the victory of the emperor Augustus in the naval battle of Actium (31 BC) was predicted by the haruspices on the basis of an enlarged, double gall bladder; by contrast, the absence of a pyramidal process gave advance warning of the death of the consul Marcus Marcellus in the battle against Hannibal (208 BC); this ominous portent also foretold the emperor Caligula his imminent murder (41 AD) and the emperor Claudius his death by poisoning (54 AD) without, however, being able to prevent these assassinations.

▶ From the Babylonian and Assyrian civilizations to the fall of the Roman Empire — more than 2,000 years — hepatoscopy was firmly established in human belief. It influenced the lives and determined the major decisions of important people, and thus also affected the fate of entire nations and civilizations.

1.2 Mythological-speculative medicine

1.2.1 Liver as the seat of inner emotions

The Egyptian Papyrus Ebers (ca. 1550 BC) is one of the oldest known medical documents. It contains the first descriptions of the liver in a speculative medical sense and regards it as the seat of inner emotions: *"Four vessels lead to the liver, supplying it with air and water, and, being overfilled with blood, influence the occurrence of all sorts of illness"*; or: *"The wrath of the heart results from ebullition of parts of the liver and rectum."*

The Babylonians' medical concept of the liver, based on detailed knowledge of hepatoscopy, was likewise purely speculative. For them, the liver was the seat of emotions, feelings, desires and sexual potency. (11)

Further references to the liver as the seat of emotional life are found in the Old Testament, for example in the lamentations of Jeremiah (Lamentations 2, 11): *"Mine eyes do fail with tears, my bowels are troubled, my liver is poured upon the earth because of the misery of the daughter of my people ..."*

The Greeks similarly perceived the liver as the seat of feelings and rage as well as of the soul. In his "Timaios", Platon (427–347 BC) described the liver as the location of the "desiring soul", which he subordinated to the "rational soul" of the head. (3) Horatius designated the liver as the organ of love (12), whereas Juvenalis saw it as the seat of anger. (14)

The significance of the liver (and bile) in emotional life is reflected to the present day in the form of **familiar quotations** such as: „*eine Laus über die Leber gelaufen*" (German) (literally: a louse has crawled over his liver; meaning: something is biting him); „*frei von der Leber weg reden*" (German) (literally: to speak straight from the liver; meaning: to speak one's mind); „*sich gelb und grün ärgern*" (German) (literally: to be yellow and green with anger; meaning: to be black with anger); „*die Galle hochkommen lassen*" (German) (literally: it rouses my bile; meaning: it makes me angry or indignant). The possession of "liver spots" (German: „Leberflecken") was attributed to the immoral tendencies of the bearer.

1.2.2 Liver and mythology

Mythology dominated the Greeks' medical concept of the liver. Hesiod (8th century BC) and Aischylos (525–456 BC) wrote of **Prometheus**, who was fastened to a rock in the Caucasus mountains by the gods: As a punishment for his having brought back the gift of fire to the mortals, he was chained to a rock, and an eagle came every day to eat away at his liver, which regenerated itself each night (4) (s. fig. 1.11) — **the first record of the regenerative capacity of the liver!** • Such a fate also befell Tityos, the son of Gaea, on whose liver two vultures fed in the underworld (Odyssey 11, 576–578): *"And I saw Tityos, son of magnificent Gaea, lying on the ground. Over nine roods he stretched, and two vultures sat, one on either side, and tore his liver, plunging their beaks into his bowels, nor could he beat them free. For he had offered violence to Leto, the glorious wife of Zeus."*

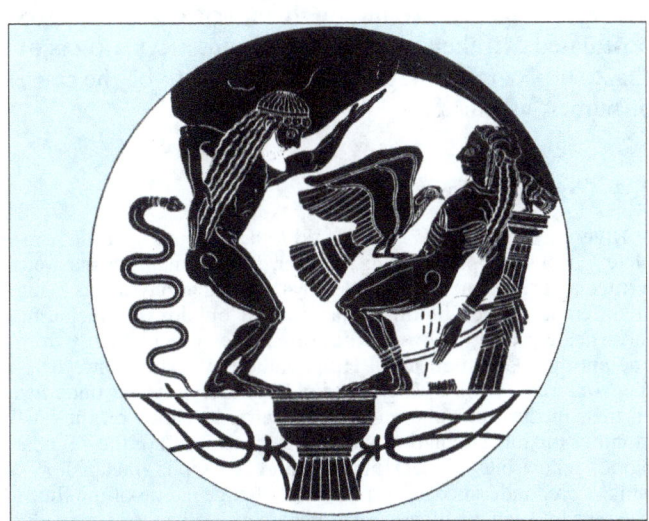

Fig. 1.11: An eagle devours the liver of Prometheus, who is tied fast and unable to escape; the liver regenerated each night (left: his brother Atlas) (Laconic kylix, 555 BC; Vatican Museums, Rome)

▶ Here we have two examples showing liver regeneration in antiquity. Interestingly, no other organ was attributed such regenerative capacity!

The position of the liver in the right upper abdomen and its close proximity to the diaphragm are described by Homer, and a stab wound in the liver was regarded as a fatal injury. Only when one had taken possession of an enemy's liver was the latter deemed truly dead. Thus Hecuba, craving revenge for her dead son Hektor, demanded the liver of Achilles (Iliad 24, 212). This conception is illustrated throughout the epic (Iliad 11, 579; 13, 412; 17, 349) and particularly in the twentieth stanza (Iliad 20, 469): *"... but he smote him upon the liver with his sword, and forth his life slipped, and the dark blood welling therefrom filled his bosom; and darkness enfolded his eyes as he swooned."*

1.3 Natural-philosophical medicine

In the 5th and 6th centuries BC, "logos" began to supersede "mythos" in liver research, as in other fields.

DIOGENES OF APOLLONIA (ca. 430 BC) described a symmetrical vascular supply system, in which spleen and liver were regarded as a paired double organ. He named the major blood vessel leading from the liver to the right axilla and hand *"hepatitis"* and that connecting the spleen with the left hand *"splenitis"*. Bleeding of the vein running from the right arm to the royal *("basilikos")* inner organ was the recommended treatment for liver disease; this vein is still known as basilic vein even today.

EMPEDOKLES OF AGRIGENT (490−430 BC) viewed the liver as the central organ of both the vascular system and nutrition. The liver was generally accepted as being the site of *biligenesis*, although PHILOLAOS OF CROTON postulated extrahepatic bile production. ANAXAGORAS OF CLAZOMENAE (500−428 BC) believed bile to be the cause of numerous illnesses.

1.4 Corpus Hippocraticum

▶ HIPPOCRATES (460−377 BC) is said to be the author of the complete Corpus Hippocraticum; however, several manuscripts were written and subsequently compiled by many other physicians living at different periods of time. The medical opinions − including those dealing with the liver − thus often diverge significantly from one another. Common to all Hippocratic physicians, however, is the *"Doctrine of the Fluids"* (cardinal humours), which underlies all their medical postulations. Good health depended on the harmonious mixing, circulation and effects (**"eucrasia"**) of the 4 fluids: blood, yellow bile (choler), mucous, and black bile (melancholy), while a preponderance of or qualitative change in one of the fluids (**"dyscrasia"**) led to illness. Treatment consisted in restoring the "life-balance" (**diaita**", i.e. Greek for "dietetics").

▶ The **liver** was held to derive from the transformation of liquid blood into a solid, rigid mass. It comprised five lobes, with the gall bladder lying over the 4th lobe. The conception of the sacrificial priests regarding the anatomy of the liver, while known to the Hippocratic physicians, was not further developed medically, yet the few technical terms deriving from these sacrificial priests were subsequently adopted. In accordance with the doctrine of DIOGENES, the vein of the liver was designated *"hepatitis phleps"*; it roughly corresponds to the superior vena cava with its extension to the vein of the right arm. The liver was viewed as the central point of the entire venous system; the intrahepatic branches of a blood vessel were described, and the course of a vein from the navel to the liver(!) was determined. The excretion of bile into the intestine and into the urine was also known.

The Hippocratic physicians used **abdominal palpation** to diagnose a liver disease and already recognized as **symptoms** jaundice, dropsy, decolourized and foul-smelling stools, fever, itching, rumbling of the intestine and upper abdominal pain. Liver pain was believed to derive directly from a folding over of the hepatic lobe. Jaundice, according to their interpretation, resulted from the inundation of the body with bile due to dyscrasia. Dropsy was regarded as a consequence of a melting of the liver. To this excellent collection of symptoms was added the observation that dark stools (tarry stools!) presaged imminent death. Echinococcal infection of the liver was also mentioned. • Indeed, one impressive conclusion was that the consumption of *raw ox liver soaked in honey* was the correct **treatment** for liver disease and night blindness (= vitamine A therapy). A liver abscess was to be opened with a red-hot knife (= cautery).

1.5 Platon of Athens

Platon (427−377 BC) described the main part of his medical knowledge and understanding, which was based on the Sicilian school, in his "Timaios" (s.p. 5). He defined the liver as "dense, smooth and sweet" (!) with a "touch of bitterness" (!). He explained bile as "old blood which is born of meat broken down in the liver". Moreover, he recognized not only the hepatic porta, but also the portal vein as a vessel with a large lumen. For him, the spleen appears to be a cleansing organ for the liver; the accumulation of harmful substances in the spongy spleen caused splenomegaly.

1.6 Aristoteles of Stagira

ARISTOTELES OF STAGIRA (384−322 BC) introduced a new epoch in liver research by the establishment of a comparative approach to anatomy and physiology. He recognized that the human liver most closely resembled bovine liver. For him, liver and spleen resulted from blood coagulation at the extreme end of the vessels. He described the extrahepatic bile ducts for the first time and disputed the Hippocratic concept that bile was one of the cardinal fluids of the body and that it caused disease. Bile seemed to him to be an irrelevant secretion. He was the first to distinguish between the hepatic arteries and veins with their open intrahepatic endings and also differentiated the portal vein within the venous system; he introduced the term aorta. ARISTOTELES regarded the task of the liver to be the digestion of food ("pepsis") and the cleansing of the blood, the latter function being supplemented by the lungs. • The liver and lungs were thus conceived as being complementary excretory organs of the body. The functioning of the liver was considered decisive for a person's life span.

1.7 Alexandrian School of Medicine

HEROPHILUS OF CHALCEDON (310−250 BC) already distinguished two hepatic lobes. Although he still believed that the venous vessels originated from the liver, he was the first to describe the portal vein system and to recognize its significance as the draining site of all resorbent intestinal veins. In addition, he detected mesenterial lymph nodes and lymphatic vessels.

ERASISTRATUS OF CHIOS (ca. 300–250 BC) coined the term *"parenchyma"* (i.e. poured out beside) for liver tissue, based on the belief that it was formed by coagulation of the blood released from the hepatic vessels. For him, however, liver parenchyma was a completely useless structure. He also described for the first time the *"choledochos"*, which he believed absorbed the redundant and rather harmful bile (transported into the liver with the portal vein blood) from the intrahepatic bile ducts, and conducted it away. This separation of bile from blood in the liver was allegedly effected by the different viscosities of the two fluids and the different diameters of the adjacent (!) intrahepatic bile ducts and blood vessels. Stoppage of the bile flow would lead to jaundice (obstructive icterus!) and inflammation of the liver. He attributed the dropsy commonly associated with liver disease to a hardening of the liver, which he termed *"skirros"*: this compressed the intrahepatic vessels, diverting the flow of the watery fluid into the abdomen. Based on this surmise, he rejected the practice of puncturing an ascites (= paracentesis) as being an unnecessary and non-causal therapeutic measure (!). Contrary to this idea, the Hippocraticians regarded the softening of the liver as being the cause of ascites.

1.8 Roman Medicine

CELSUS (ca. 30 BC–50 AD) is well known for his eight volumes of *"De Medicina"*, which have been preserved to the present. A. C. CELSUS reviews the entire field of medicine of that time and introduces precise Latin terminology. He described four liver lobes (whereas the Hippocraticians still postulated five lobes). He also supplied an impressive description of liver surgery, which – because of the organ's richness in blood – was already being performed using red-hot ("cautery") knives (!). He termed dropsy *"ascites"* and linked it not only to liver disorders, but also to diseases of the spleen and general bad health (carcinoma?); he regarded paracentesis to be a good measure. Considering the liver to be the "royal" organ, he named jaundice *"morbus regius"*: the diet prescribed for liver patients was so complicated that only royalty could afford such a costly therapy. He recommended bed rest and "psychotherapy" for treating jaundice: *"One should have a good bed in a tasteful room, seek relaxation and good humour, and take heart from the comforting pleasure which will relieve the soul."*

PLINIUS THE ELDER (23–79 AD) based his ideas on the Corpus Hippocraticum. He advocated treating liver diseases by means of wolf's liver with honey or donkey's liver with parsley and honey. • CAELIUS AURELIANUS (5th century AD) was the first to recommend the treatment of liver diseases using poultices and laxatives, which is still known in modern times. He also described the discolouration of urine associated with jaundice.

RUFUS OF EPHESUS (1st–2nd century AD) differentiated the portal vein system and the veins and arteries of the liver. However, he clearly rejected the existence of the "splenitis phleps" (which was seen as the reason for phlebotomy). He also regarded yellow bile as a waste product and black bile as the dark sediment of the blood. He even distinguished between febrile and obstructive icteru as well as a haematogenic form, whereby blood was converted into bile. He deduced that the term *"icterus"*, already used at that time for jaundice, derived from the bright yellow eyes of the pine marten (ictis). The skin colour of the jaundiced patient was also compared to a yellow stone (ikterios lithos) and to a yellowish-green lizard as well as to a yellow bird called the golden oriole (ikteros), the sighting of which by a jaundiced patient would effect a cure while at the same time killing the bird (as documented about 50 years earlier by PLINIUS THE ELDER: Nat. Hist. 30, 93). (1, 8, 16, 18, 19)

1.9 Aretaios of Cappadocia

ARETAIOS (2nd century AD) described the forming of blood in the liver from intestinally resorbed food. Thus, the liver is built up from coagulated blood. He likewise maintained that bile was generally derived from the liver, although this could also happen extrahepatically. The entire food intake had to pass through the liver before being given over to the body as a whole. ARETAIOS described the vascular system of the liver with afferent and efferent vessels, which in antiquity was unknown for any other organ. He detected the superior and inferior vena cava. Due to the blood-richness of the liver, operations could only be carried out with the help of a cautery knife. His description of obstructive icterus was the best of that time. He differentiated between hepatic and extrahepatic icterus.

1.10 Galenos of Pergamon

GALENOS OF PERGAMON (131–201 AD) compiled the body of medical knowledge that had accumulated since the 5th century BC, and which was in places completely contradictory, into an immense work. He supplemented and corrected this by a wealth of his own investigations. GALENOS (s. fig. 1.12) thus created a phenomenal, self-contained medical system that enjoyed dogmatic validity for over 1,500 years.

▶ GALENOS described the anatomy of the **liver** in greater detail than had ever been done before. In addition to separating the hepatic arteries from the veins, he recognized both the ramifications of the intrahepatic vessels and the capillary junctions of the portal vein system and hepatic veins. The conception of the liver as the origin of the venous system was retained. Liver parenchyma was held to derive from the solidification of blood under the influence of body heat. Having detected no morphological differentiations, GALENOS described the fine structure of the liver as "simple". The organ was thought to be a vegetative centre controlled by the brain via the liver nerve (vagus) — a view previously put forward by PLATON in his "Timaios". He also adopted to a great extent the Platonic doctrine regarding the "trinity of the soul", according to which the "psyche epithymetike" was to be found in the liver. The nutritive, or vegetative, liver was said to be superior to all the other abdominal organs: the essential life forces ("dynameis physikai") likewise originated here. The excretory organs — spleen, gall bladder and kidneys — were allegedly responsible for cleansing the liver. The metabolism of the liver was thus described as being directed by **four vegetative forces**: the *attracting force* drew the nutrient fluids from the intestine, the *retaining force* held the chylus in the liver vessels, the *transforming force* mediated the transformation of the nutrient substances into blood, and the *expelling force* propelled the blood through the hepatic veins to the other body organs. Thus the gall bladder *attracted* bile from the liver via extremely fine intrahepatic bile ducts with minute openings which terminated (!) in the liver; the *retaining* force facilitated the accumulation of bile in the gall bladder, and the *expelling* force drove it into the intestine. The liver was considered the source of heat generation which warmed the stomach like a saucepan, making it the site of the first "pepsis". The nutrient fluids thus generated flowed into the mesenteric and portal veins, where they were thought to undergo a second "pepsis". The parenchyma allegedly produced blood from the transformed and by now blood-like chylus.

into bile, e.g. after a poisonous animal bite. *These ideas are almost identical to the modern pathogenic concepts of mechanically, toxically or haemolytically induced icterus.*

GALENOS' morphological and pathophysiological conceptions based on animal experiments served as unchallenged dogma for over 1,000 years. • ***He may justifiably be regarded as the founder of scientifically orientated hepatology.***

2 Liver research in the Middle Ages

Arabian medicine: Liver research in the following centuries was generally stagnant and bereft of new ideas. It is true that Arabian medicine led by RHAZES (865–926) underwent a revival and that AVICENNA (980–1037) supplied a compendium on the art of Galenic and Arabian medicine in his five-volume *"Canon medicinae"* — nevertheless, Arabian medicine did not contribute any new morphological or physiological findings to the body of knowledge regarding the liver.

Anatomia Mundini: It is not known in which way the famous anatomists of that time — HEROPHILOS and ERASISTRATOS (s. p. 6) as well as GALENOS (s. p. 7) — obtained their knowledge about the human body. All previous descriptions regarding the anatomy of the liver were recorded in 1316 by MONDINO DE LUZZI (Bologna) in his *"Anatomia Mundini"*.

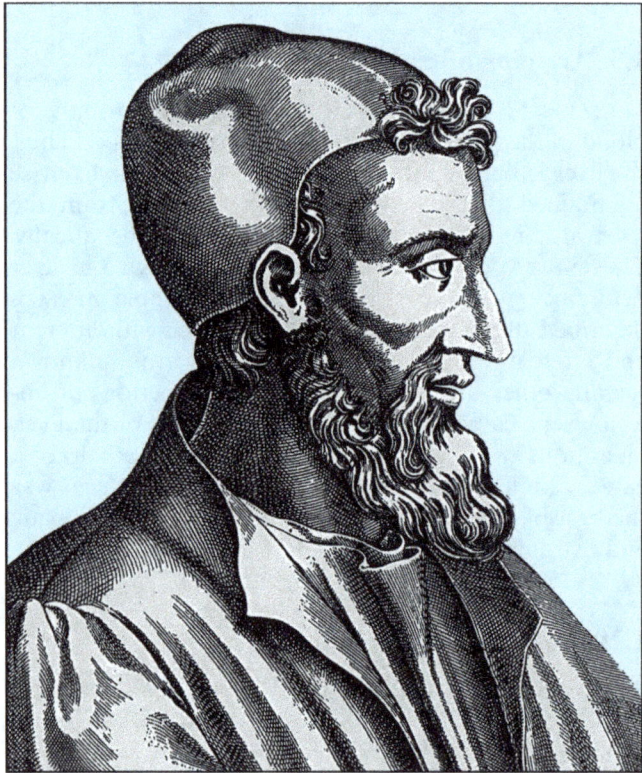

Fig. 1.12: GALENOS OF PERGAMON (131–201 AD) (129–199 AD?) (Medical Academy Paris; photo by René Jacques, Paris)

▶ GALENOS was the first to ligature the liver veins of live animals in the interests of liver research. He held the opinion that further biological reactions must occur in the liver parenchyma. He also recognized the peristalsis-stimulating effect of yellow bile (!). Following the older description of RUFUS OF EPHESUS, GALENOS differentiated various **forms of icterus**: (*1.*) icterus could occur as a result of inflammation, hardening or compression of the choledochus, (*2.*) icterus could develop at the crisis of a feverish illness, (*3.*) obstruction of the excretion of bile from the liver could cause jaundice, and (*4.*) icterus could result from the transformation of blood

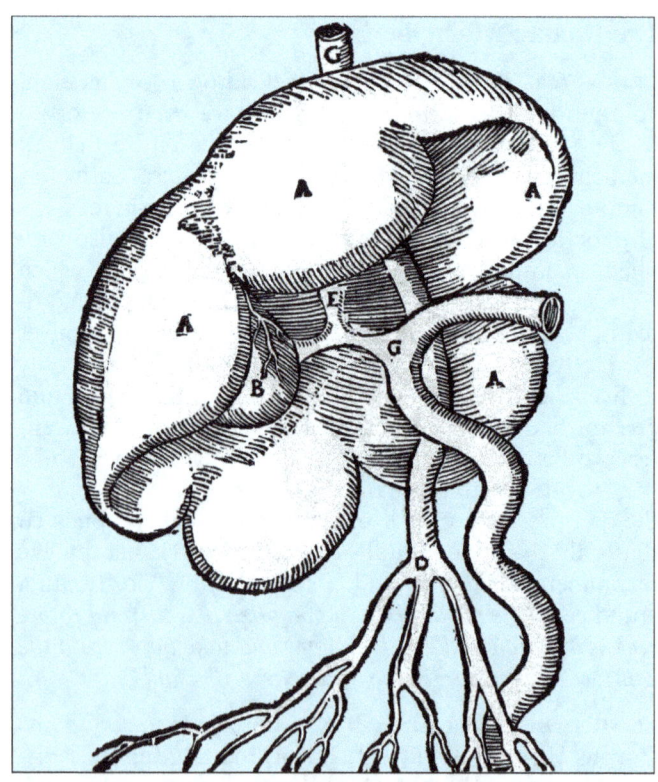

Fig. 1.13: Visceral surface of the multiple-lobed liver (A), with the gall bladder (B), portal vein (D), bile duct, bile system (C, E) ("Anatomia Mundini", 1316) (MONDINO DE LUZZI, Bologna)

This work is based on autopsies which he carried out for the very first time in public in 1306 and 1315. This unprecedented textbook of anatomy served as a canon for almost two centuries. (s. fig. 1.13)

LEONARDO DA VINCI (1452–1519) was perhaps the greatest universal genius in the history of mankind. In the field of hepatology, he studied the portal vein system, intrahepatic vessels and bile-duct system in an excellent manner. He did not publish his first-rate observations, which therefore remained unknown for a long time.

PARACELSUS (1493–1541): The many bitter attacks by Theophrastus Bombastus of Hohenheim, known as PARACELSUS, against the doctrines of GALENOS and AVICENNA heralded the end of the first epoch of liver research (ca. 2000 BC – ca. 1500 AD). PARACELSUS also initiated the era of iatric chemistry. He regarded the liver as the site of chemical and material transformations, particularly the processing of nutrient and metabolic "mercurial" substances. The emphasis was no longer on the "digestio" but on the "separatio" of substances inside the liver. (s. fig. 1.14) (s. pp XIX, 83, 923)

In his book *"De origine morborum ex tartaro"* (1531), PARACELSUS described the role of the liver as follows:

> *"... because the liver is a source of many diseases, and is a noble organ that serves many organs, almost all of them: so it suffers, it is not a small suffering, but a great and manifold one."*

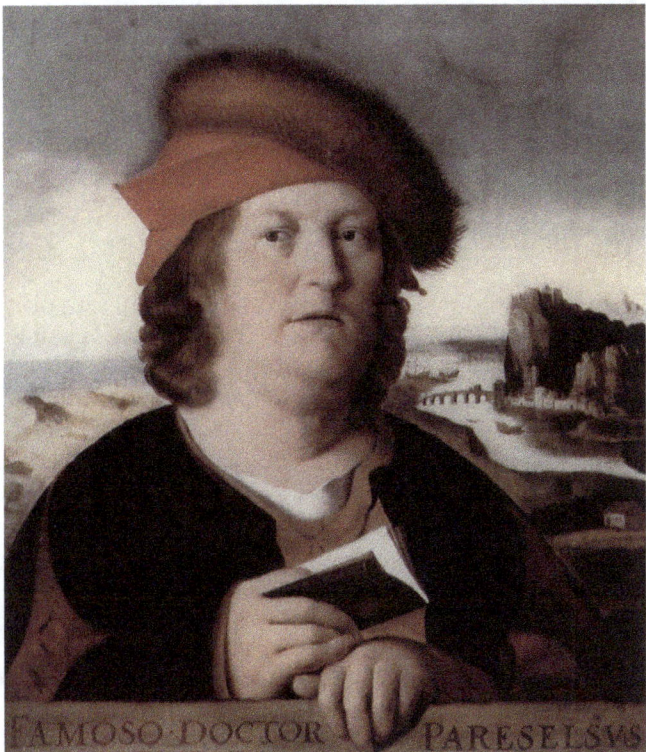

Fig. 1.14: PARACELSUS (1493–1541) (Jan van Scorel, Louvre Museum, Paris; colour photo by Laniepce, Paris)

VESALIUS (1514–1564): An anatomical and historical demarcation line between the ancient and the more modern and scientific doctrine was drawn in 1543 with the publication of *"De corporis humani fabrica libri septem"* by A. VESALIUS, who thus became the founder of contemporary anatomical science. He introduced a uniform Latin nomenclature. (25) Supported by careful investigations, the morphology of the liver and its blood vessels was presented in exact detail for the first time in the seventh book. (s. fig. 1.15) The previously held belief that the liver comprised four or five distinct lobes was discredited. His idea was to differentiate between the right and left lobe as well as between the quadrate and caudate process; he also described the falciform ligament. In addition, he discovered that the vena cava did not originate in the liver. The Galenic dogma that the liver is the origin of the venous system was rejected. He did, however, adopt the Galenic concepts of liver function and recognized the foetal connection between the portal vein and the inferior vena cava (1561), later termed the *ductus venosus Vesalii*, and not *"Arantii"*.

Remember that G. C. ARANZI did not discover the D. venosus until 1564.) (see quot. 18: vol. I/p. 67!)

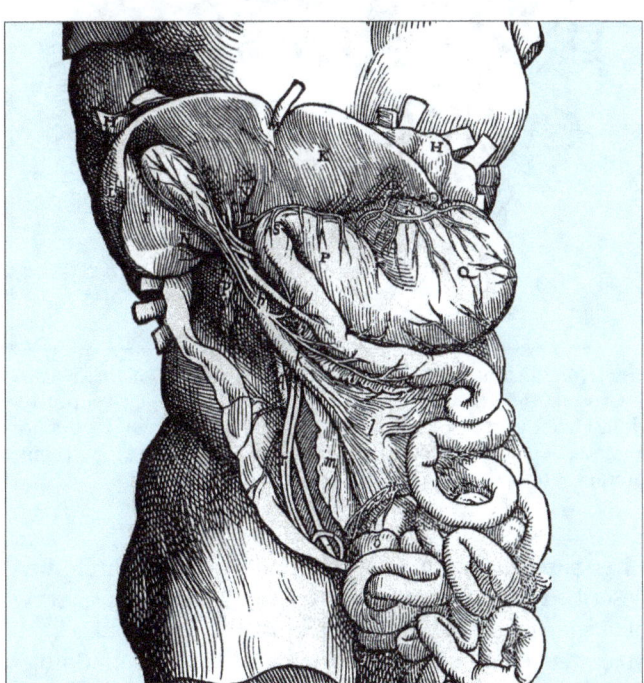

Fig. 1.15: Illustration of the human visceral liver surface by A. VESALIUS, 1543 (25)

Blood circulation: With the new doctrine of the blood circulatory system by W. HARVEY (1578–1657), the old hepatological theory collapsed. The arteries were now regarded as nutrition-bearing vessels. The liver was no longer deemed the site of blood production, but was integrated in the venous arm of the blood circulatory system. It was seen as a point of collection and storage for chylus and nutrients (1628).

GLISSON (1597−1677): In 1654 F. GLISSON published the first comprehensive monograph on the liver, which was to serve as an authoritative research work of reference for the next two centuries. (9) The inner structure of the liver, characterized by its intrahepatic vascular vessels, the differentiation of liver segments (!) through the large branches of the portal vein, the terminal regions of the blood capillaries and bile capillaries as functional pathways and the dynamics of the bile flow were all described in detail in *"Anatomia hepatis"*. (s. fig. 1.16) "Glisson's capsule" was recognized as branching, tree-like intrahepatic connective tissue. The portal vessels, which are surrounded by connective tissue, are termed portal trias ("Glisson's triangle") (1659). GLISSON found nerves only in the liver capsule, and not in the parenchyma. The role of the liver parenchyma was regarded as that of separating the bile from the blood by mechanisms of "affinity".

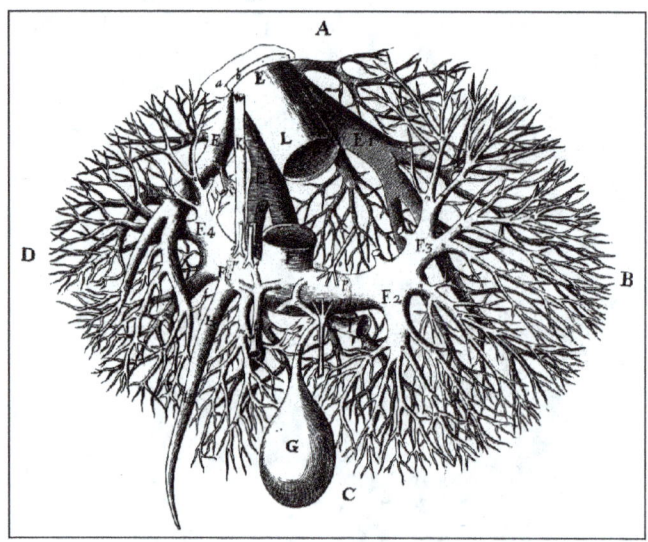

Fig. 1.16: Illustration of the blood and bile vessels of the liver by F. GLISSON, 1654 (A: dorsal region, B: right aspect, C: ventral region, D: left aspect, E: hepatic veins, H: umbilical vein, K: duct of ARANTIUS, G: gall bladder, I: bile duct, F: portal vein) (9) (Univ. Library, Freiburg)

Liver parenchyma, now at the forefront of research, was described in the pig by J.J. WEPFER (1664) as consisting of a gland comprising innumerable liver "lobules". M. MALPIGHI (1666) discovered the grapelike "out-budding" structure of the parenchyma into "lobuli" and "glandulosi acini". He defined the latter as the smallest functional unit of the organ, with each acinus having a branch of an afferent and an efferent vein as well as a bile-duct terminus. M. F. X. BICHAT (1771−1802) considered the liver parenchyma to be a special tissue in terms of function and morphology. In addition, he suspected that the liver had far more capabilities than had previously been assumed.

Bile began to assume increasing importance in theories on the processes of metabolism: it was defined as an alkaline secretion and the paramount digestive fluid by J.B. VAN HELMONT (1579−1644). J. JASOLINUS (1654) made a distinction between gall-bladder bile and liver bile, which was subsequently confirmed by J. BOHN (1697) as well as by H. BOERHAAVE (1708), who also recognized the role of bile in the digestion of fats. M. MALPIGHI had already established the thickening of bile in the gall bladder as early as 1687. In 1710 A. BORELLI described the enterohepatic circulation of bile through the portal vein system. The ligation of the hepatic artery by M. MALPIGHI and J. BOHN, and of the portal vein by H. BOERHAAVE, led to the conclusion that the liver, rather than the gall bladder, was the organ of biligenesis.

Lymphatic vessels: With the discovery of the intestinal lymphatic vessels by C. ASELLI (1622), of the thoracic duct by J. PECQET (1651), of the separate nature of the chylus vessels and lymphatic systems by T. BARTHOLIN (1653) and of the exact description of the hepatic lymph vessels by O. RUDBEK (1653), the liver came to be regarded as an "excretory organ" which removed bile and other aqueous fluid (T. BARTHOLIN: *"lympha"*) from the blood. PECQET recognized that nutrients reach the thoracic duct via the lacteal ducts and are then fed into the venous system before the right heart.

Connective tissue: It appears that J. WALEUS (1640) was the first to describe connective tissue in the liver, namely in the area surrounding the vessels. • M. MALPIGHI (who is considered the founder of microscopic anatomy) detected connective tissue between the acini in 1666.

Nervous system: The innervation of the liver was described by TH. WILLIS (1621−1675).

HALLER (1708−1777): No doubt the most significant milestone text in the field of liver research was *"Elementa physiologiae corporis humani"* published in 1764 by ALBRECHT VON HALLER. (s. fig. 1.17)

In *Volume 6* of this immense encyclopaedia, HALLER presented a comprehensive picture of 18th century **hepatology**. His work was so advanced that it was to form the indispensable basis of liver research up to modern times. All previous findings and conclusions dating back to antiquity were critically reviewed; dogmatic and speculative hypotheses and outmoded results were rejected and sound findings, mostly proven in experiments of his own, confirmed to yield a balanced, all-embracing account of the field of hepatology. It is important to mention that the theory of haematopoiesis in the liver was finally refuted. The main task of the liver was seen in the formation of bile, which was regarded as an indispensable digestive substance. HALLER was the first to describe the variants of the hepatic artery the pathophysiology of obstructive jaundice and the insensitivity to pain of the liver parenchyma.

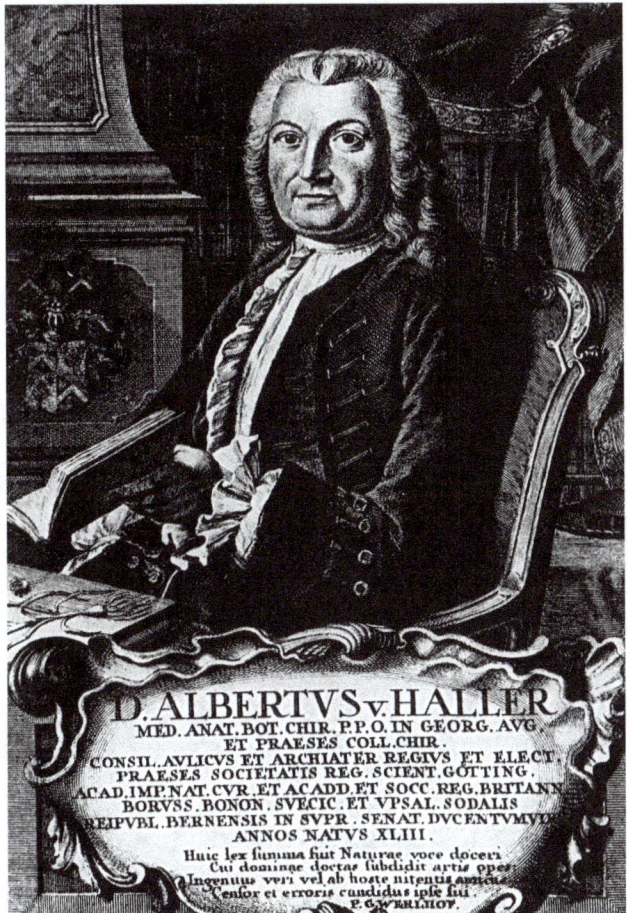

Fig. 1.17: ALBRECHT VON HALLER (1708–1777) (Nat. Library Bern; photo by Boissonnas, Geneva)

3 Liver research up to modern times

In subsequent years, a series of landmark findings substantially furthered the science of hepatology. The use of the microscope brought greater insight into the morphology of liver diseases. As a result of refined methods of chemical investigations, the liver was recognized as a *"chemical laboratory"* and as the *"site of intermediary metabolism"*. (6, 16, 18, 20, 26)

1757 Proof of crystallization of bile acid compounds by P. RAMSAY.

1775 Discovery of bile cholesterol by B. G. F. CONRADI (published in 1783) – apparently postdating the earlier description of this substance by F. P. L. POULLETIER DE LA SALLE.

1789 First mention of green or yellow "bile pigments" by A. F. FOURCROY.

1796 S. TH. SÖMMERING defined the total mass of the liver lobule as "acinus" on the grounds that it was composed solely of vessels (cf. M. MALPIGHI, 1666).

1815 C. B. ROSE confirmed a decrease of urea concentration in the urine in chronic liver disease and postulated the synthesis of urea in the liver.

1816 M. E. CHEVREUL reconfirmed the presence of cholesterol in both bile and gallstones (1824) and termed this compound "cholesterol".

1817 F. MAGENDIE postulated the detoxifying function of the liver.

1824 L. GMELIN described cholic acid (= glycocholic acid) as well as the bile pigments "brown bile" and "green bile" arising from oxidation processes. Inauguration of "Gmelin's test". Bile acid chemistry begins.

1826 Proof of cholic acid and taurin in the bile by F. TIEDEMANN and L. GMELIN.

1828 F. WÖHLER demonstrated the artificial synthesis of urea from ammonia.

1833 Description of the hexagonal architecture of the liver lobule and of the anastomoses of the fine bile capillaries by F. KIERNAN. (s. fig. 1.18)

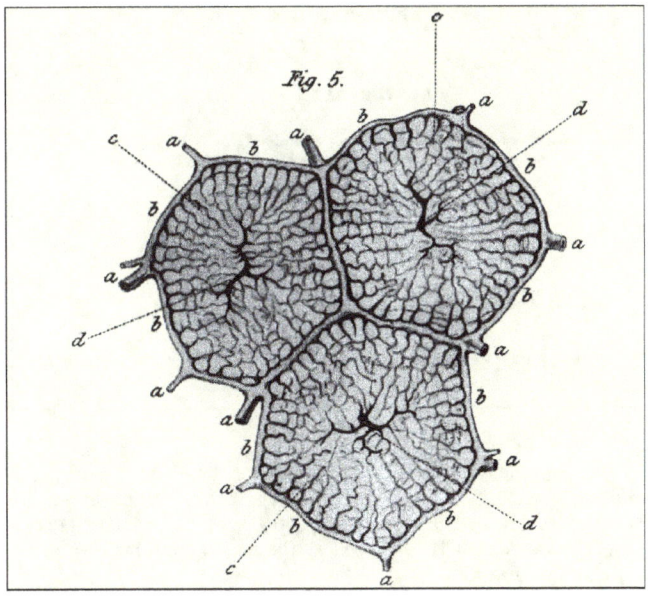

Fig. 1.18: Illustration of liver lobules and vessels by F. KIERNAN, 1833 (a, b: interlobular veins, c: intralobular vein plexus, d: intralobular branch of the central hepatic vein) (15)

1837 Discovery of the liver cell with its core by J. E. PURKINJE, later by J. HENLE (1838), also by F. DUJARDIN and G. VERGER, but probably already discovered at an earlier time by M. DUTROCHET (1824).

1839 Description of the intralobular connective tissue by E. HALLMANN.

1840 The "green bile" described by L. GMELIN is designated "biliverdin" by J. J. BERZELIUS.

1841 J. HENLE describes the bile canaliculi in the liver lobules as simple, unwalled intracellular spaces.

1842 J. LIEBIG postulated the liver's role in intermediary metabolism; bile production was described as one part of protein and carbohydrate metabolism, and the synthesis of urea in the liver was accepted.

1844 J. MÜLLER localized the site of bile synthesis in the liver

1846 Detection of haematopoiesis in the foetal liver by A. KÖLLIKER.

Dr. Hans Eppinger

KLINIK

DER

LEBERKRANKHEITEN

VON

Dr. FRIED. THEOD. FRERICHS,

ordentlichem Professor der medicinischen Klinik an der Königl. Friedrich-Wilhelms-Universität. Geheimem Medicinal-Rath und vortragendem Rathe im Ministerio der geistlichen, Unterrichts- und Medicinal-Angelegenheiten in Berlin.

IN ZWEI BÄNDEN.

ERSTER BAND.

Mit einem Atlas von 12 sorgfältig colorirten Stahlstich-Tafeln in Royal-Quart und zahlreichen in den Text eingedruckten Holzstichen.

ZWEITE VERBESSERTE AUFLAGE.

BRAUNSCHWEIG,

DRUCK UND VERLAG VON FRIEDRICH VIEWEG UND SOHN.

1861.

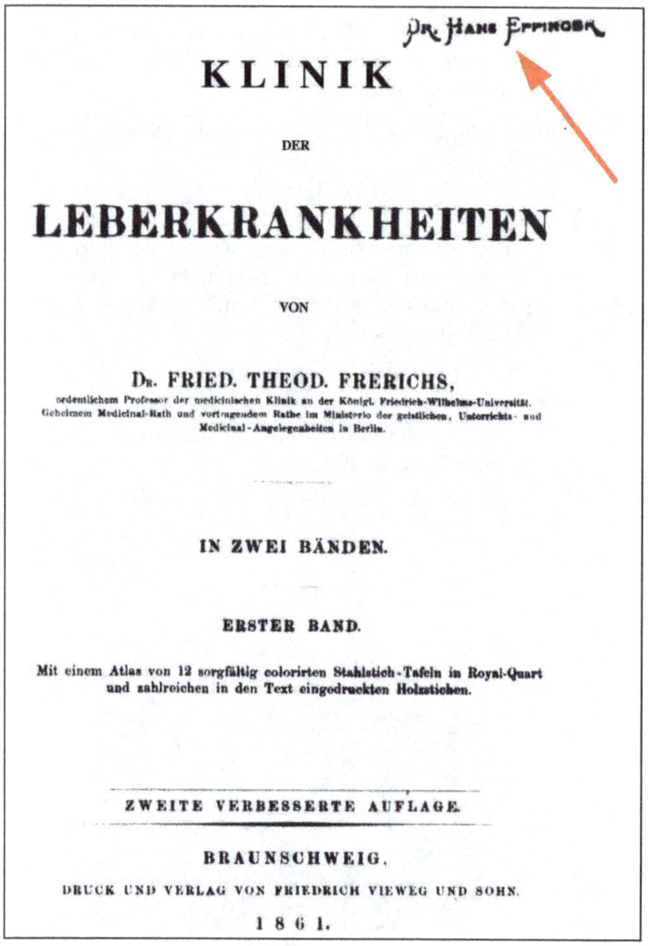

Fig. 1.19: Front page of the outstanding textbook „Klinik der Leberkrankheiten" by F. Th. Frerichs (1819–1885): two volumes (1st ed. 1858, 2nd ed. 1861) Verlag Vieweg, Braunschweig/ Germany; 416 and 549 pages respectively. (s. fig. 5.1!). – **(Personal possession of H. Eppinger! – Purchased from his estate)** • *(private property)*

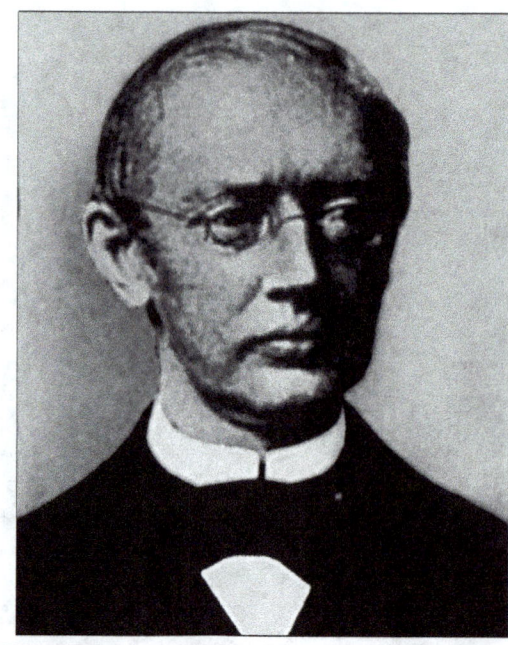

Fig. 1.20: Portrait of Friedrich Theodor Frerichs from 1862, the founder of modern liver pathology

1847 R. Virchow described "Hämatoidin" and the extrahepatic synthesis of bile pigments from haematoidin in old haematomas (s. Galenos: "blood turns to bile").

1848 Detection of 2 paired bile acids by A. Strecker: the taurin-containing cholic acid and the glycine-containing cholic acid, respectively designated taurocholic and glycocholic acid by C.G. Lehmann in 1854.

1848 Description of bile microcapillaries in peripheral hepatic lobules by J. Gerlach.

1848 Sugar synthesis (= glycogen) in the liver identified by C. Bernard and C.L. Barresvil.

1854 Description of hepatocellular trabeculae by J. Gerlach.

1855 F. Führer and H. Ludwig postulated the synthesis of urea from erythrocytes.

1857 C. Bernard was the first to demonstrate glycogen in the liver. • He became the *founder of modern liver physiology.*

1858 Publication of *„Klinik der Leberkrankheiten"* (s. fig. 1.19) by F. Th. Frerichs (1819–1885). • He became the *founder of modern liver pathology.* (s. fig. 1.20)

1863 The "brown bile" (described by L. Gmelin) is termed "bilirubin" by G. Städeler (originally termed "bilirubrin" in 1844 by E.A. Platner).

1866 E. Hering proposed that the bile capillaries were bounded solely by liver cells and that the parenchyma had a structure of little plates rather than a trabecular form.

1868 M. Jaffé isolated "urobilin" and urobilinogen from urine (corresponding to stercobilin in the stool).

1869 E. Ponfick first described the Kupffer cells and their phagocytic activity, which was more extensively documented by J. Peszke in 1874 and by K.W. von Kupffer in 1876.

1870 First description of the enterohepatic bile circulation by M. Schiff.

1871 B. Maly demonstrated the hydrolytic conversion of bilirubin to urobilin in the intestine.

1871 Detection of stercobilin by C. Vanlair and V. Masius.

1880 First blind hepatic biopsy performed by P. Ehrlich.

1882 W. von Schröder demonstrates ureagenesis in the liver.

1884 Ch. Th. Billroth carried out the first surgical treatment of a refractory ascites using hepatopexia.

1887 F. von Müller discovered urobilinogen in urine.

1890 Confirmation of the existence of perivascular lymphatic vessels by J. Disse ("Disse's space"), which had already been proposed by Th. MacGillavry in 1864.

1890 Demonstration of the blood supply to the liver through the portal vein according to the double-flow principle by F. Glenard.

1891 Description of the lattice fibres and their demarcation by elastic fibre and collagenous connective tissue by A. Oppel.
1892 S. Minot coined the term "sinusoid" to describe the blood capillaries leading in a radial fashion to the central vein of the lobule.
1893 Demonstration of "meat intoxication" following an experimental shunt operation by J. Pawlov.
1894 G. Banti performed the first surgical treatment of bleeding varices by resection of the short gastric veins with splenectomy (Note: G. Banti had already reduced portal venous volume by splenectomy in 1874).
1903 M. Vidal performed the first portocaval shunt surgery on a human subject (= end-to-side anastomosis).
1903 W. Schlesinger described the detection of urobilin in urine. • In the same year, O. Neubauer found that Ehrlich's reagent (dimethylaminoazobenzaldehyde) together with urobilinogen results in reddening.

▶ For further historical details, see the respective chapters!

The above selection of pioneering work links up with modern hepatology, which has developed from biochemistry, histology and histochemistry — and is based on biomolecular and microstructural research methods.

The current **4th epoch** of liver research may later be known as **"biomolecular hepatology"**. *Not only examination techniques based on biochemistry, histology and imaging, but also the therapy of liver disease will increasingly be determined by biomolecular research.*

References:

1. **Baumann, E.D.:** Über die Erkrankungen der Leber im klassischen Altertum. Janus 1931; 35: 153–168; 185–206
2. **Blecher, G.:** De extispicio capita tria. Töpelmann, A., Gießen, 1905, Fig. 2, Tab. 2
3. **Cahill, K.M.:** Platonic concepts of hepatology. Arch. Intern. Med. 1963; 111: 819–822
4. **Chen S.N., Th., P.S.Y. Chen:** The myth of Prometheus and the liver. J. Roy. Soc. Med. 1994; 87: 754–755
5. **Contenau, G.:** La médécine en Assyrie et en Babylonie. Paris 1938, 114–115, 137, 220, 235–269
6. **Franken, F.H.:** Die Leber und ihre Krankheiten. Zweihundert Jahre Hepatologie. Enke, Stuttgart, 1968, 247 pp.
7. **Giglioli, G.Q.:** L'arte etrusca. S.A. Fratelli Treves, Milano, 1935, Fig. 1, Tab. 298
8. **Glenard, R.:** Le foie dans l'anquité. Aesculape 1924; 14: 25–28
9. **Glisson, F.:** Anatomia hepatis. Typis Du-Gardianis. London, 1654
10. **Güterbock, H.G.:** Die Texte aus der Grabung 1935 in Bogazköy. Mitt. Dtsch. Orient-Ges., Berlin 1935; 73: 29–39
11. **Hagen, H.:** Die physiologische und psychologische Bedeutung der Leber in der Antike. Diss. Bonn, 1961
12. **Horaz:** Epistulae. Ep. 18, 73
13. **Jastrow, M.:** Bildermappe zur Religion Babyloniens und Assyriens. Töpelmann, A., Gießen, 1912, Tafel Nr. 34, 102
14. **Juvenal:** Satirae. Sat. 1, 45; cf. 6, 648
15. **Kiernan, F.:** The anatomy and physiology of the liver. Philos. Transact. Royal Soc. London 1833; 123: 711 (fig. XXIII, 5)
16. **Kluge, F.:** Die Leber und ihre Krankheiten: Ein historischer Rückblick. Leber Magen Darm 1997; 27: 15–22
17. **Langlotz, E.:** Griechische Vasen. Obermetter, München, 1932, Tafel Nr. 175, 507
18. **Mani, N.:** Die historischen Grundlagen der Leberforschung. Band 1: Die Vorstellungen über Anatomie, Physiologie und Pathologie der Leber in der Antike. Schwabe, Basel, 1965. Band 2: Die Geschichte der Leberforschung von Galen bis Claude Bernard. Schwabe, Basel, 1967
19. **Meythaler, F., Pietsch, W.:** Anschauungen über die Bedeutung von Leber und Galle im Altertum bis Galen. Med. Welt 1936; 10: 431–434
20. **Pressel, A.:** Die Lebermittel der alten Medizin. Diss. Univ. Jena, 1936, 80 pp.
21. **Rutten, M.:** Trente-deux modèles de foies en argile inscrits provenant de Tell-Hariri (Mari). Rev. Assyr. 1938; 35: 36–70
22. **Sigerist, H.E.:** A history of medicine. Vol. I: Primitive and archaie medicine. New York 1951
23. **Stieda, L.:** Über die ältesten bildlichen Darstellungen der Leber. Anatom. Hefte 1900; 15: 675–720
24. **Tillyard, E.M.W.:** The hope vases. Cambridge, Univ. Press., 1923, Fig. 26
25. **Vesalius, A.:** De corporis humani fabrica libri septem. Oporin, Basel, 1543, Fig. 12
26. **Vorwahl, H.:** Die Leber in der Volksmedizin. Dtsch. Med. Wschr. 1928; 54: 1769–1770

2 Morphology of the Liver

		Page:
1	*Embryology of the liver*	16
1.1	Liver stem cells	17
2	*General anatomy of the liver*	17
2.1	Topography	18
2.2	Form and variants	18
2.3	Segmental subdivisions	19
3	*Structure and histology of the liver*	20
3.1	Intrahepatic vascular system	20
3.1.1	Hepatic artery	20
3.1.2	Portal vein	21
3.1.3	Hepatic vein	21
3.1.4	Biliary system	21
3.1.5	Lymph vessels	22
3.2	Stroma of the liver	22
3.2.1	Capsule of the liver	22
3.2.2	Perivascular connective tissue	23
3.2.3	Lattice fibre network	23
3.2.4	Portal tract	24
3.3	Sinusoidal cells	24
3.3.1	Endothelial cells	24
3.3.2	Kupffer cells	24
3.3.3	Ito cells	24
3.3.4	PIT cells	25
3.4	Hepatocytes	25
3.5	Biliary epithelial cells	26
4	*Nervous system*	26
5	*Hepatic lobules and acinus*	26
5.1	Central vein lobule	26
5.2	Portal vein lobule	27
5.3	Liver acinus	27
6	*Subcellular structures*	29
6.1	Cytoplasm	29
6.2	Cell nucleus	29
6.3	Organelles	30
6.4	Membrane	31
6.5	Cytoskeleton	32
	• References (1−79)	32

(Figures 2.1−2.19; table 2.1)

2 Morphology of the Liver

1 Embryology of the liver

> The development of the fertilized ovum during the first 18 days is defined as **blastogenesis** • After that, **embryogenesis** begins (lasting up to the 56th day): during this phase, the organs and organ systems are formed. • The period from the 56th day until birth is known as **fetogenesis**.

From the 18th day of gestation (with an embryo length of 2.5 mm) **hepatogenesis** begins with a thickening of the endoplasmic epithelium in the region of the caudal foregut. (The foregut is the future duodenum.) This endodermal area subsequently opens up into the liver groove. As from the 22nd day of gestation (with an embryo length of 3−4 mm), the groove widens into a diverticular recess with a cranial and caudal region. From the cranial part of the diverticulum, the liver is formed with the intrahepatic bile ducts. From the caudal part of the diverticulum, the gall bladder, ductus cysticus and ductus choledochus are formed.

▶ The *onset of hepatogenesis* is dependent on FGF1 and FGF2. Further FGFs of the 22 members of the FGF family have other functions during the later stages of hepatogenesis. In addition, bone morphogenetic protein (BMP) helps to induce liver development within the ventral endoderm. Important sources of signalling molecules are also found in heart and transverse septum mesenchyma.

Hepatoblasts (= primitive hepatocyte precursor cells) develop from the endodermal outgrowths of the cranial diverticulum and sprout into the mesenchymal tissue of the transverse septum. They form plates which are five to six liver cells thick (= *muralium multiplex*). The plates invade the transverse septum and surround preexisting spaces, from which the sinusoids subsequently develop. The hepatoblasts proliferate along these sinusoidal spaces, similar to a guide rail. (17) **Sinusoids** develop in situ. As the embryo continues to grow together with an increase in parenchymal proliferation, the endothelium-lined spaces become better defined. Finally, small vessels appear. In the sinusoidal endothelium, large intercellular gaps can be found, which allow the passage of haematopoietic cells. During the 8th−10th gestation week, hepatic haematopoiesis begins. In the course of postnatal life, the liver cell plates are reduced to a thickness of two cells (= *muralium duplex*); after the fifth year of life, the liver has a thickness of just one cell (= *muralium simplex*). From the 29th day of gestation, the formation and secretion of α_1-fetoprotein begins in the hepatoblasts (it is repressed immediately after birth).

The mesenchymal framework of the transverse septum forms the stroma, capsule and mesothelium of the liver; the mesoderm on the surface becomes its peritoneal cover. As the liver invades the transverse septum, the mesenterium is split into two membranes: the lesser omentum and the falciform ligament. As from the 6th week, the liver expands due to its rapid growth, into the abdominal cavity. At this point, the two liver lobes are already recognizable. The embryo now has a length of 10 mm.

In the 6th embryonic week, the **canaliculi** begin to develop between three to seven neighbouring parenchymal cells (the embryo is now in the 10 mm stage). Bile duct epithelia form in the vicinity of the portal vein branches; they are derived from hepatoblasts (i.e. of hepatocytogenic origin). These ductular cells are seen as a kind of cuff around the "portal" ramifications and thus create a double-layered epithelial sleeve, the so-called **ductal plate** (J.A. HAMMAR, 1926). • As from the 12th embryonic week, remodelling of the ductal plate into the interlobular bile ducts takes place, whereby surplus bile ducts are degraded. Bile secretion commences after the 16th week. Principally, the formation of the bile ducts is completed by the 28th embryonic week. Cholangiogenesis is accompanied by the expression of various keratin profiles, e.g. type 7, 8, 18 and 19. (8, 60)

▶ However, the intrahepatic bile-duct system is still immature at birth; that means the final development of the smallest ramifications takes place during the first few neonatal weeks. At this stage, the intrahepatic biliary system is most susceptible to noxae, which can lead to paucity or even atresia of the bile ducts. (s. p. 696)

The **Ito cells** appear in the 6th to 8th week of gestation. **Kupffer cells** develop as from the 3rd embryonic month; they are most probably derived from primitive macrophages built up in the yolk sac or from haematopoietic stem cells.

Already in the 6th week (= 10 mm stage), the first haematoblasts appear, and the liver begins to assume the task of **haematopoiesis**. In the 7th week (= 12 mm stage), the first blood-forming islands develop. They invade all the hepatic parenchyma, but are more pronounced in the right lobe of liver. The maximum activity of haematopoiesis is evident in the 6th and 7th month; after that, it is repressed, as the bone marrow becomes haematopoietic. At birth, the foetal liver contains only a few disseminated islands, which disappear in the first weeks of life. Lymphocytic cells are detectable as from the 14th week of gestation.

The vitelline (= omphalomesenteric) veins form a capillary plexus. Anastomotic capillaries connect the vitelline venous plexus with the umbilical veins. In the 6 mm embryo, a large venous trunk develops in the sinusoidal system and shunts blood directly from the umbilical vein to the inferior vena cava. The **duct of Arantius** persists until birth, when it atrophies; 10 to 20 days later, it leaves as a vestige the ligamentum venosum. In reality, the ductus venosus should be called duct of Vesalius, because VESALIUS recognized this anastomosis in 1561, whereas ARANTIUS did not make his observation until 1564. (s. p. 9) The segment of the umbilical vein between the umbilicus and the liver regresses into a fibrous cord, the round ilgament (= lig. teres hepatis). The definitive vascular pattern of the liver is established around the 6th week (= 17 mm stage). The initially paired umbilical vein changes markedly; the right vein and the proximal portion of the left umbilical vein rapidly disappear. (78)

1.1 Liver stem cells

R. VIRCHOW founded **"cellular pathology"** in 1858. He postulated that illnesses resulted from disturbances of the cells. Later, **"cellular therapy"** developed, whereby missing or malfunctioning cells are replaced by intact cells. • This is accomplished by the healthy organism itself with the help of various body cells; however, only cells of the same type can be renewed: thus they are only unipotent in terms of *"reparative medicine"*.

> **Stem cells** are cells which reveal no or only slight differentiation; they are not yet predetermined for their later function in the growing organism. Stem cells possess two fascinating capabilities: (*1.*) they are able to multiply in an unlimited fashion and to regenerate continuously; (*2.*) they are able to produce highly differentiated progenitor cells.

Adult stem cells are detectable during an individual's whole life, e.g. in bone marrow, in the brain and liver, but also initially in the umbilical cord. Their task is to replace necrotic tissue by differentiating into cells of the same tissue (= *reparative medicine*). During the process, they may lose the ability to divide, but can also fulfil tissue-specific tasks. Since the cells only differentiate into cell types of the same tissue, they must be regarded as *multipotent*.

▶ In 1963, J. TILL et al. detected multipotent blood stem cells in the bone marrow of mice. These stem cells were capable of forming leukocytes, erythrocytes, monocytes and thrombocytes.

Embryonic stem cells exist in two forms: (*1.*) stem cells which are only found in the *blastomere stage* up to the first segmentation: this consists of a cell cluster (= morula) with 50−150 cells in a phase 4−5 days after fertilization of the ovum. These stem cells are *totipotent* (= omnipotent), i.e. it is still possible for all of the approximately 210 cell forms in the human being to develop from these cells. (*2.*) Stem cells in the *blastocyst stage* are *pluripotent*, i.e. it is possible for all types of body cells of the three germ layers (endoderm, mesoderm, ectoderm) to develop from these cells − however, they cannot become placenta cells. If no stimuli are given for cell-specific differentiation, the embryonic stem cells will divide and each daughter cell will remain pluripotent. Due to their unique capacity to combine unlimited expansion and pluripotency, these cells must be seen as a possible source for *"regenerative medicine"* and tissue replacement in cases of injury or disease.

▶ In 1998, J. THOMSON was the first investigator to isolate embryonic stem cells from a seven-day-old human embryo, which had been fertilized in vitro, and to use them for culturing several cell lines.

Liver stem cells: In 1958, J.W. WILSON and E.H. LEDUC postulated the presence of liver stem cells (LSC) for the first time. They are considered to be genuine and participate in the normal turnover of the liver parenchyma. Such LSCs (7−15 μm) have multilineage differentiation potential and self-renewal capability, similar to the cells of the cranial and caudal diverticulum after the 6th week of gestation. • In addition, so-called **oval cells** can be found. They are formed from terminal periductular cells. The population comprises immature small cells with a scant cytoplasm and ovoid nuclei. Such cells can differentiate into hepatocytes and biliary epithelial cells. In the case of severe liver injury, the regenerative potential of the stem cells and/or oval cells is activated. In the adult liver, both LSC and oval cells are able to replace parenchymal loss. Apparently, specific signalling substances are required for stimulating the regeneration mechanism. An important stem cell growth factor is G-CSF (= granulocyte-colony stimulating factor). • A **third population** of stem cells with hepatic potential is found in the bone marrow. It was possible to transform these stem cells into hepatocytes. However, it remains unclear in what way these three stem cell populations work together to replace parenchyma. (14, 51, 56, 79)

There are three different mechanisms for **regeneration** of the liver: (*1.*) transdifferentiation of LSCs into hepatocytes and biliary epithelial cells, (*2.*) proliferation of oval cells as so-called liver progenitor cells, and (*3.*) division of hepatocytes. The last mentioned process is of less importance with regard to regeneration following resection, but more so concerning loss of function of the liver parenchyma.

▶ Each hepatocyte can divide at least 30 times. After 60% resection, the liver regenerates without any problem within 1−2 weeks in the animal model. Such 60% resections can be repeated several times after a corresponding ten-day regeneration period. The normal turnover in terms of continued proliferation of hepatocytes and biliary epithelial cells begins in the portal zone and "streams" towards the central veins (77). In the case of severe injury of the liver, including loss of parenchyma, this process is enhanced in a carefully steered manner.

2 General anatomy of the liver

The liver is the largest solid organ in the body. • The **weight** of a normal liver comprises about 1/18 of the newborn child's body weight (approx. 5%) and about 1/50 of the adult's body weight (2.3−3%), varying in men from 1,500−1,800 g and in women from 1,300−1,500 g. The relatively larger weight in infancy is mainly due to an enlargement of the left lobe. The weight of the liver relative to body weight decreases from 3% to 2% with age. With regard to **size,** the liver is on average 25−30 cm in width, 12−20 cm in length and 6–10 cm in thickness. The **surface** is smooth and shiny. The **colour** of the liver is brownish red. The lobular structure can be seen distinctly upon close inspection. The **position** is intraperitoneal (with the exception of the area nuda and the gall-bladder bed). (s. fig. 2.1) Due to the suction of the lung, the position of the liver depends on the position of the diaphragm; the respiratory displacement of the liver is approx. 3 cm. (s. fig. 4.3)

2.1 Topography

The topography of the liver is characterized by the (smaller) *left lobe* and the (about six times larger) *right lobe*, which are separated by the (translucent) *falciform ligament*. This peritoneal duplicature splits dorsad into a right and left coronary ligament of liver; both terminate in the left and right triangular ligament; the right part finally ends as the hepatorenal ligament. (s. figs. 2.1, 2,5; 16.4)

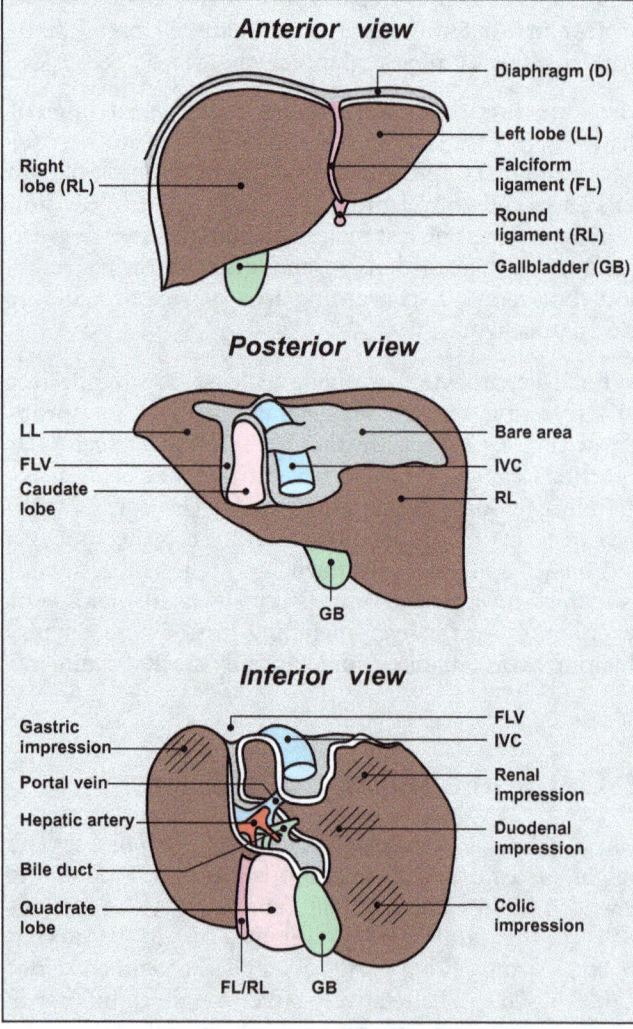

Fig. 2.1: Views of the liver: anterior, posterior, inferior. (LL = left lobe, RL = right lobe, D = diaphragm, GB = gall bladder, FLV = fissure for ligamentum venosum, RL = round ligament (= lig. teres), IVC = inferior vena cava, FL = falciform ligament)

The *round ligament* (= lig. teres) is a remnant of the umbilical vein of the foetus. It runs in the free edge of the falciform ligament (during the time of foetal development, it actually joins the left branch of the portal vein) and is often coated by drop-shaped mesenteric fat tissue. The *ligamentum venosum* is a slender remnant of the duct of Arantii in the foetus. (s. p. 9!) • On the inferior liver surface – separated by the portal vein – are the *quadrate lobe* (lying anteriorly between the gall bladder and round ligament) and the *caudate lobe* with papillary tubercle and caudate process (lying posteriorly along the inferior vena cava in front of the hepatic porta). This *hilum of the liver* in the centre of the inferior liver surface consists of the proper hepatic artery, portal vein, common hepatic duct, lymph vessels, and hepatic nerve plexus. These are held together by the perivascular fibrous capsule. (s. fig. 2.1)

With its convex **diaphragmatic surface**, the liver, which faces forwards and upwards, abuts the arch of the diaphragm and the anterior abdominal wall. It bears a flat cardiac impression. This diaphragmatic surface is differentiated into the *pars libera* (covered with peritoneum) and the *pars affixa* (= area nuda). • The **visceral surface** inclines both backwards and downwards. The superior and inferior surfaces form together the sharp liver margin (*margo inferior*). The inferior surface may show impressions caused by adjacent organs (gaster, colon, kidney, duodenum, gall bladder) and the posterior surface shows a *fissure* for the ligamentum venosum. (s. fig. 2.1)

2.2 Form and variants

The **shape** of the liver resembles largely that of a pyramid lying at a slant with its base towards the right side of the body. The exterior form can vary greatly. (s. p. 2)

Variations in form: In the first instance, *genetic factors* are responsible for variations. Additional *internal causative factors* worthy of mention include changes due to portal vein thrombosis, haemocongestion, cardiac cirrhosis, thesaurismosis, fibrosis and atrophy. *External causative factors* include impression effects caused by pillar of diaphragm, costal arch, xiphoid process and wearing tight belts or laced corsets. (37) • Chronic coughing may lead to mostly parallel *cough furrows* on the convexity of the right lobe, – one to six in number. (33) • *Zahn's furrows* can appear on the right surface of the liver; they generally run sagittally and are caused by hypertrophic columns as a result of chronic lung emphysema and also (more rarely) congenital factors. (s. fig. 2.2) • The posterior surface of the liver occasionally has furrows, known as *rima coeci Halleri*. A branch of the portal vein always extends beneath their bed (J. HYRTL, 1873). • A tongue-shaped projection of the right (or more rarely the left) lobe of liver adjacent to the gall bladder is known as *Riedel's lobe* (I. RIEDEL, 1888). This condition may be congenital or arise due to the traction of a gall bladder enlarged by stones. Ried-

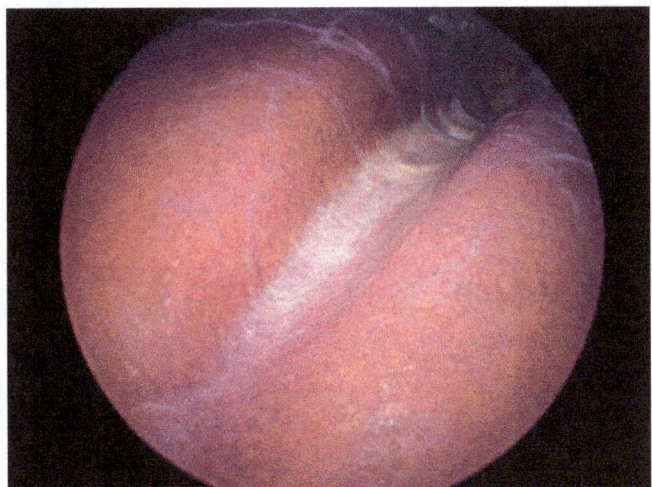

Fig. 2.2: Zahn's furrow: diagonal craniocaudal impression of a hypertrophic diaphragm contour. Along the bottom of the furrow, there is a capsular fibrosis

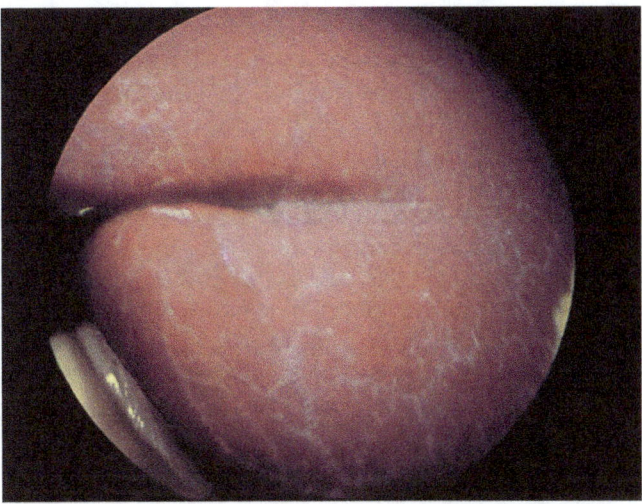

Fig. 2.3: Reticular fibrosis of the liver surface in chronic persistent hepatitis B with a so-called "simian cleft" (s. figs. 31.22; 35.5)

el's lobe is more frequent in women. It is not deemed to be a true accessory lobe. It is easily mistaken for other tumours in this area. • *Fissures* (also called "simian cleft") (s. figs. 2.3; 31,22; 35.5) – which may give rise to a hepar succenturiatum (= accessory lobe) (13) or hepar lobatum – are without clinical significance.

Variations in position: An interposition of intestinal loops (generally transverse colon) between liver and diaphragm is termed *Chilaiditi syndrome*. It is the result of hepatoptosis. • Any noticeable *relaxation of diaphragm* due to congenital muscular aplasia in the region of the right diaphragm leads to displacement of the right liver lobe into the right thoracic space. (68)

Accessory lobe: This anatomical abnormality is rare and without clinical significance. Torsions are rare findings. Up to 16 accessory lobes have been reported in a single patient. They are usually located on the inferior surface of the liver. (s. fig. 2.4) Therefore they are generally detected only during the course of imaging examinations, surgery or autopsy. In case of suspicion, diagnostic laparoscopy is indicated. Often an accessory lobe may contain its own blood, bile and lymph vessels. (13, 30, 38)

Lobar atrophy: Atrophy may develop as a result of disturbances in the portal blood supply or biliary drainage of a lobe. It is generally possible to differentiate between the two aetiologies with the help of scintigraphic methods. • Likewise, lobar atrophy (the left liver lobe is most frequently affected) may develop following necrosing processes of the parenchyma, such as those caused by acute virus hepatitis (s. figs. 21.13; 22.16), intoxications and chemoembolization, or in cases of severe inanition as well as in marked cirrhosis (s. figs. 35.1, 35.17). Compensatory hypertrophy of the opposite lobe is usually in evidence. (20, 21, 76)

Lobar agenesis: In most cases, agenesis affects the right lobe. This very rare abnormality is mostly associated

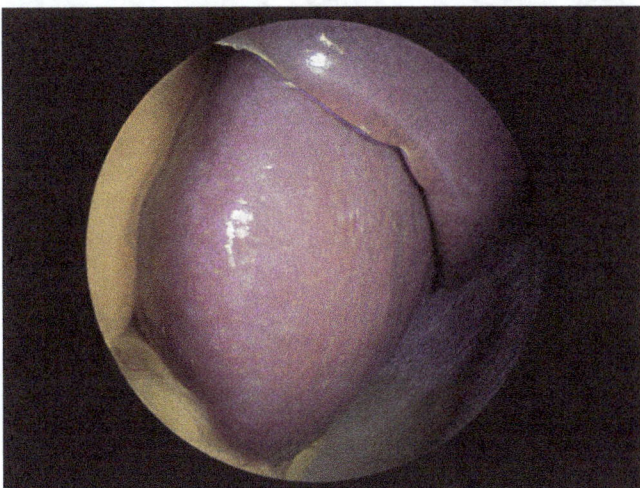

Fig. 2.4: Accessory lobe on the inferior surface of the right lobe of liver. Here shown in chronic hepatitis B

with other congenital malformations, especially of the biliary system. The unaffected liver lobe will generally develop compensatory hypertrophy. (25, 39, 47)

2.3 Segmental subdivisions

The boundaries regarding physiological topography are marked by the distribution pattern of the portal vein, the hepatic artery and the bile ducts, or according to the origin of the three large hepatic veins. The result is a clear and precise subdivision of the liver in the sense of a functional lobulation into 12 segments (3 main segments, each with 4 subsegments) or 9 segments, respectively. The essential findings are based on the investigations of C.H. HJORTSJÖ (1948, 1951), C. COUINAUD (1954, 1957), S.C. GUPTA et al. (1977, 1981), H. BISMUTH (1982), and A. PRIESCHING (1986). (s. figs. 2.5; 40.4)

Rex-Cantlie's line (H. REX, 1889; J. CANTLIE, 1898), running from inferior vena cava to gall bladder, forms the boundary between the two portal distribution areas and thus between the right lobe (right portal vein) and the left lobe (left portal vein) of liver (= *double-flow principle of the portal vein*). Additionally, however, the left part of the right lobe of liver (segment II 1—4, so-called *"centre of the liver"*) is supplied by both branches of the portal vein. Consequently, segment II 3 (equivalent to segment IV) would correspond to the quadrate lobe, segment II 2 to the caudate process, and segment II 1,2 (or I) to the caudate lobe. The caudate lobe, which is situated in the posterior medical part of the right lobe, is also termed segment I. It contains portal venous blood from the right and left portal vein; the venous blood runs off directly into the retrohepatic inferior vena cava, and not into the hepatic veins. (s. figs. 2.5; 40.4)

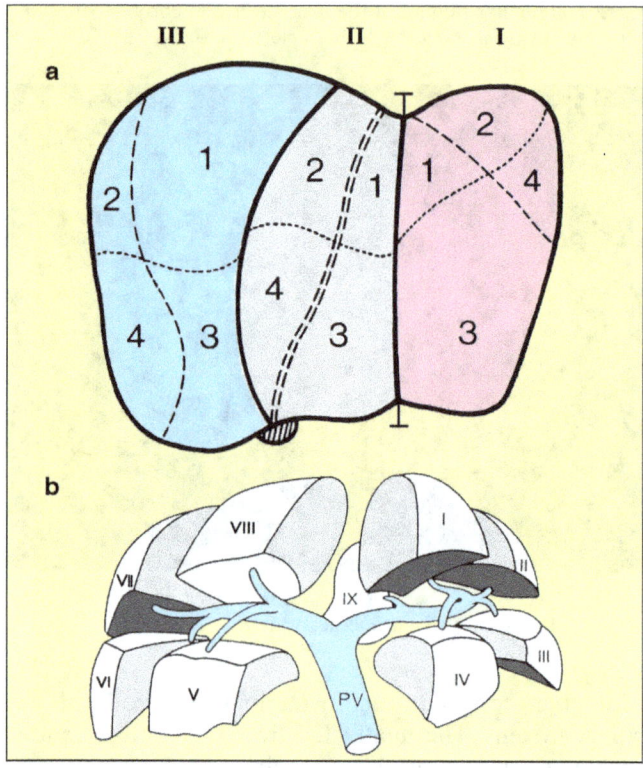

Fig. 2.5: Segmentation of the liver. • **a:** *Left lobe* (I, 1—4): 4 segments; "centre of the liver" (II): quadrate lobe (II, 3): caudate lobe (II, 1,2) and caudate process (II, 2); *right lobe* (III, 1—4): 4 segments. • Rex-Cantlie's line (===) as functional division between both liver lobes runs between II 2,4 and II 1,3. Topographically, the liver lobes are separated by the falciform ligament (⊢——⊣) between I 1,3 and II 1,3. • **b:** The liver can be divided into 9 segments (I—IX) according to the ramifications of the portal veins. Segments II/III, I/IV, V/VIII and VI/VII are also combined into double segments

The "portal segments" and the "hepatovenous segments" are, however, subject to considerable individual variations with respect to their size and the position of their boundaries. This point must always be considered in cases of hepatectomy. For this reason there is, as yet, no general agreement concerning the designation of the segments. (19, 67)

3 Structure and histology of the liver

In terms of structure and histology, it is possible to divide the liver into **four tissue systems:** (*1.*) intrahepatic vascular system, (*2.*) stroma, (*3.*) sinusoidal cells, and (*4.*) hepatocytes.

3.1 Intrahepatic vascular system

3.1.1 Hepatic artery

The **common hepatic artery** is a branch of the coeliac trunc (= *Haller's tripod*), from which the splenic artery, the phrenic artery and the left gastric artery emerge. In about 18% of cases there is a second hepatic artery leading out of the left gastric artery and in about 10% of cases there is a second hepatic artery leading out of the superior mesenteric artery. The common hepatic artery extends into the proper hepatic artery. Prior to this point, the gastroduodenal artery and the right gastric artery branch off. The course and the ramification of the hepatic artery are "normal" only in about 55% of cases! (57) These frequent vessel abnormalities are of great importance in surgery. • The pressure in the hepatic artery amounts to 100 mm Hg, with a pressure-dependent autoregulation of the blood flow (increase of pressure = decrease of blood flow, and vice versa).

In the hepatic porta, the **proper hepatic artery** divides into the *right branch* (from which the cystic artery emerges) and the *left branch* (from which a "middle hepatic artery" occasionally emerges). The branches of the hepatic artery run close to the portal veins and may even (rarely) coil round them in places. An arterial sphincter is located prior to the further division of the hepatic artery into smaller branches. • There are anastomoses between the arterial branches and the hepatic vein. By way of an arteriolar sphincter (45), the *interlobular arteries* branch into *intralobular arterioles*, supplying the lobules of the liver with arterial blood. The arterial blood enters the sinusoids either through terminal branches or through arterioportal anastomoses and mixes with the portal blood. The pressure in the hepatic arterioles is 30—40 mm Hg. (36, 45, 57)

The blood of the hepatic artery supplies **five regions** of the liver: (*1.*) peribiliary vascular plexus as the greatest arteriolar compartment, (*2.*) interstitium of the portal fields, (*3.*) vasa vasorum of the portal vein, (*4.*) vasa vasorum of the hepatic vein, and (*5.*) liver capsule.

▶ **Hepatic blood flow** amounts to ca. 1,200 ml/min in women and ca. 1,800 ml/min in men, depending on the prevailing physiological conditions. Of this blood, 70—75% are supplied by the portal vein and 20—25% by the hepatic vein. The oxygen supply is secured by the hepatic artery at 20 vol. % and the portal vein at 16—17 vol. %. • The **blood content** is equivalent to 25—30%

of liver weight. The liver blood volume accounts for 10–15% of the total blood content of the body – an extremely high proportion.

▶ **Oxygen consumption** of the liver amounts to 6 ml/minute/100 g wet weight. The acino-peripheral region (zone 1) has the best supply of oxygen (mainly aerobic metabolism), whereas the centroacinar region (zone 3) has the most oxygen-deficient blood (mainly anaerobic metabolism). A decrease in liver blood supply generally occurs whilst standing, during sleep, when fasting, and in old age. Oxygen extraction in the liver amounts to approx. 40%; any additional requirement of oxygen is (initially) met by a considerable increase in oxygen extraction of up to 95%. The regulation of the blood flow in the sinusoids is influenced in different ways: (*1.*) neural factors (adrenergic and dopaminergic receptors), (*2.*) anatomical mechanisms, and (*3.*) vasoactive substances (e.g. endothelin, CO, NO, adenosine).

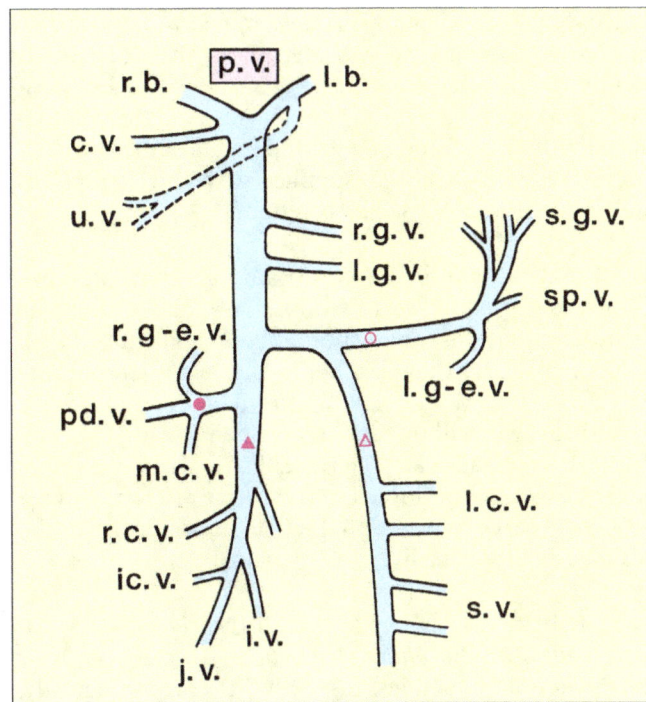

Fig. 2.6: Diagram of the portal vein: p.v. = portal vein, r.b. = right branch, l.b. = left branch; c.v. = cystic vein; u.v. = umbilical vein; r.g.v. = right gastric vein, l.g.v. = left gastric vein; sp.v. ○ = splenic vein, s.g.v. = short gastric veins, l.g-e. v. = left gastro-epiploic vein; ● = gastrocolic trunc; r.g-e.v. = right gastro-epiploic vein, pd.v. = pancreaticoduodenal vein, m.c.v. = middle colic vein; ▲ = superior mesenteric vein, r.c.v. = right colic vein, ic.v. = ileocolic vein, j.v. = jejunal veins, i.v. = ileal veins; △ = inferior mesenteric vein, l.c.v. = left colic vein, s.v. = sigmoid veins

3.1.2 Portal vein

The portal vein is formed posterior to the pancreatic isthmus by coalescence of the superior mesenteric vein and splenic vein. The inferior mesenteric vein enters at a point not far from this junction. The portal vein then runs through the hepatoduodenal ligament and absorbs venous blood from the ventricular coronary vein. • At the porta hepatis, the portal vein divides into the *right branch* (which takes in the cystic vein as well as one or two veins from the caudate lobe) and the *left branch*, into which flow the paraumbilical veins, extending through the round ligament, and the ventroflexal ramus, emerging from the left sagittal fossa. (s. fig. 2.6) • The branches of the portal vein extend (by further branching and reduction in the lumen) into the portal tracts. Here they merge with the *interlobular veins*, which generally divide into two *conductor veins* (= venulae interlobulares). The conductor veins divide into *distributor veins* and continue as Y-shaped *terminal branches* (= venulae afferentes). The portal blood passes through the periportal limiting plate of hepatocytes, entering the **sinusoids** through venous inlets. This means that the blood of the portal vein flows only into the sinusoids. Terminal branches of the arteries join up with the sinusoids separately. The outflow of sinusoidal mixed blood (75% from the portal vein, 25% from the hepatic artery) occurs via venous capillaries in the *central hepatic vein* (or *terminal hepatic vein*). The venous blood from the capillaries of the portal tract flows off either through the distributor veins or directly into the sinusoids. The difference in pressure between portal veins and hepatic veins is more important for the sinusoidal supply of blood than are the respective absolute values. (36) • These radicular portal veins, which originate in the portal fields, have therefore also been described as the *"inner root of the portal veins"* (H. ELIAS et al., 1949).

3.1.3 Hepatic vein

The hepatic vein emerges from the *central hepatic vein* in the centre of the lobule. It runs at an acute angle into the *sublobular vein*. From the confluence of the sublobular veins, *collecting veins* are formed which fuse to form five *trunk veins*: the right and left superior hepatic vein as well as the right, left and intermediate hepatic vein (the latter two forming a common trunk in 60–70% of cases). The hepatic veins progress intersegmentally; they receive branches from adjacent segments. This group of superior hepatic veins drains into the *inferior vena cava* at the posterior surface of the liver below the diaphragm. • By contrast, the group of inferior hepatic veins (= accessory hepatic veins) is very varied in terms of number, diameter and draining sites.

3.1.4 Biliary system

The *bile canaliculus* is formed as a bile capillary by means of a groove-like canal in the intercellular space, bounded by 2 adjacent liver cells. The bile canaliculi have no walls of their own, but are surrounded by a special zone of the cell membrane (so-called *pericanalicular ectoplasm*). Their diameter amounts to 0.5–1.0 μm. They are interconnected and form an extensive polygonal network. The surface area of the bile capillaries is increased by *microvilli*, which show great functionally determined variability. The canalicular membrane constitutes 10% of the total plasma membrane in the hepatocytes. Similar to the pericanalicular ectoplasm, the hepatocytes contain contractile microfilaments and other components of the cytoskeleton. These canaliculi are supplied with carrier proteins and enzymes to control bile secretion. (2, 34)

The canaliculi continue into an ampulla-like extension known as *Hering's canal* (E. HERING, 1866). This area can be regarded equally as the end point of the canaliculi and the beginning of the ductules, hence the term *intermediate ductule* is used (M. CLARA, 1930). From here the bile ducts have their own wall of cuboidal epithelial cells. They are 7–20 μm in diameter. Their designation as *preductules* has been generally adopted. (54) Because of their extreme proneness to damage, the preductules are described as the "Achilles' heel of the liver" (L. ASCHOFF, 1932).

The preductules merge either with the *cholangioles* (M. CLARA, 1934) or the *biliferous ductules* (H. ELIAS, 1949) or the perilobular ductules, respectively. Morphologically, it is generally not possible to distinguish between preductules and ductules. Thus both structures are subsumed under the term "cholangioles" or "terminal bile ducts". The ductules are followed by the *interlobular bile ducts* with a diameter of >50 μm. They run through the connective tissue wedges of the portal tracts (= Glisson's triangles). These interlobular bile ducts (15–100 μm) anastomose with each other. The larger septal (100–400 μm) and segmental (0.4–0.8 mm increasing to 1.0–1.5 mm) bile ducts continue into the *right* and *left hepatic duct*, which unite at the hepatic porta to form the *common hepatic duct*. The latter confluences directly afterwards with the cystic duct, thus forming the *common bile duct* (= ductus choledochus). (34, 49, 75)

3.1.5 Lymph vessels

The liver forms more *lymph* than any other organ of the body (0.4–0.6 mg/kg BW/min). Lymph capillaries take up lymph from **Disse's space** (J. DISSE, 1890) and thereafter from **Mall's space** (F.P. MALL, 1906), which lies between the limiting plate and the portal connective tissue. Disse's space is also considered to be the main source of lymph. In addition, lymph capillaries commence in the adventitia of sublobular veins and run close to the hepatic veins as far as the paracaval lymph nodes. Lymph vessels possess valves which permit the lymph to flow only in one direction. Lymphatic vessels are present in all portal fields. They are found exclusively in the perivascular connective tissue and in the capsule of the liver. (s. fig. 16.4) • Drainage is effected by the *hepatic lymph nodes* in the area of the porta hepatis. Lymph reaches the *thoracic duct* via large valved lymphatic trunks and interconnected lymph nodes. Thus it enters the systemic circulation. (22, 64)

3.2 Stroma of the liver

The term **stroma** comprises the interstitial connective tissue of an organ. • In the liver, **four types of tissue structure** are differentiated: (*1.*) capsule of the liver, (*2.*) perivascular connective tissue, (*3.*) Glisson's portal tract, and (*4.*) reticular network.

▶ This **extracellular matrix** (ECM) is a dynamic concentration of complex macromolecules. (66) Besides mechanical functions, the components of ECM also have important physiological tasks; therefore they have bidirectional contacts with the liver cells. These *matrix components* include: collagens, elastin, glycosaminoglycanes, proteoglycanes, and glycoproteins. • In the liver, there are mainly **collagens** I, III (= large fibrils), IV (= net structure), and V, VI (= small fibrils). The non-fibrillar collagen type XVIII is found in the perisinusoidal space and in the basal membranes. The Ito cells are deemed the main producers of ECM. The biosynthesis of collagen comprises the intermediate steps of pre- and procollagen. The half-life of liver collagen amounts to approx. 30 days. The *degradation of collagen* occurs through matrix-metalloproteinases, which are mainly formed in the Ito cells. During the degradation process, hydroxyproline develops, which in turn is either oxidized in the liver into CO_2 and H_2O (ca. 75%) or excreted in the urine (ca. 25%). Thus the *excretion rate of hydroxyproline* in the urine is an indicator for collagen metabolism. • **Elastin** gives the hepatic structures their elasticity. Connective tissue cells secrete the precursor proelastin, which is converted into elastin; the latter then combines with collagen and glycoproteins to form elastic fibres. Degradation takes place with the help of elastase and metalloproteinases. α_1-antitrypsin is a specific inhibitor of elastase. • **Proteoglycanes** are the main component of ECM. They consist of a central protein strand with long, unbranched carbohydrate side chains (= glycosaminoglycan). This group also contains hyaluronic acid. Proteoglycans are hydrophylic and can bind cations. They are mainly built up from Ito cells and broken down by lysosomal hydrolases. • **Adhesive glycoproteins** (= *nectins*) ensure contact between ECM, hepatocytes and non-parenchymal cells. They comprise fibronectin, laminin, nidogen, tenascin and indulin. • The numerous heterogeneous components of the ECM are closely interwoven and communicate bidirectionally with the liver cells by means of special substances, so-called *integrins*.

3.2.1 Capsule of the liver

The capsule of the liver (A. von HALLER, 1764) is 43–76 μm thick. It consists of the endothelial coating (= serosa) and a network of collagenous and elastic fibres. The capsule and the falciform ligament contain sensitive phrenicoabdominal branches of the phrenic nerve, which vary in extent (algesia or shoulder pain may thus accompany liver biopsy). Moreover, blood and lymph vessels as well as rudimentary bile ducts (which may become enlarged in the case of portal hypertension, ascites or cholestasis) are present in the capsule. The small blood vessels of the capsule anastomose with branches of the portal vein, yet not with the hepatic veins. The inner surface of the capsule is intimately connected to the liver parenchyma, particularly in the area of the interlobular connective tissue.

3.2.2 Perivascular connective tissue

The perivascular fibrous capsule (F. GLISSON, 1654) commences in the hepatic porta as a tree-like branching framework of connective tissue surrounding the interlobular vessels. It also surrounds the central hepatic vein and its small tributaries, which are joined to the parenchyma by radial fibres as well as being established in the portal tracts. This prevents a suction-induced collapse of the venous vessels as a result of respiration-dependent negative pressure in the pleural cavity. The perivascular connective tissue, known as *Glisson's capsule*, extends fine secondary trabeculae into the parenchyma. They contain the intralobular biliary, lymphatic and blood capillaries.

3.2.3 Lattice fibre network

The reticular network consists mainly of *lattice fibres* (O. OPPEL, 1891) which lie on the hepatic cell plates and serve as a mechanical support for the sinusoids and also as a directrix in hepatocyte regeneration. The microvilli of the hepatic cells extend through this lattice fibre network into **Disse's space** (J. DISSE, 1890). In general, this space is not visible in vivo, and thus the sinusoid wall appears to abut directly onto the hepatocytes. However, it constitutes about one third of the entire extracellular space in the liver, which itself accounts for 15–20% of the liver volume and 2–4% of the liver parenchyma. It is via Disse's space that the exchange of different substances between liver and blood takes place. The width of Disse's space varies between 0.2–1.0 μm, depending upon the resorptive and secretory capacity of the hepatocytes. Fluid, protein and particles up to 100 nm may, however, enter this perisinusoidal space (increasingly in hypoxia) and be drained off. The space itself lies between the trabeculae and the sinusoids. It is thought to be connected to Mall's space, but no direct connection from Mall's space into the lymph vessels within the periportal region has so far been demonstrated. (s. figs. 2.7–2.9)

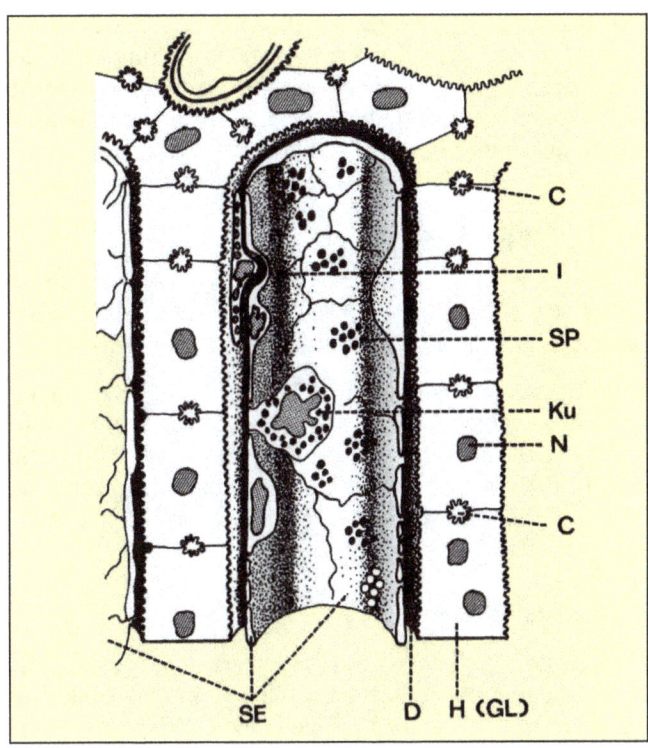

Fig. 2.8: Spatial relationship of sinusoid and hepatic cells: hepatocytes (H) in the form of boundary lamella (BL), cell nucleus (CN), canaliculus (BC), Disse's space (D), endothelial cells (E), sieve plate (SP), Kupffer cell (K), Ito cell (I). The cellular interchange area is increased by microvilli (modified from D. SASSE, 1986)

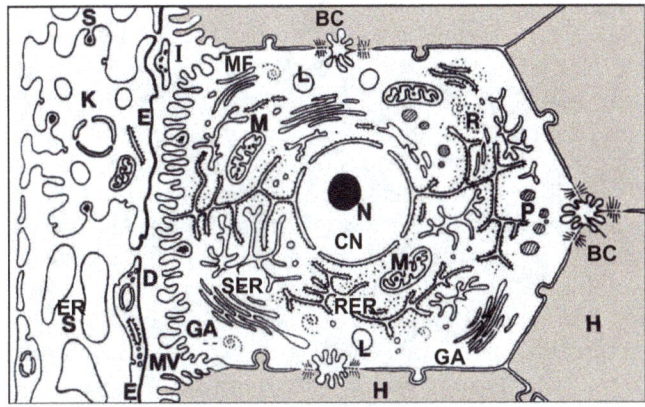

Fig. 2.9: Liver cell and sinusoidal cells with organelles and polarized membrane compartments: hepatocytes (H), sinusoids (S), Disse's space (D), erythrocytes (ER), endothelial cells (E), Kupffer cells (K), Ito cells (I), microvilli (MV), canaliculus (BC), nucleolus (N), tight junctions (tj), cell nucleus (CN), mitochondria (M), smooth endoplasmic reticulum (SER), rough endoplasmic reticulum (RER), Golgi apparatus (GA), lysosomes (L), peroxisomes (P), ribosomes (R), microfilaments (MF) (modified from L. COSSEL) (s. figs. 2.16–2.18)

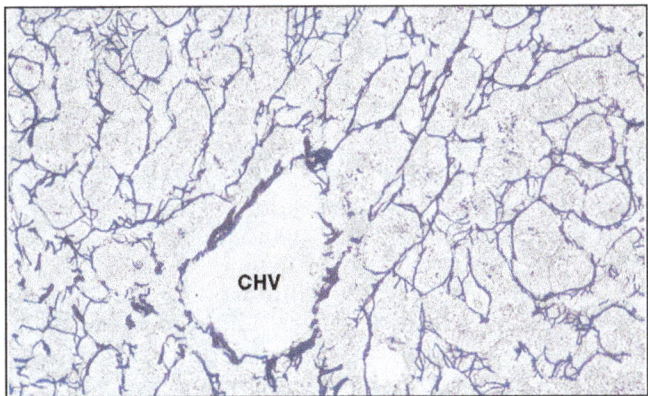

Fig. 2.7: Reticular fibre network with central hepatic vein (CHV) (Gomori's reticulin stain)

3.2.4 Portal tract

In the *portal tract* (= Glisson's triangle, portal field) (F. GLISSON, 1659), the perivascular connective tissue with its enclosed (and protected) radicles of the portal veins, the hepatic arterioles, bile ducts, lymph vessels and nerve fibres terminates in the connective tissue covering of the perivascular fibrous capsule. Any lymphocytic infiltrations as well as occasional isolated histiocytic or monocytic forms which are embedded in this area are considered to be physiological. The continuous line of hepatocytes immediately bordering the portal tract is designated *limiting plate*. (s. figs. 2.8, 2.10, 2.12)

3.3 Sinusoidal cells

Four different *mesenchymal cell types* are subsumed under the term **sinusoidal cells:** (*1.*) endothelial cells, (*2.*) Kupffer cells, (*3.*) Ito cells, and (*4.*) PIT cells.

Although the sinusoidal cells (31 million/mg liver) make up only a relatively small proportion of the liver volume (6.3%), they constitute 30–40% of the total cell number. The total surface area of their plasma membranes is 26.5% of the total membrane surface of all liver cells. (3, 5, 29, 43, 53, 55, 59) (s. figs. 2.8, 2.9)

3.3.1 Endothelial cells

Endothelial cells constitute the greatest proportion (70%) of the sinusoidal cells. These are flat cells, the nuclei of which camber the cell body. With their slim nuclear branches, they are in loose connection with both the neighbouring endothelial cells and the microvilli of the hepatocytes. They are located on a fine layer of extracellular matrix. Their proportion of the total cell number is 15–20%, but they make up only 2.8% of the liver volume. They form a continuous lining of the **sinusoids** which, however, possesses numerous intercellular spaces (0.1–0.5 µm) (S. MINOT, 1892). The sinusoids (with a total surface area of 400 m²) are 4–15 µm wide and 350–500 µm long. Here portal blood combines with arterial blood. The entry and exit of blood is controlled by sinusoidal sphincters. (36, 73) Compared to the capillaries of other organs, sinusoids show fundamental structural differences. They are interspersed with **pores** which have a basic diameter of 0.1 µm, actively variable in width. When grouped together, such pores are known as *sieve plate*. (s. fig. 2.8) There are also larger pores (0.5 µm), so-called *fenestrae*. The smaller pores, the fenestrae and the intercellular spaces are essential for the process of filtering the components of the blood; they have scavenger functions (52) and regulate the exchange of fluid and material between the blood in the sinusoids and the hepatocytes. In addition, they are of great importance for the balance of lipids, cholesterol, and vitamin A. Endothelial cells also form and secrete cytokines (e.g. Il 1, 6, IF, α-TNF), matrix components (e.g. collagens, fibronectin) and growth factors (e.g. HGF, IGF, FGF) as well as vasoactive substances (e.g. NO, endothelin). • The cells themselves can be damaged or even completely destroyed by the effect of toxins, alcohol, hypoxia, viruses or increased pressure in the sinusoids. In this case, the hepatocytes are completely "naked" and exposed to all attacks. The endothelial cells are stabilized by a network of lattice fibres. • Because of their structural and functional characteristics, the endothelial cells, Disse's space and the so-called vascular hepatocyte pole are subsumed under the term *"perisinusoidal functional unit"*. (44)

3.3.2 Kupffer cells

The stellate cells initially determined by K. W. von KUPFFER (1876) by means of the gold chloride method were actually Ito cells located in Disse's space. It was not until 1898 and 1899 that the sinus macrophages were described by von KUPFFER again – though at this point not sufficiently differentiated from the gold-reactive fat-storing cells.

Kupffer cells constitute about 25% of the sinusoidal cells. They make up 8–12% of the total liver cells and 2.1% of the liver volume. Their overall number/mg of liver amounts to 31,000, the half-life being 12.4 days. They probably derive from monocytes and are released by stem cells in the bone marrow. Thus they belong to the mononuclear phagocytosis system (MPS) (R. VAN FURTH et al., 1970). Kupffer cells can multiply by mitosis. Their villiform surface (fuzzy coat) and irregular, mostly star-shaped form led to the designation "stellate cells". They are randomly distributed in the sinusendothelium, but occur three to four times more frequently in the periportal region than in the perivenous zone. They connect with adjacent cells or spaces by means of ramifications and through pores. Their cytoplasm contains numerous organelles. Charged Kupffer cells may be flushed out with sinusoidal blood. • *Phagocytosis* can be seen as the most important function of Kupffer cells. Apart from the cells at the base of the pulmonary vascular bed, they have the greatest intravascular phagocytic capacity. Further functions include (*1.*) *pinocytosis*, (*2.*) discharge of *signal substances* (e.g. cytokines, growth factors, erythropoietin, eicosanoids) or proteins and/or enzymes, and (*3.*) *clearance* of toxins, antigens, antigen-antibody complexes and purines. The phagocytosis and clearance of Kupffer cells is reduced through alcohol and drugs (e.g. mitomycin, α-methyldopa). (29, 53, 55, 62, 69) (s. p. 69) (s. figs. 2.8, 2.9)

3.3.3 Ito cells

Ito cells (T. ITO, 1951) are also known as fat-storing cells, hepatic stellate cells or lipocytes. These long-lived cells, 5–10 µm in size with long thin strands, lie in Disse's space (s. figs. 2.8, 2.9) and contain numerous cytoplasmic fat droplets as well as an abundance of vitamin A (= retinol ester). The retinol esters of the chylomicrons are absorbed by the hepatocytes and hydrolyzed into retinol. The latter is either passed to the blood by means of RBP or transported to Ito cells and stored. In the fat droplets of Ito cells, about 75% of the liver retinoids are present in the form of retinol esters. These fat droplets are characteristic of Ito cells; they represent vacuolized cisterns of RBP. Ito cells constitute about 3—8% of the total liver cell number and 1.4% of the volume of the liver, occurring in a proportion of one Ito cell to 12—20 liver cells. Zone 3 of the acinus has the highest number. Ito cells are involved in the regulation of the width of the sinusendothelium, the microvascular tone and the regeneration of cells. They contain numerous filaments and organelles for protein synthesis, but cannot themselves produce RBP. Moreover, they are capable of transformation into myofibroblasts. Ito cells are able to synthesize and secrete collagen types I, III and IV, fibronectin, laminin, or other substances. Unlike fibroblasts, Ito cells can express desmin. Hence they may play an important part in fibrogenesis, particularly in pathological intralobular fibrosis. (4, 7, 16, 29, 55, 58, 70)

3.3.4 PIT cells

PIT cells were first demonstrated in the sinusoidal wall in rats (E. WITTE et al., 1970). Later on, these lymphocytes with large granules and rod-cored vesicles were also found in the human liver, particularly in the sinusoids and in Disse's space. Due to their pseudopodia, they are variable. The proportion of PIT cells to Kupffer cells is 2:10. They are natural killer cells and destroy tumour cells or foreign cells as well as necrosed cells. It is not clear whether they have any additional "endocrine" function. Because of the strongly polarized distribution of their granulae, they could justifiably be classified as APUD cells. (6, 28, 29, 55, 65, 72)

3.4 Hepatocytes

▶ Hepatocytes were discovered by M.H. DUTROCHET, who recognized "cellules vesiculaires agglomerées" in liver tissue in 1824. • This **first description** was confirmed and expanded by F. KIERNAN (1833), J. HENLE (1836) and J.E. PURKINJE (1837) — they also discovered the liver cell nucleus.

Hepatocytes are **polygonal epithelial cells** with six or more faces corresponding to their individual position in the overall cell structure. The plate-like, overlapping hepatocyte formations build a three-dimensional system. With the reduction in weight of the liver from 3% to 2% relative to body weight with increasing age, there is also a corresponding decrease in the absolute number of hepatocytes. The usual life span of hepatocytes is at least 150—200 days; they perish as so-called *oncocytes* ("moulting"). This *programmed death* of the old hepatocytes is designated **apoptosis**. As yet, there is no reliable information available regarding the normal life span of human hepatocytes. It is determined on the one hand by genetic factors and on the other hand by exogenous factors, which differ in nature and scope of influence. In rats, a life span of 191 to 453 days was established for hepatocytes.

Proportion of liver volume	80%
Proportion of total cell number	60—65%
Number of liver cells	300 billion
Number of hepatocytes per g of liver	171 million
Diameter of hepatocytes	20—40 μm
Proportion of hyaloplasm in cell volume	54,9%
Lifespan of hepatocytes	150 (—200) days
Mitosis rate per 10,000—20,000 liver cells	1
Membrane surface of hepatocytes and organelles (s. p. 26)	33,000 m^2

Hepatocytes show a varying content of carrier, receptor and channel proteins. They have a clearly contoured cell membrane which is divided into three compartments defined by morphological and functional **cellular polarization.** (*1.*) About 37% of the external area of the hepatocyte membrane is *sinusoidal surface* (= basolateral) the absorptive and secretory function of which is increased sixfold by numerous microvilli; they lie in Disse's space. Some even protrude through the fenestrae into the sinusoids and thereby have direct contact with the blood. On the sinusoidal membrane, there are invaginations with vesicles underneath. (*2.*) About 15% of the outer hepatocyte membrane consist of canaliculi, termed *canalicular surface* (= apical). This area is the secretory pole of the cell. (*3.*) The remaining 50% of the external hepatocyte membrane constitute the smooth *intercellular fissure,* which is connected with Disse's space. This fissure is sealed from the canaliculi by *tight junctions* (= zonula occludens), allowing only an exchange of water and cations to take place. The adjacent adhesion areas of the neighbouring hepatocytes, the *intermediate junctions* (= zonula adhaerens) and the *desmosomes* (= macula adhaerens), are sealed by membrane proteins. These last two connecting structures are known collectively as adhering junctions. Thus, desmosomes link neighbouring hepatocytes, whereby the cytoskeleton is involved. They are distributed in an irregular fashion on the lateral membrane and help to stabilize the hepatocyte structure. Actually, they contain *gap junctions* (= maculae communicantes) which form tube-like connections between adjacent hepatocytes and so facilitate the intercellular exchange. When cell death occurs, the gap junctions of neighbouring cells, as dynamic structures, close down in order to prevent the progression of cell death. (s. figs. 2.8—2.10, 2.16)

Three **zonal areas** can also be differentiated in hepatocytes based on ultrastructural and functional differences (9, 32, 35, 59): (*1.*) *vascular zone* (supranuclear), (*2.*) *lateral zone*, and (*3.*) *biliary zone* (adjacent to the bile capillaries). • They each have a different stock of *organelles.* (s. p. 30)

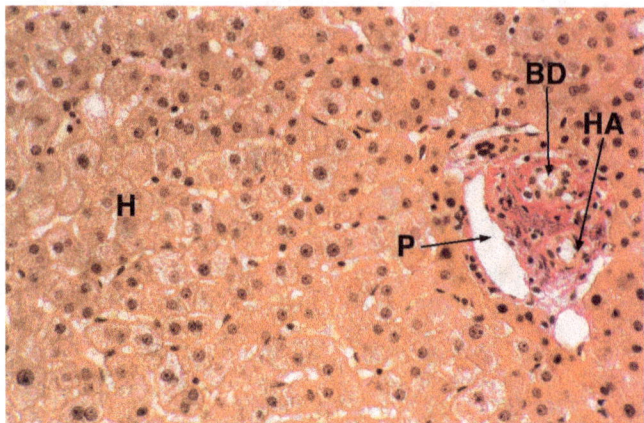

Fig. 2.10: Normal hepatic tissue. H = hepatocytes, P = portal vein, BD = bile duct, HA = hepatic arteriole (EvG)

3.5 Biliary epithelial cells

Biliary epithelial cells are organ-typical. They constitute some 3.5% of all hepatic cells. Depending on the size of the biliary ducts in which they are located, they show distinct histological and histochemical variations. In comparison with hepatocytes, biliary epithelial cells contain fewer mitochondria and less ER; there is a complete absence of cytochrome P 450. They are rich in cytoskeleton and contain Golgi apparatus and vesicles. The round-to-oval nuclei lie in the basal cytoplasm. These biliary cells probably play a role in biligenesis. (63) The epithelial cells of the intermediate ductules are also regarded as stem cells for the liver parenchyma.

4 Nervous system

The hepatic nerves consist of fibres of the sympathetic ganglia Th_5–Th_9 and the postganglionic fibres of the coeliac ganglion the vagus and the right phrenic nerve. At the porta hepatis, they form one plexus around the hepatic artery and another plexus around the portal vein plus biliary duct. With the vessels, the nerves reach the liver and "terminate" in the portal fields, where they regulate biliary and vascular structures. Also in the perisinusoidal space, there is a fine neural network which is in direct contact with hepatocytes and Ito cells. The nerves contain adrenergic (aminergic), cholinergic and peptidergic fibres; the function of peptidergic innervation is unknown. This most finely ramified hepatic nervous system influences haemodynamics, the metabolism of hepatic cells, and the motility of the biliary ducts. The liver parenchyma itself is not sensitive to pain as it contains no sensory nerves. The liver capsule and the falciform ligament are innervated by sensitive phrenicoabdominal branches of the phrenic nerve. (1, 5, 61) • *A transplanted and therefore* **denervated liver** *shows that innervation is not essential for the function of the organ. This remarkable phenomenon cannot yet be explained.*

5 Hepatic lobules and acinus

▶ The term **parenchyma** referring to the liver tissue was coined by ERASISTRATOS. The **liver lobules** were first described in the pig in 1664 by J.J. WEPFER (using microscopic techniques) while the lobular structure was confirmed by M. MALPIGHI in 1666. The term **acinus** was coined by S.Th. SÖMMERING in 1796. • However, it was F. KIERNAN (1833) who first gave a classic definition of the lobule in pig liver ("hepatic lobule"). Today, such anatomical clarity can only be found in the livers of the camel, polar bear and seal. (s. fig. 1.18)

▶ KIERNAN's description of the acinus provided the basis for subsequent definitions, such as *"biliary lobule"* (CH. SABOURIN, 1888), *"portal unit"* (F.P. MALL, 1906), *"hepaton"* (R. RÖSSLE, 1930) and *"synergid of the liver"* (H. SIEGMUND, 1943). In 1848 J. GERLACH had recognized that liver cells were arranged in bands (columns). • Not until a hundred years later did H. ELIAS (1949) describe the arrangement of liver cells in the form of plates as muralium simplex or lamina hepatis, with internal cavities (= lacunae). (11) (s. fig. 2.11) • E.H. BLOCH (1970) considered the "single sinusoidal unit" to be a functional unit of the liver, the main component of which is a sinusoid lying sandwich-like between the hepatocyte trabeculae. • T. MATSUMOTO et al. (1979) suggest an angioarchitectural concept. The portal corner region with septal ramifications is seen as the basic structure of the primary hepatic lobule. In the parenchyma, *vascular septa* are postulated, i.e. terminal ramifications of the portal vein which join up with the sinusoids directly. (In 1997, W. EKTAKSIN et al. described them as inlet venules.) (s. fig. 2.12)

Total number of hepatic lobules	1.0–1.5 million
Depth of hepatic lobules	1.5–2.0 mm
Diameter of hepatic lobules	1.0–1.3 mm

5.1 Central vein lobule

The classic central vein lobule accords with the traditional description of *lobular structure* (F. KIERNAN, 1833; H. EPPINGER, 1937; H. ELIAS, 1949). The hepatic lobule resembles a hexagon with portal tracts at the corners. It consists of radially arranged columns (or plates) of 15–25 liver cells placed between the limiting lamellae and the central vein, the axis of which they are also aligned with. This particular arrangement of the hepatocyte plates does not occur until after birth and is due to the suction effect of the right ventricle. The lobule is limited by the surrounding periportal fields. The hollow spaces between the liver cell plates form a labyrinth, in which the sinusoids and Disse's space are located. The *limiting plate* (W.H. HARRIS, 1942) or *limiting lamella* (H. ELIAS, 1949) consists of smaller, basophilic and glycogen-free liver cells with a nucleus which is richer in chromatin. As a unicellular liver plate, it lies perpendicular to the remaining liver cell plates. It is penetrated only by capillaries. As it is limited on the periportal side by Mall's space, it can only be reached by peripheral sinusoidal blood on the lobular side. Due to its optimal blood supply, the limiting plate proves itself to be a particularly resistant layer of liver cells. It constitutes a dividing wall between parenchyma and mesenchyma. This lobular structure thus shifts the periportal fields with the supplying branches of the hepatic artery and portal vein to the periphery and the central vein to the centre of the lobule, which results in centripetal blood flow. The bile flows centrifugally towards the periphery. (s. figs. 1.18; 2.11−2.13)

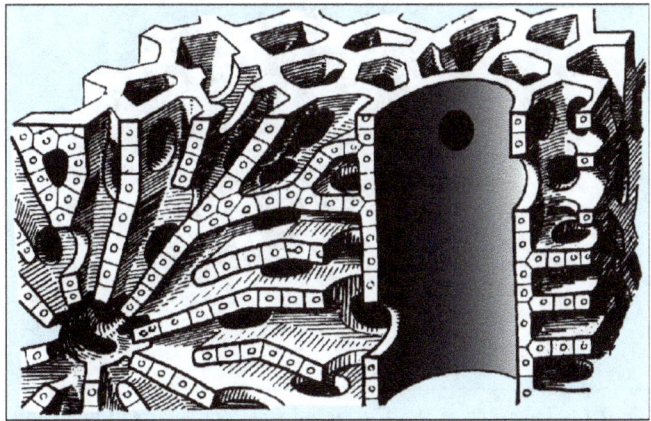

Fig. 2.11: Diagram of the traditional ("classic") hepatic lobule according to the lobular structure (F. KIERNAN, 1833) (s. fig. 1.18) and as stereogram (H. ELIAS, 1949): the liver cell columns run radially from the limiting plate to the central vein (11) (s. fig. 2.16)

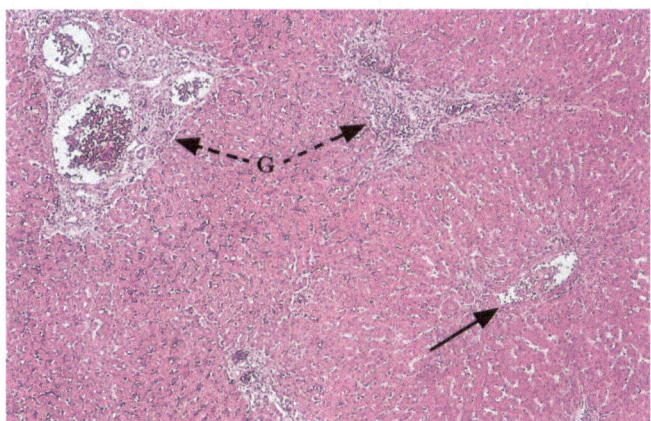

Fig. 2.12: Hepatic lobules with central vein (↑) and Glisson's triangles (G --→). Slight distortion of the lobular architecture (HE)

5.2 Portal vein lobule

The portal vein lobule was first recognized in the description of the "portal unit" given by F. P. MALL (1906). It resembles a hexagon. The periportal field constitutes the axis at the centre while the central veins form the limiting points. (s. fig. 2.13) The glandular character of the liver is the main criterion of differentiation of the portal vein lobule. Thus the direction of blood flow is from the centre towards the periphery (centrifugal) and the direction of bile flow from the periphery towards the centre (centripetal). It could also be demonstrated that the lobule periphery is enclosed by basket-like ramifications of the portal vein (= *corbicula portalis*). (74) This further emphasizes the significance of the hepatic lobule.

5.3 Liver acinus

The functional and microcirculatory hepatic unit forms the basis for assessing the hepatic acinus (A. M. RAPPAPORT, 1954). (40−42) The portal vascular bundle, with the terminal branches of the hepatic artery and portal vein diverging fan-shaped after penetrating the lobules, is at the centre of the *acinar structure*. These vessels represent the central axis for the circular blood supply of the related liver parenchyma. This area is roughly the shape of a rhombus, the outer angles of which are formed by the two *central veins* of the adjacent lobules while the diagonal corresponds to the (arterial and portal) *terminal vessels*. The central vein at the periphery of the acinus, to which the sinusoids extend radially, drains off the venous blood; it is generally known as the *terminal hepatic venule* (= terminal hepatic vein). (s. p. 21) The liver acinus also serves as *secretory unit* for the transport of bile. In the acinus, the blood flow occurs centrifugally and the flow of bile centripetally. Three or more acini together form a so-called complex acinus. • This zonal model has been modified according to more recent findings, so that zones 1 to 3 do not surround the terminal afferent vessels in an onion-like way, but are now arranged in circular form around the vessels. (31) (s. figs. 2.13−2.15)

The zones of the acinus differ in their blood supply, corresponding to the distance of the hepatic cells from the periportal field and terminal blood vessels respectively. **Zone 1** has the best supply of oxygen and substrates; it comprises the (lobule-peripheral) parenchyma adjacent to the limiting lamella. Toxins are most damaging in zone 1. **Zone 2** corresponds to the intermediate area with a reduced supply of blood. **Zone 3,** which has the poorest blood supply, is located near the central vein, i.e. at the end of the microcirculatory system of the liver. Having the lowest oxygen supply, this area has the least resistance to damaging influences, e.g. oxygen deficiency, and it has the lowest regenerative capacity. It has also been postulated that the two halves of zone 2 can be added to zones 1 and 3 respectively, because zone 2 has no separate functional boundaries of its own. (18) • **Zones A, B, C** form concentric circles round the periportal field, which have a similarly decreasing quality of blood supply. Thus zone C1 is better supplied than, for example, C3, A2 or A3, i.e. the optimal blood supply does not only depend on proximity to the periportal field, but also on proximity to the terminal distributory branches of the blood vessels or to the limiting lamella. (s. figs. 2.13−2.15)

In correspondence with the oxygen gradient in zones 1 to 3 and A to C, there is a metabolic and enzymatic "zoning" of the hepatocytes. W. EGER had already described "functional zones" in 1954. (10) They have subsequently undergone reclassification as acini, although they were initially considered to be part of the lobular structure. This chemomorphology of the acinus is designated the **metabolic heterogeneity** of hepatocytes (K. JUN-

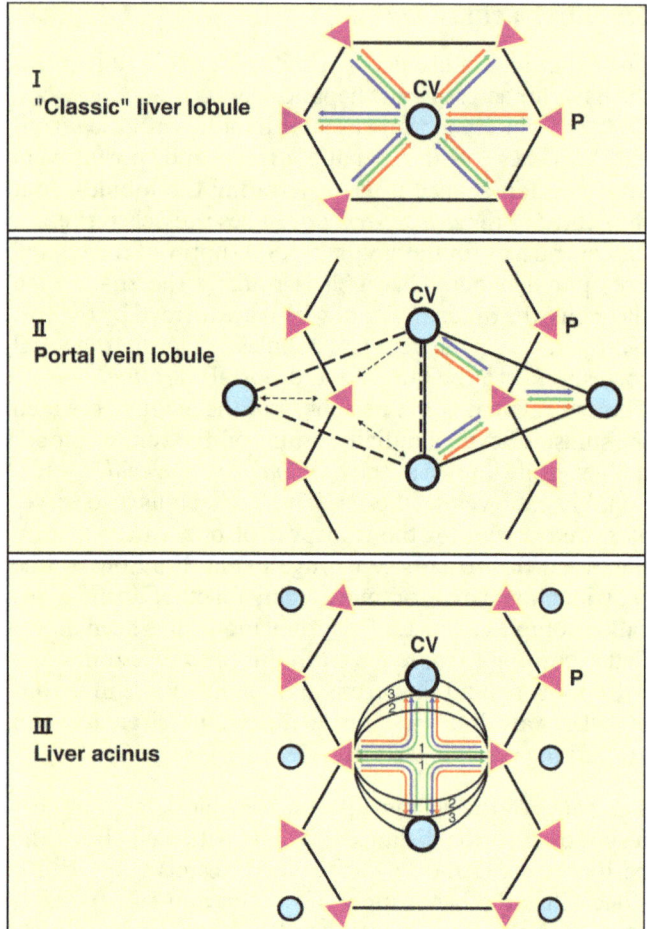

Fig. 2.13: Diagram of the classic hepatic lobule (I), the portal vein lobule (II) and the hepatic acinus (III): CV = central vein (○), P = portal tract (▶). Flow direction: venous blood (= blue arrow), arterial blood (= red arrow) and bile (= green arrow), with the microcirculatory acinus zones 1, 2, 3. • (cf. W. EKATAKSIN et al., 1992: the microvascular unit is regarded as an area in which all liver cells receive blood from a common terminal vessel)

GERMANN et al., 1978). (15, 18, 26, 27, 31, 63) (s. p. 36) Thus different metabolic processes are found in the periportal region (zone 1) and in the perivenous area (zone 3). Additionally, zones 1 to 3 are equipped with a very varied stock of enzymes, which does not, however, remain constant. There is also an **ultrastructural heterogeneity.** In zone 1, Kupffer cells, microvilli, mitochondria, lysosomes and the Golgi structures are more numerous than in zone 3, and the lumen of the bile capillaries is larger. (35) By contrast, there is less smooth endoplasmic reticulum in zone 1 than in zone 3 (15,700 μm³ against 21,600 μm³ per cell). The fenestration of the sinus-endothelium increases continuously from zone 1 to zone 3. (24) • Enzyme content and metabolic capacity of the hepatocytes depend on *microcirculatory variability* (caused endogenously or exogenously) and can vary considerably in the individual acinus areas.

Strong arguments have, however, been put forward against metabolic heterogeneity, at least against the concept of rigid zoning. The columns of the hepatocytia

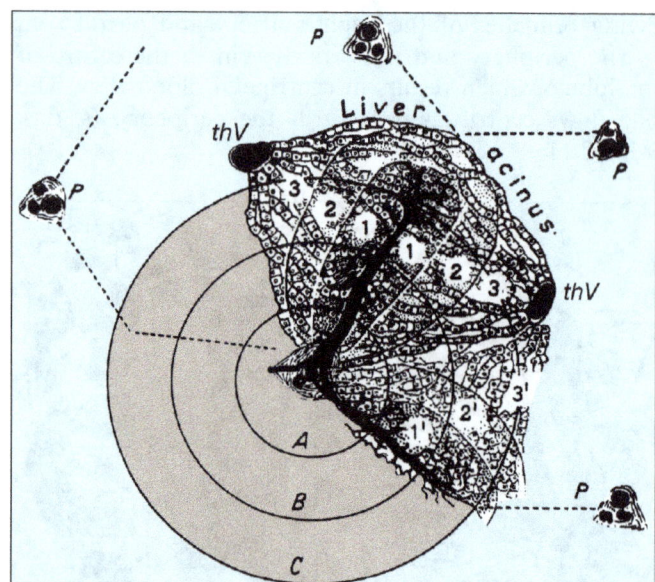

Fig. 2.14: Diagram of the functional (microcirculatory) liver unit ("simple acinus") (A.M. RAPPAPORT, 1960, 1963): terminal hepatic vein (thV), periportal field (P), zones of different blood supply A, B, C and 1, 2, 3. Zone 1 (afferent zone): zone richest in O_2, nutrients and hormones. Zone 3 (efferent zone): zone poorest in O_2, nutrients and hormones, but enriched with CO_2 and metabolites from zones 1 and 2. (Direction of blood flow is from 1 to 3 and from A to C)

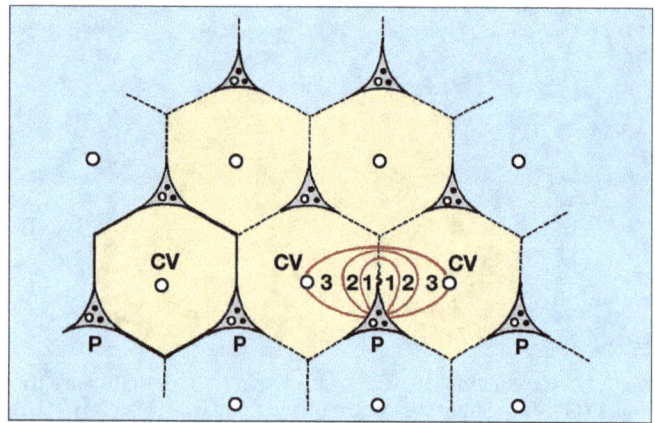

Fig. 2.15: Diagram of the liver lobule and the acinus arranged like a clover leaf around the portal field according to the acinar structure (modified from D. SASSE, 1986): central hepatic vein (CV) or terminal hepatic vein, periportal field (P). Circulatory and metabolically different zones: zone 1 (periportal), zone 2 (intermediate), zone 3 (perivenous)

the separate zones proved to be variable with regard to staining characteristics as well as enzyme content. Surprisingly, it could be unequivocally shown that a clear cellular multiplication occurs in the peripheral, i.e. in the periportal, zone and that the hepatocytes formed here are displaced towards the central vein. The hepatocytes migrate through all three zones at a speed of 1.44 μm/day, which is 0.32% of the diameter of the acinus (*"streaming liver"*). (77) From this it can be established that hepatocytes adopt the respective zonal differentiation during their migration from zone 1 to zone 3 and that the individual hepatocyte also receives the complement of enzymes typical for the respective zones during its spatial displacement. • With regard to their *metabolic capacities*, hepatocytes are thus pluripotent: their zonal position, the variability of microcirculation and their ability to migrate interzonally may possibly decide which metabolic functions are fulfilled directly and which are "deferred" from zone to zone.

The morphological unit is the **liver lobule.** With regard to the histological evaluation of a liver biopsy specimen, the use of this *lobular structure* is imperative to pathologist and clinician alike.

On the basis of the acinar concept, the **liver acinus** can be seen as a *"structural + microcirculatory + functional unit"*, which is nevertheless subject to the blood flow and the variability of the same.

6 Subcellular structures

Liver cells comprise the cell nucleus (= *karyoplasm*) and the cell body (= *cytoplasm*). Hepatocytes and sinusoidal cells have various types of *organelles* in their eosinophilic cytoplasm, such as endoplasmic reticulum, Golgi apparatus, lysosomes, mitochondria, peroxisomes, ribosomes, centrioles and kinetosomes. Numerous and diverse metabolic processes take place with their help. Almost all cytoplasmic structures of liver cells are continuously renewed (up to twice daily). (23, 28, 32, 35, 46, 50, 55) (s. figs. 2.9, 2.16–2.18) (s. tab. 2.1)

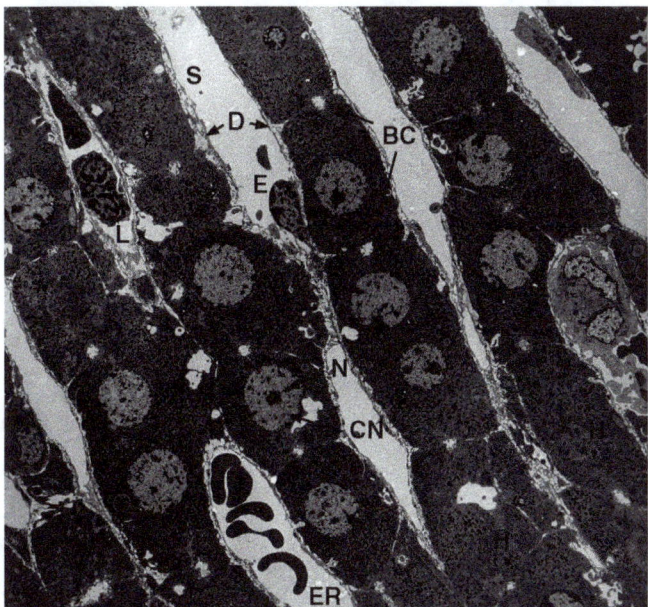

Fig. 2.16: Hepatocytes (H) in the form of cellular trabeculae with biliary capillaries (BC), cell nucleus (CN) and nucleolus (N); sinusoids (S) with leucocyte (L), endothelial cell (E) and erythrocytes (ER); Disse's space (D); × 1,980 (s. figs. 2.10–2.12)

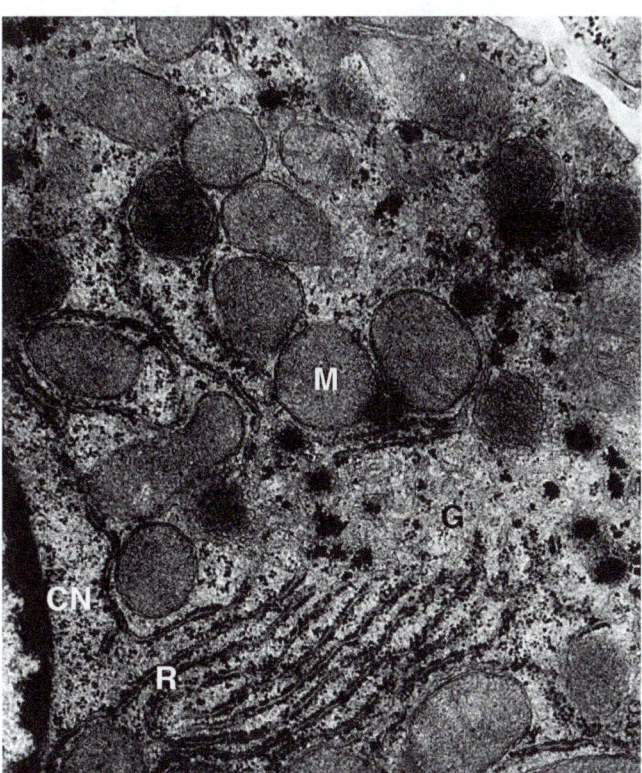

Fig. 2.17: Hyaloplasm of the hepatocyte: glycogen granules (G), mitochondria (M), rough endoplasmic reticulum with ribosomes (R); edge of the cell nucleus (CN); × 32,000 (s. fig. 2.9)

6.1 Cytoplasm

The cytoplasm of the cell is designated *hyaloplasm* in electron microscopy and *cytosol* in biochemistry. It constitutes about 51% of the cell volume and shows a microtubular lattice. (s. fig. 2.17) Basophilia, caused by ribonucleic acid, is the histochemical index for increased functional activity of the hepatocytes. The smooth endoplasmic reticulum is responsible for the pale eosinophilic colouring of the cytoplasm. Together with the cell membrane, the hyaloplasm is also involved in the formation of microvilli, pseudopodia, etc. • The watery solution of the hyaloplasm contains a mixture of molecular components. Of these, the proteins with about 10,000 different forms (15–20% of the weight, 10 billion protein molecules) are by far the most important. Further, glycogen granula in high numbers as well as pigments and lipid droplets can be found. Water loss from the hepatocytes gives rise to so-called *dark liver cells* (= shrinkage, with catabolic signal); conversely, water retention gives rise to so-called *hydropic liver cells* (= swelling, with anabolic signal). Indeed, the latter term cannot really be defined as such since numerous changes in the cells are involved.

6.2 Cell nucleus

The nucleus of the liver cell has one or two nucleoli. (s. fig. 2.18) Its proportion of the cell volume is 6%. About 20–25% of liver cells have two nuclei, presumably as a sign of increased cell activity. Number, size, nuclear pat-

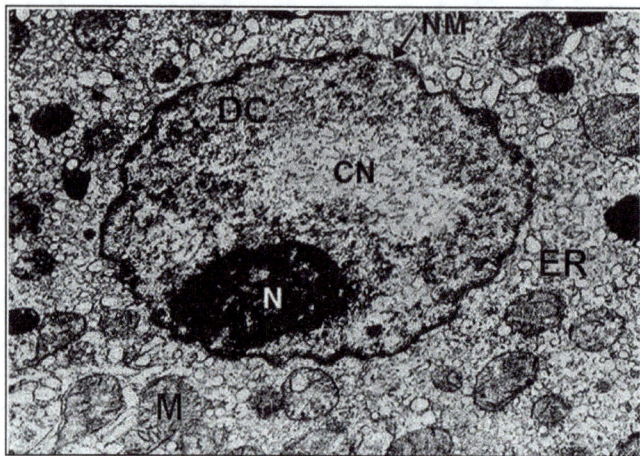

Fig. 2.18: Nucleus, nucleolus and hyaloplasm of the liver cell (20): cell nucleus (CN), marginal nucleolus (N), electron-dense dark nuclear capsule (DC), undulating nuclear membrane with (partial) fusion of the two membranes (NM), endoplasmic reticulum (ER), mitochondria (M); × 14,600

tern or nuclear changes are very varied due to diverse influences (e.g. age, nutrition, physiological "moulting") – above all in pathological processes. About 10–44% of the nuclei are diploid, 55–80% are tetraploid and 5–6% are octoploid. Increasing polyploidy is deemed a precancerous phase. The nucleus has a bilaminar "nuclear membrane" (D. W. Fawcett, 1955). The inner nuclear membrane is connected to the heterochromatin, while the outer layer is joined via membrane eversions to the endoplasmic reticulum it is covered with ribosomes. Between the two membranes is the 20–70 nm wide perinuclear cavity, which is connected to the spatial system of the rough endoplasmic reticulum. • The inner structure of the nucleus is non-homogeneous due to granules and the thread-like form of the chromatin; the latter constitutes the main component of the nucleus. This comprises chromosomes which contain genetic information in the form of DNA (deoxyribonucleinic acid). With approx. 3×10^9 nucleotides per nuclei, this information is incredibly tightly packed. The DNA is firmly attached to histones (nucleosomes). RNA transcription occurs in the interphase nucleus, and DNA is reduplicated prior to cell division. In the metabolically activated nucleus, RNA substances are concentrated in the nucleolus, in which the ribosomes are synthesized. It is chiefly the non-activated, non-despiralized chromatin in the form of heterochromatin which is deposited in the nuclear periphery, so that a dark nuclear capsule can be differentiated. Number and size of the nucleoli are dependent upon various influences. The exchange of substances and the transfer of genetic or metabolic information between nucleus and cytoplasm occur predominantly through (*1.*) diffusion, (*2.*) cell membrane pores (diameter ca. 10 nm), and (*3.*) pinocytosis.

6.3 Organelles

Various tiny structures, so-called organelles, are embedded in the cytoplasm, where they make numerous cell functions possible. (s. fig. 2.9) (s. tab. 2.1) • The enzyme-

	Membrane surface in proportion to total hepatocyte membrane surface	Proportion of hepatocyte cell volume	Number per hepatocyte	Function
1. Rough endoplasmic reticulum (RER)	35%	13%	1	Synthesis of proteins, glucose-6-phosphatase, triglycerides, coagulant factors, *etc.*
2. Smooth endoplasmic reticulum (SER)	16%	7,7%	1	Biotransformation; synthesis of steroid hormones, phospholipids, bilirubin conjugation, cholesterol, bile acids, glucose metabolism, *etc.*
3. Golgi apparatus	7%			Secretion of lipoprotein, bile acids, glycoprotein synthesis, protein glycolization
4. Mitochondria	39%	18–22%	1,700–2,200	Protein secretion, haem synthesis, transport and degradation functions, cellular energy generation (ATP), oxidative phosphorylation, urea synthesis, gluconeogenesis, liponeogenesis, ketogenesis, β-oxidation of fatty acids, citric acid cycle, respiratory chain, *etc.*
5. Lysosomes	0.4%	2%	200–300	Degradation of "foreign" macromolecules in the cell by means of hydrolytic enzymes, deposition of copper, ferritin, lipofuscin, bile pigment, *etc.*
6. Peroxisomes	0.4%	1,3%	400–1,000	Oxidative degradation processes by means of peroxidases, catalase, xanthine oxidase, degradation of long-chain fatty acids, antioxidative function, bile acid synthesis, alcohol metabolism, purine metabolism, *etc.*

Tab. 2.1: Numerical and functional summary of the most important organelles (adapted from B. Alberts et al., 1983) (s. figs. 2.9, 2.17)

rich **mitochondria** have an outer and an inner membrane, with the latter forming creases (= cristae). The outer membrane is relatively permeable for small molecules. However, the inner membrane (which surrounds the matrix) must use specific transport proteins to enable protons, calcium, phosphate and so on to pass. Energy-rich substrates are transformed into ATP in the mitochondria. The enzymes which are responsible for fatty-acid degradation and the citric-acid cycle can be found in the matrix. The inner membrane also contains the enzymes of the so-called respiratory cycle. An enormous number of energy-providing reactions and metabolic processes take effect at this site. They have a round-to-oval shape with a diameter of about 1 µm. There are 1,000(–2,200) mitochondria per liver cell (18–22% of the liver cell volume). They generally lie in the vicinity of the rough ER and are able to move within the cell. Multiplication occurs through division. Their half-life is 9–10 days. (s. figs. 2.17, 2.18) • The **endoplasmic reticulum** (= about 20% of the liver cell volume) consists of a smooth (SER) (40%) and a rough (RER) (60%) portion. The rough surface is due to ribosomes (9–10 million/liver cell); it is also known as ergastoplasm (identical to the basophilic granulae). (s. fig. 2.17) The SER contains microsomes. It forms tubules and vesicles as well as being the site of the cytochrome P 450 systems. • The **Golgi complex** is generally found between the cell nucleus and the canaliculus and consists of four to six cisternae. This membrane system, which is formed from lamellar vesicles, communicates with the smooth ER. It is primarily concerned with the intracellular transport of various substances, but also with processes of degradation and excretion. • The **lysosomes** (200–300/liver cell) lie predominantly close to the canaliculus. They are organelles for the digestion and storage of cellular and noncellular (also exogenous) material. Lysosomes contain hydrolytic enzymes, mainly proteases (= lysosomal enzymes) and acid phosphatase. • The **peroxisomes** (= microbodies) are enzyme-rich and oxidative-reactive structures. They are round to oval in shape and 0.2–1.0 µm in size. The liver cell contains 400–1,000 peroxisomes.

6.4 Membrane

Hepatocytes, like the essential organelles, are surrounded by membranes which differ in their function and structure. The membrane of the hepatocytes consists of lipids (52–54%), proteins (44–46%) and carbohydrates (2–4%). The latter are structural, antenna-like docking points for tissue-specific receptors. (s. fig. 2.19) The membrane surface area of 3×10^5 million liver cells and their organelles is 33,000 m², i.e. *a surface area that is 5 times larger than that of a football field* (inner membrane surface area = 24,000 m²). • The basolateral (sinusoidal) proportion of the hepatocyte membrane

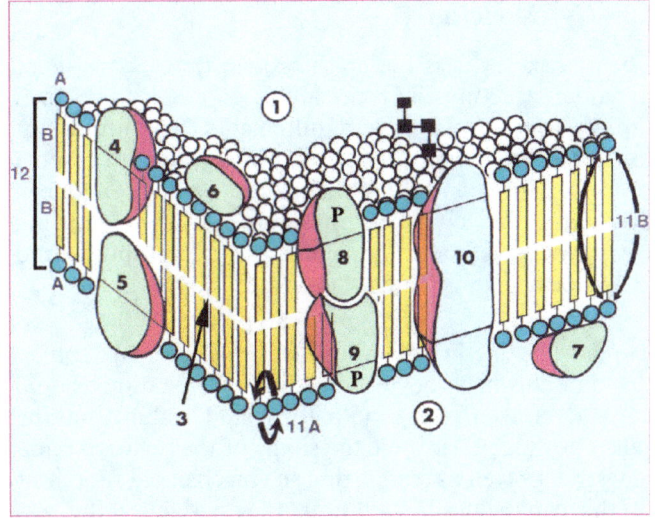

Fig. 2.19: Diagram of the plasma membrane showing its integral proteins (fluid mosaic model) (adapted from S. J. Singer et al., 1972 and H. Knüfermann, 1976). • 1: external aqueous milieu, 2: internal aqueous milieu, 3: fracture plane of the apolar membrane layer, 4: externally orientated intrinsic protein (ectoprotein), 5: internally orientated intrinsic protein (endoprotein), 6: external extrinsic protein, 7: internal intrinsic protein, 8, 9: membrane-penetrating proteins with hydrophobic interactions in the inside of the membrane (P = polar region), 10: membrane pervaded by glycoprotein with sugar residues (■-■), 11: lateral diffusion (A) and flip-flop (B), 12: hydrophilic region (A) and hydrophobic region (B) of the bilayer membrane

amounts to approx. 85%, the apical (canalicular) proportion to approx. 15%. • The membranes consist of a double layer (bilayer) of choline phospholipids, into which cholesterol, proteins, glycolipids and glycoproteins are incorporated with "systematic variability". This specific structure makes possible the enormous number of membrane-related functions. The hydrophilic parts of the phospholipid molecules form the outer and inner boundaries of the membrane, while the hydrophobic parts are directed towards its interior. The bilayer membrane is a liquid crystalline system (= *fluidity of the membrane*) allowing lateral movement (= *lateral diffusion*) of the proteins and phospholipids deposited in this area. In addition, the phospholipids can change position between the layers (= *flip-flop*). (71) The side of the sinusoidal cell turned towards the hepatic lacuna carries numerous microvilli, increasing the surface area of the cell membrane. (48) The form and number of the microvilli not only depend upon the functional condition of the liver cell, but also upon damaging effects. • The hepatocyte membrane has multiple and existential *functions* such as (*1.*) mechanical and chemical protection, (*2.*) demarcation of neighbouring cells, (*3.*) link with the extracellular matrix, (*4.*) contact and interaction with neighbouring cells, (*5.*) signal exchange between intracellular and extracellular space, (*6.*) transport mechanisms, (*7.*) enzymatic reactions, (*8.*) anchoring of the cytoskeleton.

6.5 Cytoskeleton

The cytoskeleton, made up of protein fibres, consists of dynamic structures with the ability to adapt their form rapidly to any respective requirements. It is important for the overall organization of the cell (e.g. transport processes, organelle movement, cell polarity, and cell division). The cytoskeleton comprises the following *components:* (*1.*) actin filaments, (*2.*) microtubules, and (*3.*) intermediate filaments. (12) (s. fig. 2.9)

Thread-like **actin filaments** (microfilaments) spread through the hepatocytes, creating a three-dimensional network and ensuring both form and stability of the cell. They also guarantee the shape of the microvilli and fenestrae as well as supporting the mechanical functions of the canaliculi. In addition, they influence the viscosity of the cytoplasm. Cytochalasin A depolymerizes actin with lumen enlargement of the canaliculi, thus causing cholestasis; in this way phalloidin both stabilizes and inhibits the bile flow. • The tube-like **microtubules** consisting of tubulin also form a network within the cell. They serve the targeted transport of subcellular substrates or organelles, and they are important for the mitotic mechanisms involved in cell division. • The **intermediate filaments** also have a tubular structure and, in addition to their stabilizing functions, probably serve the intracellular transport of materials, too. • **Microtrabeculae** have also been postulated (possibly as a special form of actin filaments), forming a three-dimensional cytoplasmic meshwork, in which enzymes may also be deposited. The microtrabeculae form a dynamic lattice and in this way are connected with all organelles, microtubules and filaments as well as with the nuclear and cellular membranes. Various "motor proteins" produce a diverse range of motilities at the cellular and subcellular level. • This gives rise to the **cytoplast,** the vital functional unit of the liver cell.

References:

1. **Akiyoshi, H., Gonda, T., Terata, T.:** A comparative histochemical and immunohistochemical study of aminergic, cholinergic, and peptidergic innervation in rat, hamster, guinea pig, dog and human livers. Liver 1998; 18: 352–359
2. **Arias, I.M., Che, M., Gatmaitan, Z., Levelle, C., Nishida, T., Pierre, M.S.:** The biology of the bile canaliculus, 1993. Hepatology 1993; 17: 318–329
3. **Atermann, K.:** The parasinusoidal cells of the liver: a historical account. Histochem. J. 1982; 18: 279–305
4. **Ballardini, G., Degli Espoti, S., Bianchi, F.B., Bandiali, L., de Giorgi, A., Faccani, L., Biocchini, L., Busacchi, C.A., Pisi, E.:** Correlation between Ito cells and fibrogenesis in an experimental model of hepatic fibrosis. A sequential stereological study. Liver 1983; 3: 58–63
5. **Bioulac-Sage, P., Lafon, M.E., Saric, J., Balabaud, C.:** Nerves and perisinusoidal cells in human liver. J. Hepatol. 1990; 10: 105–112
6. **Bouwens, L., Wisse, E.:** PIT cells in the liver. Liver 1992; 12: 3–9
7. **Burt, A.D.:** Pathobiology of hepatic stellate cells. J. Gastroenterol. 1999; 34: 299–304
8. **Crawford, J.M.:** Development of the intrahepatic biliary tree. Semin. Liver Dis. 2002; 22: 213–226
9. **David, H., Reinke, P.:** Der vaskuläre Pol des Hepatozyten: Struktur, Funktion und Pathologie. Zbl. Allg. Path. Path. Anat. 1986; 132: 83–98
10. **Eger, W.:** Zur Pathologie des zentralen und peripheren Funktionsfeldes des Leberläppchens. Zbl. Allg. Path. Path. Anat. 1954; 91: 255–267
11. **Elias, H.:** A reexamination of the structure of the mammalian liver. II. The hepatic lobule and its relation to the vascular and biliary system. Amer. J. Anat. 1949; 85: 379–456
12. **Feldmann, G.:** The cytoskeleton of the hepatocyte. Structure and functions. J. Hepatol. 1989; 8: 380–386
13. **Fellbaum, Ch., Beham, A., Schmid, Ch.:** Isolierte Nebenleber (Hepar succenturiatum) am Gallenblasenhals. Fallbericht mit Literaturübersicht. Wien. Klin. Wschr. 1987; 99: 825–827
14. **Forbes, S., Vig, P., Poulson, R., Thomas, H., Alson, M.:** Hepatic stem cells. J. Pathol. 2002; 197: 510–518
15. **Gebhardt, R.:** Metabolic zonation of the liver: regulation and implications for liver function. Pharm. Ther. 1992; 53: 275–354
16. **Gressner, A.M., Bachem, M.G.:** Cellular sources of noncollagenous matrix proteins: role of fat-storing cells in fibrogenesis. Semin. Liver Dis. 1990; 10: 30–46
17. **Grompe, M.:** The origin of hepatocytes. Gastroenterology 2005; 128: 2158–2160
18. **Gumucio, J.J., May, M., Dvorak, C., Chianale, J., Massey, V.:** The isolation of functionally heterogeneous hepatocytes of the proximal and distal half of the liver acinus in the rat. Hepatology 1986; 6: 932–944
19. **Gupta, S.C., Gupta, C.D., Gupta, S.B.:** Hepatovenous segments in the human liver. J. Anat. 1981; 133: 1–6
20. **Hadjis, N.S., Blumgart, L.H.:** Editorial: Clinical aspects of liver atrophy. J. Clin. Gastroenterol. 1989; 11: 3–7
21. **Ham, J.M.:** Lobar and segmental atrophy of the liver. World. J. Surg. 1990; 14: 457–462
22. **Henriksen, J.H., Horn, T., Christoffersen, P.:** The blood-lymph barrier in the liver. A review based on morphological and functional concepts of normal and cirrhotic liver. Liver 1984; 4: 221–232
23. **Holle, G.:** Die gegenwärtigen Vorstellungen über den Feinbau der Leber. Acta Hepato-splen. 1961; 8: 253–264
24. **Horn, T., Henriksen, J.H., Christoffersen, P.:** The sinusoidal lining cells in "normal" human liver. A scanning electron microscopic investigation. Liver 1986; 6: 98–110
25. **Inoue, T., Ito, Y., Matsuzaki, Y., Okauchi, Y., Kondo, H., Horiuchi, N., Nakao, K., Iwata, M.:** Hypogenesis of right hepatic lobe accompanied by portal hypertension: case report and review of 31 Japanese cases. J. Gastroenterol. 1997; 32: 836–842
26. **Jungermann, K., Katz, N.:** Functional hepatocellular heterogeneity. Hepatology 1982; 2: 385–395
27. **Jungermann, K., Katz, N.:** Functional specialization of different hepatocyte populations. Physiol. Rev. 1989; 69: 708–764
28. **Kaneda, K.:** Liver-associated large granular lymphocytes. Morphological and functional aspects. Arch. Histol. Cytol. 1989; 52: 447–459
29. **Karpen, S.J., Crawford, Y.M.:** Cellular and molecular biology of the liver. Curr. Opin. Gastroenterol. 1999; 15: 184–191
30. **Khan, A.M., Hundal, R., Manzoor, K., Dhuper, S., Korsten, M.A.:** Accessory liver lobes: A diagnostic and therapeutic challenge of their torsions. Scand. J. Gastroenterol. 41; 2006: 125–130
31. **Lamers, W.H., Hilberts, A., Furt, E., Smith, J., Jonges, G.N., van Noorden, C.J., Gaasbeek Janzen, J.W., Charles, R., Moorman, A.F.M.:** Hepatic enzymic zonation: a reevaluation of the concept of the liver acinus. Hepatology 1989; 10: 72–76
32. **Lapp, H.:** Die submikroskopische Organisation der Leberzelle. Münch. Med. Wschr. 1963; 105: 1–12
33. **Loeweneck, H.:** Anatomische Varianten der Lebergebilde. Chirurg 1972; 43: 345–350
34. **Ludwig, J., Ritman, E.L., LaRusso, N.F., Sheedy, P.F., Zump, G.:** Anatomy of the human biliary system studied by quantitative computer-aided three-dimensional imaging techniques. Hepatology 1998; 27: 893–899
35. **Ma, M.H., Biempica, L.:** The normal human liver cell. Cytochemical and ultrastructural studies. Amer. J. Path. 1971; 62: 353–376
36. **McCuskey, R.S.:** Morphological mechanisms for regulating blood flow through hepatic sinusoids. Liver 2000; 20: 3–7
37. **Philips, D.M., La Brecque, D.R., Shirazi, S.S.:** Corset liver. J. Clin. Gastroenterol. 1985; 7: 361–368
38. **Pujari, B.D., Deodhare, S.G.:** Symptomatic accessory lobe of liver with a review of the literature. Postgrad. Med. J. 1976; 52: 234–236
39. **Radin, D.R., Colletti, P.M., Ralls, P.W., Boswell, W.D., Halls, J.M.:** Agenesis of the right lobe of the liver. Radiology 1987; 164: 639–642
40. **Rappaport, A.M., Borowy, Z.J., Lougheed, W.M., Lotto, W.N.:** Subdivision of hexagonal liver lobules into a structural and functional unit; role in hepatic physiology and pathology. Anat. Rec. 1954; 119: 11–34
41. **Rappaport, A.M.:** The structural and functional unit in the human liver (liver acinus). Anat. Rec. 1958; 130: 673–687
42. **Rappaport, A.M.:** The microcirculatory hepatic unit. Microvasc. Res. 1973; 6: 212–228
43. **Reinke, P.:** Die Nichthepatozyten der Leber-Struktur, Funktion und Bedeutung für pathologische Prozesse der Leber. Z. Klin. Med. 1986; 41: 811–816
44. **Reinke, P., David, H.:** Struktur und Funktion der Sinusoidwand der Leber. ("Die perisinusoidale Funktionseinheit"). Eine Übersicht. Z. Mikrosk.-anat. Forsch. 1987; 101: 91–136
45. **Rhodin, J.A.G.:** The ultrastructure of mammalian arterioles and precapillary sphincters. J. Ultrastruct. Res. 1967; 18: 181–223
46. **Riede, U.N., Sasse, D.:** Quantitative topography of organelles in the liver. A combined histochemical and morphometric analysis. Cell. Tiss. Res. 1981; 221: 209–220
47. **Sato, N., Kawakami, K., Matsumoto, S., Toyonaga, T., Ishimitsu, T., Nagafuchi, K., Miki, T., Shiozaki, H.:** Agenesis of the right lobe of the liver: report of a case. Jpn. J. Surg. 1998; 28: 643–646

48. **Schachter, D.:** Fluidity and function of hepatocyte plasma membranes. Hepatology 1984; 4: 140–151
49. **Schmidt, H., Guttmann, E.:** Die Verzweigungen der großen intrahepatischen Gallenwege in der röntgenologischen Darstellung (Analyse des Cholangiogramms). Fortschr. Röntgenstr. 1954; 81: 283–296
50. **Schulze, H.-U., Staudinger, Hj.:** Struktur und Funktion des endoplasmatischen Retikulum. Naturwissenschaften 1975; 62: 331–340
51. **Sigal, S.H., Brill, S., Fiorino, A.S., Reid, L.M.:** The liver as a stem cell and lineage system. Amer. J. Physiol. 1992; 263: G 139–G 148
52. **Smedsrod, B., Pertoft, H., Gustafson, St., Laurent, T.C.:** Scavenger functions of the liver endothelial cell. Biochem. J. 1990; 266: 313–327
53. **Smedsrod, B., de Bleser, P.J., Braet, F., Lovisetti, P., Vanderkerken, K., Wisse, E., Geerts, A.:** Cell biology of liver endothelial and Kupffer cells. Gut 1994; 35: 1509–1516
54. **Steiner, J.W., Carruthers, J.S.:** Studies on the fine structure of the terminal branches of the biliary tree. I. The morphology of normal bile canaliculi, bile pre-ductules (Ducts of Hering) and bile ductules. Amer. J. Path. 1961; 38: 640–649
55. **Stockert, R.J., Wolkoff, A.W.:** Cellular and molecular biology of the liver. Curr. Opin. Gastroenterol. 2001; 17: 205–210
56. **Strain, A.J., Crosby, H.A., Nijjar, S., Kelly, D.A., Hubscher, S.G.:** Human liver-derived stem cells. Semin. Liver Dis. 2003; 23: 373–383
57. **Takasaki, S., Hano, H.:** Three-dimensional observations of the human hepatic artery (Arterial system in the liver). J. Hepatol. 2001; 34: 455–466
58. **Tanuma, Y., Ito, T., Shibasaki, S.:** Further electronmicroscope studies on the human hepatic sinusoidal wall with special reference to the fat-storing cell. Arch. Histol. Jap. 1982; 45: 263–274
59. **Teutsch, H.F.:** The molecular microarchitecture of human liver. Hepatology 2005; 42: 317–325
60. **Tietz, P.S., LaRusso, N.F.:** Cholangiocyte biology. Curr. Opin. Gastroenterology 2005; 21: 337–343
61. **Tiniakos, G.D., Lee, J.A., Burt, A.D.:** Innervation of the liver: morphology and function. Liver 1996; 16: 151–160
62. **Toth, C.A., Thomas, P.:** Liver endocytosis and Kupffer cells. Hepatology 1992; 16: 255–266
63. **Traber, P.G., Chianale, J., Gumucio, J.J.:** Physiologic significance and regulation of hepatocellular heterogeneity. Gastroenterology 1988; 95: 1130–1143
64. **Trutmann, M., Sasse, D.:** The lymphatics of the liver. Anat. Embryol. 1994; 190: 201–209
65. **Vanderkerken, K., Bouwens, L., De Neve, W., van den Berg, K., Baekeland, M., Delens, N., Wisse, E.:** Origin and differentiation of hepatic natural killer cells (PIT cells). Hepatology 1993; 18: 919–925
66. **Van Eyken, P., Desmet, V.J.:** Cytokeratins and the liver. Liver 1993; 13: 113–122
67. **Van Leeuwen, M.S., Noordzij, J., Fernandez, M.A., Hennipman, A., Feldberg, M.A.M., Dillon, E.H.:** Portal venous and segmental anatomy of the right hemiliver: observations based on three-dimensional spiral CT rendering Amer. J. Roentgenol. 1994; 163: 1395–1404
68. **Vogl, A., Small, A.:** Partial eventration of the right diaphragm (congenital diaphragmatic herniation of the liver). Ann. Intern. Med. 1955; 43: 63–82
69. **Wake, K., Decker, K., Kirn, A.:** Cell biology and kinetiky of Kupffer cells in the liver. Int. Rev. Cytol. 1989; 118: 173–192
70. **Weiner, F.R., Giambrone, M., Czaja, M.J., Shah, A., Annoni, G., Takahashi, S., Eghbali, M., Zern, M.A.:** Ito-cell gene expression and collagen regulation. Hepatology 1990; 11: 111–117
71. **White, J.M.:** Membrane fusion. Science 1992; 258: 917–924
72. **Wisse, E., van't Noordende, J.M., van der Meulen, J., Daems, W.T.:** The PIT cell: description of a new type of cell occuring in rat liver sinusoids and peripheral blood. Cell. Tiss. Res. 1976; 173: 423–435
73. **Wisse, E., De Zanger, R.B., Charles, K., van der Smissen, P., McCuskey, R.S.:** The liver sieve: considerations concerning the structure and function of endothelial fenestrae, the sinusoidal wall and the space of Disse. Hepatology 1985; 5: 683–692
74. **Wünsche, A., Preuss, F.:** Pfortaderkörbchen um Leberläppchen beweisen die Läppchengliederung der Leber. Acta Anat. 1986; 125: 32–36
75. **Yoshida, J., Chijiiwa, K., Yamaguchi, K., Yokohata, K., Tanaka, M.:** Practical classification of the branching types of the biliary tree: an analysis of 1,094 consecutive direct cholangiograms. J. Amer. Coll. Surg. 1996; 182: 37–40
76. **Yoshiura, K., Sawabe, M., Esaki, Y., Tanaka, Y., Naitoh, M., Kino, K., Tsuru, M., Fukazawa, T.:** Extreme right lobar atrophy of the liver. A rare complication of autoimmune hepatitis. J. Clin. Gastroenterol. 1998; 26: 334–336
77. **Zajicek, G., Oren, R., Weinreb, M. jr.:** The streaming liver. Liver 1985; 5: 293–300
78. **Zhao, R., Duncan, S.A.:** Embryonic development of the liver. Hepatology 2005; 41: 956–967
79. **Zheng, Y.W., Taniguchi, H.:** Diversity of hepatic stem cells in the fetal and addult liver. Semin. Liver Dis. 2003; 23: 337–348

3 Biochemistry and Functions of the Liver

		Page:
1	*Metabolic functions of the liver*	36
2	*Regulatory metabolic mechanisms*	36
3	**Bilirubin metabolism of the liver**	37
4	**Porphyrin metabolism of the liver**	38
5	**Bile acid metabolism of the liver**	39
5.1	Biosynthesis of bile acids	39
5.2	Enterohepatic circulation of bile acids	40
5.3	Functions of bile acids	41
5.4	Composition and secretion of bile	41
6	**Protein metabolism of the liver**	42
6.1	Biochemistry of amino acids	42
6.2	Protein synthesis and catabolism	44
7	**Carbohydrate metabolism of the liver**	44
7.1	Glycogenesis and glycogenolysis	45
7.2	Gluconeogenesis and glucolysis	45
8	**Lipid metabolism of the liver**	46
8.1	Classification of lipoproteins	46
8.2	Regulation of lipoproteins	48
8.3	Cholesterol metabolism	49
9	**Hormone metabolism and the liver**	49
9.1	Classification of hormones	50
9.2	Effector hormones and the liver	50
9.3	Steroid hormones and the liver	50
9.4	Thyroid hormones and the liver	51
10	**Vitamin metabolism and the liver**	51
10.1	Classification of vitamins	51
10.2	Mechanisms of vitamin action	51
10.2.1	Fat-soluble vitamins	51
10.2.2	Water-soluble vitamins	52
11	**Trace elements and the liver**	53
11.1	Iron	54
11.2	Copper	54
11.3	Zinc	55
11.4	Selenium	55
11.5	Manganese	55
11.6	Chromium	56
11.7	Cobalt	56

		Page:
12	**Biotransformation and detoxification**	56
12.1	Foreign compounds (xenobiotics)	56
12.2	Metabolization of xenobiotics	56
12.3	Mechanisms of metabolic detoxification	57
12.4	Biotransformation	57
12.4.1	2-phase reaction	57
12.4.2	Enzyme adaptation	58
13	**Ammonia detoxification and bicarbonate neutralization**	61
13.1	Urea cycle	61
13.2	Glutamine cycle	62
13.3	Bicarbonate neutralization	63
14	**Alcohol uptake and degradation**	64
14.1	Endogenous alcohol synthesis	64
14.2	Exogenous alcohol uptake	64
14.3	Alcohol absorption	65
14.4	Biochemical parameters	65
14.5	Alcohol degradation	66
15	**Reticuloendothelial system**	69
15.1	Systematics and nomenclature	69
15.2	Functions of the hepatic RES	69
16	**Radicals and antioxidants**	70
16.1	Definition	70
16.2	Formation and importance of free radicals	71
16.3	Balance between formation and inactivation	71
16.4	Scavengers and antioxidants	72
16.5	Pathophysiology	72
16.6	Lipid peroxidation	73
17	**Cellular transport processes**	73
17.1	Passive transport	73
17.2	Active transport	74
17.3	Vesicular transport	74
	● References (1–95) (Figures 3.1–3.16; tables 3.1–3.25)	74

3 Biochemistry and Functions of the Liver

1 Metabolic functions of the liver

▶ The morphological and functional integrity of the liver is vital to the health of the human organism. This essentially depends upon constant maintenance of the numerous biochemical functions of the liver and the diverse metabolic processes occurring in the hepatocytes and sinusoidal cells. • *The liver ensures that approximately* **70 partial functions** *within* **12 major metabolic areas** *proceed either continuously or in biological (e.g. circadian) rhythms, or vary according to specific requirements.* (s. tab. 3.1)

1. Acid-base balance
2. Alcohol degradation
3. Amino acid and protein metabolism
4. Bile acid metabolism
5. Bilirubin metabolism
6. Biotransformation and detoxification
7. Carbohydrate metabolism
8. Hormone metabolism
9. Lipid and lipoprotein metabolism
10. Porphyrin metabolism
11. Trace elements and the liver
12. Vitamin metabolism

▶ *About 500 separate biochemical processes occur in one single liver cell!*

Tab. 3.1: Essential biochemical metabolic functions of the liver

Metabolic processes utilize a variety of differing and contrasting biochemical routes to enable synthesis of degradation and activation or deactivation of substances; in addition, they facilitate cellular uptake and excretory mechanisms. Moreover, there are various links between different metabolic pathways and functional processes. Intermediate chemical products generated in the course of metabolic reactions may be taken up by other pathways or cycles. Substrates are shifted between subcellular structures, and the metabolic end-products of one process are often used as the original substrate for new syntheses.

A general picture of the intricate complexity of various cycles, biochemical pathways and metabolic reactions within the liver has been presented in **two posters.** (25)*

---

*) 1. *Holldorf, A. W., Krahl-Mateblowski, U., Mateblowski, M., Wütherich, S.*: Pathways of metabolism in liver. (9th Ed., 1992)
2. *Reutter, W., Geilen, Ch., Baum, O.*: Metabolic pathways in the liver cell. (6th Ed., 1998)

2 Regulatory metabolic mechanisms

The intricate network of biochemical reactions occurring within the restricted volume of the liver cell requires subtly controlled metabolic regulatory mechanisms. (28) These occur on **four levels:** (*1.*) at the molecular level, (*2.*) within the organelles, (*3.*) at the cellular level, and (*4.*) at the organ level.

(*1.*) *Regulation* may occur at the **molecular**:
- through negative feedback, whereby the end-product of a metabolic reaction inhibits the activity of the enzyme which determines the speed of reaction. This affords a rapid adaptation of specific chemical reactions in response to alterations in metabolic conditions;
- through changes in the actions of activators and inhibitors;
- through modulation of enzyme activities;
- through changes in the rate of enzyme synthesis or degradation.

(*2.*) *Regulation* can take place within the **organelles**:
- Protein synthesis occurs in the ribosomes of the rough endoplasmic reticulum – by contrast, the process of protein degradation occurs in the lysosomes.
- Fatty acids are synthesized in the smooth endoplasmic reticulum, but they are broken down in the mitochondria.

(*3.*) *Regulation* may be effected at the **cellular level**:
- Hepatocytes display *metabolic heterogeneity* according to their zonal location within the acinus. (38) (s. p. 28) Specific chemical processes thus proceed exclusively or predominantly in the hepatocytes of the periportal or the perivenous zones. The zonally segregated reactions may also be regulated separately. It seems that, under certain conditions, metabolic processes are also "shifted" from one zone of the acinus to another.
- Hepatocytes interact closely with the sinusoidal cells and Kupffer cells (e.g. in the breakdown of erythrocytes and the degradation of pyrimidine nucleotides).
- Hepatocytes and sinusoidal cells are influenced by vegetative nerve fibre endings in Disse's space.

(*4.*) *Regulation* of metabolic processes may be achieved through biochemical interactions at the **organ level**:
- between the liver and the musculature
- between the liver and the kidneys
- between the liver and the endocrine system
- between the liver and the intestine

Zonal heterogeneity

Although hepatocytes appear to be relatively uniform under the light microscope, they display structural heterogeneity when viewed under an electronic microscope and functional heterogeneity on a metabolic level. (s. p. 28) This heterogeneous zoning provides optimum control and prevents futile cycles. However, the zones have no clear-cut boundaries and merge freely with each other. (9, 26, 38−40, 42) (s. tab. 3.2)

Periportal zone (zone 1)	Perivenous zone (zone 3)
Hepatocytes smaller Mitochondria larger Golgi membrane ↑ Golgi glycogen ↑ Smooth ER ↓ Lysosomes ↓	Hepatocytes larger Mitochondria smaller Golgi membrane ↓ Golgi glycogen ↓ Smooth ER ↑ Lysosomes ↑
Fenestrae ↓ Kupffer cells ↑ larger Ito cells ↑ PIT cells ↑	Fenestrae ↑ Kupffer cells ↓ smaller Ito cells ↓ PIT cells ↓
− gluconeogenesis − β-oxidation of fatty acids − urea synthesis from amino acids − glutamine hydrolysis − amino acid degradation − mitochondrial carbonic anhydrase − bile acid-dependent fraction − glycogen synthesis from lactate or amino acids − glycogen degradation − O₂ uptake − cholesterol synthesis − citrate cycle − respiratory chain reactions − pigment deposition	− glycolysis − liponeogenesis − glutamine synthesis − glutamate transport − cytosolic carbonic anhydrase − bile acid-independent fraction − glycogen synthesis from glucose − glycogen degradation to lactate − biotransformation − ketogenesis

Tab. 3.2: Morphological heterogeneity of liver cells and organelles as well as metabolic heterogeneity of hepatocytes according to their respective zonal location in the acinus (s. pp 27, 28)

Bile acids are channelled from the sinusoids periportally via transport systems with low affinity and high capacity, and in the perivenous area via transport systems with high affinity and low capacity. The bile acids are therefore excreted with decreasing concentration from the periportal to the perivenous area.

Intrahepatic biliary epithelium plays a contributory role in functional heterogeneity. The absorption and secretory processes along the bile ducts fulfil different functions. Such cholangiocytic heterogeneity can be detected in various reactions to different forms of damage. (42)

In addition to the regulatory mechanisms listed above, metabolic processes may be altered at the cellular and subcellular levels by further **influencing factors**, such as hormones, vitamins, trace elements and the autonomic nervous system. • *The liver requires ca. 340 kcal/day in order to carry out all its functions adequately.*

3 Bilirubin metabolism of the liver

▶ The complete structure of bilirubin was described as an open tetrapyrrole derivative of haem by H. Fischer in 1935.

Bilirubin is an organic anion. It is mainly (ca. 80 %) derived from the degradation of ageing erythrocytes in the spleen, liver (hepatocytes, Kupffer cells), kidneys and bone marrow. Approximately 36.2 mg bilirubin are produced from 1 g haemoglobin. The daily output of bilirubin is 250−350 mg (3.8 ± 0.6 mg/kg BW).

The oxidation of **haem**, a complex consisting of iron and protoporphyrin derived from haemoglobin, is effected by haem oxygenase to produce **biliverdin IXα**. This is subsequently converted to **bilirubin IXα** by biliverdin reductase. The reaction speed is governed by the haem oxygenase. This enzyme complex contains the inducible cytochrome P 450, which accelerates bilirubin production when the haemoglobin level is elevated. A small proportion of bilirubin (20−30%) is produced from the degradation of other metalloporphyrins. (s. fig. 3.1)

Bilirubin − an apolar, water-insoluble lipophile substance − is potentially toxic. It is bound to serum albumin and transported to the sinusoidal membrane of the liver cell as a **bilirubin-albumin complex**. (s. fig. 3.1) The binding capacity of albumin is exceeded only at a serum bilirubin concentration of >4−5 mg/dl. In the case of decreased albumin binding (e. g. in acidosis) or oversaturated binding capacity, there is a danger of toxic cell damage due to the diffusion of unbound bilirubin into the cells (in some cases accompanied by kernicterus). Neonates and premature babies are at particular risk because of their immature blood-cerebrospinal fluid barrier. Albumin-bound bilirubin can function as an antioxidant to intercept free radicals and/or O₂ radicals. (84) (s. tab. 3.25)

The precursory peak or **shunt bilirubin** (10−20%) is formed during the first three days of life from the breakdown of erythrocyte precursors in the bone marrow. A smaller proportion originates from haemoproteins in the liver. In increased erythropoiesis or in dyserythropoiesis, the proportion of precursory bilirubin is raised. • Albumin is bound to the sinusoidal surface of the cell membrane (by a specific receptor?), and detachment of bilirubin follows. Subsequently, nonspecific membrane glycoproteins mediate the active **bilirubin uptake** (even against a concentration gradient) into the liver cell. • **Binding of the bilirubin** to the Y protein (= ligandin, identical to glutathione-S transferase) is effected in the cytosol of the liver cell, preventing both movement of bilirubin from the cytosol into the cellular organelles and its diffusion back into the bloodstream. With a higher bilirubin concentration and a saturation of the Y protein, bilirubin is bound to the Z protein (= fatty acid-binding protein). It has a lower affinity with, but a larger capacity for bilirubin than ligandin. (5, 77)

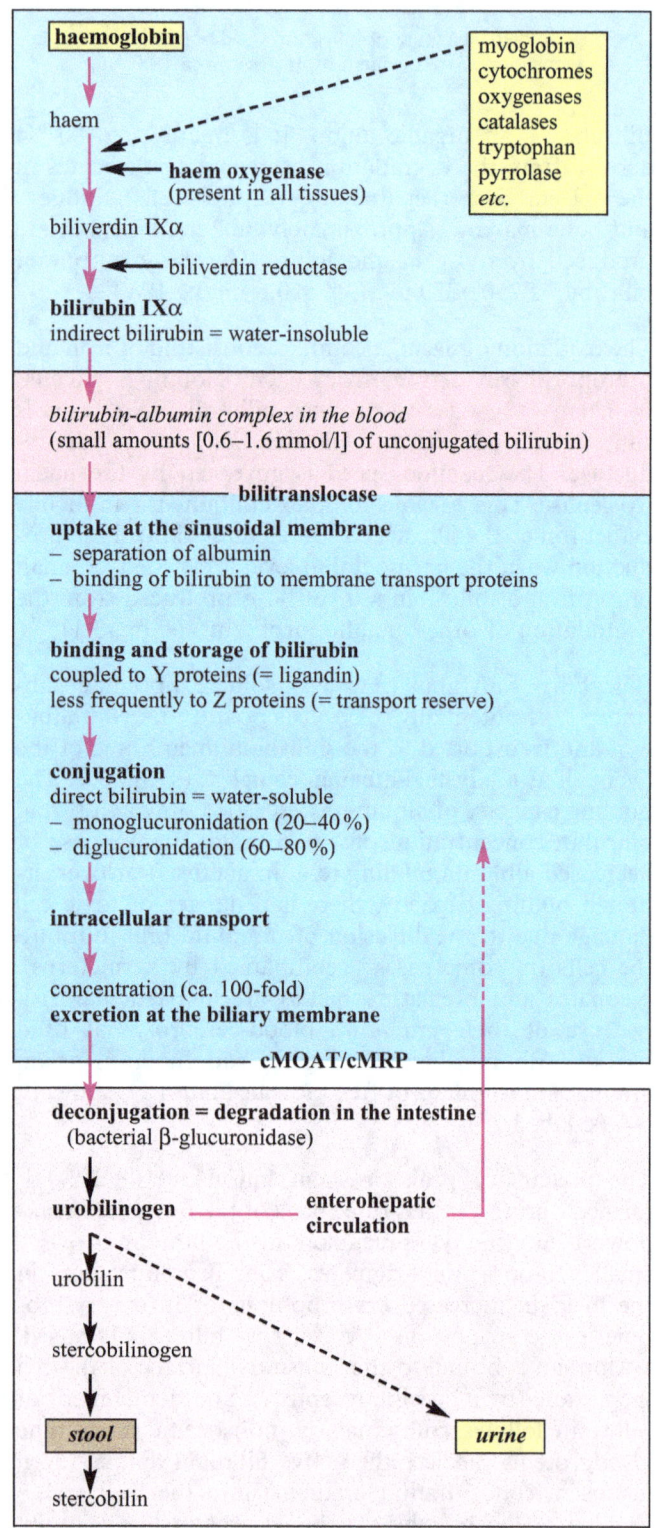

Fig. 3.1: Diagram showing bilirubin metabolism

The **conjugation** of bilirubin occurs in the SER, mediated by microsomal enzymes: bilirubin is esterified with glucuronic acid through the action of UDP-glucuronyltransferase (localized in the q 37 area of chromosome 2) to produce monoglucuronide. The subsequent diglucuronidation takes place in the RER. (s. fig. 3.1) The conjugation converts **indirectly reacting** (lipophilic, unconjugated, water-insoluble, primary) bilirubin to **directly reacting** (water-soluble, conjugated, secondary) bilirubin, which is consequently eliminated via the bile and urine. The conjugated form of bilirubin is normally present in the blood in 3−10% of the total serum bilirubin. A small amount of bilirubin is covalently bound to protein, a proportion of which reaches the serum as **δ-bilirubin** (half-life in serum is 14 days). • The *intracellular transport* of bilirubin is effected via the microtubules of the Golgi apparatus and also by means of passive diffusion processes in the cytosol.

Active **excretion** occurs in the canaliculi at the canalicular membrane, albeit independently of bile acids, by means of nonspecific transport proteins (mainly by MOAT), but is independent of bile acids; during this process bilirubin is found in 100-fold concentrations. Various substances compete with the bilirubin excretory process for this nonspecific carrier system. Bilirubin is transported together with cholesterol, bile acids and phospholipids in mixed micelles or vesicles. Bilirubin diglucuronide is discharged into the intestine together with the bile. Absorption is neither possible from the gall bladder nor from the intestine; in general, no enterohepatic reabsorption of bilirubin takes place. The glucuronic acid moieties are released by the action of β-glucuronidase from enteric bacteria, and bilirubin is converted into colourless, stereoisomeric **urobilinogen** by bacterial reductases. Oxidation of urobilinogen gives rise to **urobilin** and **stercobilin,** which, together with their degradation products, are responsible for the brown colour of the stools. A portion of the urobilinogen (ca. 1%) is reabsorbed, transported through the portal vein back to the liver and re-excreted via the bile (= *enterohepatic circulation*). A small proportion of the urobilinogen in the blood is eliminated from the body in the urine (1.0−3.5 mg/day; 1.7−5.9 μmol/day). Some 70−470 μmol (40−280 mg) stercobilin are excreted in the stools daily. (s. fig. 3.1) *(see chapter 5.6.1; 12)*

4 Porphyrin metabolism of the liver

Porphyrins represent the prosthetic groups of haemoproteins (haemoglobin, myoglobin, cytochromes, oxygenases, catalases, peroxidases, etc.). The chemical parent compound of the porphyrins is the tetranuclear pyrrolic dye, porphin. • The capacity for **haem synthesis** is common to almost all cells, but is especially important in the erythrocyte precursors for the synthesis of haemoglobin and in the hepatocytes for the synthesis of hepatic haemoproteins. Haem synthesis mainly takes place in the bone marrow (80–85%) and in the liver (ca. 15%). Two-thirds of the haem synthesized in the liver are required for the formation of cytochrome P 450. Daily production of haem amounts to ca. 300 mg (0.7–1.6 µmol/kg BW), of which only 1% is excreted unused in the urine and stools. The action of oxygen gives rise to the strongly red-fluorescing (λ_{max} = 366 nm) porphyrins. (s. fig. 7.10) • Haem synthesis begins in the mitochondria, then progresses through a series of cytosolic reactions before being completed again in the mitochondria. (s. fig. 3.2) The porphyrinogens represent colourless intermediate products. Each step in this process is enzymatically controlled. • The **regulation** of haem synthesis is highly efficient, whereby 3 enzymes play key roles: (*1.*) δ-aminolaevulinic acid synthase, (*2.*) uroporphyrinogen synthase, and (*3.*) ferrochelatase. The most crucial enzyme is δ-aminolaevulinic acid synthase, whose activity is subject to negative feedback control by the end-product haem – i.e. haem controls its own rate of synthesis. Porphyrins are irreversible oxidation products. With the exception of protoporphyrin, they are not utilized for other purposes, but are excreted. Under pathological conditions, they are stored in cells. Some intermediate products are eliminated in the stool (e.g. protoporphyrin IX) and others in the urine (e.g. coproporphyrin III, uroporphyrin I). (s. tab. 3.3) • Important **inducers** of δ-aminolaevulinic acid synthase include: barbiturates, sulphonamides, oestrogens, androgens, alcohol and fasting. *(see chapter 31.15)*

	µmol/24-hour urine
δ-aminolaevulinic acid	1.9–49.0
porphobilinogen	0.5–7.5
	µmol/24-hour urine
uroporphyrin	4–30
coproporphyrin	20–120
tricicarboxyporphyrin	0–2
heptacarboxyporphyrin	0–4
	µmol/g stool
uroporphyrin	1–5
coproporphyrin	5–37
protoporphyrin	20–150

Tab. 3.3: Reference values of porphyrins and their precursors in urine and the stool for differential diagnosis of porphyria

5 Bile acid metabolism of the liver

5.1 Biosynthesis of bile acids

▶ The complete structure of the bile acids was elucidated by H. WIELAND in 1932.

The **primary bile acids** are formed in the hepatocytes as liver-specific degradation products of cholesterol due to the action of microsomal, peroxisomal and mitochondrial enzymes; they are linked to cytosolic proteins. The initial enzyme in the biosynthesis, **cholesterol-7α-hydroxylase**, is also the rate-determining one. This enzyme, a cytochrome P 450 mixed-function oxidase, is localized in the SER. Its enzymatic activity is regulated by a *negative feedback* mechanism, in which bile acids re-enter the liver after passage through the enterohepatic circulation. After a possible second hydroxylation, the enzymatic removal of side chains as well as the introduction of a carboxylic group take place in the mitochondria. (s. fig. 3.3) • Two primary bile acids are thus synthesized. Twice as much cholic acid (1 mmol) as chenodeoxycholic acid is produced (1 mmol corresponds to 0.4 g free bile acid). The two bile acids represent 60–90% of the total bile acid production:

1. **Cholic acid** (ca. 40%)
   (3α-,7α-,12α-trihydroxy-5β-cholanic acid)
2. **Chenodeoxycholic acid** (ca. 40%)
   (3α-,7α-dihydroxy-5β-cholanic acid)

Biosynthesis of the two primary bile acids is followed by conjugation of their carboxylic group with the amino group of either glycine or taurine, mediated by a cytoplasmic enzyme. By means of this conjugation, the primary bile acids, which initially are barely water-soluble, become anions and are thus rendered hydrophilic. In this way **four conjugated bile acids** are formed:

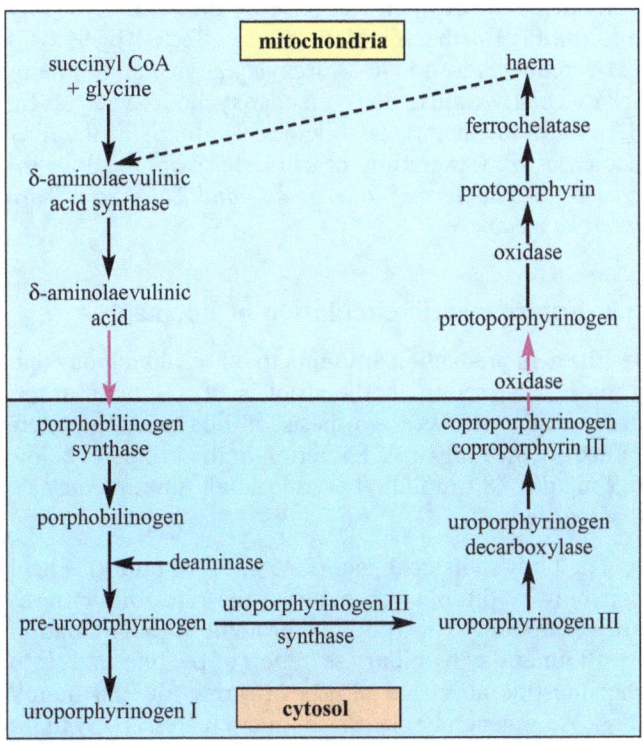

Fig. 3.2: Diagram showing porphyrin metabolism with haem synthesis in the liver (0.7–1.4 µmol/kg body weight per day = ca. 10–20% of total haem synthesis) (s. tab. 3.3)

1. Glycocholic acid	24%
2. Taurocholic acid	12%
3. Glycochenodeoxycholic acid	24%
4. Taurochenodeoxycholic acid	12%
= ca. 72% conjugated primary bile acids	

1. Glycodeoxycholic acid	16%
2. Taurodeoxycholic acid	8%
3. Glycolithocholic acid	0.7%
4. Taurolithocholic acid	0.3%
= ca. 25% conjugated secondary bile acids	

▶ The **secondary bile acids** result from the activity of anaerobic intestinal microorganisms in the ileum, caecum and colon. (s. fig. 3.3) • *Deconjugation*, with the subsequent release of free bile acids, is a prerequisite for these reactions. This is followed by 7α-dehydroxylation of cholic acid and chenodeoxycholic acid to yield deoxycholic acid and lithocholic acid, respectively. 7α-dehydrogenation and oxidation of chenodeoxycholic acid also yield ketolithocholic acid:

1. **Deoxycholic acid**
   (3α-,12α-dihydroxy-5β-cholanic acid)

2. **Lithocholic acid**
   (3α-hydroxy-5β-cholanic acid)

3. **Ketolithocholic acid**
   (3α-hydroxy-7keto-5β-cholanic acid)

▶ The **tertiary bile acids** are formed in the liver as well as in the gut. (s. fig. 3.3) • Intestinally absorbed lithocholic acid is enzymatically converted to sulpholithocholic acid in the liver. Ketolithocholic acid is transformed to (hypercholeretic) ursodeoxycholic acid in both the intestine and the liver. When passing through the canaliculi, UDC is partly reabsorbed by epithelial cells and returned to the liver via the blood circulation (= *cholehepatic shunt*). (37) The latter is chemically and structurally identical to chenodeoxycholic acid, of which it is deemed to be the 7β-epimer:

1. **Sulpholithocholic acid**
   (3-sulphohydroxy-5β-cholanic acid)

2. **Ursodeoxycholic acid** (2–5%)
   (3α-,7β-dihydroxy-5β-cholanic acid)

The bile acids may be further modified by **enzymatic reactions.** The enzymes involved have been found in the liver, intestine and kidney. By their action, conjugated and unconjugated primary or secondary bile acids may become bound to sulphuric acid, glucuronic acid or glucose. A further improvement in water-solubility can be obtained by **sulphation** or **glucuronidation**.

Regulation of the biosynthesis of bile acids is predominantly achieved through feedback by the respective daily loss quota. Further regulations are effected by HMG-CoA reductase and 7α-hydroxylase, which are themselves chiefly adjusted by ursodeoxycholic acid. (s. fig 3.3) With advancing age, bile acid synthesis in the liver decreases and excretion of cholesterol in the bile increases. • *The terms "bile acids" and "bile salts" are interchangeable.*

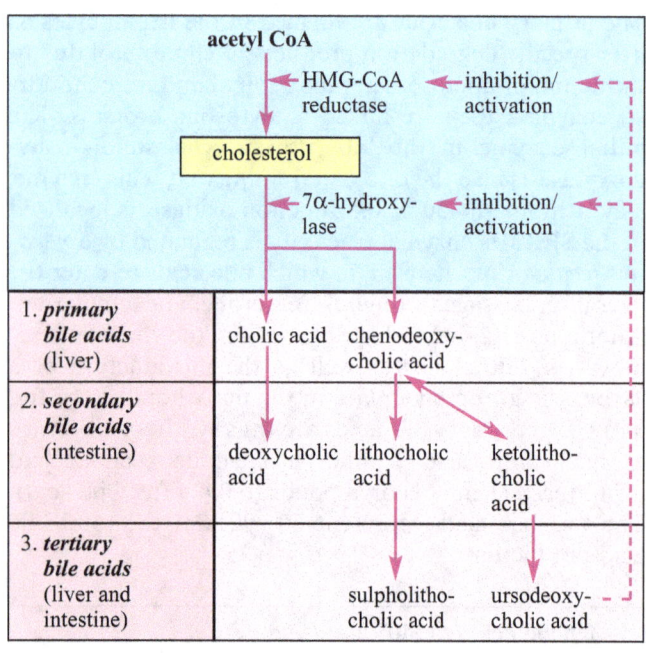

Fig. 3.3: Biosynthesis of primary, secondary and tertiary bile acids

5.2 Enterohepatic circulation of bile acids

▶ **Bile acid production** amounts to 400–500 mg/day (ca. 1 mmol). Excretion in the stool is of a similar order; accordingly, renewed synthesis of bile acids is determined by the daily loss. Excretion in the urine lies below 0.5 mg/day (8 μmol/day) – this small amount may be disregarded.

▶ The body's **bile acid pool** (2–5 g, 5–10 mmol) is held constant by the balance between the rates of synthesis and excretion. This pool is brought into circulation 3–10 times/day by biliary secretion of the bile acids into the intestine at a rate of 12–24 g/day (30–60 mmol/day). As a general rule, the pool circulates 2(–3) times per meal. Approximately 95% of the intestinal bile acids are reabsorbed. The hourly uptake of bile acids by the liver is in the order of 450 μmol (180 mg).

The secondary bile acids become partially (30–50%) absorbed in the intestine and, following reconjugation with glycine or taurine in the liver, are excreted into the canaliculi. The bile thus contains a mixture of primary and secondary bile acids. Deoxycholic acid as a secondary bile acid is likewise an "end-product"; it enters the enterohepatic circulation without further modification. • Conjugation of the secondary bile acids in the liver yields the following **four conjugated bile acids:**

Circulation of the bile acids is guaranteed by several **metabolic pump systems** in such a way that they are also transported against a concentration gradient. (1, 10, 15, 19, 28, 33, 45, 51, 54, 64, 74, 83, 86)

(1.) **Bile acid uptake** at the *sinusoidal membrane surface* is achieved actively by several Na^+-dependent (NTCP) as well as Na^+-independent (OATP) carrier proteins and passively by facilitated "biological" diffusion or free "physical" diffusion processes.
(2.) **Bile acid release** occurs at the *biliary membrane surface* in the canaliculi either actively, facilitated by ATP-driven carrier glycoproteins such as MRP2 (also called cMRP or MOAT) and BSEP (identical to cBAT), or by exocytosis of intracellularly derived mixed vesicles, or with the help of a potential-dependent membrane carrier.
(3.) **Bile acid uptake** at the *mucosal surface* of the enterocytes proceeds actively either through Na^+-dependent carrier systems in the ileum or by free diffusion in the ileum and colon.

▶ The gall bladder and upper small intestine serve as **mechanical stores** with the ability to drive the circulation of the bile pool by peristaltic action. • The bile acids become bound chiefly to albumin or HDL for **transport in the blood**. Incorporation into HDL is effected by apolipoproteins A_1 and A_2. • **Uptake into the hepatocytes** is mediated by a membrane-specific transport system, which comprises polypeptides and glycoproteins with strong affinities for bile acids. This influx process is predominantly an active transport mechanism against an electrochemical gradient. Energy is supplied by Na^+/K^+-ATPase. • **Intracellular transport** of bile acids to the biliary pole of the hepatocytes follows after their binding to cytosolic proteins: "free" bile acids would be damaging to subcellular structures because of their amphiphilic nature and detergent activity. As in the case of bilirubin, vesicles of the endoplasmic reticulum and of the Golgi apparatus as well as of the cytoskeleton are involved in transcellular transport.

All bile acid transport systems possess a high **reserve capacity,** the potential of which greatly exceeds the normal maximum secretion level. Bile acid cross-over from the enterohepatic into the peripheral circulation arises only in the case of massive disturbances in secretion (e. g. in cholestasis). The approx. 1% proportion of bile acids present in the peripheral system remains constant, both pre- and post-prandially. The first-pass elimination of bile acids from the portal blood reaches 70–90%, depending on their type and conjugation status. The bile acids have a half-life of two to three days.

5.3 Functions of bile acids

The essential **functions of bile acids** are found in cholesterol metabolism, digestion and resorption of fats in the intestine, and regulation of bile flow. (s. tab. 3.4)

Conjugated bile acids have amphiphilic properties in that all their hydrophilic groups lie on one side of the molecule and their hydrophobic (lipophilic) groups on the opposite side. This explains their capacity for **micelle formation.** Owing to their internally orientated hydrophobic groups, such bile acid micelles are able to take up water-insoluble compounds (cholesterol, triglycerides, fat-soluble vitamins, etc.) and then keep them in "solution" in the aqueous milieu by means of their outwardly orientated hydrophilic groups. On attaining a critical size, the disk shape of the micelle is transformed into a bubble-like structure (= vesicle, liposome). The micelle may also serve as an excretory mechanism for heavy metals such as copper and mercury.

1. **Cholesterol metabolism**
    a. reduction in excess cholesterol
        - through degradation of cholesterol to bile acids
        - by solubilization of cholesterol in the bile
    b. regulation of cholesterol synthesis in the liver and intestine
    c. regulation of cholesterol output into the bile
        - 3α-,7α-bile acids inhibit secretion
        - 3α-,12α-bile acids increase secretion
2. **Digestion and resorption of dietary fats**
    a. by formation of micelles
    b. by stabilization and activation of enzymes (e. g. pancreatic lipase, phospholipase A_2, pancreatic cholesterol esterase)
3. **Effects on the bile flow due to osmotic water movement**
4. **Effects on bile secretion**
    a. monohydroxy bile acids function cholestatically
    b. dihydroxy and trihydroxy bile acids have a choleretical effect
5. **Emulsification of fat-soluble vitamins**
6. **Stimulation of intestinal motility**

Tab. 3.4: Functions of bile acids

5.4 Composition and secretion of bile

Primary bile, already containing various compounds (= solutes) collected during transcellular transport, is formed by osmotic filtration at the canalicular membrane of the hepatocytes. It is yellow to orange in colour. Paracellular incorporation of further solutes into the bile occurs via the intercellular gap and the tight junctions. The **canalicular bile flow** comprises two fractions:

(1.) The **bile acid-dependent fraction** (250 ml) is formed chiefly in the periportal acinus. (s. tab 3.2) There is a linear relationship between bile acid excretion and bile flow. Osmotic filtration of water and inorganic ions is proportionally elevated (dependent upon bile salt concentration). Other secretory mechanisms or pump systems may also be activated by bile acids.

(2.) The **bile acid-independent fraction** (200 ml) is to be found in the absence or near absence of bile acids. This fraction is formed chiefly in the perivenous acinus. (s. tab. 3.2) However, Na^+/K^+-ATPase, glutathione and an active bicarbonate transporter also play an important role. Likewise, the prostaglandins A_1, E and E_2 stimulate the production of this fraction.

The bile acid uptake capacity at the sinusoidal membrane is 8–10 times higher than the secretion rate at the canalicular membrane. Approximately 450 ml **canalicular bile** are formed daily, each fraction constituting half of this total. Secretion of bile into the canaliculi is further assisted by microfilaments. In the case of loss of microfilament function, the canaliculi become broadened and immobile, thereby also inhibiting the bile flow.

This volume of secretion is supplemented in the ductules by ca. 150 ml **ductular bile,** resulting in a daily production of ca. 600 ml. Bile formation is lower at night than during the day. The most important constituents of *liver bile* are the bile acids, phospholipids, proteins, cholesterol and bilirubin. The term **bile lipids** includes cholesterol, bile salts and phospholipids. How cholesterol is excreted into the gall bladder is not yet known, nor have any cholesterol-specific transport systems been detected. Cholesterol is primarily broken down into bile acids. (see above) (s. tab. 3.5)

Bile acids (bile salts) (3–45 mM)			67%
Phospholipids (150–800 mg/dl)			22%
Protein, IgA, IgM, glutathione			5%
Cholesterol (80–200 mg/dl)			4%
Bilirubin (1–2 mM)			0.3%
Electrolytes (Na^+, K^+, Ca^{++}, HCO_3^-)			
Water	90–95%	pH	6.2–8.5
Solutes	5–10%	Spec. gravity	0.995–1.008

Tab. 3.5: Composition of ductular bile (so-called liver bile)

6 Amino acid and protein metabolism of the liver

The body contains approx. 14,000 g protein in total. There is a turnover of 600–700 g/day of the amino acid pool. The musculature has the highest rate of protein synthesis. The protein synthesized here is retained for exclusive use in the muscles. In relation to its weight, the liver generates more protein than the musculature: the synthesis rate amounts to 120 g/day, whereby 70–80% of these proteins are released by the hepatocytes, so that only 20–30% remain available for their own use. Plasma protein turnover is 25 g/day, that of the total tissue protein approx. 150 g/day. Amino acid turnover and protein synthesis proceed rapidly and continuously.

6.1 Biochemistry of amino acids

Human protein metabolism is essentially dependent on 20 amino acids. These amino acids lend themselves to various **classification criteria,** which also give hints regarding their *biochemical functions*:

1. according to their **metabolic characteristics** into ketogenic and glucogenic amino acids;
2. according to their **chemical structure** into α-, β- and γ-amino acids;
3. according to their **configuration** into D- and L-amino acids;
4. according to their **isoelectric point** into neutral, acidic and basic amino acids as well as amphoteric amino acids;
5. according to the **polarity** of their side chains into polar amino acids (with neutral + hydrophilic side chains) and nonpolar amino acids (with neutral + hydrophobic side chains) as well as those carrying basic + hydrophilic side groups (e.g. aspartate, glutamate) or those carrying basic + hydrophobic side groups (e.g. arginine, histidine, lysine);
6. according to their **biosynthesis** in the human organism into 8 essential, 10 non-essential and 2 semi-essential amino acids.

Essential amino acids are indispensable in that the body is incapable of replacing them simply by using its own synthesizing facilities: they must either be supplied in adequate quantities from outside or generated by degradation of body proteins. • **Non-essential amino acids** are synthesized in the liver, muscles, kidneys and intestine. Only the synthesis of arginine from ornithine and the hydroxylation of phenylalanine to tyrosine are liver-specific reactions.

The division between **branched-chain amino acids** (isoleucine, leucine, valine) and the group of **aromatic amino acids** (methionine, phenylalanine, tryptophan, tyrosine) is of clinical relevance. (s. tab. 3.6) (s. fig. 3.4)

The **amino acid pool** (600–700 g) is distributed among the musculature (80%), the liver (15%) and the plasma (5%). The proportion of free amino acids merely amounts to about 0.5% of the total amino acids contained in the body proteins. Of this amount, 300–500 g are used daily for protein synthesis, and approx. 2 g are used for the synthesis of other N-containing compounds (e.g. purines, porphyrins, pyrimidines); a further 120–130 g are degraded per day. • This daily amino acid consumption is replaced from *three sources*, so that the amino acid pool is maintained at a constant level: (*1.*) 70–100 g should be contained in the diet, (*2.*) 300–500 g derive from protein degradation, and (*3.*) 30–40 g are replenished from the biosynthesis of non-essential amino acids. The essential amino acids released by proteolysis are utilized as rapidly and completely as possible in the neosynthesis of proteins (= *recycling of essential amino acids*).

The **degradation** of essential amino acids proceeds primarily in the liver – only the three branched-chain amino acids (isoleucine, leucine, valine) are broken down in the muscles. Non-essential amino acids are degraded in the liver and muscles (but also in other organs). This is effected by transamination and oxidative deamination. (16) • The *C-skeleton,* an intermediate product in amino acid degradation, is used for energy production in the citric acid cycle. *Ketoplastic amino acids* serve to produce energy while *glucoplastic amino acids* guarantee gluconeogenesis. (s. fig. 3.4)

The **amino group** is excreted to a minor extent as ammonia. Because of its toxicity, ammonia must be rapidly converted into a nontoxic derivative. This is achieved by the binding of ammonia either to α-ketoglutarate or to a PO_4 ion to produce glutamate or carbamylphosphate, respectively. Both compounds are subsequently channelled into the urea cycle. A third alternative metabolic pathway is the coupling of ammonia to glutamate to yield glutaminic acid, which is then eliminated in the urine. The *"temporary ammonia detoxification"* takes place in both the liver and the musculature as well as in other organs. The *"definitive ammonia detoxification"* is, however, a liver-specific reaction in the urea cycle. (s. p. 61)

Biochemistry and Functions of the Liver

Amino acids	essential AA	semi-essential AA	non-essential AA	BCAA	AAA	polar AA	ketogenic AA	glucogenic AA
Alanine			+			+		+
Arginine		+						+
Asparagine			+			+		
Aspartate			+					+
Cysteine			+			+		+
Glutamine			+			+		
Glutamate			+					+
Glycine			+			+		+
Histidine		+						+
Isoleucine	+			+		+	+	
Leucine	+			+		+	+	
Lysine	+							
Methionine	+				+	+		
Phenylalanine	+				+	+	+	
Proline			+			+		+
Serine			+			+		+
Threonine	+					+		
Tryptophan	+				+	+		
Tyrosine			+		+	+	+	
Valine	+			+		+		+

Tab. 3.6: Classification of the 20 important (essential and non-essential) amino acids (AA = amino acid; BCAA = branched-chain amino acid; AAA = aromatic amino acid)

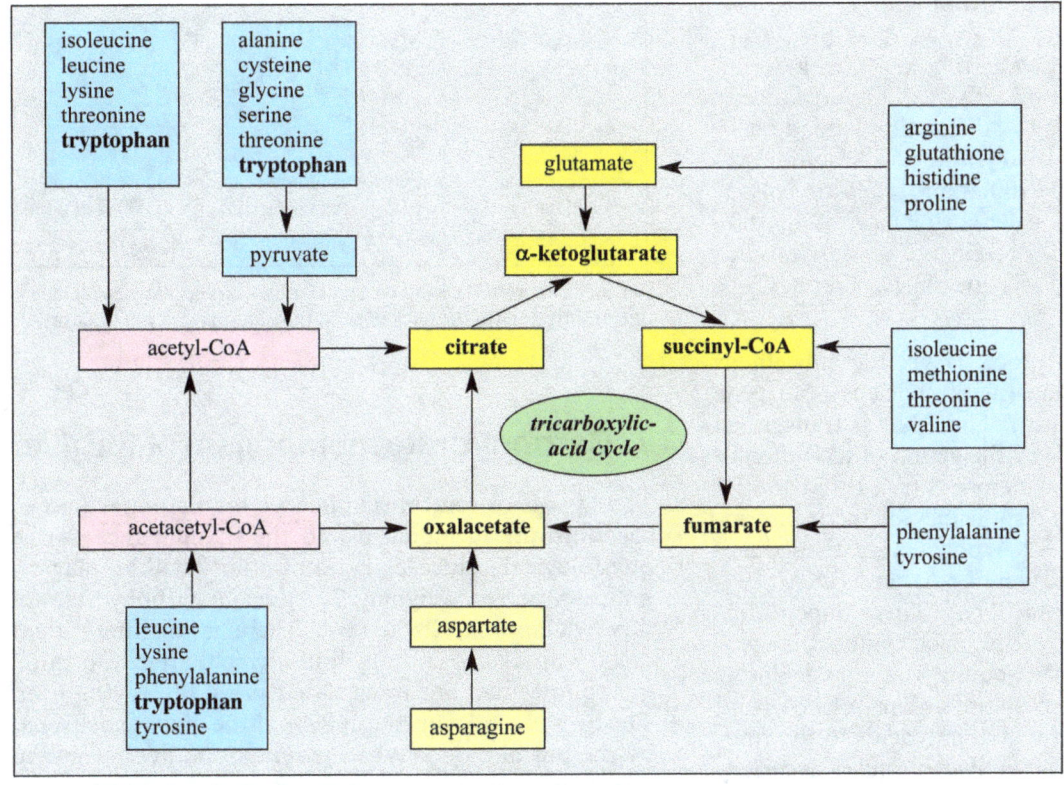

Fig. 3.4: Transfer of carbon skeletons from the amino acids into the tricarboxylic-acid cycle via intermediates (G. Rehner, H. Daniel, 1999)

▶ Dietary protein deficiency, especially a lack of essential amino acids, has a long-term effect on regulatory mechanisms. **Tryptophan** plays a significant role here. A deficiency of tryptophan leads to decreased protein synthesis, which is reversible solely by dietary supplementation of tryptophan even during inanition. The tryptophan effect occurs rapidly following the stimulation of nuclear RNA synthesis. (80) (s. fig. 3.4)

The **glucose-alanine cycle** between the liver and the musculature is particularly significant. In muscle tissue, ammonia is generated during the degradation of amino acids (particularly the branched-chain amino acids). The transfer of ammonia to pyruvate yields alanine, which is then transported through the bloodstream to the liver. Here, the C-skeleton of alanine is liberated for use in glucose synthesis via pyruvate, while the amino-N of alanine is incorporated as ammonia into the urea cycle. Glucose is released from the liver back to the muscle tissue. Up to 60–70% of the alanine released from the muscles are derived from glucose.

The **regulation** of amino acid metabolism is achieved by feedback mechanisms. The varying concentrations of amino acids in the portal blood are balanced in the liver, whereby there is a negative feedback in relation to the amino acid output of the intestine. The degradation and synthesis of amino acids (and consequently also of proteins) are kept constant. A circadian rhythm operates in this instance. Only the branched-chain amino acids pass through the liver unmetabolized, irrespective of their concentration in the portal blood. • The synthesis of amino acids and proteins is regulated by various *hormones*: glucagon inhibits protein synthesis, while stimulation is effected by insulin, somatotrophin, TSH and glucocorticoids. Besides metabolites and hormones, vitamins (B1, B2, B6, biotin, ascorbic acid) also regulate the metabolism of amino acids.

6.2 Protein synthesis and catabolism

The word "protein" (derived from the Greek term "proteuo" = "I take first place") was first introduced by J.J. BERZELIUS in 1838. • A distinction is made between globular and fibrillar proteins. Amino acid chains with a length of 2–100 amino acids are called peptides, and those with a length of more than 100 amino acids are called proteins. The derivatives, which result from proteolysis, are called peptones.

Hepatic **protein synthesis** proceeds via the subcellular stages of gene transcription (in the nucleus) and gene translation (in the cytoplasm). The DNA is transcribed into various types of RNA by the action of the different DNA-dependent RNA polymerases I (A), II (B) and III (C). RNA polymerase I is responsible for the transcription of ribosomal RNA, RNA polymerase II mediates the transcription of messenger RNA, and RNA polymerase III forms transcriptal RNA. These three different RNA types move out of the nucleus into the cytoplasm. Here the **ribosomes** acquire the genetic information needed for protein synthesis via mRNA, and tRNA transports the activated amino acids to the ribosomes, which are themselves activated (and if necessary replicated) by rRNA. (s. figs. 2.9, 2.17; 3.5)

Proteins destined for secretion from the liver cell collect as "bound polysomes" on the endoplasmic reticulum, which is thus recognizable as *rough endoplasmic reticulum* (RER). From here the proteins are transported to the Golgi apparatus, where they are either stored or "processed", but are also available for secretion. Protein synthesis in the hepatocytes is also controlled by colloid osmotic pressure.

More than 100 plasma proteins are synthesized in the liver cell, the majority being **glycoproteins.** About 15 of the glycoproteins (including C-reactive protein, fibronectin, α_2-macroglobulin) belong to the *acute-phase-reaction* group. • Numerous **transport proteins,** including prealbumin (= transthyretin), albumin (66), ceruloplasmin, haemopexin, haptoglobin, retinol-binding globulin, thyroxine-binding globulin, transcobalamin, transcortin and transferrin are synthesized in the liver.

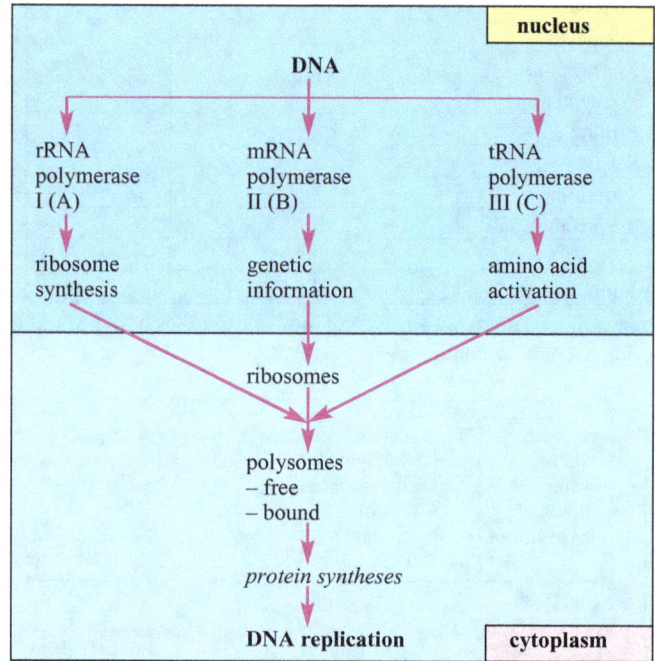

Fig. 3.5: Diagram showing protein synthesis in the liver cell by means of transcription (in the nucleus) and translation (in the cytoplasm)

7 Carbohydrate metabolism of the liver

The liver is of central significance for the regulation of carbohydrate metabolism and the maintenance of the physiological glucose concentration within narrow limits. A person weighing 70 kg has a carbohydrate reserve of approx. 2,500 kcal. There is an intermittent dietary uptake of carbohydrates which, after resorption in the intestine, are transported primarily to the liver. The liver can take up about 87% of the glucose delivered by the portal blood. When required, the liver is able to release glucose from its stored carbohydrate reserves to compensate for any deficiency and maintain the normal blood sugar value. The adjustment of blood sugar concentration, which is responsible for all intermediary metabolic processes, is regulated by the interplay between insulin and its antagonists, such as glucagon and adrenalin. Thyroxine, glucocorticoids and STH are also involved in this regulatory system. (s. fig. 3.6)

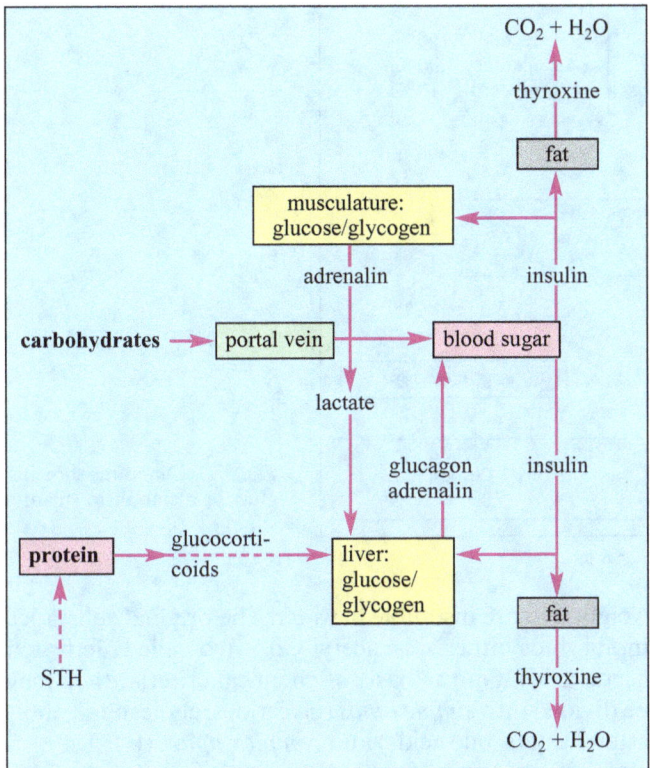

Fig. 3.6: Regulation of carbohydrate metabolism in the liver and musculature as well as its relationship to protein and fat metabolism

Moreover, the liver fulfils functions in the pentose-phosphate cycle as well as in the metabolism of galactose, fructose and sorbitol. • Thus the liver contributes in four different ways to the maintenance of **glucose homoeostasis** within the context of carbohydrate metabolism: (*1.*) glycogenesis, (*2.*) glycogenolysis, (*3.*) gluconeogenesis, and (*4.*) glucolysis. • *The liver therefore functions as a glucostate* (K. JUNGERMANN, 1986).

7.1 Glycogenesis and glycogenolysis

The postprandial glycogen content of the liver is 65–80 g/kg liver wet weight (= 5–8% of total liver weight). This reserve is sufficient to maintain glucose homoeostasis in the organism for up to 10 hours or, in conjunction with gluconeogenesis, up to 20 hours. In periods of fasting, the glycogen content sinks to 0.1%, but rises to >10% when a high-carbohydrate diet is consumed. Some 250–350 g glycogen are stored in the muscles, but this is solely for utilization by the muscle tissue. The total amount of glycogen in the body is 400–500 g. Glucose, fructose and galactose are available as initial basic substances. Fructose and galactose are converted to glucose in the liver and may then be channelled into glycogenesis. The metabolization of fructose is insulin-dependent, whereas that of galactose is insulin-independent.

▶ The **uptake** of glucose by the perivenous hepatocytes is effected in relation to its respective concentration and carried out by insulin-independent glucose transporter isoform (GLUT 2, and possibly GLUT 1). To little is known about the function of GLUT 1,

which is present in the perivenous scavenger cells. It is mainly found in centroacinar hepatocytes and has a high glucose affinity at low capacity. GLUT 4 can be found on adipocytes and skeletal muscle cells. • In the first instance, the liver allows most of the incoming glucose to pass through to the peripheral organs for utilization; it is only the returning 3-carbon moieties which are subsequently incorporated into glycogen (= **glucose paradox**) (J.D. MCGARRY et al., 1987). Glucose is converted by glucokinase to glucose-6 phosphate and glucose-1 phosphate. This leads to the synthesis of UDP glucose (= *activated glucose*), from which **glycogen** is formed. Once glycogen has reached saturation level, the remaining glucose is broken down into lactate. When lactate is transported via the blood stream, it is taken up together with alanine by the periportal hepatocytes, which are then able to form glycogen by means of gluconeogenesis.

▶ In **hypoglycaemia**, a protein phosphorylase is activated by glucagon and adrenalin via cyclic AMP. Glycogenesis is inhibited and **glycogenolysis** is stimulated: glycogen is converted by glycogen phosphorylase to glucose-1 phosphate, which is converted to glucose-6 phosphate. This leads to the release of **free glucose**. *Glucose-6 phosphate is therefore the key activator in glucose metabolism.*

7.2 Gluconeogenesis and glucolysis

The extracellular **glucose pool** is 110 mmol (= 20 g) in a volume of 28 litres, giving a concentration of 5 mmol/l. (s. fig. 3.7) • *Glucose* is able to cross the plasma membranes freely and enter the liver cells independently of insulin. It is capable of taking part in metabolism only after phosphorylation (by hexokinase or glucokinase). • Glucokinase activity is regulated according to the blood sugar level in the portal vein. The physiological glucose concentration is thus maintained within a range of 2.5 mmol/l (= 45 mg/dl) to 7.77 mmol/l (= 140 mg/dl). Glycogenolysis in the liver releases glucose at a rate of 26 mmol/hr in the resting state. This is supplemented by 13 mmol/hr from gluconeogenesis. These 39 mmol are released hourly into the extracellular glucose pool. The CNS receives 20 mmol/hr, i.e. more than twice as much as the muscles (9.4 mmol/hr) and the erythrocytes (8.3 mmol/hr). The glucose entering intermediary metabolism serves as an energy source, but is also incorporated into the pentose-phosphate cycle and glycogen synthesis. A total of 38 mmol/hr (6.8 g) glucose are consumed, and 39 mmol (= 7.0 g) are simultaneously liberated. Glucose, as glucose-6 phosphate, may be channelled into various metabolic pathways, e.g. into the pentose-phosphate cycle, into glycolysis with pyruvate and/or lactate as end-products, or into the citrate cycle with degradation into CO_2, H_2O and energy (ATP). Aerobic glycolysis produces 38 mol ATP.

Gluconeogenesis is activated when the glycogen reserves are exhausted. There are three alternative substrates available in the liver cells for glucose synthesis:

1. *Lactate* (60%)
   = from anaerobic glycolysis
2. *Amino acids*, mainly alanine (30%)
   = from proteolysis
3. *Glycerol* (10%)
   = from lipolysis in the fatty tissue

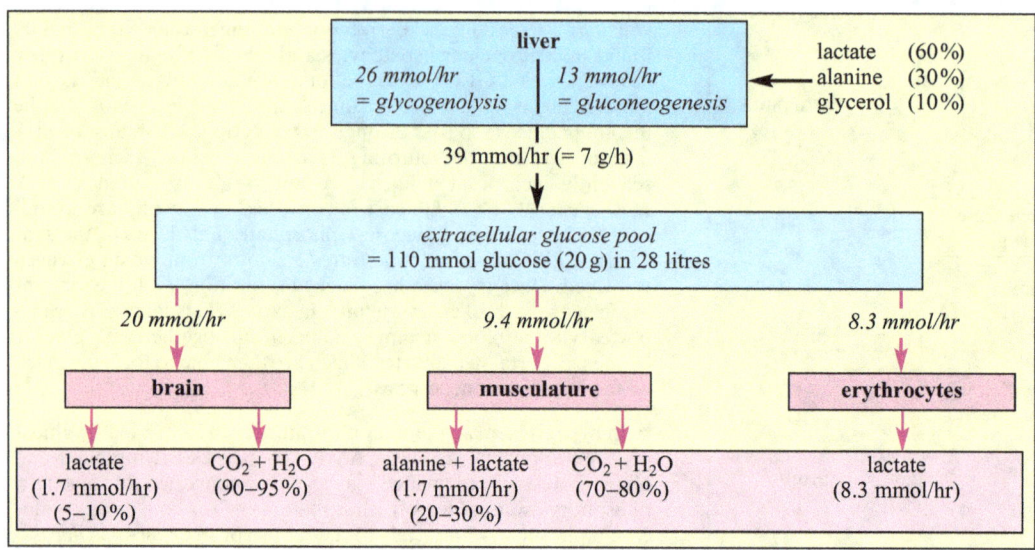

Fig. 3.7: Diagram showing glucose metabolism (fasting state)

Gluconeogenesis enables the liver to produce at least 240 g glucose per day. This amount can be used up by erythrocytes and the nervous system in two days of fasting. Most amino acids required for gluconeogenesis during fasting originate from the degradation of proteins in muscle tissue and visceral organs (including the liver). Fatty acids are no longer available for gluconeogenesis because the acetyl residues which are produced in their β-oxidation are completely metabolized in the citrate cycle. Gluconeogenesis is an energy-rich process which is increased in the short term by glucagon, adrenaline and acetyl-CoA or in the long term by glucocorticosteroids, but it is inhibited by insulin. The key enzymes of glycolysis are activated by insulin, and a catabolic metabolism is converted to an anabolic one. The hormone amyline, a peptide made up of 37 amino acids, is secreted by β-cells together with insulin. Although it raises glucose levels slightly, it considerably increases the lactate level, which is then used in gluconeogenesis. (71)

Ketogenesis is an important metabolic function in the liver. It is the result of an increase in lipolysis in the fatty tissue, with a rise in fatty acids. Insulin inhibits ketogenesis, whereas it is accelerated by fasting as well as by glucagons and insulin deficiency. Ketones (acetacetate, 3-hydroxybutyrate, acetone) are synthesized by means of β-oxidation from acetyl-CoA, assuming the production of this substance exceeds the amount required by the hepatocytes (and glucose metabolism is simultaneously reduced). The liver itself does not require any ketones: acetone is expired, whereas 3-hydroxybutyrate and acet-acetate serve as a source of energy. Ketonaemia can lead to metabolic acidosis and electrolyte shifts.

8 Lipid metabolism of the liver

Fats and fat-like compounds of varying chemical structures are classified as **lipids**. They have a low molecular weight and are insoluble in water. The original substance in fat biosynthesis is acetyl-CoA (so-called activated acetic acid). On the basis of chemical criteria, they may be divided into *simple lipids* (glycerides, cholesterol, cholesterol esters, bile acids) and *complex lipids*. (14)

The liver has a variety of **functions** in lipid metabolism: (*1.*) uptake, oxidation and transformation of free fatty acids, (*2.*) synthesis of plasma lipoproteins, (*3.*) transformation of lipoproteins, (*4.*) catabolization of LDL, VDL and chylomicron remnants, and (*5.*) secretion of enzymes for lipoprotein metabolism. (14) (s. tab. 3.7)

Simple lipids		
cholesterol esters	(ca. 225 mg/dl)	32.7%
free cholesterol	(ca. 65 mg/dl)	9.0%
triglycerides	(ca. 170 mg/dl)	24.0%
free fatty acids		1.0%
bile acids		0.3%
Complex lipids		
glycerophospholipids	(ca. 200 mg/dl)	29.0%
sphingolipids		4.0%

Tab. 3.7: Distribution of simple and complex lipids in the plasma

8.1 Classification of lipoproteins

Lipoproteins are macromolecules comprising proteins (= apolipoproteins, apoproteins) and lipids. They transport water-insoluble lipids in the blood, with the exception of the albumin-bound free fatty acids. Only short-chain fatty acids are dissolved in plasma. The lipoproteins are formed in the liver and in the mucosa of the small intestine. (13)

Lipoprotein **characteristics** depend on the varying proportions of protein and lipid present. Lipids are of lower density (<0.9 g/ml) than proteins (>1.28 g/ml), giving a range of lipoprotein densities from 0.9 to 1.21 g/ml. • Lipoprotein **classification** is made according to the respective densities as determined by ultracentrifugation or according to their electrophoretic migration.

Chylomicrons are synthesized from exogenously derived triglycerides with *long-chain fatty acids* (C_{16}–C_{20}) after their cleavage and re-esterification in the intestinal mucosa. The *medium-chain fatty acids* (C_{10}–C_{14}) and the *short-chain fatty acids* (C_4–C_8) are transported through the portal vein directly to the liver. Chylomicrons have a particle size of up to 1,000 nm and consist of 98% lipids and 0.5–2.5% proteins. Their density is <0.95 g/ml. The function of the chylomicrons is the transport of exogenous triglycerides in the lymph and blood. Their contents are released to the tissues via the capillaries (by the action of hepatic triglyceride lipase and lipoprotein lipase). They are taken up by the liver as cholesterol-rich "remnants" and degraded in the lysosomes. (s. fig. 3.8)

Very low density lipoproteins (VLDL) are synthesized in the liver cell at the contact area of the smooth and rough endoplasmic reticulum and, to a very minor degree, in the mucosa of the small intestine. They have a particle size of 30–80 nm and consist of 90% lipids and 8–13% proteins. Their density is <1.006 g/ml. The predominant apolipoproteins are B, C III, and E. They are designated as pre-beta lipoproteins on the basis of their electrophoretic migration. The main function of VLDL is the transport of triglycerides of endogenous origin. (s. fig. 3.8)

Low density lipoproteins (LDL$_2$) are formed from VLDL in the plasma (by the action of lipoprotein lipase) via *intermediate density lipoproteins* (LDL$_1$ or IDL). If no VLDL is secreted, there is no synthesis of LDL. Insulin and oestrogen increase VLDL secretion. They display a particle size of ca. 20 nm and consist of 75% lipids and 20–30% proteins. They have densities of <1.063 g/ml. The predominant apolipoproteins are A I and A II. According to their electrophoretic migration, they are classified as beta-lipoproteins. The function of LDL is the transport of cholesterol and cholesterol esters. Cell surface LDL receptors take up LDL-bound cholesterol (50–60%) according to cellular requirements. In the event of increased LDL availability, scavenger cells (e.g. macrophages) can also act to clear away cholesterol, independently of the LDL receptors. (s. fig. 3.8)

High density lipoproteins (HDL$_{2,3}$) are formed in the liver and small intestine. A minor proportion of the HDL appears to derive from triglyceride-rich lipoproteins in the plasma. HDL have a particle size of 5–15 nm and appear initially as disk-shaped bodies which, after uptake of lipids and lipoproteins, develop in the blood to spherically shaped molecules. They comprise ca. 50% lipids and 45–55% proteins. Their density is <1.21 g/ml. They are designated α_1-lipoproteins based on their electrophoretic migration. HDL transport cholesterol esters derived from the action of lecithin-cholesterol-acetyl transferase (LCAT). They are further differentiated into HDL$_{2a}$, HDL$_{2b}$ and HDL$_3$ on the basis of their varying densities and protein moiety. (14, 27) (s. fig. 3.8)

Fatty-acid synthesis is primarily carried out by means of acetyl-CoA cocarboxylase from acetyl-CoA in the cell plasma. In each case, the synthesized fatty acid can be extended by attaching acetyl residues (the opposite can be achieved using β-oxidation) (14). (s. fig. 3.9)

Lipogenesis, the synthesis of lipids from carbohydrate via acetyl-CoA, occurs almost exclusively in the liver cells and the fatty tissue. (s. fig. 3.9) • According to *lipid topogenesis* (4), the enzymes involved in triglyceride and phospholipid synthesis are localized on the cytoplasmic

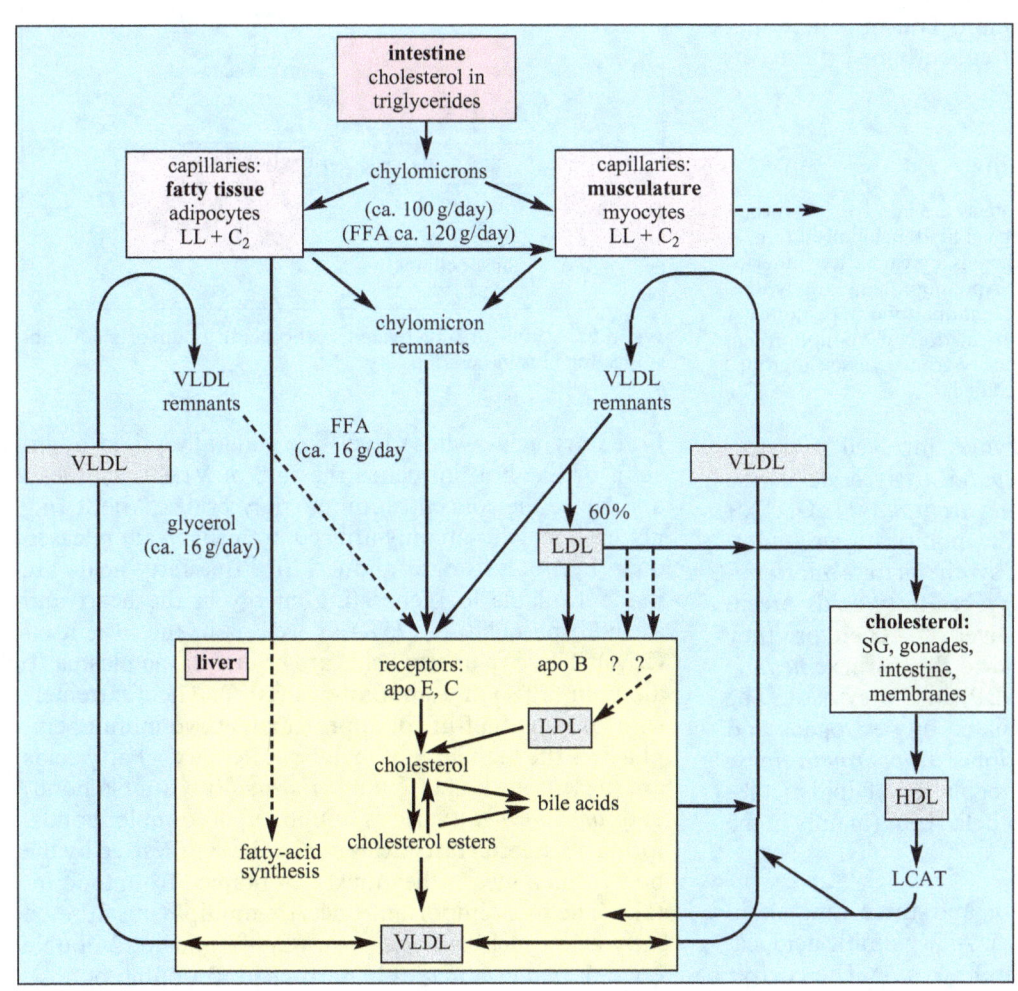

Fig. 3.8: Diagram showing the metabolic exchange of lipids between intestine, fatty tissue, musculature and liver (FFA = free fatty acids, LL = lipoprotein lipase, C_2 = apoprotein, SG = suprarenal gland)

surface of the endoplasmic reticulum. The level of hepatic synthesis is regulated primarily by the *insulin-glucagon quotient*, as described by R.H. UNGER in 1971.

▶ The mechanism of **oxidative energy generation** in the liver is mainly the result of *fatty-acid degeneration*. This process begins when the fatty acids are activated. It is followed by β-oxidation (= constant splitting of two carbon units until the carbon chain has been completely broken down) in the mitochondria. The acetyl-CoA which is produced can be channelled into the citrate cycle by means of oxaloacetation or used in other biosyntheses. Beta-oxidation of the fatty acids produces (apart from H_2O and CO_2) a total of 44 mol ATP from 1 mol of a C_6-fatty acid (by comparison, one molecule of glucose produces "only" 32 mol ATP). Another, albeit insignificant, means of fatty-acid degeneration is possible with the aid of α- or φ-oxidation. Peroxisomes are also involved in β-oxidation. The latter produces acetyl-CoA, which is subsequently oxidized to CO_2 in the citrate cycle. • *Amino acids* (e.g. alanine, isoleucine, leucine, serine) may provide a further source of energy via pyruvate or acetyl-CoA.

Energy can likewise be generated by means of *fructose* and *ethanol oxidation*. The partial pressure of oxygen falls from 13 % (centroacinar) to 6 % (perivenous) due to progressive oxygen consumption. Thus it is here that hypoxic cell damage can most frequently be expected.

8.2 Regulation of lipoproteins

▶ Up to now, 13 different **apolipoproteins** are known to be necessary for the maintenance of physiological lipid metabolism (e.g. A I-IV, B 100, C I-III, E). As a result, there is a great variety in terms of their biochemistry and function. Apolipoproteins are synthesized predominantly in the rough endoplasmic reticulum. A further form of classification and regulation of apolipoprotein types is possible according to four density groups, or seven groups if HDL_{2a}, HDL_{2b} and HDL_3 are included.

The liver synthesizes two enzymes involved in intraplasmic lipid metabolism: *hepatic triglyceride lipase* (HTL) and *lecithin-cholesterol-acyltransferase* (LCAT). • The liver is further involved in the modification of circulatory lipoproteins as the site of synthesis for *cholesterol-ester transfer protein* (CETP). • Free fatty acids are in general potentially toxic to the liver cell. Therefore they are immobilized by being bound to the intrinsic *hepatic fatty acid-binding protein* (hFABP) in the cytosol. The activity of this protein is stimulated by oestrogens and inhibited by testosterone. • Peripheral *lipoprotein lipase* (LPL), which is required for the regulation of lipid metabolism, is synthesized in the endothelial cells (mainly in the fatty tissue and musculature).

Triglycerides consist of glycerol and three long-chain fatty acids (ca. 45% oleic acid, ca. 26% palmitic acid, ca. 16% linolic acid). They contain 9.5 kcal/g. The correct biochemical term is triacylglycerol. The total fat content in a person of standard weight provides an energy reservoir of approx. 110,000 kcal. Triglycerides are synthesized from fatty acids and glycerol in lipocytes and hepatocytes. They carry no electrostatic charge and are thus designated *neutral fats*. The liver synthesizes approx. 57 mmol (= 50 g) triglycerides, which are released as VLDL bodies. There is normally no storage in the hepatocytes. VLDL triglycerides are transported to the white fatty tissue, where they are enzymatically split to allow storage of the resulting fatty acids as triglycerides in the adipocytes. Degradation of triglycerides stored in the fatty tissue is effected by means of lipase and hormone activity (catecholamines, ACTH, glucagon). (s. fig. 3.9)

Phospholipids are a heterogeneous group of lipids, consisting mainly of phosphatidylcholine (ca. 67%), sphingomyelin (ca. 21%), lysolecithin (ca. 7%) and phosphatidylethanolamine (ca. 4%). Each of these constituents has a separate fatty-acid composition. (14) (s. fig. 3.9)

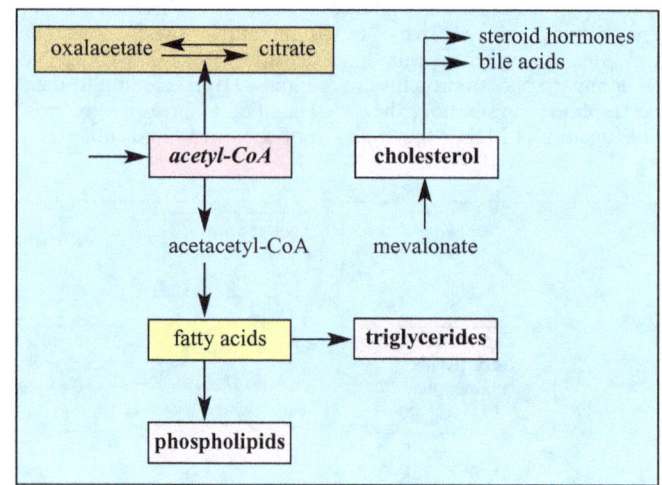

Fig. 3.9: Acetyl-CoA (activated acetic acid) as an original substance for biosynthesizing fats

Free fatty acids, whose levels are generally raised by insulin or alcohol, influence the rate of VLDL synthesis and hence the concentration of triglycerides. About 16 g glycerol, which is mainly utilized in the liver, are released daily by lipolysis, and about 120 g free fatty acids are made available for generating energy in the heart and skeletal musculature (75%) as well as in the liver itself (25%). These free fatty acids are bound in the plasma to albumin (50%) and lipoproteins (50%). Their extremely short plasma half-life of approximately two minutes emphasizes the high level of metabolic activity. • Fatty acids are present in the plasma in *saturated* (no double bond) and *unsaturated* (various numbers of double bonds) forms. • **Essential fatty acids** cannot be synthesized by the body, which means they must be obtained from food intake. The most important ones are multiple unsaturated fatty acids such as *linolic acid* (C_{18}-fatty acid, 2 double bonds), *linolenic acid* (C_{18}-fatty acid, 3 double bonds),

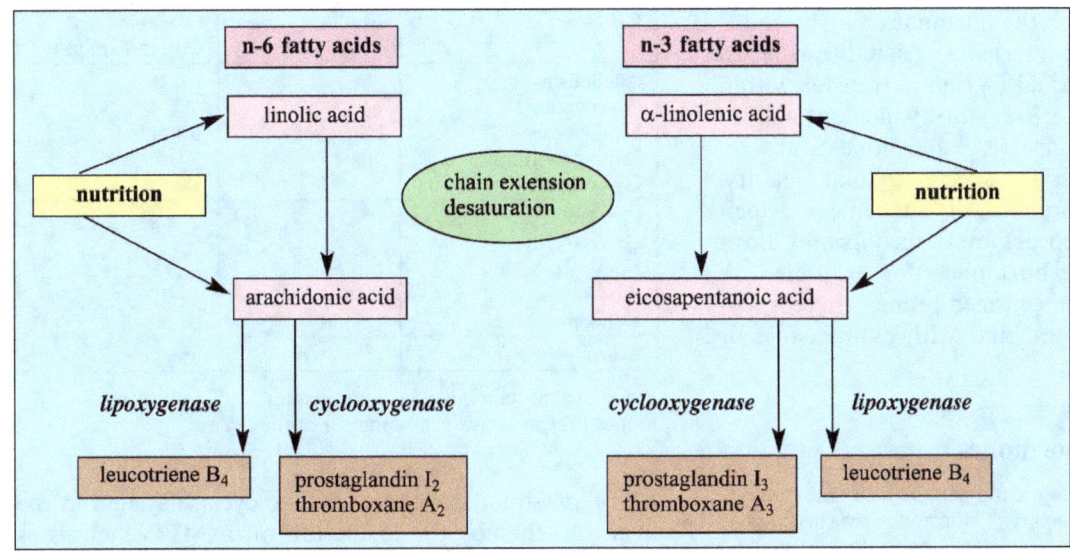

Fig. 3.10: Synthesis of eicosanoids (leucotriene B_4, B_5, prostaglandin I_2, I_3, and thromboxane A_2, A_3) from ω-3 and ω-6 fatty acids

and *arachidonic acid* (C_{20}-fatty acid, 4 double bonds). Their prime function is to act as precursors for the synthesis of eicosanoids. (s. fig. 3.10)

▶ Arachidonic acid is of particular importance, being the initial compound for **eicosanoid biosynthesis.** Prostaglandins, prostacyclins and thromboxanes are synthesized from the eicosanoids via the *cyclo-oxygenase pathway.* • The important mediators of inflammation – such as leukotrienes and leukotetraenes – are synthesized via the *lipoxygenase pathway.* (s. fig. 3.10)

8.3 Cholesterol metabolism

Cholesterol is formed in the liver (85%) and intestine (12%) – this constitutes 97% of the body's cholesterol synthesis of 3.2 mmol/day (= 1.25 g/day). Serum cholesterol is esterized to an extent of 70–80% with fatty acids (ca. 53% linolic acid, ca 23% oleic acid, ca 12% palmitic acid). The cholesterol pool (distributed in the liver, plasma and erythrocytes) is 5.16 mmol/day (= 2.0 g/day). Homocysteine stimulates the production of cholesterol in the liver cells as well as its subsequent secretion. Cholesterol may be removed from the pool by being channelled into the bile or, as VLDL and HDL particles, into the plasma. The key enzyme in the synthesis of cholesterol is *hydroxy-methyl-glutaryl-CoA reductase* (HGM-CoA reductase), which has a half-life of only three hours. Cholesterol is produced via the intermediate stages of mevalonate, squalene and lanosterol. • *Cholesterol esters* are formed in the plasma by the linking of a lecithin fatty acid to free cholesterol (by means of LCAT) with the simultaneous release of lysolecithin. (s. figs. 3.8, 3.9) (s. tab. 3.8)

▶ Endogenous consumption, degradation and elimination of cholesterol are kept in balance metabolically by dietary intake, endogenous synthesis and intestinal reabsorption. Cholesterol is an important substance for the structure and function of biomembranes. Moreover, it is the initial substrate for the biosynthesis of bile acids, vitamin D_3 and steroid hormones. (s. tab. 3.8)

Cholesterol supply/day	Cholesterol consumption/day

1. From the diet
    = 300–400 mg
	1. Incorporation into VLDL,
	    HDL = 1,000 mg

2. From endogenous synthesis
    – liver   1,000 mg
    – intestine   200 mg
    – tissue   50 mg
	2. Biochemical degradation
	    – bile acids 350 mg
	    – hormones 50 mg
	    – vitamin D_3 10 mg

3. From intestinal reabsorption
    = 300–500 mg
	3. Excretion
	    – intestine 500 mg
	    – skin 100 mg

Tab. 3.8: Cholesterol balance (supply/consumption per day) under normal conditions

9 Hormone metabolism and the liver

In minute amounts, **hormones** engender specific biochemical *"primary reactions"* through cellular metabolic processes, which subsequently trigger *"secondary reactions"* through physiological processes.

Hormone **synthesis** takes place in special cells or tissues either in the form of precursors with storage potential (= **prohormones**) or in the form of stored or continuously secreted substances in an active state (= **hormones**). Synthesis, release and activation of the hormones are under the strict control of a regulatory system, which itself responds according to a variety of endogenous and exogenous stimuli.

Inactivation of the hormones occurs mainly due to enzymes (in the kidney, plasma and target cell) and in the liver as a result of proteolytic or redox reactions. The liver contributes to the maintenance of **hormonal homoeostasis**. Liver diseases may thus affect the hormone regulation in different ways, giving rise to various and sometimes long-lasting disorders.

In the endocrine system the **signal substances** are called *hormones*, in the nervous system they are known as *neurotransmitters*, and in the immune system *cytokines*. •

Signals transferred through the hormones may be endocrinal, neuroendocrinal, paracrinal (= signal transfer to adjacent cells) and autocrinal (= signal transfer within the individual cell itself). • *Receptors*, which are able to *detect* and *bind* a substance (e.g. hormones), are required to transmit signals for special cellular activity, including that of hormones. All substances which specifically bind with receptors are termed *ligands*. Both glycoprotein and peptide hormones, for example, are bound to receptors on the cell membrane, whereas steroid and thyroid hormones bind with cytoplasmic or nuclear receptors.

9.1 Classification of hormones

Proteohormones, steroid hormones and peptide hormones are differentiated as per **chemical structure**. • Hormones are classified as *neurosecretory* (e.g. hypothalamus), *glandular* (endocrine glands) or *aglandular* according to **source tissue**. Aglandular hormones are also known as tissue hormones: they are synthesized in special cells located in specific organs. • Hormones can be differentiated according to **transport characteristics** into unbound hormones and hormones which are coupled to a carrier protein. • A further classification is based on **principal functions**. (s. tab. 3.9)

1. **Water-salt balance-regulating hormones**
   - renin, angiotensin, aldosterone, *etc.*
   - mineralocorticoids
   - atrial natriuretic peptides
   - vasopressin
2. **Effector hormones**
   - catecholamines (adrenalin, noradrenalin, dopamine)
   - insulin, glucagon
3. **Personality-differentiating hormones**
   - ACTH, STH, TSH, TRH, FSH, LH, PL, MSH
   - thyroxine (T_4), triiodothyronine (T_3)
   - androgens, oestrogens, gestagens, progesterones
   - glucocorticoids
4. **Calcium phosphate metabolism-regulating hormones**
   - parathormones, 1,25 dihydroxycholecalciferol, calcitonin
5. **Gastrointestinal hormones**
   - bombesin, cholecystokinin-pancreozymin, enterogastrones, gastrin, GIP, motilin, neurotensin, secretin, somatomedin, somatostatin, substance P, VIP

Tab. 3.9: Classification of hormones according to their principal biological functions

9.2 Effector hormones and the liver

The so-called effector hormones (insulin, glucagon, catecholamines) evoke an extremely fast response. Within a short time, a rapid and lasting redirection of the metabolism can be attained. Catecholamines are degraded in the liver and, following sulphation or glucuronidation, are eliminated as metabolites in either the bile or urine.

Insulin stimulates glucose uptake in both the musculature and the fatty tissue. Structural modification of STH, with a concomitant enhancement of its activity, is effected by insulin. The storage of amino acids in the muscles is also increased. (s. tab. 3.10)

Criteria	Insulin	Glucagon, Catecholamines
Anabolism Glycogenesis Lipogenesis Protein synthesis Glycolysis	Increased	Inhibited
Catabolism Glycogenolysis Lipolysis Proteolysis Ketogenesis	Inhibited	Increased
Gluconeogenesis	Inhibited	Increased

Tab. 3.10: Metabolic effects of insulin and contra-insulin hormones (glucagon, catecholamines) in the liver

Glucagon stimulates the adenylate cyclase system in the liver and thereby the formation of cAMP, which gives rise to important metabolic changes. (s. tab. 3.10) • Furthermore, there is a consequent decline in cholesterol synthesis, improvement in alanine membrane transport, activation of the enzymes of the urea cycle and stimulation of amino acid degradation.

9.3 Steroid hormones and the liver

Glucocorticoids, androgens, oestrogens and gestagens belong to the group of biologically active steroid hormones. The biogenesis of all steroid hormones involves the key compound cholesterol. (s. tab. 3.11)

Glucocorticoids
1. Increase in gluconeogenesis
2. Increase in protein synthesis
3. Regulation of amino acid metabolism
   - increase in amino acid degradation in muscle tissue
   - increase in amino acid uptake by the liver
4. Improved efficiency of urea synthesis
5. Inhibition of phagocytic activity of Kupffer cells

Androgens
1. Increase in haem synthesis
2. Stimulation of specific protein syntheses
3. Increased activity of cytochrome P 450
4. Decrease in hFABP

Oestrogens
1. Increase in hFABP
2. Increase in δ-aminolaevulinic acid with decrease in porphyrin decarboxylase
3. Increase in protein synthesis
4. Stimulation of phagocytic activity of Kupffer cells
5. Inhibition of cytochrome P 450 subtypes
6. Increase in lithogenicity of the bile
   - increase in cholesterol excretion
   - decrease in bile acid excretion
   - decrease in secretion of bile

Progesterone
1. Induction of haem synthesis
2. Limited stimulation of protein synthesis
3. Substrate-dependent (inhibitory or stimulatory) regulation of the cytochrome P 450 complex

Tab. 3.11: Significant effects of steroid hormones in the liver

Likewise, elimination of the steroid hormones occurs almost exclusively via the liver (after glucuronidation and sulphation) into the bile or urine. They are only excreted in a free form in minute amounts via the urine, intestine or skin. There are numerous important interactions between the liver and steroid hormones.

9.4 Thyroid hormones and the liver

Conversion of 70% of the total T_4 (thyroxine) to T_3 (3,5,3-triiodothyronine) occurs in the liver: 20% of the T_4 input are catabolized in the liver cells, and the remaining 10% follow various metabolic pathways. About 30% of the T_4 and 50% of the T_3 are stored in the hepatocytes due to binding to specific proteins. The more active hormone T_3 is involved in numerous metabolic reactions in the liver. (s. tab. 3.12)

1. Increase in protein synthesis
2. Increase in gluconeogenesis
3. Increase in ketogenesis
4. Increase in amino acid uptake
5. Regulation of bile acid metabolism
   - increase in bile acid synthesis
   - increase in biliary cholesterol excretion
   - increase in bile flow
6. Increased turnover of vitamin K-dependent clotting factors
7. Increase in size and number of mitochondria
8. Hypertrophy of the smooth endoplasmic reticulum

Tab. 3.12: Metabolic effects of T_3 in the liver

10 Vitamin metabolism and the liver

10.1 Classification of vitamins

Vitamins are vital (= *vita*) and mainly nitrogenous substances (= *amines*) of low-molecular weight. They must be present in the diet as "essential" components. A few vitamins (e. g. A, K, B_1, B_5, B_{12}, folic acid, biotin) are formed in the intestine by bacteria. Plants constitute the main source of exogenous vitamin supply. In a biochemical context, the principal biocatalytic effect of vitamins consists in substituting cofactors of enzymes which have undergone metabolic degradation.

Water-soluble vitamins are readily absorbed under physiological conditions. They are transported to the intra- and extracellular fluid and act as coenzymes in a number of enzyme reactions in protein, nucleinic acid and energy metabolism. They are readily excreted via the kidney. (s. tab. 3.13)

Fat-soluble vitamins require the simultaneous presence of lipids and bile acids for their absorption. In order to be transported to the liver, they are bound to lipoproteins of the chylomicrons. Fat-soluble vitamins are stored in the liver or fatty tissue, often in large amounts and for prolonged periods of time. From there they become available to the intermediary metabolism for complex tasks. Vitamins A and D are secreted from the liver cells by means of carrier proteins. By undergoing biotransformation, fat-soluble vitamins become metabolically inactive as well as water-soluble and are thus capable of being excreted. (s. tab. 3.13)

10.2 Mechanisms of vitamin action

Vitamins are involved in a variety of ways in almost all processes of the intermediary metabolism taking place in the liver. An understanding of the major mechanisms of action provides insight into the possibilities of disturbance and the occurrence of symptomatological dysfunctions in liver diseases.

10.2.1 Fat-soluble vitamins

Vitamin A: Both vitamin A_1 (= *retinol*) and A_2 (= *3-dehydroretinol*) occur in nature. Like their derivatives, they are classed under the term *axerophtol*. The major provitamin is *β-carotin*. Vitamin A is stored as a lipoglycoprotein complex in the fat-storing cells of the liver. It is released when necessary by being coupled with a retinol-binding protein (RBP) and is then transported to the cells which require vitamin A. In the case of zinc deficiency the rate of RBP synthesis is markedly increased, and as a result serum retinol concentration is reduced. Retinol deficiency can be compensated by zinc substitution. The daily requirement is approx. 1 mg.

Biological actions:
- involvement in the synthesis of glycoproteins, glycolipids and proteoglycane
- stabilization of the cellular and subcellular membranes
- involvement in the production of steroid hormones

Vitamin D: *Calciferol* is taken up from the food as vitamins D_2 (= *ergocalciferol*) and D_3 (= *cholecalciferol*). In skin exposed to UV radiation, vitamin D_2 is formed from the provitamin ergosterol, and vitamin D_3 from the provitamin 7-dehydrocholesterol. 25-hydroxycholecalciferol (= *calcidiol*) is formed in the liver, 1,25-dihydroxycholecalciferol (= *calcitriol*) is produced in the kidney. The synthesis rate in the liver is controlled through the respective cholecalciferol concentration. Transport in serum is effected by a D-binding protein (DBP) identical to Gc-globulin. Oestrogen and pregnancy are known to cause an increase in DBP. (6)

Biological actions:
- involvement and control in regulating intra- and extracellular calcium concentrations

Vitamin E: *Tocopherol* is the umbrella term for all derivatives of the tocoltrienol and tocotrienol type that are similar in their mode of action. Of these derivatives, α-tocopherol is the most effective. Only a small part of the vitamin E supply is absorbed (20−40%), the process being facilitated by the presence of nutritional lipids, bile and pancreatic secretion, and medium-chain triglycerides. No transport protein for vitamin E is known.

Biological actions:
- protection of vitamin A and β-carotin
- protection of unsaturated fatty acids in biomembrane phospholipids (= antioxidant towards oxygen and hydroxyl radicals)
- influence on cholesterol metabolism
- influence on nucleinic acid metabolism

Vitamin K: Vitamin K_1 (= *phylloquinone*), of plant origin, and vitamin K_2 (= *menaquinone*), synthesized by bacteria, are naturally occurring vitamins. Vitamin K is the only fat-soluble vitamin acting as a coenzyme. Furthermore, synthetic K vitamins exist (K_3-K_7); of these, K_3 (= *menadione*) and K_4 (= *menadiol*) are the most significant. The vitamin is stored in the liver only in small quantities. About 50% of the daily requirement is covered by intestinal bacterial synthesis. No intermediary degradation of vitamins K_1 and K_2 is known. The synthetic menadione (K_3) and its derivatives are converted into K_2 in the microsomal fraction of the liver cells. Vitamin K_3 competes with the excretion of bilirubin in the biotransformation process; depending on the dosage, it may have toxic effects. • *Parenteral application of K_1 and K_2 in patients with cirrhosis may cause a paradoxical fall in the clotting factors with an increase in toxic metabolites and additional liver damage* (G. Mandel et al., 1980).

Biological actions:
- stimulation of the production and secretion of the coagulation factors II, VII, IX and X as well as of the two inhibitors, protein C and protein S
- influence on bone mineral metabolism via osteocalcin

Vitamin F: Essential fatty acids (e. g. unsaturated *linolic acid, linolenic acid, arachidonic acid*) are also known collectively as vitamin F. They belong to the group of vitamin-like agents. Exogenous supply is necessary.

Biological actions:
- constituent of phospholipids in all biomembranes
- constituent of prostaglandin precursors
- influence on the mitochondrial metabolism

10.2.2 Water-soluble vitamins

Vitamin B_1: Vitamin B_1 was discovered in 1926 by Jansen and Donath, who synthesized it in its crystalline form from rice bran. It was initially called *aneurine* due to its antipolyneuropathic effect. Because it contains sulphur, Windaus correctly renamed it *thiamine* in 1932, a term by which it is still known today. The structure of this vitamin was described by Williams and Grewe in 1936. It is made up of pyrimidine and thiazole. Thiamine occurs in nature as free thiamine and in the form of thiamine monophosphate, diphosphate and triphosphate. A maximum amount of 8–15 mg is absorbed daily in the proximal portion of the small intestine. In the case of oversupply, thiamine is neither stored nor intestinally absorbed. A regular intake, with a daily requirement of about 1 mg, is necessary. The major coenzyme is thiamine pyrophosphate (TPP). Thiamine deficiency may be caused by malnutrition, impaired absorption, alcoholism, antithiamines or a lack of magnesium. • *Magnesium is an important cofactor for the coenzyme thiamine pyrophosphate.*

Biological actions:
- as cocarboxylase it is crucial to carbohydrate metabolism and the citric acid cycle
- involvement in the pentose phosphate cycle
- involvement in the formation of acetylcholine

Vitamin B_2: It is also termed *riboflavin* or *lactoflavin*. Vitamin B_2 was isolated from eggs by Kuhn and György in 1933 (= ovoflavin) and from whey (= lactoflavin) by Ellinger and Kochara in the same year. After being found in animal organs and plants (= hepatoflavin), it became known as riboflavin. Its structure was described by Kuhn and Karrer in 1935. The riboflavin coenzymes, such as flavine mononucleotide (FMN) and flavine adenine dinucleotide (FAD), are taken up with food, converted into riboflavin and absorbed in the intestine. They are reconverted as FMN and FAD in tissue cells, mainly hepatocytes. No storage of vitamin B_2 takes place.

Biological actions:
- involvement in the transformation of amino acids into keto acids
- involvement in the breakdown of saturated fatty acids by β-oxidation
- involvement in the synthesis of long-chain fatty acids
- influence on the inactivation of biogenic amines to imines and subsequently to ammonia
- component of xanthine oxidase, glutathione reductase, aldehyde dehydrogenase, microsomal flavoprotein monooxygenase, and membrane-related NADPH granulocyte oxidase

Vitamin B_5: *Niacin* (= nicotinic acid) and *niacinamide* (= nicotinamide) are supplied in the diet and converted in the body into the coenzymes nicotinamide-adenine dinucleotide (NAD) and nicotinamide-adenine dinucleotide phosphate (NADP). These coenzymes are important in tissue respiration. Nicotinic acid can also be formed from tryptophan via kynolin acid.

Biological actions:
- component of the electron carriers $NAD^+/NADH$ and $NADP^+/NADPH$ (thus it acts as a coenzyme for several oxidoreductases)
- histamine antagonist

Vitamin B_6: Three substances are classed under the term *pyridoxine* or *adermine: pyridoxol, pyridoxal* and *pyridoxamine*. Pyridoxine was isolated by various study groups in 1938. Its structure was described by Folkers and Kuhn in 1939. Pyridoxal and pyridoxamine were discovered by Snell in 1942. Pyridoxal phosphate and pyridoxamine phosphate are biologically active substances. • Intestinal absorption of B_6 is dose-dependent and not limited. In alcoholism, a deficiency of vitamin B_6 is encountered in 20–30% of cases, whereas the respective percentage is 50–70% in alcoholic cirrhosis. Vitamin B_6 is an important coenzyme for transaminases, which transfer amino groups from amino acids to keto acids. In

Water-soluble vitamins	Fat-soluble vitamins	Acting as a coenzyme	Not acting as a coenzyme	Vitamin-like agents
B_1	A	B_1	A	Essential fatty acids (F)
B_2	D	B_2	C	Carnitine (T)
B_6	E	B_6	D	Bioflavonoids (P)
B_{12}	K	B_{12}	E	Inosite
		K		
Biotin (H)		Biotin (H)		
Pantothenic acid		Pantothenic acid		
Niacin (PP)		Niacin (PP)		
Folic acid (M)		Folic acid (M)		
		Ubiquinone (Q)		

Tab. 3.13: Classification of vitamins and vitamin-like agents

this way, biochemical pathways between the citric acid cycle and carbohydrate and amino acid metabolisms are created. (92)

Biological actions:
- coenzyme for numerous enzymes
- influence on the metabolism of steroid hormones
- activation of δ-aminolaevulinic acid synthase
- involvement in lipid metabolism
- involvement in the synthesis and metabolism of amino acids
- involvement in the formation of nicotinamide from tryptophan
- involvement in serotonin synthesis

Vitamin B_{12}: This vitamin was isolated for the first time in 1948 by Folkers and Smith. Its structure was described by various study groups in 1955. Substances with a central cobalt atom in a modified porphyrin ring are called *cobalamins*. The major forms are: cyanocobalamin (B_{12}), hydroxocobalamin (B_{12a}), aquacobalamin (B_{12b}), nitrosocobalamin (B_{12c}), and methylcobalamin. The coenzyme of vitamin B_{12} is 5-desoxyadenosylcobalamin. Its "gastric intrinsic factor vitamin B_{12} complex" is absorbed in the lower ileum, from where it passes into the portal vein. Transcobalamin I, II and III are available as transport proteins. Transcobalamin II constitutes the principal extracellular transport protein, whereas transcobalamin I and III are intracellular storage proteins. In the cells, the coenzyme is mainly found; in the plasma, methylcobalamin predominates. Approx. 1 mg (of the body's total content of 2–5 mg) is stored in the liver. Vitamin B_{12} excreted in the bile is reabsorbed (70%) and channelled into the enterohepatic circulation.

Biological actions:
- involvement as a coenzyme in amino acid and nucleinic acid metabolism
- involvement in DNA and protein synthesis
- conversion of methylmalonyl-CoA into succinyl-CoA for lipid and porphyrin synthesis

Vitamin M: Vitamin M is also called pteroylglutaminic acid or *folic acid*. It was isolated from yeast extract by Wills in 1930. Its structure was described by Angier in 1946. Folic acid is made up of pteridine + p-aminobenzoic acid + glutamic acid. There are several known derivatives, called *folates*, which are capable of mutual restructuring. The coenzyme *tetrahydrofolic acid*, which plays a role in many biochemical reactions, is formed with the help of B_{12}. Around 50% of total body folate are stored in the liver. A folate-binding protein (FBP) is available for transport. Folate undergoes enterohepatic circulation. The release of folate from the liver cells is stimulated by alcohol, which increases urine excretion. Folate deficiency (e.g. in the case of alcohol abuse) is accompanied by the development of macrocytosis.

Biological actions:
- influence on the intermediary metabolism of homocysteine, histidine and serine
- promotion of the biosynthesis of nucleinic acids
- involvement as a coenzyme in porphyrin synthesis

Vitamin H: In the liver, *biotin* participates as a prosthetic group in carboxylases and transcarboxylases. It is found in the free form as well as covalently linked with protein.

Biological actions:
- involvement in fatty acid synthesis
- involvement in gluconeogenesis
- effect on amino acid metabolism
- involvement in the urea cycle
- promotion of purine synthesis
- promotion of transfer-RNA synthesis

Vitamin C: *Ascorbic acid* is the most important redox substance of cell metabolism. The body contains 2–5 g, the major part being stored in the liver and muscles. Intestinal absorption (80–90%) is an active, sodium-dependent process. The transport of ascorbic acid in the blood probably takes place as an ascorbic acid-albumin complex. Cellular uptake is stimulated by insulin.

Biological actions:
- influence on the hydroxylation of proline and lysine residues in collagen synthesis
- promotion of the synthesis of noradrenaline from dopamine
- involvement in the hydroxylation of steroid hormones
- incorporation of iron into ferritin
- sulphate donor in the sulphation of proteoglycanes
- antioxidant effect

Vitamin T: *Carnitine* is a trimethylbetaine encountered in nearly all tissues, above all in the musculature.

Biological actions:
- involvement in fatty acid transport
- involvement in mitochondrial fatty acid oxidation
- involvement in transmethylation
- influence on the effect of thyroxine

11 Trace elements and the liver

Trace elements are micronutritive elements occurring in minute, species-specific quantities (<0.01% of body mass or $<10^{-6}$ g/g BW). These inorganic bioelements are subdivided into essential and non-essential (accidental) trace elements. (s. tab. 3.14)

Essential		Non-essential	
Chromium	Cr	Aluminium	Al
Cobalt	Co	Barium	Ba
Copper	Cu	Bismuth	Bi
Fluorine	F	Cadmium	Cd
Iodine	I	Caesium	Cs
Iron	Fe	Gold	Au
Manganese	Mn	Lead	Pb
Molybdenum	Mo	Silver	Ag
Nickel	Ni	Titanium	Ti
Selenium	Se		
Silicon	Si		
Tin	Sn		
Vanadium	V		
Zinc	Zn		

Tab. 3.14: Essential and non-essential trace elements in the human body

The results of investigations available so far have demonstrated that the liver assumes a central role in preserving the **homoeostasis** of trace elements. Liver diseases may also lead to persistent disturbances in the metabolism of trace elements, which are of clinical significance and may require therapeutic steps. (52, 60)

Essential trace elements are vital substances, the deficiency of which leads to specific abnormalities of the structural or biochemical type. These disorders can be prevented or eliminated by supplementation of the respective element. They are important components of enzymes, chromoproteins or hormones. In humans, 14 trace elements are recognized as "essential". (s. tab. 3.14)

For many of these elements, the mechanisms of intestinal absorption, transport in the blood, intracellular uptake, especially by the liver cells, and the question of their storage or elimination are still not fully understood. • It should be considered that trace elements may also have **toxic effects** if given in overdosage or in the case of increased accumulation in the body due to insufficient excretion.

11.1 Iron

Of the body's daily iron uptake, 1−2 mg are absorbed in the duodenum and proximal jejunum. Resorption is pH-dependent; Fe^{3+} is insoluble at a pH value of >4. Vitamin C enhances iron resorption (= reduction of iron and formation of a soluble iron-ascorbat chelate). DCT 1 (= divalent cation transporter) serves as a mucosa transporter and also supports mucosal transport of zinc, copper, cobalt, etc. Iron facilitates O_2 transport and the transfer of electrons.

In the intracellular space, iron is stored as both ferritin (ca. 47%) and haemosiderin (ca. 12%) as well as in the form of an iron-transit pool (ca. 27%). (20) Iron metabolism is of utmost importance for the organism and is characterized by the following **values**:

> **Total body iron content:** 4−5 g (0.07−0.09 mol)
> (men: 50 mg/kg BW, women: 35 mg/kg BW)
> − 60−65% in haemoglobin (ca. 2.5 g)
> − 10% in myoglobin (ca. 0.5 g)
> − 20−30% as depot iron (ca. 1.0 g)
>   (bone marrow, liver, spleen)
> − 5% in enzymes
>   (e.g. cytochrome, catalase, peroxidase, enolase, succinate dehydrogenase, certain hydroxylases, and ribonucleotide reductase)

Transferrin is mainly synthesized in the hepatocytes. There are about 20 known variants. Iron is transported by transferrin (approx. 30% of transferrin is saturated with iron). With the help of a membrane receptor, the iron-transferrin complex is taken up and released in the liver cell, where it is immediately bound (because of its toxicity) to ferritin. The liver cells take up iron predominantly from transferrin, to a lesser degree also from haptoglobin, haemopexin, lactoferrin and circulating ferrin. Transferrin, which is mainly formed in the hepatocytes, may also bind and transport, in decreasing order, chromium, copper, manganese, cobalt, cadmium, zinc and nickel. The half-life of transferrin is 1−2 hours, which is very short in view of its total blood concentration of 3−4 mg. Approximately 0.4 g ferritin iron is stored in the liver. In the case of transferrin deficiency, its bacteriostatic and fungistatic effects are also reduced.

Transferrin without iron saturation is known as **apotransferrin**. (29, 60, 61)

Lactoferrin can only be distinguished from transferrin immunologically. It is an iron transport protein which is formed in granulocytes and glandular epithelia.

Ferritin neutralizes the intracellular toxicity of iron and effects its water-solubility. It is formed in the RES (as well as at the polysomes of the liver cells) and degraded the lysosomes. The serum ferritin value corresponds to the total amount of mobilizable depot iron in the body.

Haemosiderin is also an iron-protein complex, assumed to be formed from ferritin. In the case of iron overload in the body, more haemosiderin than ferritin is formed, which is then stored in the intracellular space. Haemosiderin can be demonstrated biochemically using the Berlin blue reaction. *(see chapters 5.5.2 and 31.17)*

Haemopexin is a protein which is formed in the hepatocytes. It facilitates the intracellular transport of both haem and iron while preventing the loss of haem-Fe via the kidneys. With increasing diminution of the synthesis capacity of the liver, there is a corresponding decrease in the serum level of haemopexin.

11.2 Copper

The body's total content of copper is calculated to be 80−150 mg (1.5−2.35 mmol). Of this amount, 10−15% are found in the liver. In the liver cells, copper is encountered in the cytoplasm, nucleus, mitochondria and microsomes. The daily copper requirement in the diet is 3−5 mg. Copper is excreted at 2−4% in the urine and at 80% in the bile; consequently, the serum level of copper is increased in cholestasis. Copper levels can also be raised by the influence of oestrogens as well as by an increased oral intake of zinc. • **Ceruloplasmin** is an α-globulin and belongs to the acute phase protein group. It is able to reoxidize iron and can therefore be termed ferrioxidase; it also facilitates the transfer of iron into transferrin. For transport in the blood, 95% are bound to ceruloplasmin, whereas 5% are bound to albumin or free amino acids. The biological effect of copper consists in activating copper-dependent enzymes needed for several cellular metabolic actions. (12, 24, 60, 90) *(see chapters 5.6.5 and 31.16)*

> *Biological actions:*
> − oxidation of Fe^2 to Fe^3
> − cross-linkage of collagen and elastic fibres
> − metabolism of catecholamines (by monoamine oxidase)
> − metabolism of keratin and pigment (by tyrosinase)
> − conversion of superoxide radicals into O_2 and H_2O_2 (by zinc-copper superoxide dismutase)
> − involvement in the intracellular respiratory chain (by mitochondrial cytochrome C-oxidase)
> − activation of phosphatases

11.3 Zinc

The normal zinc content of the body amounts to 20–30 mmol (1.3–2.0 g). The daily dietary requirement is 10–15 mg. In the blood, zinc is bound to α_2-macroglobulin, albumin or amino acids, and a small amount is also bound to transferrin. Zinc is crucial to a variety of enzyme reactions. This applies especially to the liver. More and more attention has therefore been paid to the role of zinc in liver disease in recent years. Six enzyme groups (hydrolases, isomerases, ligases, lyases, oxidoreductases and transferases) with a total of 35 **zinc metalloenzymes** are listed. (88) • *Almost 200 enzyme reactions in the body are zinc-dependent!*

1. **Increased zinc requirement**
   - Infections, burns, stress
   - Pregnancy
   - Surgical procedures
   - Tumour disease
2. **Insufficient alimentary supply of zinc**
   - Abuse of laxatives
   - Alcoholism
   - Nutrition poor in zinc
3. **Reduced intestinal absorption**
   - Colitis, Crohn's disease
   - Inhibition of absorption by starch, phosphate and calcium as well as by phytic acid (in the case of a vegetarian diet)
   - Intestinal bypass
   - Sprue, pancreatic insufficiency
   - Wilson's disease
4. **Altered zinc distribution**
   - Acute and chronic hepatitis
   - Alcoholic liver disease
   - Autoimmune diseases
   - Inflammatory processes, infections
   - Liver cirrhosis
   - Malignant diseases
   - Pharmacons (glucocorticoids, contraceptives, antimetabolites, chelate formers)
5. **Increased zinc excretion**
   - Alcoholism, alcoholic liver diseases
   - Diabetes mellitus
   - Diarrhoea
   - Liver cirrhosis
   - Pharmacons
   - Renal diseases, diuretics
   - Severe hepatitis
   - Surgical procedures

Tab. 3.15: Aetiology of absolute and relative zinc deficiency

Zinc assumes a special role in the intrahepatic formation of retinol-binding protein, which is essential for the release of vitamin A into the blood. Zinc deficiency results in a decrease in RBP. Furthermore, as a part of ADH, zinc is crucial for alcohol degradation in the hepatocytes and for enzyme activation in the detoxification of ammonia in the urea cycle. (s. fig. 3.12!)

The metabolism of zinc is influenced by hormones, stress situations, lipopolysaccharides, toxins, oxygen radicals, lipid peroxidations, etc. This may lead to fluctuations in the zinc concentration, mainly due to the induction of **metallothioneine** (MT), which is a transport and intracellular depot protein. One third of this protein consists of cysteine, which binds zinc, copper, cadmium, cobalt and mercury. This protects the body from toxic heavy metal ions (e. g. cadmium and mercury). The induction of MT thus also leads to increased (yet reversible) binding of zinc, which feigns zinc deficiency. It cannot be excluded that altered zinc distribution might eventually result in lower zinc levels in the body. This can be caused by various factors. (60, 70, 88) (s. tab. 3.15)

Biological actions:
- influence on carbohydrate, protein and lipid metabolism
- influence on alcohol metabolism
- influence on epithelial differentiation
- stabilization of biological membranes
- receptor binding of insulin
- influence on the production of testosterone
- influence on the metabolism of vitamin A
- influence on the immune system
- influence on blood formation
- influence on the urea cycle

11.4 Selenium

Selenium is taken up in the body in both an inorganic and organic form. The body's selenium amounts to 10–15 mg or 0.12–0.19 mmol (= 5 mmol/kg wet weight). The estimated daily requirement is 20–100 µg. The serum concentration (normal: 50–120 µg/l) is regulated through renal elimination (normal: 10–50 µg/l). Inorganic selenium is bound to VLDL and LDL, while organic selenium is bound to amino acids. (57, 60, 89) • Selenium deficiency occurs particularly in alcoholism and liver cirrhosis. This may set up a vicious circle leading to further liver cell necrosis. Selenium is incorporated into cysteine and thus becomes an essential component of both glutathione peroxidase and phospholipid-hydroxyperoxide-glutathione peroxidase. These enzymes play an important role as radical scavengers in the prevention of lipid peroxidation in the area of the biomembranes. Selenium is deemed to have a protective effect in fulminant hepatitis and an inhibitory effect on the formation and growth of malignant tumours. • **5-deiodase** is a further selenium-containing enzyme involved in the formation of triiodothyronine.

11.5 Manganese

The amount of manganese in the liver contains 24 µmol/kg BW, which is equivalent to approximately 10% of the body's manganese depot (0.2–0.36 mmol). It is bound to transferrin for transport in the blood. (60)

Acetyl-CoA decarboxylase, alkaline phosphatase, aminopeptidases, arginase, carboxypeptidase A, enolase, glucokinase, hyaluronidase, mevalonatekinase, pyruvate decarboxylase and superoxide dismutase are regarded as manganese metalloenzymes or manganese-dependent enzymes. • Thus the formation of glucose from lactate, the synthesis of triglycerides and the formation of cholesterol are positively affected, and the synthesis of mucopolysaccharides is promoted. Superoxide dismutase is important for the elimination of superoxide-anion radicals (O_2^-) through the formation of H_2O and O_2.

11.6 Chromium

The chromium content of the liver amounts to 1 µmol/kg BW, which corresponds to 1% of the body's total quantity of ca. 100 µmol. Chromium is bound to transferrin and α-globulin for transport in the blood. (59)

▶ The **biological effect** of chromium is based on the binding of insulin with the cell membrane (together with nicotinic acid and glutathione), where it is at the same time partly responsible for insulin activity. In chromium deficiency (e.g. due to stress), glucose tolerance is reduced. In diabetics requiring insulin, the urinary loss of chromium is increased. The *linkage* of chromium + nicotinic acid + glutathione is called the **glucose tolerance factor.** An increase in blood sugar leads to an augmented formation of this factor in the liver cells — insofar as this is still possible with limited liver function. Chromium has a stimulating effect on RNA synthesis. It is involved in lipoprotein metabolism.

11.7 Cobalt

Inorganic cobalt is transported in the blood by albumin and transferrin; it is taken up by the liver. The serum concentration amounts to 1.9–7.6 mmol/l. An increased value is a sign of liver cell necrosis (e.g. acute hepatitis). Its biological significance is attributed to its position as a central atom in vitamin B_{12} and its involvement in the release of renin and erythropoietin.

12 Biotransformation and detoxification

The **elimination** of endogenous and exogenous substances from the body is necessary if they: (*1.*) do not serve the production of energy, (*2.*) are not needed for the maintenance of structure, or (*3.*) cannot be stored without causing harm. • Therefore *gaseous substances* are excreted via the lungs and *water-soluble substances* are excreted via the kidney or (through bile) in the faeces. However, *fat-soluble foreign substances* cannot be excreted in an unchanged state.

Exogenous and endogenous substances which may cause damage to the body must be broken down and/or detoxified and made water-soluble, so that they are capable of being excreted in the stool or urine. This especially applies to lipophilic or corpuscular substances which cannot be excreted and may therefore accumulate in the body at potentially toxic levels. • *The liver is the central organ for the degradation and/or detoxification of superfluous and harmful substances as well as their excretion from the body.*

Of the twelve metabolic functions shown in table 3.1, both the biotransformation and the detoxifying function are of major relevance. Disturbance of one or several of the other metabolic fields may be hazardous and is often associated with complications — any breakdown of the detoxifying function, however, leads to cell necrosis and liver failure, and thus death.

12.1 Foreign compounds (xenobiotics)

The term **xenobiotics** comprises firstly substances which trigger defence mechanisms in the organism and secondly exogenous substances which contaminate or burden and thus damage the ecological systems of the organism itself or the environment. Xenobiotics are therefore substrates which may also be defined as potentially hepatotoxic substances. (s. tab. 3.16)

```
1. Alcohol
2. Chemicals
3. Drugs
4. Heavy metals
5. Endogenous toxic metabolic products
6. Toxins:   a. plant toxins
             b. animal toxins
             c. bacterial toxins
```

Tab. 3.16: Xenobiotics or potentially hepatotoxic substances

▶ Xenobiotics may be present in *water-soluble* (hydrophilic) or in *fat-soluble* (lipophilic) form. However, they are also taken up in the body as *gaseous* substances and *corpuscular-insoluble* substrates (e.g. heavy metals). Any xenobiotics reaching the liver must be rendered inactive and harmless, i.e. capable of being excreted.

Hydrophilic xenobiotics enter the cell at the sinusoidal side of the hepatocyte membrane by means of transport systems using carrier proteins. These carrier proteins exhibit no or only low substrate specificity, so that various endogenous and also exogenous substances can be transported through the cell membrane. Competition between these substances for carrier proteins may lead to mutual inhibition of the transport mechanism.

Lipophilic xenobiotics are superior in number (about 70–80%). Because of their high solubility in fats — thus also in the phospholipid double layer of the cellular and subcellular membranes — these substances rapidly (and without hindrance) reach the liver cells and organelles according to the laws of nonionic diffusion.

12.2 Metabolization of xenobiotics

The detoxifying function of the liver was established by F. MAGENDIE as early as 1817. For the conversion of endogenous and exogenous toxic substances, the term **detoxification** was introduced. Later, however, a **change of metabolization** was demonstrated, meaning not only that foreign substances are detoxified by the liver, but that atoxic substances may become toxic after undergoing metabolization in the liver (*"toxication"*), e.g. the insecticide parathion, or the conversion of CCl_4 into highly reactive radicals, or the carcinogenicity of benzpyrene, aflatoxin and nitrosamine. As a result of dysregulation of cellular metabolic processes, toxic metabolites may also be produced (*"biotoxometabolites"*) which are not normally metabolites of the parent compound. • Furthermore, it was noted that some therapeutically active substances were converted in the liver into inactive metabolites (*"inactivation"*) and some inactive medical substances, such as prodrugs (e.g. cyclophosphamide), into active metabolites (*"activation"*). Moreover, during their liver passage, active substances were found to be weakened or even potentiated in their activity (*"change of activity"*). (s. fig. 3.11)

Based on the individual variability in the behaviour of the liver cell towards foreign substances and drugs, the thesis was put forward that both the effectiveness as well as the side-effects of medicaments are genetically determined (A.G. MOTULSKY, 1957). As a result, the term **pharmacogenetics** (F. VOGEL, 1959) was introduced to define clinically relevant, hereditary differences in the effects of drugs which lead to abnormal reactions in patients (due to genetic polymorphism). (17, 21, 91)

Moreover, major *influences on the metabolism* of xenobiotics in the liver due to nutritional factors as well as through interactions with chemicals and alcohol have been reported. Distinct age and gender-related differences have also been noted. (s. tab. 3.18) • *The glucuronidation capacity of the liver can be measured by means of* **4-methylumbelliferone** (H.-D. KUNTZ, 1983). (46–49)

Any foreign substances in the gastrointestinal tract — even in high concentrations — are directly transported to the liver because of its topographic position and functional role. At the same time, several (superfluous and occasionally harmful) substances also travel to the liver via the haematogenous system. • *The liver is constantly required to clear such substances from the body.*

12.3 Mechanisms of metabolic detoxification

Due to the multiplicity of substances to be eliminated, both *substrate-specific* and *substrate-nonspecific* mechanisms are necessary. The liver is thus capable of eliminating a maximum number of foreign substances with little biomolecular effort. By means of its nonspecific elimination systems, the liver is generally able to cope metabolically with the daily variety of foreign substances as well as with "newly formed" ones. (s. tab. 3.17)

If these elimination systems are overburdened or their functions are disturbed, the extent to which the metabolism can be relieved of unnecessary or harmful substances may be more or less limited. This leads to accumulation and eventually produces toxic effects of substances which, in normal quantities, would be well tolerated and readily eliminated.

---

1. **Biotransformation**
   – 2-phase reaction
   – enzyme adaptation
2. **Ammonia detoxification and bicarbonate neutralization**
   – urea cycle/glutamine cycle
   – bicarbonate neutralization
3. **Alcohol degradation**
4. **Reticuloendothelial system**
5. **Radical scavengers and antioxidants**

Tab. 3.17: Important (substrate-specific and substrate-nonspecific) mechanisms of metabolic clearance

12.4 Biotransformation

The term **biotransformation** is defined as biochemical changes in a substance through autometabolic processes. In this way, lipophilic substances can be converted into water-soluble (= excretable) metabolites in the liver.

▶ *Lipid-soluble, non-excretable substances* (if subject to glomerular filtration) are almost completely reabsorbed from the primary urine by renal tubules, with the result that they are hardly ever excreted via the kidney. This might involve the danger of accumulations of lipophilic xenobiotics in the body, especially in fatty tissue. Therefore hydrophilization of these substances (with the associated feature of being excretable in the bile or urine) is required.

The enzyme systems involved in biotransformation are largely **substrate-nonspecific**. Therefore, they are not only able to convert exogenous or endogenous lipophilic substances into water-soluble metabolites, but also to intervene in the metabolism of endogenous substances (e.g. bile acids, hormones). These enzymes are mainly localized **structure-bound** in the biomembranes or found **non-structure-bound** as soluble enzymes. About 5% of the total protein reserves of the liver are needed for the biotransformation of enzymes.

This biotransformation process takes place principally in the liver, i.e. in the *smooth endoplasmic reticulum*, partly also in the *mitochondria*. The kidneys, lungs, intestine, muscles, spleen and skin are involved to a lesser degree in biotransformation. Through hydrolysis and reduction, the intestinal flora may also play a role in this metabolic process. • Biotransformation is limited by the hepatic blood flow (= *flow-limited elimination*) and by the capacity of microsomal enzyme systems (= *capacity-limited elimination*).

12.4.1 2-phase reaction

Biotransformation of xenobiotics takes place in two phases. In **phase I** (= *functionalization reactions*), reactive groups are either activated or inserted into the substance molecule, thus providing the lipophilic molecule with a functional hydrophilic group. (In phase II, a hydrophilic residue is added to this group; transferases hereby catalyze the conjugation with an endogenous substance.) • Phase I effects the insertion of reactive (polar) groups (such as −OH, −COOH, −SH, −NH$_2$) by means of four chemical processes: oxidation, reduction, hydrolysis, hydration.

> **Oxidation reactions** (or hydroxylation) by *oxidases* (= removal of hydrogen or electrons) and *dioxygenases* (= insertion of the 2 atoms of the oxygen molecule into the foreign substance) as well as by *monooxygenases* (= insertion of one oxygen atom into the foreign substance and reduction in the other oxygen atom to H$_2$O) are of great significance in biotransformation. • Here the conversion of xenobiotics may be accomplished via various enzymatic pathways by means of *oxidation*: (*1.*) aromatic amines, (*2.*) aliphatic chains, (*3.*) alcohol and aldehydes, (*4.*) oxidative N-desalkylation, (*5.*) oxidative O-desalkylation, (*6.*) oxidative desamination, (*7.*) S-oxidation, (*8.*) N-oxidation, and (*9.*) S-O-exchange.

Cytochrome P 450: The drug-metabolizing enzymes responsible for the breakdown of xenobiotics (B. B. BRODIE, 1967) exhibit mainly oxidative properties. In particular, the microsomal mixed-function monooxygenases are worth mentioning. They contain the haemprotein cytochrome P 450 consisting of a complex of various isoenzymes. The name cytochrome P 450 signifies that reduced cytochrome has a carbon-monoxide difference spectrum with 450 nm maximum absorption (R.W. ESTA-BROOK et al., 1975). CYP enzymes are found in the smooth ER and, after high-speed centrifugation, in the microsomal fraction. The highest levels of CYP activity are seen in centroacinar zone 3 and the lowest in periportal zone 1. Biliary epithelia, endothelial cells and Kupffer cells contain no cytochrome P 450. Up to now, 57 functional CYP genes and 33 pseudogenes arranged into 18 families and 42 subfamilies are known, including 1A1, 1A2, 2A6, 2A7, 1B1, 2B1, 2B4, 2B6, 2B7, 2C3, 2C6−2C9, 2C11, 2C18, 2C19, 2D1, 2D6, 2E1, 3A1, 3A4, 3A5, 3E1, 4A1, 4B1, 5A1 and others (= number of the enzyme group, letter of the enzyme subgroup, number of the respective enzyme species). Cytochrome P 450 enzymes are ubiquitous. They are found in bacteria, plants and animals. The approx. 500 known cytochrome P 450 genes have developed from a common gene, which probably originated 3.0−3.5 billion years ago. (65) • Furthermore, a *flavoprotein* (= hydrogen transfer agent) and an *NADPH-cytochrome-C reductase* (= hydrogen donor) exist. One oxygen atom is needed for the oxidation of the respective substrate, the second oxygen atom serves the oxidation of hydrogen to water. The high degree of hereditary biochemical individuality in biotransformation is achieved through these diverse oxidative reactions. (93)

The range of microsomal enzymes includes *epoxide hydratase*. This is required for the degradation of epoxides, which may originate as aliphatic or aromatic decomposition products from the metabolism of foreign substances. The precursors of these biotoxometabolites are hydroperoxides, formed, for example, from arachidonic acid by means of lipoxygenase activity. Epoxides are capable of provoking toxic, mutagenic, antigenic, carcinogenic and other effects (= *chemical lesion*).

Reduction: Phase I can also be accomplished by means of reductions. The reductive enzymes are localized both in the microsomes and the cytosol. They trigger the enzymatic transformation of ketones, aldehydes, sulphoxides, nitrolinkages and azolinkages, etc. The intestinal flora also contributes to the reductive metabolism of foreign substances.

Hydrolysis: This is of minor significance in biotransformation. Amidases and glycosidases are the important enzymes in this process. Intestinal bacteria with hydrolytic activity split mainly phase II metabolites in the large intestine, with the result that absorbable catabolites then enter the enterohepatic circulation.

> Through the metabolic stages of phase I alone, substances can be made water-soluble and thus capable of being excreted via the kidney.

In **phase II** (= *conjugation reactions*), the foreign substance molecule or a metabolite formed in phase I conjugates with an endogenous substance by means of specific transferases. The resulting, mostly acidic conjugation products are highly hydrophilic and readily excreted in the urine and/or bile. Most of these conjugates are biologically inactive and thus literally "detoxicated". Some conjugates are rehydrolized to the initial substance and reabsorbed in the intestine. • Phase II, with its enzyme reactions, occurs (like phase I) in the endoplasmic reticulum. For the conjugation process, various substances can be used as *endogenous ligands:*

Endogenous ligands
1. Activated glucuronic acid (by glucuronosyl transferase)
2. Activated sulphuric acid (by sulphotransferase or thiosulphate-S transferase)
3. Activated acetic acid (by N-acetyl transferase)
4. Amino acids (glycine, glutamine, taurine) (by transacylase)
5. S-adenosyl methionine (by transmethylase)
6. Mercapturic acid derivatives (by glutathione-S transferase)

Phase II is adequate for biotransformation if the initial substance possesses a group with binding ability, i.e. phase I is no longer needed for the activation or insertion of a reactive group.

Sometimes neither phase I nor phase II is required for the elimination of a foreign substance: the given substance is firstly taken up by the liver cells due to its low lipophilicity, but can nevertheless be excreted adequately via the kidneys despite its low hydrophilicity.

12.4.2 Enzyme adaptation

In the course of evolution and during the short life-span of every human being, it was − and still is − necessary for the performance of enzyme systems involved in biotransformation to adapt permanently to the requirements of life. This enzyme adaptation is achieved by **four mechanisms:**

1. Enzyme induction
2. Enzyme inhibition
3. Activation of an inactive enzyme
4. Reduction in enzyme breakdown

Changes in the enzyme activities involved in biotransformation may be caused by various **factors**. These can be both variable and non-variable in nature with individually different modes of influence. (s. tab. 3.18) (s. fig. 3.11)

Variable factors	Non-variable factors
1. Protein content of nutrition 2. Pharmacons 3. Chemicals 4. Alcohol 5. Constituents of tobacco smoke 6. Heavy metals 7. Pregnancy 8. Diseases etc.	1. Genetics 2. Gender 3. Age

Tab. 3.18: Variable and non-variable factors influencing the biochemical mechanisms involved in the metabolism of foreign substances

Enzyme induction is of the greatest importance. Xenobiotics may lead to an increase in biotransformation enzymes. Various foreign substances induce different enzyme systems, resulting in various types of enzyme inductions. (93) Initially, enzyme induction can only be detected using electron microscopy. In more intensive and longer-lasting induction, proliferation of the *smooth endoplasmic reticulum* (SER) becomes more clearly visible microscopically. (s. figs. 2.9; 21.2) This is accompanied by a rise in γ-GT in serum, as this enzyme is formed there and produced in higher amounts corresponding to increased proliferation of the SER. (s. p. 103)

▶ *Viewed from this angle, a rise in γ-GT is a "physiological" process, i.e. criterion for increased enzyme induction or sign of adaptation to the requisite (and accomplished) enhancement in biotransformation performance.*

▶ *Membrane hyperplasia:* The proliferation rate of the SER may have developed to such an extent that cell volume grows by up to 50%; this can increase the weight of the liver and cause hepatomegaly. *(see chapter 11)*

In response to enzyme induction, various **metabolic processes** may occur:

(*1.*) Biotransformation or degradation capacity is increased, and thus the plasma half-life is shortened. This is achieved by endogenous active substances (e.g. steroid hormones), essential substances (e.g. vitamin D) and foreign substances (especially drugs) as well as by changes in the enzyme inducer.

(*2.*) With lower activity of the catabolites towards the initial substance, the effect is weakened; with higher activity of the metabolite, the effect is potentiated.

(*3.*) As a result of the activation of foreign substances, adverse effects or chronic toxicity — even cancerogenicity — may occur.

(*4.*) **Biotoxometabolites:** Owing to their chemical binding to cellular proteins, metabolites of foreign substances may be unexpectedly converted into biotoxometabolites. These *chemical lesions* constitute irreversible changes to essential cell components. The main cause of cellular biotoxication are free radicals or epoxides, such as are produced in the course of oxidative and reductive metabolic processes. A lack of radical scavengers (catalase, superoxide dismutase, glutathione, vitamins C and E, etc.) and an overload or disturbance regarding the respective detoxification pathways may lead to a dangerous increase in such biotoxometabolites. This involves the danger of the unpredictable appearance of allergens, antigens, carcinogens, mutagens or toxins, and possibly antivitamins. (s. fig. 3.11)

Alcohol plays an important role in the metabolism of foreign substances and is responsible for numerous interactions with drugs. A special type of cytochrome P 450 (P 450 II E 1) is induced by the chronic intake of alcohol. This subtype may influence other drug-metabolizing enzyme systems and possibly account for the carcinogenicity of dimethylnitrosamine in the gastrointestinal tract. • The cellular endowment of other organs with cytochrome P 450 may — in the case of corresponding activation of specific enzyme systems and with formation of such biotoxometabolites — lead to carcinogenesis in the respective organ.

Enzyme inhibition may be triggered by a number of foreign substances. Such a process, in turn, results in an inhibition of biotransformation and thus in a prolongation of the effects of drugs and xenobiotics as well as of the inhibitor. A reduction in enzyme activity occurs in response to an inhibition of synthesis or an increase in breakdown induced by foreign substances. It can likewise be conditioned by the fact that several substances are competing for the enzyme-binding site. In administering drugs to elderly people, it should be considered that cytochrome P 450-dependent enzyme reactions get slower with age, thus making dose adjustments necessary.

The major **types** of enzyme inducers are: (*1.*) phenobarbital (*2.*) methylcholanthrene, and (*3.*) anabolic steroid. (s. tab. 3.19)

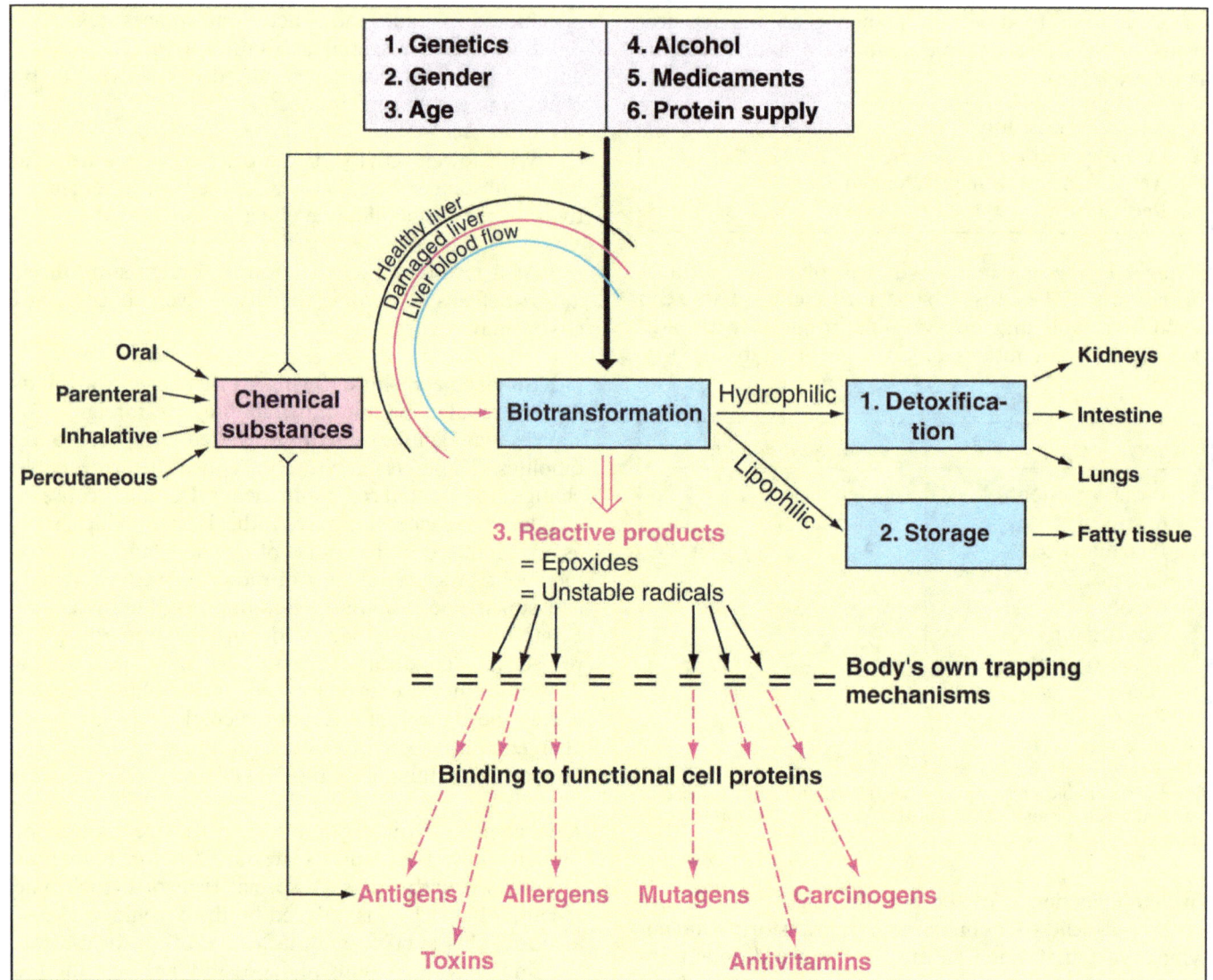

Fig. 3.11: Diagram showing the biotransformation of foreign substances and their influencing factors as well as the development of reactive products and biotoxometabolites

Effect of induction	Phenobarbital type	Methylcholan-threne type
– Microsomal proteins	++	(+)
– Cytochrome P 450	++	++
– Cytochrome P 448	(+)	++
– NADPH cytochrome-C reductase	++	∅
– NADPH-cytochrome P 450 reductase	++	∅
– Glucuronyl transferase	(+)	++
– Steroid metabolism – Acceleration of metabolism – Bile secretion	+ by several active substances ++	∅ by only a few active substances ∅
Liver weight	++	(+)
Onset of effect	after 2–3 days	after 12–24 hours

Tab. 3.19: Effects of enzyme inducers of the phenobarbital and methylcholanthrene types (+ = increased or accelerated, (+) = slightly increased, ∅ = not increased or not accelerated)

▶ The knowledge of biotransformation currently available raises the following issue, which up to now may not have been given the attention it deserves: owing to the considerable *individual variability* of drug metabolization (= *pharmacogenetics*) with multiple influencing factors, it might be problematic in **clinical studies** to administer the same drug dosage to all participants and to obtain comparable equivalent results for the drug under study. • Both the therapeutic efficacy and side effects of a drug may vary greatly in different patients, even with similar plasma concentrations.

▶ This might further explain the potential divergency of clinical study results – and possibly also the potential "inefficacy" of a drug or an "adverse drug reaction".

13 Ammonia detoxification and bicarbonate neutralization

13.1 Urea cycle

▶ As early as 1815, C.B. Rose had assumed the synthesis of urea to be localized in the liver. In 1858 A. Heynsius observed that the concentration of urea was higher in the liver than in all other organs. • In 1868 E. Stadelmann found patients with liver disease to have markedly increased blood levels of ammonia compared with normal individuals.

Ammonia: NH_3 is a colourless gas. It is freely soluble in water, whereby ammonium is formed. Ammonia forms in the liver after degradation of protein, amino acids, nucleinic acids and biogenic amines, and in the kidney by tubular hydrolysis of glutamine.

Ammonium: NH_4^+ is free NH_3 dissolved in water. It is defined as the sum of free NH_3 and ionized NH_4^+, which is in a pH-dependent dissociation balance with NH_3, i.e. alkalosis shifts the balance towards free ammonia. With a normal blood pH value of 7.4, more than 90% of the ammonium are available as NH_4^+.

The **formation of ammonium** is a continuous metabolic process. The highest amount of about 4 g/day (= 0.23 mol/day) is formed in the *colon*, a lower production of ammonium takes place in the *small intestine* from glutamine. Furthermore, 20% of the urea formed in the intestine are rehydrolyzed to ammonium. A total of 300–500 mmol ammonia are produced daily in the intestinal tract; thus the concentration of NH_4^+ is 5–10 times higher in the portal vein than in the peripheral blood. • The *liver* produces a higher amount of NH_4^+ from the degradation of protein and amino acids which, however, is directly detoxified in the urea cycle. • A considerable amount of ammonia is also formed in *muscle*, depending on muscular action. • In the *kidneys*, 30–40 mmol ammonium are produced daily by the tubular hydrolysis of glutamine (with the help of glutaminase) and passed into the blood. In potassium deficiency and alkalosis, the renal formation of ammonia is markedly increased. • *Helicobacter pylori* also produces ammonium: this pathogen carries urease molecules on its surface. These split the urea, which is amply formed in the contents of the stomach, into ammonium and hydrogen carbonate. Depending on the number of pathogens and the amount of urea, large concentrations of ammonium accumulate. As a result, the gastric acid is neutralized in its microenvironment by helicobacter, so that the pathogen gains time to penetrate the mucosa.

▶ With the degradation of (e.g.) *100 g protein, 20 g ammonia* are formed. It is freely diffusible and thus toxic. Therefore it must be rapidly dissolved in water and converted into nondiffusible ammonium. The higher intracellular concentration of protons causes NH_4^+ to accumulate in the cell. (s. fig. 3.15)

An increase in freely diffusible, and thus toxic, ammonia may be due to a dissociation imbalance with ammonium as well as inadequate detoxification of NH_3 and NH_4^+. The question of the toxicity of ammonia, especially **neurotoxicity**, has not been fully explained with regard to its pathogenesis. Proposed potential **causes** include: (*1.*) damage to the mitochondria, (*2.*) disturbance or insufficiency of major liver cell functions, (*3.*) increase in the permeability of the blood-liquor barrier, and (*4.*) dysregulation of neurotransmitters and their receptors.

The **detoxification of ammonium** must be balanced with the formation of ammonium in order to avoid toxic concentrations in the blood. The urinary elimination rate is 20–40 mmol/day (= 1.9 g). • The detoxification of ammonium takes place in the liver-specific urea cycle. The skeletal muscles and the brain are involved in ammonium detoxification via the glutamine cycle.

The *urea cycle*, also called *ornithine cycle*, was first described by H.A. Krebs and K. Henseleit in 1932. (quot. 46) The principle of ammonia detoxification in the urea cycle is based on the conversion of ammonium and bicarbonate in the mitochondria under ATP consumption into carbamoyl phosphate (by means of carbamoyl phosphate synthetase). It enters the urea cycle, which is localized mainly – yet with a low affinity for ammonium – in the periportal zone of the liver lobule. In the urea cycle alone, about two thirds of the amino nitrogen of ammonia are irretrievably lost to the organism (= *definitive ammonia detoxification*). (s. fig. 3.12)

With increasing dysfunction of the liver, the enzymes responsible for the urea cycle display a marked loss of activity. Some of these enzymes are zinc-dependent (s. fig. 3.12); a decrease in enzyme activity is therefore evident in zinc deficiency. (s. tab. 3.15)

The remaining third of the ammonia is trapped by the peripheral hepatocytes (= scavenger cells) due to their high affinity. By means of glutamine synthetase, glutamine is formed as a nontoxic transport form of ammonia. At the same time, it also serves to activate the urea cycle (= *temporary ammonia detoxification*). (s. fig. 3.13)

▶ **Urea cycle:** *Carbamoyl phosphate synthetase* is of decisive importance in the detoxification process. However, it requires a relatively high concentration of NH_4^+. An increase in enzyme activity (and thus in urea synthesis) is not only rapidly achieved by an elevation in NH_4^+, but also by ATP and *ornithine*. N-acetylglutamate serves as a further enzyme activator, becoming active within one hour. In the long term (within 3–7 days), glucocorticoids and glucagon cause an increase in carbamoyl phosphate synthetase activity. • From the hepatocyte cytosol, NH_4^+ travels to the mitochondria, where it is enzymatically restructured into carbamoyl phosphate. NH_4^+ may also be formed in the mitochondria through glutamine splitting. The mitochondrial linkage of *carbamoyl phosphate* and ornithine leads, by means of ornithine carbamoyl transferase, to the formation of *citrullin*. This reaches the cytosol and combines, under ATP consumption, with aspartate (by means of argininosuccinate synthetase) to form *argininosuccinate*. The latter is split (by means of argininosuccinate lyase) into arginine and fumarate. *Fumarate* enters the citric acid cycle. *Arginine* is split (by means of arginase) into ornithine and *urea* – a reaction reported by A. Kossel and H.D. Dakin as early as 1904. (quot. 46) *Ornithine* again reaches the mitochondria to be reincorporated in the cycle. (s. fig. 3.12)

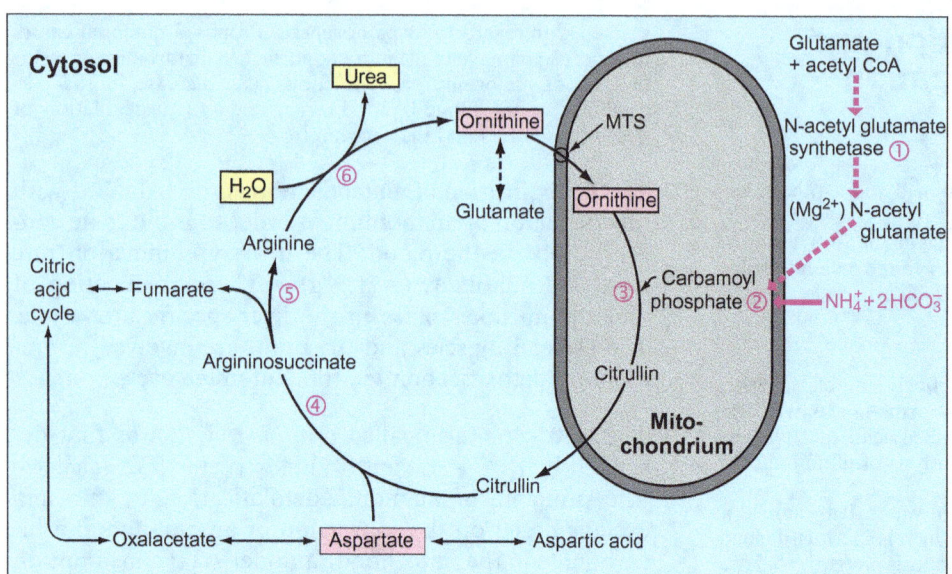

Fig. 3.12: Diagram showing the ammonia detoxification process in the urea cycle (= ornithine cycle) (H. A. Krebs, K. Henseleit, 1932) (A. L. Lehninger, 1979)

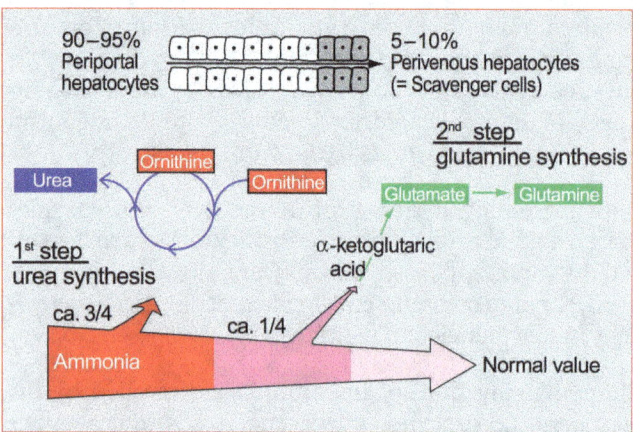

Fig. 3.13: Diagram showing the urea and glutamine cycle in the liver acinus

As a rule, 2 mol bicarbonate are required for the synthesis of 1 mol urea. The amount of urea eliminated in the urine is approximately 500 mmol/day (ca. 30 g). Normally, only about 25% of the capacity of the urea cycle are used. It is therefore virtually impossible for hyperammonaemia to be a sequela to isolated NH_4^+ hyperproduction alone. • In patients with liver cirrhosis, the capacity for urea synthesis is reduced by approximately 80%, i.e. there is a considerable decrease in ammonia detoxification in the periportal field, predominantly due to a function loss on the part of the perivenous scavenger cells.

Alkalosis and hypokalaemia (possibly caused by secondary hyperaldosteronism or use of diuretics) shift the dissociation constant towards free, toxic NH_3. By contrast, ammonia is considered — in a process resembling a vicious circle — to be a secondary stimulus for aldosterone production. • Thiazide diuretics in particular put an overload on the detoxification capacity of the scavenger cells. This is because of an insufficient supply of bicarbonate for carbamoyl phosphate synthetase reaction due to diuretic-induced inhibition of the mitochondrial carboanhydrase.

13.2 Glutamine cycle

▶ In **glutamine synthesis**, glutamate is initially formed by the binding of NH_4^+ to α-ketoglutaric acid, which is converted into glutamine through ATP-dependent amidation by means of glutamine synthetase. This synthetase is found in the microsomes and mitochondria of the hepatocytes as well as of the muscle and brain cells. Glutamine synthesis is not a liver-specific process. *Glutamine constitutes the non-toxic transport form of NH_4^+ between the tissues.* Glutamine synthesis and glutamate transport take place in the *perivenous* zone, whereas the glutaminase reaction occurs in the *periportal* zone (= **intercellular glutamine cycle**).

The *glutamine cycle* and the urea cycle are economically sequenced. The *urea cycle* localized in the periportal field requires a high concentration of NH_4^+, which is likewise available in the sinusoidal blood of that area. Through the glutaminase reaction, which is also localized in the periportal field, an additional amount of NH_4^+ is released by glutamine splitting for stimulation of urea synthesis (= high capacity with low affinity). • By contrast, glutamine synthetase shows a high affinity for NH_4^+, so that even small amounts of ammonium, which have escaped the urea cycle, are "temporarily" detoxified by the *glutamine synthesis* taking place in the perivenous blood (= low capacity with high affinity). Only 8% of the perivenous hepatocytes are needed for fixation of residual ammonia. (s. fig. 3.13)

The glutamine formed in the *liver* is released into the systemic circulation. Through arterial blood, the *brain* is also supplied with ammonium (approximately 10% of the plasma concentration). Detoxification is effected via glutamine synthesis. The glutamine formed in the brain enters the blood circulation. In the *muscles*, ammonium is also converted into glutamine through the pathway of glutamine synthesis and passed into the blood. Glutamine travels from the blood to the *kidneys*, where it is

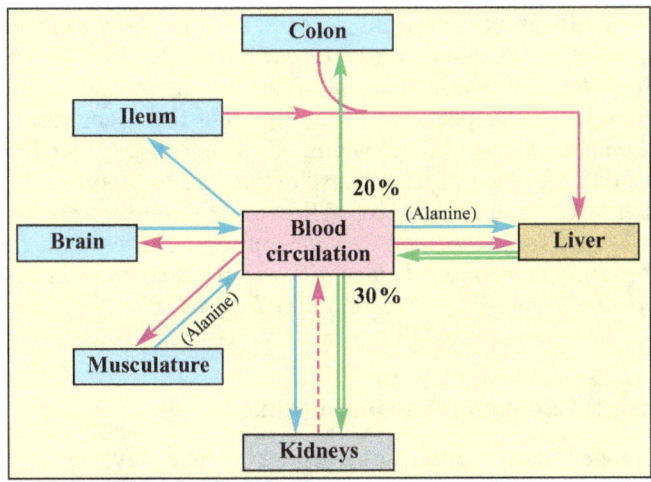

Fig. 3.14: Schematic diagram showing ammonium metabolism and the organs which are involved via the blood circulation (blue = glutamine, red = NH_4^+, green = urea)

split into glutamate and ammonia by glutaminase. NH_3 is excreted in the urine. Glutamine is also released into the *small intestine*, where it serves as the main source of energy for mucosal cells. The ammonia liberated by splitting is transported as NH_4^+ through the portal vein to the liver for detoxification. (s. fig. 3.14) • NH_4^+ is rapidly converted into a *nontoxic form*. This is done by (*1.*) transfer to a ketonic acid with formation of a corresponding amino acid, (*2.*) formation of carbamoyl phosphate, and (*3.*) formation of the acid amide of glutaminic acid (= *temporary ammonia detoxification*). The nitrogen from the acid amide group of glutamine remains in the metabolism for various syntheses. This group of acid amides is therefore called the *ammonium storage group*.

13.3 Bicarbonate neutralization

A high amount of bicarbonate is constantly being produced in the body. Degradation of 100 g protein yields approximately 1 mol bicarbonate (= 61 g). Bicarbonate neutralization takes place via the urea cycle too, as the synthesis of 1 mol urea requires 2 mol bicarbonate. Besides the lungs and kidneys, the liver therefore also plays an important role in acid-base metabolism and is partly responsible for pH homoeostasis.

The pH value in the portal vein drops in the case of increased urea synthesis. This decrease corresponds to the consumption of HCO_3^-. At the same time, intrahepatic and extrahepatic glutamine synthesis is reduced. When the pH value falls in the blood, corresponding amounts of bicarbonate must be made available for the compensation of *metabolic acidosis*. This amount of HCO_3^- is then not available for urea synthesis, which results in a curbing of the urea cycle. Additionally, the glutaminase reaction is reduced, and there is a decline in the intramitochondrial production of bicarbonate as a result of decreased carbonic anhydrase activity, with a further curbing of the urea cycle. At the same time, an increase is observed in hepatic glutamine synthesis, and (by augmentation of the pH-regulated glutamine degradation in the kidneys) the definitive urinary elimination of surplus NH_4^+ is achieved (= *renal ammoniogenesis*) − without simultaneously influencing the acid-base metabolism. • The rise in the blood pH value is followed by an increase in urea synthesis: in *metabolic alkalosis*, the uptake of NH_4^+ and HCO_3^- by the mitochondria is enhanced with an elevated consumption of bicarbonate for increased urea synthesis. In the mitochondria, CO_2 is converted spontaneously or by carbonic anhydrase into H-ions and bicarbonate.

Thus the **bicarbonate buffer** in the liver with its components CO_2 and HCO_3^- is also used for maintaining pH homoeostasis. The various cellular and subcellular compartments can only keep their own specific pH values constant provided the pH value of the extracellular space is not subject to major fluctuations. A constant balance between the formation and excretion of CO_2 and HCO_3^- must therefore be guaranteed. • **Bicarbonate neutralization** takes place, energy-driven and irreversibly, in the urea cycle. In this

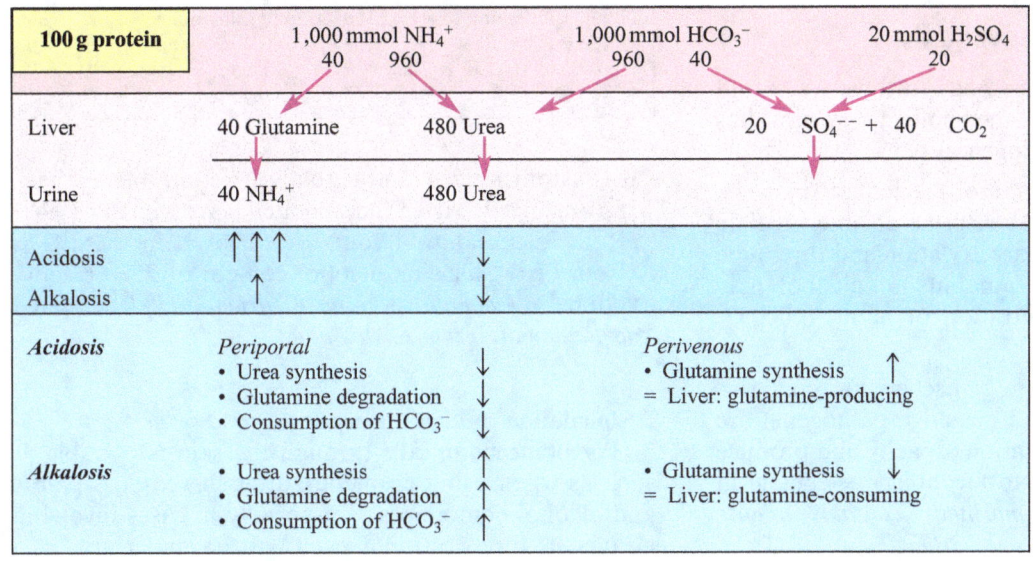

Fig. 3.15: Tabular survey of catabolites of 100 g protein and their hepatic and renal metabolic pathways, including excretion in the urine under normal metabolic-acidosic and metabolic-alkalotic conditions. (If no other units are specified, the data are in mmol)

context, HCO_3^- is considered to be a relatively strong base, whereas NH_4^+ is regarded as a weak acid.

The following mean metabolic values apply to the **degradation of 100 g protein**: ca. 1,000 mmol NH_4^+, ca. 1,000 mmol HCO_3^-, 20 mmol SO_4^{--} and 3 mol CO_2 (0.5 mol CO_2/day are additionally formed in urea synthesis and sulphuric acid neutralization). Some 40 mmol HCO_3^- are buffered by 20 mmol H_2SO_4. • The amounts of 960 mmol NH_4^+ and 960 mmol HCO_3^- give a total of 480 mmol urea reaching the kidneys. Furthermore, 40 mmol NH_4^+ are transferred as *glutamine* from the liver to the kidneys, where they are again split to give 40 mmol NH_4^+. (s. fig. 3.15)

The **acid-base metabolism** is influenced by the pH- and HCO_3^--regulated switchover of ammonium detoxification from urea to glutamine formation. In acidosis, bicarbonate is conserved by curbing hepatic urea synthesis; in alkalosis, however, bicarbonate is consumed by enhancing hepatic urea synthesis. (1, 30, 31)

14 Alcohol uptake and degradation

Alcohol is the designation for hydrocarbons in which the H-atoms are substituted by one or several hydroxyl groups (−OH).

> According to the **number of OH groups**, a subdivision is made into *6 alcohol types*: 1-valent (= alcohols), 2-valent (= glycols), 3-valent (= glycerins), 4-valent (= erythritols), 5-valent (= pentitols), and 6-valent (= hexitols).
> According to the **binding type of the OH group**, a distinction is drawn between primary (−CH$_2$−OH), secondary (=CH−OH) and tertiary (≡C−OH) alcohols.
> The **nomenclature** follows two principles: (*1.*) the ending "ol" is added to the name of the paraffin hydrocarbon (e.g. methanol), or (*2.*) the name of the corresponding alkyl group is placed before the word alcohol (e.g. methyl alcohol).

The term "alcohol" which is generally applied in medicine corresponds to the chemical compound ethanol or ethyl alcohol. Its empirical formula is either **C_2H_5OH** or **CH_3-CH_2-OH**.

14.1 Endogenous alcohol synthesis

Alcohol may be formed in the body in three ways, and therefore a cellular alcohol-metabolizing system has evolved in the course of phylogenesis:

1. Under physiological conditions, alcohol may be formed in **intermediary metabolism** as an intermediate product, e.g. in pyruvate decarboxylation and threonine degradation. Here minimal amounts of alcohol may arise (blood alcohol concentration of about 0.0009−0.001‰).

2. Some **intestinal bacteria** (e.g. Escherichia coli, salmonellae, and especially gram-negative pathogens) are also equipped with a fermentation capacity and produce small amounts of alcohol. No alcohol is detectable in the stool, however. *Blood normally contains minute quantities of alcohol (on average 0.012 g/l).*

3. Endogenous intestinal fermentation may occur in the case of an excessive intake of carbohydrates in the diet (e.g. fruit juices, farinaceous food, raw fruit and vegetables), in the presence of certain **intestinal fungi** (e.g. *Candida species* [C. albicans, C. tropicalis, C. stellatoidea, C. glabrata, C. parapsilosis, C. guilliermondii, C. kefyr, C. robusta, etc.] as well as *Saccharomyces cerevisiae* and some types of *Torulopsis* and *Trichosporum*). *In this way, amounts of alcohol corresponding to a blood alcohol level of 0.15−0.30‰ may be produced.*

14.2 Exogenous alcohol uptake

Exogenous alcohol uptake occurs in three ways:

1. **Oral** consumption of alcohol in various forms:
   − alcoholic beverages
   − alcoholic home remedies
   − alcohol contained in drugs
   − alcohol contained in food (e.g. kephir, bread)
   − alcohol-"free" fruit juices are allowed to have an alcohol content of up to 0.5% by volume due to fermentation in the bottle
   − alcohol-"free" beers have an alcohol content of up to 0.4% by volume
   − alcohol produced from fruit, e.g. intestinal fermentation of the durian (*Durio Zibethinus*).

Too little attention has been paid to the alcohol content of **drugs,** or the respective content has generally been considered negligible. In this context, we found the following relevant data: In the 1993 *"Rote Liste"**, 902 drugs had an alcohol content of between 5% and >81% by volume; the corresponding figure for 1996 was 854 out of 11,714 preparations (= 7.3%).

* "Rote Liste" (= "Red List": German Pharmaceutical Directory)

Red List	1993	1996		1993	1996
−10% in volume =	147	114	51−60% in volume =	121	161
11−20% in volume =	166	196	61−70% in volume =	72	90
21−30% in volume =	121	127	71−80% in volume =	3	6
31−40% in volume =	126	130	>81% in volume =	10	10
41−50% in volume =	133	147	no data =	3	−

> It is astonishing − and actually irresponsible − that 15 (out of 89) "liver therapeutics" given in the 1994 „Rote Liste" and 14 (out of 95) given in the 1997 „Rote Liste" have an alcohol content of 25−66% in volume. • *Alcoholics who have "dried out" should pay particular attention to this point!*

2. **Inhalation** of alcohol vapour.
3. **Percutaneous** uptake through the skin is possible − such as when using cosmetics, after-shave, gloss paints and alcohol compresses − especially in cases involving an increased resorption capacity of the epidermis.

14.3 Alcohol absorption

Only small amounts of alcohol are absorbed by the oral mucosa. About 20 to 30% are absorbed in the stomach and 70 to 80% in the duodenum and the upper section of the small intestine. The extent and speed of absorption are influenced by various factors. (69) (s. tab. 3.20)

Increased gastric ADH activity and/or inhibition of absorption
1. Full stomach
2. Kind of food
– rich in proteins, rich in fats
– rich in fibre
3. Slow drinking
4. Low alcohol concentration
5. Pyloric stenosis
Reduced gastric ADH activity and/or acceleration of absorption
1. Empty stomach
2. Kind of alcoholic beverage
– sweet or hot
– carbonated
3. Rapid drinking
4. High alcohol concentration
5. Gastric resection

Tab. 3.20: Factors influencing the absorption of alcohol

Due to a number of **influencing factors,** the amounts of alcohol absorbed per time unit vary greatly in the individual case. Thus the rate of hepatocyte exposure to alcohol is also influenced. Furthermore, different absorption rates occur depending on the mental state (e. g. balanced mood, aggressive excitation, exhaustion accompanied by resignation) and the physical condition (e. g. resting, carrying out heavy work).

Absorption of alcohol in the gastrointestinal tract takes place far more rapidly than its degradation. As a result, accumulation of alcohol, even at toxic levels, readily occurs. Alcohol is completely absorbed in the upper gastrointestinal tract and transported to the liver via the portal vein. Thereafter, alcohol dissolves in the body fluids and is distributed to all organs depending on their water content. On average, the body's water content amounts to 65%, the average water content of blood being 83%. When a diffusion balance has been achieved between the blood and the tissues (after about 45–90 minutes), the alcohol concentration in the blood is 1.27 times higher than in the body tissues. Five minutes after its uptake, it is already detectable in the blood. Maximum concentrations are reached after 30–60 minutes. In obese people, blood alcohol levels are considerably higher than in persons of normal weight.

14.4 Biochemical parameters of alcohol uptake

The **caloric value** of alcohol is 7.1 cal/g (= 29.7 kJ). In the case of alcoholic beverages with calorie-containing ingredients, it is necessary to add the calories for carbohydrates (4.0 cal/g) and, if applicable, for protein (4.0 cal/g) as well as for fat (9.0 cal/g). • The **quantity** of alcohol should be determined using enzymatic or chromatographical methods. (s. tab. 3.21)

Beverage	Alcohol content (vol. % per beverage)	Alcohol content (grams/litre per beverage)
export, pils, weissbier	4–6	32.0–48.0
bockbier, doppelbock	6–9	48.0–72.0
apple wine	4–6	32.0–64.0
sparkling wine	5–12	76.0–96.0
champagne	5–12	76.0–96.0
white wine	9–12.5	72.0–100.0
red wine	9.5–12.5	76.0–100.0
sherry, vermouth	17–20	136.0–160.0
advocaat, cherry brandy	20–25	160.0–200.0
herbal liqueur	30–37	240.0–296.0
corn schnapps,	32–38	256.0–304.0
calvados, gin, brandy	38–40	304.0–320.0
whisky, aquavit, cognac	40–44	320.0–352.0
vodka, rum	40–55	320.0–440.0
balm spirit	79	632.0

Tab. 3.21: Alkohol content in vol. % and grams per litre for a variety of beverages

The biochemical concentration is always based on pure alcohol in grams. (s. tab. 3.21) The amount ingested in grams (A) is calculated from the volume % of the drink multiplied by the specific weight of the alcohol (0.8):

$$\text{vol. \%} \times 0.8 = \text{amount of alcohol contained in grams/100 ml alcoholic beverage}$$

Example: Beer with 5 % volume alcohol contains 5 grams, i.e. 50 grams alcohol/litre. As alcohol is lighter than water, this is multiplied by 0.8. Therefore 50 x 0.8 = 40 grams alcohol/litre.

Conversely, alcohol volume percentage (vol. %) can also be calculated from the alcohol-gram content per litre:

$$\text{alcohol grams/litre} \times 1.25 = \text{vol. \%}$$

The **blood alcohol concentration** (BAC) is the balance between absorbed and eliminated amounts of alcohol. Fatty tissue takes up little alcohol and is incapable of degrading it. Here the various factors influencing absorption are not considered. (s. tab. 3.20) The BAC is calculated using *Widmark's formula* (E. M. P. WIDMARK, 1922):

$$A = c \times p \times r$$

whereby A represents the amount of alcohol (in g), c the blood alcohol concentration (in ‰), p the body weight (in kg), and r a reduction factor of 0.7 for men and 0.6 for women.

The **alcohol level** (‰) is given in grams of ethanol per 1,000 ml blood and is calculated on the basis of the following formula:

$$c = \frac{A}{p \times r}$$

Example: One glass of beer of 0.2 l and with 5% alcohol in volume contains 8 g pure alcohol. In the case of a man weighing 70 kg this corresponds to a ratio of 8:49 (70 x 0.7) = 0.16‰.

14.5 Alcohol degradation

The capacity to degrade alcohol is, to a high degree, genetically determined. Approximately 90% are degraded by the liver. A small percentage (<10%) is also metabolized in the stomach by means of gastric alcohol dehydrogenase. The ADH activity of the gastric mucosa is reduced in women, in old age, following administration of cimetidine and after gastric resection as well as in cases of chronic alcohol abuse (more markedly so in women than in men). Up to 8% are eliminated unchanged via the lungs and the skin, whereas around 1% is excreted in the urine. Some 10–15% are degraded enzymatically by the gastric mucosa and around 80% by the liver. Alcohol elimination increases considerably in the case of chronic alcohol consumption.

The metabolization rate of alcohol amounts to 1.9–3.2 mmol × kg^{-1} × hr^{-1}, i.e. 88–146 mg alcohol/kg BW/hr for a single intake in a healthy organism; the maximum degradation capacity is about 240 g alcohol/24 hr. Following completed absorption and diffusion balance between blood and tissues, alcohol is degraded in a linear manner at a constant reaction speed. The maximum degradation of alcohol in men with a body weight of 70 kg is calculated to be 168 g within 24 hours, the corresponding value for women being 143 g. At a rough estimate, 0.7–1 g alcohol/hr is broken down per 10 kg BW, meaning that the blood alcohol level is reduced by 0.10–0.15‰ per hour. In the case of protein deficiency (<20–25 g protein/day), the degradation capacity is reduced by 28–49%. This is demonstrated in fasting (36 hours) with a 43% decrease in the degradation rate, which is attributable to the associated increase in fatty acid oxidation. (8, 69, 78, 86)

The **lethal concentration** is 4.2–4.8 g/l (although, in individual cases, people have survived higher concentrations). The **lethal dose** is 2.5–3.5 g/kg BW when alcohol ingestion occurs over a period of 1–2 hours (e.g. in a drinking bet) or 300–800 g alcohol in total, depending on the individual case. (s. fig. 28.6!)

The **consumption of oxygen** for alcohol degradation in the liver is very high: approximately 75% (in alcohol intoxication 85% and more) of the hepatocyte O$_2$-uptake is used for the oxidative metabolization of alcohol. Therefore the hepatocytes are in a state of relative hypoxia. This may lead to a severe disturbance in many physiological processes of intermediary metabolism. The period of oxygen-consuming alcohol degradation is thus associated with increased vulnerability of the liver cell to further damaging factors.

A total of **three enzyme systems**, which can be differentiated by column chromatography, are available in the liver cells for alcohol degradation. These enzyme systems differ with regard to hepatocellular localization and biochemical properties. (s. tab. 3.22)

1. Alcohol dehydrogenase (ADH)
2. Microsomal ethanol-oxidizing system (MEOS)
3. Catalase

Criteria	ADH	MEOS	Catalase
Intracellular localization	Cytosol	Endoplasmic reticulum	Peroxisomes
Cofactor pH optimum	NAD 11	NADPH; O$_2$ 6.9–7.5	H$_2$O$_2$ 5.5
Substrate specificity – Methanol – Ethanol – Propanol – Butanol – Pentol	 ++ +++ ++++ ++++ ++++	 ++ ++++ +++ ++ +	 ++++ ++++ (+) ∅ ∅
Increase in enzyme activity following chronic consumption of alcohol	∅	++++ (♂ > ♀)	∅

Tab. 3.22: Localization-related and biochemical differences of the three enzyme systems responsible for alcohol degradation

1. **Alcohol dehydrogenase** (ADH) is of great relevance for alcohol degradation. It is not available before the 3rd year of life and is localized in the cytosol of the hepatocyte, predominantly in the centre of the liver lobule. ADH is a zinc-dependent enzyme; in cases of *zinc deficiency* (as caused by alcohol abuse in particular), there is a loss of activity with further diminution of alcohol metabolization. So far, five isoenzymes (ADH$_{1-5}$) with additional subgroups have been identified; in the meantime, another gastric ADH isoenzyme has been detected in the gastric mucosal cells. The activity of gastric ADH depends, for example, on gender, age, drug intake and potential colonization with Helicobacter pylori. • An "atypical ADH$_{2.2}$" (with three to six times higher activity) occurs in Europeans in 5–20% of cases, the respective frequency for East Asians (e.g. Japanese, Chinese, Koreans) being 80–98%. The increased occurrence of the *"flushing syndrome"* in these races is based on this "atypical ADH" and on a genetic reduction in the ALDH$_1$ isoenzyme. (s. tab. 3.23) (s. p. 69) (8, 55, 72)

ADH 4 and ADH 5 can only rarely be demonstrated. Both possess a low affinity with alcohol; they are therefore of no importance for degradation purposes. ADH 4 is only found in the gastric mucosa. It is to be noted that cimetidine and ranitidine inhibit the ADH of the liver and the gastric mucosa, thus elevating the blood alcohol level. This is, however, not the case with famotidine. • In patients with liver disease, ADH activity is reduced — and therefore alcohol degradation as well.

ADH also oxygenates methanol into toxic formaldehyde. Consequently, ethanol should be administered in order to inhibit the breakdown of methanol in cases of methanol intoxication.

Class	Allele	Localization
I	ADH 1 ADH 2.1 ADH 2.2 ADH 2.3 ADH 3.1 ADH 3.2	liver, stomach liver, stomach liver, stomach liver, stomach liver, stomach liver, stomach
II	ADH 4	liver, stomach
III	ADH 5	liver, stomach
IV		stomach

Tab. 3.23: Isoenzymes of ADH in the liver and in gastric mucosa

Saturation of the enzyme ADH is already achieved at a blood alcohol concentration of 0.5‰, with full enzyme activity occurring at 0.2–0.5‰. Thus a maximum rate of alcohol degradation is reached at these relatively low concentrations. • There is no *induction of the enzyme ADH* following chronic alcohol consumption. Higher alcohol concentrations as well as protein deficiency, sexual hormones, thyroidal hormones, etc. may even cause a decrease in ADH activity.

ADH catalyzes the oxidation process in the cytosol of the hepatocyte, forming a complex of ethanol, ADH and NAD^+. The reaction consists in transferring the hydrogen from the ethanol molecule to NAD^+ with parallel formation of acetaldehyde.

$$CH_3-CH_2-OH + NAD^+ \longrightarrow CH_3-CHO + NADH + H^+$$

In a subsequent and likewise NAD-dependent reaction, the highly toxic acetaldehyde is converted to acetic acid in the mitochondria by way of aldehyde dehydrogenase (ALDH). The resulting NADH is then reoxidized. (55, 72) (s. fig. 3.16)

$$CH_3-CHO + NAD^+ + H_2O \longrightarrow CH_3-COOH + NADH + H^+$$

The speed of alcohol degradation by ADH is determined by the **reoxidation rate** of NADH to NAD. The metabolization of 1 mol alcohol yields 2 mol $NAD + H^+$. This leads to a massive shift in the redox status of the liver cell in favour of reduction. Alcohol degradation would cease if NADH were not continuously reoxidized. Thus the degradation of alcohol is limited by all NADH-oxidizing processes taking place in the hepatocyte. The reoxidation of NADH, i.e. the removal of alcohol hydrogen, occurs through the oxidation of hydrogen to water in the mitochondrial respiratory chain, whereby energy is produced. An inhibition of the respiratory chain by specific inhibitors almost completely stops the degradation of alcohol. Acetic acid is released into the blood, where it is converted to acetyl CoA in the extrahepatic tissues. It is included in the citric acid and fatty acid cycles as well as in cholesterol synthesis, or is oxidized to CO_2. • *Acetic acid is the final product of alcohol degradation.* (s. fig. 3.16)

Alcohol hydrogen is transferred via the *malate-aspartate cycle* from the cytosol to the *mitochondrial respiratory chain*. The passage of 1 mol-reducing equivalents is effected by transporting 1 mol malate and 1 mol glutamate into the mitochondria and simultaneously removing 1 mol α-ketoglutarate and 1 mol aspartate from the mitochondria. In this way, cytosol hydrogen enters the respiratory chain, which is functionally embedded in the citric acid cycle.

2. The **microsomal ethanol-oxidizing system** (MEOS) (C. S. Lieber, L. M. DeCarli, 1968, 1970) is the second enzyme system involved in alcohol degradation (10–20%). It is localized in the endoplasmic reticulum, mainly in perivenous hepatocytes. Men invariably show higher MEOS activity than women, but many other factors (nutrition, age) are involved. With regard to its localization and its mixed-function oxidation system of cytochrome P 450 and cytochrome P 450 reductase, MEOS corresponds to the biotransformation system for the breakdown of foreign substances. **CYP 2E1** is a relatively alcohol-specific isoenzyme, which breaks down large quantities of alcohol into hepatotoxic acetaldehyde. Further isoenzymes are 1A2, 2A6, 2B6, 2D6, and 3A4. • MEOS is usually localized in centroacinar hepatocytes, where there is already minimal O_2 partial pressure. Consequently, the large amount of O_2 required to break down the alcohol triggers alcohol-toxic liver damage in the centre of the lobule. As a cofactor, MEOS requires molecular oxygen plus NADPH. Moreover, it contains phospholipids, whose role is not known. Normally, alcohol degradation via MEOS plays a minor role because of the lower substrate affinity involved. MEOS becomes increasingly active, however, with regular alcohol consumption and higher alcohol levels in the blood (>0.5‰). (s. fig. 3.16)

$$CH_3-CH_2-OH + NADPH + H^+ + O_2 \longrightarrow CH_3-CHO + NADP^+ + 2H_2O$$

MEOS is induced by chronic alcohol consumption, so that both the degradation of alcohol and the metabolization of foreign substances (and drugs) are accelerated with regular alcohol ingestion; some industrial solvents and carcinogens are also more highly activated. This is only possible, however, if no alcohol is present in the body during the uptake of foreign substances because that would result in a competitive inhibitory effect. Thus alcohol consumers have an increased metabolization capacity for foreign substances when sober (= *higher dose*

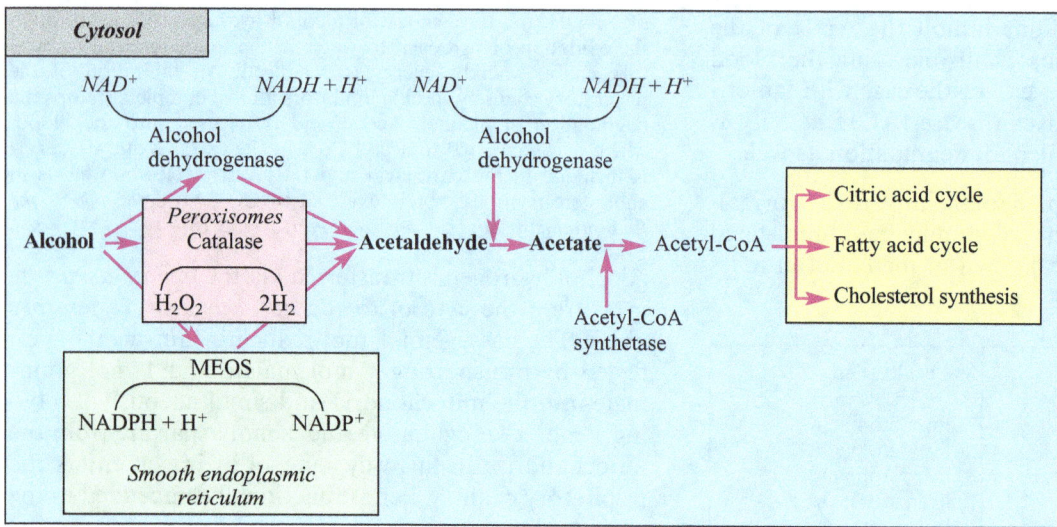

Fig. 3.16: Diagram showing alcohol degradation in the liver cell by means of alcohol dehydrogenase (ADH), catalase and the microsomal-ethanol oxidizing system (MEOS) as well as by aldehyde dehydrogenase (ALDH)

tolerance), which is due to increased induction of MEOS, whereas the breakdown of foreign substances is slowed down under alcohol consumption (= *higher dose sensitivity*). Enzyme induction sets in after two to three days of alcohol intake, even in the case of higher concentrations, and persists for up to three weeks after discontinuing consumption. ADH and MEOS metabolize alcohol to acetaldehyde: both enzyme systems have their own specific reaction and activity. For alcohol oxidation, MEOS does not require ADH either in an obligatory or in a facultative sense. Accelerated metabolization of foreign material due to increased MEOS activity may also lead to the formation of *biotoxometabolites*. (s. p. 59) (s. figs. 3.11, 3.16)

3. **Catalase** (D. KEILIN et al., 1945) is localized in the peroxisomes; alcohol is oxidized via intermediate steps to xanthine by xanthine oxidase. This releases H_2O_2, which is deactivated with the help of glutathione and then split into oxygen and water. This peroxidase reaction degrades alcohol to acetaldehyde. (11) However, in the case of chronic alcohol consumption, glutathione is bound to acetaldehyde with the result that the released H_2O_2 can intensify lipid oxidation. (s. fig. 3.16)

$$CH_3-CH_2-OH + H_2O_2 \longrightarrow CH_3-CHO + 2H_2O$$

Catalase activity only occurs in alcohol concentrations of >1‰, with alcohol acting as a hydrogen donor. Chronic alcohol intake has no effect on catalase activity. The reaction time is determined by the amont of H_2O_2 available. Oxidative alcohol degradation by catalase (approx. 2%) is of little importance under physiological conditions. It differs greatly from ADH and MEOS. (s. tab. 3.22)

All three oxidative pathways of alcohol degradation lead to the formation of **acetaldehyde** within the cytosol of hepatocytes, preferably in the perivenous area. But around 20% of Kupffer cells are also damaged by the acetaldehyde. These then release highly reactive cytotoxins into the extracellular space, which may lead to endotoxinaemia. The oxidation of alcohol to form acetaldehyde and its reduction to an acetate require NAD as a cofactor, which is then reduced to NADH. Permanent overloading of the system shifts the NAD/NADH ratio towards NADH, i.e. hepatic redox status. • This is the major cause of numerous hepatocellular *metabolic disorders* such as (1.) reduced activity of the tricarboxylic cycle, (2.) reduced fatty acid oxidation, (3.) reduced gluconeogenesis, (4.) increased triglycerine synthesis, and (5.) lactic acidosis. • Acetaldehyde is a reactive molecule.

Biochemical effects of acetaldehyde:
– covalent bond with phospholipids and proteins
– alkaloid-like complex formation
– release of prostaglandins
– separation of pyridoxal-6-phosphate from the protein bond
– peroxidation of lipids
– binding to cellular membranes
– stimulation of collagen synthesis in Ito cells
– inhibition of fatty acid oxidation
– inhibition of lipoprotein secretion from the liver cell
– immunogenic effectiveness
– membrane damaged by lipid peroxidation
– suppression of oxidative phosphorylation
– shift in redox status (NAD/NADH)
– deactivation of glutathione
– diminished leukocytic defence mechanisms

Toxic acetaldehyde resulting from alcohol oxidation is almost completely oxidized to acetate in the liver cell by **aldehyde dehydrogenase** (ALDH). For this purpose, various NAD-dependent ALDH isoenzymes are available. Isoenzyme II is bound to the mitochondrial matrix, while isoenzymes I, III and IV are found in the cytosol as well as in the microsomes and, to a lesser degree, in the mitochondria. They also exhibit biochemical differences. Acetaldehyde can be oxidized either by ALDH or by xanthine oxidase during the formation of acetate from H_2O_2, with the potential appearance of lipid peroxidations. Following chronic intake of alcohol, the activity of mitochondrial ALDH is reduced with an increase in acetaldehyde, partly due to diminished NADH reoxidation in the mitochondria. A genetically determined $ALDH_2$ deficiency, first discovered in the Japanese with an incidence of about 50% (H. W. GOEDDE et al., 1979), is considered to be a further cause of alcohol intolerance in the form of catecholamine-induced vasodilation with potential dysphoric symptoms (*"flushing syndrome"*) (s. p. 66). Increased production of acetaldehyde may also be attributed to microsomal enzyme induction of MEOS. (s. fig. 3.16)

▶ Increased acetaldehyde concentrations in the liver cell lead to severe morphological damage, especially in the mitochondria and the cytoskeleton, and to increased lipid peroxidations.

15 Reticuloendothelial system

▶ As early as 1893, M. PAVLOV had established in his clinical investigations that the liver had an antitoxic function: following a ligature of the portal vein, the blood was led past the liver, which resulted in toxication symptoms in the form of fever and nephritis. • *In 1924 the term "reticuloendothelial system" (RES) was coined by L. A. ASCHOFF.* He used this term to describe a widely distributed cellular functional system in the organism, composed of sessile and circulating macrophages of mesenchymal origin. These cells had a marked phagocytic capability for particulate material. The RES was demonstrable in the liver in particular. • Thus 30 years after the first observation made by PAVLOV, the significance of the liver as an important defence system was confirmed.

15.1 Systematics and nomenclature

The macrophages stored in the *reticuloendothelial system* are found in the CNS as microglia, and in the spleen, lymph nodes, thymus, tonsils and bone marrow in the form of reticulum cells. They occur as sinus wall cells in the spleen and bone marrow, but mainly in the liver in the form of sinusendothelial, Kupffer, Ito and PIT cells. (s. p. 24) About 90% of the total RES are localized in the liver.

Microphages develop from eosinophilic and neutrophilic granulocytes; they are capable of phagocytizing small particles (especially bacteria). • The *monocytary system* is localized in the connective tissue of nearly all organs. It consists of sessile histiocytes and mobile macrophages. Both cellular types may originate from blood monocytes, which are also part of this system.

▶ Based on morphological and functional criteria, it was suggested that the term "reticuloendothelial system" should be replaced by the designation **"reticulohistiocytary system" (RHS)** or the term **"mononuclear-phagocytizing system" (MPS)** (H.L. LANGEVOORD et al., 1970). This designation has not been widely accepted, however, so that the term **"reticuloendothelial system" (RES)** is still mainly used.

15.2 Functions of the hepatic RES

The total blood flow from the vessels of the splanchnic bed through the portal vein as well as the chyle and lymph flow through the thoracic duct must pass the liver. The same applies to the systemic blood flow. Therefore, the liver is indeed the central organ for checking the blood for foreign particles and substances as well as for endogenous substances which must be eliminated for physiological reasons. For these vital functions, the RES cells are provided with special **capabilities** (2, 43, 58, 63, 67, 79, 82):

1. Marked capability for phagocytosis
2. Marked capability for pinocytosis
3. Release of signal substances (cytokines, eicosanoids)
4. Endotoxin clearance
5. Abundance of enzymes
6. Capability for storing substances
7. Synthesis of the platelet-activating factor (PAF)
8. Synthesis of matrix components (collagenase, fibronectin, proteoglycans)

1. Filter function: The sinusendothelial cells are equipped with numerous pores of various diameters, depending on their different functions. Larger molecules and particles are hereby filtered out and kept away from the liver parenchyma.

2. Phagocytosis function: Owing to the favourable localization of the Kupffer and sinusendothelial cells in the sinusoidal blood flow, they are able to phagocytize any foreign colloidal or particulate substrates, endogenous macromolecules, altered erythrocytes, autologous altered protein, tumour cells, tissue particles, immune complexes, bacteria, fungi, etc. For this purpose, Kupffer cells are equipped with a special surface-ciliated border and stellate branches, which act as mechanical trapping mechanisms. Moreover, they carry specific receptors for carbohydrate components as well as for the Fc part of the IgG molecule and for complement C_3. They also possess lysosomal enzymes, yet in much lower amounts than do the sinusendothelial cells. The degradation of bilirubin and haemoglobin as well as the transport of iron take place in Kupffer cells. The intensity of hepatic phagocytosis shows a reverse correlation with the rate of blood flow in the liver, which is of clinical significance. Tumour cells, which are intensively phagocytized by Kupffer cells, provoke liver metastases to a lesser extent than do less phagocytized tumour cells. Exogenous structures are submitted to very intensive phagocytosis by the RES — as are higher molecular weight foreign proteins.

3. Metabolization of foreign substances: Sinusendothelial cells are also capable of endocytosis and, due to their extensive enzyme equipment, in a perfect position to metabolize different kinds of foreign substances. They have a good stock of acid phosphatase, acid DNase, β-N-acetylglucosaminidase, β-glucuronidase, arylsulphatase (A, B), cholesterol esterase, collagenases, etc.

4. Clearance function: Sinusendothelial cells assume a clearance function regarding *connective-tissue macromolecules* (e. g. mucopolysaccharides) through endocytosis and enzymatic breakdown. The clearance of bigger molecules takes place more rapidly than that of smaller ones. Mucopolysaccharides (e. g. components of coagulation, of blood groups and of immune substances) are constantly produced in the intermediary metabolism. It is imperative to clear such substances from the blood. The biosynthesis of mucopolysaccharides in the endoplasmic reticulum is stimulated by androgens and STH, and is inhibited by glucocorticoids. • The RES plays a special role in the breakdown of polypeptide- and polysaccharide-containing *fibrinolysis activators* (e. g. tissue plasminogen activator). Insufficient breakdown of these substances is a major cause of impaired hepatogenic haemostasis. • Its capacity to remove *antigens* from the blood circulation means that the liver is the central organ for nonspecific defence processes. Bacteria, viruses and macromolecules, which generally pass from the gastrointestinal tract through the portal vein into the sinusoidal blood, may function as antigens. Likewise, immune complexes are taken up and eliminated by the RES. However, hepatocytes are also able to eliminate antigens and immune complexes by means of their IgG-Fc and C_3 receptors. Although the phagocytosis capacity of Kupffer cells is 14 times higher than that of hepatocytes, the liver contains twice as many hepatocytes as Kupffer cells. RES cells and hepatocytes form a barrier against antigens and immune complexes. The liver indirectly participates in humoral and cellular immune reactions by means of this phagocytosis of antigenic substances. (58, 75, 79)

5. Elimination of endotoxins: Bacterial lipopolysaccharides moving from the intestine through the portal vein to the liver are detoxified in the RES (especially by Kupffer cells) under physiological conditions. Hepatocytes are also capable of taking up and detoxicating endotoxins. In the case of reduced clearance function of the RES and augmented formation of endotoxins or their increased influx into the bloodstream, endotoxinaemia with secondary liver cell damage may occur. (63)

6. Metabolization of lipoproteins: The hepatic RES assumes an important role in the clearance of cholesterol esters and lipoproteins. The uptake of lipoproteins by Kupffer cells is 3–4 times higher than by liver cells, even though the absolute uptake capacity of liver cells is naturally much higher due to their being twice as numerous. The hepatic endothelial cells bind to their surface chylomicrons, VLDL, LDL and HDL, all of which contain apolipoprotein E. These cells also exhibit lipase and cholesterol esterase activity. Under pathological conditions, Kupffer cells may take up cholesterol esters in amounts high enough for conversion into so-called *foam cells*. Blockage of the hepatic RES leads to a decline in lipoprotein clearance, potentially resulting in hyperlipoproteinaemia. Moreover, Ito cells are able to store lipids.

Influence on the RES: The activity of the RES may be intensified by **opsonins** (A. E. WRIGHT et al., 1903). Opsonins are endogenous substances which can attach themselves to bacteria, fungi, foreign bodies, immune complexes, etc. and thus promote their phagocytosis. Fibronectin (so-called "molecular adhesive"), which is formed in liver cells (and possibly also in RES cells), is a major opsonin. The group of opsonins further comprises the immunoglobulins G, M, C_{3b} and C_5. Glucans, zymosan and oestrogens also enhance the activity of the RES, whereas higher concentrations of alcohol, glucocorticoids and endotoxins cause an inhibition in its activity.

Production of signal substances: Kupffer cells also secrete substances influencing the metabolism of liver cells. The synthesis of **acute phase proteins** is stimulated accordingly. In this connection, it is particularly worth mentioning the *antiproteases*, which are able to interrupt proteolytic reaction cascades. Such reactions are triggered in inflammatory processes or tissue lesions by *proteases* formed in the liver. • Potential overactivity of these reaction cascades is prevented by the antiproteases produced by Kupffer cells. Thus the liver itself is capable of controlling these reactive processes. The ideal localization and morphology of hepatic RES cells facilitate optimum functional interplay.

This cooperation not only exists between the sinusoidal cells, but also with the hepatocytes: (*1.*) endothelial and Kupffer cells complement each other through various mechanisms of endocytosis and different pathways of enzymatic clearance; (*2.*) as a double barrier, they protect the liver cells from toxic and undesired substances, even to the extent of "self-sacrifice"; (*3.*) they intervene in the metabolism of liver cells with self-produced substances; (*4.*) they send "signal substances" like cytokines (e. g. interferons) and eicosanoids (e. g. leukotrienes) to the liver cells for independent control of biochemical and biomolecular reaction cascades.

▶ Hepatic RES is of great relevance both under physiological and pathological conditions. In the past 10 years, an array of experimental results yielding further knowledge of the RES have become available – yet, many questions remain unanswered or are under discussion. Moreover, there are hardly any procedures for measuring RES functions in a clinical setting. Nevertheless, the RES might offer various possibilities for targeted therapeutic approaches.

16 Radicals and antioxidants

16.1 Definition

H_2O_2 is produced by superoxide dismutase or peroxisomal oxidases. It is, in fact, not a radical. However, due to its immense ability to penetrate biological membranes, H_2O_2 may well have a direct damaging effect on many biological systems. It is above all a precursor of hydroxyl radical. H_2O_2 is reduced by catalase and glutathione-peroxidase activity.

Radicals and **reactive oxygen intermediates** (ROI), or activated oxygen species, are atomic or molecular substrates formed during the reduction of oxygen in the body. In their outer molecular surface, they carry one or several unpaired electrons. Consequently, they are highly reactive — but also short-lived. Their half-life ranges between 10^{-9} (HO˙) and 10 seconds. The small amounts of incidentally released superoxides are usually inactivated by high concentrations of protective enzymes (SOD, glutathione peroxidase, catalase) contained in the mitochondria. Superoxide anion radicals are one of the chief sources of oxygen toxicity. They are mainly formed in the electron transport chain of the mitochondria and endoplasmic reticulum. As so-called free radicals, they are available in a chemically free form. As unstable, highly reactive molecules, radicals are able to capture an electron from adjacent stable molecules in order to stabilize their own atomic structure. The adjacent molecule concerned is thus turned into a radical itself: the process starts anew and a chain reaction (e.g. lipid peroxidation) sets in. This chain reaction is only interrupted when the radical encounters another radical or when it is rendered harmless by an antioxidant. Hydroxyl radical (HO˙), which is produced by water hydrolysis, is the most reactive of all free oxygen radicals. It can react with almost every organic molecule. In their capacity as prooxidants, the reactive oxygen intermediates are both free radicals and non-radical molecules. Several types of radicals are of relevance in biological systems. (s. tab. 3.24)

HO˙	hydroxyl radical
RO˙	alkoxyl radical
$^1O_2$	singlet oxygen
$O_2^{˙-}$	superoxide radical
$HO_2˙$	perhydroxy radical
H_2O_2	hydrogen peroxide
ROO˙	peroxyl radical
NO˙	nitric oxide radical
L˙	fatty acid alkyl radical
LO˙	fatty acid alkoxyl radical
LOO˙	fatty acid peroxyl radical

Tab. 3.24: Radicals and reactive oxygen species

16.2 Formation and importance of free radicals

Mitochondria constitute the main source of oxygen in the cell. This is principally effected by the respiratory chain in the inner mitochondrial membrane. Moreover, the additional formation of cellular oxygen takes place through the transport of electrons in the nuclear membranes and microsomes. Eosinophilic granulocytes are believed to be active in creating oxygen radicals. Cytochrome P 450 yields reactive oxygen intermediates. Thus it can be seen that the presence of oxygen in virtually all cellular structures allows the ubiquitous formation of oxygen radicals to take place. • Exogenous sources of free radicals include UV radiation, X-rays, tobacco smoke, organic solvents, pesticides, etc. (s. tab. 3.24) (22, 36, 56)

$$\text{Haber-Weiss reaction: } O_2^{˙} + H_2O_2 \longrightarrow OH^{˙} + OH + O_2$$

$$\text{Fenton reaction: } Fe^{2+} + H_2O_2 \longrightarrow Fe^{3+} + OH˙ + OH^-$$

All oxygen-reducing metabolic processes are accompanied by the development of reactive oxygen intermediates, which have a high level of efficacy. Their formation is therefore a prerequisite for a variety of specific cellular metabolic processes. This applies especially to biomolecular reactions relating to phagocytosis and biotransformation, the metabolism of arachidonic acid, collagen, iron, purine, neurotransmitters and histamine, the blood coagulation system, enzymatic activities of flavoproteins, iron-sulphur proteins, quinones, etc. In many reactions, one to two oxygen atoms are inserted into the carbon skeleton of metabolic intermediates by way of monooxygenases or bioxygenases. This process is catalyzed by a reductant. The catalytic enzyme activity of oxygenases is most probably influenced by reactive oxygen intermediates.

> The view is held that the **origin of life** in the universe ca. 3.5 billion years ago is attributable to the formation of radicals: amino acids and nucleotides may well have been formed from simple reduced components of the primitive atmosphere, assuming free radicals were generated through solar radiation (D. HARMANN, 1986).

16.3 Balance between formation and inactivation

The *biological necessity* regarding the presence of reactive oxygen intermediates to ensure the smooth course of multiple biomolecular metabolic processes is undisputed. The prerequisite is, however, that the concentration of both prooxidants and free radicals is kept (under physiological conditions) within the required cellular "normal range" by a subtle coupling mechanism between formation and inactivation. This is accomplished by morphologically and functionally intact biological membranes and by a physiological inactivation system of enzymatic and non-enzymatic mechanisms (= *antioxidants*). These antioxidants are either formed endogenously or are supplied by an exogenous route. The *antioxidative capacity* is the total of all endogenous and exogenous defence mechanisms; this process guarantees the oxidative balance.

Maintaining a physiological equilibrium (= concentration) of cell-formed reactive oxygen intermediates by means of highly sensitive regulation mechanisms is a fundamental process of biomolecular homoeostasis.

16.4 Scavengers and antioxidants

Scavengers are substances which bind and eliminate free radicals at the *right* moment, in the *right* concentration, with *high* selectivity and with a *stoichiometric* reaction.

Antioxidants are substances which keep oxygen radicals or "reactive oxygen intermediates" (ROI) under control by means of subtle time- and concentration-specific inactivation. This can be the result of enzymatic or non-enzymatic processes. The most important antioxidants in this respect are catalase, superoxide dismutase and glutathione peroxidase as well as DNA repair enzymes (such as DNA glycosylases, endonucleases and DNA ligases) in close cooperation with p53.

Antioxidants were used by the Egyptians for the **preservation of corpses** of high-ranking persons (E.E. CROSS et al., 1987). • The use of scavengers (e.g. 2-mercaptoethylamine) has also been reported to **prolong the lives** of mammals by up to 30% (E.L. SCHNEIDER et al., 1985).

It was not until thirty years after the copper-containing protein erythrocuprein was discovered (T. MANN, D. KEILING, 1939) that its enzymatic nature was proved. At that time, this protein was shown to convert superoxide radicals into molecular oxygen and H_2O_2 (J.M. MCCORD, 1969; I. FRIDOVICH, 1969); it was FRIDOVICH who coined the term *superoxide dismutase* (SOD). This presumably most important of antioxidants accelerates the conversion of superoxide radicals 10,000 times more effectively than spontaneous dismutation.

1. $O_2^\bullet + O_2^\bullet + 2H^+ \xrightarrow{SOD} H_2O_2 + O_2$

2. Catalase reaction: $H_2O_2 + H_2O_2 \longrightarrow 2H_2O + O_2$

Antioxidants participate in various reaction steps in the elimination of reactive oxygen species. Such intervention is possible due to their varying chemical structures and capabilities. A number of different substances have been recognized as more or less potent antioxidants. (s. tab. 3.25). In addition, the following drugs may also act as scavengers: *indomethacin, acetylsalicylic acid, penicillamine* and *allopurinol* (which blocks the xanthine oxidase reaction and prevents the formation of $O_2^\bullet$ and H_2O_2) as well as *deferoxamine* (which inhibits hydroxyl radicals in Fenton's reaction). Antioxidants have a synergistic effect, i.e. they display a mutual reinforcing action, but they cannot replace each other. Thus hydrogen superoxide is eliminated by catalase and the reduction in organic peroxides is catalyzed by glutathione peroxidase through *reduced glutathione* (= GSH). (7, 76, 81, 82, 84)

3. $2\,GSH + H_2O_2 \longrightarrow GSSG + H_2O + H_2O$

To ensure a physiological balance between the formation and the inactivation of free radicals − or reactive oxygen species − numerous substrates (such as enzymes, vitamins, provitamins, trace elements, transport proteins, amino acids) must always be available in adequate quantities and in an active form.

Endogenous antioxidants	Exogenous antioxidants
catalases glutathione peroxidases glutathione reductases glutathione transferases superoxide dismutases	β-carotene N-acetylcysteine polyphenols sulphides vitamin C vitamin E
albumin α-lipoic acid bilirubin coenzyme Q10 coeruloplasmin glutathione transferrin uric acid, *etc.*	flavonoids (Carduus marianus, Ginkgo biloba, Quercetin, *etc.*)
	Adjuvant substances
	manganese selenium zinc, *etc.*

Tab. 3.25: Substrates acting as scavengers (endogenous and exogenous antioxidants) or adjuvant substances

16.5 Pathophysiology

Depending on the metabolic status within the various compartments of the cell, fluctuations in the concentration of radicals or reactive oxygen species may occur.

Continued **reduction** or cessation in the formation of oxygen radicals (especially in the area of the mitochondria, nuclear membranes or microsomes) is eventually fatal to the cell. • An uncontrolled *increase* in the cellular formation of superoxide dismutase (as is found in mental disease, trisomy 21, etc.) may also entail dangerous disturbances in the cellular oxygen balance. • Moreover, a *change* in the physicochemical properties of superoxide dismutase under pathological conditions, which may lead to reduced enzyme activity and altered cell compartments, is being discussed as a further influencing factor.

An **increase** in free radicals or reactive oxygen species is encountered in various diseases or metabolic disorders. This may lead to changes in cell metabolism and/or enhanced nonspecific reactions, and even cell death.

▶ The augmented formation of free radicals and their reduced inactivation are discussed as *pathogenetic factors*, e.g. irradiation, sunburn, autoimmune diseases, collagenoses, inflammatory (especially bacterial and viral) processes, operations, severe traumatization, myocardial ischaemia, intestinal ischaemia, colitis, haemoglobinopathies, atherosclerosis, haemorrhagic shock, cerebrovascular insult, Parkinson's disease, cataractogenesis, retrolental fibroplasia, chemical intoxication (e.g. CCl_4, smog, paraquat, adriamycin) and carcinogenesis – as well as the body's ageing process, which is due among other things to extreme physical activity, alcohol abuse and smoking. So-called **free radical diseases** are directly or indirectly caused by oxidative stress.

▶ Moreover, the occurrence of fluorescing *pigments* in the form of lipofuscin, ceroid and porphyrin (as found in Wilson's disease, haemochromatosis, Dubin-Johnson-Sprinz syndrome, porphyria cutanea tarda and abuse of analgesics – as well as pigmentation in old age) is a reliable sign of excessive free-radical formation in the cell.

From the biomolecular viewpoint, increased concentrations of radicals lead to hazardous biological reactions, e.g. (*1.*) lipid peroxidation, (*2.*) oxidation of SH- and NH_2-groups in proteins, and (*3.*) hydroxylation of nucleic acids with modification of DNA. • Radicals cause oxidative changes and damage by withdrawing electrons from other molecules. • **Oxidative stress** *is defined as an imbalance between free-radical formation and antioxidative capacity.* Oxidative stress causes oxidation of mitochondrial NAD(P)H and produces ROS in the mitochondria. This increases free CA^{++} levels in the mitochondria and activates the serine proteases, which can kill the cell. Direct damage to the hepatocytes by ROS may trigger so-called inflammatory factors and cause more cellular damage. • Low GSH levels in hepatocytes render them particularly vulnerable to oxidative stress. (18, 36, 73, 87) (s. p. 408)

16.6 Lipid peroxidation

In lipid peroxidation, unsaturated fatty acids are peroxidized in the biological membranes of cells and their organelles. This leads to chain breaks in fatty acids with insertion of hydrophilic groups and cis-trans-isomerization. Membrane-bound proteins are damaged. Lipid radicals (L˙) are transformed into unstable lipid-peroxy radicals (L00˙). • Lipid peroxidation markers include *malondialdehyde* and *4-hydroxynonenal*. (18, 34, 73, 87) (s. figs. 2.19; 21.12)

Further sequelae to lipid peroxidation include inhibition of membrane-bound, phospholipid-dependent sodium-potassium ATPase and calcium ATPase with various changes in the electrolyte milieu, especially calcium overloading of the cell with subsequent cell damage and cell death as well as inhibition of adenylate cyclase. This results in loss of function in the mitochondria and microsomes. Damage to the DNA leads to enzyme defects or impaired enzyme synthesis, which triggers more metabolic changes. This also causes a cellular overload with calcium and subsequent activation of proteases, which in turn affect other enzyme systems in such a way that indeed further radicals are produced instead of the usual degradation products being formed. (s. fig. 21.12)

The data currently available on the formation of radicals and antioxidants have also contributed to clarifying various pathophysiological relationships in the field of hepatology. The hazardous interplay between the increased formation of free radicals, the occurrence of lipid peroxidation and cell damage – in the sense of a vicious circle – has provided a better understanding not only of the mechanisms causing toxic and inflammatory damage to liver cells, but also of cell death.

17 Cellular transport processes

The functioning of a cell (hepatocytes included) depends essentially on the orderly and targeted transport of molecules. This applies equally to absorption into the cell, intracellular transport, and discharge from the cell, whereby individual substances may either remain unaltered or undergo biochemical changes. The most important substances required by liver cells are water, electrolytes, trace elements, proteins, lipids, carbohydrates, bile salts, and bilirubin. The structure of the **cell membrane** and its functional capacities are key factors in these transport processes. (5, 15, 24, 28, 33, 35, 41, 44, 45, 53, 54, 61, 62, 64, 68, 90, 94) (s. p. 31) (s. fig. 2.19)

Cellular transport primarily occurs with the help of (*1.*) ionic channels, (*2.*) carrier proteins, (*3.*) pumps, and (*4.*) vesicles. These transport processes may be in the form of active, passive or vesicular mechanisms.

17.1 Passive transport

Passive transport through the cell membrane rarely requires any form of energy. It takes place along electrochemical gradients through either free or facilitated diffusion.

Free diffusion: This process is the simplest form of transport through the cell membrane. It is, however, only possible for small molecules (e.g. water, urea, and dissolved gases such as oxygen, carbon dioxide, ammonia). Molecules are transported from areas of high concentration to areas of low concentration until equilibrium is achieved. No energy is required here. This process is not exposed to any form of competitive inhibition.

Facilitated diffusion: Large molecules (e.g. glucose, protein, organic ions) cannot diffuse across the cell membrane barrier unaided. Mechanisms in the form of channels or transport proteins (= carriers) are therefore required to enable molecules to penetrate the impermeable membrane when entering and leaving the cell. These mechanisms sometimes require energy and may be exposed to competitive inhibition. Each of the *ion channels* contains a special channel protein with water-filled pores through which the molecules can diffuse. A selection filter distinguishes between the individual ions such as Ca^{++}, Na^+, K^+, and Cl^-. These ion channels can alter their permeability by opening or closing. There are also water channels. • *Transport proteins* are part of the cell membrane (ectoproteins, endoproteins, membrane-penetrating proteins). (s. fig. 2.19) They facilitate the substrate-specific passage through the membrane. In order to carry out this function, they are activated by physical, chemical or hormonal stimulants. However, these carriers can also be blocked by inhibitors. If the carrier system becomes overloaded, its transport capacity is reduced and the process slows down. Individual substances are bound to specific transport proteins during their passage through the membrane.

Uniporter		Transport of 1 substance in one direction
Cotransporter	*Symporter*	Transport of 2–3 substances stoichiometrically in one direction (= *positive plus-coupling*)
	Antiporter	Transport of 2–3 substances in the opposite direction (= *negative plus-coupling*)

17.2 Active transport

Active transport through the cell membrane always requires energy. This is derived from splitting ATP. Transport takes place against an electrochemical gradient, i.e. in an "uphill" movement. • *Primary active transport* occurs when ATP splitting is directly linked to the transport process (as is the case with Na^+/K^+-ATPase). This can involve three different ATPase groups (known as P-, V- and F-ATPases). (53) The Na^+/K^+-ATPase consists of an essential ion pump which is found in all body cells. It acts as an antiporter. With each pump cycle 2 K^+ are transferred into the cell and 3 Na^+ are removed. This transport process uses up 30–70 % of the cell's energy capacity and is subject to competitive inhibition. It can be activated and displays substrate specificity as well as saturation kinetics. • *Secondary active transport* occurs when ATP splitting is part of another reaction (e.g. Na^+/glucose transport in intestinal mucosa) instead of being directly coupled with the transport process. • *Pumps* ensure active transport; the proteins involved are likewise ATPases, which split ATP hydrolytically on the inner side of the membrane. Each pump has a separate function, e.g. ion pumps, peptide pumps and pharmaceutical pumps.

17.3 Vesicular transport

Vesicular transport denotes the transport of macromolecules inside hepatocytes in the form of vesicles encased in a membrane. There are four forms of absorption and release: (*1.*) exocytosis, (*2.*) endocytosis, (*3.*) transcytosis, and (*4.*) diacytosis. (19, 23)

Exocytosis: Macromolecules are transferred from cytoplasmic secretory vesicles to the extracellular space; for this purpose the vesicles fuse with the cell membrane. After its contents have been released into the extracellular space, the vesicle frees itself from the external cell membrane and returns to the cytoplasm for the next transport sequence (= recycling). This process requires energy and is Ca^{++}-dependent. Exocytosis can be triggered by an external stimulus. This is then called *controlled exocytosis*. If there is no external stimulus, it is known as *constitutive exocytosis*.

Endocytosis: The term endocytosis denotes the *internalization* (= encasing) of molecules inside vesicles. This can take place in the form of *pinocytosis* (= fluid-phase endocytosis), whereby the molecules remain in a detached state with no membrane binding. It can also occur in the form of adsorptive endocytosis, whereby the molecules are bound to membrane receptors by a ligand and the whole complex is transported into the cell.

Transcytosis: In this process, the vesicles are moved from one cell pole to another without their contents changing.

Diacytosis: In this process, a part of the intact and internalized ligand receptor complex returns to the cell surface.

These vascular transport mechanisms within the hepatocytes require an intact cytoskeleton. This is because the transport of the membrane-encased vesicle keeps close to the cytoskeleton structures.

Motor proteins (e.g. microtubular kinesin, cytoplasmic dynein) move the vesicles. This requires energy from ATP. Vesicular transport also involves other cytoplasmic factors and is influenced by other effects (e.g. Ca^{++}, cAMP, C-protein kinases).

References:

1. **Atkinson, D.E., Camien, M.N.:** The role of urea synthesis in the removal of metabolic bicarbonate and the regulation of blood pH. Curr. Top. Cell. Reg. 1982; 21: 261–302
2. **Baas, J., Senninger, N., Elser, H.:** Das retikuloendotheliale System. Eine Übersicht über Funktion, Pathologie und neuere Meßmethoden. Z. Gastroenterol. 1994; 32: 117–123
3. **Bahar, R.J., Stolz, A.:** Bile acid transport. Gastroenterol. Clin. North Amer. 1999; 28: 27–58
4. **Bell, R.M., Ballas, L.M., Coleman, R.A.:** Lipid topogenesis. J. Lipid Res. 1980; 22: 391–403
5. **Berk, P.D., Stremmel, W.:** Hepatocellular uptake of organic ions. Progr. Liver Dis. 1986; 8: 125–144
6. **Bikle, D.P., Gree, E., Halloran, B., Haddad, J.G.:** Free 1,25-dihydroxy-vitamin D in serum from normal subjects, pregnant subjects and subjects with liver disease. J. Clin. Invest. 1984; 74: 1966–1971

7. **Bors, W., Saran, M.:** Radical scavenging by flavonoid antioxidants. Free Radic. Res. Commun. 1987; 2: 289–294
8. **Bosron, W.F., Li, T.K.:** Genetic determinations of alcohol and aldehyd dehydrogenases and alcohol metabolism. Semin. Liver Dis. 1981; 1: 179–188
9. **Bouwens, L., De Bleser, P., Vanderkerken, K., Geerts, B., Wisse, E.:** Liver cell heterogeneity: functions of non-parenchymal cells. Enzyme 1992; 46: 155–168
10. **Boyer, J.L.:** Bile duct epithelium: frontiers in transport physiology. Amer. J. Physiol. 1996; 270: 1–5
11. **Bradford, B.U., Enomoto, N., Ikejima, K., Rose, M.L., Bojes, H.K., Forman, D.T., Thurman, F.G.:** Peroxisomes are involved in the swift increase in alcohol metabolism. J. Pharm. Exper. Ther. 1999; 288: 254–259
12. **Bremner, J.:** Involvement of metallothioneins in hepatic metabolism of copper. J. Nutr. 1987; 117: 19–24
13. **Calvert, G.D., Abbey, M.:** Plasma lipoproteins apoproteins and proteins concerned with lipid metabolism. Adv. Clin. Chem. 1985; 24: 218–298
14. **Canbay, A., Bechmann, L., Gerken, G.:** Lipid metabolism in the liver. Zschr. Gastroenterol. 2007; 45: 35–41
15. **Chignard, N., Mergey, M., Veissiére, D., Parc, R., Capeau, J., Poupon, R., Paul, A., Housset, C.:** Bile acid transport and regulating functions in the human biliary epithelium. Hepatology 2001; 33: 496–503
16. **Christensen, H.E.:** Role of amino acid transport and countertransport in nutrition and metabolism. Physiol. Rev. 1990; 70: 43–70
17. **Clark, D.W.J.:** Genetically determined variability in acetylation and oxidation. Therapeutic implications. Drugs 1985; 29: 342–375
18. **Comparti, M.:** Biology of disease: lipid peroxidation and cellular damage in toxic liver injury. Lab. Invest. 1985; 53: 599–623
19. **Crawford, J.M.:** Role of vesicle-mediated transport pathways in hepatocellular bile secretion. Semin. Liver Dis. 1996; 16: 169–189
20. **De Silva, D.M., Askwith, C.C., Kaplan, J.:** Molecular mechanisms of iron uptake in eukaryotes. Physiol. Rev. 1996; 76: 31–47
21. **Eichelbaum, M.:** Genetische Polymorphismen des oxidativen Arzneimitteltelstoffwechsels. Therapeutische und toxikologische Implikationen. Internist 1983; 24: 117–127
22. **Elstner, E.F.:** Oxygen radicals – biochemical basis for their efficacy. Klin. Wschr. 1991; 69: 949–956
23. **Enrich, C., Pol, A., Calvo, M., Pons, M., Jäckle, St.:** Dissection of the multifunctional "receptor-recycling" endocytic compartment of hepatocytes. Hepatology 1999; 30: 1115–1120
24. **Ettinger, M.J., Darwish, H.M., Schmitt, R.C.:** Mechanism of copper transport from plasma to hepatocytes. Fed. Proc. 1986; 45: 2800–2804
25. **Falk Foundation e. V.:** Freiburg 79108/Germany (available).
26. **Gebhardt, R.:** Metabolic zonation of the liver: regulation and implications for liver function. Pharmac. Ther. 1992; 53: 275–354
27. **Genschel, J., Schmidt, H.H.J.:** HDL metabolism. Zschr. Gastroenterol. 2001; 39: 321–327
28. **Hagenbuch, B., Meier, P.J.:** Sinusoidal (basolateral) bile salt uptake systems in hepatocytes. Semin. Liver Dis. 1996; 16: 129–136
29. **Halliday, J.W., Powell, L.W.:** Ferritin metabolism and the liver. Semin. Liver Dis. 1984; 4: 207–216
30. **Häusinger, D.:** Organization of hepatic nitrogen metabolism and its relation to acid-base homeostasis. Klin. Wschr. 1990; 68: 1096–1101
31. **Häussinger, D.:** Liver regulation of acid-base balance. Min. Electr. Metab. 1997; 23: 249–252
32. **Hendriks, H.F.J., Verhoofstad, W.A.M.M., Brower, A., de Leeuw, A.M., Knook, D.L.:** Perisinusoidal fat-storing cells are the main vitamin A storage sites in rat liver. Exp. Cell Res. 1985; 160: 138–149
33. **Hofmann, A.F.:** Bile acid secretion, bile flow, and biliary lipid secretion in humans. Hepatology 1990; 12 (S): 17–25
34. **Horton, A.A., Fairhurst, S.:** Lipid peroxidation and mechanisms of toxicity. CRC Crit. Rev. Toxicol. 1987; 18: 27–79
35. **Jäger, W., Wilcox, H.G., Bitterle, T., Berr, F.:** Intracellular supply of phospholipids for biliary secretion: evidence for a nonvesicular transport component. Biochem. Biophys. Res. Comm. 2000; 268: 790–797
36. **Jaeschke, H.:** Reactive oxygen and mechanisms of inflammatory liver injury. J. Gastroenterol. Hepatol. 2000; 15: 718–724
37. **Yoon, Y.B., Hagey, L.R., Hofmann, A.F., Gurantz, D., Michelotti, E.L., Steinbach, J. H.:** Effect of side-chain shortening on the physiologic properties of bile acids: Hepatic transport and effect on biliary secretion of 23-nor-ursodeoxycholate in rodents. Gastroenterology 1986; 90: 837–852
38. **Jungermann, K.:** Metabolic zonation of liver parenchyma. Semin. Liver Dis. 1988; 8: 329–341
39. **Jungermann, K., Katz, N.:** Functional spezialization of different hepatocyte populations. Physiol. Rev. 1989; 69: 708–764
40. **Jungermann, K., Kietzmann, T.:** Oxygen: modulator of metabolic zonation and disease of the liver. Hepatology 2000; 31: 255–260
41. **Kamisako, T., Gabazza, E.C., Ishihara, T., Adachi, Y.:** Molecular aspects of organic transport across the plasma membrane of hepatocytes. J. Gastroenterol. Hepatol. 1999; 14: 405–412
42. **Kanno, N., LeSage, G., Glaser, S., Alvaro, C., Alpini, G.:** Functional heterogeneity of the intrahepatic biliary epithelium. Hepatology 2000; 31: 555–561
43. **Knolle, P.A., Gerken, G.:** Local control of the immune response in the liver. Immunol. Rev. 2000; 174; 21–34
44. **Kullak-Ublick, G.A.:** Regulation of organic anion and drug transporters of the sinusoidal membrane. J. Hepatol. 1999; 31: 563–573
45. **Kullak-Ublick, G.A., Stieger, B., Hagenbuch, B., Meier, P.J.:** Hepatic transport of bile salts. Semin. Liver Dis. 2000; 20: 273–292
46. **Kuntz, E.:** Die Aufklärung der Harnstoffsynthese in der Leberzelle vor 60 Jahren. Zum Gedenken an H. A. Krebs und K. Henseleit. In: Die hepatische Enzephalopathie. Aspekte der Diagnose und Behandlung. E. Kuntz (Hrsg.) Univ. Verlag Jena, 1992, 5–8
47. **Kuntz, H.-D.:** Glukuronidierungskapazität der Leber. Fortschr. Med. 1987; 105: 149–152
48. **Kuntz, H.-D., Femfert, U., May, B.:** Leber und Alter. Einfluß des Lebensalters auf Leberfunktion und Arzneimittelmetabolismus. Dtsch. Med. Wschr. 1987; 112: 757–759
49. **Kuntz, H.-D., Femfert, U., May, B.:** Pharmakokinetik von 7-Hydroxy-4-Methyl-2-H-benzofuran-2on als Funktionsprüfung für die Glukuronidierungskapazität der Leber. Verh. Dtsch. Ges. Inn. Med. 1983; 89: 630–633
50. **Kuntz, H.-D., Femfert, U., May, B.:** Biotransformation und biliäre Exkretion von Methylumbelliferon bei Patienten mit chronischer Stauungsleber. Verh. Dtsch. Ges. Inn. Med. 1984; 90: 1853–1856
51. **LeSage, G., Glaser, S., Alpini, G.:** Regulatory mechanisms of ductal bile secretion. Dig. Liver Dis. 2000; 32: 563–566
52. **Lindner, M.C.:** Other trace elements and the liver. Semin. Liver Dis. 1984; 4: 264–276
53. **Lomri, N., Fitz, J.G., Scharschmidt, B.F.:** Hepatocellular transport: role of ATP-binding cassette protein. Semin. Liver Dis. 1996; 16: 201–210
54. **Love, M.W., Dawson, P.A.:** New insights into bile acid transport. Curr. Opin. Lipid. 1998; 9: 225–229
55. **Lundquist, F.:** Acetaldehyde and aldehyde dehydrogenases: central problem in the studies of alcoholism. Eur. J. Clin. Invest. 1983; 13: 183–184
56. **McCord, J.M.:** The superoxyde free radical: its biochemistry and pathophysiology. Surgery 1983; 94: 412–414
57. **Medina, D., Morrison, D.:** Current ideas on selenium as a chemopreventive agent. Path. Immunopath. Res. 1988; 7: 187–199
58. **Mehal, W.Z., Azzaroli, F., Crispe, N.:** Immunology of the healthy liver: old questions and new insights. Gastroenterology 2001; 120: 250–260
59. **Mertz, W.:** Chromium, an ultra trace element. Chem. Scripta 1983; 21: 71–83
60. **Milman, N., Laursen, I., Podenphant, I., Asnaes, S.:** Trace elements in normal and cirrhotic human liver tissue. I. Iron, copper, zinc, selenium, manganese, titanium and lead measured by X-ray fluorescence spectrometry. Liver 1986; 6: 111–117
61. **Morgan, E.H., Baker, E.:** Iron uptake and metabolism by hepatocytes. Fed. Proc. 1986; 45: 2810–2816
62. **Müller, M., Jansen, P.L.M.:** The secretory function of the liver: new aspects of hepatobiliary transport. J. Hepatol. 1998; 28: 344–354
63. **Nagashima, I.:** Experimental study on endotoxinemia and reticuloendothelial system in hepatectomized cirrhotic rats. J. Japan. Surg. Soc. 1991; 92: 551–561
64. **Nathanson, M.H., Boyer, J.L.:** Mechanisms and regulation of bile secretion. Hepatology 1991; 14: 551–565
65. **Nebert, D.W., Russell, D.W.:** Clinical importance of the cytochromes P 450 (review). Lancet 2002; 360: 1155–1162
66. **Ockner, R.K., Weisiger, R.A., Gollan, J.L.:** Hepatic uptake of albumin bound substances: albumin receptor concept. Amer. J. Physiol. 1983; 245: 413–418
67. **Okada, S., Ohto, M., Kuniyasu, Y., Higashi, S., Arimizu, N., Uematsu, S.:** Estimation of the reticuloendothelial function by positron emission computed tomography (PET) study in chronic liver disease. (jap.) Japan. J. Gastroenterol. 1990; 87: 90–99
68. **Olkonen, V.M., Ikonen, E.:** Genetic defects of intrazellular-membrane transport. New Engl. J. Med. 2000; 343; 1095–1104
69. **Oneta, C.M., Simanowski, U.A., Martinez, M., Allali-Hassani, A. Parés, X., Homann, N., Conradt, C., Waldherr, R., Fiehn, W., Coutelle, C., Seitz, H.K.:** First pass metabolism of ethanol is strikingly influenced by the speed of gastric emptying. Gut 1998; 43: 612–619
70. **Pattison, S.E., Cousins, R.J.:** Zinc uptake and metabolism by hepatocytes. Fed. Proc. 1986; 45: 2805–2809
71. **Pilkis, S.J., Granner, D.K.:** Molecular physiology of the regulation of hepatic gluconeogenesis and glycolysis. Ann. Rev. Physiol. 1992; 54: 885–909
72. **Pocker, Y.:** Bioinorganic and bioorganic studies of liver alcohol dehydrogenase. Chem. Biol. Interact. 2001; 130: 383–393
73. **Poli, G., Albano, E., Dianzani, M.U.:** The role of lipid peroxidation in liver damage. Chem. Phys. Lipids 1987; 45: 117–142
74. **Prall, R.T., LaRusso, N.F.:** Biliary tract physiology. Curr. Opin. Gastroenterol. 2000; 16: 432–436
75. **Reynoso-Paz, S., Coppel, R.L., Mackay, I.R., Bass, N.M., Ansari, A.A., Gershwin, M.E.:** The immunobiology of bile and biliary epithelium. Hepatology 1999; 30: 351–357
76. **Robak, J., Gryglewski, R.J.:** Flavonoids are scavengers of superoxide anions. Biochem. Pharmacol. 1988; 37: 837–841
77. **Rosenthal, P., Pincus, M., Fink, D.:** Sex- and age-related differences in bilirubin concentrations in serum. Clin. Chem. 1984; 30: 1380–1382
78. **Seitz, H.K., Korsten, M.A., Lieber, C.S.:** Ethanol oxidation by intestinal microsomes: increased activity after chronic ethanol administration. Life Sci. 1979; 25: 1443–1448
79. **Seki, S., Habu, Y., Kawamura, T., Takeda, K., Dobashi, H., Ohkawa, T., Hiraide, H.:** The liver as a crucial organ in the first line of host defense: the roles of Kupffer cells, natural killer (NK) cells and NK 1.1 Ag+T cells in T helper 1 immune response. Immunol. Rev. 2000; 174: 35–46
80. **Sidransky, H., Murty, C.N., Verney, E.:** Nutritional control of protein synthesis. Studies related to tryptophan-induced stimulation of nucleocytoplasmatic translocation of mRNA in rat liver. Amer. J. Pathol. 1984; 117: 298–309
81. **Sies, H.:** Strategies of antioxidant defense. Eur. J. Biochem. 1993; 215: 213–219

82. **Smedsrod, B., Pertoft, H., Gustafson, St., Laurent, T.C.:** Scavenger functions of the liver endothelial cell. Biochem. J. 1990; 266: 313–327
83. **Solaas, K., Ulvestad, A., Soreide, O., Kase, B.F.:** Subcellular organization of bile acid amidation in human liver: a key issue in regulating the biosynthesis of bile salts. J. Lipid Res. 2000; 41: 1154–1162
84. **Stocker, R., Glaze, A. N., Ames, B. N.:** Antioxidant activity of albumin-bound bilirubin. Proc. Nat. Acad. Sci. 1987; 84: 5918–5922
85. **Stricker, B.H.C.:** Hepatic injury by drugs and environmental agents. Liver Ann. 1986; 5: 419–482
86. **Suchy, F.J., Ananthanarayanan, M.:** Bile salt excretory pump: Biology and pathobiology. J. Pediatr. Gastroenterol. Nutr. 2006; 43: (Suppl. 1); 10–16
87. **Suter, P.M., Schutz, Y., Jequier, E.:** The effect of ethanol on fat storage in healthy subjects. New Engl. J. Med. 1992; 326: 983–987
88. **Ungemach, F.R.:** Pathobiological mechanisms of hepatocellular damage following lipid peroxidation. Chem. Phys. Lipids 1987; 45: 171–205
89. **Vallee, B.L., Galdes, A.:** The metallobiochemistry of zinc enzymes. Adv. Enzymol. 1984; 56: 283–430
90. **Voigtmann, R.:** Selen. Dtsch. Med. Wschr. 1993; 118: 1094–1095
91. **Vulpe, C.D., Packman, S.:** Cellular copper transport. Ann. Rev. Nutr. 1995; 15: 293–322
92. **Weber, W.W., Hein, D.W.:** N-Acetylation pharmacogenetics. Pharmacol. Rev. 1985; 37: 25–79
93. **Wilson, G.E., Davis, R.E.:** Clinical chemistry of vitamin B_6. Adv. Clin. Chem. 1983; 23: 1–68
94. **Wolf, C.R., Moll, E., Friedberg, T., Oesch, F., Buchmann, A., Kuhlmann, W.D. Kunz, H.W.:** Characterization, localization and regulation of a novel phenobarbital-inducible form of cytochrome P 450, compared with three further P450-isoenzymes, NADPH P450-reductase, glutathione transferases and microsomal epoxide hydrolase. Carcinogenesis 1984; 5: 993–1001
95. **Wolkoff, A.W.:** Hepatocellular sinusoidal membrane organic anion transport and transporters. Semin. Liver Dis. 1996; 16: 121–127

Diagnostics in Liver Diseases
4 Clinical findings

		Page:
1	*Elements of liver diagnostics*	78
1.1	Diagnostic targets	79
1.2	Diagnostic pillars	79
1.3	Diagnostic accuracy	80
2	*Clinical findings*	80
2.1	*Anamnesis*	80
2.2	*Palpation*	81
2.2.1	Palpation of the liver	81
2.2.2	Palpation of the spleen	83
2.3	*Percussion*	83
2.3.1	Percussion of the liver	83
2.3.2	Percussion of the spleen	83
2.3.3	Ascites	83
2.3.4	Meteorism	83
2.4	*Inspection*	83
2.4.1	Chvostek's body type	84
2.4.2	Facies cirrhotica	84
2.4.3	Parotid enlargement	84
2.4.4	Hair changes	84
2.4.5	Jaundice	84
2.4.6	Spider naevus	84
2.4.7	Palmar/plantar erythema	85
2.4.8	Telangiectases	86
2.4.9	White nails	86
2.4.10	Muehrke's nail lines	86
2.4.11	Paper money skin	86
2.4.12	White spots on the skin	86
2.4.13	Smooth red tongue	86
2.4.14	Liver tongue	87
2.4.15	Lacquered lips	87
2.4.16	Gynaecomastia	87
2.4.17	Dupuytren's contracture	87
2.4.18	Pigmentation and striae	88
2.4.19	Inflammatory erythematous stigmata	88
2.4.20	Xanthelasmas and xanthomas	89
2.4.21	Scratch marks in pruritus	89
2.4.22	Eye changes	89
2.4.23	Drumstick fingers	90
2.4.24	Testicular atrophy	90
2.4.25	Cutaneous and mucosal haemorrhages	90
2.4.26	Vein dilatation	91
2.5	*Hepatic foetor*	91
2.6	*Fatigue*	91
2.7	*Auscultation*	92
3	*Liver check list*	92
	• References (1–48)	93
	(Figures 4.1–4.22; tables 4.1–4.3)	

4 Clinical findings

1 Elements of liver diagnostics

In the case of a disease, the basic requirement for systematic and appropriate therapy is the diagnosis. (34)

▶ When translated, the Greek word **"diagnosis"** means *"decision"*, *"differentiation"* or *"assessment"*. • A disease is identified by the information gained from the patients themselves (= *auto-anamnesis*) or their personal environment (= *external anamnesis*) as well as from diverse examination results (= *findings*).

The term **diagnosis** includes the nosological and systematic designation of a clinical picture and the sum total of the results, which provide a basis for medical action and therapeutic success.

The term **diagnostics** covers all measures aimed at identifying the development of a disease and ultimately producing a diagnosis.

A diagnosis should be *rational* (= *in terms of intellect*), that is to say logical and targeted. At the same time, however, the way it is arrived at must be *efficient and economical* (= *expedient*), i.e. financially viable (cost effective for the health service) as well as acceptable in terms of the strain it puts on the individual patient. • For this reason, economical and efficient diagnostics is by definition rational.

A rational diagnostic procedure is always economical and efficient when carried out at the hospital or in the doctor's surgery – even though it may be more expensive in individual cases. • Economical and efficient diagnostics must never become irrational!

These two basic requirements for rational and economical diagnostics are likewise true for detailed diagnosis (19) – even if a **detailed diagnosis** understandably entails greater reflection and higher costs. With a detailed diagnosis, however, particularly an **early diagnosis**, the therapeutic measures applied can be better targeted, more appropriate and indeed more successful – and ultimately less cost-intensive. (s. fig. 4.1)

▶ Each diagnostic step and each detailed diagnosis presents certain **difficulties** in terms of methodology and theory:

1. Emergency therapy may be urgently required **prior to** diagnosis.
2. Diagnostics may be **limited:**
   a. because examination techniques are (still) insufficiently developed,
   b. because of inadequate equipment for examination purposes,
   c. because they are refused by the patient.
3. All too often there is, unfortunately, a tendency to apply examination techniques on a broad and cost-intensive scale, and indeed "irrationally".

▶ In 1979 J. E. HARDISON drew up a *list of arguments* that are used to explain this kind of behaviour in medical practice, and which are equally applicable today (14):

1. the excuse that "everything has been done";
2. the excuse that if something is not done immediately, it will never be done at all;
3. the excuse that more has to be undertaken under inpatient conditions than at the doctor's surgery;
4. the academic excuse – as if there were such a thing as an academic or a non-academic diagnosis;
5. the father-mother excuse: "If it were my father or mother, I would do it like that";
6. the precluding excuse: "Well, perhaps we'll find something we never even thought of";
7. the legal excuse: "If we don't carry out the examination, we could be sued".

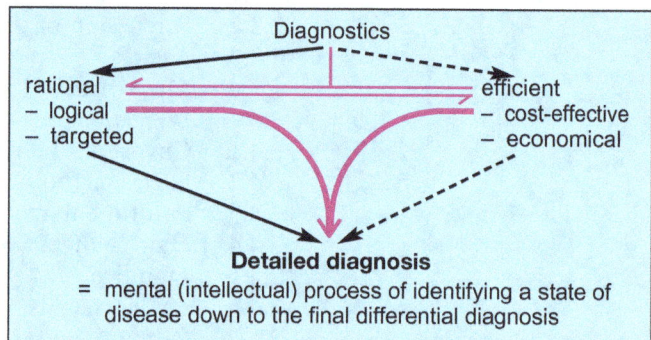

Fig. 4.1: Elements of diagnostics

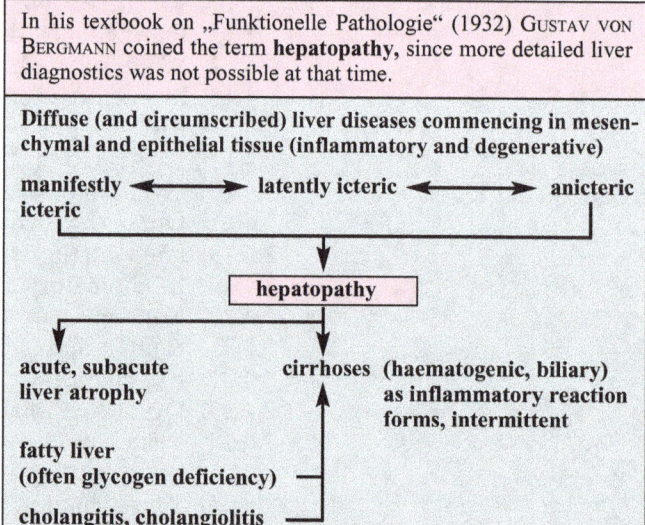

1st hepatological principle

The term "hepatopathy", coined by GUSTAV VON BERGMANN in 1932, and the expression "liver parenchymal damage", which has also been employed occasionally, should only be used to describe the so-called "prediagnostic stage" of liver disease.

In any form of suspected "hepatopathy", the preliminary steps towards reaching a **diagnosis** and ultimately the **detailed diagnosis**, whether at the doctor's surgery or at the hospital bedside, should always proceed rationally and economically by means of step-by-step systematic examination.

The impressive, almost "99%" certainty of present-day liver diagnostics is the outcome of the coordination of all available examination techniques that have meanwhile been perfected — in conjunction with the further development of sensitive and specific procedures.

1.1 Diagnostic targets

The seven main diagnostic questions (s. tab. 4.1) can be answered in nearly all cases using four sets of examinations (s. fig. 4.2) — provided all the necessary diagnostic channels can be applied. By repeatedly reviewing the activity and the function of the liver, it is possible to make reliable statements on the course of the disease, the success of therapy and the prognosis.

▶ In this context, **check lists** simplify and accelerate the examination procedure. It is most important that no key factors are forgotten and nothing is undertaken unnecessarily. (19) (s. figs. 4.22; 5.2; 15.3; 35.10) (s. tab. 29.7) • In addition, a **step-by-step programme** subdivided into minimum, necessary and maximum requirements (s. tab. 5.23) together with logically constructed **flow diagrams** (s. figs. 9.4; 13.7; 16.10, 16.17; 19.15; 22.9–12) facilitate the required rational and economical *"step-by-step diagnostics"*.

2nd hepatological principle

It is not **"what is done"** in terms of numerous examinations and chemical laboratory parameters that is ultimately decisive, but the clinical **interpretation** of the findings and the clinical consequences which result from that.

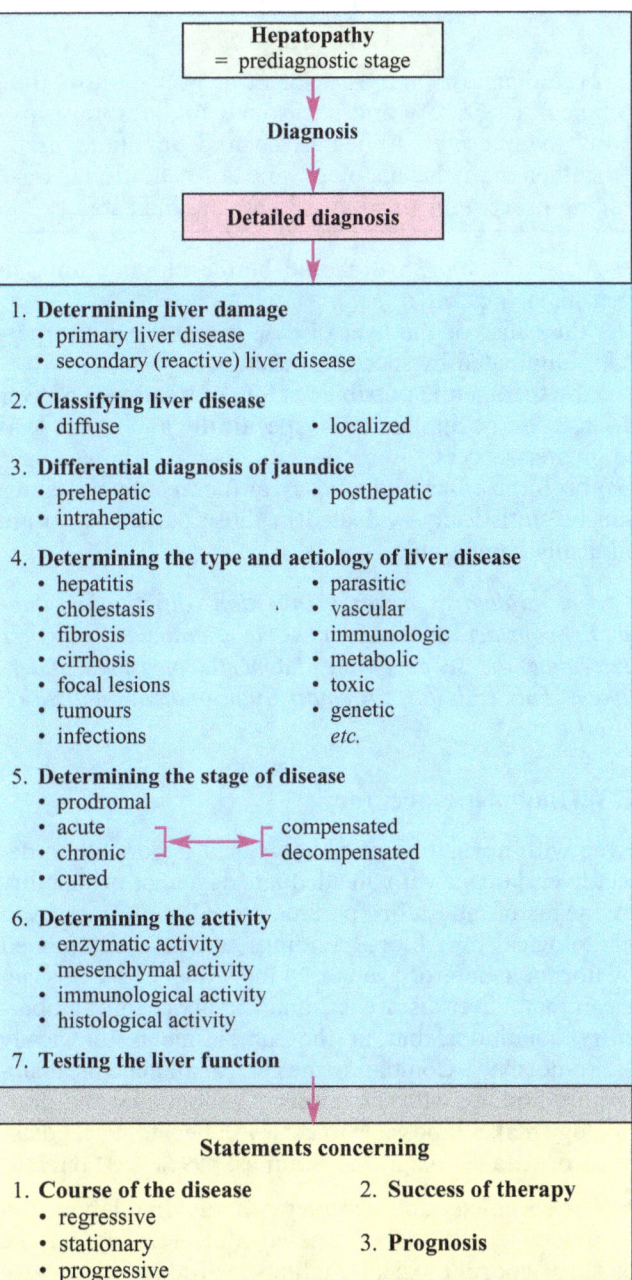

Tab. 4.1: Diagnostic targets and other relevant aspects in liver diseases

1.2 Diagnostic pillars

The target of a detailed diagnosis is generally achieved using various and mutually complementary examination techniques. Diagnostic methods in liver disease are founded on four diagnostic pillars, which are applied stepwise and nearly always provide the basis for an exact and detailed diagnosis. Complex or invasive techniques are only used in cases where they are clearly indicated. If the various examination procedures are inadequately coordinated and the results improperly interpreted, it is, unfortunately, all too easy to obtain "false-positive" or "false-negative" results. (19) (s. fig. 4.2)

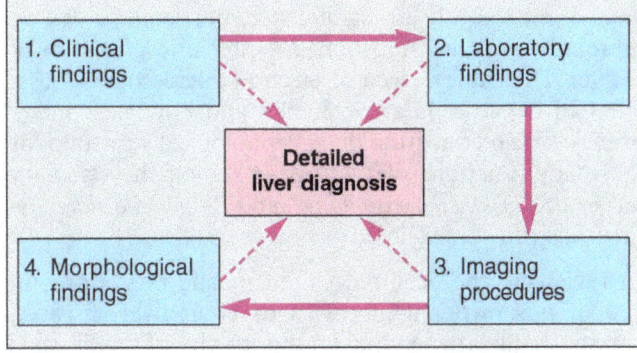

Fig. 4.2: Diagnostic pillars for detailed diagnosis in liver diseases

> *3rd hepatological principle*
>
> In the diagnosis and assessment of liver disease, the clinical, laboratory and ultrasound findings must always be interpreted integratively and simultaneously, together with the histology and any additional imaging procedures (insofar as these are indicated).

Clinical findings	30%
Laboratory parameters	81−96%
Ultrasonography	60−75%
Histology	82−95%
Laparoscopy	78−88%
Laparoscopy + histology	97%

Tab. 4.2: Accuracy of diagnostic procedures in various liver diseases (E. KUNTZ, 1987) (s. tab. 5.11)

▶ A *detailed diagnosis* should be the ultimate aim, so that in each case:
(*1.*) the cause of the liver disease is identified and perhaps eliminated by successful therapy;
(*2.*) the therapeutic possibilities for the treatment of liver disease can be applied more specifically and hence lead to greater success;
(*3.*) both the effect and efficacy of therapeutic measures can be statistically evaluated in those patients who are clinically comparable.

The hepatological issues in question, differential diagnostic considerations and possible therapeutic outcome determine the scope of the diagnostic measures undertaken. This calls for systematization and rationalization at all times.

> *4th hepatological principle*
>
> Up to now, no single examination method exists (be it a clinical, laboratory chemical, morphological or imaging procedure) which, in itself, allows a global statement to be made regarding a particular type of liver disease or liver dysfunction.

1.3 Diagnostic accuracy

Even with normal bioptic histology, it is possible to detect liver damage with an adequate degree of probability by means of laboratory parameters. • By contrast, even pathological liver biopsy findings can be accompanied by normal laboratory values. In individual cases, this can mean that a liver disease is "mute" under chemical laboratory conditions, but at the same time histologically "false-normal". Combining the clinical and chemical laboratory findings with the results of sonography and morphology makes it possible to achieve a hepatological diagnosis or detailed diagnosis of almost **"99%" certainty**.

▶ The **specificity** and **accuracy** of individual laboratory parameters used to be assessed almost solely on the basis of morphological findings. • Today, exact procedures are available for hepatological detailed diagnosis which provide excellent sensitivity and specificity (especially in the fields of serology and immunology). But they have by no means ousted the histological examination of the liver. On the contrary, **histology** has gained enormously in significance, particularly due to more advanced methods and a better interpretation of results. The same is true of **electron microscopic** assessment of hepatocellular organelles and biological membranes, which constitute the morphological substrate for the many functions of the liver. • Hence, the **visionary target** of *"organelle pathology"* and *"organelle diagnostics"* has proved feasible.

In reviewing the accuracy of diagnostic procedures in 520 of our own patients with different liver diseases, varying results (depending on the severity of the disease) were found. (s. tab. 4.2)

2 Clinical findings

At the forefront of liver diagnostics are the tried and tested methods of *anamnesis, inspection, palpation* and *percussion* or even *auscultation*. These specific medical examinations can be regarded as a safety net in daily routine diagnostics. Within the scope of the many examinations that take place at the doctor's surgery, these basic medical skills help to filter out patients with "suspected hepatopathy". Ascertaining the clinical findings is deemed to be the *1st diagnostic pillar* and, as such, constitutes the commencement of any diagnostic procedures focused on the liver. (s. fig. 4.2)

2.1 Anamnesis

The anamnesis is of particular significance for the clinical findings − and *is usually the first step towards establishing a diagnosis.*

Determining whether there has been any history of hepatobiliary disease in the *family* and establishing the geographic and ethnic origin of the patient are both key anamnestic factors. • It must be ascertained whether the *disease* has occurred suddenly, developed gradually, or simply not been noticed up to now. • It is also important to determine whether this is a *primary* or *secondary* liver disorder (the latter is a concomitant reaction which has occurred during a systemic illness or other organic disease). The anamnestic search for the cause of the infection in the patient should take into account viral, bacterial, parasitic and mycotic diseases. *(see chapters 22−26)* (s. tab. 4.1)

Anamnestic evidence of *alcoholism* or *drug abuse* and also personal questions relating to *sexual habits* should be handled with extreme care and sensitivity. Once one has gained the patient's trust, it is considerably easier to obtain the relevant details. • It is essential to establish whether the patient has been exposed to any *foreign sub-*

stances (medicines, herbal remedies, aphrodisiacs, chemicals). This can be done with the aid of the **check list** which we have been using for many years. (s. tab. 29.7) *(see chapters 29 and 30)*

It is mainly "targeted" **questioning** which sheds light on the possibility of liver disease.

> ▶ **Questions:**
> *"Targeted"* (i.e. specific) questions are most likely to lead to the *"target"*:
> – previous diseases of the liver or biliary tract?
> – previous operations?
> – previous blood transfusions (blood products)?
> – particular eating habits?
> – metabolic diseases (diabetes, gout, hyperlipidaemia, etc.)?
> – consumption of alcohol?
> – intake of medicaments?
> – occupation- or hobby-related liver noxae?
> – drug abuse?
> – journeys abroad?
> – sexual habits?
> – hereditary liver diseases?

Another group of anamnestic findings is based on the patient's subjective **complaints**. However, patients suffering from liver disorders frequently fail to recognize symptoms by themselves.

> ▶ **Complaints:**
> • Fatigue (*"pain of the liver"*), decline in performance and productivity, weariness, affective lability, nervousness, lassitude, sleeping disorders, lack of concentration (s. p. 91)
> = *such as can be witnessed in many harassed people today as "neurasthenic syndrome".*
> • Abdominal pain, repletion, flatulence, nausea, loss of appetite, indigestion, food intolerance, loss of weight
> = *such as are found in various abdominal diseases.*
> • Epigastric pain, nausea, vomiting, intolerance regarding fatty foods or smoking and alcohol, pruritus, constipation, meteorism
> = *such as occur in cholecystopathy.*
> • Stenocardia, vertigo, tachycardia, hypotonia, circulatory disorders
> = *such as are found in cardiovascular diseases.*
> • Fever, arthralgia, myalgia, muscle cramps
> = *such as are often witnessed in infectious diseases.*
> • Impotence, amenorrhoea, nosebleeds, bleeding gums, tendency to haematoma, night blindness
> = *which can also lead to a wrong diagnostic conclusion.*

This wide range of very different subjective ailments makes it clear that there are no typical symptoms and that it is not possible to draw any conclusions on the basis of such complaints as to the severity of the liver disease. Here the constellation of the symptoms and findings (as well as the time when they first appeared and their duration) can provide more information than is available from merely one symptom or finding.

The most frequent, yet **non-specific complaints** mentioned by liver patients are fatigue, languor, repletion, flatulence, epigastric pressure, lack of appetite, nausea, various forms of intolerance, pruritus and impotence. • *Information* on dark-coloured urine, discoloured stools, haematemesis, cutaneous haemorrhages or tarry stools are important signs of hepatobiliary disease. (s. fig. 4.22)

2.2 Palpation

2.2.1 Palpation of the liver

> *"One good feel of the liver is worth any two liver function tests"* (F.M. Hanger, jr., 1971).

Determining liver size is the *"simplest"* and *"cheapest"* liver function test and, chronologically speaking, also the *"first"*. (s. fig. 4.3) (9, 21, 26–29, 31, 32, 35–37)

> ▶ Every enlarged or hard liver must be considered pathological – until counter-evidence is produced by laboratory values and ultrasonography and, if necessary, by means of histology or laparoscopy.

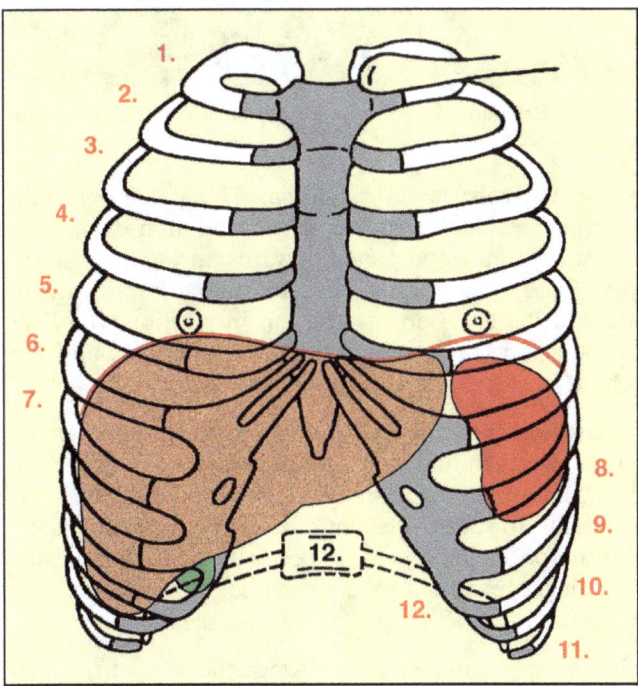

Fig. 4.3: Contours of the liver (brown) and spleen (red) and part of the gall bladder (green) in the right and left hypochondrium (costae verae 1–7; costae spuriae 8–10; costae fluctuantes 11–12)

Sliding palpation: Liver size, consistency and surface as well as tenderness on pressure can be determined by sliding palpation. The lower edge of the liver is perceptible by touch at the costal arch in the mid-clavicular line. It crosses the epigastrium and ends at the left costal arch on the level of the parasternal line. Under palpation, the liver edge was felt to be deeper than shown by the scan, and only in 60% of all cases did palpation of the liver edge correlate with the scan. (32)

Bimanual ventral palpation: The finger tips of both hands are pressed inwards 1—2 cm, flat and parallel to each other below the costal arch. Upon deep inspiration, the size of the liver can be determined by the caudal shift of the liver margin. (s. fig. 4.4)

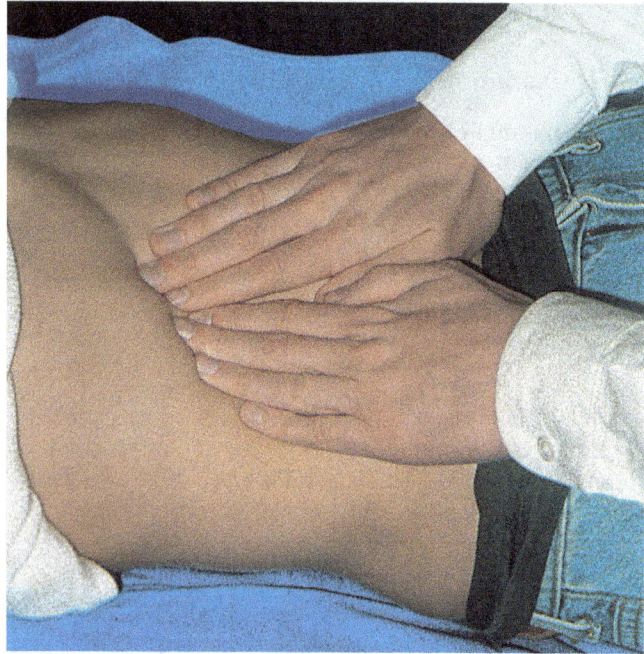

Fig. 4.4: Palpation of the liver: bimanual ventral palpation (GILBERT's technique)

Bimanual ventrodorsal palpation: The palpating right hand presses deep into the right costal arch during the expiratory phase and moves upwards during the inspiratory phase — taking the skin and tissue layers with it. Because it moves downwards on inspiration, the liver can be better felt by the left hand when pressing up from behind in a ventral direction. (s. fig. 4.5)

Hepatomegaly can easily be mimicked under palpation by phrenoptosis in lung emphysema, ptosis of the liver, asthenic habitus and an enlarged Riedel's lobe. (s. p. 18) • It is difficult to state the extent of liver enlargement exactly in terms of "finger breadths" below the costal arch: when 120 "finger breadths" were compared, they were found to range from 1.3 to 2.4 cm. (32) *(see chapter 11)*

Liver atrophy can be assumed when the edge of the liver is elevated due to meteorism or in the Chilaiditi syndrome. • However, the liver may also shrink or no longer be palpable due to increasing liver atrophy in acute viral

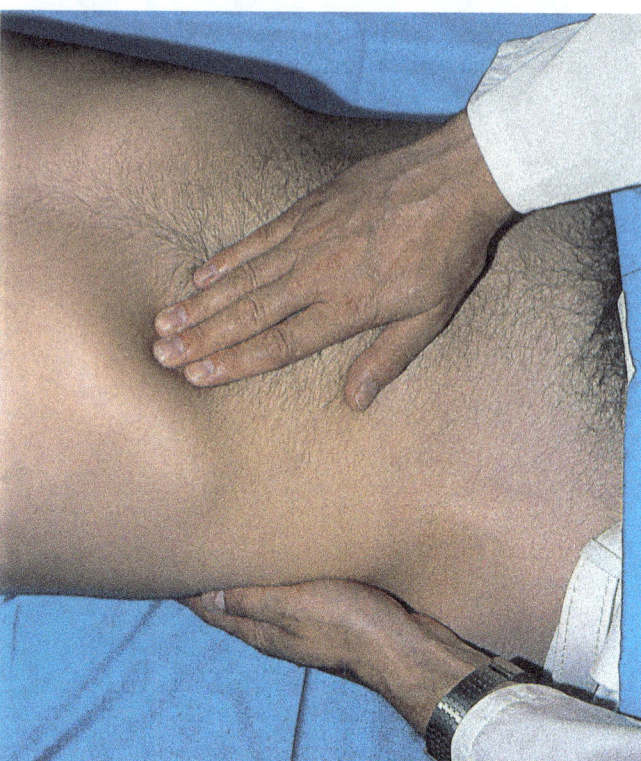

Fig. 4.5: Palpation of the liver: bimanual ventrodorsal palpation (CHAUFFARD's technique)

hepatitis or liver cirrhosis. Thus, a diminished liver can be a more severe condition (generally with a poorer prognosis) than an enlarged liver (e.g. fatty liver).

During palpation, the **liver surface** proves to be smooth, humped or roughly noduled. The consistency of the liver is perceptible as soft, firm or hard. It is important to point out that the firmer the liver, the larger it appears to the palpating hand.

In a normal liver, the **liver edge** feels relatively sharp and insensitive to pain; the surface is smooth and the consistency is soft. In liver cirrhosis, the edge of the liver is sharp and hard; the consistency is firm. In acute hepatitis, the edge of the liver, which tends to be rounded, and the clearly enlarged liver are painful under pressure. • *Hepatomegaly*, caused for example by a fatty liver, displays a rounded liver edge with little or no sensitivity to pressure, whereas in congestive liver, the blunt liver edge proves to be very painful on palpation. • There is admittedly a slight chance of confusing the edge of the liver with *tendinous inscriptions*, but the latter are not displaced in relation to the skin and tissue layers during respiration.

Pain on palpation mainly points to capsular tension as a result of an enlarged liver (acute viral hepatitis, fatty liver, congested liver). In general, the metastatic liver is likewise painful. *Liver abscesses* may cause (frequently severe) pain on tapping. The liver parenchyma itself is insensitive to pain, although pain receptors are found sporadically in the walls of the portal and arterial vessels or in interlobular connective tissue.

2.2.2 Palpation of the spleen

Palpation of the spleen should always accompany palpation of the liver. It is carried out with the patient in a semidextral recumbent position, the knees bent and the arms lying flat at the sides of the body. Normally, the spleen is not palpable.

Splenomegaly is perceptible by touch at the costal arch in the inspiratory phase. This can be accomplished in particular during ventrodorsal palpation when the physician's right hand works from the back towards the (not too deeply) palpating left hand. An enlarged spleen is easily perceptible due to its "downward and inward" movement (in contrast to the left lobe of liver). • *Sensitivity to pressure* of the enlarged spleen points to an inflammation. *(see chapter 11)*

The following **technique** can also be used to detect an enlargement of the spleen: the examining physician, standing to the left of the patient (who is positioned as described above), palpates with the finger tips of the left hand below the costal arch in order to detect the enlarged spleen during the inspiratory phase.

2.3 Percussion

2.3.1 Percussion of the liver

Percussion also enables the size of the liver to be established; hepatic dullness (in cm) is determined by the localization of the so-called liver-lung margin and the lower liver edge, as measured on the right mid-clavicular line (MCL). During this procedure, the lower lung margin is subjected to light percussion, whereas the upper margin, i.e. lung-liver margin, is determined by heavy percussion. This gives the superficial dullness, i.e. *absolute liver dullness*, which is usually deemed to represent the *size of the liver*. Experience shows that the rounded top of the liver can be assumed to be about 5 cm higher than revealed by percussion. The size of the liver seems to be smaller with percussion than with ultrasound. Determining the liver size upwards is, however, of no genuine clinical significance, since hepatomegaly develops "downwards" in the area of least resistance. • Percussible determination of the **normal liver size** has produced mean values of $10-12$ cm (9 ± 2 cm in women, 11 ± 2 cm in men) (E. HAFTER, 1962; J. NAFTALIS et al., 1963; H.A. KÜHN et al., 1979). (7, 21, 26−29, 31, 32, 35−37)

Once the percussion technique has been mastered, the **relative liver dullness** can also be more closely defined within the area of superficial dullness as a zone with a resonance on percussion resembling that of the thigh, i.e. the cranial part of the liver covered by the lung. This is the only way of determining the true size of the liver "upwards". • The size of the **left lobe of liver** is determined by percussion above *Traube's space*, which is narrowed in terms of percussion from the right due to an increase in size of the left lobe of liver.

Scratch auscultation is another way to determine the liver size or the lower liver edge. The stethoscope is placed on the epigastrium, i.e. above the liver; the finger tip strokes ("scratches") the midclavicular line in a cranial to caudal direction at intervals of approx. 1 cm parallel to the presumed edge of the liver; when the liver margin is crossed, the scratching noise in the stethoscope fades and finally disappears. However, this technique is not deemed to be reliable. (18, 42)

2.3.2 Percussion of the spleen

Percussion of the spleen is difficult and is carried out by tapping gently at various points on the anterior axillary line. The upper spleen margin lies about $10-15$ cm above the left costal arch. The **absolute splenic dullness** (so-called spleen width) is about 6 to 7 cm; it lies between 9th and 11th rib. The splenic width established by percussion corresponds to the anterior lower two thirds of the spleen, i.e. adjacent to the thoracic wall. The upper third of the spleen is covered by the lung. When the spleen is subjected to percussion, variations in the shape of the thorax, diaphragm status and intestinal loops are evident (cf. liver percussion).

2.3.3 Ascites

Ascites can be recognized by the wide protuberance of the abdomen with moderate bulging of the abdominal flanks and spreading of the navel. Examination by percussion produces *tympanic intestinal resonance* in the upper area and typical *dullness in the flanks*. Small ascites (about 1 litre) is determined in the *knee-elbow position*, whereby dullness is detected in the lower abdominal region. The *fluctuation wave* is an impressive sign: a short hard surge of the fluid swell against the palpating hand is virtually conclusive. *(see chapter 16)*

2.3.4 Meteorism

Meteorism presents as a pointed arching of the abdomen at navel level. This condition is likewise associated with tympanic resonance; however, the dullness in the flanks is missing.

> ▶ It would be a tremendous loss if, on account of ultrasound methods, palpation and percussion of the liver and spleen were inadequately learned, inappropriately performed and no longer mastered as a basic examination technique for interpretative purposes.

2.4 Inspection

> *"Even though you read and learn so much, your learning does not mean that you know; let your eyes be your professors!"* PARACELSUS (s. pp XIX, 9, 923)

Hardly any other organ of the body causes such a wide variety of externally discernible changes to the skin and mucosa as the diseased liver. Inspection of the body gives diagnostic clues regarding the presence of a liver disease or special maladies of the liver. Examination of the liver-diseased patient produces various findings concerning the whole body and the skin as well as the mucosa, nails and eyes. These signs are summarized under the term **skin stigmata in liver diseases** (German: *Leber-Haut-Zeichen"*; H. KALK, 1955, 1957). (4, 16, 17, 25) (s. tab. 4.3)

1. Chvostek's body type	14. Liver tongue
2. Facies cirrhotica	15. Lacquered lips
3. Parotid enlargement	16. Gynaecomastia
4. Hair changes	17. Dupuytren's contracture
5. Jaundice	18. Pigmentation and striae
6. Spider naevus	19. Erythematous stigmata
7. Palmar erythema	20. Xanthelasmas and xanthomas
8. Telangiectases	21. Scratch marks in pruritus
9. White nails	22. Eye changes
10. Muehrke's nail lines	23. Drumstick fingers
11. Paper money skin	24. Testicular atrophy
12. White spots on the skin	25. Cutaneous haemorrhages
13. Smooth red tongue	26. Vein dilatation

Tab. 4.3: Skin stigmata in liver diseases (check list: s. fig. 4.22)

2.4.1 Chvostek's body type

The habitus described by F. CHVOSTEK (1922) is frequently found in alcohol-related cirrhosis. In the male, it is characterized by the absence of secondary hair on the chest and abdomen as well as of axillary hair, and by a horizontal, female-like boundary of the pubes and a lengthening of the distance between xiphoid process and navel. *"Abdominal baldness"* (which means *effemination* with changes in the pattern of body hair) is a typical finding. The incidence is given as approx. 70%. These changes are often accompanied by thick hair-covering of the head growing down onto the forehead, and bushy eyebrows. • In women suffering from alcoholic cirrhosis, the pubic and axillary hair may also be largely absent, and the mammae may be atrophic.

2.4.2 Facies cirrhotica

Patients with liver cirrhosis often show typical facial skin stigmata: the colour is a pallid yellowish grey, mostly with patchy pigmentation due to the greater deposition of melanin. Spider naevi and reticular telangiectases are found. The skin frequently appears shrivelled, wrinkled and prematurely aged.

2.4.3 Parotid enlargement

Parotid enlargement is occasionally found in cirrhotic patients, especially in alcohol-related cirrhosis (M. SPOSITO, 1942). An enlarged parotid is not painful. (11, 48)

2.4.4 Hair changes

Apart from the *hypotrichosis* of primary and secondary pubic hair, already described in Chvostek's body type, cirrhosis patients occasionally show an absence of frizziness in pubic hair. • In kwashiorkor, the hair becomes light in colour and straggly, and loses its frizzy appearance with simultaneous hypotrichosis.

Localized *hypertrichosis* is found in Chvostek's body type in the form of noticeably bushy eyebrows. It is also, however, found in porphyria cutanea tarda in the area around the zygomatic arch and lateral to the eyes, as well as on the forearm and lower leg, mostly in the form of short, compact hairs.

▶ Hypertrichosis (particularly of the lanugo type) is also described as the **paraneoplastic syndrome**, above all in cases of carcinoma of the intestinal tract or the digestive organs (*Herzberg-Potjan-Gebauer syndrome*, 1969).

2.4.5 Jaundice

In the case of increased serum bilirubin levels of 1.8 – 2.0 mg/dl, diffusion is effected through the blood capillaries, and bilirubin accumulates in the connective tissue, mainly in elastin. (s. p. 37) In its subsiding phase, jaundice is therefore still visible for longer periods even when serum bilirubin values are normal. • Initially, *scleral icterus* develops, which is easily recognizable in daylight when serum bilirubin values are > 2 mg/dl. (s. p. 89) This subicterus is likewise witnessed in the conjunctiva and occasionally on the oral mucosa at the boundary between the soft and hard palate as well as on the periumbilical abdominal skin. (33, 42) • In fully developed *jaundice*, colours range from straw-coloured yellow through bright yellow to greyish yellow as well as reddish yellow and greenish yellow. Icteric discoloration of the skin is frequently darker in the upper than in the lower part of the body. *(see chapter 12)*

Verdin icterus is deemed to be the prototype of obstructive jaundice, particularly in long-standing courses of the disease; **melas icterus** displays a greyish green hue; **rubin icterus** (rust-coloured) is mainly regarded as a sign of hepatocellular jaundice, whereas **flavine icterus** is more likely to occur in cases of haemolysis (TH. BRUGSCH, 1930). Such systematization of the icteric forms in terms of pathogenesis is, however, unreliable and obsolete, since the differences in colour mainly correlate with the duration of the jaundice and the level of serum bilirubin.

2.4.6 Spider naevus

▶ These arterial telangiectases were observed in liver disease by V. HANOT and A. GILBERT in 1890, by A. GILBERT and M.C. HERRSCHER in 1903 and by F. PARKES-WEBER in 1904. • Such spiders were first described in pregnant women by D. CORBET in 1914. Spiders evident in liver disease were the focus of renewed attention in the nineteen-thirties (J. STEINMANN, 1935; N. FIESSINGER, 1936; H. EPPINGER, 1937).

The term spider naevus (Latin: naevus araneus) is also known as liver star, liver spider, vascular spider or spider naevi. (17, 20, 25, 30)

Spider naevi consist of a central arterial vessel, about the size of a pinhead, from which minute, steadily narrowing capillaries, similar to a spider's legs, lead off radially. A passage into the veins, however, cannot be discerned. The central artery winds its way upwards out of the subcutis with an ampulla-like dilatation directly under the epidermis. From the morphological point of view, the course of the vessel can be divided into five sections (G. A. MARTINI, 1964). The central arterial telangiectasis, often button-like and occasionally even clearly protruding, can be seen to pulsate. Spiders occur as solitary or multiple stigmata. (s. fig. 4.6)

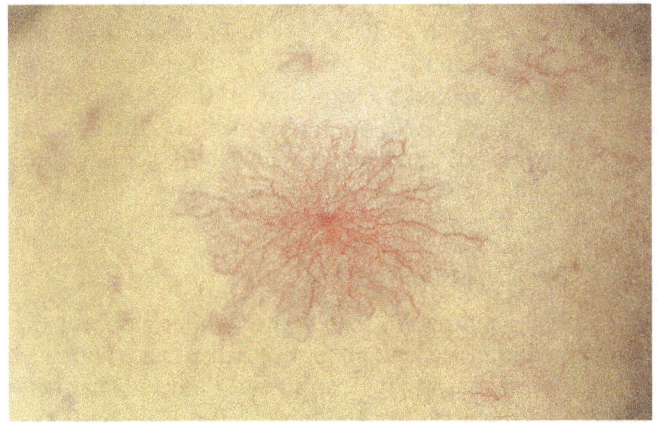

Fig. 4.6: Spider naevus in liver cirrhosis in the ventral side of the left shoulder

The size of the areola of spiders ranges from just a few millimetres up to 2 cm, or even more. When pressed with a glass spatula, the radiating areola disappears and the small pulsating central vessel remains visible, but also disappears if more pressure is applied. Removing the pressure leads to a swift filling of the central vessel and the peripheral vascular areola. The spider can have a narrow white marginal rim. • The most common sites are nose, forehead, zygomatic arch, neck, throat, shoulders, chest and back as well as the extensor sides of the arms and dorsum of the hand. Hence, this localization of the spider naevi corresponds to the area of influence of the superior vena cava, the region of the excitation erythema, the projection fields of the trigeminus core region as well as the phrenic dermatomes (C_3 and C_4) and the neighbouring dermatomes (C_5 to C_8).

The spider naevi occur as segmental reflexes, depending on visceral affections. This would explain why they "blossom" and reoccur when the liver condition deteriorates, and fade when the liver condition improves. The occurrence and rapid appearance of fresh spiders can be considered as an unfavourable sign, such as is observed, for example, in serious virus hepatitis or in the development of primary liver cell carcinoma.

Aetiopathogenesis: W. B. BEAN (1942) assumed the cause of spiders was increased oestrogen blood levels. Other aetiopathogenic factors include the activation of vasoactive ferritin and vasoactive histamine or the presence of bradykinin and endotoxins. Consequently, the altered haemodynamics in chronic liver disease in the sense of a hyperdynamic circulation would also affect the dermatome areas, specified above as preferred sites. • Spider naevi are found not only in liver disease, but also in pregnancy, collagen disorders, hyperthyroidism as a paraneoplastic symptom, lead poisoning, vitamin deficiency conditions or following the intake of oestrogen and similar hormone preparations.

2.4.7 Palmar/plantar erythema

Palmar erythema (erythema palmare symmetricum, "liver palms"), frequently observed (60−75%) in chronic liver disease, was initially described by H. J. CHALMERS in 1899. It becomes manifest as diffuse or patchy reddening of the palms up to the start of the wrist joint; it is particularly evident on the balls of the small finger and thumb as well as on the finger tips and finger joints. The affected area is clearly outlined against the rest of the hand surface. The centre of the palm is generally free of erythema. The hands are warm − corresponding to the vasodilatation and increased circulation. Palmar erythema varies in its intensity: during sporadic deterioration in the course of the disease, it can be more pronounced, and when the liver findings improve, it can fade. (s. fig. 4.7) • Occasionally, the soles of the feet are also affected and show *plantar erythema*. (16)

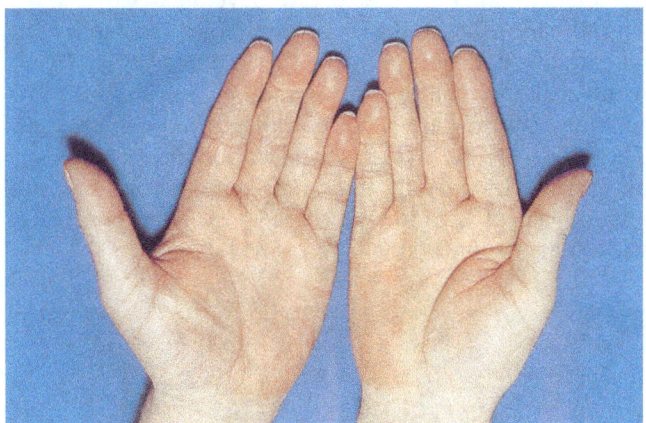

Fig. 4.7: Palmar erythema in liver cirrhosis

Morphology: No morphological changes of the cutis are witnessed. The blood capillaries are irregularly distributed and of differing length; however, they meander greatly in their path with arch-shaped dilatation of the final loop. The blood flow is rapid and jerky.

▶ **Differential diagnosis:** Palmar erythema is also found in pregnancy, in hyperthyroidism, collagen diseases, endocarditis, long-standing feverish conditions, tuberculosis, diabetes mellitus, malignant tumours, chronic polyarthritis and in cases of malnutrition − as well as in healthy people.

Aetiopathogenesis: As with spider naevi, the capillary dilatation causing palmar erythema is attributed to an increased oestrogen content of the blood, a rise in bile acids or endotoxins and an activation of vasodilating substances with more numerous arteriovenous shunts as well as a hypercirculatory syndrome. Portal hypertension is seen as an important codeterminant. • The "blossoming" of spider naevi and palmar erythema is also observed in the phenomenon of *haemodynamic-related resistance to diuretics*.

Incomplete spider naevi are known to develop within a palmar erythema: they do not possess a central artery. The combination of these two liver skin stigmata is frequently found in decompensated liver cirrhosis and in highly active chronic hepatitis.

2.4.8 Telangiectases

Apart from spider naevi, reticular telangiectases are frequently witnessed, particularly in alcoholic liver disease. They appear as tiny, bluish red vessels, in general symmetrically positioned on the cheeks, but also on the nose, forehead and neck. Those parts of the skin that are exposed to light are predominantly affected. The arterial and venous capillary loops are dilated.

2.4.9 White nails

White nails is the term, which is generally used to describe a light pink/silvery-white enlargement of the nail lunula. (41) Ultimately, the entire nail plate is coloured a diffuse lacklustre white, except for a narrow, normal-coloured rim. The lunula of the thumb, the colour of which resembles frosted glass, can also spread and eventually take up the entire nail. The nails frequently have *longitudinal grooves*. Fully developed white nails actually look as though they have been coated with mother-of-pearl nail varnish. In the majority of cases, white nails occur after long-standing liver cirrhosis (10 to 20 years); they are hence considered to be a late sign. The cause of the whitish discoloration is attributed to air bubbles in the nail resulting from a disorder in the metabolism of keratin. White nails are often combined with "paper money skin". (4, 25, 41) (s. fig. 4.8)

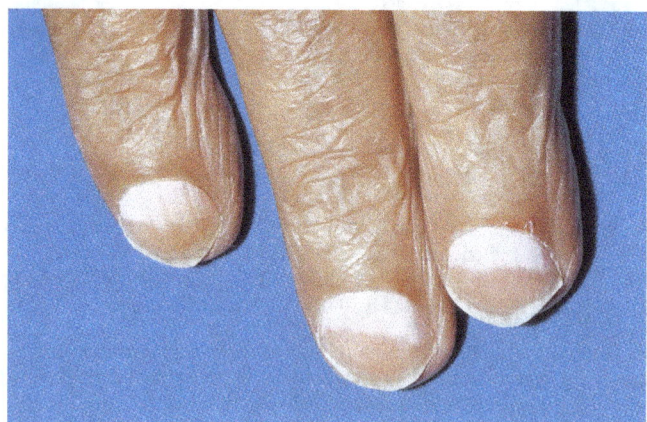

Fig. 4.8: White nails and paper money skin in liver cirrhosis

2.4.10 Muehrke's nail lines

These are white lines running across the nail plate parallel to the lunula. They were first observed by C.R. MUEHRKE (1956). Instead of being contained in the actual nail, the lines are set in the nail bed. This is thought to be caused by severe prolonged hypalbuminaemia (<2.2 g/dl), especially in cases of cirrhosis or nephrotic syndrome. This finding is, however, relatively rare. (24)

2.4.11 Paper money skin

The skin of the chronic liver patient often resembles so-called *parchment skin*: it appears prematurely aged, shrivelled, wrinkled, dry and atrophic — mostly greyish yellow in colour. (s. figs. 4.8, 4.19; 20.1) In contrast, partially atrophic, slightly reddened skin areas that have the appearance of a fading exanthema can occasionally be seen. Within these areas of the skin, there are fine, linear telangiectases, scattered at random, resembling delicate fibres. For this reason, the term *paper money skin* was coined (W.B. BEAN, 1945). These changes are mostly found around the neck down to the chest area, on the cheeks, behind the ears and on the surface of the hands and fingers. Exposure to sun and wind renders the appearance of paper money skin more pronounced. It is frequently combined with spider naevi.

2.4.12 White spots on the skin

Liver-disease patients often display white spots on the skin, which are the size of a lentil (sometimes as large as 0.5–1.0 cm in diameter). They can be detected chiefly in the area of the arms, on the back and on the buttocks. Upon cooling of the skin, white spots appear or become more pronounced, so that a cold-related vasocontraction is assumed to be the causative factor. In the predilection area of the spider naevi, the white spotting of the skin is usually deemed to be a preliminary stage of liver star: within the round white spot, a central red dot is formed, from which the typical spider naevus develops with a white areola.

Vitiligo: Vitiligo (caused by functional failure of the melanocytes) sometimes occurs in primary biliary cirrhosis or autoimmune hepatitis.

2.4.13 Smooth red tongue

A *smooth red tongue*, first described by H. KALK (1955) (16), is raspberry-coloured. It is moist and more or less atrophic. There is no coating of the tongue, nor can any independent capillary changes or venous stasis be detected. The red colour is often in contrast to the yellowish or greyish yellow skin colouring. The tongue changes mainly develop parallel to the course of the cirrhosis: upon clinical improvement, the raspberry shade changes into the normal reddish grey colour of the tongue, which regains its coating. These changes of the tongue occur relatively rapidly as the condition improves or deteriorates. In cases with significant hepatic dysfunction, the smooth red tongue generally remains unchanged. Its cause is assumed to be metabolic cell dysfunction or hyperergic-allergic phenomena. (15) • There is often *angular cheilosis* with rhagades (perlèche, angulus infectiosus), such as can be witnessed in vitamin B_2 deficiency, diabetes mellitus, iron deficiency, infections, etc. (s. fig. 4.9)

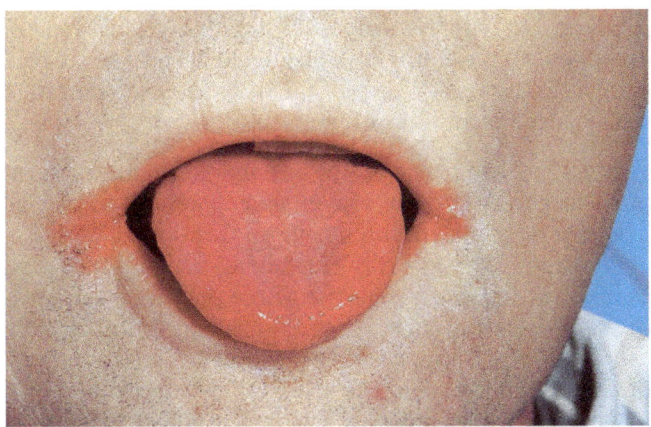

Fig. 4.9: Smooth red tongue with angular cheilosis in liver cirrhosis

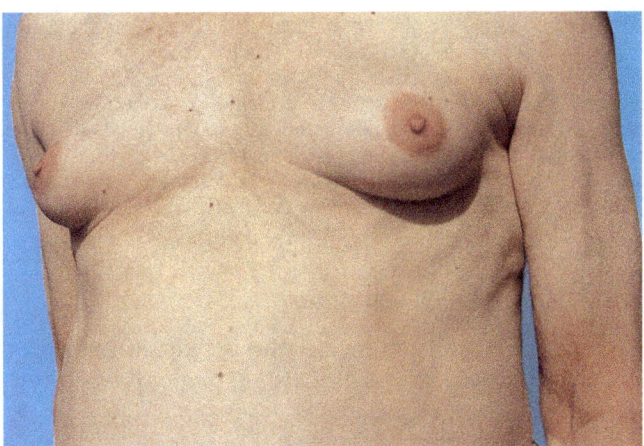

Fig. 4.10: Gynaecomastia in liver cirrhosis

2.4.14 Liver tongue

A so-called congested tongue or "liver tongue" (R. PANNHORST et al., 1957) is voluminous due to the accumulation of fluid and displays tooth marks at the edges. It often has a deep median vertical groove and several small furrows or fissures. Corresponding to its occurrence with (or due to) portal hypertension, it is bluish purple in colour and its undersurface displays greatly distended veins. (15)

2.4.15 Lacquered lips

A smooth red tongue is often combined with a peculiar reddish colouring and smoothness of the lips, known as lacquered lips. They are also one of the late signs of cirrhosis, mainly with a necrotic course of the disease.

2.4.16 Gynaecomastia

In cases of gynaecomastia, the male mammary gland is enlarged. Within the increased volume of the breast, a firm, circumscribed and relatively well-defined tissue mass can be felt, which is usually sensitive to pressure. Apart from the enlargement of the mammary gland, which causes the patient mental as well as physical distress, spontaneous and sometimes sharp pain occurs. Occasionally, a serous or milk-like secretion is discernible. Gynaecomastia can also be unilateral. It occurs most frequently in alcoholic cirrhosis. (s. fig. 4.10)

The **cause** of gynaecomastia is generally attributed to inadequate inactivation of oestrogen or decreased production of testosterone (e.g. due to a lack of zinc in chronic alcoholism). Likewise of causative significance are the increased prolactin plasma level and a greater degree of response on the part of the mammary gland tissue. (6, 8, 25)

Differential diagnosis: Gynaecomastia is also found as a persistent pubertal condition and in adiposity. It is always important to exclude other causes such as testicular tumours, hypogonadism, corticoadrenal tumours, bronchial carcinoma, etc. • Gynaecomastia can also occur as a result of treatment with *spironolactone*, which is often indicated in cirrhosis patients – however, when the medicament is no longer taken, this finding is reversible.

2.4.17 Dupuytren's contracture

The term Dupuytren's contracture (F. PLATTER, 1614; G. DUPUYTREN, 1832) denotes a hardening of the palmar fascia in the connective tissue, with firm band-like connections extending as far as the periosteum and even into the outermost skin layers. The preferred site is the distal ulnar quadrant of the flat of the hand. Severe flexion contractures, especially of the 4th and 5th fingers, ultimately develop. (s. fig. 4.11)

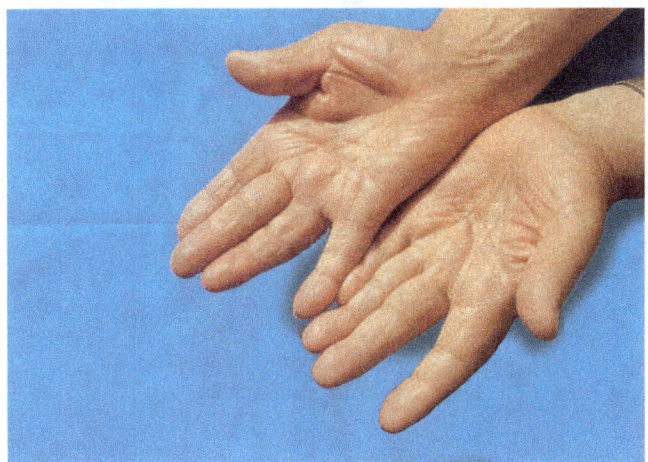

Fig. 4.11: Dupuytren's contracture in liver cirrhosis

Whereas Dupuytren's contracture is only found in about 2% of the population, it is detectable in about 30% of all cirrhosis patients, mainly bilaterally. Men are affected in 90% of cases and thus far more often than women. The disease generally commences unilaterally. Men are frequently affected in their younger years, whereas in women, the disease commences later and takes a more rapid course. There is a greater tendency towards recurrence of the disease after surgery than after radiological treatment. In cirrhosis patients, contracture occurs predominantly in combination with palmar erythema. There also seems to be a correlation between contracture and spider naevi. (2, 12, 23, 25)

At present, there are only hypothetical explanations for the **cause** of the contracture and its correlation with liver cirrhosis. A genetic factor probably plays a part, possibly also in combination with genuine epilepsy. Its more frequent incidence in alcoholic cirrhosis points to a disorder in collagen metabolism as a pathogenic factor. Evidently, the platelet-derived growth factor (PDGF) which is produced, causes the connective tissue to proliferate and contract. PDGF stimulates the formation of prostaglandin E., which likewise changes the fibroblast contractility. (40)

2.4.18 Pigmentation and striae

Patients suffering from **liver cirrhosis** frequently display a brownish discoloration of the skin, predominantly due to the deposition of melanin.

In **haemochromatosis**, a pronounced brownish pigmentation is found due to the deposition of haemosiderin and melanin in the skin (= *bronze diabetes*), particularly in the lines of the palm. (s. fig. 4.12) Other predilection sites with distinctive slate-grey pigmentation are the axillae and the inguinal or lumbar region. Occasionally, a brownish ring-shaped discoloration is seen on the proximal fraction of the nail plate.

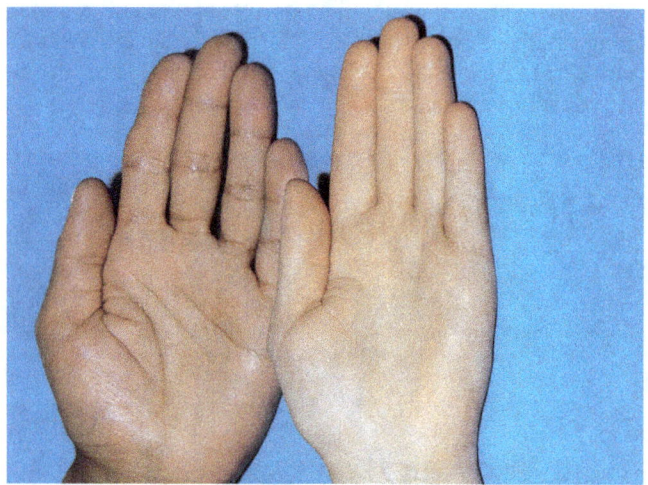

Fig. 4.12: Pigmentation of the lines of the palm in haemochromatosis (left) – in comparison with a normal hand

Wilson's disease is occasionally accompanied by an argyric-like discoloration of the *skin* (greyish brown to bluish grey). The fingernails often display skyblue-coloured lunulae (A.G. BEARN et al., 1958). (46)

Primary amyloidosis can cause the skin to turn reddish brown. • In **Gaucher's disease**, greyish brown pigmentation can develop, similar to chloasma uterinum. This symmetric pigmentation sometimes extends upwards from the foot to the knee. • In **kwashiorkor**, dark red blotches are sometimes found in the inguinal and peri-umbilical area. • In **hamartoma** of the liver, a greyish brown skin pigmentation of the acanthosis nigricans type has been described. In the axillae, the skin is thickened and its texture has a greater consistency; it is also more fissured. • **Juvenile cirrhosis** (= lupoid hepatitis) often produces dark purple stripes on the hips, gluteal region and thighs of the young women affected. These striae run parallel to the tension lines of the skin. They can fade due to skin atrophy and loss of pigmentation.

Where the skin is exposed to sunlight, **porphyria cutanea tarda** displays a greyish brown, maculate or even patch-like area of pigmentation, resulting from the deposition of melanin. The skin can be changed in the same way as in sclerodermatitis. Because of the photosensitivity of the skin, sporadic subepidermal blisters or pimples with encrusted skin lesions are formed, as a result of which the skin injures easily. The scars take the form of whitish, irregularly circumscribed blotches. (s. fig. 4.13) Periorbitally deposited melanin pigment is a typical feature.

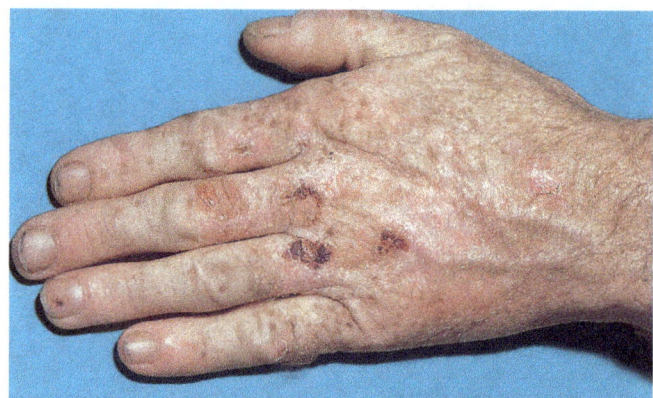

Fig. 4.13: Back of the hand in porphyria cutanea tarda

Butterfly sign: Hypopigmentation in the form of butterfly-shaped areas of skin on the back, located on either side of the spine, are sometimes seen in patients with cholestatic jaundice. (44)

2.4.19 Inflammatory erythematous stigmata

Erythema diffusum hepaticum can be observed in patients suffering from acute liver insufficiency. It is manifested as diffuse plate-shaped erythema of the face, extending up to the hair line. Occasionally, it can also be detected in the region of the jugulum and sternum. Minute red dots are frequently observed within the erythema. These become more prominent as the erythema fades away. Should reddish-coloured telangiectases occur in this area, the picture of paper money skin emerges. (s. figs. 4.8, 4.19)

Exanthemas are prodromal skin symptoms in acute viral hepatitis (5–20% of cases). They appear as urticaria, scarlatinoid or morbilliform exanthemas as well as varicella and erythematous multiform rashes.

Acrodermatitis papulosa eruptiva infantum (*Gianotti-Crosti syndrome*) can occur in children with acute viral hepatitis B. This is a lichenoid-papuloid skin rash on the face and limbs, which breaks out suddenly. The skin stigmata take 2–8 weeks to disappear. (s. p. 439)

2.4.20 Xanthelasmas and xanthomas

Xanthelasmas can be found at the corners of the eye or periorbitally, above all in cases of biliary cirrhosis due to primary biliary cholangitis (CDNC). (1) They display a yellow, reddish yellow to brownish yellow colouring and are sharply circumscribed, sometimes as large as a fingernail, sometimes arranged in stripes. They can be flat (*xanthelasma planum*) or, due to cholesterol deposits, appear as raised bulges or tubers (*xanthelasma tuberosum*). (s. fig. 4.14)

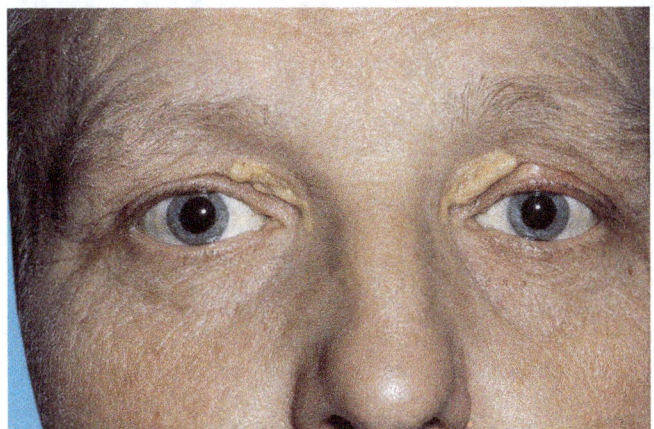

Fig. 4.14: Xanthelasmas in biliary cirrhosis as a result of primary biliary cholangitis

Xanthomas (*xanthoma tuberosum*) display a straw-like yellow through to greyish yellow hue. These are round, well circumscribed, plaque-like raised or papuloid deposits in the skin, which predominantly occur on the extensor sides of the extremities, the elbow and knee area, the external ear, parts of the buttocks and back, occasionally also on the hands and soles of the feet. They can appear in cholestatic liver diseases, particularly in biliary cirrhosis as a result of CDNC. Their occurrence depends on the lipid and cholesterol content of the blood. (1) These changes are considered to be late symptoms. (s. p. 243) (s. figs. 4.15, 4.16)

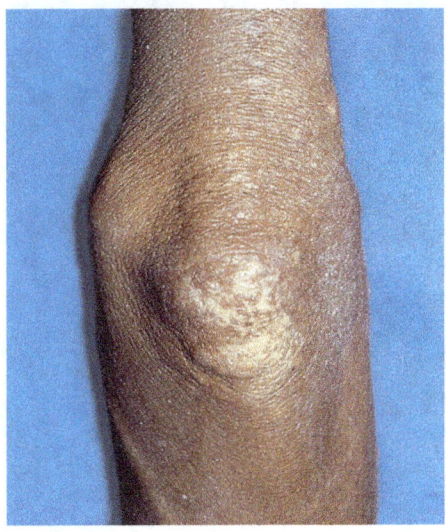

Fig. 4.15: Xanthoma on the elbow in biliary cirrhosis as a result of primary biliary cholangitis

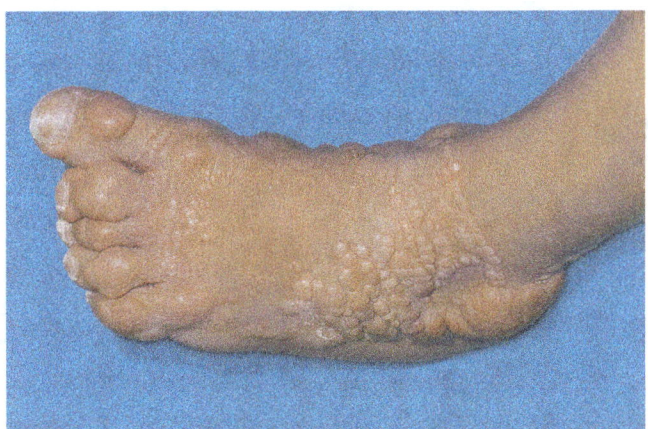

Fig. 4.16: Multiple xanthomas in chronic cholestasis due to congenital biliary tract atresia

2.4.21 Scratch marks in pruritus

Scratch marks as the outcome of an often unbearable pruritus are found in the form of stripe-like excoriations, blood-encrusted skin lesions, dot-like erosions or secondary papuloid dermatitis, lichenification and bacterially superinfected scratch wounds. There may still be some visible signs of scarring and pigmentation. (s. p. 243) (s. fig. 13.3)

When **pruritus** occurs in systemic disease without any initial changes of the skin, it is known as pruritus sine materia. This condition includes the cholestatic liver diseases and liver hamartoma that accompany pruritus in up to 70 % of cases. It is often in itself a cardinal symptom, with the itching mostly commencing in the palms of the hands and on the soles of the feet; in the evening and during the night, it is considerably more pronounced. Itching does not correlate with the degree of severity of cholestasis. In cases of unbearable itching, psychosomatic disorders and reactive depression or thoughts of suicide can appear. (3)

▶ The pathophysiology of pruritus has not yet been fully resolved. It can be assumed that the free nerve endings of the unmyelinated C-fibres in the dermis and epidermis serve as nocireceptors. These are activated directly by mechanical or thermal stimuli and indirectly via chemical, pruritogenic substances. The latter include: histamines, serotonin, proteases, prostaglandins (D2, E2), kinins, substance P, neurokinin A, etc. It is not known, which substances(s) can cause pruritus with cholestasis. The pathogenetic role of the bile acids is still in discussion (e.g. enhanced values of individual or combined bile acids, a shift in the relationship between bile acids). It seems certain that a greater opioidergic tonus prevails in cholestatic liver disease. Hence, pruritus could be caused by the epidural or intrathecal administration of opioids, but also eliminated by opioid-receptor antagonists.

2.4.22 Eye changes

Scleral icterus occurs from a serum bilirubin level of 1.6–1.8 mg/dl upwards. At the same time, the conjunctiva is icterially discoloured. Jaundice is based on the affinity of the elastic fibres for bilirubin. (s. fig. 4.17)

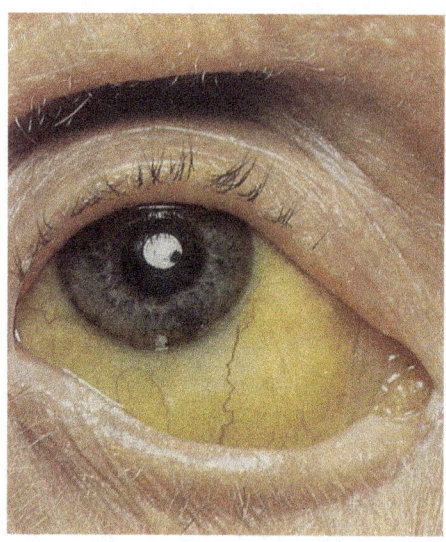

Fig. 4.17: Scleral icterus in akute viral hepatitis A

Kayser-Fleischer corneal ring (B. Kayser, 1902; B. Fleischer, 1903) occurs in Wilson's disease. It has also been observed in alcoholic liver disease. (47) Deposits of copper compounds form a brownish green corneal ring of 1–3 mm in width near the limbus. It can be identified at an early stage by slit-lamp examination. (s. fig. 4.18) • Individual radiating, greenish brown **sunflower cataracts** are sporadically detectable in Wilson's disease.

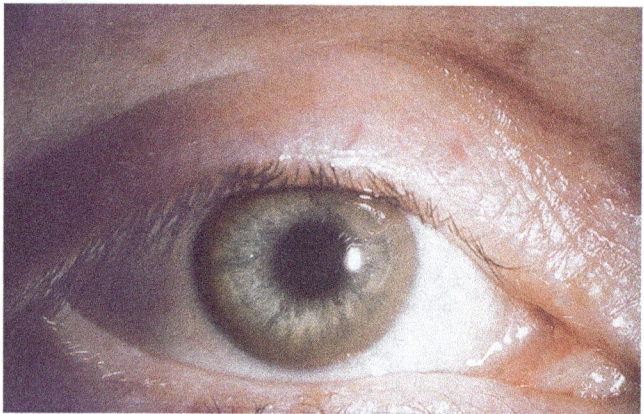

Fig. 4.18: Kayser-Fleischer corneal ring in Wilson's disease

Pingueculae present as wedge-shaped, yellowish deposits on both sides of the pupilla and are observed in Gaucher's disease. • **Retraction of the eyelid** (= Darlrymple's sign) and **infrequent blinking** (= Stellwag's sign), such as in hyperthyroidism, are also found in cirrhosis patients.

2.4.23 Drumstick fingers

Drumstick fingers can be observed in chronic liver patients with a hepatopulmonary syndrome. *(see chapter 18)* These changes are due to increased blood supply to the distal phalanges and the opening of arteriovenous anastomoses with relative hypoxia of the tissue as well as a more extensive formation of connective tissue between nail and bone. • The exaggerated convexity found in **hour-glass nails** can be a preliminary stage of drumstick fingers. Occasionally, a combined occurrence of finger clubbing and white nails is observed (= *hypertrophic osteoarthropathy*). (s. fig. 4.19) (s. p. 342)

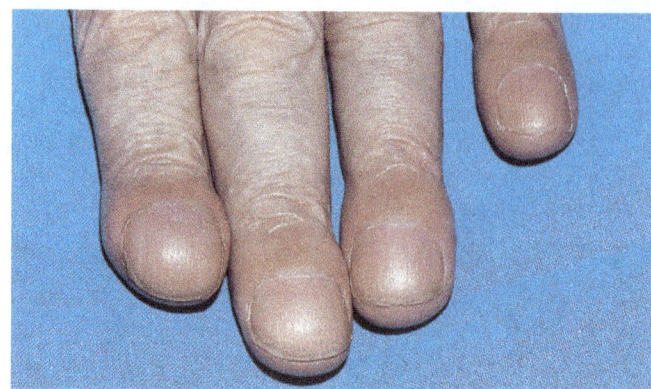

Fig. 4.19: Drumstick fingers and hour-glass nails in liver cirrhosis (and moderate paper money skin: s. figs. 4.8; 20.1)

2.4.24 Testicular atrophy

Considerable endocrine disorders may be present at times in cirrhosis patients. Progressive testicular atrophy with impotence and eunuchoidism (hypogonadism, "abdominal baldness", Chvostek's habitus) can occur. Fully developed testicular atrophy appears regularly in haemochromatosis.

2.4.25 Cutaneous and mucosal haemorrhages

Cutaneous and mucosal haemorrhages can occur in both liver insufficiency and liver cirrhosis. They appear as *suggilations* (coin-sized haemorrhagic foci) (s, figs. 4.20, 20.1), *purpurae* (small maculae) (s. fig. 20.2) or *vibices* (streak-like markings) as well as more extensive *ecchymoses* (circumscribed haemorrhagic foci >3 mm in size) and *petechiae* (pinpoint-sized capillary haemorrhagic foci) or as *suffusions* (confluent haemorrhagic foci, generally without sharp circumscription).

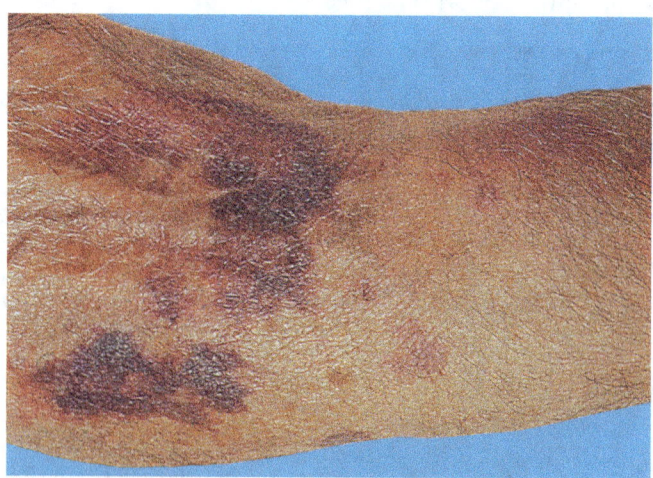

Fig. 4.20: Cutaneous haemorrhages (confluent and streak-like) on the lower part and wrist of the left arm in a patient with cirrhosis (s. figs. 20.1, 20.2)

The haemorrhages are spontaneous or occur as a result of skin punctures or traumatism. Causative factors include greater fragility of the vessels, defective anchoring of the smallest subcutaneous vessels, increased hydrostatic pressure when standing, and coagulaopathy.

2.4.26 Vein dilatation

Clearly *recognizable veins* in the chest and abdominal area in approx. 40% of cases are a visible sign of portal hypertension with collateral veins. (s. fig. 4.21)

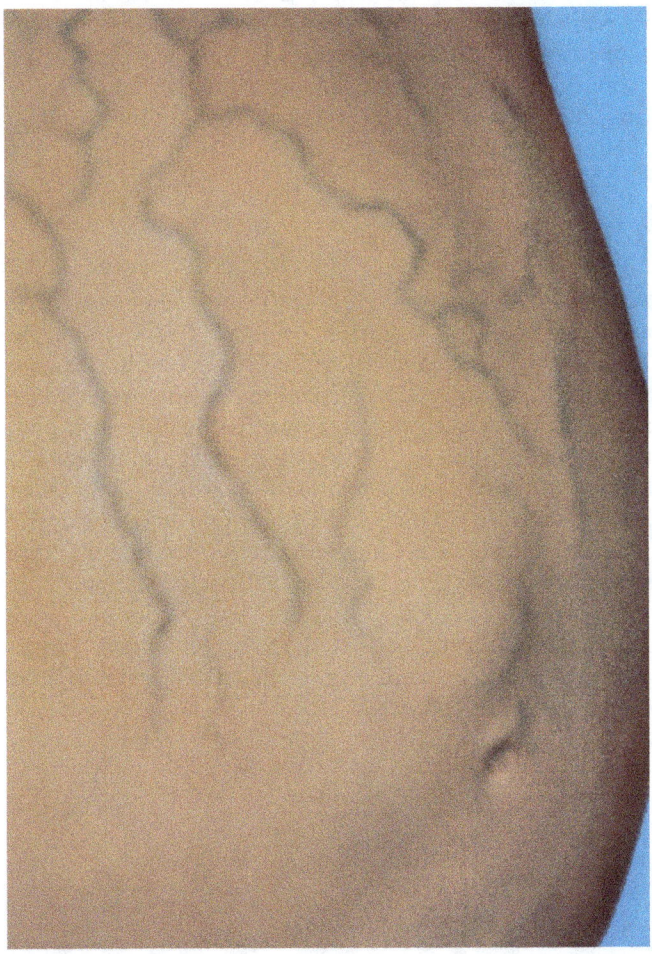

Fig. 4.21: Vein dilatation and tortuosity in the abdominal wall of a cirrhotic patient suffering from ascites and jaundice

Caput Medusae: Excessive forms of vein dilatation can develop in the abdominal skin, such as *vein convolutions* or *Medusa's head* (M. A. SEVERINO, 1632); the latter is also known as *Cruveilhier's sign* (J. CRUVEILHIER, 1829). It develops in portal hypertension, with the result that after the obstructed umbilical vein has been reopened, collaterals are formed over the paraumbilical veins (so-called Sappey's veins). Subsequently, visible venectasiae radiate out from the navel, like the snakes on the head of the gorgon Medusa. • A similar venectasia can also be seen in the area of the epigastric and superficial thoracic veins (*Cruveilhier-von Baumgarten syndrome*). (s. fig. 7.4) • Caput Medusae is also formed as a result of a persistent and malformed umbilical vein with hypoplasia as well as in thrombosis of the intrahepatic branches of the portal vein. It even occurs in children and juveniles (*Cruveilhier-von Baumgarten disease*). With caput Medusae, the umbilical vein remains open or is reopened, or the paraumbilical veins are dilated without change in the blood pressure. • Thus a prehepatic block (portal vein or splenic vein thrombosis) can never cause a caput Medusae because it never affects the umbilical vein. (s. pp 254, 265, 861) (s. fig. 14.13)

2.5 Hepatic foetor

There can be a pronounced increase in methionine and its derivatives in acute liver failure or in serious cases of cirrhosis. From these substances, mercaptans are formed in the colon (e. g. methandiol, ethandiol, dimethyldisulphide). The cause of the *sweetish aromatic smell* of the expiratory air ("fresh-raw liver") known as hepatic foetor (F. UMBER, 1926; L. SCHIFF, 1946) is deemed to be volatile *dimethylsulphide*, a derivate of methanethiol. (39) Its concentration does not correlate with the degree of encephalopathy or hepatic insufficiency, but with the intensity of the portosystemic shunts. • *Trimethylamine* is also suspected of being a causative factor. (22) (s. pp 275, 383)

2.6 Fatigue

In patients with liver disease, fatigue is the most commonly encountered symptom; it has a significant impact on the quality of life. This complex symptom encompasses a range of complaints, such as weariness, exhaustion, lack of concentration, lassitude, lethargy, malaise, drowsiness and sleeping disorders. The frequency of fatigue in patients with different forms of liver disease is variable; the highest incidence is actually found in cholestasis (65–85%), followed by autoimmune hepatitis, drug-induced liver diseases and chronic hepatitis B or C; it is observed less often in acute viral hepatitis. Remarkably, it has often been possible to detect antibodies to serotonin or gangliosides or phospholipids. • No specific therapies are currently available. CNS stimulants, including modafinil, have been discussed; sometimes, nocturnal therapy with low-dose amitriptyline or fluoxetine shows a slight response. In a recent clinical trial, the 5-HT3 receptor antagonist ondansetron appeared to have a limited effect on fatigue in PBC patients. (38)

▶ Central fatigue results from altered neutrotransmission within the brain and is, therefore, often associated with depression and anxiety. Experimental and clinical attention is focused on behavioural activation, arousal and locomotor activity; it would appear that basal ganglia, the brain stem and the limbic system, as well as higher cortical centres, are involved in central fatigue. The condition may result from a defective central release of CRH, which is the most potent activator of the hypothalamic-pituitary adrenal (HPA) axis. Serotonin plays an important role by activating a larger number of receptor subtypes. Interestingly, CRH and serotonin (probably 5-HT1.A) are intimately interrelated. The hypofunction of the HPA axis has also been intensively discussed in relation to the development of central fatigue in liver disease. Other possible causes include the dopaminergic and cannabinoid system. In this context, increased cytokine levels may be a connecting link between liver disease and disorders of the neurotransmitter systems. (38)

2.7 Auscultation

Although auscultation of the abdomen is less important, this method of examination should be performed in certain diagnostic situations. Vascular sounds can occur in the form of arterial bruit or venous hum.

1. Arterial bruit: A systolic rushing sound synchronized with the heart beat indicates increased arterial blood flow. This often barely audible sound is easier to discern if one listens for arterial bruit and feels the patient's pulse at the same time. • It is sometimes heard where aneurysm or stenosis is present in large arteries (e.g. coeliac artery, hepatic artery) as well as in arteriovenous malformations, highly vascularized liver tumours, pronounced acute alcohol hepatitis, 1–2 days after liver biopsy resulting from temporary arteriovenous fistula, or in twisted arteries in cirrhosis. It is seldom found in healthy persons. (10, 13, 45)

2. Venous hum: LAENNEC (1819) was the first to describe the sound which one could hear coming from the veins of patients with cirrhosis. In France this sound phenomenon was termed "bruit de diable" (BOUILLAUD, 1835). The German term "Nonnensausen" is believed to have been introduced by von MERING (1901) in his textbook on internal medicine. It is derived from the noise made by a children's humming-top and is therefore best translated as "humming-top murmur". • Pronounced portal collateral circulation may cause a constant rushing sound due to increased blood flow. This hum mainly occurs between the navel and xiphoid. It is heard frequently and distinctly in the Cruveilhier-von Baumgarten syndrome as well as in venous convolutions on the surface of the abdomen and in the centre of the (extremely rare) caput Medusae. The noise increases when the patient inhales or is in a standing position. (5)

3. Friction rub: A respiratory friction sound above the liver is an indication of perihepatitis. This inflammation of the liver occurs in tumours, liver abscesses or bacterial perihepatitis (e.g. *Fitz-Hugh-Curtis syndrome*) and, in rare cases, temporarily after a liver biopsy. • Perisplenic rubbing is occasionally discernible after splenic infarction. When pressure is applied to the stethoscope, the rubbing sound increases.

3 Liver check list

A *liver check list* provides a swift and clear method of ensuring that all important **clinical findings** can be "ticked off" in the patient's file. This list comprises the ten most important subjective ailments, the twelve most important liver skin stigmata and the nine most important clinical findings. *One glance is enough to review the total findings of the liver patient; moreover, documentation itself involves a minimum of time and effort.* Over the years, such a check list has proved its value in numerous practitioners' surgeries and outpatient departments. It ensures that nothing is "forgotten" or "overlooked" and (particularly during the first check-up) enables a simple, yet extensive, documentation of hepatologic findings to be drawn up. (s. fig. 4.22)

Liver check list of clinical findings				Name				Date			
Anamnesis **10 most important complaints**				**Skin stigmata in liver diseases** **12 most important skin stigmata**				**Clinical findings** **9 most important clinical findings**			
	∅	+	++		∅	+	++		∅	+	++
1. Fatigue				1. Jaundice				1. Liver palpation			
2. Weariness				2. Spider naevi				2. Dark urine			
3. Repletion				3. Palmar erythema				3. Acholic stools			
4. Flatulence				4. Smooth red tongue				4. Bleeding			
5. Inappetence				5. Lacquered lips				5. Hepatic foetor			
6. Nausea				6. Gynaecomastia				6. Testicular atrophy			
7. Intolerances				7. Paper money skin				7. Splenic palpation			
8. Itching				8. White nails				8. Oedemas, ascites			
9. Impotence				9. Chvostek's habitus				9. Handwriting test (signature)			
10. Upper abdominal pressure				10. Dupuytren's contracture							
				11. Scratch marks							
				12. Haemorrhages							

Fig. 4.22: Liver check list of clinical findings (s. fig. 4.2) with the 10 most important subjective complaints, the 12 most important skin stigmata in liver diseases, and the 9 most important clinical findings (19) (s. fig. 5.2)

References:

1. **Ahrens, E.H. jr., Kunkel, H.G.:** The relationship between serum lipids and skin xanthomata in eighteen patients with primary biliary cirrhosis. J. Clin. Invest. 1949; 28: 1565–1574
2. **Attali, P., Ink, O., Pelletier, G., Vernier, C., Jean, F., Moulton, L., Etienne, J.-P.:** Dupuytren's contracture, alcohol consumption, and chronic liver disease. Arch. Intern. Med. 1987; 147: 1065–1067
3. **Bergasa, N.:** The pruritus of cholestasis. J. Hepatol. 2005; 43: 1078–1088
4. **Berman, J.E., Lamkin, B.C.:** Hepatic disease and the skin. Dermatol. Clin. 1989; 7: 435–448
5. **Bloom, H.J.G.:** Venous hums in hepatic cirrhosis. Brit. Heart J. 1950; 12: 343–350
6. **Braunstein, G.D.:** Gynecomastia. New Engl. J. Med. 1993; 328: 490–495
7. **Castell, D.O., O'Brien, K.D., Muench, H., Chalmers, T.C.:** Estimation of liver size by percussion in normal individuals. Ann. Intern. Med. 1969; 70: 1183–1189
8. **Cavanaugh, J., Niewoehner, C.B., Nuttall, F.Q.:** Gynecomastia and cirrhosis of the liver. Arch. Intern. Med. 1990; 150: 563–565
9. **Cerlek, S., Sirracki, J., Brzovic, S., Krasulja, D., Mostovac, B.:** How frequently is a palpable liver to be found during systematic examination of an apparently healthy population? Acta Hepato-splenol. 1971; 18: 397–402
10. **Clain, D., Wartnaby, K., Sherlock, S.:** Abdominal arterial murmurs in liver disease. Lancet 1966 II: 516–519
11. **Dutta, S.K., Dukehart, M., Narang, A., Latham, P.L.:** Functional and structural changes in parotid glands of alcoholic cirrhotic patients. Gastroenterology 1989; 96: 510–518
12. **Evans, R.A.:** The etiology of Dupuytren's disease. Brit. J. Hosp. 1986; 36: 198–199
13. **Goldstein, L.I.:** Enlarged, tortuous arteries and hepatic bruit. J. Amer. Med. Ass. 1968; 206: 2518–2520
14. **Hardison, J.E.:** To be complete. New Engl. J. Med. 1979; 300: 193–194
15. **Jacoby, H., Phlippen, R.:** Beziehungen der Zungenveränderungen bei Leberzirrhose und chronischer Hepatitis zur Mikrozirkulation und Leber-Struktur. Med. Welt 1967; 18: 613–617
16. **Kalk, H.:** Über Hauterscheinungen und über das Symptom der „roten, glatten Zunge" bei Leberinsuffizienz. Dtsch. Med. Wschr. 1955; 80: 955
17. **Kalk, H.:** Über Hautzeichen bei Lebererkrankungen. Dtsch. Med. Wschr. 1957; 82: 1637–1641
18. **Karobath, H., Redtenbacher, M.:** Kratzauskultation der Leber: Wert als Untersuchungsmethode. Leber Magen Darm 1974; 4: 352–355
19. **Kuntz, E.:** Seminar Hepatologie. Diagnostik der Leberkrankheiten. Mkurse Ärztl. Fortbild. 1977; 27: 542–545, 585–587, 630–635, 690–693, 732–735, 782–785, 821–823, 854–857. – 1978; 28: 35–38, 70–72, 107–110, 147–148, 182–184, 219–220, 257–258, 299–302, 343–344, 384–386, 427–428
20. **Martini, G.A.:** Über Gefäßveränderungen der Haut bei Leberkranken. Zschr. Klin. Med. 1955; 153: 470–526
21. **Meidl, E.J., Ende, J.:** Evaluation of liver size by physical examination. J. Gen. Intern. Med. 1993; 8: 635–637
22. **Mitchell, S., Ayesh, R., Barrett, T., Smith, R.:** Trimethylamine and foetor hepaticus. Scand. J. Gastroenterol. 1999; 34: 524–528
23. **Moorhead, J.J.:** Dupuytren's contracture: Review of the disputed etiology, 1831–1956. N. Y. J. Med. 1956; 56: 3686–3703
24. **Muehrcke, R.C.:** The finger-nails in chronic hypoalbuminaemia. A new physical sign. Brit. Med. J. 1956; 1327–1328
25. **Müting, D., Sperr, K., Müting, Chr., Perisoara, A.:** Leberhautzeichen: Ihre Bedeutung für Diagnose und Prognose von chronischen Leberkrankheiten. Dtsch. Ärztebl. 1985; 82: 1780–1785
26. **Naftalis, J., Leevy, C.M.:** Clinical estimation of liver size. Amer. J. Dig. Dis. 1963; 8: 236–243
27. **Naylor, C.D.:** Physical examination of the liver. J. Amer. Med. Ass. 1994; 271: 1859–1865
28. **Niederau, C., Sonnenberg, A., Fritsch, W.-P., Strohmeyer, G.:** Bestimmung der Lebergröße in der klinischen Routine. Dtsch. Med. Wschr. 1983; 108: 1599–1601
29. **Peternel, W.W., Shaffer, J.W., Schiff, L.:** Clinical evaluation of liver size and hepatic scintiscan. Amer. J. Dig. Dis. 1966; 11: 346–350
30. **Pirovino, M., Linder, R., Boss, Ch., Köchli, H.P., Mahler, F.:** Cutaneous spider nevi in liver cirrhosis: capillary microscopical and hormonal investigations. Klin. Wschr. 1988; 66: 298–302
31. **Riemenschneider, P.A., Whalen, J.P.:** Relative accuracy of estimation of increased liver and spleen by radiologic and clinical methods. Amer. J. Roentgen. Rad. Ther. Nucl. Med. 1965; 94: 462–468
32. **Rosenfield, A.T., Laufer, I., Schneider, P.B.:** The significance of a palpable liver. A correlation of clinical and radioisotope studies. Amer. J. Roentgen. 1974; 122: 313–317
33. **Ruiz, M.A., Saab, S., Rickman, L.S.:** The clinical detection of scleral icterus: observations of multiple examiners. Mil. Med. 1997; 162: 560–563
34. **Salter, R.H.:** Diagnosis before treatment? Lancet 1985/I 863–864
35. **Sapira, J.D., Williamson, D.L.:** How big is the normal liver? Arch. Intern. Med. 1979; 139: 971–973
36. **Skrainka, B., Stahlhut, J., Fulbeck, C.L., Knight, F., Holmes, R.A., Butt, J.H.:** Measuring liver span. Bedside examination versus ultrasound and scintiscan. J. Clin. Gastroenterol. 1986; 8: 267–270
37. **Sullivan, S., Krasner, N., Williams, R.:** The clinical estimation of liver size: a comparison of techniques and an analysis of the source of error. Brit. Med. J. 1976; 2: 1042–1043
38. **Swain, M.G.:** Fatigue in liver disease: pathophysiology and clinical management Can. J. Gastroenterol. 2006; 20: 181–188
39. **Tangerman, A., Meuwese-Arends, M.T., Jansen, J.B.M.:** Cause and composition of foetor hepaticus. Lancet 1994; 343: 483.
40. **Terek, R.M., Jiranek, W.A., Goldberg, M.J., Wolfe, H.J., Alman, B.A.:** The expression of platelet-derived growth-factor gene in Dupuytren contracture. J. Bone Joint Surg. 1995; 77: 1–9
41. **Terry, R.:** White nails in hepatic cirrhosis. Lancet 1954/I: 757–759
42. **Theodossi, A., Knill-Jones, R.P., Skene, A., Lindberg, G., Bjerregaard, B., Holst-Christensen, J., Williams, R.:** Inter-observer variation of symptoms and signs in jaundice. Liver 1981; 1; 21–32
43. **Tucker, W.N., Saab, S., Rickman, L.S., Mathews, W.C.:** The scratch test is unreliable for detecting the liver edge. J. Clin. Gastroenterol. 1997; 25: 410–414
44. **Venecie, P.Y., Cuny, M., Samuel, C., Bismuth, H.:** The "butterfly" sign in patient with primary biliary cirrhosis. J. Amer. Acad. Dermatol. 1988; 19: 571–572
45. **Watson, W.C., Williams, P.B., Duffy, G.:** Epigastric bruits in patients with and without celiac axis compression. A phonoarteriographic study. Ann. Intern. Med. 1973; 79: 211–215
46. **Whelton, M.J., Pope, F.M.:** Azure lunules in argyria. Corneal changes resembling Kayer-Fleischer rings. Arch. Intern. Med. 1978; 121: 267–269
47. **Williams, E.J., Gleeson, D., Burton, J.L., Stephenson, T.J.:** Kayser-Fleischer like rings in alcoholic liver disease: A case report. Eur. J. Gastroenterol. Hepatol. 2003; 15: 91–93
48. **Wolfe, S.J., Summerskill, W.H.J., Davidson, C.S.:** Parotid swelling, alcoholism and cirrhosis. New Engl. J. Med. 1957; 256: 491–495

Diagnostics in Liver Diseases
5 Laboratory diagnostics

		Page:
1	*Four epochs of laboratory liver diagnostics*	96
2	*Difficulties of laboratory liver diagnostics*	96
3	***Prerequisites for correct laboratory findings***	97
3.1	Preanalytical phase	97
3.2	Analytical phase and assessment	98
4	***Selection criteria for liver tests***	98
5	***Assessment of hepatocellular integrity***	99
5.1	Enzyme diagnostics	99
5.1.1	GPT (ALT)	102
5.1.2	GOT (AST)	102
5.1.3	Glutamate dehydrogenase (GDH)	102
5.1.4	Lactate dehydrogenase (LDH)	103
5.1.5	Gamma-glutamyl transferase (γ-GT)	103
5.2	Iron and ferritin	104
5.3	Zinc	105
6	***Disorders of excretion***	105
6.1	Bilirubin	105
6.2	Bile pigments in the urine	106
6.3	Bile acids	107
6.4	Enzymatic markers of cholestasis	107
6.4.1	Alkaline phosphatase (AP)	107
6.4.2	Leucine arylamidase (LAP)	108
6.4.3	5′-Nucleotidase (5′-NU)	108
6.5	Copper	108
6.6	Cholesterol	108
7	***Disorders of synthesis capacity***	109
7.1	Cholinesterase (ChE)	109
7.1.1	Diagnostic accuracy using enzymes	109
7.2	Coagulation factors	110
7.2.1	Fibrinogen and factor VIII	110
7.2.2	Quick's value	111
7.2.3	Antithrombin III (AT III)	111
7.3	Dysproteinaemia and hypalbuminaemia	111
7.4	Lipoprotein X (LP-X)	112
7.5	α_1-foetoprotein (AFP)	112
8	***Disorders of metabolism***	113
8.1	Ammonia	113
9	***Diagnostics of liver functions***	113
9.1	Galactose elimination capacity (GEC)	114
9.2	Indocyanine green test (ICG)	114
9.3	Aminopyrine ^{14}C breath test	115
9.4	Antipyrine test	115
9.5	Caffeine elimination test (CET)	115
9.6	Monoethylglycinexylidide test (MEGX)	115
9.7	Sorbitol clearance	116
9.8	(99 m) Tc-Membrofenin	116
9.9	Bengal rose ^{131}iodine test	116
9.10	Bromsulphalein test	116
10	***Assessment of mesenchymal reaction***	116
10.1	Gamma globulins	116
10.2	Immunoglobulins	116
10.3	Procollagen-III-peptide (P-III-P)	118
11	***Serological diagnostics of viral hepatitis***	118
11.1	Hepatitis A virus (HAV)	118
11.2	Hepatitis B virus (HBV)	119
11.3	Hepatitis C virus (HCV)	121
11.4	Hepatitis D virus (HDV)	122
11.5	Hepatitis E virus (HEV)	123
11.6	Other hepatitis viruses	123
12	***Immunological diagnostics***	123
12.1	System of antibodies	124
12.2	ANA	124
12.3	LMA	125
12.4	SMA	125
12.5	LKM	125
12.6	AMA	126
12.7	SLA/LP	126
12.8	pANCA	127
12.9	Antihistone-2B	127
12.10	Anti-GOR	127
13	***Biochemical algorithmic diagnostics***	127
	• References (1–124) (Figures 5.1–5.15; tables 5.1–5.23)	128

5 Laboratory diagnostics

1 Four epochs of laboratory liver diagnostics

First epoch

► In the two volumes of the classical textbook of hepatology by F. Th. Frerichs „Klinik der Leberkrankheiten" ("Clinical aspects of liver diseases"; 1858, 1861), there is no mention of laboratory diagnostics. (s. figs. 1.19, 1.20) • According to our knowledge, laboratory diagnostics was first presented in 1923 by G. Lepehne in his book „Die Leberfunktionsprüfungen, ihre Ergebnisse und ihre Methodik" ("Liver function tests, their results and methods"). This monograph initiated the **1st epoch of biochemical liver diagnostics.** The laboratory field was again addressed by H. Eppinger in 1937 in his textbook „Die Leberkrankheiten" ("Liver diseases") consisting of 52 pages; enzyme tests, however, were not mentioned. (s. fig. 5.1)

DIE
LEBERKRANKHEITEN

ALLGEMEINE UND SPEZIELLE PATHOLOGIE
UND THERAPIE DER LEBER

VON

PROF. DR. HANS EPPINGER
VORSTAND DER I. MEDIZINISCHEN UNIVERSITÄTSKLINIK IN WIEN

MIT 111 ZUM TEIL FARBIGEN ABBILDUNGEN

WIEN
VERLAG VON JULIUS SPRINGER
1937

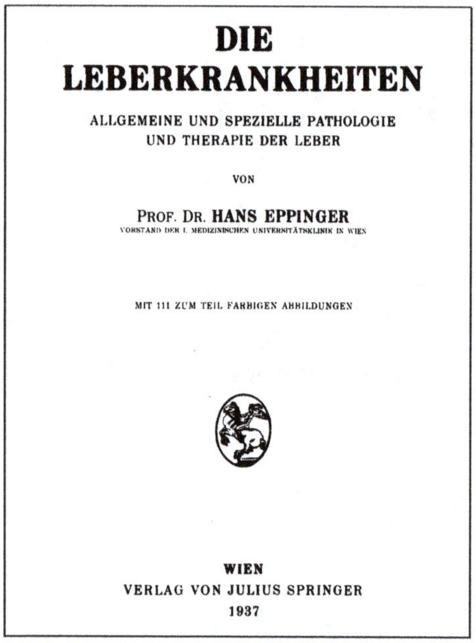

Fig. 5.1: H. Eppinger (1879–1946): „Die Leberkrankheiten" ("Liver diseases"), publisher J. Springer, Wien, 1937, 801 pages *(private property)* (s. fig. 1.19!)

Second epoch

► The introduction of alkaline phosphatase (1933), cholinesterase (1938), aldolase (1954), transaminases (1955), γ-GT (1961) and GDH (1962) into liver diagnostics marked the onset of the **2nd epoch**, the **era of enzymochemistry.** • The resulting understanding with regard to the biochemistry of the liver appeared so fascinating to the hepatologists of that time that enzyme diagnostics was classified as *"biochemical biopsy"* (F. Wroblewski et al., 1956). • In his monograph „Leberfunktionsproben" ("Liver function tests"), H. Schaefer (1951) listed 171 liver tests, including alkaline phosphatase and cholinesterase. An up-to-date presentation of biochemical diagnostics was given by I. Magyar (1961) in his textbook „Erkrankungen der Leber und der Gallenwege" ("Diseases of the liver and biliary tract"). Up to that time, ca. 200 "liver tests" were known.

Third epoch

► The discovery of the Australian antigen by B. S. Blumberg et al. (1965) using serological techniques can be considered as the onset of the **3rd epoch** of laboratory liver diagnostics. With the advent of modern techniques in **serology and immunology,** liver diagnostics has improved tremendously.

Fourth epoch

► The fourth epoch of liver research is based on biomolecular and microstructural methods. This **4th epoch** may some day become known as **biomolecular hepatology.** (s. p. 13!)

2 Difficulties of laboratory liver diagnostics

In order to evaluate the results of biochemical tests within a hepatological context in an adequate manner, one has to be aware of some *fundamental issues*:

(*1.*) Owing to the liver's large functional reserve capacity as well as to its outstanding regenerative ability, morphological damage may evade biochemical detection, i. e. the damage may remain "biochemically silent".

(*2.*) A great number of liver tests are nonspecific, and their results are pathological in other diseases as well. It is therefore necessary to consider the specificity, sensitivity and clinical validity of the respective tests when setting up the diagnostic procedure.

(*3.*) In a variety of liver diseases, it often happens that only certain partial functions or cellular structures are impaired; this impairment can differ widely in intensity and extent in the individual patient. Therefore, when applying only a few biochemical tests, pathological changes may well be overlooked. For the detection of hepatocellular damage or disorders of hepatic functions, a variety of examination methods will have to be employed in order to provide a comprehensive assessment derived from the various single findings.

(*4.*) With increasing duration of liver or biliary tract diseases, but also with the simultaneous appearance of complications, biochemical findings become more and more ambiguous and misleading.

In order to give due consideration to these facts and reduce the uncertainties of liver diagnostics, a large number of function tests with a multitude of modifications were developed. However, the application of such **"batteries of tests"** or **"liver test arrays"** as well as **"shotgun investigations"** did not only result in unnecessary discomfort for patients and staff alike, but also in the uneconomical use of laboratory testing. Furthermore, these tests failed to improve liver diagnostics.

3 Prerequisites for correct laboratory findings

We usually assume that laboratory findings are correct. However, we tend to overlook the wide range of factors which might influence the measured value considerably. • *Therefore, it is absolutely essential to ensure the reliability of laboratory findings.*

During *(1.) sample collection, (2.) sample transport, (3.) sample preparation*, and *(4.) sample processing* (including *storage*), laboratory findings may be exposed to a multitude of influencing factors, thus allowing serious mistakes to occur. (1)

In order to obtain accurate laboratory values, **three steps** are necessary, each requiring continuous monitoring and control: *(1.)* preanalytical phase, *(2.)* analysis, and *(3.)* analytical assessment.

3.1 Preanalytical phase

Mistakes leading to an incorrect laboratory value mostly occur in the preanalytical phase — since there is no "quality management" at this point, as there is in the later phase of analysis and analytical assessment.

Influencing factors: Factors affecting haemanalysis values include:
(1.) Food intake: An empty stomach strictly means no consumption of food or alcohol (and preferably of nicotine as well) 10−12 hours prior to blood collection. (1)
(2.) Time of day: The most favourable time to take the blood sample is between 7 and 9 o'clock in the morning. (8)
(3.) Body position: The blood sample should be taken when the patient is in a sitting or lying position — following a 10-minute resting period. (1)
(4.) Physical activity: No previous physical strain.
(5.) Drugs: Medication must be reported to the laboratory; it should only be administered after the blood sample is taken.
(6.) Further possible influencing factors: Body weight, temperature, circadian rhythms, climate and altitude as well as various diagnostic examinations. (1, 2, 7, 8)

Blood sample collection: It is important to take the blood sample under standardized conditions (1, 3, 7):
(1.) Venous stasis with 40−50 (max. 60) mm Hg.
(2.) No pumping of the fist.
(3.) If possible, syringe with needle No. 1 — downward insertion of the needle at an angle of approximately 30°.
(4.) Gentle aspiration, blood collection at a slow and constant rate; if the blood flow stops, syringe should be slightly rotated.
(5.) Stasis of the vein should not exceed two to three minutes.
(6.) Respective instructions regarding the collection of different types of samples (serum, plasma, citrated and EDTA blood) have to be observed.
(7.) After removing the needle, do not bend the arm, but elevate it — this will empty the vein and avoid bleeding as well as preventing haematoma.

Haemolysis: Haemolysis has a negative influence on the reliability of certain laboratory values, such as an *elevation* of LDH, GOT, GPT and potassium as well as a *decline* of alkaline phosphatase, γ-GT and bilirubin. (6) Haemolysis has to be avoided in all cases.

In artificially induced haemolysis, haptoglobin is normal; however, in intravasal haemolysis, it is reduced or hardly detectable. • **Colour reactions** such as bilirubinaemia, hyperlipidaemia and discoloration of serum by medication or i.v. diagnostic substances can also distort laboratory values. (1, 4)

▶ **Specimen identification:** The sample must not be dispatched until it has been labelled correctly and the appropriate form for specimen identification has been enclosed. Mistakes made during identification (mismatching of names or samples) can be the source of considerable misjudgements or delays and may also cause grave errors with possible legal consequences.

▶ **Specimen transport:** The sample must reach the laboratory in the shortest time possible and the mode of transport should not change laboratory findings in any way. Precise regulations have therefore been established for transportation. When mailing samples, the results may alter within the course of two days by as much as 10%. (1, 7)

Specimen stability: The stability of a sample is of relevance for the preanalytical phase as well as for phases 2 and 3 (analysis and analytical assessment), which are performed exclusively in the laboratory. (5) When stored in a refrigerator (4°C) in closed containers, only a minor loss of *serum enzyme activity* is to be expected after 3−5 days — this increases slightly at room temperature (20−25°C). • The *substrates* necessary for biochemical liver diagnostics will remain stable for several days under identical conditions (exception: ammonia with a maximum of 2 hours). (s. tab. 5.1)

Loss of enzyme activity	4°C	20−25°C
Alkaline phosphatase	0%	(10%)
Cholinesterase	0%	(0%)
GDH	5%	(15%)
GOT	8%	(12%)
GPT	10%	(17%)
γ-GT	0%	(0%)
LAP	0%	(0%)
LDH	8%	(2%)

Stability of substrates	4°C	20−25°C
Ammonia (in hours!)	2	(−)
Autoimmune antibodies	14	(5)
Cholesterol	6	(6)
Copper	14	(14)
Electrophoresis	6	(6)
Hepatitis serology	14	(5)
Immunoglobulins	7	(3)
Iron	7	(4)
Neutral fats	3	(−)
Potassium	14	(14)
Protein	6	(6)
Sodium	14	(14)

Tab. 5.1: Loss of enzyme activity (in %); stability of substrates (in days) during storage of serum in a refrigerator (4°C) and at room temperature (20−25°C)

Scope of duties: The following tasks are a mandatory part of the *preanalytical phase*; they require strict observation in order to obtain reliable laboratory values:

1. Adequate preparation of the patient
2. Standardized collection of the blood sample
3. Knowledge of influencing factors
4. Correct labelling (sample + accompanying form)
5. Transportation of the sample
6. Storage of the sample

- inflammatory
- necrotizing
- degenerative
- proliferative
- accumulative
- fibrogenic

These forms of morphological damage lead to the appearance of certain **biochemical disorders** of varying intensity and in several combinations. (s. tab. 5.3)

3.2 Analytical phase and assessment

During the phase of **analysis** (phase 2), substrates are determined using reliable (standardized) methods. • During the phase of **analytical assessment** (phase 3), the performance (= reliability) of the methods is assessed. • **Criteria for reliability** are (*1.*) *precision*, (*2.*) *accuracy*, (*3.*) *specificity and sensitivity*, and (*4.*) *upper and lower limits of detection*. In addition, (*5.*) the *plausibility* of a finding is also assessed. • **Standard values for quality control** demonstrate the degree of seriousness of having wrong findings and simultaneously limit the respective maximum error value. In clinical chemistry, **precision** (= exactness of measured values or congruence of repeated measurements) and **accuracy** (= deviation from nominal values) are imperative. Measuring values for the various biochemical parameters are specified at different levels.

4 Selection criteria for liver tests

▶ After the introduction of modern biochemical techniques (such as enzyme diagnostics, serology and immunology) into hepatology, only a few of the numerous liver function tests have prevailed. Hepatic diagnostics has been "streamlined" and completely redeveloped. Only the determination of bilirubin, serum iron and urinary bile pigments has remained from the first epoch.

Assessment scale: It is necessary to use various biochemical tests to obtain a reliable, differentiated and economical liver diagnostic schedule. (9–11) • *Such tests should complement one another in their diagnostic informativeness, but at the same time they should overlap as little as possible.* • For selecting the biochemical tests, various **criteria** are applied as an assessment scale. (s. tab. 5.2)

I.	II.
1. Specificity	1. Costs involved
2. Sensitivity	2. Practicability
3. Clinical reliability	3. Inconvenience to the patient
	4. Influencing factors

Tab. 5.2: Selection criteria used as an assessment scale for biochemical hepatic tests

Morphological lesions: Hepatocytes and biliary capillaries respond to damage with structural disorders of their membranes and organelles. Electron microscopic differentiation of these lesions may yield additional diagnostic possibilities *("pathology of organelles")*. (14) • Depending on the nature and intensity of the damage as well as the duration of exposure, *morphological lesions* appear in various forms and also in combination:

1. **Disorders of hepatocellular integrity**
   - GPT (ALT), GOT (AST), GDH, LDH, γ-GT
   - Iron
   - Zinc
   - Vitamin B_{12}
2. **Excretory disorders**
   - Bilirubin
   - Bile pigments (in urine)
   - Bile acids
   - AP, LAP, 5′-NU, γ-GT
   - Copper
   - Cholesterol
   - Indocyanine green test (ICG)
   - Bengal rose test
3. **Disorders of synthesis capacity**
   - Cholinesterase (ChE)
   - Clotting factors
   - Antithrombin III (AT III)
   - Albumin
   - LP-X, LCAT, lipoprotein
   - $α_1$-foetoprotein (AFP)
   - Transport proteins
   - Glycoproteins
   - Binding and carrier proteins
4. **Disorders of metabolic performance**
   - Ammonia
   - Galactose test (GEC)
   - Free phenols (in serum and urine)
5. **Disorders of biotransformation**
   - Bilirubin glucuronization
   - Aminopyrine ^{14}C breath test
   - Caffeine elimination test (CET)
   - 4-Methylumbelliferone test
6. **Disorders of hepatic blood perfusion**
   - Indocyanine green test (ICG)
7. **Elevation of mesenchymal reactions**
   - γ-globulins
   - Immunoglobulins A, G, M
   - Copper
   - Procollagen-III-peptide (P-III-P)
8. **Changes in serology and immunology**
   - Virus serology
   - Autoantibody
   - Tumour marker
   - Lymphocyte transformation
   - Leucocyte migration

Tab. 5.3: Most common biochemical reactions and dysfunctions of the liver together with related laboratory parameters

Liver-function tests: There is no single biochemical method which provides a global statement on the hepatic function itself. (s. p. 113) Here the term **liver-function tests**

should be limited to those tests *which make possible the assessment of a specific liver function!* • Thus the elevation of indicator enzymes (GPT, GOT, GDH), which point to a disorder of hepatocellular integrity, cannot be designated as a test of liver function any more than, for example, the elevation of alkaline phosphatase can be described as an indicator of biliary diseases. • *With these liver-function tests, only a small number of the various hepatic functions are recorded. The common (endogenous and exogenous) function tests can, in general, merely indicate a disorder of a certain partial hepatic function.*

> *5th hepatological principle*
> Rational and reliable liver diagnostics requires the simultaneous application of certain liver tests for ascertaining important parameters of cellular integrity and essential liver functions. In some cases, they have to be complemented by further specific tests.

Liver check list: On the basis of their biochemical or biomolecular classification, essential laboratory results are systematically classed in five groups in a liver check list. (13) (s. fig. 5.2) (see also fig. 4.22!)

Graduated programme: This check list facilitates a rational and step-by-step diagnosis as well as a detailed biochemical classification and interpretation of findings. Depending on the diagnostic issue, only single specific parameters are applied and possibly complemented "stepwise" in the form of a graduated programme (= algorithm). (12, 13) (s. tab. 5.23)

▶ Both the decline in enzyme activity and the change in measured values of substrates are comparatively low during storage in a refrigerator. (s. tab. 5.1) The patient's serum should therefore be stored for three to four days in order to determine the additional values required *("step-by-step")* without inconvenience and loss of time to the patient, without additional demands on the staff and without extra material costs.

5 Assessment of hepatocellular integrity

5.1 Enzyme diagnostics

Enzymes: As high-molecular proteins, enzymes are essential components of cellular ultrastructures. Enzymes are synthesized on demand, following the same mechanism as other proteins. Within the human organism, more than 1,000 enzymes are known, although only 50 have been utilized for diagnostic purposes so far. • As biocatalysts, enzymes facilitate biochemical processes in a specific direction and at an appropriate pace without undergoing modifications themselves. Due to their protein structure, they possess a high substrate specificity, thereby allowing a multitude of simultaneous metabolic processes to take place. In order to be effective, some enzymes rely on cofactors, prosthetic groups or coenzymes. The nomenclature of enzymes is derived from the reaction they catalyze, or their specific substrate, by adding the suffix "-ase". Historic denotations for enzymes also exist.

Categories: The enzymes are divided into 6 major categories: *(1.) oxidoreductases, (2.) transferases, (3.) hydrolases, (4.) lyases, (5.) isomerases,* and *(6.) ligases.* Each enzyme is characterized by an **EC number** (= Enzyme Commission), which is further subdivided by means of points. (s. tab. 5.4)

Check list of biochemical findings								Name				Date					
Hepatocellular damage				**Cholestasis**				**Hepatic function**				**Mesenchymal activity**				**Immunology**	
	∅	+	++		∅	+	++		∅	+	++		∅	+	++		∅	+	++
GPT				alkaline phosphatase				indirect bilirubin				γ-globulin				HA antibody			
																HBs antigen			
GOT				LAP				cholin-esterase								HBs antibody			
																HBc antibody			
GDH				γ-GT				Quick's value				IgA				HBe antigen			
																HBe antibody			
γ-GT				5′-nucleo-tidase				albumin				IgG (AB)				HBV DNA			
																HCV antibody			
LDH				bile acids				bile acids				IgM (AB)				HDV antibody			
																HEV antibody			
				GDH				fibrinogen								ANA			
																AMA			
				direct bilirubin				ammonia				copper				SMA			
																SLA			
iron/ferritin				cholesterol				indocyanine green test				procollagen-III-peptide				LKM			
																ANCA			
zinc				copper				galactose								α_1-foetoprotein			

Fig. 5.2: List of essential biochemical findings and the respective "hepatic diagnostic evaluation" (2nd diagnostic pillar; s. fig. 4.2) according to their principal biochemical or biomolecular classification (s. fig. 4.22) (s. tab. 5.23)

Hepatobiliary enzymes: Each organ possesses a typical quantitative and, to some extent, qualitative distribution of enzymes resulting in a cellular profile of enzymes, which is termed the **enzyme pattern.** Thus within the hepatocytes and the biliary ducts, the liver also possesses a characteristic distribution of enzymes with gradually varying specificity. This specificity of essential hepatobiliary enzymes is of importance for the diagnosis of hepatobiliary diseases. (24) (s. tab. 5.4)

1. Glutamic pyruvic transaminase (= Alanine aminotransferase)	GPT ALT	2.6.1.2	+++
2. Glutamic oxaloacetic transaminase (= Aspartate aminotransferase)	GOT AST	2.6.1.1	+
3. Glutamate dehydrogenase	GDH	1.4.1.3	++
4. Gamma-glutamyl transferase	γ-GT	2.3.2.2	++
5. Lactate dehydrogenase	LDH	1.1.1.27	+
6. Cholinesterase	ChE	3.1.1.8	+++
7. Phosphohexoisomerase	PHI	5.3.1.9	+
1. Alkaline phosphatase	AP	3.1.3.1	+++
2. Leucine arylamidase (= Leucine aminopeptidase)	LAP	3.4.11.1	++
3. Gamma glutamyl transferase	γ-GT	2.3.2.2	++
4. 5'-Nucleotidase	5'-NU	3.1.3.5	++

Tab. 5.4: Seven essential hepatocellular and four biliary diagnostic enzymes together with their respective terminology, abbreviations, EC code and specificity (+ → +++)

▶ The (ubiquitous) enzyme **phosphohexoisomerase** (PHI) is also found within hepatocytes. Elevated activity is observed in malignancies, and thus this enzyme can be used to monitor the course and therapy of these diseases. Particularly in metastasizing liver cell carcinoma, PHI exhibits the most reliable elevation of enzymes, as compared to GOT and GPT (84%: 50%: 30%) (M. K. Schwartz, 1973). • Although both (mitochondrial) **ornithine carbamoyltransferase** (OCT) and (cytoplasmic) **sorbitol dehydrogenase** (SDH) possess a high hepatocellular specificity, they play no part in diagnostics. Likewise, the assessment of **isocitrate dehydrogenase** (ICDH) as a marker of centroacinar necrosis (17), **aldolase** (ALD) and **alcohol dehydrogenase** (ADH) is unnecessary during the course of enzyme diagnostics in hepatobiliary diseases.

Classification: The classification of the hepatobiliary enzymes essential for enzyme diagnostics is based on their characteristic nature – i.e. *excretory, secretory* and *indicator enzymes.* (s. tab. 5.5) They are located predominantly within the liver cells and the biliary ducts as well as within the hepatic lobules. The speed of **enzyme elimination** does not depend on the blood enzyme levels, but follows an exponential curve. This allows the computation of the **half-life** of enzymes within the plasma, which is not influenced either by gender or age and is a typical enzyme characteristic. The velocity of enzyme elimination is largely constant. (s. tab. 5.5) However, in chronic diseases of the liver, it is known, for example, that GPT is usually eliminated faster than GOT despite its longer half-life.

Normal levels: Under normal conditions and during physiological "moulting", hepatocytes leak minor quantities of enzymes, which are detectable in the serum as

Indicator enzymes	GPT, GOT, GDH, LDH
Secretory enzymes	ChE
Excretory enzymes	AP, LAP, γ-GT, 5'-NU
Unilocular	
Cytoplasm	GPT, LDH
Mitochondria	GDH
Endoplasmic reticulum	γ-GT, ChE
Bilocular	
Cytoplasm	cGOT (20%)
Mitochondria	mGOT (80%)
Periportal (zone 1)	GPT, LDH, AP
Pericentral (zone 3)	GDH, ADH
Zones 1–3	GOT

half-life	in hours	half-life	in days
LDH_5	10 ± 2	γ-GT	3–4
GOT	13 ± 1	AP	3–7
GDH	16 ± 2	ChE	<10
GPT	47 ± 10	LAP	<10

Tab. 5.5: Schematic differentiation of hepatocellular enzymes according to their type and preferred localization within the liver cell or the liver lobule as well as their half-life

"normal values". Due to inflow (= enzyme secretion from the liver cell) and outflow (= enzyme elimination), these values are kept largely constant within a normal range.

Elevation of enzyme values: The liver contains approx. 400 U GPT/g protein and 500 U GOT/g protein. In increased permeability of or damage to the liver cell membrane – referred to as low-grade disorders of cellular integrity – cytoplasmic enzymes (GPT, GOT, γ-GT, LDH) enter the plasma. Only during cellular necrosis – resulting in the destruction of mitochondria and the endoplasmic reticulum – do localized enzymes (GDH, γ-GT, GOT) enter the bloodstream. These enzymes then become elevated to levels which are considered to be pathological. One gram of liver tissue contains approx. 171 million hepatocytes. (s. p. 25) *Damage to the cellular membranes of only 1 gram of liver parenchyma (with a normal wet weight of the liver of ca. 1,500 g) results in an increase in the serum enzyme activity of GPT to pathological levels. With corresponding liver cell necrosis, GOT and GDH respond in the same fashion with a measurable increase in activity. If the liver loses only $1/1000$ of its cell enzymes, there is a rise in the respective enzyme activity in the serum by a factor of 2.* The enzyme content in the hepatocytes can be up to 10,000 times higher than in the serum. Hence, there is a genuine correlation between the nature and intensity of hepatocellular damage and the increase in activity of free cytoplasmic as well as bound mitochondrial enzymes.

Enzyme distortion: A shift in the normal enzyme pattern is usually termed enzyme distortion. It is possible to derive various kinds of *information* from the prevailing enzyme pattern:

1. The less distorted the enzyme pattern within the serum, the more profound is the underlying necrotic hepatocellular damage, i.e. the enzyme profile within the serum corresponds to that within the hepatocytes: LDL > GOT > GPT > GDH.

2. The more distorted the enzyme pattern, the more chronic is the course of the disease.

3. The severity and type of cell damage (inflammatory or necrotizing) are determined by the relation between enzymes localized in the cytoplasm and the mitochondria.

4. The level of enzyme values supplies information on the extent of the hepatic parenchymal damage.

5. The relative half-life of enzymes is indicative of the duration of the disease (acute, chronic).

6. The relation between cholinesterase and indicator enzymes gives insight into the stage of a chronic liver disease.

▶ The cell-integrity enzymes GPT (ALT), GOT (AST) and GLDH cannot be regarded as *liver-function tests* (LFT) because they are not markers of a specific liver function. (s. p. 113) Therefore, the term "LFT" is a *misnomer* and should not be used for these enzymes!

Enzyme ratios: In hepatocellular damage, the serum GPT value generally exceeds the GOT value, the so-called *inflammatory type*. Only during cellular necrosis with associated destruction of mitochondria does the GOT activity exceed that of GPT, because the mitochondrial portion of GOT then leaks into the serum. This constitutes the basis for the **DeRitis ratio** (F. DeRitis et al., 1956). The course of disease is more severe (i.e. more necrotic) and the respective prognosis more serious if the GOT/GPT ratio exceeds 1, the so-called *necrotizing type*. In chronic active hepatitis C, a value of >1 correlates closely with the extent of fibrosis and the development of cirrhosis. (30) This ratio may be >2 in alcoholic or malignant liver diseases and it may be >4 in fulminant hepatitis. • In hepatological diagnostics, further **ratios** can be applied as additional parameters. (s. tabs. 5.6, 5.7)

Transaminases: The transaminases catalyze the reversible transformation of α-ketoacids into amino acids. Frequently, the two transaminases GPT (= *glutamic pyruvic transaminase*) (or ALT = *alamine transaminase*) and GOT (= *glutamic oxaloacetic transaminase*) (or AST = *aspartate transaminase*) are used in enzyme diagnostics (F. DeRitis et al., 1955; F. Wroblewski et al., 1955). (s. tab. 5.4) While GOT is distributed evenly, the GPT concentration continuously decreases from periportal to pericentral in the acinus. These are the basic parameters in the diagnosis and follow-up of hepatocellular disease. If the cause of elevated transaminases remains unclear, liver biopsy is indicated. (19, 22, 23, 26, 29, 31)

▶ *Generally, the elevation of transaminases is a reliable marker of hepatocellular damage, particularly of the inflammatory or necrotizing type* (s. tab. 5.6).

GOT/GPT ratio (= DeRitis ratio)	
1. **Inflammatory type**	GOT < GPT = <1
2. **Necrotizing type**	GOT > GPT = >1
– in severe alcoholic or malignant liver disease	GOT > GPT = >2
γ-GT/GOT ratio	
1. Acute viral hepatitis	= <1
2. Toxic hepatitis Chronic persistent hepatitis	= <2
3. Chronic hepatitis Acute alcoholic hepatitis Cirrhosis	= 2–3
4. Alcoholic cirrhosis Acute obstructive jaundice	= 3–6
5. Biliary cirrhosis Chronic obstructive jaundice	= >6
6. Liver carcinoma. Liver metastases	= >12
(GPT + GOT)/GDH ratio	
1. Severe toxic/inflammatory damage of perivenous parenchyma	= <10
2. Liver metastases	= <10
3. Obstructive jaundice Necrotic episode in acute hepatitis Acute intoxication, liver carcinoma	= <20
4. Biliary cirrhosis	= 20–30
5. Acute episode in chronic hepatitis or in liver cirrhosis	= 30–40
6. Cholestasis	= 30–50
7. Acute viral hepatitis Acute alcoholic hepatitis	= >50

Tab. 5.6: Enzyme ratios (using optimized tests) as additional "cheap" and "fast" enzyme parameters of differential diagnosis of liver diseases (13, 18, 30)

LDH/GOT ratio	
1. Haemolytic jaundice	= >12
2. Hepatocellular jaundice	= <12
GPT/GDH ratio	
1. Obstructive jaundice	= <10
2. Hepatocellular jaundice	= >10

Tab. 5.7: Enzyme ratios as additional support for the differential diagnosis of hyperbilirubinaemia

Extrahepatic causes of increased transaminases include: (*1.*) cardiac infarction, (*2.*) severe tachycardia, (*3.*) muscular diseases, (*4.*) pulmonary embolism, (*5.*) hypo-/hyperthyreosis, (*6.*) coeliac disease, (*7.*) heatstroke, (*8.*) hyperthermia, (*9.*) excessive physical exercise, (*10.*) long-term fasting, (*11.*) above-average protein intake, (*12.*) haemolysis, and (*13.*) long-term venous stasis.

Macroenzymes are characterized by a high molecular weight and therefore have a delayed clearance. For this reason, they cause false-positive increases of certain liver cell enzymes. *Type 1 macroenzymes* result from the formation of antigen-antibody complexes, using GPT, GOT, γGT and AP. *Type 2 macroenzymes*, result from oligomerization, using γGT, AP, LAP and 5'-NU.

In unresolved elevation of the transaminases (possibly also of other hepatobiliary enzymes), percutaneous liver biopsy will supply a normal result in up to 10% of cases. (20) This *"histological normality"* is, however, not necessarily representative of the entire liver! (s. pp 150, 168) (s. figs. 7.8) *Any histological findings should be limited exclusively to the individual biopsy punch. Consequently, the localized findings obtained by the pathologist should not be automatically related by the hepatologist to the liver as a whole.*

5.1.1 GPT (ALT)

GPT possesses a sensitivity of 83%, with a specificity of 84% relating to nonhepatic diseases and 97.8% relating to healthy subjects. • According to our own investigations, elevation of GPT as a **"screening enzyme"** was demonstrated in 81% of 520 patients with very different liver diseases. (13) (s. tabs. 4.2; 5.11)

▶ *Elevated GPT is the most sensitive indicator of hepatocellular damage. An exclusive rise in GPT is, as a rule, of hepatocellular origin.*

However, it is not possible to detect the cause of hepatocellular damage, nor to differentiate primary liver disease from a secondary hepatic reaction (e.g. in various inflammatory processes). Moreover, the chronicity of a liver disease, or its respective stage, cannot be determined by virtue of elevated GPT values. • Serum GPT may also be increased due to obesity, extreme physical strain, persisting tachycardia, hyperthyroidism, long-term fasting, excessive protein intake and blood collection. Slightly elevated GPT values may occur in the second trimester of pregnancy. (15) In the absence of clinical findings, a continuous elevation of GPT (and also of GOT) is found with the appearance of macroenzyme-1 immune complexes.

Determination of GPT has proved to be a reliable marker for the follow-up of a precisely diagnosed inflammatory liver disease and the so-called asymptomatic HBsAg-carrier state as well as for the screening of blood donors. In extensive hepatocellular damage, the elevation of GPT is accompanied by a corresponding increase in the GOT value.

▶ *False-normal GPT* values are often found – despite the presence of liver damage – in: (*1.*) haemochromatosis, (*2.*) ileo-jejunal bypass, (*3.*) marked (e.g. alcohol-induced) deficiency of pyridoxal phosphate (B_6), (*4.*) severe loss of liver parenchyma, and (*5.*) during the terminal stages of liver disease with exhaustion and/or blockage of hepatocellular enzyme synthesis caused by toxins. • In "healthy" persons, slightly elevated GPT values were detected in 0.5% of cases.

Normal GPT value (37 °C) *) s. p. 128	
Women < 34 U/l	Men < 45 U/l

5.1.2 GOT (AST)

The diagnostic sensitivity of GOT (71%) is significantly lower than that of GPT. This is understandable, since it is only the cytoplasmic portion of the GOT (20%) which will enter the blood if the liver cell membrane is damaged – a factor which arithmetically also reduces the sensitivity. The isolated elevation of GOT is not to be expected in liver diseases – except for false-normal GPT due to B_6 deficiency. GOT is mainly present in the heart and skeletal muscles, but is also found in the kidney, brain, pancreas and lung. Diseases of these organs are accompanied by respective increases in GOT. An elevation of GOT values may also occur as a result of haemolysis, strenuous physical exercise and prolonged venostasis during blood collection. Distinctly elevated levels were found in hypoxic hepatitis. (21, 32) As a rule, pregnancy shows a normal GOT value. (15) In hepatology, the main purpose of determining GOT is to complement GPT values. Beyond this, the GOT value can be applied for the determination of *enzyme ratios* as an additional parameter in the differential diagnosis of liver diseases. (20, 26, 29, 31, 92) (s. tabs. 5.6, 5.7).

▶ Determination of **mitochondrial GOT** (mGOT = 80%) is recommended as an additional laboratory parameter for the detection of persistent **alcohol abuse**, particularly in those cases where GDH measurements are inconclusive. Mitochondrial GOT (mGOT) serves as a fatty acid-binding protein (FABP). This might help to explain the increased uptake of fatty acids in hepatocytes due to alcohol abuse.

▶ The **decline in transaminases** to "normal" levels – with a continued deterioration of the active liver disease – and sometimes even to (extremely) subnormal concentrations is a fatal sign. Excessive enzyme deprivation, with a simultaneous marked reduction in cholinesterase activity, is commonly regarded as a *final sign of laboratory chemistry, indicating the imminent death of the liver-diseased patient.*

Any determination of **elevated transaminases** requires remeasurement after 14 days (or earlier) because:

(*1.*) after normalization, there will be no further consequences (e.g. the condition was caused by a secondary hepatic reaction to an infection),

(*2.*) a marked increase is indicative of the development of acute viral hepatitis or progressive intoxication, both of which have to be clarified,

(*3.*) a persistent elevation requires further diagnostic steps for final differentiation of the active liver disease.

Normal GOT value (37 °C) *) s. p. 128	
Women < 31 U/l	Men < 35 U/l

5.1.3 Glutamate dehydrogenase (GDH)

GDH effects the oxidative deamination of glutamate. Extensive GDH activity is found only in the liver – it is very low in the heart, kidney, brain, lung, and skeletal muscles. In hepatocytes, it is present as a mitochondrial enzyme. Therefore, it only enters the blood after extensive cellular damage with subsequent destruction of the mitochondria. Centrolobular (zone 3) GDH activity is 1.8 times higher than that found in the periphery of the liver lobule. This region represents the final stretch of the sinusoidal supply pathway. Hepatocytes located at this site are therefore particularly prone to hypoxia and toxins. (16) This results in a more pronounced elevation of GDH with a respective decline in the GPT + GOT/ GDH ratio. (18, 30) (s. tab. 5.6) • GDH is unsuitable as a "screening enzyme" since the respective sensitivity is only 47%. In combination with GPT and GOT, it can, however, yield the most reliable assessment of hepatocyte integrity.

A marked **elevation of GDH** is found in stages of extensive alcohol-induced steatosis, in primary biliary cirrhosis, during the development of liver cell carcinoma due to cirrhosis (with an increase in activity comparable to that of γ-GT and AP), in benign obstructive jaundice (with a decline in elevated GDH and transaminase values after approx. one week even though there is simultaneous persistence of cholestasis enzymes) as well as in acute incomplete obstructive biliary flow. Regression of acute viral hepatitis or progression of a chronic inflammatory liver disease is indicated more reliably by GDH than by transaminases. • During *acute cholestasis,* possibly with loss of gallstones through the bile duct, GDH is markedly elevated. This clear rise in GDH is a reliable parameter for diagnosing biliary-induced colic on the right side, because kidney stones can now be ruled out. (13) • *Extremely high GDH values* (up to 1,000 U/l and higher) are found in severe toxic liver cell necrosis (as induced by halothane, amanita phalloides, etc.), during acute right heart failure, severe respiratory insufficiency, circulatory failure, immunological rejection after liver transplantation, and abrupt impairment of the hepatic circulation. (16)

Normal GDH value (37°C) *) s. p. 128	
Women <5 U/l	Men <7 U/l

5.1.4 Lactate dehydrogenase (LDH)

LDH is a cytoplasmic enzyme which catalyzes the oxidation of lactate into pyruvate. It consists of **five isoenzymes.** As a ubiquitous enzyme and constituent of almost all tissues, LDH enters the blood circulation even in minor cell and tissue damage. The *isoenzymes LDH_4 and LDH_5* are predominantly located in the liver, cardiac muscle and malignant tissues. After severe damage of the liver parenchyma, these isoenzymes may become elevated. The half-life of LDH_5 is very short (10 ± 2 hours).

A marked *elevation* of total serum LDH is most obvious in liver metastases and obstructive jaundice. This explains why a considerable increase in LDH activity, in particular that of isoenzymes 4 and 5, can be detected in malignant ascites. An increase in LDH (in the absence of haemolysis) and low transaminase activity are reliable markers of hepatitis mononucleosa: this is due to virocytes secreting large quantities of LDH into the serum. • For the differential diagnosis of haemolytic and hepatocellular jaundice, the *LDH/GOT ratio* is helpful as an additional parameter. (s. tab. 5.7)

Normal LDH value (37°C) *) s. p. 128	
Women <247 U/l	Men <248 U/l

5.1.5 Gamma-glutamyl transferase (γ-GT)

Gamma-GT is found in the liver, bile ducts, kidney, pancreas, epididymis, heart, lung, small intestine, bone marrow, salivary glands, thymus, spleen, and brain. The kidney has the highest specific activity of γ-GT, with a concentration 25 times greater than that of the liver. The heterogeneity of γ-GT was described in 1965 (F. Kokot et al.). Eleven isoenzymes are known today. (25)

▶ Gamma-GT catalyzes the transfer of the glutamyl residues of various peptides. It is the key enzyme of the **glutamate cycle,** and it is also active in the regulation of **glutathione metabolism.** • Due to a strong enrichment in the endothelial cells and pericytes of the cerebral capillaries, γ-GT seems to exert an important **protective and detoxifying function** at the blood-brain barrier (e.g. metabolization of foreign substances via the mercapturic acid pathway).

There is *no γ-GT activity* in muscle, bone and erythrocytes. Despite high γ-GT activity in kidneys, nephropathies do not result in γ-GT elevations. During pregnancy, γ-GT activity is normal or the serum values may show a declining tendency from the second trimester onwards. • In the liver, γ-GT is found in the membranes of hepatocytes and bile duct epithelia. The periphery of the liver lobule has the highest γ-GT activity. Gamma-GT passes from the liver into the bile and is then excreted partly by the kidneys in the urine. (s. tabs. 5.4, 5.5)

Elevation of γ-GT was introduced into liver diagnostics by E. Szczeklik et al. in 1961. Elevated values can be attributed to *two causes*: (*1.*) enhanced de-novo synthesis and (*2.*) damage to the liver cell membrane. • The enhanced de-novo synthesis occurs as a result of an induction of the biotransformation enzyme system by foreign, pharmaceutical or chemical substances as well as by cholestasis or bile acids. Three-fold (or higher) rises cannot as a rule be attributed to a sole induction. • Enhanced de-novo synthesis may also be triggered by augmented cellular regeneration, which leads to an increase in the activity of a foetal form of γ-GT. Thus elevated γ-GT is often still detected during the phase of restoration after acute viral hepatitis even if other indicator enzymes have already returned to normal levels. The higher γ-GT level therefore does not only hint at persisting cellular damage, but is also indicative of the stage of regeneration and thus of the (histologically) prevailing posthepatitic "vulnerable" phase. Likewise, enhanced regeneration after cirrhosis can be accompanied by elevated γ-GT. (13, 25, 26, 33)

▶ Enhancement of the γ-GT activity – without an associated increase in GPT – can usually be explained as *enhanced induction* or *cellular regeneration*. In both of these cases, this can be seen as a *"physiological" process of adaptation in order to fulfil a more demanding task*. (s. p. 59)

Even minor *hepatocellular damage* results in the release of membrane-bound γ-GT in connection with simultaneous leakage of GPT (the low concentration of the associated GOT portion is not detectable at this point). Gamma-GT is known to be a sensitive indicator of hepatocellular damage. Normal γ-GT excludes a liver disease in 90–95% of cases.

In *hepatobiliary diseases*, the sensitivity and specificity of γ-GT is 95%, since γ-GT is also located in cholangiocytes. In individuals with a healthy liver, the specificity is 74%, in overall healthy individuals it is 95%. • In cholestasis, the sensitivity of γ-GT is six times that of AP and nine times that of LAP. • Obstruction of bile flow can be the cause of isolated γ-GT elevation in fatty liver.

Alcohol-induced liver damage elevates γ-GT. The level of elevation depends on various endogenous (including genetic) and exogenous factors. Alcohol induction, such as can be measured by elevated γ-GT, only occurs after prolonged *regular* alcohol abuse and disappears only after *rigorous abstinence for several weeks*. Yet, γ-GT is not alcohol-specific. Some 20–30% of alcoholic patients even have normal γ-GT values.

▶ It is factually wrong and not justifiable to base the assessment of persistent alcohol abuse (particularly in cases involving legal decisions, e.g. drinking and driving) *solely* upon elevated γ-GT levels. • The "possibility" of an alcohol-induced γ-GT elevation has to be made "probable" in each individual case by applying further laboratory tests, by means of psychological testing and by ensuring that all other causes of γ-GT elevation have been ruled out.

Elevation of γ-GT is found in cholestasis, liver cirrhosis, viral hepatitis, fatty liver, porphyria, toxic liver damage, pancreatitis and pancreatic cancer, myocardial infarction, nephrotic syndrome, diabetes mellitus, right heart failure, obesity (28), nicotine abuse, and brain tumours. There is a good correlation of γ-GT with CEA in colon cancer, involving a metastatic spread to the liver – an increase in γ-GT in neoplastic disease is likewise supportive of the diagnosis of hepatic metastases.

A permanent rise in γ-GT due to liver cirrhosis suggests *primary liver cell carcinoma*. The sensitivity of isoenzyme II was very high at 90%; this parameter therefore proved more reliable for diagnosis and follow-up than AP isoenzyme-1, α₁-foetoprotein or α₁-antitrypsin. Isoenzyme-2 of gamma-GT is seen as the best marker in the early stages of primary liver cell carcinoma. (33)

A **decline in γ-GT** to subnormal levels can be observed during oestrogen administration and from the second trimester of pregnancy onwards (15) as well as with excessive consumption of coffee. • In haemolysis, false-low values may be found.

Normal values of γ-GT may be the result of "cellular moulting" or of regular but still individually differing inductions within the biotransformation process caused by toxins. (s. p. 59) Normal values of γ-GT in women may also be brought about by hormonal action (e.g. decline in enzymatic activity through oestrogens).

Normal γ-GT value (37°C) *) s. p. 128	
Women < 38 U/l	Men < 55 U/l

5.2 Iron and ferritin

Hepatocytes are involved in iron metabolism in two ways: they are the site of transferrin synthesis, and they represent the most important site in the storage of iron in the form of ferritin or haemosiderin. Hence, the level of iron in the serum depends on the ability of the hepatocyte to store iron and to synthesize transferrin. *(see chapters 3.11 and 31.17)*

The first observation of **hypersideraemia** in an icteric liver disease was made by A. WARBURG and H. A. KREBS (1927). In 1939 G. HEMMELER used the determination of serum iron to differentiate hepatocellular jaundice from obstructive jaundice, because the latter regularly reveals a normal iron value.

Structural hepatocellular damage causes iron to leave the cell and subsequently results in an increase in serum iron. After diffuse liver damage has worn off, the elevated serum iron level takes a relatively long time to return to normal. This leads to the conclusion that hepatocellular damage is terminated (detectable in the return of enzymatic activities to normal) before the hepatocyte regains the ability to store iron.

The **range of variation** in iron values primarily depends on age, gender and nutrition. In addition, there are distinct circadian variations: in the evening, the iron value is lower than in the morning. Day-to-day changes are also evident (varying RES activity?). • Considerable **interference factors** are possible during the collection of a blood sample: (*1.*) for the determination of iron, an iron-free needle has to be employed, (*2.*) any excessive venous stasis results in elevated iron values, (*3.*) contamination can also be caused by ferrous syringes, and (*4.*) haemolysis has to be avoided.

Ferritin shows a direct and quantitative correlation to the iron stored in the RES. It therefore represents a useful indicator of the total concentration of stored iron in the organism. The liver is the organ with the highest ferritin concentration. Thus ferritin levels below 15 µg/l are always an indicator of depletion of the iron depot – with or without associated anaemia. Ferritin is equally important for monitoring therapeutic measures concerning the restoration or reduction of the iron depot. The iron value decreases in severe liver diseases as well as in neoplasms, and there is no longer a correlation with the iron stored, whereas serum ferritin levels start to increase. (27) • For the differentiation of primary (idiopathic) haemochromatosis from the more frequent secondary haemosiderosis, the **deferoxamine test** has proved to be reliable.

> **Method:** After emptying the bladder, deferoxamine (one vial of 500 mg) is injected (i.m.) and urine is collected for exactly six hours with subsequent determination of iron excretion. Iron levels of > 4 mg are deemed characteristic of primary haemochromatosis, while iron levels of < 2 mg are regarded as normal, or caused by secondary haemosiderosis. • This test can also be executed as follows: 10 mg/kg BW deferoxamine (i.m.) with urine collection for 24 hours, whereby the haemochromatosis value is > 10 mg iron and the normal value is < 2 mg iron.

Elevated iron, which usually corresponds to increased ferritin, is found *primarily* in idiopathic haemochromatosis and *secondarily* in acute viral hepatitis, liver cell necrosis and necrotic episodes, alcoholic liver diseases, porphyria cutanea tarda, oestrogen administration, etc.

Reduced iron is found in infections or chronic inflammations, in neoplasms as a *distributive disorder* (i.e. shift of the serum iron pool to the macrophages), or as *iron deficiency* (i.e. due to reduced iron intake or a decline in transferrin synthesis). Iron deficiency can also appear during liver cirrhosis due to occult bleeding.

Normal iron value *) s. p. 128	
Women 23–134 µg/dl	Men 35–168 µg/dl
Normal ferritin value	
Women 9–140 µg/l	Men 18–360 µg/l
Normal transferrin value	
Women 1.9–4.4 mg/l	Men 2.2–5.0 mg/l
Iron-transferrin saturation	
16–45%	

5.3 Zinc

Zinc is an important trace element. *Zinc deficiency* or a disorder of *zinc distribution* plays an increasingly important role in hepatology: hypoproteinaemia, reduction in the urea synthesis or disturbance of cell-mediated immunity may be the result. (s. p. 55) (s. tab. 3.15)

The first description of zinc deficiency in a patient with alcoholic cirrhosis (B. L. VALLÉE et al., 1956) has meanwhile been confirmed by numerous investigations. In cases where zincuria is initially elevated and subsequently reduced, the decreased zinc levels may be used for diagnosis and at the same time indicate therapeutic substitution.

Normal zinc value *) s. p. 128	
Serum	0.6–1.2 mg/l
Urine	0.15–0.8 mg/24 hr

6 Disorders of excretion

Within a certain degree of hepatocellular damage, liver cell functions remain completely or widely intact; at least, no impaired partial functions are yet detectable under clinical conditions. As liver damage progresses, however, numerous cellular functions become increasingly affected, so that clinically relevant disorders are now evident. Thus impairment of the hepatic excretory capacity can be taken as a criterion of parenchymal damage.

▶ There are two metabolic functions which are affected by **disorders of excretion,** both of which take place predominantly in the *smooth endoplasmic reticulum:*

(*1.*) **Endogenous clearance** excretes physiological metabolites in a timely manner and in quantitatively appropriate proportions (e.g. bilirubin, enzymes, bile pigments, bile acids).

(*2.*) **Exogenous clearance** eliminates ingested substances within a certain period of time and in a certain quantity (e.g. foreign substances used in diagnostics).

6.1 Bilirubin

Under normal conditions, 250–300 mg bilirubin are produced per day. Primary, albumin-bound, unconjugated and therefore water-insoluble bilirubin is conjugated in the liver to become water-soluble; it can now be eliminated by the kidneys. (s. p. 37)

The differentiation between **indirect bilirubin** (= primary, albumin-bound, water-insoluble/fat-soluble form) and **direct bilirubin** (= secondary, conjugated, water-soluble/fat-insoluble form) using diazobenzolsulfonic acid was introduced by A. A. HIJMANS VAN DEN BERGH (1918). Direct bilirubin is detected "directly" by way of diazotization, while indirect serum bilirubin can only be determined after extraction with alcohol or in the presence of an accelerator (caffeine, sodium acetate) by way of the diazo reaction. (s. p. 38) • Direct bilirubin consists of two fractions: bilirubin monoglucuronide and bilirubin diglucuronide. Besides these water-soluble bilirubin fractions, serum also contains **delta bilirubin** as a third water-soluble form (half-life is 18 days). Thus together with indirect bilirubin, **total bilirubin** consists of four fractions. The serum level for indirect bilirubin is computed from the difference between total and direct bilirubin. There is no direct bilirubin, but a normal level of < 0.3 mg/dl is "faked" when using conventional methods of detection. The excretory capacity of the liver regarding bilirubin is twice the physiologically required level. This is why the serum bilirubin level is only seen to be elevated after substantial disturbance of excretory hepatic functions (e.g. bilirubinuria is recognized earlier than bilirubinaemia). • The concentration of total bilirubin may be slightly higher in men than in women, with a normal age-related peak between the ages of 20 and 25. The value of bilirubin is not influenced by pregnancy.

A *false-pathological elevation* of the bilirubin concentration can be induced by fasting (>24 hrs.), intense muscular activity, haemolysis and certain drugs (e.g. antibiotics, propranolol, methyldopa and oestrogen).

A *false-pathological decrease* of the bilirubin concentration can be induced by the displacement of bilirubin from albumin-binding sites due to pharmaceutical substances or xenobiotics. This leads to an increased migration of bilirubin into the tissue, causing the bilirubin concentration to decline. A decrease in the serum bilirubin value is also found in pregnancy. (15) Intensive exposure to sunlight similarly reduces the serum bilirubin concentration (up to 30% loss).

▶ **Hyperbilirubinaemia** is a clinical symptom. *Scleral icterus* becomes evident if bilirubin exceeds 1.6–1.8 mg/dl, while clinical *icterus* is diagnosed at levels of >2.5 mg/dl. (s. p. 84) Congenital (hereditary) hyperbilirubinaemias are primary disorders of bilirubin metabolism. Hyperbilirubinaemias are divided into pre-, intra- and posthepatic jaundice. • The diagnostic *sensitivity* and *specificity* of hyperbilirubinaemia for the detection of a liver disease is low. The *prognostic value* is equally low with certain exceptions, e.g. alcoholic hepatitis, primary biliary cirrhosis or mechanical obstruction of bile ducts. • Prehepatic (haemolytic) jaundice can be differentiated from hepatic jaundice using the LDH/GOT ratio in addition to other parameters. • Differential diagnosis of posthepatic (mechanical) and intrahepatic (hepatocellular) jaundice is facilitated by the GPT/GDH ratio. (s. tab. 5.7) • Mechanical jaundice is demonstrated in most cases either by a value of less than 20 in the GPT+GOT/GDH ratio or by a value of more than 6 in the γ-GT/GOT ratio. (s. tab. 5.6) *(see chapter 12)*

Normal bilirubin value *) s. p. 128
Total bilirubin <1.2 mg/dl
Indirect bilirubin 0.3–1.1 mg/dl

6.2 Bile pigments in the urine

The various bile pigments urobilinogen, urobilin and stercobilin (along with related polymers) are produced in the intestine. They are excreted predominantly in the faeces, while a minor portion (10–15%) is reabsorbed into the **enterohepatic circulation** by hepatocytes. Minor quantities of bile pigments (<2%) enter the main bloodstream to be excreted as water-soluble substances via the kidneys in the urine (1.0–3.5 mg/day). • Normally, **bilirubin** is not detectable in the urine. Bilirubinuria can occur in hepatobiliary diseases, with bilirubin regularly appearing in its conjugated (water-soluble) form. The condition is often identified prior to the detection of icterus. Jaundice without parallel bilirubinuria suggests unconjugated hyperbilirubinaemia.

The determination of **urobilinogen** based on the aldehyde reaction (which is non-specific for urobilinogen) was established by P. Ehrlich (1901). (s. pp 12, 13, 38) Excretion of urobilinogen in the urine is influenced by a number of factors. Since urobilinogenuria only occurs in relatively serious disorders of the hepatobiliary system, it is only of minor diagnostic relevance. • A *lack of urobilinogen* in the urine in an icteric patient points to complete obstructive jaundice. Even after total cessation of bile production due to severe liver disease or destruction of the intestinal flora, urobilinogen may also be absent. (s. fig. 5.3) (s. tab. 5.8)

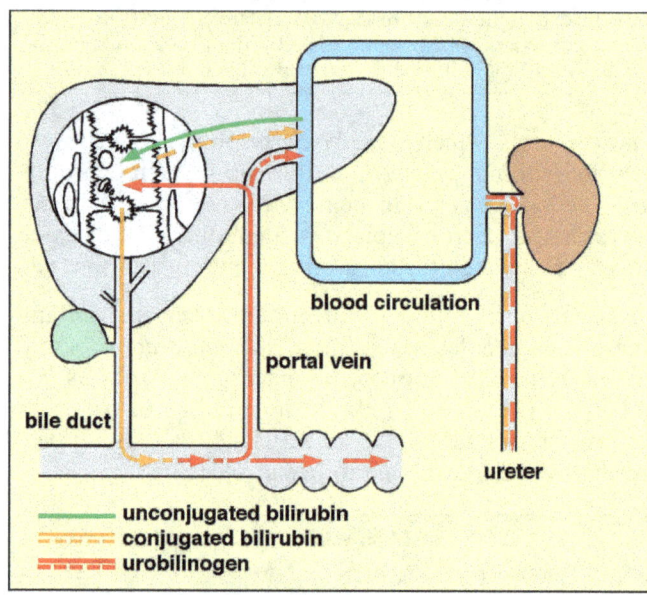

Fig. 5.3: Enterohepatic circulation and excretion of bile pigments

Bilirubinuria
1. Hepatocellular damage with increased membrane permeability
2. Disorder of bilirubin excretion
3. Intrahepatic bile obstruction
4. Extrahepatic obstructive jaundice
Prehepatic urobilinogenuria   = *severely overstrained functional hepatic capacity*
1. Significant elevation of bilirubin production (haemolysis, *etc.*)
2. Significant increase in intestinal urobilinogen production (ileus, enterocolitis, *etc.*)
Hepatic urobilinogenuria   = *severely limited functional hepatic capacity*
1. Severe liver disease
2. Collateral hepatic circulation (cirrhosis, portal vein thrombosis, occlusion of hepatic vein, *etc.*)

Tab. 5.8: Causes of bilirubinuria and urobilinogenuria

Urine test strips: Commercially available urine test strips are reliable in detecting urobilinogenuria and bilirubinuria. When performed as a routine screening test, the urine may occasionally reveal a positive reaction. *Bilirubinuria* and/or *urobilinogenuria* are attributable to various causes. (s. tab. 5.8)

6.3 Bile acids

The liver is the sole organ for the synthesis, conjugation, transport, excretion and reabsorption of bile acids. Therefore, bile acids assume a key role as a test of **endogenous hepatic function,** since they may suggest (*1.*) hepatocellular damage, (*2.*) excretory disorders of the liver, (*3.*) decrease in synthesis capacity, and (*4.*) existence of portosystemic shunts. The determination of bile acids can indeed be extremely useful in the diagnosis and follow-up of liver diseases. Elevated values are accepted as a sensitive and early sign of **cholestasis** and thus constitute a precise liver-specific parameter. (34, 37, 75) *(see chapters 3.5 and 13)*

▶ Previous difficulties concerning the method of determination were overcome through the introduction of a reliable **enzymatic dye test,** with a specificity for 3-α-hydroxy groups and a precision of ± 5–8%. There is no age- or gender-dependent range of variation. Half-life is 2–3 days.

The *sensitivity* of values determined two hours after food consumption seems to be higher than that after fasting. The fasting value is, however, preferred for the sake of reproducibility. In liver diseases, the postprandial increase in serum values can be several times higher than after fasting. In healthy individuals, however, fasting values are only exceeded by 50–70%. The elevation of bile acids in the serum is reflected by an increase in their excretion in the urine (normal < 8 μmol/day). The elevated level of bile acids returns to normal at a relatively slow pace.

The *specificity* of bile acid determination in liver diseases is high, particularly in those with a cholestatic component. The *sensitivity* has been determined as 89%. Congruence with liver histology was found to be 83% after fasting and 96% in postprandial patients. The sequence for *diagnostic accuracy* was determined as: bile acids (fasting) > ICG test > GPT > AP > bilirubin.

Normal bile acid value *) s. p. 128	
Total bile acids	
– fasting	1.0–6.0 μmol/l
– postprandial (2 hrs)	6.0–9.0 μmol/l

6.4 Enzymatic markers of cholestasis

The term "enzymatic markers of cholestasis" comprises alkaline phosphatase, leucine aminopeptidase (or leucine arylamidase) as well as 5′-nucleotidase and γ-glutamyl transferase. *(see chapter 13)*

6.4.1 Alkaline phosphatase (AP)

Alkaline phosphatase (W. M. ROBERTS, 1933) catalyzes the biochemical splitting of phosphoric acid ester. • AP is found in the liver, bone, kidney, intestine, lung and placenta. A *Regan isoenzyme* can be detected as an ectopic variation of placental AP in tumour patients (10–30% of cases). The AP of the liver is located in the cytoplasm and in the membranes, primarily at the biliary pole. Placental AP is also present in the liver. The AP of bile duct epithelia is not elevated in healthy individuals. The serum activity of AP is predominantly due to the isoenzymes of the liver and osteoblasts; only 14% are of renal origin. Half-life is 3–7 days.

The **increase in AP activity** is stimulated by bile acids. A rise in bile acids, which is considered to be the most sensitive and earliest marker of cholestasis, precedes any elevation in AP. The latter derives from enzyme synthesis with increased secretion into the blood. Under pathological conditions, bile duct AP is formed, which is a sensitive marker for hepatobiliary diseases, cholestasis and space-occupying lesions of the liver. The *sensitivity* is 80–100% in cholestatic diseases. AP activity is usually higher in obstructive jaundice and cholangitis than in intrahepatic obstructions, and it is highest in the "vanishing bile duct disease" or in complete obstruction. (13, 36, 38) (s. tabs. 5.9; 13.2–13.4)

1. Bone diseases with osteoblast activity (Paget's disease, rachitis, osteomalacia, bone tumours, aseptic bone necrosis, fracture healing)
2. Autoimmune vasculitis Polymyalgia rheumatica (*typical:* AP ↑↑ and blood sedimentation rate ↑↑↑)
3. Renal diseases (diabetic glomerular sclerosis, acute tubular necrosis, hypernephroid carcinoma)
4. Tumours, particularly bronchial carcinoma, M. Hodgkin
5. Hyperthyroidism
6. Congestive liver
7. Hyperparathyroidism
8. Leukaemia, lymphoma, multiple myeloma
9. Drugs, chemicals
10. Hyperphosphatasaemia
11. Intestinal ischaemia, coeliac disease
12. Hyperlipidaemia
13. Acromegaly
14. Cystadenoma of the pancreas
15. Sarcoidosis *etc.*

Tab. 5.9: Differential diagnosis of elevated alkaline phosphatase (s. tabs. 13.2–13.4)

Elevated AP values are normally found in *periods of growth,* after *fractures* (= activity of osteoblasts and chondroblasts), during the last trimester of *pregnancy* (15), and in *healing processes* (= activation of fibroblasts). An *extremely fatty diet* can increase the isoenzyme of intestinal AP in persons of blood group B or 0. (Osteoporosis shows normal AP values!) • Augmented AP values can also be expected in *diverse diseases* such as congenital (39) or transitional hyperphosphatasaemia, cardiac infarction, renal insufficiency, chronic obstructive pulmonary disease and pancreatopathy. As a rule, AP is markedly increased in healthy women over 65 years. (s. tab. 5.9)

A **decrease in AP activity** is found in congenital hypophosphatasaemia, hypothyreosis, cachexia, haemolysis, pernicious anaemia and fulminant hepatitis due to Wilson's disease as well as in zinc and magnesium deficiency or after intake of oestrogen, clofibrate and anticoagulants. A decline in AP activity during the last trimester of pregnancy points to an impending miscarriage.

> **Normal AP value (37 °C)** *) s. p. 128
> Women 55–105 U/l   Men 40–130 U/l
> Adolescents 100–400 U/l

6.4.2 Leucine arylamidase (LAP)

Leucine arylamidase (= leucine aminopeptidase) is a ubiquitous enzyme, mainly localized in the liver and bile ducts as well as in the pancreas, breast, intestine and kidney. During pregnancy (as from 2nd trimester), LAP increases. Arylamidases are predominantly localized in the cytoplasm, while aminopeptidases are found in the microsomes of hepatocytes. LAP splits aminoterminal amino acids off from peptides. High LAP activities are detectable in the epithelia of the bile ducts.

Elevated LAP values are found predominantly in biliary and cholestatic diseases – in accordance with AP. In liver diseases due to alcohol abuse, LAP values are exhibited both more frequently and with higher values than AP. In hepatitis mononucleosa, LAP is generally also more clearly elevated than AP. Significant increases in LAP are found in pancreatic and breast cancer as well as in collagenoses of the vascular type. LAP is not found in bone: there is no evidence of elevated LAP in bone diseases. Normal LAP in connection with an increase in AP consequently rules out hepatobiliary diseases and requires further investigation. In these cases, parallel determination of AP and LAP is advisable.

> **Normal LAP value** *) s. p. 128
> Women 16–32 U/l   Men 20–35 U/l

6.4.3 5′-Nucleotidase (5′-NU)

5′-NU is membrane-bound and can be found in the liver, brain, heart, blood vessels, pancreas and intestine. It is not yet understood why this enzyme does not increase in bone disease, periods of growth or pregnancy. Even in hepatocellular damage (e.g. acute or chronic hepatitis), it is also normal or only slightly elevated. (35)

Elevation of 5′-NU is found in cholestasis, biliary diseases and liver tumours (in 80–90% of metastases). It not only precedes, but also persists longer than AP. The value and accuracy of 5′-NU can be compared to those of LAP. For this reason 5′-NU, like LAP, can be utilized for the causal differentiation of elevated AP, particularly during pregnancy. However, determination of 5′-NU is rarely carried out due to the high expenditure and greater effort required for this method.

> **Normal 5′-NU value** *) s. p. 128
> 3–26 U/l

6.5 Copper

Copper, another endogenous substance excreted with bile, has recently received increasing attention. It has important functions within the organism. (s. p. 54)

Elevation of serum copper is found in cholestasis, obstructive jaundice, primary biliary cholangitis, malignant tumours, kwashiorkor, exocrine pancreatic insufficiency, during the last trimenon of pregnancy and after administration of oestrogens. • A *decrease* in serum copper is typical of Wilson's disease. In some rare cases, it is caused by familial benign hypocupraemia and nutritional deficiency in neonates.

The simultaneous determination of serum iron allows the differentiation of various **iron-copper constellations**, which facilitates differential diagnosis. (s. tab. 5.10)

Liver disease	Iron	Copper
Acute viral hepatitis, acute hepatic damage	↑	N
Mechanical jaundice – early stage	N	N
– late stage	N	↑
Chronic hepatitis, cirrhosis, scarred liver	N–↑	
Primary biliary cirrhosis	N	↑
Carcinoma	↓	↑
Haemochromatosis	↑	N
Wilson's disease	N	↓

Tab. 5.10: Types of iron-copper constellations in some liver diseases (N = normal)

> **Normal copper value** *) s. p. 128
> Women 68–169 µg/dl   Men 56–111 µg/dl

6.6 Cholesterol

▶ As early as 1862, A. FLINT described **hypercholesterolaemia** in liver disease, particularly in cholestatic forms.

Elevation of cholesterol is found in fatty liver, particularly under diabetic metabolic conditions. A rather marked increase in cholesterol can be observed in all forms of cholestasis; differentiation between intra- or extrahepatic cholestasis, however, is not possible. This elevation of cholesterol in obstruction is due to an enhanced synthesis of cholesterol in hepatocytes and intestinal walls as well as to the retention of bile lipids. Marked elevations of cholesterol are detectable in primary biliary cirrhosis and in cholesterol storage disease. A pronounced increase in cholesterol is also found in Zieve's syndrome (L. ZIEVE, 1958).

Decrease in cholesterol synthesis is found in severe hepatic parenchymal damage, particularly in cirrhosis.

Normal cholesterol value *) s. p. 128
≤ 200 mg/dl

7 Disorders of synthesis capacity

The more damage there is to the liver parenchyma, the more intense and varying are the disorders of synthesis capacity. This predominantly affects the synthesis of cholinesterase, coagulation factors, albumin, α_1-foetoprotein and lipoproteins.

7.1 Cholinesterase (ChE)

Pseudocholinesterase (W. ANTOPOL et al., 1938) represents the total activity of roughly 18 genetically determined variants. It is synthesized in the ribosomes and/or in the rough endoplasmic reticulum. This is also the site of synthesis of the coagulation factors and albumin, thus indicating a close correlation between cholinesterase and these two partial functions. Cholinesterase is released as an inactive secretory enzyme into the bloodstream, where it is activated. Half-life is 10 days. Under physiological conditions, the activity of serum ChE is held constant within a normal range. During pregnancy (as from 2nd trimester), ChE activity declines.

A **decline in ChE** activity is found in a number of diseases and/or in connection with damaging effects. The reduction in enzymatic activity correlates with the restricted synthesis capacity of the hepatocytes. (41)

(*1.*) *Liver diseases:* severe acute (necrotic) hepatitis, chronic hepatitis, chronic alcoholic liver damage, liver cirrhosis, cardiac liver, liver abscess, liver tumours and liver metastases, toxic liver damage, etc. • A severe and, above all, constant reduction in ChE activity (e. g. < 500 U/l) is usually suggestive of an unfavourable prognosis and the foreseeable moment of "liver death".
(*2.*) *Medicaments:* cytostatic substances, contraceptives, streptokinase, parasympathicomimetics, glucocorticoids, etc.

(*3.*) *Inflammatory processes:* enteritis, colitis, tuberculosis, trichinosis, polymyositis, infectious diseases, burns, irradiation, etc.
(*4.*) *Tumours:* carcinomas, Hodgkin's disease, leukoses
(*5.*) *Postoperative stress syndrome*
(*6.*) *Administration of albumin*
(*7.*) ChE activity is significantly reduced in malignant or tuberculous *pleural effusion* and *ascites*. (42)
(*8.*) *Diseases* such as hypothyreosis, malabsorption, kwashiorkor and pernicious anaemia.

An **elevation of ChE** activity can be detected in fatty liver, obesity, diabetes mellitus, exudative enteropathy, nephrotic syndrome, hyperthyroidism, Meulengracht's icterus, chronic obstructive jaundice, etc. *Specificity* in liver diseases is 61%, and *sensitivity* is 49%. In cirrhosis, however, sensitivity is 88%; normal ChE therefore widely excludes cirrhosis. In connection with other hepatobiliary enzymes, ChE can be useful in the diagnosis and assessment of the course of liver disease. There is a very good correlation of ChE activity with coagulation factors in liver diseases; however, the correlation is less significant with albumin synthesis.

Normal ChE value (37 °C) *) s. p. 128	
Women 3.93–10.8 U/l	Men 4.62–11.5 U/l

7.1.1 Diagnostic accuracy using enzymes

Clinical and enzymatic data of 520 of our patients suffering from various liver diseases were evaluated to assess the diagnostic accuracy of each method. (s. tab. 4.2)
• In the detection of "hepatopathy", application of 3–7 hepatobiliary enzymes yielded a sensitivity of 95–97%. (13) (s. tab. 5.11)

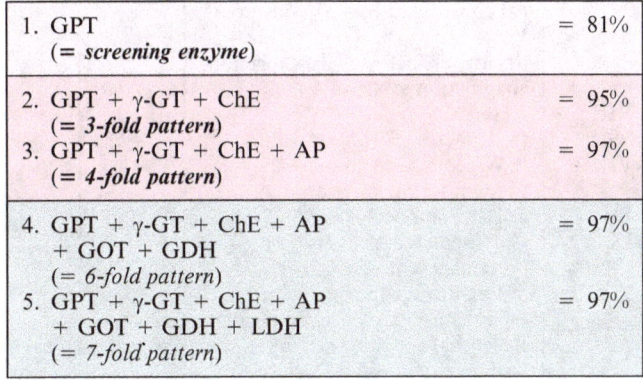

Tab. 5.11: Diagnostic accuracy in the detection or exclusion of hepatopathy using 7 hepatobiliary enzymes in 520 patients suffering from various liver diseases (13)

Threefold pattern: GPT + γ-GT + ChE was successful as a hepatological check-up; the **fourfold pattern** (including AP) proved completely reliable. Individual cases may require the inclusion of *GDH* (or *bile acids*). Utilization of enzyme ratios can further improve diagnostic accuracy. (s. tabs. 5.6, 5.7)

7.2 Coagulation factors

Coagulation factors I, II, V, VII, IX – XIII are synthesized in hepatocytes. To a minor extent, factor I is also synthesized in the intrahepatic RES, while factor VIII is formed exclusively in the RES. Formation of factors II, VII, IX and X as well as of the two inhibitor proteins C and S depends very much on vitamin K, the absence of which will cause the synthesis to decline. Factors I, V, XI, XII and XIII are formed without the mediation of vitamin K. • Proteolytic enzymes convert coagulation factors into active factors in the plasma. (s. tab. 5.12)

The following **inhibitors** are synthesized in the liver, independently of vitamin K: AT III, protein C inhibitor, C_1-esterase inhibitor, α_2-macroglobulin, histidine-rich glycoprotein, etc.

▶ The coagulation factors become effective within a proteolytic **cascade system**. This cascade consists of an interconnected exogenous (extrinsic) and endogenous (intrinsic) coagulation system as well as an activating pathway. Coagulators and inhibitors are finely regulated by positive and negative feedback mechanisms to ensure **homoeostasis of haemostasis**. (s. fig. 19.1) Disorders affecting this system can lead to serious complications. (s. fig. 19.2) (s. tab. 5.13)

Coagulation factors are proteins with varying but usually short half-lives. (s. tab. 5.12) Their determination allows the assessment of hepatic function. However, the respective half-life has to be considered. Disorders of coagulation factors are therefore important functional parameters in liver diseases – both in severe acute and in chronic cases. • In some cases, there may be a lack of coagulation factors, which is predominantly and primarily caused by a disorder of the hepatocyte synthesis capacity. • This lack can also be due to other *causes*: (*1.*) accelerated catabolism, (*2.*) altered biosynthesis of inhibitors, (*3.*) production of "abnormal" factors, and (*4.*) increased demand due to intravasal coagulation.

7.2.1 Fibrinogen and factor VIII

In frequent cases, *fibrinogen* is found to be initially elevated in liver diseases and only declines as a result of greatly impaired synthesis or severe inflammatory processes (shortening of half-life). • *Factor VIII* shows an atypical reaction: its level is either normal or even slightly elevated in liver diseases, possibly due to enhanced RES activity. (s. tab. 5.13)

Factor	Synonym	Site of synthesis hepatocyte	RES/extrahepatic	Vitamin K dependency	Half-life
I	Fibrinogen (= substrate of thrombin)	+	+	∅	4–6 days
II	Prothrombin (= zymogen of thrombin)	+		+	2–4 days
III	Thromboplastin (= activator of F VII)		+		
IV	Calcium^{2+}				
V	Proaccelerin (= cofactor of F II activator)	+		∅	12–15 hours
VI	Accelerin (= constituent of F II activator)				
VII	Proconvertin (= trigger factor of the exogenous coagulation system)	+		+	2–5 hours
VIII C	AHG-A (= cofactor of F X activator)				
VIII	v. Willebrand factor (= connecting endothelial cells/thrombocytes)		+	∅	10–18 hours
IX	Christmas factor (AHG-B) (= constituent of F X activator)	+		+	10–30 hours
X	Stuart-Prower factor (= constituent of F II activator)	+		+	20–42 hours
XI	Rosenthal factor (AHG-C) (= constituent of F IX activator)	+		∅	10–30 hours
XII	Hageman factor (= trigger factor of the endogenous coagulation system)	+		∅	2–4 days
XIII	Laki-Lorand factor (= fibrin-stabilizing factor)	+		∅	4–6 days
XIV	Fletcher factor (= prekallikrein)				
XV	Fitzgerald factor (= activator of F XII)				

Tab. 5.12: Classification and synonyms of coagulation factors, their site of synthesis, vitamin K dependency and half-life (as far as is known)

	Acute hepatitis	Acute hepatic failure	Chronic hepatitis, Cirrhosis	Obstructive jaundice, Cholestasis, Primary biliary cirrhosis
Fibrinogen	↓	↓	N-↓↓	N-↑
Quick's value, Thrombin time	↓ (↑)	↓↓ ↑↑	N-↓↓ N-↑	N-↑ N-↑
Antithrombin III	(↓)	↓↓	N-↓↓	N-↑

Tab. 5.13: Changes of some parameters of the coagulation system in liver diseases (N = normal) (s. tabs. 19.1; 35.4)

7.2.2 Quick's value

Quick's value is referred to as a global test for the determination of thrombin formation (from prothrombin) and fibrin formation in the presence of fibrinogen, calcium^{2+} and thromboplastin (= *thromboplastin time*). This simple test screens factors II, V, VII, IX and X (previously referred to as prothrombin complex). A decline in any of these factors extends the thromboplastin time, i.e. Quick's value (in %) will decline (A. J. QUICK et al., 1933). • Quick's value is rather insensitive, which is understandable in the light of the complexity of the coagulation system with the widely varying half-lives of its factors (2 hours to 4 days). Specificity also is low. Quick's value (like ChE activity) is known to be a sensitive parameter of hepatocyte protein synthesis. It is valuable in acute hepatitis, intoxication or necrotic episodes for the diagnosis of an impending coagulative disorder. Quick's value is useful in the follow-up of chronic liver diseases and can be helpful in making prognostic inferences, particularly when combined with ChE. (s. tab. 5.13)

Koller's test (F. KOLLER, 1961) differentiates between a lack of coagulation factors due to hepatocellular damage or due to vitamin K deficiency. This test facilitates the differential diagnosis between hepatocellular and mechanical jaundice as well as between liver diseases and bile-duct diseases. The *advantages* are: simple to perform, hardly any side-effects, low in costs.

> **Method:** Intravenous administration of 10 mg vitamin K in cases with a Quick's value of <70%. Diagnostically, a return to normal levels of >75% within 24 hours excludes liver disease, but favours vitamin K deficiency. A non-increase in the value indicates liver disease, since the synthesis of factors II, VII, IX and X does not depend on the administration of vitamin K.

Colombi index (in %) is the sum of factors II, V and VII (A. COLOMBI et al., 1967). The lower the index, the more serious is the liver disease (<150 = serious, <80 = very serious). With a Colombi index of <70, the prognosis of consumptive coagulopathy is poor. (s. fig. 19.2)

Normal value *) s. p. 128	
Thrombin time	16 – 24 sec
Quick's value	70 – 130%
Fibrinogen	180 – 350 mg/dl

7.2.3 Antithrombin III (AT III)

Antithrombin III is formed in the hepatocytes as an α_2-globulin. It serves as a physiological **inhibitor of serin proteases** in the coagulation system and thus inhibits activating factors IIa, IXa, Xa, XIa and XIIa. As the name implies, AT III is most effective as an inhibitor of thrombin. Half-life is 2–3 days.

A *reduction* in AT III activity (<70%) can no longer compensate coagulation processes when the activity of the procoagulator is normal or augmented: this increases the impending danger of thrombophilic diathesis (e.g. thrombosis of oesophageal varices with subsequent peptic ulceration). AT III is a specific marker of consumptive coagulopathy. Application of contraceptives causes AT III activity to decline (with genetic predisposition = approx. 1:5,000), which is paralleled by an increase in factors II, VII, IX, X and XII (= *hypercoagulopathy*). • An *elevation* of AT III activity (>120%) is found in cholestasis and obstructive jaundice. This leads to hypocoagulopathy with the danger of bleeding. (s. tab. 5.13)

Normal AT III value *) s. p. 128	
Activity	80–130%
Concentration	0.74–1.26 U/ml
	220–350 mg/l

7.3 Dysproteinaemia and hypalbuminaemia

Albumin is synthesized in the liver cell. The rate of synthesis is 12–17 g/day (150–250 mg/kg BW), which can be enhanced three to four times due to a loss of albumin. The albumin pool of the organism is approx. 500 g. Half-life is 18–21 days. Albumin is determined as a part of serum electrophoresis either quantitatively (g/l or g/dl, respectively) or as a relative percentage (rel. %). Concentrations of globulins are also quantified in this way.

Dysproteinaemia is a quantitative or qualitative change in protein fractions in the pherogram. These changes predominantly occur together with increases or decreases in certain proteins, such as acute phase proteins, immunoglobulins, haemostasis parameters, prealbumin-transferrin group and antibodies. Dysproteinaemia can therefore be detected in a number of diseases. A direct diagnosis based on dysproteinaemia or on protein constellations is not possible. There is no hyperalbuminaemia per se (except in exsiccosis). However, *statements* can be made regarding: (*1.*) clarification of the stage of activity of a disease, (*2.*) assessment of the course of a disease, and (*3.*) assignment to specific classes of diseases (e. g. gammopathies). (s. p. 116)

Hypalbuminaemia: For clinical evaluation of hypalbuminaemia, three *essential factors* have to be considered: (*1.*) the long half-life, which can conceal intermittent disorders of synthesis for two to three weeks, (*2.*) the respective size of the plasma distribution space, which is inconsistent in liver diseases, and (*3.*) a certain depressing effect on albumin synthesis exerted by the enhanced formation of γ-globulins in the RES. Thus albumin is reduced in *cirrhosis* due to an elevated distribution volume in haemodilution, particularly in association with ascites. Since the half-life is also prolonged in cirrhosis, a reduction in the rate of synthesis by 50% only lowers the serum albumin by 20%. This has to be taken into account when assessing the albumin value in patients suffering from cirrhosis. The diminished synthesis of albumin coincides with the loss of liver parenchyma. A reduction in albumin by 10 g/l is equivalent to a loss of approx. 30 g protein. • Due to the long half-life of albumin, severe acute liver diseases exhibit a decline in albumin only during the later course. Hypalbuminaemia can also be expected in chronic liver diseases, liver tumours, autoimmune diseases, liver abscesses, infectious diseases of the liver, kwashiorkor, etc. Higher sensitivity is revealed by the *prealbumin* value in simultaneous and close correlation with galactose EC. The half-life is approximately two days and thus considerably shorter than that of albumin. (43) A reduction in albumin with a parallel elevation of β-globulin is found in cholestasis and primary biliary cirrhosis. Albumin can also decline during pregnancy or due to the intake of contraceptives.

> **Normal albumin value** *) s. p. 128
> 3.7−5.9 g/dl   56−68 rel.%
> **Normal prealbumin value**
> 25−45 mg/dl

7.4 Lipoprotein X (LP-X)

LP-X was detected by D. Seidel et al. in 1969 during the course of a **cholestasis syndrome** as an abnormal lipoprotein with a low portion of protein (6%) as well as a high content of cholesterol (22%) and phospholipids (66%). The increase in the LDL fraction in cholestasis (G. B. Phillipps, 1960) was linked to the appearance of LP-X. However, it probably imitates an increase in LDL. LP-X develops in the plasma during cholestasis as a result of the fact that lipoproteins, which are normally excreted with the bile, flow back into the blood and become transformed. *(see chapter 13)*

LP-X can be detected in *cholestasis* in 90% of patients. Its sensitivity is equivalent to the activities of AP, LAP and γ-GT; however, it is believed to possess a better correlation with liver histology. It cannot be used to differentiate between intra- and extrahepatic cholestasis. Since the normalization of LP-X levels precedes the normalization of cholestasis enzymes, an earlier hint is given of a regressive course of cholestasis. In biliary cirrhosis caused by CDNC, LP-X is, as a rule, considerably elevated. (44)

7.5 α₁-foetoprotein (AFP)

> ▶ The oncofoetal antigen α_1-foetoprotein was described in 1963 (G. Abelev et al.) before being detected in 1964 for the first time by Y. S. Tatarinov in a patient suffering from liver carcinoma. The glycoprotein AFP is formed in the **foetal liver** and is biochemically identical to the tumour AFP of hepatocytes. The (physiologically) elevated AFP in the neonate will slowly and steadily decline to reach normal adult levels by the tenth month.

In **normal hepatocytes** of the adult, AFP is not formed; minute quantities in the serum (as normal levels) result from cellular growth during the course of "moulting". There is no age- or gender-specific influence on AFP levels. Its half-life is 3−6 days.

Elevation of AFP is found predominantly in *primary liver cell carcinoma*: sensitivity can be as high as 90−95%, specificity is approx. 80%. The magnitude of this value correlates with the tumour volume (or the tumour AFP concentration) and with the extent of dedifferentiation. After successful resection of the tumour, elevated AFP levels decline to normal levels in relation to their half-life. The persistence of elevated levels is indicative of the existence of tumour remnants. Values in excess of 180 µg/l suggest the existence of a primary liver cell carcinoma. Elevated levels should be re-assessed after 2−3 weeks. In 60% of cases, values exceed 100 µg/l, in 50% they exceed 1,000 µg/l, and in 40% even 10,000 µg/l; values of >2,000 µg/l are virtually conclusive. Elevation is also found during acute necrotic episodes of chronic hepatitis B, whereby such cases frequently develop into cirrhosis and liver cell carcinoma. In a metastatic liver AFP is elevated in some 30% of cases, whereas in gastrointestinal tumours this value is approx. 20%. During regeneration, e. g. in cirrhosis, moderately increased AFP levels (ca. 25%) are detectable, just as occasional temporary elevations are found in liver diseases in general. (40)

The *determination* of AFP is indicated for (*1.*) regular supervision of high-risk groups (HBsAg-positive cirrhosis, haemochromatosis, alcoholic cirrhosis), with more frequent controls as the duration of disease increases, (*2.*) early diagnosis of primary liver cell carcinoma, (*3.*) monitoring the success of surgical interventions, and (*4.*) postoperative follow-up. *(see chapter 37)*

> **Normal AFP value** *) s. p. 128
> <10 µg/l

8 Disorders of metabolism

8.1 Ammonia

▶ Ammonia is formed in the cell or by bacteria during various deamidization reactions of amino acids. A certain quantity (ca. 25%) of ammonia is produced in the intestine by bacteria or through enzymatic action in the intestinal mucosa during protein degradation. This mean value of *intestinal ammonia production* is elevated under normal conditions as a result of the increased consumption of meat or fish and reduced during a predominantly lactovegetarian protein diet. Production of ammonia is raised by physical work; a similar effect is possible in constipation.

The **determination of ammonia** in blood is carried out enzymatically, which is considered to be specific, precise and simple. (45) *Serious mistakes* can easily occur during the preanalytical phase of ammonia determination, making it imperative to comply with the "standardized" method of obtaining a blood sample. (s. p. 97) EDTA blood should be taken with the addition of sodium borate and L-serine. Furthermore, elevated serum γ-GT activity and increased thrombocytes cause the ammonia level to rise, as does cigarette smoking prior to blood collection. Even minor haemolysis (e.g. in the event of prolonged transport) will spoil the blood for ammonia determination, since the ammonia concentration of erythrocytes is three times that found in plasma. Besides these interfering factors, ammonia concentration is influenced by (*1.*) the metabolic performance of the urea cycle, (*2.*) the extrahepatic formation and elimination of ammonia, and (*3.*) the acid-base status.

Owing to the multitude of factors interfering with the ammonia concentration as well as to the multifactorial pathogenesis of hepatic encephalopathy (HE), it is understandable that there is no correlation between the levels of ammonia and the prevailing HE stage. Nevertheless, a *hyperammonia syndrome* is generally presumed if concentrations in the venous or arterial plasma reach 135–170 µg/dl. A value of > 150 µg/dl can be attributed to coma stage I. Here, the arterial ammonia level correlates better with HE than do the values found in venous blood. (s. pp 61, 274)

> The **ammonia tolerance test** (C. van Caulaert et al., 1932; E. Kirk, 1936) is carried out with the oral administration of 4–5 g ammonium acetate or 3 g ammonium chloride. Normally, there is no significant elevation of ammonia levels after 30, 60 and 120 minutes. In hepatic cirrhosis and in portacaval anastomosis, there is a clear elevation with delayed normalization. (46)

> **Normal ammonia value (plasma)** *) s. p. 128
> Women 19–65 µg/dl   Men 27–90 µg/dl

9 Diagnostics of liver functions

Principle: The principle behind quantitative diagnosis of liver functions is to administer defined test substances with known hepatic mechanisms of elimination with a view to gaining information on single hepatocellular processes for the assessment of certain *partial functions* of the liver. Such substances help to determine liver metabolism, excretion, biotransformation and hepatic perfusion. (13, 57, 61, 69, 73, 81) (s. tab. 5.14)

> 1. **Metabolic function**
>   - Galactose elimination capacity
>   (T. Stentam, 1946; N. Tygstrup, 1963)
>   - Antipyrine elimination
>   (E. S. Vesell, 1968)
>   - Ammonia tolerance test
>   (C. van Caulaert et al., 1932; E. Kirk, 1936)
>   - Tryptophan tolerance test
>   (M. Rössle et al., 1983)
>   - Methionine tolerance test
>   (K. Schreier, H. Schönsee, 1952)
> 2. **Excretory function**
>   - Indocyanine green test
>   (L. J. Fox, 1957)
>   - Aminopyrine ^{14}C breath test
>   (G. W. Hepner, E. S. Vesell, 1975)
>   - Bromsulfophthaleine
>   (S. M. Rosenthal, E. C. White, 1925)
>   - Bengal rose test
>   (G. V. Taplin, O. M. Meredith, 1958)
> 3. **Biotransformatory function**
>   - Antipyrine clearance test
>   (E. S. Vesell, 1968)
>   - Caffeine elimination test (= demethylization)
>   (E. Renner et al., 1983)
>   - 4-Methylumbelliferone (= glucuronization)
>   (H.-D. Kuntz, 1982)
> 4. **Hepatic perfusion**
>   - Indocyanine green test
>   (J. Caesar et al., 1961)
>   - Sorbitol clearance
>   (G. Molino et al., 1986)

Tab. 5.14: Test substances with various mechanisms of elimination and their applications for assessing partial liver functions

Indications: The application of direct tests of (quantitative) liver functions follows the indications listed below:

> 1. detection of previously unknown enzymatically inactive liver diseases
> 2. functional characterization of acute and chronic liver diseases
> 3. assessment of the course of chronic liver diseases
> 4. monitoring of recovery
> 5. specific issues
>   – detection and extent of toxic damage
>   – therapy trials
>   – assessment of prognosis
>   – indication for shunting
>   – indication for transplantation

Endogenous functional values (e.g. albumin, cholinesterase, Quick's value, bile acids) as well as **exogenous test substances** (e.g. galactose, indocyanine green, MEGX and aminopyrine ^{14}C) allow the reliable clinical evaluation of "liver function". • The quantitative diagnostics of hepatic function cannot be obtained by any other method of assessment (as yet) — not even through imaging or through histology. It is, however, to be expected that in future a more reliable statement regarding metabolic liver function will be possible.

▶ For the **assessment of the course** of chronic liver diseases, valuable results are supplied by defined exogenous test substances, which can determine the prognosis of a disease or the right time for a surgical intervention. In the absence of enzymatic features, the course of chronic hepatitis, hepatic fibrosis or chronic toxic damage can best be determined with the aid of specific functional tests. The course of compensated cirrhosis can also be most reliably supervised using quantitative methods of assessment. • Endogenous and exogenous factors may have unpredictable effects on the results of liver function tests, which leads to an interindividual variation range in reference values. However, intraindividual reproducibility is good, making it possible to assess the progress of each patient more accurately.

9.1 Galactose elimination capacity (GEC)

▶ Galactose was introduced by R. BAUER in 1906 as a test substance for the assessment of hepatic function. • We have presented the continuous **methodological development** of this liver function test up to the contemporary intravenous injection of galactose in excess substrate. (62)

The galactose test assesses the ability of the hepatocyte to convert galactose to glucose. A healthy liver metabolizes 500 – 600 mg galactose per minute. Roughly 90% of parenterally administered galactose is metabolized in the liver — independently of hepatic perfusion. GEC correlates with the "viable liver cell volume" (60) and is therefore a reliable measure of the metabolic function of the liver. Prior to determination of GEC, 24-hour alcohol abstinence is necessary. (47, 50, 58, 60, 62, 67, 69, 76)

Method: The principle of GEC involves the intravenous administration of galactose in excess substrate in order to assess the maximum rate of hepatic metabolization. This requires a galactose concentration of 0.5 g/kg BW (serum concentration of >45 mg/dl for at least 45 minutes), which is injected within 4–5 minutes as a 40% pyrogen-free sterile galactose solution. The bladder has to be emptied immediately prior to the injection and subsequently the urine has to be collected for exactly five hours to assess the respective galactose excretion (in grams). Blood samples are taken from the fingertip (or from the cubital vein into an EDTA test tube) at 5, 25 and 45 minutes after injection. We have reported in detail on how to conduct this method as well as on the analysis of GEC. (60, 62)

The *advantages of GEC* are obvious: (*1.*) there is no interference with bilirubin, haemolysis or hyperlipidaemia, (*2.*) neither a disorder of hepatic excretion nor a change in perfusion will alter the result, (*3.*) there are generally no side effects, (*4.*) blood samples can be taken from the fingertip as well as from the vein, (*5.*) laboratory analysis is easy to perform, (*6.*) costs for the test are low, and (*7.*) quantitative assessment of the degree of severity of a liver disease is possible:

Degree of severity of the decrease in function	
6 – 7 mg/kg BW/min	= low
5 – 6 mg/kg BW/min	= medium
4 – 5 mg/kg BW/min	= high
< 4 mg/kg BW/min	= very high

Normal GEC value *) s. p. 128
> 7 mg galactose/kg BW/min

9.2 Indocyanine green test (ICG)

Indocyanine green was introduced by J. CAESAR et al. in 1961 as a liver function test. • Anionic tricarbocyanine dye is referred to as an *ideal test substance*: (*1.*) there have been no reports of any incidents so far, and even paravenous injection is tolerated; (*2.*) it is excreted unchanged by hepatocytes in the bile as there is no biotransformation — this is why ICG clearance is valid as a measure of hepatocellular uptake and transport processes; (*3.*) there is no interference with drugs (except rifamycin), haemolysis, bilirubin (up to approx. 4 mg/dl) or hyperlipidaemia; (*4.*) the substance is not subject to the enterohepatic circulation; (*5.*) the rapid elimination, which depends on hepatic perfusion ("flow-limited"), allows the calculation of the hepatic flow volume as a whole based on ICG clearance; (*6.*) the method is simple to perform. (51, 55, 61, 67, 74, 81)

The optimal *dosage* of ICG seems to be 0.5 mg (= 0.1 ml)/kg BW. Its half-life is 2.7 ± 0.6 minutes and its plasma disappearance rate (PDR) is $25.6 \pm 4.5\%$ (PDR is the elimination per minute as a percentage of the dosage). The injection of ICG has to be carried out quickly (within 10 seconds). Taking a new syringe and the other arm, blood samples are taken after 3, 6 and 9 minutes; the time for collecting the blood sample should not exceed 30 seconds. Samples have to be analyzed immediately. The absorption maximum is at 772 (or 805) nm in the spectral photometer. • According to the literature and in the light of our own experience, the *clinical significance* of the ICG test is to be rated very highly. There is a close correlation between the Child-Pugh classification of cirrhosis and both ICG and the aminopyrine breath test. The ICG test has also proved effective for assessing liver function in PBC as well as in the resected and/or transplanted liver. As yet, however, the high costs unfortunately prevent wider application.

Normal ICG value *) s. p. 128
Half-life < 3.5 minutes

9.3 Aminopyrine ^{14}C breath test

Features of the test substance aminopyrine (dimethylaminopyrine) are: (1.) rapid and complete intestinal resorption, (2.) low protein binding, and (3.) almost exclusive metabolization by the liver. The aminopyrine test is known to be non-invasive, methodologically simple and quick to perform. Of importance is a resting period for the patient of at least 30 minutes prior to the intravenous administration of ^{14}C-aminopyrine in a dosage of 1.5 µCi. Depending on the liver function, radiation exposure of the patient corresponds to 0.6–2.5 mrem (= 1–2 thorax X-rays). The test is also influenced by numerous medicaments and alcohol as well as any alteration in the basal metabolic rate. The procedure finishes with a triple breath test at ten-minute intervals.

Principle: After the test substance has been demethylated by the microsomal enzyme system of the SER (the labelled carbon atoms are catabolized to $^{14}CO_2$. The velocity of demethylation can be measured by determining the $^{14}CO_2$ value in expired air. Catabolization of aminopyrine is enhanced with elevated activity of the cytochrome P 450 and reduced accordingly due to the loss of liver cell volume. The metabolization is independent of perfusion. Exposure to radiation is minimal.

A number of studies have demonstrated the value of the aminopyrine test. There is a close correlation with histology and prognosis of current liver diseases as well as with the estimation of the operative risk in patients suffering from cirrhosis. Accelerated aminopyrine dissimilation due to toxin-induced microsomal enzyme activation may reveal alcohol or drug abuse even without recognizable liver damage. (48, 64, 67, 68, 72, 78)

Normal value *) s. p. 128	
Oral	>7% $^{14}CO_2$ within 2 hrs
Parenteral	0.6–1.0 mol $^{14}CO_2$ within 30 min

9.4 Antipyrine test

Antipyrine is oxidized through biotransformation, independently of perfusion, predominantly in the microsomes, and is excreted after hydroxylation and conjugation. Following oral administration (15 or 18 mg/kg BW, respectively), the metabolic clearance ability of the liver (metabolic capacity of the microsomal monooxygenase system) can be assessed by computation of the concentration curve and the plasma half-life (after 3 and 24 hours). The serum half-life and plasma clearance are significantly enhanced/decreased, depending on the reduction in liver function. There is a close correlation with the GEC as well as with Quick's value. (54, 80)

9.5 Caffeine elimination test (CET)

Caffeine is completely absorbed within the intestine, and about 97% is metabolized selectively by the liver – more or less independently of perfusion – by way of microsomal demethylation (E. RENNER et al., 1984). After intravenous administration of 125 mg caffeine – equivalent to one to two cups of coffee – a plasma caffeine increase was detected in liver patients, corresponding to the limited demethylation capacity via paraxanthin. The prolongation of half-life and the limitation of plasma clearance were clearly altered in patients suffering from cirrhosis. The result can be influenced by age, smoking, contraceptives and numerous medicaments, etc. The test shows no side effects, it is cost-favourable and easy to carry out. (52, 63, 66, 79) • The caffeine breath test has proved useful in a clinical study. (75)

Normal CET value *) s. p. 128	
Half-life	<4–6 hrs
PC	<2 ml/kg BW/min

9.6 Monoethylglycinexylidide test (MEGX)

MEGX is a metabolite of lidocaine. Cytochrome P 450-dependent metabolization is measured 15 and 30 minutes after i.v. application of lidocaine (1 mg/kg BW, for 2–3 min) (M. OELLERICH et al., 1987, 1989). The blood sample is taken from the contralateral arm. The basic value (zero value) is subtracted from the MEGX value after 15 and 30 minutes. The MEGX test is influenced by numerous medicaments and substances, since lidocaine-metabolizing CYP 450 3A4 is subject to genetic polymorphism. Such disturbances together with multifarious side effects hinder wider clinical application. • Following liver transplantation, the primary transplant function was correctly predicted in about 85% of cases and primary transplant failure in about 66%. A further study with 69 transplant patients yielded a prognostic sensitivity of 73% and a specificity of 78%. In chronic hepatitis or cirrhosis, the MEGX test showed a good correlation with the severity of disease and proved to be a valuable prognostic criterion of assessment. (56, 77) A comparison between the MEGX test and the aminopyrine or galactose test, however, showed a broad range of values in minor liver diseases (46 ± 23 ng/ml) as well as in cirrhosis (19 ± 11 ng/ml), whereby the aminopyrine test exhibited a better correlation with the increase in severity than did the MEGX test. (70) The metabolic capacity is sufficiently representative for the functional reserve of the liver. (49)

Normal MEGX value *) s. p. 128	
15 min (µg/l):	30 min (µg/l):
Women: 25–60	41–70
Men: 42–90	58–98

9.7 Sorbitol clearance

The D-sorbitol test (G. MOLINO et al., 1986) is considered a reliable measure for blood flow in liver parenchyma, i.e. liver plasma flow. A 40% sorbitol solution is administered via perfusor i.v. within three hours (= 7.5 ml/hr or 50 mg sorbitol/min). There are no side effects. The test is cost-favourable, but time-consuming. • Between 120th and 180th minute urine is collected and blood samples are taken, the latter in 10-minute intervals. (59, 71)

9.8 (99 m) Tc-Membrofenin

A significant correlation was found between the uptake of 85 MBq mebrofenin (i.v. injection) and the 15-minute clearance rate of IC_G-G15. (53)

9.9 Bengal rose ^{131}iodine test

This method tests the excretory function of the liver (exogenous clearance), with no metabolization of the substance in the liver. In addition, this test might possibly reveal insufficient parenchymal storage. The Bengal rose test cannot be applied in the icteric patient. For clinical hepatology, this test is of minor importance.

9.10 Bromsulphalein test

Owing to various disadvantages and side effects, this test (S. M. ROSENTHAL et al., 1925) is no longer available today — although it was a helpful diagnostic tool in the past.

10 Assessment of mesenchymal reaction

Elevation of indicator enzymes (particularly GPT, GOT and GDH) in the sense of hepatocellular damage is labelled **"enzymatic activity"**. • Quantitative changes of gamma globulins, immunoglobulins, serum copper and procollagen-III-peptide can be suggestive of the mesenchyma being involved in the liver disease. An enhancement of the mesenchymal reaction can be subsumed under the term **"mesenchymal activity"**.

Any thorough detailed laboratory diagnosis should test and clinically interpret the enzymatic activity as well as the mesenchymal activity.

10.1 Gamma globulins

Chronic liver diseases are generally associated with an increase in γ-globulins, which is indicative of the effects of the chronic process on the liver mesenchyma. (100)

Synthesis: Synthesis of γ-globulins occurs in the RES, plasma cells and lymph nodes. The sinusoids of the liver comprise an abundance of globulin-forming cells. Under normal conditions, however, the proportion of γ-globulins synthesized in these cells is low. The half-life of γ-globulins is between 5 and 23 days. The liver only degrades some 30% of γ-globulins.

Cause of γ-globulinaemia: Antibodies directed against tissue antigens, particularly bacterial antigens of the intestinal tract, are believed to be the cause of γ-globulinaemia. Furthermore, toxins (particularly endotoxins) entering the reticuloendothelial system of the liver via the portal vein are essential causal factors. These substrates stimulate the globulin-forming cells, causing them to multiply and increase their synthesis: each cell will now produce a greater number of γ-globulins. Basically, the cause of polyclonal hypergammaglobulinaemia is the persistence of antigen stimulation due to deficient RES function as well as non-specific generalized immunological ("mesenchymal") hyperreactivity.

Elevation: An increase in γ-globulins is found during the late stage of acute or subacute diseases as well as in chronic inflammatory processes and malignomas. • Such an increase can thus be observed to a varying extent during the course of active viral hepatitis, in chronic persistent hepatitis, in chronic toxic or chronic inflammatory liver damage, and particularly in cirrhosis. A characteristic merger of the β- and γ-peaks (so-called "bridging" or "shoulder") can be found occasionally in cirrhosis. The increase in γ-globulins does not provide any diagnostic hints, but it is still useful for the assessment of the course of a liver disease. • It is noteworthy that γ-globulinaemia exerts a certain *depressor effect* on albumin synthesis. The administration of lactulose or paromomycin, for example, for enhanced intestinal detoxification can therefore serve as an initial therapy to minimize the formation and transport of intestinal toxins via the portal vein to the liver RES. (91)

> Normal γ-globulin value *) s. p. 128
> 5.8–15.2 g/l
> 9–19 rel.%

10.2 Immunoglobulins

The **humoral** and **cellular immune systems** function jointly as an acquired defence against infection. Whether the humoral or the cellular defence system is predominantly used depends in the individual case on the nature of the pathogen or the foreign body, the reactivity of the organism and the mode of infection. The humoral immune response proceeds via the B-lymphocytes and plasma cells, while the cellular immune response is mediated via the T-lymphocytes. The haematopoetic stem cells mature into B-lymphocytes and are transformed to plasma cells. They in turn synthesize IgM, but can also "switch" to produce IgA and IgG. (90)

In decreasing concentrations, **serum immunoglobulins** consist predominantly of IgG, IgA and IgM with their subclasses G_{1-4}, A_{1-2} and M_{1-2}. Quantitative changes of immunoglobulins are only partially detected using electrophoresis: the γ-globulin fraction consists predominantly of IgG, while IgA and IgM are detectable in the β- or β/γ-fraction. Catabolization of IgG depends on the respective immunoglobulin concentration, while IgM and IgA are catabolized independently of the serum level. The half-life of IgG is 9–23 days, of IgA 6 days and of IgM 5 days.

There is no known immunoglobulin constellation which is found exclusively in liver diseases and which possesses real diagnostic value in itself. Except for the extent of the parenchymal damage, the course and prognosis of liver diseases are, however, clearly influenced by the intrahepatic mesenchymal reaction. Immunoglobulins thus make possible an assessment of "mesenchymal activity" in the persisting presence of antigen. In liver diseases, an inhomogeneous polyclonal gammopathy is regularly found, with certain immunoglobulin patterns being suggestive of certain liver diseases and courses. This **immunogram** (13) is a valuable tool in the follow-up of diffuse liver diseases and can be used for prognostication. (s. tab. 5.15)

In **acute viral hepatitis A,** there is a marked increase in IgM during the course of six to eight weeks and a subsequent slight increase of IgG. As of the second week of disease, the IgM level declines faster than the slightly elevated IgG level, with normalization of IgM after four weeks. A persistent elevation of IgM and IgG or a marked elevation of IgG is suggestive of persistent (protracted) hepatitis. • Apart from an increase of IgM, **acute viral hepatitis B and C** are associated with a stronger and earlier increase in IgG than in viral hepatitis A. Normalization of IgG and IgM values occurs more slowly than in hepatitis A. Normal values of IgG are mostly reached only after six months. There are no differences between the icteric and the anicteric form.

There is a marked elevation of IgM in **chronic persistent hepatitis** with normal or only slightly elevated IgA. A continuing rise in IgG would be suggestive of a progression to chronic active hepatitis.

Chronic active hepatitis is associated with a strong elevation of IgG with normal or slightly elevated IgM and IgA. Marked elevations of IgG and IgA — with a strong parallel rise in the blood sedimentation rate (BSR), in γ-globulin values and in total protein — are found in autoimmune hepatitis. These considerable increases in IgG reflect the degree of mesenchymal inflammation with plasma cell infiltration, which is why this form is also referred to as the so-called *"hyper-γ-globulinaemic chronic hepatitis"*. Chronic inflammatory liver diseases are therefore characterized inter alia by marked IgG elevations and only minor IgM increases, even if histology has not yet detected the chronicity of the process. The elevation of IgM, along with IgG, is indicative of the infectious agent still being active within the organism. Cholestatic forms usually exhibit an elevation of IgG.

Chronic steatohepatitis reveals only slight elevations of IgA and IgG. A pronounced increase in IgA is usually suggestive of an alcoholic or drug-induced cause. Elevation of IgA and IgG are laboratory markers for the development of cirrhosis.

Primary biliary cholangitis or primary biliary cirrhosis are both characterized by strong elevations of IgM. Only occasionally (in 20−30% of cases) is there also an elevation of IgG in immunologically and clinically more active forms. IgA values only show a slight increase during the late course.

In **drug-induced liver damage,** a similar immunological mechanism is conceivable: the respective medicament acts as a hapten, and an endogenous protein turns into an autoantigen. In hypersensitivity reactions, IgE can increase.

Liver cirrhosis shows an elevation of all three classes of immunoglobulins, which is also the cause of the fusion of the β- and γ-fractions ("bridging"). *(see chapter 35)*

Normal immunoglobulin value *) s. p. 128			
IgG	92−207	U/ml	= 77%
	800−1,800	mg/dl	
IgA	54−264	U/ml	= 14%
	90−450	mg/dl	
IgM	60−250	mg/dl	= 9%
IgE	0−100	U/ml	

Immunoglobulins			Liver disease
IgA	IgG	IgM	
Normal			• No mesenchymal or autoaggressive activity detectable • No infectious agent detectable
(↑)	(↑) ↑ ↑	↑↑ ↑ − ↑↑ ↑ ↑	1. Acute viral hepatitis 2. Subsiding acute viral hepatitis 3. Stage of complete recovery from acute viral hepatitis 4. Protracted acute viral hepatitis
N−(↑)	↑↑ ↑	↑ − ↑↑ ↑ − ↑↑	1. Conversion of protracted viral hepatitis to chronic aggressive hepatitis 2. Chronic persistent hepatitis
N−(↑) N−(↑) ↑ − ↑↑ ↑↑ − ↑↑↑	↑↑ − ↑↑↑ ↑↑ ↑↑ ↑↑	N−↑ N−(↑) N−(↑) N−(↑)	1. Chronic aggressive hepatitis 2. Autoimmune hepatitis 3. Tendency to develop cirrhosis 4. Additional alcoholic damage
N−(↑) (↑) ↑ − ↑↑ ↑↑ − ↑↑↑	N−(↑) (↑) (↑)−↑ ↑	N−(↑) (↑) (↑) ↑	1. Fatty degeneration of the liver (stages I, II) 2. Chronic hepatitis of fatty liver (stage III) 3. Alcoholic chronic hepatitis of fatty liver 4. Alcoholic cirrhosis
↑ − ↑↑ ↑ − ↑↑	↑ − ↑↑ (↑)−↑ ↑↑	(↑)−↑ ↑↑↑ ↑ − ↑↑	1. Liver cirrhosis 2. Primary biliary cholangitis or cirrhosis 3. Deterioration of the prognosis in cirrhosis

Tab. 5.15: Immunogram of various liver diseases

10.3 Procollagen-III-peptide (P-III-P)

A **normal liver** contains roughly 7–9 mg collagen per gram wet weight. Types I, II and IV are detectable in comparable concentrations. With increasing **fibrosis,** especially type I and type III collagen contents rise in the liver. In advanced stages of long-term disease, synthesis of type I prevails. • The chronic inflammatory process of a liver disease activates the connective tissue metabolism with significant elevation of monoamine oxidase and collagen peptidase serum levels. Of all the metabolites of collagen metabolism, the N-terminal propeptide of procollagen III exhibits the best correlation with fibrosis activity. The activity of proteoglycan and glycoprotein metabolisms (and therefore also of lysosomic enzymes) is detected most reliably with the N-acetyl-β-D-glucosaminidase. The lysosome release also reflects the **mesenchymal activity.** • Procollagen III is initially synthesized in parenchymal cells, Ito cells and fibroblasts; it is then secreted into the extracellular space. Here propeptides are split off, whereby the concentration of the separated P-III-P is used as a direct measure for the amount of collagen synthesized and deposited extracellularly. The collagen monomers formed are deposited as collagen fibrils in the connective tissue and some of the P-III-P is discharged into the blood. Further **fibrosis markers** are: P-I-CP, type IV collagen and prolylhydroxylase.

Procollagen-III-peptide was detected by H. ROHDE et al. in 1978. The results of P-III-P determination in liver diseases were presented by the same research group in 1979. P-III-P determination is less important for diagnosis, but it facilitates monitoring the course of a liver disease with respect to the current degree of fibrosis. This makes it possible to obtain information on the *activity* (= connective tissue formed per unit of time) and *reversibility* of liver fibrosis. Thus there is a good correlation between P-III-P concentrations and the histomorphometrically estimated fibrosis activities.

▶ Patients with chronic congestive liver or alcoholic cirrhosis exhibited distinctly elevated P-III-P values. In long-lasting, slightly active posthepatitic cirrhosis, P-III-P has only limited value, since type I collagen is predominantly elevated in these cirrhotic forms. Increasing levels of P-III-P are an early and sensitive marker of veno-occlusive diseases. In chronic hepatitis, P-III-P values are often elevated. Sensitivity is 94% for the differential diagnosis of chronic active and chronic persistent forms, whereby this value cannot substitute the histological result. The favourable response to cortisone treatment in chronic hepatitis was allegedly detectable at an earlier stage in the decline in P-III-P values than in the activity of transaminases. In the progression of primary biliary cholangitis, P-III-P may, in certain cases, be a better marker than histology. There were also marked elevations of P-III-P serum values in extrahepatic cholestasis and schistosomiasis. P-III-P elevations were likewise detectable in progressive drug-induced liver damage, chronic liver congestion, and enhanced mesenchymal activity in the progression of alcoholic fatty liver to chronic steatohepatitis. (82–89)

> Normal P-III-P value *) s. p. 128
> 3–16 μg/dl
> 0.3–0.8 U/ml

11 Serological diagnostics of viral hepatitis

Numerous viruses are able to cause acute viral hepatitis. **Primary hepatotropic viruses** lead to a completely independent form. • **Secondary hepatotropic viruses** lead to systemic infection (with various organs being affected) as well as simultaneous and often predominant concomitant hepatitis. • **Tropical virus infections** may at times trigger inflammatory concomitant reactions of the liver. This requires differential diagnosis for epidemiological and clinical reasons as well as to comply with legal regulations (= *notifiable disease*). (s. tab. 5.16)

> **Primary hepatotropic viruses**
> 1. Hepatitis A virus
>   – Picorna virus
> 2. Hepatitis B virus
>   – Hepadna virus
> 3. Hepatitis C virus
>   – Flaviviridae group
> 4. Hepatitis D virus
>   – Delta viroid
> 5. Hepatitis E virus
>   – Caliciviridae group
> 6. Hepatitis G virus
>   – Flaviviridae group
> 7. Molecular, partially identified
>   – Hepatitis non-A, non-E virus
>   – Hepatitis GBV (A–C)
>
> **Secondary hepatotropic viruses**
> 1. Herpes viruses
>   – Epstein-Barr virus
>   – Herpes simplex viruses
>   – Human herpes viruses
>   – Varicella-Zoster virus
>   – Cytomegalovirus
> 2. Enteroviruses
>   – Coxsackie virus
>   – Echovirus
> 3. Rubella virus
> 4. Paramyxoviruses
> 5. Adenoviruses
>
> **Exotic hepatotropic viruses**
> 1. Togaviridae viruses
>   a. Alpha viruses
>   – Semliki Forest viruses
>   b. Flavi viruses
>   – Yellow fever virus
>   – Dengue virus
>   – Kyasanur Forest virus
> 2. Filo viruses
>   – Marburg virus
>   – Ebola virus
> 3. Bunya viruses
>   – Hanta virus
>   – Rift Valley fever
> 4. Arena viruses
>   – Lassa virus

Tab. 5.16: Pathogens of acute viral hepatitis as independent or concomitant disease (s. tab. 23.1!)

11.1 Hepatitis A virus (HAV)

▶ The uncoated hepatitis A virus was discovered in the stools of afflicted patients with the help of immunoelectron microscopy by S. M. FINESTONE et al. in 1973. This RNA virus (27–32 nm) belongs to the family of Picornaviridae. It is a spherical particle of icosahedral symmetry (= a polyhedron limited by 20 triangular faces). The RNA possesses functional and structural regions, encoding three enzymatically active peptides (P1 to P3) and four structural proteins (VP1 to VP4). Whereas VP1 to VP3 are easily recognizable from the outside, also for the immune system, VP4 is concealed on the inner side. The genome consists of positive, linear single-stranded RNA with 7,478 nucleotides. It possesses one open reading frame (ORF) with both a 5'NCR and a 3'NCR (non-coding region). The ORF translates a polyprotein, which is degraded into structural protein P1 as well as into non-structural proteins P2 and P3. From P1 and RNA, immature viral particles originate. With the help of the enzymatic degradation into the four capsid proteins VP1–VP4, mature viruses develop. (s. p. 426) (s. fig. 5.4)

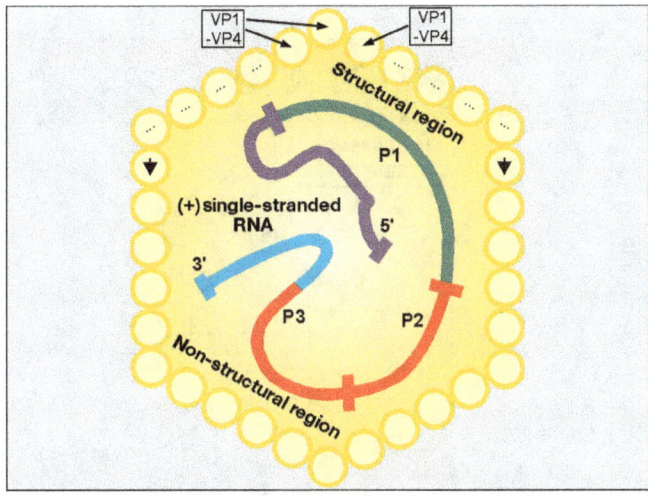

Fig. 5.4: Structure of the hepatitis A virus. It consists of 60 capsomeres, which as a whole form the capsid

11.2 Hepatitis B virus (HBV)

▶ The hepatitis B virus is a coated, circular, double-stranded DNA molecule, with a (+) partial overlapping strand; the minus strand has a length of approx. 3.2 kilobases. This virus with a diameter of 42 nm is classified as a hepadnavirus of the orthohepadnavirus family. HBV is also referred to as **Dane particle** after its discoverer (D.S. DANE et al., 1970). (s. pp 121, 422) It consists of a coat and a nucleocapsid. The **virus coat** is made up of the "s" (= antigen surface), which was discovered as a so-called Australian antigen by R.S. BLUMBERG et al. in 1965. (99) (s. p. 422) It comprises a large (l), medium (m) and small (s) protein. The **nucleocapsid** with a diameter of 27 nm contains the "c" (= core) antigen and the "e" (= envelope) antigen, which is a protein subunit of the core. Thus four **open reading frames** S, C, P and X code for the viral proteins HBsAg, HBeAg and HBxAg as well as for DNA polymerase. Replication of the DNA is effected by reverse transcriptase. There are two regions called DR1 and DR2 (= direct repeat) as well as two regions called Enh1 and Enh2 (= enhancer of the replication). • Eight genotypes are known. (s. fig. 5.6) *(see chapter 22.4!)*

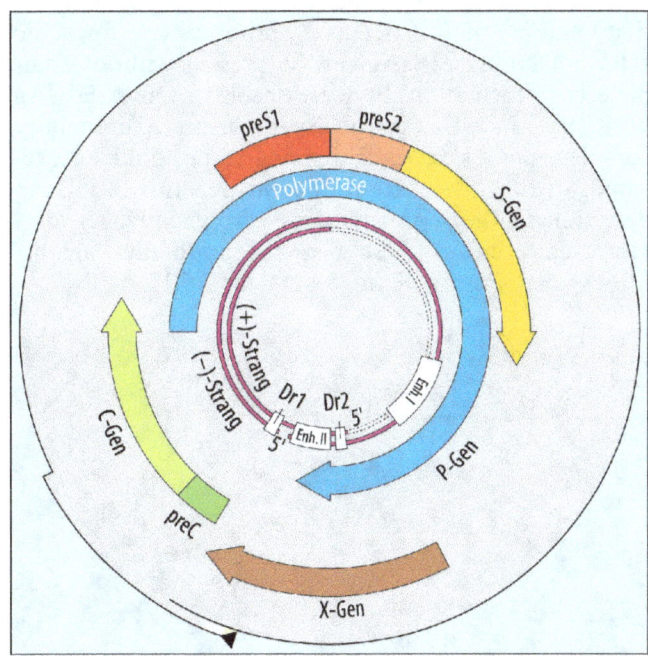

Fig. 5.6: Scheme of genome organization of HBV: a (−) singular strand and a partial overlapping (+) strand with direct repeat regions (DR 1, DR 2) and replication enhancer regions (Enh 1, Enh 2); there are four open reading frames, namely S, P, X and C, with the coding areas for the different HBV proteins (S, pre S1, pre S2 for the three surface proteins s, m and l, P = DNA polymerase, X = X protein, pre C for the HBe antigen and C for the HBc antigen); the nucleocapsid HBc encircles the genome HBV

Virus RNA is infectious. HAV multiplies within the cytoplasm of hepatocytes. • Approximately 2 to 3 weeks after infection, the viruses appear in the stool, but disappear after 4 to 5 weeks, thereby terminating the infectivity. As of the 4th week, HAV antibodies (anti-HAV) of the IgM and IgG type appear in the serum as **serological markers.** (s. fig. 5.5) Acute hepatitis A has a high IgM titre, whereas an infection occurring several months earlier can be recognized by a high IgG titre. • Once the infection has been overcome, the elevated IgG titre remains for life. Immunity is permanent. Renewed rises in titre (= *booster effect*) are possible after recurrent HAV contacts. The HAV vaccine induces equal IgM and IgG immune responses. By means of quantitative determination of the total anti-HAV, it is possible, for example, to differentiate between passive immunization and (acute or past) HAV infection. HAV RNA can be detected with the help of hybridization tests, and HAV with the help of PCR. (92, 100, 110) *(see chapter 22.3!)*

Besides the complete HBV, there are other DNA-free **HBs particles**, which are detectable in serum as so-called redundant surface material. These particles present as *spheres* or *tubular filaments*. The spherical particles have a diameter of 22 nm, whereby the length of the tubules is variable. Both particles are non-infectious since they possess no precursor polypeptide to bind to the hepatocyte receptor. • The relation of infectious viruses to non-infectious particles is about 1 : 1,000. (s. p. 432) (s. fig. 5.9!)

HBsAg particles contain a common **determinant "a"**, which is coded by the S gene. Apart from that, there are four other distinguishable *subtypes* d, y, w and r, which

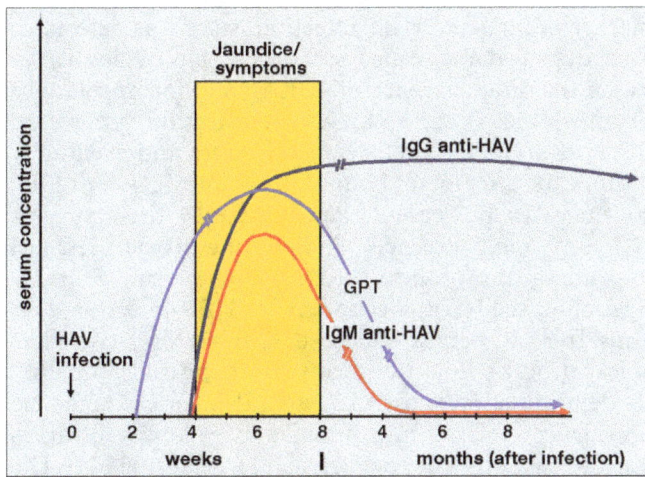

Fig. 5.5: Scheme of the immune status during the course of acute viral hepatitis A

seem to be of merely epidemiological significance. This results in four constellations *adw, adr, ayw* and *ayr*, all of which are detected by the serological HBsAg test. (92–94, 97, 98, 105–107, 110) **HBsAg** is identical to the Australian antigen (see above); HBsAg can be demonstrated histochemically in the cytoplasm and on the membranes of the hepatocytes as well as in the serum. Hepatocytes containing HBsAg appear as **ground-glass cells** in normal histology. (s. pp 402, 432) (s. figs. 5.7, 22.8) • After an incubation period of two to six months, HBsAg appears as the earliest serological marker in the serum – two to five weeks prior to the onset of clinical symptoms. Highest values are reached with the manifestation of the disease, followed by a gradual and steady decline to negativity within three to six months in a favourable course. This reduction in titre cannot be observed in cases with a tendency towards chronicity. HBsAg is neither carrier nor proof of infectivity and is not accepted as a "primary test" for acute HBV infections. HBsAg can be present without complete virus formation. In questionable or minor HBsAg positivity as well as in cases with suspected immunity complexes, an HBsAg-confirming test should be executed. In 20–25% of cases of acute hepatitis B, HBsAg detection in the serum remains permanently negative. However, even in these patients, antibodies against HBsAg can appear. (s. fig. 5.8) (s. tabs. 5.17, 5.18)

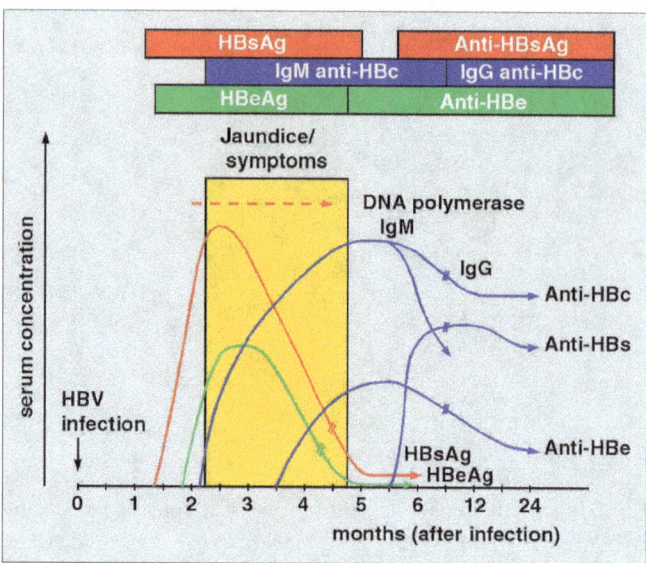

Fig. 5.8: Scheme of the immune status during the course of viral hepatitis B

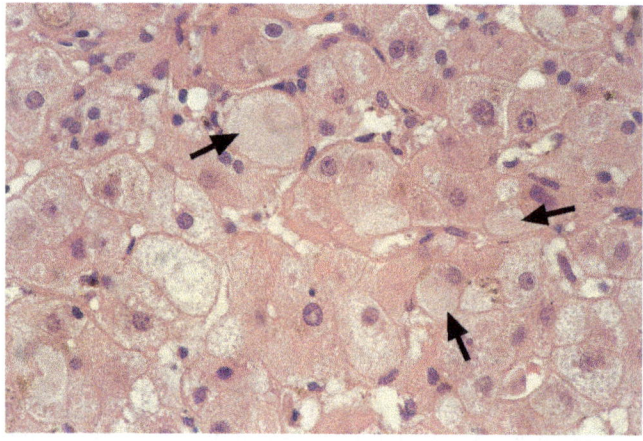

Fig. 5.7: Ground-glass hepatocytes (see arrows) in chronic hepatitis B virus infection (HE) (s. figs. 22.7, 22.8)

HBV mutants: During the infection, HBV can mutate. Such mutants may multiply and cause reinfection, even in the presence of anti-HBs. There are, for example, pre-core mutants (which prevent HBeAg secretion), X gene mutants, pre-S/S gene mutants ("immune escape mutant") and YMDD mutants of the polymerase gene (especially during lamivudine therapy). (s. p. 433) • Despite successful B vaccination, mutated HBV strains have the potential for eliciting a virus B infection!

HBeAg (L.O. MAGNIUS et al., 1972) is detectable in serum together with HBsAg, or shortly afterwards. This condition is present in the nuclei of the hepatocytes and can be demonstrated by immunoelectron microscopy in the endoplasmic reticulum and cytosol. HBeAg is a subcomponent or a degradation product of HBcAg. It is a marker for replicating HBV, i.e. viraemia, and as such it is proof of infectivity. HBeAg normally disappears at the peak of the disease, generally prior to HBsAg turning negative. Persistence for more than 12 weeks indicates a transition to chronic hepatitis. With the appearance of HBV mutants, which do not form pre-C protein, no HBeAg is produced: disappearance of HBeAg with positive HBsAg is not to be interpreted as a favourable course with the infection being overcome, but as suspected formation of mutants.

HBcAg is also found in the nuclei of the hepatocytes, but it is not present in the serum in its free form. (s. p. 433) (s. fig. 22.8)

Anti-HBc is the earliest immunological response to HBV antigens. Initially, there are high concentrations of IgM anti-HBc. This is known to be the most reliable marker of an acute HBV infection, since it is detectable even during the so-called serological gap (which is between the disappearance of HBsAg and the appearance of anti-HBs). (s. fig. 5.8) As the infection progresses, the IgM antibody level steadily declines and eventually disappears after 6 to 12 months, while IgG anti-HBc continues to be present. Persistent IgM titres suggest (*1.*) continuing presence of replicating HB viruses, (*2.*) impending transition to chronic hepatitis, and (*3.*) reactivation of the HBV infection. After HBV infection, IgG anti-HBc will persist and be detectable for a considerable period of time (for many years, possibly for life). Its determination is useful as a marker for the epidemic prevalence of HBV in a population – however, this is not the case with the determination of anti-HBs. • The positive detection of anti-HBc on its own allows various *interpretations*: (*1.*) anti-HBs has disappeared after an infection long passed while IgG anti-HBc is still present, (*2.*) IgM anti-HBc has again appeared after reinfection, (*3.*) anti-HBc is already being produced, but HBsAg is forming immune complexes with anti-HBs, and (*4.*) there is a "smouldering" or "silent" hepatitis (e.g. in drug addicts, in cases of haemodialysis or in immunocompromised patients). Although very small amounts of HBsAg are actually found in all cases, they are not detectable, with the result that anti-HBs remains subliminal and only anti-HBc appears. (93) Differential diagnosis between "late immunity" and "smouldering" hepatitis can generally be accomplished via HBV DNA determination (possibly PCR). • Infection with HBV through an exclusively anti-HBc-positive carrier (e.g. by blood transfusion) is possible.

Anti-HBs is formed after the disappearance of HBsAg and a subsequent "serological gap" of five to six months following the infection. (s. fig. 5.8) This gap can be extended by several weeks if the appearance of anti-HBs is delayed. Sufficiently high titres of antibodies ensure immunity against HBV reinfection. Anti-HBs is detectable for many years. Some 10−15% of patients do not form any antibodies and remain HBsAg carriers.

Anti-HBe develops with the disappearance of HBeAg in the serum. This serum conversion occurs roughly at the peak of the clinically manifest disease. Detection of anti-HBe is a favourable sign and suggests cessation of (clinically relevant) infectivity. Even this extremely short-lived HBV antibody may nevertheless be present for several years. (s. fig. 5.8)

HBV DNA is found in serum as long as there are replicating HB viruses. The sensitivity of *dot-blot hybridization* is in the range of 1 picogram HBV DNA (= 1 billionth of a gram, i.e. 3×10^4 to 3×10^5 virus particles). • Meanwhile, a most sensitive method for the qualitative detection of HBV DNA has been developed: in-vitro gene amplification, also known as *polymerase chain reaction (PCR)* (K. B. MULLISS, 1985). This technique allows the detection of 1 femtogram HBV DNA (= 1 trillionth of a gram, i.e. 3×10^1 to 3×10^2 HBV particles, approx. 10−100 viruses/ml). Given this incredible sensitivity, it is doubtful whether such a minimal quantity of viruses has any clinical relevance. • *After all, with the PCR method it was possible to confirm the persistence of replicable HB viruses in 100% of HBeAg-positive patients, in 80% of individuals with anti-HBe and in 57% of "healthy" HBsAg carriers.* • The detection of HBV DNA as the most sensitive marker of virus replication and, as such, proof of infectivity has replaced the determination of DNA polymerase. In routine diagnostics, however, a quantitative test should be used. There are different procedures, e.g. membrane hybridization (dot-blot, slot-blot), branched DNA hybridization.

HBV replication occurs in hepatocytes and extrahepatic cells (i.e. in bone marrow, kidney, pancreas, thymus, spleen, lymph nodes and endothelium). Results of the highly sensitive PCR should therefore be interpreted with caution in each individual case. (s. fig. 5.9)

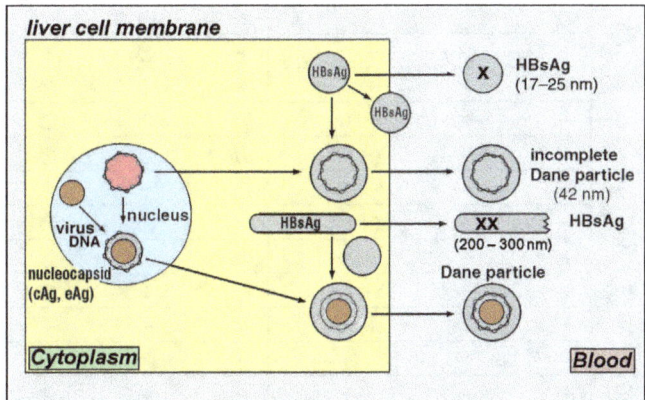

Fig. 5.9: Scheme of HBV replication in hepatocytes (or in extrahepatic cells) with incomplete, non-infectious HBsAg particles in the serum in the form of spheres (x) and tubular filaments (xx)

11.3 Hepatitis C virus (HCV)

▶ In 1989 molecular biological methods helped to demonstrate a hepatitis C virus which was identified as the pathogen in 90% of hepatitis non-A-non-B (Q. L. CHOO et al.). (96) The same research group also developed an anti-HCV test (G. KUO et al., 1989). This marker was positive in 70−92% of patients with posttransfusion hepatitis and in 58−79% of patients with sporadic NANB hepatitis. *(see chapter 22.5!)*

The enzyme immunoassay (EIA) of the *1st generation* determined antibodies against a non-structural protein (C 100) of the NS4 region with a sensitivity of 70%. • The *2nd generation* of the anti-HCV test is carried out with a mixture of core (C 22), NS 3 (C 33) and NS 4 (C 100) antigens. • The *3rd generation* possesses in addition the proteins of NS 5. The latter is best suited for the detection of RNA. This meanwhile established third generation test has achieved a significant improvement in the reliability of results. • In suspected HCV infection, an anti-HCV test is required. Anti-HCV titres were detected in 20−40% of patients with acute hepatitis C at the onset of the disease; after three months, this was the case in 70−90%. In patients with extremely low HCV viraemia, anti-HCV may even be missing. Anti-HCV antibodies are also detectable in the urine and saliva. • Positive antibody titres were found with relatively high frequency in alcoholic cirrhosis, autoimmune hepatitis and PBC as well as in drug addicts. • A positive test does not reveal whether there is still an active infection or whether recovery has been reached. Over the years, anti-HCV can disappear from the serum. (s. p. 448)

A positive anti-HCV test should be confirmed by means of the **RT-PCR test** or quantitative **hybridization test**, e.g. branched-DNA hybridization, amplicor technique. With the help of these procedures, it is possible to detect HCV RNA within just one week following infection. (95, 96, 99, 102, 104, 110)

	Anti-HBc	IgG	IgM	HBsAg	Anti-HBs	HBeAg	Anti-HBe	HBV DNA	HDV Ag	Anti-HDV
1.	Ø			+	Ø	Ø	Ø	+		
2.	Ø			+	Ø	+	Ø	+		
3.	+	(+)	+	+	Ø	+	Ø	+		
4.	+	+	+	+	Ø	Ø	+	+		
5.	+	+	(+)	Ø	Ø	Ø	+	(+)/Ø		
6.	+	+	(+)	Ø/(+)	Ø	Ø	+	Ø		
7.	+	+		Ø	+	Ø	+	Ø		
8.	+	+	(+)	Ø	Ø	Ø	Ø	+		
9.	+	+	+	+	Ø	Ø	Ø	+		
10.	+	+	(+)	+	+*	Ø	Ø	(+)		
11.	+	+	+	+	+*	+	Ø	+		
12.	+	+		+	Ø	Ø	Ø/+	Ø/(+)		
13.	+	+		+	+*	Ø	Ø/+	Ø/(+)		
14.	+	+	+	+	Ø	Ø	+*	+		
15.	+	+	(+)	+	Ø	Ø	+*	(+)		
16.	Ø			Ø	+	Ø	Ø	Ø		
17.	+	+	+	+	Ø	+	Ø	+	+	Ø/(+)
18.	+	+	(+)	O	Ø	Ø	+	(+)/Ø	+	Ø/(+)
19.	+	+		Ø	+	Ø	+	+	Ø	+
20.	+	+		Ø	+	Ø	+/Ø	Ø		

Tab. 5.17: Constellations of serological findings and their clinical interpretation during the course of HBV and HDV infection or HBV vaccination (* = immune complex) (98, 105–107, 110) (s. tab. 5.18)

11.4 Hepatitis D virus (HDV)

Hepatitis delta virus is a viruoid from the plant kingdom. It needs a helper virus (e.g. HBV) for replication. The hepadnavirus HBV delivers its coat protein to complete a pathogen, which then penetrates the hepatocytes. • So far, three genotypes of HDV are known. Compared to genotypes 2 and 3, genotype 1 more often leads to a severe or fulminant course as well as the development of HCC. (s. fig. 22.18) *(see chapter 22.6)*

Serological diagnosis is effected by determining HDAg and/or anti-HDAg, with parallel positive HBsAg. Acute infections and chronic diseases are confirmed serologically by IgM and IgG anti-HDV. The detection of HDV RNA is possible using PCR. Infection with HDV can occur as coinfection or superinfection. • The *coinfection* is paralleled by positive IgM anti-HBc, HBeAg and HBV DNA as well as IgM anti-HDV. • The *superinfection* usually has the following constellation: predominantly positive IgG anti-HBc, anti-HBe and IgG anti-HD, usually with negative HBV DNA. • After an HDV infection has been cured, anti-HDV disappears from the serum, making recognition of a previous delta hepatitis virtually impossible. (s. tabs. 5.17, 5.18) (s. fig. 22.18)

During the course of HBV or HDV infection, a multitude of serological findings are obtained. A clinical *interpretation of such serological constellations* is necessary for each single case, since this will yield an essential understanding of the stage and course of disease, infectivity, prognosis or serological cure. In single cases, unequivocal interpretations can be further clarified by determining titre levels or IgM antibodies.

Constellations of serological findings

1. Early, presymptomatic phase of acute already infectious hepatitis B (= late incubation period)
2. Onset of manifestation phase
3. Acute hepatitis B
4. Subsiding hepatitis B; persisting infectivity
5. Recent hepatitis B infection; "diagnostic window"; low or no virus persistence or infectivity; probability of immunity to reinfection (development of anti-HBs can be delayed for a period of 4 to 6, or even 12 months)
6. Phase of convalescence/stage of recovery; immunity to reinfection; no infectivity
7. Previous infection; immunity; no sign of infectivity
8., 9. Previous infection with subclinical or chronic course; infectivity; reactivated chronic hepatitis B
10., 11. Chronic course of hepatitis B with varying activity; simultaneous infection with infectivity; high-risk situation
12., 13. "Healthy" HBV carrier status with varying infectivity; varying immune response; varying threshold of detectability of markers
14., 15. "Ill" HBV carrier status; infectivity; subsiding infection
16. Outcome of active immunization
17. Acute HBV/HDV coinfection
18. Chronic HBV infection with HDV superinfection
19. Subsiding HBV/HDV coinfection with negativity of HDV and persisting infectivity
20. Previous HBV infection long passed; immunity

Tab. 5.18: Serological markers allow differentiation of hepatitis B infection (s. fig. 5.9) (s. tab. 5.17)

11.5 Hepatitis E virus (HEV)

Until recently, the entire virus group of NANB hepatitis was thought to be transmitted parenterally; in the meantime, however, an enterally transmitted hepatitis E virus has been identified. It is a single-stranded RNA virus with a diameter of 32–34 nm, which has so far been classified as a calicivirus. (111) According to virological investigations (E. V. Koonin et al., 1992), it possesses great similarity with the RNA of rubella viruses (of the Togaviridae group). This could also explain the similar consequences of rubella viruses and HEV for both the pregnant woman and the embryo. The viral genome was isolated from the stool of patients, whereas the viral antigen was detected in the liver of infected chimpanzees. In a self-experiment, HEV was transmitted, inducing acute viral hepatitis E (A. Chauhan, 1993). Cultivation in cell cultures has not been possible. In the meantime, cloning and sequencing has been successfully performed and a test developed for the detection of *IgM* and *IgG anti-HEV*. (101, 109, 111) *(see chapter 22.7)*

11.6 Other hepatitis viruses

As is commonly known, it has been possible to isolate parenterally transmitted HCV and enterally transmitted HEV of the hepatitis non-A-non-B group. However, further types of viruses seem to exist. *The previous NANB group has proved to be a reservoir for several types of viruses (e.g. HFV, HGV, GBV).*

Thus a virus particle was detected which was provisionally labelled *virus F* (**HFV**). • In a further case, another virus was differentiated as *virus G* (**HGV**). • In 1992 the research group of G. Berencsi discovered **yellow fever virus antibodies** in the serum of patients with transfusion hepatitis, although these Hungarian patients had never been in contact with yellow fever. The yellow fever-positive sera (following transfusion hepatitis) turned out to be negative with regard to all other hepatitis viruses. Such a hepatitis virus, cross-reacting with attenuated yellow fever viruses, actually seems to be the cause of further, still unknown, forms of posttransfusion hepatitis. *(see chapter 22.8–13)*

12 Immunological diagnostics

Autoimmunity is essential in each individual – and normally it does exist. Natural autoreactive antibodies ensure **immunological homoeostasis.** The immune system is well-equipped to fulfil its tasks of distinguishing between endogenous and exogenous structures.

Invasion of the organism by infectious or exogenous agents triggers a multitude of cellular **defence reactions** which are intended to help eliminate the foreign agents. The different interactions between the defence reactions of the immune system and the foreign agent cause varying clinical symptoms as well as varying courses of disease.

▶ Chronic liver disease, particularly that of viral origin, can therefore be caused by a **weakened immune system.** In contrast, autoimmune-induced chronic liver disease is attributable to an **overreaction of the immune system:** the immune system has lost its ability to distinguish between substances of an endogenous and exogenous (or secondary modified endogenous) nature. This leads to immune reactions against endogenous structures and usually also to autoimmune hepatitis. The ability to differentiate exogenous from endogenous applies to both T and B lymphocytes. The balance between helper and suppressor T cells ensures the functional efficacy of the immune system. The maturation process of B lymphocytes into specific antibody-producing plasma cells is supported by helper T cells.

A disorder of this homoeostasis can induce the **production of autoantibodies** or the activation of autoantigen-specific T lymphocytes. This leads to antigen-antibody reactions. These autoantibodies react with subcellular structures; they are only partly disease-specific and only organ-specific in single cases. There seems to be a certain genetic disposition for immunologically abnormal reactions or immune deficiencies. (130) • In some liver diseases, such autoantibodies are found with a characteristic frequency or concentration as well as in certain combinations. This condition not only facilitates a differential diagnosis, but also leads to findings of therapeutical value. So far, no specific antibody could be determined as the cause of a liver disorder. However, autoantibodies play a pathogenic role in several courses of disease. Most antibodies detected in hepatology can also be observed in other diseases without liver involvement. • *Antibodies are occasionally found at low titre levels and even in healthy (particularly elderly) individuals as well as in asymptomatic patients.*

The **detection of autoantibodies** is facilitated by: (*1.*) immunofluorescence in tissue sections, (*2.*) immunodiffusion, (*3.*) counterelectrophoresis, (*4.*) enzyme immunoassay, (*5.*) radio-immunoassay, and (*6.*) immunoblotting.

The most important and most widely applied screening method regarding antibodies in the serum is **indirect immunofluorescence microscopy.** This is carried out on frozen sections of isolated cells or tissue which are incubated with the diluted serum of the patients. After further incubation with an antihuman antigen marked with a fluorescent dye, a microscopic examination is performed with the help of light of a given wavelength. Then, any fluorescent glow indicates where antihuman antigen has recognized autoantibodies, which are bound to cell or tissue antigens. The detection threshold lies at ca. 100 ng antibodies/ml serum.

Circulating immune complexes form in the presence of a quantitative excess of antigens (or antibodies) as small, still soluble particles, which are distributed by the blood in the body, and which penetrate vascular walls or tissues. Here they can initiate multiple damaging mechanisms and even so-called **immune complex diseases**. In primary biliary cholangitis and primary sclerosing cholangitis, increased circulating immune complexes were observed. They can be detected by the *Raji-cell test* and the *C-1-q-binding assay*. • When positive, the determination of the **rheumatoid factor**, described for the first time by K. MEYER in 1922 *in patients with liver cirrhosis*, may also suggest circulating immune complexes.

12.1 System of antibodies

▶ The autoantibodies known in hepatology are classified in **two groups:** (*1.*) *nonorgan-specific antibodies* and (*2.*) *organ-specific antibodies*. Some of them can be characterized by additional subtypes, which allows more detailed differential diagnosis (e.g. immunological mixed forms, overlap with systemic collagenoses) and prognostic statements. (s. tab. 5.19) • *Of the more than 100 autoantibodies known to date, some have proved useful for the diagnostic and prognostic assessment of various hepatobiliary diseases.*

I. Non-organ-specific antibodies
1. *Antibodies against mitochondria (AMA)* 　Subtypes:　anti-M_1 to anti-M_9
2. *Antibodies against nuclear antigens (ANA)* 　– homogeneous　　– circular 　– speckled　　　– nuclear 　Subtypes: 　Anti-ds-DNA　　Anti-Sm 　Anti-ss-DNA　　Anti-SSA 　Antihistone　　　Anti-SSB 　Anti-U1-nRNP　　Anti-Scl-70 　Anticentromeres 　Human nuclear antigen (HNA), etc.
3. *Antibodies against histone-2B (IgA type) (AHA)*
4. *Antibodies against smooth muscles (SMA)* 　Subtype:　Antiactin
5. *Antibodies against microsomes (LKM)* 　Subtypes:　Anti-LKM_{1-3} 　　　　　　Anti-MFR_{1-2}
6. *Antibodies against granulocytes (ANCA)* 　– cANCA = cytoplasmatic ANCA 　– pANCA = perinuclear ANCA
7. *Antibodies against the cytoskeleton:* 　Subtypes: 　Anti-intermediary filaments 　Antimicrofilaments 　Antimicrotubuli
8. *Antibodies against ribosomes*
9. *Antibodies against basal cells*
10. *Antibodies against reticulin*
11. *Antibodies against polyalbumin*
II. Organ-specific antibodies
1. *Antibodies against liver membrane antigens (LMA)*
2. *Antibodies against liver cytoplasm antigens (SLA)*
3. *Antibodies against biliary duct epithelia*
4. *Antibodies against biliary duct canaliculi*
5. *Antibodies against liver ribosomes*

Tab. 5.19: Autoantibodies and their subtypes in chronic hepatobiliary diseases

There are chronic autoimmune-associated liver diseases with and without cholestasis which are negative in virus serology. With the help of selected autoantibodies, a detailed laboratory diagnosis can be achieved. (114, 116, 119, 120, 123, 124) (s. tabs. 5.19−5.21; 32.1) *(see chapter 32)*

12.2 Antinuclear antibodies (ANA)

Evidently, ANA (first described by G.J. FRIOU et al. in 1957) belong to the natural autoantibodies which are continuously stimulated by a still unknown mechanism (possibly a persisting agent) in certain diseases. However, this antibody phenomenon is inconsistent and neither organ- nor disease-specific. ANA can be visualized by immunofluorescence in cryostat tissue sections of the rat liver and rat kidney as a *homogeneous* (s. fig. 5.10), *speckled* (s. fig. 5.11), circular or nuclear fluorescence pattern. This allows conclusions to be drawn as to the specificity of antinuclear antibodies and in some cases as to the nature of the underlying disease as well.

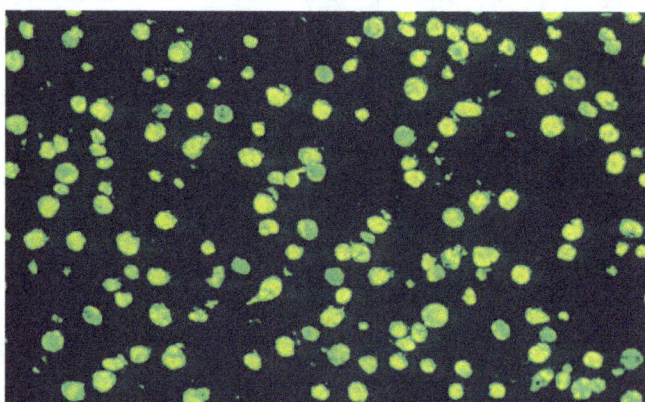

Fig. 5.10: Antinuclear antibodies (ANA) with homogeneous fluorescence pattern, here in chronic autoimmune hepatitis

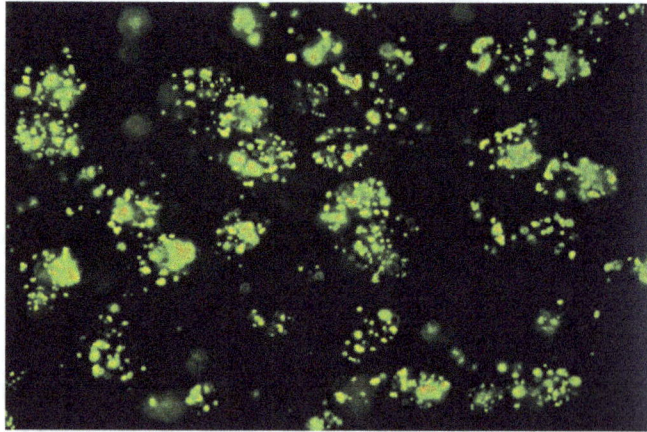

Fig. 5.11: Antinuclear antibodies (ANA) with speckled fluorescence pattern, here in PBC

To a varying extent, ANA are detectable in chronic active hepatitis (CAH), in mixed forms of CAH/PBC and particularly in lupoid hepatitis (autoimmune hepatitis type I) (in 80−100%) as well as in oxyphenisatin-induced CAH. Clinically relevant titres start at a serum dilution of 1:80. Level of the titre, pattern of fluorescence and in particular interaction with the complement system are relevant for the pathogenic valence of ANA. The determination of ANA and SMA is indicated when autoimmune hepatitis is in question.

In the case of a positive reaction, further differentiation of antigen specificity should follow. In the case of a negative reaction together with sufficient clinical suspicion, immunological diagnostics must be extended to include antibodies against microsomes (LKM), ribosomes and the cytoskeleton. (s. tabs. 5.20; 32.1)

12.3 Liver membrane antibodies (LMA)

Heterogeneous autoantibodies of the IgG class against liver cell membrane were detected using immunofluorescence (W. B. STORCH, 1973; U. HOPF et al., 1976). These antibodies are of no essential importance for clinical or differential diagnosis. In addition to that, their detection is a rather painstaking procedure (requiring hepatocytes of a perfused liver). • Likewise, **anti-LPS** has lost its importance, since it is an impure antigen fraction. • The *asialoglycoprotein receptor* has now been identified as an antigen of anti-LPS. Antibodies against these receptor proteins generally seem to correlate with the activity of chronic hepatitis.

12.4 Antibodies against smooth muscles (SMA)

Antibodies against smooth muscle antigens (SMA) were first detected by G. D. JOHNSON et al. in 1965. They are found in various viral and toxic forms of hepatitis as well as in PBC and PSC (40–70 % of cases). However, they are extremely heterogeneous. These antibodies react with structures of the cytoskeleton. Actin is the most important target antigen in liver diseases. SMA are not species-specific, but organ-specific. The frequency of SMA does not increase with age. In general, they have a low titre. They are best detected in the muscular layer of arteries and arterioles. High titres of antibodies of the IgG class and of the anti-actin subtype are found predominantly in autoimmune CAH (type I, rarely type III) and in mixed forms of CAH/PBC (80% of cases). A high titre and sole occurrence is typical of SMA-positive CAH. (s. tabs. 5.20; 32.1) (s. fig. 5.12)

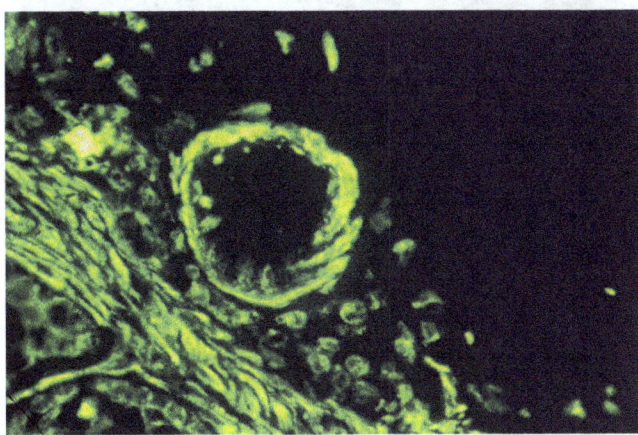

Fig. 5.12: Antibodies against smooth muscles (SMA) in autoimmune chronic active hepatitis

12.5 Antibodies against liver-kidney microsomes (LKM)

Autoantibodies against liver-kidney microsomal antigen (LKM) – also known as antigen against endoplasmic reticulum (AER) – were discovered in 1973 and termed LKM 1 by both M. RIZZETTO et al. and W. B. STORCH. • In the meantime, five subtypes have been differentiated. Autoimmune hepatitis type II is classified as anti-LKM 1 subtype. The accepted target antigen is a membrane lipoprotein of the rough and smooth endoplasmic reticulum – in this context, it is cytochrome P 450 2D6. This rarely detectable antibody is often found in high titres in younger patients with chronic aggressive hepatitis. (113) • LKM 2 antibodies have so far only been found in drug-related hepatitis caused by the diuretic agent tienyl acid (J. C. HOMBERG et al., 1984). Interestingly, LKM 3 anti-

	ANA	LKM	LP(SLA)	SMA	LMA	AMA	pANCA	AHA
1. Chronic active hepatitis (CAH)	Ø–(+)	Ø	Ø	Ø–(+)	Ø–(+)	Ø	Ø	Ø
2. Autoimmune hepatitis (AIH) • "lupoid" AIH (type 1) • LKM-positive AIH (type 2) • SLA-positive AIH (type 3) • SMA-positive AIH (type 4)	+++ Ø Ø Ø	Ø–(+) +++ Ø Ø	Ø–(+) Ø +++ Ø–+	++ Ø Ø +++	++ Ø Ø Ø–+	Ø–(+) Ø Ø Ø–+	Ø–+ Ø Ø Ø	+ Ø Ø Ø
3. Primary biliary cholangitis (PBC)	Ø–(+)	Ø	Ø	Ø–(+)	Ø	+++	Ø	++
4. Mixed forms of CAH/PBC	+	Ø	Ø–+	+	+	++	Ø	Ø
5. Primary sclerosing cholangitis	Ø–(+)	Ø	Ø	Ø	Ø	Ø	++	Ø
6. Alcohol-induced CAH	(+)	Ø	Ø	Ø	Ø	(+)	Ø	+
7. Drug-induced CAH	+	+++	Ø	Ø–(+)	Ø–(+)	(+)	Ø	Ø

Tab. 5.20: Autoimmune-associated hepatobiliary diseases and their possible autoantibody constellations (s. tab. 33.1)

bodies were found in chronic hepatitis D (O. Crivelli et al., 1983). (s. tabs. 5.20; 32.1) (s. fig. 5.13)

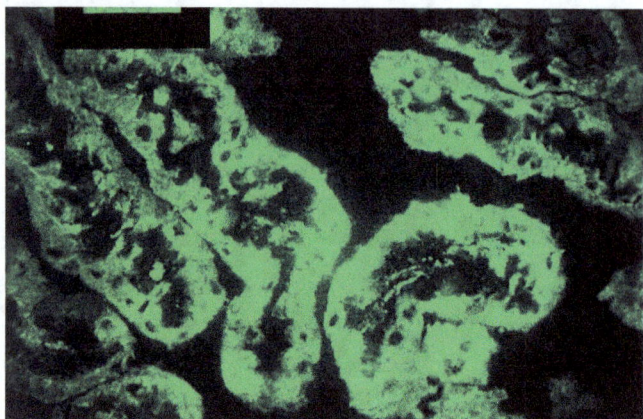

Fig. 5.13: Antibodies (type 1) against microsomes from liver and kidney (LKM) or against endoplasmic reticulum (AER). Antigenic substrate: kidney. Green fluorescence of the cytoplasm, particularly in the third segment of proximal tubules. The distal tubules are negative (40 x) (124)

12.6 Antibodies against mitochondria (AMA)

AMA are heterogeneous nonorgan-specific as well as organ-specific antibodies against antigens of the inner and outer mitochondrial membrane. They were discovered in 1965 (J.G. Walker et al.). These antibodies are visualized in liver and kidney tissue using immunofluorescence. • Various research groups have meanwhile identified nine different **AMA subtypes** associated with different diseases. These antibodies against subtypes have therefore achieved diagnostic and prognostic relevance. (s. tab. 5.21) The diagnosis of a PBC constellation showing a progressive tendency should lead to more intensive therapeutic measures. (112, 116, 121) (s. fig. 5.14)

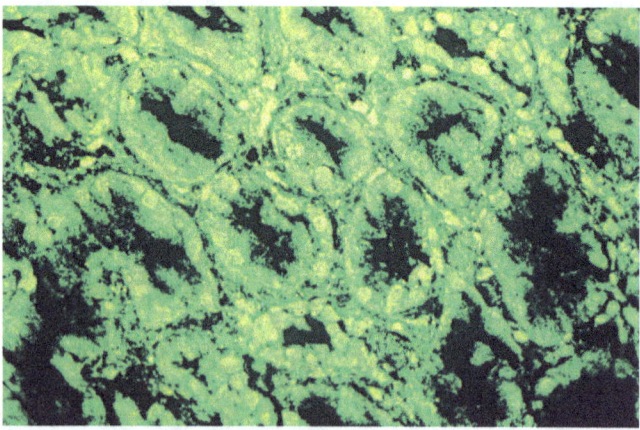

Fig. 5.14: Antibodies against mitochondria (AMA) in primary biliary cirrhosis (diffuse cytoplasmic fluorescence of renal tubuli with additional antibodies against nuclei)

In primary biliary cholangitis, AMA were found in 95–100% of cases at high titres (>1:100). They usually belong to the IgG class and are directed mainly against the M_2 antigen of the inner mitochondrial membrane. (121) Pyruvate dehydrogenase (PDH), branched-chain ketoacid dehydrogenase (BCKD) and ketoglutarate dehydrogenase (KGD) have meanwhile been identified as autoantigens. AMA also appear in chronic inflammatory liver diseases, in particular in cholestatic forms. "Mixed forms" of primary biliary cirrhosis and CAH always have to be considered. (s. tab. 5.20) • AMA of the subtype M_5 are detectable in collagenoses. • In hepatitis induced by iproniacid, AMA of the subtype M_6 were frequently found. Since iproniacid was taken off the market, M_6 antibodies have no longer been detected. • A significantly elevated AMA titre often presents an early sign of primary biliary cholangitis, long before clinical or laboratory symptoms become manifest. In suspected PBC, subtypes (anti-M_2, anti-M_9, anti-M_4 and anti-M_8) should be differentiated when AMA are positive. (s. tabs. 5.21; 32.1)

AMA specificity	Incidence	Antigen specificity
anti-M_1	syphilis (stage II)	iMM
anti-M_2	primary biliary cholangitis (PBC)	iMM
anti-M_3	pseudolupus	oMM
anti-M_4	active PBC, CAH, AIH	miC
anti-M_5	collagenoses	oMM
anti-M_6	drug-induced CAH	oMM
anti-M_7	cardiomyopathies, AIH	iMM
anti-M_8	PBC: unfavourable prognosis	oMM
anti-M_9	PBC: favourable prognosis	mcC

1. **AMA+, anti-M_2+**
   – confirmation of diagnosis of PBC
2. **AMA+, anti-M_2+, anti-M_9+**
   – stages I and II, predominantly stationary course, favourable prognosis
3. **AMA+, anti-M_2+, anti-M_8+**
   – progressive course, unfavourable prognosis
4. **AMA+, anti-M_2+, anti-M_4+, anti-M_8+**
   – progressive course, cholestatic CAH, less favourable prognosis

Tab. 5.21: Classification of AMA subtypes according to their presumed antigenic specificity and in relation to various diseases (iMM = interior mitochondrial membrane, oMM = outer mitochondrial membrane, miC = mitochondrial internal compartment, mcC = mitochondrial cytoplasmic compartment) • *In other studies, AMA profiles were not confirmed as prognostic parameters*

12.7 Antibodies against soluble liver protein (SLA/LP)

These antibodies, detected by M.P. Manns et al. in 1987, are targeted against soluble cytoplasmatic liver protein as the target protein (SLA). (118) They are likely to be the antibodies described earlier by P.A. Berg (1981), which are directed against a liver-pancreas antigen (**LP**). Anti-SLA-positive patients are always anti-LP-positive as well. The antigens are neither species-specific nor organ-specific, but characteristic of the existence of an immunologic disorder, the (re-)occurrence of which can point to a new episode of disease. Anti-SLA or anti-LP are presumably antibodies against cytosol, as first described by W. B. STORCH (1975). (123, 124) These antibodies may be an additional subgroup of AIH (type 3). (s. tab. 5.20) Other antibodies are generally detectable only in low titres and frequency. In about 25% of cases, merely SLA antibodies are present.

12.8 Antibodies against granulocytes (pANCA)

Perinuclear antineutrophilic cytoplasmatic antibodies (pANCA) react mainly with the target antigen myeloperoxidase, but also with other antigens. An atypical form of pANCA is xANCA, which does not react with myeloperoxidase. This is a combination of cANCA and pANCA, also described as "snowdrift pattern". The antibodies are seen as markers of primary sclerosing cholangitis (75−85%) as well as of colitis ulcerosa and panarteriitis nodosa. In Crohn's disease, pANCA are detectable in less than 10% of cases. pANCA are found in 25−30% of relatives. Their presence in AIH type 1 is helpful in differentiating pANCA-negative AIH type 2. (115, 116, 122) (s. fig. 5.15)

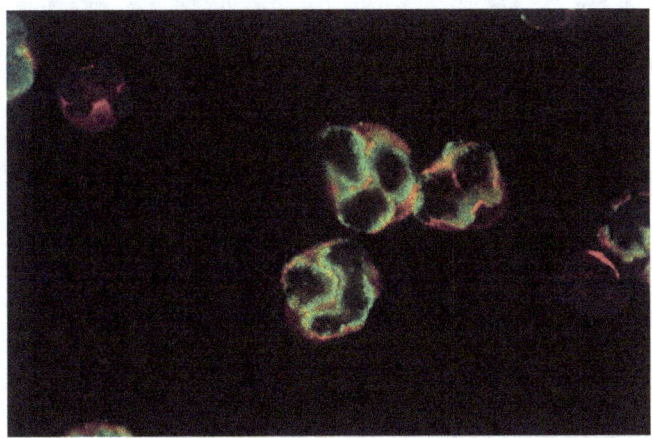

Fig. 5.15: Antibodies against perinuclear antigens of granulocytes (pANCA). Antigenic substrate: granulocytes. Counter-staining with Evans blue. Green fluorescence of the perinuclear cytoplasm of the granulocytes, red colouring of the lymphocytes (100 x) (124)

12.9 Antihistone-2B

Antihistone antibodies of the IgA type are significantly correlated with PBC and AIH, occasionally with alcoholic liver diseases. The antihistone antibody is a nuclear antigen. (121) (s. tabs. 5.20; 32.1)

12.10 Anti-GOR

The anti-GOR antibody (S. MISHIRO et al., 1990) is frequently detected in the early stage of viral hepatitis C. For more information about the *"term GOR"*, see page 659! (s. tab. 32.1) *(This information was given personally by S. MISHIRO!)*

In borderline cases, **immunological confirmation** is always required, even if only 10−15% of chronic liver diseases are of *autoimmune pathogenesis*. • Apart from that, liver diseases are quite frequently superimposed by immunological *epiphenomena*, just as there can be an overlap with *collagenoses*.

13 Biochemical algorithmic diagnostics

From a biochemical viewpoint, **three forms of activity** can be differentiated in hepatobiliary diseases: (*1.*) *enzymatic activity*, (*2.*) *mesenchymal activity*, and (*3.*) *serological and immunological activity*. (s. tab. 5.22)

1. **Enzymatic activity**
   • GPT ↑, GOT ↑, GDH ↑, γ-GT ↑
2. **Mesenchymal activity**
   • γ-globulins ↑
   • immunoglobulins A, G, M ↑
   • copper ↑
   • procollagen-III-peptide ↑
3. **Immunological activity**
   • hepatitis antigens/antibodies +
   • immunoglobulins A, G, M ↑
   • autoantibodies +
4. **Histological activity**

Tab. 5.22: Four forms of activity of hepatobiliary diseases

These do not necessarily correlate with one another − in fact, they may even be present to a markedly different degree, or they may not be detectable at all. Such differentiated observations and interpretations of biochemical findings provide a better insight into the pathophysiological process and course of hepatobiliary diseases. Based on the morphological findings, the pathologist may add *histological activity* as a fourth form of activity with varying degrees of intensity. (s. p. 714)

▶ In the case of suspected hepatobiliary disease, **algorithmic biochemical diagnostics,** structured step-by-step, has proved to be efficient and economical for diagnosis or differential diagnosis. The biochemical mosaic becomes all the clearer, the more mutually complementary and separate puzzlestones are inserted. The confirmation of a hepatobiliary disease by means of clinical and biochemical (as well as sonographic) findings is equally possible in the doctor's surgery and under clinical conditions. During this procedure, biochemical parameters have to be utilized in a targeted manner *(and therefore economically)*, adapted according to the relevant issue and extended from a minimum programme into the programme required. Hereby, enzyme-screening schemes and enzyme ratios may be of additional diagnostic help. Only single cases require parameters taken from the maximum programme. (s. tab. 5.23)

	Minimum	Necessary	Maximum
1. **Enzymatic activity**	GPT, γ-GT	→ GOT, GDH	→ LDH
2. **Synthesis capacity**	ChE, Quick's value	→ albumin	→ ammonia, galactose EC
3. **Excretion capacity**	AP, bile pigments in the urine	→ bilirubin; LAP	→ bile acids, iron, copper, cholesterol, indocyanine green, LP X
		Enzyme-screening scheme **Enzyme ratios**	
4. **Mesenchymal activity**	γ-globulins	→ immunoglobulins, A, G, M	→ procollagen-III-peptide, copper
5. **Immunological activity**	HBs antigen, HBc antibody, HA antibody, AMA	→ HBs antibody, ANA	→ HBe antigen, HBe antibody, HBV DNA, HDV, HCV antibody, SMA, LMA, α_1-foetoprotein *etc.*

*) With regard to clinical assessment, the respective normal values depend on the reference value of every laboratory

Tab. 5.23: Biochemical algorithmic programme for the diagnosis or differential diagnosis of hepatobiliary diseases (12, 13) (s. tabs. 5.6, 5.7, 5.11, 5.15, 5.17, 5.20, 5.21)

References:

Correct laboratory diagnostics

1. **Fiedler, G.M., Thiery, J.:** The incorrect laboratory result. Part 1: Pre- and postanalytical phase. Internist 2004; 43: 315–332
2. **Harm, K., Dieckvoss, E., Nagel, H.-H., Voigt, K.D.:** Alters- und Geschlechtsabhängigkeit klinisch-chemischer Kenngrößen. Lab. Med. 1981; 5: 134–141
3. **Junge, B., Hoffmeister, H., Feddersen, H.-M., Röcker, L.:** Standardisierung der Blutentnahme. Einfluß der Stauung auf 33 Blut- und Serumbestandteile. Dtsch. Med. Wschr. 1978; 103: 260–265
4. **Keller, H., Staber, G.:** Arzneimittel-Interferenzen bei klinisch-chemischen Tests. Lab. Med. 1983; 7: 164–171
5. **Massarat, S., Herbert, V.:** Haltbarkeit der Serumenzyme beim Versand. Dtsch. Ärztebl. 1977; 74: 1909–1910
6. **Sonntag, O.:** Haemolysis as an interference factor in clinical chemistry. J. Clin. Chem. Clin. Biochem. 1986; 24: 127–139
7. **Thomas, L.:** Blutentnahme und Probentransport. Dtsch. Ärztebl. 1991; 88: 1873–1877
8. **Wisser, H., Knoll, E.:** Tageszeitliche Änderungen klinisch-chemischer Meßgrößen. Ärztl. Labor 1982; 28: 99–108

Selection criteria for liver tests

9. **Blum, H.E., Weizsäcker, von, F.:** Rationelle klinisch-chemische Diagnostik hepatobiliärer Erkrankungen. Internist 1991; 32: 239–243
10. **Chopra, S., Griffin, P.H.:** Laboratory tests and diagnostic procedures in evaluation of liver disease. Amer. J. Med. 1985; 79: 221–230
11. **Irrgang, B., Adam, N., Pätzold, K., Przybylski, F.:** Zur Testauswahl für ein labordiagnostisches Stufenprogramm zur gezielten Unterstützung der Diagnostik von Lebererkrankungen. Z. Klin. Med. 1990; 45: 2223–2227
12. **Kuntz, E.:** Aktuelle laborchemische Leberfunktionsdiagnostik. Münch. Med. Wschr. 1972; 114: 781–788, 830–835
13. **Kuntz, E.:** Rationelle Diagnostik der Leberkrankheiten. Fortschr. Med. 1987; 105: 297–299, 335–336, 377–378, 419–420, 433–434, 454–456, 552, 593–594, 641–642, 660–662
14. **Popper, H., Medline, A.:** Die "Organellen-Pathologie". Ihre Bedeutung bei der Beurteilung von Leberfunktionsproben. Münch. Med. Wschr. 1969; 111: 1569–1574

Hepatocellular integrity

15. **Bacq, Y., Zarka, O., Bréchot, J.-F., Mariotte, N., Vol, S., Tichet, J., Weill, J.:** Liver function tests in normal pregnancy: a prospective study of 103 pregnant women and 103 matched controls. Hepatology 1996; 23: 1030–1034
16. **Chemnitz, G., Schmidt, E., Schmidt, F.W., Lobers, J.:** Diagnostische und prognostische Bedeutung massiv erhöhter Glutamat-Dehydrogenase-Aktivität im Serum. Dtsch. Med. Wschr. 1984; 109: 1789–1793
17. **Chung, Y.H., Jung, S.A., Song, B.C., Chang, W.Y., Kim, J.A., Song, I.H., Kim, J.W., Choi, W.B., Shong, Y.K., Lee, Y.S., Suh, D.J.:** Plasma isocitrate dehydrogenase as a marker of centrilobular hepatic necrosis in patients with hyperthyroidism. J. Clin. Gastroenterol. 2001; 33: 118–122
18. **Cohen, J.A., Kaplan, M.M.:** The SGOT/SGPT ratio – an indicator of alcoholic liver disease. Dig. Dis. Sci. 1979; 24: 835–838
19. **Craxi, A., Almasio, P.:** Diagnostic approach to liver enzyme elevation. J. Hepatol. 1996; 25 (suppl. 1): 47–51
20. **Daniel, S., Ben-Menachem, T., Vasuderan, G., Ma, C.K., Blumenkehl, M.:** Prospective evaluation of unexplained chronic liver transaminase abnormalities in asymptomatic and symptomatic patients. Amer. J. Gastroenterol. 1999; 94: 3010–3014
21. **Johnson, R.D., O'Connor, M.L., Kerr, R.M.:** Extreme serum elevations of aspartate aminotransferase. Amer. J. Gastroenterol. 1995; 90: 1244–1245
22. **Kamath, P.S.:** Clinical approach to the patient with abnormal liver test results. Mayo Clin. Proc. 1996; 71: 1089–1096
23. **Kew, M.C.:** Serum aminotransferase concentration as evidence of hepatocellular damage. Lancet 2000; 355: 591–592
24. **MacNamara, E., Goldberg, D.M.:** Serum enzymes and enzyme profiles in the diagnosis of liver and biliary tract disease. Surv. Dig. Dis. 1985; 3: 165–186
25. **Nemesanszky, E., Lott, J.A.:** Gamma-glutamyltransferase and its isoenzymes: progress and problems. Clin. Chem. 1985; 31: 797–803
26. **Pratt, D.S., Kaplan, M.M.:** Evaluation of abnormal liver enzyme results in asymptomatic patients. New Engl. J. Med. 2000; 342: 1266–1271
27. **Prieto, J., Barry, M., Sherlock, S.:** Serum ferritin in patients with iron overload and with acute and chronic liver disease. Gastroenterology 1975; 68: 525–533
28. **Puukka, K., Hietala, J., Koivisto, H., Anttila, P., Bloigu, R., Niemelä, O.:** Additive effects of moderate drinking and obesity on serum γ-glutamyl transferase activity. Amer. J. Clin. Nutr. 2006; 83: 1351–1354
29. **Sherwood, P., Lyburn, I., Brown, S., Ryder, S.:** How are abnormal results for liver function tests dealt with in primary care? Audit of yield and impact. Brit. Med. J. 2001; 322: 276–278
30. **Sheth, S.G., Flamm, St.L., Gordon, F.D., Chopra, S.:** AST/ALT ratio predicts cirrhosis in patients with chronic hepatitis C virus infection. Amer. J. Gastroenterol. 1998; 93: 44–48
31. **Skelly, M.M., James, P.D., Ryder, S.D.:** Findings on liver biopsy to investigate abnormal liver function tests in the absence of diagnostic serology. J. Hepatol. 2001; 35: 195–199
32. **Whitehead, M.W., Hawkes, N.D., Hainsworth, I., Kingham, J.G.C.:** A prospective study of the causes of notably raised aspartate aminotransferase of liver origin. Gut 1999; 45: 129–133
33. **Xu, K., Meng, X.-Y., Wu, J.-W., Shen, B., Shi, Y.-C., Wei, Q.:** Diagnostic value of serum γ-glutamyl-transferase isoenzyme for hepatocellular carcinoma: a 10-year study. Amer. J. Gastroenterol. 1992; 87: 991–995

Disorders of excretion

34. **Cravetto, C., Molino, G., Biondi, A.M., Cavanna, A., Avagnina, P., Frediani, S.:** Evaluation of the diagnostic value of serum bile acid in detection and functional assessment of liver diseases. Ann. Clin. Biochem. 1985; 22: 596–605
35. **Fukano, M., Amano, S., Hazama, F., Hosoda, S.:** 5'-nucleotidase activities in sera and liver tissues of viral hepatitis patients. Gastroenterol. Japon. 1990; 25: 199–205
36. **Komoda, T., Koyama, I., Nagata, A., Sakagishi, Y., DeSchryver-Kecskemeti, K., Alpers, D.H.:** Ontogenic and phylogenic studies of intestinal, hepatic, and placental alkaline phosphatases. Gastroenterology 1986; 91: 277–286
37. **Mannes, G.A., Thieme, C., Stellard, F., Wang, T., Sauerbruch, T., Paumgartner, G.:** Prognostic significance of serum bile acids in cirrhosis. Hepatology 1986; 6: 50–53
38. **Moss, D.W.:** Alkaline phosphatase isoenzymes. Clin. Chem. 1982; 28: 2007–2016
39. **Rosalki, S.B., Foo, A.Y., Dooley, J.S.:** Benign familial hyperphosphatasaemie as a cause of unexplained increase in plasma alkaline phosphatase activity. J. Clin. Pathol. 1993; 46: 738–741

Disorders of synthesis capacity
40. Bisceglie, A.M., Hoofnagle, J.H.: Elevations in serum alpha-fetoprotein levels in patients with chronic B-hepatitis. Cancer 1989; 64: 2117–2120
41. Brown, S.S., Kalow, W., Pilz, W., Whittacker, M., Woronick, C.L.: The plasma cholinesterase: A new perspective. Adv. Clin. Chem. 1981; 22: 1–123
42. Kuntz, E.: Die Bestimmung der Serumcholinesterase-Aktivität bei Kranken mit unspezifischen, tuberkulösen und malignen Lungenveränderungen. Med. Welt 1964; 2466–2477
43. Rondana, M., Milani, L., Merkel, C., Caregaro, L., Gatta, A.: Value of prealbumin plasma levels as liver test. Digestion 1987; 37: 72–78
44. Walli, A.K., Seidel, D.: Role of lipoprotein-X in the pathogenesis of cholestatic hypercholesterolemia. J. Clin. Invest. 1984; 74: 867–879

Disorders of metabolism
45. Barsotti, R.J.: Measurement of ammonia in blood. J. Pediatr. 2001; 138 (Suppl.): 11–19
46. Castell, D.O.: The ammonia tolerance test: an index of portal hypertension. Gastroenterology 1965; 49: 539–543

Diagnostics of liver functions
47. Aebli, N., Reichen, J.: Prognostische Wertigkeit der seriellen Bestimmung der Galactose-Eliminationsgeschwindigkeit bei chronisch-aktiver Hepatitis. Schweiz. Med. Wschr. 1991; 121: 970–976
48. Armuzzi, A., Candelli, M., Zocco, M.A., Andreoli, A., de Lorenzo, A., Nista, E.C., Miele, L., Cremonini, F., Cazzato, I.A., Grieco, A., Gasbarrini, G., Gasbarrini, A.: Review article: breath testing for human liver function assessment. Aliment. Pharmacol. Ther. 2002; 16: 1977–1996
49. Arrigoni, A., Gindro, T., Aimo, G., Cappello, N., Meloni, A., Benedetti, P., Molino, G.P., Verme, G., Rizzetto, M.: Monoethylglycinexylidide test: a prognostic indicator of survival in cirrhosis. Hepatology 1994; 20: 383–387
50. Bergstrom, M., Soderman, C., Eriksson, L.S.: A simplified method to determine galactose elimination capacity in patients with liver disease. Scand. J. Clin. Lab. Invest. 1993; 53: 667–670
51. Burns, E., Triger, D.R., Tucker, G.T., Bax, N.D.S.: Indocyanine green elimination in patients with liver disease and in normal subjects. Clin. Sci. 1991; 80: 155–160
52. Cheng, W.S.C., Murphy, T.L., Smith, M.T., Cooksley, W.G.E., Halliday, J.W., Powell, L.W.: Dose-dependent pharmacokinetics of caffeine in humans: relevance as a test of quantitative liver functions. Clin. Pharmacol. Ther. 1990; 47: 516–524
53. Erdogan, D., Heijnen, B.H.M., Bennink, R.J., Kok, M., Dinant, S., Straatsburg, I.H., Gouma, D.J., van Gulik, T.M.: Preoperative assessment of liver function: a comparison of (99 m) Tc-Mebrofenin scintigraphy with indocyanine green clearance test. Liver Internat. 2004; 24: 117–123
54. Grieco, A., Castellano, R., Matera, A., Marcoccia, S., Di Rocco, P., Ragazoni, E., Vecchio, F.M., Gasbarrini, G.: Antipyrine clearance in chronic and neoplastic liver diseases: a study of 518 patients. J. Gastroenterol. Hepatol. 1998; 13: 460–466
55. Hemming, A.W., Scudamore, Ch.H., Shackleton, Ch.R., Pudek, M., Erb, S.R.: Indocyanine green clearance as a predictor of successful hepatic resection in cirrhosis patients. Amer. J. Surg. 1992; 163: 515–518
56. Huang, Y.-S., Lee, S.-D., Deng, J.-F., Wu, J.-C., Lu, R.-H., Lin, Y.-F., Wang, Y.-J., Lo, K.-J.: Measuring lidocaine metabolite – monoethylglycinexylidide as a quantitative index of hepatic function in adults with chronic hepatitis and cirrhosis. J. Hepatol. 1993; 19: 140–147
57. Jalan, R., Hayes, P.C.: Quantitative tests of liver function. Aliment. Pharmacol. Ther. 1995; 9: 263–270
58. Keiding, S.: Galactose clearance measurements and liver blood flow. Gastroenterology 1988; 94: 477–481
59. Keiding, S., Engsted, E., Ott, P.: Sorbitol as a test substance for measurement of liver plasma flow in humans. Hepatology 1998; 28: 50–56
60. Kuntz, H.-D., May, B.: Die Galaktose-Eliminationskapazität. Aussagekraft und klinische Bedeutung. Med. Welt 1983; 34: 646–648
61. Kuntz, H.-D., May, B.: Quantitative Leberfunktionsdiagnostik. Münch. Med. Wschr. 1983; 125: 678–680
62. Kuntz, H.-D., Kuntz, E.: Intravenöse Galaktose-Belastung als Leberfunktionsprobe. Fortschr. Med. 1983; 101: 999–1004
63. Lewis, F.W., Rector, W.G.: Caffeine clearance in cirrhosis. The value of simplified determinations of liver metabolic capacity. J. Hepatol. 1992; 14: 157–162
64. Lotterer, E., Högel, J., Gaus, W., Fleig, W.E., Bircher, J.: Quantitative liver function tests as surrogate markers for end-points in controlled clinical trials: a retrospective feasibility study. Hepatology 1997; 26: 1426–1433
65. Marchesini, G., Fabbri, A., Bugianesi, E., Bianchi, G.P., Marchi, E., Zoli, M., Pisi, E.: Analysis of the deterioration rates of liver function in cirrhosis, based on galactose elimination capacity. Liver 1990; 10: 65–71
66. McDonagh, J.E., Nathan, V.V., Bonavia, I.C., Moyle, G.R., Tanner, A.R.: Caffeine clearance by enzyme multiplied immunoassay technique: a simple, inexpensive, and useful indicator of liver function. Gut 1991; 32: 681–684
67. Merkel, C., Gatta, A., Zoli, M., Bolognesi, M., Angeli, P., Iervese, T., Marchesini, G., Ruol, A.: Prognostic value of galactose elimination capacity, aminopyrine breath test, and ICG clearance in patients with cirrhosis. Comparison with the Pugh score. Dig. Dis. Sci. 1991; 36: 1197–1203
68. Merkel, C., Bolognesi, M., Bellon, S., Bianco, S., Honisch, B., Lampe, H., Angeli, P., Gatta, A.: Aminopyrine breath test in the prognostic of patients with cirrhosis. Gut 1992; 33: 836–842
69. Merkel, C., Marchesini, G., Fabbri, A., Bianco, S., Bianchi, G., Enzo, E., Sacerdoti, D., Zoli, M., Gatta, A.: The course of galactose elimination capacity in patients with alcoholic cirrhosis: possible use as a surrogate marker for death. Hepatology 1996; 24: 820–823
70. Meyer-Wyss, B., Renner, E., Luo, H., Scholer, A.: Assessment of lidocaine metabolite formation in comparison with other quantitative liver function tests. J. Hepatol. 1993; 19: 133–139
71. Molino, F., Cavanna, A., Avagnini, P., Ballare, M., Torchio, M.: Hepatic clearance of D-sorbitol. Noninvasive test for evaluating functional liver plasma flow. Dig. Dis. Sci. 1987; 32: 753–758
72. Monroe, P.S., Baker, A.L., Schneider, J.F., Krager, P.S., Klein, P.D., Schoeller, D.: The aminopyrine breath test and serum bile acids reflect histologic severity in chronic hepatitis. Hepatology 1982; 2: 317–322
73. Moseley, R.H.: Evaluation of abnormal liver function tests. Med. Clin. N. Amer. 1996; 80: 887–906
74. Mukherjee, S., Rogers, M.A., Buniak, B.: Comparison of indocyanine green clearance with Child's-Pugh score and hepatic histology: A multivariate analysis. Hepato-Gastroenterol. 2006; 53: 120–123
75. Park, G.J.H., Katelaris, P.-H., Jones, D.B., Seow, F., Le Couteur, D.G., Ngu, M.C.: Validity of the (13)C-caffeine breath test as a noninvasive quantitative test of liver function. Hepatology 38; 2003: 1227–1236
76. Salerno, F., Borroni, G., Moser, P., Sangiovanni, A., Almasio, P., Budillon, G., Capuano, G., Murala, M., Marchesini, G., Bernardi, M., Marenco, G. Molino, G., Rossaro, L., Solinas, A., Ascione, A.: Prognostic value of the galactose test in predicting survival of patients with cirrhosis evaluated for liver transplantation. A prospective multicenter Italian study. J. Hepatol. 1996; 25: 474–480
77. Testa, R., Caglieris, S., Risso, D., Arzani, L., Campo, N., Alvarez, S., Giannini, E., Lantieri, P.B., Celle, G.: Monoethylglycinexylidide formation measurement as a hepatic function test to assess severity of chronic liver disease. Amer. J. Gastroenterol. 1997; 92: 2268–2273
78. Urbain, D., Muls, V., Thys, O., Ham, H.R.: Aminopyrine breath test improver long-term prognostic evaluation in patients with alcoholic cirrhosis in Child class A and B. J. Hepatol. 1995; 22: 179–183
79. Wang, T., Kleber, G., Stellaard, F., Paumgartner, G.: Caffeine elimination: a test of liver function. Klin. Wschr. 1985; 63: 1124–1128
80. Williams, S.J., Farrell, G.C.: Serial antipyrine clearance studies defect altered hepatic metabolic function during spontaneous and interferon-induced changes in chronic hepatitis B disease activity. Hepatology 1989; 10: 192–197
81. Zoedler, T., Ebener, C., Becker, H., Roeher, H.D.: Evaluation of liver function tests to predict operative risk in liver surgery. HPB Surgery 1995; 9: 13–18

Mesenchymal reaction
82. Bayerdörffer, E., Lamerz, R., Fliege, R., Köpcke, W., Mannes, G.A.: Predictive value of serum procollagen-III-peptide for the survival of patients with cirrhosis. J. Hepatol. 1991; 13: 298–304
83. Bell, H., Raknerud, N., Orjaseter, H., Haug, E.: Serum procollagen III peptide in alcoholic and other chronic liver diseases. Scand. J. Gastroenterol. 1989; 24: 1217–1222
84. Beukers, R., Zanten, van, R.A.A., Schalm, S.W.: Serial determination of type III procollagen amino propeptide serum levels in patients with histologically progressive and non-progressive primary biliary cirrhosis. J. Hepatol. 1992; 14: 22–29
85. Fayol, V., Hassanein, H.I., El-Badrawy, N., Ville, G., Hartmann, D.J.: Aminoterminal propeptide of type III procollagen: a marker of disease activity in schistosomal patients. Eur. J. Clin. Chem. Clin. Biochem. 1991; 29: 737–741
86. Lotterer, E., Gressner, A.M., Kropf, J., Grobe, E., Knebel, von, D., Bircher, J.: Higher levels of serum aminoterminal type III procollagen peptide, and laminin in alcoholic than in nonalcoholic cirrhosis of equal severity. J. Hepatol. 1992; 14: 71–77
87. Müller, A., Krombholz, B., Pott, G., Machnik, G., Vollandt, R., Reinhardt, M., Jorke, D.: Collagen peptidase and type III procollagen peptide serum levels in chronic liver diseases. Clin. Chim. Acta 1991; 197: 59–66
88. Niemelä, O., Risteli, J., Blake, J.E., Risteli, L., Compton, K.V., Orego, H.: Markers of fibrogenesis and basement membrane formation in alcoholic liver disease. Relation to severity, presence of hepatitis, and alcohol intake. Gastroenterology 1990; 98: 1612–1619
89. Trinchet, J.-C., Hartmann, D.J., Pateron, D., Laarif, M., Callard, P., Ville, G., Beaugrand, M.: Serum type I collagen and N-terminal peptide of type III procollagen in chronic hepatitis. J. Hepatol. 1991; 12: 139–144
90. Vuitton, D.A., Seillès, E., Cozon, G., Rossel, M., Bresson-Hadni, S., Revillard, J.P.: Secretory immunoglobulin A in hepatobiliary diseases. Dig. Dis. 1991; 9: 78–91
91. Wolf, P.L.: Interpretation of electrophoretic patterns of serumproteins. Clin. Lab. Med. 1986; 6: 441–455

Serological diagnostics
92. Berasain, C., Betés, M., Panizo, A., Ruiz, J., Herrero, J.I., Civeira, M.-P., Prieto, J.: Pathological and virological findings in patients with persistent hypertransaminasaemia of unknown aetiologie. Gut 2000; 47: 429–435

93. **Blum, H.E., Weizsäcker, von, F.:** Der HBsAg-negative, anti-HBc/anti-HBs-positive Patient. Internist 1991; 32: 262–266
94. **Blumberg, B.S., Alter, H.J., Visnich, S.:** A "new" antigen in leukemia sera. J. Amer. Med. Ass. 1965; 191: 541–546
95. **Caldwell, St.H., Jeffers, L.J., Ditomaso, A., Millar, A., Clark, R.M., Rabassa, A., Reddy, K.R., De Medina, M., Schiff, E.R.:** Antibody to hepatitis C is common among patients with alcoholic liver disease with and without risk factors. Amer. J. Gastroenterol. 1991; 86: 1219–1223
96. **Choo, Q.L., Kuo, G., Weiner, A.J., Overby, L.R., Bradley, D.W., Houghton, M.:** Isolation of a cDNA clone derived from a blood-borne Non-A, Non-B viral hepatitis genome. Science 1989; 244: 359–361
97. **Gerber, M.A., Thung, S.N.:** Molecular and cellular pathology of hepatitis B. Lab. Invest. 1985; 52: 572–590
98. **Grob, P.J.:** Hepatitisserologie: Anwendung und Interpretation. Therapeut. Umschau 1992; 49: 287–301
99. **Houghton, M., Weiner, A., Han, J., Kuo, G., Choo, Q.L.:** Molecular biology of the hepatitis C viruses: implications for diagnosis, development and control of viral disease. Hepatology 1991; 14: 381–388
100. **Najarian, R., Caput, D., Gee, W., Potter, S.J., Renard, A., Merryweather, J., van Nest, G., Dino, D.:** Primary structure and gene organization of human hepatitis A virus. Proc. Nat. Acad. Sci. 1985; 82: 2627–2631
101. **Ray, R., Aggarwal, R., Salunke, P.N., Mehrotra, N.N., Talwar, G.P., Naik, S.R.:** Hepatitis E virus genome in stools of hepatitis patients during large epidemic in North India. Lancet 1991; 338: 783–784
102. **Reyes, G.R., Purdy, M.A., Kim, J.P., Luk, K.-C., Young, L.M., Fry, K.E., Bradley, D.W.:** Isolation of a cDNA from the virus responsible for enterically transmitted non-A, non-B hepatitis. Science 1990; 247: 1335–1339
103. **Rizzetto, M., Verme, G.:** Delta hepatitis-present status. J. Hepatol. 1985; 1: 187–193
104. **Roggendorf, M.:** Hepatitis-C-Virus. Dtsch. Med. Wschr. 1990; 115: 352–354
105. **Seelig, H.P.:** Polymerase-Kettenreaktion und Hepatitis B. Dtsch. Med. Wschr. 1993; 118: 277–279
106. **Shiina, S., Fujino, H., Kawabe, T., Tagawa, K., Unuma, T., Yoneyama, M., Ohmori, T., Suzuki, S., Kurita, M., Ohashi, Y.:** Relationship of HBsAg subtypes with HBeAg/anti-HBe status and chronic liver disease. Part II: Evaluation of epidemiological factors and suspected risk factors of liver dysfunktion. Amer. J. Gastroenterol. 1991; 86: 872–875
107. **Shiina, S., Fujino, H., Uta, Y., Tagawa, K., Unuma, T., Yoneyama, M., Ohmori, T., Suzuki, S., Kurita, M., Ohashi, Y.:** Relationship of HBsAg subtypes with HBeAg/anti-HBe status and chronic liver disease. Part I: Analysis of 1744 HBsAg carriers. Amer. J. Gastroenterol. 1991; 86: 866–871
108. **Strobel, E., Schöniger, M.:** False-positive hepatitis serology after administration of immunoglobulins. Dtsch. Med. Wschr. 2006; 131: 1325–1327
109. **Velazquez, O., Stetler, H.C., Avila, C., Ornelas, G., Alvarez, C., Hadler, S.c., Bradley, D.W., Sepulveda, J.:** Epidemic transmission of enterically transmitted non-A, non-B hepatitis in Mexico, 1986–1987. J. Amer. Med. Ass. 1990; 263: 3281–3285
110. **Weston, S.R., Martin, P.:** Serological and molecular testing in viral hepatitis: an update. Can. J. Gastroenterol. 2001; 15: 177–184
111. **Yarbourgh, P.O., Tam, A.W., Fry, K.E., Krawczynski, K., McCaustland, K.A., Bradley, D.W., Reyes, G.R.:** Hepatitis E virus: identification of type-common epitopes. J. Viral. 1991; 65: 5790–5797

Immunological diagnostics

112. **Berg, P.A., Klein, R.:** Antimitochondrial antibodies in primary biliary cirrhosis and other disorders: definition and clinical relevance. Dig. Dis. 1992; 10: 85–101
113. **Czaja, A.J., Manns, M.P., Homburger, H.A.:** Frequency and significance of antibodies to liver/kidney microsome Type 1 in adults with chronic active hepatitis. Gastroenterology 1992; 103: 1290–1295
114. **Czaja, A.J., Homburger, H.A.:** Autoantibodies in liver disease. Gastroenterology 2001; 120: 239–249
115. **Duerr, R.H., Targan, S.R., Landers, C.J., LaRusso, N.F., Lindsay, K.L., Wiesner, F.H., Shanahan, F.:** Neutrophil cytoplasmatic antibodies: a link between primary cholangitis and ulcerative colitis. Gastroenterology 1991; 100: 1385–1391
116. **Klein, R., Berg, P.A.:** Autoantikörper bei chronischen Lebererkrankungen: klinische und diagnostische Relevanz. Klin. Lab. 1993; 39: 611–626
117. **Laskin, C.A., Vidins, E., Blendis, L.M., Soloninka, Ch.A.:** Autoantibodies in alcoholic liver disease. Amer. J. Med. 1990; 89: 129–133
118. **Manns, M., Kyriatsoulis, A., Gerken, G., Staritz, M., Meyer zum Büschenfelde, K.-H.:** Characterisation of a new subgroup of autoimmune chronic active hepatitis by autoantibodies against a soluble liver antigen. Lancet 1987/I 292–294
119. **Manns, M.P., Meyer zum Büschenfelde, K.-H.:** Nature of autoantigens and autoantibodies in autoimmune hepatitis. Springer Semin. Immunopath. 1990; 12: 57–65
120. **Meyer zum Büschenfelde, K.-H., Lohse, A.W., Manns, M., Poralla, T.:** Autoimmunity and liver disease. Hepatology 1990; 12: 354–363
121. **Penner, E., Müller, S., Zimmermann, D., Van, M.H.V.:** High prevalence of antibodies to histones among patients with primary biliary cirrhosis. Clin. Exper. Immunol. 1987, 70: 47–52
122. **Seibold, F., Slametschka, D., Gregor, M., Weber, P.:** Neutrophil autoantibodies: a genetic marker in primary sclerosing cholangitis and ulcerative colitis. Gastroenterology 1994; 107: 532–536
123. **Storch, W.B.:** New autoantibodies and their antigens in autoimmune diseases. Cell. Molec. Biol. 1997; 43: 337–344
124. **Storch, W.B.:** Immunofluorescence in clinical immunology. A primer and atlas. Birkhäuser (Basel), 2000

Diagnostics in Liver Diseases
6 Sonography

		Page:
1	***Physical principles***	132
1.1	Basic information	132
1.2	Echo types	132
1.3	Artefacts	133
2	***Special sonographic techniques***	133
2.1	Sonography-guided puncture	133
2.2	Doppler sonography	133
2.3	Endoscopic ultrasonography	135
2.4	Ultrasound contrast media	135
2.5	Sonographic elastography	135
3	***Examination of the liver***	136
3.1	Section planes	136
3.2	Normal findings	136
3.3	Indications	137
3.4	Limitations and complementary procedures	137
4	***Diffuse liver diseases***	138
4.1	Congestive liver	138
4.2	Fatty liver	138
4.3	Hepatitis	139
4.4	Liver cirrhosis	139
4.5	Portal hypertension	139
4.6	Obstruction of hepatic veins	140
4.7	Jaundice	140
4.8	Portal vein thrombosis	141
4.9	Ascites	141
5	***Circumscribed liver diseases***	141
5.1	Echofree lesions − cyst, abscess	141
5.2	Hypoechoic lesions − adenoma, focal fat reduction, haematoma, FNH, lymphadenopathy	142
5.3	Hypoechoic lesions − haemangioma, NRH, echinococcus, HCC, metastasis, focal fat accumulation	143
6	***Examination of the spleen***	145
	• References (1−118) (Figures 6.1−6.21; tables 6.1−6.6)	146

6 Sonography

> **Ultrasonography is today a routine examination measure in the diagnosis of hepatobiliary diseases.**

After years of experience with ultrasonography (US), a well-trained sonographer will produce highly reliable results in the field of liver imaging. • The method neither inconveniences nor harms the patient. Thus there is a broad range of indications for examination by ultrasonography in patients with hepatobiliary diseases. There are no contraindications. Specific diagnostic statements, however, are rarely possible.

1 Physical principles

1.1 Basic information

▶ **Mechanical oscillations of > 18,000 Hz are referred to as ultrasound.** • In solid bodies, sound waves spread longitudinally as well as transversally; in fluids, gases or body tissue, however, waves only spread longitudinally. The average **velocity of sound conduction** (v) in tissues is approximately 1,540 m/sec.

	v (m/sec)	reflection
Air	331	99.88%
Fat	1,470	0.12%
Water	1,492	0.00%
Muscle	1,568	0.48%
Liver	1,570	0.30%
Bone	3,600	46.00%

Ultrasonic waves are generated by a piezoelectric crystal and emitted via a sound-conductive medium. These waves are reflected, broken, dispersed and absorbed by boundary layers. The piezoelectric crystal also acts as a sound-wave receiver and registers the modified ultrasonic waves (= *reciprocal piezoelectric effect*). They are then converted into an electric signal and displayed by means of oscilloscopic imaging.

Sound waves of identical phasing touch each other and serve as reciprocal reinforcement (= interference). The spatial dispersion of the regions with intensification and diminution is known as **interference pattern**. To a large extent, this determines the sonographic picture. • Contrary to the A mode *(= amplitude mode)*, the B mode does not show the amplitudes as deflections (= peaks), but as dots of light. The brightness of the dots corresponds proportionally to the intensities of the electric signals, i.e. intensity of the echo. In other words, the stronger the signal, the brighter the dot of light *(= brightness mode)*. • The sound field is composed of a slim, bundled near field and a diverging far field; precise scanning is only possible in the bundled near field.

This process will result in wavelengths of 0.1 to 1.5 mm in the **diagnostic frequency range** of 1 to 20 MHz. The 3.5 MHz range has proved suitable for abdominal sonography. A 5 MHz transducer will increase the resolution (0.6 mm axially, 1.2 mm laterally), but will also decrease the depth of penetration (10 cm) of sound waves. • Resolution in tissue is approx. 1 mm towards the sound beam (= axial) and 2–6 mm perpendicular to the axis of the sound beam (= lateral). This means that resolution depends on ultrasonic frequency and focus. An increase in ultrasonic frequency produces higher resolution and greater penetration depth. • A **linear scanner** applies parallel sound waves, while a **sectorial scanner** emits waves of a focal or curved source. • Both of these techniques rapidly produce images at a rate of 30/sec (= *real time*). This allows (*1.*) direct monitoring of internal physical motion and (*2.*) mobile handling of the transducer for **dynamic portrayal** and analysis of the image. In this way, the image can be frozen at any stage for documentation purposes, or the process of examination can be videotaped. (1)

1.2 Echo types

The sonographic technique is based on *reflection*; it works by measuring and portraying differences of impedance. Variations in *acoustic characteristics* of structures and tissues constitute the basis of sonographic differentiation.

The product of sonic speed in the respective tissue, together with the specific tissue density, yields the **acoustic impedance**. Each medium has its own value with regard to sonic resistance. • The partition between two media of different acoustic impedance is termed **acoustic interface** (which should not be confused with anatomical interface). The magnitude of difference of impedance determines the acoustic effectiveness of this interface. • Continuous technical development in grading the degrees of brightness of image points has made it possible to define the **different shades of grey** between the two extremes of reflection, black and white. With contemporary devices, 256 different shades of grey (scale of brightness) can be shown. The single dots of light appear in straight rows. Various organs, including the liver, exhibit characteristic shades of grey. Connective tissue, fat deposition, liquids, air or cellular infiltration will each alter the **grey scale.** This has considerably improved the differentiation of both the organs and the findings − thus a more exact diagnosis is guaranteed. (1)

Ultrasound impulses emitted into the body are reflected by interfaces, so that boundaries of organs are received as **contour echoes,** whereas internal heterogenicities of organs are received as **structure echoes.** Analysis of the echo structure is seen as a specific feature of ultrasonography. The sonic energy reflected by interfaces is visible on the screen in the form of bright spots. • As a rule, the echo represents an acoustic interface within a solid structure. Sonography differentiates between various zones: (*1.*) **hyperechoic**, (*2.*) **isoechoic**, (*3.*) **hypoechoic**, and (*4.*) **echofree**. Echofree areas point to the absence of acoustic interfaces, which as a rule corresponds to a "liquid" consistency. (s. figs. 6.4, 6.11)

▶ *The terms "hypodense", "isodense" and "hyperdense" depict pathological changes observed in CT.* For physical reasons, they are reserved for CT examinations and should not be used in sonography. (s. p. 179)

1.3 Artefacts

Sonographic artefacts may at times impede the assessment considerably. (42) Artefacts are mainly associated with the method applied and hence can often be eliminated simply by changing the examination technique. The occurrence of artefacts is largely fostered by extensive differences in acoustic impedance within a particular substrate, especially in the abdomen. In some 5% of cases, artefacts render sonographic examination impossible. They may appear in **multiple forms:**

1. amplification artefacts	5. mirror artefacts
2. arched artefacts	6. precursory artefacts
3. artificial sedimentation	7. reverberation echoes
4. contour aberrations	8. shadow zones

Given their manner of generation, but also in diagnostic terms, some artefacts can be of help to an experienced examiner, and possibly even provide additional information on the characteristics of the tissue.

2 Special sonographic techniques

2.1 Sonography-guided puncture

Liver changes of uncertain aetiology, whether of a diffuse or local nature, require histological clarification. This is particularly important if therapeutic consequences or prognostic statements are to be derived. For this purpose, the following possibilities exist: (*1.*) **fine-needle biopsy** with cytological or microbiological examination (3, 11, 22, 23, 73, 90) or (*2.*) **thick-needle biopsy** with histological or histochemical evaluation. (8, 58, 92) For diagnostic and especially for therapeutic purposes, there is also (*3.*) **puncture** of lesions (cysts, abscesses) with the possible placement of a *drainage* and the application of antibiotic lavage, the *injection* of cytostatics or alcohol into the tumour region or the injection of substances to promote the *sclerosing of cysts.* (s. tab. 7.3)

Fine-needle biopsy: The external diameter of the customary fine needle is < 1 mm (18−22 gg). A *Chiba needle* is generally used, although this is only suitable for obtaining cytological material. Diagnostic assessment of the bioptic material requires special experience of cytology. • Using the *incisive biopsy cannula* (diameter ca. 1 mm), a narrow biopsy cylinder can be extracted, which is processed and assessed in the usual histological or immunohistochemical manner. As opposed to Chiba cytology, this bioptic method allows a more reliable assessment of the benignancy or malignancy of a liver tumour. As a rule, the shortest biopsy channel is the best. In suspected haemangioma or subcapsular tumour, it is advisable to use a longer and self-tamponing channel.

For assessing focal hepatic alterations, it is preferable to use needles with which one can obtain cytological and histological material in one session, namely with the help of fine-needle technology (e. g. Trucut bioptic gun, 21 G). A further development is to be seen in the self-activating vacuum needle, which, as a fine needle, ensures a high degree of accuracy in obtaining tissue for histological examination. Use of the Chiba needle, which was widespread in the past, now tends to be less common.

> **Method:** *There are three ways of proceeding:*
>
> (*1.*) **Free puncture:** Puncture or biopsy needle and sound transducer are not connected mechanically.
>
> (*2.*) **Linked puncture:** Biopsy is performed using *needle forceps* attached to the side of a sound transducer. The passage of the needle and the targeted focus are shown on a monitor using a sight line. The puncture path is at an angle (adjustable as required) to the propagation of sound, i.e. the sound follows a different path from the biopsy needle.
>
> (*3.*) **Linked puncture with central perforation** of the linear sound transducer. Needle and sound follow the same route. The visibility of the needle is not as good as when the biopsy needle is introduced into the sound field from the side.

Contraindications include coagulation disorders, superficial hyperechoic foci (e. g. haemangioma), massive ascites, obesity, vascular aneurysm, portal hypertension, obstructive jaundice and hydatid cysts. Care should also be taken not to damage any previously unknown structures along the path of the biopsy needle.

Possible **complications** are (*1.*) bleeding, (*2.*) spread of tumour cells into the puncture channel (0.05%), (*3.*) mismanaged biopsy as well as possible injury or perforation of other organs, (*4.*) spread of infectious material from abscesses, and (*5.*) bile peritonitis. The frequency of these complications is approximately 0.5% and the lethality approximately 0.08%. *Hepatic haematoma* resulting from puncture can be detected by ultrasonography, provided it is large enough and subsequently monitored in the follow-up. (43, 76) Occurrence of pain in the region of the liver after puncturing is a strong indication for ultrasonography.

Thick-needle biopsy: Percutaneous "blind" biopsy, formerly used in Menghini's technique, is today considered obsolete; it has been replaced by **sonography-assisted liver biopsy.** As a consequence, the safety of biopsy has been significantly improved. (s. p. 156)

2.2 Doppler sonography

The **Doppler effect** (J. Ch. Doppler, 1842) signifies that light moving towards the measuring instrument appears increasingly blue, i. e. it has shorter wavelengths and higher frequencies, whereas light moving away from the measuring instrument appears increasingly red. • The Doppler frequency shift depends on the speed of the erythrocytes (= **c**ontinuous **w**ave Doppler) as well as on the direction and frequency of the emitted signal (= **p**ulse **w**ave Doppler). In the one-dimensional process, the blood vessel is hit by a single sound wave coming in at a certain angle, and flow velocity is then measured in the direction taken by the sound wave. Very high speeds develop in stenosis. The above process is applied in spectral Doppler sonography.

Colour-encoded Doppler sonography (CEDS): The introduction of CEDS in 1987 can be attributed to a combination of 2D Doppler sonography with real-time greyscale sonography. Both the volume and the direction of the blood flow are represented semiquantitatively by way of colour encoding (with different shades of brightness). The method is dependent upon the relationship between the vascular course and the transducer (red = blood flow towards the probe, blue = blood flow away from the probe). (5) (s. fig. 6.1) • The portal vein blood flow is centripetal and slightly pulsatile; the mean velocity of flow has been measured as 15.2 ± 2.6 cm/sec, representing a flow volume of 693 ± 235 ml/min. (s. fig. 6.2)

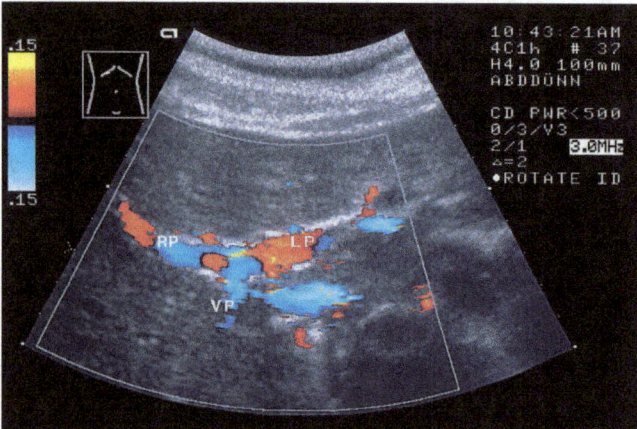

Fig. 6.1: Portal vein (PV) and division into the right (RP) and left (LP) portal vein trunk (subcostal section)

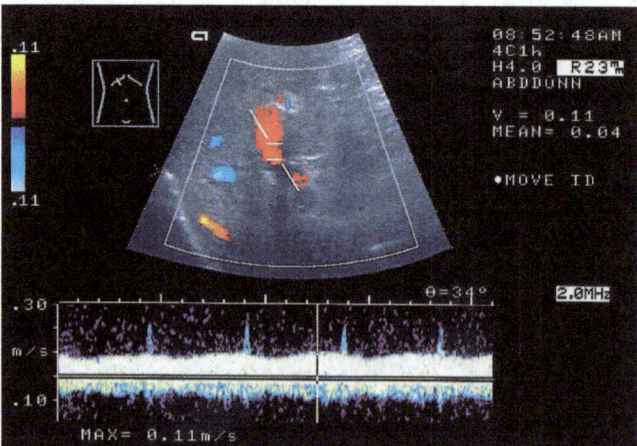

Fig. 6.2: Portal vein flow depicted by means of spectral analysis (velocity of flow = 11 cm/sec); hepatopetal flow is shown in red

The volume increases slightly during expiration, but significantly after eating (880 ± 269 ml/min). Portal hypertension is most reliably determined by measuring the flow volume prior to and following a test meal. (48) • In the case of suspected pathological findings in the area of the splanchnic vessels, colour-encoded Doppler sonography is indicated. This method will incorporate the portal vein system, hepatic veins, splenic vein, superior mesenteric vein and coeliac artery as well as the arterial vascular system. (s. tab. 6.1) (s. figs. 6.17, 6.18; 14.13; 35.15)

1. Signs of liver cirrhosis
2. Diagnosis of portal hypertension (with detection of hepatofugal flow as well as the slowing down of blood flow in the portal vein)
3. Confirmation of collateral circulation (e.g. umbilical vein, veins of the gall-bladder wall) or flow reversal with centrifugal refluxes
4. Unclear splenomegaly
5. Suspected partial or complete thromboses of the splenic-portal vascular bed
6. Budd-Chiari syndrome or veno-occlusive disease
7. Vascular system in liver tumours, tumour compression
8. Diagnosis of focal hepatic lesions (low or high number of blood vessels)
9. Assessment of a portosystemic shunt
10. Gastrointestinal bleeding of unknown cause
11. Internal or external head of Medusa
12. Assessment of the portal vein system before and after liver transplantation
13. Variations or malformations in the portal vein system (or visceral arteries)
14. Suspected Cruveilhier-von Baumgarten syndrome
15. Suspected cavernous transformation (formation of multiple venous collaterals close to the hepatic porta)
16. Therapeutic assessment of the vascularization of liver tumours after surgical interventions, chemo-embolization or parenteral chemotherapy

Tab. 6.1: Indications for colour-encoded Doppler sonography

Duplex sonography combines three different techniques: B mode with cw-pw-Doppler. Using this procedure, it is possible to measure the blood flow directly or (more commonly) indirectly, i.e. place-specific spectral analysis of a defined sample volume. By contrast, colour-encoded duplex sonography is an area-related representation depicting flow (or non-flow), flow direction, haemodynamics and perfusion pattern. It is not possible to show capillary flow, such as is found in tumours with special angio-architecture. (17, 39, 59, 63, 79, 81, 93, 96)

Power Doppler sonography (= transparent energy mode) shows flow intensity without any indication of flow direction. This process is highly sensitive in determining perfusion; thus very slow flow rates and tiny flow volumes or deeply-set vessels can also be detected. (15, 77)

2.3 Endoscopic ultrasonography

Endoscopic ultrasonography (EUS) promises greater accuracy as it involves placing a specialized sound transducer directly on the liver by means of laparoscopy or surgery.

Laparoscopic ultrasonography: As early as 1975, D. LOOK et al. showed the gall bladder, using the A-scan mode of ultrasonography via the laparoscope. In 1980 Y. FURUKAWA et al. described laparoscopic ultrasonography by employing the B-scan mode. Initially, optic lenses were employed, before being substituted later by linear probes. In 1989 F. FORNARI et al. reported on the laparoscopic application of a rotating sectorial scanner. (98) Here a linear sound transducer (7 MHz) attached to a rigid shaft by means of a flexible segment produced optimum results. This routine has the advantage of a wider scope of motility and improved orientation inside the gas-filled abdomen − without significant additional inconvenience to the patient. • Laparoscopic ultrasonography not only detects intrahepatic foci − with the possibility of targeted biopsy − but it also allows better matching of a focal lesion with the respective segment, together with more reliable preoperative tumour staging. • This procedure is also of advantage for the intraoperative application of ultrasonography in the detailed search for intrahepatic foci as well as in the intraoperative depiction of segmental borders. (97−107)

Intraductal ultrasonography (IDUS): This technique involving flexible miniature ultrasound probes with a diameter of approximately 1.5−2.0 mm (7.5−20 MHz) will expand the diagnostic spectrum concerning pathological processes in the larger bile ducts. The choledochus can usually be examined up to the hepatic duct. The identification rate of malignant or benign findings is high (accuracy 92%, sensitivity 90%, and specificity 93%). (108−112)

2.4 Ultrasound contrast media

Contrast media were originally applied to enhance insufficient echoes. In connection with the development of special technical devices, it is now possible to detect the presence of very small quantities of contrast media (i.e. low blood volume and passage of contrast medium through the vascular system can be quantified). A contrast medium consists of a shell with enclosed air or chemical gas. The latter possesses a longer contact phase. The shell can be hard (e.g. galactose particles, albumin) or flexible (e.g. phospholipids). These microbubbles (2−10 μm) act as a potent reflector for the ultrasound beam, intensifying the backscatter signal. Depending on the perfusion phase (arterial, portal venous, capillary), this leads to an enhancement of different liver structures. Some contrast media contain a special tissue affinity, which means that these substances are enriched in the tissue at the end of the vascular phase (e.g. RES of liver or spleen). Hyper- or hypovascularized lesions can therefore be differentiated into an arterial or portal venous phase in a reliable way. The application of microbubbles is an important measure in staging and controlling cancer patients as well as in monitoring local ablative therapy. (9, 10, 16, 89)

2.5 Sonographic elastography

▶ Based on sonographic measuring of elasticity by R.M. LERNER et al. (1987), M. SANADA et al. (2000) reported on first measurements of elasticity in patients with chronic hepatitis or cirrhosis. They found out that the average velocity of low-frequency waves in the liver of these patients was higher than in healthy persons. Methodological progress had already led to the development of D2-transient elastography by L. SANDRIN et al. (1991) − this is a combination of ultrasound (5 MHz) and low-frequency (50 Hz) elastic waves. Initial investigations with sonoelastography in chronic hepatitis C showed a good correlation with the histological degree of fibrosis (113). This good correlation of "quantifiable, dynamic, transient elastography" with the degree of fibrosis could be confirmed in further trials. (114−118) It is to be expected that in the near future more technical and methodological improvements will follow and that they will be well accepted in hepatology. • The transducer head transmits low-frequency sound waves (1 cm/sec), which deform the liver. The extent of the deformation indicates the stiffness of the liver, so that the degree of fibrosis can be quantified. The hard and more inelastic the liver, the faster the waves pass through it and the higher the values are, i.e. the more extensive is the fibrosis. The liver cylinder which is focused during the measurement has a length of 4 cm and a width of 1 cm, i.e. about 1% of the total volume of the liver (with liver biopsy, only 1/50,000 of the liver is available for analysis). The elasticity value is given in kilo-Pascal (kPa). A value of 3−10 kPa is seen as normal (with today's technology).

Various **sonographic procedures** can be applied in medical examinations, depending on the specific tasks and objectives. (s. tab. 6.2)

---

1. Conventional sonography
2. Doppler sonography
   − duplex sonography
     (combination of 2D conventional sonography with 1D Doppler sonography)
   − colour-encoded sonography
     (combination of real-time grey-scale sonography with 2D colour-encoded real-time Doppler sonography)
   − Doppler-power sonography
   − contrast-enhanced ultrasound
3. 3D Doppler sonography
4. Sonographic elastography

Tab. 6.2: Sonographic examination procedures

3 Examination of the liver

3.1 Section planes

The ultrasonographic examination of the liver is performed on the basis of section planes. This investigation is best carried out by adhering to a well-established system. Movement, i.e. repositioning the transducer, should be reduced in favour of tilting and requiring the patient to breathe in deeply. (s. fig. 6.3)

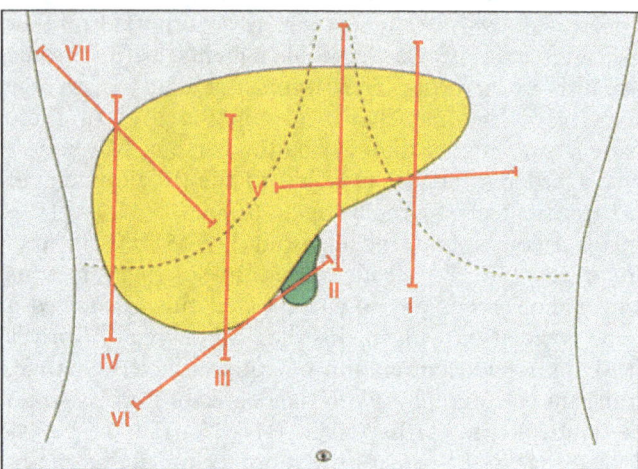

Fig. 6.3: Section planes in the sonographic examination of the liver: longitudinal sections (I-IV), transverse section (V), subcostal section (VI), intercostal section (VII)

With the help of these planes, it is possible to display numerous anatomical formations and structures. (s. tab. 6.3)

1. *Longitudinal sections I, II*	size, shape and internal structure as well as motility and compressibility of the left lobe of liver
2. *Longitudinal sections III, IV*	size, shape and internal structure as well as motility and compressibility of the right lobe of liver; gall bladder, hepatic porta, portal vein, inferior vena cava, common hepatic duct
3. *Transverse section V*	hepatic porta, falciform ligament, left lobe of liver
4. *Subcostal section VI*	internal structure of the right lobe of liver with portal vein, portal vein branches and hepatic veins; gall bladder, intrahepatic bile ducts
5. *Intercostal section VII*	right lobe of liver with subphrenic region

Tab. 6.3: Sonographic diagram of hepatobiliary structures and formations using five section planes

3.2 Normal findings

Liver assessment is based on sonographic anatomy as well as on external, internal and dynamic criteria. Evaluation of sonographic results must allow for variations in body height, body weight, shape of the thorax, habitus and age. (28, 30, 72, 80) The normal liver parenchyma reveals equal or marginally higher echogenicity than the (right) renal parenchyma. (57) From the age of 60–65, the liver loses up to a third of its weight ("senile atrophy", F. Th. Frerichs, 1858). (s. tabs. 6.4, 6.5) (s. fig. 6.4)

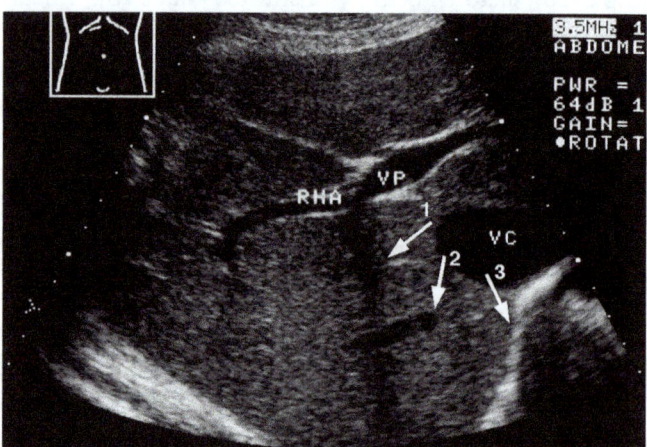

Fig. 6.4: Normal liver with portal vein (VP), inferior vena cava (VC) and right branch of the portal vein (RHA). Subcostal plane: 1 = left branch of VP; 2 = right branch of hepatic vein; 3 = cranial diaphragm

1. **External criteria** • Shape (dorsal and ventral contour) • Margin (inferior border of the liver) • Surface • Size (measuring of the right liver lobe in the MCL) • Position (e.g. downward displacement due to pulmonary emphysema) 2. **Internal criteria** • Circumscribed alterations • Internal structure • Sound conduction • Vascular structures • Anatomical segmentation 3. **Dynamic criteria** • Compressibility • Pain upon palpation • Respiration-related motility • Vascular pulsations

Tab. 6.4: Criteria for the sonographic examination of the liver

Close to the **round ligament**, the lower liver margin is somewhat drawn in and rounded off. There is a circular-to-oval, precisely circumscribed hyperechoic change of structure, marking the border between the right and left lobe of liver. The higher the fatty tissue content of the round ligament of the liver, the more striking this normal finding appears to be. (s. p. 179!) Dorsal to this finding, a shadow zone may be generated by the absorption of sound waves due to connective tissue present at this site.

Likewise, the structure of the **falciform ligament** as shown by ultrasonography must be observed and correctly interpreted. (33) (s. figs. 6.5; 8.1!)

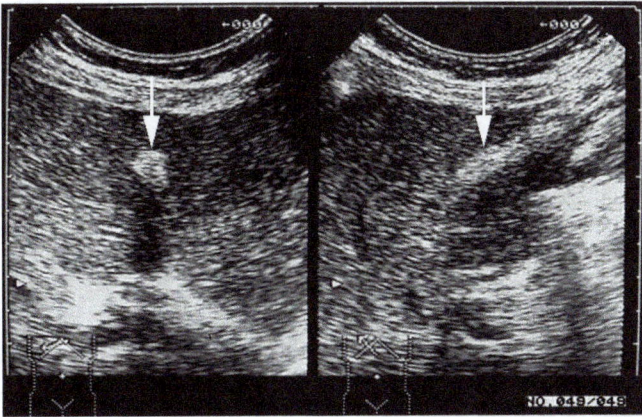

Fig. 6.5: Falciform ligament of the liver: transverse and longitudinal image (simulating "liver metastasis" with concomitant rectal carcinoma) (s. fig. 8.1!)

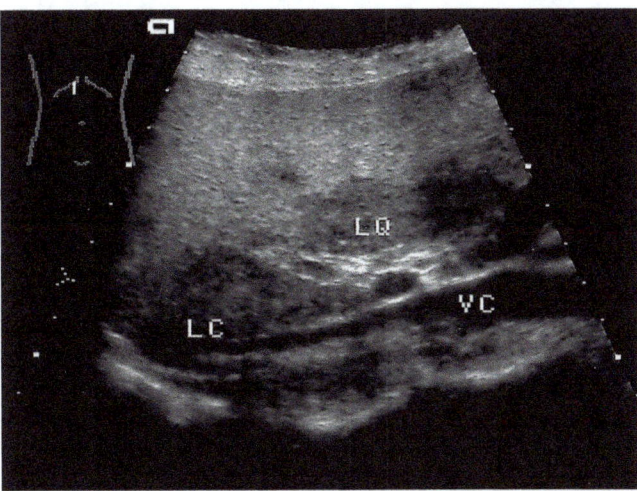

Fig. 6.6: Hypoechoic caudate lobe (LC) (= segment I) ventral of the vena cava (VC) and hypoechoic quadrate lobe (LQ) (= segment IV)

Size	12 ± 3 cm in the MCL (vertical) 9 ± 1 cm in depth
Shape	wedge-shaped
Margin	right $\leq 75°$, left $\leq 45°$, sharp-edged
Surface	smooth, slightly concave
Contour	dorsally and ventrally extended
Internal structure	fine homogeneous reflexes; somewhat more echogenic than the kidney parenchyma, slightly less echogenic than the pancreas; rather "dark" and "sharply contrasted"; the area of the caudate lobe is usually more hypoechoic
Quadrate lobe	43 ± 8 mm
Liver veins	easily depictable as far as the periphery, <6 mm, no wall echoes, lumen fluctuations during Valsalva's manoeuvre
Portal vein	mostly <12 mm, ventral to the inferior vena cava, marked wall echoes, branching distribution from the hepatic porta, no respiratory modulation
Hepatic artery	branching with pulsations in the hepatic porta
Bile ducts	thin, bright reflex bands, mostly demonstrable (<4 mm; $<50\%$ of the accompanying portal vein branch)
Ductus choledochus	≤ 7 mm; following cholecystectomy and in old age ≤ 11 mm

Tab. 6.5: Normal ultrasound findings of the liver. (The liver is an organ rich in variation and thus the figures given should be seen merely as points of reference to be treated individually)

The *caudate lobe* (= segment I) and the *quadrate lobe* (= segment IV) are distinguished from the liver in form and hypoechoic structure. (s. figs. 6.6) The papillary process of the caudate lobe may be misinterpreted as being a space-occupying proliferation. (38) • An enlarged *Riedel's lobe* shaped like a tongue (variation of the norm) can extend as far as the pelvic region. • Sonographic definition of liver segments — e.g. using laparoscopic sonography — has proved valuable in surgical procedures. (24, 41, 71) (s. p. 135)

3.3 Indications

In the case of suspected liver or biliary diseases, US is always indicated. Sonography has become a routine examination technique. (50) (s. tab. 6.6)

1. Diffuse liver diseases	
• diagnostic confirmation	++
• detection of complications	++
• differentiation	+
• malignant degeneration	(+)
2. Circumscribed liver diseases	
• diagnostic confirmation	+ − ++
• follow-up monitoring	+ − ++
• biopsy aid	+++
• differentiation	+
• diagnosis by exclusion	(+)
3. Jaundice and cholestasis	
• differentiation	++
4. Endoscopy or surgery	
• prior clarification	++
• follow-up examination	++
5. Screening after abdominal trauma	++
6. Assessment of portal veins and hepatic veins	+
7. Liver biopsy	
• targeted biopsy	+++
• targeted fine-needle biopsy	+++
8. Perihepatic lymphadenopathy	+

Tab. 6.6: Indications for sonography of the liver with regard to accuracy or validity: $+++$ = very high ($>90\%$), $++$ = high ($>70\%$), $+$ = moderate ($>50\%$), $(+)$ = minimal

3.4 Limitations and complementary procedures

The results presented so far in the literature concerning the sensitivity and specificity of ultrasonography undoubtedly reflect the success of the respective investigators following **many years of experience.** *The accuracy of such results should, however, always be seen in relative terms, and any general statements made in this connection should be qualified to obtain a more realistic mean value.*

▶ Diagnostic expectations regarding ultrasonography in liver diseases are often exaggerated. Hence, the **critical interpretation** of results is all too often neglected, and false-positive or false-negative conclusions are drawn all too hastily. Even when there is the slightest doubt in interpreting findings, the examination should be carried out again: **repeated investigations** improve accuracy.

Under optimal conditions, **focal lesions** of a diameter of 5 mm upwards can be identified. Liver metastases at varying stages are only detectable in 50—60% of cases. • If the assessment of focal hepatic changes is not possible with ultrasonography — even after colour-encoded duplex sonography — the indication for **computer tomography** (CT) is given. Indeed, the new *spiral CT generation* with i.v. injection of contrast medium provides excellent vascular representation. The differentiation of focal and malignant as well as vascular alterations of the liver is thus achieved in a way previously not thought possible. • **Magnetic resonance imaging** (MRI) has gained increasing importance since the introduction of T_2 contrast medium (iron-[II, III]-oxides) as well as of *MRI angiography*; this imaging technique now needs to be redefined from the hepatological point of view. • For the differential diagnosis of focal nodular hyperplasia versus adenoma, a **scintiscan** is indicated. • *If diagnostic explanation has not been provided by means of these complementary examinations, the indication for* **laparoscopy** *with targeted biopsy (possibly with forceps biopsy) has to be considered.* (s. tab. 7.11)

4 Diffuse liver diseases

▶ *A normal sonographic finding does not necessarily rule out a diffuse liver disease (30% of cases).* • *The morphologically normal liver exhibits 20—25% false-positive ultrasonographic findings in terms of a diffuse liver disease. Indeed, in 35—40% of all ultrasound findings in the liver, results can be classified as diffuse parenchymal processes.* • *Ultrasonography is no substitute for histology!*

The **increase in echogenicity** (i. e. increase in density) of a homogeneous, frequently coarsened structure with decreased sound conduction in the form of a "structurally dense liver" is a reliable indicator of a diffuse liver disease. This increase in intensity and frequency of echoes yields the image of a *"bright (white) liver"* (e. g. fatty liver, haemachromatosis). A diffuse liver disease can also be accompanied by a **decrease in echogenicity**, which is why the hypoechoic liver is known as a *"dark liver"* (e. g. acute liver congestion, acute viral hepatitis, amyloidosis). (s. fig. 6.7)

▶ In terms of ultrasonography, various liver diseases appear as diffuse changes in the parenchyma. They usually exhibit uncharacteristic findings. In cases where the diagnosis is uncertain, particularly after employing CT, liver biopsy (or laparoscopy) is then indicated:

1. acute hepatitis	6. congestive liver
2. chronic hepatitis	7. systemic haematological diseases
3. fatty liver	8. liver cirrhosis
4. metabolic diseases	9. granulomatous liver diseases
5. infectious diseases	10. diffuse metastatic spread

▶ Neither subclassification nor aetiological classification of the various diffuse diseases of the liver is possible by means of ultrasonography. There are, however, criteria and constellations of findings which are typical of some forms of disease. (6, 32, 36, 52, 78, 83)

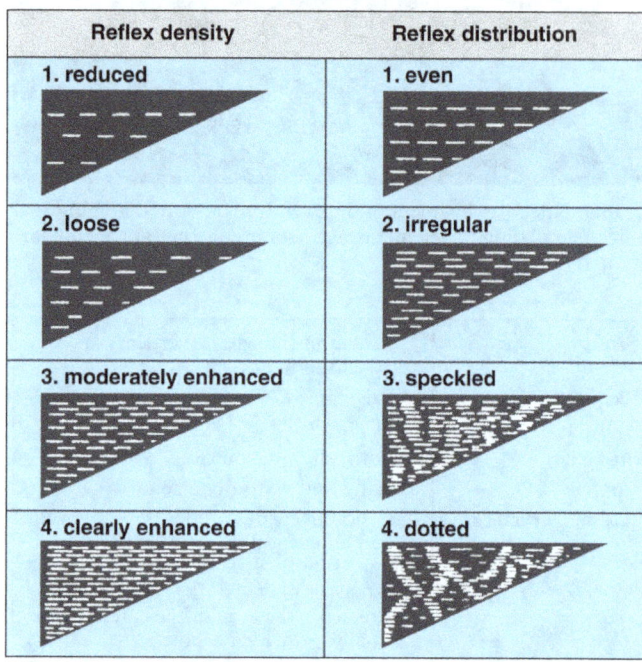

Fig. 6.7: Structural changes in the hepatic parenchyma with regard to reflex density and reflex distribution

4.1 Congestive liver

The congestive liver is enlarged and tender on pressure. The contours are rounded. Echogenicity is weak. The hepatic veins are dilated (normal diameter of the right hepatic vein is < 6 mm) and may be traced to the periphery. The inferior vena cava is widened and no longer exhibits the typical respiration-dependent double pulsation. • Characteristic of chronic congestive liver is the rise in echogenicity, so that during the progressive course of the disease, the findings may resemble those of micronodular cirrhosis. (s. fig. 39.5) *(see chapter 39.1)*

4.2 Fatty liver

The markedly enhanced echogenicity of the fatty liver ("bright liver" or "large white liver") is due to the high number of water-to-fat interfaces. (s. fig. 6.8) False-positive findings occur in roughly 20% of cases. In decreasing hepatic steatosis (< 30%), the sensitivity of recognition is reduced accordingly. Sonographically, a fatty deposit is evidenced in > 20% of hepatocytes in about 90%

of cases. There is a good correlation between ultrasonography and histological results, as there is between hypertriglyceridaemia and diabetes. The liver volume measured by ultrasonography is elevated, a fact which is also suggested by the rounded liver margin. The interior structure is inhomogeneously coarsened (in contrast to the kidney parenchyma), sound conduction continuously decreases dorsad, and hepatic veins are poorly imaged. In pronounced fatty liver, the portal vein can be dilated due to portal hypertension. In 20−30% of cases, the sonographic findings are mistaken for liver fibrosis, haemochromatosis, micronodular cirrhosis, chronic hepatitis C, thesaurismoses and systemic diseases. Occasionally, the distribution of fat shows focal or regional disorders, e.g. focal fat reduction (s.p. 142) or focal fat accumulation (s. p. 144). In a pathogenetic context, there may be regional differences in blood supply. • An *acute fatty liver of pregnancy* usually produces a normal sonographic image. *(see chapter 31.3, 31.6)*

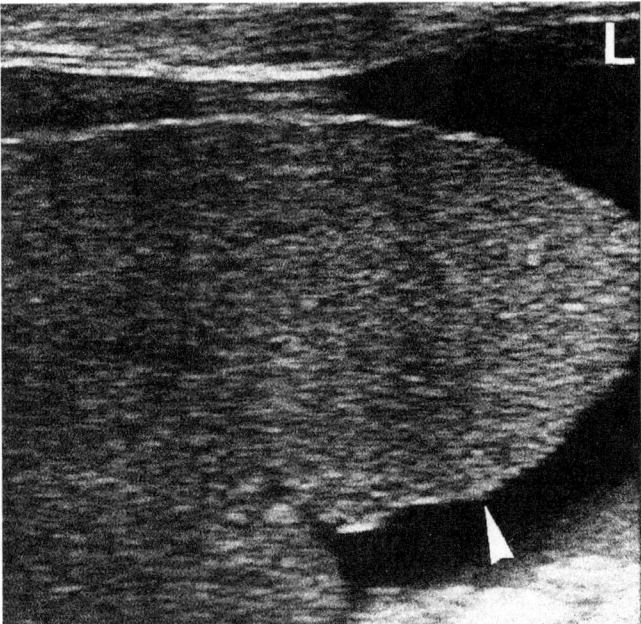

Fig. 6.9: Liver cirrhosis with ascites (longitudinal section): the left lobe of liver is rounded and plump; intrahepatic vessels are reduced. Irregular and inhomogeneous structure. Clear undulatory limitation (arrow) on the underside caused by nodular transformation. Wide hypoechoic fringe due to ascites

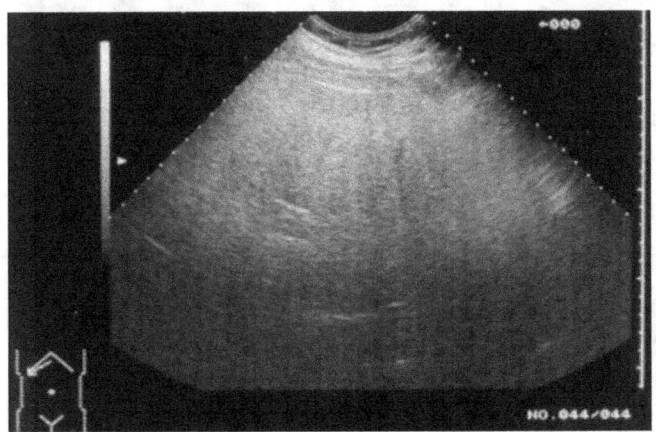

Fig. 6.8: Pronounced fatty liver (so-called *"bright white liver"*)

4.3 Hepatitis

Sonographically, acute hepatitis shows an enlarged liver with reduced echogenicity; the portal vessels appear more pronounced. In up to 50% of cases, a thickening of the gall-bladder wall (= oedema) is found; this may be mistaken for acute cholecystitis. As a rule, the lymph nodes are swollen, especially those in the hepatic porta (mostly with a diameter of more than 17 mm).

4.4 Liver cirrhosis

Sonographic findings in liver cirrhosis are polymorphic on account of the vastly differing individual hepatic structures (loss of parenchyma, regenerative nodes, connective tissue, fat depositions, compressed hepatic veins, splenomegaly, collateral circulation, etc.). (s. figs. 6.9, 6.10) *(see chapter 35)*

The size of the cirrhotic liver varies between hepatomegaly, normal findings and atrophy. The regular proportion of both liver lobes may have changed, resulting in an asymmetric enlargement or reduction of the liver. As a rule, ultrasonography shows the left lobe of liver to be affected to a greater extent and to be larger than the right lobe. The surface appears finely or roughly coarsened − particularly when applying a 5 or 10 MHz transducer. The contours can be seen as rounded edges and are frequently shaped like a bird's head. Echogenicity is increased with reduced sound conduction. • The quadrate lobe (= segment IV) often shows a reduced diameter (<30 mm). • Since the caudate lobe is less affected by this cirrhosis-related transformation due to its own special blood supply, it appears enlarged, it is strikingly hypoechoic and its contours are clearly delineated − a finding which always points to cirrhosis. (s. p. 137) • There is often a thickening of the gall-bladder wall (>4 mm). Prominent arteries may represent the *"pseudo double-barrelled-gun phenomenon"*. (cf. fig. 6.11) Occasionally, the liver arteries become corkscrew-like. The arterial blood flow is generally increased, whereas the blood flow in the portal vein is decreased. • The Doppler perfusion index (DPI) is usually increased. In cases of pronounced cirrhosis, sensitivity is 85−90% and specificity is 80−95%. (2, 9, 30, 40, 53, 70, 84, 94, 95, 96)

4.5 Portal hypertension

Detection of portal hypertension is of crucial importance in the diagnosis of cirrhosis. Sensitivity is 76−80% and specificity is 100%. The following findings may be present: *(1.)* dilation of the portal vein (>1.5 cm), *(2.)* calibre leap between the extrahepatic and intrahepatic segments of the portal vein in the hepatic porta (so-called *portal vein amputation*), (*3.*) dilation of the splenic vein (>1.5 cm), (*4.*) widening of the hepatic artery, (*5.*) splenomegaly with contact between the liver and spleen, (*6.*) dilation and/or rigid calibre of the superior mesenteric vein, (*7.*) detection of collateral vessels, particularly in the spleen and hepatic porta as well as in the anterior wall of the stomach, (*8.*) thickening of the stomach wall to >22 mm (66) and of the gall-bladder wall (67), and (*9.*) recanalization of the umbilical vein (s. fig. 6.10), which can be traced back to the umbilical region (= *Cruveilhier-von Baumgarten syndrome*). Highly-sensitive colour-encoded duplex sonography is useful in identifying small collateral vessels. There is often an increase in systolic and diastolic blood flow in the hepatic artery as well as a decrease in blood flow in the area of the portal vein. (s. fig. 7.4) (31, 84) *(see chapter 14)*

(< 8 cm/sec) without undulations; in some cases a pendula flow is found. The resistance index in the hepatic artery propria is > 0.75. (34) *(see chapter 39.2.2)*

4.7 Jaundice

Diagnostic accuracy in differentiating between obstructive and nonobstructive jaundice can be achieved in up to 90% of cases. (s. tab. 12.1) • Ultrasonography will reveal the cause of an *obstruction* in 30–60% of patients and localize this occlusion in almost all cases. (s. fig. 25.8!) Ultrasound shows the congested intrahepatic bile ducts as resembling vessels which run parallel to the portal vein branches and are mostly found in a ventral

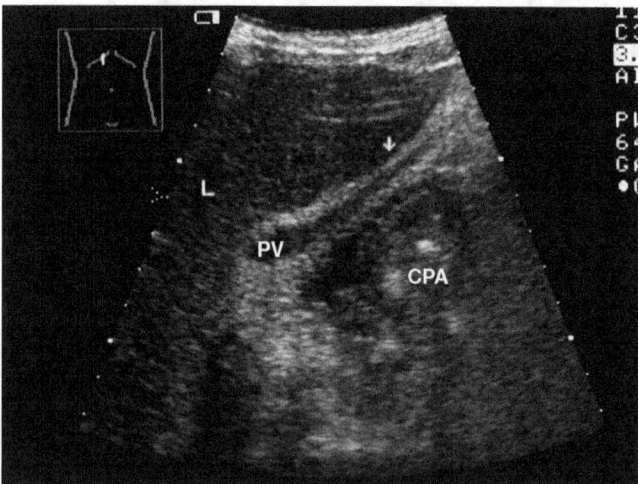

Fig. 6.10: Alcohol-induced cirrhosis with recanalized umbilical vein (= hypoechoic band: see arrow); (PV = left branch of the portal vein; CPA = cockade of pyloric antrum) (s. fig. 14.12)

4.6 Obstruction of hepatic veins

The **Budd-Chiari syndrome** is discernible by the total obstruction of hepatic veins or by their diminished lumen. The residual lumen of a vein often shows hyperechoic thrombotic material. The echogenicity of the liver parenchyma is stage-dependent. Sometimes membraneous webs of varying lengths consisting of hyperechoic structures with acoustic shadows are visible in the lumen of the inferior vena cava. The liver is enlarged. Due to its own venous drainage system, the caudate lobe (= segment I) is noticeably augmented (normal 6.8 ± 1.3 cm) and usually presents a hypoechoic structure. In most cases, ascites is also present. (7, 64) *(see chapter 39.2.1)*

The **veno-occlusive disease** is characterized by an acute obliteration of the small intrahepatic terminal veins. Sonographically, hepatomegaly, an hypoechoic reflection pattern and a thickening of the gall-bladder wall are evident. Typically, there is a flow rate in the portal vein

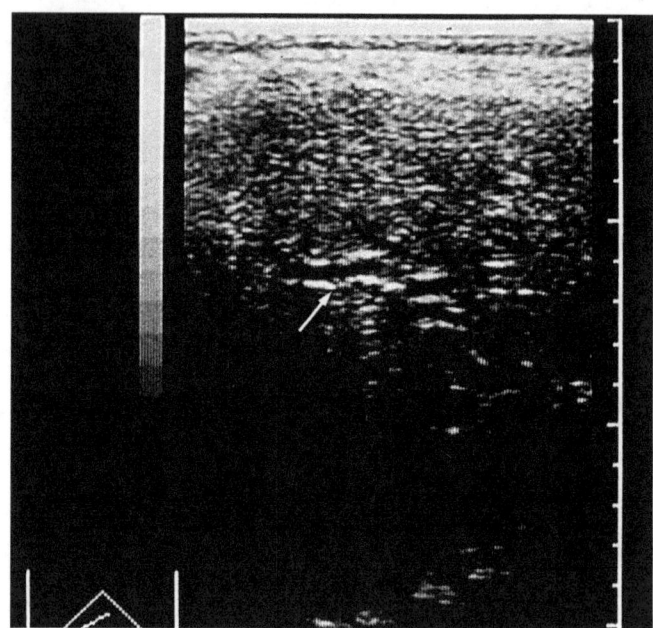

Fig. 6.11: Double-barrelled-gun phenomenon in obstructive jaundice (see arrow)

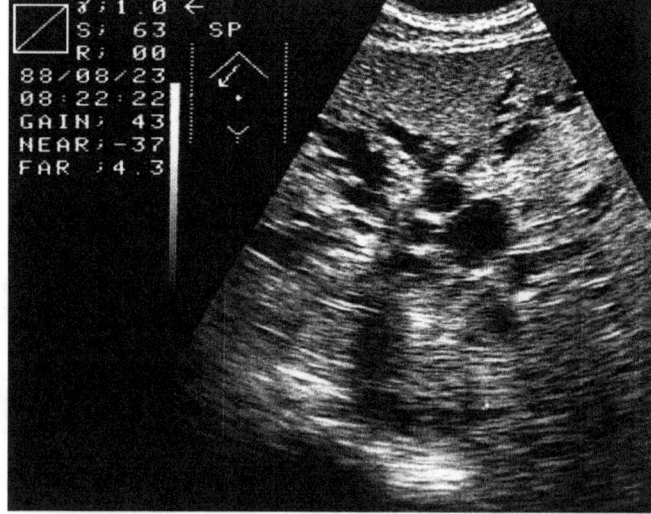

Fig. 6.12: Blockage and dilation of the intrahepatic bile ducts (*"lakeland plain"*) in obstructive jaundice

position (so-called *"double-barrelled-gun phenomenon"*). (s. fig. 6.11) • These congested bile ducts can also take on a *"lakeland plain"* appearance. (s. fig. 6.12) Close to the hepatic porta, dilated bile ducts may also appear in a radial pattern (so-called *"wheelspoke phenomenon"*). An extrahepatic occlusion is generally easier to recognize if there is a change in the lumen of the common bile duct when Valsalva's manoeuvre is applied. (60) *(see chapter 12)*

4.8 Portal vein thrombosis

Portal vein thrombosis with gradual or incomplete obstruction merely produces anastomoses and develops asymptomatically. After complete obstruction, ultrasonography will show paraportal, angiomatous anastomoses, mainly in the hepatic porta (= *cavernous transformation*). (85) Splenomegaly is seen with a normal-sized liver. The portal vein is not detectable. Echogenicity is variable and depends on the age of the thrombus. • Colour duplex sonography has become of paramount importance in portal vein system diagnostics. *(see chapter 39.3.3)*

4.9 Ascites

Ascites can be diagnosed even in small quantities (< 200 ml). Given a favourable location (preferred sites), it is possible to detect fluid volumes of < 50 ml. • Typical preferred sites include Douglas' space and the so-called *Morrison's pouch*. In the latter condition, the inferior surface of the right lobe is anterior to the colon and posterior to the perirenal fatty tissue, from which it is separated by a peritoneal recess. Here a small amount of ascitic fluid generally collects, which can be detected sonographically at an early stage. • Ascites coats abdominal organs, especially the liver and the spleen, and is shown as an echofree fringe zone. (s. fig. 6.9) Occasionally, intestinal loops float freely in the ascitic fluid, revealing the mesenteric attachment (so-called *"sea-anemone phenomenon"*). In addition, concomitant pleural effusion may be visible as an echofree zone above the diaphragm. Similarly, pericardial effusion can appear as an echofree zone at the cardiac apex. As a result of adhesions, ascites is possibly discernible in honeycomb-like compartments of various shapes and sizes. (91) *(see chapter 16)*

5 Circumscribed liver diseases

Focal changes are detected by ultrasonography with a sensitivity of 60–95%. The frequency of focal hepatic lesions is 3 to 5% (up to 10%) of all ultrasonic scans. Sonography does not allow a distinction to be made between benign and malignant lesions. (10, 18, 35, 52, 62, 65, 75, 88, 90) • Focal changes in echogenicity give rise to an *inhomogeneous hepatic pattern*. Such changes can be caused by focal intrahepatic lesions, vascular abnormalities, protrusions of the liver surface or circumscribed congestion of the bile ducts. The greater the difference in acoustic characteristics and the clearer the demarcation between focal changes and the surrounding liver parenchyma, the easier it becomes to detect such a focus by means of ultrasonography. Calcium-dense foci of a diameter of 3–5 mm, cystic formations of 5–8 mm and solid foci of 5–10 mm can therefore be identified. Such irregular permeation of the liver with different tissue structures will result in a homogeneously irregular image in ultrasonography, resembling a diffuse liver disease. • Detection of small foci close to the capsule is easier if a 5 MHz transducer is used.

Focal lesions develop due to various morphological structures or aetiopathogenetic conditions; in the further course, they may be subject to secondary changes (bleeding, liquefaction, necrosis, etc.) as well as late sequelae (neovascularization, septa, scars, calcification, etc.). Therefore, in each individual patient, a wide range of sonographic findings is to be expected, with varying echogenicities. Nevertheless, it may useful, for didactic reasons, to classify focal lesions as being echofree, hypoechoic, isoechoic and hyperechoic, depending on the initial and predominant echogenicity. It is, however, important to observe closely the possible changes in echogenicity due to various factors which may arise in the future course with regard to the relevant area.

5.1 Echofree lesions

Echofree lesions are: (*1.*) cysts, (*2.*) abscesses as well as necrotic colliquation of metastases, and (*3.*) fresh or reliquefied haematomas. (43, 76) • Caroli's syndrome (74), Osler's syndrome (85) and peliosis hepatis (49) may be assigned to this class as well. These echofree lesions exhibit distal sound amplification. (s. fig. 9.4)

Cysts are typically echofree, round, with a smooth, thin, limiting wall; they show a distal amplification of echo. Sometimes, there is a small "lateral shadowing" as an artefact. Sizes of 0.5 cm and more can be identified using ultrasound. The prevalence of (dysontogenetic) congenital hepatic cysts in the general population is 3–5%. They are mostly found in the right liver lobe, more frequently in women than in men, and are multiple in around 25% of cases. The cysts are usually 1–3 cm in size. However, they develop at differing rates and can grow to as much as 20 cm in diameter. When they reach a certain size, the cysts may have suppression effects within the liver itself and also on adjacent organs. Bleeding into the cysts can cause internal sedimentary echoes in the cyst lumen. (12) (s. figs. 6.13; 36.11–36.13)

In autosomal dominant *polycystic liver disease* (86), varying numbers of different-sized cysts are found in the liver and in the kidneys, sometimes also in the pancreas and the spleen. Liver vessels frequently become shifted and may be difficult to recognize. The overall frequency is 0.5–0.8%. (s. figs. 8.6; 36.14) *(see chapter 36.4.14.1)*

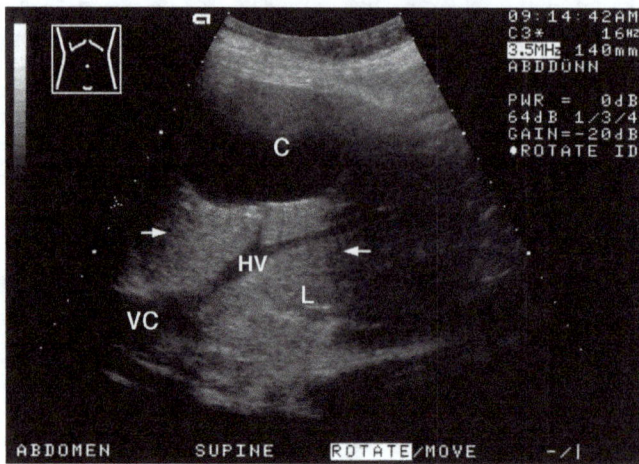

Fig. 6.13: Liver cyst. (C = cyst; HV = hepatic vein; VC = inferior vena cava; L = right lobe of liver; arrows = hyperechoic area below the cyst) (s. figs. 8.6; 36.9)

Abscesses display fine interior echoes, irregular shapes and blurred walls. An abscess may appear initially as an echofree, liquid-filled lesion, but also as an isoechoic structure. Later, in cases of cicatrization, it can become more reflective and even hyperechoic. Using colour-encoded duplex or contrast media, it may be possible to detect a central area without blood supply, but with highly vascularized surroundings. Gas-filled abscesses cause stronger reflections. There are repetitive echoes (so-called *"comet-tail phenomenon"*).

Differentiation between an amoebic and pyogenic abscess is not possible with sonography. In the light of the multiple aspects of ultrasound findings regarding abscesses, a three-type classification system has been drawn up in line with the respective internal structures, which has been broken down further into types IIIb, IV and V. (61, 82) (s. figs. 6.14; 9.2; 25.1) *(see chapter 27)*

5.2 Hypoechoic lesions

▶ The following lesions may be initially (or as a result of effects in the disease process) hypoechoic: (*1.*) metastases, (*2.*) liver cell carcinoma, (*3.*) adenomas, (*4.*) focal nodular hyperplasia, (*5.*) abscesses, (*6.*) haematomas, (*7.*) early liver infarction, (*8.*) foci showing reduced fatty infiltration, (*9.*) lymphomas, and (*10.*) lipomas. • In individual cases, differentiation between a benign and a malignant structural defect may cause considerable difficulties. (53) (s. fig. 9.4)

Adenomas are encapsulated epithelial tumours. Frequency is generally < 0.5%; in women and in patients with glycogenosis, it is higher. They have a smooth wall, are variable in size and appear round-to-oval. Adenomas are solitary (right more than left) and can be both hypoechoic or (more rarely) hyperechoic − this is possibly due to bleeding within the adenoma. They contain no biliary ducts or portal veins. Therefore, contrast media does not enter during the portal venous phase. *(see chapter 36.4.1)*

Focal reduction of fat in a fatty liver appears as a hypoechoic area and is predominantly found close to the gall bladder or the caudate lobe. Mostly it has a triangular shape, and there is a vascular association. In rare cases, it shows a round shape. (14) (s. figs. 6.15, 6.16)

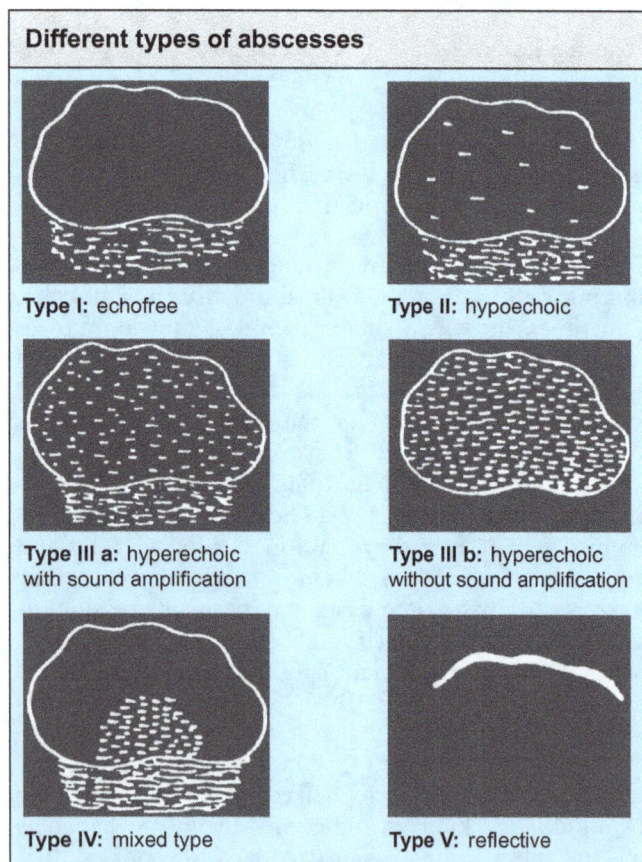

Fig. 6.14: Synoptic view of five different types of abscesses as shown by means of sonographic examination

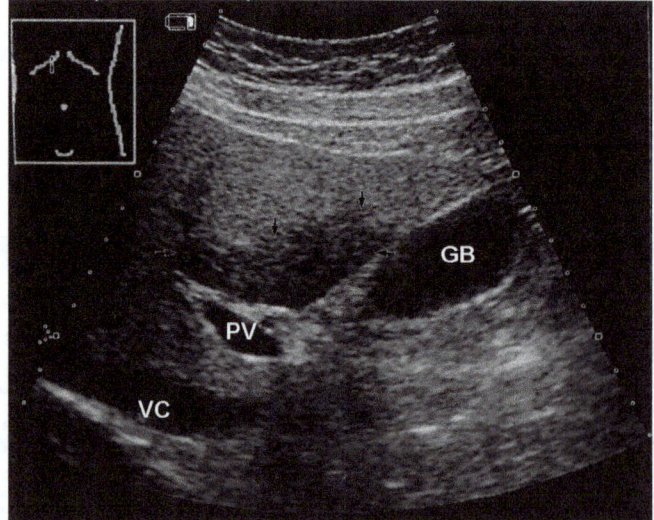

Fig. 6.15: Focal reduction of fat in a fatty liver: hypoechoic, triangular shape (see arrow) near to the right branch of the portal vein (PV) and the gall bladder (GB); (VC = inferior vena cava)

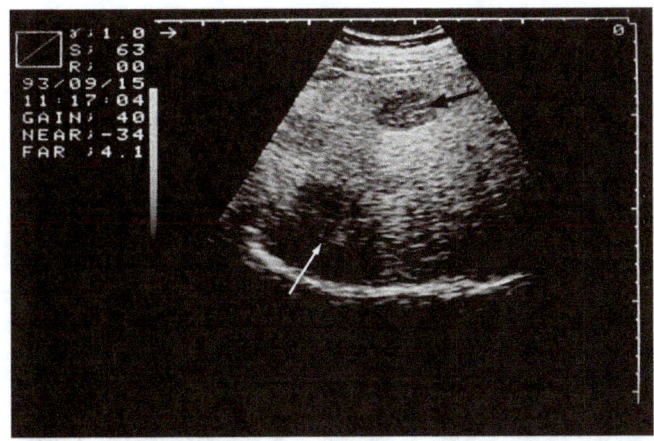

Fig. 6.16: Focal reduction of fat in a fatty liver: hypoechoic round shape (see arrows)

Focal nodular hyperplasia – as a benign hepatocellular tumour in terms of vascular deformation – is mostly hypoechoic, but sometimes also isoechoic. Occasionally, it can be differentiated as a protruding contour or a pediculate liver tumour. Compression of the surrounding liver tissue may be the cause of a visible "capsule", which actually has no anatomical structure of its own. At a size of >3 cm, fibrous septa and arteries can resemble a typical *wheelspoke pattern*, often with a clearly visible central core. • The blood circulation within the tumour can be visualized by means of contrast medium: early arterial hyperperfusion is usually in evidence. As a hypervascularized lesion, FNH sometimes has afferent arteries, which may surround the lesion like a basket. (s. fig. 6.17) *(see chapter 36.4.2)*

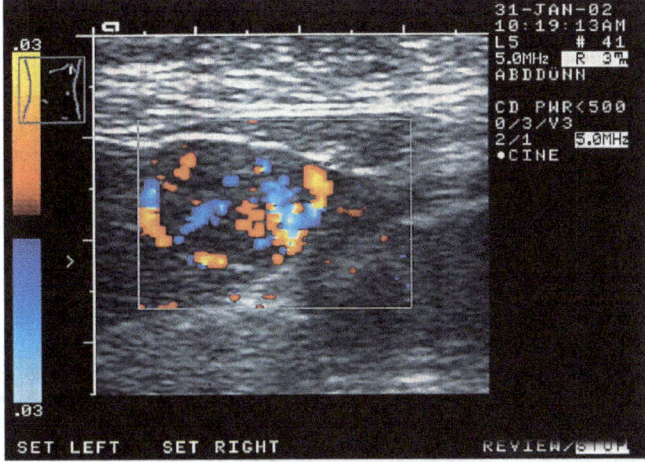

Fig. 6.17: FNH: hypervascularized internal structure with hyperechoic star-shaped scar (= *wheelspoke pattern*)

Macronodular **tuberculosis** (46), **granulomatosis** of the liver (54) and particularly **liver metastases** may likewise appear as focal liver diseases with differing echogenicity. **Haematomas** are initially hyperechoic, but turn hypoechoic when they liquefy within a few days, and even become echofree at a later stage. "Older" haematomas usually revert to being hyperechoic. (43, 76)

Lymphadenopathy: Enlarged abdominal lymph nodes are frequently detectable in acute viral hepatitis (A–D) and chronic hepatitis (B, C) – occasionally also in autoimmune hepatitis, primary biliary cirrhosis and primary sclerosing cholangitis. (13) Lymphadenopathy corresponds to the histological stage of chronic hepatitis C. (20) Sonographic determination of perihepatic lymphadenopathy, predominantly in the hepatoduodenal ligament (51, 107), is not regarded as a pathognomonic sign of an underlying malignant disease.

5.3 Hyperechoic lesions

Hyperechoic lesions may be (*1.*) metastases, (*2.*) liver carcinoma, (*3.*) cholangiocarcinoma, (*4.*) haemangioma, (*5.*) hamartoma, (*6.*) nodular regenerative hyperplasia, (*7.*) old haematoma, (*8.*) focal accumulation of fat, (*9.*) echinococcus alveolaris, (*10.*) scarring, (*11.*) calcification (s. fig. 9.4), and (*12.*) aerobilia (s. fig. 33.6).

Haemangioma is the most common benign finding and usually detected incidentally as a homogeneous and sometimes circular focal lesion. It is found in solitary or multiple (10–30%) form. Frequency is eight times higher in women than in men. The preferred localization is close to the diaphragm or larger vessels. It does not produce any biochemical variations from the norm. Occasionally, there is an afferent and efferent vessel. • The *typical haemangioma* (80–90%) has a diameter of 1–4 cm; it is uniformly hyperechoic (a white tumour like a "snowball"). It forms a clearly defined, yet irregularly shaped ("lobulated") surface with a distal amplification of sound. Such a haemangioma is often found close to a hepatic vein. It has no halo. A centripetal filling in a high-flow haemangioma (like the CT "iris diaphragm phenomenon") can be detected using echo contrast media. In a small number of cases (<0.5%) it may happen that a malignant tumour is hidden beneath the image of a haemangioma, and thus goes unnoticed. (45) (s. figs. 6.18; 36.7–36.10)

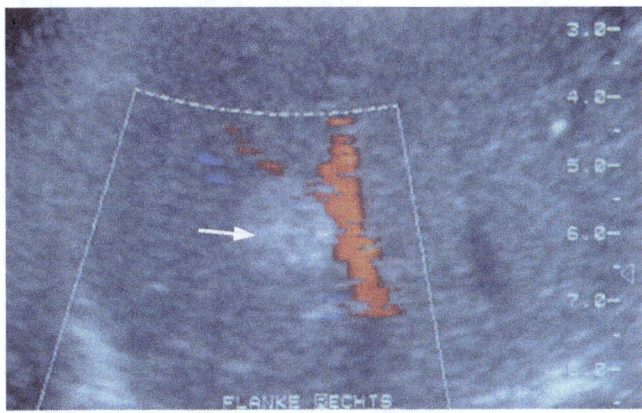

Fig. 6.18: Typical haemangioma: hyperechoic density like a white tumour ("*snowball*") (see arrow) near to a hepatic vein (= red-coloured) (s. figs. 8.5, 8.9; 36.6, 36.7)

The *atypical haemangioma* is indistinctly circumscribed and usually larger than 4 cm. The inhomogeneous hyperechoic internal structure is caused by multiple acoustic interfaces (blood-filled cavernous spaces, bleedings, thrombosis, organized tissues, etc.). In certain cases, large haemangiomas exhibit the *"chameleon phenomenon"*: when the patient assumes a different position, they change their echogenicity. (89) *(see chapter 36.4.4)*

Nodular regenerative hyperplasia is also deemed to be a benign hyperechoic structural deficiency. The multiple foci resemble grapes in their appearance and are found in the direct vicinity of vessels, possibly causing portal hypertension. They are 1−3 cm in size and may easily be confused with metastases. *(see chapter 36.4.3)*

Echinococcus alveolaris is a solid and irregularly shaped focus. Inside, small cysts can be differentiated. Such foci exhibit infiltrating growth and can imitate a malignant process. (19) *(see chapter 25.2.3.2)* • *Hydatid cysts* often comprise daughter cysts with a doubling of the wall contour. The echo image may be extremely heterogeneous. The cyst walls are sometimes hyperechoic and thicker (with occasional calcification); they mostly show a smooth contour. (19, 47) A typical finding is the presence of smaller daughter cysts inside the mother cyst, e.g. honeycomb pattern in type IIb or III. (s. figs. 25.15, 25.16) For purposes of sonographic classification, it has proved beneficial to have five categories. (19)

Focal accumulation of fat is predominantly found either near to the falciform ligament of the liver or to the portal branches as well as in segment IV. It appears as an irregularly limited hyperechoic focus, which is often difficult to classify by differential diagnosis and can even be misinterpreted as being malignant. Blood vessels run normally. (27, 68, 87) (s. figs. 8.2−8.4)

Hepatocellular carcinoma is five times more frequent in men than in women. Hypoechoic as well as hyperechoic structural defects are observed, with a variety of different sound qualities present in a single tumour. The carcinoma may appear as a solitary or multiple phenomenon, at times also infiltrating diffusely. HCC can be differentiated from regeneration nodes by enhanced early arterial perfusion of the contrast medium. However, there is a "chaotic" vascular pattern (as opposed to that observed in FNH). The rate of detection is 35−40% for tumours of <1 cm and approx. 90% for tumours of >1−2 cm in diameter. When applying endoscopic or intraoperative ultrasonography (s. p. 135), the respective values are 86% and 98%! Hepatocellular carcinoma most frequently develops in cases of liver cirrhosis (ca. 75%) or haemochromatosis (ca. 20%), which further complicates the diagnostic process when using ultrasonography. (8, 21, 25, 53, 88, 89) (s. fig. 6.19) *(see chapter 37.3)*

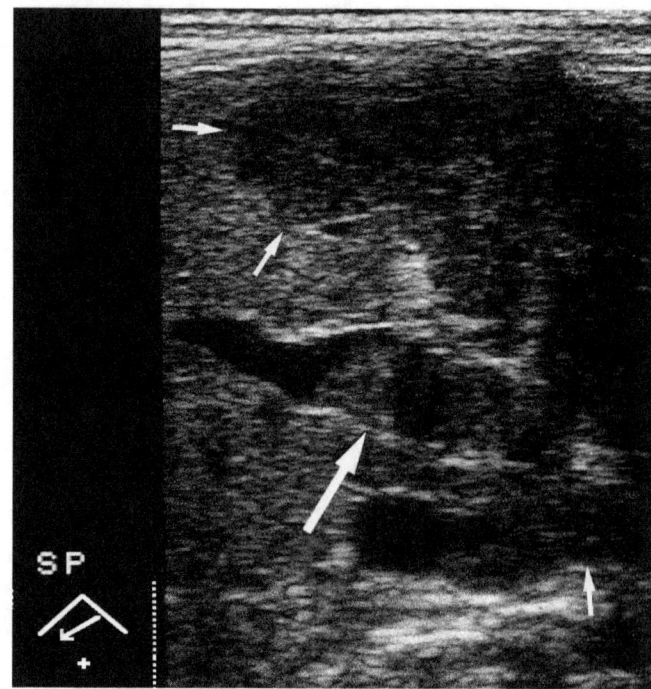

Fig. 6.19: Hepatocellular carcinoma (subcostal section) with extended hypoechoic carcinoma (small arrows). Infiltration of the intrahepatic portal vein (large arrow) as a pathognomonic sign of liver cell carcinoma

Liver metastases are depicted with extreme variability under ultrasonography. They occur mostly as multiple and less frequently as solitary tumours. The spread of multiple small metastases is the cause of a diffuse heterogeneous echoic pattern in large parts of the liver without any distinct focal findings. The *echoic pattern* of liver metastases varies between hypoechoic and hyperechoic − even within a single metastasis. This spectrum of variation depends largely on the vascularity and/or respective development of the tumour. Occult metastases can be detected by measuring the Doppler perfusion index (DPI). (44) Occasionally, there are separate hypoechoic and hyperechoic structural deficiencies with and without a halonated (hypoechoic) margin, possibly due to the varying age of the tumour with its intermittent metastatic spread. In some cases, signs of infiltration are found in the adjacent liver tissue, biliary tract and vessels. The hypoechoic fringe embracing a more hyperechoic centre (the so-called "halo") is termed *"target phenomenon"*. By contrast, the *"bullseye phenomenon"* displays a hyperechoic fringe and a hypoechoic or echofree (i.e. liquid) centre due to central colliquation of a metastasis. (s. fig. 6.20) Calcified metastases (particularly of a mucinous colorectal carcinoma) are hyperechoic with sound extinction. (s. figs. 37.29, 37.30) Hyperechoic metastases are often found in rectal or colon carcinoma, while hypoechoic metastases are more often identified in mammary, pancreatic and bronchial carcinoma. • *There is no relation between the sonographic criteria of a metastasis and the localization or cell type of the primary tumour.*

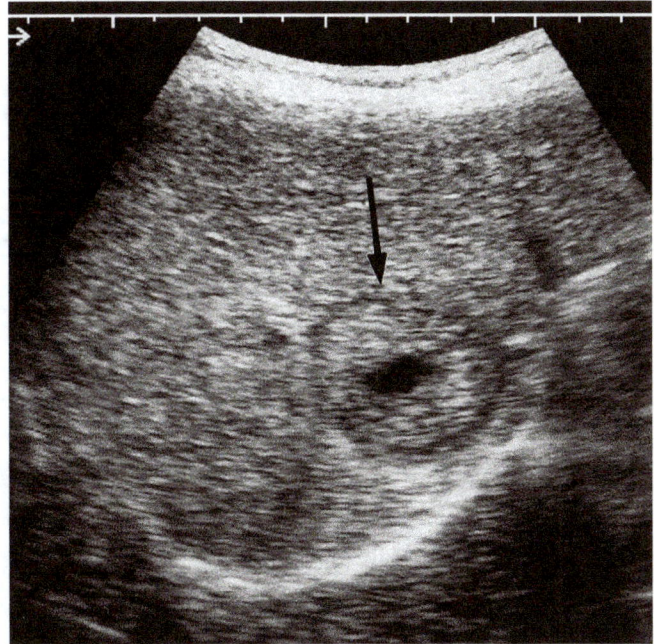

Fig. 6.20: Liver metastasis (subcostal section): hypoechoic fringe (arrow); wide, more hyperechoic margin and hypoechoic central colliquation (*"bullseye"*). Structural inhomogeneity of the remaining hepatic segments

▶ Humps on the surface of the liver, displacement or compression of intrahepatic vessels as well as bile ducts with cholestasis are all known to be important signs of a tumour. Central necrosis, bleeding, indistinct outlines and the formation of branches in the vicinity are signs of a high degree of malignancy or rapid tumourous growth. • The precision of detection regarding metastases by means of ultrasonography ranges from 44% to more than 90%, with a sensitivity of 40–80% and a specificity of 62–100%. Accuracy does not only depend on the size and location of metastases, but also on the type of the primary tumour. Metastases of 0.5 cm upwards are detectable by ultrasonography. Tumourous foci in the left lobe of liver (as well as subphrenic or right-sided foci) are easily overlooked. In addition, differentiation between haemangioma or colorectal metastasis may prove difficult in some cases. (4, 50, 88, 89, 99) *(see chapter 37.10)*

This synopsis of circumscribed structural defects shows that solid focal alterations may be hypoechoic or hyperechoic as well as benign or malignant. • It is important to emphasize the fact that the real value of ultrasonography is the actual detection and not the definite specific diagnosis of such focal findings!

The strategy which is generally applied in the diagnostic clarification of a suspected **"liver tumour"** is shown in detail at a later point in a **flow diagram.** (s. p. 204) (s. fig. 9.4)

6 Examination of the spleen

The spleen is hidden underneath the left costal arch. Examination of the normal spleen ($4 \times 7 \times 13$ cm) using ultrasonography (from the left side, through the intercostal window) is therefore quite difficult. The hump of the spleen may be covered by aeriferous lung segments in the phrenicocostal sinus. The weight of the spleen depends on its respective blood content as well as on the anatomy and gender of the individual; it varies from 120 to 200 g. The pole of the spleen has a length of up to 13 cm, and the spleen has a diameter of up to 5 cm; in advanced age, the values become lower. The echogenicity is fine and homogeneous; the pattern can be either looser or more dense than that of the liver, but markedly more echogenic than the kidney. The wheelspoke pattern is characterized by the segmental vessels (arteries, veins). An accessory spleen is found in up to 10% of cases. The following pathological focal lesions should be mentioned: cysts, infarctions, haemangiomas, splenomas, lipomas; malignant processes are rare. Additional investigations with the help of contrast media or colour-encoded duplex sonograhy might sometimes be useful. The normal spleen may show indentations or even flaps. Variable sectioning facilitates the determination of the size of the spleen in **splenomegaly.** (s. figs. 6.21; 11.1)

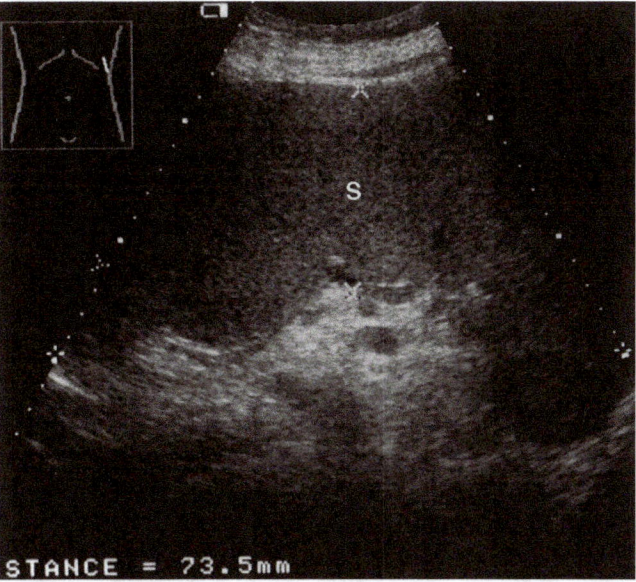

Fig. 6.21: Splenomegaly (S) in chronic myeloplastic leukaemia (length = 21 cm, depth = 7.4 cm)

The most useful parameter for the diagnosis of splenomegaly using sonography is a splenic width of >5 cm (80% accuracy) or >7 cm (100% sensitivity). The length of the spleen in splenomegaly (>13 cm) is used for diagnostic orientation. In long-standing splenomegaly, the echo structure is coarsened. In liver cirrhosis, the spleen is as a rule significantly enlarged. *However, the absence of splenomegaly in individual cases excludes neither portal hypertension nor cirrhosis, since the release of pressure may have been effected via collateral vessels. Patency of the splenic vein or the portal vein excludes thrombosis as a cause of splenomegaly. (see chapter 11)*

References:

1. **Abbitt, P.L.:** Ultrasonography-update on liver technique. Radiol. Clin. N. Amer. 1998; 36: 299–307
2. **Aubé, C., Oberti, F., Korali, N., Namour, M.-A., Loisel, D., Tanguy, J.-Y., Valesia, E., Pilette, C., Rousselet, M.C., Bedossa, P., Rifflet, H., Maiga, M.Y., Penneau-Fontbonne, D., Caron, C., Cales, P.:** Ultrasonographic diagnosis of hepatic fibrosis or cirrhosis. J. Hepatol. 1999; 30: 472–478
3. **Badea, R., Badea, Ch., Galtar, N., Cracium, C., Marin, M., Buchen, M.:** Die Bedeutung der aspirativen Feinnadelbiopsie in der Präzisierung ultraschalldiagnostizierter Lebertumoren. Untersuchungen an 165 Patienten. Z. Klin. Med. 1991; 46: 1489–1493
4. **Becker, D., Strobel, D., Hahn, E.G.:** Tissue harmonic imaging and contrast harmonic imaging. Improving the diagnosis of liver metastasis. Internist 2000; 41: 17–23
5. **Blank, W., Braun, B.:** Gewebsdiagnostik durch Dopplersonographie. Bildgebung 1995; 62 (Suppl. 1): 31–35
6. **Bleck, J.S., Gebel, M., Manns, M.P.:** Quantitative sonography. Clinical role and perspectives. Internist 2000; 41: 10–16
7. **Bolondi, L., Gaiani, S., Li Bassi, S., Zironi, G., Bonino, F., Brunetto, M., Barabara, L.:** Diagnosis of Budd-Chiari syndrome by pulsed Doppler ultrasound. Gastroenterology 1991; 100: 1324–1331
8. **Bolondi, L., Gaiani, S., Benzi, G., Rigamonti, A., Fusconi, F., Barbara, L.:** Ultrasonography and guided biopsy in the diagnosis of hepatocellular carcinoma. Ital. J. Gastroenterol. 1992; 24: 46–49
9. **Bolondi, L., Correas, J.M., Lencioni, R., Weskott, H.P., Piscaglia, F.:** New perspectives for the use of contrast-enhanced liver ultrasound in clinical practice. Dig. Liver Dis. 2007; 39: 187–195
10. **Brannigan, M., Burus, P.N., Wilson, S.R.:** Blood flow patterns in focal liver lesions at microbubble-enhanced US. Radiographics 2004; 24: 921–935
11. **Buscarini, L., Fornari, F., Bolondi, L., Colombo, P., Livraghi, T., Magnolfi, F., Rapaccini, G.L., Salmi, A.:** Ultrasound-guided fine-needle biopsy of focal liver lesions: techniques, diagnostic accuracy and complications. A retrospective study on 2091 biopsies. J. Hepatol. 1990; 11: 344–348
12. **Caremani, M., Vincenti, A., Benci, A., Sassoli, S., Tacconi, D.:** Ecographic epidemiology of non-parasitic hepatic cysts. J. Clin. Ultrasound 1993; 21: 115–118
13. **Cassani, F., Zoli, M., Battoni, L., Cordiani, M.R., Brunori, A., Bianchi, F.B., Pisi, E.:** Prevalence and significance of abdominal lymphadenopathy in patients with chronic liver disease: an ultrasound study. J. Clin. Gastroenterol. 1990; 12: 42–46
14. **Caturelli, E., Squillante, M.M., Andriulli, A., Cedrone, A., Cellerino, C., Pompili, M., Manoja, E.R., Rapaccini, G.L.:** Hypoechoic lesions in the "bright liver": a reliable indicator of fatty change. A prospective study. J. Gastroenterol. Hepatol. 1992; 7: 469–472
15. **Cedrone, A., Pompili, M., Sallustio, G., Lorenzelli, G.P., Gasbarrini, G., Rapaccini, G.L.:** Comparison between color power Doppler ultrasound with echo-enhancer and spiral computed tomography in the evaluation of hepatocellular carcinoma vascularization before and after ablation procedures. Amer. J. Gastroenterol. 2001; 96: 1854–1859
16. **Cosgrove, D.O., Blomley, M.J.K., Jayaram, V., Nihoyannopoulos, P.:** Echo-enhancing (contrast) agents. Ultrasound Quart. 1998; 14: 66–75
17. **D'Alimonte, P., Cioni, G., Cristani, A., Ferrari, A., Ventura, E., Romagnoli, R.:** Duplex-Doppler ultrasonography in the assessment of portal hypertension. Utility of the measurement of maximum portal flow velocity. Radiology 1993; 17: 126–129
18. **Delorme, S., Kaick, van, G.:** Sonographie fokaler Leberveränderungen. Praktische Hinweise für die Differentialdiagnostik. Radiologe 1992; 32: 198–206
19. **Didier, D., Weiler, S., Rohmer, P., Lassegue, A., Deschamps, J.P., Vuitton, D., Miguet, J.P., Weill, F.:** Hepatic alveolar echinococcosis: correlative US and CT study. Radiology 1985; 154: 179–186
20. **Dietrich, C.F., Stryjek-Kaminska, D., Teuber, G., Lee, J.H., Caspary, W.F., Zeuzem, S.:** Perihepatic lymph nodes as a marker of antiviral response in patients with chronic hepatitis C infection. Amer. J. Roentgenol. 2000; 174: 699–704
21. **Dodd, G.D., Miller, W.J., Baron, R.L., Skolnick, M.L., Campbell, W.L.:** Detection of malignant tumours in end-stage cirrhotic livers: efficacy of sonography as a screening technique. Amer. J. Roentgenol. 1992; 159: 727–733
22. **Dumas, O., Roget, I., Coppéré, H., David, A., Richard, P., Barthélémy, C., Veyret, C., Audigier, J.-C.:** Etude comparée des données de la cytoponction à l'aiguille fine et des aspects échographiques des formations tumorales hépatiques en fonction des circonstances de découverte. A propos de 206 patients. Gastroenterol. Clin. Biol. 1990; 14: 67–73
23. **Edoute, Y., Tibon-Fisher, O., Ben Haim, S., Malberger, E.:** Ultrasonically guided fine-needle aspiration of liver lesions. Amer. J. Gastroenterol. 1992; 87: 1138–1141
24. **Frank, W.:** Die Darstellung der Lebersegmente im Ultraschall. Radiologe 1992; 32: 189–197
25. **Gaiani, S., Volpe, L., Piscaglia, F., Bolondi, L.:** Vascularity of liver tumours and recent advances in Doppler ultrasound. J. Hepatol. 2001; 34: 474–482
26. **Gharbi, H.A., Hassine, W., Brauner, M.W.:** Ultrasound examination of the hydatid liver. Radiology 1981; 139: 459–465
27. **Giorgio, A., Francica, G., Aloisio, T., Tarantino, L., Pierri, P., Pellicano, M., Buscarini, L., Livraghi, T.:** Multifocal fatty infiltration of the liver mimicking metastatic disease. Gastroenterol. Internat. 1991; 4: 169–172
28. **Gladisch, R., Elfner, E., Schlauch, D., Filser, T., Heene, D.L.:** A simple technique for sonographic estimation of liver volume. Z. Gastroenterol. 1988; 26: 694–698
29. **Georg, C., Schwerk, W.B., Georg, K.:** Splenic lesions: sonographic patterns, follow-up, differential diagnosis. Eur. J. Radiol. 1991, 13: 59–66
30. **Goyal, A.K., Pokharna, D.S., Sharma, S.K.:** Ultrasonic diagnosis of cirrhosis: reference to quantitative measurements of hepatic dimensions. Gastrointest. Radiol. 1990; 15: 32–34
31. **Goyal, A.K., Pokharna, D.S., Sharma, S.K.:** Ultrasonic measurements of portal vasculature in diagnosis of portal hypertension. A controversial subject reviewed. J. Ultrasound 1990; 9: 45–48
32. **Hartmann, P.C., Oosterveld, B.J., Thijssen, J.M., Rosenbusch, G.J., Berg, van den, J.:** Detection and differentiation of diffuse liver disease by quantitative echography. A retrospective assessment. Invest. Radiol. 1993; 28: 1–6
33. **Hillman, B.J., D'Orsi, C.J., Smith, E.H., Bartrum, R.J.:** Ultrasonic appearance of the falciform ligament. Amer. J. Roentgenol. 1979; 132: 205–206
34. **Hommeyer, St.C., Teefey, S.A., Jacobson, A.F., Higano, C.S., Bianco, J.A., Colacurcio, C.J., McDonald, G.B.:** Venoocclusive disease of the liver; prospective study of US evaluation. Radiology 1992; 184: 683–686
35. **Jang, H.J., Lim, H.K., Lee, W.J., Kim, S.H., Kim, K.A., Kim, E.Y.:** Ultrasonographic evaluation of focal hepatic lesions: comparison of pulse inversion harmonic, tissue harmonic, and conventional imaging techniques. J. Ultrasound Med. 2000; 19: 293–299
36. **Joseph, A.E.A., Saverymuttu, S.H., Al-Sam, S., Cook, M.G., Maxwell, J.D.:** Comparison of liver histology with ultrasonography in assessing diffuse parenchymal liver disease. Clin. Radiol. 1991; 43: 26–31
37. **Kennedy, J.E., ter Haar, G.R., Wu, F., Gleeson, F.V., Roberts, I.S., Middleton, M.R. Crauston, D.:** Contrast-enhanced ultrasound assessment of tissue response to high-intensity focused ultrasound-ultrasound Med. Biol. 2004; 30: 851–854
38. **Korn, M.A., Mostbeck, G.H., Tscholakoff, D.:** Der Processus papillaris des Lobus caudatus–sonographische Fehlbewertung als Raumforderung. Ultraschall 1991; 12: 197–200
39. **Körner, Th.:** Die abdominelle Duplexsonographie zur Diagnostik von Thrombosen der Pfortader und der Milzvene–eine prospective Studie. Endoskopie heute 1995; 8: 5–7
40. **Ladenheim, J.A., Luba, D.G., Yao, F., Gregory, P.B., Jeffrey, R.B., Garcia, G.:** Limitations of liver surface US in the diagnosis of cirrhosis. Radiology 1992; 185: 21–24
41. **Lafortune, M., Madore, F., Patriquin, H., Breton, G.:** Segmental anatomy of the liver: a sonographic approach to the Couinaud nomenclature. Radiology 1991; 181: 443–448
42. **Laing, F.C.:** Commonly encountered artefacts in clinical ultrasound. Semin. Ultrasound 1983; 4: 27–43
43. **Lankisch, P.G., Thiele, E., Mahlke, R., Lübbers, H., Riesner, K.:** Prospective study of the incidence of ultrasound-detected hepatic hematomas 2 and 24 hours after percutaneous liver biopsy. Z. Gastroenterol. 1990; 28: 247–250
44. **Leen, E., Goldberg, J.A., Angerson, W.J., McArdle, C.S.:** Potential role of Doppler perfusion index in selection of patients with colorectal cancer for adjuvant chemotherapy. Lancet 2000; 355: 34–37
45. **Leifer, D.M., Middleton, W.D., Teefey, S.A., Menias, C.O., Leahy, J.F.:** Follow-up of patients at low risk for hepatic malignancy with a characteristic hemangioma at US. Radiology 2000; 214: 167–172
46. **Levine, C.:** Primary macronodular hepatic tuberculosis: US and CT appearances. Gastrointest. Radiol. 1990; 15: 307–309
47. **Lewall, D.B., McCorkell, S.J.:** Hepatic echinococcal cysts: Sonographic appearance and classification. Radiology 1985; 155: 773–775
48. **Limberg, B.:** Duplexsonographische Diagnose der portalen Hypertension bei Leberzirrhose. Einfluss einer standardisierten Testmahlzeit auf die portale Haemodynamik. Dtsch. Med. Wschr. 1991; 116: 1384–1387
49. **Lloyd, R.L., Lyons, E.A., Levi, C.S., Bristowe, J.R.B., Schollenberg, J.:** The sonographic appearance of peliosis hepatis. J. Ultrasound Med. 1982; 1: 293–294
50. **Lygidakis, N.J., Makuuchi, M.:** Clinical application of preoperative ultrasonography in liver surgery. Hepato-Gastroenterol. 1992; 39: 232–286
51. **Lyttkens, K., Forsberg, L., Hederstroem, E.:** Ultrasound examination of lymph nodes in the hepatoduodenal ligament. Brit. J. Radiol. 1990; 63: 26–30
52. **Marn, C.S., Bree, R.L., Silver, T.M.:** Ultrasonography of liver: technique of focal and diffuse disease. Radiol. Clin. North Amer. 1991; 29: 1151–1170
53. **Mikami, N., Ebara, M., Yoshikawa, M., Ohto, M.:** Relationship between ultrasound-findings of low-echoic nodule of hepatic parenchyma in liver cirrhosis and development of hepatocellular carcinoma. (Japan.) Japon. J. Gastroenterol. 1990; 87: 1010–1019
54. **Mills, P., Saverymuttu, S., Fallowfield, M., Nussey, S., Joseph, A.E.A.:** Ultrasound in the diagnosis of granulomatous liver disease. Clin. Radiol. 1990; 41: 113–115

55. **Nino-Murcia, M., Ralls, P.W., Jeffrey, R.B., Johnson, M.:** Color flow Doppler characterization of focal hepatic lesions. Amer. J. Roentgenol. 1992; 159: 1195–1197
56. **Numata, K., Tanaka, K., Mitsui, K., Morimoto, M., Inoue, S., Yonezawa, H.:** Flow characteristics of hepatic tumors at color Doppler sonography: correlation with arteriographic findings. Amer. J. Roentgenol. 1993; 160: 515–521
57. **Osawa, H., Mori, Y.:** Sonographic diagnosis of fatty liver using a histogram technique that compares liver and renal cortical echo amplitudes. J. Clin. Ultrasound 1996; 24: 25–29
58. **Papini, E., Pacella, C.M., Rossi, Z., Bizzarri, G., Fabbrini, R., Nardi, F., Picardi, R.:** A randomized trial of ultrasound-guided anterior subcostal liver biopsy versus the conventional Menghini technique. J. Hepatol. 1991; 13: 291–297
59. **Platt, J.F., Ellis, J.H., Rubin, J.M., Merion, R.M., Lucey, M.R.:** Renal duplex Doppler ultrasonography: a noninvasive predictor of kidney dysfunction and hepatorenal failure in liver disease. Hepatology 1994; 20: 362–369
60. **Quinn, R.J., Meredith, Ch., Slade, L.:** The effect of the Valsalva maneuver on the diameter of the common hepatic duct in extrahepatic biliary obstruction. J. Ultrasound Med. 1992; 11: 143–145
61. **Ralls, P.W., Colletti, P.M., Quinn, M.F., Halls, J.:** Sonography findings in hepatic amebic abscess. Radiology 1982; 145: 123–126
62. **Rubaltelli, L., Savastano, S., Cellini, L., Zambotti, B., Marchioro, U.:** Hyperechoic pseudotumors in segment IV of the liver. J. Ultrasound Med. 1997; 16: 569–572
63. **Sabba, C., Ferraioli, G., Buonamico, P., Berardi, E., Antonica, G., Taylor, K.J., Albano, O.:** Echo-Doppler evaluation of acute flow changes in portal hypertensive patients: flow velocity as a reliable parameter. J. Hepatol. 1992; 15: 356–360
64. **Sakugawa, H., Higashionna, A., Oyakawa, T., Kadena, K., Kinjo, F., Saito, A.:** Ultrasound study in the diagnosis of primary Budd-Chiari syndrome (obstruction of the inferior cava) (Japan.). Gastroenterol. Japon. 1992; 27: 69–77
65. **Salo, J., Bru, C., Vilella, A., Gines, P., Gilabert, R., Castells, A., Bruguera, M., Rodes, J.:** Bile-duct hamartomas presenting as multiple focal lesions on hepatic ultrasonography. Amer. J. Gastroenterol. 1992; 87: 221–223
66. **Saverymuttu, S.H., Corbishley, C.M., Maxwell, J.D., Joseph, A.E.:** Thickened stomach–an ultrasound sign of portal hypertension. Clin. Radiol. 1990; 41: 17–18
67. **Saverymuttu, S.H., Grammatopoulos, A., Meanock, C.I., Maxwell, J.D., Joseph, A.E.:** Gallbladder wall thickening (congestive cholecystopathy) in chronic liver disease: a sign of portal hypertension. Brit. J. Radiol. 1990; 63: 922–925
68. **Scott, W.W. jr., Sanders, R.C., Siegelman, S.S.:** Irregular fatty infiltration of the liver: diagnostic dilemmas. Amer. J. Radiol. 1980; 135: 67–71
69. **Seno, H., Konishi, Y., Wada, M., Fukui, H., Orazaki, K., Chiba, T.:** Endoscopic ultrasonograph evaluation of vascular structures in thge gastric cardia predicts esophageal variceal recurrence following endoscopic treatment. J. gastroenterol. Hepatol. 2006; 21: 227–231
70. **Simonovsky, V.:** The diagnosis of cirrhosis by high resolution ultrasound of the liver surface. Brit. J. Radiol. 1999; 72: 29–34
71. **Smith, D., Downey, D., Spouge, A., Soney, S.:** Sonographic demonstration of Couinaud's liver segments. J. Ultrasound Med. 1998; 17: 375–381
72. **Soyupak, S.K., Narli, N., Yapicioglu, H., Satar, M., Aksungur, E.H.:** Sonographic measurements of the liver, spleen and kidney dimensions in the healthy term and preterm newborns. Europ. J. Radiol. 2002; 43: 73–78
73. **Spamer, C., Brambs, H.-J., Koch, H.K., Gerok, W.:** Benign circumscribed lesions of the liver diagnosed by ultrasonically guided fine-needle biopsy. J. Clin. Ultrasound 1986; 14: 83–88
74. **Stellamor, K., Hruby, W.:** Ultraschalldiagnostik beim Caroli-Syndrom–Die Methode der Wahl. Ultraschall 1982; 3: 84–86
75. **Strobel, D., Krodel, U., Martus, P., Hahn, E.G., Becker, D.:** Clinical evaluation of contrast-enhanced color Doppler sonography in the differential diagnosis of liver tumors. J. Clin. Ultrasound 2000; 28:1–13
76. **Sugano, S., Sumino, Y., Hatori, T., Mizugami, H., Kawafune, T., Abei, T.:** Incidence of ultrasound-detected intrahepatic hematomas due to Tru-Cut needle liver biopsy. Dig. Dis. Sci. 1991; 36: 1229–1233
77. **Sumi, N., Yamashita, Y., Mitsuzaki, K., Yamamoto, H., Urata, J., Nishiharu, T., Takahashi, M.:** Power Doppler Sonography assessment of tumor recurrence after chemoembolization therapy for hepatocellular carcinoma. Amer. J. Roentgenol. 1999; 172: 67–71
78. **Tchelepi, H., Ralls, P.W., Radin, R., Grant, E.:** Sonography of diffuse liver disease. J. Ultrasound Med. 2002; 21: 1023–1032
79. **Teichgräber, U.K.M., Gebel, M., Benter, T., Manns, M.P.:** Duplexsonographische Charakterisierung des Lebervenenflusses bei Gesunden. Ultraschall in Med. 1997; 18: 267–271
80. **Thiel, van, D.H., Hagler, N.G., Schade, R.R., Skolnick, M.L., Pollitt Heyl, A., Rosenblum, E., Gavaler, J.S., Penkrot, R.J.:** In vivo hepatic volume determination using sonography and computed tomography. Gastroenterology 1985; 88: 1812–1817
81. **Tincani, E., Cioni, G., Cristani, A., D'Alimonte, P., Vignoli, A., Abbati, G., Ventura, P., Romagnoli, R., Ventura, E.:** Duplex Doppler ultrasonographic comparison of the effects of propranolol and isosorbide-5-mononitrate on portal hemodynamics. J. Ultrasound 1993; 21: 525–529
82. **Trautmann, M., Weinke, Th., Held, Th, Ruhnke, M., Lufft, H.:** Multiple Amoebenleberabszesse: Sonographische Diagnostik und ultraschallgezielte Punktion. Ultraschall. Med. 1990; 11: 142–145
83. **Trigaux, J.P., Beers, van, B., Melange, M., Buysschaert, M.:** Alcoholic liver disease value of the left-to-right portal vein ratio in its sonographic diagnosis. Gastrointest. Radiol. 1991; 16: 215–220
84. **Vilgrain, V., Lebrec, D., Menu, Y., Scherrer, A., Nahum, H.:** Comparison between ultrasonographic signs and the degree of portal hypertension in patients with cirrhosis. Gastrointest. Radiol. 1990; 15: 218–222
85. **Volk, B.A., Schölmerich, J., Billmann, P., Gerok, W.:** Vaskuläre Erkrankungen der Leber: kavernöse Pfortadertransformation, M. Osler und Budd-Chiari-Syndrom. Ultraschall 1984; 5: 117–121
86. **Wan, S.K.H., Cochlin, D.L.:** Sonographic and computed tomographic features of polycystic disease of the liver. Gastrointest. Radiol. 1990; 15: 310–312
87. **Wang, S.S., Chiang, J.H., Tsai, Y.T., Lee, S.D., Lin, H.C., Chou, Y.H., Lee, F.Y., Wang, J.S., Lo, K.J.:** Focal hepatic fatty infiltration as a cause of pseudotumors: ultrasonographic patterns and clinical differentiation. J. Clin. Ultrasound 1990; 18: 401–409
88. **Wernecke, K., Vassallo, P., Bick, U., Diederich, S., Peters, P.E.:** The distinction between benign and malignant liver tumors on sonography: value of a hypoechoic halo. Amer. J. Roentgenol. 1992; 159: 1005–1009
89. **Wilson, S.R., Burns, P.N., Muradali, D., Wilson, J.A., Lai, X.:** Harmonic hepatic US with microbubble contrast agent: initial experience showing improved characterization of hemangioma, hepatocellular carcinoma, and metastases. Radiology 2000; 215: 153–161
90. **Won, H.J., Han, J.K., Lee, K.H., Kim, K.W., Ybon, C.J., Kim, Y.J., Park, C.M., Choi, B.I.:** Value of four-dimensional ultrasonographically guided biopsy of hepatic masses. J. ultrasound Med. 2003; 22: 215–220
91. **Yeh, Hsu-Chong, Wolf, B.S.:** Ultrasonography in ascites. Radiology 1977; 124: 783–790
92. **Zins, M., Vilgrain, V., Gayno, S., Rolland, Y., Arrivé, L., Denninger, M.-H., Vullierme, M.-P., Najmark, D., Menu, Y., Nahum, H.:** US-guided percutaneous liver biopsy with plugging of the needle track: a prospective study in 72 high-risk patients. Radiology 1992; 184: 841–843
93. **Zironi, G., Gaiani, S., Fenyves, D., Rigamonti, A., Bolondi, L., Barbara, L.:** Value of measurement of mean portal flow velocity by Doppler flowmetry in the diagnosis of portal hypertension. J. Hepatol. 1992; 16: 298–303
94. **Zoli, M., Cordiani, M.R., Marchesini, G., Abbati, S., Bianchi, G., Pisi, E.:** Ultrasonographic follow-up of liver cirrhosis. J. Clin. Ultrasound 1990; 18: 91–96
95. **Zizka, J., Elias, P., Krajina, A., Michl, A., Loji,, M., Ryska, P., Maskova, J., Hulek, P., Safka, V., Vanasek, T., Bukac, J.:** Value of Doppler sonography in revealing transjugular intrahepatic portosystemic shunt malfunction: a 5-year experience in 216 patients. Amer. J. Roentgenol. 2000; 175: 141–148
96. **Zoller, W.G., Wagner, D.R., Zentner, J.:** Effect of propranolol on portal vein hemodynamics in patients with liver cirrhosis: assessment by duplex sonography. Z. Gastroenterol. 1993; 31: 425–428

Laparoscopic/surgical ultrasonography
97. **Bönhof J.A., Frank, K., Loch, E.G., Linhart, P.:** Laparoscopic sonography. Ann. Radiol. 1985; 28: 16–18
98. **Brüggemann, A., Neufang, T., Lepsien, G.:** Laparoskopische Sonographie. Überlegungen zur Sondengestaltung anhand der Literatur und eigener Untersuchungen. Ultraschall Klin. Prax. 1993; 8: 44–47
99. **Charnley, R.M., Morris, D.L., Dennison, A.R., Amar, S.S., Hardcastle, J.D.:** Detection of colorectal liver metastases using intraoperative ultrasonography. Brit. J. Surg. 1991; 78: 45–48
100. **Cozzi, P.J., McCall. J.L., Jorgensen, J.O., Morris, D.L.:** Laparoscopic vs open ultrasound of the liver: an in vitro study. HBP Surg. 1996; 10: 87–89
101. **Foley, E.F., Kolecki, R.V., Schirmer, B.D.:** The accuracy of laparoscopic ultrasound in the detection of colorectal cancer liver metastases. Amer. J. Surg. 1998; 176: 262–264
102. **Foroutani, A., Garland, A.M., Berber, E., String, A., Engle, K., Ryan, T.L., Pearl, J.M., Siperstein, A.E.:** Laparoscopic ultrasound vs triphasic computed tomography for detecting liver tumours. Arch. Surg. 2000; 135: 933–937
103. **Fukuda, M., Hirata, K., Mima, S.:** Preliminary evaluation of sonolaparoscopy in the diagnosis of liver diseases. Endoscopy 1992; 24: 701–708
104. **Lo, C.-M., Lai, E.C.S., Liu, C.-L., Fau, S.-T., Wong, J.:** Laparoscopy and laparoscopic ultrasonography avoid exploratory laparotomy in patients with hepatocellular carcinoma. Ann. Surg. 1998; 227: 527–532
105. **Mills, W.F.A., Paterson-Brown, S., Garden, O.J.:** Laparoscopic contact hepatic ultrasonography. Brit. J. Surg. 1992; 79: 419–420
106. **Nieven van Dijkum, E.J., de Wit, L.T., van Delden, O.M., Kruyt, P.M., van Lanschot, J.J.B., Rauws, E.A.J., Obertop, H., Gouma, D.J.:** Staging laparoscopy and laparoscopic ultrasonography in more than 400 patients with upper gastrointestinal carcinoma. J. Amer. Coll. Surg. 1999; 189: 459–465
107. **Roethlin, M., Largiader, F.:** The anatomy of the hepatoduodenal ligament in laparoscopic sonography. Surg. Endoscopy 1994; 8: 173–180

Intraductal sonography
108. **Farrell, R.J., Agarwal, B., Brandwein, S.L., Underhill, J., Chuttani, R., Pleskow, D.K.:** Intraductal US is a useful adjunct to ERCP for distinguishing malignant from benign biliary strictures. Gastrointest. Endosc. 2002; 56: 681–687
109. **Hyodo, T., Hyodo, N., Yamanaka, T., Imawari, M.:** Contrast-enhanced intraductal ultrasonography for thickened bile duct wall. J. Gastroenterol. 2001; 36: 557–559
110. **Inui, K., Yoshino, J., Okushima, K., Miyoshi, H., Nakamura, Y.:** Intraductal EUS. Gastrointest. Endosc. 2002; 56 (S.): 58–62
111. **Songür, Y., Temucin, G., Sahin, B.:** Endoscopic ultrasonography in the evaluation of dilated common bile duct. J. Clin. Gastroenterol. 2001; 33: 302–305
112. **Tamada, K., Inui, K., Menzel, J.:** Intraductal ultrasonography of the bile duct system. Endoscopy 2001; 33: 878–885

Sonographic elastography

113. **Coletta, C., Smirne, C., Fabris, C., Toniutto, P., Rapetti, R., Minisini, R., Pirisi, M.:** Valiue of two noninvasive methods to detect progression of fibrosis among HCV carries with normal aminotransferases. Hepatology 2005; 42: 838–845
114. **Colli, A., Fraquelli, M., Andreoletti, M., Marino, B., Zuccoli, E., Conte, D.:** Severe liver fibrosis or cirrhosis: accuracy of US for detection. Analysis of 300 cases. Radiology 2003; 227: 89–94
115. **Corpechot, C., El Naggar, A., Poujol-Robert, A., Ziol, M., Wendum, D., Chazouilleres, O., de Lédinghen, V., Dhumeaux, D., Marcellin, P., Beaugrand, M., Poupon, R.:** Assessment of biliary fibrosis by transient elastography in patients with PBC and PSC. Hepatology 2006; 43: 1118–1124
116. **Foucher, J., Chanteloup, E. Vergniol, J., Castera, L., Le Bail, B., Adhoute, X. Bertet, J., Couzigou, P., de Ledinghen, V.:** Diagnosis of cirrhosis by transient elastograph (FibroScan): A prospective study. Gut 2006; 55: 403–408
117. **Gomez-Dominguez, E., Meindoza, J., Rubio, S., Moreno-Monteagudo, J.A., Garcia-Buey, L., Moreno-Otero, R.:** Transient elastography. A valid alternative to biopsy in patients with chronic liver disease. Aliment. Pharm. Therap. 2006; 24: 513–518
118. **Sandrin, L., Fourquet, B., Hasquenoph, J.-M., Yon, S., Fournier, C., Mal, F., Christidis, C., Ziol, M., Poulet, B., Kazemi, F., Beaugrand, M., Palau, R.:** Transient elastography : a new noninvasive method for assessment of hepatic fibrosis. Ultrasound Med. Biol. 2003; 29: 1705–1713

Diagnostics in Liver Diseases
7 Liver biopsy and laparoscopy

		Page:
1	*Liver biopsy*	150
1.1	Historical development	150
1.2	*Indications*	151
1.3	Contraindications	152
1.4	*Technique of liver biopsy*	152
1.5	Postpuncture complaints	153
1.6	Complications	154
1.7	Frequency of complications	155
1.8	Liver biopsy in children	155
1.9	Outpatient liver biopsy	156
1.10	*Transjugular liver biopsy*	156
1.11	*Transfemoral liver biopsy*	156
1.12	Ultrasound- or CT-guided biopsy	156
2	*Laparoscopy*	157
2.1	Historical development	157
2.2	Definition of laparoscopy	158
2.3	*Indications*	158
2.4	Exploratory laparoscopy	158
2.5	Contraindications	159
2.6	*Technique of laparoscopy*	161
2.7	Course of examination	162
2.7.1	Assessment of the portal vessels	163
2.7.2	Assessment of the spleen	163
2.7.3	Tumour staging	163
2.7.4	Fever of unknown aetiology	164
2.7.5	Assessment of the lymphatic vessels	164
2.7.6	Ascites of unknown aetiology	164
2.8	*Photographic documentation*	164
2.9	*Directed biopsy*	165
2.10	UV fluorescence	166
2.11	Extrahepatic findings	166
2.12	Complications	167
2.13	Frequency of complications	167
2.14	*Diagnostic validity*	168
3	*New technical progress*	170
4	*Synopsis and recommendation*	170
	• References (1−315)	171
	(Figures 7.1−7.18; tables 7.1−7.16)	

7 Liver biopsy and laparoscopy

1 Liver biopsy

Exceptions apart, it is impossible or nearly impossible to meet the essential target of a *detailed diagnosis* for hepatobiliary disease without histological sampling. Morphological diagnostics is based on **three examination methods,** the diagnostic relevance of which can be improved with a number of *additional techniques.* (s. tab. 7.1)

Examination methods

1. **Liver biopsy**
  a. percutaneous biopsy
    − ultrasound-guided biopsy
  obsolete: percussion-guided biopsy
  b. *rare:* • transjugular venous biopsy
        • transfemoral venous biopsy
2. **Laparoscopy**
  a. without biopsy
  b. with guided thick needle biopsy
  c. with guided fine needle biopsy
  d. with guided forceps biopsy
3. **Fine needle biopsy**
  a. ultrasound-guided
  b. computer tomography-guided

Additional techniques

1. Photodocumentation for *every* laparoscopy
2. UV-light examination of *each* liver biopsy specimen
3. Special morphological processing
  a. various staining techniques
  b. histochemical methods
  c. immunohistochemical stains
  d. immunofluorescence examinations

Tab. 7.1: Morphological examination methods and additional techniques for the clarification of hepatobiliary diseases

▶ *For this reason, the aim should always be a combination of clinical, laboratory, sonographic and morphological diagnostics.* This is important because morphological changes in the liver can remain concealed from clinical and laboratory detection − just as striking laboratory findings are not necessarily reflected in the bioptic material. • Moreover, *liver bioptic material is not always representative* of the underlying liver disease or the actual normality of the liver parenchyma − whereas an increase of GPT in the individual case always points to liver cell damage. • Even if sonography is deemed to be a routine examination in clarifying hepatobiliary diseases, *it cannot provide any histological statement.*

1.1 Historical development

▶ In cases of purulent echinococcus, puncture of the liver was carried out by Récamier as early as 1825 and by Stanley in 1833. In 1844, the diagnostic opportunities of liver biopsy were discussed in France by A.G.M. Vernois. • In his book "On diabetes" (1884), F.Th. Frerichs reported on the **first liver biopsy**, which was carried out by P. Ehrlich in Berlin in 1880. This publication included illustrations of the biopsy instruments used and the liver tissue removed. • In 1895 L. Lucatello reported on liver biopsy as a method of diagnosis, the cytomaterial being examined as smear or teased-out preparation. Using the thicker needle developed by F. Schupfer (1907), successful liver and spleen biopsies were carried out, so that the tissue cylinder could be assessed histologically as well. (134) A. Josefson (1920) also succeeded in performing liver biopsies in some cases. (73) A. Bingel (1923) (8) and J. Olivet (1926) (111) reported from the same hospital on systematically performed liver biopsies. • A **new aspiration method** with modified biopsy needles was presented by I. Silverman (1938, 1954) (138) as well as by P. Iversen and K. Roholm (1939). (67) Yet even this new technology failed to help liver biopsy achieve full recognition as a clinical method despite the fact that W. Kofler (1940) had termed liver biopsy "a useful and clinically important examination method" on the basis of over 100 specimens. (77) • The following years witnessed more publications on this examination method. (3, 5, 31, 46, 106, 124, 151, 163−165) *Nevertheless, liver biopsy was almost completely excluded from the world of clinical diagnosis.* (s. tab. 7.2)

First performance of liver biopsy		
1880	P. Ehrlich	Berlin[1]
1895	L. Lucatello	Roma[2]
1907	F. Schupfer	Firenze[2]
1923	A. Bingel	Braunschweig[1]
Second stage in method development		
1926	J. Olivet	Marburg[1]
1935	P. Huard et al.	Paris[7]
1938	I. Silverman	New York[3]
1939	E. Baron	New York[3]
1939	P. Iversen et al.	Kobenhavn[4]
1940	W. Kofler	Wien[5]
1943	J.H. Dible et al.	London[8]
Third stage as Menghini technique		
1957	G. Menghini	Perugia[2]
1958	G. Menghini	Perugia[2]
Ultrasound- and CT-guided biopsy		
1964	Wang Hsin-Fang et al.	Shanghai[6]
1972	S.N. Rasmussen et al.	Hjallerup[4]
1976	J.R. Haaga et al.	Cleveland[3]
1983	L. Greiner et al.	Wuppertal[1]

Tab. 7.2: Historical development of percutaneous liver biopsy (1 = Germany; 2 = Italy; 3 = USA; 4 = Denmark; 5 = Austria; 6 = China; 7 = France; 8 = Great Britain) (city names are given in the original language)

▶ In 1957 (not 1958 as is usually and wrongly quoted!) G. Menghini presented the first report on a new biopsy method: using thin-walled, small calibre needles with a sharply slanting bevel and without a trocar, it was possible to puncture the liver in a split second (so-called *"one-second needle biopsy"*). (101) This new concept brought acclaim and led finally to the application of liver biopsy worldwide. • **In this way, Menghini biopsy marked the birth of histological liver diagnostics.**

1.2 Indications

▶ The *first* and most important *prerequisite* for avoiding complications is a precise indication. • This differs from case to case — and the relative importance of the indication (weighting) varies individually from "minimal" to "absolutely necessary".

Percutaneous liver biopsy ranks highly as a diagnostic method. The experience gained over many years in all sorts of locations has culminated in an exact definition and confirmation of the specific indication. (11, 14, 18, 23, 42, 49, 64, 65, 71, 72, 81, 84, 87, 91, 104, 107, 108, 117, 125, 133, 136, 139, 142, 144, 146, 148, 153, 157, 164, 165, 169, 170, 173) (s. tab. 7.3)

The **indication** for carrying out a liver biopsy is in principle given if:

(*1.*) a definitive diagnosis cannot be drawn up based on anamnesis together with clinical, laboratory and sonographic findings or other imaging procedures (65, 139),

(*2.*) it is likely to provide significant information concerning the patient with regard to therapy or prognostics on the basis of morphological findings,

(*3.*) during the course of laparoscopy, further important findings are likely to be found from a biopsy,

(*4.*) laparoscopy is indeed indicated, but it poses a greater risk and therefore has to be converted into a non-contraindicated liver biopsy,

(*5.*) additional morphological clarification can be acquired without any difficulty during a cholecystectomy, particularly with suspected concomitant hepatobiliary disease,

(*6.*) it is necessary to identify and assess diseases in the transplanted liver, such as acute and chronic (so-called ductopenic) rejection reactions, inflammatory or vascular processes as well as recurrence of the basic disease,

(*7.*) there is fever of unknown aetiology with liver involvement, whereby diagnostic clarification may be attempted by means of bacterial cultures. (62, 95)

▶ Furthermore, histological immuno- or histochemical processing of the liver material procured by biopsy is of extremely high value for gaining new scientific insight.

▶ It must, however, be considered that a biopsy punch of 1.5–3.0 cm in length is proportionate to approx. 1/50,000th of the normal liver volume (J. VOLMER et al., 1981). For histological assessment, the punch should be > 1.5 cm long and include at least four portal fields; the weight of such a bioptate generally amounts to 20–30 mg. The smaller the sample, the more difficult is the histological assessment; at a length of < 1.5 cm diagnos-

1. Unclarified cholestasis
2. Unclarified non-obstructive jaundice
3. Unclarified laboratory results
4. Acute hepatitis
   • with anicteric course
   • with atypical course
   • with issues relating to differential diagnosis
   • to check course and therapy
   • to furnish proof of healing
   • to detect posthepatic sequelae
5. Chronic hepatitis (27, 117)
   • validation of diagnosis
   • to ascertain the degree of activity and fibrosis
   • with issues relating to differential diagnosis
   • prior to interferon therapy
   • to check course and therapy
6. Toxic liver damage
   • validation of diagnosis
   • to ascertain the extent of liver damage
   • to control course and therapy
7. Fatty liver (NALD, ALD)
8. Thesaurismosis and metabolic diseases
   e.g. haemochromatosis (90), porphyria (15)
   • for differential diagnosis
   • to ascertain the extent of liver damage
   • to check course and therapy
9. Suspected infectious liver damage
   • in viral, bacterial or parasitic liver damage
   • in AIDS (97, 128)
10. Suspected granulomatous liver diseases
11. Histological assessment
    • prior to commencement of potentially hepatotoxic medication
12. Targeted biopsy (US, CT) in space-occupying lesions
13. Condition after liver transplantation (22, 44, 141, 155)

Tab. 7.3: Indications for liver biopsy — unless definitive validation is possible by other procedures. • *The diagnostic significance of an indication is different in each individual case and can be categorized in steps ranging from "of little significance" through to "very important" or "absolutely necessary"*

tic reliability drops to < 60%, at a length of < 0.5 cm it is only 20–40%. • It must also be considered that a liver disease is not necessarily expressed evenly, so that the biopsy punch may indeed suffer from a certain degree of unreliability. (96) Above all, this applies to chronic hepatopathy. The varying expressivity of chronic hepatitis was already detected in 1962 (!) by L. WANAGAT (s.p. 189). • It must furthermore be considered *that in the case of percutaneous biopsy, only a limited area in the right lobe of liver can be reached.* (s. fig. 7.8) Thus histological findings should actually be limited to this biopsy site alone. In every laparoscopy with non-distinct focal lesion or insufficiently diffuse expressivity, we have always taken one (or two) bioptates from the right as well as the left lobe of liver. *We have often discussed the variability in biopsy findings with a pathologist, and occasionally the pathologist even had doubts as to whether the bioptates were indeed taken from the same patient!* The reduced reliability of a percutaneous biopsy sample has been repeatedly referred to in the literature (1, 6, 63, 94, 96, 136, 143, 165) – *but too little attention is paid to this fact!*

1.3 Contraindications

▶ The *second* important *prerequisite* for avoiding complications is to exclude contraindications. (s. tab. 7.4)

1. *Clotting disorders*
2. *Cardiac insufficiency*
3. *Respiratory insufficiency*
4. *Cerebral insufficiency*
5. Thoracic empyema (right), subphrenic abscess (right), pleuropneumonia (right)
6. Purulent cholangitis
7. Obstructive jaundice and cholestasis with dilated bile ducts
8. Portal decompensated liver cirrhosis
9. Ascites
10. Peritonitis
11. Focal liver findings
    - Polycystic liver
    - Echinococcosis
12. Increased bleeding tendency
    - Leukaemic infiltrates of the liver
    - Osteomyelosclerosis
    - Amyloidosis of the liver
    - Haemangioma
    - Adenoma
    - Malignant foci
13. Anatomic features
    - Liver positioned on edge (transverse rotation of liver)
    - Diaphragmatic hernia (right)
    - Diaphragmatic paresis (right)
    - Diaphragmatic relaxation (right)
    - Severe pulmonary emphysema
    - Chilaiditi syndrome
    - Situs inversus
14. Lack of cooperation on the part of the patient

Tab. 7.4: Contraindications for percutaneous liver biopsy

Threshold values for **blood coagulation** may only be taken as guidelines. They have to be critically assessed in each individual case. Recommendations for percutaneous biopsy in hospitalized patients are: (*1.*) Quick's value >60%, (*2.*) bleeding time <3(−4) minutes, and (*3.*) thrombocytes >100,000, although the function of the thrombocytes is more important than their mere number. • Even with reduced coagulation parameters, biopsy can still be carried out following the administration of vitamin K, fresh frozen plasma, etc.

We regard **stasis in dilated bile ducts** as a contraindication of biopsy, although there are controversial views in the literature concerning this point. (105, 146) The risk of biliary complications should not be underestimated, especially since new examination techniques have indeed made such risky biopsies unnecessary. By contrast, even excessive jaundice (> 20mg/dl) is per se no contraindication. • We are also against percutaneous biopsy in **ascites**. Laparoscopic biopsy with visual monitoring involving almost complete removal of the ascites does not lead to any complications if haemostasis is guaranteed. • Moreover, with **focal liver lesions**, we principally give preference to laparoscopy with targeted biopsy over percutaneous biopsy. • This also applies in the event of suspected **amyloidosis**, as the amyloidotic tissue is brittle and can easily split under biopsy, causing considerable afterbleeding. Therefore laparoscopically directed biopsy is recommended in such cases. • With **dialysis** patients, liver biopsy should occur 1 day after dialysis; prior to biopsy, the administration of desmopressine is useful.

1.4 Technique of liver biopsy

▶ The *third* important *prerequisite* for avoiding complications is the correct performance of the biopsy coupled with adequate experience of the investigating physician. (11, 23, 49, 86, 91, 107, 130, 156)

Instruments
− Biopsy needle with a blunt pin within its shaft (also available as a disposable needle): diameter usually 1.40 mm or possibly 1.60 mm (when faced with a potentially greater puncturing risk, the diameter should be 1.20 mm)
− Syringe (10 ml), best fitted with a Luer-Lock and containing 2 to 3 ml isotonic (0.9%) NaCl solution; syringe (5 ml) with 3 to 6 ml local anaesthetic (e.g. 1% to 2% lidocaine)
− Incision lancet to perforate the skin
− Thin injection needle for skin anaesthesia, thicker and longer needle for bathyanaesthesia
− Glass dish with 2−3 ml 0.9% NaCl solution
− Sterile pads and first-aid dressing

Both classical and modified types of biopsy needles are available: *suction needles* (e.g. Menghini, Klatskin, and Jamshidi) and *cutting needles* (e.g. Vim-Silverman and Trucut) as well as *spring-loaded needles*. (11, 25, 86, 120, 125, 153, 157)

Preparation of the patient
(*1.*) *Correct briefing* of the patient including written consent to the biopsy;
(*2.*) *Examination of blood coagulation* (see above);
(*3.*) *Premedication:* atropine (1 ml/0.5 mg s.c.) about 15 minutes prior to the biopsy (beware of atropine contraindications!).

Prior to percutaneous liver biopsy, it is not necessary to perform either a chest X-ray or a cholecystography, or to determine the blood group. *These examinations are of no practical significance.*

Preparation of the biopsy
(*1.*) *Location of the biopsy:* Liver biopsy can be carried out in the patient's room, in the ward examination room or in the endoscopy department. The medicaments and appliances required for possible emergency treatment must be available.
(*2.*) *Positioning of the patient:* The patient (fasted condition) lies on his/her back, turned slightly to the left (established technique

in line with G. MENGHINI), the right arm stretched over the head (or right hand under the head). To stabilize the position, a pillow may be tucked underneath the right lumbar region. • During the biopsy, the patient stays in his/her own (normal) bed (= no postbioptic repositioning, which is psychologically advantageous!).

(*3.*) *Site of puncture:* Prior to carrying out a percutaneous liver biopsy, a *sonographic examination* of the liver (for focal processes) as well as of the adjacent organs (to rule out morphological anomalies) should be effected. This can be carried out directly prior to the biopsy or a few hours to one week preceding the biopsy. The suitable puncture site is established directly prior to the biopsy by ultrasound and subsequently marked (possibly by the print of a fingernail). The puncture site as determined by percussion clearly differs in 13% of cases to that determined by sonography. The puncture canal is transthoracic in the 6th or 7th intercostal space. The abdominal (i.e. subcostal) method is only acceptable in a markedly enlarged liver. It is as a rule safe with sonographic monitoring even under outpatient conditions. (114, 126) This *ultrasound-guided biopsy* (52) does not call for sonography during the actual performance of the puncture. (114, 115, 172) • **Percussion-guided liver biopsy is considered obsolete today!**

(*4.*) *Disinfection of the skin.*

(*5.*) *Anaesthesia:* Skin wheal as large as a thumb nail; anaesthesia of the intercostal space through to the (painful) peritoneum: this is the site for the anaesthetic depot.

(*6.*) *Perforation of the skin* with a lancet.

(*7.*) *Attempted apnoea:* 4–6 sec after normal expiration. • *An experienced physician can carry out the biopsy in a split second at the end of an expiration phase, so that the patient need not be asked to hold his breath and is thus not subject to "expectation anxiety"!*

Slow (extrahepatic) phase
(*1.*) Examination of the needle: its diameter, sharpness and in particular ultimate strength.

(*2.*) Insertion of the needle.

(*3.*) Injection of 0.5 to 1.0 ml 0.9% NaCl solution (to clear the needle) after penetration of the intercostal fascia.

(*4.*) Apnoea at the end of normal expiration.

(*5.*) Aspiration: retraction of injection plunger, whereby the direction of puncture is dorsocranial towards the xiphoid.

Rapid (intrahepatic) phase
Puncture involving a swift, straight movement forwards and backwards without rotation and without sideways deviation (2 to 4 cm penetration depth depending on the body volume), immediate withdrawal of needle with syringe in aspiration position. • *This phase normally takes a maximum of 0.5 seconds.*

▶ The swiftness of the intrahepatic puncture phase reduces the danger of bleeding. For this reason, a **modified puncture technique** with the Menghini needle has become established practice: this involves a straight, forward movement, effected in a split second and performed *at the same time* as rapid aspiration suction followed by immediate withdrawal of the needle with continuing suction – *a customary method of biopsy, which we have also found to be most satisfactory.* With an experienced operator, the intrahepatic phase can be reduced to <1/10 second and, at the same time, aspiration suction can be remarkably increased.

Intrahepatic biopsy is performed as swiftly as possible using standard instruments (available as a disposable set with a Menghini needle); this ensures the "shooting" of the biopsy needle into the liver after release of the spring tension (based on the principle of the spring-loaded needle). Today's high-speed biopsy sets are obtainable with needles of varying diameters; they allow comfortable one-hand operating techniques and enable penetration shots with adjustable depth (e. g. 15 or 20 mm).

Handling the bioptic material
Placing a pin in the needle ensures that the **puncture cylinder** stays in the needle lumen, so that it is not aspirated into the syringe. It is thus guaranteed that the still intact specimen (2 to 3 cm long) can be ejected with the rest of the NaCl solution into the Petri dish with 0.9% NaCl solution. The biopsy material obtained usually amounts to 20–30 mg (up to 70 mg). • The frequency of "unsuccessful" biopsy is 0.4–0.6%.

The biopsy material should be observed under **UV fluorescence** (366 nm; so-called Wood light) to rule out porphyria. (s. fig. 7.10) Only when UV-fluorescence assessment has been carried out can the biopsy material be fixed in the formalin solution. A short written description of the biopsy material should then be made. • Depending on the individual diagnostic issue in question, the material is prepared in compliance with **special regulations** (frozen section, electron microscopy, RNA detection, etc).

Aftercare of the patient
Positioning of the patient on the right side with the elbow against the site of biopsy. This position should be maintained for about two hours (66).

Bed rest for 24 hours; as from the 8th hour, bed rest can be semistrict. This is, however, not generally called for in the literature. (102, 130)

Control of pulse rate and blood pressure every quarter of an hour for up to two hours; from then on, every half hour through to the 6th hour.

1.5 Postpuncture complaints

▶ Postpuncture complaints can be observed in 5–10% of patients. They are found more frequently in anxious patients and – it would appear – especially when no parasympathetic blocking agent in the form of atropine has been administered. All these ailments are unpleasant, but harmless. Occasionally, symptomatic measures are required.

(*1.*) **Upper abdominal pain:** Traction at the falciform ligament due to the puncture as well as a subcapsular haematoma can lead to slight pain.

(*2.*) **Pain in the right shoulder** and possibly cervicalgia on the right side due to irritation of the phrenic nerve.

(*3.*) **Respiratory pain** as a result of a subcapsular haematoma.

(*4.*) **Vagus shock:** Irritation of the pleura or peritoneum due to stimulation of the vagus nerve can result in a vagal (or peritoneal) shock: bradycardia, a drop in blood pressure, practically instantaneous violent pain in the right upper abdomen, guarding of abdominal muscles, weak pulse – the patients are pale, they sweat and hardly dare to breathe. • Such a situation appears threatening for both the patients and their environment – however, during more than 30 years of experience, we have only observed one such "dangerous" event. We would rate this as being the positive outcome of *basic premedication with atropine*. Because of the rare contraindications of atropine premedication on the one hand and the very unpleasant event of a vasovagal reaction on the other hand, we would always recommend such a procedure.

▶ Vagus shock might also be caused by **postbioptic biliary leakage** with acute irritation of the serosa. H. THALER observed this event 19 times in 7,500 biopsies; we have noticed it just once with 4,124 biopsied patients. This would suggest that bile-related acute irritation of the serosa is only likely to be the cause of a peritoneal shock in rare cases.

1.6 Complications

Each invasive examination procedure is limited by its own risks and complications. These depend on a variety of **influencing factors.** (s. tab. 7.5) In every case, the physician must examine whether influencing factors are involved in a complication and if so, what they are, how they should be assessed and to what extent they can be avoided in future. • *There is no doubt that many of the complications cannot be attributed to the method of liver biopsy itself! (This is also true of laparoscopy!)*

▶ Disregard of contraindications ▶ Incorrect or uncritical evaluation of the indication
1. **Influence exercised by the investigating physician** • perfection of method • continuous acquisition of experience • manual dexterity 2. **Influence exercised by the patient** • mental state • anatomical features 3. **Influence exercised by existing disease(s)** • underlying disease • secondary diseases 4. **Instrumentation and personnel** – optimal – limited – insufficient

Tab. 7.5: Factors that influence frequency and severity of complications in liver biopsy and laparoscopy

Causes of morbidity and mortality as a result of percutaneous liver biopsy have been assigned to a variety of circumstances. (14, 26, 42, 44, 57, 59, 70, 85, 87, 116, 118, 151, 153, 156, 173) (s. tabs. 7.5, 7.6)

Puncture of the gall bladder (with impending bile peritonitis) is practically always due to a faulty technique in performing the biopsy and is only rarely caused by an anomaly in the position of the gall bladder; such an anomaly is usually detected in prebioptic sonography. • **Puncture of the adjacent organs** is usually harmless and only rarely leads to complications. • Subsequent **bleeding** is mostly observed within the first 2 hours and only rarely during the following 6 hours. Depending on the localization and severity of the bleeding, this effect can develop "asymptomatically" through to "dramatically". More pronounced bleeding is to be expected in about 0.2% of patients. (16, 37, 58, 78, 93, 99, 100, 120, 123, 140, 152) • Different investigators have noted **intrahepatic haematomas** in 1.1%, in 4%, in 7% and even in 23% of cases. Application of the Menghini needle yielded the best results. Such haematomas are usually not significant, since they are resorbed spontaneously. (50, 79, 102, 122, 135, 147, 149) • Likewise without clinical significance and generally unnoticed are **a.v. fistulas,** found in about 5% of cases. (68, 92, 110, 112, 121) Occasionally, **haemobilia** occurs as a result of an arterioportal fistula (detectable today by means of MRCP), rendering embolization necessary in individual cases. This event was even observed up to 10 days after liver biopsy. (2, 40, 60, 82, 83, 92, 110, 140) • A **pneumothorax** is a very rare occurrence and in itself harmless due to the rapid resorption of the gas used in laparoscopy. (113, 137) • A **haematothorax** has also been seen in rare cases. (118)

1. **Puncture of the gall bladder** (46) 2. **Puncture of adjacent organs** • frequent: kidneys, colon, lung • less often: pancreas, small intestine, adrenal gland 3. **Haematoma** • intrahepatic • subcapsular 4. **Bleeding** • early bleeding • late bleeding (98, 123, 171) 5. **Arteriovenous fistula** • intrahepatic (possibly with haemobilia) • intrarenal (possibly with haematuria) 6. **Haemothorax** (118) 7. **Biliary leakage** (53, 118) • peritoneal shock • bile peritonitis (85, 127, 151) • biliary pleural effusion (119) • haemocholascos • bilhaemia (160) • bile embolism (28) 8. **Pneumothorax** (113, 137) • pleural effusion (118) 9. **Breakage of biopsy needle** (118) 10. **Infection** • sepsis (118) • liver abscess • subphrenic abscess (7) 11. **Anatomical variants**

Tab. 7.6: Causes of morbidity and lethality after percutaneous liver biopsy (with some additional references)

There are only isolated reports of **late bleeding** (4th to 13th day). This may be attributed to late fibrinolysis of the thrombus in the area of the biopsy canal. These reports do not, however, exclude more obvious causes, e. g. abdominal press, traumatization, rupture of a subcapsular haematoma, influence on blood coagulation. • Late bleeding occurred in some 61% of patients within the first 2 hours, in 21% during the following 8 hours (= 82%) and in 14% within the following 14 hours; i.e. 96% of the complications were noticed in the course of the first day. (118) The frequency of complications does not depend on the length of postbioptic bed rest. (130)

In the case of suspected postbioptic bleeding or biliary leakage, **emergency laparoscopy** is indicated as the primary possibility after previous abdominal sonography and before exploratory laparotomy is deemed necessary. The diagnosis can generally be clarified by means of laparoscopy, and the bleeding or biliary leakage can be managed. (177, 256)

1.7 Frequency of complications

▶ The **literature** available to us does not provide adequate confirmation of the high lethality rate of 1% following "blind" liver biopsy in the pre-Menghini era as published by I. Snapper in 1951. In a summary covering 18,894 directed as well as non-directed liver biopsies (D. Gemsjäger, 1957), lethality was 0.17%. In other compiled statistics relating to 15,274 biopsies, lethality was put at 0.22%. (173) A. Terry observed a lethality rate of 0.07% and a morbidity rate of 0.32% in 7,532 biopsies. (151) In another study comprising 13,150 liver biopsies, the lethality rate was 0.21% (H. Lüdin, 1955). The calculations of L. Schiff (1951) register no fatal cases at all. (133) Other publications may be referred to in this respect. (59, 116, 156)

> Since the introduction of Menghini's technique in 1957 (101), the risk of complications has been reduced to one quarter and lethality to one tenth.

One of the first major compilations of statistics was made by H. Thaler in 1964: in 23,382 biopsies, the lethality rate was 0.017% and the complication rate 0.10%. (153) In evaluating 79,381 liver biopsies, H. Lindner (1967) calculated a lethality rate of 0.015% and a morbidity rate of 0.34%. (85) In 19,563 liver biopsies, E. Wildhirt registered no fatal cases with a morbidity rate of 0.089%. (170) In a multicentre study carried out by F. Piccionino et al., 68,276 liver biopsies were recorded during the period 1973–1983 with a lethality rate of 0.009% and a morbidity rate of 0.21%. In this study, the Vim-Silverman and Trucut needle types proved to have the highest risk rate (0.31% to 0.34%). (118) Severe complications were found in 0.57% of cases by J.F. Cadranel et al. (14) • Among *4,124 of our own biopsies* (Menghini needle), we registered no cases of death whatsoever from 1961 to 1987; the complication rate was 0.15% (s. tab. 7.7).

▶ In 1990 D.B. McGill et al. reported on the evaluation of 9,212 liver biopsies with an amazingly high complication rate (99): 10 cases of severe bleeding proved fatal (0.11%), whereas 22 cases (0.24%) could be managed. In malignant liver tumours, the frequency of bleeding with lethal outcome was 0.40% and the frequency of arrest of bleeding 0.57%. In patients without liver tumours, there was a lethal bleeding risk rate of 0.04% and nonlethal rate of 0.16%. Only the needle types Trucut, Vim-Silverman and Jamshidi had, however, been used here. • The lethality rate of

Morbidity				
Thaler, H.*	(1964)	23,382	23	= 0.98%
Lindner, H.*	(1967)	79,381	273	= 0.34%
Wildhirt, E.	(1981)	19,563	16	= 0.082%
Piccionino, F.*	(1986)	68,276	141	= 0.21%
Kuntz, E.	(1987)	4,124	6	= 0.15%
Eisenburg, J.	(1988)	35,000	6	= 0.017%
		229,726	465	= 0.20%
Lethality				
Thaler, H.*	(1964)	23,382	4	= 0.017%
Lindner, H.*	(1967)	79,381	12	= 0.015%
Wildhirt, E.	(1981)	19,563	—	—
Piccionino, F.*	(1986)	68,276	6	= 0.009%
Kuntz, E.	(1987)	4,124	—	—
Eisenburg, J.	(1988)	35,000	—	—
		229,726	22	= 0.001%

Tab. 7.7: Frequency of liver biopsy complications broken down into morbidity and lethality (* = compiled statistics). • The results of E. Wildhirt and J. Eisenburg are particularly worth noting

0.10% found by G.H. Millward-Sadler et al. (1985) is also unusually high (7–10 times higher compared to other published data).

A closer look at the publications, however, often reveals that some *contraindications* and *problem situations* (e.g. ascites, amyloid degeneration, liver tumours, leukaemia, obstructive jaundice) were not heeded. Likewise, *inadequacies* in applying the various methods may be responsible for complications. Biopsy needles with a larger diameter of >1.6 mm (e.g. Vim-Silverman, Jamshidi) were also found to involve greater risks.

> Given the correct indication (s. tab. 7.3), due attention to possible contraindications (s. tab. 7.4) and continuous experience on the part of the investigating physician (s. tab. 7.5), an upper limit of about **0.30%** for **morbidity** and about **0.01%** for **lethality** should be set for ultrasound-guided liver biopsy. Any higher frequency of complications is unacceptable.

1.8 Liver biopsy in children

Indications and contraindications in children are the same as in adults. In general, the diameter of the needle should not exceed 1.2 mm. Premedication is advisable to ensure a smooth (and hence low-risk) biopsy. • D. Feist et al. (1972) reported on 385 biopsies with just one complication (no fatal cases) (38), and H. Thaler (1979) observed only 2 minor complications in 764 biopsies (154), while M.B. Cohen et al. (1992) reported a lethality rate of 0.60%, slight complications in 11.7% and serious events in 4.5% of cases. (24) A.O. Scheinmann et al. found complications in 6.83% of cases, of which 2.4% were severe; lethality was 0.4%. (132) Liver biopsies have also been successfully carried out in children under outpatient conditions. (51)

1.9 Outpatient liver biopsy

▶ Many investigators have reported in the **literature** on their wide experience concerning outpatient liver biopsy. (21, 34, 35, 41, 47, 70, 76, 88, 103, 161, 168) E. RICHTER et al. (1972), K. TEUBNER (1975) and H. THALER (>4,000 complication-free outpatient biopsies!) have also reported on this subject. Additional statements have been made by R. DECKING (1991) (29), the latter following recommendations issued by the "Patient Care Committee" (W. H. JACOBS et al., 1989). More recent results obtained by A. GIGER et al. (1993) (48) and S. VIVAS et al. (1998) further advocate this method. The Jamshidi needle also proved to be low in risk.

We have acquired *our own experience* with 318 outpatient biopsies, included in our total number of 4,124 biopsies — we observed no complications whatsoever in these 318 patients. (s. tab. 7.7) • Evaluation of the publications quoted and our own experience show that the **frequency of complications** tends to be even lower than in hospitalized patients. This is probably due to the fact that only very experienced physicians perform outpatient biopsies and that indications and contraindications are heeded with greater stringency.

Isolated instances of *objections* to outpatient biopsies are neither objectively nor legally justifiable, provided the necessary criteria are duly observed. Besides the paramount requirement concerning the qualification of the investigating physician, we have always been in favour of and have insisted on *"restricted indications with expanded contraindications"*. In contrast to percutaneous liver biopsy under hospital conditions, outpatient percutaneous biopsy calls for *normal blood coagulation parameters*. • We have extended the list of **contraindications** (s. tab. 7.4) to include some additional points. (s. tab. 7.8)

---
1. Previous intake of acetylsalicylic acid or other substances which affect blood coagulation
2. Unclear diagnostic conception
3. Inadequate prediagnostics
4. Biopsies at the request of a general practitioner
5. Diameter of needle in excess of 1.6 mm
6. Patient-related problems
   - long or complicated journey home
   - unsuitable means of transport
   - lack of telephone contact
   - lack of monitoring at home
   - unreliability on the part of the patient

Tab. 7.8: Additional contraindications for outpatient liver biopsy (complementary to table 7.4)

There are differing recommendations concerning the direct **monitoring time** following a biopsy. Due to the fact that most complications occur within the first 3 hours, an initial monitoring period of *6 hours* may be considered adequate; contact observation of the patient is imperative, while the pulse rate and blood pressure are taken (and charted!) every 15 minutes during the first hour and subsequently every half hour. However, we have always adhered to a 6–8 hour monitoring period because of clinical factors. **Transport** of the patient to his home must always be "passive" (i.e. with family members or friends, possibly by taxi).

Both the patient and the accompanying person must be given a careful **briefing.** Upon the occurrence of symptoms, the hospital where the biopsy was performed is to be informed immediately by telephone (for this reason the patient always has to be given the telephone number and name of the emergency doctor in writing). In such a case, the local practitioner should not be consulted — so as to avoid any loss of time! The emergency physician at the hospital has to be informed of the name and residence of the biopsied patient, so that he is "prepared" for a telephone call at all times. • Should the biopsy have been carried out at a specialist surgery, it is advisable to inform an emergency physician at a nearby hospital of the name and residence of the patient — upon the occurrence of complications, the patient should be taken immediately to that hospital (and not to the local practitioner's surgery!).

1.10 Transjugular liver biopsy

Transjugular venous liver biopsy was first described by W. HANAFEE et al. in 1967. It has been successfully performed (monitoring by ECG!) with few complications in high-risk patients (e. g. ascites, bleeding tendency, severe adiposity, massive intra-abdominal adhesions), both adults and children. Furthermore, the biopsy material obtained by this method (albeit shorter than in percutaneous biopsy) has generally been rated as adequate for assessment. The modified 15 G or 16 G Ross needle, but also an 18 G automated core biopsy needle, are considered preferable over the Trucut needle. The technique is deemed to be safe and reliable, and the complication rate is acceptable. (s. tab. 7.9) (4, 12, 13, 20, 30, 32, 33, 43, 45, 56, 69, 80, 98, 109, 129, 131, 162, 175)

---
1. Neck haematoma
2. Pneumothorax
3. Transient Horner syndrome
4. Transient trachyphonia
5. Passing abdominal pain
6. Passing fever
7. Cardiac arrythmias
8. Intrahepatic a.v. fistula
9. Perforation of the liver capsule
10. Cardiac arrest

Tab. 7.9: Complications of transjugular liver biopsy (mortality rate 0.1–0.5%)

1.11 Transfemoral liver biopsy

The technique of transfemoral liver biopsy using flexible forceps was described by M. W. MEWISSEN et al. in 1988. Some studies have shown this to be just as safe and efficient as the transjugular method. (75, 80, 89, 150)

1.12 Ultrasound- or CT-guided biopsy

The first **ultrasound-guided liver biopsy** (using the A technique) was carried out by WANG HSIN-FANG et al. in 1964 to diagnose and treat liver abscesses. (s. tab. 7.2)

Ultrasound-guided Menghini biopsy was recommended in 1983 as an alternative to percussion-guided biopsy. (52) • *Today, it is deemed the method of choice.* (19, 25, 35, 54, 56, 72, 88, 115, 158, 169, 172, 174) (s. tab. 7.2)

Ultrasound-guided fine-needle biopsy was introduced by A. LUNDQUIST in 1971. It is deemed to be a low-risk method for the sampling of cytological material and is almost indispensable for differential diagnosis between benign and malignant foci. (10) Its sensitivity is 60—80% and its specificity higher than 90%. This form of biopsy can also be applied in the treatment of abscesses. The use of cutting biopsy needles (involving greater risks) even makes it possible to sample liver tissue for histological assessment. There are many reports on the biopsy technique as well as on the results and complications involved. (9, 17, 28, 36, 39, 61, 74, 145, 166, 257) Up to now, reports have been received on 10 fatal cases subsequent to fine-needle puncture of abdominal organs — six of them as a result of liver biopsy. • Spreading of tumour cells via the bloodstream or lymphatic system can be more or less ignored. The genesis of vaccination metastases and spreading of tumour cells or infectious material into the biopsy canal is considered rare. • Even if the commonly used fine needle with a cutting surface of 22 G only has a diameter of 0.7 mm (cf. Menghini needle with 17 G and Jamshidi needle with 15 G), the possibility of afterbleeding, though seldom, must still be considered. (58; quot. 166) • The evaluation of 11,700 abdominal fine-needle biopsies by T. LIVRAGHI et al. (1983) yielded a complication rate of 0.55%; serious complications occurred in 0.05% of patients. The frequency of pronounced bleeding given by M. GEBEL et al. (1986) was 1.5—2.5%, depending on the tumour type. (quot. in 166) (s. p. 133)

CT-guided liver biopsy was reported for the first time by J. R. HAAGA et al. in 1976. Biopsy of *focal lesions of the liver* may also be carried out with the help of CT guidance. (19, 55, 74, 159, 167)

2 Laparoscopy

2.1 Historical development

▶ The first laparoscopy following a pneumoperitoneum was reported by the surgeon GEORG KELLING from Dresden at a lecture given in Hamburg on 23.9.1901. He presented this method of examination, using the term **coelioscopy**. (quot. 235) In the same year (1901), DIMITRI EDLER VON OTT also described this technique in St. Petersburg, calling it **ventroscopy**. (269) • The name **laparoscopy** originates from HANS CHRISTIAN JACOBAEUS, who in 1910 reported on the examination of the abdominal cavity using Nitze's cystoscope following pneumoperitoneum placement. (226) In the USA, this method was termed **organoscopy** (B. M. BERNHEIM, 1991) (182), **peritoneoscopy** (B. H. ORNDOFF, 1920) (268), and **abdominoscopy** (O. STEINER, 1924) (292). The first atlas of laparoscopy was published by R. KORBSCH in 1927, based on his own experience since 1921. (238) Following these publications, laparoscopy was adopted in numerous countries as a new method of examination. (s. tab. 7.10)

▶ The **3rd developmental stage** of laparoscopy is linked to the name of H. KALK, who (commencing in 1923/1924) systematically revised the technique of laparoscopy in Frankfurt and brought out the first publication on the subject in 1929. (229) His experience has been documented in papers dating back to the years 1935 (Indications and dangers) (230), 1942 (Introduction to photolaparoscopy), 1943 (Directed liver biopsy under laparoscopic vision) as well as 1948, 1953 and 1955. • The clinicians N. HENNING (Leipzig), C. FERVERS (Solingen) who became the first to carry out adhesiolysis (1933), J. C. RUDDOCK (Los Angeles) and E. B. BENEDICT (Boston) were also involved in this development phase. (s. tab. 7.10)

▶ It was only the consistent work of H. KALK which gave laparoscopy its worldwide high status. (252) • Further perfecting of laparoscopy, attributable to K. BECK, W. BRÜHL, J. EISENBURG, H. HENNING, H. LENT, H. LINDNER, W. SIEDE, L. WANNAGAT and E. WILDHIRT — to name but a few of the German schools of thought — resulted in laparoscopy becoming an integral part of clinical diagnostics. With continual further development of medical technology, important additional techniques have been rendered possible.

First performance of laparoscopy		
1901	G. KELLING *(coelioscopy)*	Dresden[1]
1901	D. EDLER VON OTT *(ventroscopy)*	St. Petersburg[2]
New description of laparoscopy		
1910	H. CH. JACOBAEUS *(laparoscopy)*	Stockholm[3]
1911	B. M. BERNHEIM *(organoscopy)*	Baltimore[4]
1920	B. H. ORNDOFF *(peritoneoscopy)*	Chicago[4]
1921	R. KORBSCH (1927: 1st atlas of laparoscopy)	Oberhausen[1]
1924	O. STEINER *(abdominoscopy)*	Atlanta[4]
Third phase of "laparoscopic discovery"		
1923/24	H. KALK	Frankfurt[1]
1928	N. HENNING	Leipzig[1]
1934	J. C. RUDDOCK	Los Angeles[4]
1939	E. B. BENEDICT	Boston[4]
Fourth laparoscopic development phase		
since 1980	*laparoscopic surgical procedures*	
since 1980	*laparoscopic sonography*	
since 1995	*exploratory mini-laparoscopy*	

Tab. 7.10: Historical development of laparoscopy (a selection of important steps) (1 = Germany; 2 = Russia; 3 = Sweden; 4 = USA)

After 1950 there was an enormous worldwide increase in the number of laparoscopic examinations. Statistics from H. LINDNER et al. (1976) reflect this with 141,981 laparoscopies in European countries. (249) The highest level of laparoscopic examinations (between 1970 and 1980) was estimated as being in excess of one million!

The introduction of new methods into hepatological diagnostics (virus serology, sonography, CT, MRT, to name just a few) has led to a reduction in the frequency of laparoscopic examinations since 1975. Even in hospitals with very high laparoscopy figures, frequency has been reduced to about 10%. (219) This *"laparoscopic slump"* is also obvious in our own statistics. (243)

2.2 Definition of laparoscopy

> Laparoscopy is a low-risk instrumental examination technique for the abdominal cavity with a high degree of diagnostic relevance and low personnel input.

Laparoscopy, like the terms **coelioscopy, ventroscopy, organoscopy, peritoneoscopy** and **abdominoscopy** (s. tab. 7.10), actually means an *"endoscopy of the abdomen"* and not only of the *"liver"* — unfortunately, such a "hepatoscopy" was all too often performed on its own. *(see page 2 for further details on the term "hepatoscopy")*

2.3 Indications

Morphological findings are deemed to be an essential part of detailed diagnosis in liver diseases. Yet the results of percutaneous liver biopsy lead all too easily (e. g. with focal findings) and to a somewhat high percentage (e. g. with liver cirrhosis, chronic virus hepatitis C) to misinterpretations. *Non-directed liver biopsy does not always make it possible to detect changes which are representative of the entire liver.* Additionally, in 1–2% of cases, the material yield does not necessarily suffice for histological assessment. (s. p. 168)

Assessment of the liver surface can often be the decisive starting point for diagnosis and histological interpretation. Furthermore, laparoscopy makes it possible to inspect the entire abdominal cavity. As a result, indications for exploratory laparoscopy are significantly extended. Yet modern imaging procedures can quite often produce false-negative results as well. In individual cases, laparoscopy (possibly with directed biopsy) can be taken as a method of reference. This is also true for other specific issues, such as **congenital anomalies**. (285)
• With the introduction of imaging procedures and their perfected methods, the indication list with regard to laparoscopy has changed. Based on the information found in the literature as well as on **our own experience with 6,000 laparoscopies (1955–1987)** (243), indications for exploratory laparoscopy are given for many hepatobiliary diseases. (185, 188, 189, 194, 196, 199, 204, 206, 219, 234, 243–245, 247, 249, 250, 254, 263, 264, 272, 281, 289, 293, 298, 303, 310) (s. tab. 7.11)

2.4 Exploratory laparoscopy

> The arguments put forward by G. KELLING (1923) apply just as much today as they did in the past — exploratory laparoscopy of the abdominal cavity is one of the most important aims of laparoscopy. (235) (s. tab. 7.12) • In working towards a diagnosis, it is a fundamental principle that exploratory laparoscopy should be given priority over exploratory laparotomy. (189, 196, 204, 209, 234, 243, 244, 280, 281, 299)

---

1. Chronic hepatitis (227, 243, 273, 301)
   – for differential diagnosis
   – for morphological differentiation
2. Unclarified hepatomegaly and/or increasing liver consistency
3. Unclarified splenomegaly (243)
4. Unclarified rise in liver enzymes
5. Unclarified occupation of abdominal space
6. Unclarified gall bladder findings (236, 243)
7. Unclarified abdominal symptoms (240, 282)
   – adhesions (178, 223, 243)
   – suspected tuberculous peritonitis (184, 222)
   – suspected carcinomatous peritonitis (191, 243)
   – appendicitis (187, 296, 308)
8. Suspected liver cirrhosis (192, 220, 261, 266, 276)
   – differential diagnosis (212, 243)
   – assessment of further complications (232, 294)
   – demarcation of a scarred liver (243, 294)
9. Suspected focal liver lesions (190, 243, 246)
   – adenoma, echinococcosis, haemangioma (243), focal nodular hyperplasia (195, 225, 243), tuberculosis (243), sarcoidosis (243), Hodgkin's disease (243, 283, 312), liver abscess (221), *etc.*
10. Suspected malignant tumours
    – primary liver cell carcinoma (214, 231, 251)
    – malignancy in haemochromatosis
    – gall-bladder carcinoma (200, 241)
    – liver metastases (186, 191)
    – abdominal metastatic spread (243)
11. Suspected parasitic disease
12. Fever of unknown aetiology (218, 239, 289)
13. Ascites of unknown aetiology (198, 277)
14. Cholestasis of unknown aetiology (267, 286)
15. Clarification of systemic diseases
16. Tumour staging: "pre-look" prior to surgery, "second look" after carcinoma surgery
17. Assessment of indication for transplantation
18. Suspected lack of one liver lobe (243)
19. Emergency laparoscopy (177, 256)
    – in postbioptic bleeding
    – in postbioptic biliary leakage
    – following blunt abdominal trauma
20. Vascular processes
    – peliosis hepatis (225, 290)
    – Budd-Chiari syndrome (183)
    – Osler disease (291)

Tab. 7.11: Indications for (exploratory) laparoscopy — where it is not possible to guarantee a definitive diagnosis by means of other procedures. • *The diagnostic significance of an indication is individual and different in each case and can be categorized in steps ranging from "of little significance" through to "very important" or "absolutely necessary"*

In calling for **quality assurance** in diagnostics, it is not possible to do without the relevant accuracy and significance of laparoscopy. For this reason, the indications outlined have to be reviewed in each individual case. They can either be viewed more stringently or interpreted more widely; their diagnostic significance may be greater or less, depending on the respective case. (s. tab. 7.11)

Laparoscopy is always indicated if an abdominal clinical picture has not been clarified or a hepatobiliary disease could not be defined by non-invasive or minimally invasive procedures (such as sonography, CT, ERC, scintigraphy, MRI). (234, 243, 281) (s. tab. 7.12)

Main targets of laparoscopy
Assessment of:
1. liver and gall bladder
2. spleen
3. peritoneum, omentum, ligaments, free diaphragmatic areas
Secondary targets of laparoscopy
Assessment of:
1. free stomach wall areas, intestine, appendix
2. female minor pelvis in a head-down position (uterus, ovaries, tubes)
3. hernial orifices
To a limited extent — pancreas — kidneys

Tab. 7.12: Organ-related examination targets (main and secondary) in exploratory laparoscopy

▶ With considerably less inconvenience to the patient, exploratory laparoscopy offers a better view of the minor pelvis through to the subphrenic space than can be provided by exploratory laparotomy with the limitations imposed by incision. Adhesions can also be viewed better with the help of laparoscopy as compared to laparotomy.

▶ Time and personnel involved as well as the costs of nursing are all far lower with exploratory laparoscopy than with laparotomy. In the vast majority of cases, exploratory laparoscopy renders exploratory laparotomy superfluous. Above all, this is true for the detection of nonoperable carcinomas.

▶ When examining women, every laparoscopy should include an inspection of the minor pelvis in the head-down position.

▶ Each abnormal or pathological finding is to be recorded by photographic documentation. A surgeon or gynaecologist should be consulted in assessing specific findings relating to his field.

▶ With selected patients, *outpatient laparoscopy* has proved to be a safe and cost-saving (approx. 30% less expensive) method with follow-up monitoring of three to four hours under hospital conditions. (297)

Mortality risk is given as being about 0.1% (−0.2%) for exploratory laparoscopy, whereas exploratory laparotomy has a lethality rate of about 2.5% − i.e. roughly 20 times higher! In advanced carcinomas, the lethality rate is as high as 50% for exploratory laparotomy versus 7.4% for laparoscopy.

The strategy generally applied in a diagnostic clarification in the case of suspected **"liver tumour"** is outlined later in a **flow algorithm**. (s. p. 204) (s. fig. 9.4)

2.5 Contraindications

Attention must be paid to clotting disorders, cardiac and coronary insufficiency, severe cardiac arrhythmia, serious hypertension, respiratory insufficiency and purulent peritonitis as possible contraindications. The same is true of Bekhterev's disease and cerebral insufficiency (depending on the respective severity). Despite a wide range of indications, the list of contraindications (except hepatogenic clotting disorders) only covers severe extrahepatic diseases. In these cases, it is the treatment of the condition which is of paramount importance and not the diagnostic clarification of abdominal or hepatobiliary diseases. (217, 233, 244, 255, 262) (s. tab. 7.13)

Relative contraindications: Given the technical experience of the physician and the implementation of adjuvant measures, certain contraindications can be categorized as relative, and accordingly overcome; in such cases, however, a greater risk is to be expected. • *Pronounced adhesions, extreme adiposity and severe meteorism are reasons for greater restraint and due caution.* (s. tab. 7.13)

Absolute contraindications
1. Clotting disorders
2. Cardiac and coronary insufficiency, arrhythmia
3. Severe hypertension
4. Respiratory insufficiency
5. Bacterial peritonitis
6. Large hiatus hernia
Relative contraindications
7. Bekhterev's disease
8. Cerebral insufficiency
9. Pronounced adiposity
10. Severe meteorism
11. Massive adhesions

Tab. 7.13: Absolute and relative contraindications for laparoscopy

Adhesions are not deemed to be general contraindications, yet in some cases they do involve considerable technical difficulties and a higher risk of complications

– e.g. as a result of the perforation of adherent bowel loops or of the stomach. (178, 228, 274) This was also shown by three of our own cases with a bland course of disease. (243) Another factor to be feared is the puncturing of vessels in the area of the adhesions, particularly in the presence of portal hypertension with "spontaneous Talma" effect. (s. p. 163) (s. figs. 7.5; 14.11). We observed this event in 4 cases, all of which could be well managed. (243) *"Extensive adhesions will always be the worst enemy of laparoscopy"* (H. KALK, 1929). (229) • With suspected postoperative adhesions, above all in the laparoscopic working area, we have occasionally carried out a lateral X-ray examination after placement of the pneumoperitoneum. The relevance of such an examination should, however, not be overestimated. (s. fig. 7.1) This *"diagnostic method using X-ray with a gas-filled abdominal cavity"* was described for the first time by O. GOETZE in 1918. • Nevertheless, it must be clearly emphasized that abdominal adhesions are also present in a considerable percentage of patients who have not undergone surgery in the abdominal cavity. These **spontaneous adhesions** can be found in all areas of the abdomen (14.6% of cases) and are due to trauma, intestinal inflammations, pancreatitis or cholecystitis. (306) • Photographic documentation is an absolute necessity in the case of adhesions! • Frequently, symptoms related to adhesions in themselves constitute an *indication for laparoscopy.* In the course of establishing a differential diagnosis for unclarified abdominal discomfort (nausea, vomiting, etc.), it may be necessary, after ruling out all other possibilities, to consider a painful adhesion-related **"serosa syndrome".** (243, 244) By means of an exploratory probe, the pain characteristics familiar to the patient can indeed often be triggered and then localized in the area where the adhesions exist. (s. figs. 7.2, 7.3) • In the case of **adhesiolysis** (C. FERVERS, 1933), free adhesive bridles can be severed by thermocautery, and occasionally relief from pain is achieved. • Sail-like adhesions can be carefully "fenestrated" by thermocautery in order to advance the laparoscope into areas which have hitherto been out of sight. In retrospective evaluation, we applied *thermocautery* in 120 cases (243): 87 times to fenestrate and improve visibility and 33 times as adhesiolysis for therapeutic reasons in cases of previously indeterminate abdominal pain. Almost all of these 33 patients had been through extensive diagnostic procedures, often over a number of years, with multiple courses of therapy. *One of these patients with pericholecystitic adhesions (an example of which is shown in figure 7.3) had been unsuccessfully treated for almost three years (even psychotherapeutically), but after adhesiolysis, she was ultimately freed from her discomfort.*

> ▶ In cases of unclarified abdominal pain – *after* all other diagnostic steps have failed – exploratory laparoscopy should constitute the next step *before* commencing psychotherapy!

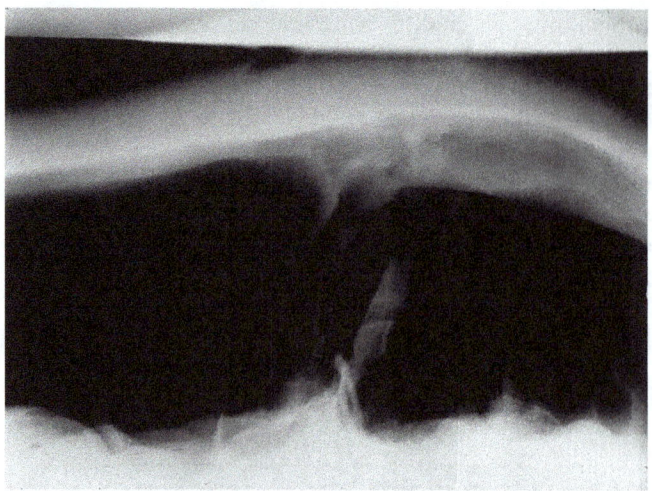

Fig. 7.1: Pneumoperitoneum with pronounced cord-like or sail-like adhesions in the abdominal cavity (X-ray from the side)

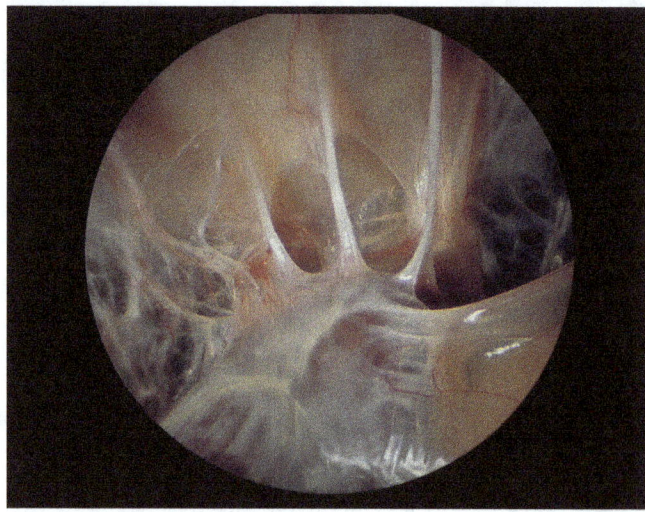

Fig. 7.2: Extensive postoperative adhesions and bridles

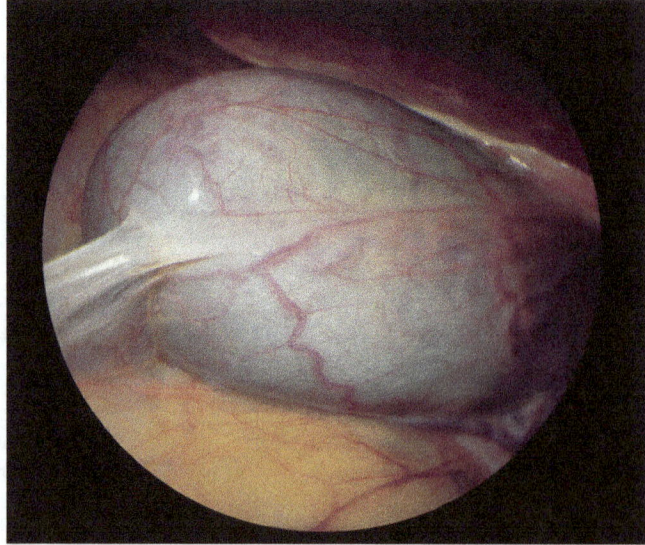

Fig. 7.3: Pericholecystitic adhesions causing years of abdominal pain ("serosa syndrome") – *without* previous operative intervention in the abdominal cavity

Adiposity is undoubtedly a laparoscopic problem. The abdominal walls can be enormously rich in fat, and the fatty mass is often deposited in the abdominal omentum. Sometimes excessively long instruments are required (such as anaesthesia needles, Veres needle). In two of our own cases, we were only able to carry out the examination under tremendous difficulty because the trocar was too short. The highest reported weight of a patient undergoing laparoscopy is 160 kg. (217)

Hernias likewise do not constitute a general contraindication. (217) In numerous cases, we have observed no complications. (243) • Large hiatus hernias are, however, an accepted contraindication.

Advanced age is not in itself a contraindication. The patients were above 80 years in 0.3–0.7% of cases. In our group of patients (243), 11 men and 8 women (0.32%) were older than 80, of whom 5 (0.08%) were aged between 85 and 90 years. There were no complications. Nevertheless, in cases of advanced age, indications should be viewed critically.

Children can undergo laparoscopy without particular difficulty. (207, 310) The youngest child was an infant aged 14 days (H. SELMAIR et al., 1973). We ourselves experienced no problems in examining 9 children aged between 5 and 14 years. (243) Laparoscopy is performed under general anaesthesia. With older children (as in our own cases), neuroleptic analgesia or an individual sedation is sufficient. Hepatosplenomegaly, jaundice, metabolic diseases, tumours, chronic hepatitis and portal hypertension are some of the indications.

2.6 Laparoscopic technique

Once the indications have been drawn up and critically considered, and possible contraindications weighed up, the *briefing of the patient* follows (on the day prior to laparoscopy) and the *patient's written consent* is obtained. All further measures are then taken. (s. tab. 7.14)

Sterility and **asepsis** are imperative for all instruments used and for the places where they are deposited (e.g. instrument trolley). We also recommend the use of sterile drapes as well as sterile surgical gowns (caps and masks are not required) after having disinfected the patient's abdomen. Once the photographic documentation has been completed (using reflex camera, Polaroid, video, etc.), gloves and drapes should be changed. Even though experience has shown the risk of infection to be extremely low for the patient, and although the sterility and asepsis aimed at are not guaranteed in certain working sequences, we still advocate, as a matter of principle, that *laparoscopy should be carried out under conditions that are largely sterile*.

Premedication

It is advisable to prepare anxious patients with sedation (e.g. doxepin 10 mg) on the evening prior to laparoscopy. For premedication

1. *Sonography*
2. *Blood coagulation tests*
   – *Quick's value, thrombocyte count, bleeding time*
3. *Possibly ECG, pulmonary function*

4. **Preparation for laparoscopy**
   - patient under fasting conditions (ca. 12 hours, avoiding gas-forming vegetables)
   - voiding of the bladder
   - stabilizing and protecting a possible hernia with an external adhesive bandage
   - with men, shaving of the abdominal area
   - premedication
     – promethazine (50 mg) + pethidine (50 mg) i.m.
     or:
     promethazine (50 mg) + doxepin (25 mg)
     or:
     midazolam (0.05–0.1 mg/kg BW)
     (i.m., some 20–30 minutes prior to laparoscopy)
     or:
     midazolam (initially 1.0–2.5 mg) slowly i.v., up to 5 mg total dose
     – atropine (0.5 mg) s.c. about 15 minutes earlier
     (After administration of triflupromazine, we occasionally observed extrapyramidal side-effects; for this reason we ceased using this substance.)
   - positioning of the patient: precisely, comfortably, with wrists and knees fixed loosely to an operating table which can be tilted on all sides
     – padded support of the ulnaris nerve
     – support of the greater trochanter from the side
   - positioning of neutral electrode for coagulation, generally on the right thigh
   - sterile draping of the patient
   - disinfecting the abdomen

Tab. 7.14: Preparation for laparoscopy

purposes, the following drugs have proved to be suitable (s. tab. 7.14): pethidine (50 mg) + atropine (0.5 mg), or hydromorphone (2 mg) + atropine (0.5 mg), or midazolam (individual dosage upwards of 1 mg) + atropine (0.5 mg). • *We would recommend the administration of atropine in principle and not only if vagovasal reactions occur.* (s. pp 152, 153)

Local anaesthesia

Local anaesthesia is effected as intracutaneous skin wheal using a thin needle, whereas for bathyanaesthesia a long injection needle has to be applied. Lidocaine is recommended as an anaesthetic (0.5 or 1.0%). With the continuous injection of anaesthetic, a sharp pain is reached in the peritoneum, where a preperitoneal depot is then placed.

Veres cannula

▶ A description of the **Veres needle** was published by J. VERES in 1938. (300) *His name was, however, wrongly printed as Veress in this publication – the correct spelling of his name is "Veres" and the correct pronunciation is "veresch".* • After a stab incision with the tip of the scalpel (i.e. lancet), the needle is inserted against abdominal muscular pressure on the part of the patient. The resistance of both fascia and peritoneum can be felt clearly. A hollow internal cannula with a rounded end stays retracted within the Veres needle during penetration. As soon as the peritoneum has been penetrated, the blunt stylet springs out of the sharp cannula in the peritoneal cavity, and a double clicking sound of the Veres needle is audible. The free position of the needle is checked by the rapid injection of 10–20ml physiological NaCl solution. (s. fig. 7.18)

Pneumoperitoneum

The point of placement used for the pneumoperitoneum is the so-called **Kalk's point** (this is the later site of insertion for the laparoscope) or the **Monro-Richter line** in the left lower abdominal region (this is the connecting line between the umbilicus and the left anterior superior iliac spine). In the third outer quarter of the line (or at the lateral tertiary point) is the "classical point" for abdominal puncture as well as for the pneumoperitoneum. • Even if a later, second anaesthesia is required for the laparoscope, we consider it useful to maintain the functional capacity of the Veres cannula throughout the whole procedure *as a possible insufflation channel that can be used if required – without discomfort to the patient.* • As a variation on the above-mentioned points of insertion, sites can also be selected below and to the left of the umbilicus. • In 1918 O. Goetze (Halle) introduced an **automatic needle** for producing the pneumoperitoneum. (s. fig. 7.1) (s. tab. 7.15)

Insufflation

Insufflation with nitrous oxide (N_2O, i.e. laughing gas) is now carried out by an **automatic-charting N_2O gas insufflator**. The free inflow of nitrous oxide is detectable by auscultation as an even, gentle noise above the Veres needle. After insufflation of the first 300 to 500 ml nitrous oxide, the liver dullness fades, and after a further 1 to 2 litres N_2O, a tympanitic percussion sound is generally ascertained. (259, 288, 312) • From the beginning of the slow and evenly maintained process of insufflation, it is advisable to shake the vertically held Veres needle so as to remove any fragments of the omentum which may have been speared. At the same time, fragments which might be caught up between the needle and the stylet can be removed by retraction and forward thrusting of the blunt stylet. Under constant observation of the filling pressure (10 to 20 mm Hg), the required N_2O amount is introduced (3 to 5 litres, in certain cases even more) and the insufflator then switched over to automatic refill. Intraperitoneal pressure is now 10–12 mm Hg. The abdominal walls should be evenly raised. • *CO_2 is painful and therefore unsuitable for exploratory laparoscopy!*

1. Formation of emphysema
   - skin emphysema
   - preperitoneal emphysema
   - omentum emphysema
   - mediastinal emphysema
   - scrotal emphysema
2. Injuries from insertion
   - laceration of intestine
   - laceration of blood vessels
   - laceration of an ovarian cyst
3. Circulatory disorders
   - collapse
   - arrhythmia
   - cardiac arrest

Tab. 7.15: Possible complications in producing the pneumoperitoneum or inserting a trocar

Insertion of the trocar

The site of insertion for the trocar is **Kalk's point**: 2–3 cm to the left of and above the umbilicus at the medial edge of the *rectus abdominis*. Further to the left, laterally, there is some danger due to the proximity of the superior epigastric artery, and further to the right, above the umbilicus, there is a certain risk of injuring the round ligament and the umbilical vein as well as the gall bladder. The right lower abdominal region in the area of *McBurney's point* is also to be avoided regarding the insertion of the trocar. • With ascites and adiposity, the navel moves caudad (with gynaecological cystoma, craniad), which must be considered when selecting the point of insertion. In hepatomegaly, splenomegaly and tumours, or with operation scars, the normal site of insertion should be varied accordingly. (s. tab. 7.15)

Local anaesthesia is effected in the same way (see above). After some gas has penetrated the syringe sheath, either spontaneously or after slight suction, the depth of the gas-dome and the free lateral mobility is checked with the anaesthesia needle. The **incision** is horizontal, 1.0–1.5 cm in length (subcutis and muscles must not be severed!). The **insertion of the trocar** (s. fig. 7.17) is carried out under abdominal muscular pressure on the part of the patient in the inspiration phase and by exerting considerable left-right rotating pressure. A finger of the guiding hand placed along the shaft of the trocar acts as an **"emergency brake"**. After perforation of the peritoneum by the trocar (perceived by the sudden feeling of penetration into a free space and an audible outflow of gas from the tap), the trocar tip is withdrawn and the tap closed.

▶ *We most definitely prefer a trocar (11 mm ⌀) with a conical, tapering tip* (N. Henning, 1950) *as opposed to the three-edged tip.* (s. fig. 7.17) With the three-edge tipped trocar, we experienced pronounced venous bleeding of the abdominal wall, which, however, could be overcome conservatively.

The sterile **side-view laparoscope,** which has been slightly warmed, is then introduced under direct vision. (s. fig. 7.17) Subsequently, the insufflation tube is removed from the Veres cannula and fitted to the trocar. It has proved beneficial to leave the closed Veres needle (ready for use) in its position throughout the procedure of laparoscopy.

Staff requirements

Apart from the endoscopist (with intensive-care experience), a further physician should attend the laparoscopy (if possible). Two nurses trained in intensive care are required to assist. This staff constellation has proved optimal. (243)

Monitoring by apparatus

The patient is monitored by means of blood pressure measurement, ECG, and pulse oximeter. A trolley with emergency equipment must always be at hand in the endoscopy room. Further, the possibility of electrocoagulation should be given in case there is delayed bleeding. • Consideration must be given to a number of **dangers** which can be involved in producing the pneumoperitoneum or inserting a trocar. (176, 181, 197, 208, 244) (s. tab. 7.15)

2.7 Course of examination

Initial inspection focuses on the position of the Veres needle and, if necessary, an adjustment is made. • To ensure correct examination, an established **inspection schedule** has proved useful. When such a schedule is applied as a matter of routine, important findings or additional information will not be overlooked. • With *extreme changes in position*, vertigo, nausea, respiratory distress and a tendency to collapse may be observed, but these symptoms rapidly ease off once the body position has been normalized. • Altogether, the examination procedure entails four different positions. In this way, optimal results can be obtained.

Position 1	All-round view of the entire abdominal cavity in a supine position (= peritoneum, omentum, bowel loops, adhesions).
Position 2	Inspection of the right upper abdomen with the upper body raised in left rotation (= right lobe of liver, gall bladder, round ligament, falciform ligament, duodenum).
Position 3	Inspection of the left upper abdominal region with the upper body raised in right rotation (= left lobe of liver, spleen, round ligament, falciform ligament, phrenicocolic ligament, stomach, diaphragm with oesophageal foramen, pancreas).
Position 4	Inspection of the minor pelvis in a head-down position and in right and left rotation (= coecum, appendix, uterus, Fallopian tubes, ovaries, hernial orifices).

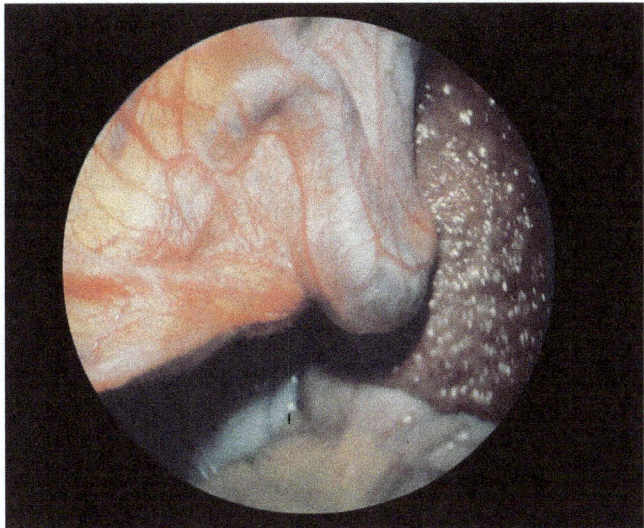

Fig. 7.4: Cruveilhier-von Baumgarten syndrome in alcohol-induced cirrhosis

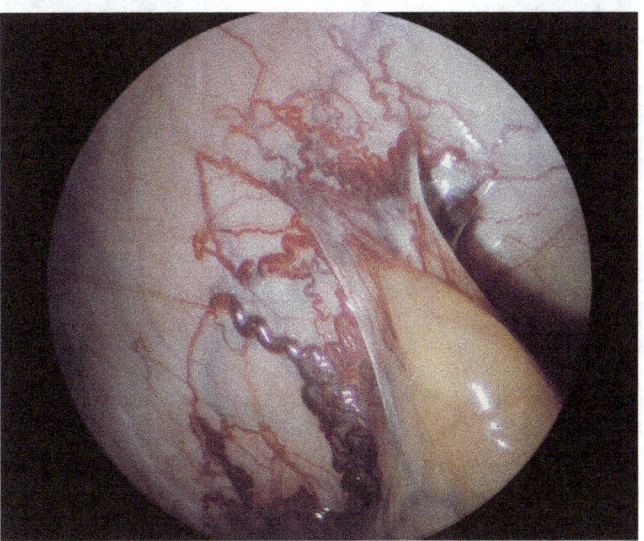

Fig. 7.5: Portal hypertension with pronounced collateral circulation in an area with adhesions (*"spontaneous Talma"* effect)

2.7.1 Assessment of the portal vessels

The development of *portal hypertension* is detectable at a very early stage by the dilatation of small venous vessels in the greater omentum, at the serosa of the stomach, at the parietal peritoneum and, in particular, at the round ligament and falciform ligament. A further increase in portal hypertension produces tortuosity of the dilatated fine calibre veins. • *Collateral circulatory pathways* ultimately develop, mostly noticeable at the phrenicocolic ligament, round ligament and falciform ligament with a progredient recanalization of the umbilical vein (s. figs. 6.10; 14.12; 35.14) and paraumbilical veins (= *Cruveilhier-von Baumgarten syndrome*) (s. fig. 7.4) as well as in an area with adhesions (*"spontaneous Talma"* effect). (s. pp 160, 264) (s. figs. 7.5; 14.11)

2.7.2 Assessment of the spleen

Each laparoscopy should aim at a visual assessment of the spleen in terms of (*1.*) size, (*2.*) colour, (*3.*) shape, and (*4.*) identifiable *spleen diseases*. Special mention has to be made of capsular fibrosis, hyalinosis ("sugar-coated spleen"), tumours (e.g. Hodgkin's disease, retothelial sarcoma), tuberculosis, splenic cysts, splenic infarction (s. fig. 35.10) and splenic haematoma. Given appropriate positioning, the spleen is visible in 80% of cases. In the event of myeloproliferative diseases, a biopsy of the spleen (e.g. by means of the Menghini technique) may possibly provide a definitive diagnosis. (s. pp 145, 261) (s. figs. 11.1; 14.7) (*see chapter 11*)

2.7.3 Tumour staging

In 1979 T. HALD et al. reported on the importance of laparoscopy in the staging of tumours of the efferent urinary tract. In 30–60% of cases, imaging procedures do not allow the inoperability of liver tumours to be recognized. Preoperative staging by means of laparoscopy showed a sensitivity of 78% and a specificity of 100%. Some 70% of the liver surface can be assessed (as can parts of the underside of the liver when the lobes are lifted). After the noninvasive staging procedure (= recording of TNM classification and other prognostic factors) has been performed, laparoscopy should be used to evaluate operability. (244) • It is also possible for metastases to develop in liver cirrhosis; this was confirmed in 11.4% of cases. (315) • Despite careful preliminary examinations, it was only laparoscopic staging which rendered the detection of peritoneal metastases possible in 9.1% (202), 35% (305) and 40% (242) of cases, whereupon inoperability was established. • After surgery on ovarian cancer, peritoneal metastases can be expected frequently due to lymphogenic factors — in 22% of cases, this could only be detected by means of laparoscopy. (202) • In tumour staging after application of the available imaging methods in patients with oesophagus and/or gastric cardia cancer, metastases could actually be detected by means of laparoscopy in 24% (201) to 76% (307) of cases. (210, 242, 260, 265, 278) • In patients with pancreatic carcinoma, the laparoscopic detection rate for abdominal metastases varied from 24% to 42%. (179, 279, 304, 305) • In 23—38% of cases, an unnecessary laparotomy could be avoided. (179, 265, 278, 305) Laparoscopy is the best method for the detection of metastases of the omentum and/or peritoneum. (180, 191, 209, 213, 228, 243, 248, 312) (s. figs. 7.6; 37.33—37.35)

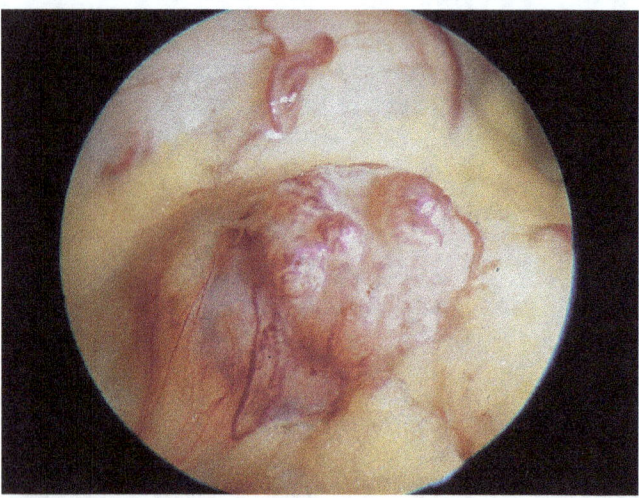

Fig. 7.6: Metastasis of a malignant melanoma in the area of the greater omentum (it is as a rule not detectable with US or CT) (s. figs. 37.35, 37.36)

2.7.4 Fever of unknown aetiology

It is not always possible to link the symptom of "fever" to a specific disease. In such cases, laparoscopy provides valuable diagnostic aid in differentiating the respective changes of the liver in order to detect rare and otherwise unidentifiable diseases. (218, 239, 289) • This was impressively demonstrated by *one of our own cases of small nodular liver tuberculosis detected by laparoscopic (and histological) diagnostics, which had been preceded by sojourns at two hospitals and unsuccessful implementation of all diagnostic possibilities.* (244) (s. figs. 24.2, 24.5) (s. p. 761!) In view of the "uncertainty" inherent in unexplained febrile conditions with liver enzyme activity, we consider percutaneous liver biopsy to be too dangerous and too unreliable in its outcome. Using laparoscopy, it was possible to explain the cause of fever (after ineffective application of every other examination method) in 37% (with the involvement of the abdominal organs in up to 94%) (218) and in 66% of cases. (289)

2.7.5 Assessment of the lymphatic vessels

The transparent-white lymphatic vessels, which normally are not (or hardly) identifiable, allow the lymph to flow to the falciform ligament in a deltoid manner. Visible lymphatic vessels are in general deemed to be congested and hence are indirectly suggestive of liver disease. Congested lymphatic vessels appear as blue-grey/silver-grey pathways, often displaying fine fibrotic introsusceptions. In cases of jaundice, the lymphatic vessels take on a distinct yellowish/brownish colour. With pronounced dilation, segmentation of the walls is evident. (s. figs. 7.7; 16.4)

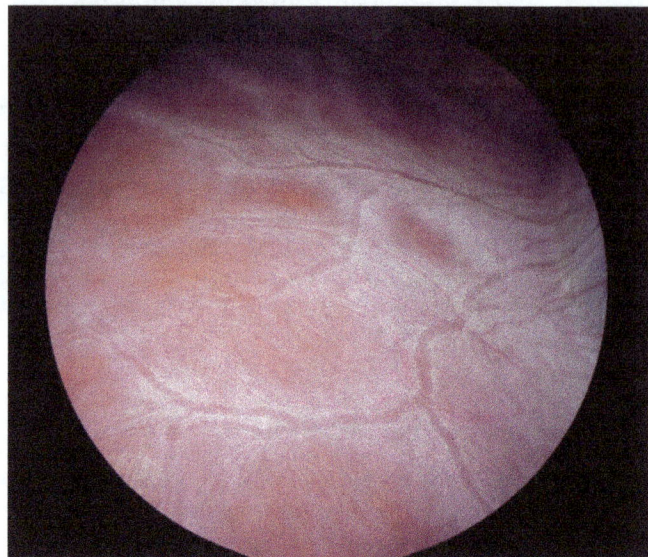

Fig. 7.7: Congested lymphatic vessels in the area of the medial part of the right lobe of liver (insertion of the left falciform ligament can be clearly identified) with partial vessel wall segmentation. Here in chronic toxic hepatitis

2.7.6 Ascites of unknown aetiology

According to our knowledge, the explanation of the aetiology of ascites goes back to O. E. Nadeau et al. (1925) and S. M. Fierst et al. (1975). After the unsuccessful application of all diagnostic procedures available today, laparoscopy ascertained the cause of ascites in 86% of cases. (198, 277) (s. figs. 16.9; 37.25)

2.8 Photographic documentation

Each pathological or interesting finding should be documented by colour photography. Laparoscopy without photographic documentation would be rather like *an X-ray examination without the X-ray picture*. However precisely a particular finding might be described, it never convinces in the same manner as a coloured photo can. Written findings and colour photography must complement one another (cf. physician's obligation to keep records!).

▶ It would be of great benefit to the **pathologist** if a colour Polaroid shot was enclosed with each sample of laparoscopic material obtained by liver biopsy — in addition to laboratory values, diagnostic issue in question and description of the liver surface. In evaluating the liver biopsy, the pathologist should be aware of the traditional dual assessment of an organ: *macroscopy + histology*.

Documentation of findings is facilitated by **reflex camera** and **Polaroid camera** for coloured photos. Various zoom ranges are used with extracorporeal flash. The film material should be highly sensitive and fine-grained. The photos should be sharply focused close-ups of the main subject. The middle ray of light should be directed vertically, and not tangentially. For photolaparoscopy, the sterile drape of the patient is covered with an extra sterile slit drape, so that the nonsterile photographic techniques can be carried out on top of it. Once the photos have been taken, the slit drape is removed and new sterile gloves are put on.

2.9 Directed biopsy

Providing there are no contraindications, each laparoscopy should incorporate a directed liver biopsy (H. KALK et al., 1943). This is mainly performed by making a *second incision* in the right upper abdominal region below the costal arch in the area of the right liver lobe, as a rule using a *Menghini needle*. (309)

(1.) In cases of **cirrhosis** and pronounced **fibrosis** or **scarred liver**, the danger of bleeding can be greater than the benefit of additional histological information. Moreover, use of the Menghini needle only produces crumbly liver fragments from the cirrhosis (rich in connective tissue), which are not reliable in their histological relevance (compare the fragments of fibrotic liver in chronic porphyria cutanea tarda as shown in figure 7.10!). Even without a biopsy of the cirrhosis, the requirement for objective documentation of all important findings is fully satisfied by coloured photographs. (s. figs. 7.15, 7.16)

(2.) Unclear structures can be punctured with a fine needle initially as an exploratory procedure (consistency? cyst? blood vessel?) before the Menghini needle is used. Reports have been written, for example, on the laparoscopic diagnosis of Budd-Chiari syndrome (183), liver abscesses (221), peliosis hepatis (225, 290), FNH (195, 225), Osler's disease (291), and unclarified cholestasis. (267, 286)

(3.) In all cases of doubt, or when findings of the right and left lobe of liver differ, both lobes should be biopsied (possibly at two different sites): the right lobe by using the customary second puncture, the left lobe by using a particularly long Menghini needle inserted through the operating laparoscope.

(4.) It should be noted that findings in the area of the right lobe of liver can usually be checked later by percutaneous biopsy — whereas this is not possible in the case of the left lobe.

(5.) With all difficult cases, there is a possibility of taking a second or third biopsy punch to produce a greater histological yield (e.g. in cases of granulomatous changes, haemochromatosis).

(6.) The *site of puncture* must be easy to observe. The *direction of the puncture* should be as diagonal as possible to the liver surface, mainly in the lateral (or medial cranial) part of the right lobe of liver. (s. fig. 7.8) When puncturing the left lobe, thought must be given to its significantly smaller diameter (and the danger of "piercing through").

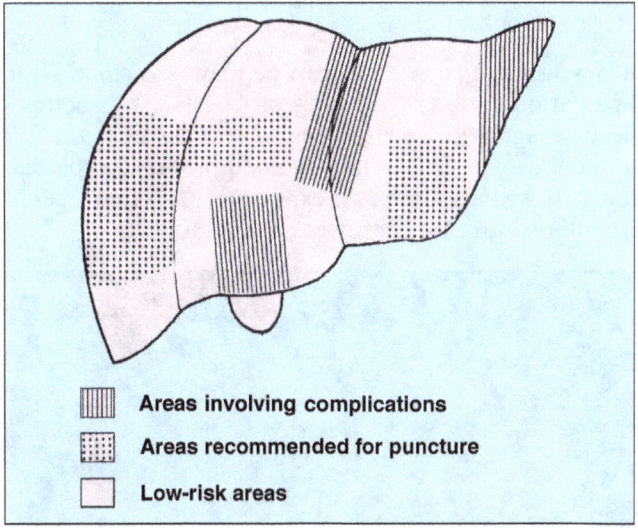

Fig. 7.8: Recommended, low-risk and contraindicated areas of puncture for liver biopsy

In cirrhosis and fibrosis, the biopsy needle used will either be the **Vim-Silverman** needle or the **Trucut** needle. Adequate tissue can thereby be obtained for assessment. Because of the increased bleeding tendency connected with these needle types, the diameter should not exceed 1.6 mm (which is generally not required anyway). The liver is punctured tangentially, mainly in the lateral area of the right lobe. Subsequent to the puncture, the stylet is removed, the outer cannula advanced, the inner needle sheath pushed forwards in a rotating movement out of the outer cannula before both are finally withdrawn together.

With circumscribed liver findings, the liver biopsy can mostly be carried out using **Robbers' forceps** (H. ROBBERS et al., 1951) (= double-spoon forceps with both lancet jaws opening). By reason of the very shallow and diagonal setting of the biopsy, there is less danger of bleeding and biliary leakage. • Occasionally, certain findings call for **combined tissue biopsy** by means of needle biopsy and forceps biopsy of the liver and/or forceps biopsy in the area of the remaining abdominal cavity.

Aftercare for each point of puncture should be continued until the bleeding has definitively stopped and delayed biliary leakage can be ruled out. Upon termination of laparoscopy, the site of puncture and the abdominal cavity as well as the point of exit of the Veres cannula must be checked for signs of bleeding. The Veres cannula should be withdrawn under observation.

Bleeding after liver biopsy generally stops spontaneously and definitively. Compression of the low-angle puncture canal (20–30°) with a (bulbous) probe can help in this respect. Further methods of arresting the bleeding include local application of thrombin solution, electrocoagulation, Heather method, BICAP technique (s. p. 357), fibrin glue injection (295), positioning of a gelatine cylinder (211), argon-plasma coagulation, and arterial embolization. (83, 112)

Biliary leakage (s. fig. 7.9) can be managed canal with a palpation probe or drawing off the bile by suction. Electrocoagulation is also deemed reliable, as is the introduction of a drain through an appropriately placed trocar. It was also our own experience (243) that operative intervention was not necessary. (118)

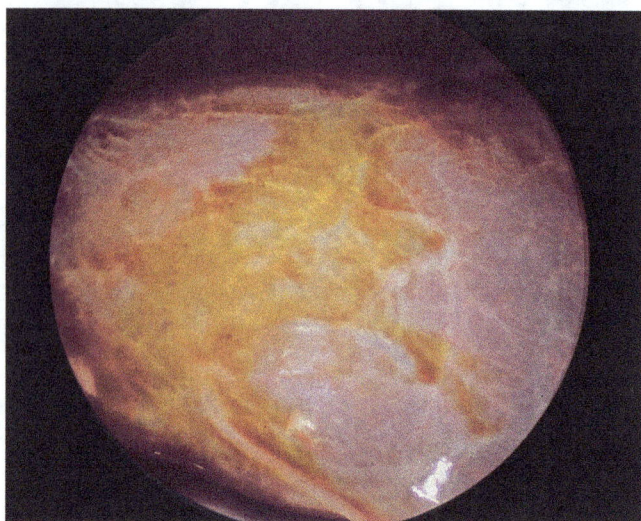

Fig. 7.9: Biliary leakage from biopsy canal after puncture

2.10 UV fluorescence

Porphyria cutanea tarda and chronic hepatic porphyria are characterized by porphyrin fluorescence in the liver cell. For every 1,000 biopsies, there are three to five red fluorescent liver specimens. Unfortunately, such UV examinations of the biopsy material are not carried out regularly. In an indeterminate diagnosis, red fluorescence can confirm chronic hepatic porphyria that has hitherto remained unidentified. (s. fig. 7.10)

After being extracted, each **biopsy specimen** should be examined in a dish with physiological NaCl solution under **UV light (366 nm)** for a period of some 15 minutes so as not to overlook the typical red fluorescence of **chronic hepatic porphyria:** *types A* and *B* only show isolated red fluorescent spots in the liver sample, *type C* (as a clinically latent form) already displays a net-like red fluorescence and *type D* (as a manifest form) a homogeneous distribution of red fluorescence. (s. fig. 7.10) • The pathologist will notice the uncharacteristic liver changes, but is not able to attribute their genesis to porphyria. (15) For this reason, chronic liver disease sometimes remain unexplained and hence "cryptogenic".

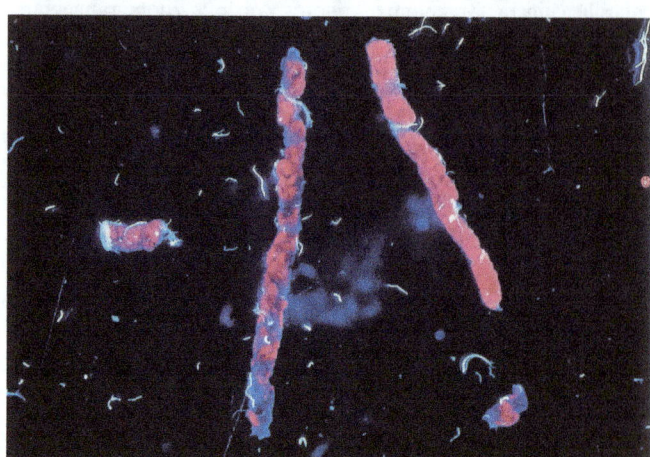

Fig. 7.10: Red fluorescent liver specimen in porphyria cutanea tarda (type D)

2.11 Extrahepatic findings

The diagnostic yield of unexpected, even surprising, extrahepatic findings is quite high at 5–10%. Among our 5,992 laparoscopies, we noted 452 such findings (= 7.5%): e.g. adhesions (s. figs. 7.1–7.3), peritoneal tuberculosis (184, 222) (s. fig. 7.11), and carcinosis (191) (s. figs. 7.6; 37.33–37.35), diverse malignomas (s. fig. 7.12), Fitz-Hugh-Curtis syndrome (s. fig. 24.2), endometriosis, myomas, ovarian cysts, Stein-Leventhal syndrome (s. fig. 7.13), Hodgkin's disease (s. fig. 38.8), chronic appendicitis, echinococcus, and so on. (243) • In cases of unexplained pain in the abdomen, laparoscopy is indicated as a last resort for clarification of the complaints. (244, 282) This is necessary above all in differential diagnosis between gynaecological disease and appendicitis. (187, 240, 308) In suspected appendicitis, appendectomy frequently proved to be the wrong decision: in 23% of cases involving young women, a gynaecological cause of complaint was found; however, in older patients (> 50 years), appendicitis was actually detected in 92–96% of cases. (187) • The clinical picture of an acute abdomen could be clarified in > 85% of cases by means of exploratory laparoscopy. (177, 256, 282) • *The opportunity of clarifying unexplained symptoms by exploratory laparoscopy should be made use of whenever possible.* At this early point, it is of no importance whether the ultimate explanation or definition of findings proves to be clinically relevant in the individual case, or is without significance. (219, 241)

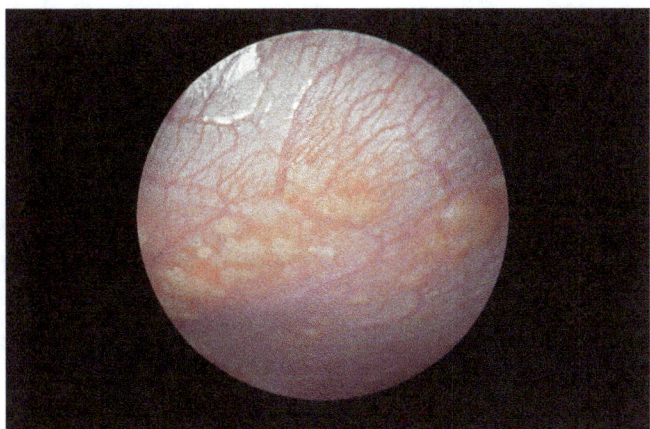

Fig. 7.11: Peritoneal tuberculosis: fever of unknown aetiology in a severe course of disease

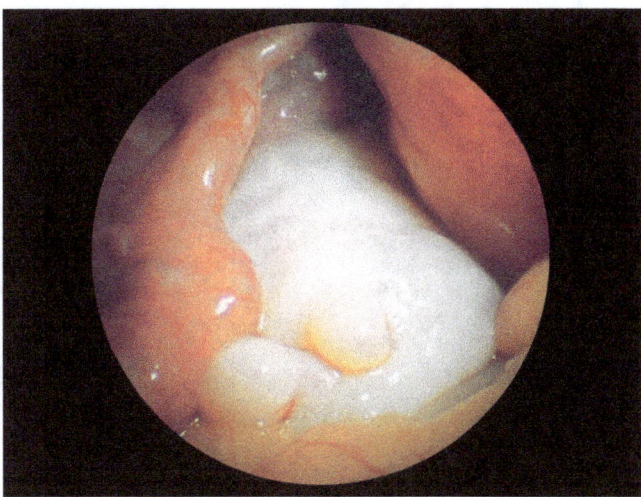

Fig. 7.13: Stein-Leventhal syndrome: white, thickened capsule of the right ovary. Clinical suspicion of pronounced liver damage due to hormone therapy

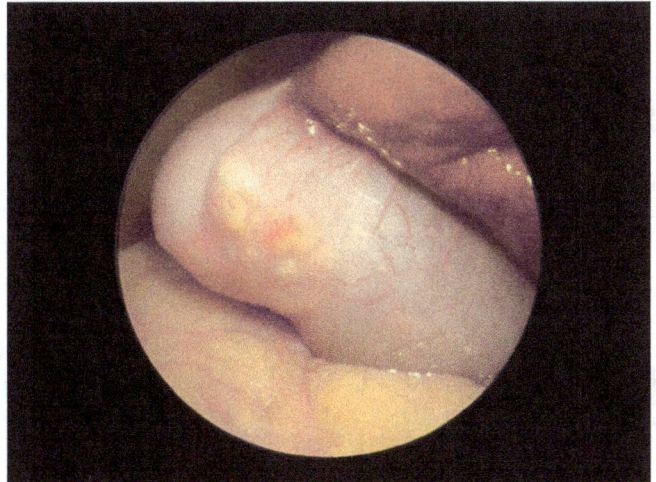

Fig. 7.12: Gall-bladder carcinoma: clinical and radiological suspicion of "cholecystopathy"

2.12 Complications

The type and frequency of complications involved in laparoscopy are determined by the same **influencing factors** as were outlined for the complication rate of percutaneous liver biopsy. (s. tab. 7.5) These factors should be considered critically and without bias.

The most frequent complication by far is **bleeding**. If this cannot be stopped conservatively, it may require surgery – or it can even prove lethal. Injuries may occur during the insertion of the *Veres cannula* and the *trocar* when vessels and varices in the abdominal wall and omentum as well as abdominal vessels have been pierced. Isolated cases of bleeding have been reported after injury to the spleen – which is perhaps understandable in splenomegaly, but nevertheless avoidable. *Liver puncture* (as well as *forceps biopsy* in the case of pathological abdominal findings) can be a further cause of bleeding, above all in cirrhosis or liver tumours.

Other *severe complications* worth mentioning include: perforation of hollow organs (gall bladder, colon, stomach, small intestine, ovarian cysts), emphysema formation due to gas insufflation, circulatory and cardiac arrhythmia, respiratory arrest, rupture of the spleen (203) and injury to the spleen (253), as well as the complications occasionally occurring with liver biopsy (haemobilia (275), haematoma, a. v. fistula (284), biliary leakage, sepsis (205), etc.). (176, 185, 206, 217, 233, 255, 262, 271) The (disturbing) occurrence of bradycardia is not usually evident when atropine is administered as routine premedication. (s. p. 161) • Among our own 5,992 laparoscopies, we recorded 58 complications (0.97%), yet no instance of death. In five cases of bleeding, operative treatment was required (0.08%). (243)

▶ During laparoscopy, we routinely maintain an intravenous *drip*. This has proved beneficial for additional sedation as well as in those cases where complications occur; it can therefore be recommended as a general principle.

2.13 Frequency of complications

Compiled statistics and publications involving a larger number of patients provide an overview of the frequency of complications and cases of death. (s. tab. 7.16) In 17 laparoscopy series covering 46,364 patients, a complication rate of 0.149% and a lethality of 0.054% were established. (262) • Occasionally, the complication rate was somewhat higher in centres with more frequent examinations: it is indeed possible that the greater the experience on the part of the physician, the more likely it is that risks are taken in evaluating contraindications. • With a decrease in the number of laparoscopies performed, however, it must be expected that laparoscopic experience will also decline, so that the incidence of complications will (unfortunately) rise – a fact which might be blamed all too easily on laparoscopy itself. Neither of these extreme situation-related developments can be ac-

Author	Total number	Complications n	%	Cases of death n	%
Brühl, W. (1966)*	63,845	1,595	2.49	19	0.029
Look, D. (1975)*	21,387	336	1.57	3	0.014
Paolaggi, J. A. et al. (1976)*	34,597	176	0.51	33	0.09
Silvis, St. E. et al. (1976)	4,404	31	0.70	1	0.02
Wittmann, J. et al. (1979)	2,322	7	0.30	1	0.04
Takemoto, T. et al. (1980)*	31,652	300	0.95	24	0.076
Manenti, A. et al. (1980)*	3,000	49	1.66	4	0.133
Henning, H. et al. (1985)*	46,364	69	0.15	25	0.054
Kuntz, E. (1987)	5,992	58	0.97	–	–
Marti-Vicente, A. et al. (1992)	8,915	54	0.60	10	0.11
Vargas, C. et al. (1995)	1,715	39	2.15	1	0.06
	224,193	2,665	1.19	121	0.054

Tab. 7.16: Frequency of laparoscopic complications and cases of death (* = compiled statistics)

cepted. • Some of the complications observed in the past (193, 230, 271, 293) should not really be expected today, given modern technical possibilities. Some statistics not only included severe complications, but also harmless ones, a fact which explains the differences in percentages. • The frequency of *more severe complications* is **0.15—0.80%,** the *total rate* of significant complications can be put at **< 1.0%.** Based on compiled statistics, the lethality rate is up to **0.07%.** • Some **0.08—0.2%** of complications required *operative intervention.* • Registration of all complications (even slight or harmless events) resulted in a complication rate of 3.0% (255) and 4.87% (217). • In 6,000 laparoscopies of our own, the complication rate was 0.97%, with a mortality rate of 0%. (243) • Out of 20,000 laparoscopies, the largest number ever registered in one hospital, E. WILDHIRT reported just 2 cases of death (0.01%). • The largest number of laparoscopies to be performed in a single hospital is believed to be over 50,000 (R. LLANIO et al., Habana/Cuba) *(personal communication).*

2.14 Diagnostic validity

The accuracy of histological diagnosis depends on (*1.*) the *biopsy specimen* being large enough (> 1.5 cm, 5—10 portal fields) as well as being definitively assessable (1, 63, 94, 143, 165) and (*2.*) whether the specimen can be deemed to be *representative for the liver* — bearing in mind that the usual weight of a biopsy punch amounts to 20—30 mg (i. e. 1/75,000 to 1/50,000) of the total liver. • It depends equally on the *hepatological experience* of the investigating pathologist and on the findings available to him (possibly including a Polaroid photograph of the liver!). • It was shown in a study that when the histological result was double-checked by a pathologist with extensive experience in hepatology, there was complete agreement only in 34.4%, considerable discrepancy in 28.0% and slight discrepancy in 37.6% of cases. (6)

Diffuse liver diseases: Histological findings of the biopsy specimen are generally considered to be representative for the given liver disease. The accuracy of percutaneous bioptic diagnosis is 80 to 100%. • The colour of the biopsy specimen, which varies from pale yellow (fatty liver) to greenish-black (metastasis of melanoma), may give a hint of the respective underlying disease. (s. fig. 7.14) (27, 104, 106, 108, 212, 227, 247, 273, 301, 303)

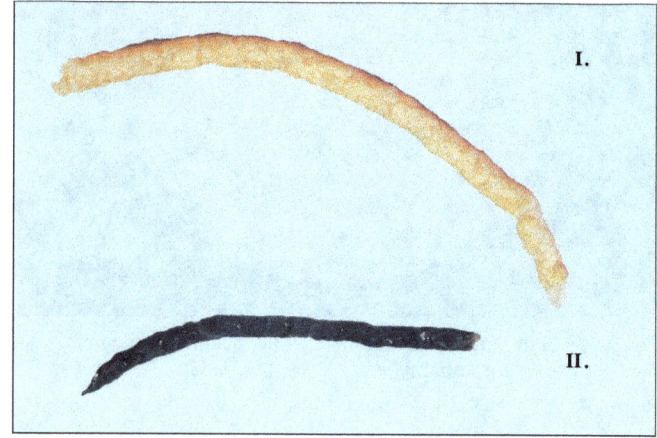

Fig. 7.14: Liver biopsy specimens: I. in fatty liver (pale yellow), II. in a metastasis of a malignant melanoma (greenish-black) (s. fig. 7.10)

Focal liver diseases: Biopsy material cannot be guaranteed as being representative in every case. A higher degree of diagnostic accuracy can be achieved by a two- to threefold liver biopsy in the course of a laparoscopic-bioptic examination of both lobes of liver. The same is true for peliosis hepatis (225, 270), granulomas and chronic hepatitis C, for example. (117)

▶ **Cirrhosis:** In cases of cirrhosis, consideration must be given to the fact that the condition relates to the entire liver — yet not necessarily to each lobular area. For this reason, micronodular cirrhosis is generally better targeted (95%) than macronodular cirrhosis (60%). (84) Under certain circumstances, the biopsy of a large regenerative node can lead to the (understandably) wrong diagnosis of a "practically normal liver parenchyma". *Consequently, the false-negative rate with percutaneous biopsy of cirrhosis lies between 9.3% and 51%* (84, 192,

220, 227, 237, 243, 261, 270, 276, 301, 302, 314) and can even be as high as 80% if the yield is smaller than 5 mm. (63) This high error rate is caused by the Menghini needle slipping off the cirrhotic connective tissue and penetrating the neighbouring soft regenerations. The Menghini technique usually only produces *crumbly fragments* of a cirrhotic liver, since fibrous tissue septa remain in the liver, rather like the panicles of a stripped leaf. Such fragments generally suggest the presence of cirrhosis, even if the pathologist is unable to make a definitive diagnosis. (s. figs. 7.15, 7.16) • *A percutaneous bioptic diagnosis of cirrhosis is not acceptable because of the wide margin of error and the greater risks involved with the biopsy. Laparoscopy with its additional techniques – now deemed to be the gold standard – ought to be performed instead.* • The diagnosis of liver cirrhosis, and its differentiation from fibrosis and scarred liver, can as a rule be reliably established by looking closely at the surface of the liver ("glance diagnosis"). Findings should also be documented by colour photography. (s. figs. 14.3; 16.4, 16.5; 21.9; 24.2, 24.5; 31.22; 32.5; 33.4; 35.2, 35.4, 35.8, 35.17, and others)

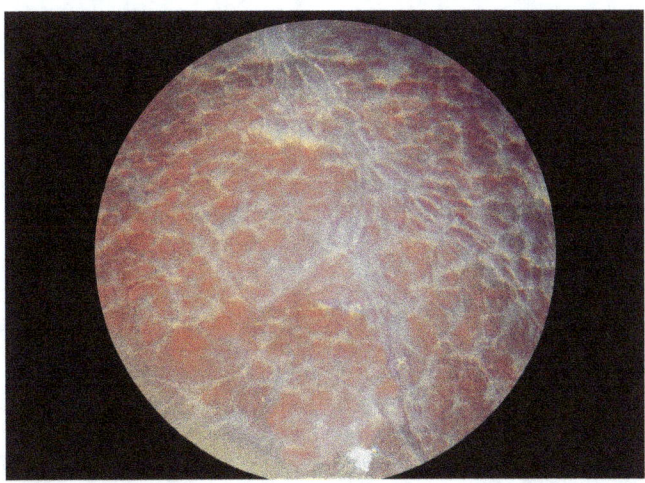

Fig. 7.16: Inactive, micronodular (drug-related) cirrhosis with fine pathways of connective tissue; clinically and histologically definable as "liver fibrosis" (sonographically no signs of portal hypertension)

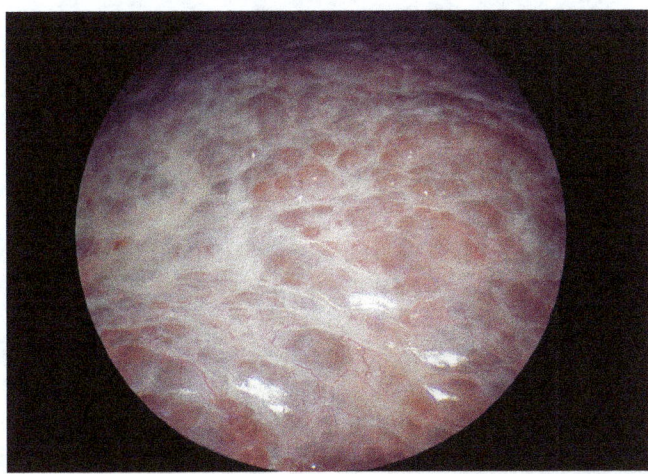

Fig. 7.15: Active, micronodular, in part moderately nodular (alcohol-related) cirrhosis with pronounced pathways of postnecrotic connective tissue

Due to their cutting action (which differs from the Menghini technique), **Vim-Silverman** and **Trucut needles** produce a sufficiently large and almost intact cirrhosis tissue sample. As a consequence, the false-positive results can be brought down to below 10%. Nevertheless, the risk of subsequent bleeding is clearly higher. For this reason, the diameter of the needle should definitely not exceed 1.6 mm.

▶ The combined examination with **laparoscopy** and **directed biopsy** (thick- or fine-needle biopsy or use of Robbers' forceps) yields the greatest diagnostic accuracy at 97–100%. This has been impressively confirmed in *children* as well. • Foci not visible by laparoscopy can be detected by ultrasound- or CT-guided biopsy and fine-needle puncture. Occasionally, an existing liver disease cannot be differentiated morphologically, simply because biopsy is contraindicated.

▶ Laparoscopy is particularly significant in differentiating between **benign** or **malignant foci,** such as adenoma with malignant degeneration (s. fig. 29.14), haemangioma (s. figs. 36.8, 36.9), focal nodular hyperplasia (s. fig. 29.12), Hodgkin's disease (313) (s. fig. 38.8), carcinoma in cirrhosis (232) (s. fig. 37.9), metastases in the area of the liver, ligaments or serosa (s. figs. 37.24, 37.33, 37.34, 37.35), etc. Exploratory laparotomy, which was mostly used in the past, is now obsolete. • In such cases, there is no need to perform "one-second needle biopsy" – just **"one-second glance diagnosis"** might well be fully sufficient for an exact assessment. *(see chapters 36 and 37)*

▶ The **cost factor** must likewise be considered; in Germany, for example, laparoscopy is very reasonable at about 75 US dollars as compared to scintigraphy (approx. 130 US dollars), CT (approx. 240 US dollars) and MRT (approx. 400 US dollars).

▶ From the point of view of hepatological **detailed diagnosis,** it is necessary to carry out liver biopsy, laparoscopy or fine-needle biopsy, depending on the diagnostic issue in question. They are part of the diagnostic routine of a clinical hepatologist. A high degree of experience resulting from the routine performance of laparoscopy also guarantees a maximum of diagnostic findings in combination with a minimum of complications. • In this connection, a **laparoscopic training programme** has proved most useful. (272, 299) Such programmes might help in future to revive laparoscopy as a routine method of investigation – even under outpatient conditions.

3 New technical progress

▶ With the help of fibre optics it has been possible to develop much smaller instruments with a diameter of 2 mm (max. 2.75 mm) – so-called **mini-laparoscopy**. (s. fig. 7.18) Clinically speaking, this revolutionary technique has stood the test in an excellent manner. (224) This also applies to the field of hepatology, especially concerning high-risk patients. (215, 216, 258, 287) The lighting conditions are still not completely satisfactory and illumination is often insufficient. Up to now, only prograde optics have been available (cf. **conventional laparoscopy** with side-vision and angle optics). (s. fig. 7.17) Nevertheless, we now have a minimally invasive, elegant and safe technique for exploratory laparoscopy and targeted biopsy at our disposal. This new technique will signify the renaissance of laparoscopy, probably also under outpatient conditions.

▶ The introduction of **laparoscopic sonography** has opened up new diagnostic possibilities. (s. p. 135) (s. tab. 7.10) This applies above all to the detection of intrahepatic metastases, lymphnodular metastases and changes in the vascular system. In 46% of patients, new insight was gained, which led to a modification of therapy in 40% of cases. (210) In 10% of patients, intrahepatic metastases, some with a diameter of <1 cm, were discovered with the help of this technique, even in segments 3 and 4 (H. Foroutani et al., 2000).

▶ It is to be expected that by means of **light-induced fluorescence diagnostics**, further improvements in the differentiation of morphological findings will be achieved in the future.

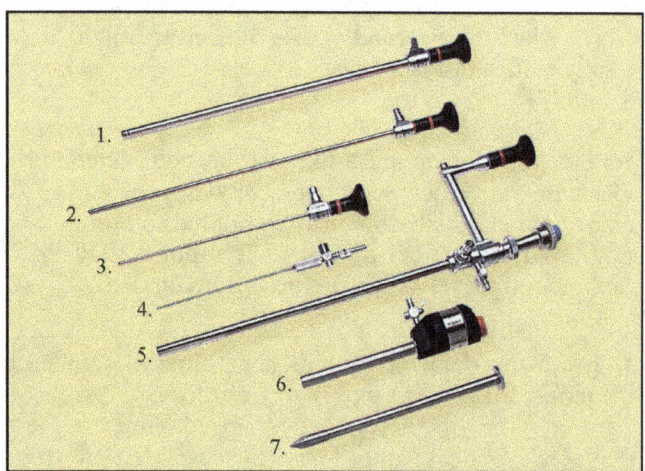

Fig. 7.17: *Conventional laparoscopy equipment:* (*1.*) laparoscope, ⌀ 10 mm, distortion-free, angle of view 0°, working length 300 mm; (*2.*) laparoscope, ⌀ 5.3 mm, distortion-free, angle of view 25°, working length 300 mm; (*3.*) laparoscope ⌀ 3.5 mm, working length 180 mm; (*4.*) Veres cannula including Luer connector, working length 120 mm; (*5.*) operating laparoscope, ⌀ 10 mm, distortion-free, with right-angled eyepiece, 5 mm working channel, with detachable automatic instrument valves, angle of view 0°, working length 265 mm; (*6.*) trocar sleeve, with insufflation tap and magnetic-ball valve, metal sleeve standard, straight distal tip, working length 100 mm; (*7.*) trocar, pyramidal tip (autoclavable)

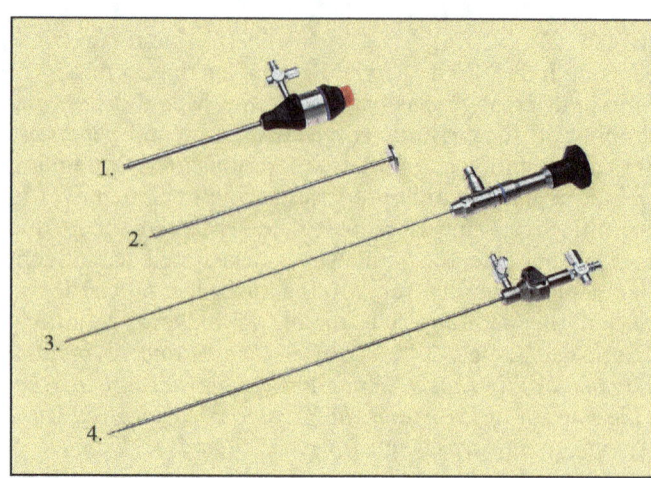

Fig. 7.18: *Mini-laparoscopy equipment:* (*1.*) trocar sleeve, ⌀ 5.5 mm, with insufflation tap and magnetic-ball valve; (*2.*) trocar, conical tip; (*3.*) minifibre laparoscope, ⌀ 2 mm, angle of view 0°, working length 270 mm; (*4.*) Veres cannula, ⌀ 2.3 mm, with outer sheath, working length 270 mm (autoclavable)

4 Synopsis and recommendation

During laparoscopy, there is something like personal contact with the pathological finding. For me, in the course of more than 6,000 laparoscopies, this feeling was always an enrichment regarding the relationship between doctor and patient.

No other procedure provides a finding which is so true to colour and so impressive in detail as that performed by the eye of the laparoscopist.

Only laparoscopy makes it possible to carry out targeted (or occasionally multiple) biopsy in both liver lobes. Particularly in chronic hepatitis, such a procedure improves diagnostic safety considerably, because this disease is often not equally pronounced in all parts of the liver. Furthermore, the small area which can be accessed by percutaneous biopsy is not necessarily representative of the liver as a whole!

As a rule, numerous findings pertaining to liver surface, peritoneum, omentum and ligaments are easily recognized with the laparoscopic eye; in most cases, they can be attributed to a corresponding diagnosis and histologically verified with the help of targeted biopsy. This is simply not possible with other procedures.

Using Robbers forceps, the laparoscopist is able to extract optimal tissue for the pathologist from small focal lesions of the liver surface, which is not possible with percutaneous biopsy or imaging-guided biopsy. The search for metastases by means of all available methods can be improved by laparoscopy to a considerable extent. This may be of decisive importance for later therapy.

The risks involved in laparoscopy when carried out by an experienced team are minimal; statistically speaking, they are "less than making the journey to the hospital by car" (this also applies to imaging techniques).

The costs of laparoscopy are in every respect (acquisition, maintenance, personnel, clinical application) far lower than with CT, MRT, etc.

▶ Every department of hepatology really ought to have an experienced laparoscopy team! The indication for laparoscopy is given in those cases where no certain diagnosis has been reached by means of imaging procedures – provided, of course, that there is a good chance of success. All findings should be archived with the help of photodocumentation and verified histologically by means of biopsy. The ultimate aim is to achieve a combined assessment based on macroscopic and microscopic morphology.

References:

Leberbiopsie

1. **Amaral, J.G., Schwartz, J., Chait, P., Temple, M., John, P., Smith, C., Taylor, G., Connolly, B.:** Sonographically guided percutaneous liver biopsy in infants: A retrospective review. Amer. J. Roentgenol. 2006; 187: 644–649
2. **Asselah, T., Condat, B., Sibert, A., Rivet, P., Lebray, P., Bernuau, J., Benhamou, J.P., Erlinger, S., Marcellin, P., Valla, D.:** Haemobilia causing acute pancreatitis after percutaneous liver biopsy: Diagnosis by magnetic resonance cholangiopancreatography. Europ. J. Gastroenterol. Hepatol. 2001; 13: 877–879
3. **Axenfeld, H., Brass, K.:** Klinische und bioptische Untersuchungen über den sogenannten Icterus catarrhalis. Frankfurt. Z. Pathol. 1942; 57: 147–236
4. **Azoulay, D., Raccuia, J.S., Roche, B., Reynes, M., Bismuth, H.:** The value of early transjugular liver biopsy after liver transplantation. Transplant. 1996; 61: 406–409
5. **Baron, E.:** Aspiration for removal of biopsy material from the liver. Arch. Intern. Med. 1939; 63: 276–289
6. **Bejarano, P.A., Koehler, A., Sherman, K.E.:** Second opinion pathology in liver biopsy interpretation. Amer. J. Gastroenterol. 2001; 96: 3158–3164
7. **Ben-Itzhak, J., Bassan, H.M.:** Subphrenic abscess following percutaneous liver needle biopsy. Israel J. Med. Sci. 1983; 19: 356–358
8. **Bingel, A.:** Über die Parenchympunktion der Leber. Verh. Dtsch. Ges. Inn. Med. 1923; 35: 210–212
9. **Bissonnette, R.T., Gibney, R.G., Berry, B.R., Buckley, A.R.:** Fatal carcinoid crisis after percutaneous fine-needle biopsy of hepatic metastasis: case report and literature review. Radiology 1990; 174: 751–752
10. **Borzio, M., Borzio, F., Macchi, R., Croce, A.M., Bruno, S., Ferrari, A., Servida, E.:** The evaluation of fine-needle procedures for the diagnosis of focal liver lesions in cirrhosis. J. Hepatol. 1994; 20: 117–121
11. **Bravo, A.A., Sheth, S.G., Chopra, S.:** Liver biopsy. New Engl. J. Med. 2001; 344: 495–500
12. **Brenard, R., Horsmans, Y., Rahier, J., Druez, P., Descamps, C., Geubel, A.:** Transjugular liver biopsy. An experience based on 500 procedures. Acta Gastroenterol. Belg. 1997; 60: 138–141
13. **Bruzzi, J.F., O'Connell, M.J., Thakore, H., O'Keane, C., Crowe, J., Murray, J.G.:** Transjugular liver biopsy: assessment of safety and efficacy of the Quick-Core biopsy needle. Abdom. Imag. 2002; 27: 711–715
14. **Cadranel, J.F., Rufat, P., Degos, F.:** Practices of liver biopsy in France: Results of a prospective nationwide survey. Hepatology 2000; 32: 477–481
15. **Campo, E., Bruguera, M., Rodes, J.:** Are there diagnostic histologic features of porphyria cutanea tarda in liver biopsy specimens? Liver 1990; 10: 185–190
16. **Cash, J.M., Swain, M., di Bisceglie, A.M., Wilder, R.L., Crofford, L.J.:** Massive intrahepatic hemorrhage following routine liver biopsy in a patient with rheumatoid arthritis treated with methotrexate. J. Rheumatol. 1992; 19: 1466–1468
17. **Caturelli, E., Squillante, M.M., Andriulli, A., Siena, D.A., Cellerino, C., de Luca, F., Marzano, M.A., Pompili, M., Rapaccini, G.L.:** Fine-needle liver biopsy in patients with severely impaired coagulation. Liver 1993; 13: 270–273
18. **Caturelli, E., Giacobbe, A., Facciorusso, D., Bisceglia, M., Villani, M.R., Siena, D.A., Fusilli, S., Sqillante, M.M., Andriulli, A.:** Percutaneous biopsy in diffuse liver disease; increasing diagnostic yield and decreasing complication rate by routine ultrasound assessment of puncture site. Amer. J. Gastroenterol. 1996; 91: 1318–1321
19. **Charboneau, J.W., Reading, C.C., Welch, T.J.:** CT and sonographically guided needle biopsy: current techniques and new innovations. Amer. J. Roentgenol. 1990; 154: 1–10
20. **Chau, T.N., Tong, S.W., Li, T.M., To, H.T., Lee, K.C., Lai, J.Y., Lai, S.T., Yuen, H.:** Transjugular liver biopsy with an automated trucut-type needle: comparative study with percutaneous liver biopsy. Europ. J. Gastroenterol. Hepatol. 2002; 14: 19–24
21. **Chawla, Y.K., Ramesh, G.N., Kaur, U., Bambery, P., Dilawari, J.B.:** Percutaneous liver biopsy: a safe outpatient procedure. J. Gastroenterol. Hepatol. 1990; 5: 94–95
22. **Chezmar, J.L., Keith, L.L., Nelson, R.C., Plaire, J.C., Hertzler, G.L., Bernardino, M.E.:** Liver transplant biopsies with a biopsy gun. Radiology 1991; 179: 447–448
23. **Chuah, S.Y., Moody, G.A., Wicks, A.C.B., Mayberry, J.F.:** A nationwide survey of liver biopsy–is there a need to increase resources, manpower and training? Hepato- Gastroenterol. 1994; 41: 4–8
24. **Cohen, M.B., A-Kader, H.H., Lambers, D., Heubi, J.E.:** Complications of percutaneous liver biopsy in children. Gastroenterology 1992; 102: 629–632
25. **Colombo, M., del Ninno, E., de Franchis, R., de Fazio, C., Festorazzi, S., Ronchi, G., Tommasini, M.A.:** Ultrasound- assisted percutaneous liver biopsy: superiority of the true-cut over the Menghini needle for diagnosis of cirrhosis. Gastroenterology 1988; 95: 487–489
26. **Conn, H.O.:** Liver biopsy: increased risks in patients with cancer. Hepatology 1991; 14: 206–209
27. **Czaja, A.J., Carpenter, H.A.:** Sensitivity, specificity, and predactibility of biopsy interpretations in chronic hepatitis. Gastroenterology 1993; 105: 1824–1832
28. **Decker, R., Hofmann, W., Buhr, H.:** Galleembolie der Lunge nach intraoperativer Leberfeinnadelbiopsie. Fallbericht und Literaturübersicht. Chirurg 1985; 56: 666–669
29. **Decking, R.:** Die perkutane Leberbiopsie bei ambulanten Patienten. Z. Gastroenterol. 1991; 29: 311–312
30. **De Hojos, A., Loredo, M.L., Martinez-Rios, M.A., Gil, M.R., Kuri, J., Cardenas, M.:** Transjugular liver biopsy in 52 patients with an automated Trucut-type needle. Dig. Dis. Sci. 1999; 44: 177–180
31. **Dible, J.H., McMichael, J., Sherlock, S.:** Pathology of acute hepatitis: aspiration biopsy studies of epidemic, arsenotherapy and serum jaundice. Lancet 1943; 245: 402–408
32. **Dinkel, H.-P., Wittchen, K., Hoppe, H., Dufour, J.-F., Zimmermann, A., Triller, J.:** Transjugular liver core biopsy : indications, results and complications. Fortschr. Röntgenstr. 2003; 175: 1112–1119
33. **Donaldson, B.W., Gopinath, R., Wanless, I.R., Phillips, M.J., Cameron, R., Roberts, E.A., Greig, P.D., Levy, G., Blendis, L.M.:** The role of transjugular liver biopsy in fulminant liver failure: relation to other prognostic indicators. Hepatology 1993; 18: 1370–1374
34. **Douds, A.C., Joseph, A.E.A., Finlayson, C., Maxwell, J.D.:** Is day case liver biopsy underutilised? Gut 1995; 37: 574–575
35. **Duchmann, J.-C., Joly, J.-P.:** Ponction échoguidée ambulatoire en pathologie tumorale abdominale. Etude de 131 cas. Gastroenterol. Clin. Biol. 1996; 20: 258–262
36. **Edoute, Y., Tibon-Fisher, O., Ben Haim, S., Malberger, E.:** Ultrasonically guided fine-needle aspiration of liver lesions. Amer. J. Gastroenterol. 1992; 87: 1138–1141
37. **Ewe, K.:** Bleeding after liver biopsy does not correlate with indices of peripheral coagulation. Dig. Dis. Sci. 1981; 26: 388–393
38. **Feist, D., Rossner, J.A., Stefan, H.:** Indikationen und Ergebnisse der percutanen Leberbiopsie im Kindesalter. Mschr. Kinderheilk. 1972; 120: 491–498
39. **Fornari, F., Filice, C., Rapaccini, G.L., Caturelli, E., Cavanna, L., Civardi, G., di Stasi, M., Buscarini, E., Buscarini, L.:** Small (≤ 3 cm) hepatic lesions. Results of sonographically guided fine-needle biopsy in 385 patients. Dig. Dis. Sci. 1994; 39: 2267–2275
40. **Forné, M., Panés, J., Viver, J.M., Marco, C.:** Hemobilia por fistula arteriovenosa hepaticoportal secundaria a biopsia hepatica. Revision de la literatura. Gastroenterol. Hepatologia 1989; 12: 349–354
41. **Frank, R., Leodolter, I.:** Praktische Erfahrungen mit der ambulanten Leberbiopsie. Wien. Klin. Wschr. 1966; 78: 756–758
42. **Froehlich, F., Lamy, O., Fried, M., Gonvers, J.J.:** Practice and complications of liver biopsy. Results of a nationwide survey in Switzerland. Dig. Dis. Sci. 1993; 38: 1480–1484
43. **Furuya, K.N., Burrows, P.E., Phillips, M.J., Roberts, E.A.:** Transjugular liver biopsy in children. Hepatology 1992; 15: 1036–1042
44. **Galati, J.S., Monsour, H.P., Donovan, J.P., Zetterman, R.K., Schafer, D.F., Langnas, A.N., Shaw, B.W.jr., Sorrell, M.F.:** The nature of complications following liver biopsy in transplant patients with Roux-en-Y choledochojejunostomy. Hepatology 1994; 20: 651–653
45. **Gamble, P., Colapinto, R.F., Stronell, R.D., Colman, J.C., Blendis, L.:** Transjugular liver biopsy: a review of 461 biopsies. Radiology 1985; 157: 589–593
46. **Gamble, R.D., Sullivan, B.H. jr.:** Needle biopsy of the liver. Clinical evaluation of 323 biopsies; report of two cases of accidental biopsy of the gallbladder. Gastroenterology 1953; 24: 394–404

47. Garcia-Tsao, G., Boyer, J.L.: Outpatient liver biopsy: how safe is it? Ann. Intern. Med. 1993; 118: 150–153
48. Giger, A., Reichen, J.: Die Leberbiopsie bei ambulanten Patienten. Schweiz. Med. Wschr. 1993; 123: 1474–1481
49. Gilmore, I.T., Burroughs, A., Murray-Lyon, I.M., Williams, R., Jenkins, D., Hopkins, A.: Indications, methods, and outcomes of percutaneous liver biopsy in England and Wales: an audit by the British Society of Gastroenterology and the Royal College of Physicians of London. Gut 1995; 36: 437–441
50. Glaser, J., Mann, O., Siegmüller, M., Pausch, J.: Prospective study of the incidence of ultrasound-detected hepatic hematomas due to percutaneous Menghini needle liver biopsy and laparoscopy–guided Silverman needle biopsy. Ital. J. Gastroenterol. 1994; 26: 338–341
51. Gonzalez-Vallina, R., Alonso, E.M., Rand, E., Black, D. D., Whitington, P.F.: Outpatient percutaneous liver biopsy in children. J. Pediatr. Gastroenterol. Nutrit. 1993; 17: 370–375
52. Greiner, L., Franken, F.A.: Die sonographisch assistierte Leberbiopsie – Ablösung der blinden Leberpunktion? Dtsch. Med. Wschr. 1983; 108: 368–372
53. Grijm, R., Tytgat, G.N., van der Schoot, J.B., van Royen, E.: Bile leakage after liver biopsy and its diagnosis by HIDA-scan. Neth. J. Med. 1984; 27: 408–411
54. Gunneson, T.J., Menon, K.V.N., Wiesner, R.H., Daniels, J.A., Hay, J.E., Charlton, M.R., Brandhagen, D.J., Rosen, C.B., Porayko, M.K.: Ultrasound-assisted percutaneous liver biopsy performed by a physician assistant. Amer. J. Gastroenterol. 2002; 97: 1472–1475
55. Ha, H.K., Sachs, P.B., Haaga, J.R., Abdul-Karim, F.: CT- guided liver biopsy: an update. Clin. Imag. 1991; 15: 99–104
56. Habdank, K., Restrepo, R., Ng, V., Connolly, B.L., Temple, M.J., Amaral, J., Chait, P.G.: Combined sonography and fluoroscopic guidance during transjugular hepatic biopsies performed in children: A retrospective study of 74 biopsies. Amer. J. Roentgenol. 2003; 180: 1393–1998
57. Hederström, E., Forsberg, L., Floren, C.-H., Prytz, H.: Liver biopsy complications monitored by ultrasound. J. Hepatol. 1989; 8: 94–98
58. Hertzanu, Y., Peiser, J., Klin, H.: Massive bleeding after fine needle aspiration of liver angiosarcoma. Gastrointest. Radiol. 1990; 15: 43–46
59. Hjelms, E., Pedersen, T.: Komplikationer ved 583 lever-biopsier a.m. Menghini. Nordisk Med. 1970; 84: 978–981
60. Hodgson, R.S., Taylor-Robinson, S.D. Jackson, J.E.: Haematochezia in Crohn's disease caused by late-onset haemobilia following percutaneous liver biopsy (case report). Eur. J. Gastroenterol. Hepatol. 2004; 16: 229–232
61. Hollerbach, S., Willert, J., Topalidis, T., Reiser, M., Schmiegel, W.: Endoscopic ultrasound-guided fine-needle aspiration biopsy of liver lesions: Histological and cytological assessment Endoscopy 2003; 35: 743–749
62. Holtz, T., Moseley, R.H., Scheiman, J.M.: Liver biopsy in fever of unknown origin. A reappraisal. J. Clin. Gastroenterol. 1993; 17: 29–32
63. Holund, B., Poulsen, H., Schlichting, P.: Reproducibility of liver biopsy diagnosis in relation to the size of the specimen. Scand. J. Gastroenterol. 1980; 15: 329–335
64. Huard, P., May, J.M., Joyeux, B.: La ponction biopsie du foie et son utilité dans le diagnostic des affections hepatiques. Ann. Anat. Path. Norm. Med.-chir. 1993; 12: 1118–1124
65. Hultcrantz, R., Gabrielsson, N.: Patients with persistent elevation of aminotransferases: investigation with ultrasonography, radionucleide imaging and liver biopsy. J. Intern. Med. 1993; 233: 7–12
66. Hyun, C.B., Beutel, V.J.: Prospective randomized trial of post-liver biopsy recovery positions – Does positioning really matter? J. Clin. Gastroenterol. 2005; 39: 328–332
67. Iversen, P., Roholm, K.: On aspiration biopsy of the liver, with remarks on its diagnostic significance. Acta Med. Scand. 1939; 102: 1–16
68. Jabbour, N., Reyes, J., Zajko, A., Nour, B., Tzakis, A.G., Starzl, T.E., van Thiel, D.H.: Arterioportal fistula following liver biopsy. Three cases occurring in liver transplant recipients. Dig. Dis. Sci. 1995; 40: 1041–1044
69. Jackson, J.E., Adam, A., Allison, D.J.: Transjugular and plugged liver biopsies. Clin. Gastroenterol. 1992; 6: 245–258
70. Janes, Ch.H., Lindor, K.D.: Outcome of patients hospitalized for complications after outpatient liver biopsy. Ann. Intern. Med. 1993; 118: 96–98
71. Jenkins, D., Gilmore, I.T., Doel, C., Gallivan, S.: Liver biopsy in the diagnosis of maligny. Q. J. Med. 1995; 88: 819–825
72. Joly, J.-P., Khouani, S., Decrombeque, C., Razafimahaleo, A., Sevestre, H., Capron, J.-P.: La ponction-biopsie hépatique échoguidée pourrait remplacer la ponction-biopsie à l'aveugle dans les hépatopathies diffuses. Gastroenterol. Clin. Biol. 1995; 19: 703–706
73. Josefson, A.: Diagnosis through small particles. Acta Med. Scand. 1920; 53: 770–773
74. Kettenbach, J., Blum, M., El-RaBadi, K., Langenberger, H., Happel, B., Berger, J., Ba-Ssalamah, A.: Perkutane Leberbiopsie. Übersicht über verschiedene Verfahren. Der Radiologe 2005; 45: 44–54
75. Khosa, F., McNulty, J.G., Hickey, N., O'Brien, P., Tobin, A., Noonan, N., Keeling, P.W.N., Kelleher, P.P., McDonald, G.S.A.: Transvenous liver biopsy via the femoral vein. Clin. Radiol. 2003; 58: 487–491
76. Knauer, C.M.: Percutaneous biopsy of the liver as a procedure for outpatients. Gastroenterology 1978; 74: 101–102
77. Kofler, W.: Die Leberpunktion als brauchbare und wertvolle klinische Untersuchungsmethode. Z. Klin. Med. 1940; 138: 744–755
78. Kowdley, K.V., Aggarwal, A.M., Sachs, P.B.: Delayed hemorrhage after percutaneous liver biopsy. Role of therapeutic angiography. J. Clin. Gastroenterol. 1994; 19: 50–53
79. Lankisch, P.G., Thiele, E., Mahlke, R., Lübbers, H., Riesner, K.: Prospective study of the incidence of ultrasound-detected hepatic hematomas 2 and 24 hours after percutaneous liver biopsy. Z. Gastroenterol. 1990; 28: 247–250
80. Lebrec, D., Goldfarb. G., Degott, C., Rueff, B., Benhamou, J.-P.: Transvenous liver biopsy. An experience based on 1000 hepatic tissue samplings with this procedure. Gastroenterology 1982; 83: 338–340
81. Leeuwen, van, D.J., Wilson, L., Crowe, D.R.: Liver biopsy in the mid-1990s: questions and answers. Semin. Liver Dis. 1995; 15: 340–359
82. Levinson, J.D., Olsen, G., Terman, J.W., Cleaveland, C.R., Graham, C.P.jr., Breen, K.J.: Hemobilia secondary to percutaneous liver biopsy. Arch. Intern. Med. 1972; 130: 396–400
83. Lichtenstein, D.R., Ducksoo Kim, Chopra, S.: Delayed massive hemobilia following percutaneous liver biopsy: treatment by embolotherapy. Amer. J. Gastroenterol. 1992; 87: 1833–1838
84. Lindenfelser; R., Breining, H.: Diagnostische Zuverlässigkeit der Leberpunktion bei Zirrhose. Med. Klin. 1970; 65: 2021–2025
85. Lindner, H.: Das Risiko der perkutanen Leberbiopsie. Med. Klin. 1971; 66: 924–929
86. Lindner, H.: Die Technik der perkutanen Leberbiopsie nach Menghini. Dtsch. Med. Wschr. 1971; 96: 1766–1770
87. Lindner, H.: Grenzen und Gefahren der perkutanen Leberbiopsie mit der Menghini-Nadel: Erfahrungen bei 80.000 Leberbiopsien. Dtsch. Med. Wschr. 1967; 92: 1751–1757
88. Lindor, K.D., Bru, C., Jorgensen, R.A., Rakela, J., Bordas, J.M., Gross, J.B., Rodes, J., McGill, D.B., Reading, C.C., James, E.M., Charboneau, J.W., Ludwig, J., Batts, K.P., Zinsmeister, A.R.: The role of ultrasonography and automatic-needle biopsy in outpatient percutaneous liver biopsy. Hepatology 1996; 23: 1079–1083
89. Lipchik, E.O., Cohen, E.B., Mewissen, M.W.: Transvenous liver biopsy in critically ill patients: adequacy of tissue samples. Radiology 1991; 181: 497–499
90. Ludwig, J., Batts, K.P., Moyer, T.P., Baldus, W.P., Fairbanks, V.F.: Liver biopsy diagnosis of homozygous hemochromatosis: a diagnostic algorithm. Mayo Clin. Proc. 1993; 68: 263–267
91. Lüning, M., Schröder, K., Wolff, H., Kranz, D., Hoppe, E.: Percutaneous biopsy of the liver. Cardiovasc. Intervent. Radiol. 1991; 14: 40–42
92. Machicao, V.I., Lukens, F.J., Lange, S.M., Scolapio, J.S.: Arterioportal fistula causing acute pancreatitis and hemobilia after liver biopsy. J. Clin. Gastroenterol. 2002; 34: 481–484
93. Mahal, A.S., Knauer, C.M., Gregory, P.B.: Bleeding after liver biopsy: how often and why? Gastroenterology 1979; 76: 1192
94. Maharaj, B., Maharaj, R.J., Leary, W.P., Naran, A.D., Cooppan, R.M., Pirie, D., Pudifin, D.J.: Sampling variability and its influence on the diagnostic yield of percutaneous needle biopsy of the liver. Lancet 1986/I: 523–525
95. Malchow, H., Röllinghoff, W.: Die Bedeutung der Leberbiopsie bei der Diagnostik unklarer Fieberzustände. Internist 1975; 16: 436–443
96. Malik, A.H., Kumar, K.S., Malet, P.F., Jain, R., Prasad, P., Ostapowitz, G.: Correlation of percutaneous liver biopsy fragmentation with the degree of fibrosis. Alimen. Pharm. Therap. 2004; 19: 545–549
97. Marano, B.J.jr., Bonanno, C.A.: Liver biopsy in patients with immunodeficiency syndrome. Amer. J. Gastroenterol. 1993; 88: 2139
98. McAfee, J.H., Keefe, E.B., Lee, R.G., Rösch, J.: Transjugular liver biopsy. Hepatology 1992; 15: 726–732
99. McGill, D.B., Rakela, J., Zinsmeister, A.R., Ott, B.J.: A 21-year experience with major hemorrhage after percutaneous liver biopsy. Gastroenterology 1990; 99: 1396–1400
100. McVay, P.A., Toy, P.T.C.Y.: Lack of increased bleeding after liver biopsy in patients with mild hemostatic abnormalities. Amer. J. Clin. Pathol. 1990; 94: 747–753
101. Menghini, G.: a) Un effetto progresso nella tecnica della puntura-biopsia del fegato. Rass. Fisiopat. Clin. Ter. 1957; 29: 756–773. • b) One-second needle biopsy of the liver. Gastroenterology 1958; 35: 190–199
102. Minuk, G.Y., Sutherland, L.R., Wiseman, D.A., MacDonald, F.R., Ding, D.L.: Prospective study of the incidence of ultrasound-detected intrahepatic and subcapsular hematomas in patients randomized to 6 or 24 hours of bed rest after percutaneous liver biopsy. Gastroenterology 1987; 92: 290–293
103. Montalto, G., Soresi, M., Carroccio, A., Bascone, F., Tripi, S., Aragona, F., di Gaetano, G., Notarbartolo, A.: Percutaneous liver biopsy: A safe outpatient procedure? Digestion 2001; 63: 55–60
104. Morisod, J., Fontolliet, C., Haller, E., Gardiol, D., Hofstetter, J.R., Gonvers, J.J.: Place actuelle de la biopsie dans le diagnostic des maladies hepatiques. Schweiz. Med. Wschr. 1988; 118: 125–133
105. Morris, J.S., Gallo, G.A., Scheuer, P.J., Path, M.R.C., Sherlock, S.: Percutaneous liver biopsy in patients with large bile duct obstruction. Gastroenterology 1975; 68: 750–754
106. Moyer, J.H., Wurl, O.A.: Liver biopsy: Correlation with clinical and biochemical observations. Amer. J. Med. Sci. 1951; 221: 28–37
107. Muir, A.J., Trotter, J.F.: A survey of current liver biopsy practice patterns. J. Clin. Gastroenterol. 2002; 35: 86–88
108. Ness, van, M.M., Diehl, A.M.: Is liver biopsy useful in the evaluation of patients with chronically elevated liver enzymes? Ann. Intern. Med. 1989; 111: 473–478
109. Neuerburg, J., Günther, R.W.: Transvenous liver biopsy. Fortschr. Röntgenstr. 1999; 170: 521–527

110. Okuda, K., Musha, H., Nakajima, Y., Takayasu, K., Suzuki, Y., Morita, M., Yamasaki, T.: Frequency of intrahepatic arteriovenous fistula as a sequela to percutaneous needle puncture of the liver. Gastroenterology 1978; 74: 1204−1207
111. Olivet, J.: Die diagnostische Leberparenchympunktion (Lpp.). Med. Klin. 1926; 22: 1440−1443
112. Ormann, W., Starck, E., Pausch, J.: Arterielle Embolisation einer arterio-venösen Fistel mit Hämobilie nach Leberblindpunktion. Z. Gastroenterol. 1991; 29: 153−155
113. Ortmans, H.: Unbemerkte Pneumothoraxentstehung nach perkutaner Leberbiopsie. Leber Magen Darm 1972; 2: 231−233
114. Papini, E., Pacella, C.M., Rossi, Z., Bizzarri, G., Fabbrini, R., Nardi, F., Picardi, R.: A randomized trial of ultrasound-guided anterior subcostal liver biopsy versus the conventional Menghini technique. J. Hepatol. 1991; 13: 291−297
115. Pasha, T., Gabriel, S., Therneau, T., Rolland Dickson, E., Lindor, D.: Cost-effectiveness of ultrasound-guided liver biopsy. Hepatology 1998; 27: 1220−1226
116. Perrault, J., McGill, D.B., Ott, B.J., Taylor, W.F.: Liver biopsy: complications in 1000 inpatients and outpatients. Gastroenterology 1978; 74: 103−106
117. Perrillo, R.P.: The role of liver biopsy in hepatitis C. Hepatology 1997; 26: 57−61
118. Piccinino, F., Sagnelli, E., Pasquale, G., Giusti, G.: Complications following percutaneous liver biopsy. A multicentre retrospective study on 68.276 biopsies. J. Hepatol. 1986; 2: 165−173
119. Pisani, R.J., Zeller, F.A.: Bilious pleural effusion following liver biopsy. Chest 1990; 98: 1535−1537
120. Plecha, D.M., Goodwin, D.W., Rowland, D.Y., Varnes, M.E., Haaga, J.R.: Liver biopsy: effects of biopsy needle caliber on bleeding and tissue recovery. Radiology 1997; 204: 101−104
121. Preger, L.: Hepatic arteriovenous fistula after percutaneous liver biopsy. Amer. J. Röntgenol. 1967; 101: 619−620
122. Raines, D.R., Heertum, van, R.L., Johnson, L.F.: Intrahepatic hematoma: a complication of percutaneous liver biopsy. A report on the incidence of postbiopsy scan defects. Gastroenterology 1974; 67: 284−289
123. Reichert, C.M., Weisenthal, L.M., Klein, H.G.: Delayed hemorrhage after percutaneous liver biopsy. J. Clin. Gastroenterol. 1983; 5: 263−266
124. Ricketts, W.E., Kirsner, J.B., Palmer, W.L., Sterling, K.: Observations on the diagnostic value of liver biopsy, tests of hepatic function, and electrophoretic fractionation of serum proteins in asymptomatic portal cirrhosis. J. Lab. Clin. Med. 1950; 35: 403−407
125. Röcken, C., Meier, H., Klauck, S., Wolff, S., Malfertheiner, P., Roessner, A.: Large-needle biopsy versus thin-needle biopsy in diagnostic pathology of liver diseases. Liver 2001; 21: 391−397
126. Rossi, P., Sileri, P., Gentileschi, P., Sica, G.S., Forlini, A., Stolfi, V.M., de Majo, A., Coscarella, G., Canale, S., Gaspari, A.L.: Percutaneous liver biopsy using an ultrasound-guided subcostal route. Dig. Dis. Sci. 2001; 46: 128−132
127. Ruben, R.A., Chopra, S.: Bile peritonitis after liver biopsy: nonsurgical management of a patient with an acute abdomen. A case report with review of the literature. Amer. J. Gastroenterol. 1987; 82: 265−268
128. Ruijter, T.E.G., Eeftinck Schattenkerk, J.K.M., van Leeuwen, D.J., Bosma, A.: Diagnostic value of liver biopsy in symptomatic HIV-1-infected patients. Eur. J. Gastroenterol. Hepatol. 1993; 5: 641−645
129. Sada, P.N., Ramakrishna, B., Thomas, C.P., Govil, S., Koshi, T., Chandy, J.: Transjugular liver biopsy: a comparison of aspiration and trucut techniques. Liver 1997; 17: 257−259
130. Satsangi, J., Ireland, A., Bloom, St., Trowell, J.M., Lindsell, D.R.M., Chapman, W.G.: The effect of bed rest and operator experience on the incidence of complications after liver biopsy. Europ. J. Gastroenterol. Hepatol. 1993; 5: 173−176
131. Sawyerr, A.M., McCormick, P.A., Tennyson, G.S., Chin, J., Dick, R., Scheuer, P.J., Burroughs, A.K., McIntyre, N.: A comparison of transjugular and plugged-percutaneous liver biopsy in patients with impaired coagulation. J. Hepatol. 1993; 17: 81−85
132. Scheimann, A.O., Barrios, J.M., Al-Tawil, Y.S., Gray, K.M., Gilger, M.A.: Percutaneous liver biopsy in children: Impact of ultrasonography and springloaded biopsy needles. J. Pediatr. Gastroenterol. Nutrit. 2000; 31: 536−539
133. Schiff, L.: The clinical value of needle biopsy of the liver. Ann. Intern. Med. 1951; 34: 948−967
134. Schupfer, F.: De la possibilité de faire "intra vitam" un diagnostic histo-pathologique précis des maladies du foie et de la rate. Sém. Méd. (Paris) 1907; 27: 229−230
135. Scott, D.A., Netchvolodoff, C.V., Bacon, B.R.: Delayed subcapsular hematoma after percutaneous liver biopsy as a manifestation of warfarin toxicity. Amer. J. Gastroenterol. 1991; 86: 503−505
136. Sheela, H., Seela, S., Caldwell, C., Boyer, J.L., Jain, D.: Liver biopsy − Evolving role in the new millennium (review). J. Clin. Gastroenterology. 2005; 39: 603−610
137. Shiraki, K., Hamada, M., Sugimoto, K., Ito, T., Murata, K., Fujikawa, K., Takase, K., Nakano, T., Tameda, Y.: Pneumothorax after diagnostic laparoscopy (case report). Hepato-Gastroenterol. 2002; 49: 1033−1035
138. Silverman, I.: A new biopsy needle. Amer. J. Surg. 1938; 40: 671−672 • Improved Vim-Silverman biopsy needle. J. Amer. Med. Ass. 1954; 155: 1060−1061
139. Skelly, M.M., James, P.D., Ryder, S.D.: Findings on liver biopsy to investigate abnormal liver function tests in the absence of diagnostic serology. J. Hepatol. 2001; 35: 195−199
140. Smith, T.P., McDermott, V.G., Ayoub, D.M., Suhocki, P.V., Stackhouse, D.J.: Percutaneous transhepatic liver biopsy with tract embolization. Radiology 1996; 198: 769−774
141. Snover, D.C., Sibley, R.K., Freese, D.K., Sharp, H.L., Bloomer, J.R., Najarian, J.S., Ascher, N.L.: Orthotopic liver transplantation: a pathological study of 63 serial liver biopsies from 17 patients with special reference to the diagnostic features and natural history of rejection. Hepatology 1984; 4: 1212−1222
142. Solis Herruzo, J.A.: Current indications of liver biopsy. Rev. Esp. Enferm. Dig. 2006; 98: 122−139
143. Soloway, R.D., Baggenstoss, A.H., Schoenfield, L.J., Summerskill, W.H.J.: Observer error and sampling variability tested in evaluation of hepatitis and cirrhosis by liver biopsy. Amer. J. Dig. Dis. 1971; 16: 1082−1086
144. Sorbi, D., McGill, D.B., Thistle, J.L., Therneau, T.M., Henry, J., Lindor, K.-D.: An assessment of the role of liver biopsies in asymptomatic patients with chronic liver test abnormalities. Amer. J. Gastroenterol. 2000; 95: 3206−3210
145. Spamer, C., Brambs, H.-J., Koch, H.K., Gerok, W.: Beningn circumscribed lesions of the liver diagnosed by ultrasonically guided fine-needle biopsy. J. Clin. Ultrasound 1986; 14: 83−88
146. Spellberg, M.A., Bermudez, F.: Value and safety of percutaneous liver biopsy in obstructive jaundice. Amer. J. Gastroenterol. 1977; 67: 444−448
147. Spinzi, G., Imperiali, G., Terruzzi, V., Minoli, G.: Ematomi epatici da epatobiopsia secondo Menghini. Min. Gastroenterol. Dietol. 1992; 38: 207−210
148. Strik, W.O.: Erfahrungen mit der perkutanen Leberbiopsie nach Menghini. Med. Klin. 1964; 59: 1051−1055
149. Sugano, S., Sumino, Y., Hatori, T., Mizugami, H., Kawafune, T., Abei, T.: Incidence of ultrasound-detected intrahepatic hematomas due to Tru-Cut needle liver biopsy. Dig. Dis. Sci. 1991; 36: 1229−1233
150. Teare, J.P., Watkinson, A.F., Erb, S.R., Mayo, J.R., Connell, D.G., Weir, I.H., Owen, D.A., Wolber, R., Morris, D.C.: Transfemoral liver biopsy by forceps: a review of 104 consecutive procedures. Cardiovascul. Intervent. Radiol. 1994; 17: 252−257
151. Terry, R.: Risks of needle biopsy of the liver. Brit. Med. J. 1952; 1: 1102−1105
152. Terjung, B., Lemnitzer, I., Dumoulin, F.L., Effenberger, W., Brackmann, H.H., Sauerbruch, T., Spengler, U.: Bleeding complications after percutaneous liver biopsy. An analysis of risk factors. Digestion 2003; 67: 138−145
153. Thaler, H., Javitz, J.: Leberbiopsie. Internist 1970; 11: 364−374
154. Thaler, H.: Die Stellung der Nadelbiopsie in der Diagnostik kindlicher Lebererkrankungen. Leber Magen Darm 1979; 9: 253−258
155. Thiel, van, D.H., Gavaler, J.S., Wright, H., Tzakis, A.: Liver biopsy. Its safety and complications as seen at a liver transplant center. Transplant. 1993; 55: 1087−1090
156. Tobkes, A.I., Nord, H.J.: Liver biopsy: review of methodology and complications. Dig. Dis. 1995; 13: 267−274
157. Vargas-Tank, L., Martinez, V., Jiron, M.I., Soto, J.R., Armas-Merino, R.: Tru-cut and Menghini needles: different yield in the histological diagnosis of liver disease. Liver 1985; 5: 178−181
158. Vautier, G., Scott, B., Jenkins, D.: Liver biopsy: blind or guided? Brit. Med. J. 1994; 309: 1455−1456
159. Verbecke, C.S., Bohrer, M.H., Wetzl, E.: Computertomographisch gesteuerte Feinnadelbiopsie. Neue Dimensionen der bioptischen Diagnostik. Dtsch. Med. Wschr. 1993; 118: 1389−1394
160. Verhille, M.S., Munoz, S.J.: Acute biliary-vascular fistula following needle aspiration of the liver. Gastroenterology 1991; 101: 1731−1733
161. Vivas, S., Palacio, M.A., Rodriguez, M., Lomo, J., Cadenas, F., Giganto, F., Rodrigo, L.: Ambulatory liver biopsy: complications and evolution in 264 cases. Rev. Esp. Enferm. Dig. 1998; 90: 179−182
162. Vlavianos, P., Bird, G., Portmann, B., Westaby, D., Williams, R.: Transjugular liver biopsy: use in a selected high risk population. Europ. J. Gastroenterol. Hepatol. 1991; 3: 469−472
163. Volwiler, W., Jones, C.M.: The diagnostic and therapeutic value of liver biopsies−with special reference to trocar biopsy. New Engl. J. Med. 1947; 237: 651−656
164. Wagoner, G., Ulevitch, H., Gall, E.A., Schiff, L.: Biopsy of needle-specimens of liver tissue. Amer. J. Clin. Pathol. 1951; 21: 338−341
165. Waldstein, S.S., Szanto, P.B.: Accuracy of sampling by needle biopsy in diffuse liver disease. Arch. Pathol. 1950; 50: 326−328
166. Weiss, H., Weiss, A., Schöll, A.: Tödliche Komplikation einer Feinnadelbiopsie der Leber. Dtsch. Med. Wschr. 1988; 113: 139−142
167. Welch, T.J., Sheedy II, P.F., Johnson, C.D., Johnson, C.M., Stephens, D.H.: CT-guided biopsy: prospective analysis of 1000 procedures. Radiology 1989; 171: 493−496
168. Westaby, D., MacDougall, B.R., Williams, R.: Liver biopsy as a day-case procedure: selection and complications in 200 consecutive patients. Brit. Med. J. 1980; 281: 1331−1332
169. Whitmire, L.F., Galambos, J.T., Phillips, V.M., Sewell, C.W., Erwin, B.C., Torres, W.E., Gedgaudas-McClees, R.K., Bernardino, M.E.: Imaging guided percutaneous hepatic biopsy: diagnostic accuracy and safety. J. Clin. Gastroenterol. 1985; 7: 511−515
170. Wildhirt, E., Möller, E.: Erfahrungen bei nahezu 20.000 Leberblindpunktionen. Med. Klin. 1981; 76: 254−256

171. **Wildhirt, E.:** Zur Frage der Spätkomplikationen nach Leberbiopsie. Münch. Med. Wschr. 1970; 112: 1234–1237
172. **Younossi, Z. M., Teran, J.C., Ganiats, T.G., Carey, W.D.:** Ultrasound-guided liver biopsy for parenchymal liver disease. An economic analysis. Dig. Dis. Sci. 1998; 43: 46–50
173. **Zamcheck, N., Klausenstock, O.:** Liver biopsy. The risk of needle biopsy. New Engl. J. Med. 1953; 249: 1062–1069
174. **Zins, M., Vilgrain, V., Gayno, S., Rolland, Y., Arrivé, L., Denninger, M.-H., Vullierme, M.-P., Najmark, D., Menu, Y., Nahum, H.:** US-guided percutaneous liver biopsy with plugging of the needle track: a prospective study in 72 high-risk patients. Radiology 1992; 184: 841–843
175. **Zwiebel, F.M., Holl, J., Kleber, G.:** Transjuguläre Leberpunktion. Bildgebung 1993; 60: 161–168

Laparoskopie

176. **Adamek, H.E., Maier, M., Benz, C., Huber, T., Schilling, D., Riemann, J.F.:** Schwerwiegende Komplikationen der diagnostischen Laparoskopie. Med. Klin. 1996; 91: 694–697
177. **Agresta, F., Michelet, I., Coluci, G., Bedin, N.:** Emergency laparoscopy. A community hospital experience. Surg. Endosc. 2000; 14: 484–487
178. **Arndt, H.J., Creutzfeld, W.:** Abdominalschmerzen durch Adhäsionen und ihre laparoskopische Beseitigung. Dtsch. Med. Wschr. 1976; 101: 395–398
179. **Arnold, J.C., Schneider, A.R.J., Zöpf, T., Riemann, J.F.:** Laparoscopic tumor staging—a safe method in the hands of internists. Klinikarzt 2001; 30: 142–146
180. **Babineau, T.J., Lewis, W.D., Jenkins, R.L., Bleday, R., Steele, G.D.jr., Forse, R.A.:** Role of staging laparoscopy in the treatment of hepatic malignancy. Amer. J. Surg. 1994; 167: 151–155
181. **Berg, K., Wilhelm, W., Mertzlufft, F.:** Herz-Kreislauf- Funktion während Laparoskopien. Dtsch. Med. Wschr. 1995; 120: 1561–1567
182. **Bernheim, B.M.:** Organoscopy: cystoscopy of the abdominal cavity. Ann. Surg. 1911; 52: 764–767
183. **Bhargava, D.K., Arora, A., Dasarathy, S.:** Laparoscopic features of the Budd-Chiari-Syndrome. Endoscopy 1991; 23: 259–261
184. **Bhargava, D.K., Shriniwas, Chopra, P., Nijhawan, S., Dasarathy, S., Kushwaha, A.K.S.:** Peritoneal tuberculosis: laparoscopic patterns and its diagnostic accuracy. Amer. J. Gastroenterol. 1992; 87: 109–112
185. **Birchler, R., Gonvers, J.J., Hofstetter, J.R.:** 2000 laparoscopies, un nouveau bilan. Praxis 1984; 73: 683–685
186. **Bleiberg, H., La Meir, E., Lejeune, F.:** Laparoscopy in the diagnosis of liver metastases in 80 cases of malignant melanoma. Endoscopy 1980; 12: 215–218
187. **Borgstein, P.J., Gordijn, R.V., Eijsbouts, Q.A.J., Cuesta, M.A.:** Acute appendicitis—a clear-cut case in men, a guessing game in young women: a prospective study on the role of laparoscopy. Surg. Endosc. 1997; 11: 923–927
188. **Boyce, H.W.:** Diagnostic laparoscopy in liver and biliary disease. Endoscopy 1992; 24: 676–681
189. **Boyd, W.P., Nord, H.J.:** Diagnostic laparoscopy. Endoscopy 1998; 30: 189–197
190. **Brady, P.G., Goldschmid, S., Chappel, G., Slone, F.L., Boyd, W.P.:** A comparison of biopsy techniques in suspected focal liver disease. Gastrointest. Endosc. 1987; 33: 289–292
191. **Brady, P.G., Peebles, M., Goldschmid, S.:** Role of laparoscopy in the evaluation of patients with suspected hepatic or peritoneal malignancy. Gastrointest. Endosc. 1991; 37: 27–30
192. **Bruguera, M., Bordas, J.M., Mas, P., Rodes, J.:** A comparison of the accuracy of peritoneoscopy and liver biopsy in the diagnosis of cirrhosis. Gut 1974; 15: 799–800
193. **Brühl, W.:** Zwischenfälle und Komplikationen bei der Laparoskopie und gezielten Leberpunktion. Ergebnis einer Umfrage. Dtsch. Med. Wschr. 1966; 91: 2297–2299
194. **Buffet, C., Pelletier, G., Etienne, J.P.:** Que reste-t-il des indications de la laparoscopie en 1983? Gastroenterol. Clin. Biol. 1983; 7: 134–140
195. **Cano-Ruiz, A., Martin-Scapa, M.A., Larraona, J.L., Gonzales-Martin, J.A., Moreno-Caparros, A., Garcia-Plaza, A.:** Laparoscopic findings in seven patients with nodular regenerative hyperplasia of the liver. Amer. J. Gastroenterol. 1985; 80: 796–800
196. **Cardi, M., Muttillo, I.A., Amadori, L., Petroni, R., Mingazzini, P., Barillari, P., Lisi, D., Bolognese, A.:** Superiority of laparoscopy compared to ultrasonography in diagnosis of widespread liver diseases. Dig. Dis. Sci. 1997; 42: 546–548
197. **Catarci, M., Carlini, M., Gentileschi, P., Santoro, E.:** Major and minor injuries during the creation of pneumoperitoneum – a multicenter study on 12,919 cases. Surg. Endosc. 2001; 15: 566–569
198. **Chu, C.-M., Lin, S.-M., Peng, S.-M., Wu, C.-S., Liaw, Y.- F.:** The role of laparoscopy in the evaluation of ascites of unknown origin. Gastrointest. Endosc. 1994; 40: 285–289
199. **Crantock, L.R.F., Dillon, J.F., Hayes, P.C.:** Diagnostic laparoscopy and liver disease: experience of 200 cases. Aust. N. Z. J. Med. 1994; 24: 258–262
200. **Dagnini, M., Marin, G., Patella, M., Zotti, S.:** Laparoscopy in the diagnosis of primary carcinoma of the gallbladder. Gastrointest. Endosc. 1984; 30: 289–291
201. **Dagnini, G., Caldironi, M.W., Marin, G., Buzzaccarini, O., Tremolada, C., Ruol, A.:** Laparoscopy in abdominal staging of esophageal carcinoma. Report of 369 cases. Gastrointest. Endosc. 1986; 32: 400–402
202. **Dagnini, G., Marin, G., Caldironi, M.W., Piccigallo, E., Miola, E.:** Laparoscopy in staging, follow-up, and restaging of ovarian carcinoma. Gastrointest. Endosc. 1987; 33: 80–83
203. **Dancygier, H., Jacob, R.A.:** Splenic rupture during laparoscopy. Gastrointest. Endosc. 1983; 29: 63.
204. **De Groen, P.C., Rakela, J., Moore, S.C., McGill, D.B., Burton, D.D., Ott, B.J., Zinsmeister, A.R.:** Diagnostic laparoscopy in Gastroenterology. A 14-year experience. Dig. Dis. Sci. 1987; 32: 677–681
205. **Domingo, M., Grau, J., Vazquez, A., Diez, J., Coll, J., Vivancos, J.:** Septic shock and bacteremia associated with laparoscopic guided liver biopsy, report on two cases. Endoscopy 1989; 21: 240–241
206. **Drèze, Ch., Delforge, M., Demoulin, J.C., Fontaine, F., Gillard, V.:** La laparoscopy en 1992. Une experience de 37 années. Rev. Med. Liege 1992; 47: 384–414
207. **Esposito, C., Garipoli, V., Vecchione, R., Raia, V., Vajro, P.:** Laparoscopy – guided biopsy in diagnosis of liver disorders in children. Liver 1997; 17: 288–292
208. **Feig, B.W., Berger, D.H., Dougherty, T.B., Dupuis, J.F., Hsi, B., Hickey, R.C., Ota, D.M.:** Pharmacologic intervention can reestablish baseline hemodynamic parameters during laparoscopy. Surgery 1994; 116: 733–741
209. **Fermelia, D., Berci, G.:** Diagnostic and therapeutic laparoscopy. An entity often overlooked by the surgeon. Surg. Endosc. 1987; 1: 73–77
210. **Feussner, H., Omote, K., Fink, U., Walker, S.J., Siewert, J.R.:** Pretherapeutic laparoscopic staging in advanced gastric carcinoma. Endoscopy 1999; 31: 342–347
211. **Friedrich, K., Henning, H.:** Laparoskopische Blutstillung nach Leberbiopsie durch Installation eines Gelatine- Zylinders. Z. Gastroenterol. 1987; 25: 726–730
212. **Friedrich, K., Henning, H.:** Stellenwert der Laparoskopie in der Diagnostik der chronischen nichteitrigen destruierenden Cholangitis. Z. Gastroenterol. 1986; 24: 364–374
213. **Gaisford, W.D., Berci, G.:** Peritoneoscopy: Preferred alternative to surgical exploration. Gastrointest. Endosc. 1978; 24: 197.
214. **Gandolfi, L., Muratori, R., Solmi, L., Rossi, A., Leo, P.:** Laparoscopy compared with ultrasonography in the diagnosis of hepatocellular carcinoma. Gastrointest. Endosc. 1989; 35: 508–511
215. **Helmreich-Becker, I., Gödderz, W., Mayet, W.J., Meyer zum Büschenfelde, K.-H., Lohse, A.W.:** Die Minilaparoskopie in der Diagnostik chronischer Lebererkrankungen. Endoskopie heute 1997; 10: 195–200
216. **Helmreich-Becker, I., Meyer zum Büschenfelde, K.-H., Lohse, A.W.:** Safety and feasibility of a new minimally invasive diagnostic laparoscopy technique. Endoscopy 1998; 30: 756–762
217. **Henning, H.:** The Dallas report on laparoscopic complications. Gastrointest. Endosc. 1985; 31: 104–105
218. **Henning, H.:** Value of laparoscopy in investigating fever of unexplained origin. Endoscopy 1992; 24: 687–688
219. **Henning, H.:** Renaissance laparoskopischer Techniken in der Diagnostik von Abdominalerkrankungen. Internist 1993; 34: 208–211
220. **Herrerias, J.M., Perez, F., Osorio, M., Garrido, M.:** Discrepancias entre el diagnostico laparoscopico e histologico en la cirrhosis hepatica. Rev. Esp. Enf. Apar. Dig. 1974; 92: 709–714
221. **Hitanant, S., Trong, D.T.-N., Damrongsak, C., Chinapak, O., Boonyapisit, S., Plengvanit, U., Viranuvatti, V.:** Peritoneoscopy in the diagnosis of liver abscess. Experience with 108 cases during a 10-year period. Gastrointest. Endosc. 1984; 30: 234–236
222. **Hossain, J., Al-Aska, A.K., Al Mofleh, I.:** Laparoscopy in tuberculous peritonitis. J. Roy. Soc. Med. 1992; 85: 89–91
223. **Hübner, A., Buchmann, K.:** Die Bedeutung intraabdomineller Verwachsungen für die Laparoskopie. Z. Ges. Inn. Med. 1980; 35: 255–257
224. **Humke, U., Siemer, S., Bonnet, L., Gebhardt, T., Uder, M., Ziegler, M.:** Verwirklichung minimaler Invasivität durch ein neues Instrumentarium für die Laparoskopie im Kindesalter. Urologe 1996; 36: 372–377
225. **Izumi, S., Nishiuchi, M., Kameda, N., Nagano, S., Fukunishi, T., Kohro, T., Shinji, Y.:** Laparoscopic study of peliosis hepatis and nodular transformation of the liver before and after renal transplantation: natural history and aetiology in follow-up cases. J. Hepatol. 1994; 20: 129–137
226. **Jacobaeus, H.C.:** Über die Möglichkeit, die Zystoskopie bei Untersuchung seröser Höhlungen anzuwenden. Münch. Med. Wschr. 1910; 58: 2090–2092
227. **Jalan, R., Harrison, D.J., Dillon, J.F., Elton, R.A., Finlayson, N.D.C., Hayes, P.C.:** Laparoscopy and histology in the diagnosis of chronic liver disease. Q. J. Med. 1995; 88: 559–564
228. **John, T.G., Greig, J.D., Crosbie, J.L., Miles, W.F.A., Garden, O.J.:** Superior staging of liver tumors with laparoscopy and laparoscopic ultrasound. Ann. Surg. 1994; 220: 711–719
229. **Kalk, H.:** Erfahrungen mit der Laparoskopie (Zugleich mit Beschreibung eines neuen Instrumentes). Zschr. Klin. Med. 1929; 111: 303–348
230. **Kalk, H.:** Indikationsstellung und Gefahrenmomente bei der Laparoskopie. Dtsch. Med. Wschr. 1935; 61: 1831–1833
231. **Kameda, Y., Shinji, Y.:** Early detection of hepatocellular carcinoma by laparoscopy: yellow nodules as diagnostic indicators. Gastrointest. Endosc. 1992; 38: 554–559
232. **Kameda, Y., Asakawa, H., Shimomura, S., Shinji, Y.:** Laparoscopic prediction of hepatocellular carcinoma in cirrhosis patients. J. Gastroenterol. Hepatol. 1997; 12: 576–581
233. **Kane, M.G., Krejs, G.J.:** Complications of diagnostic laparoscopy in Dallas. A 7-year prospective study. Gastrointest. Endosc. 1984; 30: 237–240
234. **Karnam, U.S., Reddy, K.R.:** Diagnostic laparoscopy: an update. Endoscopy 2002; 34: 146–153
235. **Kelling, G.:** Zur Coelioskopie. Arch. Klin. Chir. 1923; 126: 226–229

236. **Kestenholz, P.B., von Flüe, M., Harder, R.:** Gallenblasenagenesie bei Erwachsenen: Eine laparoskopische Diagnose. Chirurg 1997; 68: 643–645
237. **Klegar, E.K., Marcus, S.G., Newman, E., Hiotis, S.P.:** Diagnostic laparoscopy in the evaluation of the viral hepatitis patient with potentially resectable hepatocellular carcinoma. HPB. 2005; 7: 204–207
238. **Korbsch, R.:** Die Laparoskopie nach Jakobaeus. Berlin. Klin. Wschr. 1921; 58: 696–698
239. **Kortsik, C., Winckelmann, G., Beck, K., Lütke, A.:** Was leistet die Laparoskopie bei der Klärung von Fieber unbekannter Ursache? Dtsch. Med. Wschr. 1987; 112: 1657–1660
240. **Kresh, A.J., Seifer, D.B., Sachs, L.B., Barrese, I.:** Laparoscopy in 100 women with chronic pelvic pain. Obstetr. Gynec. 1984; 64: 672–674
241. **Kriplani, A.K., Jayant, S., Kapur, B.M.L.:** Laparoscopy in primary carcinoma of the gallbladder. Gastrointest. Endosc. 1992; 38: 326–329
242. **Kriplani, A.K., Kapur, B.M.L.:** Laparoscopy for pre- operative staging and assessment of operability in gastric carcinoma. Gastrointest. Endosc. 1991; 37: 441–443
243. **Kuntz, E.:** 30 Jahre Erfahrungen bei 6000 Laparoskopien (1955–1986). Fortschr. Med. 1987; 105: 521–524
244. **Kuntz, E.:** Der aktuelle Stellenwert der Laparoskopie in der Hepatologie. Med. Welt 1999; 50: 42–47
245. **Kurtz, W., Strohm, W.D.:** Indikationen, Kontraindikationen, Voruntersuchungen und Nachsorge bei der Laparoskopie. Therapiewoche 1981; 31: 5214–5220
246. **Leuschner, M., Leuschner, U.:** Diagnostic laparoscopy in focal parenchymal disease of the liver. Endoscopy 1992; 24: 689–692
247. **Leuschner, U., Leuschner, M., Strohm, W.D., Hübner, K., Kurtz, W., Hagenmüller, F.:** Laparoskopie und Blindpunktion in der modernen Leberdiagnostik. Leber Magen Darm 1981; 11: 245–250
248. **Lightdale, C.J.:** Laparoscopy for cancer staging. Endoscopy 1992; 24: 682–686
249. **Lindner, H., Henning, H.:** Die Laparoskopie als diagnostische Methode. Internist 1976; 17: 214–219
250. **Lindner, H.:** Die diagnostische Sicherheit von Laparoskopie und perkutaner Leberbiopsie. Med. Welt 1968; 19: 1503–1513
251. **Lo, C.-M., Lai, E.C.S., Liu, C.-L., Fan, S.-T., Wong, J.:** Laparoscopy and laparoscopic ultrasonography avoid exploratory laparotomy in patients with hepatocellular carcinoma. Ann. Surg. 1998; 227: 527–532
252. **Lytinski, G., Schaeff, B., Paolucci, V.:** Zum 100. Geburtstag von Heinz Kalk. Der Durchbruch der Laparoskopie. Z. Gastroenterol. 1995; 33: 594–597
253. **Mahlke, R., Bogusch, G., Lankisch, P.G.:** Splenic lesion as a complication of laparoscopy. Case report. Z. Gastroenterol. 1992; 30: 795–797
254. **Mansi, C., Savarino, V., Picciotto, A., Testa, R., Canepa, A., Dodero, M., Celle, G.:** Comparison between laparoscopy, ultrasonography and computed tomography in widespread and localized liver diseases. Gastrointest. Endosc. 1982; 28: 83–85
255. **Marti-Vicente, A., Garcia, V., Toro, H., Seres, I., Enriquez, J., Vilardell, F.:** Accidentes y complicaciones de la laparoscopia. Revision de 8915 casos. Rev. Esp. Enf. Dig. 1992; 82: 411–417
256. **Merkel, R., Zillessen, E.:** Die Notfall-Laparoskopie. Krankenhaus Arzt 1986; 59: 355–356
257. **Mortensen, M.B., Durup, J., Pless, T., Plagborg, G.J., Ainsworth, A.P., Nielsen, H.O., Hovendal, C.:** Initial experience with new dedicated needles for laparoscopic ultrasound-guided fine-needle aspiration and histological biopsies. Endoscopy 2001; 33: 585–589
258. **Nader, A.K., Jeffers, L.J., Reddy, R.K., Molina, E., Leon, R., Lavergne, J., Schiff, E.R.:** Small-diameter (2 mm) laparoscopy in the evaluation of liver disease. Gastrointest. Endosc. 1998; 48: 620–623
259. **Neuhaus, S.J., Gupta, A., Watson, D.I.:** Helium and other alternative insufflation gases for laparoscopy–a review. Surg. Endosc. 2001; 15: 553–560
260. **Nieven van Dijkum, E.J., de Wit, L.T., van Delden, O.M., Kruyt, P.M., van Lanschot, J.J.B., Rauws, E.A.J., Obertop, H., Gouma, D.J.:** Staging laparoscopy and laparoscopic ultrasonography in more than 400 patients with upper gastrointestinal carcinoma. J. Amer. Coll. Surg. 1999; 189: 459–465
261. **Nord, H.J.:** Biopsy diagnosis of cirrhosis: blind percutaneous versus guided direct vision techniques: a review. Gastrointest. Endosc. 1982; 28: 102–104
262. **Nord, H.J.:** Complications of laparoscopy. Endoscopy 1992; 24: 693–700
263. **Nord, H.J., Boyd, W.P.jr.:** Diagnostic laparoscopy. Endoscopy 1996; 28: 147–155
264. **Nord, H.J.:** What is the future of laparoscopy and can we do without it? Z. Gastroenterol. 2001; 39 (Suppl. 1): 41–44
265. **O'Brien, M.G., Fitzgerald, E.F., Lee, G., Crowley, M., Shanahan, F., O'Sullivan, G.C.:** A prospective comparison of laparoscopy and imaging in the staging of esophagogastric cancer before surgery. Amer. J. Gastroenterol. 1995; 90: 2191–2194
266. **Orlando, R., Lirussi, F., Okolicsanyi, L.:** Laparoscopy and liver biopsy: further evidence that the two procedures improve the diagnosis of liver cirrhosis. A retrospective study of 1003 consecutive examinations. J. Clin. Gastroenterol. 1990; 12: 47–52
267. **Orlando, R., Sawadogo, S.:** La laparoscopie dans la cholestase. Acta Endoscop. 1990; 20: 537–543
268. **Orndoff, B.H.:** The peritoneoscopy in diagnosis of diseases of the abdomen. J. Radiol. 1920; 1: 307–325
269. **Ott, D. (Edler von Ott):** Ilumination of the abdomen (ventroscopia) (in Russian). J. Akush. Zhensk. Boliez. 1901; 15: 1045–1049
270. **Pagliaro, L., Rinaldi, F., Craxi, A., Di Piazza, S., Filippazzo, G., Gatto, G., Genova, G., Magrin, S., Maringhini, A., Orsini, S., Palazzo, U., Spinello, M., Vinci, M.:** Percutaneous blind biopsy versus laparoscopy with guided biopsy in diagnosis of cirrhosis. A prospective, randomized trial. Dig. Dis. Sci. 1983; 28: 39–43
271. **Paolaggi, J.-A., Debray, C.:** Accidents de la laparoscopie. Enquete nationale. Ann. Gastroenterol. Hepatol. (Paris) 1976; 12: 335–343
272. **Phillips, R.S., Reddy, K.R., Jeffers, L.J., Schiff, E.R.:** Experience with diagnostic laparoscopy in a hepatology training program. Gastrointest. Endosc. 1987; 33: 417–420
273. **Picciotto, A., Ciravegna, G., Lapertosa, G., Celle, G.:** Percutaneous or laparoscopic needle biopsy in the evaluation of chronic liver disease? Amer. J. Gastroenterol. 1984; 79: 567–568
274. **Pickert, H., Henning, H.:** Laparoskopie nach Bauchoperationen. Med. Klin. 1965; 60: 1852–1856
275. **Pohle, W., May, B., Bohle, H., Fritze, E.:** Das Hämobilie- Syndrom. Seltene Komplikation nach gezielter Leberpunktion. Med. Welt 1977; 28: 125–126
276. **Poniachik, J., Bernstein, D.E., Reddy, K.R., Jeffers, L.J., Coelho-Little, M.-E., Civantos, F., Schiff, E.R.:** The role of laparoscopy in the diagnosis of cirrhosis. Gastrointest. Endosc. 1996; 43: 568–571
277. **Porcel, A., Alcain, G., Moreno, M., Amaya, A., Guillen, P., Martin, L.:** Value of laparoscopy in ascites of undetermined origin. Rev. Esp. Enferm. Dig. 1996; 88: 485–489
278. **Possik, R.A., Franco, E.L., Pires, D.R., Wohnrath, D.R., Ferreira, E.B.:** Sensitivity, specificity, and predictive value of laparoscopy for the staging of gastric cancer and for the detection of liver metastases. Cancer 1986; 58: 1–6
279. **Reed, W.P., Mustafa, I.A.:** Laparoscopic screening of surgical candidates with pancreatic cancer or liver tumors. Surg. Endosc. 1997; 11: 12–14
280. **Sackier, J.M., Berci, G., Paz-Partlow, M.:** Elective diagnostic laparoscopy. Amer. J. Surg. 1991; 161: 326–331
281. **Saeian, K., Reddy, K.R.:** Diagnostic laparoscopy: an update. Endoscopy 1999; 31: 103–109
282. **Salky, B.A., Edye, M.B.:** The role of laparoscopy in the diagnosis and treatment of abdominal pain syndromes. Surg. Endosc. 1998; 12: 911–914
283. **Sans, M., Andreu, V., Bordas, J.M., Llach, J., López-Guillermo, A., Cervantes, F., Bruguera, M., Mondelo, F., Montserrat, E., Terés, J., Rodés, J.:** Usefulness of laparoscopy with liver biopsy in the assessment of liver involvement at diagnosis of Hodgkin's and non-Hodgkin's lymphomas. Gastrointest. Endosc. 1998; 47: 391–395
284. **Sato, M., Ishida, H., Konno, K., Komatsuda, T., Hamashima, Y., Naganuma, H., Ohyama, Y.:** Longstanding arterioportal fistula after laparoscopic liver biopsy. Abdom. Imag. 1999; 24: 383–385
285. **Sato, S., Watanabe, M., Nagasawa, S., Niigaki, M., Sakai, S., Akagi, S.:** Laparoscopic observations of congenital anomalies of the liver. Gastrointest. Endosc. 1998; 47: 136–140
286. **Schier, F., Waldschmidt, J.:** Experience with laparoscopy for the evaluation of cholestasis in newborns. Surg. Endosc. 1990; 4: 13–14
287. **Schneider, A.R.J., Benz, C., Adamek, H.E., Jakobs, R., Riemann, J.F., Arnold, J.C.:** Minilaparoscopy versus conventional laparoscopy in the diagnosis of hepatic diseases. Gastrointest. Endosc. 2001; 53: 771–775
288. **Sharp, J.R., Pierson, W.P., Bradey III, C.E.:** Comparison of CO_2- and N_2O-induced discomfort during peritoneoscopy under local anesthesia. Gastroenterology 1982; 82: 453–456
289. **Solis-Herruzo, J.A., Benita, V., Morillas, J.D.:** Laparoscopy in fever of unknown origin – study of seventy cases. Endoscopy 1981; 13: 207–210
290. **Solis-Herruzo, J.A., Colina, F., Munoz-Yagüe, Castellano, G., Morillas, J.D.:** Reddish-purple areas on the liver surface: the laparoscopic picture of peliosis hepatis. Endoscopy 1983; 15: 95–100
291. **Solis-Herruzo, J.A., Garcia-Cabezudo, J., Santalla-Pecina, F., Duran-Aguado, A., Olmedo-Camacho, J.:** Laparoscopic findings in hereditary haemorrhagic teleangiectasia (Osler-Weber-Rendu disease). Endoscopy 1981; 13: 137–139
292. **Steiner, O.P.:** Abdominoscopy. Surg. Gyn. Obstetr. 1924; 38: 266–269
293. **Stiefel, G.E.:** Über die Gefahren, Kontraindikationen und Indikationen der Laparoskopie, der gezielten und der blinden Leberbiopsie. Schweiz. Med. Wschr. 1961; 91: 97–105
294. **Tameda, Y., Yoshizawa, N., Takase, K., Nakano, T., Kosaka, Y.:** Prognostic value of peritoneoscopic findings in cirrhosis of the liver. Gastrointest. Endosc. 1990; 36: 34–38
295. **Thiele, H., Berg, P.L., Frick, B., Kalk, J.-F.:** Fibrinkleberinjektion – eine neue Methode zur Blutstillung nach laparoskopischer Leberbiopsie. Dtsch. Med. Wschr. 1989; 114: 1196–1198
296. **Tytgat, S.H.A., Bakker, X.R., Butzelaar, R.M.J.M.:** Laparoscopic evaluation of patients with suspected appendicitis. Surg. Endosc. 1998; 12: 918–920
297. **Ünal, G., van Buuren, H.R., de Man, R.A.:** Laparoscopy as a day-case procedure in patients with liver disease. Endoscopy 1998; 30: 3–7
298. **Vander Velpen, G.C., Shimi, S.M., Cuschieri, A.:** Diagnostic yield and management benefit of laparoscopy: a prospective audit. Gut 1994; 35: 1617–1621
299. **Vargas, C., Jeffers, L.J., Bernstein, D., Reddy, K.R., Munnangi, S., Behar, S., Scott, C., Parker, T., Schiff, E.R.:** Diagnostic laparoscopy: a 5-year experience in a hepatology training program. Amer. J. Gastroenterol. 1995; 90: 1258–1262
300. **Veress, J.:** Neues Instrument zur Ausführung von Brust- oder Bauchpunktionen und Pneumothoraxbehandlung. Dtsch. Med. Wschr. 1938; 41: 1480–1481

301. **Vido, I., Wildhirt, E.:** Korrelation des laparoskopischen und histologischen Befundes bei chronischer Hepatitis und Leberzirrhose. Dtsch. Med. Wschr. 1969; 94: 1633–1637
302. **Vido, I., Winckler, K.:** Diagnose der Leberzirrhose anhand laparoskopischer und histologischer Befunde. Med. Klin. 1972; 67: 400–402
303. **Vogel, H.-M., Scherer, K., Look, D.:** Comparative studies of laparoscopy, histology and gray-scale echotomography in diffuse diseases of the liver. Endoscopy 1980; 12: 166–174
304. **Vollmer, C.M., Drebin, J.A., Middleton, W.D., Teefey, S.A., Linehan, D.C., Soper, N.J., Eagon, C.J., Strasberg, S.M.:** Utility of staging laparoscopy in subsets of peripancreatic and biliary malignancies. Ann. Surg. 2002; 235: 1–7
305. **Warshaw, A.L., Tepper, J.E., Shipley, W.U.:** Laparoscopy in the staging and planning of therapy for pancreatic cancer. Amer. J. Surg. 1986; 151: 76–80
306. **Watanabe, M., Tanaka, S., Ono, M., Hamamoto, S., Nagaki, M., Uchida, Y., Akagi, S., Kinoshita, Y.:** Laparoscopic observations of hepatic capsular abnormalities: non-postoperative adhesions and hepatic capsules thickening. Gastrointest. Endosc. 1999; 50: 664–666
307. **Watt, I., Stewart, I., Anderson, D.:** Laparoscopy, ultrasound, and computed tomography in cancer of the oesophagus and gastric cardia: a prospective comparison for detecting intra-abdominal metastases. Brit. J. Surg. 1989; 76: 1036–1039
308. **Whitworth, C.M., Whitworth, P.W., Sanfillipo, J., Polk, H.C.:** Value of diagnostic laparoscopy in young women with possible appendicitis. Surg. Gynec. Obstetr. 1988; 167: 187–190
309. **Wildhirt, E.:** Laparoskopie und Leberbiopsie. Wien. Med. Wschr. 1970; 120: 66–69
310. **Wildhirt, E., Selmair, H.:** Ergebnisse der Laparoskopie im Kindesalter. Endoscopy 1970; 2: 209–212
311. **Wildhirt, E.:** The diagnostic value of laparoscopy – a prospective study. Tokai J. Exp. Clin. Med. 1981; 6: 223–227
312. **Wurst, H., Finsterer, U.:** Pathophysiologische und klinische Aspekte der Laparoskopie. Anästhes. Intensivmed. 1990; 31: 187–197
313. **Zornig, G., Emmermann, A., Peiper, M., Richter, M., Weh, H.J.:** Staging-Laparoskopie beim Morbus Hodgkin. Vollwertige Alternative zur Staging-Laparotomie. Dtsch. Med. Wschr. 1993; 118: 1401–1404
314. **Zotti, S., Papaleo, E., Marin, G., Patella, M., Bergamo, S., Caldironi, M.W., Cecchetto, A., Dagnini, G.:** Laparoscopy and liver biopsy in the morphological diagnosis of cirrhosis: concordance and diagnostic validity. Ital. J. Gastroenterol. 1981; 13: 14–17
315. **Zotti, S., Piccigallo, E., Rampinelli, L., Romagnoli, G., Tufano, A., Dagnini, G.:** Primary and metastatic tumors associated with cirrhosis. Gastrointest. Endosc. 1986; 32: 91–95

Diagnostics in Liver Diseases
8 Radiological diagnostics

		Page:			Page:
1	*Computer tomography*	178	3	*Angiography*	186
1.1	Principle	178	3.1	Arteriography	187
1.2	Hounsfield units	178	3.1.1	Indications	187
1.3	Contrast media	179	3.1.2	Contraindications	187
1.4	Normal liver	179	3.1.3	Complications	187
1.5	Contraindications	179	3.1.4	Focal lesions	188
1.6	Indications	180	3.1.5	Diffuse liver diseases	188
1.7	Diffuse liver diseases	180	3.1.6	Therapeutic infusion	188
1.7.1	Fatty liver	180	3.2	Portography	189
1.7.2	Liver cirrhosis	181	3.2.1	Indications	189
1.7.3	Haemochromatosis	181	3.2.2	Direct splenoportography	189
1.8	Focal liver lesions	181	3.2.3	Indirect splenoportography	190
1.8.1	Benign liver tumours	181	3.2.4	Omphaloportography	190
1.8.2	Vascular lesions	182	3.2.5	Percutaneous transhepatic portography	190
1.8.3	Hepatic cysts	182	3.3	Phlebography	190
1.8.4	Inflammatory liver lesions	183	4	*Cholangiography*	191
1.9	Malignant liver tumours	183	4.1	Indirect cholangiography	191
1.10	Bile duct obstruction	183	4.1.1	Intravenous cholangiography	191
1.11	Surgical therapy	183	4.1.2	Spiral CT and MRCP	191
2	*Magnetic resonance imaging*	184	4.2	Direct cholangiography	191
2.1	Principle	184	4.2.1	ERC	191
2.2	Advantages	184	4.2.2	PTC	193
2.3	Disadvantages	184	4.2.3	TVC	194
2.4	Normal liver	184	4.2.4	PTCS	194
2.5	Diffuse liver diseases	185	4.2.5	Intraoperative cholangiography	194
2.6	Focal liver lesions	185	4.2.6	Postoperative cholangiography	194
				• References (1–191)	195
				(Figures 8.1–8.15; tables 8.1–8.10)	

8 Radiological diagnostics

A definite diagnosis is often not obtained in liver disease despite the combined use of the **mainstays of diagnostics:** (*1.*) *clinical findings*, (*2.*) *laboratory examination data*, and (*3.*) *ultrasonography*. Possibly, even (*4.*) *morphological analysis* has been unproductive or was not indicated at all. This raises the question of using special radiological and nuclear medical examination techniques. • Diagnostic problems may arise, especially with regard to the following **issues:**

- Identification of intrahepatic foci
- Clarification of the benignancy or malignancy of focal liver lesions
- Differentiation of vascular-related liver diseases
- Detection of alterations regarding the bile ducts
- Differential diagnosis of mechanical jaundice
- Assessment of portal hypertension
- Extent of collateral vessels
- Unclarified diffuse alterations of the liver
- Control following liver trauma
- Staging of malignant tumours
- Checking indications for surgical intervention
- Examination before and follow-up after LT

Different **radiological procedures** are available for clarifying these diagnostic issues. (s. tab. 8.1)

1. Computer tomography (CT)
2. Magnetic resonance imaging (MRI)
3. Arteriography
4. Portography
5. Phlebography
6. Cholangiography

Tab. 8.1: Radiological procedures used in the diagnosis of hepatobiliary diseases

These various imaging techniques (s. tab. 8.1) — as well as some nuclear medicine-based methods (*see chapter 9*) — enable key features of benign and malignant tumours to be recognized, including (*1.*) vascularity, (*2.*) internal structure, (*3.*) hepatocyte functions, (*4.*) biliary tract, (*5.*) bile secretion, (*6.*) calcification, and (*7.*) Kupffer cell activity.

1 Computer tomography

▶ Tomography was developed by A.E.M. BOCAGE and registered as a French patent in the same year. It was further developed in the form of transversal (and axial) tomography by H. VIETEN (1936) and registered as a German patent. A research team headed by A. GEBAUER presented a device for use in clinical practice in 1945.

▶ The **introduction** of computer tomography (CT) into medicine by G. N. HOUNSFIELD in 1971 (skull CT) and as computerized transverse axial scanning (tomography) in 1973 was a revolutionary event comparable with the discovery of X-rays by W. C. RÖNTGEN in 1895. (15) • As early as 1975, the first normal CT scan of the upper abdomen was reported (R.J. ALFIDI et al.) (1), and in the same year, the first pathological findings from abdominal diseases (relating to the liver) were also presented (D. SCHELLINGER et al., 1975). (38)

1.1 Principle

In computer tomography, the attenuations of many finely focused X-rays are measured by detectors and converted to electrical signals. These values are transmitted to a computer. Subsequently, the absorption value of each image point is calculated and displayed in a complex digital image. The transmission of X-rays through the body occurs in the form of fan beams and is recorded by a rotating detector fan (3rd CT generation). The 4th CT generation features a static detector crown, spanning 360 degrees, around which the X-ray source continually rotates. (9) • More advanced spiral CT facilitates spiral scanning, permitting continuous imaging of the analyzed area while the patient holds his/her breath. This provides accurate anatomical data without respiratory artefacts and with optimum exploitation of the CM bolus. (3, 5, 6, 10, 12)

In contrast to ultrasonography, which is based on the recording and imaging of the reflection of sound waves between tissues with varying acoustic impedance, the radiological signal is produced by **differences in absorption.** • With the **radiation doses** used (100–140 kv), the absorbed dose of energy corresponds to 0.013 Gy (1.3 rad) per tomographical slice. By using many finely focused X-rays, the dose is largely restricted to the body layer to be imaged. Therefore, only a relatively low scatter of radiation has to be taken into consideration. The radiation exposure of a CT scan is comparable to that of a plain radiograph of the abdomen.

With consecutive tomograms, the thickness of each section of the body is 5-8-10 (−12) mm. In individual cases, additional thin-section tomograms of 1 mm can be obtained. Resolution is 1×2 mm in the hepatic area, with an accuracy in attenuation values of up to 0.5%. In this way, the values for a particular cross-section and their spatial distribution are visualized in a scan. This results in blur-free, anatomically precise imaging of a layer of the body in an axial plane. CT scans provide satisfactory information if an object diameter of 1.5 to 3.0 mm is resolved with a density gradient of 0.5% to the surrounding area at an integral dose of 10 mGy.

1.2 Hounsfield units

The attenuation values are given in Hounsfield units (HU), the density scale ranging from −1,000 (= air) through 0 (= water) to +1,000 (= bone). These 2,000 shades of brightness are recorded by the computer, but are not perceived by the human eye. Due to the technical possibility of choosing only a small part of the Hounsfield scale and shifting it within an organ section, smaller differences in density can be more easily detected. Thus within certain limits, CT is indeed able to provide information about the kind of lesion involved. The special value of CT lies in the possibility of determining the density of various tissues, e.g. the structure of fatty tissue is identifiable. This option helps with the differential diagnosis of space-occupying processes (benign vs. malignant). There may be slight fluctuations in the normal Hounsfield units caused by *small vessels* included in the measuring volume. • The terms **hypodense**, **isodense** and **hyperdense** are used to describe pathological changes. (s. p. 132)

1.3 Contrast media

(*1.*) A major improvement in the diagnostic power from **native CT** is achieved by the use of contrast media (CM) (1.0–1.5 ml/kg BW; 1–5 ml/sec), transported via the kidney or in the bile. The CM is administered as i.v. infusion using programmable infusiomates or in the form of i.v. or intra-arterial bolus-triggering. With the conventional CT apparatus (which has a short scanning period of 0.7–5.0 seconds), i.v. administration of a CM bolus (if necessary, with additional i.v. infusion of CM) has proved most effective with regard to the subsequent rapid imaging (4–8 pictures during the first minute) of **dynamic-sequential CT**. This provides detailed assessment of CM dispersion in the intravascular and extravascular areas. (25) The differences in density between the various organs and between the normal liver parenchyma and pathological tissue structures are markedly accentuated. Furthermore, the arterial phase, enhancement of the parenchyma and the phase of venous drainage are recorded simultaneously. • The value of **cine CT** with extremely short scanning periods (7 pictures per second) has not yet been defined with respect to liver diagnostics.

(*2.*) Application of **CT arteriography** (CTA) through the hepatic artery or **CT arterioportography** (CTAP) corresponding to indirect splenoportography (i.e. via the superior mesenteric artery or splenic artery) is considered to be the most efficient procedure in the diagnosis of focal liver lesions. However, it has the disadvantage of being an invasive method. Exact indications (above all for preoperative use) have been defined. • *Modern spiral CT (SCTA or SCTAP) with i.v. injection of contrast medium facilitates excellent angiographic tissue reconstruction on an outpatient basis.* (6) • The development of **multidetector-row CT** (MDCT) has improved liver imaging considerably. With 40–60 row-scanners, true isotropic imaging with a z-axis resolution of 0.3–0.6 mm has become possible. (39)

1.4 Normal liver

The normal liver is characterized by smooth contours and a homogeneous density of 1.068 ± 0.005 g/cm^3. The absorption values are 60 ± 6 HU (or 64 ± 5 HU). Major vessels are delineated as hypodense areas with values of 40–45 HU. The bile ducts near the hilus are occasionally recognized by their hypodensity (5–15 HU); imaging is improved by using a biliary contrast material. CT permits good visualization of the gall bladder. The density of a normal liver is either the same as or up to 8 HU higher than that of the spleen. In some cases, the segments can be delineated.

Volumetry: Using CT, it is possible to determine the size, shape and volume of the liver with considerable accuracy. Hepatic volumetry can be performed with high-level reliability (deviation ± 5–10%). (48)

Falciform ligament: Reduction in the density values in the area of the falciform ligament is explained in the literature by fat deposition. (s. fig. 8.1) • **In more than 6,000 laparoscopies, I have never observed any fat deposition at the areas of attachment of the falciform ligament** (neither in the liver nor at the abdominal wall) or on the transparent ligament itself. (s. fig. 16.4!) • I did, however, frequently find mesenteric fatty tissue along the *round ligament*. In addition, **intrahepatic fat deposits under the falciform ligament are not known either to the anatomist or the pathologist**. • This finding is probably the round ligament, which is occasionally rich in fat, or regional (pathological?) fatty degeneration, as shown in figures 8.3 and 8.4. (s. p. 136)

▶ *Up to now, such (oval) fat deposition has been interpreted by the radiologist as being a falciform ligament (s. fig. 8.1) – this viewpoint must now be reconsidered. It should in any case be noted that the falciform ligament is totally devoid of fat!*

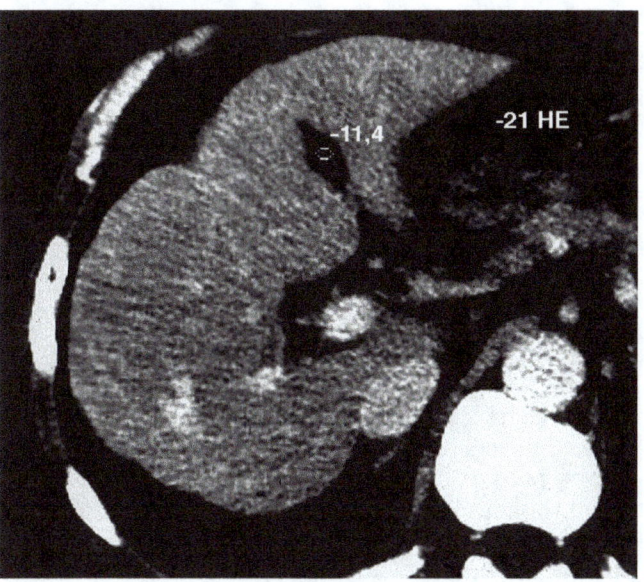

Fig. 8.1: Frequently recorded reduction in density in the area of the falciform ligament (here: 11.4 HU) resembling "fatty tissue" (possibly a round ligament?) (s. p. 136)

1.5 Contraindications

Contraindications include (*1.*) pregnancy, especially in the early stages, (*2.*) known contrast-medium intolerance (restricted to native CT), and (*3.*) renal insufficiency (in which only native CT may be used). With creatinine levels of >1.5 mg/dl, the administration of contrast material is only advisable after consulting an experienced nephrologist. (*4.*) In existing hyperthyreosis (latent or manifest), the thyroid gland must be blocked with sodium perchlorate and even treated with carbimazole if necessary — because of the application of a CM which contains iodine (ca. 300 mg/ml). • A *relative contraindication* applies to diabetics treated with the oral antidiabetic metformin hydrochloride, as this compound competes with the CM in the kidney for elimination. The drug should be discontinued two days prior to the administration of the contrast medium.

1.6 Indications

The indication for the use of CT is only given after a careful (and as far as possible repeated) ultrasonographic examination. Due to the considerable amount of technical equipment required and the high costs involved as well as the radiation exposure associated with this method, CT is not a routine examination procedure. Clinical indications should be assessed thoroughly and must in themselves be justified. (9) (s. tab. 8.2)

1. Primary liver tumours
    - primary liver cell carcinoma (5, 11, 18, 23, 28, 30, 31)
    - haemangiopericytoma, -endothelioma
    - cholangiocarcinoma (55)
    - cystadenocarcinoma (4)
2. Secondary liver tumours
    - metastases (22, 39, 50, 53, 57)
3. Benign liver tumours
    - cysts (51)
    - abscesses
    - adenoma, FNH (2, 23, 24, 26, 34, 37, 42, 52)
    - haemangioma (17, 32, 35, 40, 54)
    - echinococcus (8)
    - tuberculosis (19, 21)
    - lipoma
4. Parenchymal disorders (29)
    - focal fatty infiltration (13, 36, 40, 45, 56)
    - cirrhosis (49)
    - haemochromatosis (20, 29)
    - primary sclerosing cholangitis (7)
5. Mechanical jaundice (47)
6. Condition following liver trauma (33, 41)
    - haematoma
    - rupture
7. Caroli's syndrome (16, 44)
8. Prior to and after liver transplantation (43)
9. Fasciola hepatica (14)
10. Unknown ascites
11. Splenomegaly
12. Budd-Chiari syndrome (27)
13. Portal vein system (46)
14. Interventional measures
    - punctures, drainage tubes
    - chemoembolization

Tab. 8.2: Indications for computer tomography in hepatobiliary diseases (with some references)

1.7 Diffuse liver diseases

1.7.1 Fatty liver

In correlation with fatty infiltration, the fatty liver shows a *diffuse reduction in density* with decreased Hounsfield units. The fatty liver appears much darker than the spleen (= *grey liver*). Hepatomegaly with smooth contours is visible. The parenchyma is isodense or hypodense compared with the vessels and bile ducts, which is why (depending on the degree of fatty infiltration) there is a reversal of density (= *negative scan*). A linear correlation exists between the extent of the fatty infiltration and the decrease in the density recorded. An increase in the relative fat content by 10% leads to a reduction in density of 17(−20) HU. • With fatty degeneration of about 80%, the density is decreased to approx. −50 HU. CT may be useful in controlling the course of a fatty liver, a scan through the middle of the liver being sufficient for this purpose. Dif-

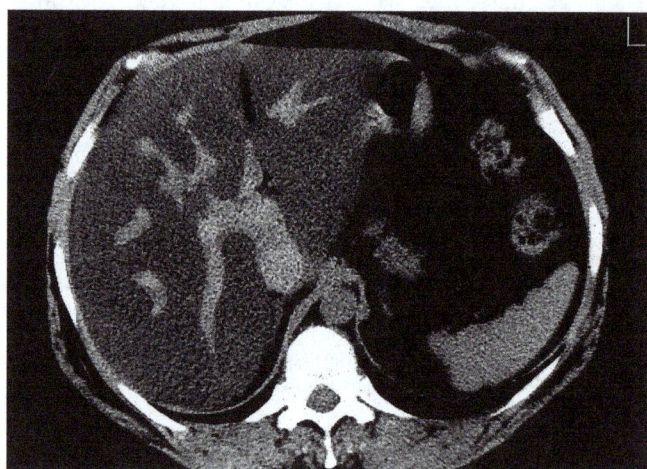

Fig. 8.2: Pronounced, toxic fatty liver following cytostatic chemotherapy with recorded values of between −9.9 and −1.1 HU. The liver is homogeneously dark (compared to the bright spleen). The vessels appear brighter (values of between +40 and +50 HU)

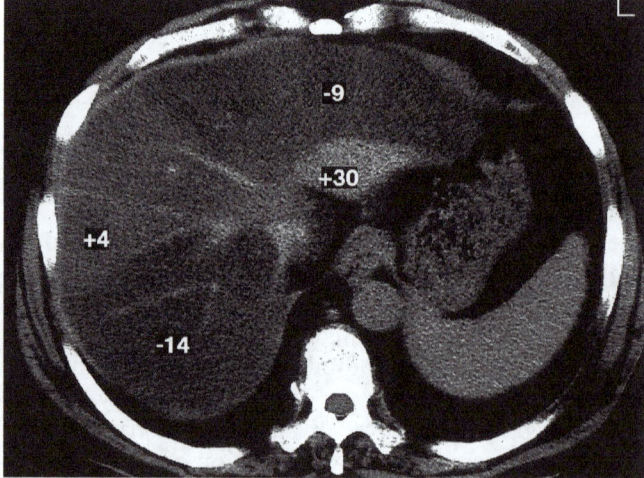

Fig. 8.3: Pronounced focal (regional) fatty degeneration of the liver of varying intensity: both visual and confirmed by Hounsfield units (−14, −9, +4, +30). Native CT, normal value +65 HU

ferentiation between hepatocellular *fatty infiltration* and *fatty liver* is not feasible with CT. The detection rate for diagnosing a fatty liver by means of CT is 85–95%. (s. fig. 8.2) • Besides being diffuse and homogeneous, the fatty liver may also exhibit regional (lobular or segmental) *focal fatty infiltration* of varying degrees. (s. figs. 8.3, 8.4) (cf. figs. 6.12, 6.13) Occasionally, focal infiltration is only barely, or not at all, distinguishable from a malignant tumour. Here MRI is an important additional procedure. (13, 36, 40, 45, 56) *(see chapter 31.3)*

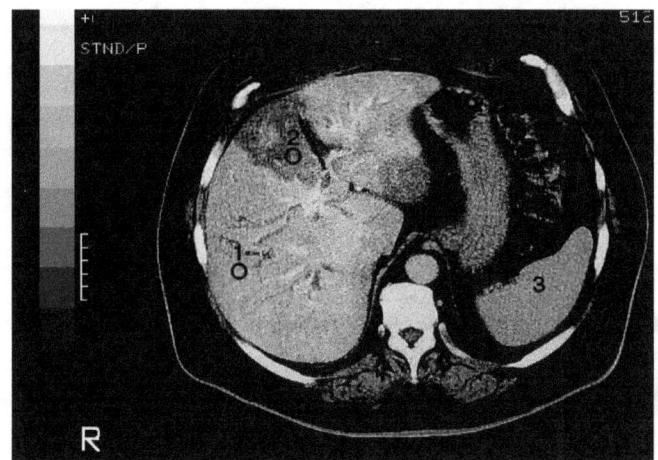

Fig. 8.4: Segmental fatty degeneration of the liver (2 = 37.3 HU) following application of CM compared to liver parenchyma of normal density (1 = 68.5 HU), and the spleen (3)

1.7.2 Liver cirrhosis

As a rule, liver cirrhosis exhibits absorption values which are no different from those of a normal liver. Advanced stages show an enlargement of the caudate lobe and possibly also of the left lobe as well as alterations in form or shrinkage of the right lobe (or both lobes) with fine to coarse nodular irregularities on the surface. In some cases, an increase in density of up to 60–70 HU is verifiable. Usually, splenomegaly and further signs of portal hypertension are present. • Hypodense foci may indicate HCC and should be examined with the aid of contrast medium or MRI. (7, 29, 46, 49)

1.7.3 Haemochromatosis

Haemochromatosis leads to an increase in the density of the liver parenchyma, which correlates with the accumulation of iron. CT scans reveal a remarkably dense and bright liver parenchyma with density values of up to +140 HU (so-called *"white liver"*). The deposition of 1 g iron results in a rise in density of 1 HU. (20) CT densitometry clearly facilitates effective control of therapeutic success in this storage disease. It is not possible, however, to differentiate pronounced secondary haemosiderosis. • *Hyperdense values* are also found in long-term **gold therapy,** in **glycogen thesaurismosis** and **M. Wilson,** or in chronic **arsenic poisoning.**

1.8 Focal liver lesions

Even by means of computer tomography (like ultrasonography), a definitive distinction cannot be made between primary and secondary or benign and malignant liver tumours, except in the case of liver lipoma. However, differentiation is greatly improved by using contrast medium and CT angiography. Radiomorphological identification of focal lesions with a diameter of < 0.3 – 0.8 cm is not (yet) possible, even with the aid of more sophisticated appliances: geometric resolution and density resolution have their limits. The density analysis of focal findings will thus only yield reliable information if the diameter of the focal lesion is within the range of the twofold thickness of the section plane used. Compared to liver parenchyma, most focal lesions are hypodense. *Hyperdense values* (see above) are encountered with calcifications and occasionally also with fresh bleeding and scar tissue. (2, 12, 18, 23)

The **sensitivity** of CT for the confirmation of focal lesions is 84–96%, with a **specificity** of 86–100%. Differentiation between intra- and extrahepatic obstruction was successful in 77–97% of cases; the location of the obstruction was clarified in 79–98%, and the aetiology of the obstruction was established in up to 76% of cases.

1.8.1 Benign liver tumours

1. **Adenoma** is not characterized by any specific features in CT. Density varies between hypodense and slightly hyperdense. The contours are smooth. Following the administration of CM, brief and homogeneous accumulation mostly occurs in the adenoma with the appearance of an initially hypodense margin, which is enhanced in the late phase as a hyperdense border. However, contrast medium which is transportable in the bile cannot enter the adenoma, because it does not contain any biliary structures. An adenoma is frequently distinguished from FNH by evidence of necrotizing areas or sites of fresh bleeding; the latter are recognizable as hyperdense areas. (24, 26, 52)

2. **Focal nodular hyperplasia (FNH)** is distinctly circumscribed, usually round or oval in shape and isodense to slightly hypodense. As a rule, a predominantly hyperdense, central scar zone with stellate septa consisting of connective tissue is visible. Following application of CM (by i.v. infusion), equal concentrations are seen in the liver parenchyma and hepatic tumour, so that the latter may easily pass undetected. In contrast, following i.v. bolus injection of CM, a short, marked and homogeneous enhancement occurs, except in the central cicatricial area. • By means of hepatobiliary sequential scintigraphy, the diagnosis of FNH can be confirmed, particularly with regard to its differentiation from adenoma. (26, 34, 37, 42, 52) (s. p. 202)

3. **Cavernous haemangioma** is hypodense; in some cases, small hyperdense calcified foci are seen within the generally thrombotic centre. The contours of the haemangioma are usually smooth. Density is 35–55 HU. *Bolus injection of CM* is an important diagnostic tool. In the early phase (10–30 seconds), increased, predominantly irregular or garland-form enhancement is observed in the periphery, followed within a few minutes by a slow centripetal increase in density up to isodense values (so-called *"iris-diaphragm phenomenon"*). In the late phase (>10–15 minutes), even hyperdense values may be recorded with a parallel decrease in the density of the surrounding liver parenchyma. (s. fig. 8.5) Haemangiomas with a diameter of >1.0 cm can usually be diagnosed. Thrombotic or fibrotic processes within the haemangioma make differential diagnosis more difficult. (17, 32, 35, 40, 54) • *In our opinion, percutaneous fine-needle biopsy is not advisable!*

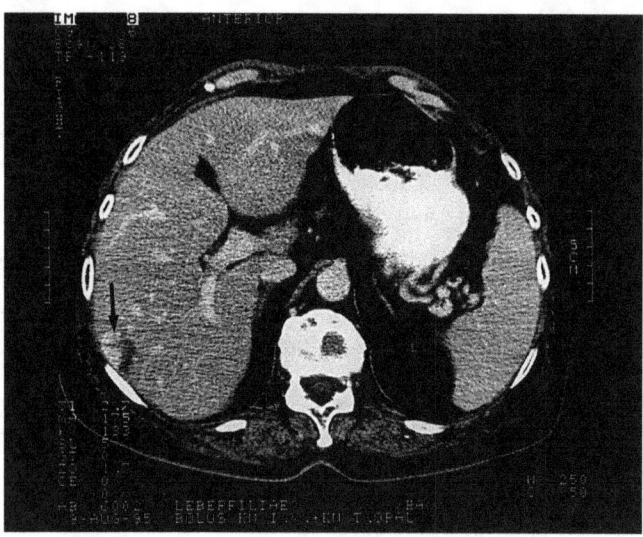

Fig. 8.5: Haemangioma (see arrow). Dynamic CT (contrast-enhanced); portal venous phase (s. figs. 6.18; 8.9; 36.7–36.9)

1.8.2 Vascular lesions

1. **Hepatic haematoma** mostly appears as a well-defined hypodense area; branching is seen in some cases. Intrahepatic haematomas are predominantly round-oval, whereas subcapsular haematomas are mainly crescent-shaped. Depending on their persistence, haematomas have different density values: initially, they are slightly hypodense (40–50 HU), but moderately hyperdense values can already be recorded after a few hours following the reabsorption of plasma. The values become more hypodense (10–20 HU) with increasing lysis and exceed 80 HU in the presence of calcification. Connective tissue generally shows values ranging from 50 to 60 HU.

2. **Liver injury:** Fresh bleeding can be reliably differentiated from a long-standing haemorrhage by CT, which is of importance in cases where surgical procedures are being considered. (33, 41)

3. **Liver infarction** generally leads to a sharply delineated, in most cases triangular, hypodense area, possibly extending up to the liver surface.

4. **Budd-Chiari syndrome** may be imaged in CT as hypodense zones; the findings are not reliable. (27) A definitive diagnosis can be obtained by angiography or MRI.

1.8.3 Hepatic cysts

1. **Dysontogenetic cysts** are solitary or multiple. They are clearly distinguishable from their surroundings, have smooth walls and are readily recognizable by their hypodense (water-equivalent) density values (0–20 HU). In the case of bleeding into the cyst, higher density values are recorded. (This also applies to infections of the cyst fluid or the occurrence of mucous contents.) Following i.v. application of CM, the cyst exhibits no increase in density (in contrast to metastases). A cystic liver is usually associated with cystic kidneys or cystic pancreas. (51) (s. figs. 6.13; 8.6; 36.11–36.14)

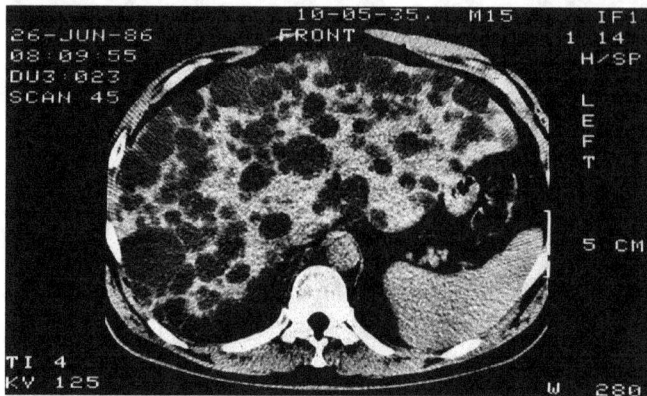

Fig. 8.6: Pronounced dysontogenetic cystic liver and cystic kidney

2. **Echinococcus cysticus** is generally visualized as a multilocular septate cyst with embedded secondary cysts. Both primary and secondary cysts are surrounded by inflammatory granular tissue. During the subsequent course of the disease, calcium deposition is seen in the cystic wall. The application of CM results in mural enhancement. The resulting demarcation of the cysts within the liver is relatively sharp. (8) (s. p. 510)

3. **Echinococcus alveolaris** presents a totally different picture: during the exocystic development of secondary cysts, the parasite gives the impression of growing in an infiltrative, destructive manner. CT scans reveal vaguely outlined, hypodense lesions of a cyst-like nature with nodular calcification (in most cases). Following the application of CM, an inhomogeneous increase in density is observed within the perifocal inflammation. Echinococcus alveolaris is, therefore, easily confused with malignant tumours. (s. p. 512)

4. **Caroli's disease** presents with multiple tubular structures, which correspond to focal cystic dilations of large interlobular bile ducts. The reduced density values of

these ectatic structures in CT are bile-equivalent. Intravenous application of a biliary CM provides the definitive diagnosis. Both portal fibrosis and portal hypertension are present. (16, 44) (s. pp 697, 785)

5. **Choledochal cysts** are congenital, segmental dilations of the larger intrahepatic bile ducts and/or the common bile duct. Diagnosis is obtained by i.v. administration of a biliary contrast medium. Choledochal cysts are frequently combined with tumours, so that additional corresponding signs of biliary obstruction may be verified by means of CT.

1.8.4 Inflammatory liver lesions

1. **Liver abscesses** are mostly (approx. 80%) localized in the right lobe of liver. A pyogenic abscess is visible as a hypodense lesion (0–30 HU) corresponding to the suppurative material with relatively sharp contours. It is surrounded by a hyperdense rim, caused by the well-vascularized granulation tissue. Should a perifocal oedema be present, it may produce an additional hypodense rim. Following the application of CM, an increase in the density of the hyperaemic and hyperdense abscess wall is observed, whereas the density of the abscess remains unchanged. Gas formations inside an abscess caused by anaerobes are easily recognizable on a CT scan. The success rate for detection is 95%. (s. figs. 6.14; 9.2; 25.1; 27.1) *(see chapter 27)*

2. **Macronodular tuberculosis** as screened by CT may be very problematic with respect to its differentiation from benign or even malignant liver tumours. (19, 21)

1.9 Malignant liver tumours

Most malignant liver tumours are hypodense; the difference in value to normal liver parenchyma is usually 15–25 HU. Evidence of hepatic malignancy is obtained by CT, especially by CTAP, in approx. 85% of cases with tumours of >0.5 to 1.0 cm in diameter. (50, 53)

1. **Hepatocellular carcinomas** are extremely variable on CT scans because of their different forms of growth. Morphologically, they appear as (*1.*) isolated masses, (*2.*) multinodular infiltration, or (*3.*) diffuse parenchymatous infiltration. In addition to the mainly hypodense areas, hyperdense regions are also distinctly visible. The often somewhat irregular and slightly blurred, but nevertheless clearly hypodense border shows marked enhancement under CM. Space-occupying lesions, hitherto unrecognizable, may become discernible at this point. Evidence of hypodense areas in liver cirrhosis always strongly suggests primary liver carcinoma. Segmental or lobar decreases in density as a result of frequently occurring infiltrations of the portal vein indirectly suggest the presence of a tumour. Lymph node metastases can also be detected. It is much easier to recognize involvement of the vascular system with the help of CTAP or spiral CT. Depending on the size and location of the hepatocellular carcinoma, contour bulging is also observed. The sensitivity is approx. 75%. CT is an indispensable feature in planning surgery. (5, 28, 30, 31)

2. **Liver metastases** are frequently multiple. They vary in size and are usually hypodense. In contrast to liver parenchyma, they display relatively sharp contours, with a difference in density of at least 10–15 HU. In fatty liver, metastases may even appear hyperdense. Liver metastases are mainly supplied by arterial blood. Therefore i.v. (or even intra-arterial) bolus injection of CM produces the best diagnosis: the metastasis shows increased CM enrichment during the short hypervascular phase; additionally, a peripheral margin forms as a result of the increased concentration of CM. Metastases of 5–10 mm can be detected. Data in the literature confirm a *sensitivity* of 65–91% (in breast cancer up to 100%) and a *specificity* of 81–92%, giving a detection rate of 80–85%. Proof of metastases clearly depends on the histology of the primary tumour; the best diagnostic results are obtained in breast and colon carcinomas. (22, 40, 50, 53, 57)

3. **Malignant lymphomas** may appear in the liver as focal, hypodense lesions. By contrast, diffuse impairment of the periportal region is only demonstrable with CT using special CM. Additionally, extrahepatic lymphomas can be detected at the same time.

1.10 Bile duct obstruction

Obstruction of a large bile duct leads to dilated intrahepatic bile ducts, which appear on CT scans as ramified linear or rounded structures with bile-equivalent density. Their luminal diameter increases progressively in the direction of the hilus. (47) Segmental dilation of the bile ducts may be indicative of a tumour. A dilation of the bile duct of >9 mm points to a peripheral obstruction, mostly near the papilla of Vater.

1.11 Surgical therapy

Pre- and post-therapy CT examinations must be carried out in resections and transplants as well as arterial ligatures, embolization therapy with or without chemotherapy, and also regional chemotherapy. Haematomas, seromas and abscesses can occur around the edge of the resection; compensatory hypertrophia from the residual parenchyma can be identified if no complications occur. After a transplant, hypodensities may point to complications (e.g. necrosis, infarctions, rejection foci). Portal veins enhanced by accompanying hypodense lines are a sign of rejection. Postoperative fluid in the abdomen can also be easily detected using ultrasound and computer tomography. Thromboses in the hepatic artery are discernible with the aid of dynamic CT.

The strategy generally applied in diagnostic clarification in a case of suspected **"liver tumour"** is shown later in a **flow diagram.** (s. p. 204) (s. fig. 9.4)

2 Magnetic resonance imaging

▶ Magnetic resonance imaging (MRI) – also known as magnetic resonance tomography (MRT) – was introduced into medical diagnostics by P.C. LAUTERBUR in 1973.

2.1 Principle

The production of a strong magnetic field induces alignment of the protons along this magnetic field. The homogeneous alignment is perturbed by appropriate high-frequency signals. The protons are diverted and set in a spinning motion. As a result of their efforts to return to the original position, energy is released, which is registered as a signal, calculated by computer analysis and converted to images. The resulting MR signal is dependent on hydrogen nuclei in the object and on the tissue-based time constants T_1 and T_2, i.e. the signals can deviate from the norm (= **isointensive**) by being either **hypointensive** or **hyperintensive**. In this way, (1.) tissues with different proton density values can be distinguished, (2.) concentrations of body-own elements (C, F, N, P) can be determined, and (3.) chemical compositions of certain tissue areas are clarified by means of supraconductive apparatus with magnetic fields of 0.5–2.0 tesla (T).

Four parameters are thus imaged in MRI by means of mathematical calculations: (1.) *proton density,* (2.) *relaxation time T_1* (= binding force between the nuclear spin grate and the surrounding molecular grate), (3.) *relaxation time T_2* (= binding effect between the various nuclear spins), and (4.) *flow velocity.*

Two types of appliance are used: (1.) resistance (or iron) magnets and (2.) supraconductive magnets.

Paramagnetic substances such as manganese or gadolinium compounds (Gd-DTPA, Gd-EOB-DTPA, Gd-BOPTA, Gd-DOTA of Mn-DPOP) are used as i.v. contrast media. They are absorbed by the hepatocytes, so that healthy liver tissue appears lighter on T_1 images ("whitener" effect). These substances are excreted via the biliary and renal system. • **Superparamagnetic particles of iron oxides** (SPIO) is a new contrast medium for exact localization of focal liver lesions and for differentiation of normal and pathological regions. The 3–5 nm iron oxide nuclei grow to a size of 45–60 nm due to the polysaccharide sheath. They are principally absorbed by the RES (but also collect temporarily in the extravascular space). These iron oxide nuclei are broken down into lysosomes and taken into normal iron storage; the respective iron uptake corresponds to the average nutritional intake of two to three days. Healthy liver tissue appears as dark areas in T_2 images ("darkener" effect). This shows that CM is also stored in the fatty liver and FNH. Foci of up to 2–3 mm can be detected. Hepatic metastases appear extremely "light" compared to the "black" parenchyma. (62, 84, 89, 97, 103, 122)

2.2 Advantages

These techniques can be used to achieve a very *sharp contrast between various tissues.* This permits better differentiation and characterization of normal or pathological tissues, compared with ultrasonography and CT.

• A great advantage of MRI is the possibility of imaging not only transverse *cross-sections* (as is the case with CT), but also *longitudinal sections* of various planes (e.g. sagittal and coronary) in the hepatic area – without changing the patient's position. Topographic analysis and the interpretation of findings are hence less complicated than with CT. The thickness of the section planes is usually 10 mm. • MRI is also capable of differentiating static from flowing conditions and calculating the *flow rate* in various vascular areas. • Furthermore, the concentration of certain *elements* and the *proton density* can be measured. MRI is thus a valuable diagnostic tool in certain situations, serving to supplement CT and at the same time replacing intra-arterial angiography or scintigraphy. • A further major advance is the development of **MR angiography** – which may well prove to be a (better) alternative to invasive catheter angiography. (99)

2.3 Disadvantages

The use of first-generation MRI was associated with certain problems, e.g. **artefactual images** caused by respiratory movement, cardiac action, vascular pulsation and intestinal peristalsis. The introduction of turbo-spin-echo-pulse sequences, however, led to a drastic shortening of recording periods, so that artefacts due to breathing and peristalsis are now rare. It is important that the patient breathes normally and is in a resting position. In addition to the reduction in recording periods with modern apparatus, the time needed for reconstruction has been shortened thanks to new computer imaging techniques (polytomography, 3D-layer batch). • Thought should be given in this respect to the **physical stress** experienced by the patient through a static magnetic field, temporally varying magnetic fields and high-frequency fields in the megahertz range. No clinically significant damage has been reported if attention is paid to the contraindications. • In individual cases, the time spent in the magnetic tunnel may, however, cause **mental distress.** Sometimes this claustrophobia requires sedative premedication. In order to suppress **intestinal peristalsis,** administration of spasmolytics or glucagon (0.5 to 1.0 mg i.v.) is recommended. • The operators should be aware of potential **contrast-medium incidents.** In practice, however, such adverse reactions are rarely seen.

Contraindications are internal *ferromagnetic objects* in the body, e.g. implants, clips, splinters and especially cardiac pacemakers. Through their electromagnetic effects, they may cause biomolecular disturbances, and even cellular damage. Based on the current level of knowledge and the developmental stage of the technical equipment and contrast media, it is advisable that *pregnant women* and *nursing mothers* as well as *epilepsy patients* be generally excluded from MRI examinations (however, such contraindications become relative in the face of a strong indication).

2.4 Normal liver

On MRI scans, a normal liver generally produces a picture similar to that obtained by CT. The parenchyma appears as a homogeneous area with relatively high signal intensity (T_1). The portal and liver veins are easily differentiated as signal-free or low-signal structures. With prolonged echo-time, the signal intensity of the liver veins also increases. (s. fig. 8.7) shows a clear increase in signal intensity. Regeneration nodes are distinguishable because the T_1 and T_2 signal is weaker here than in cirrhotic tissue. So-called siderotic nodes are found in 25% of cases ($T_2 \downarrow$). Malignant foci do not contain any iron. This results in "nodes within nodes", where malignant growth occurs in a regeneration node. (86, 92, 93, 96, 107)

Haemochromatosis: Due to the accumulation of iron in the liver cells, the relaxation time T_2 is much shorter and the signal intensity weaker. This can also be determined quantitatively. Depending on the iron content, the liver appears dark grey to black. (s. fig. 8.8) The detection rate is 100% at an iron concentration of 1 mg/g liver tissue. An iron-free node may suggest HCC. • *Haemosiderosis* with iron deposition in the RES is characterized by similar, yet less marked findings. A fall in signal intensity is discernible when the iron content/g in the liver tissue has almost quadrupled. (58, 64, 78, 91, 94, 113)

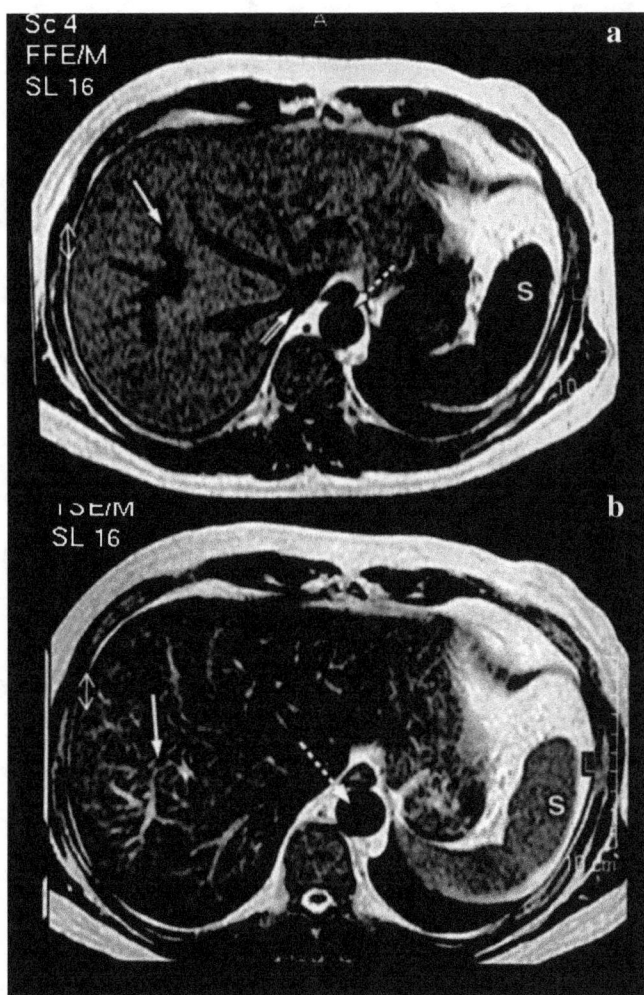

Fig. 8.7: Normal MRI: **a)** T_1-weighted scan; **b)** T_2-weighted scan. • Branches of the portal vein (→), aorta (--▶), spleen (S), inferior vena cava (⇒) with stellate ramifications of the hepatic veins

2.5 Diffuse liver diseases

Acute hepatitis: In the early stages of the disease, the T_2-scan shows an increase in signal intensity, whereas a prolongation of T_1 tends to be observed before the occurrence of liver cell necrosis.

Fatty liver: Fatty infiltration into liver cells is not detected by MRI, even though fatty tissue shows high signal intensity on spin-echo imaging. The water associated with the (hyperdense) fatty liver may lead to a signal reduction during the T_1-time, whereby the plus and minus variations in signal intensity result in an indifference, which corresponds to normal liver tissue; T_1 and T_2 thus remain unchanged. Only markedly T_1-weighted scans exhibit increased signal intensity. MRI is an important method in searching for (hypodense) metastases in a (hyperdense) fatty liver. (39, 89) (s. p. 138, 180)

Cirrhosis: Like CT, MRI also portrays cirrhosis-related changes in liver size and shape, irregular superficial contours, dilated portal vessels and collaterals (generally also reversal of portal flow) as well as splenomegaly. As a result of the enhanced blood engorgement, the spleen

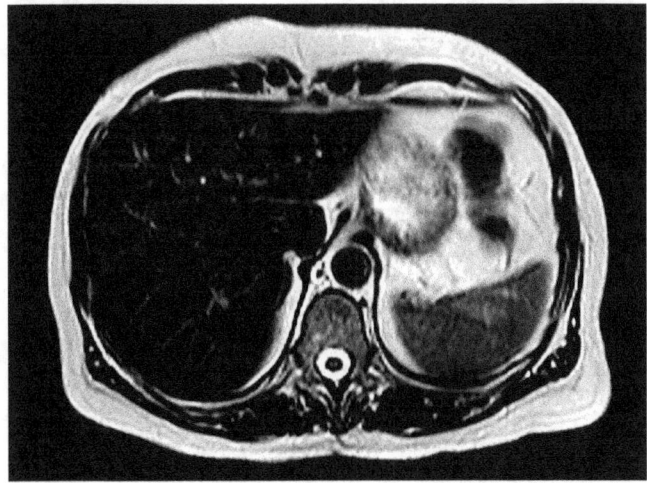

Fig. 8.8: Haemochromatosis: characteristically weakened signal (or even signal elimination) in a T_2-weighted scan due to disturbances in the magnetic field caused by iron deposition in the liver

Primary biliary cirrhosis: In correspondence with the extent of copper deposition in the liver, the relaxation times T_1 and T_2 are shortened, with a distinct decrease in signal intensity. (121)

Others: Further study results are available relating to amyloidosis (29, 111), primary sclerosing cholangitis (73), peliosis hepatis (105), Budd-Chiari syndrome (29, 60, 108), schistosomiasis (29, 79), biliary tract diseases (75, 82, 120), echinococcosis (69, 71) and adenoma. (67, 74)

2.6 Focal liver lesions

Focal liver lesions of >2 mm in diameter are detectable in MRI. In addition, the specificity of MRI is higher than can be achieved by means of CT examination. (2, 29, 61, 62, 89, 97, 106, 119)

Cavernous haemangioma: The visualized findings consist of a roundish, homogeneous high-signal (T_2-weighted *"light bulb"*) area and a well defined hypointense to isointense (T_1-weighted) area. (s. fig. 8.9) Usually, no internal structures are visible. The imaging effect is best accomplished following i.v. administration of Gd-DTPA on the T_1-weighted scan with centripetal contrast-medium enhancement. Because of the paramagnetic component of methaemoglobin, the signal intensity may be more pronounced, although it is usually reduced in a T_1-weighted scan. (63, 76, 83, 87, 101, 110, 114, 116)

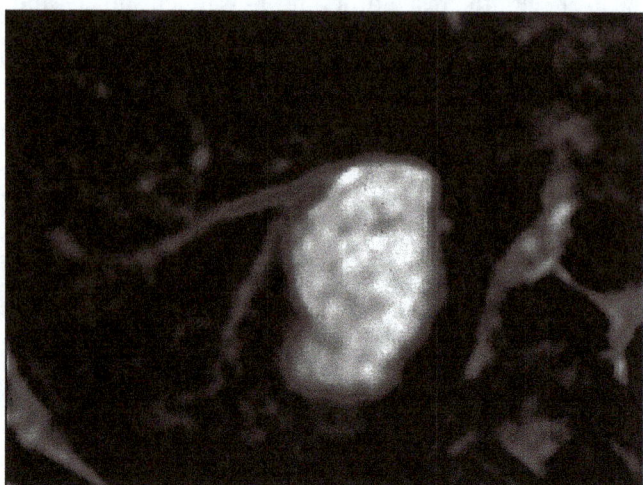

Fig. 8.9: Cavernous haemangioma: a large (2.5 × 4.2 cm) hyperintense (white) lobular focus with an afferent vessel (T_2-weighted scan; transverse) (s. figs. 6.15; 8.5: 36.6)

Focal nodular hyperplasia: On MRI scans (as with CT), FNH shows the characteristic central venous star. Otherwise, the signal intensity of FNH is homogeneously isointense (T_1) or slightly hyperintense (T_2). Immediately following the i.v. administration of CM (Gd-DTPA), a distinct but rapidly fading enhancement is observed. (65, 95, 100, 102, 110, 118)

Malignant tumours: Due to their prolonged relaxation times, malignant tumours are sharply demarcated from the liver parenchyma. On T_1-weighted scans they are low-signal, on T_2-weighted scans they are high-signal areas. Differentiation of tumour tissue from central necrosis is possible. Intrahepatic, tumour-induced vascular displacements as well as capsular structures and perifocal oedema can be demonstrated. This is characterized by an intact ring of enhancement on hepatic arterial dominant-phase images. There is sometimes a peripheral or heterogeneous washout of contrast agent in the hepatic venous phase or a washout leading to hypointensity, even in hypervascular metastasis. It is not (yet) possible to define the tumour type. Moreover, differentiating malignant tumours from adenomas (67, 74) and haemangiomas (76, 87, 101) or from focal fatty infiltration (39) is problematic. The success rate for differentiating patients devoid of liver tumours from those with metastatic liver is 87% (CT: 84%) with a specificity of 98% (CT: 91%). (70, 97) • Proof of metastases (23, 29, 39, 66, 70, 72, 76, 87, 101, 102, 117, 119) (s. fig. 8.10) or hepatocellular carcinomas (29, 66, 68, 80, 81, 85, 90, 96, 98,

112) is obtained in 85–95% of cases. Study results in patients with cholangiocarcinoma (77), mesenchymal tumours (104, 109) and plasmocytoma are also available. Small-nodular carcinosis in the omentum or peritoneum (without concomitant ascites) and subcapsular hepatic metastases (< 5 mm) remain undetected with US, CT or MRI – they can only be found using laparoscopy.

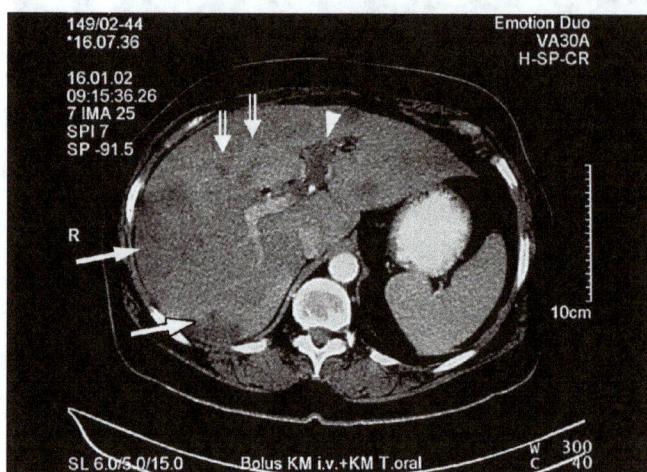

Fig. 8.10: Multiple metastases of a pancreatic carcinoma (↑); numerous focus-like signs of aerobilia (⇑); thrombosis of the left portal vein (▲)

Hepatic cysts: Cysts are visualized on the T_1-weighted scan as low-signal (= black) and on the T_2-weighted scan as homogeneously high-signal (= bright), closely circumscribed, focal lesions. An increase in signal intensity on the T_1-weighted scan suggests bleeding into the cysts.

Hepatic abscesses: An abscess is displayed as low-signal in the T_1 image and signal-intensive in the T_2 image. The perifocal oedema cannot be separated from the lesion. Gadolinium CM can be used to visualize a thick abscess wall in the T_1 image. Gas appears hypodense and cannot be differentiated from prior bleeding. • Treatment of such abscesses is easily monitored.

Portal veins: There are reports on MRI visualization of large intrahepatic portovenous shunts (59), collaterals in the portal vein (92, 115) and VOD staging. (88)

> The strategy generally applied in diagnostic clarification in a case of clinical suspicion of **"liver tumour"** is shown later in a **flow diagram.** (s. p. 204) (s. fig. 9.4)

3 Angiography

For clarifying vascular liver diseases and alterations of vessels associated with liver diseases (especially tumours), angiographic procedures are available, should CEDS, CT and MRI yield no definitive diagnosis. With the help of contrast media, they make possible the imaging of the afferent arterial or portal vessels and the efferent veins in the area of the liver. (s. tab. 8.3)

Arteriography
1. Coeliac artery (coeliac trunc HALLERI) (s. fig. 8.11)
2. Selective arteriography
   - common hepatic artery
   - superior mesenteric artery
   - splenic artery
   - right/left hepatic artery

Portography
1. Direct splenoportography
   - percutaneous (s. fig. 8.12)
   - laparoscopic
2. Indirect portography
   - splenoportography via the splenic artery
   - portography via the superior mesenteric artery (s. fig. 8.11)
3. Omphaloportography (s. fig. 8.13)
4. Transhepatic portography

Phlebography
1. Cavography
2. Phlebography of the hepatic veins
3. Transhepatic phlebography

Tab. 8.3: Angiographic liver examination methods which are possible in principle, but which are now partially obsolete

3.1 Arteriography

▶ Selective arteriography uses a transfemoral catheter technique (S.I. SELDINGER, 1953; P. ÖDMAN, 1959). (s. fig. 8.11) • The catheter may also be introduced into the axillary artery. Superselective CM visualization of hepatic arteries via the proper hepatic artery shows blood vessels down to the sixth division; the smallest depictable diameter is approx. 0.5 mm. Imaging of the arteries is effected by nonionic iodine-containing contrast medium at a reduced flow rate (20−30 ml, 6−8 ml per second). Using this infusion technique, 8 to 12 angiograms can be produced within a period of approx. 12 seconds. In this way, both the early arterial phase and the parenchymal phase as well as the venous phase can be recorded. Visualization of the CM-filled blood vessels is effected by (*1.*) *conventional film angiography* which has been replaced by digital subtraction angiography, (*2.*) *digital subtraction angiography* (DSA) using an image-intensifying TV link instead of the X-ray film, (*3.*) *CT arterioportography*, or (*4.*) *MRI angiography* and meanwhile *whole body MR arteriography* using gadolinium. (133)

3.1.1 Indications

Focal liver lesions of > 1.0−1.5 cm in diameter are usually detectable. Even hypervascular foci with a diameter of > 0.5 cm are visible when using the infusion technique. In 75−90% of cases, a normal arterial blood supply is guaranteed via the proper hepatic artery. Alterations relating to the hepatic arteries can be angiographically confirmed in virtually 100% of cases. Vascular anomalies (10−20%) are of no clinical significance. Knowledge of their existence may, however, be important in surgical procedures. Variations in the location and shape of the liver and changes in the region of the caudate lobe and quadrate lobe are also recognizable. Despite the initial use of noninvasive imaging methods, and possibly laparoscopy, hepatic arteriography is still indicated in some situations, especially for the purpose of *angiotherapy*. (123, 124, 128, 135, 136, 141, 145, 147, 148, 151, 157) (s. tab. 8.4)

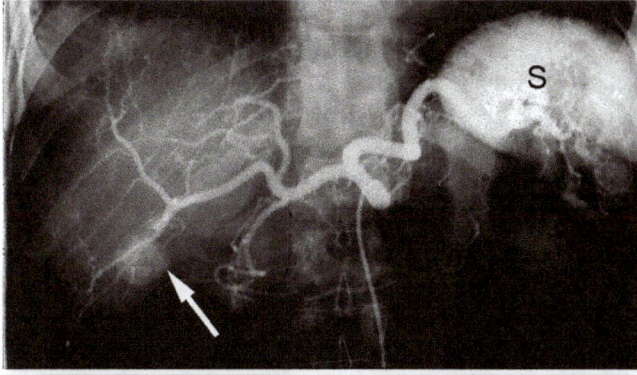
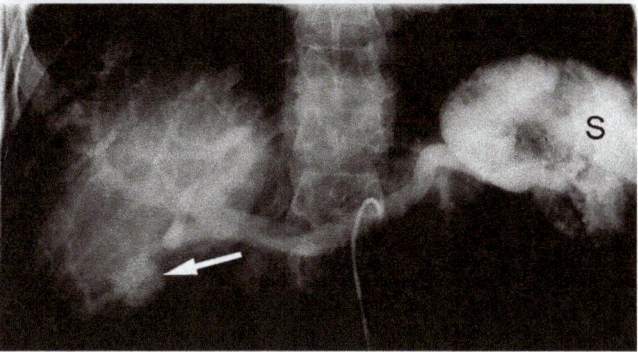

Fig. 8.11: Arterioportography: coeliacography with good visualization of the branches of the coeliac trunk including the fine ramifications. Small hypervascularized haemangioma (↑); S = spleen. (The pancreatic vessels are also visible.) • Normal depiction of the portal vessels in the venous phase

1. Vascular anomalies, stenoses or aneurysms
2. Preoperative study of vascular blood supply
3. Haemobilia
4. Arteriovenous fistula
5. Occlusive (including posttraumatic) embolization
6. Angiotherapy within the framework of a transjugular intrahepatic portosystemic stent shunt (TIPS)
7. Treatment of liver tumours
   - chemoinfusion, chemoperfusion, chemoembolization

Tab. 8.4: Possible indications for hepatic arteriography if modern contrast-medium-based CEDS, CT and MRI fail to provide reliable information, or if angiotherapy is indicated

3.1.2 Contraindications

Hepatic arteriography is contraindicated in cases of severe *coagulation disorders*. Cut-off values are deemed to be: Quick's value of > 60%, thrombocytes of > 100,000, and bleeding time of < 3 minutes. These figures only serve as a guide; a more careful assessment must be made in each individual case. • In the presence of *renal failure*, the use of contrast media, and thus arteriography, is contraindicated.

3.1.3 Complications

With strict heparinization, the incidence of serious complications is below 1%. A lethality rate of 0.06% has been reported. Arterial puncture is associated with certain risks relating to the introduction of a guide wire or catheter (thrombosis, formation of haematomas, arteriovenous fistula) and to the catheter itself (damage to the vascular wall, thrombosis, vascular perforation). Intolerance reactions to the contrast medium may also occur (in 3—5% of cases). With DSA, however, the complication rate decreases.

3.1.4 Focal lesions

In the diagnosis of focal liver lesions, angiography is no longer of any real practical value. The angiogram of focal liver lesions is usually nonspecific. • *With regard to its indications, hepatic arteriography has lost importance as a diagnostic tool, but has become more valuable as a therapeutic approach.* • Hypervascular foci and foci situated in the peripheral liver sections are identified more reliably than those in the central areas. The intermediary region between the right and left lobe of liver shows less vascularization; additional vascular supply variants are seen here more often. In hypervascular tumours, the success rate for detection is >90%. This is further improved by the use of angio-CT.

Primary malignant liver tumours with a predominantly hypervascular blood supply mainly comprise carcinomas and sarcomas. Depending on the vascularization of the tumour, the parenchymal phase shows areas that are lower in CM density and others with increased CM density (*"pooling"*). Where there is insufficient blood flow, this pooling often results in patchy images. • The *criteria of malignancy* are neovascularization, irregular outline, "vascular break-offs", "blood lakes" as a result of dilated vessels, early discharge of contrast material via arteriovenous anastomoses in pathological veins, vascular occlusions, increase in the calibre of nutritive hepatic arteries, reduced intratumoural circulation, corkscrew-shaped arteries of different calibres, and vascular displacements (stretching, spreading or arciform displacement of arteries). Cholangiocellular carcinomas and the hepatocellular carcinomas related to liver cirrhosis are mainly hypovascular. For this reason, they are hardly recognizable. (130, 139, 144, 149—151)

Secondary malignant liver tumours, such as metastases of adenocarcinomas, are also hypovascular and therefore usually not identifiable by arteriography. In contrast, the metastases of malignant goitre, hypernephroid carcinoma, insulinoma and chorionepithelioma are hypervascular and therefore readily visible.

Benign focal lesions usually lead to a smoothly curved displacement of arteries (and veins). In the parenchymal phase, they show more or less sharply delineated filling defects. (132, 145, 156)

In 80—90% of cases, *focal nodular hyperplasia* shows a typical, radial (spoke-like) arrangement of coiled vessels in the area of the tumour, which originate from a circular artery. Occasionally, fine a.v. shunts are present. The smooth-edged lesion is hypervascular. The parenchymal phase, with its homogeneous concentration of contrast medium, allows the lesion to be clearly demarcated from healthy liver tissue. (156) • *Hepatic adenoma* is generally hypervascular. Displaced vessels are frequently visible.

A nutritive vessel extends into the tumour from the periphery. Neovascularization and irregularities of the vessels may be shown, which complicates differential diagnosis with regard to malignancy. In the parenchymatous phase, the tumour exhibits marked enhancement. (156) • The *cavernous haemangioma* shows late filling of the hollow spaces; the contrast medium initially accumulates in the form of lacunes at the margin of the tumour. Patchy, blurred outflows of contrast material subsequently appear in the whole tumour area. The contrast medium persists for an extremely long period of time into the parenchymatous phase. No arteriovenous fistulas are detected. (129) • Intrahepatic *haematomas* lead to separation of the major vessels with vascular break-offs and extravasations. Arteriovenous shunts may occur. There is no visualization of the parenchyma. • *Haemobilia* is characterized by an arteriobiliary flow of CM with imaging of the intra- and extrahepatic bile ducts. (142) • *Echinococcus alveolaris* with its invasive and multilocular growth produces an image similar to that seen in malignant liver tumours. At the periphery, irregular, often twisted and stenotic or occluded arteries and small CM extravasations are visible. In the parenchyma, contrast medium-free areas as well as occasional CM enhancement can be detected.

3.1.5 Diffuse liver diseases

Arteriography is not a suitable method for diagnosing **liver cirrhosis.** It may only be used in special situations (e. g. planned surgical procedures). In liver cirrhosis, the arteries appear dilated in some cases or take the form of narrow vessels; mostly, the arterial presentation is sparse. At the periphery, the arteries often follow a spiral course. The parenchymal phase exhibits an inhomogeneous, patchy image; regions with connective tissue appear hypovascular. Regeneration nodes can resemble benign liver tumours in arteriograms. In advanced stages of cirrhosis, the hepatic artery may dilate as a result of increased arterial flow, with a subsequent reversal of the flow in the gastroduodenal artery. The latter is therefore no longer visible in coeliacography. In patients with cirrhosis showing dilation of the hepatic artery and a reversed blood flow in the gastroduodenal artery, the blood circulation and functions of the liver are better than in patients without this "steal effect". *Such a finding may be an important criterion when considering a portacaval shunt operation.* (123, 127, 141, 143)

3.1.6 Therapeutic infusion

In traumatic bleeding in the area of the liver, haemostasis may be performed within the framework of diagnostic arteriography by means of embolization. Arterial access likewise facilitates embolization and cytostatic treatment of liver tumours (following angiographic insertion of the catheter). (s. tab. 8.4)

3.2 Portography

▶ In animal experiments, a contrast medium was first injected percutaneously into the spleen by S. ABEATICI et al. in 1951 in order to visualize the portal circulation by means of X-ray. This method was later introduced into clinical practice as direct splenoportography by J.L. LEGER (1951) and R. BOULVIN et al. (1951).

Portography is defined as the radiological visualization of the portal vein and its various afferent branches as well as their distribution in the liver. (s. tab. 8.3) It facilitates not only the direct measurement of portal pressure, but also the exact localization of portal flow obstruction and thus the differentiation between prehepatic, intrahepatic or posthepatic block. The prehepatic block can be located at the edge of the splenic and/or portal vein. Blood flow is predominantly in a hepatopetal direction. Central blocks are frequently the result of an infection in the umbilical vein during early childhood. (s. p. 190) This usually leads to cavernous transformation of the veins in the hepatoduodenal ligament and the formation of periportal veins. An intrahepatic block results in hepatofugal blood flow. Portal high pressure can be recognized in the early stages by a widening of the left gastric vein (> 5−6 mm). For surgical planning in portal hypertension, knowledge of portal vascular morphology and haemodynamics is a major prerequisite. • Shunt function, blood flow to the liver and collateral circulation are accurately displayed with the aid of indirect mesenteric and splenic portography. In more difficult cases, the shunt can be monitored using a direct probe via the inferior vena cava. (128, 137)

Impressive images of portal arteries and hepatic veins can be produced by MR angiography. (131, 152) Nowadays, CM-supported MRA is the method of choice in monitoring the portal artery system (primarily before and after TIPS insertion). (152)

3.2.1 Indications

Ultrasound and, more particularly, colour-encoded Doppler sonography are the methods of choice for the diagnostic study of the portal venous system. • Equivocal findings are an indication for contrast-medium CT or MRI, both of which provide superior angiographic images following i.v. injection of an appropriate CM − this is equally possible on an outpatient basis. • Portographic examination techniques should only be used in special instances which are not sufficiently clarified by these imaging procedures. The various techniques may have different indications in individual cases. The appropriate method should be carefully selected; this depends to a large extent on patient-related considerations. (s. tabs. 8.3, 8.5)

1. Differentiation of various forms of portal hypertension, with measurement of blood pressure if necessary
2. Checking on the possibility of anastomosis in portal vessels
3. Detection of spontaneous splenorenal shunts
4. Proof of collateral flow in bleeding oesophageal varices
5. Follow-up after shunt operation
6. Suspected Budd-Chiari syndrome
7. Identification of the morphological course of hepatitis (with variations between the single segments)

Tab. 8.5: Potential indications for portography if modern contrast-medium CEDS, CT and MRI fail to provide reliable findings

3.2.2 Direct splenoportography

1. **Laparoscopic splenoportography** has three **advantages** over the percutaneous technique (153): (*1.*) splenic puncture is performed under visual control, (*2.*) the procedure can be repeated several times during the same examination, and (*3.*) complications are rare. • The **examination** itself is not subject to time pressure, thus permitting measurement of the "standing" blood column with imaging up to ten minutes and longer following the injection of contrast medium. The needle is inserted from the medial splenic margin 4−5 cm deep into the caudal or medial segment, axially and in the segmental central line. The correct positioning of the needle in the spleen can be checked by the **decholine test,** which also provides information on the portal circulation. With open arterial crus and simultaneously closed venous crus or with both vascular crura open (filling and flow phases), pseudoarterial afterbleeding lasting for ten minutes or longer may occur, which spontaneously ceases when there is a change in phase from filling to emptying. Coagulation measures are advisable in prolonged secondary haemorrhage.

2. **Laparoscopic transhepatic retrograde splenoportography** allows early diagnosis of portal hypertension by segmental portography of the liver. The puncture cannula is correctly positioned in a portal vessel when the injected contrast medium is distributed like the crown of a tree and the measured portal pressure (normal 8−15 mmHg) exceeds the pressure of the hepatic vein (normal: 4−8 mmHg). • **Direct splenography using laparoscopy also allows identification of different morphological alterations in various segments!** (153, 154) *Particular consideration must be given to this factor when assessing a liver biopsy specimen.* • With laparoscopic angiography, both *segmental portography* and *segmental arteriography* have proved effective. (155)

3. **Percutaneous splenoportography** has lost its importance. Should a direct procedure be indicated, laparoscopic splenoportography is a possible alternative. Recently, a **new technique** has been described. (134) • The percutaneous splenic puncture is performed using a thin needle under screen control, with the needle directed at the splenic hilus. The pressure of the splenic pulp can be measured directly in order to estimate the portal vein pressure. Contrast medium is injected manually or by a special device. From this depot in the red pulp, the splenic vein, the portal vein and the intrahepatic branches of the portal vein are contrasted within a few seconds. (s. fig. 8.12) • *Complications* resulting from percutaneous splenoportography include afterbleeding from the spleen, bilateral rupture of the spleen, arterial aneurysms and a.v. shunts − these complications are serious in nature, but rare. • *Contraindications* for the procedure should be carefully observed. (s. tab. 8.6)

1. Clotting disorders
2. Ascites
3. Adhesions, especially perisplenic adhesions
4. Inoperability with respect to a shunt procedure
5. Splenic diseases (cysts, tumours, leukaemia, *etc.*)

Tab. 8.6: Contraindications for direct (particularly percutaneous) splenoportography

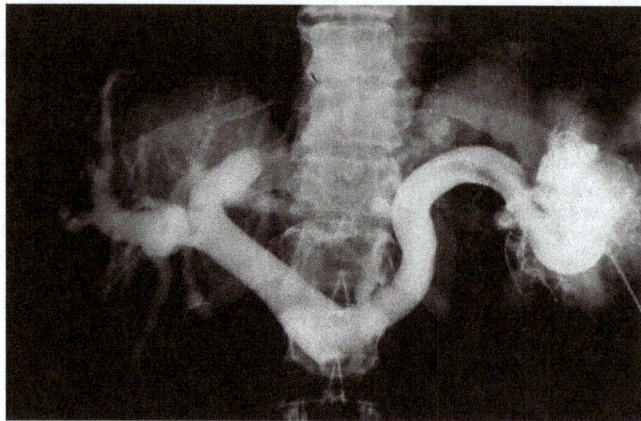

Fig. 8.12: Use of direct percutaneous splenoportography in portal hypertension

3.2.3 Indirect splenoportography

Except where there are individual unresolved diagnostic issues, direct portography has been replaced by arteriography. Using selective arteriography, the same examination yields (in 80−90% of cases) an indirect splenoportogram through the splenic artery and an indirect portogram via the superior mesenteric artery. In addition, the hepatofugal collaterals are shown, so that it is possible to assess the hepatic block and the direction of the blood flow. Portal pressure cannot be measured by means of this technique. • Following injection of a contrast medium into the coeliac trunk, the CM flows through the splenic artery into the spleen and returns through the splenic vein. Thus, in addition to the arterial system, the portal vein with its extra- and intrahepatic branches is also visible. (126) (s. fig. 8.11) • The *contraindications* and *complications* valid for any transfemoral catheterizations apply equally to indirect splenoportography. The low frequency of complications together with a good diagnostic yield make indirect splenoportography useful in clarifying specific issues. • In the case of severe **splenomegaly,** the attempt to visualize the splenic vein via the splenic artery usually fails, even with high doses of contrast medium of 60−80 ml − the CM simply "sinks into" the large spleen. In these cases, direct splenoportography is the method of choice.

3.2.4 Omphaloportography

Umbilical portography was first described by D. G. DUVINER in 1954 and introduced into clinical use by O. GONZALES GARBALHAES in 1959. The umbilical vein consists of a right branch (which is totally obliterated postpartum) and a left branch (the cranial portion of which is closed, whereas the section in the vicinity of the liver is only sealed by endothelium); the latter is frequently preserved as a residual channel. The omphaloportographic **technique** is based on the surgical opening (at a point 5−7 cm above the umbilicus) and bouginage of the umbilical vein, with the subsequent insertion of a catheter. The probe is successful in 90% of cases. The (specially shaped) catheter can be inserted as far as the splenic or mesenteric vein. By injecting a contrast medium, the portal venous system is successfully imaged. (s. fig. 8.13) Visualization of single portal branches may be attempted using special catheters. Portal vein pressure can be measured directly. **Indications** are rare. It is, however, possible to determine the pressure in the portal vein directly (e.g. prior to shunt operations). (138) In the case of suspected apudomas, blood samples can be taken from the splenic vein for hormone analysis. It is also possible to use high-dosage chemotherapy (e.g. in colorectal liver metastases). In a laparotomy, omphaloportography may be useful for clarifying certain issues in isolated cases. (s. tab. 8.7) • Potential **complications** include perforation, thrombosis and infection. The complication rate is 10−15%. (138, 146)

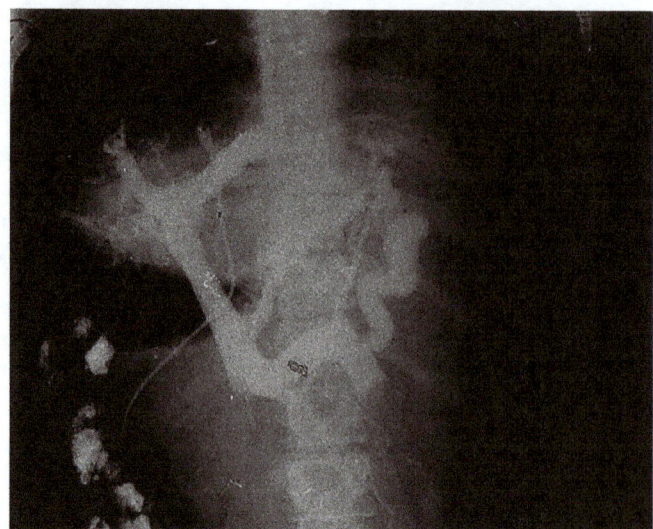

Fig. 8.13: Use of omphaloportography in portal hypertension

1. Preoperative diagnosis prior to liver resection or shunt operation
2. Status after thrombosis of the splenic vein or after splenectomy
3. Suspected "pseudo-obstruction" of the portal vein
4. Use of an extracorporeal makeshift vessel
5. Diagnosis directly from portal blood
   (e.g. measurement of portal pressure, apudoma)
6. Therapeutic instillation into portal blood
   (e.g. targeted high-dose chemotherapy in colorectal liver metastases)

Tab. 8.7: Indications for omphaloportography which are possible in principle, but now largely obsolete

3.2.5 Percutaneous transhepatic portography

This method was developed as an alternative to laparoscopic transhepatic portography. Some 40 ml of CM are usually injected at a rate of 10 ml/sec. It is a difficult technique, takes more time and involves greater risks. This method allows the portal pressure to be measured. After positioning the catheter with the aid of a guide wire, any branch of the portal vein can be visualized in a superselective manner following application of CM. This method can also be used to take blood samples from various veins for the purpose of hormone analysis. If oesophageal variceal bleeding occurs, targeted obliteration of the coronary vein is possible. Existing collaterals, including splenorenal connections, can be visualized. The frequency of severe complications (e.g. bile peritonitis, bleeding) is 2−3%.

3.3 Phlebography

The venous system of the liver can also be shown by X-ray. (s. tab. 8.3) Such radiological methods have their specific diagnostic yields and thus their own indications. (125, 131, 140, 158)

1. **Cavography** may be useful in patients with suspected Budd-Chiari syndrome or anomalies of the hepatic veins as well as prior to liver transplantation and in clarifying the aetiology of a posthepatic block. Cavography can be performed both through the femoral vein and inferior vena cava and through the arm or jugular vein via the right atrium and superior vena cava.

2. **MDCT venography** with a 16-row scanner provides detailed anatomical information in the evaluation of the three main branches of the hepatic vein. This is very important both for the donor and the recipient before LDLT, but also before and after LT. MDCT venography is a valuable diagnostic tool in other entities such as BCS, TIPS, intrahepatic venous shunt or hepatic venous involvement in the case of different tumours. (158)

3. **Transvenous hepatophlebography** is based on experimental studies in dogs and on initial clinical experience (A.M. RAPPAPORT, 1951). This radiological method for imaging the hepatic veins was introduced into clinical practice by G. TORI in 1953. Selective hepatography introduces a catheter through the femoral vein (also via the median cubital vein or jugular vein) into a hepatic vein.

4. **Percutaneous transhepatic hepatophlebography** involves a typical puncture of the liver with a needle from the right midaxillary line to enter a hepatic vein. Pressure measurement and CM injection ensure that the position of the needle or the catheter is correct. Thrombosis of the portal vein is an absolute contraindication, which is why indirect splenoportography must be carried out prior to percutaneous hepatophlebography. Serious complications occur in 1.5−4.0% of cases.

4 Cholangiography

Visualization of the bile ducts can be accomplished indirectly or by means of various direct methods. (s. tab. 8.8)

Indirect cholangiography
1. Intravenous injection
2. Intravenous infusion
3. Spiral CT
4. MRI cholangiography

Direct cholangiography
1. Endoscopic retrograde
2. Percutaneous transhepatic
3. Transvenous
4. Intraoperative
5. Postoperative via drain

Tab. 8.8: Indirect and direct methods of cholangiography

4.1 Indirect cholangiography

In terms of the success rate, conventional X-ray diagnosis of the efferent bile ducts cannot be entirely replaced by (stress-free, easy-to-repeat, technically uncomplicated and less costly) ultrasonography. For example, for diagnosing choledocholithiasis, *i.v. cholangiography* and *tomography* are much more efficient (90−92%) than sonography (67%). The use of (invasive) ERC, however, provides three to four times more reliable diagnostic information than does i.v. cholangiography (V. MYLLYLÄ et al., 1984). Furthermore, ultrasonography or i.v. cholangiography (as a rule in conjunction with tomography or MRCP) produces a noninvasive, but inadequate assessment of the intrahepatic bile ducts. In this respect, the methods of direct cholangiography are infinitely superior. • The use of i.v. cholangiography is restricted due to severe damage to the liver cells (GPT, GOT > 150 U/l), increased serum bilirubin (> 3 mg/dl) or cholestasis (AP > 300 U/l). It is further limited by the high technical requirements in individual cases (tomography, infusion cholangiography). • In the case of significant sonographic findings in the area of the bifurcation of the cystic duct and common bile duct (e.g. suspected *Mirizzi syndrome*), consideration should first be given to i.v. cholangiography (with tomography) and then to ERC. Intravenous cholangiography is also indicated for noncongested bile ducts and in cases where ERC has proved unsuccessful. (164, 178)

4.1.2 Spiral CT and MRCP

Biliary secretion of CM under **spiral CT** is used to produce 3D models of the biliary tract, enabling 70−75% of intraductal concrements to be detected. Malignant and benign processes were diagnosed in 75% and 93% of cases. (182) In cholestasis, the biliary tract could also be visualized without the use of CM. (190)

The introduction of **MR cholangiography** by B.K. WALLNER et al. (1991) represents a significant development in this field. (187) If CM is not used, the biliary passages in the biliary tract are visualized by distinct T_2-weighted sequences in a coronary display. More rapid gradient systems have further improved display quality (161, 180); here it was possible to achieve comparable results to those obtained in MRC and ERC. (159, 169, 181, 186)

4.2 Direct cholangiography

The use of direct cholangiography is indicated (*1.*) if alterations in the area of the efferent bile ducts could not be clarified by ultrasound and i.v. cholangiography or (*2.*) if the use of i.v. cholangiography is contraindicated, not indicated or likely to be inadequate. Various direct cholangiographic methods are available depending on individual pathological situations and diagnostic issues. (188) (s. tab. 8.8)

4.2.1 ERC

▶ First described by W.S. McCUNE et al. (1968) and I. OI et al. (1969), endoscopic retrograde cholangiography (ERC) is now a valuable and standardized examination method.

Indications: Due to the continuous improvement of ERC (better diagnostic value and reduced complication rate), a number of indications have now been established. (s. tab. 8.9)

1. Suspected mechanical obstruction
   - choledocholithiasis
   - bile-duct tumour
   - bile-duct stricture
   - compression of a bile duct, *etc.*
2. Unresolved hepatobiliary diseases
   - primary sclerosing cholangitis
   - chronic (possibly recurrent) cholangitis
   - intrahepatic gallstones
   - parasitic diseases, *etc.*
3. Prior to surgical procedures on bile ducts
4. Postoperative epigastric symptom complex
5. Negative or unresolved cholangiography
6. Suspected bile-duct anomalies, papillomatosis
7. Suspected congenital intrahepatic bile-duct cysts (Caroli's disease)
8. Follow-up biliodigestive anastomosis
9. Suspected acute biliary pancreatitis
10. Contrast-medium intolerance

Tab. 8.9: Indications for endoscopic retrograde cholangiography

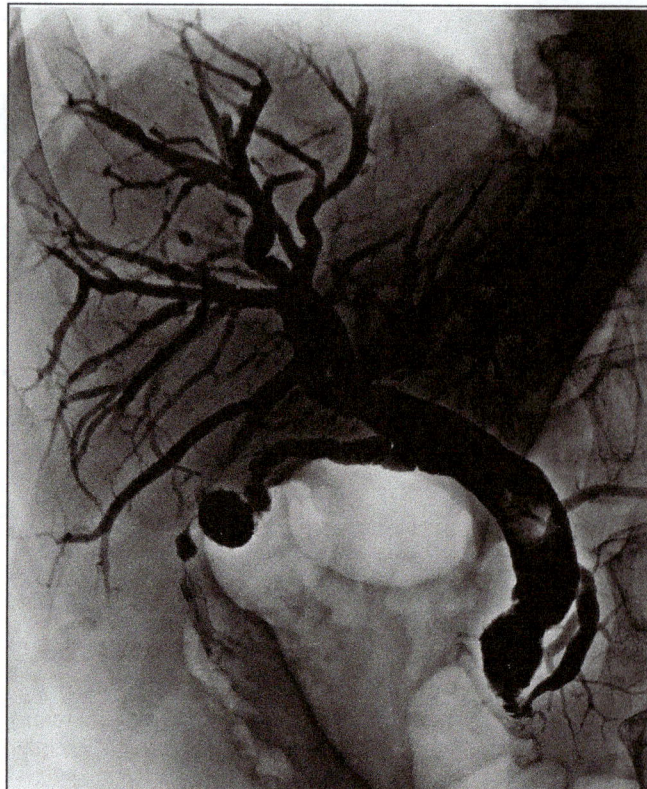

Fig. 8.14: Use of ERC in obstructive jaundice induced by a large biliary concrement, with congested extrahepatic and intrahepatic bile ducts. Secondary findings: shrunken gall bladder with a cholecystocholic fistula

1. Endoscopy of the bile duct allows parasitological (e.g. proof of larvae or eggs), bacteriological or cytological *analysis of the bile* in hepatobiliary issues.

2. A number of other new *therapeutic procedures* have developed against the background of ERC, including the transpapillary insertion of stents for palliative bridging of ductal stenosis.

3. In cases of *mechanical jaundice,* not only the location of the obstruction in the biliary tract is determinable, but usually the type and extent of the (partial or complete) obstruction as well. As a result, a decision can often be taken during the same examination concerning causal or palliative treatment. The coagulation parameters should be within a range which renders papillotomy, stone extraction or tissue biopsy possible without danger to the patient. (s. fig. 8.14)

4. The clarification of *hepatobiliary diseases* is an important indication for ERC. (s. tab. 8.9) • Suppurative cholangitis related to mechanical flow obstruction in a bile duct is a clear indication for ERC, whereby appropriate therapeutic measures (e.g. papillotomy, stone extraction, insertion of tubes or stents) should be carried out at the same time. Septic cholangitis is considered to be an emergency indication. • For diagnosing primary sclerosing cholangitis, ERC is the method of choice. Complete visualization of the intrahepatic biliary system ought to be possible with this method.

Success rate: The success rate for visualizing the biliary tract is 95%, whereas in patients with gastric resection (Billroth II) and Braun's anastomosis, the success rate is only 30–40%. Ultrasonography permits the differentiation between intra- and extrahepatic cholestasis in 75–80% of patients, whereas with ERC the rate is 90–95%. For identifying the type of obstruction, ERC shows even better success rates (89% vs. 58%). On the whole, this method provides a definitive diagnosis in biliary tract disorders in 78–93% of cases. (160, 162, 166, 169, 172, 174, 177, 181, 184, 185)

Contraindications: Fundamentally, there are no absolute contraindications to ERC when performed by an experienced endoscopist, except in the case of uncooperative patients. • Clotting disorders, however, call for special caution when applying this method in view of its invasive nature. With organ decompensation, especially cardiac or respiratory insufficiency, or severe arrhythmia, ERC is generally not the primary method for hepatobiliary diagnosis. In cases of oesophageal varices, an intraabdominal increase in pressure due to retching during the examination may promote or cause variceal bleeding. With high-risk patients, antibiotics should be given as a prophylaxis. The patients must be informed of the increased risk associated with the examination.

Complications: Complications include pancreatitis (0.8–1.0%), cholangitis and sepsis (0.6–0.8%), adverse reactions to premedication and contrast media (0.4–0.6%), and instrument-induced injuries (0.2%). The frequency of bacteriaemia is 15%. An increase in pancreatic enzymes is observed in 15–20% of patients, whereas a rise in transaminases, γ-GT and AP only occurs in isolated cases. Increases in enzymes are mainly found with injections involving high-viscosity CM, larger doses or excessive pressure. • *Sepsis* can develop after injection of CM into a congested biliary tract. Therefore, in this situation, parallel papillotomy and decompression drainage are required together with peri-interventional prophylactic antibiotics. • The complication rate is altogether 1.0−2.3%; the frequency of cardiopulmonary complications in older patients is 8% (166). Lethality is 0.1%.

4.2.2 PTC

▶ The method of percutaneous transhepatic cholangiography (PTC) was first described by H. BURCKHARDT et al. in 1921 and by P. HUARD et al. in 1937, and revived by R.F. CARTER et al. in 1952. Routine use was recommended by F. GLENN et al. in 1962. • After the development of a thin and flexible puncture needle (Y. TSUCHIYA, 1969) and using a Chiba needle (K. OKUDA et al., 1974), PTC became a widely used clinical method. (174)

Indications: The indications for PTC have become increasingly limited in favour of ERC, since preference is given to the visualization of the biliary tract through the major duodenal papilla (= physiological access) over invasive and non-physiological transhepatic access. Moreover, the rate of complications regarding PTC is clearly higher than with ERC. • *Obstructive jaundice* not clarified by ERC is an indication for diagnostic PTC. However, the higher success rate of approx. 90% for ERC in clarifying obstructive jaundice, compared with approx. 70% for PTC, makes ERC the method of choice. PTC is also indicated if drainage of congested bile is necessary and recommended for preoperative diagnosis or drainage before operations on bile ducts, above all in the area of the hepatic hilus. PTC may also be applied in cases involving nondilated bile ducts where suspected biliary obstruction could not be clarified by i.v. cholangiography and ERC. (s. fig. 8.15) The use of PTC as an operation channel for therapeutic measures in the biliary system is of great importance in a wide range of diseases, e.g. stone extraction, bile-duct dilation, antibiotic rinsing in suppurative cholangitis, electroresection and intraluminal radiation. • With dilated bile ducts, the puncture is successful in >95% and with nondilated bile ducts in 50(−70)% of cases. No more than five attempts at puncture should be made. With a correctly positioned needle in a bile duct, the CM only flows slowly and in a mediocaudal direction, remaining in the vessel once the injection has been stopped. (168, 174, 183, 189)

Technique: PTC is relatively easy to carry out and requires minimal technology. It is performed under sonographic or X-ray control. The target is the liver hilus where it joins with larger bile ducts at the level of the 12th intercostal space, three "finger breadths" from the right margin of the 12th thoracic vertebra. The *target technique of OKUDA* has proved useful for determining the correct position and direction of the puncture. (176) • Rapid flow of the CM with a tree-like ramification shows that the needle is located in a branch of the portal vein; some blood escapes from the cannula. Should the CM flow rapidly towards the inferior vena cava, the needle is positioned in a branch of the hepatic vein. Fine and irregular vessels depicted with a slowing down of the mediocaudal flow of the CM suggest a filling of the lymphatic vessels. After administration of the contrast medium and removal of the needle, it is possible, by altering the patient's position, to ensure adequate filling of the intrahepatic bile ducts and gall bladder; when the upper part of the body is raised, the bile duct (= d. choledochus) is also well visualized. One drawback is the general inability to assess the biliary situation distal to the occlusion (comparable with ERC cranial to the occlusion) if this point cannot be visualized due to the fact that the CM was not able to pass the obstruction.

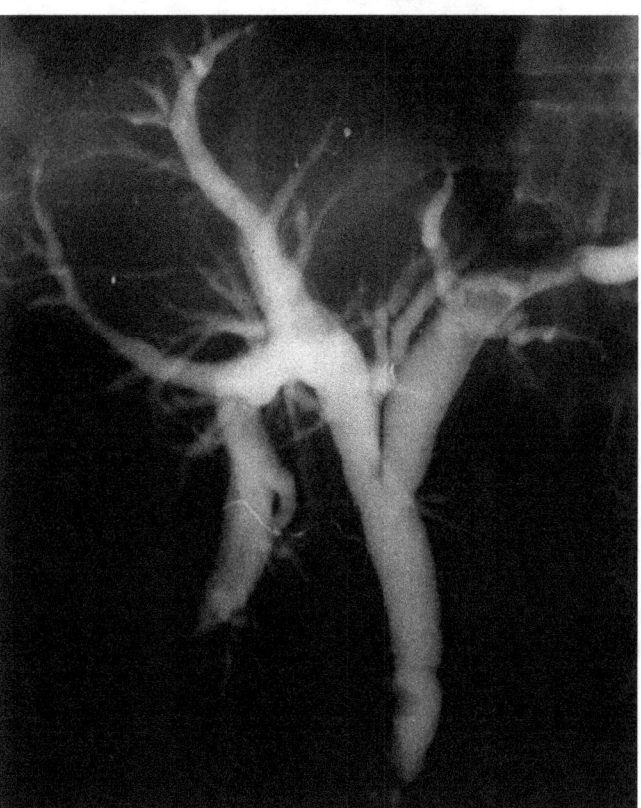

Fig. 8.15: Use of percutaneous transhepatic cholangiography in benign papillary stenosis. Hard fibrotic tissue after repeated passing of gallstones associated with colics over a period of three years. Treatment: papillotomy

Contraindications: Contraindications include clotting disorders, echinococcus cyst, marked ascites, liver abscess, liver metastases and cirrhosis.

Complications: In 3−6% of cases, complications occur; compiled statistics showed a frequency of up to 10.2% and 13.2%. In 3.4% of cases, a surgical procedure was required. The main complications are bilious peritonitis, haemorrhage, haemobilia, cholangitis and sepsis. Lethality was 0.06−0.08% − even 0.9%. There is a risk of piercing unidentified abscesses, tumours and metastases along the transhepatic route. The gall bladder must also be circumvented. A long intrahepatic course of the puncture channel is designed to ensure greater safety with regard to biliary leakage. Even in cases of incomplete obstruction, biliary decompression (which can be achieved for example by aspirating bile prior to injecting the CM or by rinsing) is advisable in order to avert dangerous increases in pressure in the bile ducts. As far as possible, the amount of CM should not exceed 20–40 ml. Prophylactic antibiotics are recommended.

Laparoscopic transhepatic cholangiography (LTC)
This technique, as described by M. ROYER in 1952, is a PTC variant. Although it entails fewer complications, the success rate is also reduced, since the length of the intrahepatic puncture channel is only 3 cm. The puncture is performed at a point approx. 3 cm away from the falciform ligament and 5 cm cranial to the edge of the liver, with a puncture angle of 45°.

4.2.3 TVC

Transvenous cholangiography (TVC) was described by W. HANAFEE et al. in 1967 as a transjugular form of direct cholangiography. In this procedure, a catheter is introduced through the right jugular vein into a hepatic vein; by transhepatic advancing of the catheter, a bile duct is punctured with an improved Ross needle. This method was modified by R. GÜNTHER (1975), who used the right subclavian vein as the site of access. (168) Catheterization through a basilic or cubital vein (I. F. HAWKINS jr. et al., 1976) is not considered to be of any advantage. TVC is more complicated than PTC in terms of time and instruments. The success rate for congested bile ducts is 65–93% for cases of non-congestion 10–69%. There is no need to prepare for surgery. TVC is only indicated in exceptional cases. • The *complication rate* is 8.9% (mild complications 5.5%, serious incidents 3.4%), with a lethality of 0.4%. The main complications are intraperitoneal bleeding, subcapsular liver haematoma, haemobilia, bilihaemia and sepsis. No bile peritonitis has been reported so far. • *Contraindications* include acute cholangitis, hepatic echinococcus and liver abscess.

4.2.4 PTCS

Percutaneous transhepatic cholangioscopy (PTCS) is indicated (*1.*) to clarify the benignancy or malignancy of bile-duct stenoses, (*2.*) to visualize the biliary tract by X-ray using a guide wire and a catheter positioned by the endoscopist's naked eye, and (*3.*) to perform lithiotripsy of bile duct stones and remove any local obstruction of bile flow. The examination is carried out with a percutaneously placed biliocutaneous fistula, which is stable enough after eight to ten days to permit insertion of a cholangioscope. Endoscopic evaluation is carried out under continuous rinsing with a physiological NaCl solution. (173)

4.2.5 Intraoperative cholangiography

Intraoperative cholangiography was introduced into biliary diagnosis by P. L. MIRIZZI in 1932. Since then, this technique has been under development and it is (still) used as an indispensable, additional intraoperative diagnostic tool in borderline cases. Interventions in the area of the gall bladder or bile ducts are generally unacceptable without the possibility of a cholangiographic examination of the biliary tract. (163, 165, 170, 175, 179, 188)
• Intraoperative cholangiography should be reserved for resolving special issues. (s. tab. 8.10)

1. Length and width of the common bile duct
2. Choledocholithiasis
3. Hepaticolithiasis
4. Examining the biliary tract for
– anomalies   – ligatures
– breaks   – contour irregularities
– fistulas   – intraoperative injuries
– stenoses
5. Examining the major duodenal papilla
6. Examining the pancreatic duct, if necessary

Tab. 8.10: Indications for intraoperative cholangiography

Several **methods** are available for intraoperative cholangiography. These are used prior to or after opening the common bile duct: (*1.*) direct cholangiography consisting of puncture of the bile duct by a sharp cannula, (*2.*) cholangiography through the cystic duct, whereby a blunt and curved button cannula or a Nélaton's catheter is inserted by stab incision through the cystic duct (which is situated under the ligatures) into the bile duct, (*3.*) transvesical cholangiography, including the introduction of a special trocar cannula into the fundus of the gall bladder, and (*4.*) cholangiography after choledochotomy by means of a blocker catheter or a double-balloon T-catheter. • Using these methods, the bile ducts can be shown by X-ray in both the direction of the liver and the duodenum. (191)

4.2.6 Postoperative cholangiography

Postoperative cholangiography is an indispensable follow-up prior to removing the drain. This method is aimed at confirming surgical success and obtaining proof of an undisturbed bile flow into the duodenum. The examination, performed with the patient in a head-down position, also enables visualization of the intrahepatic bile ducts, so as to exclude the presence of small residual concrements. The injection of contrast medium can be combined with the simultaneous measuring of pressure. Imaging is performed during consecutive stages of biliary filling.

Synopsis

Since the discovery of X-ray by W. C. RÖNTGEN (1895), several radiological examination methods have been developed. They have also been used in the field of hepatology with great instrumental subtlety and manual skill. These methods have proved irreplaceable in the imaging of vessels and bile ducts. • The development of CT and MRI – in particular helical CT and MRI cholangiography – constitutes a breakthrough in radiology once held to be inconceivable.

▶ The introduction of various contrast-medium techniques not only in sonography (CEDS) but also in CT and MRI has led to rapid changes in the field of radiological diagnosis in hepatology. • *Particularly in the visualization of portal, venous and arterial vessels, fascinating angiographic tissue reconstruction has become possible, even on an outpatient basis.* • Similarly, with respect to the differentiation of tissue structures, more detailed information, which was long deemed beyond reach, can now be obtained. It is to be expected that even cellular metabolic processes will be shown by imaging techniques in the future – an absolutely fascinating idea!

It was therefore seen as a matter of great importance in this chapter to follow the **path of radiological diagnosis in hepatology**, tracing the course of the examination methods hitherto applied (and now deemed in part to be out of date and obsolete) through to those techniques still undergoing development.

References:

Computer tomography

1. **Alfidi, R.J., Haaga, J., Meaney, T.F., McIntyre, W.J., Gonzalez, L., Tarar, R., Zelch, M.G., Boller, M., Cook, S.A., Jelden, G.:** Computed tomography of the thorax and abdomen; a preliminary report. Radiology 1975; 117: 257–264
2. **Barakos, J.A., Goldberg, H.I., Brown, J.J., Gilbert, T.J.:** Comparison of computed tomography and magnetic resonance imaging in the evaluation of focal hepatic lesions. Gastrointest. Radiol. 1990; 15: 93–101
3. **Bluemke, D.A., Fishman, E.K.:** Spiral CT of the Liver. Amer. J. Roentgenol. 1993; 160: 787–792
4. **Choi, B.I., Lim, J.H., Han, M.C., Lee, D.H., Kim, S.H., Kim, Y.I., Kim, C.:** Biliary cystadenoma and cystadenocarcinoma: CT and sonographic findings. Radiology 1989; 171: 57–61
5. **Choi, B.I., Lee, H.J., Han, J.K., Choi, D.S., Seo, J.B., Han, M.C.:** Detection of hypervascular nodular hepatocellular carcinoma: value of triphasic helical CT compared with iodized-oil CT. Amer. J. Roentgenol. 1997; 168: 219–224
6. **Dillon, E.H., van Leeuwen, M.S., Fernandez, M.A., Mali, W.P.T.M.:** Spiral CT angiography. Amer. J. Roentgenol. 1993; 160: 1273–1278
7. **Dodd, G.D.I., Baron, R.L., Oliver, J.H.I.:** End-stage primary sclerosing cholangitis: CT findings of hepatic morphology in 36 patients. Radiology 1999; 211: 357–362
8. **El-Tahir, M.I., Omojola, M.F., Malatani, T., Al-Saigh, A.H., Ogunbiyi, O.A.:** Hydatid disease of the liver: evaluation of ultrasound and computed tomography. Brit. J. Radiol. 1992; 65: 390–392
9. **Federle, M.P., Blachar, A.:** CT evaluation of the liver: Principles and techniques. Semin. Liver Dis. 2001; 21: 135–145
10. **Freeny, P.C.:** Helical computed tomography of the liver: Techniques, applications and pitfalls. Endoscopy 1997; 29: 515–523
11. **Furuse, J., Maru, Y., Yoshino, M., Mera, K., Sumi, H., Sekiguchi, R., Sataka, M., Hasebe, T., Ochiai, A.:** Assessment of arterial tumor vascularity in small hepatocellular carcinoma. Comparison between color Doppler ultrasonography and radiographic imagings with contrast medium: dynamic CT, angiography, and CT hepatic arteriography. Eur. J. Radiol. 2000; 36: 20–27
12. **Hänninen, E.L., Vogl, T.J., Felfe, R., Pegios, W., Balzer, J., Clauss, W., Felix, R.:** Detection of focal liver lesions at biphasic spiral CT: randomized double-blind study of the effect of iodine concentration in contrast materials. Radiology 2000; 216: 403–409
13. **Halvorsen, R.A., Korobkin, M., Ram, P.C., Thompson, W.M.:** CT appearance of focal fatty infiltration of the liver. Amer. J. Roentgenol. 1982; 139: 277–281
14. **Hodler, J., Meier, P.:** Leberbefall bei Fasciola hepatica: Sonographie und CT. Fortschr. Röntgenstr. 1989; 151: 740–741
15. **Hounsfield, G.N.:** Computerized transverse axial scanning (tomography): Part 1. Description of system. Brit. J. Radiol. 1973; 46: 1016–1022
16. **Inui, A., Fujisawa, T., Suetmitsu, T., Fujikawa, S., Ariizumi, M., Kagimoto, S., Kinoshita, K.:** A case of Caroli's disease with special reference to hepatic CT and US findings. J. Pediatr. Gastroenterol. Nutr. 1992; 14: 463–466
17. **Itai, Y., Araki, T., Ohtomo, K., Kokubo, T., Yoshida, H., Minami, M., Yashiro, N.:** Well-defined dense and continuously spreading enhancement on single level dynamic CT of the liver: a characteristic sign of hepatic cavernous haemangioma. Fortschr. Röntgenstr. 1989; 151: 697–701
18. **Jones, E.C., Chezmar, J.L., Nelson, R.C., Bernardino, M.E.:** The frequency and significance of small ≤ 15 mm) hepatic lesions detected by CT. Amer. J. Roentgenol. 1992; 158: 535–539
19. **Kawamori, Y., Matsui, O., Kitagawa, K., Kadoya, M., Takashima, T., Yamahana, T.:** Macronodular tuberculoma of the liver: CT and MR findings. Amer. J. Roentgenol. 1992; 158: 311–313
20. **Klöppel, R., Reinhardt, M., Lieberenz, S., Fuchs, M., Winnefeld, K., Machnik, G.:** Untersuchungen zur diagnostischen Wertigkeit der CT bei der Siderophilie (primäre idiopathische Hämochromatose). Gastroenterol. J. 1989; 49: 122–125
21. **Levine, C.:** Primary macronodular hepatic tuberculosis: US and CT appearances. Gastrointest. Radiol. 1990; 15: 307–309
22. **Lundstedt, C., Ekberg, H., Hederström, E., Tranberg, K.-G.:** The accuracy of computed tomography of the liver in colo-rectal carcinoma. Clin. Radiol. 1990; 42: 335–339
23. **Lüning, M., Koch, M., Abet, L., Wolff, H., Wenig, B., Buchali, K., Schöpke, W., Schneider, Th., Mühler, A., Rudolph, B.:** Treffsicherheit bildgebender Verfahren (Sonographie, MRT, CT, Angio-CT, Nuklearmedizin) bei der Charakterisierung von Lebertumoren. Fortschr. Röntgenstr. 1991; 154: 398–406
24. **Lüning, M., Simon, C., Dewey, Ch., Decker, T., Sperling, P.:** CT diagnosis of hepatic adenoma. Eur. J. Radiol. 1987; 7: 30–36
25. **Marchal, G., Baert, A.L.:** Dynamic CT of the liver. Radiologe 1992; 32: 211–216
26. **Mathieu, D., Bruneton, J.N., Drouillard, J., Pointreau, C.C., Vasile, N.:** Hepatic adenomas and focal nodular hyperplasia: dynamic CT study. Radiology 1986; 160: 53–58
27. **Mathieu, D., Vasile, N., Menu, Y., van Beers, B., Lorphelin, J.M., Pringot, J.:** Budd-Chiari syndrome: dynamic CT. Radiology 1987; 165: 409–413
28. **Miller, W.J., Federle, M.P., Campbell, W.L.:** Diagnosis and staging of hepatocellular carcinoma: comparison of CT and sonography in 36 liver transplantation patients. Amer. J. Roentgenol. 1991; 157: 303–306
29. **Mortele, K.J., Ros, P.R.:** Imaging of diffuse liver disease. Semin. Liver Dis. 2001; 21: 195–212
30. **Murakami, T., Kim, T., Takamura, M., Hori, M., Takahashi, S., Federle, M.P., Tsuda, K., Osuga, K., Kawata, S., Nakamura, H., Kudo, M.:** Hypervascular hepatocellular carcinoma: detection with double arterial phase multi-detector row helical CT. Radiology 2001; 218: 763–767
31. **Numata, K., Tanaka, K., Kiba, T., Saito, S., Ikeda, M., Hara, K., Tanaka, N., Morimoto, M., Iwase, S., Sekihara, H.:** Contrast-enhanced, wide-brand harmonic gray scale imaging of hepatocellular carcinoma: correlation with helical computed tomographic findings. J. Ultrasound Med. 2001; 20: 89–98
32. **Päivänsalo, M., Lähde, S., Jalovaara, P.:** Computed tomography of hepatic haemangiomas: a chance for a definite diagnosis. Bildgebung 1991; 58: 29–32
33. **Poletti, P.A., Mirvis, S.E., Shanmuganathan, K., Killeen, K.L., Coldwell, D.:** CT criteria for management of blunt liver trauma: correlation with angiographic and surgical findings. Radiology 2000; 216: 418–427
34. **Procacci, C., Fugazzola, C., Cinquino, M., Mangiante, G., Zonta, L., Bergamo Andreis, J.A., Nicoli, N., Pistolesi, G.F.:** Contribution of CT to characterization of focal nodular hyperplasia of the liver. Gastrointest. Radiol. 1992; 17: 63–73
35. **Quinn, St.F., Benjamin, G.G.:** Hepatic cavernous hemangiomas: simple diagnostic sign with dynamic bolus CT. Radiology 1992; 182: 545–548
36. **Raptopoulos, V., Karellas, A., Bernstein, J., Reale, F.R., Constantinou, C., Zawacki, J.K.:** Value of dual-energy CT in differentiating focal fatty infiltration of the liver from low-density masses. Amer. J. Roentgenol. 1991; 157: 721–725
37. **Rogers, J.V., Mack, L.A., Freeny, P.C., Johnson, M.L., Sones, P.J.:** Hepatic focal nodular hyperplasia: angiography, CT, Sonography, and scintigraphy. Amer. J. Roentgenol. 1981; 137: 983–990
38. **Schellinger, D., Di Chiro, G., Axelbaum, S.P., Twigg, H.L., Ledley, R.S.:** Early clinical experience with the ACTA scanner. Radiology 1975; 114: 257–261
39. **Schima, W., Kulinna, C., Ba-Ssalamah, A., Grünberger, T.:** Multidetector computed tomography of the liver. Radiologe 2005; 45: 15–23
40. **Schörner, W., Neumann, K., Langer, M., Heim, T., Keck, H., Felix, R.:** Zur Differentialdiagnostik von Lebermetastasierung und regionaler Leberverfettung: Vergleich von CT und MRT. Fortschr. Röntgenstr. 1991; 154: 628–633
41. **Schweizer, W., Becker, Ch., Tanner, S., Schaeppi, B., Huber, A., Blumgart, L.H.:** Die Bedeutung der Computertomographie (CT) für die konservative Behandlung des Lebertraumas. Schweiz. Med. Wschr. 1993; 123: 577–581
42. **Shamsi, K., De Schepper, A., Degryse, H., Deckers, F.:** Focal nodular hyperplasia of the liver: radiologic findings. Abdom Imaging 1993; 18: 32–38
43. **Shyn, P.B., Goldberg, H.I.:** Abdominal CT following liver transplantation. Gastrointest. Radiol. 1992; 17: 231–236
44. **Sood, G.K., Mahapatra, J.R., Khurana, A., Chaudhry, V., Sarin, S.K., Broor, S.L.:** Caroli disease: computed tomographic diagnosis. Gastrointest. Radiol. 1991; 16: 243–244

45. Tang-Barton, P., Vas, W., Weissman, J., Salimi, Z., Patel, R., Morris, L.: Focal fatty liver lesions in alcoholic liver disease: a broadened spectrum of CT appearances. Gastrointest. Radiol. 1985; 10: 133–137
46. Taylor, C.R.: Computed tomography in the evaluation of the portal venous system. J. Clin. Gastroenterol. 1992; 14: 167–172
47. Teefey, S., Baron, R.L., Schulte, S.J., Patten, R.M., Molloy, M.H.: Patterns of intrahepatic bile duct dilatation at CT: correlation with obstructive disease processes. Radiology 1992; 182: 139–142
48. Van Thiel, D.H., Hagler, N.G., Schade, R.R., Skolnick, M.L., Pollitt Heyl, A., Rosenblum, E., Gavaler, J.S., Penkrot, R.J.: In vivo hepatic volume determination using sonography and computed tomography. Validation and a comparison of the two techniques. Gastroenterology 1985; 88: 1812–1817
49. Vignaux, O., Legmann, P., Coste, J., Hoeffel, C., Bonnin, A.: Cirrhotic liver enhancement on dual-phase helical CT: comparison with noncirrhotic liver in 146 patients. Amer. J. Roentgenol. 1999; 173: 1193–1197
50. Vlachos, L., Trakadas, S., Gouliamos, A., Lazarou, S., Mourikis, D., Ioannou, R., Kalovidouris, A., Papavasiliou, C.: Comparative study between ultrasound, computed tomography, intra-arterial digital subtraction angiography, and magnetic resonance imaging in the differentiation of tumors of the liver. Gastrointest. Radiol. 1990; 15: 102–106
51. Wan, S.K.H., Cochlin, D.L.: Sonographic and computed tomographic features of polycystic disease of the liver. Gastrointest. Radiol. 1990; 15: 310–312
52. Welch, T.J., Sheedy II, P.F., Johnson, C.M., Stephens, D.H., Charboneau, J.W., Brown, M.L., May, G.R., Adson, M.A., McGill, D.B.: Focal nodular hyperplasia and hepatic adenoma: comparison of angiography, CT, US, and scintigraphy. Radiology 1985; 156: 593–595
53. Wernecke, K., Rummeny, E., Bongartz, G., Vassallo, P., Kivelitz, D., Wiesmann, W., Peters, P.E., Reers, B., Reiser, M., Pircher, W.: Detection of hepatic masses in patients with carcinoma: comparative sensitivities of sonography, CT, and MR imaging. Amer. J. Roentgenol. 1991; 157: 731–739
54. Whitehouse, R.W.: Computed tomography attenuation measurements for the characterization of hepatic haemangiomas. Brit. J. Radiol. 1991; 64: 1019–1022
55. Yamashita, Y., Takahashi, M., Kanazawa, S., Charnsangavej, C., Wallace, S.: Parenchymal changes of the liver in cholangiocarcinoma: CT evaluation. Gastrointest. Radiol. 1992; 17: 161–166
56. Yates, C.K., Streight, R.A.: Focal fatty infiltration of the liver simulating metastatic disease. Radiology 1986; 159: 83–84
57. Zocholl, G., Kuhn, F.-P., Augustin, N., Thelen, M.: Diagnostische Aussagekraft von Sonographie und Computertomographie bei Lebermetastasen. Fortschr. Röntgenstr. 1988; 148: 8–14

Magnetic resonance imaging
58. Andersen, P.B., Birgegard, G., Nyman, R., Hemmingsson, A.: Magnetic resonance imaging in idiopathic hemochromatosis. Eur. J. Haematol. 1991; 47: 174–178
59. Araki, T., Ohtomo, K., Kachi, K., Monzawa, S., Hihara, T., Ohba, H., Ainoda, T., Kumagai, H., Uchiyama, G.: Magnetic resonance imaging of macroscopic intrahepatic portal-hepatic venous shunts. Gastrointest. Radiol. 1991; 16: 221–224
60. Arita, T., Matsunaga, N., Kobayashi, H.: Budd-Chiari syndrome: peripheral abnormal intensity of the liver on magnetic resonance imaging. Clin. Radiol. 2000; 55: 640–642
61. Barakos, J.A., Goldberg, H.I., Brown, J.J., Gilbert, T.J.: Comparison of computed tomography and magnetic resonance imaging in the evaluation of focal hepatic lesions. Gastrointest. Radiol. 1990; 15: 93–101
62. Ba-Ssalamah, A., Happel, B., Kettenbach, J., Dirisamer, A., Wrba, F., Längle, F., Schima, W.: MRI of the liver. Clinical significance of nonspecific and liver specific MRI contrast agents. Radiologe 2004; 44: 1170–1184
63. Birnbaum, B.A., Noz, M.E., Chapnick, J., Sanger, J.J., Megibow, A.J., Maguire, G.Q. jr., Weinreb, J.C., Kaminer, E.M., Kramer, E.L.: Hepatic hemangiomas: diagnosis with fusion of MR, CT, and Tc-99m-labeled red blood cell SPECT images. Radiology 1991; 181: 469–474
64. Bonkovsky, H.L., Rubin, R.B., Cable, E.E., Davidoff, A., Rijcken, T.H.P., Stark, D.D.: Hepatic iron concentration: noninvasive estimation by means of MR imaging techniques. Radiology 1999; 212: 227–234
65. Butch, R.J., Stark, D., Malt, R.A.: Magnetic resonance imaging of hepatic focal nodular hyperplasia. J. Comput. Assist. Tomogr. 1986; 10: 874–877
66. Caudana, R., Morasna, G., Pirovano, G.P.: Focal malignant hepatic lesions: MR imaging enhanced with gadolinium benzyloxy-propionictetra-acetate (BOPTA) – preliminary results of phase II clinical application. Radiology 1996; 199: 513–520
67. Coombs, R.J., Woldenberg, L.S., Skeel, R.T., Bishara, H.M., Merrick, H.W.: Magnetic resonance imaging of hepatic adenoma. Clin. Imag. 1990; 14: 44–47
68. Dalla Palma, L., Pozzi-Mucelli, R.S.: Computed tomography and magnetic resonance imaging in diagnosing hepatocellular carcinoma. Ital. J. Gastroenterol. 1992; 24: 87–91
69. Davolio Marani, S.A., Canossi, G.C., Nicoli, F.A., Alberti, G.P., Monni, S.G., Casolo, P.M.: Hydatid disease: MR imaging study. Radiology 1990; 175: 701–706
70. Demas, B.E., Hricak, H., Goldberg, H.I., Margulis, A.R.: Magnetic resonance imaging diagnosis of hepatic metastasis in the presence of negative CT studies. J. Clin. Gastroenterol. 1985; 7: 553–560
71. Duewell, S., Marincek, B., Schulthess, von, G.K., Ammann, R.: MRT und CT bei alveolärer Echinokokkose der Leber. Fortschr. Röntgenstr. 1990; 152: 441–445
72. Fretz, C.J., Stark, D.D., Metz, C.E., Elizondo, G.,Weissleder, R., Jong-Her Shen, Wittenberg, J., Simeone, J., Ferrucci, J.T.: Detection of hepatic metastases: comparison of contrast-enhanced CT, unenhanced MR imaging, and iron oxide-enhanced MR imaging. Amer. J. Roentgenol. 1990; 155: 763–770
73. Fulcher, A.S., Turner, M.A., Franklin, K.J.: Primary sclerosing cholangitis: evaluation with MR cholangiography–a case-control study. Radiology 2000; 215: 71–80
74. Gabata, T., Matsui, O., Kadoya, M., Takashima, T., Ueda, Y., Komatsu, Y., Sasaki, M.: MR imaging of hepatic adenoma. Amer. J. Roentgenol. 1990; 155: 1009–1011
75. Gillams, A.R., Lees, W.R.: Recent development in biliary tract imaging. Gastrointest. Endosc. Clin. N. Amer. 1996; 6: 1–15
76. Goldberg, M.A., Saini, S., Hahn, P.F., Egglin, T.K., Mueller, P.R.: Differentiation between hemangiomas and metastases of the liver with ultrafast MR imaging: preliminary results with T_2 calculations. Amer. J. Roentgenol. 1991; 157: 727–730
77. Hamrick-Turner, J., Abbitt, P.L., Ros, P.R.: Intrahepatic cholangiocarcinoma: MR appearance. Amer. J. Roentgenol. 1992; 158: 77–79
78. Hayes, A.M., Jaramillo, D., Levy, H.L., Knisely, A.S.: Neonatal hemochromatosis: diagnosis with MR imaging. Amer. J. Roentgenol. 1992; 159: 623–625
79. Herborn, C.U., Narin, B., Ruehm, S.G.: Schistosomia mansoni in the liver. Magnetic resonance images. Röfo. 2002; 174: 495–496
80. Hirai, K., Aoki, Y., Majima, Y., Abe, H., Nakashima, O., Kojiro, M., Tanikawa, K.: Magnetic resonance imaging of small hepatocellular carcinoma. Amer. J. Gastroenterol. 1991; 86: 205–209
81. Honda, H., Onitsuka, H., Murakami, J., Kaneko, K., Murayama, S., Adachi, E., Kanematsu, T., Sugimachi, K., Masuda, K.: Characteristic findings of hepatocellular carcinoma: an evaluation with comparative study of US, CT, and MRI. Gastrointest. Radiol. 1992; 17: 245–249
82. Irie, H., Honda, H., Tajima, T., Kuroiwa, T., Yoshimitsu, K., Makisumi, K., Masuda, K.: Optimal MR cholangiopancreatographic sequence and its clinical application. Radiology 1998; 206: 379–387
83. Itai, Y., Ohtomo, K., Furui, S., Yamauchi, T., Minami, M., Yashiro, N.: Noninvasive diagnosis of small cavernous hemangiomas of the liver: advantage of MRI. Amer. J. Roentgenol. 1985; 145: 1195–1199
84. Ito, K., Mitchell, D.G., Matsunaga, N.: MR imaging of the liver: techniques and clinical applications. Eur. J. Radiol. 1999; 32: 2–14
85. Ito, K., Mitchell, D.G., Gabata, T., Hann, H.-W.L., Kim, P.N., Fujita, T., Awaya, H., Honjo, K., Matsunaga, N.: Hepatocellular carcinoma: association with increased iron deposition in the cirrhotic liver at MR imaging. Radiology 1999; 212: 235–240
86. Ito, K., Mitchell, D.G., Gabata, T.: Enlargement of hilar periportal space: a sign of early cirrhosis at MR imaging. J. Magn. Reson. Imag. 2000; 11: 136–140
87. Itoh, K., Saini, S., Hahn, P.F., Imam, N., Ferrucci, J.T.: Differentiation between small hepatic hemangiomas and metastases on MR images: importance of size-specific quantitative criteria. Amer. J. Roentgenol. 1990; 155: 61–66
88. Jansen, T.L.T.A., de Vries, R.A., Kesselring, F.O.H.W., Meijer, J.W.R.: Magnetic resonance imaging in the staging of hepatic veno-occlusive disease. Eur. J. Gastroenterol. Hepatol. 1994; 6: 453–456
89. Johnson, C.D.: Magnetic resonance imaging of the liver: current clinical applications. Mayo Clin. Proceed. 1993; 68: 147–156
90. Kadoya, M., Matsui, O., Takashima, T., Nonomura, A.: Hepatocellular carcinoma: correlation of MR imaging and histopathologic findings. Radiology 1992; 183: 819–825
91. Kim, M.J., Mitchell, D.G., Ito, K., Hann, H.W.L., Park, Y.N., Kim, P.N.: Hepatic iron deposition on MR imaging in patients with chronic liver disease: correlation with serial serum ferritin concentration. Abdom. Imag. 2001; 26: 149–156
92. Kim, M.-J., Mitchell, D.G., Ito, K.: Portosystemic collaterals of the upper abdomen: review of anatomy and demonstration on MR imaging. Abdom. Imag. 2000; 25: 462–470
93. Koslow, S.A., Davis, P.L., DeMarino, G.B., Peel, R.L., Baron, R.L., van Thiel, D.H.: Hyperintensive cirrhotic nodules on MRI. Gastrointest. Radiol. 1991; 16: 339–341
94. Kreeftenberg, H.G. jr., Mooyart, E.L., Huizenga, J.R., Sluiter, W.S., Kreeftenberg, H.G.: Quantification of liver iron concentration with magnetic resonance imaging by combining T1-, T2-weighted spin echo sequences and a gradient echo sequence. Neth. J. Med. 2000; 56: 133–137
95. Kreft, B., Steudel, A., Harder, T., Bockisch, A., Jakschik, J.: Qualitative und quantitative kernspintomographische Befunde der fokal nodulären Hyperplasie der Leber. Fortschr. Röntgenstr. 1990; 152: 649–653
96. Krinsky, G.A., Lee, V.S., Theise, N.D., Weinreb, J.C., Rofsky, N.M., Diflo, T., Teperman, L.W.: Hepatocellular carcinoma and dysplastic nodules in patients with cirrhosis: prospective diagnosis with MR imaging and explantation correlation. Radiology 2001; 219: 445–454
97. Laing, A.D.P., Gibson, R.N.: MRI of the liver. J. Magn. Reson. Imag. 1998; 8: 337–345
98. Lalonde, L., Beers, van, B., Jamart, J., Pringot, J.: Capsule and mosaic pattern of hepatocellular carcinoma: correlation between CT and MR imaging. Gastrointest. Radiol. 1992; 17: 241–244
99. Lavelle, M.T., Lee, V.S., Rofsky, N.M., Krinsky, G.A., Weinreb, J.C.: Dynamic contrast-enhanced three-dimensional MR imaging of liver

parenchyma: source images and angiographic reconstructions to define hepatic arterial anatomy. Radiology 2001; 218: 389–394
100. Lee, M.J., Saini, S., Hamm, B., Taupitz, M., Hahn, P.F., Seneterre, E., Ferrucci, J.T.: Focal nodular hyperplasia of the liver: MR findings in 35 proved cases. Amer. J. Roentgenol. 1991; 156: 317–320
101. Lombardo, D.M., Baker, M.E., Spritzer, C.E., Blinder, R., Meyers, W., Herfkens, R.J.: Hepatic hemangiomas vs metastases: MR differentiation at 1,5 T. Amer. J. Roentgenol. 1990; 155: 55–59
102. Mahfouz, A.-E., Hamm, B., Taupitz, M., Wolf, K.-J.: Hypervascular liver lesions: differentiation of focal nodular hyperplasia from malignant tumors with dynamic gadolinum-enhanced MR imaging. Radiology 1993; 186: 133–138
103. Mahfouz, A.-E., Hamm, B., Taupitz, M.: Hepatic magnetic resonance imaging: new techniques and contrast agents. Endoscopy 1997; 29: 504–514
104. Marti-Bonmati, L., Ferrer, D., Menor, F., Galant, J.: Hepatic mesenchymal sarcoma: MRI findings. Abdom. Imag. 1993; 18: 176–179
105. Maves, C.K., Caron, K.H., Bisset, G.S., Agarwal, R.: Splenic and hepatic peliosis: MR findings. Amer. J. Roentgenol. 1992; 158: 75–76
106. Mueller, G.C., Hussain, H.K., Carlos, R.C., Nieghiem, H.V., Francis, I.R.: Effectiveness of MR imaging in characterizing small hepatic lesions: Routine versus expert interpretation. Amer. J. Roentgenol. 2003; 180: 673–680
107. Murakami, T., Kuroda, C., Marukawa, T., Harada, K., Wakasa, K., Sakurai, M., Monden, M., Kasahara, A., Kawata, S., Kozuka, T.: Regenerating nodules in hepatic cirrhosis: MR findings with pathologic correlation. Amer. J. Roentgenol. 1990; 155: 1227–1231
108. Noohe, T.C., Semelka, R.C., Woosley, J.T., Pisano, E.D.: Ultrasound and MR findings in acute Budd-Chiari syndrome with histopathologic correlation. J. Comput. Assist. Tomogr. 1996; 20: 819–822
109. Ohtomo, K., Araki, T., Itai, Y., Monzawa, S., Ohba, H., Nogata, Y., Hihara, T., Koizumi, K., Uchiyama, K.: MR imaging of malignant mesenchymal tumors of the liver. Gastrointest. Radiol. 1992; 17: 58–62
110. Petersein, J., Dewey, Ch., Lüning, M., Schnackenburg, B., Wenig, B., Koch, M., Schneider, T., Mühler, A.: Quantitative Auswertung der dynamischen MRT mit Gd-DTPA: Vergleich von Hämangiomen und fokalen nodulären Hyperplasien der Leber. Radiolog. Diagnost. 1992; 33: 95–100
111. Rafal, R.B., Jennis, R., Kosovsky, P.A., Markisz, J.A.: MRI of primary amyloidosis. Gastrointest. Radiol. 1990; 15: 199–201
112. Rofsky, N.M., Weinreb, J.C., Bernardino, M.E., Young, S.W., Lee, J.K.T., Noz, M.E.: Hepatocellular tumors: characterization with Mn-DPDP-enhanced MR imaging. Radiology 1993; 188: 53–59
113. Siegelman, E.S., Mitchell, D.G., Outwater, E., Munoz, S.J., Rubin, R.: Idiopathic hemochromatosis: MR imaging findings in cirrhotic and precirrhotic patients. Radiology 1993; 188: 637–641
114. Stark, D.D., Felder, R.C., Wittenberg, J., Saini, S., Butch, R.J., White, M.E., Edelman, R.R.: Magnetic resonance imaging of cavernous hemangioma of the liver: tissue specific characterization. Amer. J. Roentgenol. 1985; 145: 213–222
115. Taylor, C.R., McCauley, T.R.: Magnetic resonance imaging in the evaluation of the portal venous system. J. Clin. Gastroenterol. 1992; 14: 268–273
116. Tung, G.A., Vaccaro, J.P., Cronan, J.J., Rogg, J.M.: Cavernous hemangioma of the liver: pathologic correlation with high-field MR imaging. Amer. J. Roentgenol. 1994; 162: 1113–1117
117. Vassiliades, V.G., Foley, W.D., Alarcon, J., Lawson, T., Erickson, S., Kneeland, J.B., Steinberg, H.V., Bernardino, M.E.: Hepatic metastases: CT versus MR imaging at 1,5 T. Gastrointest. Radiol. 1991; 16: 159–163
118. Vilgrain, V., Fléjou, J.-F., Arrivé, L., Belghiti, J., Najmark, D., Menu, Y., Zins, M., Vullierme, M.-P., Nahum, H.: Focal nodular hyperplasia of the liver: MR imaging and pathologic correlation in 37 patients. Radiology 1992; 184: 699–703
119. Vlachos, L., Gouliamos, A., Kalovidouris, A., Trakadas, S., Lygidakis, N., Matsaidonis, D., Papadopoulos, A., Papavasiliou, C.: Differential diagnosis of space-occupying lesions of the liver with MR imaging. Hepato-Gastroenterol. 1992; 39: 461–465
120. Vogl, T.J., Hammerstingl, R., Schnell, B., Eibl-Eibesfeldt, B., Peqios, W., Lissner, J.: Magnet-Resonanz-Tomographie des hepatobiliären Systems: Indikation, Limitationen und Ausblick. Bildgebung 1992; 59: 195–199
121. Wenzel, J.S., Donohoe, A., Ford, K.L., Glastad, K., Watkins, D., Molmenti, E.: Primary biliary cirrhosis: MR imaging findings and description of MR imaging periportal halo sign. Amer. J. Roentgenol. 2001; 176: 885–889
122. Zech, C.J., Schoenberg, S.O., Herrmann, K.A., Dietrich, O., Menzel, M.I., Lanz, E., Wallnöfer, A., Helmberger, T., Reiser, M.F.: Modern visualization of the liver with MRI. Current trends and future perspectives. Radiologe 2004; 44: 1160–1169

Angiography
123. Aspestrand, F., Kolmannskog, F.: CT and angiography in chronic liver disease. Acta Radiol. 1992; 33: 251–254
124. Blumke, D.A., Fishman, E.K.: Spiral CT arterial portography of the liver. Radiology 1993; 186: 576–579
125. Cavaluzzi, J.A., Sheff, R., Harrington, D.P., Kaufmann, St.L., Barth, K., Maddrey, W.C., White, R.I.jr.: Hepatic venography and wedge hepatic vein pressure measurements in diffuse liver disease. Amer. J. Roentgenol. 1977; 129: 441–446
126. Düx, A., Bücheler, E., Thurn, P.: Die indirekte Splenoportographie: Methodik, Indikationen und Ergebnisse. Fortschr. Röntgenstr. 1967; 106: 183–197
127. Finucci, G., Bellon, S., Merkel, C., Mormino, P., Tirelli, M., Gatta, A., Zuin, R.: Evaluation of splanchnic angiography as a prognostic index of survival in patients with cirrhosis. Scand. J. Gastroenterol. 1991; 26: 951–960
128. Foley, W.D., Stewart, E.T., Milbrath, J.R., San Dretto, M., Milde, M.: Digital subtraction angiography of the portal venous system. Amer. J. Roentgenol. 1983; 140: 497–499
129. Freeny, P.C., Vimont, T.R., Barnett, D.C.: Cavernous hemangioma of the liver: ultrasonography, arteriography, and computed tomography. Radiology 1979; 132: 143–148
130. Garbagnati, F., Spreafico, C., Marchiano, A., Salvetti, M., Segura, C., Piragine, G.: Staging of hepatocellular carcinoma by ultrasonography, computed tomography, and angiography: the role of CT combined with arterial portography. Gastrointest. Radiol. 1991; 16: 225–228
131. Goldberg, M.A., Yucel, E.K., Saini, S., Hahn, P.F., Kaufmann, J.A., Cohen, M.S.: MR angiography of the portal and hepatic venous system: preliminary experience with echoplanar imaging. Amer. J. Roentgenol. 1993; 160: 35–40
132. Goldstein, H.M., Neiman, H.L., Mena, E., Bookstein, J.J., Appelman, H.D.: Angiographic findings in benign liver cell tumors. Radiology 1974; 110: 339–343
133. Goyen, M., Ruehm, St.G., Debatin, J.F.: Whole-body MR angiography for arterial screening. Med. Klin. 2002; 97: 285–289
134. Jain, R., Sawhney, S., Sahni, P., Taneja, K., Berry, M.: CT portography by direct intrasplenic contrast injection: a new technique. Abdom. Imag. 1999; 24: 272–277
135. Komori, K., Sonoda, T., Ikeda, Y., Kanematu, T., Sugimachi, K.: Demonstration of hepatic artery aneurysma by subtraction angiography. Amer. J. Gastroenterol. 1991; 86: 1650–1653
136. Langer, R., Langer, M., Scholz, A., Neuhaus, P., Astinet, F., Ferstl, F.J., Felix, R.: Stellenwert der Angiographie und radiologischen Intervention vor und nach Lebertransplantation. Fortschr. Röntgenstr. 1991; 155: 416–422
137. Lindberg, C.G., Lundstedt, C., Stridbeck, H., Tranberg, K.G.: Accuracy of CT arterial portography of the liver compared with findings at laparotomy. Acta Radiol. 1993; 34: 139–142
138. Mateev, B., Wirbatz, W., Kiessling, J., Wittbrodt, S., Eichhorn, H.-J.: Die Katheterisierung der V. portae über die V. umbilicalis (transumbilikale Portohepatographie). Fortschr. Röntgenstr. 1969; 110: 178–191
139. Merine, D., Takayasu, K., Wakao, F.: Detection of hepatocellular carcinoma: comparison of CT during arterial portography with CT after intra-arterial injection of iodised oil. Radiology 1990; 175: 707–710
140. Meves, M., Apitzsch, D.E.: Die Lebervenenangiographie zum Nachweis von intrahepatischen Tumoren. Fortschr. Röntgenstr. 1976; 125: 247–251
141. Oberstein, A., Kauczor, H.U., Mildenberger, P., Ibe, M., Teifke, A., Rieker, O., Gerken, G., Thelen, M.: Triphasic spiral CT scanning in the diagnosis of liver diseases: comparison with CT arteriography and CT arterioportography. Fortschr. Röntgenstr. 1996; 164: 449–456
142. Okazaki, M., Ono, H., Higashihara, H., Koganemaru, F., Nozaki, Y., Hoashi, T., Kimura, T., Yamasaki, S., Makuuchi, M.: Angiographic management of massive hemobilia due to iatrogenic trauma. Gastrointest. Radiol. 1991; 16: 205–211
143. Ono, N., Toyonaga, A., Nishimura, H., Hayabuchi, N., Tanikawa, K.: Evaluation of magnetic resonance angiography on portosystemic collaterals in cirrhotic patients. Amer. J. Roentgenol. 1997; 92: 1515–1519
144. Pavone, P., Marsili, L., Albertini Petroni, G., Cardone, G., Cisternino, S., Di Girolamo, M., Passariello, R.: Arteriography in diagnosing hepatocellular carcinoma. Ital. J. Gastroenterol. 1992; 24: 92–94
145. Pollard, J.J., Nebesar, R.A., Mattoso, L.F.: Angiographic diagnosis of benign diseases of the liver. Radiology 1966; 86: 276–283
146. Schwartz, D.S., Gettner, P.A., Konstantino, M.M., Bartley, C.L., Keller, M.S., Ehrenkranz, R.A., Jacobs, H.C.: Umbilical venous catherization and the risk of portal vein thrombosis. J. Pediatr. 1997; 131: 760–762
147. Stiglbauer, R., Barton, P., Jantsch, H., Pichler, W., Schurawitzki, H., Mühlbacher, F.: Angiographie nach Lebertransplantation. Fortschr. Röntgenstr. 1990; 153: 357–361
148. Stulberg, H.J., Bierman, H.R.: Selective hepatic arteriography. Normal anatomy, anatomic variations, and pathological conditions. Radiology 1965; 85: 46–55
149. Takahashi, K., Saito, K., Tamura, K., Honda, M., Touei, H., Sakai, O., Kawashima, Y., Kuji, T., Ohtani, M., Kawamoto, T., Ohsawa, T.: Hepatic neoplasms: detection with hepatoportal subtraction angiography – a new technnique of DSA. Radiology 1990; 177: 243–248
150. Takayasu, K., Shima, Y., Muramatsu, Y., Goto, H., Moriyama, N., Yamada, T., Makuuchi, M., Yamasaki, S., Hasegawa, H., Okazaki, N., Hirohasi, S., Kishi, K.: Angiography of small hepatocellular carcinomas: analysis of 105 resected tumors. Amer. J. Roentgenol. 1986; 147: 525–529
151. Tomczak, R., Zeitler, H., Rilinger, N., Pfeifer, T., Häberle, H.J., Leibing, U., Friedrich, J.M.: Stellenwert der Portangiographie bei der Verlaufskontrolle der lokoregionären Chemotherapie. Fortschr. Röntgenstr. 1992; 157: 552–554
152. Vosshenrich, R., Fischer, U., Grabbe, E.: MR angiography in portal hypertension. State of the art. Radiologe 2001; 41: 868–876
153. Wannagat, L.: Die laparoskopische Splenoportographie. Klin. Wschr. 1955; 33: 750–758.

154. **Wannagat, L.:** Das intrahepatische Splenoportogramm bei der Hepatitis. Med. Klin. 1962; 57: 853–857
155. **Wannagat, L.:** Splenoportographie und Segmentangiographie der Leber. Dtsch. Ärztebl. 1977; 2279–2286
156. **Welch, T.J., Sheedy II, P.F., Johnson, C.M., Stephens, D.H., Charboneau, J.W., Brown, M.L., May, G.R., Adson, M.A., McGill, D.B.:** Focal nodular hyperplasia and hepatic adenoma: comparison of angiography, CT, US, and scintigraphy. Radiology 1985; 156: 593–595
157. **Zajko, A.B., Bron, K.M., Starzl, Th.E., van Thiel, D.H., Gartner, J.C., Iwatsuki, S., Shaw, B.W.jr., Zitelli, B.J., Malatack, J.J., Urbach, A.H.:** Angiography of liver transplantation patients. Radiology 1985; 157: 305–311
158. **Zhang, L.J., Qi, J., Shen, W.:** 16-slice CT hepatic venography. Abdom. Imag. 2006; 31: 308–314

Cholangiography
159. **Alcaraz, M.J., De la Morena, E.J., Polo, A., Ramos, A., De la Cal, M.A., Mandly, A.G.:** A comparative study of magnetic resonance cholangiography and direct cholangiography. Rev. Espan. Enferm. Digest. 2000; 92: 433–438
160. **Bilbao, M.K., Dotter, C.T., Lee, T.G., Katon, R.M.:** Complications of endoscopic retrograde cholangiopancreatography (ERCP). A study of 10.000 cases. Gastroenterology 1976; 70: 314–320
161. **Bret, P.M., Reinhold, C.:** Magnetic resonance cholangiopancreatography. Endoscopy 1997; 29: 472–486
162. **Carr-Locke, D.L.:** Overview of the role of ERCP in the management of diseases of the biliary tract and the pancreas. Gastrointest. Endosc. 2002; 56: (Suppl.): 157–160
163. **Corlette, M.B. jr., Schatzki, St., Ackroyd, F.:** Operative cholangiography and overlooked stones. Arch. Surg. 1978; 113: 729–734
164. **Dawson, P., Adam, A., Benjamin, I.S.:** Intravenous cholangiography revisited. Clin. Radiol. 1993; 47: 223–225
165. **Famos, M., Stadler, P., Schneekloth, G.:** Die selektive intraoperative Cholangiographie. Helv. Chir. Acta 1989; 56: 897–901
166. **Fisher, L., Fisher, A., Thomson, A.:** Cardiopulmonary complications of ERCP in older patients. Gastrointest. Endosc. 2006; 63: 948–955
167. **Flamm, C.R., Mark, D.H., Aronson, N.:** Evidence-based review of ERCP: introduction and description of systematic review methods. Gastrointest. Endosc. 2002; 56 (Suppl.): 161–164
168. **Günther, R., Georgi, M., Schaeffer, H.J.:** Transvenöse Cholangiographie und perkutane transhepatische Feinnadelcholangiographie. Dtsch. Med. Wschr. 1980; 105: 255–262
169. **Hintze, R.E., Adler, A., Veltzke, W., Abou-Rebyeh, H., Hammerstingl, R., Vogl, T., Felix, R.:** Clinical significance of magnetic resonance cholangiopancreatography (MRCP) compared to endoscopic retrograde cholangiopancreatography (ERCP). Endoscopy 1997; 29: 182–187
170. **Kakos, G.S., Tompkins, R.K., Turnipseed, W., Zollinger, R.M.:** Operative cholangiography during routine cholecystectomy. A review of 3012 cases. Arch. Surg. 1972; 104: 484–488
171. **Kiesslich, R., Holfelder, M., Will, D., Hahn, M., Nafe, B., Genitsariotis, R., Daniello, S., Maeurer, M., Jung, M.:** Interventional ERCP in patients with cholestasis. Degree of biliary bacterial colonization and antibiotic resistance. Zsch. Gastroenterol. 2001; 39: 985–992
172. **Kuntz, H.D., May, B.:** Endoskopisch-retrograde Cholangiographie bei primären Lebererkrankungen. Med. Welt 1984; 35: 116–119
173. **Maier, M., Kohler, B., Benz, C., Korber, H., Riemann, J.F.:** Perkutane transhepatische Cholangioskopie (PTCS) – eine wichtige Ergänzung in Diagnose und Therapie von Gallenwegserkrankungen. Z. Gastroenterol. 1995; 33: 435–439
174. **Matzen, P., Malchow-Moller, A., Lejerstofte, J., Stage, P., Juhl, E.:** Endoscopic retrograde cholangiopancreatography and transhepatic cholangiography in patients with suspected obstructive jaundice. A randomized study. Scand. J. Gastroenterol. 1982; 17: 731–735
175. **Merrill, J.R.:** Operative cholangiography by direct puncture of the common bile duct. Surg. Gynec. Obstetr. 1984; 158: 331–334
176. **Okuda, K.:** Thin needle percutaneous transhepatic cholangiography – Historical review. Endoscopy 1980; 12: 2–7
177. **Ponchon, T., Pilleul, F.:** Diagnostic ERCP (review). Endoscopy 2002; 34: 29–42
178. **Rasenack, U., Laubenberger, Th.:** Bedeutung der intravenösen Cholangiographie. Dtsch. Med. Wschr. 1984; 109: 1927–1930
179. **Rolfsmeyer, E.S., Bubrick, M.P., Kollitz, P.R., Onstad, G.R., Hitchcock, C.R.:** The value of operative cholangiography. Surgery 1982; 154: 369–371
180. **Schumacher, K.A., Wallner, B., Weidenmaier, W., Friedrich, J.M.:** Biliäre Obstruktion: MR-Cholangiographie mit einer schnellen Gradientenecho-Sequenz (2D CE-Fast). Fortschr. Röntgenstr. 1991; 155: 332–336
181. **Soto, J.A., Barish, M.A., Yucel, E.K., Siegenberg, D., Ferrucci, J.T., Chuttani, R.:** Magnetic resonance cholangiography: comparison to endoscopic retrograde cholangiopancreatography. Gastroenterology 1996; 110: 589–597
182. **Stockberger, S.M., Sherman, S., Kopecky, K.K.:** Helical CT cholangiography. Abdom. Imaging 1996; 21: 98–104
183. **Teplick, St.K., Flick, P., Brandon, J.C.:** Transhepatic cholangiography in patients with suspected biliary disease and nondilated intrahepatic bile ducts. Gastrointest. Radiol. 1991; 16: 193–197
184. **Topazian, M., Kozarek, R., Stoler, R., Vender, R., Wells, C.K., Feinstein, A.R.:** Clinical utility of endoscopic retrograde cholangiopancreatography. Gastrointest. Endosc. 1997; 46: 393–399
185. **Vilgrain, V., Erlinger, S., Belghiti, J., Degott, C., Menu, Y., Nahum, H.:** Cholangiographic appearance simulating sclerosing cholangitis in metastatic adenocarcinoma of the liver. Gastroenterology 1990; 99: 850–853
186. **Vitellas, K.M., Enns, R.A., Keogan, M.T., Freed, K.S., Spritzer, C.E., Baillie, J., Nelson, R.C.:** Comparison of MR cholangiopancreatographic techniques with contrast-enhanced cholangiography in the evaluation of sclerosing cholangitis. Amer. J. Roentgenol. 2002; 178: 327–334
187. **Wallner, B.K., Schumacher, K.A., Weidenmaier, W., Friedrich, J.M.:** Dilated biliary tract: evaluation with MR cholangiography with a T_2-weighted contrast-enhanced fast sequence. Radiology 1991; 181: 805–808
188. **Wamsteker, E.J.:** Updates in biliary endoscopy. Curr. Opin. Gastroenterol. 2006; 22: 300–304
189. **Zajko, A.B., Bron, K.M., Campbell, W.L., Behal, R., van Thiel, D.H., Starzl, Th.E.:** Percutaneous transhepatic cholangiography and biliary drainage after liver transplantation: a five-year experience. Gastrointest. Radiol. 1987; 12: 137–143
190. **Zeman, R.K., Berman, P.M., Silverman, P.M., Cooper, C., Garra, B.S., Patt, R.H., Ascher, S.M.:** Biliary tract: three-dimensional helical CT without cholangiographic contrast material. Radiology 1995; 196: 865–867
191. **Zimmermann, H.-G.:** Intraoperative Gallenwegsdiagnostik. Chirurg 1981; 52: 440–444

Diagnostics in Liver Diseases
9 Scintigraphic diagnostics

		Page:
1	*Principle*	200
2	***RES scintigraphy***	200
2.1	Liver cirrhosis	200
2.2	Budd-Chiari syndrome	201
2.3	Focal liver lesions	201
3	***Hepatobiliary sequential scintigraphy***	201
3.1	Cholestasis	202
3.2	Focal nodular hyperplasia	202
3.3	Hepatic adenoma	202
3.4	Biliary leakage	202
3.5	Liver blood flow	202
3.6	Diffuse liver disease	203
3.7	Hepatocellular carcinoma	203
3.8	Neuroendocrine tumour	203
4	***Erythrocyte scintigraphy***	203
4.1	Haemangioma	203
5	***Positron emission tomography***	203
6	***Flow diagram in suspected "liver tumour"***	204
	• References (1–43)	205
	(Figures 9.1–9.4; tables 9.1–9.3)	

9 Scintigraphic diagnostics

▶ In 1951 examination of the liver using radionuclides was rendered possible through the development of an **automatic scanner** (B. CASSEN et al.). In the same year, liver scintigraphy was also introduced by R. L. WIELAND. The first proof of liver metastases was obtained in animal experiments in 1953 by means of ^{131}I-albumin (E. YUHL et al.). As early as 1954, liver scintigraphy was applied in the clinical setting (L. STIRRETT et al.). Since 1955, several ^{131}I-labelled substances excreted through bile, such as rose bengal (G. V. TAPLIN et al.), later also bromsulphane, have become available for functional assessment in hepatology. In 1958 G. V. TAPLIN et al. reported on their own clinical experience. • The development of the **scintillation camera** was a further major advance (H. O. ANGER et al., 1959). Using the scintillation camera, sequential images could be taken in rapid succession. In 1971 C. WINKLER et al. were the first investigators to use a scintillation-camera process-control computer system for studying the hepatic blood flow. • The following **radionuclides** were available: ^{198}aurum (L. STIRRETT et al., 1954; H. N. WAGNER et al., 1961), ^{99m}technetium (P. V. HARPER et al., 1964), ^{133}xenon (J. R. REES et al., 1964), and ^{113}indium (A. A. GOODWIN et al., 1966).

Indications for scintigraphic methods may be given in specific situations: (1.) to evaluate certain partial liver functions, (2.) to clarify special issues when other imaging techniques (including laparoscopy) are not feasible, and (3.) to differentiate between benign and malignant tissue. The most commonly used short-lived radionuclide ^{99m}technetium (with a physical half-life of six hours) is associated with a strongly limited and justifiable radiation dose (total body < 1 mGy = 0.1 rad; screened organ 10–20 mGy = 1–2 rad). ^{99m}Tc may be marked both with colloids (proof of storage by Kupffer cells) and with erythrocytes (proof of perfusion and venous pooling); HIDA derivatives are tracers that can be excreted by hepatocytes and canaliculi. (s. tab. 9.1)

Colloids	storage capacity of Kupffer cells and of the RES (e.g. ^{99m}Tc sulphur or albumin colloids)
Iminodiacetate derivatives	uptake, transformation and excretion by the hepatocytes (e.g. IDA, HIDA, DISIDA)
Galactosyl neoglycoalbumin	hepatocyte-specific ligand
Erythrocytes	pooling and perfusion (e.g. ^{99m}TcO$_4$)
Homotaurocholic acid	bile flow (e.g. ^{75}Se HCA)
Carcinoma antibodies	immunoscintigraphy in colorectal liver metastases (e.g. ^{99m}Tc AB CEA)

Tab. 9.1: Various radionuclides with their main characteristics and functions

Contraindications for scintigraphic investigations include pregnancy and lactation as well as intolerance to mucinous antibodies.

▶ The great value of nuclear medical examinations lies in the fact that the test results (including those produced by static scans) reflect biological functions. Furthermore, such sophisticated methods are generally helpful in defining the benignancy/malignancy and structural origin of the respective focal lesion.

1 Principle

The term scintigraphy describes the production of a planar, two-dimensional image showing the distribution of radioactivity in an organ in which a radioactive substance has been stored. Depending on the radionuclide used, **information** regarding the hepatic area is obtained on (1.) functional capacity of the RES, (2.) hepatocellular function, (3.) biliary excretion kinetics, and (4.) hepatic blood flow. (4, 8, 11, 12, 20, 22, 28, 38, 39) • The **images** taken by means of high-resolution large-area gamma-cameras are (1.) (static) liver scans or (2.) (dynamic) sequential scans. • Further technical and diagnostic improvements comprise: *positron emission tomography* (**PET**) and *single photon emission computer tomography* (**SPECT**).

2 RES scintigraphy

^{99m}**Tc-colloid:** In the RES of the liver (as well as of the spleen and bone marrow), 80–90% of the radio-labelled colloids are usually taken up. This procedure is therefore also termed **static colloid scintigraphy**. Colloid particles of 200–1000 nm are usually taken up in the liver RES. The size and shape of the organ can be determined. Areas of the RES with reduced or no uptake of radioactivity appear as defective, i.e. silent or cold zones ("negative scan"). • The **extent of uptake** of the radiocolloids is reflected by different *shades of colour*, ranging from dark red ("hot") through yellow, light green, dark green, blue-green and blue to blue-black ("cold"). Multiple accumulations are a rare occurrence. These storage defects do not have any specific significance. • *Further evidence of centrally located defects is obtained by carrying out additional SPECT scintigraphy.* (36)

2.1 Liver cirrhosis

Following the administration of 100–200 MBq ^{99m}Tc-sulphur colloid intravenously, liver cirrhosis is characterized by a reduction in the uptake of radioactivity in the liver and an increased uptake by the spleen and bone marrow. Colloidal uptake in the liver is thus a valuable parameter for assessing any functional loss of the hepatic RES and for evaluating the residual parenchyma which is still functioning. The phagocytic capacity of the hepatic RES is closely related to the sinusoidal blood flow, the reduction of which is a result of the development of collaterals in the area of the hepatic sinusoids — this is an early sign of portal hypertension.

Scintigraphic proof of cirrhosis is based on (*1.*) enlarged rectangular liver, (*2.*) reduced and patchy uptake of radioactivity by the hepatic RES ("mottled liver"), (*3.*) shift in the maximum activity from the right to the left lobe of liver, and (*4.*) increased uptake by the spleen and bone RES. • The recorded scintigraphic findings permit *assessment of the course* of liver cirrhosis and provide information on focal complications such as (*1.*) occlusion of the branches of the portal vein with locally impaired perfusion and (*2.*) development of hepatocellular carcinoma.

▶ Thus the liver and the spleen form an anatomical and functional unit by being interlinked not only through the lienoportal vascular system, but also through the reticuloendothelial system. (s. fig. 9.1) *(see chapter 35)*

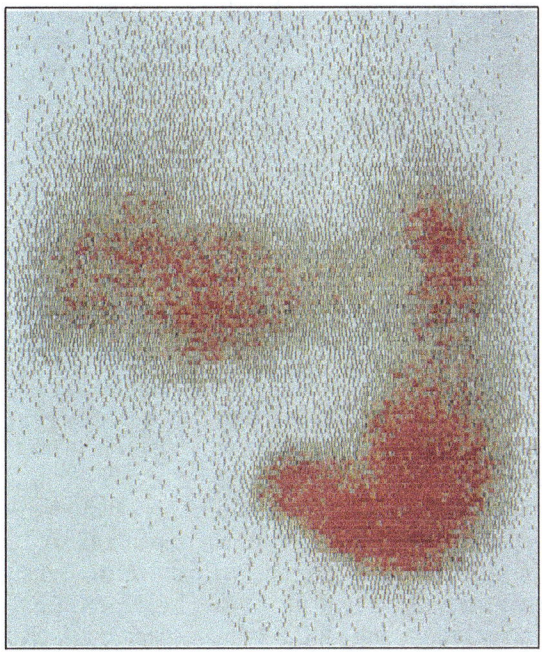

Fig. 9.1: Liver cirrhosis: diffuse decrease in the uptake of radioactivity by the liver with a markedly increased uptake by the clearly enlarged spleen (= colloid shift)

2.2 Budd-Chiari syndrome

In the Budd-Chiari syndrome, the central area of the liver shows a normal or even higher concentration of radioactivity, whereas the peripheral regions of both lobes of liver exhibit reduced or even no uptake ("hot spots" and multiple focal storage defects). Only the caudate lobe shows increased activity; due to its separate venous flow, it is not functionally affected by hepatic vein thrombosis. (27)

2.3 Focal liver lesions

Focal lesions with a diameter of > 1.5 cm can be detected with a sensitivity of > 80% and are visible as circumscribed storage defects, e. g. in the case of amoebic abscesses. (s. figs. 6.11; 9.2; 25.1) FNH is a liver tumour with maintained or even increased phagocytosis activity. • The nuclear medical diagnosis of *metastases* is now obsolete, having been replaced by more efficient imaging techniques. (s. fig. 9.3) (5, 9, 11, 23, 28, 30, 41) • If necessary, immune scintigraphy using antibodies (e.g. ^{99m}Tc-AB-CEA) may be applied in colorectal liver metastases. In HCC diagnosis, use of ^{99}Tc-anti-alpha fetoprotein produces a sensitivity of 90−95% in SPECT.

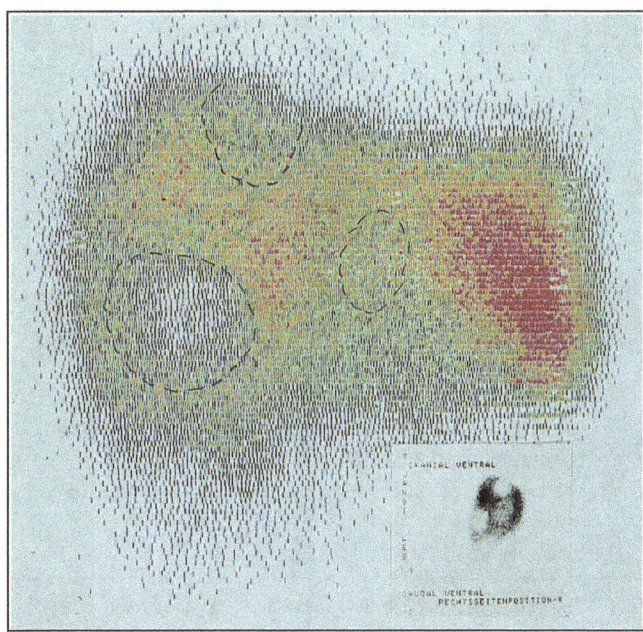

Fig. 9.2: Amoebic abscesses: storage defects and indistinct liver contours with hepatomegaly (s. fig. 25.1)

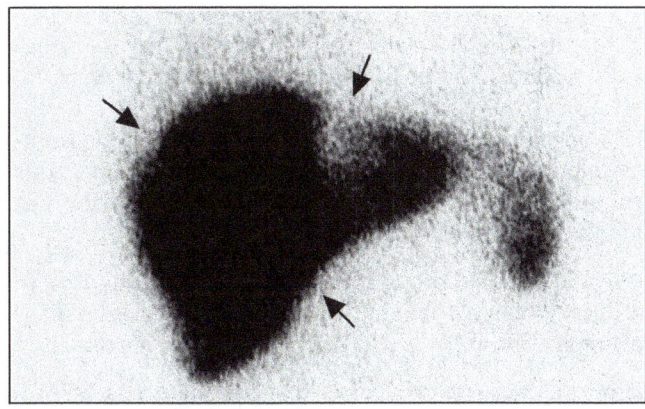

Fig. 9.3: Liver metastases: Anterior view during scintigraphy using Tc^{99m}-S-colloid (100 MBq): three foci in the right lobe of liver in colon carcinoma

3 Hepatobiliary sequential scintigraphy

^{99m}**Tc-iminodiacetic acid derivatives** (IDA, HIDA, DISIDA, BIDA) usually reach their maximum concentration in the hepatocytes 2−5 minutes after i.v. injection and are then excreted into the bile ducts. After 30−45 minutes, the radioactive substance has largely been cleared from the liver. (4, 14, 26) • ^{99m}Tc-mebrofenin correlates well with the ICG clearance test. It provides information of segmental functional liver tissue, which is of additional use when planning liver resection. (8) (s. tab. 9.2)

> 1. Examination of the hepatic perfusion of focal lesions
> 2. Evaluation of radionuclide uptake by hepatocytes (parenchymal phase): assessment of liver function (34)
> 3. Detection of biliary obstruction, such as in cholestatic syndrome with and without jaundice − search for (posttraumatic or postoperative) biliary leakage (e. g. following liver transplantation)
> 4. Examination of bilio-digestive anastomosis
> 5. Monitoring runoff after papillotomy
> 6. Follow-up after liver transplantation
> 7. Differential diagnosis of neonatal jaundice (below 10−12 mg/dl) vs. neonatal biliary atresia
> 8. Contrast-medium intolerance
> 9. Acute cholecystitis (exact visualization of the gall bladder excludes acute cholecystitis)
> 10. Focal nodular hyperplasia

Tab. 9.2: Indications for hepatobiliary sequential scintigraphy

3.1 Cholestasis

Differentiation between obstructive and parenchymatous cholestasis is possible in >90% of cases. A serum bilirubin level of up to 30 mg/dl is not seen as a methodological impediment to sequential scintigraphy. In incomplete obstruction with nondilated bile ducts, this technique provides more information than can be obtained using ultrasound. (17, 19)

^{75}SeHCAT: The homotaurocholic acid test using ^{75}Se to evaluate the hepatobiliary function (e. g. in the bile-acids losing syndrome) is also worth mentioning here. (42)

Scintigraphic assessment of **liver transplants** is helpful (e.g. perfusion, rejection, bile-duct obstruction or bile leakage). (29)

3.2 Focal nodular hyperplasia

FNH is the second most frequent benign hepatic tumour. It is a pseudotumorous regenerative node, most frequently occurring in women. Four-phase cholescintigraphy using ^{99m}Tc-IDA is currently the best method of detection. In 80−90% of cases, perfusion is good with hypervascular tumours of >2−3 cm in diameter. This results in initial enhancement of the FNH. However, the tracer cannot be discharged into the bile ducts quickly enough, because in FNH they only consist of irregular proliferations. This results in tracer retention in the excretion phase (so-called "trapping") in FNH, whereas the surrounding liver parenchyma is already tracer-free. Preserved colloid uptake by the RES is typical, whereas occasional uptake is deemed pathognomonic. • In 10−20% of cases, no intact RES is available in FNH. Thus the latter is scintigraphically "cold". (14, 40)

3.3 Hepatic adenoma

Hepatic adenoma consists of atypical, strand-like hepatocytes. It is characterized by normal perfusion and an extensive absence of Kupffer cells as well as irregularity of the bile ducts. Scintigraphically, it is possible to demonstrate that there is no elimination of iminodiacetates from the adenoma and that uptake of the radioactive tracer is prolonged compared with the normal liver parenchyma ("trapping" on IDA scans). (40) No colloidal albumin or ^{99m}Tc-colloid is taken up − this allows differentiation of an adenoma from focal nodular hyperplasia. • The additional use of the SPECT technique increases sensitivity.

3.4 Biliary leakage

Hepatobiliary sequential scintigraphy has proved useful in tracing biliary leakage, especially when it is posttraumatic or postoperative. With the help of this method, it is possible to demonstrate pathognomonic extrahepatic nuclide accumulation in the traumatized areas. A biliary leakage of 0.5 ml/min can be easily detected. Sensitivity and specificity are as high as 100%. This procedure is used as an initial screening modality in suspected biliary leakage. (29, 32, 42)

3.5 Liver blood flow

^{99m}Tc-DTPA: Arterial perfusion accounts for 20−40% of the circulation; in portal hypertension, cirrhosis causes arterial perfusion to increase to over 60%. In portal vein thrombosis, only an arterial curve is visible. Liver metastasis usually displays relatively high arterial perfusion. In (rare) occlusions of the hepatic artery, only a portal venous curve is visible. When a bolus injection of 400 MBq ^{99m}Tc-diethylenetriamine pentaacetic acid (DTPA) is applied, scintigraphy is able to reveal a biphasic time-activity curve. The initial increase of activity is produced by the arterial influence and the second peak by the portal venous inflow. Both curves can be evaluated quantitatively. (38) • Perfusion scintigraphy may be useful in the case of liver trauma, TIPS, hypervascularized hepatic tumours and partial liver resection as well as after liver transplantation.

3.6 Diffuse liver disease

99mTc-NGA: Hepatic binding protein (HBP) found on the hepatocyte surface can bind desialylated glycoproteins with terminal galactose residues. There is a close correlation between a change in HBP activity due to liver trauma and an increase in bonding inhibitors in plasma. • Galactosyl-neoglycoalbumin (NGA) belongs to a group of hepatocyte-specific tracers, whose accumulation is dependent upon HBP bonding; this can be measured scintigraphically using ^{99m}Tc-NGA (D.R. VERA et al., 1984). The lysosomes mark the end of the tracer take-up in the hepatocytes (> 90 %). • The first clinical findings in cases of liver trauma were reported on by the same group (R.C. STADALNIK et al., 1980). Results of the investigation into liver cirrhosis and HCC were presented later. It has not yet been possible to obtain any substantial findings in diffuse liver damage using conventional tracer methods. However, use of the hepatocyte-specific tracer ^{99m}Tc-NGA can be helpful in assessing liver injury and recovery. (16, 34, 37)

3.7 Hepatocellular carcinoma

^{67}**Gallium:** The uptake of ^{67}gallium by HCC is greater than in normal liver tissue. It is possible to differentiate foci in cirrhosis with the help of this radionuclide. In the case of a focus measuring more than 2 cm, specificity is 91% and sensitivity is 96%. This method should also be used for detecting early recurrent HCC. The tracer ^{67}gallium is, however, non-specific, since it is also taken up by non-hepatocyte-derived tumours and inflammatory lesions. (33) • Colloid scintigraphy and IDA derivates are not significant in HCC diagnosis.

3.8 Neuroendocrine tumour

^{111}**In DTPA-DPhe-Octreotide:** Neuroendocrine tumours show a greater expression of somatostatin receptors, which can be detected by means of this marked ligand. Such a form of szintigraphy makes it possible to locate a primary tumour as well as metastases; it is also indicated to monitor therapy.

4 Erythrocyte scintigraphy

Blood pool scintigraphy using a bolus injection of 750 MBq ^{99m}Tc-labelled erythrocytes may lead to a diagnosis of intrahepatic space-occupying processes which cannot be differentiated by US or CT. This applies especially to haematomas, haemangiomas and haemangiosarcomas. The SPECT technique helps to increase sensitivity. With regard to angiographic imaging reconstruction, however, the contrast medium-based imaging techniques available today produce by far the best results.

4.1 Haemangioma

Cavernous haemangiomas are the most common form of benign liver tumours. They occur in the form of a single lesion in approx. 90% of cases. When using ^{99m}Tc-pertechnetate labelling, haemangiomas exhibit a reduced uptake of radioactivity in the early perfusion phase compared with adjacent liver tissue; in the late phase, however, an increase in uptake is detectable. This "fill in" occurs faster in small haemangiomas than in larger ones due to the lower stasis. In the latter case, scanning should be carried out at a later phase. At 2 cm, a specificity and sensitivity of up to 100% is obtainable using a high-resolution three-headed system. (42) Smaller haemangiomas (< 2 cm) can be identified by interference-free SPECT in up to 90% of cases. (15, 35) The RES, hepatocytes and bile ducts show no scintigraphic reaction. (1−3, 15, 21, 25, 43)

5 Positron emission tomography

Positron emission tomography (PET) has two significant advantages compared to single-photon emission computed tomography: (*1.*) improved spatial resolution, and (*2.*) absolute quantification of tracer take-up.

Positron emission tomography with ^{18}**F-fluoro-2-deoxy-D-glucose** (^{18}F-FDG) visualizes partial physiological and biochemical functions and thus also pathophysiological and pathobiochemical aspects at the molecular level in a nuclear medical procedure. PET may be a useful method for the differential diagnosis of hepatic foci (malignant/benign). Liver metastases of gastrointestinal tumours can be detected with significantly greater sensitivity using ^{18}F-FDG-PET. In relapse diagnosis of colorectal carcinoma, sensitivity is 93−100% and specificity 95−98%. (5, 35) Malignant melanoma takes up the most ^{18}F-FDG, enabling foci as small as 1.5 mm (as well as affected lymph nodes) to be identified with a high degree of accuracy. Hodgkin's lymphoma, which accounts for approx. 1% of all carci-

---

1. Lentodegenerative alterations in Wilson's disease
2. Biochemical changes related to hepatic encephalopathy
   − measurement of the blood-brain barrier by ^{68}Ga-DTPA
   − determination of neuroreceptors by ^{18}F-dopa, ^{11}C-dopamine, ^{11}C-serotonin
   − neurotransmitter mapping by ^{18}F in combination with metaraminol, *etc.*
3. Questions on protein synthesis
   − by means of ^{11}C-labelled methionine, leucine, phenylalanine
4. Hypoxia/necrosis markers
   − by means of ^{18}F-labelled misonidazole
5. Glucose metabolism-related activity patterns of liver cells
6. Measurable assessment of liver cell regeneration
   − by means of 2-^{11}C thymidine, *etc.*
7. Detection of hepatocellular carcinoma
   − by means of ^{11}C-acetate

Tab. 9.3: Application fields for PET scanning in (still experimental) hepatology with respective tracers

nomas, is a rare entity. In stages I and II, the 10-year survival rate is around 80%. PET has proved to be a useful tool in staging and monitoring. (6) • In the field of (still experimental) hepatology, a wide range of **scientific issues** may be amenable to PET. (s. tab. 9.3).

Tumour cells frequently display increased glycolysis. A radioactive-marked glucose derivative can therefore be taken up in the tumour cells and demonstrated using a PET scan after 40−45 minutes. The glucose cellular metabolism is measured after i.v. injection of ^{18}F-FDG. This tracer is easily absorbed by the cells before being converted by hexokinase into ^{18}F-FDG-6-phosphate which, after phosphorylation, is subsequently trapped inside the cells for a prolonged period ("metabolic trapping"). Its half-life is 110 minutes. In the field of hepatology, ^{18}F-FDG-PET has become clinically significant in staging, therapy follow-up and relapse diagnosis of liver tumours. (5, 7, 10, 13, 24, 31, 35)

^{68}**Ga DOTATOC-PET:** In PET, the gamma emitter ^{111}In is replaced by the positron emitter ^{68}Ga. This tracer is highly specific for detecting somatostatin receptors, particularly in combination with CT/PET.

^{18}**FDOPA-PET:** Neuroendocrine tumours are able to decarboxylate 5-hydroxytryptamin and L-3-4-dihydroxyphenylalanin. This tracer can therefore be used for diagnosis and monitoring therapy.

^{11}**C-acetate:** The application of ^{11}C-acetate PET led to far higher sensitivity and specificity than was the case with ^{67}Ga scintigraphy. Thus this technique may become a potential diagnostic tool. (18)

6 Flow diagram in suspected "liver tumour"

Various tumourous and pseudotumourous foci may form in the liver and hepatobiliary system. Differential diagnosis in thus more challenging. But a definitive diagnosis is necessary to be able to initiate therapeutic measures and to establish a prognosis.

> After carrying out the imaging techniques (if necessary with contrast media) *(see chapters 6, 8, 9)* and laparoscopy/biopsy *(see chapter 7)*, the strategy of establishing a diagnosis by **flow diagram** is recommended in suspected **"liver tumour"**. (s. fig. 9.4)

A flow chart should include echocomplex focuses and a distinction between single and multiple focuses. Haematoma and (especially) abscesses, are not always echofree; they may also be hypoechoic or reveal varied echoes. This must be taken into account in the diagnosis of these two conditions. Scintigraphy is becoming less significant, whereas MRI is considerably more important today. However, scintigraphy may be indicated when carrying out a differential diagnosis for adenoma and FNH. Economic constraints can make it necessary to omit some diagnostic steps regarding imaging procedures in order to produce a faster and more cost-effective diagnosis. As an alternative, targeted FNB, biopsies or laparoscopy are recommended. It may even be desirable in individual cases to obtain an earlier histological diagnosis and, if necessary, follow the flow chart in the opposite direction. • *All in all, an extremely careful and critical assessment is required, taking into account the risks, costs and benefits involved.* (s. fig. 13.2)

▶ In cases of suspected *"liver tumour"*, **ultrasonography** is the method of choice. If the type of focal process cannot be adequately identified even by very experienced investigators, sonographic monitoring should be performed within a short period of time. Even in cases where the differential diagnostic approach fails, pathological or potentially positive findings can still be obtained with a certain degree of reliability. If an exact diagnosis cannot be achieved, however, imaging techniques are then as a rule indicated. (s. fig. 9.4)

▶ In order to clarify pathological results or potentially positive findings, **computer tomography** is indicated. The use of CT may also be advisable even with negative sonographic findings if the clinical and laboratory parameters point to a focal process in the area of the liver or the biliary tract. (s. fig. 9.4)

▶ In the case of differential diagnosis of adenoma versus focal nodular hyperplasia, **scintigraphy** is indicated, whereas in the case of metastases, more reliable imaging techniques are preferred. (s. fig. 9.4)

▶ In suspected haemangioma, sonography, scintigraphy and MRI are the most efficient procedures. • In individual cases, these three imaging techniques might be interrelated with respect to diagnosis/indication. (s. fig. 9.4)

▶ Should the differential diagnosis of focal liver findings remain unresolved despite the use of imaging techniques, **laparoscopy** is indicated (possibly with targeted forceps biopsy or liver biopsy). Depending on the findings, *explorative laparoscopy* is also undertaken for the purpose of tumour staging. • Medical assessment of the clinical and sonographic findings may, in some cases, suggest laparoscopy with targeted tissue biopsy − even without previous CT − when an accurate diagnosis is required. (s. p. 158) (s. fig. 9.4)

▶ The indications for sonography-guided or CT-guided **fine-needle biopsy** (FNB) are (*1.*) contraindications to the use of laparoscopy (s. p. 149) or (*2.*) if it seems unlikely that previously unresolved findings will be clarified by laparoscopy. • In consideration of all relevant findings from sonography or CT as well as the patient's condition,

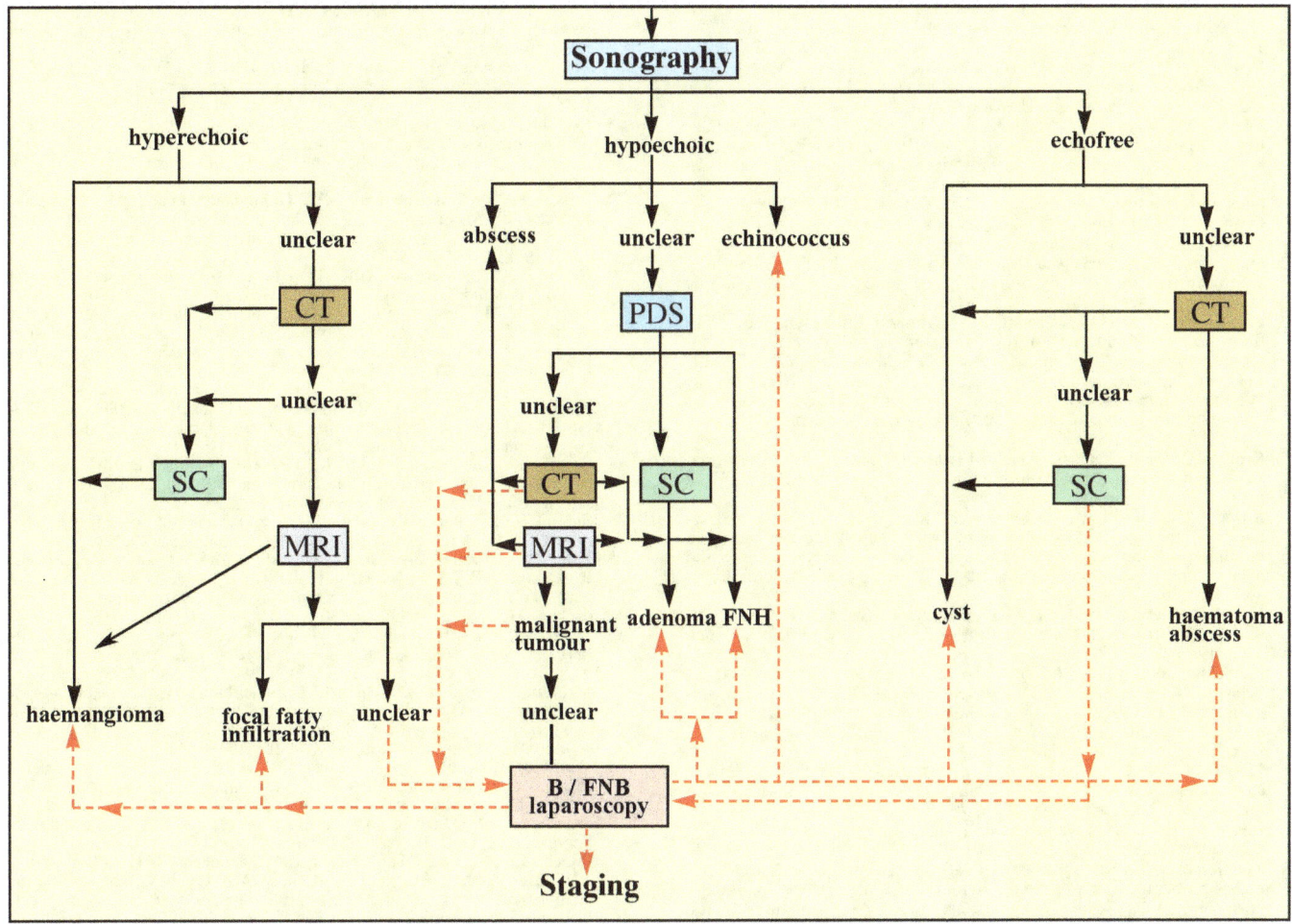

Fig. 9.4: Flow chart for use in clinically suspected "liver tumour" with positive sonographic findings. • Imaging procedures (→) which may be indicated include power-Doppler sonography (PDS), computer tomography (CT), magnetic resonance imaging (MRI) and scintigraphy (SC). • Histological diagnosis is indicated in some cases in order to confirm or exclude imaging diagnosis. (--▶)

it may be necessary in individual cases to resort to FNB as the primary approach instead of biopsy or laparoscopy. (s. fig. 9.4) • The non-availability of laparoscopy or insufficient experience with this technique are in themselves not an "indication" for percutaneous fine-needle biopsy. (s. fig. 9.4)

In view of growing financial constraints in many contries regarding the health service, the question of the cost/benefit ratio should also be taken into consideration. In the current economic situation, the **total costs** incurred for the respective examination methods can indeed be substantial.

Basically, the **prioritization of methods** within a diagnostic flow diagram should be determined by the question of whether (*1.*) use of an examination technique is indicated, (*2.*) indication applies at the given moment, and (*3.*) definitive diagnosis is likely to be obtained. • *Usually, only a definitive diagnosis allows statements to be made on therapy and prognosis!*

References:

1. **Birnbaum, B.A., Weinreb, J.C., Megibow, A.J., Snager, J.J., Lubat, E., Kanamuller, H., Noz, M.E., Bosniak, M.A.:** Definitive diagnosis of hepatic hemangiomas: MR imaging versus Tc-99m-labeled red blood cell SPECT. Radiology 1990; 176: 95–101
2. **Bradley, M., Stewart, I., Metreweli, C.:** Diagnosis of the peripheral cavernous haemangioma: comparison of ultrasound, CT and RBC scintigraphy. Clin. Radiol. 1991; 44: 34–37
3. **Brown, R.K., Gomes, A., King, W., Pusey, E., Lois, J., Goldstein, L., Busuttil, R.W., Hawkins, R.A.:** Hepatic hemangiomas: evaluation by magnetic resonance imaging and TC-99m red blood cell scintigraphy. J. Nucl. Med. 1987; 28: 1683–1687
4. **Colombo, C., Castellani, M.R., Balistreri, W.F., Seregni, E., Assaisso, M.L., Giunta, A.:** Scintigraphic documentation of an improvement in hepatobiliary excretory function after treatment with ursodeoxycholic acid in patients with cystic fibrosis and associated liver disease. Hepatology 1992; 15: 677–684
5. **De Wit, M., Bohuslavizki, K.H., Buchert, R., Bumann, D., Clausen, M., Hossfeld, D.K.:** ^{18}FDG-PET following treatment as valid predictor for disease-free survival in Hodgkin's lymphoma. Ann. Oncol. 2001; 12: 29–37
6. **Delbeke, D., Martin, W.H., Sandler, M.P., Chapman, W.C., Wright, J.K., Pinson, C.W.:** Evaluation of benign vs malignant hepatic lesions with positron emission tomography. Arch. Surg. 1998; 133: 510–516
7. **Dimitrakopoulou, A., Strauss, L.G., Clorius, J.H., Ostertag, H., Schlag, P., Heim, M., Oberdorfer, F., Helus, F., Haberkorn, U., van Kaick, G.:** Studies with positron emission tomography after systemic administration of fluorine-18-uracil in patients with liver metastases from colorectal carcinoma. J. Nucl. Med. 1993; 34: 1075–1081
8. **Erdogan, D., Heijnen, B.H.M., Bennink, R.J., Kok, M., Dinant, S., Straatsburg, I.H., Gouma, D.J., van Gulik, T.M.:** Preoperative assess-

ment of liver function: A comparison of (99m) Tc-Mebrofenin scintigraphy with indocyanine green clearance test. Liver Internat. 2004; 24: 117–123

9. **Farlow, D.C., Chapmann, P.R., Gruenewald, S.M., Antico, V.F., Farrell, G.C., Little, J.M.:** Investigation of focal hepatic lesions: is tomographic red blood cell imaging useful? World J. Surg. 1990; 14: 463–467

10. **Findlay, M., Young, H., Cunningham, D., Iverson, A., Cronin, B., Hickish, T., Pratt, B., Husband, J., Flower, M., Ott, R.:** Noninvasive monitoring of tumor metabolism using fluorodeoxyglucose and positron emission tomography in colorectal liver metastases: correlation with tumor response to fluorouracil. J. Clin. Oncol. 1996; 14: 700–708

11. **Gratz, K.F., Weimann, A.:** Diagnostik von Lebertumoren–wann ist die Szintigraphie von Bedeutung? Zbl. Chir. 1998; 123: 111–118

12. **Hultcrantz, R., Gabrielsson, N.:** Patients with persistent elevation of aminotransferases: investigation with ultrasonography, radionucleide imaging and liver biopsy. J. Intern. Med. 1993; 233: 7–12

13. **Keiding, S., Munk, O.L., Schlott, K.M., Hansen, S.B.:** Dynamic 2-[^{18}F] fluoro-2-deoxy-d-glucose positron emission tomography of liver tumours without blood sampling. Eur. J. Nucl. Med. 2000; 27: 407–412

14. **Kotzerke, J., Schwarzrock, R., Krischek, O., Wiese, H., Hundeshagen, H.:** Technetium-99m DISIDA hepatobiliary agent in diagnosis of hepatocellular carcinoma, adenoma, and focal nodular hyperplasia. J. Nucl. Med. 1989; 30: 1278–1279

15. **Krause, T., Hauenstein, K., Studier-Fischer, B., Schümichen, C., Moser, E.:** Improved evaluation of technetium-99m-red blood cell SPECT in hemangioma of the liver. J. Nucl. Med. 1993; 23: 375–380

16. **Kwon, A.H., Matsui, Y., Ha-Kawa, S.K., Kamiyama, Y.:** Functional hepatic volume measured by technetium-99m-galactosyl-human serum albumin liver scintigraphy: comparison between hepatocyte volume and liver volume by computed tomography. Amer. J. Gastroenterol. 2001; 96: 541–546

17. **Lee, A.W., Ram, M.D., Shih, W.-J., Murphy, K.:** Technetium-99m BIDA biliary scintigraphy in the evaluation of the jaundiced patient. J. Nucl. Med. 1986; 27: 1407–1412

18. **Li, S., Beneshti, M., Peck-Radosavljevic, M., Oezer, S., Grumbeck, E., Schmid, M., Hamilton, G., Kapiotis, S., Dudczak, R., Kletter, K.:** Comparison of (11)C-acetate positron emission tomography and (67) Gallium citrate scintigraphy in patients with hepatocellular carcinoma. Liver Internat. 2006; 26: 920–927

19. **Lieberman, D.A., Krishnamurthy, G.T.:** Intrahepatic versus extrahepatic cholestasis. Discrimination with biliary scintigraphy combined with ultrasound. Gastroenterology 1986; 90: 734–743

20. **Lin, E.C., Kuni, C.C.:** Radionuclide imaging of hepatic and biliary disease. Semin. Liver Dis. 2001; 21: 179–194

21. **Middleton, M.L.:** Scintigraphic evaluation of hepatic mass lesions: emphasis on hemangioma detection. Semin. Nucl. Med. 1996; 26: 4–15

22. **Neumann, M.C., Schober, O.:** Nuclear imaging investigations in the liver. Radiologe 2000; 40: 916–924

23. **Newman, J.S., Oates, E., Arora, S., Kaplan, M.:** Focal spared area in fatty liver simulating a mass. Scintigraphic evaluation. Dig. Dis. Sci. 1991; 36: 1019–1022

24. **Okazumi, S., Isono, K., Enomoto, K., Kikuchi, T., Ozaki, M., Yamamoto, H., Hayashi, H., Asano, T., Ryu, M.:** Evaluation of liver tumors using fluorine-18-fluorodeoxyglucose PET: characterization of tumor and assessment of effect and treatment. J. Nucl. Med. 1992; 33: 333–339

25. **Pink, V., Buchali, K., Lüning, M., Sydow, K., Schneider, Th., Koch, M.:** Qualification of blood pool scintigraphy for imaging diagnosis of liver hemangiomas. Radiol. Diagnost. 1991; 32: 26–31

26. **Pinos, T., Xiol, X., Herranz, R., Figueras, C., Catala, I.:** Caroli's disease versus polycystic hepatic disease. Differential diagnosis with Tc-99m DISIDA scintigraphy. Clin. Nucl. Med. 1993; 18: 664–667

27. **Powell-Jackson, P.R., Karani, J., Ede, R., Mire, H., Williams, R.:** Ultrasonic scanning and 99m Tc sulphur colloid scintigraphy in diagnosis of Budd-Chiari syndrome. Gut 1986; 27: 1502–1506

28. **Reuland, P., Kurtz, B., Müller-Schauenburg, W., Feine, U.:** Vergleichende Diagnostik fokaler Leberveränderungen mittels Computer-Tomographie und szintigraphischer Methoden. Nuklearmedizin 1991; 30: 43–54

29. **Rossleigh, M.A., McCaughan, G.W., Gallagher, N.D., Morris, J.G., Bautovich, G.J., McLaughlin, A.F., Painter, D.M., Thompson, J.F., Sheil, A.G.:** The role of nuclear medicine in liver transplantation. Med. J. Aust. 1988; 148: 561–563

30. **Rubin, R.A., Lichtenstein, G.R.:** Hepatic scintigraphy in the evaluation of solitary solid liver masses. J. Nucl. Med. 1993; 34: 697–705

31. **Ruers, T.J.M., Langenhoff, B.S., Neeleman, N., Jager, G.J., Strijk, S., Wobbes, T., Corstens, F.H.M., Oyen, W.J.G.:** Value of positron emission tomography with [F-18] fluorodeoxyglucose in patients with colorectal liver metastases: A prospective study. J. Clin. Oncol. 2002; 20: 388–395

32. **Sandoval, B., Goettler, C., Robinson, A., O'Donnell, J., Adler, L., Stellato, T.:** Cholescintigraphy in the diagnosis of bile leak after laparoscopic cholecystectomy. Amer. J. Surg. 1997; 63: 611–616

33. **Serafini, A., Jeffers, L., Reddy, K., Heiba, S., Schiff, E.:** Early recognition of recurrent hepatocellular carcinoma utilizing gallium-67 citrate scintigraphy. J. Nucl. Med. 1988; 29: 712–716

34. **Shiomi, S.:** Evaluation of hepatic functional reserve by scintigraphy with (99m) Tc–GSA (editorial). Hepatol. Res. 2005; 31: 124–126

35. **Valk, P.E., Abella-Columna, E., Haseman, M.K., Pounds, T.R., Tesar, R.D., Myers, R.W., Greiss, H.B., Hofer, G.A.:** Whole-body PET imaging with (^{18}F) Fluorodeoxyglucose in management of recurrent colorectal cancer. Arch. Surg. 1999; 134: 503–511

36. **Van Heertum, R.L., Yudd, A.P., Brunetti, J.C., Pennington, M., Gualtieri, N.:** Hepatic SPECT imaging in the detection and assessment of hepatocellular disease. Clin. Nucl. Med. 1992; 17: 948–953

37. **Virgolini, I., Müller, C., Höbart, J., Scheithauer, W., Angelberger, P., Bergmann, H., O'Grady, J., Sinzinger, H.:** Liver function in acute viral hepatitis as determined by a hepatocyte-specific ligand: ^{99m}Tc-galactosyl-neoglycoalbumin. Hepatology 1992; 15: 593–598

38. **Walmsley, B.H., Fleming, J.S., Ackery, D.M., Karran, S.J.:** Non-invasive assessment of absolute values of hepatic haemodynamics using radiocolloid scintigraphy. Nucl. Med. Com. 1987; 8: 613–621

39. **Waxman, A.D.:** Scintigraphic evaluation of diffuse hepatic disease. Semin. Nucl. Med. 1982; 12: 75–88

40. **Welch, T.J., Sheedy, P.F., Johnson, C.M., Stephens, D.H., Charboneau, J.W., Brown, M.L., May, G.R., Adson, M.A., McGill, D.B.:** Focal nodular hyperplasia and hepatic adenoma: Comparison of angiography, CT, US, and scintigraphy. Radiology 1985; 156: 593–595

41. **Wetzel, E., Loose, R., Georgi, M.:** Nuklearmedizinische Differenzierung fokaler Läsionen der Leber. Radiologe 1988; 28: 370–373

42. **Williams, W., Krishnamurthy, G.T., Brar, H.S., Bobba, V.R.:** Scintigraphic variations of normal biliary physiology. J. Nucl. Med. 1984; 25: 160–165

43. **Ziessman, H.A., Silverman, P.M., Patterson, J., Harkness, B., Fahey, F.H., Zeman, R.K., Keyes, J.W.:** Improved detection of small cavernous hemangiomas of the liver with high-resolution three-headed SPECT. J. Nucl. Med. 1991; 32: 2086–2091

Diagnostics in Liver Diseases

10 Neurological and psychological diagnostics

		Page:
1	*Brain disorders in liver diseases*	208
2	***Diagnosis of disorders in cerebral performance***	208
2.1	EEG	208
2.2	Neuropsychological test procedures	209
3	***Basic psychometric programme***	210
3.1	Psychometric test procedures	210
3.1.1	Sickness impact profile	210
3.1.2	Mechanical testing procedures	210
3.2	Psychometric test programmes	211
3.2.1	Handwriting-specimen test	211
3.2.2	Number-connection test	212
3.2.3	Line-tracing test	213
3.2.4	Star-construction test	213
3.2.5	Serial-subtraction test	213
3.2.6	Story-retelling test	214
4	***Synopsis***	214
	• References (1−51)	214
	(Figures 10.1−10.4; tables 10.1−10.10)	

10 Neurological and psychological diagnostics

▶ There are **two basic dimensions** in the way the human brain copes with everyday routine; these are known as crystalline and fluid intelligence (R.B. CATELL, 1963).

1. **Crystalline intelligence** is acquired by education and experience; it proves susceptible to disturbance at a relatively late stage in life and to a relatively small extent. • Crystalline (cognitive and verbal) intelligence implements the contents of what has been learned or acquired at an earlier stage to perform tasks or to solve problems. This verbal ("cognitive") intelligence is retained for a long time, so that any impairment of cerebral function is noticed at a relatively late stage in people who pursue mental occupations.

2. **Fluid intelligence** depends largely on the speed at which information is processed; it becomes impaired relatively early and to a greater extent. • Fluid (practical and nonverbal) intelligence is characterized by the capability for solving new problems without reference to experience or education in the course of processing information. This form of intelligence deteriorates at an early stage with any impairment of cerebral function, which is why the intelligence involved in performing practical tasks, so-called handling intelligence, is most susceptible to disturbance — it is for this reason that manual activities are primarily impaired.

▶ Many different **brain functions** are available to enable routine everyday tasks to be mastered correctly. (s. tab. 10.1)

1. Attentiveness
2. Intellectual capacity
3. Logical thinking
4. Memory for design
5. Perceptive faculty
6. Power of concentration
7. Psychomotoricity
8. Reactive capacity
9. Short-term memory
10. Spatial perception and mental comprehension of numbers or letters, *etc.*

Tab. 10.1: Brain functions important for mastering routine everyday tasks

1 Brain disorders in liver diseases

In cerebral dysfunction, it is possible for disorders to be reflected individually in differing states of intensity and in various combinations. This results in a diverse pathophysiological and clinical picture of **encephalopathy**. Such a collective term for restrictions in the function of the brain does not, however, yield any statement as to their origins or pathogenesis. Encephalopathy can be triggered by some 50—60 disorders and aetiological factors — including liver diseases. *(see chapter 15)*

Hepatic encephalopathy (HE) is defined as a functional, potentially reversible disorder of the brain in the wake of severe (either acute or chronic) liver disease. The term comprises all neurological and mental symptoms.

Diagnosis of the four clinical stages of **manifest HE** (stages I—IV) is simple and reliable. But it is important firstly to recognize **latent HE** (stages 0, 0—I), also called *subclinical hepatic encephalopathy (SHE)* or *minimal HE*. • At this stage, no clinically identifiable mental or neurological defects can be detected, nor do the laboratory parameters provide any real clues. Yet, some (still reversible) neurophysiological and neuropsychological deviations from the norm can be quantified.

Early diagnosis of HE at the **latency stage** is significant in social terms, for industrial medicine and for prognostics; therefore it is of enormous economic importance as well. The development of latent (minimal and subclinical) or subsequent manifest HE (stages I—IV) depends on various factors. • *Latent HE is seen as the "most frequent complication" in hepatology.*

2 Diagnosis of disorders in cerebral performance

It should be noted that the diagnosis of latent HE (stages 0, 0—I) can cause great **difficulties.**

Despite the considerable medical and social implications of SHE, which in objective terms are undeniable, the patient subjectively feels unchanged and free from symptoms. There are no ailments or malaise felt by the patient which point to the development of SHE, and neither the conversation with the physician nor the anamnesis are suggestive of this condition. *Verbal intelligence is not affected!*

Neither clinical findings nor laboratory parameters (including intensive and scientific tests) correlate with the stage of SHE. There are no neurological abnormalities (no hyperreflexia, tremor or asterixis, etc.). • *For the diagnosis of subclinical hepatic encephalopathy, only electroencephalographic and neuropsychological (psychometric) test procedures are available so far.*

2.1 EEG

Spontaneous EEG can occasionally show a minimal increase in slow waves and a deceleration of the basic activity below the normal alpha wave range (8—12 Hz), yet there is no correlation with the occurrence of SHE. Only with knowledge of the individual's normal state and with the help of the regular spontaneous EEG as follow-up procedure for cirrhosis can SHE be recognized in 30—50% of cases. However, this is not feasible on a regular basis. With the manifestation of HE (stages I, II), the spontaneous EEG slows down to the theta and delta wave ranges (4.0—7.5 and 1—3 Hz), which are deemed to be pathological in a waking state. Groups of relatively even waves at a rate of two or three times per second, and above all frontotemporal delta Faren rhythms, are considered to be hints of a more severe HE. (7, 18, 20, 29, 43, 44, 47)

Visually evoked potentials: In the diagnosis of SHE, neither the use of visually evoked potentials (VEP) nor acoustically or somatically evoked potentials yielded better results than the spontaneous EEG. Using these exogenously evoked potentials, functional disorders of sensory pathways are identified by assessing the P-100 wave. (2, 10, 12, 21, 26—28, 36, 43, 47, 49—51)

P-300 wave: The technique of *endogenously evoked potentials (EEP)* can be applied for the registration of stimulus assessment processes and "attention processes". The *P-300 wave* is deemed to be the electrophysiological correlate of stimulus assessment processes (E. DONCHIN, 1979). P-300 latency indicates the time required for assessment and categorization of a stimulus. About 30% (45) to 71% (16) of patients with SHE and some 70% (45) to >85% (16) of cases with stage I HE show a lengthening in the latency of the P-300 wave. The sensitivity of this test procedure for the diagnosis of SHE is therefore good. The specificity is minimal because of the widely differing origins of HE. • Determination of the P-300 wave is, however, both time-consuming and expensive, calling for specialized knowledge and experience. For this reason, the process is not suitable as a routine test. • *Nevertheless, in diagnosing SHE, assessment of the P-300 wave in an endogenously evoked EEG is seen as the most valuable neurophysiological method of examination.* (5, 11, 26, 37, 42, 48)

▶ The use of **proton MR spectroscopy,** with glutamine as a marker, has opened up new diagnostic horizons. (35)

2.2 Neuropsychological test procedures

In order to objectify disruptions in brain performance, numerous test procedures have been established in clinical psychology. With the help of these procedures, various cerebral functions can be tested. (s. tab. 10.1)

The term **psychometrics** signifies the most objective recording possible concerning mental functions and personality features with the aid of a variety of test procedures.

Quality criteria and secondary criteria: Test procedures applied in clinical psychology should fulfil the requisite **quality criteria** including (*1.*) objectivity, (*2.*) reliability, and (*3.*) validity. • Alongside these main criteria, neuropsychological test procedures should also incorporate other **secondary criteria,** such as (*1.*) standardizability, (*2.*) comparability, (*3.*) cost factor, (*4.*) usefulness, and (*5.*) sensitivity. • *Obviously, it will not always be possible to meet all of these criteria in full in every case.*

No single test is absolutely reliable or even accurate. The results of neuropsychological tests are subject to various **influences** and thus confounded by a number of factors occurring individually to differing degrees of intensity and in a variety of combinations. (s. tab. 10.2) • This no doubt explains the widely differing assessments of the frequency of SHE which are reported in the literature. An examination of several of the multiple brain functions (s. tab. 10.1) requires the skilful selection of test procedures with their respective targets.

1. **Influential factor "test procedure"**
   - desired test targets
   - suitable test combination
   - professional implementation of the test
2. **Influential factor "liver disease"**
   - severity
   - aetiology and pathogenesis
   - acute or chronic state
   - portosystemic collaterals
3. **Coexistent factors**
   - consumption of alcohol
   - cerebral noxae
   - cerebral or cerebrovascular damage
4. **Individual factors**
   - age
   - intelligence
   - social status
   - fluctuation in the course of SHE

Tab. 10.2: Factors influencing the reliability of test results and the detection of SHE frequency

Quite clearly, it is not a single test, but rather a **combination of tests,** focusing on as many different brain functions as possible, which guarantees an overall result that is meaningful.

Neuropsychological tests: Among the large number of neuropsychological tests available, several procedures are considered apt for the detection of subclinical brain disturbances. Some involve complex methods and call for specialized knowledge. Nevertheless, a few can be regarded as the *"gold standard"* for clinical issues involved in the diagnosis of SHE. (1, 6, 15, 17, 43) (s. tab. 10.3)

Test combinations: For clinical purposes, suitable test combinations can be set up on the basis of the overview given (s. tab. 10.3) and in accordance with the respective issues. Due to their feasibility and reliability, the following tests are particularly useful: (*1.*) basic intelligence test, (*2.*) multiple-choice vocabulary intelligence test, (*3.*) short test for general intelligence, (*4.*) short test for cerebral intelligence, (*5.*) attentiveness-concentration test, (*6.*) Benton test, (*7.*) syndrome short test, and (*8.*) trail-making test. • In clinical studies, the Wechsler adult intelligence scale (WAIS) is often used. (14, 38, 41) In such studies, the WAIS verbal IQ is seen to be largely undisturbed, whereas there are clear deficits in that *part of the WAIS which relates to performing practical tasks* (handling IQ), particularly in the number-symbol test and in the mosaic test. At the same time, other psychological test procedures are applied, mainly the trail-making test as well as EEG (VEP, P-300 wave).

3 Basic psychometric programme

▶ The principle of early diagnosis and early treatment of a disease together with the prevention of a progressive or complicated course are fundamental targets in everyday medical routine. *This applies especially to latent hepatic encephalopathy, which can be found in a high percentage of patients suffering from liver disease.*

Intellectual capacity
1. Hamburg-Wechsler adult intelligence test
   (D. WECHSLER, 1964); 60–90 minutes
2. Basic intelligence test
   (R. B. CATTELL et al., R. H. WEISS, 1972)
3. Multiple-choice vocabulary intelligence test
   (S. LEHRL, 1977); 5–8 minutes
4. Short test for general intelligence
   (S. LEHRL et al.); 8–10 minutes
5. Short test for cerebral intelligence
   (S. LEHRL et al.)

Powers of attention and concentration
6. Attentiveness and concentration test
   (R. BRICKENKAMP, 1968); 5 minutes
7. Revision test
   (G. MARSCHNER, 1972); 8 minutes

Memory
8. Benton test
   (A. L. BENTON, 1953)
9. Syndrome short test
   (H. EERZIGKEIT); 15 minutes
10. Mini-mental-status test
    (M. L. FOLSTEIN et al., 1975); 10 minutes
11. Wechsler memory test
    (D. WECHSLER); 45–60 minutes

Recognition of shapes
12. Visual-design-potential test
    (L. BENDER, 1946); 20 minutes

Speed of cognitive performance
13. Trail-making test (parts A and B)
    (R. M. REITAN, 1955)
14. Number-connection test (part A of trail-making test, fourfold variations)
    (H. O. CONN, 1977)

Reactive capacity
15. Measurement by technical appliances
    – speed of response
    – accuracy of response

Tab. 10.3: Neuropsychological test procedures with respective test target priorities (and average duration of test)

3.1 Psychometric test procedures

Obviously, the EEG examinations and psychological tests outlined above are not suitable for use at the doctor's surgery or in clinical routine as a screening programme for the presence of SHE. Although they meet the required quality criteria, they are time-consuming and cost-intensive, and thus unacceptable. • In the past thirty years, some 50 simple *psychometric screening tests* have been developed and reports made on their application (in a variety of combinations). (4, 6, 8–10, 14, 15, 19, 22, 23, 25, 30, 31, 34, 38, 40, 41, 43, 45) (s. tab. 10.4) • The *multiple-choice determination device* is another test which has proved its worth.

1. Alphabetic deletion test
2. Archimedes spiral test
3. Block design test
4. Circle-dotting test
5. Colour word test
6. Digit-span test
7. Dot test
8. Handwriting-specimen test
9. Line-labyrinth test
10. Line-tracing test
11. Logical inductive test
12. Memory for design test
13. Number and symbol test
14. Perceptual maze test
15. Raven's matrices test
16. Serial-subtraction test
17. Star-construction test
18. Story-retelling test
19. Tracing of geometric figures
20. Visual motor design test
21. Visual retention test
22. Word-pair retention test

Tab. 10.4: Selection of psychometric screening tests (in alphabetical order)

3.1.1 SIP

Use of a questionnaire comprising 136 questions relating to the "sickness impact profile" (SIP) indicated a marked decrease in patients' capacity to perform routine daily activities and a diminished quality of life in 27% of cases of latent HE. (9)

3.1.2 Mechanical testing procedures

With appliance-based tests, it is possible to measure both reaction time and accuracy of response.

Multiple choice determination device: Five electronically controlled coloured light pulses (yellow, red, green, blue, white) are activated in alternating sequences. Pressing a button with the same colour indicates that the test person has recognized and registered the colour both instantly and correctly. This device has proved to be a useful instrument in clinical testing environments. (14)

Posner test: This mechanical testing procedure is designed for measuring spatial-visual attention and orientation (M.I. POSNER et al., 1988). The test persons are required to sit in front of a computer monitor using a cross in the middle of the screen as a fixation point. A square is visible on either side of the cross. In the neutral position, a question mark is displayed as a cue 200 milliseconds before the stimulus (= asterisk) appears in one of the squares. In the valid position, the cue is an arrow directed towards the square where the stimulus will appear. In the invalid position, it is directed towards the opposite square. When the stimulus appears, the test person pushes a button as quickly as possible. The Posner test reveals the varying delay in reaction time in patients with cirrhosis; it does not appear to have a higher sensitivity than the number-connection test. (1)

Critical flicker frequency: The principle of flicker-fusion frequency analysis was first introduced by E. SCHAFHÄUTL in 1855 and later developed for clinical use by L. GOLDBERG in 1943. This method has since been widely used in differential diagnosis of organic brain syndromes. • It was first established in patients with latent HE in 2002. (13) The patient observes what appears to be a constant red light shining on the screen, but which is in fact flickering at a high frequency. This flickering is normally detected by the test persons above 42 light pulses/sec with individual variations. However, in patients with latent HE, this occurred below 39 pulses/sec (cutoff value), in HE stage I below 36 pulses/sec, and in stage II below 32 pulses/sec. The results are independent of the patient's education level; there is no learning effect when the test is repeated. (39)

These simple psychometric screening tests do, however, have certain **disadvantages**, which have to be considered when results are being assessed. (s. tab. 10.5)

1. Several complementary screening tests are required for the identification of SHE
2. It has not been adequately defined which functional brain areas are covered by the tests
3. Standardized test evaluation is often not possible
4. There is still no adequate basis for comparison with scientifically established test procedures in neuropsychology

Tab. 10.5: Disadvantages of psychometric testing

3.2 Psychometric test programmes

Based on the results in the literature (which also correspond to our own experience), psychometric test programmes have been developed for use in the hospital and the doctor's surgery.

1. Simple to carry out
2. Easy to assess
3. Low time factor
4. Minimal costs
5. Reproducibility
6. Semiquantitative evaluability
7. Allows examination of various functional areas or performance capacity of the brain (even if not specifically defined or differentiated)

Tab. 10.6: Requirements for psychometric test procedures relevant for application in the doctor's surgery

Such test programmes make it possible to objectify neuropsychic disturbances and hence yield semiquantitative identification of the subclinical (latent) stage (0, 0−I) as well as manifestation stage I (or I−II) of HE. These programmes can be considered relatively reliable owing to the standardized instructions for their implementation and adequate objectivity in the evaluation process. A psychometric test programme suitable for use in the doctor's surgery and at the hospital should meet the **requirements** given above. (s. tab. 10.6)

1. **PSE syndrome test** (W. HAMSTER, M. KLUCK, H. SCHOMERUS): The **short form of the test** is comprised of (*1.*) number-connection test (part A) and (*2.*) line-tracing test. The test results are converted into standard values according to age. • The **long form of the test** is made up of (*1.*) number-symbol test, (*2.*) number-connection test (part A), (*3.*) circle-dotting test, (*4.*) target-fixing test, and (*5.*) line-tracing test.

2. **Psychometric test set** (E. KUNTZ, H.-D. KUNTZ): This test set facilitates psychodiagnostic monitoring of potential liver-diseased patients, identification of SHE and control of therapeutic measures. The *four basic tests* can be evaluated in their overall assessment with even greater reliability using *supplementary tests*, which are likewise easy to implement. (19) (s. tab. 10.7)

Basic tests
1. Handwriting-specimen test
2. Number-connection test (part A)
3. Line-tracing test
4. Star-construction test

Supplementary tests
1. Serial-subtraction test
2. Story-retelling test
3. Mechanical testing procedures

Tab. 10.7: Psychometric test programme for identification and monitoring of SHE (E. KUNTZ, H.-D. KUNTZ, 1991) (19)

3.2.1 Handwriting-specimen test

The handwriting-specimen test (I. SZAM, 1977) is a simple procedure providing insight into fine motor control. Subtle changes in the handwriting are thought to be a sign of constructive apraxia, i.e. there are disturbances in carrying out learned expedient movements, although the powers of perception and mobility are still intact. The possibilities of using *medical graphology* in hepatology have been presented in detail in the literature. (24) • **Regular handwriting tests are quite correctly known as the "poor man's EEG".**

▶ In line with neurophysiological findings, the patient should write his first and last name and *not* texts, placenames or dates! *The signature constitutes a swift, habitual sequence; as a reflex action which does not involve the application of willpower,* it is considered to be a person's **graphological identity**. In the early stages of HE, fine, swift and controlled movements of the hand are impaired. The handwriting-specimen test correlates well with the number-connection test and the subtraction test. • *Impaired handwriting* is reflected in small jagged peaks, hooks, interruptions in the flow, subtle irregularities, fluctuations in pen pressure, size of the lettering, etc. The assessment is based on the subjective criteria of the physician, which is, however, perfectly adequate for hospital or surgery purposes. (s. figs. 10.1; 15.3) • In addition, the results can be graded according to the physician's personal scoring system. (s. tab. 10.8)

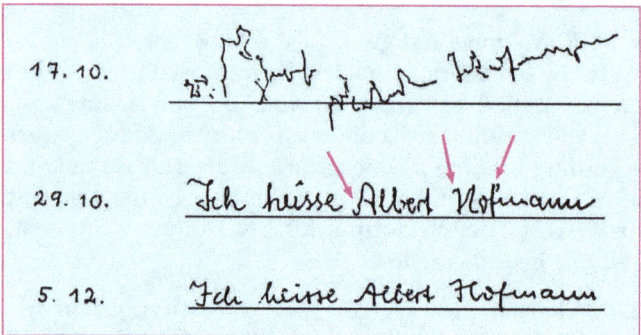

Fig. 10.1: Specimens of a patient's handwriting (first name and surname) in stage II (17 Oct.), in the SHE stage (29 Oct.) and in a normal state (5 Dec.) (s. fig. 15.2)

Changes	Score (points)	Stage of HE
not detectable	0	no HE, stage 0
very minimal or minimal	1	SHE, 0 – I
moderate	2	I, I – II
clearly evident	3	II
pronounced	4	II – III

Tab. 10.8: Assessment criteria for the handwriting-specimen test

3.2.2 Number-connection test

The **trail-making test** (R. M. REITAN, 1955) originated from the "army individual test" (1945) and the test results of S. G. ARMITAG (1946). It comprises two parts: the *number-connection test (NCT)* with numbers from 1–25 (part A) and the *number and letter combination test (NLCT)* with numbers from 1–13 and the letters A–L (part B). (32, 33) (s. fig. 10.2)

The *NCT* presented by H. O. CONN in 1977 (3) corresponds to part A of the *number-connection test* as described above; however, four different test sheets are used, each with a different arrangement of figures. In this way, a possible learning effect from sheet to sheet is ruled out. The four different test sheets are of equal difficulty and generally require the same period of time to complete. • With NCT and NLCT (parts A and B), logical thinking, powers of concentration and perception, together with the capacity to handle three-dimensional numbers and letters are assessed. Swift cognitive speed in thought processing is called for as well as the capacity to adapt. (19, 38, 46, 49)

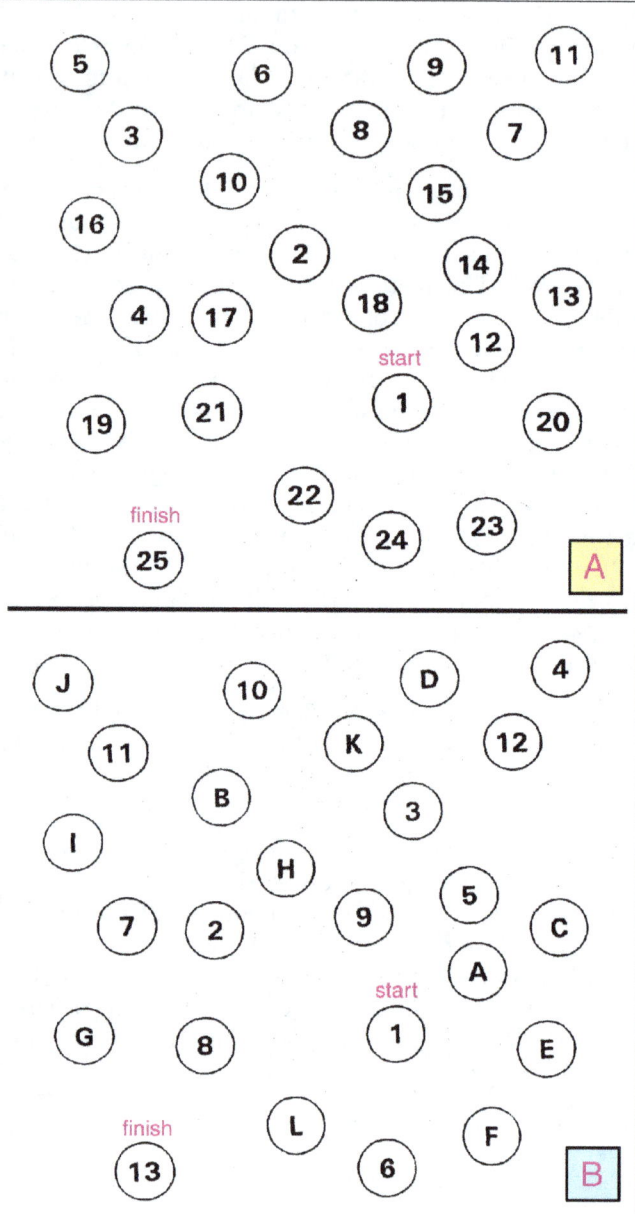

Fig. 10.2: Number-connection test (NCT; part A) and number-letter-connection test (NLCT; part B) (R. M. REITAN, 1955; H. O. CONN, 1977)

Time in seconds	Score (points)	Stage of HE
< 40	0	no HE, stage 0
41–60	1	SHE, 0 – I
61–90	2	I, I – II
91–120	3	II
> 121	4	II – III

Tab. 10.9: Assessment criteria for the number-connection test (NCT; part A)

▶ In order to complete the test, either the 25 figures in part A or the numbers 1–13 in consecutive alternation with the letters A–L in part B have to be correctly linked up by lines as quickly as possible, whereby any corrections are included in the time allotted.

If the patient is unable to complete the test within 150 seconds, it is broken off. The last correctly linked number and the respective time are noted (e.g. 17/150). The time required by the patients for part A of the number-connection test, as used by us in the psychometric examination set, allows a relatively reliable clinical interpretation to be made. In the number-connection test (part A), the **normal value** should be set at no more than 40 seconds. • The relevant score can be noted as an assessment criterion. (s. tab. 10.9)

3.2.3 Line-tracing test

The line-tracing test (LTT) is used to determine the accuracy of a person's fine motor control. A test sheet (s. fig. 10.3) shows a relatively complex "road map", 5 mm in width (corresponding to a 2.5 m wide lane). The patient is asked to trace this not-so-easy path with a pencil from start to finish, as quickly as possible, without going over the edges. The number of errors provides a semiquantitative assessment. • In addition, the respective number of points can be recorded on the score sheet. (s. tab. 10.10)

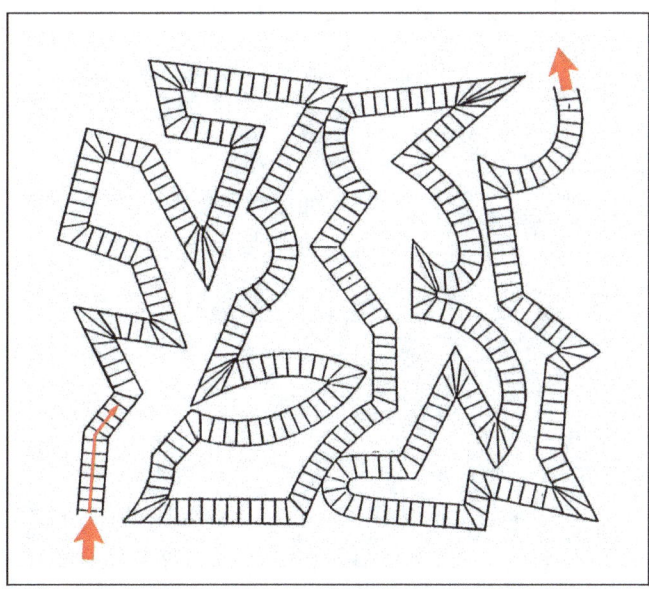

Fig. 10.3: Line-tracing test (LTT) using a difficult path, 5 mm in width (corresponding to a 2.5 m wide lane on a normal road)

3.2.4 Star-construction test

The star-construction test examines the patient's psychomotor function, recognition of shapes, and short-term memory. A test sheet (s. fig. 10.4) is presented to the patient, who is requested to look at the five-pointed star drawn on it for about ten seconds (E. A. DAVIDSON et al., 1956). (4) The test sheet is then covered or turned over. The patient is now asked to copy the star using 10 matchsticks, whereby the tips of the matches should form the pointed tips of the star. A lack of precision or errors in arranging the matchsticks and/or any confusion which arises during the test are rated as mistakes. • In addition, the respective number of points can be recorded on the score sheet. (s. tab 10.10)

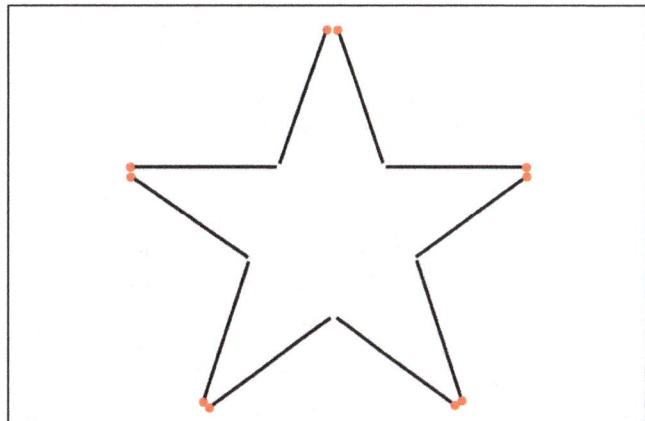

Fig. 10.4: Star-construction test (E. A. DAVIDSON et al., 1956) (4)

Number of errors	Score (points)	Stage of HE
no error	0	no HE, stage 0
0–2	1	SHE, 0 – I
3–5	2	I, I – II
6–9	3	II
> 9	4	II – III

Tab. 10.10: Assessment criteria for the line-tracing test and star-construction test

▶ The results of these four tests can be summarized by means of their score to give a **total number of points**, thereby simplifying the clinical interpretation in the individual case. (19)

The **time needed** for each test procedure (explanation, implementation and evaluation) is three to four minutes, provided the necessary test materials are already at hand (test sheets, stop-watch, pencil, matchsticks, etc.). • It is possible to have the tests carried out by trained personnel.

These simple test procedures can be executed in any surgery. A code number could be assigned as the *cost-calculation item* for health-insurance purposes. • It is neither organizationally possible, nor medically justifiable, let alone financially viable to make the implementation and assessment of these tests dependent on a specific professional qualification, such as is acquired in further education programmes. • *Every doctor is capable of carrying them out!*

If it is impossible to assess the presence of SHE with these tests, some additional, basic **supplementary tests** can be applied at the surgery. They require no test materials. The time needed for each test is three or four minutes.

3.2.5 Serial-subtraction test

With the help of the serial-subtraction test, the patients' powers of attention and concentration can be easily tested as well as their short-term memory and mental arithmetic capabilities.

From a specific initial figure selected at random (such as 100 or 110 or 130), the patient is asked to deduct another number, likewise selected at random (= subtrahend), continuing the subtraction procedure through a number of steps by "mental arithmetic" (e.g. $100-7 = ?, -7 = ?, -7 = ?$). After the third or fourth arithmetical step, a patient with SHE and a disturbed short-term memory usually no longer knows which number he/she has to deduct from which previous result. This simple test can likewise be adequately quantified for practical purposes. • *If the test is repeated, the same numbers can be taken for the same patient and the results compared. There is virtually no learning effect involved.*

3.2.6 Story-retelling test

Another psychometric supplementary test that can be used is the retelling of a story. Here the patient's short-term memory, perceptive faculties and logical thinking are tested.

The physician tells the patient the following story (lasting about one minute), which then has to be retold by the patient (also in about one minute): *"A bee flies to the brook to take a bath and falls into the water. A dove sees the bee and saves it from drowning. The dove lays the bee on a leaf to dry off. The next day, a hunter comes into the wood and takes aim to shoot at the dove. The bee flies at him and stings the hunter's hand so that his shot misfires."* It is important to note any **incorrect renderings of the plot** which are typical of SHE — e.g. the hunter or the dove drown, the dove stings the bee, the hunter shoots the bee, the dove stings the hunter, etc.

4 Synopsis

▶ Such a test programme makes screening for SHE very simple; it is reliable for both surgery and hospital purposes. The test sheets and test results should be documented and filed for an appropriate period of time. • Patients who display cerebral dysfunction during these simple tests generally show more pronounced impairment of cerebral functions when complex and specific test procedures are applied. • *Psychometric tests are highly sensitive as regards disturbances in cerebral performance, yet they have no specificity regarding underlying causes or the disease itself — for this reason they are not "specific to the liver" either.*

▶ In suspected subclinical hepatic encephalopathy, psychometric tests are extremely important for the diagnosis and cannot be substituted by other examination procedures (e.g. anamnesis, inspection, laboratory analysis, imaging techniques).

▶ The transition from the latent stage (SHE) to stage I of clinically manifest HE can be gradual, as demonstrated by the results of the psychometric tests. In this *transitional zone (SHE I)*, there may occasionally be minor neurological findings, such as hyperreflexia, fine tremor or asterixis. (s. p. 272) (s. tab. 15.5)

References:

1. **Amodio, P., Marchetti, P., Del Piccolo, F., Campo, G., Rizzo, C., Iemmolo, R.M., Gerunda, G., Caregaro, L., Merkel, C., Gatta, A.:** Visual attention in cirrhotic patients: a study on covert visual attention orienting. Hepatology 1998; 27: 1517–1523
2. **Bombardieri, G., Gigli, G.L., Bernardi, L., Ferri, R., Grassi, C., Milani, A.:** Visual evoked potential recordings in hepatic encephalopathy and their variations during branched chain amino-acid treatment. Hepato-Gastroenterol. 1985; 32: 3–7
3. **Conn, H.O.:** Trailmaking and number-connection tests in the assessment of mental state in portal systemic encephalopathy. Dig. Dis. 1977; 22: 541–550
4. **Davidson, E.A., Summerskill, W.H.J.:** Psychiatric aspects of liver disease. Postgrad. Med. J. 1956; 32: 487–494
5. **Davies, M.G., Rowan, M.J., MacMathuna, P., Keeling, P.W.N., Weir, D.G., Feely, J.:** The auditory P 300 event-related potential: an objective marker of the encephalopathy of chronic liver disease. Hepatology 1990; 12: 688–694
6. **Elsass, P., Lund, Y., Ranek, L.:** Encephalopathy in patients with cirrhosis of the liver. A neuropsychological study. Scand. J. Gastroenterol. 1978; 13: 241–247
7. **Foley, J.M., Watson, C.W., Adams, R.D.:** Significance of electroencephalographic changes in hepatic coma. Trans. Amer. Neurol. Ass. 1950; 75: 165–171
8. **Gilberstadt, S.J., Gilberstadt, H., Zieve, L., Buegel, B., Collier, R.O., McClain, C.J.:** Psychomotor performance defects in cirrhotic patients without overt encephalopathy. Arch. Intern. Med. 1980; 140: 519–521
9. **Groeneweg, M., Moerland, W., Quero, J.C., Hop, W.C.J., Krabbe, P.F., Schalm, S.W.:** Screening of subclinical hepatic encephalopathy. J. Hepatol. 2000; 32: 748–753
10. **Guedon, C., Ducrotte, P., Weber, J., Hannequin, D., Colin, R., Denis, P., Lerebours, E.:** Detection of subclinical hepatic encephalopathy with pattern reversal evoked potentials and reaction time to light: can malnutrition alter the results? Eur. J. Gastroenterol. Hepatol. 1993; 5: 549–554
11. **Hollerbach, S., Kullmann, F., Fründ, R., Lock, G., Geissler, A., Schölmerich, J., Holstege, A.:** Auditory event-related cerebral potentials (P 300) in hepatic encephalopathy. Topographic distribution and correlation with clinical and psychometric assessment. Hepato-Gastroenterol. 1997; 44: 1002–1012
12. **Johansson, U., Andersson, Th., Persson, A., Eriksson, L.S.:** Visual evoked potential – a tool in the diagnosis of hepatic encephalopathy. J. Hepatol. 1989; 9: 227–233
13. **Kircheis, G., Wettstein, M., Timmermann, L., Schnitzler, A., Häussinger, D.:** Critical flicker frequency for quantification of low-grade hepatic encephalopathy. Hepatology 2002; 35: 357–366
14. **Koch, H., Schauder, P., Schäfer, G., Dahme, B., Ebel, W., Vahldiek, B., König, F., Henning, H.:** Untersuchungen zur Diagnose und Prävalenz der latenten hepatischen Enzephalopathie. Z. Gastroenterol. 1990; 28: 610–615
15. **Korman, M., Blumberg, St.:** Comparative efficiency of some tests of cerebral damage. J. Consult. Psychol. 1963; 27: 303–309
16. **Kügler, Ch. F.A., Lotterer, E., Petter, J., Wensing, G., Ahmad Taghary, Hahn, E.G., Fleig, W.E.:** Visual event-related P 300 potentials in early portosystemic encephalopathy. Gastroenterology 1992; 103: 302–310
17. **Kuhlbusch, R., Enck, P., Häussinger, D.:** Hepatic encephalopathy: neuropsychological and neurophysiological assessment. Z. Gastroenterol. 1998; 36: 1075–1083
18. **Kullmann, F., Hollerbach, S., Lock, G., Holstege, A., Dierks, T., Schölmerich, J.:** Brain electrical activity mapping of EEG for the diagnosis of (sub)clinical hepatic encephalopathy in chronic liver disease. Eur. J. Gastroenterol. Hepatol. 2001; 13: 513–522
19. **Kuntz, E.:** Hepatische Enzephalopathie. Psychometrische Tests zur Diagnose, Bewertung und Therapiekontrolle in der Praxis. Münch. Med. Wschr. 1992; 134: 76–80
20. **Laidlaw, J., Read, A.E.:** The EEG in hepatic encephalopathy. Clin. Sci. 1963; 24: 109–120
21. **Levy, L.J., Bolton, R.P., Losowsky, M.S.:** The visual evoked potential in clinical hepatic encephalopathy in acute and chronic liver disease. Hepato-Gastroenterol. 1990 (Suppl. II); 37: 66–73
22. **Loguercio, C., Del Vecchio-Blanco, C., Coltorti, M.:** Psychometric tests and "latent" portal-systemic encephalopathy. Brit. J. Clin. Pract. 1984; 38: 407–411
23. **Loiselle, R.H., Young, K.M., McDonald, M.M.:** Four common tests of brain damage compared. Psychiatr. Commun. 1968; 10: 41–44
24. **Ludewig, R., Dettweiler, Ch., Stein Lewinson, T.:** Möglichkeiten und Grenzen der medizinischen Graphologie. Inn. Med. 1992; 47: 549–557; 1993; 48: 5–12; 1993; 48: 52–59
25. **Manganaro, M., Zardi, E.M., Ceccanti, M., Spada, S., Attilia, M.L., Pancheri, P., Biondi, M., Paga, G.:** Correlation between a psychometric

test and biochemical indices of hepatic encephalopathy in alcoholics. Hepato-Gastroenterology 2000; 47: 455–460
26. **Mehndiratta, M.M., Sood, G.K., Sarin, S.K., Gupta, M.:** Comparative evaluation of visual, somatosensory, and auditory evoked potentials in the detection of subclinical hepatic encephalopathy in patients with nonalcoholic cirrhosis. Amer. J. Gastroenterol. 1990; 85: 799–803
27. **Myslobodsky, M.S., Sharon, D., Novis, B.H.:** Pattern-reversal visual evoked potentials in hepatic cirrhosis. Hepato-Gastroenterol. 1986; 33: 145–147
28. **Nora, D.B., Amaral, O.B., Busnello, J.V., Quevedo, J., Vieira, S., da Silveira, T.R., Kapczinski, F.:** Evoked potentials for the evaluation of latent hepatic encephalopathy in pediatric liver transplant candidates. J. Pediatr. Gastroenterol. Nutr. 2000; 31: 371–376
29. **Parsons-Smith, B.G., Summerskill, W.H.J., Dawson, A.M., Sherlock, S.:** The electroencephalograph in liver disease. Lancet 1957/II: 867–871
30. **Pérez-Cuadrado Martínez, E., Silva González, C., Robles Reyes, A.:** Variabilidad y alargamiento del tiempo de reaccion en el diagnostico precoz de la encefalopatia hepatica subclinica. Rev. Esp. Enferm. Dig. 1990; 77: 29–32
31. **Rehnström, S., Simert, G., Hansson, J.A., Johnson, G., Vang, J.:** Chronic hepatic encephalopathy. A psychometrical study. Scand. J. Gastroenterol. 1977; 12: 305–311
32. **Reitan, R.M.:** The relation of the trail making test to organic brain damage. J. Consult. Psychol. 1955; 19: 393–394
33. **Reitan, R.M.:** Validity of the trail making test as an indicator of organic brain damage. Percept. Motor. Skills 1958; 8: 271–276
34. **Rikkers, L., Jenko, P., Rudman, D., Freides, D.:** Subclinical hepatic encephalopathy: detection, prevalence and relationship to nitrogen metabolism. Gastroenterology 1978; 75: 462–469
35. **Ross, B.D., Danielsen, E.R., Bluml, S.:** Proton magnetic resonance spectroscopy: the new gold standard for diagnosis of clinical and subclinical hepatic encephalopathy. Dig. Dis. 1996; 14: 30–39
36. **Sandford, N.L., Saul, R.E.:** Assessment of hepatic encephalopathy with visual evoked potentials compared with conventional methods. Hepatology 1988; 8: 1094–1098
37. **Saxena, N., Bhatia, M., Joshi, Y.K., Garg, P.K., Tandon, R.K.:** Auditory P 300 event-related potentials and number connection test for subclinical hepatic encephalopathy in patients with cirrhosis of the liver: a follow-up study. J. Gastroenterol. Hepatol. 2001; 16: 322–327
38. **Schomerus, H., Hamster, W., Blunck, H., Reinhard, U., Mayer, K., Dölle, W.:** Latent portalsystemic encephalopathy. I. Nature of cerebral functional defects and their effect on fitness to drive. Dig. Dis. Sci. 1981; 26: 622–630
39. **Sharma, P., Sharma, B.C., Puri, V., Sarin, S.K.:** Critical flicker frequency: Diagnostic tool for minimal hepatic encephalopathy. J. Hepatol 2007; 47: 63–73
40. **Shiota, T.:** Quantitative psychometric testing and subclinical hepatic encephalopathy-comparative study between encephalopathic and non-encephalopathic patients with liver cirrhosis. Acta Med. Okayama 1984; 38: 193–205
41. **Sood, G.K., Sarin, S.K., Mahaptra, J., Broor, S.L.:** Comparative efficacy of psychometric tests in detection of subclinical hepatic encephalopathy in nonalcoholic cirrhotics: search for a rational approach. Amer. J. Gastroenterol. 1989; 84: 156–159
42. **Taghavy, A., Kügler, Ch.F.A.:** The pattern flash elicited P 300-complex (PF- P 300): A new method for studying cognitive processes of the brain. Intern. J. Neuroscience 1988; 38: 179–188
43. **Tarter, R.E., Scalabassi, R., Sandford, S.L., Hoys, A.L., Carra, J.P., Thiel, van, D.H.:** Relationship between hepatic injury status and event-related potentials. Clin. Electroenceph. 1987; 18: 15–19
44. **Van der Rijt, C.C.D., Schalm, S.W.:** Quantitative EEG analysis and evoked potentials to measure (latent) hepatic encephalopathy. J. Hepatol. 1992; 14: 141–142
45. **Watanabe, A., Tuchida, T., Yata, Y., Kuwabara, J.:** Evaluation of neuropsychological function in patients with liver cirrhosis with special reference to their driving ability. Metab. Brain Dis. 1995; 10: 239–248
46. **Weissenborn, K., Rückert, N., Hecker, H., Manns, M.P.:** The number connection tests A and B: Interindividual variability and use for the assessment of early hepatic encephalopathy. J. Hepatol. 1998; 28: 646–653
47. **Weissenborn, K., Ennen, J.C., Schomerus, H., Rückert, N., Hecker, H.:** Neuropsychological characterization of hepatic encephalopathy. J. Hepatol. 2001; 34: 768–773
48. **Yang, S.-S., Chu, N.-S., Liaw, Y.-F.:** Brainstem auditory evoked potentials in hepatic encephalopathy. Hepatology 1986; 6: 1352–1355
49. **Yen, C.-L., Liaw, Y.-F.:** Somatosensory evoked potentials and number connection test in the detection of subclinical hepatic encephalopathy. Hepato-Gastroenterol. 1990; 37: 332–334
50. **Zeegen, R., Drinkwater, J.E., Dawson, A.M.:** Method for measuring cerebral dysfunction in patients with liver disease. Brit. Med. J. 1970; 2: 633–636
51. **Zeneroli, M.L., Pinelli, G., Gollini, G., Penne, A., Messori, E., Zani, G., Ventura, E.:** Visual evoked potential: a diagnostic tool for the assessment of hepatic encephalopathy. Gut 1984; 25: 291–299

Symptoms and Syndromes
11 Hepatomegaly and splenomegaly

		Page:
1	***Hepatomegaly***	218
1.1	Definition	218
1.2	Pathogenesis	218
1.2.1	Replication of cells	218
1.2.2	Enlargement of cellular structures	218
1.2.3	Augmentation of the extracellular space	218
1.2.4	Local processes	219
1.3	Causes	219
1.4	Diagnosis	219
1.4.1	Subjective symptoms	219
1.4.2	Clinical findings	219
1.4.3	Methods of examination	219
2	***Splenomegaly***	220
2.1	Normal values of the spleen	220
2.2	Definition	220
2.3	Pathogenesis and causes	221
2.4	Functional sequelae	221
2.5	Therapy	221
	• References (1–40)	221
	(Figures 11.1–11.2; tables 11.1–11.2)	

11 Hepatomegaly and splenomegaly

1 Hepatomegaly

1.1 Definition

Hepatomegaly is present if (*1.*) *palpation* locates the lower border of the right lobe of liver to be more than 2 cm (one to two finger breadths) below the left costal arch (MCL lateral to rectus abdominis) (caution: phrenoptosis), (*2.*) the absolute liver dullness on *percussion* is more than 14 cm, or (*3.*) the longitudinal diameter of the liver in the MCL is greater than approximately 15 cm in the *sonogram*.

Hepatomegaly is a cardinal symptom in a number of liver diseases or a concomitant reaction of the liver in various extrahepatic or systemic diseases. When detected, differential diagnostic clarification is always necessary.

Hepatomegaly can affect the entire liver as a *diffuse* enlargement or only a certain region of the liver as a *circumscribed* increase in volume. • Under clinical conditions, the **liver size** is ascertained by the combined application of *palpation* (to determine the inferior border of the liver) and *percussion* (to determine the border between the liver and lungs). (s. pp 81, 83) Determination of the liver size by *sonography* is considerably more precise. • It is also necessary to assess the **liver consistency** (soft, elastic, firm, compact, hard), the **liver surface** (smooth, protuberant), the **tenderness on pressure**, and the sonographically detectable **internal structure** (homogeneous, inhomogeneous, formation of foci, enlarged bile ducts or vessels). The **density** of the normal liver in the CT is 60 ± 6 HU. (s. p. 179)

1.2 Pathogenesis

1.2.1 Replication of cells

A diffuse enlargement of the liver can be caused by cell replication.

(*1.*) Replication of *hepatocytes* in the form of excessive hyperplasia can occur occasionally after extensive parenchymal necrosis or partial liver resection. However, this does not generally cause a clinically discernible form of hepatomegaly.

(*2.*) In systemic haematological diseases, the liver is usually involved in *extramedullary haematopoiesis*. This can result in hepatomegaly.

(*3.*) Diffuse enlargement of the liver can also be brought about by *lymphohistiocytic cell infiltrations*. This generally involves inflammatory reactions to viral or bacterial diseases.

(*4.*) Diffuse hepatomegaly is also expected to occur as a result of *malignant cell growth*.

1.2.2 Enlargement of cellular structures

An increase in the volume of sinusoidal cells and hepatocytes due to an enlargement of their cellular structures can be caused *actively* by proliferation or *passively* by storage processes.

(*1.*) *Endothelia* and *Kupffer cells* can be stimulated to considerable proliferation, so that in clinical terms hepatomegaly occasionally results.

(*2.*) Proliferation of the *smooth endoplasmic reticulum* due to the prolonged induction of the biotransformatory system localized at this site as a result of toxins, noxae or chemicals can bring about clinically and sonographically detectable hepatomegaly.

(*3.*) Hepatocellular *storage* of abnormal quantities of cholesterol, fat, glycogen, proteins, mucopolysaccharides, copper, iron, etc. occasionally leads to pronounced hepatomegaly. Hydropic swelling of the hepatocytes is also included in this category.

1.2.3 Augmentation of the extracellular space

Diffuse enlargement of the liver can also arise from augmentation of the extracellular space.

(*1.*) An increase in *blood* both in the sinusoids and in Disse's spaces culminates in hepatomegaly. This can be observed particularly in cases of right heart failure, constrictive pericarditis, veno-occlusive disease and the Budd-Chiari syndrome. Inflammation-related hyperaemia also occurs in acute viral hepatitis.

(*2.*) An enhanced formation of *lymph* or reduced lymph drainage can cause enlargement of the liver. Here fluid-filled *cysts* are also regarded as a possible cause of hepatomegaly.

(*3.*) A disorder of the *bile flow*, particularly in infants, leads to extensive hepatomegaly.

(*4.*) An increase in the extracellular *matrix* due to collagens, elastin, proteoglycans, glycoproteins, etc. also produces various degrees of hepatomegaly.

1.2.4 Local processes

Circumscribed enlargement of the liver is precipitated by local lesions such as cysts, abscesses, parasites (e. g. echinococcus) and benign or malignant tumours; this also results in *diffuse enlargement* of the liver in some cases.

1.3 Causes

A number of liver diseases are accompanied by an enlargement of the liver. The liver can also be involved in extrahepatic or systemic pathological diseases, possibly with the simultaneous development of hepatomegaly. Differential diagnosis is extremely varied, necessitating a broad spectrum of investigations in individual cases. (1–3, 6–8, 10, 11) (s. tab. 11.1)

---

1. **Inflammatory liver diseases**
   - acute viral hepatitis
   - acute autoimmune hepatitis
   - alcoholic hepatitis
   - concomitant hepatitis with infections
   - bacterial sepsis
   - miliary tuberculosis
   - parasitoses (e. g. echinococcus, toxocariasis)
   - HIV infection
   - liver abscess
   - bacterial cholangitis, *etc.*
2. **Chronic liver diseases**
   - chronic hepatitis
   - liver cirrhosis
   - hepatic granulomatosis, *etc.*
3. **Metabolic / toxic diseases**
   - fatty liver disease
   - hepatic porphyrias
   - amyloidosis of the liver, *etc.*
4. **Biliary diseases**
   - biliary obstruction
   - primary biliary cholangitis
   - cholestasis
   - Byler's syndrome, *etc.*
5. **Vascular liver diseases**
   - congestive liver,
   - peliosis hepatis
   - constrictive pericarditis
   - Budd-Chiari syndrome
   - veno-occlusive disease
   - arterial diseases, *etc.*
6. **Tumours**
   - benign liver tumours
   - malignant liver tumours
   - liver metastases
   - regenerative nodules
7. **Cystic liver**
8. **Congenital diseases**
   - hereditary liver storage diseases (haemochromatosis, Wilson's disease, amyloidosis, glycogenoses, lipopathies, tyrosinaemia, Zellweger's cerebrohepatorenal syndrome, fructose intolerance, α_1-antitrypsin deficiency, Burka's syndrome, galactosaemia, Mauriac syndrome, *etc.*)
   - malformations of the liver or the bile ducts
9. **Systemic haematological diseases**
10. **Systemic immunological diseases**

Tab. 11.1: Causes of hepatomegaly

1.4 Diagnosis

1.4.1 Subjective symptoms

Hepatomegaly is occasionally accompanied by a feeling of pressure or even *tenderness* in the right epigastrium. (5) This tension pain of Glisson's capsule mainly occurs with a rapid increase in the liver volume (acute viral hepatitis, acute congestive liver, etc.), whereas gradually developing hepatomegaly may be without pain. • The liver parenchyma itself is insensitive to pain. (s. pp 26, 82) Not to be associated with this is pain arising from a specific underlying disease in the liver region, which generally has no direct effect on liver enlargement, e. g. malignant tumours, cholangitis, perihepatitis.

1.4.2 Clinical findings

Hepatomegaly is easily ascertained by *palpation* and *percussion*; its size can also be well assessed. Asthenic patients may display simulated liver enlargement. (s. pp 81, 83) • In addition to the typical dextral *elevation of the diaphragm* in hepatomegaly, there is often a downward *displacement of intestinal loops* as well.

▶ *Sonography* is an indispensable investigative method for clarifying the following issues: (*1.*) differentiation between diffuse and circumscribed hepatomegaly, (*2.*) assessment of the internal structure (homogeneous or inhomogeneous), (*3.*) determination of foci, cysts, nodes, etc., and (*4.*) confirmation of hepatomegaly or detection of a simulated enlargement of the liver due to extrahepatic pathological diseases. (4, 9)

1.4.3 Methods of examination

In the majority of cases, the causality can be established on the basis of the hepatological findings or the prevailing disease. Often, however, definite clarification is only achieved by further investigative methods. • The indication for *computer tomography* (9), and perhaps also *angio-CT*, should be checked first. As non-invasive procedures, these should be given priority over bioptic methods. (s. tab. 8.2) • *Angiography* is indicated in cases where enhanced vascularity is suspected. (s. tab. 8.3)

If *biopsy* proves necessary, thought must be given to whether a fine-needle biopsy or a liver biopsy is appropriate. (s. tab. 7.3)

It should not be overlooked, however, that some indistinct liver findings can be diagnosed reliably and at little risk by *laparoscopy*, with or without biopsy. (s. tab. 7.11)

2 Splenomegaly

2.1 Normal values of the spleen

A *normal spleen* is 11 (10−14) cm in length, 7 (6−8) cm in width and 4 (3−4) cm in depth. The weight of the spleen varies greatly (< 100 g to > 250 g); a mean value of 150−170 (−180) g can be taken. • The normal diameter of the *splenic artery* is 4−5 mm, while that of the *splenic vein* is 8−14 mm with a normal mean value of about 10 mm. With a *flow rate* of 500−700 ml per minute, the blood flow through the spleen exceeds the arterial blood supply of the liver by a factor of almost 3. • The *longitudinal axis* of the spleen runs parallel to ribs 9−11 from the upper dorsal to the lower ventral.

The size and volume of the spleen are determined quite reliably by present-day methods of investigation, so that even slight increases in the size of the organ can be detected. However, in view of the wide spectrum of variation in the size of the "normal" spleen, thought must be given to the following questions: (*1.*) at what point should "splenomegaly" be diagnosed, and (*2.*) once a spleen has been classed as enlarged, should it be regarded as pathological.

Determination of the size of the spleen by *palpation* and *percussion* is most unreliable. (19) (s. p. 83) • *X-ray examination* only permits determination of the longitudinal axis in 50−90% of cases, whereas measurement of the thickness is totally inadequate, and measurement of the width is not even possible.

The values of a normal or enlarged spleen can be recorded quite reliably in a *sonogram*. (16, 18, 23, 26) Assessment is sometimes made more difficult by overlying ribs or as a result of air in the stomach or intestines. Due to the uncertain sonographic identification of the upper pole of the spleen, it seems adequate to determine the maximum width and thickness in the transverse section. *Normal values* are 4 × 7 × 11 cm (whereby the transverse diameter is 4−5 cm and the longitudinal diameter is < 11 cm). (s. p. 145)

The size of the spleen can be determined with an accuracy of ± 5% by *computer tomography*. The maximum width and thickness can be measured directly from the transverse section. The length is calculated from the difference between the upper and lower splenic poles.

Normal values are as follows: longitudinal extension 11−15 cm, longitudinal axis of the ellipsoid cross-section 7−10 cm, transverse axis 4−5 cm. The product of the normal mean values gives the *CT spleen index*, which correlates quite well with anatomical reality: 11 × 7 × 4 cm = 308 (160−440). In computer tomography, the normal density of the spleen is 46 ± 12 HU or 50 ± 8 HU.

▶ Selective *spleen scintigraphy* by chemically or heat-denatured erythrocytes and ^{197}Hg-BMHP-, ^{51}Cr- or ^{99m}Tc-labelling provides very reliable measurements.

2.2 Definition

The symptom of **splenomegaly** is defined as an enlargement of the spleen in which the normal values (4 × 7 × 11 cm) are clearly exceeded by > 2−3 cm in at least two dimensions − with a corresponding rise in the normal CT index (160−440). Sonographic reliability depends largely on spleen thickness: > 5 cm = 67%, > 6 cm = 85%, and > 7 cm = 100%. The thickness of the spleen is therefore regarded as the parameter which correlates best with clinical findings. An increase in the longitudinal diameter to well over 11 cm is also considered to be "splenomegaly". • A diameter of the splenic vein of > 10 mm is deemed pathological.

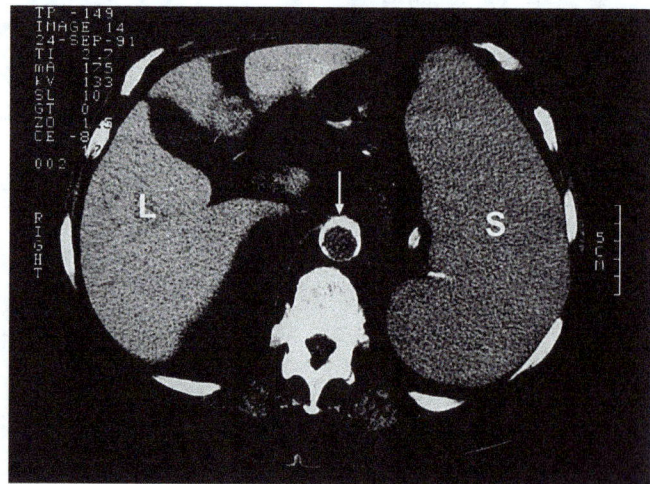

Fig. 11.1: CT (native) showing splenomegaly in non-Hodgkin lymphoma (L = liver, S = spleen, arrow = calcified aorta)

The large individual variations in the "normal" values as well as the differing results yielded by various methods of examination (palpation, sonography, CT and scintigraphy) call for greater precision in definition. Whenever the diagnosis "splenomegaly" is established, the method by which the diagnosis was obtained should be given. (s. fig. 11.1)

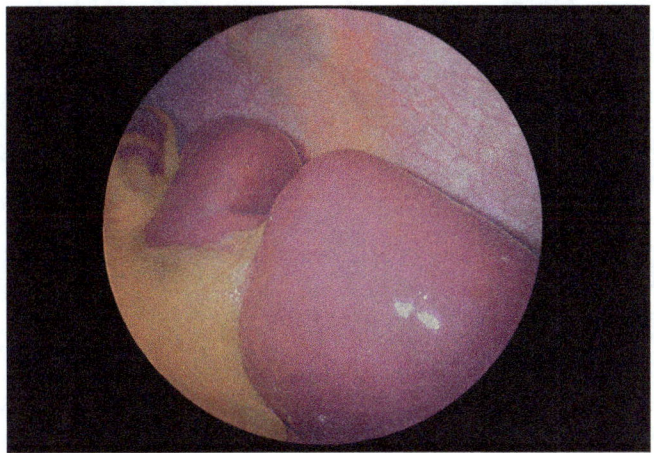

Fig. 11.2: Laparoscopy showing splenomegaly in portal hypertension due to liver cirrhosis

2.3 Pathogenesis and causes

Enlargement of the spleen can have numerous causes. It is important to rule out any possibility that the method of investigation itself could lead to splenomegaly being simulated, such as "upside-down" spleen, accessory spleen(s) or wandering spleen. The involvement of the spleen in disorders of the lymphatic and reticuloendothelial system as well as of the portal and systemic circulation explains why splenomegaly is frequently found in connection with widely differing diseases. (18, 20, 23, 34–38) (s. tab. 11.2)

Splenomegaly is very closely related to a number of liver diseases and, in particular, to the clinically recognizable involvement of the liver in a variety of pathological processes. Inclusion of the differential diagnosis of splenomegaly can, therefore, provide valuable information for the clarification of hepatological findings. (s. figs. 11.1; 11.2; 14.7; 35.10)

2.4 Functional sequelae

As a *mechanical component*, splenomegaly exerts pressure on neighbouring organs. • In addition, splenomegaly has mechanical and functional *sequelae* on the lienoportal vascular system. There is also a close relationship between splenomegaly and the quantitative or qualitative composition of the blood, which can ultimately develop into a splenogenic marrow maturation arrest. Consequently, a number of findings in liver diseases can be associated with splenomegaly or hypersplenism.

2.5 Therapy

Once the cause has been diagnosed differentially with great thoroughness, splenomegaly therapy is directed solely at the underlying disease — on the assumption that symptomatic and curative therapy options are available. (21)

Drainage disorders in the portal and systemic circulation
- Liver cirrhosis (37), liver tumours, liver echinococcosis, portal vein thrombosis, thrombosis of the splenic vein, right heart failure, Budd-Chiari syndrome, peliosis hepatis (39), *etc.*

Hepatolienal storage diseases
- Amyloidosis, fatty liver, glycogenoses, Wolman's syndrome, hyperchylomicronaemia, Wilson's disease, Zellweger's cerebrohepatorenal syndrome, Niemann-Pick disease, mucopolysaccharidoses, *etc.*

Infectious diseases
- Acute viral hepatitis, acute salmonellosis, measles, bacterial sepsis, histoplasmosis, leptospirosis, malaria, mononucleosis, Bang's disease, visceral leishmaniasis (22), rickettsioses, toxoplasmosis, tularaemia, schistosomiasis, *etc.*

Chronic infections
- Cholangitis, endocarditis lenta, malaria, eosinophilic granuloma, tuberculosis, chronic hepatitis (27), *etc.*

Collagenoses and rheumatic diseases
- Felty's syndrome, lupus erythematosus, Reiter's disease, Still's disease, Wegener's disease, histiocytosis, *etc.*

Diseases of the haematopoietic system
- Acute leucosis, chronic lymphadenosis, chronic myelosis, erythroblastosis, haemolytic anaemias, Werlhof's disease, osteomyelosclerosis, polycythaemia vera, thalassaemia, shunt hyperbilirubinaemia, *etc.*

Diseases of the lymphoreticulohistiocytic system
- Lipogranulomatosis, lymphosarcoma, Hodgkin's disease (36), Brill-Symmers disease, Waldenström's disease, *etc.*

Chronic exposure to arsenic (29, 31)

Isolated (primary) splenomegaly
- Echinococcus (13), splenic abscess (12), splenic tumours (30), splenic cysts (14, 15, 17, 24–26, 32, 33, 40), *etc.*

Non-tropical idiopathic splenomegaly
- Dacie's syndrome (J. Dacie, 1969) (28)

Tropical idiopathic splenomegaly syndrome

Tab. 11.2: Causes of splenomegaly (with some references)

References:

Hepatomegaly
1. Dockter, G., Sitzmann, F.C.: Hepatosplenomegalie im Kindesalter — vom Symptom zur Diagnose. Med. Welt 1988; 39: 1287–1292
2. Garcia Reinoso, C., Saez-Royuela, F., Gomez Rubio, M., Gomez Carrascal, C., Miranda Baiocchi, R., Hernandez Guio, C.: Formas de presentation y procedimientos diagnosticos del hemangioma hepatico gigante. Rev. Esp. Enf. Ap. Digest. 1989; 76: 617–621
3. Götz, G.F., Mathias, K., Dykgers, A.: Neuroblastom IV-S. Kasuistischer Beitrag zur Hepatomegalie. Fortschr. Röntgenstr. 1987; 147: 91–93

4. **Gosink, B., Leymaster, C.:** Ultrasonic determination of hepatomegaly. J. Clin. Ultrasound 1981; 9: 37–41
5. **Müllhaupt, B., Steuser, J., Vetter, W.:** Fettunverträglichkeit, Druck im rechten Oberbauch, Hepatomegalie. Schweiz. Rundsch. Med. (Praxis) 1990; 79: 639–642
6. **Ortega Calvo, M., Corchado Albalat, Y., Fuentes Verdera, M., Griera Borras, J.L., Martinez Manzanares, C.:** Aspectos clinicos de la hepatomegalia de estasis. Rev. Esp. Enf. Ap. Digest. 1989; 76: 612–616
7. **Schneider, J.G., Schaefer, S., Lettgen, B., Keiper, T., Nawroth, P.P., Dugl, K.A.:** Siblings with hepatosplenomegaly and lipoprotein lipase deficiency. Lancet 2002; 360: 1150.
8. **Serra, L., Poppi, M.C., Criscuolo, M., Zandomeneghi, R.:** Primary systemic amyloidosis with giant hepatomegaly and portal hypertension: a case report and a review of the literature. Ital. J. Gastroenterol. 1993; 25: 435–438
9. **Thiel, van, D.H., Hagler, N.G., Schade, R.R., Skolnick, M.L., Pollitt Heyl, A., Rosenblum, E., Gavaler, J.S., Penkrot, R.J.:** In vivo hepatic volume determination using sonography and computed tomography. Gastroenterology 1985; 88: 1812–1817
10. **Urganci, N., Arapoglu, M., Evrüke, M., Aydin, A.:** A rare cause of hepatomegaly: 3-hydroxy-3-methylglutaryl coenzyme-A lyase deficiency. J. Pediatr. Gastroenterol. Nutr. 2001; 33: 339–341
11. **Wolf, A., Lavine, J.:** Hepatomegaly in neonates and children. Pediatr. Rev. 2000; 21: 303–310

Splenomegaly
12. **Akoh, J.A., Auld, C.D.:** Splenic abscess: is conservation applicable? Brit. J. Clin. Pract. 1992; 46: 274–275
13. **Al Mohaya, S., Al-Awami, M., Vaidya, M.P., Knox-Macaulay, H.:** Hydatid cyst of the spleen. Amer. J. Trop. Med. Hyg. 1986; 35: 995–999
14. **Berquist, W.E., Diament, M., Fonkalsrud, E.W.:** Splenic cyst presenting as a gastric mass. J. Pediatr. Gastroenterol. Nutrit. 1984; 3: 805–807
15. **Burrig, K.F.:** Epithelial (true) splenic cysts. Pathogenesis of the mesothelial and so-called epidermoid cyst of the spleen. Amer. J. Surg. Pathol. 1988; 12: 275–281
16. **Caslowitz, P.L., Labs, J.D., Fishman, E.K., Siegelman, S.S.:** Nontraumatic focal lesions of the spleen: assessment of imaging and clinical evaluation. Comput. Med. Imaging Graph. 1990; 14: 133–141
17. **Dachman, A.H., Ros, P.R., Murari, P.J., Olmsted, W.W., Lichtenstein, J.F.:** Nonparasitic splenic cysts: a report of 52 cases with radiologic-pathologic correlation. Amer. J. Roentgenol. 1986; 147: 537–542
18. **Doll, M., Schölmerich, J., Spamer, C., Volk, B.A., Gerok, W.:** Klinische Bedeutung der sonographisch festgestellten Splenomegalie. Dtsch. Med. Wschr. 1986; 111: 887–891
19. **Ebaugh, F.G. jr., McIntyre, O.R.:** Palpable spleens: ten years follow-up. Ann. Intern. Med. 1979; 90: 130–131
20. **Gusberg, R.J., Peterec, S.M., Sumpio, B.E., Meier, G.H.:** Splenomegaly and variceal bleeding – hemodynamic basis and treatment implications. Hepato-Gastroenterol. 1994; 41: 573–577
21. **Guzzetta, P.C., Ruley, E.J., Merrick, H.F., Verderese, C., Barton, N.:** Elective subtotal splenectomy. Indications and results in 33 patients. Ann. Surg. 1990; 211: 34–42
22. **Horber, F.F., Lerut, J.P., Reichen, J., Zimmermann, A., Jaeger, P., Malinverni, R.:** Visceral leishmaniasis after orthotopic liver transplantation: impact of persistent splenomegaly. Transpl. Int. 1993; 6: 55–57
23. **Johnson, H.A., Deterling, R.A.:** Massive splenomegaly. Surg. Gynec. Obstetr. 1989; 168: 131–137
24. **Klee, F.E., Osswald, B.R., Wysocki, S.:** Cyst of the spleen – classical incidental diagnosis? Zb. Chir. 1996; 121: 805–816
25. **Knaut, S., Ludtke-Handjery, A., Anbuth, D.:** Die posttraumatische Milzzyste. Zentralbl. Chir. 1988; 113: 42–47
26. **Korn, M.A., Mostbeck, G.H., Tscholakoff, D.:** Duplexsonographie: Echoreiche Milzzyste oder Splenomegalie? Röntgenblätter 1990; 43: 107–108
27. **Manesis, E., Zoumboulis, P., Georgiou, S., Vardaka, J., Hadziqannis, St.:** Splenomegaly in asymptomatic chronic carriers of hepatitis B and D viruses. Eur. J. Gastroenterol. Hepatol. 1994; 6: 793–796
28. **Manoharan, A., Bader, L.V., Pitney, W.R.:** Non-tropical idiopathic splenomegaly (Dacie's syndrome). Report of 5 cases. Scand. J. Haematol. 1982; 28: 175–179
29. **Meran, J., Creutzig, A., Specht, S., Schürmeyer, Th., Brunner, G., Ranke, C., Fabel, H.:** Portale Hypertension und chronische Arsenexposition. Wien. Med. Wschr. 1989; 139: 580–584
30. **Ohta, M., Tsutsumi, Y., Tanaka, Y.:** Splenic hamartoma. Acta Pathol. Jpn. 1986; 36: 471–480
31. **Piontek, M., Hengels, K.J., Borchard, F., Strohmeyer, G.:** Nicht-zirrhotische Leberfibrose nach chronischer Arsenintoxikation. Dtsch. Med. Wschr. 1989; 114: 1653–1657
32. **Ramer, M., Diznoff, S.B., Hewes, A.C.:** Intrasplenic pancreatic pseudocyst: another cause of splenomegaly. Clin. Radiol. 1974; 25: 525–529
33. **Reynolds, M., Donaldson, J.S., Vogelzar, R.L.:** Giant iatrogenic splenic pseudocyst. J. Pediatr. Surg. 1989; 24: 700–701
34. **Schloesser, L.L.:** The diagnostic significance of splenomegaly. Amer. J. Med. Sci. 1963; 245: 118–124
35. **Schölmerich, J.:** Diagnostische Maßnahmen bei Splenomegalie. Dtsch. Med. Wschr. 1986; 111: 903–905
36. **Sekiya, T., Meller, S.T., Cosgrove, D.O., McCready, V.R.:** Ultrasonography of Hodgkin's disease in the liver and spleen. Clin. Radiol. 1982; 33: 635–639
37. **Sheth, S.G., Amarapurkar, D.N., Chopra, K.B., Mani, S.A., Mehta, P.J.:** Evaluation of splenomegaly in portal hypertension. J. Clin. Gastroenterol. 1996; 22: 28–30
38. **Waller, H.D.:** Differentialdiagnose des Milztumors. Therapiewoche 1975; 35: 4720–4732
39. **Warfel, K.A., Ellis, G.H.:** Peliosis of the spleen. Reports of a case and review of the literature. Arch. Pathol. Med. 1982; 106: 99–100
40. **Welten, C.A., Sijbrandij, E.S.:** Familial nonparasitic splenic cysts. Netherl. J. Med. 1992; 40: 236–239

Symptoms and Syndromes
12 Jaundice

		Page:
1	*Definition*	224
2	*Localization of bilirubin*	224
3	*Different shades of jaundice*	224
4	***Clinical classification of jaundice***	224
4.1	Prehepatic jaundice	226
4.2	Intrahepatic jaundice	226
4.3	Posthepatic jaundice	227
5	***Functional hyperbilirubinaemias***	227
5.1	*Neonatal and infant jaundice*	227
5.1.1	Physiological neonatal jaundice	227
5.1.2	Kernicterus	228
5.1.3	Lucey-Driscoll syndrome	228
5.1.4	Breast-milk jaundice	228
5.1.5	Blood-group incompatibility	228
5.1.6	Hereditary haemolytic anaemia	228
5.1.7	HELLP syndrome	228
5.1.8	Crigler-Najjar syndrome	229
5.2	*Jaundice in adults*	229
5.2.1	Gilbert-Meulengracht syndrome	229
5.2.2	Dubin-Johnson syndrome	230
5.2.3	Rotor syndrome	231
6	***Differential diagnosis of jaundice***	232
7	***Therapy***	233
	• References (1–80)	233
	(Figures 12.1–12.2; tables 12.1–12.7)	

12 Jaundice

> ▶ For doctor and patient alike, the phenomenon of **jaundice** evokes the idea of a disease of the liver or of the bile ducts. • Indeed, awareness of the condition of jaundice is undoubtedly as old as medical science itself. (s. pp 6, 7) • Thus ARETAIOS OF CAPPADOCIA (circa 200 AD) described icterus (jaundice) in such an exact way that his definition can be accepted even today: *"If a distribution of bile, either yellow, or like the yolk of an egg, or like safron, or of a dark-green colour, takes place from the viscus, over the whole system, the affection is called icterus".*

1 Definition

The term **jaundice** or **icterus** is used to depict the yellowish discolouring of the skin, mucous membranes and body fluids evident as a result of hyperbilirubinaemia in excess of 2.5 mg/dl, with subsequent deposition of bile pigments in tissue which is rich in elastin. In cases of severely impaired liver function or renal insufficiency, bilirubin values can rise dramatically. • The term **subicterus** is used to describe a low-grade icteric condition occurring in the region of the white sclera with a serum bilirubin value of > 1.8 mg/dl; for this reason, it is also known as *scleral icterus*. (s. pp 84, 106, 224)

> Jaundice is a **disorder in the metabolism of bilirubin** (s. p. 37); it is thus neither directly related to the bile acid metabolism (s. p. 39) nor to *cholestasis. (see chapter 13)* • **Jaundice is a symptom and not a disease. It can occur with and without cholestasis.**

2 Localization of bilirubin

Bilirubin is a hydrophobic organic anion. It shows a varied affinity to the individual tissues, so that differentiation can be made between bilirubinophilic and bilirubinophobic tissues (F. ROSENTHAL, 1930). Above all, tissue which is rich in elastin (skin, sclera, intima of the vessel wall, ligaments) absorbs bilirubin rapidly and intensively. Jaundice is thus first manifested at the sclera, where it remains detectable longest. Subsequently, the face, chest and abdomen as well as inner organs (such as the liver) and, to a lesser degree, the extremities are the most affected areas. Cartilage and nerve tissue are rarely yellow-coloured as a result of the icteric condition, and if so, only to a minor degree. The soles of the feet and palms of the hands only show slight icteric staining, if at all. • Saliva, lacrimal fluid and gastric juice are not stained icteric-yellow. Cerebrospinal fluid occasionally contains bilirubin and takes on a yellow hue, such as in hepatic coma (D. S. AMATUZIO et al., 1953) or Weil's disease (W. H. CARGILL Jr. et al., 1947).

In obstructive jaundice, bilirubin enters the lymphatic vessels, so that the lymphatic fluid is already icteric when it enters the thoracic duct. Exudates and transudates are always yellow-coloured in correlation to the serum bilirubin values, although they contain less bilirubin (in accordance with their lower protein content) than the serum itself. Due to their larger protein content, exudates are more icteric in colour than transudates. • Icteric colouring is hardly or not at all evident on paralyzed parts of the body. It would appear that bilirubin concentration also depends on normal nerve function. As a rule, jaundice is not detected in the region of an oedema (J. MEAKINS, 1927; J. H. PAGE, 1929).

3 Different shades of jaundice

▶ The respective colouring of jaundice depends on a number of different factors. The reddish shade in hepatitis patients used to be defined as **rubin jaundice**; the lemon yellow with a reddish hue observed in haemolysis was known as **flavin jaundice** (*flavus* = Latin for *yellow*) and the greenish shade observed in long-term cases of obstructive jaundice was called **verdin** or **green jaundice**. In obstructions lasting for several months, greyish-green to greenish-black tints were observed with jaundice, resulting in the term **melas jaundice** (from the Greek word *melas*, meaning *black*). (s. p. 84) • These colour differences, as interesting as they might be in the individual case, are of little help in differentiating between the various types of jaundice – *nearly every shade is possible in every single jaundice patient!*

Differential diagnosis: Jaundice has to be clearly delimited from **carotene jaundice** or **xanthodermia**, which may appear after an abundant ingestion of carrots, blood oranges and mangoes or the use of medication and cosmetic agents containing carotene. • **Lycopenaemia** can occur after an excessive ingestion of tomatoes. • A yellowing of the skin similar to that seen with increased serum bilirubin levels sometimes appears after an intake of **quinacrin** or **busulfan**.

4 Clinical classification of jaundice

> ▶ The **classification of jaundice** introduced by J. W. MCNEE (1923) still holds true today. It distinguishes between (*1.*) haemolytic, (*2.*) parenchymal, and (*3.*) obstructive. (s. p. 7) • Equally important is the classification of jaundice put forward by H. DUCCI (1947), which comprises various forms (*1.*) prehepatic, (*2.*) intrahepatic, and (*3.*) posthepatic.

Forms: In line with their *mechanisms of development* and *localization*, the various forms of jaundice can be subdivided into a well-established classification scheme consisting of three groups. (s. tab. 12.1).

1. **Prehepatic jaundice**
   = overproduction jaundice
   = repression jaundice
2. **Intrahepatic jaundice**
   a. *Dysfunction of bilirubin transport*
      - diminished bilirubin uptake in the liver cell
        = absorption jaundice
      - dysfunction of intracellular bilirubin transport (i.e. premicrosomal)
   b. *Dysfunction of bilirubin conjugation*
        = conjugation jaundice (i.e. microsomal)
      - congenital
      - postpartal
      - acquired
   c. *Dysfunction of bilirubin excretion*
        = excretion jaundice (i.e. postmicrosomal)
3. **Posthepatic jaundice**
        = obstruction or regurgitation jaundice
   a. *Extrahepatic jaundice*
   b. *Intrahepatic jaundice*

Tab. 12.1: Localization and developmental mechanisms of the various types of jaundice

Three types of bilirubin are found in the serum: unconjugated (indirect), conjugated (direct), and covalent albumin-bound bilirubin (direct). *(see chapter 3.3)*

(1.) **Unconjugated** bilirubin IXα is almost insoluble in water and therefore reversibly bound to albumin in the blood (< 1% free bilirubin remaining). Bilirubin enters the hepatocytes via transporters (= bilitranslocases) and becomes dissociated from albumin. Transport inside the hepatocytes is facilitated by the two carrier proteins, Y (= ligandin) and Z (= transport reserve).

(2.) **Conjugated bilirubin** is now formed in both rough and smooth ER, where it is conjugated with glucuronic acid. The result is a water-soluble bilirubin monoglucuronide and subsequently the respective diglucuronide. This glucuronidation process is catalyzed by uridine diphosphate-glucuronosyltransferase, which occurs as two isoenzymes. Excretion of bilirubin into the bile (20−40% as monoglucuronide, 60−80% as diglucuronide, 0.5−2.0% as unconjugated bilirubin) is actively carried out by ATP-dependent transporters (cMRP2, cMOAT). Bilirubin is transported into the bowels in mixed cells (together with bile acids, cholesterol and phospholipids). Bacterial glucuronidases then produce apolar, water-insoluble, unconjugated bilirubin, which is converted to urobilinogen by bacterial reductases.

(3.) **Delta bilirubin** is a small amount of conjugated bilirubin in the serum irreversibly bound to albumin by covalent bonding. In laboratory tests for bilirubin levels, delta bilirubin is determined together with conjugated (direct) bilirubin. • In pronounced and prolonged jaundice, the delta bilirubin level rises proportionally. The half-life of conjugated (direct) albumin-bound bilirubin is about 17 days, which is the same as albumin. This accounts for the relatively slow regression of jaundice.

Unconjugated (= indirect) hyperbilirubinaemias

1. **Bilirubin overproduction**
   - Haemolysis
   - Dyserythropoiesis
   - Jaundice from pulmonary infarction, from large haematoma, from repeated blood transfusions, occasionally in postoperative icterus
   - Repression of bilirubin from its albumin binding by endogenous or exogenous substances
2. **Diminished bilirubin uptake**
   - Long periods of fasting
   - Flavaspidic acid, rifampicin, *etc.*
   - Sepsis
   - Right heart failure
   - Portacaval shunt
   - Gilbert-Meulengracht syndrome (on occasions)
3. **Diminished bilirubin storage**
4. **Dysfunction of bilirubin conjugation**
   - Congenital disorders
     − Crigler-Najjar syndrome
     − Gilbert-Meulengracht syndrome
   - Severe neonatal icterus
   - Acquired disorders
     − medication-induced toxicity (e.g. ethinyloestradiol, gentamycin)
     − hyperthyroidism
     − hepatocellular diseases

Mainly conjugated (= direct), on occasions also combined, hyperbilirubinaemias

1. **Diminished bilirubin excretion**
   - Congenital dysfunctions
     − Dubin-Johnson syndrome
     − Rotor syndrome
2. **Dysfunctions of the hepatocytes**
   - Acquired dysfunctions
     − acute viral hepatitis
     − acute liver failure
     − liver cell necrosis in severe shock
     − chronic aggressive hepatitis
     − liver damage due to alcohol toxicity
     − pronounced storage diseases
     − severe fatty liver
     − liver cirrhosis
     − congestive liver
     − toxic liver damage
3. **Biliary obstruction**
   - Extrahepatic obstruction
   - Intrahepatic obstruction
     − mechanical
     − toxic
4. **Special forms**
   - Recurrent intrahepatic cholestasis
   - Recurrent cholestasis in pregnancy
   - Postoperative jaundice (on occasions)

Tab. 12.2: Different forms of jaundice classified in relation to the metabolic disorder of bilirubin and glucuronidation of bilirubin

Bilirubin conjugation: Another way to subdivide the different forms of jaundice is based on bilirubin conjugation, which enables all forms of jaundice to be classified into **two systems:** unconjugated and conjugated forms of hyperbilirubinaemia. This particular systematization can result in overlapping terminology or produce pathogenetic combinations. (s. tab. 12.2)

4.1 Prehepatic jaundice

Haemolytic syndrome: Prehepatic jaundice is usually generated by haemolysis. Overproduction of bilirubin results in unconjugated hyperbilirubinaemia, whereby the serum bilirubin level is rarely in excess of 5 mg/dl. *Unconjugated bilirubin* cannot pass through the kidney, so that no traces of bilirubin are detectable in the urine despite the icteric state. • The bile is pleiochromatic and lithogenic. Chronic prehepatic jaundice can give rise to cholelithiasis due to the formation of pure pigment gallstones. In severe cases of haemolysis, the *conjugated bilirubin* in the serum may also increase, so that bilirubin is now detectable in the urine. As a result of haemolysis-related hyperbilirubinaemia, increased formation and renal excretion of *urobilinogen* occur. (s. tabs. 5.8; 12.1) (s. pp 38, 106) (s. fig. 5.3)

Causes: Apart from the multicausal facets involved in the haemolytic syndrome or the disorders leading to haemolysis (e. g. erythrocyte defects, toxins, noxae, antibody-mediated or mechanical factors), other causes of prehepatic jaundice are worthy of mention:

(1.) **Dyserythropoiesis** refers to an increasing presence of abnormal erythrocyte precursors in the bone marrow and spleen (with splenomegaly, but no hepatomegaly) due to ineffective erythropoiesis and early labelled bilirubin production *(primary shunt hyperbilirubinaemia)*. Jaundice is indicated by serum bilirubin levels of 1.5–8.0 mg/dl between the ages of 20 and 30. Levels of urobilinogen in the urine are elevated, and normoplastic erythroid hyperplasia occurs in the bone marrow. Prognosis is good. (3, 10)

(2.) **Pulmonary infarction jaundice** following extensive haemorrhagic pulmonary infarction with haemolysis of the erythrocytes which have passed into the alveoli.

(3.) **Haematoma jaundice** with retrogression of large haematomas due to the fact that 1 litre of blood produces about 5 g bilirubin, which is 20 times the normal daily bilirubin production.

(4.) **Postoperative jaundice:** In some cases, postoperative hyperbilirubinaemias may also be caused by haemolysis, in particular when unconjugated bilirubin is detectable. (2, 7, 15)

(5.) **Blood transfusions:** Haemolysis is due to the shortened lifespan of transfused erythrocytes.

(6.) **Displacement of bilirubin** from its albumin bond. Various endogenous substances (e. g. long-chain fatty acids and bile acids) or exogenous compounds (e. g. medication, such as ampicillin, ajmaline, quinidine, furosemide, indomethacin, probenecid, rifampicin, sulphonamide, etc., and X-ray contrast media) can compete with bilirubin, not only with respect to its specific binding site, but also for its carrier protein.

Haemolysis: Irrespective of the aetiology and pathogenesis of haemolysis, certain *symptoms* are generally observed. (s. tab. 12.3)

1. Serum bilirubin ↑
   – mainly indirect bilirubin, seldom > 5 mg/dl
2. Urobilinogenuria +, bilirubinuria +
   – only in severe haemolysis
3. $LDH_{1,2}$ ↑
4. Haptoglobin ↓
5. LDH/GOT quotient > 12
6. Reticulocytes > 20‰
7. Splenomegaly: frequent
8. Liver biopsy: normal
   – possible detection of haemosiderin
9. Erythropoiesis in the bone marrow ↑

Tab. 12.3: General signs of haemolysis

4.2 Intrahepatic jaundice

Multiple influences may cause a disorder in the metabolism of bilirubin inside the hepatocyte. This dysfunction may be localized in the *premicrosomal, microsomal* or *postmicrosomal* region of the liver cell. (s. tab. 12.2)

(1.) **Diminished bilirubin uptake** in the liver cell may result jaundice. This is possibly caused by bile acids, medication or chemicals (e. g. vermicides such as flavaspidic acid). Extensive periods of fasting (N.A. Gilbert et al., 1907; E. Meyer et al., 1922) (< 300 calories/day, > 48 hours) and toxaemia with sepsis (14, 18, 23) can also give rise to unconjugated hyperbilirubinaemia.

(2.) **Reduced storage of bilirubin** can be caused by the bilirubin competing with exogenous substances for binding to the Y protein or with long-chain fatty acids for binding to the Z protein. Thus bilirubin may diffuse back from the liver cell into the blood.

(3.) **Dysfunction of the glucuronosyltransferase activity** is mainly attributed to congenital defects, resulting in functional, unconjugated hyperbilirubinaemias. In contrast, acquired impairment of glucuronidation as a result of medicaments (chloramphenicol, pregnanediol, testosterone, etc.) or due to hypothyroidism is deemed to be rare. This particular form of jaundice shows an increase in indirect bilirubin without occurrence of bilirubinuria. Medication-induced jaundice is rarely due to an inhibition of glucuronosyltransferase activity, because other enzyme systems in the biotransformation process (phase 2) show overlapping effects.

(4.) **Dysfunction in the secretion of bilirubin** is also a cause of jaundice. The mechanisms involved in the excretion of bilirubin into the biliary capillaries are, however, largely unresolved, and thus the starting points of the disruptive factors remain unknown. This dysfunction is a postmicrosomal regurgitation jaundice with higher levels of both unconjugated and conjugated bilirubin.

▶ *Congenital defects* include the Dubin-Johnson syndrome and Rotor syndrome. (s. tab. 12.4) Both of these diseases present a genetically determined disorder in the secretion of bilirubin.

▶ *Acquired liver diseases* (e. g. cirrhosis, liver cell necrosis in severe shock (11), pronounced toxic liver damage, cardiac congestion (11, 17), alcohol-related and medication-induced diseases of the liver) very frequently cause jaundice as a result of disorders in the secretion of bilirubin. The uptake, storage and conjugation of bilirubin are usually not impaired. A number of medicaments merely produce elevated bilirubin levels (so-called *jaundice type*). • Intrahepatic jaundice — with and without cholestasis — is most frequently attributed to acquired defects of the respective functions of the liver cell as a result of pronounced liver damage. Conjugated (sometimes even unconjugated) hyperbilirubinaemia is evident in connection with bilirubinuria and urobilinogenuria. The greater the liver damage, the higher are the frequency and degree of severity of jaundice (possibly even with additional cholestasis).

▶ *Additional cholestasis:* Isolated defects in the transport mechanisms of bilirubin not only display jaundice, but also an impairment in bile secretion. The outcome is additional intrahepatic, nonobstructive cholestasis.

4.3 Posthepatic jaundice

This form of jaundice is initiated by a *mechanical obstruction* in the region of the extrahepatic or intrahepatic bile ducts, which is why the terms "mechanical jaundice" or "obstructive jaundice" are also common. The congestion of the bile flow is either *incomplete* or *complete*. Bile stasis results in dilation of the extrahepatic and intrahepatic bile ducts, allowing *hepatomegaly* to develop. (8, 9, 16, 19) (s. tab. 12.1)

Histologically, obstructive jaundice is characterized by biliary thrombi in the canaliculi as well as the storage of bile pigments in hepatocytes and Kupffer cells. These changes are most pronounced at the centres of the lobules, since there is less chance of outflow here than in the lobular periphery.

Biochemically, a change in structure relating to the mucopolysaccharides (neuraminic acid?) and monohydroxy bile acids probably accounts for the formation of biliary thrombi. Some of the "under-hydroxylated" bile salts appear in crystalline form; the bile becomes increasingly viscous and its flow is impeded. This defect in the excretion of bile salts culminates in dysfunctions in the secretion of bilirubin, which is why bilirubin is regurgitated into the blood. The bile which accumulates in the bile ducts ultimately becomes mucous and white because of the reabsorption of bile pigments by the epithelia of the small bile ducts.

Extrahepatic obstructive jaundice is caused by stenosing processes. The region of Vater's papilla is particularly affected, for example by inflammations, stones, duodenal diverticula, carcinoma, parasites, cicatricial stenosis or adenomatosis. In this respect, special mention should also be made of carcinoma, cicatricial strictures and gallstones (s. figs. 8.14, 8.15; 33.15, 33.16), compression of the common bile duct due to a cystic duct stone (= *Mirizzi syndrome*), haemobilia, and various parasites – such as Ascaris lumbricoides (s. fig. 25.8!). All of these disorders can be found in the area of the extrahepatic bile ducts. (1, 9, 19)

Intrahepatic obstructive jaundice relates to the intrahepatic bile ducts, which can be blocked, above all *mechanically,* by inflammatory processes (cholangitis, primary biliary or primary sclerosing cholangitis), intrahepatic stones, granulomas, tumours, cysts, amyloid degeneration, eosinophilic gastroenteritis, and cystic fibrosis of the pancreas — to name but a few examples.
• In addition, biliary obstructive jaundice can also be caused by *drug-induced toxicity*, e.g. with C_{17}-substituted steroids, erythromycin estolate, chlorpromazine, chlorpropamide, ajmaline, halothane, methylthiouracil.
• Further intrahepatic forms of obstruction include recurrent intrahepatic cholestasis and recurrent cholestasis in pregnancy. (s. tab. 12.4)

Special forms: There are a multitude of factors involved in the pathogenesis of intrahepatic *benign postoperative jaundice;* hypoxia, hypotension, haemolysis, toxins, sepsis and medicaments are just a few of them. (1, 5, 6, 14, 18, 23) • Likewise, jaundice in *intensive-care patients* (1, 2, 7, 15) as well as after long-term *total parenteral nutrition* belong to this category. (1, 4)

5 Functional hyperbilirubinaemias

Hyperbilirubinaemia relates to functional disorders in the hepatocellular metabolism of bilirubin — with and without cholestasis (W. SIEDE, 1957). This means either dysfunctions regarding bilirubin conjugation (= *conjugation jaundice*) or bilirubin excretion (= *excretion jaundice*).

Unconjugated hyperbilirubinaemias

As a result of impaired bilirubin conjugation, unconjugated lipophilic bilirubin IXα increases (80–85% of the total bilirubin gives rise to an *indirect diazo reaction*). This free bilirubin passes unhindered through biological membranes and has a toxic impact on cells. Many factors may affect the various stages of the metabolic process, which is incomplete up to this point. Cholestasis is absent. (47, 62) (s. tab. 12.4)

5.1 Neonatal and infant jaundice

5.1.1 Physiological neonatal jaundice

In about 90% of all neonates, jaundice occurs after the first two to five days of life and rarely exceeds 6 mg/dl serum bilirubin. In premature infants, bilirubin levels can rise to 10–12 mg/dl. • The **cause** is related to various factors: (*1.*) reinforced degradation of haemoglobin as a result of the short erythrocyte survival span of 70–90 days (120 days in adults), (*2.*) reduction in cellular transport proteins, above all ligandin, (*3.*) deficiency of uridyltransferase and glucuronosyltransferase, and (*4.*) increasing intestinal absorption of meconium bilirubin. After about ten days, newborn jaundice subsides with

Unconjugated hyperbilirubinaemias = indirect positive diazo reaction
1. **Neonatal jaundice** *Neonatal* • Physiological neonatal jaundice • Jaundice in pyloric stenosis • Jaundice in intestinal obstruction • Blood group incompatibility • Hereditary haemolytic anaemias • Breast-milk jaundice *Connatal-hereditary* • Lucey-Driscoll syndrome • Zellweger's syndrome (s. p. 242) • Infantile Refsum's disease (s. p. 242) • Hereditary haemolytic anaemia • Dyserythropoiesis 2. **Crigler-Najjar syndrome** • Type I • Type II (= Arias syndrome) 3. **Gilbert-Meulengracht syndrome**
Conjugated (partly combined) hyperbilirubinaemias = direct positive diazo reaction
1. **Dubin-Johnson syndrome** 2. **Rotor syndrome**
Conjugated (partly combined) hyperbilirubinaemias with elevation of biliary acids *(see chapter 13)*
1. **Recurrent intrahepatic cholestasis in pregnancy** 2. **Recurrent intrahepatic cholestasis** • Benign forms – *Summerskill-Tygstrup* type – *Aagenaes* type • Progressive form – Byler's syndrome *(Clayton-Juberg type)* 3. **Idiopathic connatal or neonatal hepatitis**

Tab. 12.4: Functional, partly neonatal, partly connatal-hereditary hyperbilirubinaemias

out any further consequences. Bilirubin also acts as an antioxidant and can thus provide protection from oxygen radicals, if necessary. • Peripartal complications can, however, reinforce or prolong this state. This may occur in infantile hypothyroidism or when medication is administered directly to the infant as well as via breast milk (particularly when bilirubin is displaced from its albumin binding by drugs). In more pronounced jaundice, phototherapy and an increase in the oral intake of fluids may be advisable. (45, 48, 51, 56, 61, 71)

5.1.2 Kernicterus

Kernicterus may occur as the result of immaturity of the blood-brain barrier in *severe neonatal icterus* and can occasionally be found in *premature infants* as well, with bilirubin levels usually higher than 20 mg/dl. Unconjugated bilirubin is deposited in the basal ganglia of the hippocampus and the hypothalamus nuclei as bilirubin-phosphatidylcholine precipitate, where it gives rise to neuronal necroses. *Risk factors* (e.g. asphyxia, acidosis, hypothermia, hypoglycaemia, sepsis with lower UPT activity, and medication) promote the occurrence of the dreaded kernicterus. • In clinical terms, sucking weakness, vomiting, attacks of fever, convulsions, reflex anomalies, shrill shrieking, apathy and muscular hypotension can be observed, with subsequent muscular hypertonicity, cramps, opisthotonus, strabismus, nystagmus and apnoea. The lethality rate is about 75%. Survival is accompanied by cerebral paresis, deafness and retardation. • *Therapy* focuses on exchange blood transfusions, plasmapheresis and phototherapy (430–470 nm; 8–12 hours daily). (13, 25, 28, 63, 68, 73).

5.1.3 Lucey-Driscoll syndrome

This is a familial form of neonatal hyperbilirubinaemia (J. F. Lucey et al., 1960) (55) and can probably be attributed to the inhibitive effect of a progestagen steroid in the maternal blood serum, which impedes bilirubin conjugation. Babies show sucking weakness. Bilirubin values can be in excess of 6 mg/dl. This disorder, which occurs from approximately the second day of life onwards, regresses after two to three weeks. There is no hepatomegaly or splenomegaly; bilirubin and urobilinogen cannot be detected in the urine. The prognosis is good. In severe (extremely rare) cases, exchange blood transfusions may be indicated.

5.1.4 Breast-milk jaundice

Prolonged neonatal breast-milk jaundice is found in 0.5–1.0% of all breast-fed infants as from the fourth day and within the first two weeks of life. Bilirubin levels are drastically elevated (15–25 mg/dl). Nevertheless, this clinical picture does not generally give rise to kernicterus. Even if breast-feeding is discontinued immediately, the condition can take up to 10 weeks to regress. Possible causes are long-chain fatty acids or a pregnane derivative (pregnane-3-α-20β-diol) in the breast milk; this steroid inhibits glucuronosyltransferase activity. Apart from that, intestinal bilirubin uptake is elevated. (24, 42, 74, 75)

5.1.5 Blood group incompatibility

Rh-erythroblastosis occurs in 0.2‰ and ABO erythroblastosis in 0.6% of all pregnancies. In clinical terms, the course of the latter disease is usually more moderate. Due to severe haemolysis, unconjugated bilirubin levels rise rapidly, often reaching relatively high values. • *Therapy* includes phototherapy, exchange blood transfusions and administration of immunoglobulin (500 mg/kg BW).

5.1.6 Hereditary haemolytic anaemia

Thalassaemia, spherocytosis, sickle-cell anaemia and glucose-6-phosphate dehydrogenase deficiency are rare causes.

5.1.7 HELLP syndrome

Pre-eclampsia is characterized by hypertension, proteinuria and oedema. It develops in 3–5% of primiparas

(0.5 % in multiparas) from the second trimester of pregnancy. The liver is involved in 10—20% of cases (elevated transaminases). • **Eclampsia** is associated with additional features, such as seizures and/or coma (0.1—0.2% of pregnancies). The liver is involved in 70—90% of cases. There are elevated liver enzymes as well as portal/periportal infiltrates and cell necroses. • **HELLP syndrome** is a complication of (pre-)eclampsia. It comprises **h**aemolysis (s. tab. 12.3), **e**levated **l**iver enzymes and **l**ow **p**latelets. Usually, the HELLP syndrome develops in the third trimester, but, in about 30% of cases, it is postpartal. All patients show damage to the vascular epithelium and activation of the coagulation cascade (D-dimer is elevated in 40—50% of cases), resulting in deposition of fibrin along the sinusoids and development of microthrombi. Additionally, there are ischemic necroses of hepatocytes (partially confluent); haemorrhages and, occasionally, haematomas are observed beneath the liver capsule, with the danger of spontaneous rupture. • *Treatment* is aimed at controlling hypertension (e.g. nifedipine, because this drug also has a therapeutic effect on the liver). Prednisolone may be indicated. Delivery must be made immediately after fetal lung maturity has been determined.

5.1.8 Crigler-Najjar syndrome

> ▶ In 1952 the clinical picture of this congenital, familial, nonhaemolytic type of jaundice was described by the American paediatricians J. F. Crigler and V.A. Najjar (31).

The **cause** is a hereditary recessive (or dominant in type II) autosomal deficiency in UDP-glucuronosyltransferase. Consanguinity is common within the families affected. The gene is located on chromosome 2.

Type I: This (rare) Crigler-Najjar syndrome can be attributed to the *almost total lack* of the two isoenzymes in bilirubin UDP-glucuronosyltransferase activity as a result of (homozygous) mutations in UGT-1A1 locus. Consequently, hepatic bilirubin clearance is reduced to 1—2% of the standard rate. Bilirubin is excreted as unconjugated bilirubin IXα or in the form of polar diazo-negative metabolites. Because of the absence of conjugation, severe unconjugated hyperbilirubinaemia with bilirubin values of 18—50 mg/dl occurs during the first days of life. Within a few days, kernicterus develops with pronounced neurological disorders. (50) Stools and urine are of normal colour, the bile is colourless. The liver and spleen are not enlarged. All hepatic laboratory parameters are normal. Except for the presence of biliary thrombi, the histology of the liver is quite regular. As a result of the biliary thrombi in the dental canaliculi, the teeth can take on a yellow colouring, and enamel hypoplasia appears. • The *course of disease* is progressive and generally lethal. The mean life expectancy ranges between 6 and 18 months. Only a few of the 150—200 patients whose case histories have so far been published reached puberty. Recently, however, a successful pregnancy was observed. (36) • *Therapy* consists of exchange blood transfusions and plasma separations as well as intensive phototherapy (8—12 hours daily), possibly in combination with cholestyramine, agar, zinc and calcium carbonate or calcium phosphate. Indol-3-carbinol is also recommended as an inductor of CYP 450-1A1/-1A2. Liver transplantation may be indicated. (72)

Type II: In this Crigler-Najjar syndrome (I. M. Arias, 1962) *(Arias syndrome)* (26), glucuronosyltransferase activity is *merely reduced*, since only one isoenzyme has a (heterozygous) defect. Bilirubin conjugation is only minimally restricted. Bilirubin is largely excreted as monoglucuronide. The uptake of bilirubin into the liver cell might also be impaired. Jaundice generally occurs within the first year of life, but also during the following 20—30 years. (28) Bilirubin values fluctuate between 6 and 20 mg/dl. A more pronounced rise in bilirubin levels can be caused by various stress factors (e.g. fasting, infections, acidosis, metabolic dysfunctions). In such cases, kernicterus occasionally occurs. Like type I, type II does not display any particular stigmata: the colour of the stools and urine, the size of the liver and spleen as well as the laboratory parameters are normal. Now and again, histology displays biliary thrombi while, as with type I, hypertrophy of the smooth endoplasmic reticulum and of the Golgi apparatus is also in evidence. • The *course of disease* is more moderate, so that prognosis is usually good. Nevertheless, repeated attacks of kernicterus can culminate in permanent neurological damage (intention tremor, changes in the EEG, impaired intelligence). • As *therapy*, phenobarbital (3 × 60 mg) in combination with calcium phosphate has proved useful. Phototherapy, also in combination with albumin infusions, is likewise indicated. (13, 28, 36) Alternatively, phenytoin or phenazone can be applied. The effect is derived from the induction of the glucuronidation enzyme and the enhancement of the synthesis of the Y protein. Careful guidance of the patient is important, particularly in order to avert attacks of kernicterus. (40, 41, 45, 46, 48, 65, 71, 77)

5.2 Jaundice in adults

5.2.1 Gilbert-Meulengracht syndrome

> ▶ In 1901 A. Gilbert and P. Lereboullet described a clinical picture using the term *cholémie simple familiale*. (38, 39) The *icterus intermittens juvenilis* (59) described by E. Meulengracht in 1939 (subsequently termed familial, nonhaemolytic jaundice or constitutional hyperbilirubinaemia) proved to be identical.

The **frequency** of this harmless disorder in the metabolism of bilirubin is quite high: it affects 5—12% of the population. The syndrome is 4 times more common in men than in women. Frequency in the affected families lies between 5% and 55%. • *Genetic transmission* is dominant autosomal with differing degrees of penetrance, which accounts for the heterogeneous clinical picture. Sporadic occurrences of this syndrome have also been observed. The gene is located on chromosome 2.

The **pathogenesis** is characterized by several mechanisms: (1.) elevated production of hepatic haem bilirubin; (2.) in some 60% of the patients, minor haemolysis is evident due to a lower survival span of erythrocytes; (3.) the activity of the glucuronosyltransferase is diminished (by about one third of the norm) due to mutations in UGT-1A1 locus, and there is above all a deficiency in monoglucuronosyltransferase activity, because bilirubin monoglucuronide excretion in the bile is considerably higher than is the case in healthy persons; (4.) disorders in membrane fluidity are responsible for reduced bilirubin uptake in the hepatocytes. Ligandin and Z protein levels in the hepatocytes are reduced. • However, none of these mechanisms in itself provides an explanation for the symptoms of the Gilbert-Meulengracht syndrome.

The **subjective complaints** of the patients are reflected in irritability, moodiness, fatigue, vegetative dysfunctions, epigastric discomfort and abdominal bloating. Such complaints, however, show no correlation with the intensity of hyperbilirubinaemia. It is still not clear whether these ailments can be regarded as concomitant symptoms (= epiphenomena) or as a sequela (= hypochondriac reaction) of jaundice.

The **clinical picture** is characterized by intermittent jaundice with bilirubin levels of 1.5 to 2.5 mg/dl; there are also phases when normal values are registered. Increased bilirubin values are not only discernible after fasting and physical exercise, but also as a result of infections, alcohol consumption, menstruation, medication and severe stress. Bilirubin levels fluctuate considerably, even during the course of several days. This syndrome usually becomes manifest between the ages of 15 and 30. It is rarely found in neonates or infants. There are no further findings: liver and spleen are normal in size; urine and stools show no noticeable changes in colour; transaminases are regular, and cholestasis is not detectable. Generally, there are no signs of haemolysis, except to a slight extent in patients with higher bilirubin values. Only in 20–40% of cases is it possible to find a defect in the uptake of organic anions (e. g. indocyanine green). (57) However, reduced glucuronidation of certain medicaments was observed (e. g. acetaminophin, clofibrate, rifampicin, tolbutamide). (32) Gilbert's syndrome is only seen as a clinically significant complication when it occurs together with thalassaemia or simultaneous ingestion of ifinotecan.

The **diagnosis** is founded on: (1.) normal transaminase values, (2.) regular ultrasound findings, and (3.) an elevated level of unconjugated serum bilirubin. • The diagnosis can be confirmed by various laboratory parameters, findings or tests:

(1.) Serum values of bile acids, haptoglobin and reticulocytes are normal.
(2.) The monoglucuronide/diglucuronide quotient is elevated.
(3.) Fasting (<400 calories per day for 2 days) raises bilirubin levels to 2 (−3) times the initial value.
(4.) Maintaining a diet normal in calories yet strictly lipid-free for 2 or 3 days can cause bilirubin levels more or less to double.
(5.) Rigorous physical exercise (sports) for 1 or 2 days results in noticeably increased bilirubin values.
(6.) The nicotine acid test (50 mg nicotine acid i.v.) produces a rise in bilirubin of more than 0.9 mg/dl in excess of the initial value, measured at 4 hours after the injection. The specificity and sensitivity of this test are almost 100%. (36, 44, 66)
(7.) Administration of phenobarbital (3 × 60 mg/day) leads to a decrease (possibly normalization) in bilirubin values.

The **histology** of the liver is normal. An accumulation of intralobular bile ducts (H. Thaler, 1982) is noticeable. There may be centroacinar deposits of higher amounts of lipofuscin. An increase of five to ten times the norm is observed in the rough endoplasmic reticulum.

No **therapy** of this "cosmetic defect" is necessary. In severe cases of jaundice, administration of phenobarbital (60–180 mg/day) or rifampicin (34) may be considered. • The *harmless nature* of this congenital, purely cosmetic ailment must be pointed out to the patient. Diets or even medication are quite out of place, as are "alternative" courses of treatment. • In isolated cases, a biopsy of the liver may be required (although this is in itself not indicated) in order to provide evidence of the harmless nature of this syndrome to the patients, who are by this time often mildly neurotic and utterly convinced that their condition is chronic and can no longer be treated. (27, 32, 48, 49, 52, 54, 55, 57, 58, 60)

Conjugated (partly combined) hyperbilirubinaemias

> Conjugated hyperbilirubinaemia derives from a congenital disorder which causes decreased bilirubin excretion in the canaliculi. This is why serum bilirubin is drastically elevated during an icteric episode. More than 40% (−85%) of the total bilirubin in the serum produces a *direct diazo reaction*. Unconjugated bilirubin is also found in the blood. Bilirubin is covalently bound to albumin. Bilirubinuria and urobilinogenuria are in evidence. (47, 62) (s. tab. 12.4)

5.2.2 Dubin-Johnson syndrome

▶ The clinical picture which was first described by I. N. Dubin and F. B. Johnson (1954) (33) was observed at the same time by H. Sprinz and R. S. Nelson (1954). (74)

The **frequency** of this syndrome, which shows a recessive autosomal inheritance pattern, is characterized by ethnic differences. Over 200 confirmed reports have been published. The real number is considerably higher, since not all cases are actually diagnosed or communicated. The mutations are located on chromosome 10q 23–24. Genetic evidence of this syndrome can also be obtained from skin biopsies (= detection of MRP2 in fibroblasts).

▶ *We observed two patients who were suffering from a Dubin-Johnson syndrome, one of them in connection with acute viral hepatitis A. (s. figs. 12.1, 12.2)*

Manifestation may occur at any age, but it is usually diagnosed between the ages of 10 and 30. The disease can develop gradually or acutely, often triggered by infections, acute viral hepatitis (78), alcohol, excessive physical or mental strain, contraceptives, pregnancy, etc. • The *cause* is considered to be a dysfunction of the bilirubin transport system in the canalicular membrane of the hepatocytes. The result is a dysfunction of (conjugated) bilirubin excretion into the bile. A deficiency of MRP 2 (MOAT) is deemed to be a causative factor.

The **subjective ailments** of patients, especially in the case of icteric episodes, include fatigue, languor, inappetence, nausea, and pain on pressure in the right epigastrium – sometimes even of a colic-like nature.

The **clinical picture** is characterized by chronic or intermittent jaundice with values between 2 and 6 mg/dl, and in rare cases between 6 and 12 mg/dl. With acute icteric episodes, values can be in excess of 20 mg/dl. The proportion of conjugated bilirubin in the serum is about 60%, almost exclusively in the form of diglucuronidated bilirubin. The liver or spleen are only occasionally enlarged (50–60% or 10–15% of cases, respectively). Both the laboratory values and the bile acids in the serum are normal; cholestasis is absent. Coagulation factor VII is frequently reduced (approx. 60% of cases). In more pronounced jaundice, bilirubinuria and urobilinogenuria are in evidence. Excretion of coproporphyrin I in the urine is elevated, but that of coproporphyrin III is reduced. (35) • The oral cholecystogram is "negative", whereas the gall bladder appears normal after i.v. administration of contrast medium.

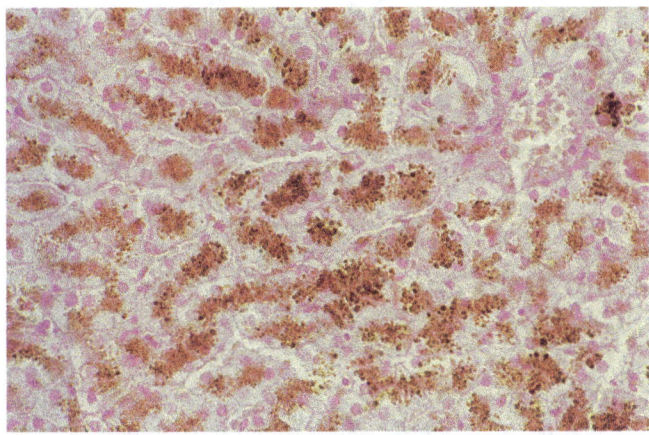

Fig. 12.1: Dubin-Johnson syndrome. (Clinically: persistent jaundice following acute viral hepatitis A.) Massive intracellular storage of lysosomal brownish pigment (Berlin blue)

Histologically, the clinical picture is characterized by the deposition of brown, coarsely grained, iron-free, melanin-like *pigments* (= ***black liver jaundice***). (s. fig. 12.2) The lipomelanin (?) is stored in the lysosomes between the cell nucleus and canaliculus, so that *pericanalicular pigment pathways* are formed. The pigment is possibly a polymerization product of catecholamines. It is detected in differing degrees of intensity and seems to fluctuate during the course of disease as well as upon regeneration of the liver cell, e.g. following acute viral hepatitis. (s. fig. 12.1) (s. p. 430)

Laparoscopically, the liver is bluish-green to bluish-black in colour (= ***black liver***). The surface is smooth and shiny, with intricate vascular multiplication; the lymphatic vessels of the capsule of the liver can appear more pronounced. (s. fig. 12.2)

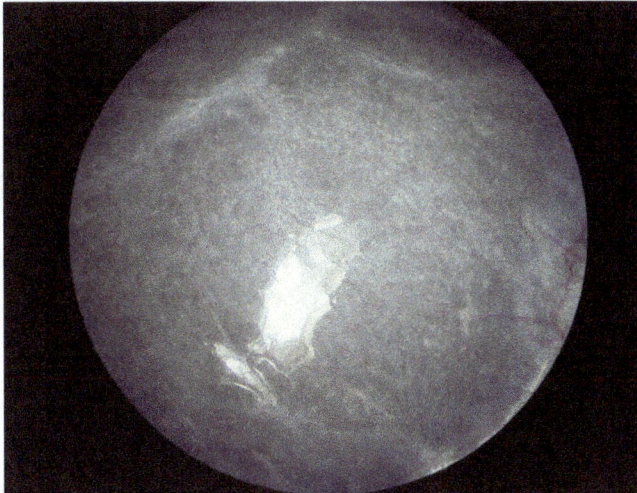

Fig. 12.2: Dubin-Johnson syndrome (so-called black liver)

Therapy is not required for this benign disease, nor is it effective. During icteric episodes, it is advisable to administer phenobarbital. The *harmless nature* of the syndrome must be explicitly pointed out to the patient, even in the case of "chronic jaundice". Stress factors, such as contraceptives, may trigger an icteric episode and should be avoided. However, there are no medical objections to pregnancy, where increased bilirubin values are often encountered. (30, 35, 43, 48, 50, 64, 69, 76, 78, 80)

5.2.3 Rotor syndrome

▶ The Rotor syndrome was first described by A. B. ROTOR et al. in 1948 (67), after G. CANALI had already reported on this form of jaundice (albeit not histologically investigated) in 1945.

This clinical picture shows a recessive autosomal inheritance pattern. In approx. 40 cases published to date (mainly concerning Filipino patients), there are no obvious signs of a gender-related preference. Conjugated hyperbilirubinaemia of this syndrome derives from a disorder of the uptake, intracellular bonding (storage) and excretion of bilirubin. Other organic anions (bromosulphophthalein, indocyanine green) are also subject to delayed excretion.

This form of jaundice is found in childhood and adolescence as conjugated hyperbilirubinaemia. Bilirubin values range between 2 and 5 mg/dl with intercurrent icteric episodes, which (as in the Dubin-Johnson syndrome) are mostly triggered by various stress factors. Bilirubinuria and urobilinogenuria may likewise appear, depending on the bilirubin values. All hepatic laboratory parameters are normal. Excretion of total coproporphyrins in the urine is elevated. (70) Oral administration of a contrast medium allows the gall bladder to be visualized. Histology of the liver shows no pathological findings; in particular, there is no pigment deposition. • *Therapeutic measures* are not necessary, and in fact none are known. Prognosis is good. Any factors that might set off an icteric episode should be avoided. (29, 48, 79, 80)

Conjugated (partly combined) hyperbilirubinaemias with impaired drainage of bile acids

The principal symptoms of this form of disease are (*1.*) largely conjugated (partly combined) hyperbilirubinaemia with **jaundice** and (*2.*) **cholestasis** with pruritus and scratch marks. • This group includes (*1.*) recurrent intrahepatic cholestasis in pregnancy, (*2.*) benign recurrent intrahepatic cholestasis (BRIC) as well as the Aagenaes form, and (*3.*) progressive familial cholestasis (PFIC) and the Byler form. *(see chapter 13)*

6 Differential diagnosis of jaundice

▶ Each case of jaundice calls for differential diagnostic clarification. The clinical spectrum ranges from the so-called cosmetic, perfectly harmless defect through to malignant obstructions. (2, 5, 8, 9, 12, 16, 20–22, 62) • *It is of the utmost importance to differentiate between nonobstructive and obstructive jaundice.*

Based on a targeted and exact *anamnesis*, subjective *complaints* by the patient and careful **physical examination** (s. tab. 12.5), it is possible in most cases to make a clear distinction between four different categories of jaundice: (*1.*) haematological, (*2.*) hepatocellular, (*3.*) biliary obstructive, and (*4.*) hereditary. (s. tabs. 12.1, 12.2, 12.4)

If there is no interference in terms of **colour reactions in the urine** due to pronounced yellowing, a preliminary categorization of the jaundice form is possible. A persistently negative urobilinogen sample, concurrent with evidence of bilirubinuria, points to a complete obstruction or serious restriction of hepatic function. A persistently positive urobilinogen reaction in the absence of bilirubinuria suggests prehepatic (haemolytic) jaundice. (s. tab. 12.6)

At the outset of clinical investigations, priority is given to determining the direct and indirect *bilirubin* reaction in the serum with the help of the diazo reaction. Other **laboratory parameters** as well as the enzyme quotients (s. tabs. 5.6, 5.7) often allow the differential diagnosis of jaundice to be made at this stage. (s. tabs. 12.6, 12.7)

▶ **Noninvasive** procedures used consecutively are ultrasound and, if necessary, computer tomography. For the diagnosis of extrahepatic jaundice, both test procedures have about the same sensitivity and specificity, yet their degree of accuracy is no greater than that obtained

1. Precise anamnesis
– Start of jaundice?   – Fluctuations in intensity?   – Relapses?   – Correlation with surgery, infusions, injections?   – Correlation with pregnancy?   – Journeys abroad?   – Occurrence of jaundice within the family?   – Alcohol abuse?   – Medication?   – Contact with chemicals?   – Pre- or coexistent hepatobiliary diseases?
2. Subjective complaints
– Pain in the right epigastrium?   – Colic?   – Lack of appetite? Loss of weight?   – Nausea?   – Itching?   – Arthralgia?   – Colour changes in stools or urine?   – Fatigue?   – Decrease in vitality?
3. Clinical results
– Hepatomegaly?   – Tenderness on pressure?   – Splenomegaly?   – Scratch marks?   – Type and intensity of jaundice?   – Skin stigmata of liver diseases?   – Hyaline cast in urine sediment?   – Stool and urine examination results?

Tab. 12.5: Important anamnestic and clinical findings for setting up a differential diagnosis of jaundice

through clinical and laboratory examinations. Laboratory diagnosis facilitates a precise differentiation between the types of hyperbilirubinaemia and their possible combination with cholestasis.

1. *Ultrasound examination* is always indicated for the clarification of jaundice. The results determine the subsequent diagnostic steps. It is important to clarify whether the bile ducts are dilated, which is a hint for obstructive jaundice. (s. tabs. 6.11, 6.12) (s. p. 140)

2. *Computer tomography* can be indicated in isolated cases, particularly in order to establish the cause of obstruction or when focal lesions are present.

The diagnostic strategy for clarification of **cholestasis** and **jaundice** is outlined later in a **flow diagram**. (s. fig. 13.7) (s. p. 247)

▶ If a particular jaundice cannot be categorized, **invasive methods** are indicated:

1. *Liver biopsy* has often proved indispensable for the differentiation and validation of unresolved prehepatic or intrahepatic jaundice. (s. tab. 7.3)

Type of jaundice	Bile	Colour of stool	Colour of urine	Urobili-nogen	Bilirubin
Prehepatic jaundice	dark	dark	normal	+	∅
Intrahepatic jaundice	light	light	dark	+	+
Posthepatic jaundice	light or ∅	acholic	dark	(+) or ∅	+

Tab. 12.6: Main colouration of duodenal bile, stools and urine as well as the results of bile pigment tests in the urine of jaundice patients (∅ = negative)

- Determination of total bilirubin with differentiation between direct (conjugated) and indirect (unconjugated) bilirubin
- Determination of cholestasis-indicating enzymes (AP, LAP, γ-GT); bile acids and bile pigments in the urine (s. tab. 12.6)
- Test for signs of haemolysis (s. tab. 12.3)
- Determination of transaminases and (possibly) enzyme quotients (s. tabs. 5.6, 5.7)
- Antimitochondrial antibodies (s. tabs. 5.20, 5.21)
- Hepatitis serology (s. tab. 5.17)
- Determination of total coproporphyrin and coproporphyrin I and III in the urine

Tab. 12.7: Important laboratory parameters for the differential diagnosis of jaundice

2. *Laparoscopy* should always be considered if the previously applied procedures have not provided any differential diagnosis.

3. *ERC* facilitates precise visualization of the bile ducts — this is also possible by means of *PTC* in cases of sonographically determined dilation of the bile ducts with suspected biliary obstruction. PTC is likewise indicated if ultrasound examination fails to produce evidence of enlarged bile ducts and/or ERC has proved inconclusive even though clinical and laboratory examinations suggest biliary obstruction. (s. pp 191, 193)

7 Therapy

Jaundice is a symptom. For this reason, there can be no standardized therapeutic concept for its treatment. Therapy is solely directed at the underlying primary cause, provided that symptom-related and curative therapeutic options are at hand.

Causal therapy: Only those forms of *obstructive jaundice* related to benign causes are open to causal treatment in the form of endoscopy (e. g. sphincterotomy) or surgery. *Operative procedures* and *interventional endoscopy* have significantly broadened the scope of therapy for mechanical jaundice, such as (*1.*) application of a stent, (*2.*) transhepatic biliary drainage, (*3.*) recanalization of strictures or stenoses, (*4.*) extraction of concrement left behind intraoperatively, and (*5.*) radiotherapy of tumour obstruction. (9, 19) • Jaundice resulting from *bacterial infection* of the bile ducts calls for the systemic and/or topical application of suitable *antibiotics*. (14, 18) •

Cholagogue agents, which are plant extracts, have become popular as supplementary therapy for stimulating bile flow, even in long-term treatment. *(see chapter 32)*

Functional hyperbilirubinaemias: These forms of jaundice do not require therapy. It is of primary importance to provide the patient with detailed information regarding the harmless nature of such disorders. • Should short-term therapy be indicated in specific cases, this can be successfully effected with phenobarbital. Both cholestyramine and cholestipol or naltrexone can be used in the treatment of pruritus. (s. p. 249) • In Crigler-Najjar type II, it may prove effective to administer phenobarbital (together with calcium phosphate), phenazone or phenytoin. With the cholestatic forms, ursodeoxycholic acid and S-adenosyl-L-methionine can be applied. • In severe cases, exchange blood transfusions or plasmapheresis as well as phototherapy (13) and possibly even liver transplantation are indicated.

References:

Jaundice
1. **Bansal, V., Schuchert, V.D.:** Jaundice in the Intensive Care Unit. Surg. Clin. North Amer. 2006; 86: 1495—1502
2. **Becker, S.D., Lamont, J.T.:** Postoperative jaundice. Semin. Liver Dis. 1988; 8: 183—186
3. **Bird, A.R., Knottenbelt, E., Jacobs, P., Maigrot, J.:** Primary shunt hyperbilirubinemia: a variant of the congenital dyserythropoietic anaemias. Postgrad. Med. J. 1991; 67: 396—398
4. **Fleming, C.R.:** Hepatobiliary complications in adults receiving nutrition support. Dig. Dis. 1994; 12: 191—198
5. **Fulop, M., Katz, S., Lawrence, Ch.:** Extreme hyperbilirubinemia. Arch. Intern. Med. 1971; 127: 254—258
6. **Greve, J.W.M., Gouma, D.J., Buurman, W.A.:** Complications in obstructive jaundice: role of endotoxins. Scand. J. Gastroenterol. 1992; 27: (Suppl. 194): 8—12
7. **Helftenbein, A., Windolf, J., Sänger, P., Hanisch, E.:** Incidence and prognosis of postoperative icterus in intensive care surgical patients. Chirurg 1997; 68: 1292—1296
8. **Iishizaki, Y., Wakayama, T., Okada, Y., Kobayashi, T.:** Magnetic resonance cholangiography for evaluation of obstructive jaundice. Amer. J. Gastroenterol. 1993; 88: 2072—2077
9. **Kauffmann, G.W., Brambs, H.-J.:** Verschlussikterus. Bildgebende Verfahren und interventionelle Radiologie. Dtsch. Ärztebl. 1988; 85: 2250—2255
10. **Klaus, D., Feine, U.:** Primäre Shunt-Hyperbilirubinämie. Dtsch. Med. Wschr. 1964; 89: 1973—1978
11. **Kuntz, H.-D., May, B.:** Veränderungen der Leberfunktion bei Schockleber und akuter Stauungsleber. Intensivmedizin 1983; 20: 17—20
12. **Matzen, P., Malchow-Moller, A., Hilden, J., Thomsen, C., Svendsen, L.B., Gammelgaard, E., Juhl, E.:** Differential diagnosis of jaundice: a pocket diagnostic chart. Liver 1984; 4: 360—371
13. **McDonagh, A.F., Lightner, D.A.:** Phototherapy and the photobiology of bilirubin. Semin. Liver Dis. 1988; 8: 272—283
14. **Miller, D.J., Keeton, G.R., Webber, B.L., Saunders, S.J.:** Jaundice in severe bacterial infection. Gastroenterology 1976; 71: 94—97
15. **Molina, E.G., Reddy, K.R.:** Postoperative jaundice. Clin. Liver Dis. 1999; 3: 477—488
16. **O'Connor, K.W., Snodgrass, P.J., Swonder, J.F., Mahoney, St., Burt, R., Cockerill, E.M., Lumeng, I.:** A blinded prospective study comparing four current noninvasive approaches in the differential diagnosis of medical versus surgical jaundice. Gastroenterology 1983; 84: 1498—1504
17. **Pierach, C.A.:** Gelbsucht bei Herzversagen. Icterus cardialis. Dtsch. Med. Wschr. 1974; 99: 1078—1084

18. **Quale, J.M., Mandel, L.J., Bergasa, N.V., Straus, E.W.:** Clinical significance and pathogenesis of hyperbilirubinemia associated with Staphylococcus aureus septicemia. Amer. J. Med. 1988; 85: 615–618
19. **Rösch, W.:** Endoskopische Verfahren zur Therapie des Verschlussikterus. Dtsch. Ärztebl. 1988; 85: 2246–2249
20. **Scharschmidt, B.F., Goldberg, H.I., Schmid, R.:** Approach to the patient with cholestatic jaundice. New Engl. J. Med. 1983; 308: 1515–1519
21. **Schölmerich, J., Spamer, C., Brambs, H.J.:** Differentialdiagnose des Ikterus. Intern. Welt 1986; 7: 1–11
22. **Vennes, J.A., Bond, J.H.:** Approach to the jaundiced patient. Gastroenterology 1983; 84: 1615–1618
23. **Zimmermann, H.J., Fang, M., Utili, R., Seff, L.B., Hoofnagle, J.:** Jaundice due to bacterial infection. Gastroenterology 1979; 77: 362–374

Functional hyperbilirubinaemia
24. **Adams, J.A., Hey, D.J., Hall, R.T.:** Incidence of hyperbilirubinemia in breast–vs. formula-fed infants. Clin. Pediatr. 1985; 24: 69–73
25. **Amit, Y., Poznansky, M.J., Schiff, D.:** Neonatal jaundice and bilirubin encephalopathy: a clinical and experimental reappraisal. Isr. J. Med. Sci. 1992; 28: 103–108
26. **Arias, M.:** Chronic unconjugated hyperbilirubinemia without overt signs of hemolysis in adolescents and adults. J. Clin. Invest. 1962; 41: 2233–2245
27. **Burchell, B., Hume, R.:** Molecular genetic basis of Gilbert's syndrome. J. Gastroenterol. Hepatol. 1999; 14: 960–966
28. **Caglayan, S., Candemir, H., Aksit, S., Kansoy, S., Asik, S., Yapiak, I.:** Superiority of oral agar and phototherapy combination in the treatment of neonatal hyperbilirubinemia. Pediatrics 1993; 92: 86–89
29. **Carre, D., Civadier, C., Foll, Y., Talarmin, B., Abgrall, J.:** Le syndrome de Rotor. A propos d'un cas. Ann. Gastroenterol. Hepatol. 1994; 30: 255–259
30. **Cosme, A., Martinez, S., Yuste, R., Alzate, L., Arenas, J.I., Gastaminza, A.:** Sindrome de Dubin-Johnson. Presentacion de tres casos. Revision de la literatura nacional. Rev. Esp. Enf. Digest. 1992; 82: 125–128
31. **Crigler, J.F. jr., Najjar, V.A.:** Congenital familial nonhemolytic jaundice with kernicterus. Pediatrics 1952; 10: 169–180
32. **De Morais, S.M.F., Uetrecht, J.P., Wells, P.G.:** Decreased glucuronidation and increased bioactivation of acetaminophen in Gilbert's syndrome. Gastroenterology 1992; 102: 577–586
33. **Dubin, I.N., Johnson, F.B.:** Chronic idiopathic jaundice with unidentified pigment in liver cells: a new clinicopathologic entity with a report of 12 cases. Medicine 1954; 33: 155–197
34. **Ellis, E., Wagner, M., Lammert, F., Nemeth, A., Gumhold, J., Strassburg, C.P., Kylander, C., Katsika, D., Trauner, M., Einarsson, C., Marschall, H.U.:** Successful treatment of severe unconjugated hyperbilirubinemia via induction of UGT 1 A1 by rifampicin (case report). J. Hepatol. 2006; 44: 243–245
35. **Frank, M., Doss, M., de Carvalho, D.G.:** Diagnostic and pathogenetic implications of urinary coproporphyrin excretion in the Dubin-Johnson syndrome. Hepato-gastroenterol. 1990; 37: 147–151
36. **Gajdos, V., Petit, F., Trioche, P., Mollet-Boudjemline, A., Chauveaud, A., Myara, A., Trivin, F., Francoual, J., Labrune, P.:** Successful pregnancy in a Crigler-Najjar type I patient treated by phototherapy and semimonthly albumin infusions (case report). Gastroenterology 2006; 131: 921–924
37. **Gentile, S., Marmo, R., Persico, M., Faccenda, F., Orlando, C., Rubba, P.:** Dissociation between vascular and metabolic effects of nicotinic acid Gilbert's syndrome. Clin. Physiol. 1990; 10: 171–178
38. **Gilbert, N.A., Lereboullet, P.:** La cholémie simple familiale. Sem. Méd. Paris 1901; 21: 241–243
39. **Gilbert, N.A., Lereboullet, P., Herscher, M.:** Les trois cholémies congénitales. Bull. Mem. Soc. Med. Hop. Paris 1907; 24: 1203–1210
40. **Gollan, J.L., Huang, S.M., Billing, B.H., Sherlock, S.:** Prolonged survival in three brothers with severe typ 2 Crigler-Najjar syndrome. Ultrastructural and metabolic studies. Gastroenterology 1975; 68: 1543–1555
41. **Green, R.M., Gollan, J.L.:** Crigler-Najjar disease type 1: therapeutic approaches to genetic liver diseases into the next century. Gastroenterology 1997; 112: 649–651
42. **Grunebaum, E., Amir, J., Merlob, P., Mimouni, M., Varsano, I.:** Breast milk jaundice: natural history, familial incidence and late neurodevelopmental outcome of the infant. Eur. J. Pediat. 1991; 150: 267–270
43. **Hashimoto, A., Uchiumi, T., Konno, T, Ebihara, T., Nakamura, T., Wada, M., Sakisaka, S., Maniwa, F., Amachi, T., Ueda, K., Kuwano, M.:** Trafficking and functional defects by mutations of the ATP-binding domains in MRP 2 in patients with Dubin-Johnson syndrome. Hepatology 2002; 36: 1236–1245
44. **Horak, J., Pokorna, B., Mertl, L., Kostihova, E., Trunecke, P.:** The nicotinic acid test in the evaluation of unconjugated hyperbilirubinemia. Z. Gastroenterol. 1989; 27: 629–632
45. **Huang, M.J., Kua, K.E., Teng, H.C., Tang, K.S., Weng, H.W., Huang, C.S.:** Risk factors for severe hyperbilirubinemia in neonates. Pediatr. Res. 2004; 56: 682–689
46. **Huang, P.W.H., Rozdilsky, B., Gerrard, J.W., Goluboff, N., Holman, G.H.:** Crigler-Najjar syndrome in four of five siblings with postmortem findings in one. Arch. Pathol. 1970; 90: 536–542
47. **Ip, S., Chung, M., Kulig, J., O'Brien, R., Sege, R., Glicken, S., Maisels, J., Lau, J.:** An evidence-based review of unportant issues concerning neonatal hyperbilirubinemia. Pediatrics 2004; 114: 130–153

48. **Jansen, P.L.M., Oude Elferink, R.P.J.:** Hereditary hyperbilirubinemia: a molecular and mechanistic approach. Semin. Liver Dis. 1988; 8: 168–178
49. **Kaplan, M., Hammerman, C., Stevenson, D.K., Vreman, H.J., Muraca, M.:** Hemolysis in Gilbert's syndrome. Hepatology 2002; 36: 764–765
50. **Kimura, A., Ushijima, K., Kage, M., Mahara, R., Tohma, M., Inokuchi, T., Shibao, K., Tanaka, N., Fujisawa, T., Ono, E., Yamashita, F.:** Neonatal Dubin-Johnson syndrome with severe cholestasis: effective phenobarbital therapy. Acta Paediatr. Scand. 1991; 80: 381–385
51. **Kivilahan, C., James, E.J.P.:** The natural history of neonatal jaundice. Pediatrics 1984; 74: 364–370
52. **Kuntz, H.-D., Femfert, U., May, B.:** Leberfunktion und Arzneimittelmetabolismus beim M. Gilbert. Z. Gastroenterol. 1986; 24: 29–30
53. **Labrune, P.H., Myara, A., Francoual, J., Trivin, F., Odievre, M.:** Cerebellar symproms as the presenting manifestations of bilirubin encephalopathy in children with Crigler-Najjar type I disease. Pediatrics 1992; 89: 768–770
54. **Lieverse, A.G., van Essen, G.G., Beukeveld, G.J.J., Gazendam, J., Dompeling, E.C., ten Kate, L.P., van Belle, S.A., Weits, J.:** Familial increased serum intestinal alkaline phosphatase: a new variant associated with Gilbert's syndrome. J. Clin. Pathol. 1990; 43: 125–128
55. **Lucey, J.F., Arias, I.M., McKay, R.J. jr.:** Transient familial neonatal hyperbilirubinemia. Amer. J. Dis. Child. 1960; 100: 787–789
56. **Maisels, J.M.:** Neonatal jaundice. Semin. Liver dis. 1988; 8: 148–162
57. **Martin, J.F., Vierling, J.M., Wolkoff, A.W., Scharschmidt, B.F., Vergalla, J., Waggoner, J.G., Berk, P.D.:** Abnormal hepatic transport of indocyanine green in Gilbert's syndrome. Gastroenterology 1976; 70: 385–391
58. **Mendez-Sanchez, N., Gonzalez, V., Flores, A., Martinez, M., Graef, A., Uribe, M.:** Delayed gastric emptying in subjects with Gilbert's syndrome. Hepato-Gastroenterol. 2001; 48: 1183–1185
59. **Meulengracht, E.:** Icterus intermittens juvenilis. (Chronischer intermittierender juveniler Subikterus). Klin. Wschr. 1939; 18: 118–121
60. **Murthy, G.D., Byron, D., Shoemaker, D., Visweswariah, H., Pasquale, D.:** The utility of rifampicin in diagnosing Gilbert's syndrome. Amer. J. Gastroenterol. 2001; 96: 1150–1154
61. **Newman, Th.B., Easterling, M.J., Goldman, E.S., Stevenson, D.K.:** Laboratory evaluation of jaundice in newborns. Amer. J. Dis. Child. 1990; 144: 364–368
62. **Nowicki, M.J., Poley, J.R.:** The hereditary hyperbilirubinaemias. Baill. Clin. Gastroenterol. 1998; 12: 355–367
63. **Ostrow, J.D., Pascolo, L., Shapiro, S.M., Tiribelli, C.:** New concepts in bilirubin encephalopathy. Europ. J. Clin. Invest. 2003; 33: 988–997
64. **Pinos, T., Constansa, J.M., Palacin, A., Figueras, C.:** A new diagnostic approach to the Dubin-Johnson syndrome. Amer. J. Gastroenterol. 1990; 85: 91–93
65. **Robertson, K.J., Clarke, D., Sutherland, L., Wooster, R., Coughtrie, M.W.H., Burchell, B.:** Investigation of the molecular basis of the genetic deficiency of UDP-glucuronosyltransferase in Crigler-Najjar syndrome. J. Inher. Metab. Dis. 1991; 14: 563–579
66. **Röllinghoff, W., Paumgartner, G., Preisig, R.:** Nicotinic acid test in the diagnosis of Gilbert's syndrome: correlation with bilirubin clearance. Gut 1981; 22: 663–668
67. **Rotor, A.B., Manahan, L., Florentin, A.:** Familial non-hemolytic jaundice with direct van den Berg reaction. Acta Med. Philipp. 1948; 5: 37–49
68. **Rubaltelli, F.F., Griffith, P.F.:** Managament of neonatal hyperbilirubinaemia and prevention of kernicterus. Drugs 1992; 43: 864–872
69. **Seligsohn, U., Shani, M.:** The Dubin-Johnson syndrome and pregnancy. Acta Hepato-Gastroenterol. 1977; 24: 167–169
70. **Shimizu, Y., Naruto, H., Ida, S., Kohakura, M.:** Urinary coproporphyrin isomers in Rotor's syndrome. A study in eight families. Hepatology 1981; 1: 173–178
71. **Sinaasappel, M., Jansen, P.L.M.:** The differential diagnosis of Crigler-Najjar disease, types 1 and 2, by bile pigment analysis. Gastroenterology 1991; 100: 783–789
72. **Sokal, E.M., Silva, E.S., Hermans, D., Reding, R., De Ville de Goyet, J., Buts, J.R., Otte, J.B.:** Orthotopic liver transplantation for Crigler-Najjar type 1 disease in six children. Transplantation 1995; 60: 1095–1098
73. **South, M., Butt, W.:** Treatment of neonatal hyperbilirubinaemia by plasmapheresis. Intensive Care Med. 1992; 18: 373–374
74. **Sprinz, H., Nelson, R.S.:** Persistent nonhemolytic hyperbilirubinemia associated with lipochrome-like pigment on liver cells: report of 4 cases. Ann. Intern. 1954; 41: 952–962
75. **Tazawa, Y., Abukawa, D., Nakagawa, M., Yamada, M.:** Abnormal results of biochemical liver function tests in breast-fed infants with prolonged indirect hyperbilirubinemia. Eur. J. Pediatr. 1991; 150: 310–313
76. **Varma, R.R., Grainger, J.M., Scheuer, P.J.:** A case of the Dubin-Johnson syndrome complicated by acute hepatitis. Gut 1970; 11: 817–821
77. **Ware, A.J., Eigenbrodt, E. Huang, P.W.H., Rozdilsky, B., Gerrard, J.W., Goluboff, N., Holman, G.H.:** Crigler-Najjar syndrome in four of five siblings with postmortem findings in one. Arch. Pathol. 1970; 90: 536–542
78. **H., Shorey, J., Combes, B.:** Viral hepatitis complicating the Dubin-Johnson syndrome. Gastroenterology 1972; 63: 331–339
79. **Wolkoff, A.W., Wolpert, E., Pascasio, F.N., Arias, I.M.:** Rotor's syndrome. A distinct inheritable pathophysiologic entity. Amer. J. Med. 1976; 60: 173–179
80. **Zimniak, P.:** Dubin-Johnson and Rotor syndromes: molecular basis and pathogenesis. Semin. Liver Dis. 1993; 13: 248–260

Symptoms and Syndromes
13 Cholestasis

		Page:
1	*Definition*	236
2	**Pathogenesis**	236
2.1	Obstructive cholestasis	236
2.2	Non-obstructive cholestasis	237
3	*Morphological changes*	237
4	**Forms of cholestasis**	238
5	**Causes of cholestasis**	238
5.1	Extrahepatic obstructive cholestasis	238
5.2	Intrahepatic obstructive cholestasis	238
5.3	Intrahepatic cholestasis	238
5.4	Genetically determined cholestasis	240
5.4.1	Primary storage diseases	240
5.4.2	Recurrent intrahepatic cholestasis in pregnancy	240
5.4.3	Benign recurrent intrahepatic cholestasis (BRIC) – Aagenaes syndrome	241
5.4.4	Progressive familial intrahepatic cholestasis (PFIC) – Byler's disease/syndrome	241
5.4.5	Zellweger's syndrome	242
5.4.6	Infantile Refsum's syndrome	242
6	**Diagnosis**	243
6.1	Anamnesis	243
6.2	Clinical findings	243
6.2.1	Fatigue	243
6.2.2	Pruritus and scratch marks	243
6.2.3	Xanthelasmas and xanthomas	243
6.2.4	Changes in biotransformation	244
6.3	Laboratory diagnostics	244
6.4	Imaging procedures	245
6.4.1	Sonography	245
6.4.2	CT and MRI	246
6.4.3	ERC, PTC and EUS	246
6.5	Liver biopsy and laparoscopy	246
7	**Clinical sequelae**	248
7.1	Abdominal complaints	248
7.2	Steatorrhoea and diarrhoea	248
7.3	Malabsorption	248
7.4	Osteopathy	248
7.5	Renal dysfunction	248
8	**Therapy**	248
8.1	Mechanical cholestasis	248
8.2	Functional cholestasis	248
	• References (1–82)	249

(Figures. 13.1–13.8; tables 13.1–13.11)

13 Cholestasis

1 Definition

Cholestasis is defined as a disorder of cholepoiesis and bile secretion as well as a mechanical or functional stoppage of the bile flow in intrahepatic or extrahepatic bile ducts − with bile components passing into the blood. • *Cholestasis can occur both with and without jaundice.*

Morphology: The morphologist uses the term cholestasis to describe the presence of bile in the hepatocytes and hypertrophic Kupffer cells (= *cellular bilirubinostasis*), particularly in the form of inspissated bile droplets and copper within the more or less dilated canaliculi (= *canalicular bilirubinostasis*). • In extrahepatic cholestasis, bile is also found within the likewise mostly dilated interlobular bile ducts (= *ductular bilirubinostasis*) as well as in the parenchyma in the form of *"bile infarcts"* or *"bile lakes"*.

Pathophysiology: The biochemist defines cholestasis as a decrease in the secretion of bile as well as a reduction in the proportion of water, together with a respective effect on the substances dissolved in it.

Clinical aspects: The clinician diagnoses cholestasis by the increase in bile acids, special enzymatic markers and cholesterol in the serum.

▶ The *principal biochemical symptom of cholestasis* is the rise in bile acids in serum (as well as changes in its spectrum) in combination with an increase in enzymatic markers of cholestasis (AP, LAP, γ-GT, 5′-nucleotidase). Cholestasis is directly related to the metabolism of bile acids. • In clinical terms, the subsequent rise in activity of enzymatic markers of cholestasis may be attributed to cholestasis, yet these enzymes are not necessarily specific to this condition. (s. p. 107)

▶ Dysfunction in the metabolism of bile acids (= *cholestasis*) is often combined with an additional dysfunction in bilirubin metabolism (= *jaundice*). The rise in bilirubin is the main biochemical and clinical symptom of jaundice; it is based on a disorder of bilirubin metabolism. Thus cholestasis is related not directly but indirectly to jaundice. • Depending on the constellation of the biochemical and clinical findings, the term *"jaundice with cholestasis"* or *"cholestasis with jaundice"* can be applied. (s. tabs. 12.1, 12.2, 12.4; 13.1) • *The main clinical sign of advanced cholestasis is pruritus.*

Various hepatobiliary diseases remain unchanged as either **cholestasis** or **jaundice**. • Often, however, a *combination of both disorders* is present from the very beginning or appears during the course of disease.

2 Pathogenesis

The liver cell is a polar unit. • The resorptive processes take place at the sinusoidal and lateral membrane, the secretory processes on the surface of the canaliculi. The cytoskeleton (microfilaments, microtubules, intracellular membranes) maintains the polar orientation of the hepatocyte. (25, 33, 42, 44, 71, 82) (s. fig. 13.1)

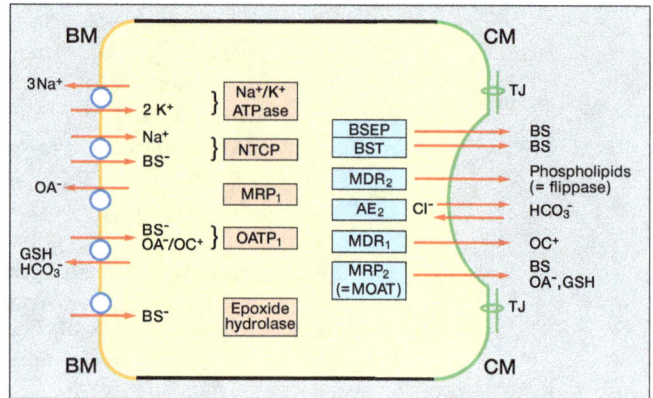

Fig. 13.1: The hepatocyte as a polar unit. • *Major hepatocellular transport systems:* CM = canalicular membrane, BM = basolateral membrane, TJ = tight junctions, BS$^-$ = bile salts, OA$^-$ = organic anions, OC$^+$ = organic cations, GSH = reduced glutathione, AE$_2$ = ATP-dependent anion exchange (Cl/HCO$_3^-$; GSH), BST = ATP-dependent bile acid transporter, NTCP = sinusoidal Na$^+$-dependent taurocholate cotransporting protein, OATP$_1$ = sinusoidal Na$^+$-independent organic anion (and cation) transporter protein, BSEP = bile salt export pump for monovalent bile salts, MRP$_2$ = canalicular multispecific organic anion transporter (= MOAT), MDR$_1$ = ATP-dependent organic cation transporter, MDR$_2$ = ATP-dependent phospholipid transporter (= flippase), MRP$_1$ = sinusoidal multidrug resistance-associated protein

2.1 Obstructive cholestasis

Obstructive cholestasis − initially often without jaundice, thereafter generally with jaundice − is caused by a mechanical impediment of the bile flow. Because of this, the bile flow is reduced and biliary stasis is generated, which, depending on the localization of the impediment, subsequently affects the bile ducts of (*1.*) the entire liver or (*2.*) only certain subzones of the liver.

Even in cases of a total obstruction with jaundice, there is no total stoppage of bile secretion due to the residual function of the hepatocytes. What happens, in fact, is that a certain form of **circulation of intrahepatic bile acids** is maintained by way of resorption processes taking place in the bile capillaries and mechanisms of regurgitation occurring at the tight junctions. This circulation of bile acids mainly runs via the periportal sections of the hepatic lobules, so that biliary thrombi are only rarely detectable here − even in cases of prolonged cholestasis. • In obstructive cholestasis, with its secondary repercussions on bile capillaries and hepatic cells, including *morphological changes,* it is probable that *functional disorders* in the polarity of the hepatocytes will ultimately appear.

2.2 Non-obstructive cholestasis

Pathogenetically, non-obstructive cholestasis is a multifactorial process. • The factors that cause intrahepatic cholestasis lead to biochemical dysfunctions and/or damage to subcellular structures, with changes in the metabolism of bile acids.

(*1.*) Various substances (taurolithocholate, ethinyl oestradiol, drugs, toxins) cause increased retention of cholesterol in cellular membranes. As a result, the permeability of hepatocellular membranes, including the tight junctions, is decreased. Hypothermia and hypoxia also disturb membrane fluidity. The osmotic pressure gradient, necessary for biliary secretion, is no longer maintained because of decreased membrane permeability.

(*2.*) Considerable dysfunction of membrane lipids is caused by a change in the double-bonding of their unsaturated fatty acids due to lipid peroxidation. More pronounced lipid peroxidations are found particularly in alcohol-induced liver damage – often accompanied by cholestasis.

(*3.*) Na^+/K^+-ATPase localized in the sinusoidal and lateral hepatocyte membrane is inhibited by cholestasis factors (chlorpromazine, oestrogens, atypical bile acids, protoporphyrin, etc.) as well as by a change in the viscosity and fluidity of the membrane. Na^+/K^+-ATPase activity works like a metabolic pump and supplies the energy needed for the cellular uptake of bile acids (along with bicarbonate and chloride).

(*4.*) Mg^{2+}-ATPase activity can likewise be inhibited in the canalicular side of the membrane by cholestatic factors (in particular bile acids). This metabolic pump transports bicarbonate and chloride into the canaliculi and is probably closely associated with the function of the microfilaments.

(*5.*) Transmembranous transport of biliary acids requires the functional competence of the carrier proteins in the sinusoidal and canalicular membrane. Cholestatic factors may also appear. Furthermore, it is possible for various substances, above all medicaments, to effect competitive inhibition of the carrier proteins in the sinusoidal wall as a result of the low substrate specificity of these proteins.

(*6.*) Intracellular transport of bile acids mainly takes place through the cytoskeleton and intracellular structures (Golgi apparatus, endoplasmic reticulum). Here, too, cholestatic factors can prove to be damaging. Microfilaments are contractile elements: not only is the intracellular transport of the bile acids disturbed, but the peristaltic activity of the canaliculi (so-called **paralytic cholestasis** within the lobules) is also reduced if the functional capacity of those microfilaments becomes diminished.

(*7.*) Shifting of the calcium gradient between the intracellular and extracellular space (normally 1 : 10,000) results in significant metabolic dysfunctions as well as cholestasis, especially in alcohol-induced liver damage.

(*8.*) Inhibition of the neosynthesis of bile acids from cholesterol leads to a decrease in the bile acid pool.

(*9.*) Monohydroxy bile acids (such as lithocholic acid produced in the intestine) are deemed to be cholestatic factors. They can, however, also be generated in the liver as a result of damage to the smooth endoplasmic reticulum, with a decrease in activity of cytochrome P 450-dependent 7α-hydroxylase: in cases of cholestasis, 3β-hydroxy-5δ-cholic acid is formed from cholesterol and converted into lithocholic acid and allo-lithocholic acid (so-called **foetal metabolic pathway of bile acids**). (10)

(*10.*) Intracellular accumulation of bile acids continues to maintain the state of cholestasis. Bile acids are detergents that cause damage to biomembranes.

Endotoxins generated in the body are broken down in the RES. Given inadequate clearance (e.g. in cholestasis) or when they are formed to excess, the state of cholestasis is reinforced. Endotoxins also lead to inflammatory reactions in the liver and are possibly the cause of complications in cases of prolonged cholestasis. (51)

The mechanisms leading to cholestasis are based on different aetiopathological factors. One single cause of cholestasis disturbs several subprocesses in the metabolism of bile acids, which in turn may trigger additional cholestatic mechanisms. Such disorders result in damage to cellular and biliary structures, leading to further dysfunctions and reinforcing cholestasis. Thus pathogenic mechanisms, acting in a synergy of addition or potentiation, set up a vicious circle culminating in cholestatis. (15, 17, 22, 33, 44, 71, 82)

3 Morphological changes

In the development of morphological damage to hepatocytes and bile capillaries, *lipid peroxidations* as well as the formation of *leukotrienes* (C4, D4, E4) play a key role, with *prostaglandin E_2* having a reinforcing effect.

▶ After only a few days, cholestasis causes potentially reversible **ultrastructural changes:**

— hydropic swelling of periportal hepatocytes,
— reinforced granulation of the cytoplasm,
— formation of Mallory's bodies,
— change in the mitochondria, formation of giant mitochondria,
— hypertrophy and subsequent reduction as well as loss of the Golgi apparatus at the canalicular pole,
— hypertrophy of the pericanalicular filaments,
— hypertrophy of the SER and RER with subsequent reduction,
— apoptosis due to bile acids.

▶ As the disease advances, **histological changes** in cholestasis can be detected by light microscopy:

— dilation of the bile capillaries due to stasis, or loss of tone in the pericanalicular microfilaments,
— flattening and ultimate loss of the microvilli at the canalicular membrane,
— formation of bile thrombi in various bile capillaries (= *cholate stasis*),
— damage to cell membranes leading to greater permeability,
— leakage at the tight junctions with subsequent paracellular regurgitation of bile into the blood,
— centroacinar, perivenular cholestasis with traces of bilirubin, and often copper, in hepatocytes and dilated canaliculi (= *bilirubinostasis*),
— biliary metaplasia of hepatocytes, linked with newly-formed bile ductules, probably caused by abnormal bile constituents (= *liver cell rosette*). This represents reversion to previous phylogenetic stages,

- uptake of biliary precipitates and components into the ductular epithelia,
- proliferation of the ductules in the portal tracts; periductal oedema,
- periportal and mesenchymal inflammatory reactions,
- widening of the portal tracts due to an increase in collagenous connective tissue; periductular sclerosis,
- hepatocytes with foamy pale cytoplasm (= *feathery degeneration*), (s. p. 246) (s. fig. 13.4)
- isolated necroses of hepatocytes (= *network necrosis*),
- extensive focal necroses of hepatocytes with the central part of each displaying a marked accumulation of bilirubin due to the fact that bilirubin has a stronger affinity for necrotic tissue (= *bile infarcts*),
- formation of bile extravasates in the parenchyma (= *bile lakes*),
- development of microabscesses,
- cell death with cellular condensation and cell shrinkage (= *apoptosis*), (17)
- development of lipid-laden macrophages (= *xanthoma cells*). (s. fig. 13.2)

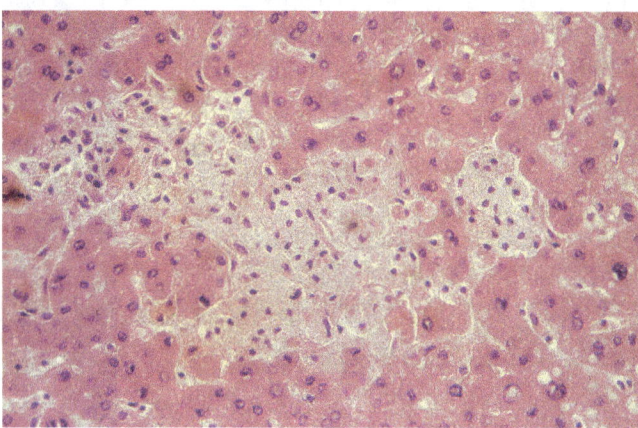

Fig. 13.2: Chronic cholestasis with granuloma-like accumulation of lipid-laden macrophages (xanthoma cells) (HE)

Persistent cholestasis with concomitant inflammatory and connective tissue reactions leads to irreversible cholestasis and, after months/years, to **biliary fibrosis** with preserved liver structure, or to (primary or secondary) **biliary cirrhosis**. (15, 17, 24, 70)

4 Forms of cholestasis

In classifying cholestasis, the *cause, localization* and *duration* of the disease as well as the involvement of *bilirubin metabolism* must be considered. Laboratory parameters of *liver cell damage* (increased activity of GPT, GOT and GDH) may be attributed to the underlying liver disease, but can also appear subsequently during the course of cholestasis-related hepatocellular damage. (s. tab. 13.1)

Concurrent **jaundice** is either due to an additional disorder of bilirubin metabolism or to mechanical biliary stasis (= if more than two-thirds of the efferent bile ducts are obstructed). During the course of its development, cholestasis may also lead to dysfunction and/or morphological damage, with subsequent jaundice.

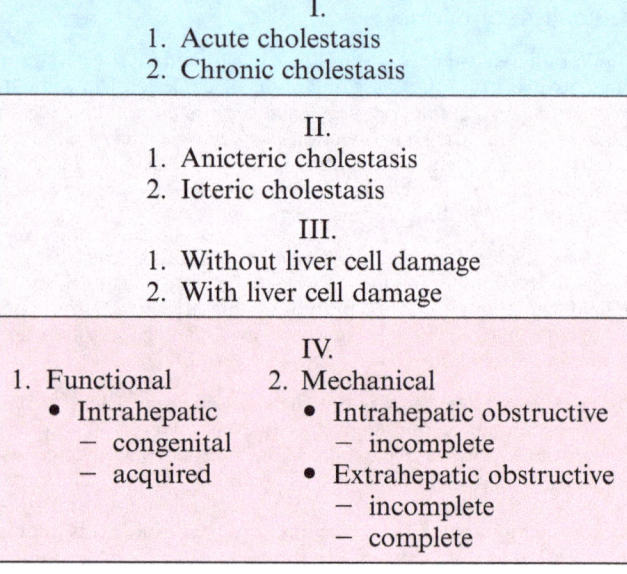

Tab. 13.1: Forms of cholestasis

5 Causes of cholestasis

There are many causes of cholestasis — *with or without jaundice* — which is why this condition proves to be an ambiguous symptom in terms of differential diagnosis.

5.1 Extrahepatic obstructive cholestasis

The bile flow is interrupted in its passage from the porta hepatis to the duodenum as a result of (*1.*) intraluminal obstruction, (*2.*) obliterating disease of the biliary duct walls, or (*3.*) compression of the extrahepatic efferent bile ducts. This form of cholestasis can be sudden in onset or progress slowly, may be transient or persistent, and occurs either as incomplete or complete obstruction with jaundice. (s. tab. 13.2) (s. figs. 8.14, 8.15; 25.8)

5.2 Intrahepatic obstructive cholestasis

This form of cholestasis is derived from a temporary or permanent obstruction of the intrahepatic bile ducts. Diffuse processes of disease can act as mechanical obstacles in the hepatic parenchyma, or major bile ducts may be subject to regional obstruction. (s. tab. 13.3)

5.3 Intrahepatic cholestasis

Intrahepatic cholestasis has numerous causes, primarily disturbing the metabolism or transport mechanisms of bile acids at various sites of action. (s. tab. 13.4) It is

Obstruction in the area of the papilla of Vater	
– inflammation	– adenomatosis
– choledocholithiasis	– choledochal cyst
– neoplasia	– parasites
– scars	– heterotopic gastric mucosa
– duodenal diverticulum	etc.
Obstruction in the area of the bile ducts	
– choledocholithiasis	– duodenal diverticulum
– neoplasia	– papillomatosis
– postoperative strictures	– haemobilia
– cicatricial distortions	– actinomycosis
– pancreatic cyst, pancreatitis	– parasites
– pancreatic carcinoma	– bile-duct atresia
– gall-bladder carcinoma	– Mirizzi syndrome
– choledochal cyst	etc.

Tab. 13.2: Causes of extrahepatic obstructive cholestasis (with or without initial jaundice; however, consecutive jaundice may develop later)

Focal changes of the liver	
– adenomas	– Hodgkin's disease (31)
– haemangiomas	– parasites
– cysts	– hepatolithiasis
– tumours	– Caroli's syndrome
– abscesses	– congenital liver fibrosis
Disseminated changes of the liver	
– sarcoidosis (60)	
– tuberculosis	
– other types of granulomatosis	
– mucoviscidosis	
Infiltrative changes of the liver	
– leukaemia	
– amyloidosis (4, 59, 81)	
– primary storage diseases	
– fatty liver	
Inflammatory proliferation of bile ducts	
– primary biliary cholangitis	
– primary sclerosing cholangitis	
– bacterial cholangitis	
– autoimmune cholangitis	
– cholangiofibromatosis (35)	
Other partially unclarified causes	
– haemobilia	
– graft-versus-host disease	
– chronic rejection reaction	
– syndromatic bile-duct hypoplasia (Alagille's syndrome) (see also tab. 13.4)	
– non-syndromatic bile-duct hypoplasia (Zellweger's syndrome) (see also tab. 13.4)	

Tab. 13.3: Causes of intrahepatic obstructive cholestasis (with some references)

Acquired causes	
Alcohol	Medicaments (s. tabs. 13.5; 29.11)
Autoimmune hepatitis	Mycotoxins
Bacterial infections	Paraneoplastic syndrome
Budd-Chiari syndrome	Parasitic infections
Chemicals	Parenteral nutrition (18, 45, 47)
Chronic hepatitis	Postoperative cholestasis
Cirrhosis	Primary biliary cholangitis
Endotoxins (51)	Primary sclerosing cholangitis
Fatty liver	Protoporphyria
Giant-cell hepatitis	Right ventricular failure
Heat-stroke	Sepsis (9, 46)
Hyperthyroidism	Virus infections (A–E, CM, EBV)
Ischaemia	Zieve's syndrome, etc.
Genetic (congenital) determination	

- Primary storage diseases *(see chapter 31)*
  – Wilson's disease, haemochromatosis, galactosaemia, glycogenosis type IV, α_1-antitrypsin deficiency, tyrosinaemia, idiopathic neonatal hepatitis, Niemann-Pick disease, Gaucher's disease, fructose intolerance, defective urea cycle, *etc.*
- Benign recurrent intrahepatic cholestasis (BRIC)
  – Aagenaes type
- Progressive familial intrahepatic cholestasis (PFIC)
  – Byler's syndrome
- Recurrent intrahepatic cholestasis of pregnancy
  – infantile Refsum's syndrome
- Alagille's syndrome *(see chapter 33.7)*
- Disorders of bile acid biosynthesis
  – disorders of side-chain catabolism
    = Zellweger's syndrome
    = (dihydroxycoprostanic acid) (DHCA)
    = (trihydroxycoprostanic acid) (THCA)
  – disorders at the steroid ring
    = defect of 7α-hydroxylase
    = defect of 3β-hydroxy-5δ-dehydrogenase/isomerase
    = defect of 3-oxo-4δ-steroid-5β-reductase

Tab. 13.4: Causes of non-obstructive intrahepatic cholestasis (with or without concurrent jaundice)

not always clear how the pathogenic mechanism triggers cholestasis. It cannot be adequately explained why one particular cause acts as a cholestatic factor in the individual case or why the same factor possibly has no effect at all. It would appear that genetic disposition is of decisive importance. Influences of everyday life (xenobiotics, drugs, alcohol, etc.), differing performances of biotransformation or coexistent diseases possibly all play a part in whether an individual cause has a cholestatic effect or not. • The *primary form* of intrahepatic cholestasis occurs without any prior disease of the liver (e. g. sepsis, whereby lipopolysacharides trigger the increase of cytokines and NO). The *secondary form* shows evidence of a previous or coexistent liver condition.

Alcohol-induced cholestasis: Alcohol is the most frequent cause of cholestasis. Concomitant jaundice is found in relatively few cases and is generally a sign of a severe course of disease. (52) (s. figs. 28.18, 28.19)

Drug-induced cholestasis: Many drugs can cause cholestasis (so-called *cholestasis type*). (s. tab. 13.5) It can be extremely difficult to pinpoint which drug has led to the condition. Interestingly, some homeopathic remedies, such as Chelidonium majus, may also cause cholestasis. Simultaneous uptake of other hepatocellular irritants can trigger or produce cholestasis. Concomitant jaundice is not usually present at first, but may develop at a later stage of disease. Many drugs cause *cholestatic hepatitis* per se or in conjunction with others. (s. tab. 29.6) As a rule, cholestasis regresses gradually after discontinuation of the drug or elimination of further irritants. It should, however, be noted that cholestasis is sometimes only diagnosed when a drug has been discontinued; with some other drugs (e.g. amoxicillin-clavulanic acid, ticlopidine), the condition may even progress until the bile ducts have completely disappeared (= *vanishing bile-duct syndrome*). (12) (s. pp 696, 700)

ACE inhibitors	Haloperidol
Amoxicillin-clavulanic acid	Imipramine
Atenolol	Ketoconazole
Azathioprine	Methyltestosterone
β-blockers	Nitrofurantoin
Benzodiazepines	Oestrogens
Busulphan	Penicillamine
Chlorothiazide	Phenylbutazone
Chlorpromazine	Phenytoin
Chlorpropamide	Phytotherapeutics
Clofibrate	Prochloperazine
Cyclosporin A	Propafenone
Danazol	Provastatine
Dicloxacillin	Sulfonamides
Disopyramide	Tamoxifen
Erythromycin	Thiabendazole
Ethambutol	Thiamazol
Floxuridine	Ticlopidine
Flurazepam	Tolazamide
Furosemide	Tolbutamide
Gold salts	Trimethoprin-sulphamethoxazole
Griseofulvin	Valproic acid
H_2 blockers	Warfarin, *etc.*

Tab. 13.5: Drugs known to cause cholestasis/cholestatic hepatitis (s. figs. 29.3, 29.4) (s. tab. 29.11)

Virus infections: *Acute viral hepatitis* (HAV, HEV, HCV) is accompanied by cholestasis in 5−20% of cases. (61) The frequency differs from country to country. It is most prevalent in those with a severe form of the disease, elderly people and women. • Cholestasis is also common in *viral infections with concomitant hepatitis*, especially due to CMV, Coxsackie virus, rubella virus, HSV (types I, II, IV), HIV, REO virus (type III), parvovirus (type B 19), and ECHO virus (types 9, 11, 14, 19).

Perinatal asphyxia: In 8−10% of asphyxiated newborns, transient cholestasis was found. The actual condition was related to the severity of neonatal stress. (24)

Others: There are many other causes of intrahepatic cholestasis that make differential diagnosis considerably more complex. (64, 70) (s. tab. 13.4)

▶ Nevertheless, jaundice does not necessarily develop as a symptom, which is why anicteric courses of the disease can also be assigned to the "cholestasis" group.

5.4 Genetically determined cholestasis

In various forms of genetically determined cholestasis, jaundice can be the most obvious primary clinical symptom leading to the clinical classification of functional hyperbilirubinaemia. • However, in most cases, pronounced cholestasis is the principal feature of the clinical picture in the diseases explained below. Many primary storage diseases, especially childhood cholestasis, can only be identified through careful differential diagnosis. Genetically determined intrahepatic cholestasis can be divided into three categories: (*1.*) bile duct defects (syndromatic or non-syndromatic), (*2.*) primary storage diseases, and (*3.*) familial intrahepatic cholestasis.

5.4.1 Primary storage diseases

When cholestasis is observed in children or young adults, a differential diagnosis is necessary to detect the possible presence of a primary storage disease. (s. tab. 13.4) Such diseases include $α_1$-antitrypsin deficiency, fructose intolerance, galactosaemia, Gaucher's disease, type IV glycogenosis, haemochromatosis, urea cycle deficiencies, Niemann-Pick disease, thyrosinaemia, and Wilson's disease. In genetically determined cholestasis, laboratory evidence of cholestasis is ultimately a secondary symptom, since primary storage diseases usually have their own specific phenotypical markers, which makes differential diagnosis easier. • *Evidence of cholestasis, with or without increased transaminases, should always be taken as a hint of a primary storage disease.*

5.4.2 Recurrent intrahepatic cholestasis in pregnancy

▶ Since the condition was first described by A. SVANBORG (1954), observations regarding both non-recurrent forms (W.C. NIXON et al., 1947) and recurrent forms (G. LUNDGREN, 1956) have been summarized under a collective term.

The disease is subject to **recessive autosomal transmission.** Given a genetic disposition (a defect in phosphatidylcholine transport (?) located on chromosome 7 q 21), a concurrent sensitivity to oestrogen, or inhibition of bile acid transport due to an increase in oestrogen/progesterone metabolites, the frequency is 1:2,000 to 8,000. There is no preference for any particular age group. The frequency is influenced by geographic, ethnic and seasonal factors. The relapse quota is 40−60%.

As a **clinical symptom,** severe *itching* (initially on the palms and soles of the feet and then all over the body), which can be intolerable at night, occurs during the 2nd or 3rd trimester. This results in pronounced sanguineous *scratch marks* (s. p. 243) • About two weeks after the onset of pruritus, *jaundice* (2−6 mg/dl) is evident in 50−70% of patients. There is conjugated hyperbilirubinaemia with bilirubinuria and urobilinogenuria in 60−80% of cases. *Laboratory biochemistry* reveals an elevation of bile acids in the serum which is 10 to 30(−100) times the standard level. Primary bile acids are usually displaced in favour of secondary forms and trihydroxylated bile acids in favour of dihydroxylated forms. AP (including placental AP) increases six to ten times, and LAP is likewise drastically elevated. Surprisingly, γ-GT is normal to subnormal, which can probably be attributed to the impact of oestrogen, especially in those pregnant women who are sensitive to this hormone. The transaminases are only moderately increased, GDH is mostly normal. There is a marked rise in cholesterol and neutral fats. Quick's value is diminished owing to disorders in the absorption of vitamin K. HLA A1 and B8 as well as BW16 are frequently detected. Steatorrhoea is often seen. Cholelithiasis is common in these women. • This syndrome is indicative of a *high-risk pregnancy*. In about 20% of cases, delivery is premature and/or the newborn is small for date; in 5–10% of cases, perinatal mortality can be expected. Fetal malformations are not to be feared. There is no danger to the mother, which is why there are no grounds for a termination of the pregnancy from this point of view. Induction of labour should, however, be considered from the 37th week onwards. (20, 32, 43, 54, 58)

Histologically, cholestasis is moderate, focal and irregular, and the biliary capillaries are dilated, displaying biliary thrombi. Bile pigments may be detectable in the liver cells. Cell necroses and signs of inflammation are absent.

Therapy involves the use of *cholestyramine* (3 x 4 g/day) or *cholestipol* (3 x 5 g/day) to alleviate and eliminate the intense itching, which is generally intolerable. *Epomediol* has also proved effective. Good results can be achieved with *ursodeoxycholic acid* (10–15 mg/kg BW/day); it was reported that high doses of UDCA (1.5–2.0 g/day) were most efficacious. There have been no reports of negative effects after application in human beings. (80) Treatment with *S-adenosyl-L-methionine* is also worth considering. Administration of *medium-chain fatty acids* and fat-soluble vitamins, in particular vitamin K, is also recommended. The prognosis is good. After delivery, the clinical picture recedes without additional consequences. Relapses can be expected in further pregnancies and after administration of oestrogen. (54)

5.4.3 Benign recurrent intrahepatic cholestasis

▶ This benign course of disease was described by W. H. J. SUMMERSKILL et al. (1959) (67) and N. TYGSTRUP (1960). (72) Since then, this form has been known as the *Summerskill-Tygstrup type*.

Benign recurrent intrahepatic cholestasis (BRIC) is subject to recessive autosomal transmission. The genetic defect is located on chromosome 18q21–q22, as in Byler's disease (PFIC 1). Up to now, publications have focused on about 100 cases. It manifests at any age, but not before the 6th–9th month of life. Even after many years without symptoms, it may be triggered by infections, toxins, allergens or other chemical substances. It begins usually with nausea, loss of appetite, abdominal pains and pruritus, followed one or two weeks later by jaundice with intermittent bilirubin values of 5–50 mg/dl. Mainly conjugated bilirubin is detectable (60–80%), covalently bound to albumin. The jaundice lasts for two or three months. On occasions, (inexplicable) coughing was observed as well as gingivitis following bilirubin decrease. Extreme fatigue is usually experienced. (34) During the icteric phase, the urine shows increased concentrations of bilirubin and urobilinogen as well as porphyrinuria, whereas stools are (largely) acholic and as such decolourized. In most cases, steatorrhoea is in evidence. Laboratory values reveal an elevation of bile acids (particularly the hepatoprotective cholic acid), AP and LAP. The transaminases are normal or moderately elevated; γ-GT shows more or less regular levels (oestrogen effect?). Quick's value can be lower due to steatorrhoea. Hepatomegaly is frequently detectable; splenomegaly is only rarely observed. Laboratory parameters may periodically improve or even normalize. The prognosis is good. Cholelithiasis is, however, frequently present. • *Histologically*, intracanalicular biliary thrombi (which are capable of regression) as well as periportal round-cell infiltrations are evident. • Bile pigment can be detected in the hepatocytes and Kupffer cells. Focal necroses are rare. Histology is normal during the disease-free period. A fine fibrosis may develop in cases of prolonged illness. (8, 11, 26, 28, 39, 49, 55, 56, 67, 73, 76)

Treatment of icteric episodes with *phenobarbital* (3 x 20–60 mg/day) together with *phototherapy* (430–470 nm, 8–12 hr/day), MARS (26, 66) and/or *plasmapheresis* is indicated. • *Cholestyramine* (3 x 4 g/day) or *cholestipol* (3 x 5 g/day) may be used to treat pruritus. Other effective antipruritics are *naloxone* (i.v.) or *naltrexone* (2–4 x 25–50 mg/day), which act as opioidergic neurotransmitters. (69) It is also possible to use the 5-HT3 antagonist *ondansetron* (i.v. or orally). (63) Refractory cholestasis pruritus has been treated successfully with *dronabinol* (50) and *sertraline*. • Administration of UCDA (22, 53), medium-chain fatty acids, PUFA (65) and fat-soluble vitamins (especially vitamin K) is recommended. (s. tab. 13.11)

Aagenaes type

This rare form, which is inherited via a recessive autosomal route, was described in 1968 as a variant of BRIC. (1, 2) The genetic defect is located on chromosome 15 q. A specific feature of this disease in neonates is giant-cell hepatitis with cholestasis. (s. p. 425) From about the sixth year of life until puberty, hypoplasia or ectasia of the lymphatic vessels with oedema are found in the lower extremities. It is not clear whether (suspected) congenital hyperplasia of lymphatic vessels in the liver is the prime cause of cholestasis. Pronounced fibrosis is often evident, whereas cirrhosis occurs rarely. About 50% of patients can expect a normal lifespan. (14)

5.4.4 Progressive familial intrahepatic cholestasis

Progressive familial intrahepatic cholestasis (PFIC) was described by R.C. JUBERG et al. (1966) (30) and R.J. CLAYTON et al. (1969) (9). This rare clinical picture was previously known as *Byler's disease* or *Juberg-Clayton type*. It comprises a heterogeneous group of patients with chronic non-recurrent cholestasis and is inherited via an autosomal recessive route. The disease was originally named after Jacob and Nancy Byler because it was first found in members of this Amish family. • The pathogenesis arises from deficiency of one or more genes that encode essential proteins required for bile secretion. This results in a bile secretion disorder and impaired bile flow. The key transport proteins have since been discovered, so that it is now possible to differentiate between *four PFIC syndromes*. (3, 11, 13, 23, 27, 75, 77)

Byler's disease: In this disorder, which is also known as *PFIC 1*, the genetic mutations are positioned on chromosome 18q21–22. The PFIC 1 defect can be found on the canalicular membrane of the hepatocytes and the apical membrane of the cholangiocytes. (16) As a result, aminophospholipid transport is impaired. This gene mutation also occurs in other epithelial body tissue, which explains the multisystem manifestation of this disorder. • The disease usually has its onset around the end of the first year of life and is characterized by pruritus and hepatomegaly as well as elevated bile acids in the serum. Gamma GT values are normal or reduced. Jaundice episodes of varying intensity together with cholestasis lead to severe malabsorption and developmental disorders. Chronic bronchitis is common in childhood. Byler's disease is generally fatal after 3-20 years. Liver cirrhosis with consequential hepatocellular carcinoma frequently develops in these patients. (9, 16, 37)

Byler's syndrome: Mutations of genes *PFIC 2–4* are associated with this syndrome and inherited via an autosomal recessive route. All these forms are characterized by non-recurrent cholestasis.

PFIC 2: This gene mutation, which is located on chromosome 2q24, impairs the canalicular bile salt export pump (BSEP), resulting in the accumulation of bile acids in hepatocytes. Laboratory tests show an increase in bile acid, AP and LAP levels with lowered gamma GT and cholesterol levels. Pruritus is common. There is histological evidence of neonatal giant cell hepatitis. Prognosis is poor.

PFIC 3: The gene mutation is located on chromosome 7q21. This produces an MDR-3 protein deficiency, resulting in anomalous secretion of phospholipids, which leaves the bile ducts unprotected against bile acids. AP, LAP and gamma GT levels are elevated and bile acid and cholesterol concentrations increase; LP-X can be detected. Pruritus and hepatomegaly also occur. Clinical symptoms appear later in life than is the case with forms 1 and 2. Histology reveals ductal proliferation with inflamed portal and periportal infiltrates, resembling primary sclerosing cholangitis.

PFIC 4: This syndrome is caused by a genetically determined 3β-hydroxy-C_{27}-steroid dehydrogenase deficiency, resulting in disturbed bile acid metabolism. There is no pruritus; bile acids and gamma GT levels are reduced, and the concentration of conjugated bilirubin increases.
• In the PFIC 4 syndrome, the combined application of cholic, chenodeoxycholic and ursodeoxycholic acid leads to good results. (78)

The **treatment** for these disorders is limited. Antipruritic agents and UDCA are indicated for itching. Good dietary management lowers the risk of malnutrition. Biphosphonates and calcium can have a positive effect on bone density. As yet, there is no medical treatment available for the often annoying chronic fatigue syndrome. • Liver transplantation may ultimately be indicated.

5.4.5 Zellweger's syndrome

This condition was first described as **cerebrohepatorenal syndrome** by P. BOWEN et al. in 1964. It was named after H. ZELLWEGER, a coauthor of the publication, who had observed two infants with such complex malformations. (6) The syndrome is an autosomal recessive genetic absence of peroxisomes in the liver and kidneys caused by mRNA mutation of peroxisome assembly factor 1. This impairs bile acid synthesis in the side chain and compromises β-oxidation of long-chain fatty acids. The peroxisome enzymes are not fully synthesized on free polysomes and thus unable to enter the peroxisomes. The absence of peroxisomes and the enzyme deficiency usually result in congenital abnormalities. • Biochemistry reveals an accumulation of long-chain fatty acids in plasma, brain and fibroblasts, a reduction in tissue plasmalogens, hyperpipecolic acidosis, and dicarboxylic aciduria. Bile acid synthesis remains at the C_{27}-bile acid stage. This often leads to damage to the mitochondria, which appear strikingly small and dense. • Clinical examination shows multiple abnormalities of the skull, face, brain and nervous system with areflexia and hypotonia; polycystic kidneys with renal insufficiency and hepatomegaly are also found. Laboratory findings include hypothrombinaemia, cholestasis, jaundice and hypersiderinaemia (with iron deposits in liver, brain and kidneys). Liver fibrosis or cirrhosis and enlarged bile ducts develop rapidly. • *Treatment* using clofibrate has not been effective. Improvements were observed after using cholic acid and chenodeoxycholic acid. However, prognosis is still poor, and most infants die after a few months. (36, 41) (s. tab. 13.4)

5.4.6 Infantile Refsum's syndrome

This rare condition was first discovered in 1937, but not reported until 1945 by S. REFSUM, who termed it *heredoataxia hemeralopia polyneuritiformis*. (57) Refsum's syndrome is caused by an autosomal recessive genetic defect in several peroxismal enzymes. It is primarily due to a phytanic acid-hydroxilase deficiency (or protein 7, which transports this enzyme into the peroxisomes). This causes an increase in phytanic acid levels in the serum, with subsequent deposition of the substance in liver, brain, kidney and skin tissues. • Clinical examination reveals neonatal cholestasis with jaundice and hepatomegaly. This disease becomes manifest in patients aged 20–30. Men and women are affected equally. *Therapy* consists of eliminating phytanic acid from the diet. Pigmentary retinopathy, peripheral polyneuritis and ataxia also occur (21). (s. tab. 13.4)

6 Diagnosis

6.1 Anamnesis

Careful anamnesis (with meticulous precision and detailed detective work) allows important information to be gathered for the distinction between intrahepatic and extrahepatic cholestasis. Questions about medication and hormone intake, chemicals (occupation, hobbies, house and garden), alcohol, teas (containing alkaloids), cosmetics, etc. as well as about fever, arthralgia, pruritus and discolouration of the stools or urine are mandatory in this context. (s. tab. 12.5) (s. p. 80)

6.2 Clinical findings

6.2.1 Fatigue

In chronic cholestasis, pronounced fatigue occurs in 65–68% of patients with PBC, which is the same frequency as in PSC and drug-induced cholestasis. In approximately half of these patients, fatigue is regarded as the most unpleasant symptom. However, fatigue has no correlation with the degree of cholestasis, liver histology or age. (34) Four possibilities are discussed with respect to pathogenesis: (*1.*) alteration of the hypothalamus-pituitary-adrenal axes, (*2.*) altered serotoninergic neurotransmission, (*3.*) an increase in interleukin-1 (IL-1), and (*4.*) decreased hypothalamic nitric oxide formation. Fatigue is a frequent symptom in chronic hepatitis C, especially in women, in whom a surprising correlation with increased plasma leptin levels was found (T. Piche et al., 2002). *Therapy* with UDCA has proved unsuccessful and the use of serotonin antagonists (5HT$_1$A), IL-1 receptor antagonists (IL-1ra) and antioxidants (34, 71) is still at an experimental stage. (s. p. 91)

6.2.2 Pruritus and scratch marks

Pruritus can occur at a very early stage – perhaps as a first sign of a cholestasis that has hitherto gone unnoticed. It is more pronounced at night and in wintertime. With a chronic course of disease, this can become excruciatingly painful and may occasionally culminate in a suicidal tendency on the part of the patient.

It is justified to assume that cholestatis-related pruritus is caused by substances that are normally excreted in the bile. Nevertheless, it has not been possible to detect a specific **causative substance** up to now. • Under experimental and clinical conditions, raised *bile acid levels* in the serum or in the skin are found both with and without pruritus – but no adequate correlation could be established. • Recent findings point to an increased *tonus of the opioid system* in the CNS (endorphins) as important in the pathogenesis. Endogenous lipophilic bile acids possibly effect the release of hitherto unknown pruritogenic substances, which stimulate opioid receptors in the CNS. It has thus been possible to eliminate pruritus straightaway and for a certain period of time using opioid antagonists (e. g. naloxone, nalmefene). (38, 62, 63, 71) (s. p. 89)

Pruritus is accompanied by **scratch marks** (s. pp 89, 240), which the tormented patient inflicts, often with great intensity, on all accessible parts of the body (*"as long as it bleeds, it doesn't itch any more"*). Fresh scratch marks on the skin alternating with older, blood-encrusted sites are characteristic of the body surface of a patient suffering from chronic cholestasis, such as primary biliary cholangitis. (s. fig. 13.3)

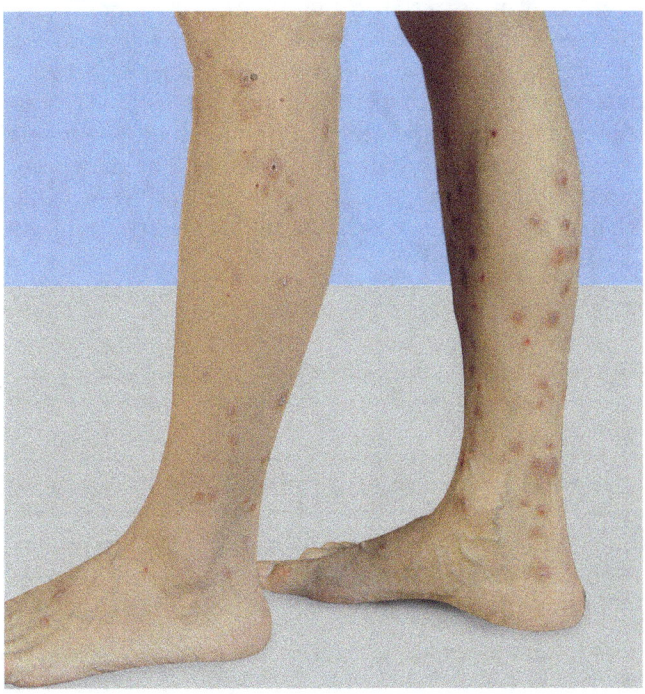

Fig. 13.3: Scratch marks resulting from pruritus in recurrent intrahepatic cholestasis

6.2.3 Xanthelasmas and xanthomas

In chronic cholestasis, xanthelasmas and xanthomas occur as a result of impaired catabolism and reduced excretion of cholesterol. Only when cholesterol levels of >400 mg/dl persist over a period of more than three months do these deposits form in the skin. Occasionally, peripheral *xanthomatous neuropathy* is observed.

Xanthelasmas are depositions, reddish-brown to yellow in colour, sharply defined, striated, up to the size of a fingernail, slightly raised (*xanthelasma planum*) or slightly humpy (*xanthelasma tuberosum*). They are most frequently found on the eyelids (*xanthelasma palpebrarum*), particularly at the inner angle of the eye.

Xanthomas appear as small nodular foci or as nodulations, mainly symmetrical, on the buttocks, elbows, knees, fingers, feet and toes, neck, tendons, and below the breast. They are reddish-brown to yellow in colour. These depositions of cholesterol are reversible – particularly with a marked reduction in the cholesterol level due to liver cirrhosis. Following transplantation of the liver, they generally disappear after one or two years. (s. p. 89) (s. figs. 4.14–4.16)

6.2.4 Changes in biotransformation

In the course of cholestasis, lower concentrations of cytochrome P 450 are found together with increased activities of some microsomal oxidases. For this reason, the biotransformation of xenobiotics can be unpredictably and permanently altered. This is largely connected with the cholestasis-associated shift in bile acids from the periportal to the intermediary and perivenous zones.

6.3 Laboratory diagnostics

Diagnosis of cholestasis is easy and accurate with the help of laboratory methods. (s. tab. 13.6) The retention of substances essential to the bile triggers biochemical changes which may also be of diagnostic significance. The visual diagnosis of subicteric conditions or jaundice can be related to hyperbilirubinaemia as well as to cholestasis with jaundice; this differentiation is possible using just a few laboratory parameters. The diagnostic methods applied must always aim to yield sufficiently reliable information on the aetiology, severity and sequelae of cholestasis.

Differentiation between obstructive ("surgical") and nonobstructive ("conservative") cholestasis is the most important diagnostic task, because this can have consequences which are of decisive importance in terms of therapy and prognosis.

1. *A rise in* **bile acids** *is the main biochemical sign of cholestasis.* For this reason, the bile acid values are well-suited for early diagnostic purposes as well as for follow-up and prognosis. The serum level can be in excess of 300 µmol/l (normal 1.0−6.0 µmol/l). (s. pp 39, 107)

In each form of cholestasis, **atypical bile acids,** such as monohydroxy bile acids, allo-bile acids, 1- or 6-hydroxylated bile acids and their sulphated or glucuronidated derivatives, are found in the serum and/or urine. In cholestasis, the increase in the neosynthesis of atypical bile acids that pass into the kidney can be seen as a compensatory mechanism which eliminates *potentially hepatotoxic bile acids* by renal clearance. The highest renal excretion quota is demonstrated by tetrahydroxy bile acids.

2. An increase in **enzymatic markers of cholestasis** is a specific laboratory sign, with *alkaline phosphatase* being of paramount importance. Normal AP activity does not necessarily exclude cholestasis! It is a ubiquitous enzyme and therefore not specific to cholestasis, which is why LAP (as well as γ-GT) ought to be determined additionally in order to confirm AP if the existence of cholestasis is uncertain. In cholestasis, γ-GT is about nine times more sensitive than LAP and about six times more sensitive than AP. The sluggish reactions of LAP are, however, far more cholestasis-specific than those of AP and γ-GT. Some forms of cholestasis demonstrate elevated AP and LAP values, yet normal γ-GT values. (s. p. 107) (s. tabs. 5.9; 13.6)

▶ These enzymes (AP, LAP, γ-GT, 5'NU) as well as Mg^{++}-*ATPase* are localized on the *canalicular side of the hepatocyte* (AP and Mg^{++}-ATPase are also detectable on the luminal surface of the ductular epithelia cells). Even under normal conditions, yet more so in cholestasis, the enzymes are released through the detergent effect of bile acids (in quantitative dependence on their concentration) and can thereby pass into the bile and blood.

3. **Serum lipids** reflect a complex picture of changes, depending on the duration and severity of the disease. A pronounced increase in *cholesterol* is observed, with a disproportionate rise in free cholesterol. The *phospholipids* are also clearly increased. Neutral fats are just slightly elevated as a rule. Detection of *lipoprotein X* is deemed to be a useful cholestasis parameter. The serum is not turbid. (s. pp 108, 112) (s. tab. 13.6)

Lipoproteins are increased and show great changes: (*1.*) clearly elevated LDH contain lipoprotein X (LP-X), (*2.*) VLDL have fewer apolipoproteins E and C, (*3.*) HDL are decreased and contain less apolipoprotein A1, yet more E, and (*4.*) LCAT activity is reduced.
• **Lipoprotein X** is a lipoprotein rich in phospholipids (ca. 60%) and cholesterol (ca. 25%), with a protein content of about 6%. It has a bilamellar discoidal structure, a diameter of 40−60 nm and a thickness of 10 nm. It is formed by the interaction of bile with blood components. LP-X inhibits the uptake of chylomicron remnants in the liver cells and supports the synthesis of cholesterol by triggering HMG-CoA reductase activity. Degradation of LP-X is effected in the RES. Despite the alleged differentiation into largely increased $LP-X_1$ in intrahepatic cholestasis and $LP-X_2$ in extrahepatic cholestasis, it is not possible to distinguish between the two forms of cholestasis in the chemical laboratory.

4. **Jaundice** does not necessarily accompany cholestasis. In severe and prolonged cholestasis, particularly if obstructive, jaundice is generally in evidence. In cholestasis, the third fraction, known as *delta bilirubin*, is largely detected by means of the diazo method. This fraction is firmly bound to albumin and can therefore only be dissociated and excreted slowly. For this reason, jaundice occurring together with cholestasis tends to subside at a significantly slower rate than the increased bile acid level in the serum. • In this case, jaundice is due to a reflux of bilirubin from the canaliculus into the blood or a bidirectional transport of bilirubin via the sinusoidal membrane. Sometimes jaundice is caused by metabolic dysfunction of the liver cells. • Bilirubin also acts as an antioxidant.

5. An increase in **GDH** often proves to be a sensitive parameter for bile stasis. In acute obstruction of the biliary tract, the GDH level rises at an early stage (*according to our own observations, up to 112 U/l on discharge of a gallstone*). • With right-side colic, a swift and pronounced increase in GDH can point to a choledochal concrement, whereas colic caused by a renal calculus has no effect on the GDH level. • A malignant obstruction shows constantly high or still increasing values, whereas GDH activity tends to decrease in benign cholestasis. (s. tab. 13.6)

6. **Quick's value** may be reduced in long-term cholestasis by vitamin K deficiency (owing to a disorder in the synthesis of clotting factors dependent on vitamin K). In this respect, the intravenous *Koller test* can facilitate the differential diagnosis between dysfunction of syn-

thesis in the liver cell or vitamin K deficiency due to impaired absorption. (s. p. 111) (s. tab. 13.6)

7. **Cholinesterase** activity continuously declines in prolonged cholestasis — pointing to an impaired synthesis capacity of the liver cells. (s. p. 109) (s. tab. 13.6)

8. The serum value for **copper** is increased. Some 80% of the absorbed copper is normally excreted via the bile in the stool. In prolonged cases of cholestasis, copper is deposited in other organs — even forming a faint Kayser-Fleischer ring on the cornea (as observed in Wilson's disease). The retained copper is not toxic. (s. p. 108)

1. Serum bile acids	↑
2. Alkaline phosphatase (AP) Leucine aminopeptidase (LAP) γ-GT 5′ nucleotidase	↑
3. Cholesterol Phospholipids Lipoprotein X	↑
4. Bilirubin	N–↑
5. GDH	N–↑
6. Quick's value, cholinesterase	↓
7. Copper, ceruloplasmin	↑
8. IgA, IgM	↑
9. Antithrombin III, haptoglobin	↑
10. Various antibodies (s. tab. 13.7)	↑

Tab. 13.6: Possible laboratory results in cholestasis (N = normal)

9. In the case of non-dilated bile ducts, further **specific laboratory parameters** may be necessary for differential diagnosis, such as electrophoresis, immunoglobulins, hepatitis serology (s. p. 118) and $α_1$-foetoprotein (s. p. 112). Determination of the AMA should always be considered. (s. p. 126) (s. tabs. 5.19–5.21; 13.7)

In cholestasis, various *antibodies* (e. g. CEA 19) may be falsely evidenced as being increased in the serum. This is because antibodies can no longer be excreted via the bile, as they usually are.

It is not possible to differentiate between intrahepatic and extrahepatic cholestasis by means of laboratory parameters.

6.4 Imaging procedures

6.4.1 Sonography

At this stage of the examination, sonography is now required to diagnose obstructive cholestasis and posthepatic jaundice and to localize the cause. In 90–95% of cases, this is done successfully; the cause can be clarified in 71–88% of cases. Ultrasound examination methods are deemed to be routine, and when aiming at the clarification of jaundice and/or cholestasis, they have a high degree of reliability. Dilated bile ducts (generally presented as a *"double-barrelled phenomenon"*) with a diameter exceeding 7–8 mm and an enlarged lumen through to the porta hepatis or papilla of Vater (extrahepatic obstruction) are clearly visible. It is usually possible to differentiate between an obstruction which is located high up in the bile duct and one which is located distally. (s. tabs. 6.4; 13.8)

Localization	Dilation		
	Gall bladder	Choledochal duct	Intrahepatic bile ducts
Extrahepatic cholestasis – proximal – distal	Ø +	Ø +	+ +
Intrahepatic cholestasis	Ø	Ø	Ø

Tab. 13.8: Ultrasound criteria for the differentiation of cholestasis (or jaundice)

Disease	M_6	AMA M_2	M_4	M_8	M_9	ANA	LMA	SMA	ANCA	AHA
Primary biliary cholangitis	Ø	+++	+	+	+	(+)	Ø	Ø	Ø	Ø
PBC/CAH	Ø	++	+	(+)	(+)	++	+	+	Ø	Ø
CAH	Ø	Ø	Ø	Ø	Ø	+++	++	++	++	Ø
Primary sclerosing cholangitis	Ø	Ø	Ø	Ø	(+)	Ø	Ø	Ø	++	Ø
Alcoholic CAH	Ø	Ø	Ø	Ø	(+)	(+)	Ø	Ø	Ø	+
Drug-induced CAH	(+)	Ø	Ø	Ø	Ø	+	Ø	+	Ø	Ø

Tab. 13.7: Possible antibody constellations in chronic cholestatic liver diseases

Criterion	Clinical and laboratory findings	Sonography	CT	MRC / ERCP, PTC
Sensitivity	95–100%	55–95%	74–76%	40–100%
Specificity	30–40%	71–96%	90–94%	90–100%

Tab. 13.9: Efficiency of diagnostic procedures in cholestasis: determination of cholestasis (= sensitivity), differentiation between intrahepatic and extrahepatic cholestasis (= specificity)

6.4.2 CT, MRI and MRC

The degree of accuracy for CT in cholestasis is 74–96% sensitivity and 90–94% specificity, which practically corresponds to that of sonography and MRI. When cholestasis is still unresolved, MRC (B. K. WALLNER et al., 1991) should be used as well. (74) (s. tab. 13.9)

6.4.3 ERC, PTC and EUS

If there is still no definitive clarification of cholestasis (even with MRC imaging), dilated bile ducts indicate an ERC or, if this is technically impossible, a PTC. Sensitivity is 60–70%, specificity is 90–95 (−100)%. The ERC should also be used to visualize non-dilated bile ducts by means of direct presentation — e.g. in cases with suspicion of destructive primary biliary or sclerosing cholangitis as well as regionally restricted intrahepatic obstruction. (s. figs. 8.14, 8.15) (s. tab. 13.9)

6.5 Liver biopsy and laparoscopy

Liver biopsy: In the case of a hitherto non-clarified differential diagnosis of cholestasis, thought should be given to percutaneous liver biopsy or laparoscopy. Although this is only indicated in isolated cases, it does promise to be successful. (s. tabs. 7.3, 7.10) • *Explorative laparotomy should not be performed!*

> Even by means of **histology**, however, it is not possible to differentiate reliably between intrahepatic and extrahepatic cholestasis.

Feathery degeneration is the term used to describe the delicate honeycomb-like, brownish streaky change of liver cells, which is due to bilirubin impregnation of the visible cytoplasmic structures. It can occur following long-term cholestasis. Cellular hydrops is evident with dilation of the endoplasmic cisternas, caused by the toxic impact of biliary acids. (s. fig. 13.4)

Eosinophilic infiltrations in the portal fields generally point to intrahepatic cholestasis. • By contrast, *ductular changes* with bile cylinders, ballooning, acidophilia of the liver cells at the lobular centres, bile infarcts, increase in the copper content, etc. are usually signs of extrahepatic cholestasis. (s. fig. 13.5) (s. tab. 13.10)

Finding	Intrahepatic cholestasis	Extrahepatic cholestasis
1. Periportal field		
– leucocytes	(+)	+/++
– eosinophilia	+++	(+)
– foam cells	(+)	+/++
– fibrosis	∅	+/++
– ductular changes	(+)	+/++
2. Bile ducts		
– dilation	(+)	+/++
– bile cast	+	+/++
3. Liver cells		
– bile pigment	+/++	+/++
– necroses	+	+/++
– fatty infiltration	(+)	+/++

Tab. 13.10: Histological findings as criteria for intrahepatic or extrahepatic cholestasis

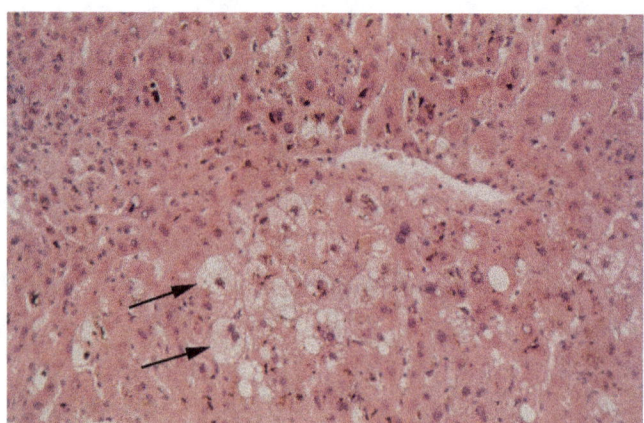

Fig. 13.4: Obstructive jaundice with feathery degeneration of hepatocytes (→) (HE)

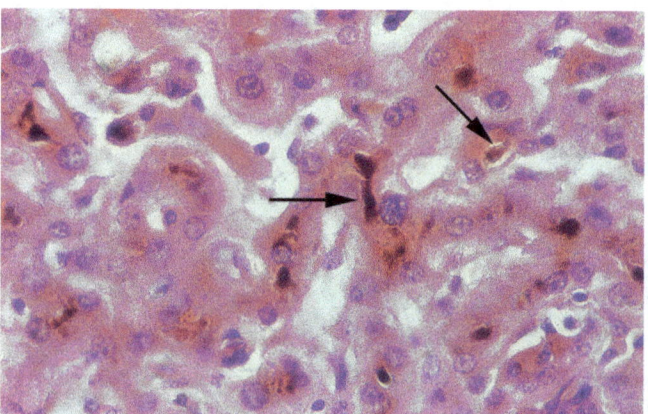

Fig. 13.5: Bilirubinostasis with bile droplets (→) in hepatocytes and canaliculi. Clinical diagnosis: extrahepatic obstructive jaundice (HE)

Laparoscopy: In laparoscopy, cholestasis is usually presented as greenish to brownish green "spotting" or as diffuse greyish green colouration of the liver surface.

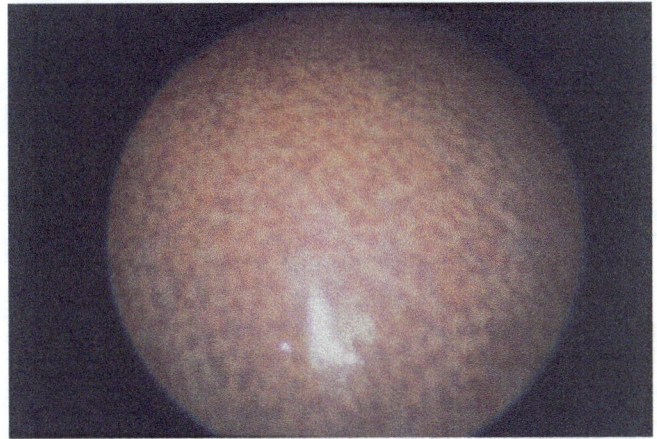

Fig. 13.6: Smooth, brownish-green sprinkled liver surface (due to azathioprine)

This greyish green colour does not always correlate with the bilirubin value (in pronounced icteric virus hepatitis, for example, the surface of the liver shows no cholestatic change). In intrahepatic obstructive cholestasis, the surface of the liver can indeed show a cholestatic discolouration, although only in the affected area. • In long-term cholestasis, however, obstructive and non-obstructive courses of the disease display clear differences: in the obstructive form, fine uneven sites increasingly appear on the liver surface, ultimately leading to granulation as well as to perivascular proliferation of connective tissue and capsular fibrosis. By contrast, in non-obstructive forms, the liver surface remains unchanged, i.e. smooth and shiny, even after weeks of cholestasis. (s. figs. 13.6; 28.18, 28.19)

The strategy of diagnosing **cholestasis** or **jaundice** is outlined in a **flow diagram**. (s. fig. 13.7)

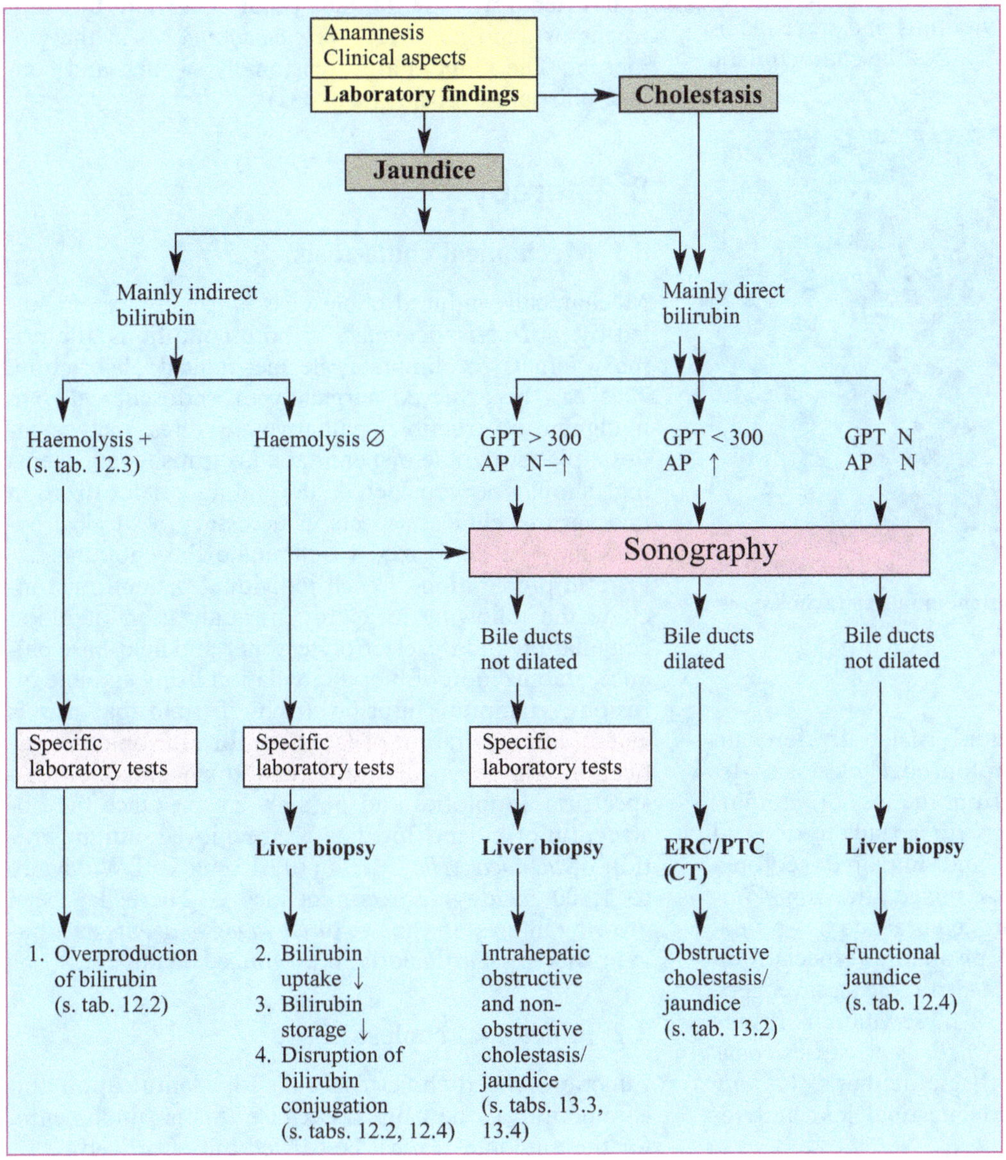

Fig. 13.7: Flow diagram of cholestasis and jaundice (N = normal, ∅ = not present) (s. fig. 9.3)

7 Clinical sequelae

In prolonged cholestasis and/or biliary deficiency in the intestine, a number of unpleasant and grave symptoms are likely to occur.

7.1 Abdominal complaints

Bile deficiency in the stools causes disturbed bacterial flora as well as insufficient digestion and absorption of nutritional fats. This leads to intestinal complaints, such as meteorism, bloating, lack of appetite, intolerance of fatty foods through to nausea and vomitus.

7.2 Steatorrhoea and diarrhoea

Biliary steatorrhoea is characterized by higher stool weight (> 200 g) and increased excretion of fat (> 7 g/day). This condition correlates with the degree of severity of cholestasis. Stools are soft and smell unpleasant. Steatorrhoea and additional *diarrhoea* lead to a loss of liquid, electrolytes, fat-soluble vitamins and trace elements. • Intestinal bile deficiency causes the characteristic *acholic stools*. (s. fig. 13.8)

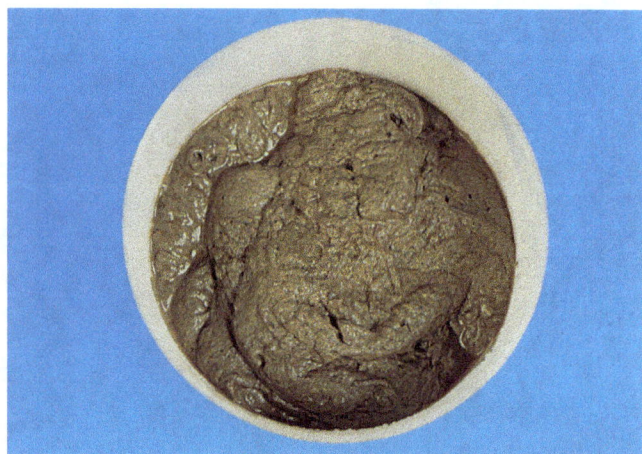

Fig. 13.8: Acholic fatty stool in recurrent intrahepatic cholestasis

7.3 Malabsorption

Steatorrhoea and diarrhoea cause malabsorption and subsequent weight loss. In prolonged cholestasis, deficiency symptoms may result from the loss of vitamins A, D, E and K. • *Vitamin A deficiency* leads to dry and atrophic skin, xerophthalmia and impaired scotopia with night blindness as well as damaged hearing. *Vitamin E deficiency* may result in cerebral ataxia, retinal degeneration, neuropathy and myopathy (especially in children). Vitamins A and E are also radical scavengers, which explains why deficiency of these vitamins results in lipid peroxidation. *Vitamin K deficiency* causes coagulative disorders with haemorrhagic diathesis. *Vitamin D deficiency* leads to increased intestinal loss and reduced absorption of calcium.

7.4 Osteopathy

Cholestasis-linked osteopathy (M. LOEPER et al., 1939), which occurs much more frequently in the form of osteoporosis than osteomalacia, can be expected in up to 50% of cases. The pathogenesis is complex. Vitamin D status can be examined by determining 25-OH-cholecalciferol in the serum. Intestinal calcium loss and reduced calcium absorption due to vitamin D deficiency are key pathogenetic factors. It is still a matter of debate whether vitamin K deficiency (which can lead to reduced osteocalcin synthesis) and deficiencies in IGF I and II (which can cause dysfunction of the osteoblasts) are possible causes of this condition. Muscle and bone pain are frequent clinical symptoms, occurring mainly in the wrists and ankles.

7.5 Renal dysfunction

Elimination of *endotoxins* is reduced owing to the restricted filtering function of the RES in cholestasis. (s. p. 69) Renal dysfunction may occur as a result of endotoxins or deposits of *IgA immunocomplexes* in the glomerula. The kidneys are occasionally swollen and contain bilirubin deposits. (s. p. 333)

8 Therapy

8.1 Mechanical cholestasis

Mechanically induced cholestasis is usually accompanied by *obstructive jaundice*. In both conditions, the primary aim is to eliminate the mechanical obstruction. This can be achieved surgically or endoscopically. In malignant obstructions, palliative measures, such as endoscopic retrograde or percutaneous transhepatic stenting, should be considered, depending on localization and various clinical aspects; if necessary, a surgical bypass may be performed to eliminate the cholestasis. • Careful preparation of each individual patient must include the following measures: normalization of blood coagulation and the electrolyte, water and acid-base balance, stabilization of blood circulation using suitable infusions, mannitol infusion (only if fluid balance is given), administration of lactulose for intestinal detoxification (in particular for endotoxinaemia), broad spectrum antibiotics and possibly zinc. • Once the obstruction of biliary flow has been removed, administration of *ursodeoxycholic acid* (10 – 15 mg/kg BW/day, up to 1,800 mg/day) is recommended. • There has been growing interest in the use of *cholagogue agents* as adjuvant therapy, particularly in prolonged treatment.

8.2 Functional cholestasis

Function-related cholestasis calls for identification and elimination of the causes. Because this is fundamental for the outcome, it must be carried out effectively.

General measures
- Reduced intake of neutral fats (< 40 g/day) with supplementary administration of medium-chain triglycerides (> 40 g/day)
- Substitution with vitamins A, D., E., K (i.m.)
- Substitution with calcium (1 g/day)
- Substitution with other electrolytes and zinc
- Short fingernails
- Increase in physical activity

Drug therapy
- Ursodeoxycholic acid (22, 53)
- S-adenosyl-L-methionine (19)
- Cholestyramine, cholestipol
- Opiate antagonists (29, 38, 62)
  - naxolone
  - naltrexone (69)
  - nalmefene (5)
- 5HT3 antagonist
  - ondansetron (63)
- Dronabinol (50)
- Serotonin reuptake inhibitor
  - sertraline (50–100 mg/day)
- Enzyme inducers
  - Rifampicin (79)
  - phenobarbital (100 mg in the evening)
  - promethazine (25–150 mg in the evening)
- Antacids
  - aluminium hydroxide
  - H_2-receptor blockers

Non-pharmaceutical therapies
- UV light (65)
- Dialysis, exchange transfusion
- MARS (26, 40, 66)

Tab. 13.11: Treatment of functional cholestasis and pruritus

General measures should include: (*1.*) reduction in the intake of neutral fats in the food (< 40 g/day) with supplementary administration of medium-chain triglycerides (> 40 g/day), (*2.*) substitution of fat-soluble vitamins A, D, E and K, (*3.*) substitution of calcium (1 g/day) as well as other electrolytes and zinc, (*4.*) reduction of scratching by constantly checking for short fingernails, and (*5.*) regular muscular activity. • Many studies using *drug therapy* have shown the effectiveness of ursodeoxycholic acid (10–15 mg/kg BW/day, up to 1,800 mg/day) (22, 53), S-adenosyl-L-methionine (1,600 mg/day) (19), cholestyramine (starting at 1 x 4 g/day and increasing to 3 x 4 and 4 x 4 g/day) and cholestipol (3 x 5 g/day) as well as rifampicin (2 x 150 mg/day, up to 2 x 300 mg/day in exceptional cases). (79) Opiate antagonists have also proved successful: naxolone (2–3 x 0.4 mg/day i.m.) or naltrexone (2–4 x 25–50 mg/day) (69) as well as the 5-HT3 antagonist ondansetron (3 x 4–8 mg/day, i.v. or orally). (63) Dronabinol has also been successfully used to treat intractable pruritus. (50) Sertraline as a selective serotonin (neuronal) reuptake inhibitor can reduce pruritus due to cholestasis with long-term efficacy. Phenobarbital (3 x 5 mg/kg BW/day and/or 100 mg in the evening) is thought to be effective through enzyme induction or direct impact on the peripheral or central nervous system. Promethazine (25–150 mg in the evening) should also be mentioned here. In some cases (especially in pregnancy cholestasis), prednisolone may be administered in the morning, gradually decreasing the dosage over a limited period. Tauroursodeoxycholic acid appears ineffective in preventing or treating total parenteral nutrition-associated cholestasis in neonates. • *Non-pharmaceutical alternatives* in the treatment of severe intractable pruritus include UV phototherapy (8–12 hours/day), dialysis or plasmaphoresis. The molecular adsorbents recirculating system (MARS) was developed as supplementary treatment in acute liver failure. This method is now being used in patients with intractable pruritus or with BRIC to produce excellent results. (s. tab. 13.11)

References:

1. **Aagenaes, O., van der Hagen, C.B., Refsum, S.:** Hereditary recurrent intrahepatic cholestasis from birth. Arch. Dis. Childh. 1968; 43: 646–657
2. **Aagenaes, O.:** Hereditary recurrent cholestasis with lymphoedema. – Two new families. Acta Paed. Scand. 1974; 63: 465–471
3. **Alonso, E.M., Snover, D.C., Montag, A., Freese, D.K., Whitington, P.F.:** Histologic pathology of the liver in progressive familial intrahepatic cholestasis. J. Pediatr. Gastroenterol. Nutr. 1994; 18: 128–133
4. **Arkenau, H.-T., Widjaja, A.:** An unusual case of cholestasis and macrohematuria in a 52-year-old patient. Med. Klin. 2002; 97: 480–483
5. **Bergasa, N.V., Alling, D.W., Talbot, T.L., Wells, M.C., Jones, E.A.:** Oral nalmefene therapy reduces scratching activity due to the pruritus of cholestasis: a controlled study. J. Amer. Acad. Derm. 1999; 41: 431–434
6. **Bowen, P., Lee, C.S.N., Zellweger, H., Lindenberg, R.:** A familial syndrome of multiple congenital defects. Bull. Hopkins Hosp. 1964; 114: 402–414
7. **Chand, N., Sanyal, A.J.:** Sepsis-induced cholestasis (review). Hepatology 2007; 45: 230–241
8. **Cissarek, T., Schumacher, B., Schwöbel, H., Sarbia, M., Neuhaus, H.:** Verlauf einer benignen rekurrierenden intrahepatischen Cholestase (Summerskill-Walshe-Tygstrup-Syndrom) über 46 Jahre. Z. Gastroenterol. 1998; 36: 379–383
9. **Clayton, R.J., Iber, F.L., Ruebner, B.H., McKusick, V.M.:** Byler disease. Fatal familial intrahepatic cholestasis in an Amish kindred. Amer. J. Dis. Child. 1969; 117: 112–124
10. **Clayton, P.T.:** Inborn errors of bile acid metabolism. J. Inher. Metabol. Dis. 1991; 14: 478–496
11. **Colombo, C., Okolicsanyi, L., Strazzabosco, M.:** Advances in familial and congenital cholestatic diseases. Clinical and diagnostic implications. Dig. Liver Dis. 2000; 32: 152–159
12. **Degott, C., Feldmann, G., Larrey, D., Durand-Schneider, A.-M., Grange, D., Machayekhi, J.-P., Moreau, A, Potet, F., Benhamou, J.-P.:** Drug-induced prolonged cholestasis in adults: a histological semiquantitative study demonstrating progressive ductopenia. Hepatology 1992; 15: 244–251
13. **Deleuze, J.-F., Jacquemin, E., Dubuisson, C., Cresteil, D., Dumont, M., Erlinger, S., Bernard, O., Hadchouel, M.:** Defect of multidrug-resistance 3 gene expression in a subtype of progressive intrahepatic cholestasis. Hepatology 1996; 23: 904–908
14. **Drivdal, M., Trydal, T., Hagve, T.A., Bergstad, I., Aagenaes, O.:** Prognosis with evaluation of general biochemistry of liver disease in lymphoedema cholestasis syndrome 1 (LCS 1/Aagenaes syndrome). Scand. J. Gastroenterol. 2006; 41: 465–471
15. **Desmet, V.J.:** Modulation of the liver in cholestasis. J. Gastroenterol. Hepatol. 1992; 7: 313–323
16. **Eppens, E.F., van Mil, S.W.C., de Vree, J.M.L., Mok, K.S., Juijn, J.A., Oude Elferink, R.P.J., Berger, R., Houwen, R.H.J., Klomp, L.W.J.:** FIC1, the protein affected in two forms of hereditary cholestasis, is localized in the cholangiocyte and the canalicular membrane of the hepatocyte. J. Hepatol. 2001; 35: 436–443
17. **Floreani, A., Guido, M., Bortolami, M., della Zentil, G., Venturi, C., Pennelli, N., Naccarato, R.:** Relationship between apoptosis, tumour necrosis factor, and cell proliferation in chronic cholestasis. Dig. Liver Dis. 2001; 33: 570–575
18. **Forrest, E.H., Oien, K.A., Dickson, S., Galloway, D., Mills, P.R.:** Improvement in cholestasis associated with total parenteral nutrition after treatment with an antibody against tumour necrosis factor alpha. Liver 2002; 22: 317–320
19. **Frezza, M., Surrenti, C., Manzillo, G., Fiaccadori, F., Bortolini, M., di Padova, C.:** Oral S-adenosylmethionine in the symptomatic treatment of intrahepatic cholestasis. A double-blind, placebo-controlled study. Gastroenterology 1990; 99: 211–215
20. **Glantz, A., Marschall, H.W., Mattsson, L.A.:** Intrahepatic cholestasis of pregnancy: Relationship between bile acid levels and fetal complication rates. Hepatology 2004; 40: 467–474
21. **Goez, H., Meiron, D., Horowitz, J., Schutgens, R.H., Wanders, R.J.A., Berant, M., Mandel, H.:** Infantile Refsum disease: neonatal cholestatic

jaundice. Presentation of a peroxismal disorder. J. Pediatr. Gastroenterol. Nutr. 1995; 20: 98−101
22. **Gores, G.J.:** Mechanisms of cell injury and death in cholestasis and hepatoprotection by ursodeoxycholic acid. J. Hepatol. 2000; 32 (Suppl. 2): 11−13
23. **Harris, M.J., Le Couteur, D.G., Arias, I.M.:** Progressive familial intrahepatic cholestasis: Genetic disorders of biliary transporters. (review). J. Gastroenterol. Hepatol. 2005; 20: 807−817
24. **Herzog, D., Chessex, P., Martin, S., Alvarez, F.:** Transient cholestasis in newborn infants with perinatal asphyxia. Canad. J. Gastroenterol. 2003; 17: 179−182
25. **Hofmann, A.F.:** Cholestatic liver disease: Pathophysiology and therapeutic options. Liver 2002; 22 (Suppl. 2): 14−19
26. **Huster, D., Schubert, C., Achenbach, H., Caca, K., Moessner, J., Beer, F.:** Successful clinical application of extracorporal albumine dialysis in a patient with benign recurrent intrahepatic cholestasis (BRIC). Z. Gastroenterol. 2001; 39 (Suppl. 2): 13−14
27. **Jacquemin, E.:** Progressive familial intrahepatic cholestasis. Genetic basis and treatment. Clin. Liver Dis. 2000; 47: 753−763
28. **Jansen, P.L.M., Müller, M.:** The molecular genetics of familial intrahepatic cholestasis. Gut 2000; 47: 1−5
29. **Jones, E.A., Neuberger, J., Bergasa, N.V.:** Opiate antagonist therapy for the pruritus of cholestasis: the avoidance of opioid withdrawal-like reactions. Quart. J. Med. 2002; 95: 547−552
30. **Juberg, R.C., Holland-Moritz, R.M., Henley, K.S., Gonzalez, C.F.:** Familial intrahepatic cholestasis with mental and growth retardation. Pediatrics 1966; 38: 819−836
31. **Kaaden, R., Zwack, K., Wienbeck, M., Klotz, E.:** Ikterische Cholestase als Frühsymptom bei Morbus Hodgkin. Dtsch. Med. Wschr. 1990; 115: 1670−1673
32. **Kondrackiene, J., Beuers, U., Kupcinskas, L.:** Efficacy and safety of ursodeoxycholic acid versus cholestyramine in ultrahepatic cholestasis of pregnancy. Gastroenterology 2005; 129: 894−901
33. **Kullak-Ublick, G.A., Meier, P.J.:** Mechanisms of cholestasis. Clin. Liver Dis. 2000; 4: 357−385
34. **Kumar, D., Tandon, R.K.:** Fatigue in cholestatic liver disease − A perplexing symptom (review). Postgrad. Med. J. 2002; 78: 404−407
35. **Kuntz, H.-D.:** Rezidivierende intrahepatische Cholestase. Münch. Med. Wschr. 1986; 128: 86−90
36. **Lazarow, P.B., Black, V., Shio, H., Fujiki, Y., Hajra, A.K., Datta, N.S., Bangaru, B.S., Dancis, J.:** Zellweger syndrome: biochemical and morphological studies on two patients treated with clofibrate. Pediatr. Res. 1985; 19: 1356−1364
37. **Linarelli, L.G., Williams, G.N., Philipps, M.J.:** Byler's disease: fatal intrahepatic cholestasis. J. Pediatr. 1972; 81: 484−492
38. **Lorette, G., Vaillant, I.:** Pruritus. Current concepts in pathogenesis and treatment. Drugs 1990; 39: 218−223
39. **Lovisetto, P., Raviolo, P., Rizzetto, M., Marchi, L., Actis, G.C., Verme, G.:** Benign recurrent intrahepatic cholestasis. A clinico-pathologic study. Res. Clin. Lab. 1990; 20: 19−27
40. **Macia, M., Aviles, J., Navarro, J., Morales, S., Garcia, J.:** Efficacy of molecular adsorbent recirculating system for the treatment of intractable pruritus in cholestasis. Amer. J. Med. 2003; 114: 62−64
41. **Maeda, K., Kimura, A., Yamato, Y., Nittono, H., Takei, H., Sato, T., Mitsubuchi, H., Murai, T., Kurosawa, T.:** Oral bile acid treatment in two Japanese patients with Zellweger syndrome. J. Pediatr. Gastroenterol. Nutr. 2002; 35: 227−230
42. **Marzioni, M., Glaser, S.S., Francis, H., Phinizy, J.L., LeSage, G., Alpini, G.:** Functional heterogeneisy of cholangiocytes. Semin. Liver Dis. 2002; 22: 227−240
43. **McDonald, J.A.:** Cholestasis of pregnancy. J. Gastroenterol. Hepatol. 1999; 14: 515−518
44. **McGill, J.M., Kwiatkowski, A.P.:** Cholestatic liver disease in adults. Amer. J. Gastroenterol. 1998; 93: 684−691
45. **Messing, B., Colombel, J.F., Heresbach, D., Chazouillres, O., Galian, A.:** Chronic cholestasis and macronutrient excess in patients treated with prolonged parenteral nutrition. Nutrition 1992; 8: 30−36
46. **Moseley, R.H.:** Sepsis associated cholestasis. Gastroenterology 1997; 112: 302−306
47. **Moss, R.L., Das, J.B., Raffensperges, J.G.:** Total parenteral nutrition-associated cholestasis: clinical and histopathologic correlation. J. Pediatr. Surg. 1993; 28: 1270−1275
48. **Nagore, N., Howe, S., Boxer, L., Scheuer, P.J.:** Liver cell rosettes: structural differences in cholestasis and hepatitis. Liver 1989; 9: 43−51
49. **Nakamuta, M., Sakamoto, S., Miyata, Y., Sato, M., Nawata, H.:** Benign recurrent intrahepatic cholestasis: a long-term follow-up. Hepat. Gastroenterol. 1994; 41: 287−289
50. **Neff, G.W., O'Brien, C.B., Reddy, K.R., Bergasa, N.V., Regev, A., Molina, E., Amaro, R., Rodriguez, M.J., Chase, V., Jeffers, L., Schiff, E.:** Preliminary observation with dronabinol in patients with intractable pruritus secondary to cholestatic liver disease. Amer. J. Gastroenterol. 2002; 97: 2117−2119
51. **Nishida, M., Tamakuma, S., Idei, T., Mochizuki, H.:** A research on the cholestasis caused by continuous endotoxemia. J. Jap. Surg. Soc. 1990; 91: 184−190
52. **Nissenbaum, M., Chedid, A., Mendenhall, Ch., Gartside, P.:** Prognostic significance of cholestatic alcoholic hepatitis. Dig. Dis. Sci. 1990; 35: 891−896
53. **Paumgartner, G., Beuers, U.:** Ursodeoxycholic acid in cholestatic liver disease: mechanisms of action and therapeutic use revisited. Hepatology 2002; 36: 525−531
54. **Paus, T.C., Schneider, G., van de Vondel, P., Sauerbruch, T., Reichel, C.:** Diagnosis and therapy of intrahepatic cholestasis of pregnancy (review). Zschr. Gastroenterol. 2004; 42: 623−628
55. **Puttermann, C., Keidar, S., Brook, J.G.:** Benign recurrent intrahepatic cholestasis−25 years of follow-up. Postgrad. Med. J. 1987; 63: 295−296
56. **Qureshi, W.A.:** Intrahepatic cholestasic syndromes: pathogenesis, clinical features and management. Dig. Dis. 1999; 17: 49−59
57. **Refsum, S.:** Heredoataxia hemeralopica polyneuritiformis − et tigligere ikke beskrevet familiaer syndrom? En forelöbig meddelelse. Nord. Med. 1945; 28: 2682−2686
58. **Reyes, H.:** Review: Intrahepatic cholestasis. A puzzling disorder of pregnancy. J. Gastroenterol. Hepatol. 1997; 12: 211−216
59. **Rubinow, A., Koff, R.S., Cohen, A.S.:** Severe intrahepatic cholestasis in primary amyloidosis. A report of four cases and a review of the literature. Amer. J. Med. 1978; 64: 937−946
60. **Rudzki, C., Ishak, K.G., Zimmermann, H.J.:** Chronic intrahepatic cholestasis of sarcoidosis. Amer. J. Med. 1975; 59: 373−387
61. **Schiraldi, O., Modugno, A., Miglietta, A., Fera, G.:** Prolonged viral hepatitis type A with cholestasis: case report. Ital. J. Gastroenterol. 1991; 23: 364−366
62. **Schirrmacher, S., Blumenstein, I., Stein, J.:** Pathogenesis and treatment of pruritus in patients with cholestasis (review). Zschr. Gastroenterol. 2003; 41: 259−262
63. **Schworer, H., Hartmann, H., Ramadori, G.:** Relief of cholestatic pruritus by a novel class of drugs: 5-hydroxytryptamine type 3 (5-HT3) receptor antagonist: effectiveness of ondansetron. Pain 1995; 61: 31−37
64. **Sevastos, N., Savvas, S.P., Rafailidis, P.I., Manesis, E.K.:** Cholestasis in acute stroke: An investigation on its prevalence and etiology. Scand. J. Gastroenterol. 2005; 40: 862−866
65. **Socha, P., Koletzko, B., Jankowska, I., Pawlowska, J., Demmelmair, H., Stolarczyk, A., Swiatkowska, E., Socha, J.:** Long-chain PUFA supplementation improves PUFA profile in infants with cholestasis. Lipids 2002; 37: 953−957
66. **Sturm, E., Franssen, C.F.M., Gouw, A., Staels, B., Boverhof, R., de Knegt, R.J., Stellaard, F., Bijleveld, C.M.A., Kuipers, F.:** Extracorporal albumin dialysis (MARS) improves cholestasis and normalizes low apo A-I levels in a patient with benign recurrent intrahepatic cholestasis (BRIC). Liver 2002; 22 (Suppl. 2), 72−75
67. **Summerskill, W.H.J., Walshe, J.M.:** Benign recurrent intrahepatic "obstructive" jaundice. Lancet 1959/II: 686−690
68. **Summerskill, W.H.J.:** The syndrome of benign recurrent cholestasis. Amer. J. Med. 1965; 38: 298−305
69. **Terg, R., Coronel, E., Sorda, J., Munoz, A.E., Findor, J.:** Efficacy and safety of oral naltrexone treatment for pruritus of cholestasis, a crossover, double blind, placebo-controlled study. J. Hepatol. 2002; 37: 717−722
70. **Trauner, M., Fickert, P., Stauber, R.E.:** Inflammatory-induced cholestasis. J. Gastroenterol. Hepatol. 1999; 14: 946−959
71. **Trauner, M., Boyer, J.L.:** Cholestatic syndromes. Curr. Opin. Gastroenterol. 2003; 19: 216−231
72. **Tygstrup, N.:** Intermittent possibly familial intrahepatic cholestatic jaundice. Lancet 1960/I: 1171−1172
73. **Ujhazy, P., Ortiz, D., Misra, S., Li, S., Moseley, J., Jones, H., Arias, I.M.:** Familiale intrahepatic cholestasis 1: studies of localization and function. Hepatology 2001; 34: 768−775
74. **Vaishali, M.D., Agarwal, A.K., Upadhyaya, D.N., Chauhan, V.S., Sharma, O.P., Shukla, V.K.:** Magnetic resonance cholangiopancreatography in obstructive jaundice. J. Clin. Gastroenterol. 2004; 38: 887−890
75. **Wang, L., Soroka, C.J., Boyer, J.L.:** The role of bile salt export pump mutations in progressive familial intrahepatic cholestasis type II. J. Clin. Invest. 2002; 110: 965−972
76. **Westermann, G., Lügering, N., August, C., Rahn, K.H., Kisters, K.:** A classic case of benign recurrent intrahepatic cholestasis (Summerskill-Walshe-Tygstrup syndrome). Med. Klin. 2000; 95: 349−354
77. **Whitington, P.F., Freese, D.K., Alonso, E.M.:** Clinical and biochemical findings in progressive familial intrahepatic cholestasis. J. Pediatr. Gastroenterol. Nutr. 1994; 18: 134−141
78. **Witzleben, C.L., Piccoli, D.A., Setchell, K.:** Case 3.A new category of causes of intrahepatic cholestasis. Pediatr. Pathol. 1992; 12 269−274
79. **Yerushalmi, B., Sokol, R.J., Narkewicz, M.R., Smith, D., Karrer, F.M.:** Use of rifampin for severe pruritus in children with chronic cholestasis. J. Pediatr. Gastroenterol. Nutr. 1999; 29: 442−447
80. **Zapata, R., Sandoval, L., Palma, J., Hernandez, I., Ribalta, J., Reyes, H., Sedano, M., Toha, D., Silva, J.J.:** Ursookoxycholic acid in the treatment of intrahepatic cholestasis of pregnancy. A 12-year experience. Liver Int. 2005; 25: 548−554
81. **Zeijen, R.N.M., Sels, J.P.J.F., Flendrig, J.A., Arends, J.W.:** Portal hypertension and intrahepatic cholestasis in hepatic amyloidosis. Netherl. J. Med. 1991; 38: 257−261
82. **Zimniak, P., Radominska, A., Lester, R.:** The pathogenesis of cholestasis. Hosp. Pract. 1990; 25: 107−125

Symptoms and Syndromes
14 Portal hypertension

		Page:
1	*Definition*	252
2	**Pathogenesis**	252
3	**Forms and aetiology**	253
3.1	Prehepatic portal hypertension	253
3.1.1	Cavernous transformation	253
3.1.2	Cruveilhier-von Baumgarten disease	254
3.1.3	Arterioportal fistulas	254
3.1.4	Portal vein thrombosis	254
3.1.5	Segmental portal hypertension	254
3.2	Intrahepatic portal hypertension	254
3.2.1	Presinusoidal block	255
3.2.2	Sinusoidal block	255
3.2.3	Postsinusoidal block	256
3.3	Posthepatic portal hypertension	257
4	**Diagnosis**	258
4.1	Anamnesis	258
4.2	Clinical findings	259
4.3	Laboratory findings	259
4.4	Sonography	259
4.5	Doppler sonography	259
4.6	Endoscopy	260
4.7	Angiography	260
4.8	CT and MRI	260
4.9	Carbon dioxide wedged venography	260
4.10	Portal pressure measurement	261
5	**Sequelae of portal hypertension**	261
5.1	Splenomegaly	261
5.2	Portacaval collateral circulation	262
5.2.1	Oesophageal and gastric varices	262
5.2.2	Anorectal varices	264
5.2.3	Intestinal varices	264
5.2.4	Abdominal wall varices	264
5.2.5	Retroperitoneal varices	265
5.2.6	Splenorenal varices	265
5.2.7	Retzius' veins	265
5.2.8	Sappey's veins	265
5.2.9	Bronchial varices	265
5.2.10	Biliary varices	265
5.2.11	Sublingual varices	265
5.3	Formation of hepatic lymphocysts	265
5.4	Portal hypertensive vasculopathy	265
5.5	Pathophysiological sequelae	266
5.6	Portal biliopathy	266
6	**Therapy**	266
6.1	Conservative treatment	267
6.2	Invasive therapy	267
	• References (1–153)	268

(Figures 14.1–14.14; tables 14.1–14.11)

14 Portal hypertension

▶ ARISTOTELES (384–322 BC) first described the portal vein within the venous system. HEROPHILOS (ca. 300–250 BC) was the first to recognize the portal vein system and its importance as the discharge zone for all resorbent intestinal veins. (s. pp 6, 7) • A description of the portal vein system with its intrahepatic branches and separate bloodstream was given by GALENUS (129–199 AD). (s. p. 8) • The independence of the portal vein circulation from the overall blood circulation was demonstrated by F. GLISSON (1597–1677). (s. p. 10)

▶ In 1905 the cause of portal hypertension was regarded by R. KRETZ as being the mechanical constriction of the hepatic veins resulting in a shunt between the arterial and venous circulation. • The term **portal hypertension syndrome** was defined by A. GILBERT and M. VILLARET (1906) and taken to encompass ascites, opsiuria, splenic tumour, haemorrhoids, gastrointestinal bleeding and the development of hepatofugal collaterals. The underlying disease consisted of cirrhosis and portal vein thrombosis. (38) • **Measurement of portal venous pressure** was taken by L. M. ROUSSELOT in 1936. Pressure measurement by puncturing oesophageal varices was first performed by P. ALLISON (1951). A. PATON et al. (1953) reported on the indirect determination of portal venous pressure with the aid of hepatic venous pressure measurements. A correlation between pressure in the portal vein and pressure in the splenic vein was established by M. ATKINSON and S. SHERLOCK (1954).

1 Definition

A persistent pressure elevation of >12 mmHg in the portal vein circulation, dilation of the portal vein to >13 mm or an increase in the portal pressure gradient of >7 mmHg (difference between the pressure of the portal vein and that of the inferior vena cava) is termed portal hypertension. At pressure values of more than 20 mmHg, collaterals generally develop. • *Portal hypertension is regarded as a systemic disease which affects a number of organ systems.*

2 Pathogenesis

The portal vein is 5–8 cm long with a diameter of 1.2 ± 0.2 (or 0.97) cm. The portal venous pressure is 3–7 (–12) mmHg. It is dependent on several *criteria*: posture, intra-abdominal pressure (e.g. coughing, compression), respiratory phase, Valsalva's manoeuvre and a number of biochemical mediators. (18)

Hepatic circulation: About 70–75% of the hepatic circulation (1,500 ± 300 ml/min, or 1.4–1.5 ml/min/1.73 m^2 body surface) pass through the portal vein (25–30% via the hepatic artery). Hepatic circulation increases after the ingestion of food, but decreases by about 30% after physical exertion as a result of sympatheticotonia. The oxygen content of portal venous blood is lower than that of arterial blood, but is significantly higher than in the rest of the venous system. The portal vein supplies about 10–12 ml O_2/min × 100 g, i.e. 50–60% of the liver's oxygen requirement. The liver is very adaptable in this respect and balances an increased or decreased oxygen supply by decreasing or increasing oxygen extraction (by almost 100%) from the portal and arterial blood. (5, 11, 81, 91) (s. pp 852, 860, 864)

Hepatic blood flow: In addition to the autoregulation of the arterial hepatic system, the hepatic blood flow is mainly regulated via neural (sympathetic) stimulation and the effects of hormones, mediators or pharmaceuticals. • Agents such as α-agonists, histamine, serotonin, noradrenaline, endothelin and angiotensin have a constrictive effect on the portal venous system. A vasodilatory effect on the arterial system is brought about by β-agonists, nitric oxide (NO) (46, 110), glucagon, prostaglandins, pentagastrin, adenosin, etc. • Under pathological conditions (e.g. lowered response to vasoconstrictors), individual factors of these biochemical regulation systems may be present to a greater or lesser extent and thereby lead to pathophysiological mechanisms. This also applies to the action of endotoxins with regard to an elevation of the portal pressure. • **Ito cells** are key targets for vasodilators: they regulate the hepatic microcirculation. (110)

Hepatic resistance: Various areas of resistance can regulate the circulation of blood in the liver: (*1.*) arterioles of the hepatic artery, (*2.*) arterioles in the region of the splanchnic vessels, (*3.*) presinusoidal portal venules, (*4.*) sinusoids and postsinusoidal sections of vessels, and (*5.*) portosystemic collaterals.

Forward-flow hypothesis: When hepatic resistance is constant, increased blood supply causes an elevation of the portal pressure. • **Backward-flow hypothesis:** This primarily requires an increase in hepatic vascular resistance. The subsequently reduced circulation of blood in the liver is compensated by increased circulation in the splanchnic vessels.

The portal hypertensive syndrome is caused by (*1.*) increased resistance in the portohepatic circulation, (*2.*) an increase in the splanchnic vein blood supply, or both.

▶ The *rise in vascular resistance* is the decisive factor and, in most cases, even the sole cause. It may be *func-*

tional and *reversible* as well as *structural* and *irreversible*. Blood flow correlates directly with vessel diameter to the 4th power, i.e. small radial changes cause large changes in vessel resistance. An increase in the blood supply leads to portal hypertension and/or respective clinical sequelae. The persistent disturbance in biochemical mechanisms which regulate the blood circulation in the liver and the impact of pathological substances may also have pathogenic effects. (21, 57, 67, 110, 119) (s. fig. 14.1)

Despite the development of *portosystemic collaterals*, which ought to lead to a fall in portal hypertension, the *hyperdynamic circulation* accompanied by splanchnic vasodilation (= increased cardiac output, decreased systemic vascular resistance, hypervolaemia, systemic arteriolar vasodilation) maintains portal hypertension in both the splanchnic and systemic vascular systems. (11, 42, 81) The hyperdynamic circulation is either the cause or the result of portal hypertension — or both. Arterial blood pressure is normal or slightly decreased.

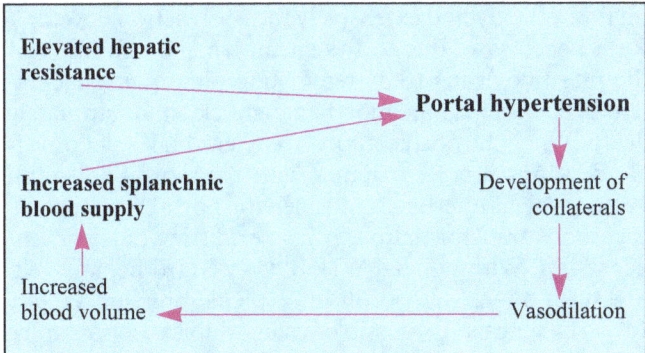

Fig. 14.1: Pathogenesis of portal hypertension

3 Forms and aetiology

Portal hypertension is classified according to the *localization* of the flow resistance. Increases in pressure in the portal vein system are rapidly transferred to the preceding vascular sections, since the portal vein does not have any venous valves. Depending on whether its localization lies before, within or beyond the liver, portal hypertension is broken down into *prehepatic, intrahepatic* and *posthepatic blocks*. The intrahepatic form is further subdivided into a presinusoidal, sinusoidal and postsinusoidal rise in resistance. Underlying *morphology* allows distinction between cirrhotic and non-cirrhotic portal hypertension. • Sometimes the aetiology is unknown (= *idiopathic, non-cirrhotic portal hypertension*). (33, 64, 66, 94, 107, 131, 133, 146, 150) (s. tab. 14.1)

3.1 Prehepatic portal hypertension

Prehepatic (non-parenchymatous) portal hypertension develops (*1.*) as a result of an increase in the portal blood supply in the form of hyperkinetic hypertension, or (*2.*) due to occlusion of the portal vein or its trunks. The frequency is 10–20%. The liver is morphologically normal, but diminished in size. Its function is not impaired. The reduced afferent portovenous flow is compensated by arterial perfusion of the liver. Ascites occurs only rarely. There are a variety of known causes for this portal block form. (s. tab. 14.2) (s. figs. 14.4, 14.5)

Phylogenetically, the portal vein is derived from several fused embryonic vessel components. Malformation can lead to *atresia* or *hypoplasia* of the portal vein and cause portal hypertension in newborns. (92, 150)

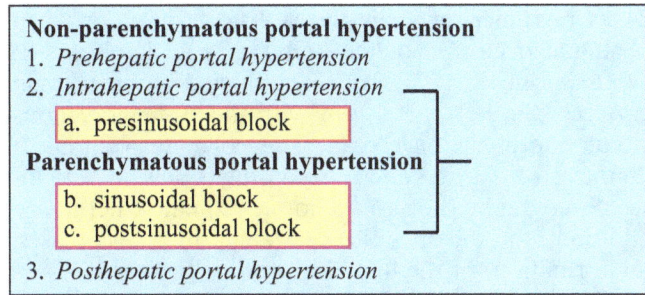

Tab. 14.1: Forms and localization of portal hypertension

Congenital or postnatal
1. Arterioportal fistulas
   = *hyperkinetic hypertension*
2. Atresia or hypoplasia of the portal vein
3. Thrombosis of the portal vein
   − encroachment of the postnatally obliterated umbilical vein on the portal vein
   − infection of the umbilical vein with phlebitis of the portal vein
4. Cruveilhier-von Baumgarten disease
5. Cavernous transformation of the portal vein

Acquired
1. Thrombophlebitis or thrombosis of the portal vein
2. Compression of the portal vein
3. Cavernous transformation of the portal vein
4. Arterioportal fistulas
   = *hyperkinetic hypertension*
5. Compression or thrombosis of the splenic vein
   = *segmental portal hypertension*

Tab. 14.2: Forms and causes of prehepatic portal hypertension

3.1.1 Cavernous transformation

The most common cause of prehepatic portal hypertension in early childhood is cavernous transformation, a primary angiomatous malformation of the portal vein (H. Breining et al., 1968; C. Marks, 1973). • In adults, septic diseases (appendicitis, pancreatitis, cholecystitis, etc.) and traumas are deemed responsible, since they trigger a slow occlusion of the portal vein (H. W. Clatsworthy, 1974). Myeloproliferative syndromes, hepatic tumours and cirrhosis are also possible causative factors. • This transformation consists of a spongy convolute of paraportal, tendril-like interlaced vascular structures in place of a single portal vein, mainly in the area of the hepatoduodenal ligament. Symptoms are abdominal pain, haematemesis, splenomegaly and oesophageal varices. Diagnosis is based on US and CT. A cavernous transformation of the portal vein usually appears sonographically as a string of bead-like varicose collaterals in the hepatoduodenal ligament. (9, 10, 122) (s. p. 861)

3.1.2 Cruveilhier-von Baumgarten disease

The **Cruveilhier-von Baumgarten disease** develops when postnatal occlusion of the umbilical vein is absent (P. VON BAUMGARTEN, 1907). An open, dilated umbilical vein connects the left portal vein with the systemic venous circulation in the navel area. This collateral vein has a diameter of >3 mm and a hepatofugal flow of >5 cm/sec. Sonography shows an echofree tubular structure. In addition to the persistence (and, in most cases, malformation) of the umbilical vein, a hypoplastic portal vein system is found. The resulting hypoplasia of the liver and its vessels culminates in portal hypertension. Typical of this condition are the massive varicose collaterals between the portal vein and the abdominal wall veins in the form of a Medusa's head (s. p. 91), a continual venous hum below the xiphoid ("bruit de diable" or "humming-top murmur") (s. p. 92), and splenomegaly. (s. p. 221) • In the **Cruveilhier-von Baumgarten syndrome**, the postnatally closed umbilical vein in the region of the round ligament is recanalized due to portal hypertension; thus the blood from the left portal branch is drained caudally. As a consequence of haemodynamically effective "shunting", flow values of >10 cm/sec can be measured.

3.1.3 Arterioportal fistulas

Hyperkinetic hypertension in the prehepatic portal vein system is caused by arterioportal fistulae with resulting increased blood flow. About 150 cases of such aneurysmal anomalies are known from the literature. (3) They occur more frequently, however, after abdominal traumas or iatrogenic interventions (e.g. liver biopsy, cholangiography, arteriography) and in the presence of malignant liver tumours. They are found mainly in the proximity of the splenic artery or mesenteric vessels. Arterial flow into the low-pressure portal region is unaffected. Oesophageal varices, splenomegaly and, in some cases, ascites develop very rapidly despite a "healthy liver" (no abnormal clinical or laboratory findings). This is followed by the subsequent development of secondary thrombosis of the portal vein as a result of fibromuscular hyperplasia of the intima and fibrosis in the portal area (= *hepatoportal sclerosis*). Clinically, a "machinery murmur" in the abdomen is discernible on auscultation. Diagnosis can be made with the aid of duplex sonography or radiological procedures.

3.1.4 Portal vein thrombosis

The most frequent cause of prehepatic portal hypertension in adults is portal vein thrombosis. Sonography displays the fresh thrombus as a hypoechoic structure in the initially dilated portal vein. (83, 95, 135) The blood flow (during the reversal phase from a hepatopetal to a hepatofugal flow) slows down due to liver cirrhosis, and this is deemed the causative factor in over 30% of cases of portal vein thrombosis. The liver function is greatly restricted. Ascites is often observed and proves difficult to treat. The presence of thrombophilia is seen as a predisposing factor. • Other causes are: thromboembolism (87), abdominal operations, traumas (63), pregnancy, collagenoses, portography, polycythaemia vera, osteomyelosclerosis, Budd-Chiari syndrome, primary hepatocellular carcinoma, hepatic echinococcus cysts (99). Septic processes (e.g. umbilical vein infection in newborns, appendicitis, diverticulitis, pancreatitis, colitis) play a major role. Tuberculosis is a rare cause. (113) (s. tab. 39.5) The severity of the clinical picture of portal vein thrombosis depends on how quickly and extensively the obstruction develops. Rapid occlusion, due to the haemorrhagic infarction of the intestine, leads to extreme abdominal pain, haematemesis, melaena, haemorrhagic shock, and ultimately death. When the obstruction is more gradual, splenomegaly develops rapidly together with paraportal collateral vessels which function as intrahepatic portal branches (= cavernous transformation), thus permitting partial compensation. With normal WHVP (= wedged hepatic vein pressure), there is a rise in intrasplenic pressure. (s. tab. 14.9) Diagnosis is possible using duplex sonography, splenoportography or modern radiological methods. Disorders of liver function are only apparent at a later stage. *Hepatoportal sclerosis* may develop. (s. p. 862)

3.1.5 Segmental portal hypertension

An increase in peripheral resistance following *thrombosis of the splenic vein* is termed segmental portal hypertension. Bleeding from gastric fundus varices is frequently found. Due to the intact liver function, bleeding from the upper gastrointestinal tract is better tolerated. Parasplenic variceal convolutes can be visualized by means of colour-encoded duplex sonography. As a rule, ascites does not occur. Pressure in the enlarged spleen is greatly elevated. The WHVP remains unchanged even with normal portal pressure. For this reason, a shunt operation is contraindicated in cases of bleeding from oesophageal or gastric fundus varices owing to segmental portal hypertension. (39, 71, 76, 117)

3.2 Intrahepatic portal hypertension

Intrahepatic portal hypertension is caused by lesions which are easy to distinguish morphologically as well as pathogenetically and which occur in the following regions: (*1.*) presinusoidal veins of the intrahepatic periportal triangles, (2.) liver sinusoids, and (3.) draining postsinusoidal veins. Pathogenic overlapping is possible, since some lesions affect both the presinusoidal and sinusoidal vascular sections simultaneously. Frequency is estimated at 70–80%. (s. figs. 14.4, 14.5)

3.2.1 Presinusoidal block

▶ The presinusoidal block is a form of non-parenchymatous portal hypertension. The WHVP is normal. There is no impairment of liver function until a later stage of the underlying disease has been reached. This type of block is caused by a congenital or acquired constriction of the lumen or by a reduction in portal venous branches within the periportal triangles. (s. tab. 14.3)

Fibrocystic liver diseases, which show an autosomal-recessive inheritance pattern, may hence cause a presinusoidal block within the clinical picture of *cholangiodysplasia*. Histological differentiation between cirrhosis and cholangiodysplastic pseudocirrhosis is very difficult. • *Congenital liver fibrosis* (D.N.S. KERR et al., 1962), an autosomal recessive disease involving the kidneys, causes an increase in presinusoidal pressure due to increased vascular resistance. *Rendu-Osler-Weber disease* and *Gaucher's disease* should also be mentioned as forms of a congenital presinusoidal block, the portal hypertension here possibly also being of sinusoidal origin. (s. tab. 14.3)

Various infectious, toxic or immunological lesions lead to a presinusoidal block in adults. From a primary endothelial lesion, endophlebitis ensues. Rich in fibres and deficient in cells, it is ultimately responsible for the obliteration and even disappearance of the portal branches. • *Obliterative portal venopathy* (N.C. NAYAK et al., 1969) with portal and periportal fibrosis and subsequent perisinusoidal sclerosis is referred to as *hepatoportal sclerosis* (W. P. MIKKELSEN et al., 1965). This is a complex disorder involving splenomegaly, hypersplenism and portal hypertension, which has also been described as non-cirrhotic portal fibrosis (J.L. BOYER et al., 1967) or idiopathic portal hypertension (K. OKUDA et al., 1982). (118) *Banti's syndrome* (8) probably fell into this group; this is, however, now an obsolete term. The WHVP and flow rates are normal and liver function is not affected. Cirrhosis may develop in cases of prolonged illness.

Thrombosis of small portal veins due to bacterial cholangitis with pericholangitis or to malignant and subsequently thrombotic processes can cause an increase in presinusoidal resistance.

Even in the early stage of *primary biliary cholangitis*, immunological or scar-related atrophy of the small portal veins is evident. (73) • In *primary sclerosing cholangitis*, these changes are only manifested once cirrhotic transformation has set in. (s. tab. 14.3)

The main cause of presinusoidal hypertension in the world is *schistosomiasis*. The eggs of the parasite are washed "embolically" into the portal veins. Thus portal hypertension is induced, whereby the rise in pressure correlates with the quantity of obstructing eggs. The WHVP is normal. In addition, a granulomatous foreign-body reaction occurs with immunologically induced eosinophilic infiltrations. This leads to pronounced portal-periportal fibrosis, in which the periportal triangles are distended with nodules and scars and incorporate the axis of the Rappaport acini (= *"pipe-stem fibrosis"*). (28, 108) (s. p. 509) (s. fig. 25.14)

Both *liver adenomas* and *nodular regenerative hyperplasia* can cause a presinusoidal block due to distortion of the portal veins. • *Wilson's disease* leads to an overlapping of presinusoidal and sinusoidal portal hypertension. • In *alcoholic cirrhosis*, there is a similar overlap of the sinusoidal and postsinusoidal forms.

Presinusoidal block
Congenital
1. Rendu-Osler-Weber disease
2. Gaucher's disease
3. Cholangiodysplasia or congenital liver fibrosis (microcystic liver), congenital polycystic disease
Acquired
1. Thrombosis of the portal venous branches (95, 135)
2. Aneurysmal dilatation of the portal vein (2)
3. Primary biliary cholangitis (73), primary sclerosing cholangitis
4. Sclerosing granulomas – schistosomiasis (28, 108) – sarcoidosis (70, 129, 134) – tuberculosis (113)
5. Toxically induced hepatoportal sclerosis/periportal fibrosis – arsenic (82, 89, 102, 105) – vinyl chloride monomers (13) – insecticides (particularly with copper sulphate) (105) – cytostatics (methotrexate, 6-mercaptopurine) (115) – immunostatic agents (azathioprine) (74) – cyanamide
6. Myeloproliferative syndromes (26, 75)
7. Collagenoses (24, 25, 54)
8. Haemoblastoses (e.g. mastocytosis)
9. Lymphoblastoses
10. Wilson's disease
11. Haemochromatosis
12. Malignant diseases
13. Liver adenoma
14. Nodular regenerative hyperplasia (86, 104, 124, 145)
15. Partial nodular transformation (116, 144)
16. Idiopathic (non-cirrhotic) presinusoidal block (146)

Tab. 14.3: Causes of elevated presinusoidal resistance in intrahepatic portal hypertension (with some references)

3.2.2 Sinusoidal block

▶ The sinusoidal block is attributed to various *pathogenic mechanisms*: (1.) compression of the sinusoids via hepatocellular storage of substances (e.g. steatosis), (2.) prolonged action of hepatotoxins with increasing collagen formation and fibrosis, (3.) disturbed passage in Disse's space (e.g. due to oedema), (4.) storage processes in the sinusoidal cells, (5.) influence of vaso-active substances on the sinusoids, and (6.) compression of the sinusoids by the formation of nodules. Increased resistance thus comes from constriction or reduction of the sinusoidal vessels. The sinusoidal block is the most common cause of portal hypertension. It is ascribed to intrahepatic parenchymal hypertension of the portal vein. Hepatomegaly is nearly always present. (s. tabs. 14.1, 14.4, 14.9) (s. figs. 14.4, 14.5)

Sinusoidal block

1. Storage of substances
   – fatty liver
   – acute fatty liver in pregnancy
   – amyloidosis (153)
   – glycogenosis type III (79)
   – Gaucher's disease
   – Niemann-Pick disease (127)
   – α_1-antitrypsin deficiency
2. Hepatotoxins
   – alcoholic hepatitis
   – vitamin A (112)
   – vinyl chloride, methotrexate
3. Severe parenchymal loss
   – acute viral hepatitis (136)
   – acute liver failure (88)
   – malaria
4. Peliosis hepatitis
5. Chronic hepatitis (69)
6. Regenerative nodes in cirrhosis
7. Formation of nodes
8. Cirrhosis

Tab. 14.4: Causes of a sinusoidal block in intrahepatic portal hypertension (with some references)

Alcohol: With regard to hepatotoxins, by far the greatest importance must be attributed to alcohol. The development of alcohol-mediated portal hypertension is complex. The increasing accumulation of fat in the hepatic cells interferes with the microcirculation, since the sinusoids become both longer and narrower as a result of fatty degeneration of the hepatocytes. In cases of fatty liver, a greater microcirculation is observed in the arterioles at the same time. Stimulation of the Ito cells is an important pathogenic factor; it induces collagenization of the perisinusoidal reticular fibres. Scar areas develop around the central veins, with perivenous sclerosis and ultimately even further obliteration of these vessels.

Vitamin A intoxication: Prolonged and marked vitamin A intoxication leads to a substantial increase in individual Ito cells. This causes constriction of the sinusoids; accompanying fatty degeneration of the hepatocytes supports the obstructive effect. The Ito cells are responsible for perisinusoidal fibrosis. The liver surface is strikingly smooth despite marked portal hypertension (often with considerable oesophageal varices). (112) (s. figs. 14.2, 14.3)

Cirrhosis: Irrespective of its aetiopathogenesis, cirrhosis always leads to portal hypertension. In addition to the principal sinusoidal factors, it is also affected by presinusoidal mechanisms. In some cases, it is not always possible to assess the pathogenic significance of individual factors. The real cause of portal hypertension lies within the sinusoids. Because of the cirrhotic conversion of the liver and the regeneration of nodes, the portal veins are nearly always compressed, allowing hypertension to build up due to the vascular resistance. The sinusoids, thereby stiffened, trigger phlebectasia in their immediate vicinity, and a compensatory increased afferent arterial flow is produced. This can be easily detected because of muscular hyperplasia of the small arteries and the occurrence of shunts between the small arteries and portal veins.

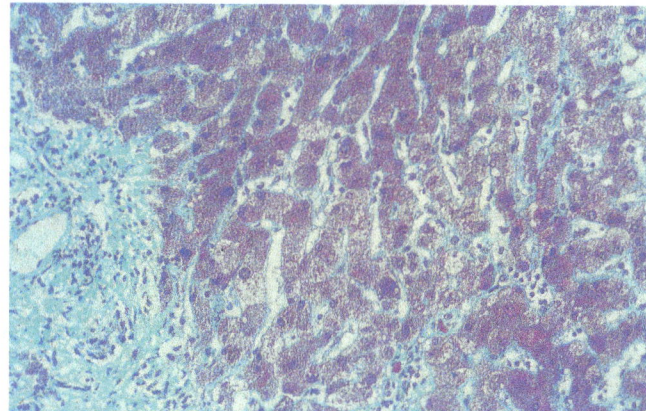

Fig. 14.2: Slight lobular inflammation. Periportal/perisinusoidal delicate fibrosis as a result of chronic vitamin A intoxication (same patient as in fig. 14.3) (Ladewig)

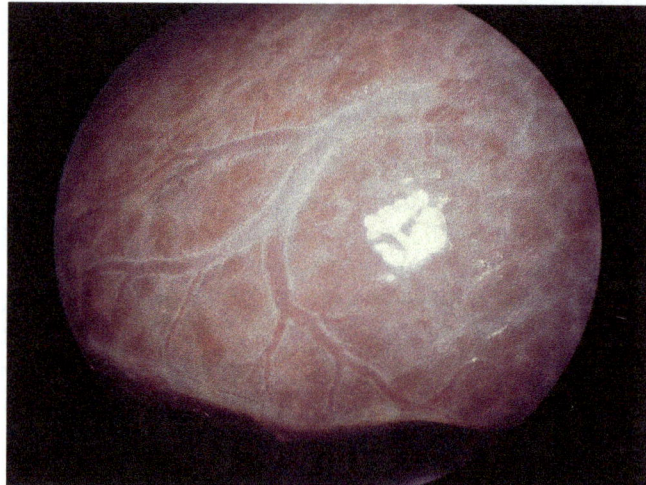

Fig. 14.3: "Smooth" cirrhosis with smooth surface and portal hypertension resulting from chronic vitamin A intoxication (same patient as in fig. 14.2)

3.2.3 Postsinusoidal block

▶ The postsinusoidal block is due to increased resistance in the hepatic veins and venules beyond the sinusoids. This block form is attributed to parenchymatous portal hypertension. (s. tabs. 14.1, 14.5, 14.9) (s. figs. 14.4, 14.5)

Liver cirrhosis is the most common cause of postsinusoidal portal hypertension. The greater resistance in this vascular zone is predominantly due to the expansive pressure caused by regenerative nodes on the small vein branches. An additional pathogenic factor is the elevated arterial blood flow to the liver. There is increasing evidence of arterioportal anastomoses. The arterial component of blood flowing to the liver can be raised by up to 80%. The blood flow from the splanchnic area is also higher. The internal pressure in the spleen and the WHVP rises in accordance with the respective stage of cirrhosis. Infiltration of portal fields, portal/periportal fibrosis and fibrous septa in cirrhosis leads to constriction and rarefaction of the portal venules and thus culminates in a presinusoidal block. For this reason, after the positioning of a portaca-

Postsinusoidal block
1. Liver cirrhosis (e.g. Wilson's disease, haemochromatosis)

2. Budd-Chiari syndrome
  • Stuart-Bras syndrome
    (veno-occlusive disease; radicular form)
    – pyrrolizidine alkaloids – contraceptives
    – cytostatic agents   – anabolic agents
    – immunosuppressants   – exposure to X-rays
                              – thorotrast
  • Chiari's disease
    (obliterative hepatic endophlebitis; truncal form)

3. Alcoholic hepatitis   Alcoholic central hyaline sclerosis
4. Partial nodular transformation of the liver (116, 145)

Tab. 14.5: Causes of a postsinusoidal block in intrahepatic portal hypertension (with some references)

val shunt, the WHVP is hardly (if at all) reduced. It is possible to ascertain the respective extent of a presinusoidal block by way of the splenosinusoidal pressure gradient.

Budd-Chiari syndrome is the term used for the clinical picture resulting from the occlusion of the hepatic veins. This occlusion may be acute or chronic, total or partial. Thrombosis of hepatic veins was first described in 1845 by G. BUDD. In 1899 H. CHIARI compiled all previously recorded observations and categorized them as an independent pathological entity. There are numerous causes: congenital anomalies of the hepatic veins, inflammatory diseases of the hepatic veins, localized or diffuse liver diseases, extrahepatic pathological processes, traumas, haematological or malignant diseases, pregnancy, myeloproliferative processes, etc. (s. p. 856)

Veno-occlusive disease (VOD) describes the occlusion of small hepatic veins and is defined as a *radicular form* of the Budd-Chiari syndrome. A variety of endotheliotoxic noxae, particularly phytotoxins, are responsible for this clinical picture. In 1951 reports were simultaneously published for the first time in South Africa (G. SELZER et al.) and Jamaica (K. R. HILL) dealing with this disease of the small venous branches, which results from chronic intoxication with pyrrolizidine alkaloids. (s. pp 562, 587) Similar morphological and clinical effects can also be caused by cytostatic agents (6-mercaptopurine, dacarbazine, thioguanine), azathioprine, contraceptives and exposure to X-rays. Since 1957, the term *Stuart-Bras syndrome* has also been used to describe the occlusion of the small hepatic veins. (s. p. 859)

Obliterative hepatic endophlebitis is also referred to as *Chiari's disease* and can be distinguished from the Budd-Chiari syndrome as its *truncal form*. It presents as primary, independent phlebitis of the large hepatic veins with secondary thrombosis. (s. tab. 14.5) In Chiari's disease, the hepatic veins are affected to differing degrees and at differing stages; this characterizes the clinical picture. Possible causes are rheumatic or paraneoplastic diseases and disorders of the immune system. Total occlusion of the hepatic veins has a dismal prognosis.

Partial occlusion results in portal hypertension with hepatosplenomegaly, ascites and oesophageal varices.

Alcoholic hepatitis also leads to a postsinusoidal block following the deposition of alcoholic hyaline in the centrilobular zone, with perivenous fibrosis and subsequent occlusion of the small veins.

3.3 Posthepatic portal hypertension

In posthepatic portal hypertension (prevalence about 5%), the flow hindrance is in the region of the inferior vena cava or the right heart. Extrahepatic processes impede the efferent flow of venous blood from the hepatic veins. Parenchymatous portal venous hypertension develops with a simultaneous elevation of pressure in the femoral vein. Liver findings correspond to the truncal form of the Budd-Chiari syndrome. (s. tabs. 14.6, 14.9) (s. figs. 14.4, 14.5)

Heart
1. Right heart insufficiency
2. Constrictive pericarditis
3. Tricuspid valve incompetence
4. Idiopathic dilative cardiomyopathy
Inferior vena cava
1. Membranous obstruction
2. Anomaly
3. Thrombosis
4. Tumours
5. Nephrotic syndrome
6. Polycythaemia vera
Hepatic veins
1. Anomaly
2. Chiari's syndrome
3. Tumours
4. Amoebic abscess

Tab. 14.6: Causes of posthepatic portal hypertension

The most frequent **cause** of posthepatic portal hypertension is *right ventricular insufficiency*. The central venous pressure is transferred to the hepatic veins and the sinusoids. • *Constrictive pericarditis* leads to a state of pronounced posthepatic portal hypertension with the early development of ascites. • Severe *tricuspid valve incompetence* also culminates in this condition. • A *membranous obstruction* of the inferior vena cava was likewise described as a genetically determined cause of posthepatic portal hypertension (S. YAMAMOTO et al., 1968). Three variants can be distinguished by angiography, depending on the different ways in which the hepatic veins are involved or whether they are affected at all. • *Thrombosis* of the inferior vena cava can develop either from thrombosis of the pelvic veins or independently in the presence of predisposing factors.

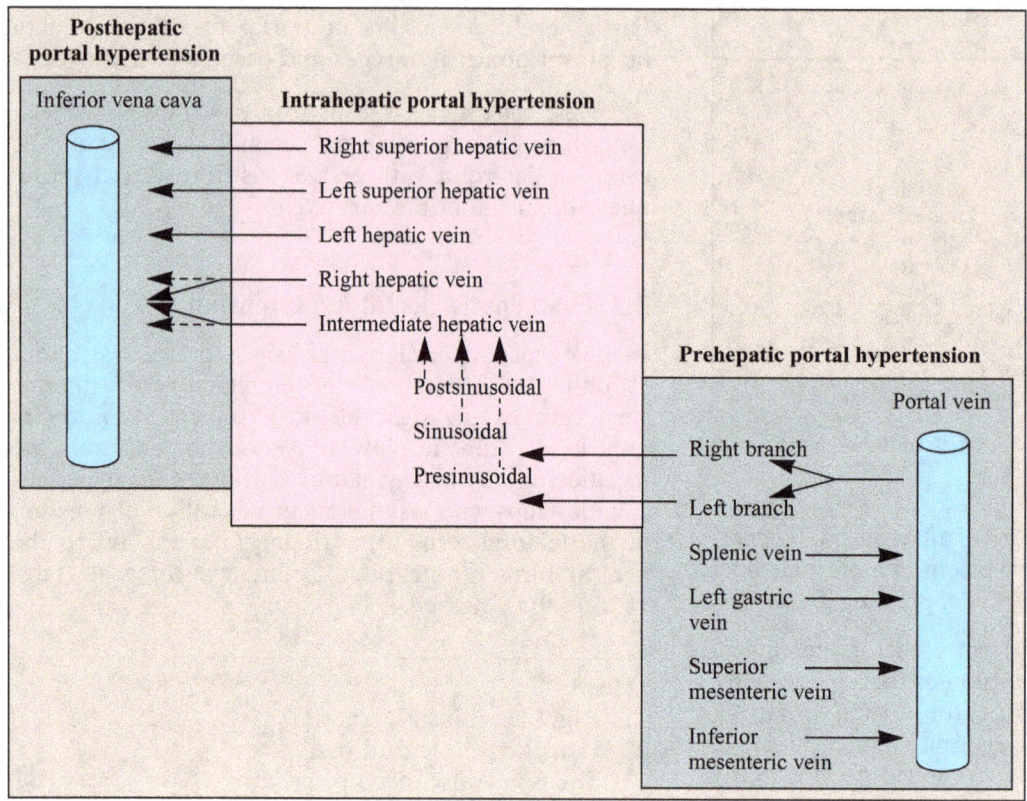

Fig. 14.4: Anatomical systematics of portal hypertension

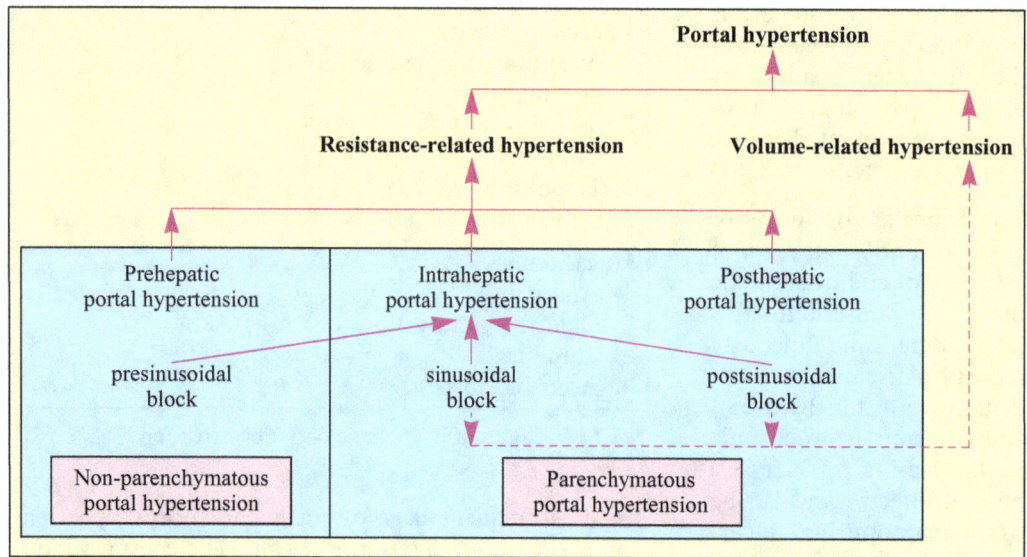

Fig. 14.5: Forms, localization and systematics of portal hypertension (resistance-related and volume-related hypertension can occur either as primary or secondary forms)

4 Diagnosis

Hypertension of the portal vein, with its numerous intrinsic or acquired causes, may not display any symptoms for several years. Portal hypertension itself is very often a concomitant symptom in a number of liver diseases. It can lead to severe or even fatal complications. For this reason, hepatological investigation frequently needs to explore (*1.*) the presence of portal hypertension, (*2.*) its aetiology, (*3.*) its severity, and (*4.*) potentially successful treatment of the underlying causes — in order to produce a favourable effect on the overall condition of the patient.

4.1 Anamnesis

Specific investigation of the patient's medical history can provide evidence of existing portal hypertension. The main *anamnestic details* given by the patient are related to various targeted questions:

- existence of a liver disease
- existence of extrahepatic diseases
- alcohol abuse
- medication
- consumption of tea containing alkaloids
- tarry stools, haematemesis, bleeding tendency, thrombophilia
- visits to tropical regions (malaria, etc.)
- oedema, abdominal pain

4.2 Clinical findings

In the physical examination, particular attention should be paid to a number of *clinical findings*:

- hepatomegaly or atrophic liver cirrhosis
- splenomegaly
- skin stigmata of liver diseases
- anorectal varices
- oedema or ascites
- epigastric pulsation
- congested neck veins
- venous patterns on the surface of the abdomen
- vessel sounds
- prolonged Q-T interval (151)

4.3 Laboratory findings

Laboratory parameters are not suitable for detecting portal hypertension. Only *thrombopenia* (< 100,000/ mm^3) should be taken as evidence of a splenomegaly due to portal hypertension; decreased *haemoglobin values* can be seen as a sign of a continuous loss of blood. Testing for *occult blood* in faeces is obligatory when portal hypertension is suspected. Elevated *ammonia values* hint at an existing shunt circulation. *Cholinesterase* provides more information on the functioning of the liver, hence facilitating a prognosis.

4.4 Sonography

Sonography provides a reliable means of detecting splenomegaly, which is often, but not always present with portal hypertension. Normal spleen findings generally rule out this condition. The sonographically based suspicion of a particular liver disease should at the same time draw attention to the possible existence of portal hypertension. Nevertheless, diagnosis cannot simply be founded on the diameter of the portal vein, since the values obtained from healthy subjects and from patients with portal hypertension overlap. The blood flow sometimes slows down even when the portal vein is normal. Furthermore, the diameter of the portal vein (and also of the splenic vein) depends on the capacity of existing collaterals. (41, 78, 142, 149) (s. tab. 14.7).

Vaginal sonography revealed rectal varices in about 50% and pararectal varices in about 80% of cases. The varices had a diameter of 2.1 – 5.5 mm. (77)

Endoscopic sonography is ideally suited for displaying intramural and perimural oesophageal varices. (125) (s. fig. 19.6) Endoscopic colour Doppler sonography is another promising procedure, particularly for demonstrating a (still) evident variceal perfusion.

4.5 Doppler sonography

Valuable information on the haemodynamics in the portal vein system can be obtained with the aid of pulsed or colour-encoded Doppler sonography – predomin-

- Splenomegaly (> 4 × 7 × 11 cm) (s. p. 220)
- Dilation of the portal vein (> 13 mm)
- Dilation of the splenic vein (> 10 mm)
- Dilation of the ventricular coronary vein (> 6 mm)
- Restricted respiratory modulation of the vascular width of up to 3 mm (increase on inspiration and decrease on exspiration) regarding the portal vein and more particularly the splenic vein and the superior mesenteric vein. • Decrease in width of the lumen by more than 50% on exhalation = absence of portal hypertension
- Jump in calibre of the portal vein
- Reversal of flow in portal vessels
- Stasis of the gall bladder and gastric walls
- Visible evidence of collaterals
- Recanalization of the umbilical vein (s. fig. 6.7)
- Cavernous transformation of the portal vein

Tab. 14.7: Sonographic criteria in portal hypertension

antly by using a transducer with 3.5 MHz. • All forms of portal hypertension can also be classified and quantified in terms of severity. • A marked deceleration of the portal flow (< 10 cm/sec) together with evidence of portosystemic collateral vessels as well as a reversal of the portal blood flow (= hepatopetal to hepatofugal), which may also occur in the splenic vein, demonstrate a severe impediment in flow capacity. In the case of portal hypertension, a hepatofugal portal flow is found in 6 – 10% of patients. A dilation of the left gastric vein of > 6 mm points to the presence of oesophageal varices, since this vein is the main collateral vessel in such cases; evidence of high hepatofugal flow (more than 15 cm/sec) represents a distinct risk of variceal bleeding. (s. p. 133)

The **Doppler effect** is produced by changes in wavelength due to the reflection of sound on moving particles (e. g. erythrocytes). Consequently, the *direction of flow* (away from or towards the sound source) as well as the *flow rate* in arterial and venous vessels can be determined. The *flow volume* is then calculated by additional sonographic measurement of the vessel diameter. It has been shown that the rate of flow is clearly dependent upon the respiratory activity, so that an increase in blood flow velocity can be determined with maximum exspiration as well as postprandially (normal value: 18 – 30 cm/sec). (30, 37)

Fibrous transformation in the structure of the liver leads to a **change in hepatic haemodynamics.** Stenosis in the region of the hepatic veins can be recognized by an increased flow rate. Yet, even in cases of marked liver fibrosis or cirrhosis, the *hepatopetal flow in the portal vein* may only be slightly lowered or even normal owing to the dilation of the portal vessels and the formation of collaterals. In cirrhosis, the arterial flow is greater than the portal flow, the rate of which is about 30% lower than in healthy persons. The *relative change (in %)* following stimulation by a **standard test meal** provides a more exact diagnosis of portal hypertension. Postprandial flow, due to digestive hyperaemia, may reach 40 cm/sec. (68, 72) In the case of a distinct reduction in the flow rate, the flow direction may be reversed (= *hepatopetal to hepatofugal*). Blood flow in the portal venous system is normally hepatopetal as opposed to pulsatile (or only slightly pulsatile) and follows an increased exspiration flow rate. • Undulating blood flow when inhaling (= hepatopetal) and exhaling (= hepatofugal) is evidence of portal hypertension. (11, 81, 91)

Congestion index (CI): This parameter is the most reliable indicator of portal hypertension. It relates the portal cross-sectional area to the portal blood flow rate. The CI ranks higher than the direct pressure level in the diagnostics of the portal system and the HVPG. These three techniques (in this order) are considered to be the *gold standard* in early diagnosis of portal hypertension. CI levels of >0.1 are associated with excessive portal pressure with >95% sensitivity and specificity. (85) Sonographic imaging of *cavernous transformation* in the portal vein usually shows beaded varicose collaterals in the hepatoduodenal ligament.

4.6 Endoscopy

▶ **Oesophagogastroscopy** is considered to be the diagnostic procedure of choice for the detection of oesophageal or gastric varices. This examination should always be extended to the antrum and the duodenum, since varices can also occur there. Endoscopy allows the detection of oesophageal varicosis at an early stage of development. It also enables an assessment to be made of the size and preferred localization of the varices as well as imaging the surface of these veins, where red spots or stripes are often found. Blackish-brown spots are due to intramucosal haemorrhage. (s. p. 263) With the aid of gastroscopy, it is also possible to identify *erosive gastropathy* caused by portal hypertension. (s. p. 265) • In combination with **coloscopy**, examination initially focuses on the presence of anorectal varices. Endoscopy of the colon frequently reveals the presence of erosive colopathy with mucosal findings similar to those in the stomach. In rare cases, colonic varices are present. • **Video capsule endoscopy** makes it possible to examine the small bowel in portal hypertension. (111)

Laparoscopy permits the very early detection of portal hypertension due to the dilation and meandering of the fine peritoneal, intestinal or gastric vessels. (93) (s. p. 163) (s. figs. 7.5; 14.6, 14.11, 14.12; 16.9)

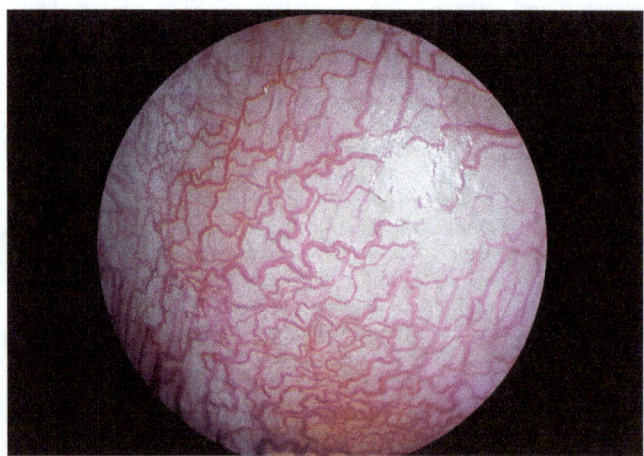

Fig. 14.6: Dilation and meandering of the fine peritoneal vessels in the initial stage of portal hypertension

4.7 Angiography

Splenoportographic procedures allow an accurate depiction of the portal vein and its afferent flow areas. Despite the development of new techniques, these methods are of importance in clarifying the cause of portal hypertension, and they are (still) deemed to be a prerequisite for operations aimed at reducing the pressure and volume in the portal venous circulation. Vessels with a diameter of < 1 cm are unsuitable for long-term patency of a shunt. Direct and indirect procedures are available. (16, 31)

In the light of a possible shunt operation, it has become more important to obtain additional information on the arterial blood supply to the liver. As regards cirrhosis with portal hypertension, **arteriographic investigations** have shown that the more the blood flow through the liver increases, the more the portal blood flow is reduced. Thus the blood flow relationship through the liver can become almost completely reversed: as little as 20% via the portal vein and as much as 80% via the hepatic arteries. Evidence of haemodynamically active stenosis in the arteries supplying the liver therefore constitutes a contraindication for shunt operations.

Direct splenoportography is the most informative procedure for visualizing the portal vein system and its collaterals. Yet this technique is costly, time-consuming and high-risk. The injection of contrast medium into the spleen is carried out either percutaneously (sonography-guided) or, preferably, by laparoscopy. It is also possible to *measure the pressure* in the portal vein system. In addition, this method ensures access to the collaterals if *radiological obliteration* is planned. (s. p. 189)

Indirect splenoportography via the femoral artery is not only very important, but also low-risk. Using radiography, the arterial branches of the abdominal aorta initially become visible, followed by the spleen, the splenic vein and the portal vein together with its afferent veins and collaterals. This procedure provides **information** on: (*1.*) localization of vascular resistance-related hypertension, (*2.*) cause of portal hypertension (in individual cases), (*3.*) patency and diameter of the respective vessel, (*4.*) extent of collateral circulation, (*5.*) hepatopetal or hepatofugal direction of flow in the portal vein, and (*6.*) shunt capacity of the splenic vein or superior mesenteric vein. (s. p. 190)

Hepatic vein phlebography via the femoral vein and the inferior vena cava facilitates visualization of the hepatic veins; it is technically simple, practically risk-free and puts little strain on the patient.

Other procedures that can be applied are indirect mesentericoportography, transjugular or transhepatic splenoportography, umbilical portography (s. p. 190) and scintigraphic splenoportography.

4.8 CT and MRI

Additional examination with CT or spiral CT may be necessary with respect to certain diagnostic questions (e. g. retroperitoneal space, CT portography). This also applies to MRI (e. g. in pronounced obesity or meteorism). Thus MRI angiography is a valuable additional diagnostic procedure. (58, 80, 128, 143)

4.9 Carbon dioxide wedged venography

Injection of carbon dioxide into a catheter in the wedged hepatic venous position facilitates excellent venography of the hepatic venous and portal venous tree. (23)

4.10 Portal pressure measurement

Vein-occlusion pressure: It is possible to measure the vein-occlusion pressure by inserting a measuring catheter through the cubital or jugular vein into a hepatic vein. Measurement can be made as free hepatic venous pressure (FHVP), whereby hepatic venous blood flows around the measuring catheter, or as wedged hepatic venous pressure (WHVP), whereby occlusion of the hepatic vein is achieved by inserting the measuring catheter into a branch of the hepatic vein or by inflating the measuring catheter balloon. The WHVP correlates closely with the portal vein pressure. Its normal value is 7–12 mm Hg. • The FHVP corresponds to the intra-abdominal pressure, which is normally 3–11 mm Hg.

Hepatovenous pressure gradient: The difference between WHVP and FHVP is used to calculate the hepatovenous pressure gradient (HVPG). This is equivalent to the portal (= sinusoidal) venous pressure. The pressure difference between the portal vein and the inferior vena cava is 1–4 mm Hg. Pressure levels of ≥ 8 mm Hg result in the formation of collateral vessels or ascites. At 12 mm Hg and higher, bleeding of the oesophageal varices occurs. The HVPG can be an important prognostic factor in terms of survival in patients with bleeding oesophageal varices. (84, 100) The examination can be carried out on an outpatient basis; this takes about 15 minutes, whereby the length of exposure to radiation is <2 minutes. Accordingly, it is possible to carry out follow-ups over a number of years. Normal WHVP values are 4–8 mm Hg. In cases of intrahepatic portal hypertension, particularly with liver cirrhosis, the WHVP corresponds to the directly measured portal venous pressure. In a prehepatic or presinusoidal block, the WHVP is normal. Posthepatic portal hypertension displays increased hepatic venous pressure. (s. tab. 14.9)

5 Sequelae of portal hypertension

The **clinical picture** of portal hypertension can vary greatly, since it is either characterized by the respective underlying disease or the symptomatology of the latter is still prevalent. • Irrespective of their aetiology and pathogenesis, all forms of long-standing portal hypertension generally lead to the same **sequelae**, albeit of differing intensity. (s. tab. 14.8)

Depending on the localization of the portal resistance, differing portal and hepatic **pressure values** and clinical findings are obtained for the five forms of portal hypertension. In this way, it is possible to gain more information for differential diagnosis. (s. tab. 14.9)

5.1 Splenomegaly

Splenomegaly following portal haemostasis (s. fig. 14.7) leads to increased haemolysis as well as leukopenia and thrombopenia. The last two conditions can also result from the sequestration of blood in the enlarged spleen or from an inhibited function of the bone marrow. Generally, these haematological findings only normalize in about 25% of cases following splenectomy or a shunt operation. It should be noted that a normal-sized spleen does not exclude portal hypertension. (36) There is no close correlation between the severity of portal hypertension and the size of the spleen. Morphological analysis reveals a thickened capsule with a firm consist-

Morphological sequelae
1. Splenomegaly
2. Portacaval collateral circulation
3. Formation of hepatic lymphocysts
4. Portal hypertensive intestinal vasculopathy
   – portal hypertensive gastropathy
   – portal hypertensive colonopathy

Haemodynamic sequelae
1. Elevated cardiac output
2. Lowered peripheral resistance
3. Elevated heart rate
4. Lowered arterial blood pressure

Pathophysiological sequelae
1. Reduced detoxification of noxae
2. Impaired biotransformation
3. Coagulation disorders
4. Hepatopulmonary syndrome
5. Endocrine and metabolic disorders
6. Disposition to bacterial infections
7. Insufficiency of lymph drainage
8. Ascites

Tab. 14.8: Characteristic morphological, haemodynamic and pathophysiological sequelae of portal hypertension

ency and dark blood oozing from the surface. An increase in fibres mainly affecting the sinus walls is the principal morphological manifestation. Sinusoids are dilated and lined with thickened epithelium. In addition to this fibroadenia, hyperplasia of the RES ensues. Haemorrhages often develop adjacent to arterioles of a Malpighian corpuscle. Splenic infarction occurs frequently. (s. fig. 35.10) • Prolonged portal hypertension sometimes leads to the formation of **Gamna-Gandy nodules.** These are brown-yellow, siderin-laden fibrous nodules within the sinus, apparently caused by microhaemorrhaging. *(see chapter 11)*

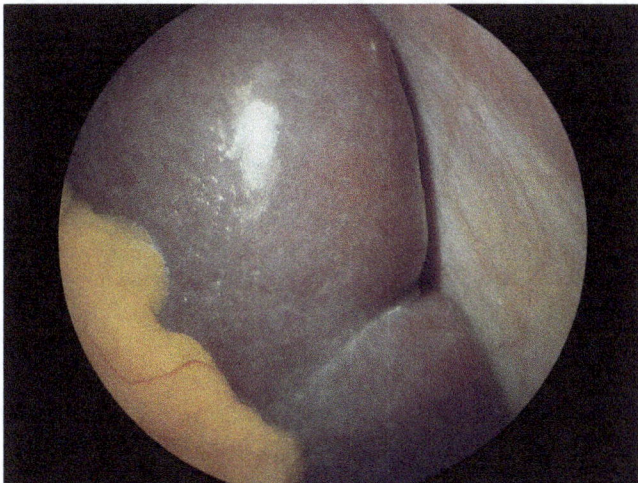

Fig. 14.7: Splenic tumour in portal hypertension following posthepatitic liver cirrhosis

Forms	Portal pressure	WHVP	Spleno-megaly	Oesophageal varices	Ascites
1. Prehepatic portal hypertension	↑	N	++	++	∅, (+)
2. Intrahepatic portal hypertension • presinusoidal • sinusoidal • postsinusoidal	↑ ↑ ↑↑	N ↑ ↑↑	+ ++ ++	++ +++ +++	(+) +++ +++
3. Posthepatic portal hypertension	↑	↑	+	++	++

Tab. 14.9: Haemodynamic and clinical findings in the 5 localized forms of portal hypertension (elevated hepatovenous pressure gradient = >9 mm Hg; increased risk of oesophageal varix bleeding = >12 mm Hg) (N = normal; ∅ = not present)

5.2 Portacaval collateral circulation

Portacaval collaterals represent the final stage of pressure-induced changes to the portal vessels. Initial *dilation* of the small portal vein branches is followed by the development of *meandering vessels*. This produces a compensating gain in vascular volume. In the long term, however, the thin-walled portal vessels are unable to withstand the elevated portal venous pressure. As a result, portacaval anastomoses form, which ultimately culminate in *varices* and frequently also in extensive *collateral circulation*. In addition to this, the portal vein itself can develop different degrees of ectasia. However, this reaction is generally accompanied by fibrosis and increased elasticity of the vessel wall. Portal hypertension leads to the dilation and reopening of veins which connect the portal vein system to the superior or inferior vena cava. Hence collateral circulation develops in the region of the oesophagus and gastric fundus as well as in the intestinal tract, retroperitoneum, lungs, spleen and kidneys, and at the anterior abdominal wall. (s. tab. 14.10) (s. figs. 7.5; 14.11, 14.12; 16.9)

Cranially draining collaterals
1. coronary gastric vein → azygous vein → short gastric veins → azygous vein
2. paraumbilical
3. portocoronary
4. portorenal
5. veins of Glisson's capsule, splenic capsule and diaphragm

Caudally draining collaterals
1. paraumbilical
2. gastrolienal
3. splenorenal
4. superior and inferior mesenteric veins → Retzius veins → ovarian/spermatic vein → haemorrhoidal venous plexus

Tab. 14.10: Possible formation of portacaval collaterals

5.2.1 Oesophageal and gastric varices

The collateral circulation described by H. Eppinger (1937) leading to the formation of oesophageal and fundic varices is still valid. (s. fig. 14.8) The hepatofugal blood flow of the portal vein passes through the coronary gastric vein to the perioesophageal venous plexus, which can form varices of the fornix or fundus. The blood is transported to the submucosal venous complex in the lower oesophagus. There are collaterals to the spleen via the short gastric veins. Anastomoses lead from the lower third of the oesophagus to the azygous and hemiazygous vein. In the central third of the oesophagus, a varicose venous plexus is formed due to stasis of the hepatopetal blood flow. From here, anastomoses run to the pericardial and intercostal veins as well as to the superior mediastinal and the diaphragmatic veins. These vessels conduct the blood to the azygous and hemiazygous veins, draining the entire blood flow into the superior vena cava. At the junction between the central and upper third of the oesophagus, the oesophageal varices disappear. This is a result of the balance of pressure with the right atrium created by the azygous vein. In line with the caudocranial blood flow, these oesophageal varices are also referred to as **"uphill"** varices (V. Buchtala, 1950) or as *type I varices*. The *pressure in the oesophageal varices* is temporarily raised by the ingestion of food and by an intra-abdominal increase in pressure (e.g. coughing, straining, lifting heavy loads). However, the pressure in the oesophageal varices is not raised in the head-down position. (35, 109, 123)

Oesophageal variceal pressure: The size of the oesophageal varices does not correlate with the magnitude of the portal venous pressure, but it does correlate with the oesophageal variceal pressure. This measurement is defined as the difference in pressure between the oesophageal lumen and the varix lumen. Measuring is done by fine-needle aspiration of a varix and the use of an extracorporeal pressure recorder. This technique is simple and reliable; it does not precipitate bleeding. Intravariceal pressure is a key factor in predicting variceal bleeding. (90) Measuring by way of a pressure sensor applied directly only yields valid results with large varices.

The **frequency**, localization and severity of oesophageal varices determine the life span of patients with portal hypertension. Oesophageal varices can be detected in about 80% of patients (i.e. some 20% of patients surprisingly do not present varices). In 90−95% of cases, the varices are located in the lower and central thirds of the oesophagus. The simultaneous occurrence of gastric fundic varices is only observed in 5−10% of patients. *Regression* of oesophageal varices (e.g. after alcohol abstinence) may occur.

The **radiographic detection** or **monitoring** of oesophageal varices using contrast medium is only carried out in rare

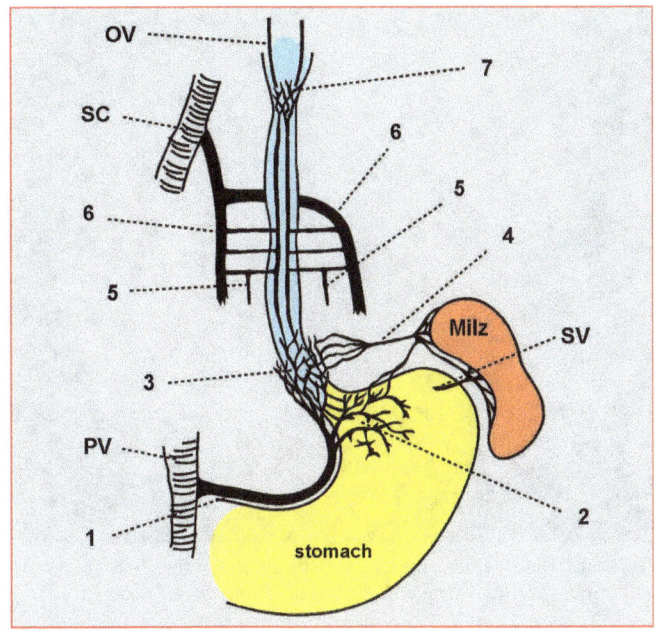

Fig. 14.8: Diagram showing the formation of oesophageal varices in portal hypertension (modified from H. Eppinger, 1937) • OV = oesophageal veins; SC = superior vena cava; SV = splenic vein; PV = portal vein; 1 = coronary gastric vein; 2 = perioesophageal venous plexus; 3 = submucous venous complex in the lower oesophagus; 4 = short gastric veins; 5 = hemiazygous vein; 6 = azygous vein; 7 = venous plexus of the central oesophagus

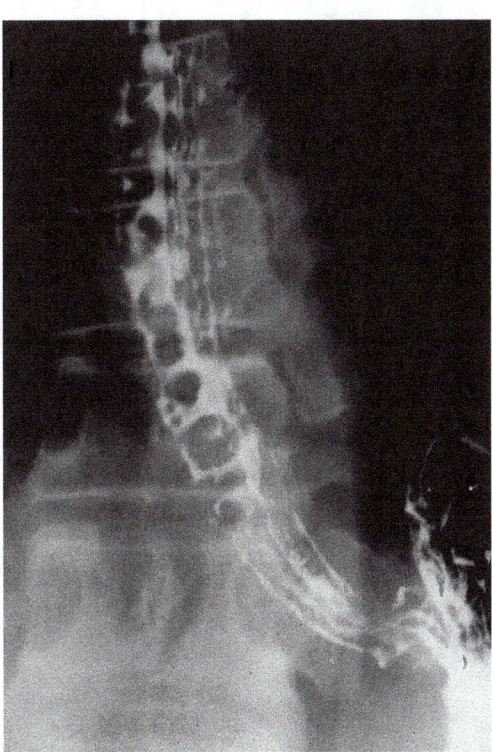

Fig. 14.9: Moderately dilated oesophagus with irregular surface. Numerous, differently sized filling defects as a result of varices

cases (after immobilizing the oesophagus by medication). During this procedure, the areas of the cardiac and fornix fundus should be carefully examined. (s. fig. 14.9)

The best method of detection is **oesophagogastroscopy.** (s. fig. 14.10) Localization, extent and severity of varices can be reliably determined with this method. (37, 121) The literature features a number of **staging schemes,** most of which have been developed empirically. (quot. 121) The main assessment *criteria* (with differing degrees of emphasis) are: length extension, vessel diameter, variations in diameter, number and colour of varices, mucosal changes (red spots, folding). Three-dimensional venous imaging (luminal prominence, length extension, diameter) can also be carried out. According to a well-accepted classification (1988), the criterion for stage I is defined as the possibility of depressing and squeezing out the varices, while stage II is characterized by the absence of this possibility. The circular enlargement of varices is defined as stage III. (s. tab. 19.6)

▶ **Downhill varices:** The downhill varices (B. Felson et al., 1964), which only occur in the proximal third of the oesophagus, are of both diagnostic and clinical significance. They were first described by M. Israelsky and H. Simchowitz in 1932. These varices do not result from portal hypertension, but are due to an elevation of pressure in the superior vena cava. This leads to a craniocaudal "downhill" blood flow. If there is an obstruction of the superior vena cava and/or the azygous vein, the blood flows from the head, neck and mediastinal region via the inferior thyroid vein and the mediastinal collat-

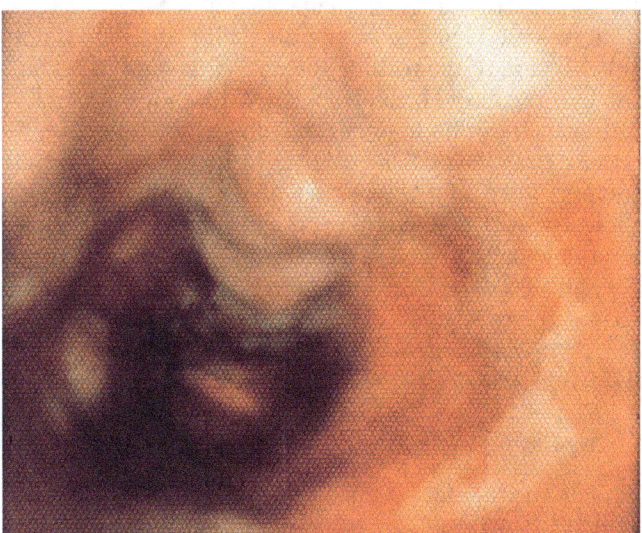

Fig. 14.10: Oesophagogastroscopy: pronounced varicosis (degree of severity III) in the lower third of the oesophagus

eral veins into the oesophageal veins and via the coronary gastric veins (hepatopetally) into the portal vein (= *type II*). Causal factors are goitre or recurrent goitre (45–60%), mediastinal fibrosis and malignant tumours with mediastinal lymph nodes (25–35%).

Type IIa is characterized by the patency of the azygous vein. Varices are only found in the upper third of the oesophagus. Retrosternal goitre has proved to be the most frequent cause. A superior vena cava syndrome is generally not detectable. • *Type IIb* is produced by the additional occlusion of the azygous vein. The entire blood volume must now be redirected to the inferior vena cava. • Although downhill oesophageal varices mainly occur in the upper third section, they often spread over the entire oesophagus in relation to the severity of the neck vein distension and the duration of the pathological condition. They are generally very pronounced and hence represent a genuine differential diagnosis of oesophageal varices in portal hypertension. The vertebral venous plexus and the thoracic veins are also used for drainage of the blood. • Bleeding from downhill oesophageal varices is rare, since (*1.*) there is a smaller blood volume with a lower pressure in the region of the superior vena cava, (*2.*) there is generally no coagulation disorder, and (*3.*) the mechanical burden in the upper oesophageal third is considerably lower. Bleeding is, however, quite possible in type IIb. • For this reason, *clarification of oesophageal varices* should always take into account the clinical picture of downhill oesophageal varices from the pathogenic and prognostic viewpoints. (27, 29)

5.2.2 Anorectal varices

Blood from the haemorrhoidal venous plexus passes via the azygous superior rectal vein into the inferior mesenteric vein and thereafter into the portal vein. By contrast, the paired middle rectal vein and inferior rectal vein discharge their blood via the iliac vein into the inferior vena cava. In portal hypertension, anorectal varices are found in the region of the rectum, the anal canal and the external anal region. • **Haemorrhoids** are distended and dislocated cavernous bodies in the rectum, which have no connection to the portal venous system. • Although haemorrhoids and anorectal varices are two different clinical pictures, it is quite possible for them to occur simultaneously. The frequency of anorectal varices (40–80%) is dependent upon the extent and duration of portal hypertension. The bleeding tendency is low (7–14%). However, there have also been reports of massive haemorrhages. (20, 40, 51, 61, 77, 97, 148) (s. tab. 14.10)

5.2.3 Intestinal varices

Varices occasionally occur in the stomach (114), duodenum (55, 140), small intestine, gall bladder (32, 78, 149) and colon (17, 40, 43, 62, 137) – excluding the transverse colon – as well as in the proximity of operative anastomoses or stomata. This generally involves collaterals between the branches of the inferior or superior mesenteric vein and small veins leading to the inferior vena cava. Colonic varices, which have not been detected endoscopically can be demonstrated by visceral angiography with a sensitivity of about 95%.

5.2.4 Abdominal wall varices

Pronounced anastomoses can develop between the mesenteric veins and the anterior abdominal wall. This is largely a result of spontaneous or postoperative adhesions (so-called *spontaneous Talma effect*). (s. figs. 7.5;

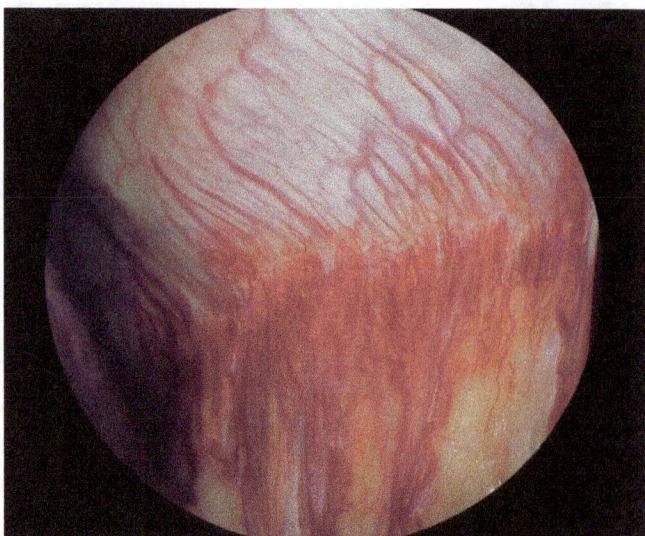

Fig. 14.11: Postoperative adhesions in the region of the abdominal wall with "spontaneous Talma effect" resulting from portal hypertension

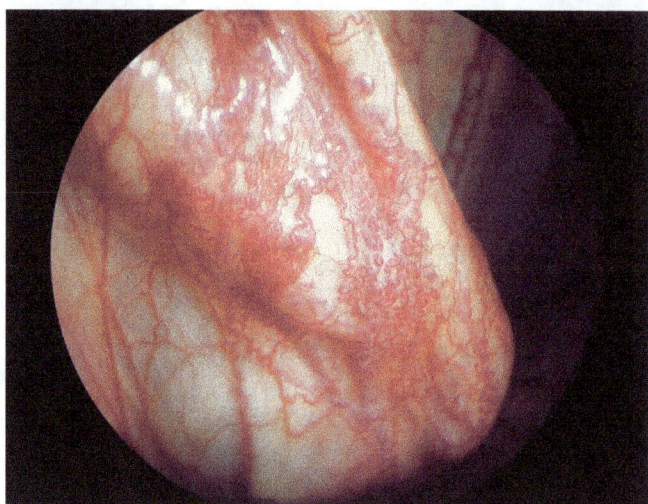

Fig. 14.12: Dilation and convolution of the small veins in the region of the round ligament (= teres) with recanalization of the umbilical vein resulting from portal hypertension (s. fig. 6.7)

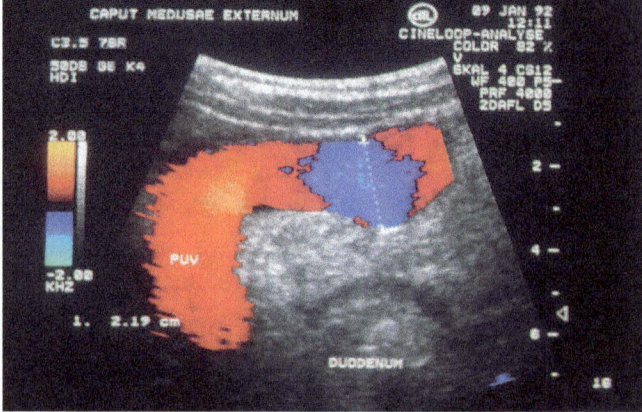

Fig. 14.13: External caput Medusae in liver cirrhosis. • The thick paraumbilical vein (diameter 2 cm) is shown subcutaneously at the exit of the vessel from Glisson's capsule. The colour-encoded vessel with a varicose enlargement at the exit point of the paraumbilical vein from Glisson's capsule is visible immediately below the ventral layers of the abdominal wall

14.11) Reopening of the umbilical vein in the round ligament (s. fig. 14.12) causes anastomoses to form with the epigastric veins in the anterior abdominal wall. (93) This can occasionally result in **caput Medusae:** radial, bluish, tortuous vessels, which are sometimes slightly raised and sometimes nodally varicose, leading from the navel to the abdominal wall. Generally, however, only a few larger collateral vessels are detectable as opposed to a complete caput Medusae. (s. p. 91) (s. fig. 14.13)

5.2.5 Retroperitoneal varices

There is a direct blood flow from the veins of the colon into the inferior vena cava via anastomoses with retroperitoneal veins.

5.2.6 Splenorenal varices

In about 5% of cases, blood passes through the short gastric veins to the splenic vein and then through other collateral veins to the left renal vein (= spontaneous splenorenal shunt).

5.2.7 Retzius' veins

Distally, the suprarenal veins and Retzius' veins provide a pathway into the inferior vena cava via the renal vein. Retzius' veins act as anastomoses between the portal vein branches in the intestinal and mesenteric regions and the branches of the inferior vena cava. (53)

5.2.8 Sappey's veins

Sappey's veins are located between the surface of the liver or spleen and the diaphragm. They are used for collateral circulation. Drainage takes place into the inferior vena cava.

5.2.9 Bronchial varices

Tracheobronchial varices with haemoptysis in alcoholic cirrhosis with portal hypertension were reported for the first time in 1994. (152)

5.2.10 Biliary varices

Biliary varices are defined by means of endosonography as serpiginous, anechoic vascular channels in and/or surrounding the extrahepatic biliary ducts as well as the gall bladder. (32, 59, 78, 98, 149) (s. p. 266)

5.2.11 Sublingual varices

Sublingual varices may be a rare source of expectorated blood in portal hypertension. (56)

5.3 Formation of hepatic lymphocysts

Particularly in intrahepatic portal hypertension, the portal vein system is relieved by an increase in hepatic lymph formation. The hepatic lymph flow is raised up to 7 ml/min (about 8 times the normal level), and the lymphatic pressure rises to 18 cm H_2O (normal value: 11.6 cm H_2O). The increase in lymphatic pressure leads to the formation of lymphocysts on the surface of the liver. Lymph, which is rich in albumin, is then able to drip from these lymphocysts into the abdominal cavity. (s. p. 297) (s. fig. 16.5)

5.4 Portal hypertensive vasculopathy

Endoscopic examination of the gastrointestinal tract often reveals erosion in the form of *portal hypertensive intestinal vasculopathy.* (48, 111, 138) These findings correlate with the degree of severity of portal hypertension. Intestinal erosion is generally the cause of a positive blood test in the faeces of patients with cirrhosis (= occult bleeding). In *portal hypertensive gastropathy* (frequency 20–30%), hyperaemic mucosa is in evidence due to dilation of the vessels and submucosal arteriovenous shunt formations. There is a mosaic-like pattern with small polygonal areas, surrounded by a whitish-yellow depressed border. Red marks (= lesions) signify a high risk of bleeding. These changes can usually be detected in the fundus, but may extend throughout the stomach. Hypoxaemia of the mucosa increases its susceptibility to aggressive elements. Numerous petechial lesions with punctiform deposits of haematinized blood are observed on the otherwise apparently intact gastric mucosa. (106, 130) Levels of prostaglandin E_2 in the mucosa are reduced. (147) (s. fig. 14.14)

About 10% of patients with cirrhosis have ulcers that bleed, whereas in 20–25% of cases, bleeding is caused by portal hypertensive gastropathy. (4, 6, 22, 34, 49, 101, 106, 120, 130, 132, 141) • Erosive vasculopathy can also be detected endoscopically in the region of the colon as *portal hypertensive colonopathy.* (12, 40, 62, 103, 126) Bleeding following vasculopathy of this kind requires local measures (e. g. laser), medication or shunting.

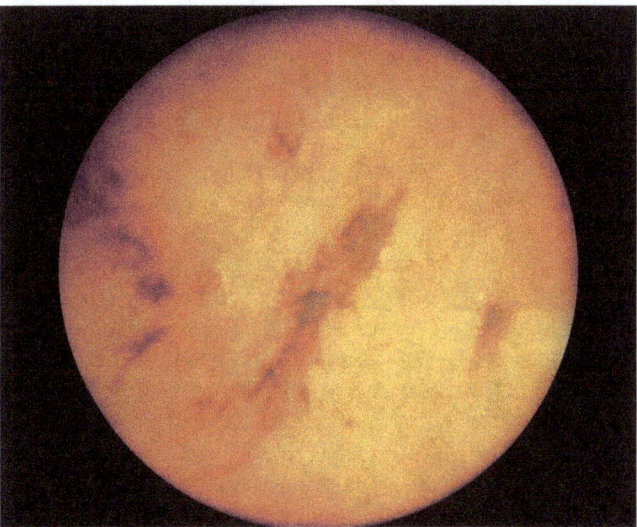

Fig. 14.14: Portal hypertensive gastropathy showing linear and patchy erosions

5.5 Pathophysiological sequelae

Portosystemic collaterals can divert up to 80% of the portal vein blood away from the liver. This initially results in haemodynamic disorders with subsequent (multifactorial) *hyperdynamic splanchnic circulation*. More and more varices develop around the bypasses in various venous areas, primarily in the form of oesophageal varices. Damage to the mucous membrane in the stomach and in the colon takes the form of hypertensive gastropathy/colopathy. Rechannelling of the umbilical vein leads to the Cruveilhier-von Baumgarten syndrome. (42) (s. tab. 14.8)

A grave consequence of collateral circulation is the reduced detoxification of exogenously administered noxae or endogenously produced toxins. This can lead to the development of latent, or eventually manifest, *hepatic encephalopathy* or neuropathy as well as to additional toxically mediated liver damage, or even liver insufficiency. • *Impairment of biotransformation* may cause unpredictable changes in the pharmacokinetics of medicaments or indeed trigger adverse drug reactions and interactions. (s. p. 57)

In addition to this, the occurrence of collateral circulation induces a protracted derangement of the numerous *RES functions*. (s. p. 69) As a result, the clearance capacities of activated coagulation products and inhibitors of the coagulation and fibrinolysis systems are reduced. Besides this, changes in the intrahepatic vascular architecture lead to a disorder of the portal microcirculation and trigger intravascular coagulation. (65) (s. p. 350) The increased RES activity results in hypergammaglobulinaemia and the subsequent inhibition of albumin synthesis. Inadequate elimination of endotoxins leads to endotoxinaemia with damage to the biological membranes, interference in hepatocellular metabolic processes, development of vasoactive substances, haemolysis, coagulopathy, etc.

Portosystemic collaterals also divert *hormones* past their target organ, the liver, with the result that they do not fully develop their activity (e.g. insulin, glucagon) or are not broken down and eliminated (e.g. aldosterone, steroids).

Portopulmonary hypertension (PPH) is defined as a secondary form of pulmonary hypertension in patients with portal hypertension. It is characterized by increased pulmonary vascular resistance in normal pulmonary capillary wedge pressure. Pulmonary hypertension typically features an anatomically fixed pulmonary vasoconstriction. The vascular changes depend on (*1.*) vasoconstriction, (*2.*) structural remodelling of the pulmonary arteries (fibroelastosis of the intima, hyperplasia of the media), and (*3.*) formation of microthrombi. Thus the histological changes are similar to those found in primary pulmonary hypertension. • Frequency of PPH in cirrhosis is 2–5%. Diagnosis is established using Doppler echocardiography and right heart catheterization. Prognosis is poor. In some patients, it was possible to improve the pulmonary blood flow by means of i.v. prostacyclin. (45, 104) *(see chapter 18)*

5.6 Portal biliopathy

Portal biliopathy as an entity was first described by S.K. SARIN et al. in 1992. This condition may be observed in portal hypertension, particularly in patients with extrahepatic portal vein obstruction. Such changes have also been reported, however, in a milder form in non-cirrhotic fibrosis, congenital hepatic fibrosis and cirrhosis.

The venous drainage of the common bile duct is guaranteed both by a paracholedochal *Petren's venous plexus* (T. PETREN, 1932; quot. 19) and a pericholedochal *Saint's venous plexus* (J.A. SAINT, 1961; quot. 19). The veins of these plexuses vary in size, but their diameter is usually no larger than 1 mm. • The development of portal hypertension leads to the opening of numerous collaterals. Likewise, the formation of varices in these plexuses may be observed. The first description of choledochal varices with subsequent compression of the common bile duct was given by A.H. HUNT in 1965. The same process causes collaterals around the gall bladder and the bile ducts.

The bile duct wall is thin and pliable, thus allowing protrusion of the varices into the lumen (a picture resembling oesophageal varices). This results in partial (and occasionally complete) bile duct obstruction, a condition which explains the usual clinical features: abdominal pain, recurrent fever, jaundice, increase of γGT and AP. It should be noted, however, that most patients are asymptomatic at onset and indeed for a long period after that. Development of choledocholithiasis is a frequent sequela. It is the cause of recurrent cholangitis, and subsequently of secondary biliary cirrhosis. Therefore, in patients with portal hypertension who show signs of biliary obstruction (clinical, biochemical, sonographical, cholangiographical), portal biliopathy may well be suspected. Sonography and MR cholangiography, if necessary ERC, are essential for establishing the diagnosis. (44)

Therapy: Asymptomatic patients do not need any treatment. With symptomatic patients, it is important to use therapeutic strategies which are directed towards the predominant symptoms. These include removal of gallstones by means of sphincterotomy (beware of varices!), antibiotics, placement of a stent, cholagogue agents, TIPS and surgical techniques. (19, 32, 59, 98, 149)

6 Therapy

The underlying cause of portal hypertension must first be found. Elimination of this cause (if possible) is even more important than treating the portal hypertension itself.

6.1 Conservative therapy

In cases of acute thrombosis, *fibrinolytic therapy* may occasionally be necessary.

Both vasodilators and vasoconstrictors can be used in the medicinal therapy of portal hypertension. However, the extensive literature available is limited almost exclusively to their use in treating oesophageal varix bleeding; less attention is paid to long-term therapy with the objective of lowering portal hypertension. The combination of β-blockers with, for example, nitrovasodilators, α-adrenergic antagonists or spironolactone leads to an additional decrease in the portal venous pressure. (7, 14, 33, 64, 119) (s. tab. 14.11)

Clonidine	= $α_2$-adrenergic agonist
Isosorbide dinitrate	= nitrovasodilator
Isosorbide-5-mononitrate	= nitrovasodilator
Molsidomine	= nitrovasodilator
Nadolol	= β-blocker (nonselective)
Prazosin	= $α_1$-adrenergic antagonist
Propranolol	= β-blocker (nonselective)
Spironolactone	= aldosterone antagonist
Terlipressin	= vasopressin derivative

Tab. 14.11: Substances for lowering portal hypertension

Propranolol, which was used for the first time by D. LEBREC et al. in 1980, brings about an approx. 50% reduction in portal venous pressure in some two thirds of patients. Dosage is established in line with the slowing-down of the heart rate (to about 25% less than that of the initial value, but not below 55/min). Propranolol also appears suitable for preventing erosive gastropathy. (6) In cases of bleeding, intravenous administration of terlipressin should be considered. (s. p. 366)

Nadolol has also been shown to reduce portal venous pressure. Gradually increasing the dosage to 2 x 1 mg/day is usually sufficient. (1)

Clonidine is an $α_2$-adrenergic agonist which is used effectively in portal hypertension at an average dosage of 0.075 – 0.3 mg/day.

Prazosin belongs to the $α_1$-adrenergic antagonist group and can be administered in portal hypertension at an average dosage of 2 – 4 mg/day.

Molsidomine is a prodrug. This substance is especially effective due to the fact that no tolerance develops. It leads to a fall in portal pressure of up to 40%, even after long-term use. Administration of this substance (e. g. 2 x 8 mg/day) is therefore recommended. (52) (s. p. 366)

Spironolactone is used as the basic medication in liver cirrhosis. By means of this therapy (upwards of 50 mg/day), it is possible to achieve a reduction in pressure in the portal system of about the same magnitude as with propranolol. (1, 60) (s. p. 312)

Ascorbic acid as an antioxidant improved the endothelium dysfunction and reduced the elevated level of malondialdehyde in patients with cirrhosis. In addition, the postprandial increase in hepatic venous pressure gradient was reduced. (50)

Total *abstinence from alcohol* (an absolute "must") can have a long-lasting beneficial effect in lowering elevated portal pressure values.

▶ These recommendations regarding medication are limited by the respective pharmacological properties, interactions and unwanted side effects. Such factors must always be taken into account. Therapeutic expectations with regard to adequate and constant reduction in portal pressure should not be set too high. Nevertheless, every possibility to reduce elevated portal venous pressure should be exploited.

6.2 Invasive therapy

In systemic diseases, *splenectomy* has to be considered. A *shunt operation* may be indicated in haemorrhage-free intervals. A proven alternative to the operative shunt is the transjugular intrahepatic portosystemic stent shunt.

Transjugular intrahepatic portosystemic stent shunt (TIPS) is available as an invasive therapy for portal hypertension. This concept has now been methodologically standardized. The success rate is extremely high. By means of balloon-expanded stents, portal decompression can be adapted to the respective situation in every single patient. The Palmaz stent can be placed with an accuracy of one millimetre; its diameter can also be adjusted in millimetre increments. The Wall stent can be used as an alternative in individual cases. **Indications** for this therapy in portal hypertension, where there is a persisting danger of variceal bleeding, are: (*1.*) lack of success with all medication therapy, including repeated sclerotherapy, (*2.*) inoperability in terms of a shunt operation, (*3.*) when a liver transplantation is not feasible, and (*4.*) bridging the time gap before an indicated liver transplantation. However, in up to 50% of patients, the period from stenosis to stenting ranges from 6 to 24 months; the stent must therefore be monitored constantly. (15, 132, 139) (s. pp 314, 320, 368, 899)

Shunt operations: Surgical shunts are only to be considered in cases where iatrogenic refractory bleeding occurs after all forms of conservative therapy have failed. A therapeutic shunt is only justified in the form of a (delayed) emergency shunt following a massive haemorrhage or as an elective shunt following bleeding. Portosystemic anastomoses are carried out in the form of a complete shunt (i. e. without maintaining residual portal perfusion) or as an incomplete shunt (i. e. maintaining residual portal perfusion with only a slight fall in the portal pressure). Portacaval end-to-side anastomosis as a complete shunt is technically the most simple and also the safest form, with the lowest risk; the thrombosis rate is less than 2%. (s. p. 370) A central total shunt is more successful in variceal bleeding or ascites (but there is a greater tendency for postoperative HE). A peripheral shunt reduces the tendency to bleed, but may cause deterioration of status in patients with ascites (however, HE is less frequent). A central shunt should not be carried out on patients who are scheduled to have a liver transplantation. There is no indication for prophylactic shunting or sclerosing of oesophageal varices before bleeding. (47, 96) (s. p. 870)

Liver transplantation not only removes the continued risk of variceal bleeding, but also eliminates the underlying liver disease causing portal hypertension. However, due to the scarcity of liver donors, limited financial resources and the life-long immunosuppression required, this major surgical intervention can only rarely be considered – perhaps in cases where a previous shunt operation or the creation of a TIPS was not possible. The survival rate for transplantation is higher than when recurrent bleeding is treated by repeated sclerotherapy (73% versus 17% after 4 years). The indication for transplantation (e.g. cirrhosis Child B or C) should be set as early as possible. (s. p. 903)

References:

1. **Abecasis, R., Kravetz, D., Fassio, E., Ameigeiras, B., Garcia, D., Isla, R., Landeira, G., Dominguez, N., Romero, G., Argonz, J., Terg, R.:** Nadolol plus spironolactone in the prophylaxis of first variceal bleed in nonascitic cirrhotic patients: a preliminary study. Hepatology 2003; 37: 359–365
2. **Alexopoulou, A., Papanikolopoulos, K., Thanos, L., Dourakis, S.P.:** Aneurysmal dilatation of the portal vein: A rare cause of portal hypertension (case report). Scand. J. Gastroenterol. 2005; 40: 233–235
3. **Aithal, G.P., Alabdi, B.J., Rose, J.D.G., James, O.F.W., Hudson, M.:** Portal hypertension secondary to arterioportal fistulae: two unusual cases. Liver 1999; 19: 343–347
4. **Albillos, A., Colombato, L.A., Enriquez, R., Oi Cheng Ng, Sikuler, E., Groszmann, R.J.:** Sequence of morphological and hemodynamic changes of gastric microvessels in portal hypertension. Gastroenterology 1992; 102: 2066–2070
5. **Alvarez, D., Mastai, R., Lennie, A., Soifer, G., Levi, D., Terg, R.:** Non-invasive measurement of portal venous blood flow in patients with cirrhosis: effects of physiological and pharmacological stimuli. Dig. Dis. Sci. 1991; 36: 82–86
6. **Aprile, L.R.O., Meneghelli, U.G., Martinelli, A.L.C., Monteiro, C.R.:** Gastric motility in patients with presinusoidal portal hypertension. Amer. J. Gastroenterol. 2002; 97: 3038–3044
7. **Banares, R., Moitinho, E., Matilla, A., Garcia-Pagan, J.C., Lampreave, J.L., Piera, C., Abraldes, J.G., de Diego, A., Albillos, A., Bosch, J.:** Randomized comparison of long-term carvedilol and propranolol administration in the treatment of portal hypertension in cirrhosis. Hepatology 2002; 36: 1367–1373
8. **Banti, G.:** Splenomegalie mit Leberzirrhose. Beitr. Path. Anat. Allg. Path. 1889; 24: 21–33
9. **Bayraktar, Y., Balkanci, F., Kayhan, B., Özenc, A., Arslan, S., Telatar, H.:** Bile duct varices or "pseudo-cholangiocarcinoma sign" in portal hypertension due to cavernous transformation of the portal vein. Amer. J. Gastroenterol. 1992; 87: 1801–1806
10. **Bayraktar, Y., Balkanci, F., Kayhan, B., Dundar, S., Uzunalimoglu, B., Kayhan, B., Telatar, H., Gurakar, A., van Thiel, D.H.:** Cavernous transformation of the portal vein: a common manifestation of Behcet's disease. Amer. J. Gastroenterol. 1995; 90: 1476–1479
11. **Benoit, J.N., Granger, D.N.:** Splanchnic haemodynamics in chronic portal hypertension. Semin. Liver Dis. 1986; 6: 287–298
12. **Bini, E.J., Lascarides, C.E., Micale, P.L., Weinshel, E.H.:** Mucosal abnormalities of the colon in patients with portal hypertension: an endoscopic study. Gastrointest. Endosc. 2000; 52: 511–516
13. **Blendis, L., Smith, P., Lawrie, B., Stephens, M.R., Evans, W.D.:** Portal hypertension in vinylchloride monomer workers. A hemodynamic study. Gastroenterology 1978; 75: 206–211
14. **Bosch, J., Abraldes, J.G., Groszmann, R.:** Current management of portal hypertension. J. Hepatol. 2003; 38 (Suppl.) 54–68
15. **Boyer, T.D., Haskal, Z.J.:** The role of transjugular intrahepatic shunt in the management of portal hypertension. Hepatology 2005; 41: 386–400
16. **Braun, S.D., Newman, G.E., Dunnick, N.R.:** Digital splenoportography. Amer. J. Roentgenol. 1985; 144: 1003–1004
17. **Bruet, A., Fingerhut, A., Eugene, C., Fendler, J.P.:** Varices intestinales et hypertension portale. Gastroenterol. Clin. Biol. 1984; 8: 725–732
18. **Burcharth, F., Bertheussen, K.:** The influence of posture, Valsalva manoeuvre and coughing on portal hypertension in cirrhosis. Scand. J. Clin. Lab. Invest. 1987; 39: 665–669
19. **Chandra, R., Kapoor, D., Tharakan, A., Chaudhary, A., Sarin, S.K.:** Portal biliopathy. J. Gastroenterol. Hepatol. 2001; 16: 1086–1092
20. **Chawla, Y., Dilawari, J.B.:** Anorectal varices – their frequency in cirrhotic and non-cirrhotic portal hypertension. Gut 1991; 32: 309–311
21. **Conn, H.O.:** Portal hypertension: history and pathogenesis. Gastroenterol. Internat. 1992; 5: 181–185
22. **D'Amico, G., Montalbano, L., Traina, M., Pisa, R., Menozzi, M., Spano, C., Pagliaro, L.:** Natural history of congestive gastropathy in cirrhosis. Gastroenterology 1990; 99: 1558–1564
23. **Debernardi-Venon, W., Bandi, J.C., Garcia-Pagan, J.C., Moitinho, E., Andreu, V., Real, M., Escorsell, A., Montanya, X., Bosch, J.:** CO_2 wedged hepatic venography in the evaluation of portal hypertension. Gut 2000; 46: 856–860
24. **DeCoux, R.E. jr., Achord, J.L.:** Portal hypertension in Felty's syndrome. Amer. J. Gastroenterol. 1980; 73: 315–318
25. **Drouhin, F., Fischer, D., Vadrot, J., Denis, J., Johanet, C., Abuaf, N., Feldmann, G., Labayle, D.:** Hypertension portale idiopathique associée à une collagénose proche du lupus érythémateux disséminé. Gastroenterol. Clin. Biol. 1989; 13: 829–833
26. **Dubois, A., Dauzat, M., Pignodel, Ch., Pomier-Layrargues, G., Marty-Double, Ch., Lopez, F.-M., Janbon, C.:** Portal hypertension in lymphoproliferative and myeloproliferative disorders: hemodynamic and histological correlations. Hepatology 1993; 17: 246–250
27. **Ehrle, U.B., Müller, M.K., Singer, M.V.:** Downhill-Varizen im Ösophagus. Ursachen und klinische Bedeutung. Dtsch. Med. Wschr. 1992; 117: 705–709
28. **Eyres, K.S., Kantharia, B., Magides, A.D., Ali, H.H., MacDonald, R.C.:** Portal hypertension due to hepatosplenic schistosomiasis: a case report and review of the literature. Brit. J. Clin. Pract. 1991; 45: 146–147
29. **Felson, B., Lessure, A.P.:** "Downhill" varices of the esophagus. Dis. Chest. 1964; 46: 740–746
30. **Fraser-Hill, M.A., Atri, M., Bret, P.M., Aldis, A.E., Illescas, F.F., Herschorn, S.D.:** Intrahepatic portal venous system: variations demonstrated with duplex and color doppler US. Radiology 1990; 177: 523–526
31. **Futagawa, S., Fukazawa, M., Horisawa, M., Musha, H., Ito, T., Sugiura, M., Kameda, H., Okuda, K.:** Portographic liver changes in idiopathic noncirrhotic portal hypertension. Amer. J. Roentgenol. 1980; 134: 917–923
32. **Gabata, T., Matsui, O., Kadoya, M., Yoshikawa, J., Ueda, K., Nobata, K., Kawamori, Y., Takashima, T.:** Gallbladder varices: demonstration of direct communication to intrahepatic portal veins by color Doppler sonography and CT during arterial portography. Abdom. Imag. 1997; 22: 82–84
33. **Gatta, A., Sacerdoti, D., Bolognesi, M., Merkel, C.:** Portal hypertension: state of the art. Ital. J. Gastroenterol. Hepatol. 1999; 31: 326–345
34. **Geraghty, J.G., Angerson, W.J., Carter, D.C.:** Erosive gastritis and portal hypertension. HPB Surgery 1992; 6: 19–22
35. **Gertsch, P., Fischer, G., Kleber, G., Wheatley, A.M., Geigenberger, G., Sauerbruch, T.:** Manometry of esophageal varices: comparison of an endoscopic balloon technique with needle puncture. Gastroenterology 1993; 105: 1159–1166
36. **Gibson, P.R., Gibson, R.N., Ditchfield, M.R., Donlan, J.D.:** Splenomegaly – an insensitive sign of portal hypertension. Aust. N. Z. J. Med. 1990; 20: 771–774
37. **Gibson, P.R., Gibson, R.N., Ditchfield, M.R., Donlan, J.D.:** A comparison of duplex Doppler sonography of the ligamentum teres and portal vein with endoscopic demonstration of gastroesophageal varices in patients with chronic liver disease or portal hypertension, or both. J. Ultrasound Med. 1992; 11: 327–331
38. **Gilbert, A., Villaret, M.:** Contribution to the study of the syndrome of portal hypertension. Compt. Rend. Soc. Biol. 1906; 60: 820–823
39. **Glynn, M.J.:** Isolated splenic vein thrombosis. Arch. Surg. 1986; 121: 723–725
40. **Goenka, M.K., Kochhar, R., Nagi, B., Mehta, S.K.:** Rectosigmoid varices and other mucosal changes in patients with portal hypertension. Amer. J. Gastroenterol. 1991; 86: 1185–1189
41. **Goyal, A.K., Pokharna, D.S., Sharma, S.K.:** Ultrasonic measurements of portal vasculature in diagnosis of portal hypertension. J. Ultrasound Med. 1990; 9: 45–48
42. **Groszman, R.J.:** Hyperdynamic circulation of liver disease 40 years later: pathophysiology and clinical consequences. Hepatology 1994; 20: 1359–1363
43. **Gudjonsson, H., Zeiler, D., Gamelli, R.L., Kay, M.D.:** Colonic varices. Report of an unusual case diagnosed by radionuclide scanning, with review of the literature. Gastroenterology 1986; 91: 1543–1547
44. **Guerrero-Hernandez, I., Weimersheimer Sandoval, M., Lopez Mendez, E., Hernandez Calleros, J., Tapia, A.R., Tiribe, M.:** Biliary structure caused by portal biliopathy. Case report and literature review. Ann. Hepatol. 2005; 4: 286–288

45. Hadengue, A., Benhayoun, M.K., Lebrec, D., Benhamou, J.-P.: Pulmonary hypertension complicating portal hypertension: prevalence and relation to splanchnic hemodynamics. Gastroenterology 1991; 100: 520–528
46. Hartleb, M., Michielsen, P.P., Dziurkowska-Marek, A.: The role of nitric oxide in portal hypertensive systemic and portal vascular pathology. Acta Gastroenterol. Belg. 1997; 60: 222–232
47. Hase, R., Hirano, S., Kondo, S., Okushiba, S., Morikawa, T., Katoh, H.: Long-term efficacy of distal splenorenal shunt with splenopancreatic and gastric disconnection for esophagogastric varices in patients with idiopathic portal hypertension. World J. Surg. 2005; 29: 1034–1037
48. Hashimoto, N., Ohyanagi, H.: Effect of acute portal hypertension on gut mucosa. Hepato-Gastroenterol. 2002; 49: 1567–1570
49. Hashizume, M., Sugimachi, K.: Classifikation of gastric lesions associated with portal hypertension. J. Gastroenterol. Hepatol. 1995; 10: 339–343
50. Hernandez-Guerra, M., Garcia-Pagan, J.C. Turnes, J., Bellot, P., Deulofeu, R., Abraldes, J.G., Bosch, J.: Ascorbic acid improves the intrahepatic endothelial dysfunction of patients with cirrhosis and portal hypertension. Hepatology 2006; 43: 485–491
51. Hosking, S.W., Smart, H.L., Johnson, A.G., Triger, D.R.: Anorectal varices, haemorrhoids, and portal hyertension. Lancet 1989/I: 349–352
52. Hüppe, D., Jäger, D., Tromm, A., Tunn, S., Barmeyer, J., May, B.: Einfluß von Molsidomin auf die portale und kardiale Hämodynamik bei Leberzirrhose. Dtsch. Med. Wschr. 1991; 116: 841–845
53. Ibukuro, K., Tsukiyama, T., Mori, K., Inoue, Y.: Veins of Retzius at CT during arterial portography: anatomy and clinical importance. Radiology 1998; 209: 793–800
54. Inagaki, H., Nonami, T., Kawagoe, T., Miwa, T., Hosono, J., Kurokawa, T., Harada, A., Nakao, A., Takagi, H., Suzuki, H., Sakamoto, J.: Idiopathic portal hypertension associated with systemic lupus erythematosus. J. Gastroenterol. 2000; 35: 235–239
55. Itzchak, Y., Glickman, M.G.: Duodenal varices in extrahepatic portal obstruction. Radiology 1977; 124: 619–624
56. Jassar, P., Jaramillo, M., Nunez, D.A.: Base of tongue varices associated with portal hypertension. Postgrad. Med. J. 2000; 76: 576–577
57. Kapoor, D., Redhead, D.N., Hayes, P.C., Webb, D.J., Jalan, R.: Systemic and regional changes in plasma endothelin following transient increase in portal pressure. Liver Transplant. 2003; 9: 32–39
58. Kim, M.J., Mitchell, D.G., Ito, K.: Portosystemic collaterals of the upper abdomen: review of anatomy and demonstration on MR imaging. Abdom. Imag. 2000; 25: 462–470
59. Kim, S., Chew, W.S.: Choledochal varices. Amer. J. Roentgenol. 1998; 150: 578–580
60. Klein, C.-P.: Spironolacton in der Behandlung der portalen Hypertonie bei Leberzirrhose. Dtsch. Med. Wschr. 1985; 110: 1774–1776
61. Kotfila, R., Trudeau, W.: Extraoesophageal varices. Dig. Dis. 1998; 16: 232–241
62. Kozarek, R.A., Botoman, V.A., Bredfeldt, J.E., Roach, J.M., Patterson, D.J., Ball, T.J.: Portal colopathy: prospective study of colonoscopy in patients with portal hypertension. Gastroenterology 1991; 101: 1192–1197
63. Kuntz, H.D., Freyberger, H., May, B.: Portale Hypertonie ohne Leberzirrhose. Zur Differentialdiagnose, Pathogenese und Klinik der posttraumatischen Pfortaderthrombose. Münch. Med. Wschr. 1985; 127: 97–99
64. LaBreque, D.R.: Portal hypertension. Clin. Liver Dis. 1997; 1: 1–24
65. Lasierra, J., Barrao, F., Cena, G., Aza, M.J., Morandeira, M.J., Barrao, M.E., Gonzalez-Gallego, J.: Changes of the fibrinolytic system in liver dysfunction: role of portal hypertension. Thromb. Res. 1992; 67: 15–21
66. Lebrec, D., Benhamou, J.-P.: Noncirrhotic intrahepatic portal hypertension. Semin. Liver Dis. 1986; 6: 332–340
67. Lebrec, D., Moreau, R.: Pathogenesis of portal hypertension. Eur. J. Gastroenterol. Hepatol. 2001; 13: 309–311
68. Lee, S.S., Hadengue, A., Moreau, R., Sayegh, R., Hillon, P., Lebrec, D.: Postprandial hemodynamic response in patients with cirrhosis. Hepatology 1988; 8: 647–651
69. Leeuwen, van, D.J., Howe, S.C., Scheuer, P.J., Sherlock, S.: Portal hypertension in chronic hepatitis: relationship to morphological changes. Gut 1990; 31: 339–343
70. Leger, L., Lemaigre, G., Prémont, M., Salmon, R., Klioua, Z., Battesti, J.-P.: Hypertension portale au cours de la sarcoidose. Trois observations dont une avec foie fibreux et hépatome malin à stroma osseux. Nouv. Presse Méd. 1980; 9: 1021–1024
71. Lenthall, R., Kane, P.A., Heaton, N.D., Karani, J.B.: Segmental portal hypertension due to splenic obstruction: imaging findings and diagnostic pitfalls in four cases. Clin. Radiol. 1999; 54: 540–544
72. Limberg, B.: Duplexsonographische Diagnose der portalen Hypertension bei Leberzirrhose. Einfluß einer standardisierten Testmahlzeit auf die portale Hämodynamik. Dtsch. Med. Wschr. 1991; 116: 1384–1387
73. Liu, G.-L., Huang, Y.-T.: Portal hypertension caused by biliary cirrhosis. Gastroenterol. Jap. 1991; 26 (Suppl. 3) 22–26
74. Lorenz, R., Brauer, M., Classen, M., Tornieporth, N., Becker, K.: Idiopathic portal hypertension in a renal transplant patient after long-term azathioprine therapy. Clin. Investig. 1992; 70: 152–155
75. Lukie, B.E., Card, R.T.: Portal hypertension complicating myelofibrosis: reversal following splenectomy. Canad. Med. Ass. J. 1977; 117: 771–772
76. Madsen, M.S., Petersen, T.H., Sommer, H.: Segmental portal hypertension. Ann. Surg. 1986; 204: 72–77
77. Malde, H., Nagral, A., Shah, P., Joshi, M.S., Bhatia, S.J., Abraham, P.: Detection of rectal and pararectal varices in patients with portal hypertension: efficacy of transvaginal sonography. Amer. J. Roentgenol. 1993; 161: 335–337
78. Marchal, G.J.F., van Holsbeeck, M., Tshibwabwa-Ntumba, E., Goddeeris, P.G., Fevery, J., Oyen, R.H., Adisoejoso, B., Baert, A.L., van Steenbergen, W.: Dilatation of the cystic veins in portal hypertension: sonographic demonstration. Radiology 1985; 154: 187–189
79. Markowitz, A.J., Chen, Y.-T., Muenzer, J., Delbuono, E.A., Lucey, M.R.: A man with type III glycogenosis associated with cirrhosis and portal hypertension. Gastroenterology 1993; 105: 1882–1885
80. Matsumoto, A., Kitamoto, M., Imamura, M., Nakanishi, T., Ono, C., Ito, K., Kajiyama, G.: Three-dimensional portography using multislice helical CT is clinically useful for management of gastric fundus varices. Amer. J. Roentgenol. 2001; 176: 899–905
81. McCormick, P.A., Burroughs, A.K.: Hemodynamic evaluation of portal hypertension. Hepato-Gastroenterol. 1990; 37: 546–550
82. Meran, J., Creutzig, A., Specht, S., Schürmeyer, T., Brunner, G., Ranke, C., Fabel, H.: Portale Hypertension und chronische Arsenintoxikation. Wien. Med. Wschr. 1989; 139: 580–584
83. Merkel, C., Bolognesi, M., Bellon, St., Sacerdoti, D., Bianco, S., Amodio, P., Gatta, A.: Long-term follow-up study of adult patients with non-cirrhotic obstruction of the portal system: comparison with cirrhotic patients. J. Hepatol. 1992; 15: 299–303
84. Meßmann, H., Holstege, A., Schölmerich, J.: Lebervenenverschlußdruckmessung. Indikation, Technik und Befunde. Dtsch. Med. Wschr. 1994; 119: 1245–1247
85. Moriyasu, F., Nishida, O., Ban, N., Nakamura, T., Sakai, M., Miyake, T., Uchino, H.: "Congestion index" of the portal vein. Amer. J. Roentgenol. 1986; 146: 735–739
86. Naber, A.H.J., van Haelst, U., Yap, S.H.: Nodular regenerative hyperplasia of the liver: an important cause of portal hypertension in non-cirrhotic patients. J. Hepatol. 1991; 12: 94–99
87. Nakanuma, Y., Ohta, G., Kurumaya, H., Tanino, M., Doishita, K., Takayanagi, N., Rin, S.: Pathological study on livers with noncirrhotic portal hypertension and portal venous thromboembolic occlusion: report of seven autopsy cases. Amer. J. Gastroenterol. 1984; 79: 782–789
88. Navasa, M., Garcia-Pagan, J.C., Bosch, J., Riera, J.R., Banares, R., Mas, A., Bruguera, M., Rodes, J.: Portal hypertension in acute liver failure. Gut 1992; 33: 965–968
89. Nevens, F., Fevery, J., van Steenbergen, W., Sciot, R., Desmet, V., de Groote, J.: Arsenic and non-cirrhotic portal hypertension. J. Hepatol. 1990; 11: 80–85
90. Nevens, F., Bustami, R., Scheys, I., Lesaffre, E., Fevery, J.: Variceal pressure is a factor predicting the risk of a first variceal bleeding. A prospective cohort study in cirrhotic patients. Hepatology 1998; 27: 15–19
91. O'Connor, M.K., MacMathuna, P., Keeling, P.W.N.: Hepatic arterial and portal venous components of liver blood flow: a dynamic scintigraphic study. J. Nucl. Med. 1988; 29: 466–472
92. Odièvre, M., Pigé, G., Alagille, D.: Congenital abnormalities associated with extrahepatic portal hypertension. Arch. Dis. Childh. 1977; 52: 383–385
93. Oelsner, D.H., Caldwell, S.H., Coles, M., Driscoll, C.J.: Subumbilical midline vascularity of the abdominal wall in portal hypertension observed at laparoscopy. Gastrointest. Endosc. 1998; 47: 388–390
94. Okuda, K., Kono, K., Ohnishi, K., Kimura, K., Omata, M., Koen, H., Nakajima, Y., Musha, H., Hirashima, T., Takashi, M., Takayasu, K.: Clinical study of eighty-six cases of idiopathic portal hypertension and comparison with cirrhosis with splenomegaly. Gastroenterology 1984; 86: 600–610
95. Okuda, K., Ohnishi, K., Kimura, K., Matsutani, S., Sumida, M., Goto, N., Musha, H., Takashi, M., Suzuki, N., Shinagawa, T., Suzuki, N., Ohtsuki, T., Arakawa, M., Nakashima, T.: Incidence of portal vein thrombosis in liver cirrhosis. An angiographic study in 708 patients. Gastroenterology 1985; 89: 279–286
96. Orozco, H., Mercado, M.A.: The evolution of portal hypertension surgery: lessons from 1000 operations and 50 years' experience. Arch. Surg. 2000; 135: 1389–1393
97. Pai, C.G., Thomas, V., Hariharan, M., Nair, K.V.: Rectal varices in extrahepatic portal hypertension. J. Gastroenterol. Hepatol. 1993; 8: 244–246
98. Palazzo, L., Hochain, P., Helmer, C., Cuillerier, E., Landi, B., Roseau, G., Gugnenc, P.H., Barbier, J.-P., Cellier, C.: Biliary varices on endoscopic ultrasonography: clinical presentation and outcome. Endoscopy 2000; 32: 520–524
99. Papadimitriou, J., Kannas, D., Papadimitriou, L.: Portal hypertension due to hydatid disease of the liver. J. Royal Soc. Med. 1990; 83: 120–121
100. Patch, D., Armonis, A., Sabin, C., Christopoulou, K., Greenslade, L., McCormick, A., Dick, R.: Single portal pressure measurement predicts survival in cirrhotic patients with recent bleeding. Gut 1999; 44: 264–269
101. Perez-Ayuso, R.M., Piqué, J.M.: Portal hypertension gastropathy. Dig. Dis. 1991; 9: 294–302
102. Piontek, M., Hengels, K.J., Borchard, F., Strohmeyer, G.: Nicht-zirrhotische Leberfibrose nach chronischer Arsenintoxikation. Dtsch. Med. Wschr. 1989; 114: 1653–1657

103. **Ponce Gonzales, J.F., Dominguez Adame Lanuza, E.D., Martin Zurita, I., Morales Mendez, S.:** Portal hypertensive colopathy: histologic appearance of the colonic mucosa. Hepato-Gastroenterol. 1998; 45: 40–43
104. **Portmann, B., Stewart, S., Higenbottam, T.W., Clayton, P.T., Lloyd, J.K., Williams, R.:** Nodular transformation of the liver associated with portal and pulmonary arterial hypertension. Gastroenterology 1993; 104: 616–621
105. **Primentel, J., Menezes, A.:** Liver disease in vineyard sprayers. Gastroenterology 1977; 72: 275–283
106. **Primignani, M., Carpinelli, L., Preatoni, P., Battaglia, G., Carta, A., Prada, A., Cestari, R., Angeli, P., Gatta, A., Rossi, A., Spinzi, G., de Franchis, R.:** Natural history of portal hypertensive gastropathy in patients with liver cirrhosis. Gastroenterology 2000; 119: 181–187
107. **Quereshi, H., Zuberi, S.J., Maher, M., Ahmed, W., Alam, S.E., Jafarey, N.A.:** Idiopathic portal hypertension: an overlooked entity. Hepatol. Res. 1998; 12: 169–176
108. **Raia, S., Caetano da Silva, L., Gayotto, L.C.C., Coutinho Forster, S., Fukushima, J., Strauss, E.:** Portal hypertension in schistosomiasis: a long term follow-up of a randomized trial comparing three types of surgery. Hepatology 1994; 20: 398–403
109. **Rigau, J., Bosch, J., Bordas, J.M., Navasa, M., Mastai, R., Kravetz, D., Bruix, J., Feu, F., Rodes, J.:** Endoscopic measurement of variceal pressure in cirrhosis: correlation with portal pressure and variceal hemorrhage. Gastroenterology 1989; 96: 873–880
110. **Rockey, D.C.:** The cellular pathogenesis of portal hypertension: stellate cell contractility, endothelin and nitric oxide. Hepatology 1997; 25: 2–5
111. **Rondonotti, E., Villa, F., Signorelli, C., de Franchis, R.:** Portal hypertensive enteropathy. Gastrointest. Endosc. Clin. North Amer. 2006; 16: 277–286
112. **Russel, R.M., Boyer, J.L., Bagheri, S.A., Hruban, Z.:** Hepatic injury from hypervitaminosis A resulting in portal hypertension and ascites. New Engl. J. Med. 1974; 291: 435–440
113. **Ruttenberg, D., Graham, S., Burns, D., Solomon, D., Bornman, P.:** Abdominal tuberculosis – a cause of portal vein thrombosis and portal hypertension. Dig. Dis. Sci. 1991; 36: 112–115
114. **Sarin, S.K., Lahoti, D., Saxena, S.P., Murthy, N.S., Makwana, U.K.:** Prevalence, classification and natural history of gastric varices: a long-term follow-up study in 568 portal hypertension patients. Hepatology 1992; 16: 1343–1349
115. **Shepherd, P., Harrison, D.J.:** Idiopathic portal hyertension associated with cytotoxic drugs. J. Clin. Pathol. 1990; 43: 206–210
116. **Sherlock, S., Feldman, C.A., Moran, B., Scheuer, P.J.:** Partial nodular transformation of the liver with portal hypertension. Amer. J. Med. 1966; 40: 195–203
117. **Shi, B.M., Wang, X.Y., Zhang, L., Yang, Z., Xu, J., Mu, Q.L. Wu, T.H.:** Regional portal hypertension diagnosed by ultrasonography: imaging findings and diagnostic value. Hepato-Gastroenterol. 2005; 52: 1062–1065
118. **Shibayama, Y., Nakata, K.:** The relation of periportal fibrosis to portal hypertension. J. Hepatol. 1990; 11: 313–317
119. **Sieber, C.C., Stalder, G.A.:** Pathophysiologische und pharmakotherapeutische Aspekte der portalen Hypertonie. Schweiz. Med. Wschr. 1993; 123: 3–13
120. **Smart, H.L., Triger, D.R.:** Clinical features, pathophysiology and relevance of portal hypertensive gastropathy. Endoscopy 1991; 23: 224–228
121. **Spech, H.J., Wördehoff, D.:** Klassifizierung von Ösophagusvarizen – endoskopische und klinische Aspekte. Leber Magen Darm 1982; 12: 109–114
122. **Spech, H.J., Pape, W.:** Kavernöse Pfortadertransformation. Dtsch. Med. Wschr. 1987; 112: 1137–1139
123. **Staritz, M., Rambow, A.:** Messung des hydrostatischen Druckes in Ösophagusvarizen. Wissenschaftliche Befunde und klinische Bedeutung. Dtsch. Med. Wschr. 1990; 115: 382–385
124. **Strohmeyer, F.W., Ishak, K.G.:** Nodular transformation (nodular "regenerative" hyperplasia) of the liver: A clinicopathologic study of 30 cases. Human Pathol 1981; 12: 60–71
125. **Sung, J.J.Y., Lee, Y.T., Leong, R.W.L.:** EUS in portal hypertension. Gastrointest. Endosc. 2002; 56 (Suppl.): 35–43
126. **Tahri, N., Ben Amor, M.M., Njeh, M., Sallemi, A., Krichen, M.S.:** Aspects coloscopiques de l'hypertension portale. Etude prospective de 31 cas. Ann. Gastroenterol. Hépatol. 1997; 33: 205–211
127. **Tassoni, J.P. jr., Fawaz, K.A., Johnston, D.E.:** Cirrhosis and portal hypertension in a patient with adult Niemann-Pick disease. Gastroenterology 1991; 100: 567–569
128. **Taylor, C.R.:** Computed tomography in the evaluation of the portal venous system. J. Clin. Gastroenterol. 1992; 14: 167–172
129. **Tekeste, H., Latour, F., Levitt, R.E.:** Portal hypertension complicating sarcoid liver disease: case report and review of the literature. Amer. J. Gastroenterol. 1984; 79: 389–396
130. **Thuluvath, P.J., Yoo, H.Y.:** Portal hypertensive gastropathy (review). Amer. J. Gastroenterol. 2002; 97: 2973–2978
131. **Tsuneyama, K., Kouda, Nakanuma, Y.:** Portal and parenchymal alterations of the liver in idiopathic portal hypertension: a histological and immunochemical study. Path. Res. Prac. 2002; 198: 579–603
132. **Urata, J., Yamashita, Y., Tsuchigame, T., Hatanaka, Y., Matsukawa, T., Sumi, S., Matsuno, Y., Takahashi, M.:** The effects of transjugular intrahepatic portosystemic shunt on portal hypertensive gastropathy. J. Gastroenterol. Hepatol. 1998; 13: 1061–1067
133. **Vakili, C., Farahvash, M.J., Bynum, T.E.:** "Endemic" idiopathic portal hypertension: report on 32 patients with non-cirrhotic portal fibrosis. World J. Surg. 1992; 16: 118–125
134. **Valla, D., Pessegueiro-Miranda, H., Degott, C., Lebrec, D., Rueff, B., Benhamou, J.P.:** Hepatic sarcoidosis with portal hypertension. A report of seven cases with a review of the literature. Quart. J. Med. 1987; 63: 531–544
135. **Valla, D., Casadevall, N., Huisse, M.G., Tulliez, M., Grange, J.D., Müller, O., Binda, T., Varet, B., Rueff, B., Benhamou, J.P.:** Etiology of portal vein thrombosis in adults. A prospective evaluation of primary myeloproliferative disorders. Gastroenterology 1988; 94: 1063–1069
136. **Valla, D., Flejou, J.F., Lebrec, D., Bernuau, J., Rueff, B., Salzmann, J.L., Benhamou, J.P.:** Portal hypertension and ascites in acute hepatitis: clinical, hemodynamic and histological correlations. Hepatology 1989; 10: 482–487
137. **Vescia, F.G., Babb, R.R.:** Colonic varices: a rare, but important cause of gastrointestinal hemorrhage. J. Clin. Gastroenterol. 1985; 7: 63–65
138. **Viggiano, T.R., Gostout, C.J.:** Portal hypertensive intestinal vasculopathy: a review of the clinical, endoscopic, and histopathologic features. Amer. J. Gastroenterol. 1992; 87: 944–954
139. **Vignali, C., Bargellini, I., Grosso, M., Passalacqua, G., Maglione, F., Pedrazzini, F., Filauri, P., Niola, R., Cioni, R., Petruzzi, P.:** TIPS with expanded polytetrafluoroethylene-covered stent: Resultats of an Italian multicenter study. Amer. J. Roentgenol. 2005; 185: 472–480
140. **Vigneri, S., Termini, R., Piraino, A., Scialabba, A., Bovero, E., Pisciotta, G., Fontana, N.:** The duodenum in liver cirrhosis: endoscopic, morphological and clinical findings. Endoscopy 1991; 23: 210–212
141. **Vigneri, S., Termini, R., Piraino, A., Scialabba, A., Pisciotta, G., Fontana, N.:** The stomach in liver cirrhosis. Endoscopic, morphological, and clinical correlations. Gastroenterology 1991; 101: 472–478
142. **Vilgrain, V., Lebrec, D., Menu, Y., Scherrer, A., Nahum, H.:** Comparison between ultrasonographic signs and the degree of portal hypertension in patients with cirrhosis. Gastrointest. Radiol. 1990; 15: 218–222
143. **Vosshenrich, R., Fischer, U., Grabbe, E.:** MR angiography in portal hypertension. State of the art. Radiologe 2001; 41: 868–876
144. **Wanless, I.R., Lentz, J.S., Roberts, E.A.:** Partial nodular transformation of liver in an adult with persistent ductus venosus. Review with hypothesis on pathogenesis. Arch. Path. Lab. Med. 1985; 109: 427–432
145. **Wanless, I.R.:** Micronodular transformation (nodular regenerative hyperplasia) of the liver: a report of 64 cases among 2500 autopsies and a new classification of benign hepatocellular nodules. Hepatology 1990; 11: 787–797
146. **Wanless, I.R.:** Noncirrhotic portal hypertension: recent concepts. Progr. Liver Dis. 1997; 14: 265–278
147. **Weiler, H., Weiler, Ch., Gerok, W.:** Decreased prostaglandin E_2 immunoactivity of gastric mucosa in portal hypertension. Netherl. J. Med. 1991; 38: 4–12
148. **Weinshel, E., Chen, W., Falkenstein, D.B., Kessler, R., Raicht, R.F.:** Hemorrhoids or rectal varices: defining the cause of massive rectal hemorrhage in patients with portal hypertension. Gastroenterology 1986; 90: 744–747
149. **West, M.S., Garra, B.S., Horti, S.C., Hayes, W.S., Cooper, C., Silverman, P.M., Zeman, R.K.:** Gall bladder varices: imaging findings in patients with portal hypertension. Radiology 1991; 179: 179–182
150. **Wilson, K.W., Robinson, D.C., Hacking, P.M.:** Portal hypertension in childhood. Brit. J. Surg. 1969; 56: 13–22
151. **Youssef, A.I., Escalante-Glorsky, S., Bonnet, R.B., Chen, Y.K.:** Hemoptysis secondary to bronchial varices associated with alcoholic liver cirrhosis and portal hypertension. Amer. J. Gastroenterol. 1994; 89: 1562–1563
152. **Ytting, H., Henriksen, J.H., Fugisang, S., Bendtsen, F., Moller, S.:** Prolonged Q-T (c) interval in mild portal hypertensive cirrhosis. J. Hepatol. 2006; 43: 637–644
153. **Zeijen, R.N.M., Sels, J.P.J.E., Flendrig, J.A., Arends, J.W.:** Portal hypertension and intrahepatic cholestasis in hepatic amyloidosis. Netherl. J. Med. 1991; 38: 257–261

Symptoms and Syndromes
15 Hepatic encephalopathy

		Page:
1	***Definition***	272
1.1	Causes of encephalopathy	272
1.2	Impaired consciousness	272
2	***Pathogenesis***	273
2.1	Preconditions	273
2.2	Hypotheses	273
2.3	Endogenous neurotoxins	274
2.3.1	Ammonia	274
2.3.2	Mercaptans and methionine derivatives	275
2.3.3	Short-chain fatty acids	275
2.3.4	Phenols and phenol derivatives	275
2.4	Amino acid imbalance	275
2.5	Disturbances of neurotransmitters	276
2.5.1	False neurotransmitters	276
2.5.2	Reduction in neurotransmitters	276
2.5.3	Increase in neurotransmitters	276
2.6	Deficiency of essential substances	277
3	*Morphological damage to the CNS*	277
4	*Causative and trigger factors*	277
5	***Clinical forms***	278
5.1	Reye's syndrome	279
5.2	Enzyme deficiency in the urea cycle	279
5.3	Pseudoportosystemic encephalopathy	279
5.4	Fulminant liver failure	279
5.5	Portosystemic encephalopathy	280
5.5.1	Subclinical (latent) form	280
5.5.2	Acute recurrent form	281
5.5.3	Chronic persistent form	281
6	*Clinical stages*	281
6.1	Coma assessment	281
7	*Diagnosis*	283
8	*Prognosis*	285
9	***Therapy***	285
9.1	Fundamental prerequisites	285
9.2	Basic therapy	285
9.2.1	Intestinal cleansing	285
9.2.2	Dietary measures	286
9.3	Standard therapy	286
9.3.1	Lactulose	287
9.3.2	Intermediates of the urea cycle	287
9.4	Branched-chain amino acids	288
9.5	Antibiotics	288
9.6	Specific or adjuvant therapy	289
9.7	Early detection and therapeutic success	289
	• References (1–157)	289
	(Figures 15.1–15.3; tables 15.1–15.6)	

15 Hepatic encephalopathy

▶ It seems that even HIPPOCRATES may have recognized a relationship between liver disease and brain disorder when he noted: *"depravedness of the brain arises from phlegm and bile"*. • One can also quote SHAKESPEARE, who wrote in Twelfth Night (1605): *"I am a great eater of beaf but I believe that does some harm to my wit."* • Such a form of "meat intoxication" was first described by N.V. ECK (1877) as being the cause of a subsequent neurologic al syndrome in dogs with a portacaval shunt, which had been fed on a diet of meat.

▶ **Cerebral symptoms in the wake of liver diseases** were already described by F. TH. FRERICHS (1861) and H.I. QUINCKE (1899) as well as over the following decades by E. POLLAK (1927), H.-J. SCHERER (1933), G. ZILLIG (1947), V. GAUSTAD (1949), R.D. ADAMS et al. (1949), J.M. WALSHE (1951), S. SHERLOCK et al. (1954), E.A. DAVIDSON et al. (1956) (22), F. ERBSLOEH (1958, 1974), G.A. MARTINI (1975) (59), and others.

Such **terms** as "hepatargy", "leucoencephalopathy", "shunt encephalomyelopathy" and "encephalomyelopathy" were put forward to classify these central nervous disorders. • The term **portosystemic encephalopathy** was introduced by S. SHERLOCK (1954). Changes in the central nervous system which occur after a long course of disease were also termed "chronic hepatoportal encephalopathy". In line with neuropsychiatric definitions, preference is given to the term "hepatic (portosystemic) encephalopathy".

1 Definition

Encephalopathy is defined as a pathological non-inflammatory brain disease resulting from heterogeneous pathological effects, which involve various neurological and/or psychic symptoms. In itself, this term says nothing about the aetiopathogenesis, nor about the respective regions of the brain affected.

Hepatic encephalopathy (HE) is defined as the totality of all cerebral dysfunctions which can occur during the course of serious – acute or chronic – liver disease. The neurological and mental symptoms, which as a rule are potentially reversible, can be observed with varying degrees of intensity and in different combinations, so that it is possible to subdivide hepatic encephalopathy into several well-defined grades of severity or distinct stages. Clinical symptomatology ranges from moderate neuropsychiatric disorders through to coma.

1.1 Causes of encephalopathy

All in all, more than 50 possible kinds of damage are known to cause encephalopathy. This large number of aetiological possibilities has to be considered when setting up the differential diagnosis, especially since symptomatology, therapy and prognosis are always determined by the respective underlying cause.

Encephalopathy can be triggered in a large number of very different ways:

(*1.*) **degenerative causes** (cerebral sclerosis, arterial hypertension, diabetes, etc.)
(*2.*) **hypoxaemia** (chronic cardiac insufficiency, constrictive pericarditis (3), respiratory insufficiency, chronic anaemia, etc.)
(*3.*) **metabolic causes** (enzymopathies, endocrine disorders, hypokalaemia, hyponatraemia, acidosis, alkalosis, exsiccosis, hypercapnia, paraproteinosis, etc.)
(*4.*) **traumatization** (Friedmann's vasomotor syndrome, boxer's encephalopathy, etc.)
(*5.*) **toxic causes** (alcohol, lead, organic solvents, bismuth, mussels contaminated with domoic acid, burn-related toxins, bilirubin [= kernicterus], vidarabine, uraemia, infectious diseases, liver insufficiency, etc.)
(*6.*) **cerebral causes** (intracranial space-occupying lesions, alcohol withdrawal syndrome, manic depression, schizophrenia, etc.)

1.2 Impaired consciousness

Consciousness is defined as the totality of mental and emotional processes perceived as current events in combination with an awareness of the subjectivity of experience. • **Quantitatively impaired consciousness** is the collective term for disturbances in awareness (= restricted vigilance). This condition is characterized by a limited readiness to show interest and concern, restricted attentiveness and impaired elements of consciousness. The activity of the ascending reticular system of the reticular formation is compromised, a condition which is generally accompanied by changes in the electroencephalogram (EEG). Moreover, disorders or loss of function are displayed in the area of the cerebral hemispheres and/or their afferent pathways, which are responsible for the subjective sensation of consciousness. • Differentiation is made between **four types** of clouded consciousness (W. HACKE, 1986):

1. Disorientation: A slight degree of impaired consciousness without clouding, yet with impediment to and deceleration of mental capacity and memory, compromised perception and reactivity (transitional psychosis).

2. Somnolence: Disorientation with additional, abnormal sleepiness, though arousal is still possible, and there can be memory gaps. • **Lethargy** is deemed to be the tendency to sleep without interruption, with greatly reduced mental/emotional responsiveness and absence of arousal reaction to normal stimuli.

3. Sopor: A condition resembling deep sleep with short-term attempts at orientation when being addressed, orderly movements of defence in reaction to pain – yet with no capability to react spontaneously.

4. Coma: Impaired consciousness of the most serious nature with long periods of profound unconsciousness and unresponsiveness to any form of address through to the absence of pain reaction and reflexes. • **Stupor** denotes total absence of physical and/or mental activity due to loss of drive, yet with full consciousness. Amimia, lack of spontaneity, unresponsiveness to external stimuli or attempts at establishing contact, and mutism are observed. • Stupor is also deemed to be unconsciousness of cerebro-organic origin, as for example in a serious transitional syndrome; it may be regarded as a physically substantiated, non-specific psychosis.

2 Pathogenesis

▶ As early as 1904, C. Neuberg and P.F. Richter reported on an increase in amino acids in the blood in cases of hepatic coma. These results were subsequently confirmed, arousing biochemical interest in this clinical picture (J. Feigl et al., 1917; F. Umber, 1922; K. Hoesch, 1931). A rise in xanthoprotein (K. Hoesch, 1931) and ammonia (E. Kirk, 1936; E.J. Conway et al., 1939) was also observed. • *Application of ammonia salts resulted in a temporary restriction of consciousness in a cirrhotic patient* (C. Van Caulaert et al., 1932). • From the wealth of results published, mention should be made of the detection of hypokalaemia and hypomagnesaemia, increases in pyruvic acid, cystine, methionine and glutamine, disruptions of the acid-base balance, and the higher levels of free amino acids in the serum. It was previously assumed that toxins absorbed by the intestine were inadequately detoxified in the diseased liver and, as such, reached the brain through the blood circulation, where they ultimately had a toxic effect (T.L. Murphy et al., 1948; D.J. Farquhar et al., 1950).

Preconditions
1. Severe (acute or chronic) liver disease
2. Portosystemic collateral circulation

Pathogenic factors
1. **Endogenous neurotoxins** ↑
   - ammonia
   - mercaptans, methionine derivatives
   - short-chain or medium-chain fatty acids
   - phenols, phenol derivatives
2. **Amino acid imbalance**
   - aromatic amino acids ↑
     - phenylalanine, tyrosine, methionine, tryptophan
   - branched-chain amino acids ↓
     - leucine, isoleucine, valine
3. **Disturbances of neurotransmitters**
   - false neurotransmitters ↑
     - octopamine, phenylethanolamine, etc.
   - excitatory neurotransmitters ↓
     - dopamine, noradrenaline
   - inhibitory neurotransmitters ↑
     - serotonin, GABA
4. **Changes in postsynaptic receptors**
   - benzodiazepine receptor activity ↑
   - picrotoxin
5. **Alterations in the blood-brain barrier**
   - change in permeability
   - compromised substrate transport

Tab. 15.1: Preconditions for hepatic encephalopathy and its development as a synergy of multiple pathogenic factors

2.1 Preconditions

The occurrence of hepatic encephalopathy (HE) is only possible under the following conditions: (*1.*) a serious (acute or chronic) **liver disease,** in which the detoxification function is significantly restricted, has to be present, and/or (*2.*) a functional or anatomic portosystemic **collateral circulation** must exist – this can be placed surgically or in the form of a TIPS (67, 84) – through which the nondetoxified portal blood bypasses the liver, so that toxic substances can reach the brain. In the presence of just one of these two conditions, the occurrence of HE can be anticipated, depending on the underlying disease. (s. tab. 15.1)

While hepatic encephalopathy is nearly always found in acute liver failure, it can only be expected in some 25–40% of patients with a portosystemic shunt. When these two preconditions coincide, as in the case of liver cirrhosis, manifest hepatic encephalopathy is found in 30–50% and a subclinical course of disease in 50–70% of patients. *In other words, the frequency, the degree of severity and the course taken by HE depend on the underlying conditions.*

2.2 Hypotheses

With respect to the correlation between liver disorders and the functions of the brain, discussion currently focuses on **five hypotheses** concerning the development of hepatic encephalopathy: (*1.*) intoxication hypothesis, (*2.*) neurotransmitter hypothesis, (*3.*) deficiency hypothesis, (*4.*) synergistic neurotoxicity, and (*5.*) hypothesis of primary gliopathy.

1. **Intoxication hypothesis:** Substances which impair or damage the functioning of the central nervous system are inadequately detoxified by the diseased liver and/or pass the liver unaltered by way of existing collateral circulatory pathways. Differentiation should be made here between (*1.*) ammonia-induced neurotoxicity and (*2.*) synergistic neurotoxic interaction between ammonia, mercaptans, short-chain fatty acids and phenols.

▶ *The so-called* **ammonia hypothesis** *was set up as early as 1952* (G.B. Phillips et al.). (71) (see above: C. Van Caulaert et al., 1932)

2. **Neurotransmitter hypothesis:** Apart from a disorder of the postsynaptic receptors, discussion centres on (*1.*) formation of false neurotransmitters such as octopamine and phenylethanolamine due to the accumulation of phenylalanine and tyrosine, (*2.*) decrease in excitatory neurotransmitters such as dopamine and noradrenaline, and (*3.*) increase in inhibitory neurotransmitters, such as GABA and serotonin.

3. **Deficiency hypothesis:** Substances which are essential to the smooth functioning of the central nervous system are not provided, or are only inadequately provided, by a seriously damaged liver. This hypothesis relates to the branched-chain amino acids as well as cellular deficits of zinc, potassium, magnesium and unsaturated fatty acids.

4. **Synergistic neurotoxicity** (L. Zieve, 1981): *None of these respective substances or mechanisms is "comagenic" in itself.* • Nevertheless, if present at the same time – even in low quantities(!) – they can cause the development of hepatic encephalopathy. The neurotoxicity of ammonia can be enhanced by these substances.

5. **Primary gliopathy:** This hypothesis (M.D. Norenberg, 1979, 1987, 1992) (68) has been backed up by recent examinations using proton MRI spectroscopy. (10, 26, 35, 51, 54, 83, 90) The cerebral detoxi-

fication of ammonia by means of glutamine formation takes place in the astrocytes. The ammonia binds with α-ketoglutarate to form glutamate or is converted enzymatically via glutamine synthetase to form glutamine. *Astrocytes are the sole cellular elements of the brain which possess glutamine synthetase for ammonia detoxification.* The markedly increased accumulation of glutamine in the glia cells is normally lowered by amino acid exchange and then equalized by the compensatory output of inositol, thus maintaining the osmotic balance. A constant surplus of ammonia (with its osmotic potency) and hence also of glutamine (with higher glutamine discharge from the CNS) will cause the glia cells to swell due to increased water intake. The elevated glutamine levels in the astrocytes cause glutamine to enter the liquor, where it is detected in high concentrations in HE patients. At the same time, there is a deficiency of glutamate at the synapse with defective glutamatergic neurotransmission. This produces an imbalance between excitatory and inhibitory activity, whereby the latter (i.e. damping effect) is predominant. *The reduction in intracerebral inositol, which functions as an osmolyte in the brain, is deemed to be the earliest sign of HE.* Swelling of the glia cells alters the cytoskeleton and compromises metabolic functions, transport properties and gene expression. • Furthermore, hypoxia, hypercapnia, benzodiazepines, electrolyte disorders, inflammatory mediators and manganese (52, 82, 93) can also cause a *swelling of the glia, so that a multifactorial pathogenesis is now given.* (s. p. 277)

2.3 Endogenous neurotoxins

The decreased hepatic metabolism of endogenous, nitrogenous neurotoxins together with their simultaneously increased formation in the intestine are generally held responsible for the development of HE. Such neurotoxins include ammonia, mercaptans, short-chain or medium-chain fatty acids, phenols, etc. (s. tab. 15.1)

2.3.1 Ammonia

Production: Ammonia is present either in its gaseous form (= NH_3) or in its ionized form (= NH_4) (i.e. dissolved in water). Ammonia is produced in the **small intestine** as a catabolite of glutamine. • In the **large intestine**, it is formed during the microbial breakdown of proteins, amino acids and urea. It is primarily Escherichia coli and Proteus mirabilis (as urease producers) which lead to the formation of ammonia. Helicobacteria in the stomach and duodenum are also urease producers, but the small amount of ammonia which they generate cannot be detected in the plasma. • Particularly during physical exercise, considerable quantities of ammonia can be discharged from the **musculature.** The forming of ammonia in the **kidney**, minimal in itself, can, however, be considerably increased by hypokalaemia and alkalosis. • In the **liver**, ammonia is produced through the breakdown of proteins and by the deamination of amino acids — and is in turn immediately detoxified. As much as 99% of the NH_3 is found in the form of NH_4^+ ions. • *Levels of >100 µmol/l in arterial blood are regarded as pathological.* (s. pp 61, 113, 890) (s. figs. 3.13, 3.14)

Detoxification: The detoxification of ammonia is effected by the synthesis of urea and glutamine in the liver. These two metabolic pathways are positioned heterogeneously in the liver acinus, i.e. they are metabolically zoned. Periportal hepatocytes detoxify ammonia with high capacity, but low affinity. In contrast, central perivenous hepatocytes (= *scavenger cells*) are free from urea cycle enzymes and specialized in the synthesis of glutamine. • *This hepatic detoxification process (urea and glutamine synthesis) is reduced by about 50% in cases of marked fatty liver and by about 80% in cases of cirrhosis* — with a simultaneous increase in hepatic glutamine synthetase activity to more than two to three times the norm. This is where the tendency towards metabolic alkalosis arises. Some 20% of the urea present is hydrolyzed by the bacterial flora of the colon, and the ammonia thus formed is again transported to the liver for detoxification. Part of the ammonia is eliminated by uptake in the muscles. Some 70—90% of the ammonia is detoxified in the urea cycle. The remainder is transformed into glutamine through glutamine synthetase and excreted in the kidney or converted back by glutaminase into glutamine, which is then available for glutamine synthesis. (s. p. 62) (s. figs. 3.12—3.15)

The extent of **hyperammonaemia** ($NH_3 \uparrow$), and possibly that of HE, hence depends on a number of factors:

> 1. nitrogenous intestinal content
> 2. change in the intestinal flora, with a greater population of colibacillus and coliform gram-negative bacilli in the colon (102) as well as helicobacter (18, 40, 61, 157), which can even ascend into the small intestine (there is no relationship between Helicobacter pylori infection, ammonia formation and HE) (s. pp 61, 66)
> 3. degree of disruption of liver function, as a result of which adequate elimination of ammonia by the urea cycle and glutamine synthesis can no longer be guaranteed
> 4. compromised urea synthesis due to congenital or acquired enzyme defects
> 5. extent of portacaval collaterals, through which portal blood, rich in ammonia, enters the circulation and hence the brain after bypassing the liver
> 6. shift in the dissociation equilibrium (pK = 8.9) as a result of metabolic alkalosis with hypokalaemia: $NH_4^+ \rightleftharpoons pH \rightleftharpoons NH_3 + H^+$
> 7. presence of hyperglucagonaemia

▶ The **neurotoxic effects of ammonia** are attributed to the direct influence of inhibitory and exhibitory neurotransmission and the indirect influence of accumulated neurotoxic metabolites of tryptophan in the brain. Thus there is a certain correlation between hyperammonaemia and HE. This general correlation is not present in specific cases or in certain phases of HE. Ammonia can pass the blood-brain barrier easily. Some 11% of the ammonia in the arterial blood is metabolized in the brain (*1.*) by binding to α-ketoglutaric acid during the formation of glutaminic acid and (*2.*) by ATP-dependent amidating of glutamate during the formation of glutamine. • Of all biochemical parameters, the **glutamine level** in the cerebrospinal fluid correlates best with the degree of severity of HE. The neurotoxic effects of ammonia might thus be attributed to the increased formation of glutamine: (*1.*) uptake of glutamine (as inactive, false neurotransmitter) into the peripheral nerve endings in place of excitatory glutamate, (*2.*) inhibition of cerebral energy metabolism, possibly in the form of an energy deficit due to compromised transport of reducing equivalents in the mitochondria or reduction in the NADH/NAD quotients in the mitochondria of the astrocytes due to ammonia (B. HINDFELT et al., 1977), (*3.*) changes in the blood-brain barrier with increased permeability for amino acids, above all tryptophan, and (*4.*) direct effects on the neuronal membranes, possibly with a change in neurotransmitter receptors. *These effects may largely be explained by the hypothesis of primary gliopathy.* • Ammonia also intervenes in the metabolism of amino acids through **glucagon** and **insulin.** Hyperammonaemia leads to increased glucagon secretion with a subsequent rise in gluconeogenesis and the resulting consumption of gluconeoplastic amino acids as well as enhanced protein catabolism. The increase in gluconeogenesis itself boosts the secretion of insulin and this in turn generates an additional uptake of **branched-chain amino acids** into the muscles, with a reduction in these amino acids in the plasma. (10, 23, 29, 31, 42–44, 58, 101)

▶ Recently, however, a correlation has been found between the pH-dependent (gaseous) partial pressure of the arterial NH_3 and the clinical degree of HE. (50) A recent study showed that ammonia levels (arterial and venous) as well as arterial and venous partial pressure of ammonia correlate with the severity of HE. It was hereby demonstrated that venous sampling is adequate for ammonia measurement. (91) Another study suggests there is no significant difference between arterial and venous ammonia levels or partial pressure of ammonia; no correlation of these three ammonia values with HE was found. (4)

The actual extent of the increase and the toxicity of non-ionized ammonia (NH_3) are influenced by several **additional factors**:

1. **Alkalosis:** Alkalosis shifts the equilibrium between NH_4^+ and NH_3 to the *non-ionized, toxic NH_3*. Only this form is able to pass the blood-brain barrier and the membrane of the cerebral cells. (34) (s. fig. 15.2)
2. **Hypokalaemia:** Hypokalaemia increases the activity of renal glutaminase, so that more ammonia is formed and transported back via the blood of the renal vein. A lack of potassium in the brain cells is in itself a further cause of serious cerebral dysfunction. (s. fig. 15.2)
3. **Aldosterone:** Hyperammonaemia acts as an additional stimulus in aldosterone formation, so that a vicious circle is created comprising hyperammonaemia → secondary aldosteronism → hypokalaemia → hyperammonaemia.
4. **Catabolism:** Increased catabolism of body protein leads to the additional formation of ammonia.
5. **Synergy:** Endogenous neurotoxins display a synergistic effect, i.e. the neurotoxic concentration of ammonia always depends on the concentration of the other endogenous neurotoxins.

▶ *Taking into account these additional factors, the mechanisms described above may explain why as yet a correlation between ammonia levels and the degree of HE has only seldom been detected.*

2.3.2 Mercaptans and methionine derivatives

Patients with HE often show an excessive (up to 30-fold) increase in methionine in the serum, CSF and brain. The administration of methionine in patients with cirrhosis may induce or aggravate HE. Methionine sulphoxim, for example, is an inhibitor of glutamine synthetase in the astrocytes. At the same time, cerebrotoxic oxidation products are found (e.g. methionine sulphoxide, methionine sulphoxim). Neurotoxic mercaptans (e.g. methanethiol, ethylmercaptan, dimethyldisulphide) are formed from methionine in the liver as well as by microbial action in the colon. It would appear that hydrogen sulphide (H_2S), and not methanethiol, is a determinant mediator. These substances are increased in the serum, CSF, brain and urine. (9) • *Dimethylsulphide* or *trimethylamine* are mainly considered to be responsible for the typical sweet odour of the **hepatic foetor** in the exspiratory air. (s. pp 91, 275, 383)

2.3.3 Short-chain fatty acids

With HE, there is often an increase in short-chain fatty acids such as propionate, butyrate, valerate and octanoate in the serum and CSF. They are formed as a result of incomplete β-oxidation of long-chain fatty acids in the intestine. They are not – or only inadequately – metabolized in the damaged liver. The neurotoxic effect is based upon inhibition of various enzymes (including enzymes of the urea cycle) and competitive inhibition in the binding of other toxins with albumin – and on the displacement of tryptophan from its binding to albumin, with a corresponding increase in free tryptophan in the serum and brain.

2.3.4 Phenols and phenol derivatives

Phenols are largely formed in the intestine from the aromatic amino acids tyrosine and phenylalanine. These amino acids are generally elevated in the early stages of HE. Phenols are detoxified in the liver by esterification with glucuronic acid and sulphuric acid. In severe cases of HE, free phenols and phenol derivatives are elevated in the serum and urine.

2.4 Amino acid imbalance

The liver plays an essential part in the metabolism of amino acids. (s. p. 42) (s. tab. 3.6) For this reason, a shift of the amino acid profile in the plasma has to be reckoned with in severe liver diseases. There is clear evidence of an *increase in aromatic amino acids* as well as a *reduction in branched-chain amino acids*. (s. tab. 15.1) Extrahepatic mechanisms (glucagon, insulin, lactate acidosis, etc.) can also effect significant changes to the amino acid spectrum. Multiple biochemical repercussions may result from this, affecting the development of HE. (8, 12, 42, 45, 49, 57, 66)

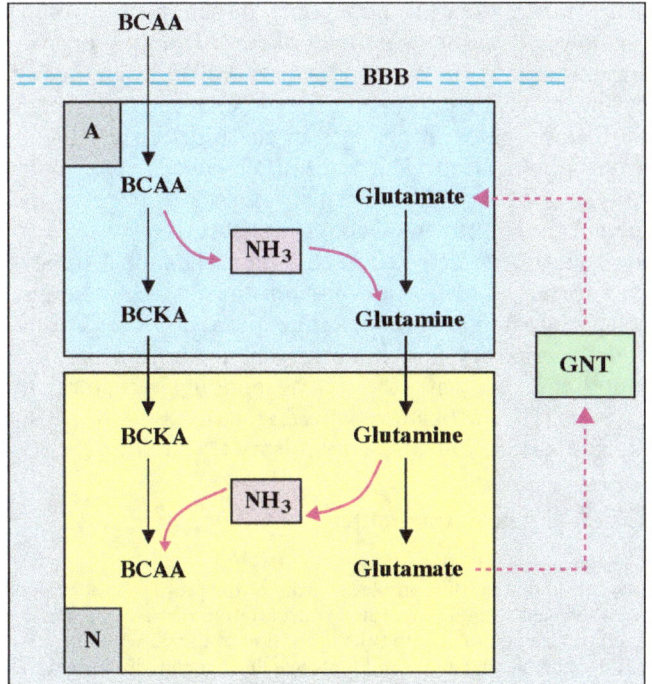

Fig. 15.1: Branched-chain amino acid cycle and glutamate cycle in the brain (A = astrozyte, N = neuron, BBB = blood-brain barrier, GNT = glutamate neurotransmitter, BCAA = branched-chain amino acids, BCKA = branched-chain keto acids) (137)

An **increase in the aromatic amino acids** *phenylalanine* and *tyrosine* occurs due to the lowered hepatic uptake of enterally released amino acids and their restricted catabolism in the liver. They are also released to a greater extent from the muscles in cases of cirrhosis with catabolism. Furthermore, phenylalanine hydroxylase activity is reduced in the cirrhotic liver. Free aromatic *tryptophan* is clearly elevated as a result of hypalbuminaemia, while the protein-bound tryptophan is simultaneously suppressed by the elevated concentration of short-chain fatty acids. Elevated cerebral tryptophan levels enhance the synthesis of serotonin. This substance, which acts as a depressant agent, causes fatigue and somnolence. Increased AAS in the brain inhibits tyrosine-3-monooxygenase and induces the formation of false neurotransmitters (e.g. octapamine, phenylethanolamine). (29, 70) • Because of bacterial putrefaction in the intestine, the volatile catabolites **indole** and **skatole** are produced from tryptophan, often giving the stools of the cirrhotic patient an intense smell.

The **reduction in the branched-chain amino acids** *leucine, isoleucine* and *valine* is caused by the higher clearance rate in HE, probably as a result of a hyperammonaemia-related increase in the secretion of insulin. These amino acids compete with the aromatic amino acids for a common carrier system through the blood-brain barrier. Because of the decrease in branched-chain amino acids, more aromatic amino acids reach the brain. This process is stimulated by ammonia. (s. fig. 15.1) (s. tab. 15.1) However, such an abnormal amino acid ratio can also be found in patients without HE.

2.5 Disturbances of neurotransmitters

Biochemical processes at the intersections (= synapses) between nerve cells as well as between nerve cells and the plasmalemma of other cells trigger the conduction of action potentials. The **synapse** comprises a pre- and postsynaptic part, separated by the synaptic gap. The neurotransmitters (noradrenaline, dopamine, serotonin, γ-amino butyric acid, etc.) are released from the presynaptic area into the synaptic gap and effect a change in permeability for ions (inflow/outflow) at the postsynaptic membrane, with changes in the bioelectrical membrane polarization. The transmitter effect is enzymatically stopped, with subsequent repolarization of the membrane. Up to now, about 80 neurotransmitter systems have been detected in the brain. The most important forms of neurotransmission are: (*1.*) GABAergic, (*2.*) glutamatergic, (*3.*) dopaminergic, and (*4.*) serotoninergic. Excitatory and inhibitory neurotransmitters are found together with their corresponding **receptors.** In cases of HE, the balance between the two systems possibly shifts in favour of the inhibitory transmitters.

2.5.1 False neurotransmitters

The **hypothesis of false neurotransmitters** (J.E. Fischer et al., 1971) (25) is founded on the complex shifting of the profile of the amino acids in the serum. The elevated concentration of *phenylalanine* in the brain leads to a boost in the formation of the false neurotransmitters phenylethylamine and **β-phenyletanolamine.** Furthermore, the intracerebral increase in phenylalanine leads to competitive inhibition of tyrosine-3-monooxygenase, which generally guarantees the enzymatic synthesis of the normal neurotransmitters dopamine and noradrenaline. A higher concentration of tryptophan also reduces the synthesis of these normal neurotransmitters while at the same time impeding the catabolism of tyrosine and stimulating the additional formation of tyrosine from phenylalanine. This high surplus of *tyrosine* is decarboxylated to tyramine and converted into the inactive and hence false neurotransmitter **octopamine** by β-hydroxylase activity. In HE, an increased concentration of tyramine may be detectable in the serum. This finding is also considered to be of significance regarding the occurrence of HE. Tyramine is formed from tyrosine by microbial action in the intestine and catabolized in the liver. Higher tyramine levels lead to increased formation of the false, inhibitory neurotransmitter octopamine. This accumulates in the synapses and severely impairs the synaptic transfer of impulses due to its very low excitatory activity. (104)

2.5.2 Reduction in neurotransmitters

The reduction of the normal neurotransmitters **dopamine** and **noradrenaline,** which trigger an excitatory effect at the synapses, is caused, among other things, by competitive inhibition of tyrosine-3-monooxygenase as a result of the higher concentration of phenylalanine. Furthermore, the increase in tryptophan leads to a reduction of these two physiological neurotransmitters, noradrenaline also being produced from dopamine by copper-containing dopamine hydroxylase. Dopamine receptors are found on neurons, which are mainly located in the substantia nigra, the reticular formation, the tegmentum of the mesolimbic system and the infundibular nerve of the hypothalamus. The reduced concentration of noradrenaline may also be responsible for peripheral vasodilation with hyperdynamic regulation of the circulation in portal hypertension. (s. p. 252) Moreover, *glutamate, aspartate* and *glycine* are also important excitatory neurotransmitters, the reduction of which (furthered by hyperammonaemia) intensifies neurodepression in cases of HE.

2.5.3 Increase in neurotransmitters

An increase in the neurotransmitters **serotonin** and **γ-amino butyric acid** (GABA) has an inhibitory effect on the neurons. Enhanced concentration of tryptophan boosts the synthesis of the physiological transmitter serotonin (5-hydroxy-tryptamine). Hence a higher concentration of serotonin in the CSF and of its metabolite 5-hydroxyindolacetate activates the serotonergic neurons. Animal experiments with serotonin antagonists brought about an improvement in HE. The increase in the postsynaptic inhibitory transmitter *γ-amino-butyric acid* observed in HE is a fundamental principle of the **GABA hypothesis** (D.F. Schafer et al., 1982). (87) GABA can be formed from glutamic acid in the presynaptic neurons and initially stored there. In reaction to specific impulses, GABA binds to postsynaptic receptors and, as a result, permeability of the membrane to chloride ions is increased with subsequent hyperpolarization of the postsynaptic membrane. GABA is either removed from the synaptic gap and broken down by enzyme action or returned to the presynaptic vesicles. GABA is also synthesized in the intestine by bacterial action. The portal vein can display a higher concentration of GABA, which is clearly decreased in line with a reduction in intestinal bacteria. GABA is broken down in the liver with the help of GABA transaminase. Patients with cirrhosis and with gastrointestinal bleeding showed increased GABA levels in the blood. The augmented GABAergic tonus can also be explained by "endogenous" benzodiazepines. The GABA levels of plasma and CSF do not correlate with HE. (6, 17, 55, 56, 60, 98) (s. tab. 15.1)

Apart from GABA, the GABA receptor also binds benzodiazepines, barbiturates, picrotoxin, etc. As regards the pathogenesis of HE, changes in the affinity and density of postsynaptic receptors play an important role for GABA as well as for other neurotransmitters. The binding of benzodiazepine to GABA receptors intensifies the effects of GABA. Consequently, there is an increase in GABA receptors – just as in zinc deficiency – together with a decrease in receptors for the excitatory neurotransmitters glutamic acid and aspartic acid, shifting the balance, once again, in favour of the inhibitory neurotransmitters. **Benzodiazepine antagonists** (e.g. flumazenil, bicuculline) have a favourable effect upon the development of HE.

2.6 Deficiency of essential substances

The energy metabolism of the brain is carried out solely by **glucose**. During this process, 5–10% of the glucose supplied is metabolized to lactate, 25–30% is directly decarboxylated by oxydative action in the tricarboxylic acid cycle for energy procurement, and 60% is converted into amino acids, mainly glutamine and glutamic acid, via α-ketoglutaric acid. (s. p. 43) In cases of cirrhosis with HE, these mechanisms of glucose metabolism are disrupted in the individual in a variety of ways. (44, 49) A pronounced **deficiency of zinc** is generally observed in cirrhosis and in alcoholic liver disease. This trace element is, however, of paramount importance to the activation of many enzyme systems, especially those of the urea cycle. Thought should thus be given to the substitution of zinc as a prophylactic measure against the development of HE. (77, 140, 155) (s. p. 55) It is advisable to ensure that the serum values of **potassium** and **magnesium** are balanced. **Unsaturated fatty acids** are also likely to be significant for the pathogenesis of HE, since they are of vital importance for the normal morphology and functioning of all biological membranes. (15)

The **outcome** of the enormous efforts made in experimental and clinical research into the pathogenesis of HE can be defined as follows: *There is a metabolic imbalance between excitatory and inhibitory neuronal activity.* (14, 23, 28, 41, 42, 69)

---

1. Up to now, no one substance can be shown to precipitate hepatic encephalopathy or coma under clinical conditions, and no single hypothesis can explain it.
2. The substances and mechanisms outlined above all have their own part to play in the development of HE. However, one of the two precursory conditions (serious liver disease and/or portosystemic collateral circulation) has to be fulfilled.
3. HE is not a metabolically homogeneous entity, but is deemed to be a multifactorial occurrence which is characterized differently in each case.
4. The multiple pathogenic possibilities interact synergistically. For this reason, successful prevention or treatment of HE is only possible if consideration is given to its multifactorial pathogenesis.

▶ *Neurotoxic ammonia indeed plays an essential, but not exclusive role in the development of HE.*

---

3 Morphological damage to the CNS

▶ As early as 1927, E. Pollak observed a "glia reaction" in Wilson's disease and other liver diseases in the form of enlarged glia elements, which he described as being poor in chromatin and with naked nuclei. This was confirmed by H.-J. Scherer in 1933.

In HE due to acute liver failure, marked *brain oedema* is predominantly evident with a spongy loosening of the tissue, capillary proliferation and a hypoxia-related loss of function of the ganglion cells (F. Erbsloeh, 1958). In 1953, R. D. Adams et al. detected diffuse hyperplasia of the astrocytes in chronic HE, with enlarged cell nuclei, yet practically without cytoplasm. Chromatine is often driven to the edge of the nucleus and vacuolated in the process. Protein concentration in the cytoskeleton is reduced. Glycogen (PAS-positive) is often deposited in the enlarged lobular, loosened nuclei of the naked astrocytes. The storage of glycogen points to considerable disruption of the cerebral metabolism, since normally no glycogen is deposited in brain cells. This form of macroglial reaction is known as *liver glia* or *Alzheimer glia type II*. Such astrocytosis is largely or even solely caused by ammonia. Furthermore, there are *changes in the ganglion cells* with the loss of Nissl's substance, distension of the cytoplasm due to the deposit of lipoproteins, and karyopyknosis. Localized failure of the ganglion cells, vascular proliferation and marrow oedema are the outcome. There is evidence of vessel-dependent blanching and softening as well as a *status spongiosus* which is largely independent of the vessels.

The morphological damage to the CNS in acute liver failure differs from that observed in chronic HE. Furthermore, the nature and localization of the damage also depend on the duration of HE as well as on its degree of severity. In chronic HE due to cirrhosis, reduction in cerebral blood flow and diminished uptake of oxygen and glucose certainly play a major role. This may well be of importance for the close correlation that exists between the astroglia — which is part of the blood-brain barrier — and the neuronal metabolism. (s. p. 273) These changes are found in the cerebral cortex and the brain stem as well as in the thalamus, putamen, pallidum and red nucleus. In the subsequent course of the disease, the spinal cord is affected in the form of damage to the axis cylinder and demyelination. Peripheral neuropathies and retrobulbar neuritis have also been observed. (10, 12, 20, 28, 90, 102) • With T_1-weighted MRI, a symmetrical hypertense globus pallidus can be demonstrated in about 70% of cirrhotic patients — even in cases without simultaneous HE. (28, 67) Such findings may be explained by the accumulation of (neurotoxic) manganese — although the reason for this manganese deposition is unclear.

4 Causative and trigger factors

In the course of serious **liver disease** (acute or chronic), the occurrence of HE must always be reckoned with. Various pathogenic factors or mechanisms can interact from case to case in a variety of ways and may spontaneously trigger this occurrence synergistically. For the most part, the pathogenetic and pathophysiological reactions are set in motion or reinforced by **trigger factors.** It is therefore clinically important to recognize and avoid them as far as possible. (s. tab. 15.2)

▶ The forming of microbial NH^+_4 in the intestinal tract is increased if the dietary **protein intake** is too high. (65, 91, 94, 95,

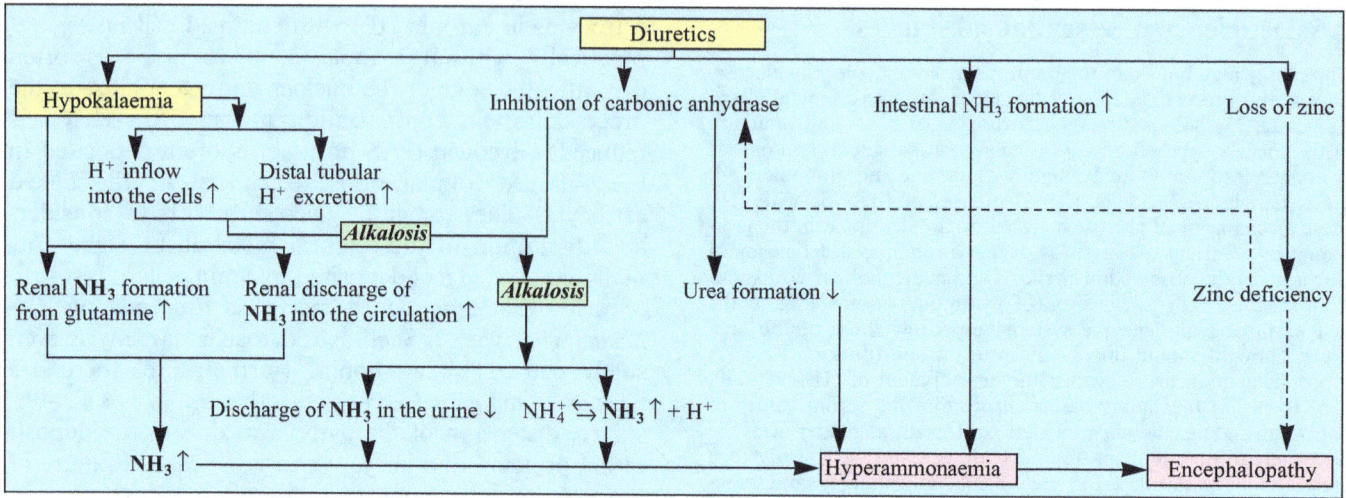

Fig. 15.2: Diagram illustrating the development of hepatic encephalopathy due to diuretics and/or hypokalaemia

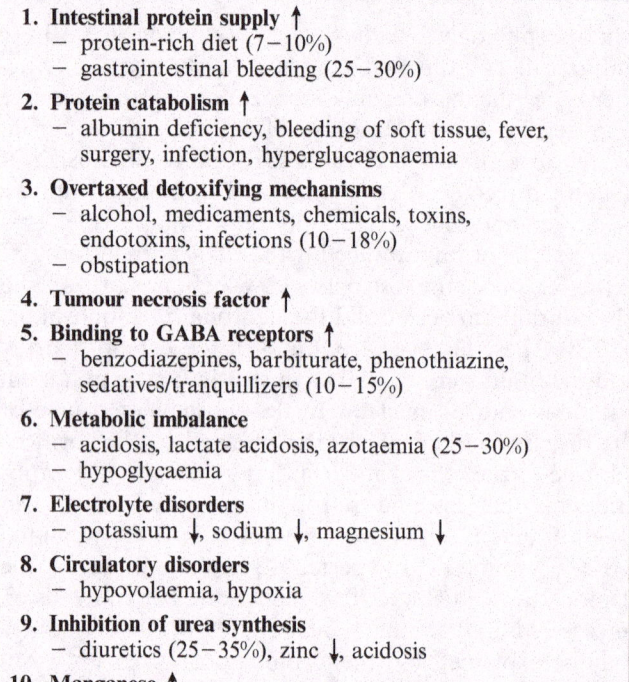

1. **Intestinal protein supply ↑**
   – protein-rich diet (7–10%)
   – gastrointestinal bleeding (25–30%)
2. **Protein catabolism ↑**
   – albumin deficiency, bleeding of soft tissue, fever, surgery, infection, hyperglucagonaemia
3. **Overtaxed detoxifying mechanisms**
   – alcohol, medicaments, chemicals, toxins, endotoxins, infections (10–18%)
   – obstipation
4. **Tumour necrosis factor ↑**
5. **Binding to GABA receptors ↑**
   – benzodiazepines, barbiturate, phenothiazine, sedatives/tranquillizers (10–15%)
6. **Metabolic imbalance**
   – acidosis, lactate acidosis, azotaemia (25–30%)
   – hypoglycaemia
7. **Electrolyte disorders**
   – potassium ↓, sodium ↓, magnesium ↓
8. **Circulatory disorders**
   – hypovolaemia, hypoxia
9. **Inhibition of urea synthesis**
   – diuretics (25–35%), zinc ↓, acidosis
10. **Manganese ↑**

Tab. 15.2: Causes of hepatic encephalopathy and hyperammonaemia (frequency in %) (s. fig. 15.2)

The **detoxifying hepatic mechanisms,** restricted in the case of severe liver disease, are overtaxed and become insufficient due to the additional *noxae*. With the presence of *obstipation*, the absorption of intestinal toxins and their transport via the portal vein are intensified, so that the diseased liver becomes subjected to an additional burden.
• The administration of sedatives or analgesics leads to **neurodepression** with additional binding to (and blocking of) GABA receptors. For this reason, these medicaments can have an unexpectedly strong impact, even in low doses and with a once-only application!

▶ **Hyperammonaemia** as well as **hypovolaemia** and **hypokalaemia** (especially when caused by diuretics) give rise to **secondary aldosteronism,** which in turn reinforces hypokalaemia, hypomagnesaemia and zinc deficiency. (s. fig. 15.2) • It is clear that additive factors also act as triggers of HE, setting in motion a vicious circle, so that a multiple and **complex process** results. • This may well explain the variety of biochemical, neuropsychiatric and clinical findings in HE. (14, 24, 41, 81) (s. tabs. 15.3, 15.5)

5 Clinical forms

The expression hepatic encephalopathy (HE) is a collective term covering **five clinical forms of disease** (H.O. CONN, 1989): (*1.*) Reye's syndrome, (*2.*) enzyme deficiency of the urea cycle, (*3.*) pseudoportosystemic encephalopathy, (*4.*) fulminant liver failure, and (*5.*) portosystemic encephalopathy. • It is not known whether the pathogenic mechanisms of these various clinical forms are identical. (s. tab. 15.3)

A **new nomenclature** of HE existing since 2002 distinguishes three forms: (*1.*) type A (= HE associated with acute liver failure), (*2.*) type B (= HE associated with portosystemic bypass without liver disease), and (*3.*) type C (= HE associated with liver cirrhosis).

112) • **Gastrointestinal bleeding** involving large quantities of plasma and erythrocyte protein is also deemed to constitute protein intake. It should be noted that 100 ml blood contain 15–20 g protein, from which large quantities of pathogenetically unfavourable aromatic amino acids and biogenic amines are formed by microbial action. The concentrations of ammonium stored in the erythrocytes are released during erythrocyte breakdown in the intestine. Occult bleeding, which is detected in the stools by chemical testing, may also cause HE. • Enhanced **protein catabolism** leads to an increase in the release of aromatic amino acids, which intervene in various pathogenic mechanisms.

▶ In the same way as diabetics have their own specific glucose tolerance threshold, all cirrhotic patients likewise have their own protein tolerance threshold.

> 1. Reye's syndrome
> 2. HE in Wilson's disease
> 3. HE in hepatic porphyria
> 4. Enzyme deficiency of the urea cycle
> 5. Pseudoportosystemic encephalopathy
> 6. Fulminant liver failure
> 7. Portosystemic encephalopathy following bypass, without liver disease
> 8. Portosystemic encephalopathy with cirrhosis
>   – subclinical (latent, minimal) form
>   – acute form
>   – acute recurrent form
>   – chronic persistent form
>   – chronic recurrent form

Tab. 15.3: Clinical forms of hepatic encephalopathy (HE)

An additional **three forms** should also be mentioned: (*1.*) deficiency of acyl-CoA dehydrogenase, (*2.*) encephalopathy in Wilson's disease, and (*3.*) encephalopathy in hepatic porphyria.

5.1 Reye's syndrome

The term Reye's syndrome (R. D. K. REYE et al., 1963; G. M. JOHNSON et al., 1963) (s. p. 606) denotes an acute, non-inflammatory syndrome with acute liver failure and encephalopathy. (7) Such a "hepatocerebral syndrome" is fatal in 30–60% of cases. It is observed in infants and children (mainly between the ages of 6 and 14 years) after feverish infection — particularly of the respiratory organs. This disease is seldom observed in adults. • The *cause* is still not completely clear, even though a virus infection (influenza A or B, Coxsackie B2, varicella), the intake of acetylsalicylic acid and mycetism are all considered to be responsible. The toxic substances, similar to those found in HE, lead to *neuronal damage* including the inhibition of neurotransmitters, brain oedema with hypoxic damage, vascular changes and demyelination. • In the region of the *liver*, severe periportal fatty degeneration is observed with cell necrosis. Examination with the electron microscope reveals marked damage to the mitochondria. (11) As a consequence, mitochondrial carbamoylphosphate synthetase is impaired, preventing ammonia from being channelled into the urea cycle. The oxidative breakdown of fatty acids in the mitochondria is also impaired. Large quantities of fat are deposited in the *visceral organs*. • The *clinical picture* commences with vomiting and fever. Stupor and tonic-clonic seizures follow, progressing into coma. Laboratory investigations show acidosis, hyperammonaemia, impaired synthesis of VLDL, hypoglycaemia, electrolyte imbalance, increased activity of transaminases and creatine phosphokinase as well as a drop in Quick's value.

A simular clinical picture can be observed in children with a deficiency of **acyl-CoA dehydrogenase**. This enzyme complex is responsible for the β-oxidation of medium-chain and long-chain fatty acids in the mitochondria without, however, causing any pathological changes.

5.2 Enzyme deficiency in the urea cycle

As a *congenital disorder*, an enzyme deficiency in the urea cycle relates to carbamoylphosphate synthetase or N-acetyl-glutamate synthetase (= hyperammonaemia type I) and ornithine carbamoyltransferase (= hyperammonaemia type II) (D. B. FLANNERY et al., 1982). (s. p. 611) This condition mainly affects the channelling of ammonium into the mitochondria and the conversion of ornithine into citrulline. (s. fig. 3.12) • Similar *acquired enzymopathies* can be expected in Reye's syndrome and in cases of zinc deficiency. Such a hyperammonaemia syndrome may also produce the clinical picture of HE.

5.3 Pseudoportosystemic encephalopathy

Pseudoportosystemic encephalopathy (pseudo-PSE) has been termed "non-ammonia-induced HE", "false liver coma" (H. KALK, 1958) or "electrolyte coma". It is mainly attributed to severe **electrolyte derangement** in the form of hypokalaemia and/or hyponatraemia (99) with a cerebro-intracellular increase in volume due to hypotonic dehydration. Hypomagnesaemia may also be present, which can likewise cause neuropsychiatric symptoms, since magnesium deficiency compromises all biochemical reactions in which ATP is involved.

Even without a simultaneous increase in nitrogenous substances, **metabolic disorders** (e. g. hypoxia, hypercapnia, hypoglycaemia) can give rise to neuropsychiatric symptoms. The primary pathogenic point of action is likely to be the damaging of the blood-brain barrier, also called the boundary structure of the glia. Here, the astrocytes and their projections encircle the blood capillaries and regulate the normal transport of substances between the blood stream and nerve cells. It is more than likely that multiple metabolic disorders or **endocrinopathies,** depending on their degree of severity or joint effect, will cause lasting damage in the area of the blood-brain barrier. (32) Neuropsychiatric symptoms with pseudo-PSE are not only to be expected in cirrhosis (as yet without any increase in nitrogenous substances), but also in other liver diseases; such symptoms likewise appear with metabolic or endocrinological disturbances. (85, 152) In this case, the clinical and laboratory findings largely reflect the underlying origins of the disease. Pseudo-PSE is thus of particular significance in the differential diagnosis of hepatic encephalopathy.

5.4 Fulminant liver failure

Fulminant liver failure is caused by an extensive loss of the liver parenchyma, resulting in severe deterioration of liver function. This clinical picture, which in most cases ends fatally, is also known as *"liver cell degeneration coma"*, *"endogenous liver coma"*, *"acute liver insuf-*

ficiency" or *"acute liver failure"*. Its causes are multiple and its pathogenesis is complex. (*see chapter 20*)

The onset is generally abrupt, sometimes even unexpected and without any hint of a previous or coexistent liver disease. A marked hepatic foetor is present at an early stage. The neuropsychiatric symptoms of FLF are largely similar to those of PSE due to chronic liver disease, especially since their pathogenesis is virtually the same, or even identical. Yet, the neuropsychiatric picture is more progressive and mostly characterized by aggressive or agitated modes of behaviour as well as screaming fits and delirious phases. The subsequent course of the disease comprises rigor, spasticity and seizures, passing into somnolence and coma. If the pupils do not react to light, this is indicative of therapy-resistant cerebral pressure due to brain oedema. (12, 20, 102)

5.5 Portosystemic encephalopathy

Portosystemic encephalopathy (PSE) develops in chronic liver diseases and/or in the wake of portosystemic circulation. Liver cirrhosis with its hepatofugal collateral circulatory pathway is thus the focus of interest in this clinical form of disease. • The term PSE is identical to *"exogenous liver coma"* or *"liver cell failure coma"*. PSE can be further subdivided according to its symptomatology and depending on its form and degree of severity. • There are three forms of PSE: (*1.*) subclinical (or latent) PSE, (*2.*) acute or acute recurrent (episodic) PSE, and (*3.*) chronic recurrent or chronic persistent PSE.

5.5.1 Subclinical (latent) form

> ▶ Subclinical (latent) PSE is founded on observations made by H. PENIN (1967), who noticed that patients with liver cirrhosis may display personality changes despite normal EEG findings. • Changes in the form of a psychosyndrome with neurasthenic features were summarized by F. ERBSLOEH et al. in 1974 as *"chronic subclinical cirrhosis-related encephalopathy"*.

With regard to an altered state of consciousness, *the subclinical form of PSE ranges between stages 0 (= normal) and I (= manifestation)*. It is to be expected, as with the majority of diseases, that the manifestation of PSE will be preceded by a stage of latency.

Despite the objective clinical importance of latent HE, the patient subjectively feels free from symptoms. No complaints or malaise point to the stage of latency, and the patient's conversation with the physician or the anamnesis (= *verbal*, i.e. *crystalline, intelligence*) does not yield any relevant clues. There are no neurological findings (hyperreflexia, asterixis, tremor, etc.), nor do examinations of the blood or CSF give any results correlating with the stage of latency.

Diagnosis of latency is extremely difficult because the patients show no clinical abnormalities and retain their verbal intelligence for a long period of time. By contrast, the *practical (fluid) intelligence* is disturbed at an early stage. No clinical findings are detectable which point to the existence of the latent stage. (s. tab. 15.4)

> 1. No subjective complaints
> 2. No clinical findings
> 3. No laboratory parameters
> 4. No neurological abnormalities
> 5. No spontaneous changes in the EEG

Tab. 15.4: Normal results in latent (subclinical) stage of PSE

Triad of HE: In 1952 G.J. GABUZDA et al. proposed the triad for identifying hepatic encephalopathy: (*1.*) mental disturbances, (*2.*) tremor, and (*3.*) EEG changes. • In this context, it seemed logical to include **neuropsychological test procedures** that had proved reliable in clinical psychology. (s. p. 209) (s. tab. 10.3) However, these test procedures, which can prove difficult to perform, are time-consuming and call for special training. Regarding scientific studies, however, neuropsychological tests are the *gold standard*. Combined use of several tests produces the most reliable diagnosis of latent HE – *even though no test is absolutely conclusive or entirely valid*. Of course, these tests provide no information on the underlying cause of encephalopathy and are consequently not "specific" to HE. The reliability of the test results depends on a number of *influential factors*, which always have to be taken into account. (s. tab. 10.2) • The fading of the myoinositol signal viewed in **proton MR spectroscopy** has proved to be a more sensitive method for the detection of latent HE. (10, 26, 35, 51, 54, 90)

The **frequency** of subclinical HE is given as 40−70% in cirrhotic patients, the different frequency rates being attributed to the way the individual influences the test procedures and to the respective underlying cause of cirrhosis. It appears that subclinical HE is most often found in alcoholic cirrhosis. A conservative estimate of the situation in Germany puts the number of cirrhotic patients at >700,000. The frequency of subclinical HE is therefore >400,000. *Hence subclinical HE is by far the most common complication associated with liver disease.* Patients suffering, for example, from severe fatty liver due to alcohol abuse show a high percentage of subclinical HE. In patients with serious liver disease, cerebral dysfunction can be detected in >80% of cases. In view of the multiple causes and factors influencing the development of HE (s. tab. 15.2) and due to its own considerable frequency, the stage of latency is of major clinical significance. (21, 27, 30, 39, 57, 74, 78, 80, 85, 86, 89, 96)

▶ The **objective disease status** (in contrast to the subjective feeling of illness!) was first demonstrated by H. SCHOMERUS et al. (1981). (88) More than 50% of clinically normal cirrhotic patients with latent HE were **unfit to**

drive; e.g. they misjudged traffic situations, braked too late, drove through red traffic lights, underestimated bends and speed. Another 25% were categorized as being only partially fit to drive. • *Note that during a so-called **blackout** (= loss of consciousness for one second), a distance of 14 metres is covered by the car without any control (!) at a speed of 50 kph (= 30 mph).*

A number of impairments, often quite severe in nature, affect the patient's **working life**: lack of concentration when operating machinery, disturbances in fine motor function during manual tasks, improper handling of equipment, uncertainties with production sequences, etc. As a result, the number of industrial accidents rises; in addition, there is greater damage to equipment or machinery and generally more production wastage.

▶ **Early diagnosis** of HE in the stage of clinical latency is of tremendous importance in daily life and at work, including fitness to drive (103); the benefits are of an economic, prognostic and prophylactic nature. In practical terms, such an early diagnosis allows a therapy to be carried out which is successful, efficient, economical and low-risk. (57) If treatment is started in time, progression to severe stages of manifest HE, with the subsequent complex and cost-intensive period of hospitalization, can be prevented. Moreover, it is imperative to avert damage to the brain cells, which may result from the chronic impact of neurotoxins. • For this reason, simple **psychometric test procedures** have been developed to identify latent HE. They do, however, have certain **disadvantages** which must be taken into account:

(1.) The cerebral functions and areas of function covered by the respective tests (s. tabs. 10.1, 10.3) are not sufficiently known or defined.

(2.) Given the varied functional disturbances in the brain (s. tabs. 10.1, 10.3), psychometrics should not rely on "one" test only.

(3.) The possibility of quantitatively reliable test evaluation is often lacking.

(4.) Various factors (s. tab. 10.2) can influence the reliability of test results.

(5.) As yet, there are neither enough comparative values available relating to normal behaviour nor sufficient results from scientifically established tests.

▶ From the publications available, we selected clinically applicable tests and compiled a **psychometric test programme** which largely complies with the general criteria for psychometric testing (s. tab. 10.5). Many years of experience have shown this programme to be appropriate. (53) A subsequent development was a *psychometric examination set*, available for use in both the practitioner's surgery and the hospital as well as in industrial and traffic medicine. This programme is simple, cheap and reliable. (1, 67, 86) (s. pp 210, 211) (s. tab. 10.6)

Critical flicker frequency: Determination of latent HE using critical flicker frequency (s. p. 211) has a sensitivity of 90–95%, a specificity of 75–80% and a diagnostic accuracy of 80–85%. This simple and relatively reliable method is independent of age and reading skills. In clinical praxis, it is already considered to be indispensable.

5.5.2 Acute recurrent form

The acute or acute recurrent form can be equated with the manifestation of portosystemic encephalopathy in chronic liver disease. It is also known as "acute episodic form". Discrete psychometric disorders usually precede the manifest picture as a *latent stage*. Manifestation includes *stages I–IV* and hence covers a wide spectrum of clinical, neurological and psychopathological symptoms. Once the liver function is stabilized and the trigger factors are eliminated, all the symptoms of this form are as a rule reversible.

5.5.3 Chronic persistent form

In 1965 M. VICTOR et al. termed this form the "non-Wilsonian type" of chronic hepatocerebral degeneration. (100) This chronic form of hepatic encephalopathy is rare. It is mainly found in patients with extended collateral circulatory pathways (19, 76), in particular after surgically created portosystemic anastomoses. At the outset, the clinical picture is similar to that of the acute recurrent form. There is evidence of irritability as well as moody or childish behaviour, indifference or depressiveness; occasionally, euphoria and talkativeness are experienced together with phases of confusion. Gradually, ataxia, choreo-athetosis, paraplegia and lancinating pains set in — similar to those of *portacaval myelopathy*. Such functional disorders are usually irreversible. The clinical picture ends in cerebral atrophy and dementia.

6 Clinical stages

In line with R. D. ADAMS et al. (1953), the next years saw the differentiation of HE into a number of stages, of which at least three, generally four or even five were defined (F. H. NETTER et al., 1957; C. TREY et al., 1970; B. RUEFF et al., 1973; S. SHERLOCK, 1975, and others). • For practical reasons, it is recommendable, and indeed clinically possible, to use just one (uniform and/or standardized) diagnostic system to categorize the stages for describing the severity of HE. The application of four stages does adequate justice to the multiplicity of the symptoms and findings and allows a patient to be assigned precisely to a standardized stage. These stages can overlap, with each one being reversible. A manifest stage of HE is one of the five criteria in the Child-Pugh classification and can be seen as a prognostic criterion.

6.1 Coma assessment

Glasgow scale: One tried and tested semiquantitative method for coma assessment is the Glasgow scale (G. M. TEASDALE et al., 1974), with a score of 3 to 15. It has a high consistency level, irrespective of the investigator ("interrogator stability"). As the severity of coma increases, the total score drops from 15 down to 3:

Criteria	Points
1. **Opening of the eyes**	
– spontaneously	4
– upon command	3
– upon pain stimulus	2
– no response	1
2. **Verbal reactions**	
– oriented and conversant	5
– confused responses	4
– inadequate responses	3
– incomprehensible sounds	2
– no response	1
3. **Motor reactions**	
– normal	6
– localized/hemilateral	5
– drawing away	4
– abnormal flexion response	3
– extensor reaction/stretching	2
– no reaction	1
	Total

Coma check-list: This Glasgow coma scale with its score points can be expediently combined with an additional *clinical coma profile*. The final result is a clinical coma check-list, which provides a basis for informative and reliable monitoring in the intensive care unit:

Name of patient	Date, time of day
1. **Pupillary reaction**	
– normal	☐
– weakened	☐
– no reaction	☐
2. **Corneal reflex**	
– normal	☐
– no reaction	☐
3. **Tendon reflexes**	
– normal	☐
– hyperreflexia	☐
– hyporeflexia	☐
– areflexia	☐
4. **Muscle tone**	
– normal	☐
– increased	☐
– diminished	☐
– slackened	☐
5. **Respiration**	
– normal	☐
– hyperpnoea	☐
– hypopnoea	☐
– apnoea	☐

▶ **Innsbruck coma scale:** This coma scale (F. GERSTEN-BRAND et al., 1984) can be used as a check-list at the bedside. The results are noted, giving the date and time of day. The highest number of points for grading a coma patient is 19. (The number of points 20–23 can be used for the waking-up period.) A sum total below 6 at the beginning of the coma and an average score below 11 during the subsequent phase point to a poor prognosis:

Name of patient		Date, time of day
Reaction to acoustic stimuli:	attention paid	3 ....
	better than extensor reflex	2 ....
	extensor reflex	1 ....
	no reaction	0 ....
Reaction to pain (pinching; edge of the trapezius muscle):	directed defence reaction	3 ....
	better than extensor reflex	2 ....
	extensor reflex	1 ....
	no reaction	0 ....
Physical posture and movement:	normal	3 ....
	better than stretching position	2 ....
	stretching position	1 ....
	slumped	0 ....
Opening of eyes:	spontaneous	3 ....
	upon acoustic stimuli	2 ....
	upon pain	1 ....
	no opening of eyes	0 ....
Pupillary width:	normal	3 ....
	narrowed	2 ....
	expanded	1 ....
	wide	0 ....
Pupillary reaction:	extensive	3 ....
	minimal	2 ....
	hardly perceptible	1 ....
	no reaction	0 ....
Ocular bulb status and movement:	eyes follow an object	3 ....
	pendular nystagmus	2 ....
	divergent, changing position	1 ....
	divergent, fixed position	0 ....
Oral automatisms:	spontaneous	2 ....
	upon external stimuli	1 ....
	none	0 ....

A categorization of the clinical picture of HE is not "liver-specific", but encompasses "encephalopathy" and its multiple aetiological aspects. Similarly, the phenomena of the individual stages do not allow conclusions to be drawn as to the type of liver coma (liver cell necrosis or functional liver cell failure). However, the course of HE with acute liver cell necrosis is more progressive and more severe.

Neurological findings: During the early stage, there is evidence of hyperreflexia, muscular hypertonicity, distortions in handwriting and speech as well as delicate flapping tremors. • A gross "flapping tremor", initially described as "wing beating" by F. TH. FRERICHS (1858) and as "asterixis" by R. D. ADAMS et al. (1949), is deemed typical of liver insufficiency. It is found in stages II and III and comprises swift bending and stretching movements of the metacarpal joints with the hands laid out flat and the wrists dorsiflexed or with outstretched dorsiflexed hands and fingers. The swift flapping movements, occurring at irregular intervals, are often accompanied by lateral spreading movements. Usually, the "flap" is bilateral; it is not synchronously bilateral, however, and mostly affects one side more than the other. (s. tab. 15.5)

EEG: For this reason, diagnostic efforts focus on the electroencephalogram. In the *spontaneous EEG*, individual cases can display a minor increase in slow waves or a slowing down of base activity below the normal alpha range (8–12 Hz). Only by knowing the individual normal status and by regularly reviewing the spontaneous EEG as a cirrhosis follow-up is it possible in 30–50% of cases to recognize features which could be interpreted as latent HE. However, this is not practicable. • The application of exogenous *visually evoked potentials* (VEP) revealed no reliable correlation either. • The determination of the **P-300 wave** as an electrophysiological correlate of endogenously stimulated potentials showed a lengthening of latency in some 30–70% of cases of subclinical HE. Although its sensitivity is high, this method is not appropriate for the initial diagnosis; for the follow-up, however, it is quite reliable. The procedure itself is very time-consuming and calls for specialized experience, which is why it is generally not suitable for routine diagnostics. • A grading system for EEG changes was developed by B. G. PARSONS-SMITH et al. in 1957. EEG evaluation has been considerably improved by computer analysis. (s. tab. 15.5) (2, 67, 86) (s. p. 208 with more references)

As from **stage I**, the base activity (normal alpha-range 8–12 Hz) slows down, there is a greater diffusion of interim waves and a symmetrical pattern of theta waves (5–8/sec). These changes generally begin at the frontotemporal region and progress posteriorly. The slowing down of the base activity can be detected in the subclinical stage of HE in 15–20% of patients. Application of exogenous visually evoked potentials (VEP) or endogenous stimuli together with evaluation of the P-300 wave made it possible for a far higher percentage (30–40% and 50–75%) of pathological EEG changes to be detected. • In **stage II**, the alpha rhythm is even more retarded (5–7/sec), the curves become flatter, and the intermittent theta waves increase. In some cases, *biphasic and triphasic potentials* are observed. • In **stage III**, the theta and theta-delta activity is accentuated and the base frequency continues to slow down (3–5/sec). Monophasic to quadriphasic complexes are observed episodically (R. G. BICKFORD et al., 1955). The individually different polymorphic waves with a high amplitude of the theta or delta type (3–5/sec and 1.5–3.0/sec, respectively) were termed "pseudoparoxysmal activities" (D. SILVERMAN, 1962). • At the beginning of **stage IV**, pseudoparoxysms were detectable as frontal or generalized occurrences, with the continued slowing down of the base frequency and prevailing delta rhythm (2–3/sec). During the further course of disease, the triphasic complexes and the pseudoparoxysms disappear. Delta and subdelta waves continue to level out, and isoelectric stretches become evident. (s. tab. 15.5)

> By means of psychometric tests, neurological/psychiatric findings and also EEG changes, an accurate assessment can be made regarding the degree of severity of HE – this guarantees a reliable follow-up, in which the efficiency of the therapy can be reviewed. (2)

▶ Defects in the cerebral functions and disturbances in the water and electrolyte balance are considered to be the earliest and most reliable signs of **commencing decompensation** in a severe liver disease, particularly cirrhosis.

▶ Clinically, the commencing decompensation can be easily diagnosed as latent hepatic encephalopathy (by means of psychometric testing) and as latent oedema (by keeping note of the increase in body weight). *These findings, recorded on a **documentation sheet**, are also of considerable importance for monitoring chronic liver patients.* (s. figs. 10.1; 15.3) (s. tab. 35.10) (s. pp 311, 767)

7 Diagnosis

Encephalopathy can occur in a number of **extrahepatic diseases**, such as toxic, metabolic or circulatory disorders, intracranial space-occupying lesions, hypothyroidism (32) and neurological/psychiatric diseases. (s. tab. 15.2) Identification of neuropsychiatric symptoms always calls for careful differential diagnosis.

Similarly, in various **liver diseases,** thought should be given to the presence of HE if neuropsychiatric disturbances occur. This is true for acute liver diseases (severe acute viral hepatitis, acute liver failure) and for severe (particularly alcohol-related) fatty liver, Wilson's disease, severe chronic hepatitis, severe infectious or parasitic liver diseases such as schistosomiasis, metastatic liver, nodular regenerative hyperplasia, and liver cirrhosis. (1, 15, 16, 21, 23, 26, 27, 38, 63, 71, 89, 96) The diagnosis of HE may prove difficult if the liver disease is (still) unknown.

A **portosystemic anastomosis** is most frequently associated with HE of differing degrees of severity. • The presence of a *surgically laid shunt* is naturally revealed during anamnesis and therefore does not constitute a diagnostic problem. (33, 37, 43, 45, 46, 56, 62, 72, 76, 82, 85)

In contrast, encephalopathic symptoms deriving from *congenital anastomoses* can render it difficult to make a differential diagnosis. (19, 47, 75)

1. Besides direct questioning of the patient, valuable information may be obtained by asking the spouse or closest relatives about possible neuropsychiatric symptoms displayed by the patient. Specific questions should be asked regarding changes in personality, working capacity, sleep behaviour, powers of concentration, capacity to register and mental reactivity. (79)

2. In all cases of suspected HE, **psychometric tests** (e. g. handwriting specimen, number-connection test B, line-tracing test, star-forming test) are a top priority. (1, 39, 53, 67, 86) (s. p. 210) (s. tab. 10.7) (s. fig. 15.3)

Date	Handwriting specimen	Body weight	Stool frequency
1.7.	Albert Hofmann	71.5	2
2.7.	Albert Hofmann	71.4	2
3.7.	Albert Hofmann	71.7	2
4.7.	Albert Hofmann	71.9	1
5.7.	Albert Hofmann	71.9 +	1
6.7.	Albert Hofmann	72.3	1

= onset of oedema
= onset of hepatic encephalopathy (subclinical/latent HE)

= beginning of outpatient therapy!

Fig. 15.3: Self-monitoring by the patient using a documentation programme for the early detection of subclinical hepatic encephalopathy or onset of oedema (s. fig. 10.1) (s. p. 311)

Stage	State of consciousness	Intellectual function	Elements of consciousness and behaviour	Neuromuscular function	Psychometric tests	EEG
0, 0-I, (sub-clinical/latent)	No abnormality	Initiative IQ ↓ concentration ↓ weakness of memory	No abnormality	Psychomotoric tests + → ++	+ → ++	No abnormality VEP (+) P 300 +
I	Disorientation absence of mind; disturbances of the sleeping-waking rhythm; exhaustability	Logical thinking ↓ serial subtraction ↓ attention ↓	Accentuated normal behaviour; depressive; irritable; euphoric; anxious; talkative; childish; restless; inability to keep one's distance	Hyperreflexia + tremor (+), + dysarthria (+), + apraxia (+), + stereotypes (+) hypertonicity	++ → +++	(+) VEP + P 300 +
II	Somnolence Lethargy	Loss of time consciousness Numeracy ↓↓ memory impairment disorientation	Reduced inhibitions; screaming; aggression; apathy; exhibitionism; inadequate or peculiar reactions; inability to keep one's distance	Asterixis (+), + dysarthria ++ apraxia ++ reflexes ++ primitive reflexes + dissociated bulbus movements hypertonicity	+++ (as far as can still be tested)	+ Deceleration
III	Sopor	Loss of orientation Sense of locality ↓ sense of position ↓ amnesia confused wandering (poriomania)	Delusions; delirious; aggressive; primitive reactions in the anal and sexual regions; confusion in the use of objects; faecal and urinary incontinence	Asterixis +, ++ tremor + stereotypes ++ (fumbling, sucking, lip smacking, etc.) nystagmus rigidity bulbar divergence pyramidal tract signs	∅	++ 3-phase waves
IV	Coma	Loss of self	∅	Spontaneous motor functions ∅ no pain stimuli loss of tonus areflexia dilated pupils opisthotonus convulsions	∅	+++ delta activity

Tab. 15.5: Diagram of the stages of hepatic encephalopathy (subclinical and latent forms and manifestation stages I–IV) as well as their respective symptomatology

The pathological outcome of these tests does not only call for further neuropsychiatric and psychological examinations, but it also means that the patient (and if the patient agrees, additionally the spouse or closest family members) must be fully informed about the situation. Due account must be taken of road safety and/or safety at the workplace in the interests of both the patient and the immediate environment. Extensive **psychological test procedures** should always be considered if generally important or even bureaucratic and legal decisions have to be taken concerning the patient.

▶ All test results and the contents of the patient briefing as well as the patient's consent or refusal must be documented by the physician and confirmed in writing by the patient or by witnesses.

3. In certain cases, the **neurological status** will be expanded on by the neurologist. In this respect, the EEG or even the initiation of visually evoked (VEP), acoustically evoked (AEP) and somatosensorily evoked (SEP) potentials may be indicated. There is often a correlation between autonomic neuropathy and the prolongation of the corrected QT interval. • Determination of the **critical flicker frequency** makes possible the best assessment of an HE 0, 0-I. (48) (s. pp 211, 281)

4. **Laboratory examinations** are of no relevance concerning diagnostic procedures focusing on HE, as interesting as it might be to determine octopamine, β-phenylethanolamine, methandiol, free phenols and tyramine in the blood and urine as well as ethandiol, dimethylsulphide, thyroid hormones and prolactin in the serum. This is also true for the detection of greater concentrations of glutamine in the CSF, which are believed to indicate the degree of severity of HE. • **Determination of ammonia** (4, 50) (s. p. 113!) in the arterial and, with less reliability, in the venous blood has *no correlation whatsoever with the degree of severity of HE*, especially since, even in a severe coma (stage IV), no hyperammonaemia is detectable in 10–15% of cases. Values of >100 µmol/l are definitely considered to be pathological. • **Breath ammonia** (measured using electrodes in collected expired air) correlates positively with **blood ammonia** levels. This method may be useful for diagnosis and follow-up in HE. (91)

5. For the differential diagnosis of HE, **computer tomography** can be important in tracing morphological changes in the brain. Interestingly, signs of atrophy were detectable in up to 50% of HE patients. CT, **magnetic resonance imaging** (26, 63) and **magnetic resonance spectroscopy** are not yet regarded as clinically significant in the diagnosis of HE.

8 Prognosis

The prognosis of HE with **acute liver failure** is generally very bad. Lethality is 80−85%; this can diminish or increase, depending on the acuteness and severity of liver cell disintegration. (1, 2, 13, 36, 97)

In **endogenous hepatic coma** (= due to loss of liver parenchyma), which in most cases develops from an existing chronic liver disease ("acute on chronic"), the prognosis is better than for acute liver failure, but nevertheless remains extremely poor. According to the information available in the relevant literature, 10−20% of patients die in stage I and 40−50% in stage II; in stages III and IV, lethality is 80−90%, the same rate as in acute liver failure. *(see chapter 20)*

In **exogenous hepatic coma** (= due to loss of liver cell function), the prognosis is somewhat better than in endogenous hepatic coma − although it is still poor: nearly all patients have a chance of survival in stage I, 60−75% in stage II, and some 30% in stages III and IV. Approximately 30% survive two to five coma phases; 10−20% of the patients have a five-year survival time following the first coma. • The prognosis depends on various influential factors:

Influential factors
1. Exogenous hepatic coma has a better prognosis than endogenous hepatic coma.
2. The size of the residual parenchyma and hence the remaining liver function is of decisive importance.
3. The aetiology of the underlying liver disease and the extent of the collateral circulatory pathways influence the prognosis in a variety of ways.
4. Advanced age and concomitant diseases render the prognosis less favourable.
5. The prognosis also depends on the trigger factors of HE being eliminated as rapidly and as completely as possible. This is particularly true of the swiftest possible elimination of blood from the intestinal tract.
6. Complications regarding cirrhosis, such as ascites, albumin deficiency, blood-clotting disorders, increasing jaundice and gastrointestinal bleeding (including occult blood), make for a considerably worse prognosis.
7. Of decisive importance is the stage at which proper treatment is initiated, so that progression can be hindered.

The best therapy results are obtained in the subclinical stage (0, 0−I) and the stage of disorientation (I). Nearly all patients can be successfully treated and brought back to the encephalopathy-free phase. • *Early diagnosis is of paramount importance for the prognosis.*

9 Therapy

Even in antiquity, it was assumed that there was a correlation between the liver and brain functions. *Normal functioning of the liver, in particular adequate detoxification, is a prerequisite for a smooth course of multiple cerebral reactions.* By contrast, decreased liver function leads to increasing impairment of the functioning of the brain. (23)

9.1 Fundamental prerequisites

▶ The treatment of subclinical hepatic encephalopathy as well as of stages I−IV explicitly calls for the *elimination of trigger factors* and other possible causes together with the avoidance of additional noxae. (s. tab. 15.2) Often these measures suffice to prevent the manifestation or progression of HE. An inadequate response to the initiated treatment should be reason enough to carry out a more thorough investigation into other possible causative factors.

▶ **Normalization of liver function** is the main aim in the treatment of hepatic encephalopathy. Basically, this can only be accomplished by overcoming the acute liver failure through intensive care procedures with subsequent restitution or by means of liver transplantation. In patients with chronic liver disease, there are in principle two long-term **treatment goals**: (*1.*) averting or eliminating factors which lead to dysfunction and/or morphological damage to the residual liver parenchyma and (*2.*) use of all possibilities in order to promote the functioning of the liver and its ultimate morphological regeneration.

▶ **Normalization of laboratory parameters** must be guaranteed: (*1.*) regulation of serum electrolytes, acid-base equilibrium and blood sugar values, (*2.*) substitution of zinc, and (*3.*) compensation of hypovolaemia. • Metabolic alkalosis should not be balanced, since it is important for the urea cycle.

These measures apply equally to all forms of hepatic encephalopathy and to all degrees of severity − and they are part of the imperative *prophylaxis* of this insidious condition.

9.2 Basic therapy

9.2.1 Intestinal cleansing

Intestinal cleansing effects the removal of nitrogenous substances and toxins from the intestine, particularly in cases of gastrointestinal haemorrhaging, increased intake of animal protein and obstipation. In HE, intestinal cleansing is always indicated, modified according to the respective degree of severity. (s. tab. 15.6).

Enemas may be necessary in acute and severe coma episodes, with highly constipated patients or in cases of massive gastrointestinal bleeding. Occasionally, a rectal enema provides adequate purgation of the rectal ampulla and the lower sections of the colon. A *high enema* should reach the entire colon up to the caecum. This is done by initially effecting insertion with the patient in a left-side position, subsequently in a supine position combined with simultaneous lifting of the lower abdomen, and finally in a right-side position. The volume used should be at least 1,000 ml. Both *sodium acetate buffers* (pH 4.5) and *lactulose* (300 ml lactulose with 700 ml water, twice a day) have proved efficacious. (147)

Oral purgatives, more reliable when applied by drip infusion via the nose and stomach, are mostly quite adequate. They have a swift and reliable effect. For example, 1,000 ml of a *10% mannite solution* with an infusion time of 60–90 minutes achieve virtually complete purgation of the intestinal tract over the following 3 or 4 hours by way of osmotic diarrhoea. In cases of gastrointestinal bleeding, the mannite solution should be supplied to the stomach via a tube until the rectal run-off liquid is clear. The isotonic *Golytely solution* (sodium hydrogen carbonate, KCl, NaCl, $NaSO_4$, polyethylene glycol) has proved most successful. Likewise, 50–100 ml of a 20 or 30% $MgSO_4$ *solution* or 2,000 ml of a 10% mannitol solution can be administered per day through a nasogastral tube. This intensive intestinal cleansing is continued by treatment with lactulose. As a rule, in subclinical HE and in stage I, oral administration of lactulose is sufficient. • *Activated charcoal* may be added (orally or rectally) to bind aromatic substances.

9.2.2 Dietary measures

The **dietary treatment** of patients with chronic liver disease *ranks highly as a therapeutic measure.* Thought must be given to the fact that the energy metabolism and the nutritive status of cirrhotic patients are at the level of long-standing inanition. • This was confirmed by the fact that a quantitatively and qualitatively adequate diet for dogs with **Eck's fistula** (= portacaval shunt) prevented the development of muscular atrophy and encephalopathy. (s. p. 272) • In patients with alcohol-related, stable liver cirrhosis, hyperalimentation improved the synthesis of proteins without the patient being exposed to the danger of HE.

The protein balance is normally in a steady state with a protein intake of 1.5 g/kg BW/day. • Although opinions differ in this respect, our own extensive experience has shown that it is advisable in HE **to restrict the protein intake** from the beginning. In subclinical HE and stages I and II, the protein quantity should be reduced to 30–40 g/day (ca. 0.4–0.6 g/kg BW). In individual cases, there may even be protein deficiency for one to three days without problems. • In stages III and IV, an optimal diet is only provided by a gastric feeding tube and i. v. solutions. (123) The oral protein intake should comprise vegetable protein and lactalbumin, especially curds, since they are best tolerated by patients exposed to the danger of HE. Vegetable proteins have less methionine and aromatic amino acids, yet more ornithine and arginine. • Cheeses containing ammonia should be avoided, as should fish, eggs and meat; blood is least tolerated. (As long ago as 1893, M. Hahn triggered "meat intoxication" with ataxia, convulsions, stupor and coma after feeding meat to *dogs with Eck's fistula*.) • An individually adjusted balance between lactalbumin products and vegetable proteins is necessary for better tolerability and general acceptance. (64, 107, 110, 115, 117, 122, 124, 148)

At intervals of three to five days, the lactovegetable protein intake is steadily increased by about 10 g, until a daily intake of 1.0–1.5 g/kg BW (in the long term up to a total of 80–100 g/day) is attained, provided this is tolerated. The **protein tolerance threshold** for lactovegetable protein and for the integration volume of animal protein can be determined with sufficient reliability by *psychometric tests.* (s. p. 210) (s. tabs. 10.6–10.9) • *All cirrhosis patients (or chronic liver patients) have their own protein tolerance threshold.* • Subsequent monitoring under outpatient conditions is carried out by the patients themselves through of self-checking, using a **documentation sheet.** (s. fig. 15.3) The use of the blood ammonia level for follow-up monitoring is unsuitable because of the sensitive pre-analysis and the low degree of reliability. • With a permanent, albeit necessary, restriction of protein intake to < 60 g/day, the protein balance can be improved by the administration of **protein compounds** (enriched with vitamins and trace elements) or **branched-chain amino acids.** *Catabolism has to be avoided at all costs!*

A **calorie intake** of 1,800–2,500 kcal/day (ca. 30 kcal/kg BW/day) is guaranteed by the adequate administration of fats (70–140 g) and carbohydrates (280–325 g). Consideration should be given to the fact that cirrhotic patients show a resistance to insulin and a glucose intolerance, with a tendency to develop a diabetic metabolic condition. For this reason, it might well be necessary to administer insulin. Carbohydrates reduce the plasma levels of ammonia and free tryptophan.

▶ **Fructose, xylitol** and **sorbitol** should not be used in view of the danger of lactate acidosis. • Restraint is likewise called for with the application of **medium-chain triglycerides,** since substances such as octanoate are only metabolized slowly and also deemed to be potentially neurotoxic.

Vitamins: In particular, water-soluble vitamins have to be provided in adequate quantities. With a carbohydrate diet and alcoholic liver disease, the daily requirement is higher. A daily intake of multivitamins, best combined with *trace elements* and *minerals,* is recommended. As a rule, liposoluble vitamins are best administered by parenteral route due to inadequate absorption. • The therapeutic significance of **zinc** (s. pp 55, 105) should always be borne in mind. (140, 142, 155)

9.3 Standard therapy

If possible, standard therapy should have an impact on both the intestine and the liver. The intestinal tract is an important source of potentially toxic protein cata-

	Latent HE	Manifest HE I–II	Manifest HE III–IV	Chronic persistent HE
Elimination of causative and trigger factors	++	++	++	++
Intestinal cleansing	+	++	++	+
Restriction or adjustment of protein intake	+	++	++	+
Lactulose	++	++	++	++
Intermediates of the urea cycle	+	+/++	+/++	+
Branched-chain amino acids	+	++	+	+
Zinc	+	++	++	+
Antibiotics	∅	++	++	∅
Flumazenil	∅	+	++	+

Tab. 15.6: Recommendations for therapy in various forms and stages of HE (∅ = not recommended, + = recommended or important in individual cases, ++ = important)

bolites and endotoxins. (s. tab. 15.1) The liver must be able to cope at all times with the requisite detoxification and the respective cellular metabolic reactions. (41, 79)

9.3.1 Lactulose

Since 1966, **lactulose** has been the therapy of choice in the treatment (and prophylaxis) of HE. (s. p. 887)

Its undisputed **efficacy** can be explained by the interaction between several pharmacological mechanisms (e.g. prevention of the absorption of ammonia or catabolic suppression of the protein metabolism of the intestinal bacteria due to a surplus of carbohydrates). As a result, ammonia and GABA (and apparently octopamine) are generated to a lesser extent in the intestine. Lactulose also has an anti-endotoxin impact and inhibits the splitting of glutamine in the mucosa of the small intestine. This inhibitory effect is also brought about by lactulose if the intestinal flora has been largely suppressed by antibiotics. (s. p. 288) Likewise detectable is an increased excretion of nitrogen in the stools. (s. tab. 15.6)

The **dosage** depends on the individual reaction and must be selected in such a way that two or three stools are purged off each day (*"never less than two, never more than three"*). With this dosage, the colon pH value lies in the required range below 6.0. Lactulose is administered in two or three single doses, each dose being adjusted in order to attain the required number of *stools*. Lactulose is deemed to be a long-term therapeutic measure, since it can (and should) be used for an unrestricted length of time, above all in patients at risk of encephalopathy. (111, 121, 128, 131, 141, 150, 151, 153)

Adverse effects are nausea, vomiting and lack of appetite (usually because of the sweet taste) as well as flatulence, meteorism and tenesmus (owing to the formation of gas in the intestine). Dehydration and electrolyte imbalance should not arise if two or three stools a day are maintained. *Compliance* on the part of the patient is considerably restricted due to the very sweet taste of lactulose. • *Pleasant in taste*, in contrast, are (*1.*) crystalline lactulose in the form of granulate, (*2.*) lactulose bound with lemon oil, and (*3.*) lactitol.

Lactitol has the same pharmacological effects, application guidelines and clinical results as lactulose, but with a better degree of acceptance in terms of taste and more rapid results. It is administered as a powder, mixed into drinks or food. The daily dosage (0.5–0.7 g/kg BW) is adjusted to the required two or three stools/day. (130, 141)

Nicotine hydroxamic acid is a urease inhibitor which reduces ammonia formation in the intestine. This substance has no systemic side effects. In a controlled double-blind study, it proved to be superior to treatment with neomycin (C. HIRAYAMA et al., 1982).

Probiotics are defined as microbial preparations of living microorganisms having a "positive" effect on the intestinal flora after oral administration (R. FULLER, 1989). Bacterial cultures such as those derived from Lactobacillus acidophilus, Lactococcus lactis, Enterococcus faecium (see below), Bifidobacterium bifidum (see below), Lactobacillus casei and Lactobacillus thermophilicum have proved reliable.

Enterococcus faecium has proved to be equivalent to treatment with lactulose in patients suffering from cirrhosis and HE stages I and II. There has been no evidence of side effects. (128)

Lactose has a laxative effect when there is lactose intolerance in the intestinal mucosa (congenital or acquired). It is still not clear whether lactose and lactulose affect the intestinal flora and its metabolism. (Certain quantities of lactose are usually contained as an additive in lactulose syrup!) (150)

Bifidum milk is a compound of bifidobacteria, lactose, lactulose, galactose and protein. The dosage is 3 × 12 to 3 × 48 g/day, always postprandial. Even with long-term treatment, there are no side effects that are worth mentioning. (128)

9.3.2 Intermediates of the urea cycle

▶ As early as 1932, H. A. KREBS and K. HENSELEIT established that of the investigated amino acids, only ornithine was able to effect a real increase in the synthesis of urea from ammonia (although arginine also displayed low efficacy). (quot. 53) • Thus it seemed possible to raise the turnover of ammonia in the metabolism process by using intermediates of the urea cycle. (s. tab. 15.6) (s. fig. 3.10) To this end, **ornithine aspartate** (oral and parenteral route), **arginine malic acid** (oral route only), **ornithine α-ketoglutarate** (only available as i.v. infusion) and **sodium benzoate** (112, 145) were used.

Urea synthesis takes place mainly in the periportal hepatocytes. **Ornithine** has a threefold effect on urea synthesis in the detoxification of ammonia: (*1.*) as a substrate of urea synthesis, (*2.*) as an activator of carbamoylphosphate synthetase, and (*3.*) as an activator of ornithine carbamoyltransferase. Together with aspartate, ornithine also reinforces *glutamine synthesis*, which serves to detoxify ammonia temporarily. Glutamine synthesis (addition of ammonia to glutamate) takes place in the perivenous hepatocytes. The influence of **aspartate** is twofold: (*1.*) as a substrate in the formation of glutamine and (*2.*) as an activator of glutamine synthesis. Glutamate, ornithine and other dicarboxylates are taken up and serve as initial substances for the synthesis of glutamine in perivenous scavenger cells. Experimental and clinical results confirm the justification as well as the success of these substances as components of HE therapy. • In therapeutical terms, **ornithine aspartate** is available as an intermediate of the urea and citric acid cycles. Depending on the severity of HE, this substance is used in granulate form or as a chewing tablet (3×3 to 3×6 g/day) or administered as a concentrated i.v. solution with $2-4 (-8) \times 5$ g/day. (73, 125, 143, 144) (s. p. 891)

Sodium benzoate: Sodium benzoate has already been successfully used to treat congenital enzymatic defects of the urea synthesis (M. L. BATSHAW et al., 1981). In HE, the administration of sodium benzoate or sodium phenylacetate (each 10 g/day) achieved clinical success equivalent to lactulose therapy in ca. 80% of cases. (112, 145) These substances (which are cheap and practically free of side effects) lead to an increased excretion of nitrogen through the conjugation of glycine and glutamine, whereby ammonium is bound as hippuric acid and excreted renally (bypassing the urea cycle).

9.4 Branched-chain amino acids

Therapeutic target: The application of branched-chain amino acids (BCAA) was based on the therapeutic target of compensating for the surplus of aromatic amino acids in order to suppress the synthesis of false neurotransmitters. Nevertheless, up to now, (*1.*) no correlation has been found between the amino acid imbalance in the plasma and the degree of severity of HE, (*2.*) no temporal correlation has been established between the normalization of the amino acid imbalance and the improvement of HE, and (*3.*) no influence has been detected on normal neurotransmitters in the CSF. These three counterarguments are, however, the subject of controversy and critical discussion.

Efficacy: The undoubtedly genuine efficacy of branched-chain amino acids cannot be explained merely by the improved metabolism of ammonia, but also by their complex influences on the metabolism of the muscles, liver and brain. The wide range of results may be the outcome of applying various test parameters as well as using different, possibly even unfavourable additives (xylitol, sorbitol, fructose, fats, etc.). Some 18 studies have been evaluated, but an ultimate assessment of the efficacy of BCAA on HE has not yet been achieved. (114)

Biochemical effects: In biochemical terms, the following effects on HE can be expected from BCAA: (*1.*) decrease in protein catabolism of the musculature and liver, (*2.*) improvement of protein synthesis in the musculature (particularly induced by leucine), (*3.*) improved urea synthesis in the liver (with higher concentrations of ornithine and N-acetylglutamate in the mitochondria), (*4.*) improvement of the nitrogen balance, (*5.*) reduction in the release of aromatic amino acids from the muscles, (*6.*) rise in glutamate and glutamine in the brain, and (*7.*) increase in oxydative phosphorylation in the brain in the form of an enhanced aspartate-malate shuttle. • Hence branched-chain amino acids are *important energy carriers*, providing a *suitable protein input* for patients insufficiently supplied with or intolerant to proteins as well as for cases of increased catabolism in latent or manifest HE.

A daily **dosage** of 0.3 g/kg BW is recommended (approx. 3×10 g). The use of BCAA has become established for latent and manifest HE. It has even been possible to render patients fit to drive again. No side effects are known. The efficacy of branched-chain amino acids as parenteral *i.v. therapy* is well validated for the severe stages II–IV of HE. The concomitant intake of arginine and ornithine aspartate has proved to be particularly effective. Fatty emulsions are to be avoided since they release tryptophan from the albumin binding and inhibit the utilization of BCAA in the musculature. (113, 116, 118, 120, 122, 127, 129, 132, 135–138, 150) (s. p. 888)

9.5 Antibiotics

Neomycin: Since 1957, neomycin, which can only be minimally absorbed in the intestine, has been successfully used to treat HE (A. M. DAWSON et al.). A *dosage* of 6–8 g/day (orally or via stomach tube) is recommended initially, with a subsequent reduction to 2–4 g/day, in three or four individual doses. A daily frequency of two or three stools should be achieved. Despite the minimal, individually variable absorption quantity (1–3% of the administered dose), ototoxicity and/or nephrotoxicity can occur as *side effects*. Moreover, when applied for longer periods or in higher doses, there is a risk of a malabsorption syndrome or intestinal bacterial superinfection as well as mycotic colonization of the intestinal tract. Neomycin should therefore only be used as *short-term therapy* in stages II–IV of HE. Treatment lasting more than one week calls for a strong indication and careful patient monitoring. Following initial treatment with neomycin, a one-day overlap with subsequent long-term lactulose treatment has proved successful. The *combined application* of neomycin and lactulose may be more effective for therapy-resistant patients because of its impact on various intestinal bacterial populations (F. R. COCKERILL et al., 1992). The principles of dosage and monitoring must be carefully observed. • The *mode of action* of neomycin is complex: production of ammonia, alanine and glutaminic acid is reduced in the intestine, absorption of ammonia is impaired, and uptake of glutamine by the mucosa cells is inhibited. (111)

Paromomycin: In place of neomycin, paromomycin can be administered in an initial dose of 3–4 g/day, with subsequent reduction to 1–2 g/day, in three or four individual doses. With regard to side effects, there seem to be certain *advantages* compared to neomycin: serum values are lower and of shorter duration, the serum plateau level area is about 2.5 times smaller, and it has a lower affinity to tissue.

Metronidazole: Up to 99% of the intestinal anaerobes that are largely responsible for the bacterial formation of ammonia are affected by metronizadole. Its efficacy corresponds to that of neomycin and paromomycin. The mode of action is still unresolved. The *dosage* is 3(−4) × 0.4 g/day with subsequent reduction to 2 × 0.4 g/day, provided two or three stools can be produced each day. When used for longer periods, peripheral neuropathies can occur. For this reason, initial treatment with metronidazole should be replaced as soon as possible by long-term lactulose therapy. (134)

Vancomycin is known as a reserve antibiotic. It has been successfully used in patients with lactulose therapy failure. (146) Above all, vancomycin reduces the bacteroides population. The recommended *dosage* is 4 × 0.5 g/day.

Rifaximin, a synthetic antibiotic drug is most effective against gram-positive and gram-negative is well as anaerobic and aerobic bacteria. If shows a very low rate of intestinal absorption and is conidered to have the best cost-benefit ratio in HE therapy. (514).

▶ When applied over a longer period of time and/or in higher doses, all of these antibiotics give rise to considerable **side effects.** Furthermore, the daily **requirement of tablets** is large, e.g. with neomycin (à 500 mg) or with paromomycin (à 250 mg), it amounts to 12−16 tablets per day. This often presents certain difficulties. The **costs** are considerable. In contrast, **lactulose** costs merely a few US dollars/day, has no or only minimal and harmless side-effects and is acceptable in usage − therefore it is the drug of choice, also in terms of expense.

9.6 Specific or adjuvant therapy

The multifactorial aetiology and complexity of the pathogenesis together with the increasingly poor prognosis in terms of irreversible brain damage or lethality substantiate the use of "obvious" **polypragmasy.** This approach is also rendered plausible because specific pathogenic factors call for appropriate polypragmatic measures. From this point of view, "liver insufficiency" requires a therapy spectrum comparable to that used for "cardiac insufficiency" or "renal insufficiency", with equally specialized or adjuvant/supportive measures. (92)

Neuropharmaceuticals: Given the neuropsychiatric symptoms of HE and considering the disorders of the neurotransmitter system, certain neuropharmaceuticals have started to attract attention. These are nootropic substances and benzodiazepine antagonists. They can be applied in patients resistant to other therapies.

Flumazenil: In 1985 the assumption that GABAergic neuroinhibition is increased in HE led to the therapeutic use of the benzodiazepine antagonist flumazenil (G. BANSKY et al.). (106) An improvement in the neuropsychiatric symptoms of HE was achieved in 66% of patients. The recommended dosage is 0.2−0.3 mg i.v. bolus, followed by 5 mg/hour as i.v. infusion. Remarkable arousal effects and unexpected long-term success (50 mg/day orally) were described even in hepatic coma. In severity stage III of HE improvement occurred in 93% of cases, and in stage IV the rate was 48%. (5, 17, 108, 109, 119, 126, 139) Recently, a meta-analysis showed that flumazenil improves clinical and electroencephalographic findings regarding HE in cirrhotic patients.

L-dopa, a precursor of the neurotransmitters norepinephrine and dopamine, was introduced into HE therapy by J.D. PARKES et al. in 1970. The results were good. As yet, there is still no accepted opinion on the use of this substance. • **Piracetam,** as a nootropic substance, led to a clear improvement in typical electrical brain activities in animals displaying hepatic damage and symptoms of encephalopathy. • Similarly, a double-blind randomized cross-over study with the nootropic agent **centrophenoxine** partly showed positive effects in psychometric testing. • **Bromocriptine,** an agonist of the dopamine receptor, was also used in 1980 for chronic hepatic encephalopathy. (133, 149) • Application of **L-carnitine** (6 g/day orally, divided into two doses, for four weeks) leads to a marked reduction of hyperammonaemia and a clear improvement in clinical symptoms of HE in cirrhotic patients.

9.7 Early detection and therapeutic success

The **early detection** of HE, if possible at the stage of latency or no later than in stage I, guarantees the best therapeutic results under outpatient conditions and thus avoids cost-intensive hospital treatment.

Elimination of the causative factors of HE, insofar as this is possible at all, is the prerequisite for successful therapy. It is necessary because HE is seen as a potentially reversible impairment of brain functions, particularly in the "precoma" stages.

▶ The various channels of pathogenetically and/or experimentally substantiated and clinically tested types of therapy applied as a **graduated therapy concept** are justified in HE − even though as a rule polypragmasy is to be viewed with some scepticism. Medication is based on the particular degree of severity of HE, the individual reaction of the patient and possible adverse effects.

References:

1. Amodio, P., del Piccolo, F., Marchetti, P., Angeli, P., Iemmolo, R., Caregaro, L., Merkel, C., Gerunda, G., Gatta, A.: Clinical features and survival of cirrhotic patients with subclinical cognitive alterations by the number connection test and computerized psychometric tests. Hepatology 1999; 29: 1662−1667

2. Amodio, P., Valenti, P., Del Piccolo, F., Pellegrini, A., Schiff, S., Angeli, P., Poci, C., Mapelli, D., Iannizzi, P., Gatta, A.: P 300 latency for the diagnosis of minimal hepatic encephalopathy: Evidence that spectral EEG analysis and psychometric tests are enough. Dig. Liver Dis. 2005; 37: 861–808
3. Arora, A., Seth, S., Acharya, S.K., Sharma, M.P.: Hepatic coma as a presenting feature of constrictive pericarditis. Amer. J. Gastroenterol. 1993; 88: 430–432
4. Barsotti, R.J.: Measurement of ammonia in blood. J. Pediatr. 2001; 138 (Suppl.): 11–19
5. Basile, A.S., Jones, E.A., Skolnick, P.: The pathogenesis and treatment of hepatic encephalopathy: evidence for the involvement of benzodiazepine receptor ligands. Pharmacol. Rev. 1991; 43: 27–71
6. Basile, A.S., Jones, E.A.: Ammonia and GABA-ergic neurotransmission: interrelated factors in the pathogenesis of hepatic encephalopathy. Hepatology 1997; 25: 1303–1305
7. Belay, E.D., Bresee, J.S., Holman, R.C., Khan, A.S., Shahriari, A., Schonberger, L.-B.: Reye's syndrome in the United States from 1981 through 1987. New Engl. J. Med. 1999; 340: 1377–1382
8. Bernardini, P., Fischer, J.E.: Amino acid imbalance and hepatic encephalopathy. Ann. Rev. Nutr. 1982; 2: 419–454
9. Blom, H.J., Ferenci, P., Grimm, G., Yap, S.H., Tangerman, A.: The role of methanethiol in the pathogenesis of hepatic encephalopathy. Hepatology 1991; 13: 445–454
10. Bosman, D.K., Deutz, N.E.P., Graaf, de, A.A., Hulst, van der, R.W.N., Eijk, van, H.M.H., Bovée, W.M.M.J., Maas, M.A.W., Jörning, G.G.A., Chamuleau, R.A.F.M.: Changes in brain metabolism during hyperammonemia and acute liver failure: results of a comparative „H-NMR spectroscopy and biochemical investigation. Hepatology 1990; 12: 281–290
11. Brown, J.K., Imam, H.: Interrelationships of liver and brain with special reference to Reye syndrome. J. Inher. Metabol. Dis. 1991; 14: 436–458
12. Bullimore, D.: The role of polyamines in hepatic encephalopathy and cerebral oedema. Europ. J. Gastroenterol. Hepatol. 1993; 5: 63–67
13. Bustamante, J., Rimola, A., Ventura, P.J., Navasa, M., Cirera, I., Reggiardo, V., Rodes, J.: Prognostic significance of hepatic encephalopathy in patients with cirrhosis. J. Hepatol. 1999; 30: 890–895
14. Butterworth, R.F.: The neurobiology of hepatic encephalopathy. Semin. Liver Dis. 1996; 16: 235–244
15. Cabré, E., Periago, J.L., Gonzalez, J., Gonzalez-Huix, F., Abad-Lacruz, A., Gil, A., Sanchez-Medina, F., Esteve- Comas, M., Fernandez-Banares, F., Planas, R., Gassull, M.A.: Plasma polyunsaturated fatty acids in liver cirrhosis with or without chronic hepatic encephalopathy: a preliminary study. J. Parenter. Enter. Nutr. 1992; 16: 359–363
16. Cadranel, J.-F., Lebiez, E., di Martino, V., Bernard, B., El Koury, S., Tourbah, A., Pidoux, B., Valla, D., Opolon, P.: Focal neurological signs in hepatic encephalopathy in cirrhotic patients: an underestimated entity? Amer. J. Gastroenterol. 2001; 96: 515–518
17. Caguin, A., Taylor-Robinson, S.D., Forton, D.M., Banati, R.B.: In vivo imaging of cerebral "peripheral benzodiazepine binding sites" in patients with hepatic encephalopathy. Gut 2006; 55: 547–553
18. Calvet, X., Nogueras, C., Roque, M., Sanfeliu, I.: Helicobacter pylori is not a risk factor for hepatic encephalopathy. Dig. Liver Dis. 2001; 33: 414–419
19. Caturelli, E., Gluttoni, G., Niro, G.A., Clemente, R., Accadia, L., Nardella, M., Andrulli, A., Anti, M.: Multiple intrahepatic vascular shunts causing hyperammoniaemic encephalopathy in a patient without liver cirrhosis. Dig. Liver Dis. 2006; 38: 347–351
20. Cordoba, J., Blei, A.T.: Brain edema and hepatic encephalopathy. Semin. Liver Dis. 1996; 16: 271–280
21. Das, A., Dhiman, R.K., Saraswat, V.A., Verma, M., Naik, S.R.: Prevalence and natural history of subclinical hepatic encephalopathy in cirrhosis. J. Gastroenterol. Hepatol. 2001; 16: 531–535
22. Davidson, E.A., Summerskill, W.H.J.: Psychiatric aspects of liver disease. Postgrad. Med. J. 1956; 32: 487–494
23. Dbouk, N., McGuire, B.M.: Hepatic encephalopathy: A review of its pathophysiology and treatment. Curr. Treat. Opt. Gastroenterol. 2006; 9: 464–474
24. Dietrich, R., Bachmann, C., Lauterburg, B.H.: Exercise-induced hyperammonemia in patients with compensated chronic liver disease. Scand. J. Gastroenterol. 1990; 25: 329–334
25. Fischer, J.E., Baldessarini, R.J.: False neurotransmitters and hepatic failure. Lancet 1971/II: 75–80
26. Geissler, A., Lock, G., Fründ, R., Held, P., Hollerbach, S., Andus, T., Schölmerich, J., Feuerbach, S., Holstege, A.: Cerebral abnormalities in patients with cirrhosis detected by proton magnetic resonance spectroscopy and magnetic resonance imaging. Hepatology 1997; 25: 48–54
27. Gitlin, N., Lewis, D.C., Hinkley, L.: The diagnosis and prevalence of subclinical hepatic encephalopathy in apparently healthy, ambulant, non-shunted patients with cirrhosis. J. Hepatol. 1986; 3: 75–82
28. Goldstein, G.W.: The role of brain capillaries in the pathogenesis of hepatic encephalopathy. Hepatology 1984; 4: 565–567
29. Grippon, P., Le Poncin-Lafitte, M., Boschat, M., Wang, S., Faure, G., Dutertre, D., Opolon, P.: Evidence for the role of ammonia in the intracerebral transfer and metabolism of tryptophan. Hepatology 1986; 6: 682–686
30. Groeneweg, M., Moerland, W., Quero, J.C., Hop, W.C.J., Krabbe, P.F., Schalm, S.W.: Screening of subclinical hepatic encephalopathy. J. Hepatol. 2000; 32: 748–753
31. Grüngreiff, K., Wolf, G., Schmidt, W., Franke, D., Kleine, F.-D.: High-affinity uptake of transmitter glutamate (GLU)in brain tissue with reference to hepatic encephalopathy (HE). Z. Gastroenterol. 1991; 29 (Suppl. 2): 95–100
32. Güven, K., Kelestimur, F., Yücesoy, M.: Thyroid function tests in non-alcoholic cirrhotic patients with hepatic encephalopathy. Eur. J. Med. 1993; 2: 83–85
33. Hashimoto, N., Ashida, H., Kotoura, Y., Nishioka, A., Nishiwaki, M., Utsunomiya, J.: Analysis of hepatic encephalopathy after distal splenorenal shunt-PTP image and pancreatic hormone kinetics. Hepato-Gastroenterol. 1993; 40: 360–364
34. Häussinger, D., Steeb, R., Gerok, W.: Metabolic alkalosis as driving force for urea synthesis in liver disease: pathogenetic model and therapeutic implications. Clin. Invest. 1992; 70: 411–415
35. Häussinger, D., Laubenberger, J., von Dahl, S., Ernst, T., Langer, H., Gerok, W., Hennig, J.: Proton magnetic resonance studies on human brain myo-inositol during hypoosmolarity and hepatic encephalopathy. Gastroenterology 1994; 107: 1475–1480
36. Hartmann, I.J.C., Groeneweg, M., Quero, J.C., Beijeman, S.J., de Man, R.A., Hop, W.C.J., Schalm, S.W.: The prognostic significance of subclinical hepatic encephalopathy. Amer. J. Gastroenterol. 2000; 95: 2029–2034
37. Held, C., Rühle, R., Steppuhn, S., Wack, R.: Fahrtauglichkeit bei Patienten mit hepatischer Enzephalopathie nach portosystemischer Shunt-Operation. Z. Gastroenterol. (Suppl. 2) 1991; 29: 107–109
38. Höckerstedt, K., Kajaste, S., Muuronen, A., Raininko, R., Seppäläinen, A.-M., Hillbom, M.: Encephalopathy and neuropathy in end-stage liver disease before and after liver transplantation. J. Hepatol. 1992; 16: 31–37
39. Homann, J., Kuntz, H.-D., Deetjen, W., Thilo-Körner, D.S., Oehler, G.: Die chronische hepatische Enzephalopathie. Med. Welt 1993; 44: 128–134
40. Huber, M., Rössle, M., Siegerstetter, V., Ochs, A., Haag, K., Kist, M., Blum, H.E.: Helicobacter pylori infection does not correlate with plasma ammonia concentration and hepatic encephalopathy in patients with cirrhosis. Hepato-Gastroenterol. 2001; 48: 541–544
41. Jalan, R., Seery, J.P., Taylor-Robinson, S.D.: Review article: pathogenesis and treatment of chronic hepatic encephalopathy. Aliment. Pharmacol. Ther. 1996; 10: 681–697
42. James, J.H., Ziparo, V., Jeppson, B., Fischer, J.E.: Hyperammonaemia, plasma aminoacid imbalance, and blood-brain aminoacid transport: a unified theory of portal-systemic encephalopathy. Lancet 1979/II: 772–775
43. Jessy, J., Mans, A.M., DeJoseph, M.R., Hawkins, R.A.: Hyperammonaemia causes many of the changes found after portocaval shunting. Biochem. J. 1990; 272: 311–317
44. Jessy, J., DeJoseph, M.R., Hawkins, R.A.: Hyperammonaemia depresses glucose consumption throughout the brain. Biochem. J. 1991; 277: 693–696
45. Joelsson, B., Aslund, U., Hultberg, B., Alwmark, A., Gullstrand, P., Bengmark, S.: Portal-systemic encephalopathy. Influence of shunt surgery and relations to serum amino acids. Scand. J. Gastroenterol. 1986; 21:900–906
46. Kardel, T., Lund, Y., Zander Olsen, P., Möllgaard, V., Gammeltoft, A.: Encephalopathy and portacaval anastomosis. Scand. J. Gastroenterol. 1970; 5: 681–685
47. Kerlan, R.K. jr., Sollenberger, R.D., Palubinskas, A.J., Raskin, N.H., Callen, P.W., Ehrenfeld, W.K.: Portal-systemic encephalopathy due to a congenital portocaval shunt. Amer. J. Roentgenol. 1982; 139: 1013–1015
48. Kircheis, G., Wettstein, M., Timmermann, L., Schnitzler, A., Häussinger, D.: Critical flicker frequency for quantification of low-grad hepatic encephalopathy. Hepatology 2002; 35: 357–366
49. Knudsen, G.M., Schmidt, J., Almdal, T., Paulson, O.B., Vilstrup, H.: Passage of amino acids and glucose across the blood-brain barrier in patients with hepatic encephalopathy. Hepatology 1993; 17: 987–992
50. Kramer, L., Tribl, B., Gendo, A., Zauner, C., Schneider, P., Ferenci, P., Madl, C.: Partial pressure of ammonia versus ammonia in hepatic encephalopathy. Hepatology 2000; 31: 30–34
51. Kreis, R., Ross, B.D., Farrow, N.A.: Metabolic disorders of the brain in chronic hepatic encephalopathy detected with H-1 MR spectroscopy. Radiology 1992; 182: 19–27
52. Krieger, D., Krieger, S., Jansen, O., Gass, P., Theilmann, L., Lichtnecker, H.: Manganese and chronic hepatic encephalopathy. Lancet 1995; 346: 270–274
53. Kuntz, E.: Hepatische Enzephalopathie. Psychometrische Tests zur Diagnose, Bewertung und Therapiekontrolle in der Praxis. Münch. Med. Wschr. 1992; 134: 76–80
54. Laubenberger, J., Häussinger, D., Bayer, S., Gufler, H., Hennig, J., Langer, M.: Proton magnetic resonance spectroscopy of the brain in symptomatic and asymptomatic patients with liver cirrhosis. Gastroenterology 1997; 112: 1610–1616
55. Levy, L.J., Losowsky, M.S.: Plasma gamma aminobutyric acid concentrations provide evidence of different mechanisms in the pathogenesis of hepatic encephalopathy in acute and chronic liver disease. Hepato-Gastroenterol. 1989; 36:494–498
56. Löscher, W., Kretz, F.-J., Karavias, T., Dillinger, U.: Marked increases of plasma gamma-aminobutyric acid concentrations in cirrhotic patients with portocaval shunts are not associated with alterations of cerebral functions. Digestion 1991; 49: 212–220

57. Marchesini, G., Zoli, M., Dondi, C., Cecchini, L., Angiolini, A., Bianchi, F.B., Pisi, E.: Prevalence of subclinical hepatic encephalopathy in cirrhotics and relationship to plasma amino acid imbalance. Dig. Dis. Sci. 1980; 25: 763−768
58. Mardini, H.A., Harrison, E.J., Ince, P.G., Bartlett, K., Record, C.O.: Brain indoles in human hepatic encephalopathy. Hepatology 1993; 17: 1033−1040
59. Martini, G.A.: Psychiatrisch-neurologische Störungen bei chronischen Leberkrankheiten. Internist 1975; 16: 20−24
60. Minuk, G.Y.: Gamma-aminobutyric acid and the liver. Dig. Dis. 1993; 11: 45−54
61. Miquel, J., Barcena, R., Boixeda, D., Fernandez, J., Lopez-San Roman, A., Martin-de-Argila, C., Ramosa, F.: Role of Helicobacter pylori infection and its eradication in patients with subclinical hepatic encephalopathy. Eur. J. Gastroenterol. Hepatol. 2001; 13: 1067−1072
62. Mohapatra, M.K., Mohapatra, A.K., Acharya, S.K., Sahni, P., Nundy, S.: Encephalopathy in patients with extrahepatic obstruction after lienorenal shunts. Brit. J. Surg. 1992; 79: 1103−1105
63. Moore, J.W., Dunk, A.A., Crawford, J.R., Deans, H., Besson, J.A.O., de Lacey, G., Sinclair, T.S., Mowat, N.A.G., Brunt, P.W.: Neuropsychological deficits and morphological MRI brain scan abnormalities in apparently health non-encephalopathic patients with cirrhosis. A controlled study. J. Hepatol. 1989; 9: 319−325
64. Mullen, K.D., Szauter, K.M., Kaminsky-Russ, K.: "Endogenous" benzodiazepine activity in body fluids of patients with hepatic encephalopathy. Lancet 1990; 336: 81−83
65. Mullen, K.D., Weber, F.L.: Role of nutrition in hepatic encephalopathy. Semin. Liver Dis. 1991; 4: 292−304
66. Müting, D., Kalk, J.-F., Wuzel, H., Flasshoff, H.J., Bucsis, L.: Störungen des Aminosäurenstoffwechsels bei Leberzirrhose ohne und mit hepatischer Enzephalopathie (HPLC-Untersuchungen an 225 Patienten). Inn. Med. 1986; 13: 137−143
67. Nolte, W., Wiltfang, J., Schindler, C., Münke, H., Unterberg, K., Zumhasch, U., Figulla, H.R., Werner, G., Hartmann, H., Ramadori, G.: Portosystemic hepatic encephalopathy after transjugular intrahepatic portosystemic shunt in patients with cirrhosis: clinical, laboratory, psychometric, and electroencephalographic investigations. Hepatology 1998; 28: 1215−1225
68. Norenberg, M.D.: Astrocytic-ammonia interactions in hepatic encephalopathy. Semin. Liver Dis. 1996; 16: 245−253
69. Odeh, M.: Endotoxin and tumor necrosis factor in the pathogenesis of hepatic encephalopathy. J. Clin. Gastroenterol. 1994; 19: 146−153
70. Ono, J., Hutson, D.G., Dombro, R.S., Levi, J.U., Livingstone, A., Zeppa, R.: Tryptophan and hepatic coma. Gastroenterology 1978; 74: 196−200
71. Phillips, G.B., Schwartz, R., Gabuzda, G.J., Dabidson, C.S.: The syndrome of impending hepatic coma in patients with cirrhosis of the liver given certain nitrogenous substances. New Engl. J. Med. 1952; 247: 239−246
72. Planas, R., Gomes-Vieira, M.C., Cabré, E., Armengol, M., Quer, J.C., Boix, J., Morillas, R., Abad-Lacruz, A., Broggi, M., Gassull, M.A.: Prognostic factors of hepatic encephalopathy after portocaval anastomosis: a multivariate analysis in 50 patients. Amer. J. Gastroenterol. 1992; 87: 1792−1796
73. Poo, J.L., Gongora, J., Sanchez-Avila, F., Aguilar-Castillo, S., Garcia-Ramos, G., Fernandez-Zertuche, M., Rodriguez-Fragoso, L., Uribe, M.: Efficacy of oral L-ornithine-L-aspartate in cirrhotic patients with hyperammonemic hepatic encephalopathy. Results of a randomized, lactulose-controlled study. Ann. Hepatol. 2006; 5: 281−288
74. Quero, J.C., Schalm, S.W.: Subclinical hepatic encephalopathy. Semin. Liver Dis. 1996; 16: 321−328
75. Raskin, N.H., Price, J.B., Fishman, R.A.: Portal-systemic encephalopathy due to congenital intrahepatic shunts. New Engl. J. Med. 1964; 270: 225−229
76. Riggio, O., Efrati, C., Catalano, C., Pediconi, F., Mecarelli, O., Accornero, N., Nicolao, F., Angeloni, S., Masini, A., Riclola, L., Attili, A.F., Merli, M.: High prevalence of spontaneous portal-systemic shunts in persistent hepatic encephalopathy. A case-control study. Hepatology 2005; 42: 1158−1165
77. Rijt, van der, C.C.D., Schalm, S.W., Schat, H., Foeken, K., Jong, de, G.: Overt hepatic encephalopathy precipitated by zinc deficiency. Gastroenterology 1991; 100: 1114−1118
78. Rikkers, L., Jenko, P., Rudman, D., Freides, D.: Subclinical hepatic encephalopathy: detection, prevalence and relationship to nitrogen metabolism. Gastroenterology 1978; 75: 462−469
79. Rink, C., Mantel, E., Haerting, J.: Ambulante Diagnose und Therapiekontrolle der porto-systemischen Enzephalopathie bei Patienten mit Leberzirrhose. Dtsch. Z. Verdau. Stoffwechselkrankh. 1985; 45: 295−301
80. Romero-Gomez, M., Boza, F., Garcia-Valdecasas, M:S., Garcia, E., Aguilar-Reina, J.: Subclinical hepatic encephalopathy predicts the development of overt hepatic encephalopathy. Amer. J. Gastroenterol. 2001; 96: 2718−2723
81. Romero-Gomez, M., Grande, L., Camacho, I., Benitez, S., Irles, J.A., Castro, M.: Altered response to oral glutamine challenge as prognostic factor for overt episodes in patients with minimal hepatic encephalopathy. J. Hepatol. 2002; 37: 781−787
82. Rose, C., Butterworth, R.F., Zayed, J., Normandin, L., Todd, K., Michalak, A., Spahr, L., Huet, P.M., Pomier Layrargues, G.: Manganese deposition in basal ganglia structures results from both portal-systemic shunting and liver dysfunction. Gastroenterology 1999; 117: 640−644
83. Ross, B., Kreis, R., Farrow, N.A., Ackerman, Z.: Metabolic disorders of the brain in chronic hepatic encephalopathy detected with H-1 MR spectroscopy. Radiology 1992; 182: 19−27
84. Sanyal, A.J., Freedman, A.M., Shiffman, M.L., Purdum, P.P., Luketic, V.A., Cheatham, A.K.: Portosystemic encephalopathy after transjugular intrahepatic portosystemic shunt: results of a prospective controlled study. Hepatology 1994; 20: 46−55
85. Sarin, S.K., Nundy, S.: Subclinical encephalopathy after portosystemic shunts in patients with non-cirrhotic portal fibrosis. Liver 1985; 5: 142−146
86. Saxena, N., Bhatia, M., Joshi, Y.K., Garg, P.K., Dwivedi, S.N., Tandon, R.K.: Electrophysiological and neuropsychological tests for the diagnosis of subclinical hepatic encephalopathy and prediction of overt encephalopathy. Liver 2002; 22: 190−197
87. Schafer, D.F., Jones, E.A.: Hepatic encephalopathy and the γ-aminobutyric acid neurotransmitter system. Lancet 1982/I: 18−20
88. Schomerus, H., Hamster, W., Blunck, H., Reinhard, U., Mayer, K., Dölle, W.: Latent portosystemic encephalopathy. I. Nature of cerebral functional defects and their effect on fitness to drive. Dig. Dis. Sci. 1981; 26: 622−630
89. Schomerus, H., Schreiegg, J.: Prevalence of latent portasystemic encephalopathy in an unselected population of patients with liver cirrhosis in general practice. Z. Gastroenterol. 1993; 31: 231−234
90. Seery, J.P., Taylor-Robinson, D.: The application of magnetic resonance spectroscopy to the study of hepatic encephalopathy. J. Hepatol. 1996; 25: 988−998
91. Shimamoto, C., Hirata, I., Katsu, K.: Breath and blood ammonia in liver cirrhosis. Hepato-Gastroenterol. 2000; 47: 443−445
92. Silva, G., Segovia, R., Ponce, R., Backhouse, C., Palma, M., Roblero, J.P., Abadal, J., Quijada, C., Troncoso, M., Iturriaga, H.: Effects of 5-isosorbide mononitrate and propranol on subclinical hepatic encephalopathy and renal functions in patients with liver cirrhosis. Hepato-Gastroenterol. 2002; 49: 1357−1362
93. Spahr, L., Butterworth, R.F., Fontaine, S., Bui, L., Therrien, G., Milette, P.C., Lebrun, L.H., Zayed, J., Leblanc, A., Pomier-Layrargues, G.: Increased blood manganese in cirrhotic patients: relationship to pallidal magnetic resonance signal hyperintensity and neurological symptoms. Hepatology 1996; 24: 1116−1120
94. Stahl, J.: Studies of the blood ammonia in liver disease. Its diagnostic, prognostic and therapeutic significance. Ann. Intern. Med. 1963; 58: 1−24
95. Strauss, E., Ferreira da Costa, M.: The importance of bacterial infections as precipitating factors of chronic hepatic encephalopathy in cirrhosis. Hepato-Gastroenterol. 1998; 45: 900−904
96. Tarter, R.E., Hegedus, A.M., van Thiel, D.H., Schade, R.R., Gavaler, J.S., Starzl, T.E.: Nonalcoholic cirrhosis associated with neuropsychological dysfunction in the absence of overt evidence of hepatic encephalopathy. Gastroenterology 1984; 86: 1421−1427
97. Tarter, R.E., Switala, J., Plail, J., Havrilla, J., Thiel, van, D.H.: Severity of hepatic encephalopathy before liver transplantation is associated with quality of life after transplantation. Arch. Intern. Med. 1992; 152: 2097−2101
98. Thirlby, R.C., Fenster, L.F., Coatsworth, J.J., Petty, F.: Reversal of chronic hepatic encephalopathy by colonic exclusion: poor correlation with blood GABA levels. Amer. J. Gastroenterol. 1990; 85: 1637−1641
99. Tien, R., Arieff, A.I., Kucharczyk, W., Wasik, A., Kucharczyk, J.: Hyponatremic encephalopathy: is central pontine myelinolysis a component? Amer. J. Med. 1992; 92:513−522
100. Victor, M., Adams, R.D., Cole, M.: The acquired (non-Wilsonian) type of chronic hepatocerebral degeneration. Medicine (Baltimore) 1965; 44: 345−396
101. Walker, C.O., Schenker, S.: Pathogenesis of hepatic encephalopathy with special reference to the role of ammonia. Amer. J. Clin. Nutr. 1970; 23: 619−632
102. Watanabe, A., Shiota, T., Tsuji, T.: Cerebral edema during hepatic encephalopathy in fulminant hepatic failure. J. Med. 1992; 23: 29−38
103. Wein, C., Koch, H., Popp, B., Oehler, G., Schauder, P.: Minimal hepatic encephalopathy impairs fitness to drive. Hepatology 2004; 39: 739−745
104. Yonekura, T., Kamata, S., Wasa, M., Okada, A., Kawata, S., Tarui, S.: Simultaneous analysis of plasma phenethylamine, phenylethanolamine, tyramine and octopamine in patients with hepatic encephalopathy. Clin. Chim. Acta 1991; 199: 91−98
105. Zieve, L.: The machanism of hepatic coma. Hepatology 1981; 1: 360−365

Therapy:
106. Bansky, G., Meier, P.J., Riederer, E., Walser, H., Ziegler, W.H., Schmid, M.: Effects of the benzodiazepine receptor antagonist flumazenil in hepatic encephalopathy in humans. Gastroenterology 1989; 97: 744−750
107. Bianchi, G.P., Marchesini, G., Fabbri, A., Rondelli, A., Bugianesi, E., Zoli, M., Pisi, E.: Vegetable versus animal protein diet in cirrhotic patients with chronic encephalopathy. A randomized cross-over comparison. J. Intern. Med. 1993; 233: 385−392
108. Bosman, D.K., Buijs, van den, C.A.C.G., Haan, de, J.G., Maas, M.A.W., Chamuleau, R.A.F.M.: The effects of benzodiazepine-receptor antagonists and partial inverse agonists on acute hepatic encephalopathy in the rat. Gastroenterology 1991; 101: 772−781
109. Cadranel, J.F., El Younsi, M., Pidoux, B., Zylberberg, P., Benhamou, Y., Valla, D., Opolon, P.: Flumazenil therapy for hepatic encephalopa-

thy in cirrhotic patients: a double-blind pragmatic randomized, placebo study. Eur. J. Gastroenterol. Hepatol. 1995; 7: 325–329
110. **Condon, R.E.:** Effect of dietary protein on symptoms and survival in dogs with an Eck fistula. Amer. J. Surg. 1971; 121: 107–113
111. **Conn, H.O., Leevy, C.M., Vlahcevic, Z.R., Rodgers, J.B., Maddrey, W.C., Seef, L., Levy, L.L.:** Comparison of lactulose and neomycin in the treatment of chronic portal- systemic encephalopathy. A double blind controlled trial. Gastroenterology 1977; 72: 573–583
112. **Del Rosario, M., Werlin, S.L., Lauer, S.J.:** Hyperammonemic encephalopathy after chemotherapy. Survival after treatment with sodium benzoate and sodium phenylacetate. J. Clin. Gastroenterol. 1997; 25: 682–684
113. **Egberts, E.-H., Schomerus, H., Hamster, W., Jürgens, P.:** Verzweigtkettige Aminosäuren bei der Behandlung der latenten portosystemischen Enzephalopathie. Eine placebo-kontrollierte Doppelblind-Cross-over-Studie. Z. Ernährungswiss. 1986; 25: 9–28
114. **Eriksson, L.S., Conn, H.O.:** Branched-chain amino acids in the management of hepatic encephalopathy: an analysis of variants. Hepatology 1989; 10: 228–246
115. **Fenton, J.C.B., Knight, E.J., Humpherson, P.L.:** Milk-and-cheese diet in portal-systemic encephalopathy. Lancet 1966/I: 164–166
116. **Freund, H., Yoshimura, N., Fischer, J.E.:** Chronic hepatic encephalopathy. Long-term therapy with a branched-chain amino-acid-enriched elemental diet. J. Amer. Med. Ass. 1979; 242: 347–349
117. **Greenberg, N.J., Carley, J., Schenker, St., Bettinger, I., Stamness, C., Beyer, P.:** Effect of vegetable and animal protein diets in chronic hepatic encephalopathy. Dig. Dis. 1977; 22: 845–855
118. **Grüngreiff, K., Kleine, F.-D., Musil, H.E., Diete, U., Franke, D., Klauck, S., Päge, I., Kleine, B., Lössner, B., Pfeiffer, K.P.:** Valin und verzweigtkettige Aminosäuren in der Behandlung der hepatischen Enzephalopathie. Z. Gastroenterol. 1993; 31: 235–241
119. **Gyr, K., Meier, R., Häussler, J., Boulétreau, P., Fleig, W.E., Gatta, A., Holstege, A., Pomier-Layrargues, G., Schalm, S.W., Groneweg, M., Scollo-Lavizzari, G., Ventura, E., Zenerolli, M.L., Williams, R., Yoo, Y., Amrein, R.:** Evaluation of the efficacy and safety of flumazenil in the treatment of portal systemic encephalopathy: a double-blind, randomized, placebo-controlled multicentre study. Gut 1996; 39: 319–324
120. **Higuchi, K., Shimizu, Y., Nambu, S., Miyabayashi, C., Takahara, T., Saito, S., Hioki, O., Kuwabara, Y., Watanabe, A.:** Effects of an infusion of branched-chain amino acids on neurophysiological and psychometric testings in cirrhotic patients with mild hepatic encephalopathy. J. Gastroenterol. Hepatol. 1994; 9: 366–372
121. **Horsmans, Y., Solbreux, P.M., Daenens, C., Desager, J.P., Geubel, A.P.:** Lactulose improves psychometric testing in cirrhotic patients with subclinical encephalopathy. Aliment. Pharmacol. Ther. 1997; 11: 165–170
122. **Horst, D., Grace, N.D., Conn, H.O., Schiff, E., Schenker, S., Viteri, A., Law, D., Atterbury, C.E.:** Comparison of dietary protein with an oral branched chain-enriched amino acid supplement in chronic portal-systemic encephalopathy: a randomized controlled trial. Hepatology 1984; 4: 279–287
123. **Keohane, P.P., Attrill, H., Grimble, G., Spiller, R., Frost, P., Silk, D.B.A.:** Enteral nutrition in malnourished patients with hepatic cirrhosis and acute encephalopathy. J. Parent. Ent. Nutr. 1983; 7: 346–349
124. **Keshavarzian, A., Meek, J., Sutton, C., Emery, V.M., Hughes, E.A., Hodgson, H.J.F.:** Dietary protein supplementation from vegetable sources in the management of chronic portal-systemic encephalopathy. Amer. J. Gastroenterol. 1984; 79: 945–949
125. **Kircheis, G., Nilius, R., Held, C., Berndt, H., Buchner, M., Görtelmeyer, R., Hendricks, R., Krüger, B., Kuklinski, B., Meister, H., Otto, H.-J., Rink, C., Rösch, W., Stauch, S.:** Therapeutic efficacy of L-ornithine-L-aspartate infusions in patients with cirrhosis and hepatic encephalopathy: results of a placebo-controlled, double-blind study. Hepatology 1997; 25: 1351–1360
126. **Laccetti, M., Manes, G., Uomo, G., Lioniello, M., Rabitti, P.G., Balzano, A.:** Flumazenil in the treatment of acute hepatic encephalopathy in cirrhotic patients: a double blind randomized placebo controlled study. Dig. Liver Dis. 2000; 32: 335–338
127. **Liersch, J., Huth, K.:** Beeinflussung der portosystemischen Enzephalopathie durch orale Zufuhr verzweigtkettiger Aminosäuren bei Patienten mit Leberzirrhose. Med. Welt 1985; 36: 448–454
128. **Loguercio, C., Abbiati, R., Rinaldi, M., Romano, A., Del Vecchio Blanco, C., Coltori, M.:** Long-term effects of Enterococcus faecium SF 68 versus lactulose in the treatment of patients with cirrhosis and grade 1–2 hepatic encephalopathy. J. Hepatol. 1995; 23: 39–46
129. **Marchesini, G., Dioguardi, F.S., Bianchi, G.P., Zoli, M., Bellati, G., Roffi, L., Martines, D., Abbiati, R.:** Long-term oral branched-chain amino acid treatment in chronic hepatic encephalopathy. A randomized double-blind casein-controlled trial. J. Hepatol. 1990; 11: 92–101
130. **Mas, A., Rodes, J., Sunyer, L., Rodrigo, L., Planas, R., Vargas, V., Castells, L., Rodriguez-Martinez, D., Fernandez-Rodriguez, C., Coll, I., Pardo, A.:** Comparison of rifaximin and lactitol in the treatment of acute hepatic encephalopathy: results of a randomized, double-blind, doubledummy, controlled clinical trial. J. Hepatol. 2003; 38: 51–58
131. **McClain, C.J., Potter, T.J., Kromhout, J.P., Zieve, L.:** The effect of lactulose on psychomotor performance tests in alcoholic cirrhotics without overt hepatic encephalopathy. J. Clin. Gastroenterol. 1984; 6: 325–329
132. **Merli, M., Riggio, O., Pieche, U., Ariosto, F., Pinto, G., Romiti, A., Varriale, M., Capocaccia, L.:** The effect of oral BCAA supplement on diurnal variations in plasma amino acid concentrations in cirrhotic patients. Nutrition 1988; 4: 351–356
133. **Morgan, M.Y., Jakobovits, A.W., James, I.M., Sherlock, S.:** Successful use of bromocriptine in the treatment of chronic hepatic encephalopathy. Gastroenterology 1980; 78: 663–670
134. **Morgan, M.H., Read, A.E., Speller, D.C.E.:** Treatment of hepatic encephalopathy with metronidazol. Gut 1982; 23: 1–7
135. **Naylor, C.D., O'Rourke, K., Detsky, A.S., Baker, J.P.:** Parenteral nutrition with branched-chain amino acids in hepatic encephalopathy. A meta-analysis. Gastroenterology 1989; 97: 1033–1042
136. **Okita, M., Watanabe, A., Nagashima, H.:** A branched-chain amino acid-supplemented diet in the treatment of liver cirrhosis. Curr. Therap. Res. 1984; 35: 83–92
137. **Platell, C., Kong, S.-E., McCauley, R., Hall, J.C.:** Branched-chain amino acids. J. Gastroenterol. Hepatol. 2000; 15: 706–717
138. **Plauth, M., Egberts, E.-H., Hamster, W., Török, M., Müller, P.H., Brand, O., Fürst, P., Dölle, W.:** Long-term treatment of latent portosystemic encephalopathy with branched-chain amino acids. A double-blind placebo-controlled crossover study. J. Hepatol. 1993; 17: 308–314
139. **Pomier-Layrargues, G., Giguère, J.F., Lavoie, J., Perney, P., Gagnon, S., Damour, M., Wells, J., Butterworth, R.F.:** Flumazenil in cirrhotic patients in hepatic coma: a randomized double-blind placebo-controlled crossover trial. Hepatology 1994; 19: 32–37
140. **Reding, P., Duchateau, J., Bataille, C.:** Oral zinc supplementation improves hepatic encephalopathy. Lancet 1984/II: 493–494
141. **Riggio, O., Balducci, G., Ariosto, F., Merli, M., Tremiterra, S., Ziparo, V., Capocaccia, L.:** Lactitol in the treatment of chronic hepatic encephalopathy – a randomized cross-over comparison with lactulose. Hepato-Gastroenterol. 1990; 37: 524–527
142. **Riggio, O., Merli, M., Capocaccia, L., Caschera, M., Zulio, A., Pinto, G., Gaudio, E., Franchitto, A., Stagnoli, R., D'Aquilino, E., Seri, S., Moretti, R., Cantafora, A.:** Zinc supplementation reduces blood ammonia and increases liver ornithine transcarbamylase activity in experimental cirrhosis. Hepatology 1992; 16: 785–789
143. **Rose, C., Michalak, A., Rama Rao, K.V., Quack, G., Kircheis, G., Butterworth, R.F.:** L-ornithine-L-aspartate lowers plasma and cerebrospinal fluid ammonia and prevents brain edema in rats with acute liver failure. Hepatology 1999; 30: 636–640
144. **Stauch, S., Kircheis, G., Adler, G., Becker, K., Ditschuneit, H., Görtelmeyer, R., Hendricks, R., Heuser, A., Karoff, C., Malfertheiner, P., Mayer, D., Rösch, W., Steffens, J.:** Oral L-ornithine-L-aspartate therapy of chronic hepatic encephalopathy: results of a placebo-controlled double-blind study. J. Hepatol. 1998; 28: 856–864
145. **Sushma, S., Dasarathy, S., Tandon, R.K., Jain, S., Gupta, S., Bhist, M.S.:** Sodium benzoate in the treatment of acute hepatic encephalopathy: a double-blind randomized trail. Hepatology 1992; 16: 138–144
146. **Tarao, K., Ikeda, T., Hayashi, K., Watanabe, A., Sakurai, A., Okeda, T., Ito, T., Karube, H., Nomoto, T., Mizuno, T., Shindo, K.:** Successful use of vancomycin hydrochloride in the treatment of lactulose resistant chronic hepatic encephalopathy. Gut 1990; 31: 702–706
147. **Tromm, A., Giga, T., Greving, I., Hilden, H., Hüppe, D., Schwegler, U., Micklefield, G.H., May, B.:** Orthograde whole gut irrigation with mannite versus paromomycine plus lactulose as prophylaxis of hepatic encephalopathy in patients with cirrhosis and upper gastrointestinal bleeding: results of a controlled randomized trial. Hepatogastroenterology 2000; 47: 473–477
148. **Uribe, M., Marquez, M.A., Ramos, G.G., Ramos-Uribe, M.H., Vargas, F., Villalobos, A., Ramos, C.:** Treatment of chronic portal-systemic encephalopathy with vegetable and animal protein diets. A controlled crossover study. Dig. Dis. Sci. 1982; 27: 1109–1119
149. **Uribe; M., Garcia-Ramos, G., Ramos, M., Valverde, C., Marquez, M.A., Farca, A., Guevara, L.:** Standard and higher doses of bromocriptine for severe chronic portal-systemic encephalopathy. Amer. J. Gastroenterol. 1983; 78: 517–522
150. **Uribe-Esquivel, M., Moran, S., Poo, J.L., Munoz, R.M.:** Invitro and invivo lactose and lactulose effects on colonic fermentation and portalsystemic encephalopathy parameters. Scand. J. Gastroenterol. 1997; 32 (Suppl. 222): 49–52
151. **Watanabe, A., Sakai, T., Sato, S., Imai, F., Ohto, M., Arakawa, Y., Toda, G., Kobayashi, K., Muto, Y., Tsujii, T., Kawasaki, H., Okita, K., Tanikawa, K., Fujiyama, S., Shimada, S.:** Clinical efficacy of lactulose in cirrhotic patients with and without subclinical hepatic encephalopathy. Hepatology 1997; 26: 1410–1414
152. **Watanabe, A.:** Portal-systemic encephalopathy in non-cirrhotic patients: classification of clinical types, diagnosis and treatment. J. Gastroenterol. Hepatol. 2000; 15: 969–979
153. **Weber, F.L. jr.:** Effects of lactulose on nitrogen metabolism. Scand. J. Gastroenterol. 1997; 32 (Suppl. 222): 83–87
154. **Williams, R., James, O.F.W., Warnes, T.W., Morgan, M.Y.:** Evaluation of the efficacy and safety of rifaximin in the treatment of hepatic encephalopathy: a double-blind, randomized, dose-finding multi-centre study. Eur. J. Gastroenterol. Hepatol. 2000; 12: 203–208
155. **Yang, S.S., Lai, Y.C., Chiang, T.R., Chen, D.F., Chen, D.S.:** Role of zinc in subclinical hepatic encephalopathy: comparison with somatosencory-evoked potentials. J. Gastroenterol. Hepatol. 2004; 19: 375–379
156. **Yoshida, T., Muto, Y., Moriwaki, H., Yamato, M.:** Effect of long-term oral supplementation with branched-chain amino acid granules on the prognosis of liver cirrhosis. Gastroenterol. Japon. 1989; 24: 692–698
157. **Zullo, A., Rinaldi, V., Hassan, C., Folino, S., Winn, S., Pinto, G., Attili, A.F.:** Helicobacter pyloric and plasma ammonia levels in cirrhotics: role of urease inhibition by acetohydroxamic acid. Ital. J. Gastroenterol. Hepatol. 1998; 30: 405–409

Symptoms and Syndromes
16 Oedema and ascites

		Page:
1	*Water and electrolyte balance*	294
2	*Definition*	295
2.1	States of hydration	295
2.2	Oedema and anasarca	295
2.3	Ascites	296
3	*Pathogenesis*	296
3.1	Oedematization	296
3.2	Formation of ascites	297
3.2.1	Mechanical factors	297
3.2.2	Biochemical factors	298
3.2.3	Increase in renal sodium retention	300
3.2.4	Theories of ascites formation	300
4	*Aetiology of ascites*	302
4.1	Differential diagnosis	302
4.2	Hepatogenic ascites	302
5	*Diagnosis of ascites*	303
5.1	Clinical findings	303
5.2	Imaging procedures	304
5.3	Laboratory diagnosis	305
6	Complications of ascites	308
7	*Spontaneous bacterial peritonitis*	308
7.1	Definition	308
7.2	Forms and frequency	308
7.3	Pathogenesis and predisposing factors	309
7.4	Clinical aspects	309
7.5	Prophylaxis and therapy	309
8	*Conservative therapy of ascites*	310
8.1	Prophylaxis	310
8.2	*Basic therapy (stage I)*	311
8.3	*Diuretic therapy (stage II)*	312
8.3.1	Pharmacology of diuretics	312
8.3.2	Side effects	314
8.3.3	Hyponatraemia	314
8.3.4	Resistance to diuretics	314
8.4	*Osmotic diuresis (stage III)*	314
8.5	*Paracentesis (stage IV)*	315
9	*Refractory ascites*	316
10	*Invasive therapeutic procedures*	316
10.1	Ascites reinfusion	316
10.2	Peritoneovenous shunt	317
10.3	TIPS	320
11	Surgical treatment	321
12	Liver transplantation	322
	• References (1–240)	323
	(Figures 16.1–16.17; tables 16.1–16.19)	

16 Oedema and ascites

1 Water and electrolyte balance

▶ **Water** is an indispensable factor of life. By means of carefully coordinated regulatory mechanisms, the *water equilibrium* and hence the reservoir of body water is held constant. It is important to keep water intake and output in balance to maintain *isovolaemia*. (s. fig. 16.1)

Water is present in a free (non-osmotically bound) state and as a chemically bound hydrate solid structure. • The **clearance** of free water is controlled by vasopressin; it is calculated from the volume of urine/minute minus the osmolal clearance. A normal daily fluid intake of 1,700–2,200 ml (25–30 ml/kg BW) in addition to some 300 ml oxidation water is balanced by a fluid discharge of approximately 1,500 ml as urine, about 100 ml in stools, roughly 600 ml as perspiration and some 400 ml as expired air. (s. fig. 16.1)

About 60% of the body's weight (ca. 55% in women) consists of water. The reservoir of body water is distributed between the **intracellular space** (ca. 40% of BW) and the **extracellular space** (ca. 20% of BW). The extracellular compartment consists of plasma fluids (ca. 4% of BW) and interstitial water (ca. 16% of BW), the latter also containing transcellular water (ca. 2.5% of BW). Because of its high degree of permeability, the body water is evenly shared between the intracellular and extracellular compartments. The water distribution between plasma and interstitium, regulated by **Starling's forces,** depends on the hydrostatic and colloidosmotic pressure gradients along the capillary walls. • **Disturbances in the excretion of water** are derived from (*1.*) an increase in ADH activity, (*2.*) a reduction in distal filtrates available in the nephron, and (*3.*) greater absorption of water in the distal nephron, independent of ADH. Disruptions in the body water pool cause changes in serum sodium or serum osmolality.

▶ **Electrolytes** are subject to dissociation into negatively charged anions and positive cations. The vital *electrolyte balance* guarantees the respective uptake and discharge and ensures the correct presence and distribution. This regulatory process is closely linked to the water equilibrium. The intracellular and extracellular spaces differ in their electrolyte content. (s. tab. 16.1)

	Plasma	Interstitial space (mval/l)	Intracellular space (mval/l)
Cations			
Sodium	142	145	10
Potassium	4	4	160
Calcium	5	5	2
Magnesium	2	2	26
	153	156	198
Anions			
Chloride	101	114	3
Bicarbonate	27	31	10
Phosphate	2	2	100
Sulphate	1	1	20
Organic acids	6	7	–
Proteins	16	1	65
	153	156	198

Tab. 16.1: Constituents of the most important electrolytes (in mval/l) in extracellular and intracellular fluid

▶ An **ionogram** of the fluid spaces compares the cation and anion content in milliequivalents, since it is not the weight, but the chem-

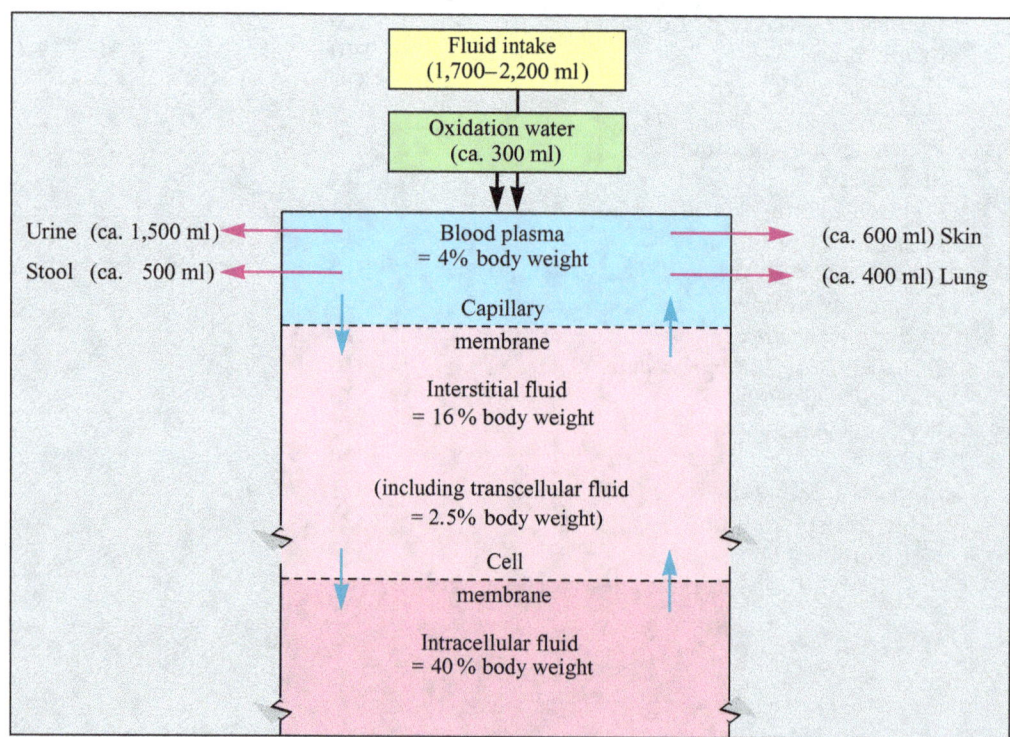

Fig. 16.1: Fluid spaces and exchange of water (blood plasma + interstitial fluid = extracellular space, intracellular fluid = intracellular space)

ical-binding potential (mval) of the ions that determines the electrochemical reactions between them. The electrolytes, which are partially integrated into the structures of the cells, do not develop any osmotic activity. For this reason, there is no osmotic gradient between the intracellular and extracellular space despite the difference in the distribution of ions (153 and 156/198 mval). • Apart from this, the ionogram also provides information on the osmotic pressure (mosmol) of the respective fluid. This value does not depend on valence, but on the number of particles dissolved in each litre of solution (= **osmolarity**; mmol/l) or per 1 kg water (= **osmolality**; mosmol/kg). All fluids with an osmolality of 285–295 mosmol/kg are isotonic with respect to plasma. (With 1-valent ions, mval, mmol and mosmol are identical; with 2-valent ions, 2 mval correspond to 1 mmol or 1 mosmol). The osmolality of urine is twofold to threefold the osmolality of serum (up to ca. 1,300 mosmol). • The normal **pH value** ranges between 7.35 and 7.45 in the extracellular fluid (blood plasma and interstitium) and between 6.8 and 7.0 in the intracellular fluid.

A number of transport systems guarantee the differing compositions of intracellular and extracellular fluid. Ion displacement gives rise to the development of concentration gradients between these two compartments. Water flows passively through the cell membranes in the direction of the hyperosmolar space. The regulatory mechanism of the so-called **Donnan equilibrium** takes effect (and generates a relative condition of ion equilibrium). To a certain extent, the compensation of osmolarity between the intracellular and extracellular spaces by way of fluid displacement in line with the **Darrow-Yanett principle** supports the homoeostasis process with the aim of maintaining iso-osmosis.

Isotonicity of the extracellular space is regulated by (*1.*) thirst mechanism, (*2.*) ADH, and (*3.*) dilution and concentration potential of the kidneys. • Maintenance of extracellular **isovolaemia** is effected by a change in renal sodium excretion. For this reason, disturbances in the sodium supply primarily result in changes in the extracellular fluid volume. • **Isohydria** is also continually regulated within the normal range.

▶ When fever occurs, the organism loses about *500 ml fluid* and some *25 mmol salts* per day for each one-degree rise in body temperature.

2 Definition

Depending on the extent of the extracellular volume, disorders of water and sodium balance are categorized as **dehydration** (= hypovolaemia) and **hyperhydration** (= hypervolaemia). In accordance with the behaviour of serum osmolality and serum sodium, hydration is subdivided into isotonic, hypotonic and hypertonic forms. Should it no longer be possible to achieve iso-osmosis owing to sustained or permanent disruptive mechanisms, the physiological regulatory processes gain ever-increasing pathophysiological significance − creating a vicious circle.

2.1 States of hydration

In the field of hepatology, three varying states of hydration are important:

(*1.*) **Isotonic dehydration** due to isotonic loss of fluid on account of diuretic therapy, diarrhoea, ascites taps or loss of blood (= extracellular space decreased, overall sodium status depressed, serum osmolality and serum sodium normal).

(*2.*) **Hypotonic dehydration** as a result of the loss of sodium from long-term diuretic therapy and from diarrhoea as well as due to inadequate sodium intake (= extracellular space decreased, intracellular space increased, overall sodium status depressed, surplus of free water, hypo-osmolality and hyponatraemia).

(*3.*) **Isotonic hyperhydration** due to hypernatraemia with generalized oedema in decompensated liver cirrhosis (= extracellular space enlarged, overall sodium status elevated, serum osmolality and serum sodium normal).

2.2 Oedema and anasarca

The term **oedema** (το οίδημα = the swelling) describes a rise in the extracellular fluid volume due to isotonic hyperhydration. Oedema is a *symptom* with multiple causes, yet no illness. • The term **anasarca** refers to a massive, generalized soaking of the subcutaneous tissue ("tissue dropsy"). (s. fig. 16.2)

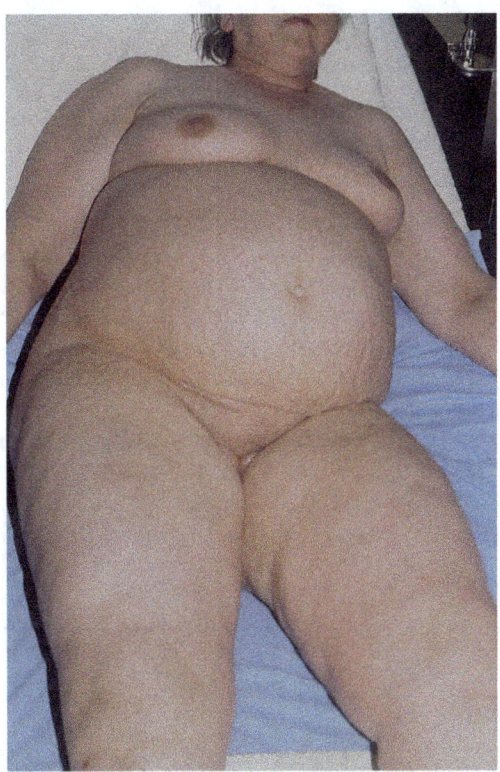

Fig. 16.2: Pronounced anasarca in portal ascites as a result of alcoholic cirrhosis

Anasarca is a circumscribed or diffuse, practically painless accumulation of serous liquid (generally poor in protein at first, but in most cases more rich in protein later on) in the skin, mucosa, parenchymal organs and nerve tissue. • The *clinical manifestation* of oedema can only be discerned during a physical examination if the enlargement of the extracellular space amounts to at least 3–5 litres. *Latent oedema* ("pre-oedema") can be identified by an increase in body weight of >1 kg within four to five days. (s. fig. 15.2)

Oedema disease: It has not yet been clarified to what extent the so-called oedema disease, a chronic generalized condition of hydration of the interstitial tissue, may be regarded as a disease in its own right.

2.3 Ascites

▶ ERASISTRATOS (ca. 300–250 BC) already recognized the connection between ascites and hepatic disease; he objected to the puncturing of ascites as being a non-causal and unnecessary measure. A. C. CELSUS (30 BC–50 AD) postulated the link between ascites and renal disease or a poor general condition (carcinoma?); he coined the term "ascites". (s. pp 6, 7) • In animal experiments, it was possible to induce ascites by means of ligature of the inferior vena cava below the diaphragm (R. LOWER, 1671). F. TH. FRERICHS (1858) observed oliguria and renal dysfunction in cirrhosis patients. In 1863 A. FLINT demonstrated that in cirrhotic patients with ascites, the morphology of the kidneys was normal – thus there must be a functional disorder in the renal area. With portal hypertension, E. H. STARLING (1884) and R. HEIDENHEIM (1891) found an increase in the lymphatic flow in the thoracic duct. • In 1943 D. ADLERSBERG et al. detected a reduced excretion of free water in cirrhosis patients with ascites. Proof of increased sodium retention was obtained by E. B. FARNSWORTH et al. in 1945. With these observations, made some 60 years ago, two essential pathophysiological findings were made in cirrhosis-induced ascites.

The term **ascites** (= hydraskos or abdominal dropsy) is defined as an accumulation of fluid in the abdominal cavity during the course of various diseases. Commensurate with the respective underlying disease, there is no homogeneity in the aetiology and pathogenesis of ascites. Hence ascites is not a disease as such, but rather a *symptom* of the advanced or severe course of an underlying disease. Generally, its prognosis is poor. The two-year rate of survival is about 50%. In liver disease or liver cirrhosis, the occurrence of ascites can give a clue to decompensation. • *Usually, ascites occurs in liver disease prior to the development of oedema.*

3 Pathogenesis

3.1 Oedematization

The **filtration pressure** (= difference between hydrostatic capillary pressure and tissue pressure) furthers the discharge of plasma fluid from the arterioles; as a result of the higher protein content of the plasma, the **colloidosmotic pressure** promotes the backflow of interstitial fluid into the venules. In the arteriole, the hydrostatic pressure is 40–45 mm Hg; it drops down to 10–15 mm Hg in the direction of the venous capillary loop. Both the colloidosmotic pressure and the tissue pressure remain unchanged at −25 to −30 mm Hg or −2 to −5 mm Hg along the arterial and venous parts of the capillaries. Consequently, an effective filtration pressure of 10–15 mm Hg is generated in the arterial capillary loop and of −10 to −15 mm Hg in the venous loop. (s. fig. 16.3)

The **pathogenesis** of oedema is derived from a change in these physical forces. The net flow from one compartment to the other is altered accordingly, as is the volume of the respective fluid space. (s. fig. 16.1) A disrupted distribution of the fluid can also be caused by damage to the capillary endothelium as a result of chemical, thermal, mechanical, toxic or immunological influences. This gives rise to a greater degree of permeability with increased protein transfer into the interstitium. • A reduction in the colloidosmotic pressure along the passage of the capillary results in less interstitial fluid being transported into the vascular lumen. (s. tab. 16.2)

1. **Deposition of interstitial liquid is augmented**
   - with increased hydrostatic capillary pressure
   - with increased permeability of the capillary endothelium
2. **Removal of interstitial fluid is restricted**
   - with depressed colloidosmotic pressure in the vascular lumen (e. g. hypalbuminaemia)
   - with augmented protein transfer into the interstitium
   - with decreased lymphatic drainage

Tab. 16.2: Causative factors of oedematization

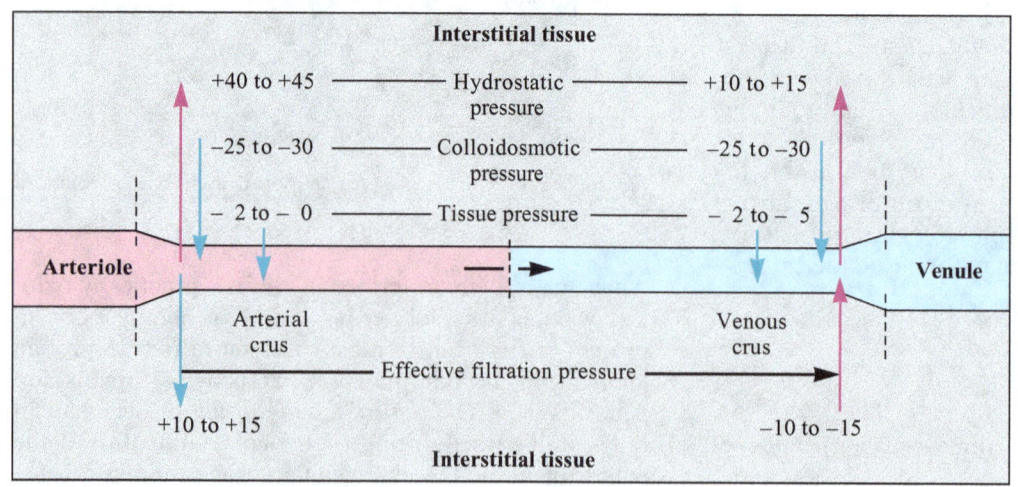

Fig. 16.3: Fluid exchange between plasma and interstitial tissue (mm Hg)

The *primary event* in oedematization is the renal retention of sodium, which provokes a greater feeling of thirst with an increase in ADH secretion. The result is renal water retention. • *A total of about 1 litre of water is retained per 140 mmol (ca. 3.3 g) sodium.*

In liver diseases involving elevated hydrostatic pressure (e. g. as a result of portal hypertension), the inflow of fluid into the interstitium is increased, whereas the return of fluid into the vascular bed is decreased due to the depressed colloidosmotic pressure (e. g. as a result of hypalbuminaemia). Likewise, a boost in capillary permeability leads to an outflow of fluid into the interstitial tissue. (2, 5, 8, 12)

3.2 Formation of ascites

3.2.1 Mechanical factors

The complex pathogenesis of ascites calls for focus on four mechanical factors. (s. tab. 16.3) The pathogenic significance of the respective factors can differ considerably in relation to the underlying diseases and at the same time vary greatly from individual to individual.

---

1. **Increase in hydrostatic pressure**
   - portal hypertension
   - narrowing of the inferior vena cava at the level of the diaphragm
   - disruption of anatomic blocking mechanisms in the hepatic veins
2. **Reduction in colloidosmotic pressure**
3. **Disturbance of capillary permeability**
4. **Insufficiency of lymphatic drainage**

Tab. 16.3: Mechanical factors in the formation of ascites

---

1. **Increase in hydrostatic pressure:** Portal hypertension due to structural changes in the liver or its vessels, with peripheral and sinusoidal impediment to the outflow of blood, leads to blood stasis in the vessels, which are dilated by pressure. This inevitably generates an increase in hydrostatic pressure. The sinusoidal increase in pressure signals a greater retention of sodium in the kidneys. Another cause of ascites is constriction of the inferior vena cava at the level of the diaphragm resulting from regeneration nodes found in cirrhosis, especially since the inflow of blood into the liver is clearly increased at the same time. Disruptions of the anatomic blocking mechanisms in the hepatic veins may constitute further mechanical causes of elevated hydrostatic pressure.

2. **Reduction in colloidosmotic pressure:** The colloidosmotic pressure in the plasma is lower in liver cirrhosis patients. This results from (*1.*) restriction in the synthesis of albumin (which is, however, only clinically manifest after three or four weeks due to the half-life of plasma albumin), (*2.*) greater loss of protein-rich fluid in the abdominal cavity, and (*3.*) dilution of the vascular volume. A critical concentration of albumin in the plasma is deemed to be about 3 g/100 ml (ca. 435 µmol/l). Below this albumin value, there is a clear correlation between portal hypertension and the formation of ascites. • *The coexistence of portal hypertension and hypalbuminaemia (critical concentration 2.5–3.0 g/dl) is an important prerequisite for the formation of ascites.*

However, the significance of the decreased colloidosmotic (oncotic) pressure is not as great as has been hitherto assumed. Nevertheless, when the hydrostatic pressure is raised at the same time, **incongruity between these two Starling forces** is created, and fluid escapes into the abdominal cavity. This process is greatly furthered by the disparity between lymph production and lymph transport. These mechanical factors (s. tab. 16.3) may effect the formation of ascites, yet they cannot produce large quantities of ascitic fluid. Such a development, however, can be expected if capillary permeability is additionally heightened due to toxic or inflammatory causes.

3. **Disturbance of capillary permeability:** Capillary permeability is increased by endotoxins, inflammations or immunological processes. As a result, the degree of permeability for protein-rich fluid is greater. For this reason, it is no longer possible to maintain a colloidosmotic pressure gradient, which is why the hydrostatic pressure (in the absence of any counteraction from the colloid-osmotic pressure) triggers an outflow of fluid into the abdominal cavity. In contrast to the sinusoids with their high potential permeability for protein-rich fluid, intestinal capillaries are only minimally pervious to protein, so that low-protein fluid passes into the abdominal cavity. Because of structural changes in the sinusoids, however, their degree of permeability to protein diminishes as the cirrhotic disease progresses.

4. **Insufficiency of lymphatic drainage:** Insufficient lymphatic drainage is of paramount pathogenic importance, which is why the theory of lymph imbalance became a subject of discussion regarding the formation of ascites. (s. p. 300) Initially, it is possible to compensate the rise in transsinusoidal lymph filtration by greater drainage via dilated lymph vessels. (s. figs. 7.7; 16.4) The normal capacity of the thoracic duct of 0.8–1.5 litres/day can thereby be raised five to ten times the standard amount and, with ascites, even to over 20 litres/day. In cases where the quantity of lymph is greater than the amount which can be removed, the lymph passes from the liver surface into the abdominal cavity (= *mechanical or mural lymph vessel insufficiency*). (s. tab. 16.4)

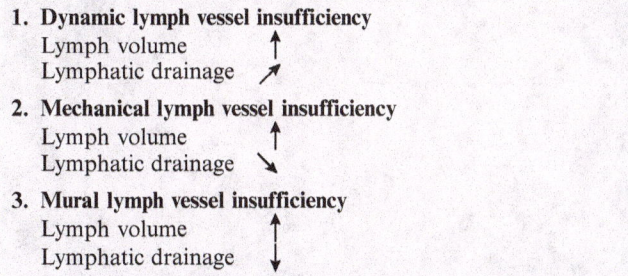

Tab. 16.4: Stages of lymph vessel insufficiency with cirrhosis (s. fig. 16.4)

▶ This development of ascites may progress through to the formation of numerous **lymphocysts** around the vascularized liver capsule and to the extravasation of protein-rich lymph, above all via ruptured lymphocysts. • *This laparoscopic finding has often been termed* **"liver weeping"**. (s. fig. 16.5)

> None of these mechanical factors can be considered "ascitogenic" in their own right. Nevertheless, they may be responsible for triggering a vicious circle in the formation of ascites due to the full impact of the mechanisms involved in elevated renal sodium and water retention.

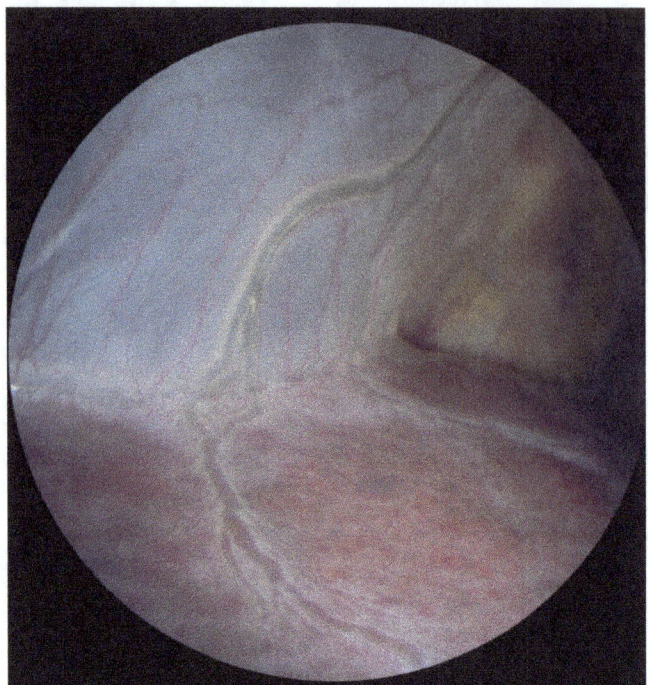

Fig. 16.4: Lymphostasis in the region of the liver capsule of the left liver lobe (lower part) and the falciform ligament

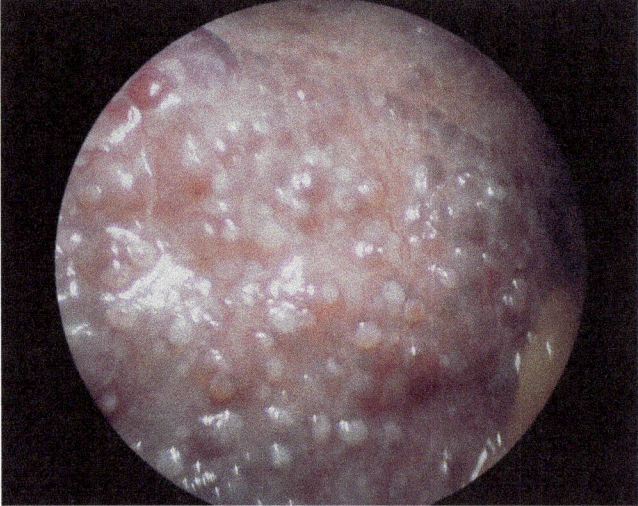

Fig. 16.5: Numerous, partially ruptured lymphocysts (light red, dot-like ruptured openings) on the liver surface with extravasation of protein-rich lymph (= *liver weeping*) in alcoholic cirrhosis

3.2.2 Biochemical factors

A great number of humoral or hormonal substances are involved in the formation of ascites, which is itself triggered by mechanical or physical factors. (s. tab. 16.5) Although the respective effects are largely known, their pathogenic significance in the formation of ascites must be rated differently in each individual case.

The **difficulty in assessment** is based on a number of *plausible reasons*, which can also explain the differing, often even controversial, examination results and the interpretations derived from them:

(*1.*) The formation of an active substance as well as its inactivation or breakdown depend on the individual functional capacity of the liver.

(*2.*) The signals necessary to activate or increase the formation of a substance or a regulatory system depend on the point in time and intensity of a specific pathophysiological situation as well as on the respective liver disease and the developmental phase of the ascites.

(*3.*) The various active substances as well as the sympathetic nervous system display a multitude of interactions, so that it is probably not so much the measuring of the individual factors that allows assessment of the respective pathophysiological situation, but rather their collective interpretation.

(*4.*) A number of individual feedback effects of the biochemical and nervous regulatory systems intervene in the various pathogenic phases, as outlined in the different ascites theories. (s. p. 300)

Renin Angiotensin II Aldosterone	↑ ↑ ↑, N
Antidiuretic hormone (ADH)	↑
Prostaglandin E$_2$ Prostacyclin Thromboxane	↓ ↓ ↑
Atrial natriuretic factor (ANF) Renal natriuretic factor (RNF)	↓, N ?
Prekallikrein Bradykinin	↓ ↓
Endotoxins	↑
Endothelin	↑
Oestrogens Prolactin	↑, ? ↑, ?
Catecholamine	↑

Tab. 16.5: Predominant changes in the concentration of biochemical factors in the blood and urine in portal ascites (N = normal)

1. **Renin-angiotensin-aldosterone system (RAAS):** The first description of aldosterone (S. A. Simpson et al., 1953) reflected awareness of its sustained effects on the electrolyte balance, which is why this hormone secreted by the adrenal cortex was originally given the name *electrocortin*. Aldosterone differs from the other adrenal cortex hormones by one "aldehyde oxygen", from which the name **ald-o-sterone** was derived. • The activity of the renin-angiotensin-aldosterone system is kept in balance by its own feedback mechanisms. Liver diseases have a lasting impact on this regulatory system by changing the formation and breakdown of the substances involved.

The **main stimuli** of the RAAS are hypovolaemia, hypotension, hypoxia, hyponatraemia, hyperkalaemia and an inadequate renal circulation, as well as upright posture or physical strain; the **ancillary stimuli** include adrenocorticotropin (ACTH), thyroxine, oestrogen, ammonia and serotonin, to name but a few. Yet the extent to which these factors play a primary or a secondary role in the individual instance of ascites formation is still not clear. • Given a half-life of aldosterone of 30—35 minutes in the circulating blood, the effect sets in within 45—60 minutes mainly at the distal tubular nephron as a sensitive regulator of sodium transport by stimulating the sodium-potassium ATPase at the interstitial cell membrane.

A **rise in aldosterone** leads to hypernatraemia (with retention of water), loss of potassium (with a hypokalaemia syndrome), loss of H-ions (with a tendency towards metabolic alkalosis) and loss of magnesium and chloride. • Angiotensin II effects a contraction of the vasa efferentia and reinforces the absorption of sodium at the proximal tubular nephron with subsequent retention of water. The serum levels of renin and aldosterone are closely correlated. The increased renin values do not depend on the degree of severity of ascites. Even with a redistribution of the intrarenal blood flow from the cortex, which is normally well-supplied with 80—90% to the renal medulla (= *shift development*), a greater release of renin results with higher aldosterone values. • Nevertheless, augmented serum values of aldosterone are only detectable in some patients with severe liver disease. This finding together with the wide fluctuation range of renin and aldosterone values as well as an absence of the circadian rhythm of the RAAS show that diverging values are found with the different phases of activity of the RAAS in the pathophysiological stages of ascites.

▶ In severe liver disease or advanced cirrhosis, the occurrence of **secondary aldosteronism** must be anticipated and initially rated as an *epiphenomenon*. Nevertheless, at a certain point, the activated RAAS can act as a signal for a boost to the renal retention of sodium and may intervene in the pathogenesis of ascites. The aldosterone value and the renal excretion of sodium are closely and inversely correlated. Yet a higher aldosterone value is not always accompanied by reinforced retention of sodium. This is indeed the case if the feedback by means of sodium is ineffective (= *escape phenomenon*). The refilling of the plasma volume may lead to normalization of the renin and aldosterone values, yet not to normalization of sodium excretion. The reduction in increased aldosterone values is usually accompanied by reinforced natriuresis and diuresis — as has been observed after bilateral adrenalectomy. (s. p. 321) Cirrhosis patients with ascites thus usually show a reduced life expectancy if the renin-plasma value is increased, whereas the prognosis is clearly better if the renin value is normal. (for further reference, see 2, 4—6)

The findings and observations described in the literature as well as the convincing efficacy of the aldosterone antagonist *spironolactone* confirm the importance of the RAAS in the genesis of renal sodium retention and hence also in the formation of ascites.

2. **Antidiuretic hormone (ADH):** In cirrhotic and ascitic patients, the ADH level is usually elevated. (s. tab. 16.5) With a reduced effective plasma volume, ADH is released by non-osmotic stimulation in the neurohypophysis and possibly broken down in the liver at a reduced rate. The plasma activity of ADH largely correlates with that of the RAAS and the sympathetic nervous system. ADH stimulates the nervous synthesis of prostaglandins. It would appear that cirrhotic patients can be divided into excretors and non-excretors as regards the suppression of ADH secretion.

3. **Prostaglandins:** As vasodilators of the renal medullary vessels, prostaglandins influence the blood volume of the kidneys as well as glomerular filtration. They counteract vasoconstriction and thus help to maintain the glomerular filtration rate (GFR), even in cases of hypotension or hypovolaemia. Prostaglandins are natriuretic and diuretic in their action. They interact with the RAAS, the ADH and the kinins as well as with the sympathoadrenal system. Prostaglandins are formed from arachidonic acid, which may, however, be reduced in cirrhotic patients. • From the clinical point of view, it is important that acetylsalicylic acid or indometacin, for example, inhibit the synthesis of prostaglandins and hence bring about a reduction in sodium excretion, urine volume and diuretic efficacy. (s. tab. 16.5)

PGE_2 promotes the renal circulation and the excretion of sodium, while $PGF_{2\alpha}$ has an inhibitive effect in this respect. (No validated information on PGD_2 is available.) Prostacyclin increases the renal circulation, whereas thromboxane gives rise to renal vasoconstriction and reduced excretion of sodium and water. The vasodilatory prostaglandins are stimulated by noradrenaline and angiotensin II in correlation with the degree of hypovolaemia and sodium retention. An important pathogenic role may well be played not only by a reduction in prostaglandin PGE_2 and an increase in thromboxane, but also by an imbalance between the individual prostaglandin fractions.

4. **Natriuretic factors:** Animal experiments and clinical investigations point to the existence of these biochemical factors. After acute volume loading in healthy volunteers, it was possible to detect substances with a natriuretic effect in the blood and urine — *yet this was not the case in cirrhotic and ascitic patients.*

▶ In 1981 the natriuretic effect of an atrial myocardial extract was described for the first time (A.J. DEBOLD et al.). Confirmation of this **atrial natriuretic factor (ANF)** as a peptide hormone was presented in 1983 (T.G. FLINN et al.). The half-life of this factor, also known by the name of *cardiodilatin*, is about three minutes. Receptors for ANF are found in the liver and the kidneys. The ANF leads to a rise in the glomerular filtration rate and in the excretion of sodium. The diuretic, natriuretic and vasodilatory effect is restricted by hypovolaemia and hypotension. The RAAS is inhibited by an i.v. injection of ANF. An increase in atrial pressure is considered to be the main stimulus for the release of ANF, whereas physical exercise, thyroxin, ADH and adrenaline prove less stimulating. In cirrhotic and ascitic patients, normal as well as significantly elevated ANF concentrations are found. This large divergence in values most probably depends on the current volume status (reduced or increased plasma volume) of the respective ascites phase. (1, 13, 193) (s. tab. 16.5)

▶ In 1989 a **renal natriuretic factor (RNF)** was detected for the first time and termed *urodilatin* (P. SCHULZ-KNAPPE et al.). As examinations have hitherto shown, urodilatin is formed in the medial nephron of the kidney and causes a distad inhibition in the absorption of water and sodium. Like ANF, its half-life is approximately three minutes. (3) • Today, *urodilatin is deemed to be important for the regulation of the water and electrolyte balance*, whereas ANF is most probably of limited significance for the excretion of sodium and its influence on sodium homoeostasis in liver cirrhosis (with or without ascites) remains unclarified. (s. tab. 16.5)

5. **Kallikrein-kinin system:** This system acts in a vasodilatory, diuretic and natriuretic manner. In cirrhotic and ascitic patients, there are lower prekallikrein and bradykinin levels as well as less renal kallikrein activity. The reduction in kallikrein excretion in the urine correlates with (*1.*) depressed glomerular filtration rate,

(*2.*) elevation of aldosterone values, and (*3.*) changes in the synthesis of prostaglandin. Nevertheless, as with ANF and RNF, there is still much to be resolved as regards the pathophysiology of cirrhotic patients with concomitant ascites. (s. tab. 16.5)

6. Endotoxinaemia: Different degrees of endotoxinaemia are often detectable in patients suffering from severe liver disease as a result of restricted hepatic endotoxin clearance. There is a correlation between endotoxinaemia and renal dysfunction, and renal blood flow is reduced. Nitrogen monoxide is also released. By reducing endotoxinaemia (after treatment with polymyxin B, for example), the diminished functional activity of the kidney improves and diuresis as well as natriuresis increase. (s. tab. 16.5)

7. Endothelin: Endothelin-1 is a polypeptide with a vasoconstrictive effect. It is generally elevated in portal ascites. The rise in endothelin correlates significantly with augmented ADH, ANF and endotoxins. It would seem to have an additional impact on the development of disrupted renal function. (20, 63) (s. tab. 16.5)

8. Sympathoadrenergic factors: Even at an early stage, the activity of the sympathoadrenal system is enhanced in cirrhotic patients due to a rise in sinusoidal pressure (probably via a glutamine-mediated *hepatorenal reflex*). As a result, the levels of **noradrenaline** and **adrenaline** rise and continue to do so as the decompensation progresses. These substances have a vasoconstrictive effect in the region of the efferent vessels and hence stimulate the retention of water and sodium. Noradrenaline values and natriuresis are closely and inversely correlated, not only because of the altered renal haemodynamics, but also through the alpha receptors situated at the proximal tubulus. Moreover, the increased activity of the sympathetic system stimulates the secretion of renin with subsequent activation of the RAAS. Due to the continuing decompensation, the greatly elevated catecholamine values might also be partly attributable to inadequate inactivation in the liver (and kidneys). (12) (s. tab. 16.5)

3.2.3 Increase in renal sodium retention

An increase in the retention of sodium occurs in the early stages of severe liver disease, particularly in liver cirrhosis, without any disruption of the water balance. This early tendency towards sodium retention can be detected using the *NaCl-tolerance test*. The retention of sodium reduces the sodium excretion rate in the urine to < 10 mval/day (normal rate: 120 to 220 mval/day). Diuresis is not primarily restricted; patients with ascites and oedema react to an excessive intake of water with an adequate excretion of diluted urine, albeit in the virtual absence of sodium excretion. The limited sodium excretion derives from increased, mainly proximal tubular reabsorption of sodium and not from diminished glomerular filtration. Overall maintenance of the liver architecture is usually accompanied by undisturbed sodium excretion, despite existing portal hypertension (such as in primary biliary cirrhosis). Marked sodium retention is, however, usually found in alcoholic-toxic cirrhosis. For this reason, such patients are not only the ones most frequently affected by ascites and oedema, but as a rule they display the most serious forms. This is probably also due to additional biochemical and hormonal factors which are present to a greater degree in patients with alcohol-related liver disease.

3.2.4 Theories of ascites formation

To explain the complex mechanisms of ascites formation, **four hypotheses** have been developed in the light of experimental and clinical findings: (*1.*) underfill theory, (*2.*) overflow theory, (*3.*) lymph imbalance theory, and (*4.*) vasodilation theory. (s. fig. 16.6)

1. Underfill theory: According to the underfill theory (S. SHERLOCK et al., 1963), the development of ascites is set off by mechanical factors and physical mechanisms ("imbalance of the Starling forces"). As a result, the effective plasma volume is reduced (= *volume deficiency concept*).

The **reduced intravasal volume** leads to a stimulation of volume receptors. In addition, the renin-angiotensin-aldosterone system and the sympathoadrenergic system are activated; the ADH level rises. This leads to a reduction in the glomerular filtration rate (GFR). The result is increased tubular sodium reabsorption, i.e. retention of sodium. Yet a reduced glomerular filtration rate is not a prerequisite for sodium retention, since this can occur even with normal GFR. • This mechanism of ascites formation through the primary reduction in the effective plasma volume is reinforced by (*1.*) growing insufficiency of the lymph vessels as a result of portal hypertension, (*2.*) decrease in peripheral resistance due to the opening of intrahepatic and systemic arteriovenous anastomoses, and (*3.*) enhanced formation or diminished breakdown of substances with a vasodilatory effect. (s. fig. 16.6)

2. Overflow theory: The overflow theory (F. L. LIEBERMANN et al., 1970) (7) is based on the principle that retention of sodium already exists as a primary event and hence causes a *volume expansion concept*.

Continuous damage to the liver architecture or a boost to the portal pressure are accompanied by a **salt-retaining signal** (with an antinatriuretic impact) being sent to the renal tubuli. Ascites formation, already triggered by the mechanical or physical factors described, is now significantly reinforced by the sodium-retaining effect with an "overflow" from the intravasal volume. The result is a further reduction in the effective plasma volume, which increasingly stimulates the volume receptors and activates the biochemical, hormonal and neural systems. (s. fig. 16.6)

▶ These two hypotheses, the *"underfill theory"* and the *"overflow theory"*, do not explain the development of ascites in each individual case. Neither do the two concepts exclude one another. They would appear to describe the respective disrupting mechanisms of the water and salt balance as being dependent on the degree of severity of the existing liver disease. • Discussion centres on the early stage of ascites formation being influenced by the overflow hypothesis, which would also explain the better efficacy of diuretics in this phase. • By contrast, the late stages of portal ascites are thought to be characterized by the theory of volume deficiency, which implies that greater therapeutic success would only be achieved by refilling the intravasal volume (once diuretic therapy has failed). (8, 10, 11)

3. Lymph imbalance theory: The lymph imbalance theory (C. L. WITTE et al., 1980) (16) contradicts the "classical" concepts of underfill and overflow. This theory is based on the idea that the disruption of the equilibrium between the extravasation of fluid from the intravasal space and its reflux into the vascular system initiates the formation of ascites; in other words, the lymph production or the actual lymph quantity can no longer be drained via the lymph vessels. (s. tab. 16.4) (s. figs. 7.6; 16.4–16.6)

The **disrupted drainage of the lymph** is attributed to (*1.*) obliterated diaphragmatic lymph vessels, (*2.*) dilated visceral lymph vessels with subsequent clearly decelerated flow velocity, and (*3.*) limited lymph kinetics at the transition between the lymphatic system and the venous system. More and more disturbances in the fluid balance between plasma and interstitium increasingly activate the adrenal hormonal systems with elevated retention of sodium and water; the lymph imbalance continues to grow.

4. Vasodilation theory: The vasodilation theory (R. W. SCHRIER et al., 1988) (14) is a variant of the underfill concept. The initial pathophysiological change in cirrhotic patients is deemed to be peripheral arterial vasodilation, in particular in the splanchnic area, with a lower degree of vascular resistance. This leads to hyperdynamic circulation with an augmented cardiac output. The opening of arteriovenous anastomoses continues to reduce the degree of peripheral vascular resistance. The subsequent

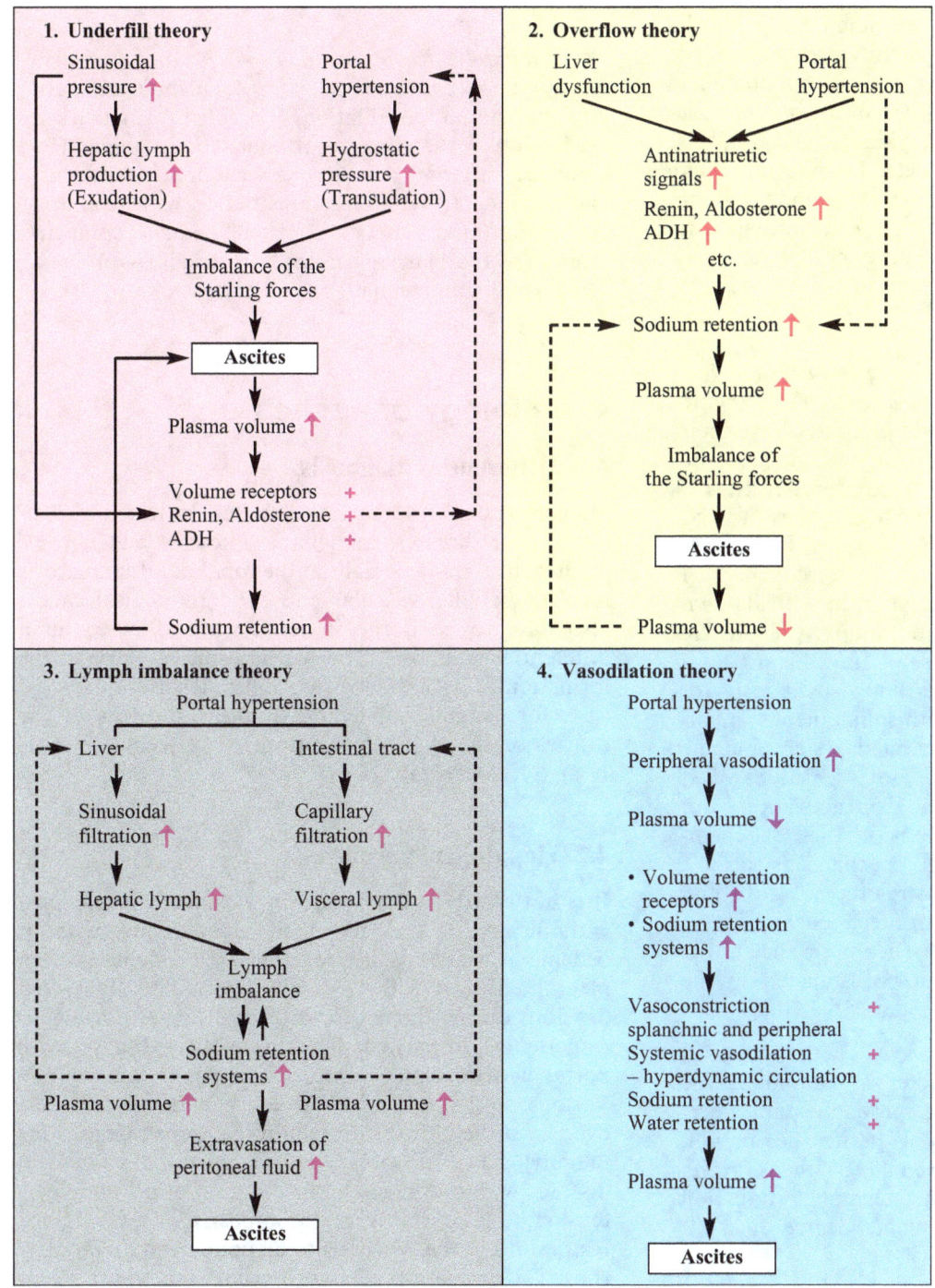

Fig. 16.6: Diagram of the main pathogenic mechanisms in the formation of ascites according to the four different theories

decrease in the effective plasma volume raises the levels of endothelin, renin, aldosterone, noradrenaline and vasopressin with subsequent renal vasoconstriction as well as the retention of sodium and water. The outcome is a further increase or a normalization of the plasma volume.
• This is why, in certain stages of ascites, the serum and urine values of these biochemical factors are (surprisingly) found to be within the normal range. (s. fig. 16.6)

Continuing deterioration of the liver disease results in renewed increase in peripheral vasodilation with a further drop in plasma volume. • Under the influence of *endotoxins* and *cytokines* (tumour necrosis factor, interleukins, etc.), *nitric oxide synthases* are expressed in the liver, blood vessels and other organs, forming large quantities of **nitric oxide** (NO). As highly potent vasodilators, nitric oxides effect a dilatation of the vessels with a reduction in the peripheral resistance. • Other **mediators of vasodilation** are prostaglandins, bradykinin, glucagon, false neurotransmitters, PAF, ANF, etc. Despite maximum activation of the sodium and water retaining systems, vasodilation and volume deficiency can ultimately no longer be offset; ascites begins to develop. (8, 9, 15)

Synopsis

Ascites formation is a complex, pathophysiological process with multifactorial pathogenesis. Severe (acute or chronic) liver diseases, mainly cirrhosis, have their own principal pathogenetic factors which give the respective starting signals at the appropriate time. • In the individual case, one of the four ascites theories hitherto discussed can explain ascites formation, whereas in other cases, the pathogenic sequences of two or three concepts are mixed, each with its own particular intensity and specific timing. • There are some hints that the early phase of ascites is predominantly accompanied by "overfilling" as a result of growing sodium retention (with simultaneous imbalance in the pressure of the vascular system and the lymphatics), while the late phase is chiefly evoked through "underfilling" (due to NO activation with simultaneous vasodilation). Some of these biochemical and sympathoadrenergic mechanisms act as mutual stimulators, inhibitors or additive factors and can even have a potentiation effect, depending on their momentary effectiveness. The importance of the respective mechanisms cannot be estimated in the individual case. (s. fig. 16.6) (s. tabs. 16.3, 16.5)

▶ *Sinusoidal portal hypertension* with increased hydrostatic pressure and decreased colloidosmotic pressure are of considerable, probably paramount importance for the onset of ascites formation. Further influencing factors could be the growing imbalance between augmented lymph production and drainage as well as the higher degree of capillary permeability.

At the same time, the elevated sinusoidal pressure values transmit biochemical signals for a compensatory retention of sodium in the renal tubules. Likewise, "functional hyperaldosteronism" occurs at an early stage and the sympathoadrenergic system is activated with its impact on splanchnic and renal haemodynamics; both events serve to counter volume deficiency and hypotension. The physiological effects of the various biochemical factors may vary under pathological conditions, depending on the respective ascitic phase; for this reason, they can be difficult to assess. Reciprocal interactions also render it more difficult to evaluate the individual factors.

▶ *Ultimately, decompensation of the water and electrolyte balance is the result of* (*1.*) splanchnic and peripheral arterial vasodilation, (*2.*) subsequent marked reduction in the effective arterial blood volume, (*3.*) increase in renin, aldosterone, vasopressin and noradrenaline, (*4.*) renal vasoconstriction with retention of sodium and water, and (*5.*) inadequate compensation of the plasma volume as a result of progressive hypalbuminaemia.

4 Aetiology of ascites

4.1 Differential diagnosis

Numerous diseases can cause ascites. In terms of *aetiology*, liver diseases, malignant processes and chronic cardiac diseases rank right at the top. Yet inflammatory, renal, metabolic, vascular and endocrinological causes also have to be borne in mind when drawing up a differential diagnosis. The mechanisms at work in the formation of ascites are often still unresolved, as is the case, for example, in hypothyroidism, diseases of the ovaries or the POEMS syndrome (P. A. Bardwick et al., 1980). (92, 154) (s. tab. 16.6)

4.2 Hepatogenic ascites

It is not clearly understood why in some cases oedema without ascites and in other cases ascites without oedema as well as ascites together with oedema or even pleural effusion without ascites occur. Ascites often develops during the course of liver disease (= *hepatogenic ascites*), in particular in chronic liver diseases with portal hypertension (= *portal ascites*). (s. tab. 16.7) • Various mechanical, biochemical and neural disorders overlap in their effects and pathways, depending on the underlying liver disease. Only rarely is ascites found in diseases with presinusoidal localization of portal hypertension (e.g. portal vein thrombosis) or with minor restrictions in the synthesis of albumin (as in biliary cirrhosis). • Formation of ascites occurs in about 50% of

1. **Liver diseases** (75–80%) (s. tab. 16.7)
   (= *portal ascites*)
2. **Malignant processes** (10–15%)
   (= *malignant ascites*)
   − abdominal tumours
   − metastases
   − Hodgkin's disease
   − leukaemia
3. **Cardiac diseases** (3–5%)
   (= *cardiac ascites*)
   − congestive cardiac insufficiency
   − constrictive pericarditis
4. **Peritonitis** (2–3%)
   (= *inflammatory ascites*)
   − through bacteria, parasites, fungal infection
   − eosinophilic peritonitis
   − postoperative starch peritonitis
5. **Pancreatic diseases** (1–2%)
   (= *pancreatic ascites*)
6. **Renal diseases** (1–2%)
   (= *renal ascites*)
   − nephrotic syndrome
   − extracorporeal dialysis
7. **Vascular diseases**
   − thrombosis of the mesenteric vein
   − obstruction of the inferior vena cava
   − peritoneal vasculitis
8. **Malnutrition**
9. **Protein-losing gastroenteropathy**
10. **Whipple's disease**
11. **Amyloidosis**
12. **Endocrinopathies**
    − hypothyroidism
    − ovarian hyperstimulation
    − syndrome of inadequate ADH secretion
    − struma ovarii
    − Meigs' syndrome
13. **Familial paroxysmal polyserositis**
14. **Formation of fistulas** (e.g. pancreatic cysts)
15. **POEMS syndrome**

Tab. 16.6: Ascites formation and various possibilities for differential diagnosis

1. Liver cirrhosis
2. Alcoholic hepatitis
3. Acute liver failure,
   severe acute viral hepatitis
4. Obstruction of the hepatic veins
   − massive fatty liver
   − cardiac liver congestion
   − Budd-Chiari syndrome
5. Neoplasia of the liver
6. Cystic liver
7. Liver fibrosis
   − sarcoidosis
   − schistosomiasis
   − syphilis
8. Arteriovenous shunts,
   arterioportal fistula
9. Portal vein thrombosis
10. Obstruction of the superior vena cava with LeVeen shunt
11. Nodular regenerative hyperplasia
12. Condition after liver transplantation

Tab. 16.7: Causes of hepatogenic or portal ascites

We were able to observe pronounced oedema, anasarca and massive ascites with concomitant signs of hepatic encephalopathy in a case of so-called **hepatitis oedematosa** *(E. GAUTIER et al., 1952). The patient was successfully treated by means of aldosterone antagonists.* (43)

5 Diagnosis of ascites

5.1 Clinical findings

Ascites may onset suddenly or slowly and unnoticed over the course of several weeks. There is a diminished tendency to sweat and the patient's skin often appears sallow and dehydrated. • With regard to the quantity of the fluid, ascites may be classified into different levels of intensity: *mild, moderate* or *tense*.

Physical methods: A *latent oedema* can be recognized by the deposition of fluid in the tissue (increase in body weight of > 1.0 kg in 4–5 days). (s. fig. 15.3) It is neither visible nor palpable. A *manifest oedema* typically shows dimpling upon digital compression. • *Ascites* without concomitant deposition of tissue fluid is generally diagnosed by a distinct increase in body weight. Detection of ascites by means of physical examination is only possible when an amount of fluid in excess of 1.5–2.0 litres is present. (30) This is best achieved when *dullness* is ascertained by percussion of the abdomen with the patient in the knee-elbow position. Larger amounts of ascitic fluid produce a typical *change in percussion sound* when the body position is altered; there is also *dullness in the flanks* and ultimately a noticeable *fluctuation wave* (i.e. ascites thrill due to excessive free fluid under tension). Reduced *movability* and/or corresponding *ele-*

all cirrhotic patients within ten years of the diagnosis being established. About half of these patients die within two years of the initial occurrence of ascites. Oedema and/or ascites develop during the course of the disease in about two-thirds of all cirrhotic patients. Statistically, alcoholic cirrhosis is most frequent.

Surprisingly, alcoholic fatty infiltration of the liver and alcoholic hepatitis often display ascites as well, mostly only discernible when applying ultrasonic methods of examination. This might suggest that certain pathogenic mechanisms in the formation of ascites (such as increase in portal pressure, structural sinus changes, and stimulation of biochemical or sympathoadrenergic factors) are favoured or become more intense as a result of alcohol (and possibly also its chemical additives). • Ascites can also occur in severe acute viral hepatitis, in which case the course of disease deteriorates considerably. (28, 43, 61)

vation of the diaphragm can also be detected by percussion. (s. p. 83) • *Meteorism* is deemed to be a precursory state of ascites *("first the wind and then the rain")*.

Puddle sign: In 1959 a very reliable physical sign was described which is present with as little as 120 ml of peritoneal fluid. This phenomenon also makes it possible to differentiate shifting dullness due to fluid-filled loops of bowel from that due to collections of free intra-abdominal fluid. The puddle sign is generally not influenced by obesity. (44)

Inspection: Pronounced cases of ascites are characterized by marked *protrusion* of the abdomen. The *umbilicus* becomes everted or bulging. The distance between the navel and the symphysis appears diminished as a result of caudal displacement of the former. With large quantities of ascitic fluid, the *abdominal skin* is taut and shiny. In long-standing cases of ascites, striae distensae, together with expanded collateral veins radiating from the navel, may be visible. Increased ascitic pressure sometimes causes a *hernia* (inguinal, femoral, umbilical or cicatricial). (s. fig. 16.7) (39, 46, 54)

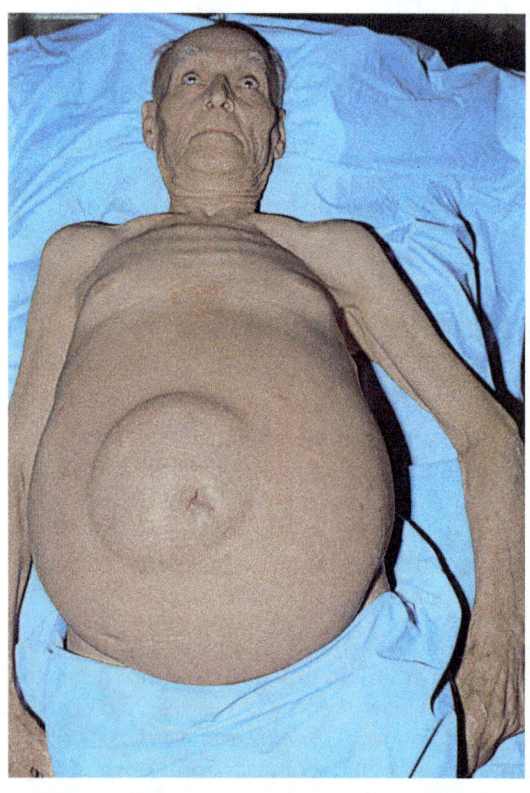

Fig. 16.7: Massive refractory ascites with large umbilical hernia. Muscular atrophy and loss of subcutaneous fatty tissue

Occasionally, *scrotal oedema* and *anasarca* are detectable. Ascites does not correlate with the incidence and extent of peripheral oedema. (s. figs. 16.2, 16.13)

5.2 Imaging procedures

Sonography: Sonography facilitates the early diagnosis of ascites (< 200 ml). If the fluid accumulates at certain preferred sites, it is possible to detect amounts of < 50 ml. In minimal and localized accumulation of fluid, sonographically guided tapping and collection of ascitic fluid as well as special examinations provide a swift and confirmed diagnosis. With massive ascites, floating intestinal loops are occasionally found, forming the so-called *sea anemone phenomenon*. (25) (s. p. 141)

Radiology: Ascites has a diffuse appearance similar to ground glass. In the individual case, various ascites-related clinical findings are observed (elevation of the diaphragm, plate-like atelectasis, cardiac rotation, hiatus hernia, distended intestinal loops, etc.). Extensive ascites may cause organ displacement (e. g. dislocation of the stomach or kidneys) or vascular compression (e. g. functional blocking of the inferior vena cava). (23, 27) The quantity of fluid can be 30 litres or more (as much as 70 litres has been recorded!). (s. figs. 16.7, 16.13)

Hepatic hydrothorax (C.S. Morrow et al., 1958) is evident during the course of liver cirrhosis with ascites in 0.4—12.0% of cases. The mean frequency is about 6%, although in two-thirds of the cases, a right-sided effusion (with the author's own patients, a bilateral effusion) was ascertained. (62) (s. fig. 16.8) • Hepatic hydrothorax is a transudate: cell count < 1,000/mm^3, protein concentration < 2.5 g/dl, total protein effusion to serum ratio < 0.5, LDH effusion to serum ratio < 2.3, serum to pleural fluid albumin gradient > 1.1 g/dl. (s. also fig. 16.9) (17, 36, 45, 50, 51, 62)

▶ Over a period of ten years (1952—1963), I examined in-patient records at the University Medical Hospital in Giessen retrospectively. On evaluation of **25,682 documented cases**, 2,534 patients were found with pleural effusion (= 9.8%) validated by radiology or autopsy. • The **frequency** of hepatogenic pleural effusion was 110 cases (= 4.3%). I found four cases of a right-sided hydrothorax and two cases of bilateral hydrothorax in 6 patients with severe *viral hepatitis*. Hydrothorax was identified in 104 patients with *cirrhosis*. • The **localization** was, however, bilateral in 69%, left-sided in 18.7% and right-sided in 12.3%. • This **controversial finding**, which contrasts with the literature, is explained by the fact that an X-ray of the thorax was taken in each case of cirrhosis and that angle effusions or minimal infrapulmonal effusions were detected by autopsy in deceased patients. *(see footnote* *)*

Causes of hepatic hydrothorax, which can occasionally appear sanguinolently as a result of the cirrhosis-related bleeding tendency, are (*1.*) congenital or acquired defects of the diaphragm (65), (*2.*) diaphragmatic lymph paths, and (*3.*) increased pressure in the azygous vein/hemiazygous vein system. With rising intra-abdominal pressure (caused by large-volume ascites, coughing, pressing, etc.), congenital or acquired gaps may form between the muscle fibres of the diaphragm. These small

---

*) *Kuntz, E.:* Pleural effusions. Differential diagnosis, clinical aspects, and therapy. Urban and Schwarzenberg, München, 1968, 207 pages, 74 figures.

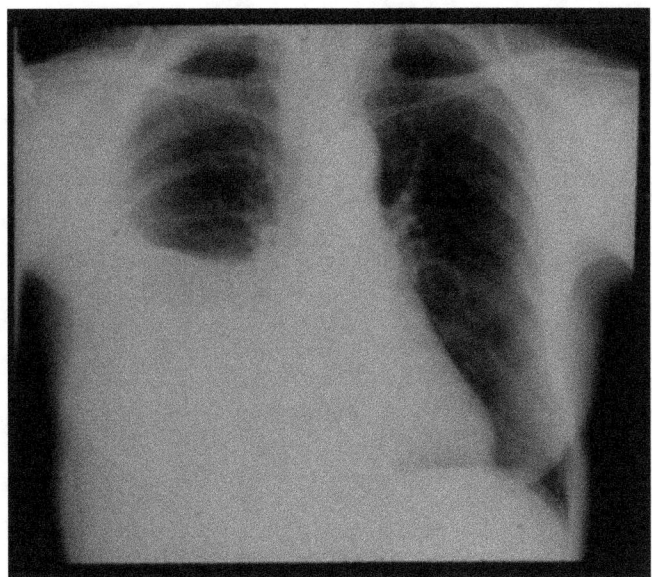

Fig. 16.8: Right-sided hepatic hydrothorax in liver cirrhosis

herniations (so-called pleuroperitoneal blebs) may rupture and allow fluid to move from the abdominal cavity into the pleural space. Occasionally, such diaphragmatic defects can be demonstrated by magnetic resonance imaging (65) or thoracoscopy. • It is clinically significant that considerable pleural effusion can even be present in liver cirrhosis *without concomitant ascites*. In cases of pulmonary complaints (e. g. dyspnoea), this possibility should be considered and investigated. (42, 53) • *Therapy* corresponds to that of ascites (s. pp 310, 312) and involves the administration of albumin. (s. p. 314) Thoracocentesis, if necessary repeated, in addition to i.v. infusion of octreotide and paracentesis (s. p. 315) is recommended. In the case of treatment failure, TIPS and eventually liver transplantation may be indicated.

Spontaneous bacterial empyema is found in 1—2% of patients with cirrhosis and ascites. The diagnosis is based on a positive bacterial test in the pleural fluid and a WBC count in excess of $250/mm^3$ (or a negative bacterial culture with a cell count exceeding $500/mm^3$) — which is analogous to spontaneous bacterial peritonitis. (95) (s. p. 308)

Computer tomography: A CT scan is only indicated in individual cases where there are problems with the differential diagnosis (e. g. in acute pancreatitis or suspected tumours). The sensitivity of fluid detection is, however, extremely high, since it is possible to demonstrate as little as 25 ml. (40)

In patients with cirrhosis, CT sometimes demonstrates a mesenteric oedema (*"misty mesentery"*). (49) Such a mesenteric, omental and/or retroperitoneal oedema can vary from a moderate infiltrative type to a pronounced oedema compressing the mesenteric vessels. (32)

Laparoscopy: Laparoscopy should be carried out in all cases which could not be clarified or precisely defined by means of clinical and biochemical laboratory examinations of the blood and ascitic fluid or using imaging procedures. (s. p. 164) If a large amount of ascitic fluid is removed by laparoscopic paracentesis, it is essential to substitute volume and protein. (s. p. 315)

Oesophagogastroscopy: An ascites-related gastro-oesophageal reflux can result in reflux oesophagitis. However, this does not provoke the onset of bleeding from oesophageal varices.

Disorders of *cerebral functions* on the one hand and of the *water and electrolyte balance* on the other hand are the earliest and most reliable hints of the onset of decompensation in severe liver disease, especially cirrhosis. • In clinical terms, they can be easily diagnosed as latent hepatic encephalopathy (by carrying out psychometric tests) and/or latent oedema (by recording the increase in body weight). • For this reason, these examination methods are also considered to be of fundamental importance in the follow-up of chronic liver disease. (s. fig. 15.3)

5.3 Laboratory diagnosis

A **diagnostic puncture** is required to withdraw ascitic fluid. In extensive ascites, this can be performed without ultrasound guidance, whereas with smaller and localized accumulations of fluid, it is always necessary to carry out ultrasound-guided puncture. The ideal entry site is deemed to be the left lower abdominal quadrant (exactly opposite McBurney's point). Prior to puncturing, the skin should be shifted tangentially over the puncture mark, leaving a Z-shaped puncture channel on removal of the needle. This guarantees more reliable protection against any postpuncture leakage of ascitic fluid. Complications are very rare. (143) The tapping of ascitic fluid is considered a safe procedure. Using a thin needle (0.4 mm in diameter) or a special puncture needle, some 50 ml fluid are withdrawn, which suffices for a wide range of laboratory investigations. However, for bacteriological or cytological examinations (possibly following centrifugation), 200—250 ml are required. Biochemical parameters are always of great importance. (24, 26, 38, 60, 66, 74) (s. fig. 16.10)

1. Colour: The impressive range of colours found in individual cases is indeed interesting, yet of no great help in the differential diagnosis. A rough definition of the various forms can be given as follows, analogous to pleural effusion *(see footnote p. 304)*:

• *serous ascites* (e.g. hepatogenic, pancreatogenic, malignant or inflammatory) can be clear or turbid, green, straw-coloured or bile-stained; (s. fig. 37.25)

• *haemorrhagic ascites* (e.g. in malignant disease). In liver cirrhosis, ascites is only rarely blood-tinged;

- *turbid ascites* (e.g. bacterially or parasitically infected, malignant or pancreatogenic, in the Budd-Chiari syndrome);
- *chylous ascites* (e.g. in cirrhosis due to impaired lymphatic drainage) has various causes: malignant disease, whipple disease, radiation, tuberculosis, intestinal lymphangiectasia. Lymphostasis can be assumed to exist if the total lipids of the ascitic fluid are twice as high as the plasma value and/or the triglyceride concentration is greater than 400 mg/dl. Therapy with orlistat has proved successful. (29, 31) (s. fig. 16.9)

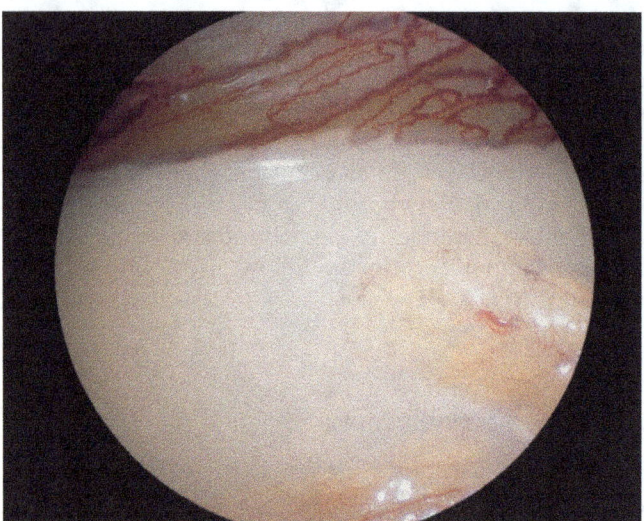

Fig. 16.9: Chylous ascites with pronounced portal hypertension as a result of posthepatitic (HBV) coarse nodular cirrhosis

2. Protein content: Depending on the protein content of the ascitic fluid or its specific gravity, differentiation is made between a transudate and an exudate. • A **transudate** is deemed to be a serous, fibrinogen-free fluid, low in cells and protein, of non-inflammatory genesis. The protein content is <2.5 g/dl (specific gravity <1,015). • An **exudate**, generally inflammatory or malignant, is rich in cells; the protein value exceeds 3.0 g/dl (specific gravity >1,016), and the bilirubin quotient (ascites : serum) amounts to more than 0.6. (35) • The **albumin gradient** (albumin value in the serum minus albumin value in ascites) is usually >1.1 g/dl in portal hypertension and <1.1 g/dl in malignant or inflammatory ascites, with a sensitivity of about 80%. (56) This gradient correlates well with the portal vein pressure. The reliability of differentiation seemed to improve with a discrimination limit of 1.5. (60) (s. fig. 16.10)

In of long-standing ascites, **protein content** can drop due to reduced permeability of the sinusoids to protein or as a result of presinusoidal obstruction. However, because of its aetiology or as a result of diuretic therapy, protein content may increase. In 15–20% of cirrhotic patients with ascites, protein values of up to 4.3 g/dl are found. • *Even with a threshold ranging between 2.5 and 3.0 g/dl, the transudate vs exudate concept does not work as well with ascites as it does with pleural effusion!* • The inconclusive information obtained from the ascites protein value sometimes becomes more reliable if the cell count is also determined. (52, 60, 74)

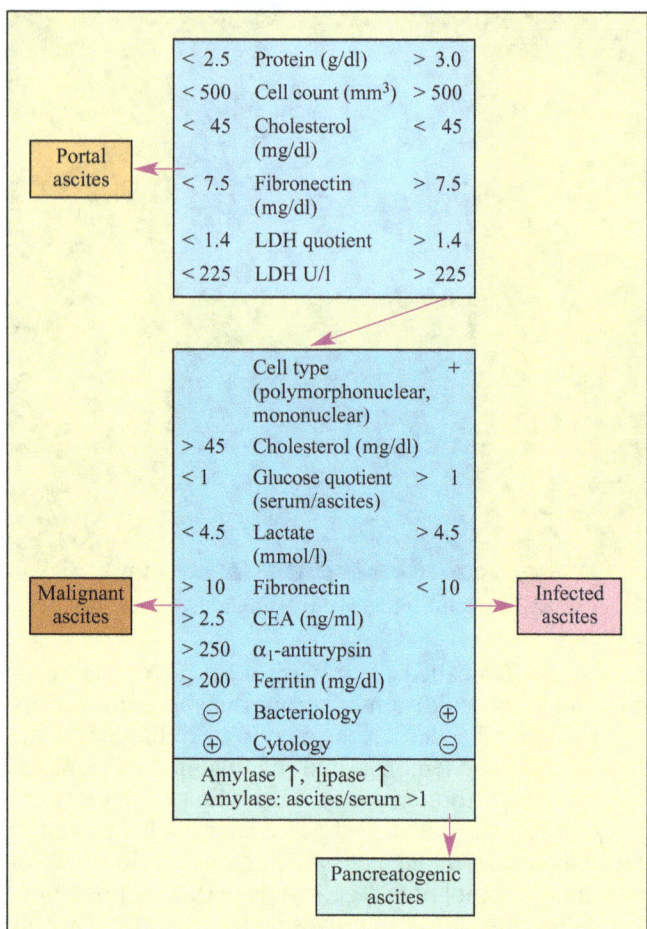

Fig. 16.10: Diagnostic steps used to differentiate between portal, infected, malignant and pancreatogenic ascites (modified from J. Schölmerich, 1990)

3. Cell count: To determine the cell count and cell type, it is advisable to use an EDTA tube (monovette) for the ascitic fluid. The cell count for a transudate is generally below 250/mm^3 and for an exudate above 1,000/mm^3. Specificity is ca. 90%, and sensitivity is ca. 60%. The absolute count is more reliable in connection with a normal or raised protein value (transudate or exudate). However, in up to 30% of cases, there were cell counts in portal ascites of >500 and in 5–20% of cases even >1,000 leukocytes/mm^3. In patients with malignant ascites, the cell count was in excess of 1,000/mm^3 in more than 50% of cases. In individual instances of hepatogenic or malignant ascites, a higher number of polymorphonuclear cells were also detected. These results make identification of spontaneous bacterial peritonitis very difficult. Evidence of **polymorphonuclear neutrophils** (>250/mm^3) suggests the presence of infected ascites. More than 80% of patients with spontaneous bacterial peritonitis show a higher value. The predominance of **lymphocytic cells** in ascites (>20% of the total leukocyte count) — with an additional ascites-blood-glucose quotient of <0.7 — suggests tuberculous peritonitis. (24, 60) In suspected tuberculosis, the Ziehl-Neelsen staining method, and possibly also PCR, is necessary.

4. Bacteriology: Ascites should be checked for aerobes and anaerobes by using haemoculture bottles. With infected ascitic fluid, the bacteriological examination yields a specificity of 100%, but a much lower sensitivity. It is possible to detect gram-negative bacteria in about 70% of cases, gram-positive microorganisms in some 25% of cases and anaerobes in about 5% of cases. In total, a bacterial infection of the ascitic fluid is present in 8—10% of cirrhotic patients. It is often hardly possible to distinguish between spontaneous and secondary bacterial peritonitis. (60, 66)

5. Cytology: Cytology has a specificity of 97—100% for the detection of malignant ascites. By contrast, the sensitivity is far lower, especially since the endothelial cells of the peritoneum are very similar cytologically to the malignant cells.

6. Cholesterol: In malignant ascites, the cholesterol level is clearly raised (R. A. ROVELSTAD et al., 1958). In differentiating the condition from portal ascites, the sensitivity is 90%, and the specificity is 95%. A threshold range of 45—48 mg/dl is deemed appropriate. Cholesterol determination is thus a valuable parameter for ascites. (41, 58) (s. fig. 16.10)

7. Fibronectin: The values of fibronectin in malignant ascites are significantly higher than in cases of portal ascites. Given a threshold value of 7.5 mg/dl, it is possible to differentiate between the two forms of ascites with a sensitivity of 100% and a specificity of more than 95%. The combined determination of cholesterol and fibronectin allows malignant ascites to be identified reliably. (33)

8. pH levels: The pH value in infected ascitic fluid is usually reduced to <7.31 by acid residues (such as lactate, oxalate, succinate and fumarate), which occur mainly in anaerobic glycolysis. With hepatogenic transudate ascites, pH levels are higher than 7.45 and the pH gradient (serum value minus ascites value) amounts to <0.10. In malignant ascites, the values are hardly any different. In isolation, the pH value and pH gradient have little meaning, whereas in connection with the protein value or cell count and cell type, they can be seen as helpful supplementary findings. (21, 55)

9. Lactate: The same assessment is true for the determination of lactate in ascitic fluid. The increase in this acid residue in infected ascitic fluid (>4.5 mmol/l) is proportional to the decrease in the pH value. Malignant ascites generally yields values of <4.5 mmol/l. (55, 60) (s. fig. 16.10)

10. LDH quotient: The LDH quotient (ascites value : serum value) is usually <1.4 in portal ascites, whereas in infected or malignant ascites, values of >1.4 are usual. The absolute discrimination value is given as being higher than 400 U/l.

11. Ferritin: The values in malignant and inflammatory ascites were regularly higher than those found in portal ascites. (60)

12. α_1-antitrypsin: The identification of α_1-antitrypsin yielded a respective specificity and sensitivity of >95% in distinguishing between portal and malignant ascites. In cases with a malignant genesis, the values were nearly always elevated to >120 mg/dl. (64)

13. Other examinations focused on the biochemical differentiation of ascites, such as determining cholinesterase, coagulant activity (22) and interleukin-6 (18) as sensitive parameters for bacterial infection as well as evaluating the receptors (p55 and p75) for the tumour necrosis factor. (19) An ascites/serum quotient for a_1-foetoprotein of >1 suggests hepatocellular carcinoma; an amylase quotient of >1 is found in pancreatitis.

▶ As early as 1964 and in later publications, it was possible to demonstrate the significance of **glycoproteins** (hexosamine, fucose, sialic acid [34], etc.) and *cholinesterase* for the detection of non-inflammatory, inflammatory or malignant disease and their follow-up as well as for the distinction between transudate and exudate in a so-called **phlogogram** (E. KUNTZ, 1964). *(see footnote on page 304)* Because of the significance and pathophysiological features of the mucopolysaccharides, appropriate biochemical parameters are likely to be of further interest. • In addition, elevated values of **hyaluronic acid** have been found in the ascitic fluid of cirrhotic patients.

Due to clinical, laboratory and therapeutic differences, it is possible to distinguish between simple and problematic ascites. The latter includes: (*1.*) recurrent ascites, (*2.*) refractory ascites, (*3.*) diuretic resistant ascites, and (*4.*) diuretic intractable ascites. (s. tab. 16.8)

	Simple ascites	Problematic ascites
Quantity	mild, moderate	tense
Manifest HE	∅	+
Natriuresis **Sodium in serum** **Albumin** **Creatinine** **Potassium in serum**	>20 mmol/day >130 mmol/l >3.5 g/dl <1.5 mg/dl 3.6—4.9 mmol/l	<10 mmol/day <130 mmol/l <3.5 g/dl >1.5 mg/dl <3.5 mmol/l >5.0 mmol/l
Diuretic therapy	mostly sufficient	insufficient

Tab. 16.8: Differentation of ascites according to its severity

The combination of several biochemical parameters in a diagnostic **stepwise approach** generally facilitates an adequately reliable differentiation between portal, infected, malignant and pancreatogenic forms of ascites. (s. fig. 16.10)

6 Complications of ascites

Ascites formation is generally accompanied by multiple complications. These mean considerable distress for the patient and constitute a genuine threat to life. Complications call for extra therapeutic measures, which are often quite complex. For this reason, emphasis should always be placed on any dangerous developments. As a rule, these are mechanical, bacterial, or metabolic in nature. (s. tab. 16.9)

Mechanical complications
1. Increased physical immobility
2. Respiratory impairment
   (= dyspnoea as a result of restrictive ventilation)
   – due to hepatic hydrothorax
   – due to an elevated diaphragm or plate-like atelectases
3. Elevated portal venous pressure
4. Compression of vessels
   – inferior vena cava syndrome
   – renal vein
5. Formation of hernias
6. Ruptured umbilical hernia
7. Dislocation of organs
   – intra-abdominal
   – cardiac rotation, diminished cardiac function
8. Promotion of a gastro-oesophageal reflux

Bacterial complications
1. Spontaneous bacterial peritonitis

Metabolic complications
1. Disturbances of electrolyte metabolism
2. Disturbances of protein metabolism, catabolism
3. Changes in pharmacokinetics
4. Hepatic encephalopathy
5. Hepatorenal syndrome

Tab. 16.9: Complications arising from ascites

Even though the mortality rate of spontaneous bacterial peritonitis can clearly be reduced by antibiotics, it still remains a very real danger for the patient. The hepatorenal syndrome has a very poor prognosis with a mortality rate of about 95%. *(see chapter 17)*

7 Spontaneous bacterial peritonitis

In severe liver diseases, particularly in cirrhosis, but also in acute viral hepatitis, bacterial infections are frequent. (70) In approx. 25% of cases, these infections are the cause of death. If there are additional complications (e.g. gastrointestinal bleeding, protein deficiency, invasive interventions, endotoxinaemia, liver metastases, continuous abuse of alcohol) culminating in a further weakening of the body's defences, the cause of death is attributable to bacterial infection in >50% of cases.

7.1 Definition

Spontaneous bacterial peritonitis (SBP) (H.O. CONN, 1964, 1971) is the term used to describe bacterially infected ascitic fluid in liver cirrhosis where the exact source or path of infection is not known. It displays a high number of polymorphonuclear neutrophils (>250/mm^3), a protein content which is usually <1.0 g/dl and a positive bacterial culture (>90%).

7.2 Forms and frequency

In terms of the number of neutrophils and the microorganisms identified, SBP can occur in ascites in **three forms** (71, 81, 82, 85, 86):

1. **Classical (complete) SBP:** >250/mm^3 polymorphonuclear neutrophils together with positive ascites culture; this constellation is the most frequent form.

2. **Culture-negative neutrocytic ascites:** <250/mm^3 neutrophils together with negative ascites culture; it appears in 4–5% of patients suffering from cirrhosis with ascites and in up to 35% of cases with suspected SBP. This form does not differ from classical SBP as regards symptomatology, clinical and laboratory findings or efficacy of the antibiotic therapy required.

3. **Culture-positive neutrophil-low ascites:** <250/mm^3 neutrophils and mostly monoculture-positive ascites; gram-positive infectious agents predominate. As a rule, this form shows an asymptomatic course and a more favourable prognosis. It is interpreted as a bland bacterial infection with good defence potential (i.e. transient colonization). Antibiotic therapy is not required, but ascites follow-up examinations are indispensable in order to initiate any necessary antibiotic treatment in good time.

Each of these three forms of SBP has to be delimited from **secondary bacterial peritonitis.** In bacterial ascites, several types of microorganisms, including fungi, can usually be identified after subculturing. The cell count exceeds 10,000/mm^3, the LDH value is elevated (>225 U/l), and the glucose concentration is <50 mg/dl.

The **frequency** of SBP is 10–25%. (69–71, 81, 96) With coexistent HE, it was found to be 36%, whereas in the absence of HE, SBP was detectable in only 10% of cases. Culture-negative ascitic fluid can be identified with SBP in up to 50% of cases and bacterascites in up to 30% of cases. (70, 87) **Relapses** occur at a rate of 43–69% per year. An ascitic protein concentration of <0.75 g/dl is considered a significant predictive factor for a relapse.

7.3 Pathogenesis and predisposing factors

▶ **Acquired immune defect syndrome in cirrhosis:** Even if pathogenesis has still not been fully resolved, it is generally attributed to various regulatory defects in the immune system (*1.*) reduction in the opsonic and bactericidal activity of the ascitic fluid, (*2.*) impaired function of the RES phagocytosis system, and (*3.*) leukocytic functional deficiency. A decrease in C_3 concentration in the ascitic fluid (<20 mg/dl) reduced the bacterial content and, according to the literature, led to the occurrence of SBP in 47% of cases within a short space of time.

▶ **Bacterial infection:** This multifactorial weakness in defence allows bacterial penetration of the ascitic fluid to be effected by (*1.*) transmural migration in portal hypertension with greater permeability of the intestinal wall, (*2.*) systemic bacteraemia in terms of haematogenic dispersion (particularly in urinary tract and bronchopulmonary infections), above all in the presence of intrahepatic and extrahepatic shunts *(portal vein bacteraemia)*, (*3.*) invasion of bacteria via the Fallopian tubes, and (*4.*) lymphatic flow into the ascitic fluid (e.g. via leaks in the lymph vessels or lymph nodes).

Predisposing factors often interact to produce a greater effect in the individual case (68, 70, 80, 81, 88):

> (*1.*) reduction in the bactericidal and **opsonic activity** (C3 < 20 mg/dl) and in the **ascitic protein value** (< 1.0 g/dl) as well as a dysfunction of the polymorphonuclear neutrophils;
>
> (*2.*) **dysfunction of the liver** (e.g. bilirubin > 3.5 mg/dl, thrombocytes <98,000/mm³) as a result of an accompanying decrease in antibodies or RES functions;
>
> (*3.*) **poor nutritional status**;
>
> (*4.*) upper gastrointestinal **bleeding** and application of balloon tamponade or variscoslerosation;
>
> (*5.*) **invasive measures** such as endoscopic or angiographic techniques or peritoneovenous shunting (some 20% of cases) with a mortality rate of about 25%;
>
> (*6.*) **infusion of vasopressin**, which leads to a deterioration in the circulation of the intestinal mucosa and hence to easier penetration by microorganisms;
>
> (*7.*) **bacterial foci** with systemic bacteraemia through arteriovenous anastomoses.

7.4 Clinical aspects

1. Pathogen detection: The decisive diagnostic criterion of SBP is the detection of the pathogen. This cannot be adequately achieved using conventional techniques. **Bedside inoculation** of 10 ml ascitic fluid per haemoculture bottle is recommended with a cultivation period of five to seven days at 37 °C, with subcultivation on days 1, 2 and 7. The yield of positive cultures is thus doubled. • Demonstration of *one* type of pathogen is considered typical for SBP (>90%), whereas determination of *several* types of pathogens or anaerobes generally suggests secondary peritonitis. • In 60–80% of cases, gram-negative aerobes are found, half of which (40–50%) are E. coli. A small fraction is comprised of Klebsiella, Citrobacter, Proteus, Enterobacter and Streptococcus (94) etc. Gram-positive microorganisms were detected in 25–30% and anaerobes in 4–6% of cases. Isolated reports have been published on the identification of Clostridia (72), Salmonella (75), Chlamydia trachomatis (78, 89) and Listeria monocytogenes (79, 84).

2. Cell count: The second important criterion of SBP is deemed to be a higher cell count (>250 polymorphonuclear neutrophils/mm³). As a result, early diagnosis is possible with a sensitivity of 92% and a specificity of 95%. A higher leukocyte count in ascitic fluid does not correlate with peripheral leukocytosis (or vice versa). Mechanical assessment of the cell count, however, also identifies lymphocytes, serosal surface cells and peritoneal macrophages. For this reason, it is imperative to distinguish the polymorphonuclear neutrophils (and possibly the number of mononuclear forms) in the ascitic fluid smear. (66, 70, 74, 96)

3. Chemical parameters: The additional determination of chemical parameters (*decreased:* fibronectin, pH value, glucose, cholinesterase, etc.; *increased:* lactate, LDH, etc.) can improve the certainty of the SBP diagnosis in individual cases and also provide a clearer picture of its severity. (74, 76, 83, 93, 96)

4. Clinical findings: In 10–50% of cases, SBP follows an *asymptomatic* course. Each sudden or inexplicable deterioration in the course of disease, manifestation or aggravation of HE, non-response to appropriate diuretic therapy, continued increase in ascites or signs of the onset of renal insufficiency all point clearly to SBP. • *Clinical symptomatology* can also develop slowly in cases of long-standing ascites. By contrast, SBP may pursue a more rapid course, with pronounced findings in the presence of existing as well as simultaneously developing ascites. (69, 70, 74, 78, 80, 86) (s. tab. 16.10)

• Fever	• Decreased bowel sounds
• Abdominal pain	• Nausea
• Abdominal guarding	• Tendency to diarrhoea
• Onset of HE	• Reduced diuresis
• Meteorism	• Arterial hypotension

Tab. 16.10: Symptoms of spontaneous bacterial peritonitis

7.5 Prophylaxis and therapy

In decompensated cirrhosis or gastrointestinal bleeding, the use of antibiotics is recommended for the prevention of SBP as well as to avert a relapse. This is especially true if predisposing factors for SBP are present. In cirrhosis with ascites, SBP occurs in about 80% of hospitalized patients within the first week. For this reason, SBP is deemed to be a *nosocomial infection* (H. O. CONN, 1987) although other investigators regard the patient's domestic surroundings as the most common site of infection. Such complications of ascites, which still have a poor prognosis despite cost-intensive therapy, should be prevented by suitable prophylactic measures.

Prevention is achieved through simply reducing the ascitic volume by means of efficient diuretic therapy, so that the total protein and complement factors in ascites rise significantly. *Paracentesis* can also be helpful if the protein deficiency is compensated at the same time. • Long-term application of *lactulose*, possibly in short-term combination with *neomycin* or *paromomycin*, is recommended. This is especially true when there are signs of an onset of hepatic encephalopathy.

Recommended *antibiotic prophylaxis* includes *neomycin* (1 g), *colistin* (1.5 million units) or *nystatin* (1 million units) four times a day. Antibiotics which have been tried and tested are *norfloxacin* (400 mg/day), *cefotaxime* and *ceftriaxone*. They result in selective intestinal decontamination as well as bactericidal action in the serum, ascitic fluid and urine. Because of the possible impact of norfloxacin on the central nervous system, special caution should be exercised during the initial stages of HE. Primary prevention with norfloxacin in high-risk patients yielded a reduction in SBP frequency from 17% to 2% and from 32% to 0%, respectively. (67, 77, 80, 82, 86, 90)

Whenever >250/mm^3 polymorphonuclear neutrophils are detected, immediate **antibiotic treatment** is called for using (*1.*) amoxicillin-clavulanic acid, (*2.*) cefotaxime (and other third generation cephalosporins), (*3.*) gyrase inhibitors such as norfloxacin, and (*4.*) aztreonam. The latter, however, does not act against gram-positive microorganisms, so that there is a danger of gram-positive proliferation. *Therapy* lasting four to five days (longer application is of no further advantage) with cefotaxime (perhaps combined with metronidazole in the possible presence of anaerobes) or amoxicillin-clavulanic acid can provide a success rate of >80%. Consequently, an *exploratory puncture* and follow-up examination of the ascitic fluid after a 48-hour antibiotic therapy is imperative. • In accordance with the **antibiogram**, it may prove necessary to change the initial antibiotics. Success is, however, usually achieved within a few days, using the substances of first choice (cefotaxime, cefoxitine, amoxicillin-clavulanic acid). Therapy results can be markedly improved through simultaneous administration of albumin (1.5 g/kg BW). (91) In order to avert a relapse, norfloxacin is recommended; this reduces the relapse rate from 68% to 20%. (71) The previously high mortality rate (some 90%) could be lowered to 40–78%, and in a recent study even to 37%. (67, 69, 73, 86, 88, 96)

Selenite: With the additional administration of selenite (e. g. 500 µg as short-term infusion), it is apparently possible to improve the survival rate even further.

8 Conservative therapy of ascites

> *"When the liver is full of water that flows off into the abdomen and the body is distended, then death is near."* (HIPPOCRATES)

Oedema and ascites call for extensive therapeutic measures. The daily life of the liver patient is additionally impaired by this condition, which may even be life-threatening. Awareness of the pathogenic factors makes it possible to apply prophylactic measures to prevent a disruption of water-electrolyte homoeostasis and to ensure appropriate therapy. (37, 47, 48, 57, 58)

In pathophysiological and prognostic terms, even ascites that can "only" be identified by ultrasonic methods is a **sign of decompensation** − either decompensation which is still latent, yet unstable, or decompensation which is slowly increasing by itself! • This latter condition ultimately calls for more severe measures (also involving more side effects) than merely moderate and cautious efforts to restore the patient to a stable state of recompensation, which should be as lasting as possible.

8.1 Prophylaxis

The principal prophylactic measures for ascites consist of a detailed consultation with the physician (preferably together with a family member) and strict *guidance* of the patient with efficient *follow-up* checks in the practitioner's surgery. (s. fig. 15.2) A major prerequisite for successful prophylactic measures is an appropriate *lifestyle* on the part of the patient regarding the disease.

▶ As far as **costs** are concerned, a one-year course of prophylactic treatment including the necessary follow-up checks and possible *early treatment of commencing water retention* is less expensive than three or four days' hospitalization. • This solely economic viewpoint is likewise true for *prophylactic measures used in hepatic encephalopathy* as well as for its early diagnosis and successful therapy at the practitioner's surgery.

The **restriction of sodium** to 7–8 g daily (or even less) is an important step. Each excessive gram of sodium which is taken up and cannot be excreted leads to a water retention of 200–300 ml. (s. tab. 16.11)

All routine activities which can be carried out in a **supine position** should indeed be performed in this way (see below). As a result, renal perfusion is improved, the sympathicotonus lessened and the tubular absorption of sodium decreased. The breakdown of aldosterone is increased by >30%, and its half-life returns more or less to normal. The central blood volume is enhanced. Removal of ascitic fluid via the subdiaphragmatic and mediastinal lymph vessels is facilitated.

Intestinal detoxification by means of lactulose, which, among other things, delays the production and/or portal uptake of endotoxins, is another important therapy step.

Should these measures prove inadequate, either because of insufficient compliance on the part of the patient or because of the advanced stage of the disease, **spironolactone** (50 mg every second day) is recommended. This dose is considered effective and sufficient (due to its longer half-life). As a rule, there are no side effects.

The patient is instructed to record his morning *body weight* (always under the same conditions) every day on a **documentation sheet** (E. KUNTZ, 1989) as well as the *frequency of stools* (e. g. under lactulose therapy) and to enter a *handwriting specimen* (usual way of writing the first and last name) every one or two days. (s. fig. 15.3)
• This documentation sheet is deemed to be a useful and efficient instrument (which can be kept as a medical record) in the control and follow-up of a chronic course of disease. An ancillary benefit is that the extent to which the patient is cooperating can also be deduced from the accuracy of the entries made. (s. p. 283)

Patients should immediately consult the doctor if their body weight rises steadily by > 1 kg in three to four days. This is *suggestive of a clinically not yet identifiable accumulation of water in the tissue* (= **latent oedema**). • Patients should also consult the doctor in the case of minor irregularities in their handwriting. Psychometric tests can be used to confirm or discount suspected cases of **latent HE**. (s. pp 211, 280) (s. fig. 15.3)

> **Self-monitoring** on the part of the patient makes it possible to identify the beginning of water accumulation in the organism (> 1 litre), a reduced lactulose effect (which is inadequate for intestinal detoxification) and/or a latent phase of hepatic encephalopathy. • In such cases, immediate **outpatient treatment** is generally reliable and swift in its therapeutic success.

> *Diuretics are not indicated as a prophylactic measure!* (because of the possible activation of RAAS)

8.2 Basic therapy (stage I)

▶ The development of **latent oedema** can be recognized by means of daily weight checks when an increase in weight of > 1 kg occurs within four days.

▶ **Latent ascites** (< 250 ml) can be determined by sonography. Detection of fluid in the abdominal cavity signals decompensation of cirrhosis and the corresponding inefficacy of prophylactic measures. Medication is recommended as part of a stepwise therapy. To start with, the prophylactic measures for ascites should be applied more intensively and consistently. Both ascites itself and its treatment harbour risks for the patient.

The earlier ascites is identified, the more successful the therapy will be, because less "aggressive" methods with minimal or no risks can be used; and, of course, the costs will also be lower. (s. tab. 16.11)

Absolute **supineness** (probably even with the head and upper body slightly lowered) promotes the excretion of water and sodium. This physical treatment significantly improves both the natriuretic and diuretic effect of a loop diuretic agent. (99, 112, 125) (s. tab. 16.11)

The aim is to break through the positive sodium balance by **restricting sodium** to ≤ 5 g/day (= 88 mmol). Natriuresis should amount to > 80 mmol/day. Given an extrarenal loss of sodium of approx. 10 mmol/day, determination of the sodium content in 24-hour urine provides a clue to the degree of compliance with the intended sodium restriction level of ≤ 5 g/day – i. e. with an excretion of < 78 mmol/day, the desired negative sodium and fluid balance is achieved. The efficacy of a low-sodium diet in the treatment of ascites is evident. *Dietary sodium restriction* is maintained by applying the following *rules:* (*1.*) preparation of food without salt, (*2.*) no extra salt to be added at the table, (*3.*) no use of baking powder, tinned food, highly salted food, mineral water or chocolate, (*4.*) no more than 0.25 l milk/day, and (*5.*) no use of medication or i. v. solutions containing sodium. • *Liquorice is prohibited!* • Certain herbal mixtures help patients to accept sodium restriction in the diet. Even food that does not taste salty may contain significant amounts of sodium (e. g. sodium nitrate, sodium phosphate). A marked restriction of sodium is accompanied by a parallel reduction in the general protein consumption; this must be averted by an adequate intake of lactovegetable proteins. • Patients should always be given **dietary advice!** (s. tab. 16.11)

Basic therapy (stage I)	
1. Sodium restriction (intake < 5 g/day)	
2. Water restriction (intake < 1,500 ml/day)	
3. Supine position	
4. Intestinal detoxification (with lactulose)	
5. Spironolactone (50–100 mg/day)	
6. Balancing of electrolytes	
7. Substitution in zinc deficiency	
8. Balancing of proteins	
Success rate	20–30%

Tab. 16.11: Basic therapy of ascites (stage I)

Normally, the daily **fluid intake** is 1,700–2,200 ml; this includes water in a bound form (e. g. fruit, yoghurt, tomatoes). If this amount is clearly reduced or exceeded, the cirrhotic patient may suffer considerable pathophysiological disturbances. From the clinical point of view, however, it is recommended to limit the fluid intake to 1,400–1,600 ml/day during this phase of therapy (in cases of hyponatraemia even to 800 ml). An increase in the dosage of **spironolactone** to 50–100 mg/day has proved effective. With this measure, a loss in weight of >1.2 kg in four days can be achieved in 15–20% of cases (= excretion of retained fluid). (s. tab. 16.11)

Follow-up checks regarding sodium, potassium, magnesium, the acid-base equilibrium and possibly zinc are required; if necessary, the status has to be duly balanced. • **Hyponatraemia** must not be "treated" by the intake of sodium, but by a further *restriction of fluid* (while monitoring sodium levels). (s. p. 314)

8.3 Diuretic therapy (stage II)

Ascites is a defined compartment of the extracellular fluid volume, which is difficult to mobilize. If the reduction in weight is inadequate after appropriate basic therapy (<1.2 kg after 4 days), stage II should be initiated with the cautious administration of diuretics. The steps already detailed for stage I are to be continued, whereby the intake of dietary sodium is restricted even further (≤3 g/day). (s. tab. 16.12)

The peritoneum has a surface area of about 2 m^2. It has the effect of a semipermeable membrane and can transport a total of 720–840 ml/day between the plasma and the peritoneal cavity. Spontaneous diuresis allows *300 ml/day* to be excreted, whereas with the use of diuretics some *500 ml/day* are possible. The presence of peripheral oedema, however, permits a loss of fluid of about *900 ml/day* (L. SHEAR et al., 1970).

The **therapeutic target** is a weight reduction of about 1.5 kg in 3 days (maximum 500 ml/day) without oedema and of 3.0 kg in 3 days (maximum 0.7–1.0 l/day) with concomitant peripheral oedema. (118)

▶ If diuretic therapy is to be low in complications, the following **prerequisites** are important: (*1.*) no electrolyte imbalance, (*2.*) no abnormality of the acid-base equilibrium, (*3.*) normal renal function, and (*4.*) no simultaneous application of non-steroidal antiphlogistics (since these inhibit the synthesis of prostaglandin and hence may cause renal dysfunction). • In line with the half-life of the diuretics, a *twice-daily administration* (morning, early evening) is more successful. The early evening diuretic dose is lower (e.g. xipamide 20 mg and *10 mg*). This serves to prevent renewed retention of fluid during the night which occurs as a result of the continuously decreasing diuretic effect of just one morning dose. It may also be necessary to administer a third low diuretic dose at midday (e.g. xipamide or torasemide 20/*10*/10 mg).

8.3.1 Pharmacology of diuretics

Of the many diuretic agents with their differing points of impact on the nephron and their respective action profiles, some preparations, even in combined application, have proved extremely successful in the treatment of portal ascites. It must be borne in mind here that liver diseases can change the pharmacokinetics of diuretics. (59, 102, 105) (s. tab. 16.12)

Never provoke abrupt diuresis. • *Never stop the use of diuretics suddenly!*

Diuretic therapy (stage II)	
1. Aldosterone antagonist	
• potassium canrenoate	(100–800 mg i.v./day)
• spironolactone	(50–400 mg/day)
2. Saluretics	
• etacrynic acid	(50–400 mg/day)
• etozolin	(200–800 mg/day)
• furosemide	(20–500 mg/day)
• torasemide	(10–40 mg/day)
• xipamide	(10–40 mg/day)
3. Sequential nephron blockade	
torasemide or xipamide combined with	(20–40 mg/day)
• butizide, *or*	(5 mg/day)
• hydrochlorothiazide, *or*	(25 mg/day)
• metolazone	(2.5–5 mg/day)
Success rate	ca. 80%

Tab. 16.12: Diuretic therapy of ascites (stage II)

1. Spironolactone (J. A. CELLA et al., 1957) is the preparation of choice. Its clinical efficacy has been substantiated in numerous studies. • The onset of effect is after 8 to 24 hours. The natriuretic/diuretic action is maintained for one or two days. A faster onset of effect is given by *potassium canrenoate*, available as an i.v. application, particularly when absorption is assumed to be impaired or if oral administration is not possible. • *Spironolactone is not primarily considered to be a diuretic agent, but more a substance with neurohumoral action.* (97, 101, 103, 106, 107, 117, 121, 123, 126; quot. 4, 5)

▶ As a specific **aldosterone antagonist,** spironolactone acts at the basolateral side of the upper-distal tubule as well as in the collecting tubule and prevents aldosterone from contacting its receptor. As a result, aldosterone-related stimulation of the sodium-potassium ATPase is inhibited at the cell membrane. For this reason, aldosterone is unable to reach the cell nucleus with its receptor complex. Synthesis of the aldosterone-induced protein, which opens the sodium canals, is prevented. The absorption of sodium is decreased and natriuresis reinforced, whereas the excretion of potassium remains normal or is diminished. In the presence of hyperaldosteronism, spironolactone is likely to be fully effective. Although aldosterone only controls some 2 (–4)% of the glomerular filtrated sodium at the tubule, a natriuretic/diuretic effect is gradually achieved. The positive effect of spironolactone on portal ascitic fluid can be attributed to an inhibition of the aldosterone-mediated absorption of sodium in the intestine, a reduction in the portal vein pressure and an increase in the synthesis of prostacyclin in the kidney. Spironolactone has no glucocorticoid impact and no influence on the metabolism of carbohydrates. • *Due to an escape effect, it does not usually cause hyperuricaemia, hyponatraemia or hyperkalaemia.* Protein binding is 98% with a bioavailability of 60–90% and a half-life of 20 hours. In cirrhosis, the pharmacokinetics of spironolactone remains unchanged. • The transtubular potassium gradient is a guide for the diuretic management of patients with cirrhosis and ascites. (47)

Action profile of spironolactone	
Natriuria ↑	Zincuria ↓
Kaliuresis none-(↓)	Hydrogen ions (in urine) ↓
Magnesiuresis none-(↓)	Chloride (in urine) ↑
Ammonia ↓	Bicarbonate (in urine) ↑
	pH value (in urine) ↑

▶ As a result of a tubular hypersensitivity to aldosterone, cirrhotic patients usually display *functional aldosteronism* in the early stages of increased sodium retention. This would explain the diuretic and natriuretic efficacy of spironolactone even in cirrhotic patients with normal aldosterone levels.

In no way do normal potassium values rule out hyperaldosteronism!

The *dosage* of spironolactone is 100 to 400 mg/day in two to three single doses. That of potassium canrenoate amounts to 100 to 800 mg/day. When therapy begins with potassium canrenoate, spironolactone should be administered orally one to two days prior to termination of the i.v. application to ensure a smooth transition, since the onset of its effect is delayed. In 25−30% of male patients, long-term application leads to (generally reversible) potency disorders and gynaecomastia.

2. Xipamide is classed as a low-ceiling diuretic with its effective dynamics and intensity ranking between furosemide and the thiazides. For this reason, there are no extreme peaks of diuresis during prolonged therapy. Calciuria is typical for loop diuretics. With portal ascites, xipamide has proved to be almost diuretically equivalent to spironolactone.

The **efficacy** of xipamide is reflected at various sites of the tubule and Henle's loop. It reaches its point of impact at the early-distal tubule − from the peritubular side. With a threshold dose of 5 mg, a dose dependency ranging between 14 and 60 mg is thus produced for the excretion of water and urine; when in excess of 80 mg, there are no further effects. The bioavailability is 73% and protein binding 98%.

A *dosage* of 20 to 40 mg xipamide per day is recommended in 1−2 (−3) single doses. For long-term therapy, it is advisable to prescribe 10 mg. Diuresis sets in after about one hour with a peak after two to eight hours. There is no rebound effect. The excretion of sodium and chloride is increased to an almost identical degree; calciuria, magnesiuresis and kaliuresis occur. For this reason, xipamide should be combined with spironolactone. Biotransformation of xipamide is clearly limited in cirrhotic patients, the half-life (7 hours) is not influenced. Xipamide passes into the ascitic fluid and reaches concentrations of 10−20% of the respective plasma level. It can even be used with restricted renal function, since it has no influence on renal haemodynamics.

3. Torasemide has proved successful in the treatment of portal ascites. The onset of effect takes between 15 and 30 minutes, and it reaches its peak after 6 to 9 hours. Torasemide has a high natriuretic and diuretic effectiveness, even with restricted renal function. Up to now, a *dosage* of 20 mg per day has been used (possibly in two single doses of 10 mg). A combination with spironolactone is very efficient. Torasemide is also available as an intravenous application. (98, 100, 113)

In terms of **efficacy,** torasemide is a high-ceiling, long-acting diuretic, which shows a linear and rapid rise in the dose-effect curve in a higher dose range. Bioavailability is 80−90%, with a protein binding of 98%. The half-life is three to four hours. The site of action is deemed to be the ascending branch of the loop of Henle. There are marked increases in the amounts of potassium, magnesium and sodium in the urine, but excretion of bicarbonate and phosphate remains constant. In cirrhosis, the half-life is lengthened to four to five hours and biotransformation is impaired. (100) Torasemide has a favourable sodium-potassium excretion quotient. It does not accumulate in renal or liver insufficiency.

4. Etacrynic acid, especially in *combination* with spironolactone and xipamide, markedly enhances natriuresis and diuresis. The *dosage* is increased as required (e. g. 1 × 25 mg or 50 mg to 2 × 50 mg per day). With a low-dose application in the form of a combined diuretic therapy, there is usually no risk of hepatic encephalopathy developing. The effect of etacrynic acid sets in at the ascending branch of the loop of Henle (active chloride transport). Renovascular resistance is lowered due to enzymatic activity, presumably as a result of a rise in the release of prostaglandin.

5. Furosemide is a high-ceiling diuretic. The onset of effect is rapid with a strong (unwanted) rebound. With a half-life of 1.5 hours, the length of impact is short (3−6 hours). The bioavailability is 65%, protein binding 70−80%. In cirrhosis, the half-life is lengthened and natriuresis is diminished. Reinforcement of potassium in the urine, alkalosis and hepatic encephalopathy are observed. Furosemide can promote enhanced formation of thromboxane in the kidneys with subsequent renal vasoconstriction. This could be the cause of renal failure in cirrhotic patients following high doses of furosemide. It only acts with intact PGE_2 synthesis, which is, however, often impaired in cirrhosis. (100, 102, 106, 117, 123, 126)

Follow-up checks: It is important to be aware of the pharmacological characteristics of diuretics and to carry out check-ups during diuretic therapy at short intervals, so that countermeasures can be initiated early enough in the event of therapeutic derailment. Intervals between check-ups as well as the diuretic dosage depend on the success of the treatment and the course of disease:

- Body weight and specimen of handwriting (daily) (s. pp 211, 311, 319) (s. figs. 10.1; 15.3)
- Urine volume (at the outset: each day)
- Electrolytes (at the outset: possibly each day)
- Serum creatinine (at the outset: possibly every 2−3 days)
- Acid-base status (at the outset: possibly every 3−4 days)

Success rate: With correctly applied diuretic therapy, the rate of success is about 80% (even in prolonged or recurring ascites).

Failure rate: If the diuretic therapy proves unsuccessful, investigation must initially focus on whether the therapeutic steps taken have been correctly implemented or whether exsiccosis with a contraction of the plasma volume has occurred as a result of excessively forced diuresis. Hypovolaemia leads to stimulation of the biochemical and sympathoadrenal regulatory systems with an occasionally deleterious effect on the course of disease.

8.3.2 Side effects

Diuretic treatment of ascites can, however, involve considerable hazards for the patient. Generally, one has to reckon with the following side effects: **encephalopathy** in 22—26% (as a result of 5—10% inhibition of carbonic anhydrase in the mitochondria of the liver cells), **hyponatraemia** in 40—50%, **azotaemia** in 20—40%, and **hypokalaemia** in up to 85% of cases. A rare event are **diuretic-associated oedemas**. (115)

Therefore, dose diuretics "as softly as possible"!

These complications occur singly or in a combined form in 30—50% of all diuretically treated patients. The more aggressive the diuretic treatment is, the more frequently these types of complications can be expected. • *Hypokalaemia*, which does not respond to potassium substitution, is possibly accompanied by (unidentified, diuretically induced) *hypomagnesaemia*, particularly in elderly patients. (122) For this reason, it may be necessary to substitute magnesium. • Thought should be given to the possibility of a *pseudo-Bartter syndrome* as a result of diuretic abuse and especially of excessive liquorice intake. • The very first signs of diuresis-related hazards call for immediate countermeasures — or even discontinuation of the diuretic therapy. *Nonsteroidal antiphlogistics are contraindicated for cirrhotic patients with ascites.*

8.3.3 Hyponatraemia

Elimination of hyponatraemia (< 125 mmol/l) is difficult. In this case, the status of body sodium is increased, and hence the body fluid as well, whereas the sodium level in the serum is lowered (= *dilutional hyponatraemia*). Treatment is effected by strictly limiting the intake of fluid (< 700—900 ml/day) and restricting salt. Albumin infusion has proved to be an effective therapy. (114, 124) • Should these measures fail to raise sodium levels in the serum and increase diuresis, i. v. administration of a hypertonic sodium chloride solution (3%) can be attempted (increasing serum sodium by no more than 1.0—1.5 mmol/l per hour and, if possible, never in excess of 130 mmol/l). This, however, automatically harbours the danger of tense ascites. For this reason, an i.v. application of furosemide should be given at the same time to promote the clearance of free water. The sodium lost in the urine (measurable in six hourly intervals after administration of a saluretic) is replaced quantitatively by the supply of NaCl. This trick produces pronounced diuresis without a "genuine" input of sodium (R. W. Schrier et al., 1973). • With intact renal function, an attempt can be made at treatment with a 5% sorbitol solution or a 10% mannitol solution. (116) Haemofiltration or i.v. application of sodium-free albumin (111) is likewise recommended. (114) • The augmented release of ADH is depressed (and sodium concentration is increased) by tolvaptan, a vasopressin-2-receptor antagonist. (127)

8.3.4 Resistance to diuretics

Resistance to diuretics occurs if the reduction in body weight ceases despite confirmed diuretic intake or if a rise in creatinine and urea restricts further diuretic application. The phenomenon of *haemodynamic resistance to diuretics* may prove problematic, i.e. the actual volume of circulating blood is reduced. (119) There is a **triad** status: (*1.*) rise in retention values, (*2.*) lower urine volume, and (*3.*) low excretion of sodium in the urine. At the same time, arterial hypotension due to pronounced peripheral vasodilation is present together with the opening of arteriovenous anastomoses. Palmar erythema or spider naevi are often seen to "blossom". (s. p. 84) The greater the peripheral vasodilation, the more pronounced is the renal vasoconstriction. As a result, it is hardly (if at all) possible for the diuretics to reach their site of action in the nephron. • Another cause of diuretic resistance is the fact that the substrate concentration required for the loop diuretics to have an effect is absent in the ascending part of Henle's loop because of the increased proximal tubular absorption of sodium — the diuretic is therefore ineffective. This renal deficiency of diuretics is wrongly equated with "resistance". *Therapy* is based on a **sequential nephron blockade**, which is achieved by combining a loop diuretic with a thiazide, e.g. torasemide (20—40 mg) (113) with butizide (5 mg), hydrochlorothiazide or metolazone as well as low-dosed ACE inhibitors. (s. tab. 16.12)

An **ornipressin infusion** and **adrenaline infusion** plus **water immersion** (up to the neck for a period of 5 hours) act on the lowered peripheral vascular resistance. • Low-dosage dopamine and prostaglandin or ANF infusions may have an effect on the increased renovascular resistance. (120) • A selective vasopressing-2-receptor antagonist induced a dose-related aquaretic response. (110)

8.4 Osmotic diuresis (stage III)

In inadequate response to diuretic therapy (stage II), osmotic diuresis is advisable in order to improve *hypoalbuminaemia* and *hypovolaemia*. (s. fig. 16.16)

Human albumin: Using i.v. application of human albumin or fresh plasma, it is possible to bring about a temporary rise in the osmotic pressure and improve the glomerular plasma flow. (91, 108) • Enlarging the plasma volume causes an increase in renal perfusion and urine excretion. • *The passage of infused human albumin into the ascitic fluid is prevented or reduced by prior administration of a plasma expander (100—200 ml) to ensure a preliminary boost to the oncotic pressure.*

Mannitol: Stimulation of osmotic diuresis is possible using mannitol (10—20% solution). (116) Mannitol is neither metabolized in the body nor reabsorbed by the tubules and is excreted almost totally through the kidney. Renal circulation and renal filtration are raised, and by reducing tubular absorption (= osmotic diuresis), water excretion is increased ("diuresis starter"). The saluretic effect is, however, relatively small. In the case of restricted renal function, application of mannitol is contraindicated. If necessary, the **mannitol test** (i. v. injection of 75 ml of a 20% solution) can be carried out beforehand. With enhanced diuresis of >40 ml/hr, the kidneys still function adequately, so that it is possible to stimulate osmotic diuresis by means of a mannitol infusion.

In the individual case, these short-term measures (possibly also reinfusion of ascitic fluid) lead to a temporary improvement of hypoalbuminaemia and hypovolaemia, so that a diuretic therapy, which has been hitherto insufficient, can nevertheless be continued and successfully completed. • *If stages I—III fail to be efficacious in eliminating ascites, paracentesis is indicated.*

8.5 Paracentesis (stage IV)

▶ Even in antiquity, attempts were made to remove ascitic fluid by abdominocentesis (ERASISTRATOS 300—250 BC, CELSUS 30 BC—50 AD). PAULUS OF AEGINA (625—690 AD) gave an exact description of ascitic fluid being tapped. • In the 16th century, PARÉ removed ascitic fluid with an inserted seton (i. e. rope made of hair) after cauterizing the abdominal wall. • In the 17th century, SANTORINI used a special instrument inserted through the navel to tap the abdominal cavity. • Figure 16.11 illustrates the **tapping of ascitic fluid** at that time (1672).

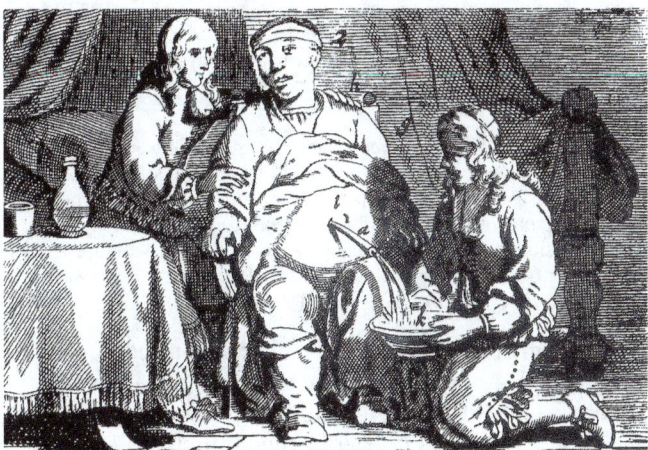

Fig. 16.11: Tapping ascitic fluid (1672) (German National Museum, Nürnberg)

Before resorting to invasive or even surgical procedures to eliminate ascites, paracentesis (stage IV) is indicated. Repeated (if necessary, daily) paracentesis can remove 1,000—4,000 ml ascitic fluid in one to two hours. The loss of complement factors possibly heightens the threat of spontaneous bacterial peritonitis — yet in view of the reduced protein content in the ascitic fluid, this danger is more likely to be diminished. Relief is provided to the portal and renal vessels. When correctly performed, complications are rare. (150) It is possible to repeat paracentesis without incurring any actual risks and to remove substantial quantities of ascitic fluid (4—6 [—23] litres) by means of a pump (132, 135, 137, 138, 140, 150) or even to evacuate a large amount of ascitic fluid almost totally. (128, 139, 141, 145, 149) Therapy is successful in about 95% of cases. Paracentesis of 6 litres of ascitic fluid removes 6×130 mmol/l sodium. Occasional circulatory dysfunction (as demonstrated by excessive activation of the RAAS) following paracentesis only rarely — or never — occurs when spironolactone and albumin substitution are applied. (s. fig. 16.17)

The following criteria are important **indications** for performing paracentesis (103, 128, 133, 141, 146, 148):

1. Lack of success or inadequate feasibility of stepwise therapy (stages I—III)
2. Extensive ascites, possibly with complications
3. Sodium excretion <10 mmol/day
4. Fractional excretion of sodium (FE_{Na}) ≤ 0.2%
5. Serum-ascites albumin gradient <1.1 g/dl
   (= serum albumin concentration minus ascites albumin concentration)

With regard to paracentesis, the following **measures** are to be considered (128, 133, 134, 136, 141, 145, 147):

1. Discontinuation of diuretic therapy some three to five days prior to paracentesis, maintenance of spironolactone (e. g. 2 to 3×50 mg/day).
2. Balancing of electrolytes, acid-base equilibrium and, if necessary, zinc substitution.
3. Replacement of sodium-free albumin (40 g or 6—8 g/litre ascitic fluid), half the amount prior to starting paracentesis; *or*: administration of 100—150 ml of a sodium-free plasma expander prior to paracentesis and prior to the replacement of albumin.
   ▶ *Prior administration of a plasma expander* raises the lowered oncotic pressure. As a result, the subsequent albumin intake is retained better in the blood stream (otherwise there is a possible danger of albumin loss from the "off-flow" into the ascitic fluid).
   ▶ Synthetic sodium-free plasma expanders are considerably (about 20 times) cheaper than albumin and equally efficient.

Results: The results of paracentesis have been good up to now: the number of successfully treated patients was higher, inpatient hospitalization was shorter, and complications were less frequent or less severe. The response to diuretic therapy improved considerably; discontinued diuretic therapy could be taken up again. (144, 145) Plasma values of renin, aldosterone and norepinephrine dropped. There was an improvement in lung volume (129, 131) and in cardiac function. (139, 142) The pressure in the oesophageal varices fell. (137) • *Paracentesis of 6 litres of ascitic fluid removes 6 × 130 mmol sodium.*

Dangers: Thought must be given to averting the following dangers deriving from repeated and/or large-scale paracentesis: (*1.*) protein loss, (*2.*) loss of electrolytes, (*3.*) hypovolaemia, (*4.*) occurrence of ascitic leakage, (*5.*) occurrence of (secondary) bacterial peritonitis, (*6.*) restricted renal function, and (*7.*) acute haemoperitoneum. (130)

An **ascites fistula** following paracentesis can be widely avoided by displacing the skin tangentially to the site of puncture, so that a *Z-shaped puncture channel* is created once the needle has been removed.

> **Danger points 1, 2 and 3 (see above) can be related to a quotation from PAULUS OF AEGINA (625–690 AD):** *"At all events, avoid any rapid evacuation of the fluid, since there are some ignorant operators who have removed the life and soul of the patient with the fluid, thereby bringing the life of the patient to an end."*

9 Refractory ascites

Before denoting ascites as refractory to conservative therapy in cases of liver cirrhosis, it is essential to rule out *what would appear to be pathogenetically or causally derived resistance to therapy.* The multiple causes of resistance to therapy must be considered in each individual case and excluded as far as possible. This can often be extremely difficult and is sometimes even impossible. (s. tab. 16.13) • Assessment of the renal cortical blood flow is facilitated by colour-encoded Doppler sonography: successful diuretic therapy of ascites requires good circulation in the renal cortex. A continuous decrease in the cortical blood flow correlates with growing therapy resistance of the ascites.

With reliable cooperation on the part of the patient, precise adherence to stepwise therapy (possibly including repeated paracentesis) and almost total exclusion of the causes of therapy resistance, it becomes clear that true **refractory ascites** or "sequestered ascites" is present in merely 5–10% of patients with portal ascites.

The prognosis of "true" refractory ascites is infaust – unless invasive measures can be applied. These would include reinfusion of ascitic fluid, peritoneovenous shunting or TIPS. Liver transplantation is the only definitive therapy. (37, 57, 120, 151–157, 170)

> 1. Unresolved cause of ascites
> 2. Excessive sodium levels in the body
>   - inadequate sodium restriction
>   - extremely high proximal reabsorption of sodium
> 3. Hypovolaemia
> 4. Absence of peripheral oedema
> 5. Excessive volume of ascitic fluid in the abdomen
>   - disturbed cardiac function
>   - compression of portal or renal vessels
> 6. Deterioration of renal function
> 7. Unfavourable diuretic effects
>   - inadequate diuretic absorption
>   - unsuitable diuretic agent
>   - incorrect dosage
>   - medication-related interactions
>   (e.g. nonsteroidal antiphlogistics, aminoglycosides)
> 8. Spontaneous bacterial peritonitis
> 9. Deterioration of liver function
>   - toxic or infection-related disorders
>   - gastrointestinal bleeding
> 10. Haemodynamic resistance to diuretics
>   - peripheral vasodilation
>   - opening of arteriovenous anastomoses
>   - relative hypotension
>   - reactive renal vasoconstriction
> 11. Portal vein thrombosis
> 12. POEMS syndrome

Tab. 16.13: Pathogenetic or causal factors which may explain apparent resistance to ascites therapy

10 Invasive therapeutic procedures

10.1 Ascites reinfusion

> ▶ In 1911 intravenous ascitic reinfusion was described as an invasive procedure to treat refractory ascites (J. GALUD). This procedure was taken up again by M. GIRARD et al. in 1949 and by R. EMMRICH et al. in 1951. In 1958 E. ADLERCREUTZ filtered the ascitic fluid prior to intraperitoneal reinfusion and thus increased its protein concentration. (158)

Methods: In the following years, various methods were developed, all of which proved their worth and led to clinical success. Central venous pressure and sodium-potassium quotient in the urine were swiftly normalized, and diuresis increased. Pathological sodium and potassium values in the serum were adjusted. Natriuresis and the concentration of ADH were not influenced. There were no electrolyte disturbances. (132, 138, 160–167, 170)

1. **Unmodified ascites:** Careful examination of the unmodified ascitic fluid prior to direct retransfusion is imperative. (s. fig. 16.10) It is likewise essential to determine the plasminogen level in the ascitic fluid.

▶ By means of an automatic infusor or a roll pump, 300–400 ml/hour are reinfused through a filter system with a pore diameter of

22 μm via a central vein catheter. Reinfusion time should be limited to 8–12 hours/day, so that a daily reinfusion quantity of 3–4 (–5) litres is achieved. Reinfusion on every second day has also proved successful. This procedure can be carried out prior to the implantation of a peritoneovenous shunt. The transport volume is varied in such a way that a good response is not accompanied by cardiopulmonary complications due to hypervolaemia. Intensive monitoring of the patient is required.

2. Modified ascites: Reinfusion of modified ascitic fluid calls for prior "desalination" or "concentration" with the later aim of "reproteinization". (159) The concentration of the reinfused protein was four to six times higher than the protein content of the ascitic fluid. Combined with diuretic therapy, up to 13 litres were removed in 24 hours. A comparative study showed no difference in efficacy or complications between the reinfusion of unmodified and ultrafiltered ascitic fluid.

Since 1960 discussion has focused on procedures for **extracorporeal dialysis** and since 1981 they have been used successfully (J. FELDMAN et al.). The **ultrafiltration** of ascitic fluid by means of haemodialysis and its subsequent reinfusion was described by E. R. HWANG et al. in 1982. Additional administration of foreign protein is not necessary. (132, 138, 163) A further development of ultrafiltration could be seen in the so-called *cascade filtration* or **double ultrafiltration.** (168) This procedure is described as safe, reliable and low in complications.

Indications: Indications and contraindications largely correspond to those of peritoneovenous shunts. For the short-term or repeated application of ascitic fluid reinfusion, the following indications can arise:

1. Refractory ascites
2. Inoperability of the patient
3. Pronounced hypovolaemia, hypotension and/or hypoalbuminaemia
4. Dilutional hyponatraemia
5. Preoperative elimination of ascites
6. Emergency situation
7. Bridging renal insufficiency that is in principle reversible

Success rate: Short-term success can be achieved in about 80% of cases, many of which also have the chance of long-term therapy success. Stage II treatment is continued parallel to the reinfusion of ascitic fluid.

Complications include clotting disorders (22, 169) and the bacterial infection of ascites.

10.2 Peritoneovenous shunt

The short-term but nevertheless relatively good clinical results achieved with the reinfusion of unmodified ascitic fluid encouraged the development of another therapeutic procedure based on a similar principle, yet with long-term efficacy. (s. fig. 16.17)

▶ Initial attempts were based on a peritoneovenous fistula with the great saphenous vein (M. RUOTTE, 1907). Later, it was the flow-controlled Spitz-Holter technique based on the principle of discharging CSF fluid from the hydrocephalus via a Holter valve (introduced by A. N. SMITH in 1962) which yielded convincing success. Consequently, a variety of pressure gradient-guided **shunt valves** were described over the following years: (*1.*) pump system of G. L. HYDE et al. (1966), (*2.*) Denver valve developed from the treatment of the hydrocephalus (W. R. WADDELL, 1971), (*3.*) LeVeen shunt (H. H. LEVEEN et al., 1974), (*4.*) Agishi valve (T. AGISHI, 1977), and (*5.*) Hakim-Cordis system (J. F. PATINO et al., 1979), based on the neurosurgical method developed by S. HAKIM et al. (1957). (171, 194)

Method: A silicone tube with roentgenopaque thread is positioned in the abdominal cavity with the intraperitoneal crus acting as an ascitic fluid collector. By means of a pressure-controlled valve, it is connected with the subcutaneously implanted section, the tip of which is introduced via the jugular vein or the subclavian vein into the superior vena cava. The ascitic fluid is forced through the valve as a result of the difference between the intraperitoneal and intrathoracic/central venous pressure. The valve only opens once this pressure gradient rises above ca. 3 cm H_2O. • Further development led to the production of pressure valves which could be operated manually by the patients themselves due to skilful surgical positioning. Each time the valve is pressed open, 4–6 ml ascitic fluid are transported. As a rule, the patient should use the pump five times per hour. In order to assess the effectiveness of a pump valve, certain **functional parameters** are applied: (*1.*) operative placement, (*2.*) opening pressure, (*3.*) pumping performance, and (*4.*) flow rate. In the light of these parameters, the Denver shunt (opening pressure 1–3 cm H_2O) is recommended as being most suitable despite its high flow rate (30–40 ml/min) because of its minimal obstruction rate and the possibility of non-operative recanalization. The decision as to which valve system is to be used must be taken in accordance with the four functional parameters described above and is ultimately made by the surgeon based on previous experience. (176, 183, 187, 201) (s. fig. 16.12)

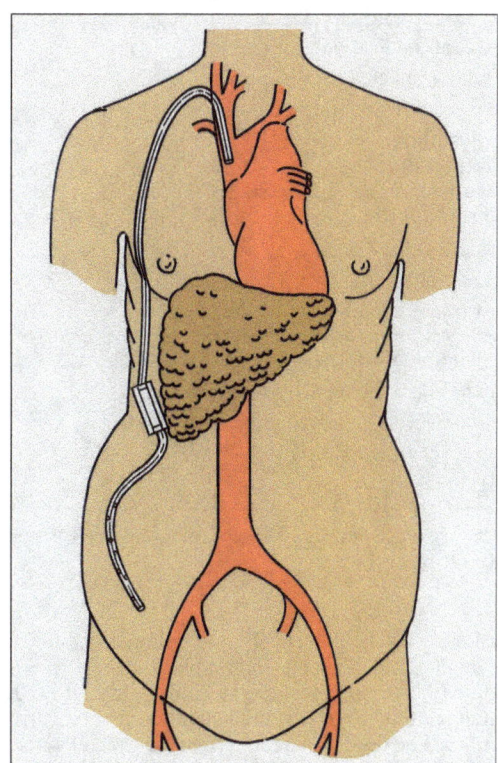

Fig. 16.12: Diagram of the positioning of a peritoneovenous shunt (with Denver valve)

Indications: The indication for a peritoneovenous shunt (PVS) must be viewed critically. (s. tab. 16.14) Before any decision is taken on the shunt implantation, the indication for TIPS or a possible *liver transplantation* must be considered and discussed with the patient. Liver transplantation provides a real opportunity to eliminate ascites permanently – generally also with a longer survival time. (181, 185, 189, 191, 202, 203)

1. Ascites in liver cirrhosis • refractory progression • conservatively treatable, albeit recurrent, condition • recurrent pleural effusions with ascites • hernia with ascites and respective complications • hepatorenal syndrome 2. Budd-Chiari syndrome 3. Chylous ascites 4. Pancreatogenic ascites 5. Refractory malignant ascites • with considerable strain on the patient

Tab. 16.14: Indications for a peritoneovenous shunt

Contraindications: Experience since 1974 with over 12,000 implanted peritoneovenous shunts has established a wide-scale consensus with respect to contraindications. Such contraindications, which are categorized as relative, have to be considered in each individual case. Successful treatment can, however, change contraindications into a correct indication, i.e. implantable condition. (s. tab. 16.15)

Absolute contraindications 1. Bacterially infected ascites, peritonitis 2. Severe general bacterial infection 3. Liver insufficiency • clotting disorders • hepatic encephalopathy (stages II–IV) • bilirubin > 10 mg/dl 4. Cardiac insufficiency 5. Respiratory insufficiency 6. Blood-tinged, highly viscous ascites
Relative contraindications 1. Increased fibrinolytic activity of the ascites 2. Previous bleeding of oesophageal varices 3. Oliguric renal insufficiency 4. Malignant ascites

Tab. 16.15: Absolute and relative contraindications for peritoneovenous shunt implantation

Complications: The frequency of postoperative complications is extremely high at 43–83% (mean complication rate 65–70%). In connection with the high postoperative mortality rate (20–22%), the question is raised as to why such simple surgery involves many complications. The **cause** can be sought in the generally poor initial condition of the patient, whose prognosis is deemed infaust anyway. Nevertheless, the opinion is also held that a considerable percentage of complications can be attributed to *avoidable mistakes.*

• Differentiation is made between **early complications** (intra- and postoperative) and (as from the first or second week) **late complications**, although no exact time spans are given. Some complications can develop at an early stage as well as at a later point in time. (173, 177, 180, 182, 186, 188, 189, 198, 201) (s. tab. 16.16)

Early complications
1. Methodological/surgical errors (10–20%) (198, 201, 206) • misplacement of venous crus • top of venous crus set at too great an angle to the vascular wall • flexion of the venous crus • venous crus too long/too short • ligature too narrow • lack of compressibility in the chamber • nuchal haematoma • injury to the recurrent nerve • pneumothorax • perforation of the coronary sinus • cardiac tamponade (due to perforation of the ventricle) 2. Fever (20–30%) 3. Clotting disorders (15–30%) (22, 184, 195) • hyperfibrinolysis • disseminated intravascular coagulation 4. Bleeding as a result of a clotting disorder 5. Fluid overload of the organism • lung oedema (178) • cardiac insufficiency • acute respiratory distress syndrome 6. Tachycardia due to misplacement of the venous crus in the right ventricle 7. Cholesterol/fat embolism in the lung 8. Bleeding of oesophageal varices (197) 9. Bacterial infection (198, 199) • wound infection • bacterial peritonitis (209) • sepsis • infection of the shunt valve • endocarditis 10. Leakage
Late complications
1. Shunt obstruction (10–20%) • fibrin-related obstruction • chyle-related obstruction (208) • thrombosis of the superior vena cava (179) • thrombosis of the jugular vein/subclavian vein • ascitic pseudocyst of the superior vena cava (205) • superior vena cava syndrome (197, 207) 2. Intestinal occlusion 3. Air embolism with intestinal perforation (190, 192) 4. Phlegmonous gastroenterocolitis (174) 5. Abdominal abscess 6. Renal failure 7. Liver insufficiency 8. Shunt wandering (177)

Tab. 16.16: Early and late complications following peritoneovenous shunt implantation (with some references)

Mortality: Since the surgical technique is well standardized and relatively simple, there is practically no *operative mortality* (0%–1.0%). In contrast, *postopera-*

tive mortality is put at 10−52% (mean mortality rate 20−22%), depending on the initial condition of the patient. The causes of death are: (*1.*) infections (27%), (*2.*) liver insufficiency (16%), (*3.*) cardiac and/or respiratory insufficiency (14%), (*4.*) consumptive coagulopathy/hyperfibrinolysis (15%), (*5.*) gastrointestinal bleeding (13%), (*6.*) renal failure (5%), and others (10%). (200, 201)

Risk reduction: The high frequency of mortality and complications can, however, be reduced markedly. It is possible to limit risks in the positioning of a PVS and in postoperative care by ensuring adherence to fundamental principles. Numerous examinations are called for prior to positioning a PVS as well as for the reinfusion of ascitic fluid. (s. tab. 16.17)

1. **Differential diagnosis of ascites** (s. fig. 16.10)
2. **Correct indication** (s. tab. 16.14)
3. **Consideration of contraindications** (s. tab. 16.15)
4. **Detailed preliminary examinations**
   − chemical laboratory values, blood coagulation values
   − plasminogen (and α$_2$-antiplasmin) in ascitic fluid
   − daily urine flow
   − daily body check
   − psychometric tests (s. p. 211)
   − Doppler ultrasonography of the jugular vein
   − central venous pressure
5. **Appropriate pre- and postoperative treatment**
   − basic and diuretic therapy (stages I and II)
   − optimal balancing of electrolytes
   − prophylactic use of antibiotics (s. pp 288, 310)
   − intestinal detoxification (s. p. 285)
   − intraperitoneal injection of dexamethasone on suspicion of increased fibrinolytic activity
   − ornithine aspartate (s. p. 287)
6. **Good cooperation on the part of the patient** (s. tab. 16.18)

Tab. 16.17: Risk reduction criteria for PVS

The determination of **plasminogen** in the ascitic fluid (with a normal value of >0.7 CTA U/ml), possibly also of α$_2$-antiplasmin (with a normal value of >0.1 IU/ml), is a priority. These values can help to estimate the risk of hyperfibrinolysis after the placing of a shunt. With a reduction in plasminogen (E. KÖTTGEN et al., 1982) to <0.7 CTA U/ml or in α$_2$-antiplasmin to <0.1 IU/ml, there is frequently a higher fibrinolytic activity of ascites (in some 40% of patients). Plasminogen activators are formed by peritoneal macrophages, the synthesis and release of which are stimulated by intestinal endotoxins. In some 50% of patients, endotoxins can be detected in ascites, yet not necessarily at the same time in the serum as well. In these cases of greater fibrinolytic activity, the injection of **dexamethasone** (16 mg) into the ascitic fluid is indicated. As a result, the synthesis of plasminogen activators in the macrophages is inhibited. Generally, the values of plasminogen and α$_2$-antiplasmin rise to within the normal range after 24 hours, so that the dangers are considerably diminished following the placement of a PVS and the subsequent infusion of ascitic fluid into the blood stream (J. SCHÖLMERICH, 1987). With inadequate response of plasminogen (>0.7 U/ml) or of α$_2$-antiplasmin (>0.1 IU/ml), the intraperitoneal administration of dexamethasone (16 mg) should be repeated. Once values have normalized, the shunt can be placed. A repetition of the intraperitoneal administration of dexamethasone may also prove necessary during the postoperative period. • **Intestinal detoxification,** which is principally desired and which can be achieved by means of *neomycin* and/or *lactulose,* serves to diminish the complication of hyperfibrinolysis by reducing the endotoxins. Where the fibrinolytic activity of ascites is increased and the efficacy of (repeatedly administered) dexamethasone proves inadequate, it is advisable to remove the ascitic fluid intraoperatively to carry out an **abdominal lavage** with a physiological NaCl solution and to instil a saline-albumin solution prior to the operative closure of the wound. • Should **clotting disorders,** in particular hyperfibrinolysis, still occur, treatment with *protease inhibitors* (e.g. aprotinin 500,000 units as bolus, then 100,000 U/hour by perfusion over 3−4 days) is required.

Antibiotics: Administration of antibiotics (e.g. cefotaxime) is advisable, starting two days prior to and continuing for about three days after shunt placement.

Compliance: Cooperation on the part of the patient is imperative for the long-term success of a peritoneovenous shunt. Some of the complications are possibly due to negligence or inadequate adherence to the principal measures required. (s. tab. 16.18)

Success of PVS: In general, a two-year survival time in ca. 50% of cirrhotic patients with ascites is considered to be a clinical success. The mortality rate for refractory ascites is almost 100% after a short period of time. • The **efficacy parameters** of PVS can be described as (*1.*) reduction in abdominal girth and body weight with improved respiratory function, physical mobility and subjective feeling of well-being, (*2.*) greater diuresis and natriuresis, (*3.*) enlargement of the intravasal fluid volume, (*4.*) increase in the renal plasma flow and glomerular filtration rate with improved creatinine clearance (172, 187), (*5.*) reduction in ADH, NAF and renin-aldosterone values (172, 175, 193, 204), and (*6.*) diminished pressure in the portal vein system.

1. Respiratory training exercises
2. Wearing of an abdominal binder
3. If a manual pump system is placed, it should be used 5−6 times per hour
4. Appropriate life-style

5. Daily weight check and handwriting test (s. pp 211, 311) (s. fig. 15.3)
6. Correct treatment in line with stages I and II
7. Polypragmatic, albeit mosaic-like, concomitant therapy for underlying ascitic disease
8. Laboratory check-ups at acceptable intervals (e.g. potassium, sodium, creatinine, haematocrit, thrombocytes, Quick's value, haemoglobin, AT III, cholinesterase, electrophoresis)
9. Physical check-ups
10. Ultrasonographic check-ups

Tab. 16.18: Necessary measures for the patient and medical check-ups after placement of PVS

▶ **Our own experience** (since 1982 at Wetzlar Hospital for Internal Medicine, including the monitoring of outpatients) is founded on the use of the LeVeen shunt (8 cases) and Denver shunt (6 cases). The patients (all suffering from alcoholic cirrhosis) were selected in line with the above criteria, examined and treated (with determination of plasminogen and application of dexamethasone, if required). The survival rate in these 14 cases amounted to 10 patients after 2 years (ca. 72%), 8 patients after 3 years (ca. 57%) and 4 patients after 4 years (ca. 29%). (s. figs. 16.13, 16.14)

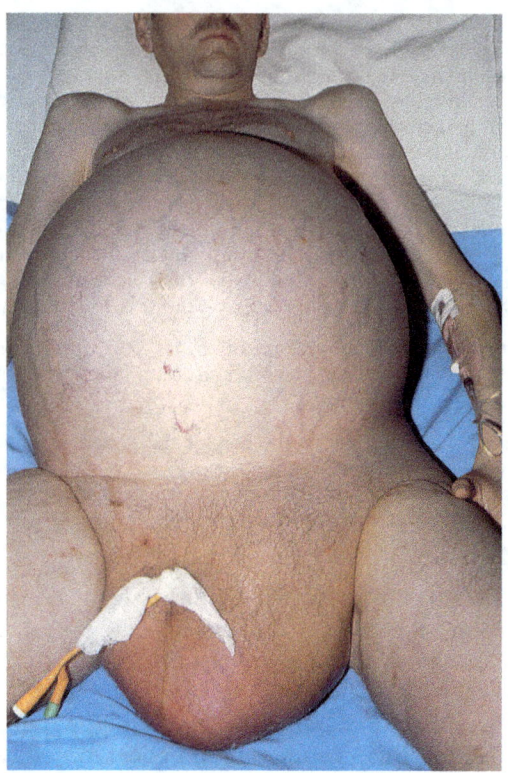

Fig. 16.13: Enormous refractory ascites in alcoholic cirrhosis. Bilateral inguinal hernia with scrotal oedema. Muscular atrophy. Hepatic encephalopathy (II−III) (same patient as in fig. 16.14)

After the positioning of a PVS, there was a **survival rate** of 40−67% after one year and 20−43% after two years, with considerably improved quality of life. It is realistic to expect that a three-year survival rate can be achieved in 30−40% of these patients nowadays. Yet this calls for close adherence to and fulfilment of the criteria on risk reduction. (s. tab. 16.17) All instructions given to the patient must be duly observed (s. tab. 16.18, points 1−5), and the medical measures taken must be appropriate to the respective situation. (s. tab. 16.18, points 6−10) • *For patients with refractory ascites, the peritoneovenous shunt or TIPS can provide real help in a situation that is otherwise hopeless!*

10.3 TIPS

On the basis of animal experiments carried out by J. RÖSCH et al. (1969, 1971), a transjugular intrahepatic portosystemic stent shunt (TIPS) was positioned for the first time in human surgery by R. F. COLAPINTO et al. in 1983. The relatively minor invasive intervention achieves a clear drop in pressure in the portal circulation with haemodynamic effects similar to side-to-side anastomosis. This technique, originally introduced for the treatment of oesophageal varicose bleeding, has since been used for refractory ascites. The success rate (i.e. complete remission of ascites) is 70−75%. The TIPS leads to a reduction in plasma renin, aldosterone and the serum-ascites albumin gradient as well as an up to fourfold increase in natriuresis (such as can be observed with PVS). With both PVS and TIPS, subsequent liver transplantation is not compromised, so that these procedures can be used both for recompensation and for bridging the time prior to a transplantation. (210) (s. pp 267, 336, 368, 899) (s. figs. 16.15, 16.16)

Method: The internal jugular vein is punctured. A catheter is introduced into the right hepatic vein. A 55 cm-long needle is pushed through the catheter. With sonographic and radiological guidance, an intrahepatic branch of the portal vein is punctured (a). The portal vein system is then viewed radiologically. The tissue tract is dilated using a balloon catheter (b), and the dilated tissue tract is laid in a metal stent splint. (s. fig. 16.15)

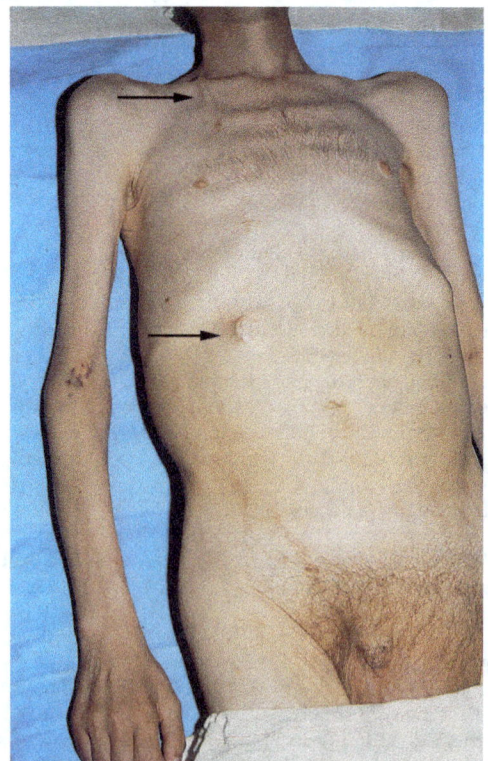

Fig. 16.14: Retrogression of ascites and oedema, increasing stabilization of biochemical and physical findings 16 weeks after placement of a LeVeen shunt (→) (survival time 45 months with two shunt recanalizations). (same patient as in fig. 16.13)

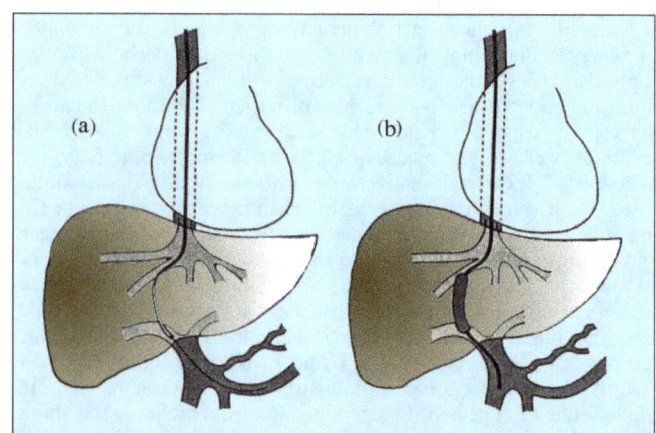

Fig. 16.15: Placement of a TIPS (according to M. RÖSSLE et al., 1989)

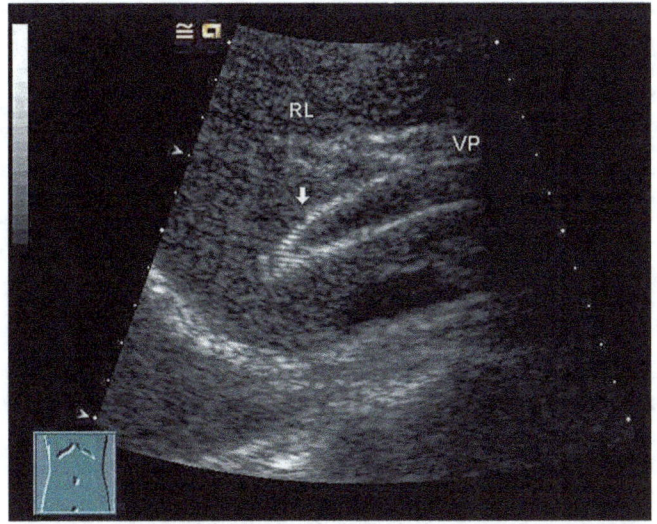

Fig. 16.16: Sonographic evidence of a TIPS (arrow) in a hypoechoic hepatic mass with the typical texture of cirrhosis (VP = portal vein; RL = right liver lobe)

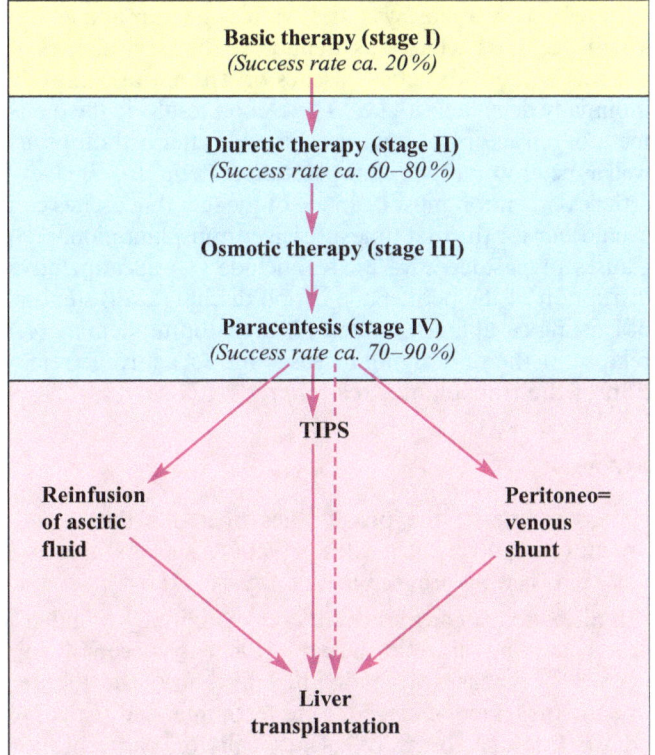

Fig. 16.17: Steps in conservative and invasive or surgical treatment for hepatogenic ascites

▶ **Underlying disease of liver cirrhosis:** This conditions does not remain stable "in itself". Actually, it causes a multitude of dysfunctions as well as disease-related conditions of deficiency and malnutrition, which impair the entire organism biochemically in a variety of ways. These factors, however, can often be permanently influenced by supporting the patient with various **therapeutic measures**. The survival time is restricted by the underlying disease. • For this reason, decision focuses on the alternatives of "optimal" conservative treatment or liver transplantation. On reviewing all clinical reports from over 100 publications available to us, it can be concluded that it is most definitely possible to improve the mortality rate and reduce the complications as well as to achieve a genuinely better quality of life while slowing down the course of disease and thus lengthening survival time. (152, 153, 210–216) (s. fig. 16.17)

11 Surgical treatment

Formerly, the possibilities of treatment were limited. At one time, 80 (–90)% of all ascites cases were considered to be refractory to therapy. Death could be expected within a short space of time. This explains the development of a multiplicity of surgical techniques – which seemed justifiable in spite of the high mortality rate (30–60%) – in order to achieve a longer survival time with a better quality of life for the individual. Despite sophisticated ideas, which indeed appeared to be logical at the time, these techniques generally proved inadequate and unfeasible in the long run. (s. tab. 16.19)

Probably the first surgical step was **hepatopexy,** as performed by CH. TH. BILLROTH in 1894. After the first **omentopexy** (or epiplopexy) was carried out by D. DRUMMOND et al. in 1896 (223) and by S. TALMA in 1898 (239), attention continued to focus on surgical ways to treat ascites. With regard to the pathophysiological aspects, the techniques can be categorized into six groups:

1. Interventions in the portal vein system
2. Interventions in the abdominal arterial system
3. Interventions in the endocrinium
4. Coating of the liver
5. Drainage operations
6. Liver transplantation

• By means of **visceropexy** (e.g. hepatopexy, omentopexy, splenopexy, rectus wick operation), an attempt was made to relieve the portal vein circulation by the gradual spontaneous development of venous collaterals and to improve the collateral circulation at the same time. (218, 223, 226, 227, 229)

• Following the first **portacaval anastomosis** on a human being carried out by E. VIDAL in 1910 (this operation had already been successfully performed on an animal by N. V. ECK in 1877), the technique was then used to treat ascites. Here, side-to-side anastomosis proved superior to end-to-side anastomosis. With the help of portacaval as well as mesocaval or splenorenal anastomosis, it was possible to achieve a sustained reduction in the portal blood flow to the liver, yet success was poor in terms of eliminating the ascites. (219)

• Likewise, an attempt was made to eliminate ascites surgically by reducing the portal and arterial blood flow to the liver. This was achieved by **arterial ligation** in the root zone of the portal vein as well as by ligation of the hepatic artery. The results were disappointing.

• In 1953 animal experiments demonstrated that bilateral **adrenalectomy** culminated in clear natriuresis, causing the ascites to disappear (J. O. DAVIS et al., 1953). This observation was confirmed in 1954 in a patient with portal ascites and bilateral adrenalectomy.

I. **Interventions in the portal vein system**
   1. Hepatopexy (CH. TH. BILLROTH, 1884)
   2. Omentopexy
      (D. DRUMMOND et al., 1896; S. TALMA, 1898)
   3. Splenectomy (I. N. RAFFERTY, 1900)
   4. Splenopexy (BUNGE, 1902)
   5. Rectus wick operation
   6. Anastomosis operation:
      – portacaval (E. VIDAL, 1910);
      – mesocaval; splenorenal
   7. TIPS (R. F. COLAPINTO et al., 1983)

II. **Interventions in the arterial system**
   1. Ligature of the hepatic artery (A. NARATH, 1909)
   2. Ligature of the splenic artery
      (R. M. MOORE et al., 1950)
   3. Ligature of the left splenic-hepatic-gastric artery (J. K. BERMAN et al., 1952)
   4. Ligature of the splenic-hepatic artery
      (J. L. MADDEN et al., 1953)
   5. Ligature of the coeliac artery (R. WANKE, 1956)

III. **Interventions in the endocrinium**
   1. Total adrenalectomy (F. G. W. MARSON, 1954)
   2. Thyroidectomy (J. W. CANTER et al., 1959)

IV. **Coating of the liver**
   1. Hepatodematosis (G. OSELLADORE et al., 1963)

V. **Drainage operations**
   1. Sapheno-peritoneostomy (M. RUOTTE, 1907)
   2. Tissue, skin (P. PATTERSON, 1910)
   3. Retroperitoneum
   4. Ureter, renal pelvis (C. FERGUSON, 1943)
   5. Urinary bladder (D. MULVANY, 1955)
   6. Ileoentectropy (C. G. NEUMANN et al., 1956)
   7. Pleuroperitoneostomy (I. EL-TOREAI, 1961)
   8. Peritoneovenous shunt (H. N. SMITH, 1962)
   9. Thoracic duct – azygous vein
      (A. E. DUMONT et al., 1963)
   10. Hepatophrenopexy (A. L. MEIER, 1970)
   11. Hepatospleno-pneumopexy (H. AKITA et al., 1980)
   12. Thoracic duct – subclavian vein
       (E. L. COODLEY et al., 1980)

VI. **Liver transplantation**

Tab. 16.19: Surgical attempts to eliminate refractory ascites (s. also tab. 19.7!)

▶ *An explanation for this success was found in the normalization of increased aldosterone values observed in ascitic dogs after adrenalectomy was performed.* (217, 228, 232) • **Thyroidectomy** (J. W. CANTER et al., 1959) proved similarly favourable in terms of its effect on ascites. (217, 220)

• **Hepatodematosis:** Both in animal experiments and in human beings, it was demonstrated that hepatodematosis can prevent the development of ascites. This coating of the liver was effected using a plastic adhesive or polyvinyl sponge. Yet this procedure had no clinical significance.

• **Other methods:** There were various attempts to **drain the ascitic fluid.** Repeated paracentesis was carried out, in which knobs or tubes with closing caps were inserted into the abdominal walls. It was recommended to channel the ascitic fluid into the skin, tissue or retroperitoneal spaces. Drainage was laid to allow the ascitic fluid to run off into the renal pelvis, ureter or urinary bladder, a procedure which was complicated, dangerous and useless. Lymphovenous anastomoses between the thoracic duct and the azygous vein or subclavian vein likewise yielded no satisfactory results. Other techniques (e.g. pleuroperitoneostomy, ileoentectropy, hepatospleno-pneumopexy, hepatophrenopexy) were interesting as regards their methodology, yet proved to be of no clinical benefit. (221, 222, 224, 225, 230–232, 233–240)

12 Liver transplantation

Transplantation of the liver essentially gives patients with refractory portal ascites a chance to start a new life. However, in the presence of large-scale ascites, the surgeon is faced with a number of specific *problems* such as overdilated and thin abdominal walls, existing hernia, spontaneous bacterial peritonitis, significant volume displacement and hypotension as a result of the complete removal of ascites, large protein losses, restricted renal function or higher consumption of erythrocyte concentrates due to more pronounced collateralization. Nevertheless, the *survival rate* of patients with refractory ascites was 91.7% after one year and 84.3% after three years, which was identical to the survival rates of patients without detectable ascites or with intraoperatively minimally detectable ascites. These good results in the treatment of refractory ascites are achievable after orthotopic as well as heterotopic liver transplantation. (s. fig. 16.17) • Nevertheless, mention must be made of the fact that ascites can even occur for the first time after liver transplantation. (234) Causes of **postoperative ascites** include (*1.*) intraoperative disruption of the perihepatic lymph discharge, (*2.*) stenosis of existing caval anastomoses, (*3.*) hypalbuminaemia, (*4.*) relapse of the underlying disease, and (*5.*) chronic rejection of the transplant. *(see chapter 40.7)*

Synopsis

This resumé of the possibilities open for the treatment of hepatogenic ascites presents a successful **step-by-step therapy programme.** (s. fig. 16.17)

In all patients, **conservative therapy** is initially founded on basic and diuretic therapy, which is successful in 60–80% of cases. In individual instances, the therapeutic measures of stage III are recommended. Apparent refractory forms of ascites call for paracentesis (stage IV), unless there are reasons against this. Some 80–90% of all patients with portal ascites can be successfully treated conservatively. Given the appropriate indication, reinfusion of ascitic fluid is also feasible.

If the results of conservative therapy (stages I–IV) are unsatisfactory, **invasive treatment** should be considered. The decision in favour of a particular procedure is determined by hepatological factors such as (*1.*) general condition and age of the patient, (*2.*) underlying disease of the ascites, (*3.*) severity of the liver disease, (*4.*) complications of the ascites, and (*5.*) secondary findings as well as additional diseases.

The above mentioned factors yield clear hints as to the indication or contraindication for a specific invasive procedure. Following this preliminary decision, an indication is evaluated together with the surgeon or radiologist. In the light of the probable three-year survival time – a period which cannot be achieved by any other surgical technique – the indication for *liver transplantation* should be a primary consideration. The problem, however, is that, given the inadequate number of donor livers available, a suitable liver cannot always be obtained, and usually not in the time required. This is why a liver transplantation should always be planned in advance, if possible.

It may indeed be necessary to postpone the transplantation or to bridge the period prior to the transplantation owing to ascites factors or other particular difficulties, including the absence of a suitable liver transplant. To this end, the *peritoneovenous shunt* and *TIPS* are suitable temporary operative steps. Indeed, it is these techniques which actually make subsequent liver transplantation possible.

Thus PVS and TIPS are principally indicated if it is not (or not yet) possible to carry out a liver transplantation.

References:

Pathogenesis

1. **Angeli, P., Caregaro, L., Menon, F., Sacerdoti, D., deToni, R., Merkel, C., Gatta, A.:** Variability of atrial natriuretic peptide plasma levels in ascitic cirrhotics: pathophysiological and clinical implications. Hepatology 1992; 16: 1389–1394
2. **Bernardi, M., Trevisani, F., Gasbarrini, G.:** Mechanisms involved in ascites formation: renin-angiotensin-aldosterone system. Gastroenterol. Internat. 1992; 5: 237–241
3. **Kentsch, M., Drummer, C., Müller-Esch, G., Gerzer, R.:** Urodilatin. Klinische Bedeutung des renalen natriuretischen Peptids. Dtsch. Med. Wschr. 1991; 116: 1405–1411
4. **Kuntz, E.:** Hepatogener (sekundärer) Aldosteronismus. Münch. Med. Wschr. 1974; 116: 1021–1030
5. **Kuntz, E.:** Störungen des Wasser- und Salzhaushaltes bei Lebererkrankungen. 1. Teil: Einführung, 2. Teil: Klinisches Bild, 3. Teil: Therapie. Münch. Med. Wschr. 1982; 124: 415–418; 447–451; 465–467
6. **La Villa, G., Salmeron, J.M., Arroyo, V., Bosch, J., Gines, P., Garcia-Pagan, J.C., Gines, A., Asbert, M., Jimenez, W., Rivera, F., Rodes, J.:** Mineralocorticoid escape in patients with compensated cirrhosis and portal hypertension. Gastroenterology 1992; 102: 2114–2119
7. **Lieberman, F.L., Denison, E.K., Reynolds, T.B.:** The relationship of plasma volume, portal hypertension, ascites, and renal sodium retention in cirrhosis: the overflow theory of ascites formation. Ann. N. Y. Acad. Sci. 1970; 170: 202–206
8. **Michielsen, P.P.:** Physiopathology of ascites in portal hypertension. Acta Gastroenterol. Belg. 1996; 59: 191–197
9. **Rahman, S.N., Abraham, W.T., Schrier, R.W.:** Peripheral arterial vasodilation hypothesis in cirrhosis. Gastroenterol. Internat. 1992; 5: 192–195
10. **Rector, W.G., Ibarra, F., Openshaw, K., Hoefs, J.C.:** Ascites kinetics in cirrhosis: relationship to plasmaoncotic balance and intensity of renal sodium retention. J. Lab. Clin. Med. 1986; 107: 412–419
11. **Reynolds, T.B.:** The history and natural history of ascites. Gastroenterol. Internat. 1992; 5: 177–180
12. **Ring-Larsen, H., Henriksen, J.H., Christensen, N.J.:** Sympathetic nervous regulation in the pathogenesis of fluid retention and ascites in patients with cirrhosis. Gastroenterol. Internat. 1992; 5: 231–236
13. **Salerno, F., Badalamenti, S., Moser, P., Lorenzano, E., Incerti, P., Dioguardi, N.:** Atrial natriuretic factor in cirrhotic patients with tense ascites. Gastroenterology 1990; 98: 1063–1070
14. **Schrier, R.W., Arroyo, V., Bernardi, M., Epstein, M., Henriksen, J.H., Rodes, J.:** Peripheral arterial vasodilation hypothesis: a proposal for the initiation of renal sodium and water retention in cirrhosis. Hepatology 1988; 8: 1151–1157
15. **Schrier, R.W., Niederberger, M., Weigert, A., Gines, P.:** Peripheral arterial vasodilation: determination of functional spectrum of cirrhosis. Semin. Liver Dis. 1994; 14: 14–22
16. **Witte, C.L., Witte, M.H., Dumont, A.E.:** Lymph imbalance in the genesis and perpetuation of the ascites syndrome in hepatic cirrhosis. Gastroenterology 1980; 78: 1059–1068

Clinical aspects

17. **Ackermann, Z., Reynolds, T.B.:** Evaluation of pleural fluid in patients with cirrhosis. J. Clin. Gastroenterol. 1997; 25: 619–622
18. **Andus, T., Gross, V., Holstege, A., Weber, M., Ott, M., Gerok, W., Schölmerich, J.:** Evidence for the production of high amounts of interleukin-6 in the peritoneal cavity of patients with ascites. J. Hepatol. 1992; 15: 378–381
19. **Andus, T., Gross, V., Holstege, A., Ott, M., Weber, M., David, M., Gallati, H., Gerok, W., Schölmerich, J.:** High concentrations of soluble tumor necrosis factor receptors in ascites. Hepatology 1992; 16: 749–755
20. **Asbert, M., Gines, A., Gines, P., Jimenez, W., Claria, J., Salo, J., Arroyo, V., Rivera, F., Rodes, J.:** Circulating levels of endothelin in cirrhosis. Gastroenterology 1993; 104: 1485–1491
21. **Attali, P., Turner, K., Pelletier, G., Ink, O., Etienne, J.P.:** pH of ascitic fluid: diagnostic and prognostic value in cirrhotic and noncirrhotic patients. Gastroenterology 1986; 90: 1255–1260
22. **Baele, G., Rasquin, K., Barbier, F.:** Coagulant, fibrinolytic, and aggregating activity in ascitic fluid. Amer. J. Gastroenterol. 1986; 81: 440–443
23. **Baer, J.W.:** Extraperitoneal mass effect by ascites under tension. Gastrointest. Radiol. 1990; 15: 3–8
24. **Bansal, S., Kaur, K., Bansal, A.K.:** Diagnosis ascitic etiology on a biochemical basis. Hepato-Gastroenterol. 1998; 45: 1673–1677
25. **Black, M., Friedman, A.C.:** Ultrasound examination in the patient with ascites. Ann. Intern. Med. 1989; 110: 253–255
26. **Boca, M., Hantak, I., Mickulecky, M., Ondrejka, P.:** Biochemical pattern of the ascitic fluid in liver cirrhosis and in neoplastic diseases. Gastroenterol. Journ. 1991; 51: 136–137
27. **Buhac, I., Flesh, L., Kishore, R.:** Intraabdominal pressure and ascitic fluid volume in decompensated liver cirrhosis. Amer. J. Gastroenterol. 1984; 79: 569–572
28. **Calvet, X., Bruix, J., Bosch, J., Rodes, J.:** Portal pressure in patients with exudative ascites in the course of acute hepatitis B. Liver 1991; 11: 206–210
29. **Cardenas, A., Chopra, S.:** Chylous ascites. Amer. J. Gastroenterol. 2002; 97: 1896–1900
30. **Catteau, E.L., Benjamin, S.B., Knuff, T.E., Castell, D.O.:** The accuracy of the physical examination in the diagnosis of suspected ascites. J. Amer. Med. Ass. 1982; 247: 1164–1166
31. **Cheng, W.S.C., Gough, I.R., Ward, M., Croese, J., Powell, L.W.:** Chylous ascites in cirrhosis: a case report and review of the literature. J. Gastroenterol. Hepatol. 1989; 4: 95–99
32. **Chopra, S., Dodd, G.D., Chintapalli, K.N., Esola, C.C., Ghiatas, A.A.:** Mesenteric, omental, and retroperitoneal edema in cirrhosis: frequency and spectrum of CT findings. Radiology 1999; 211: 737–742
33. **Colli, A., Buccino, G., Cocciolo, M., Parravicini, R., Mariani, F., Scaltrini, G.:** Diagnostic accuracy of fibronectin in the differential diagnosis of ascites. Cancer 1986; 58: 2489–2493
34. **Colli, A., Buccino, G., Cocciolo, M., Parravicini, R., Mariani, F., Scaltrini, G.:** Diagnostic accuracy of sialicacid in the diagnosis of malignant ascites. Cancer 1989; 63: 912–916
35. **Elis, A., Meisel, S., Tishler, T., Kitai, Y., Lishner, M.:** Ascitic fluid to serum bilirubin concentration ratio for the classification of transudates or exudates. Amer. J. Gastroenterol. 1998; 93: 401–403
36. **Emerson, P.A., Davies, J.H.:** Hydrothorax complicating ascites. Lancet 1995; 1: 487–488
37. **Fernandez-Esparrach, G., Sanchez-Fueyo, A., Gines, P., Uriz, J., Quinto, L., Ventura, P.-J., Cardenas, A., Guevara, M., Sort, P., Jimenez, W., Bataller, R., Arroyo, V., Rodes, J.:** A prognostic model for predicting survival in cirrhosis with ascites. J. Hepatol. 2001; 34: 46–52
38. **Gerbes, A.L., Jüngst, D., Xie, Y., Permanetter, W., Paumgartner, G.:** Ascitic fluid analysis for the differentiation of malignancy-related and nonmalignant ascites. Proposal of a diagnostic sequence. Cancer 1991; 68: 1808–1814
39. **Hurst, R.D., Butler, B.N., Soybel, D.I., Wright, H.K.:** Management of groin hernias in patients with cirrhosis. Ann. Surg. 1992; 216: 696–700
40. **Jolles, H., Coulam, C.M.:** CT of ascites: differential diagnosis. Amer. J. Roentgenol. 1980; 135: 315–322
41. **Jüngst, D., Gerbes, A.L., Martin, R., Paumgartner, G.:** Value of ascitic lipids in the differentiation between cirrhotic and malignant ascites. Hepatology 1986; 6: 239–243
42. **Kakizaki, S., Katakai, K., Yoshinaga, T., Higuchi, T., Takayama, H., Takagi, H., Nagamine, T., Mori, M.:** Hepatic hydrothorax in the absence of ascites. Liver 1998; 18: 216–220
43. **Kuntz, E.:** Hepatitis oedematosa. Med. Klin. 1975; 70:274–278
44. **Lawson, J.D., Weissbein, A.S.:** The puddle sign – an aid in the diagnosis of minimal ascites. New Engl. J. Med. 1959; 260: 652–654
45. **Lazaridis, K.N., Frank, J.W., Krowka, M.J., Kamath, P.S.:** Hepatic hydrothorax: pathogenesis, diagnosis and management. Amer. J. Med. 1999; 107: 262–267

46. **Lemmer, J.H., Strodel, W.E., Eckhauser, F.E.:** Umbilical hernia incarceration: a complication of medical therapy of ascites. Amer. J. Gastroenterol. 1983; 78: 295–296
47. **Lim, , Y.S., Han, J.S., Kim, K.A., Yoon, J.H., Kim, C.Y., Lee, H.S.:** Monitoring of transtubular potassium gradient in the diuretic management of patients with cirrhosis and ascites. Liver 2002; 22: 426–432
48. **McCullough, A.J., Mullen, K.D., Kalhan, S.C.:** Measurements of total body and extracellular water in cirrhotic patients with and without ascites. Hepatology 1991; 14: 1102–1111
49. **Mindelzun, R.E., Jeffery, R.B., Lane, M.J., Silverman, P.M.:** The misty mesentery on CT: differential diagnosis. Amer. J. Roentgenol. 1996; 167: 61–65
50. **Molina, M., Ortega, G., Vidal, L., Montoya, J.J., Perez, A., Garcia, B.:** Ascitis y derrame pleural. Estudio y seguimiento de 79 enfermos. Rev. Esp. Enf. Ap. Digest. 1989; 76: 375–378
51. **Morrow, C.S., Kantor, M., Armen, R.N.:** Hepatic hydrothorax. Ann. Intern. Med. 1958; 49: 193–203
52. **Rector, W.G., Reynolds, T.B.:** Superiority of the serum-ascites albumin difference over the ascites total protein concentration in separation of "transudative" and "exudative" ascites. Amer. J. Med. 1984; 77: 83–85
53. **Rubinstein, D., McInnes, I.E., Dudley, F.J.:** Hepatic hydrothorax in the absence of clinical ascites. Diagnosis and management. Gastroenterology 1985; 88: 188–191
54. **Runyon, B.A., Juler, G.L.:** Natural history of repaired umbilical hernias in patients with and without ascites. Amer. J. Gastroenterol. 1985; 80: 38–39
55. **Runyon, B.A., Antillon, M.R.:** Ascitic fluid pH and lactate: intensitive and nonspecific tests in detecting ascitic fluid infection. Hepatology 1991; 13: 929–935
56. **Runyon, B.A., Montano, A.A., Akriviadis, E.A., Antillon, M.R., Irving, M.A., McHutchison, J.G.:** The serum-ascites albumin gradient is superior to the exudate-transudate concept in the differential diagnosis of ascites. Ann. Intern. Med. 1992; 117: 215–220
57. **Salerno, F., Borroni, G., Moser, P., Badalamenti, S., Cassara, L., Maggi, A., Fusini, M., Cesana, B.:** Survival and prognostic factors of cirrhotic patients with ascites: a study of 134 outpatients. Amer. J. Gastroenterol. 1993; 88: 514–519
58. **Salvioli, G., Tata, C., Panini, R., Pellati, M., Lugli, R., Gaetti, E.:** Composition of ascitic fluid in liver cirrhosis: bile acid and lipid content. Europ. J. Clin. Invest. 1993; 23: 534–539
59. **Sandhu, B.S., Sanyal, J.J.:** Management of ascites in cirrhosis. Clin. Liver Dis. 2005; 9: 715–732
60. **Satz, N.:** Laborchemische Untersuchungen im Aszites. Schweiz. Med. Wschr. 1991; 121: 536–547
61. **Simmons, W.W., Warren, R.E.:** Eosinophilic pleural effusion associated with recovery from viral hepatitis A. J. Clin. Gastroenterol. 1994; 19: 143–145
62. **Strauss, R.M., Boyer, T.D.:** Hepatic hydrothorax. Semin. Liver Dis. 1997; 17: 227–232
63. **Uchikara, M., Izumi, N., Sato, C., Marumo, F.:** Clinical significance of elevated plasma endothelin concentration in patients with cirrhosis. Hepatology 1992; 16: 95–99
64. **Villamil, F.G., Sorroche, P.B., Aziz, H.F., Lopez, P.M., Oyhamburu, J.M.:** Ascitic fluid 21-antitrypsin. Dig. Dis. Sci. 1990; 35: 1105–1109
65. **Zenda, T., Miyamoto, S., Murata, S., Mabuchi, H.:** Detection of diaphragmatic defect as the cause of severe hepatic hydrothorax with magnetic resonance imaging. Amer. J. Gastroenterol. 1998; 93: 2288–2289

Spontaneous bacterial peritonitis
66. **Akriviadis, A., Runyon, B.A.:** Utility of an algorithm in differentiating spontaneous from secondary bacterial peritonitis. Gastroenterology 1990; 98: 127–133
67. **Arroyo, V., Navasa, M., Rimola, A.:** Spontaneous bacterial peritonitis in liver cirrhosis. Treatment and prophylaxis. Infection 1994; 22 (Suppl. 31): 167–175
68. **Bac, D.-J., Siersema, P.D., Mulder, P.G.H., de Marie, S., Wilson, J.H.P.:** Spontaneous bacterial peritonitis: outcome and predictive factors. Europ. J. Gastroenterol. Hepatol. 1993; 5: 635–640
69. **Bhuva, M., Ganger, D., Jensen, D.:** Spontaneous bacterial peritonitis: an update on evaluation, management, and prevention. Amer. J. Med. 1994; 97: 169–175
70. **Boixeda, D., Luis de, D.A., Aller, R., Martin de Argila, C.:** Spontaneous bacterial peritonitis. Clinical and microbiological study of 233 episodes. J. Clin. Gastroenterol. 1996; 23: 275–279
71. **Conte, D., Bolzoni, P., Bodini, P., Mandelli, C., Ranzi, M.L., Cesarini, L., Fraquelli, M., Penagini, R., Bianchi, P.A.:** Frequency of spontaneous bacterial peritonitis in 265 cirrhotics with ascites. Europ. J. Gastroenterol. Hepatol. 1993; 5: 41–45
72. **De Leeuw, P., de Mot, H., Dugernier, T., Wautelet, J., Bohy, E., Delmée, M.:** Primary infection of ascitic fluid with Clostridium difficile. J. Infect. 1990; 21: 77–80
73. **Dinis-Ribeiro, M., Cortez-Pinto, H., Marinho, R., Valente, A., Raimundo, M., Salgado, M.J., Ramalho, F., Alexandrino, P., Carneiro-de-Moura, M.:** Spontaneous bacterial peritonitis in patients with hepatic cirrhosis: evaluation of a treatment protocol at specialized units. Rev. Espan. Enferm. Dig. 2002; 94: 478–481
74. **Evans, L.T., Kim, W.R., Poterucha, J.J., Kamath, P.S.:** Spontaneous bacterial peritonitis in asymptomatic outpatients with cirrhotic ascites. Hepatology 2003; 37: 897–901
75. **Garcia, V., Vidal, F., Toda, R., Benet, A., Gonzalez, J., Roca, J.M., Richart, C.:** Spontaneous bacterial peritonitis due to Salmonella enteritidis in cirrhotic ascites. J. Clin. Gastroenterol. 1990; 12: 663–666
76. **Gitlin, N., Stauffer, J.L., Silvestri, R.C.:** The pH of ascitic fluid in the diagnosis of spontaneous bacterial peritonitis in alcoholic patients. Hepatology 1992; 2: 406–411
77. **Grangé, J.-D., Roulot, D., Pelletier, G., Pariente, É.-A., Denis, J., Ink, O., Blanc, P., Richardet, J.P., Vinal, J.P., Delisle, F., Fischer, D., Flahault, A., Amiot, X.:** Norfloxacin primary prophylaxis of bacterial infections in cirrhotic patients with ascites: a double-blind randomized trial. J. Hepatol. 1998; 29: 430–436
78. **Haight, J.B., Ockner, St. A.:** Chlamydia trachomatis perihepatitis with ascites. Amer. J. Gastroenterol. 1988; 83: 323–325
79. **Jayaraj, K., di Bisceglie, A.M., Gibson, S.:** Spontaneous bacterial peritonitis caused by infection with Listeria monocytogenes: a case report and review of the literature. Amer. J. Gastroenterol. 1998; 93: 1556–1558
80. **Kaymakoglu, S., Eraksoy, H., Ökten, A., Demir, K., Calangu, S., Cakaloglu, Y., Boztas, G., Besisik, F.:** Spontaneous ascitic infection in different cirrhotic groups: prevalence, risk factors and the efficacy of cefotaxime therapy. Eur. J. Gastroenterol. Hepatol. 1997; 9: 71–76
81. **Llach, J., Rimola, A., Navasa, M., Gines, P., Salmeron, J.M., Gines, A., Arroyo, V., Rodes, J.:** Incidence and predictive factors of first episode of spontaneous bacterial peritonitis in cirrhosis with ascites: relevance of ascitic fluid protein concentration. Hepatology 1992; 16: 724–727
82. **Llovet, J.M., Rodriguez-Iglesias, P., Moitinho, E., Planas, R, Bataller, R., Navasa, M., Menacho, M., Pardo, A., Castells, A., Cabré, E., Arroyo, V., Gassull, M.A., Rodés, J.:** Spontaneous bacterial peritonitis in patients with cirrhosis undergoing selective intestinal decontamination. J. Hepatol. 1997; 26: 88–95
83. **Mihas, A.A., Toussaint, J., Sh Hsu, H., Dotherow, P., Achord, J.L.:** Spontaneous bacterial peritonitis in cirrhosis: clinical and laboratory features, survival and prognostic indicators. Hepato-Gastroenterol. 1992; 39: 520–522
84. **Nolla-Salas, J., Almela, M., Gasser, I., Latorre, C., Salvado, M., Coll, P.:** Spontaneous Listeria monocytogenes peritonitis: a population-based study of 13 cases collected in Spain. Amer. J. Gastroenterol. 2002; 97: 1507–1511
85. **Pelletier, G., Salmon, D., Ink, O., Hannoun, S., Attali, P., Buffet, C., Etienne, J.P.:** Culture-negative neutrocytic ascites: a less severe variant of spontaneous bacterial peritonitis. J. Hepatology 1990; 10: 327–331
86. **Rimola, A., Garcia-Tsao, G., Navasa, M., Piddock, L.J.V., Planas, R., Bernard, B., Inadomi, J.M.:** Diagnosis, treatment and prophylaxis of spontaneous bacterial peritonitis: a consensus document. J. Hepatol. 2000; 32: 142–153
87. **Runyon, B.A.:** Monomicrobial nonneutrocytic bacterioascites. A variant of spontaneous bacterial peritonitis. Hepatology 1990; 12: 710–715
88. **Runyon, B.A., Antillon, M.R., McHutchison, J.G.:** Diuresis increases ascitic fluid opsonic activity in patients who survive spontaneous bacterial peritonitis. J. Hepatol. 1992; 14: 249–252
89. **Shabot, J.M., Roark, G.D., Truant, A.L.:** Chlamydia trachomatis in the ascitic fluid of patients with chronic liver disease. Amer. J. Gastroenterol. 1983; 78: 291–294
90. **Soriano, G., Guarner, C., Teixido, M., Such, J., Barrios, J., Enriquez, J., Vilardell, F.:** Selective intestinal decontamination prevents spontaneous bacterial peritonitis. Gastroenterology 1991; 100: 477–481
91. **Sort, P., Navasa, M., Arroyo, V., Aldeguer, X., Planas, R., Luiz-del-Arbol, L., Castells, L., Vargas, V., Soriano, G., Guevara, M., Gines, P., Rodes, J.:** Effect of intravenous albumin on renal impairment and mortality in patients with cirrhosis and spontaneous bacterial peritonitis. New Engl. J. Med. 1999; 341: 403–409
92. **Stepani, P., Courouble, Y., Postel, P., Mezieres, P., Tossou, H., Couvelard, A., Trophilme, D., Barbare, J.C., Bories, C.:** Portal hypertension and culture negative neutrocytic ascites in POEMS syndrome. Gastroenterol. Clin. Biol. 1998; 22: 1095–1097
93. **Storgaard, J.S., Svendsen, J.H., Hegnhoj, J., Krintel, J.J., Nielsen, P.B.:** Incidence of spontaneous bacterial peritonitis in patients with ascites. Diagnostic value of white blood cell count and pH measurement in ascitic fluid. Liver 1991; 11: 248–252
94. **Vilaichone, R.K., Mahachai, V., Kullavanijaya, P., Nunthapisud, P.:** Spontaneous bacterial peritonitis caused by Streptococcus bovis: case series and review of the literature. Amer. J. Gastroenterol. 2002; 97: 1476–1479
95. **Xiol, X., Castellvi, J.M., Guardiola, J., Sesé, E., Castellote, J., Perello, A., Cervantes, X., Iborra, M.J.:** Spontaneous bacterial empyema in cirrhotic patients: a prospective study. Hepatology 1996; 23: 719–723
96. **Zundler, J., Bode, J.C.:** Spontaneous bacterial peritonitis. Med. Klin. 1998; 93: 612–618

Conservative therapy
97. **Angeli, P., Pria, M.D., de Bei, E., Albino, G., Caregaro, L., Merkel, C., Ceolotto, G., Gatta, A.:** Randomized clinical study of the efficacy of amiloride and potassium canrenoate in nonazotemic cirrhotic patients with ascites. Hepatology 1994; 19: 72–79
98. **Applefeld, J.J., Kasmer, R.J., Hak, L.J., Dukes, G.E., Wermeling, D.P., McClain, J.:** A dose-response study of orally administered torasemide in patients with ascites due to cirrhosis. Aliment. Pharm. Therap. 1994; 8: 397–402

99. Bernardi, M., Santini, C., Trevisani, F., Baraldini, M., Ligabue, A., Gasbarrini, G.: Renal function impairment induced by change in posture in patients with cirrhosis and ascites. Gut 1985; 26: 629–635
100. Brunner, G., Bergmann, von, K., Häcker, W., Möllendorff, von, E.: Comparison of diuretic effects and pharmacokinetics of torasemid and furosemid after a single oral dose in patients with hydropically decompensated cirrhosis of the liver. Arzneim. Forsch. 1988; 38: 176–179
101. Campra, J.L., Reynolds, T.B.: Effectiveness of high-dose spironolactone therapy in patients with chronic liver disease and relatively refractory ascites. Dig. Dis. Sci. 1978; 23: 1025–1030
102. Descos, L., Gauthier, A., Levy, V.G., Michel, H., Quinton, A., Rueff, B., Fermanian, J., Frombonne, E., Durbec, J.P.: Comparison of six treatments of ascites in patients with liver cirrhosis. A clinical trial. Hepato-Gastroenterol. 1983; 30: 15–20
103. Fevery, J., Roey, van, G., Steenbergen, van, W.: Ascites: medical therapy and paracentesis. Acta Gastroenterol. Belg. 1996; 59: 198–201
104. Fogel, M.R., Sawhney, V.K., Neal, E.A., Miller, R.G., Knauer, C.M., Gregory, P.B.: Diuresis in the ascitic patient: a randomized controlled trial of three regimens. J. Clin. Gastroenterol. 1981; 3 (Suppl. 1): 73–80
105. Frakes, J.T.: Physiologic considerations in the medical management of ascites. Arch. Intern. Med. 1980; 140: 620–623
106. Fuller, R.K., Khambatta, P.B., Gobezie, G.C.: An optimal diuretic regimen for cirrhotic ascites. A controlled trial evaluating safety and efficacy of spironolactone and furosemide. J. Amer. Med. Ass. 1977; 237: 972–975
107. Gatta, A., Angeli, P., Caregaro, L., Menon, F., Sacerdoti, D., Merkel, C.: A pathophysiological interpretation of unresponsiveness to spironolactone in a stepped-care approach to the diuretic treatment of ascites in nonazotemic cirrhotic patients. Hepatology 1991; 14: 231–236
108. Gentilini, P., Casigni-Raggi, V., di Fiore, G., Romanelli, R.G., Buzzelli, G., Pinzani, M., la Villa, G., Laffi, G.: Albumin improves the response to diuretics in patients with cirrhosis and ascites: results of a randomized, controlled trial. J. Hepatol. 1999; 30: 639–645
109. Gerbes, A.L., Bertheau-Reitha, U., Falkner, C., Jüngst, D., Paumgartner, G.: Advantages of the new loop diuretic torasemide over furosemide in patients with cirrhosis and ascites. J. Hepatol. 1993; 17: 353–358
110. Guyader, D., Patat, A., Ellis-Grosse, E.J., Orczyk, G.P.: Pharmacodynamic effects of a nonpeptide antidiuretic hormone V2 antagonist in cirrhotic patients with ascites. Hepatology 2002; 36: 1197–1203
111. Hagège, H., Ink, O., Ducreux, M., Pelletier, G., Buffet, C., Etienne, J.-P.: Traitement de l'ascite chez les malades atteints de cirrhose sans hyponatrémie in insuffisance rénale. Résultats d'une étude randomisée comparant les diurétiques et les ponctions compensées par l'albumine. Gastroenterol. Clin. Biol. 1992; 16: 751–755
112. Karnad, D.R., Abraham, P., Tembulkar, P., Desai, N.K.: Head-down tilt as a physiological diuretic in normal controls and in patients with fluid-retaining states. Lancet 1987/II: 525–528
113. Knauf, H., Mutschler, E.: Liver cirrhosis with ascites: pathogenesis of resistance to diuretics and long-term efficacy and safety of torasemide. Cardiology 1994; 84 (Suppl. 2): 87–98
114. McCormick, P.A., Mistry, P., Kaye, G., Burroughs, A.K., McIntyre, N.: Intravenous albumin infusion is an effective therapy for hyponatraemia in cirrhotic patients with ascites. Gut 1990; 31: 204–207
115. Middeke, M., Pinter, W., Jahn, M., Holzgreve, H.: Diuretika-induzierte Ödeme. Dtsch. Med. Wschr. 1990; 115: 216–219
116. Pamuk, Ö.N., Sonsuz, A.: The effect of mannitol infusion on the response to diuretic therapy in cirrhotic patients with ascites. J. Clin. Gastroenterol. 2002; 35: 403–405
117. Perez-Ayuso, R.M., Arroyo, V., Planas, R., Gaya, J., Bory, F., Rimola, A., Rivera, F., Rodes, J.: Randomized comparative study of efficacy of furosemide versus spironolactone in nonazotemic cirrhosis with ascites. Relationship between the diuretic response and the activity of the renin-aldosterone system. Gastroenterology 1983; 84: 961–968
118. Pockros, P.J., Reynolds, T.B.: Rapid diuresis in patients with ascites from chronic liver disease: the importance of peripheral edema. Gastroenterology 1986; 90: 1827–1833
119. Porayko, M.K., Wiesner, R.H.: Management of ascites inpatients with cirrhosis. What to do when diuretics fail. Postgrad. Med. J. 1992; 92: 155–166
120. Rector, W.G.: Diuretic-resistant ascites. Arch. Intern. Med. 1986; 146: 1597–1600
121. Santos, J., Planas, R., Pardo, A., Durandez, R., Cabre, E., Morillas, R.M., Granada, M.L., Jimenez, J.A., Quintero, E., Gassull, M.A.: Spironolactone alone or in combination with furosemide in the treatment of moderate ascites in nonazotemic cirrhosis. A randomized comparative study of efficacy and safety. J. Hepatol. 2003; 39: 187–192
122. Sheehan, J., White, A.: Diuretic-associated hypomagnesaemia. Brit. Med. J. 1982; 285: 1157–1159
123. Stergiou, G.S., Mayopoulou-Symvoulidou, D., Mountokalakis, T.D.: Attenuation by spironolactone of the magnesiuric effect of acute furosemide administration in patients with liver cirrhosis and ascites. Miner. Electrol. Metabol. 1993; 19: 86–90
124. Tönissen, R., Kuntz, H.-D., May, B.: Pseudo-Bartter-Syndrom – medikamentös induzierter Aldosteronismus. Med. Welt 1986; 37: 1437–1439
125. Trevisani, F., Bernardi, M., Gasbarrini, A., Tame, M.R., Giancane, S., Andreone, P., Baraldini, M., Cursaro, C., Ligabul, A., Gasbarrini, G.: Bed-rest-induced hypernatriuresis in cirrhotic patients without ascites: does it contribute to maintain "compensation"? J. Hepatol. 1992; 16: 190–196
126. Van Vliet, A.A., Hackeng, W.H., Donker, A.J.M., Meuwissen, S.G.M.: Efficacy of low-dose captopril in addition to furosemide and spironolactone in patients with decompensated liver disease during blunted diuresis. J. Hepatol. 1992; 15: 40–47
127. Wong, F., Blei, A.T., Blendis, L.M., Thuluvath, P.: A vasopressin receptor antagonist (VPA-985) improves serum sodium concentration in patients with hyponatremia: a multicenter, randomized, placebo-controlled trial. Hepatology 2003; 37: 182–191

Parazentesis
128. Acharya, S.K., Balwinder, S., Padhee, A.K., Nijhawan, S., Tandon, B.N.: Large volume paracentesis and intravenous dextran to treat tense ascites. J. Clin. Gastroenterol. 1992; 14: 31–35
129. Angueira, C.E., Kadakia, S.: Effects of large-volume paracentesis on pulmonary function in patients with tense cirrhotic ascites. Hepatology 1994; 20: 825–828
130. Arnold, C., Haag, K., Blum, H.E., Rössle, M.: Acute hemoperitoneum after large-volume paracentesis. Gastroenterology 1997; 113: 978–982
131. Berkowitz, K.A., Butensky, M.S., Smith, R.L.: Pulmonary function changes after large volume paracentesis. Amer. J. Gastroenterol. 1993; 88: 905–907
132. Cadranel, J.F., Gargot, D., Grippon, P., Lunel, F., Bernard, B., Valla, D., Opolon, P.: Spontaneous dialytic ultrafiltration with intraperitoneal reinfusion of the concentrate versus large paracentesis in cirrhotic patients with intractable ascites: a randomized study. Int. J. Artif. Org. 1992; 15: 432–435
133. Fassio, E., Terg, R., Landeira, G., Abecasis, R., Salemne, M., Podesta, A., Rodriguez, P., Levi, D., Kravetz, D.: Paracentesis with dextran 70 vs. paracentesis with albumin in patients with tense ascites. Results of a randomized study. J. Hepatol. 1992; 14: 310–316
134. Garcia-Compean, D., Zacarias Villarreal, J., Bahena Cuevas, H., Garcia Cantu, D.A., Estrella, M., Garza Tamez, E., Valadez Castillo, R., Barragan, R.F.: Total therapeutic paracentesis (TTP) with and without intravenous albumin in the treatment of cirrhotic tense ascites: a randomized controlled trial. Liver 1993; 13:233–238
135. Gentile, S., Angelico, M., Bologna, E., Capocaccia, L.: Clinical, biochemical and hormonal changes after a single, large-volume paracentesis in cirrhosis with ascites. Amer. J. Gastroenterol. 1989; 84: 279–284
136. Gines, A., Fernandez-Esparrach, G., Monescillo, A., Vila, C., Domenech, E., Abecasis, R., Angeli, P., Ruiz-del-Arbol, L., Planas, R., Sola, R., Gines, P., Terg, R., Inglada, L., Vaque, P., Salerno, F., Vargas, V., Clemente, G., Quer, J.C., Jimenez, W., Arroyo, V., Rodes, J.: Randomized trial comparing albumin dextran 70, and polygeline in cirrhotic patients with ascites treated by paracentesis. Gastroenterology 1996; 111: 1002–1010
137. Kravetz, Kao, H.W., Rakov, N.E., Savage, E., Reynolds, T.B.: The effect of large volume paracentesis on plasma volume – a cause of hypovolemia? Hepatology 1985; 5: 403–407
138. Lai, K.N., Li, P.K.T., Law, E., Swaminathan, R., Nicholls, M.G.: Large-volume paracentesis versus dialytic ultrafiltration in the treatment of cirrhotic ascites. Quart. J. Med. 1991; 78: 33–41
139. Luca, A., Feu, F., Garcia-Pagan, J.C., Jimenez, W., Arroyo, V., Bosch, J., Rodes, J.: Favorable effects of total paracentesis on splanchnic hemodynamics in cirrhotic patients with tense ascites. Hepatology 1994; 20: 30–33
140. Pinto, P.C., Amerian, J., Reynolds, T.B.: Large-volume paracentesis in nonedematous patients with tense ascites: its effect on intravascular volume. Hepatology 1988; 8: 207–210
141. Planas, R., Gines, P., Arroyo, V., Llach, J., Panes, J., Vargas, V., Salmeron, J.M., Gines, A., Toledo, C., Rimola, A., Jimenez, W., Asbert, M., Gassull, A., Rodes, J.: Dextran-70 versus albumin as plasma expanders in cirrhotic patients with tense ascites treated with total paracentesis. Results of a randomized study. Gastroenterology 1990; 99: 1736–1744
142. Pozzi, M., Osculati, G., Boari, G., Serboli, P., Colombo, P., Lambrughi, C., de Ceglia, S., Roffi, L., Piperno, A., Negro Cusa, E., D'Amico, P., Grassi, G., Mancia, G., Fiorelli, G.: Time course of circulatory and humoraleffects of rapid total paracentesis in cirrhotic patients with tense, refractory ascites. Gastroenterology 1994; 106: 709–719
143. Qureshi, W.A., Harshfield, D., Shah, H., Netchvolodoff, C., Banerjee, B.: An unusual complication of paracentesis. Amer. J. Gstroenterol. 1992; 87: 1209–1211
144. Runyon, B.A., Antillon, M.R., Montano, A.A.: Effect of diuresis versus therapeutic paracentesis on ascitic fluid opsonic activity and serum complement. Gastroenterology 1989; 97: 158–162
145. Salerno, F., Badalamenti, S., Lorenzano, E., Moser, P., Incerti, P.: Randomized comparative study of hemaccel vs. albumin infusion after total paracentesis in cirrhotic patients with refractory ascites. Hepatology 1991; 13: 707–713
146. Smart, H.L., Triger, D.R.: A randomised prospective trial comparing daily paracentesis and intravenous albumin with recirculation in diuretic refractory ascites. J. Hepatol. 1990; 10: 191–197
147. Sola-Vera, J., Minana, J., Ricart, E., Planella, M., Gonzáles, N., Torras, X., Rodríguez, E., Such, J., Pascual, S., Soriano, G., Pérez-Mateo, M., Guarner, C.: Randomized trial comparing albumin and saline in the prevention of paracentesis-induced circulatory dysfunction in cirrhotic patients with ascites. Hepatology 2003; 37: 1147–1153

148. **Terg, R., Berreta, J., Abecasis, R., Romero, G., Boerr,L.:** Dextran administration avoids hemodynamic changes following paracentesis in cirrhotic patients. A safe and inexpensive option. Dig. Dis. Sci. 1992; 37: 79–83
149. **Vila, M.C., Coll, S., sola, R., Andreu, M., Gana, J., Marquez, J.:** Total paracentesis in cirrhotic patients with tense ascites and dilutional hyponatremia. Amer. J. Gastroenterol. 1999; 94: 2219–2223
150. **Wilcox, C.M., Woods, B.L., Mixon, H.T.:** Prospective evaluation of a peritoneal dialysis catheter system for large volume paracentesis. Amer. J. Gastroenterol. 1992; 87: 1443–1446

Therapie-refractory ascites

151. **Gines, P., Uriz, J., Calahorra, B., Garcia-Tsao, G., Kamath, P.S., Ruiz-del-Arbol, L., Planas, R., Bosch, J., Arroyo, V., Rodes, J.:** Transjugular intrahepatic portosystemic shunting versus paracentesis plus albumin for refractory ascites in cirrhosis. Gastroenterology 2002; 123: 1839–1847
152. **Lebrec, D., Giuily, N., Hadengue, A., Vilgrain, V., Moreau, R., Poynard, T., Gadano, A., Lassen, C., Benhamou, J.-P., Erlinger, S.:** Transjugular intrahepatic portosystemic shunts: comparison with paracentesis in patients with cirrhosis and refractory ascites: a randomized trial. J. Hepatol. 1996; 25: 135–144
153. **Loeb, J.M., Hauger, P.H., Carney, J.D., Cooper, A.D.:** Refractory ascites due to POEMS syndrome. Gastroenterology 1989; 96: 247–249
154. **Morali, G.A., Tobe, S.W., Skorecki, K.L., Blendis, L.M.:** Refractory ascites: modulation of a trial natriuretic factor unresponsiveness by mannitol. Hepatology 1992; 16: 42–48
155. **Sanyal, A.J., Genning, C., Reddy, K.R., Wong, F., Kowdley, K.V., Benner, K., McCashland, T.:** The North American study for the treatment of refractory ascites. Gastroenterology 2003; 124: 634–641
156. **Schindler, C., Ramadori, G.:** Albumin substitution to improve renal excretion function in patients with refractory ascites. – An empirical account. Leber Magen Darm 1999; 29: 183–187
157. **Velamati, P.G., Herlong, H.F.:** Treatment of refractory ascites. Curr. Treat. Opt. Gastroenterol. 2006; 9: 530–537

Ascites reinfusion

158. **Adlercreutz, E.:** Intraperitoneal infusion of ultrafiltered aszites in decompensated cirrhosis of the liver. Acta Med. Scand. 1958; 161: 9–20
159. **Amerio, A., Mastrangelo, F., Pastore, G.:** Reinfusion entsalzter und konzentrierter Aszitelösung in der Therapie der dekompensierten Leberzirrhose. Schweiz. Med. Wschr. 1972; 102: 1795–1799
160. **Arroyo, V., Mas, W., Vilardell, F.:** Clinical experience with the Rhone-Poulenc ascites reinfusion apparatus. Postgrad. Med. J. 1975; 51: 571–572
161. **Cressy, G., Jehan, P., Brissot, P., Simon, M., Gastard, J., Bourel, M.:** Utilisation thérapeutique du liquide d'ascite au cours de la cirrhose du foie. – La méthode de re-injection continue. Arch. Med. l'Ouest 1972; 4: 829–837
162. **Graziotto, A., Rossaro, L., Inturri, P., Salvagnini, M.:** R. infusion of concentrated ascitic fluid versus total paracentesis. A randomized prospective trial. Dig. Dis. Sci. 1997; 42: 1708–1714
163. **Lai, K.N., Leung, J.W.C., Vallance-Owen, J.:** Dialytic ultrafiltration by hemofilter in treatment of patients with refractory ascites and renal insufficiency. Amer. J. Gastroenterol. 1987; 82: 665–668
164. **Levy, V.G., Opolon, P., Pauleau, N., Caroli, J.:** Treatment of ascites by reinfusion of concentrated peritoneal fluid- review of 318 procedures in 210 patients. Postgrad. Med. J. 1975; 51: 564–566
165. **Parbhoo, S.P., Ajdukiewic, A., Sherlock, S.:** Treatment of ascites by continuous ultrafiltration and reinfusion of protein concentrate. Lancet 1974/I: 949–952
166. **Pearlman, D.M., Durendes, G.:** Treatment of intractable ascites by reinfusion of unmodified autogenous ascitic fluid. Surgery 1967; 62: 248–254
167. **Radvan, G.H., Chapman, B.A., Billington, B.P.:** The management of ascites using the Rhodiascit apparatus ("Paris-Pump"). Aust. N. Z. J. Med. 1981; 11: 12–15
168. **Rossaro, L., Graziotto, A., Bonato, S., Plebani, M., van Thiel, D.H., Burlina, A., Naccarato, R., Salvagnini, M.:** Concentrated ascitic fluid reinfusion after cascade filtration in tense ascites. Dig. Dis. Sci. 1993; 38: 903–908
169. **Tang, H.H., Salem, H.H., Wood, L.J., Dudley, F.J.:** Coagulopathy during ascites reinfusion: prevention by antiplatelet therapy. Gastroenterology 1992; 102: 1334–1339
170. **Volk, B.A., Schölmerich, J., Wilms, H., Hasler, K., Köttgen, E., Gerok, W.:** Treatment of refractory ascites by retransfusion and peritoneovenous shunting. Dig. Surg. 1985; 2: 93–97

Peritoneovenous shunt

171. **Agishi, T., Suzuki, T., Ota, K.:** Clinical evaluation of implanted ascites pump. Trans. Amer. Soc. Artif. Intern.Org. 1981; 27: 423–427
172. **Berkowitz, H.D., Mullen, J.L., Miller, L.D., Rosato, E.F.:** Improved renal function and inhibition of renin andaldosterone secretion following peritoneovenous (LeVeen) shunt. Surgery 1978; 84: 120–125
173. **Bernhoft, R.A., Pellegrini, C.A., Way, L.W.:** Peritoneovenous shunt for refractory ascites: operative complications and long-term results. Arch. Surg. 1982; 117: 631–635
174. **Blei, E.D., Abrahams, C.:** Diffuse phlegmonous gastroenterocolitis in a patient with an infected peritoneo-jugular venous shunt. Gastroenterology 1983; 84: 636–639
175. **Blendis, L.M., Harrison, J.E., Russell, D.M., Miller, C., Taylor, B.R., Greig, P.D., Langer, B.:** Effects of peritoneovenous shunting on body composition. Gastroenterology 1986; 90: 127–134
176. **Bories, P., Garcia Compean, D., Michel, H., Bourel, M., Capron, J.P., Gauthier, A., Lafon, A., Levy, V.G., Pascal, J.P., Quiton, A., Toumieux, B., Weill, J.P.:** The treatment of refractory ascites by the LeVeen shunt: a multicentre controlled trial (57 patients). J. Hepatol. 1986; 3: 212–218
177. **Chang, A.G.Y., Moore, J.:** Shunt migration: an unusual complication of peritoneovenous shunts. J. Clin. Gastroenterol. 1994; 19: 178–179
178. **Darsee, J.R., Fulenwider, J.T., Rikkers, L.F., Ansley, J.D., Nordlinger, B.F., Ivey, G., Heymsfield, S.B.:** Hemodynamics of LeVeen shunt pulmonary edema. Ann. Surg. 1981; 194: 189–192
179. **Dupas, J.-L., Remond, A., Vermynck, J.-P., Capron, J.-P., Lorriaux, A.:** Superior vena cava thrombosis as a complication of peritoneovenous shunt. Gastroenterology 1978; 75: 899–900
180. **Eckhauser, F.E., Strodel, W.E., Girardy, J.W., Turcotte, J.G.:** Bizarre complications of peritoneovenous shunts. Ann. Surg. 1981; 193: 180–184
181. **Epstein, M.:** Peritoneovenous shunt in the management of ascites and the hepatorenal syndrome. Gastroenterology 1982; 82: 790–799
182. **Franco, D., Cortesse, A., Castro e Sousa, F., Bismuth, H.:** Dérivation péritonéo-jugulaire dans le traitement de l'ascite irréductible du cirrhotique: résultats chez 88 malades. Gastroentérol. Clin. Biol. 1981; 5: 393–402
183. **Fulenwider, J.T., Galambos, J.D., Smith, R.B., Henderson, J.M., Warren, W.D.:** LeVeen vs Denver peritoneovenous shunts for intractable ascites of cirrhosis. A randomized, prospective trial. Arch. Surg. 1986; 121: 351–355
184. **Gibson, P.R., Dudley, F.J., Jakobovits, A.W., Salem, H.H., McInnes, I.E.:** Disseminated intravascular coagulation following peritoneovenous (LeVeen)-shunt. Aust. N. Z. J. Med. 1981; 11: 8–12
185. **Greenlee, H.B., Stanley, M.M., Reinhardt, G.F.:** Intractable ascites treated with peritoneovenous shunts (LeVeen): A 24- to 64-month follow up of results in 52 alcoholic cirrhotics. Arch. Surg. 1981; 116: 518–524
186. **Greig, P.D., Langer, B., Blendis, L.M., Taylor, B.R., Glynn, M.F.X.:** Complications after peritoneovenous shunting for ascites. Amer. J. Surg. 1980; 139: 125–131
187. **Greig, P.D., Blendis, L.M., Langer, B., Taylor, B.R., Colapinto, R.F.:** Renal and hemodynamic effects of the peritoneovenous shunt. II. Long-term effects. Gastroenterology 1981; 80: 119–125
188. **Grischkan, D.M., Cooperman, A.M., Hermann, R.E., Carey, W.D., Ferguson, D.R., Cook, S.A.:** Failure in LeVeen shunting in refractory ascites – A view from the other side. Surgery 1981; 89: 304–307
189. **Hillaire, S., Labianca, M., Borgonovo, G., Smadja, C., Grange, D., Franco, D.:** Peritoneovenous shunting of intractable ascites in patients with cirrhosis: improving results and predictive factors of failure. Surgery 1993; 113: 373–379
190. **Hirst, A.E., Saunders, F.C.:** Fatal air embolism following perforation of the cecum in a patient with peritoneovenous shunt for ascites. Amer. J. Gastroenterol. 1981; 76: 453–455
191. **Hyde, G.L., Dillon, M., Bivins, B.A.:** Peritoneal venous shunting for ascites: a 15-year perspective. Amer. Surg. 1982; 48: 123–127
192. **Jacobsen, W.K., Briggs, B.A., Thorp, R., Zemwalt, J.R.:** Air embolism in association with LeVeen shunt. Crit. Care Med. 1980; 8: 659–660
193. **Klepetko, W., Müller, C., Hartter, E., Miholics, J., Schwarz, C., Woloszczuk, W., Moeschl, P.:** Plasma atrial natriuretic factor in cirrhotic patients with ascites. Effect of peritoneovenous shunt implantation. Gastroenterology 1988; 95: 764–770
194. **LeVeen, H.H., Christoudias, G., Moon Ip, Luft, R., Falk, G., Grosberg, S.:** Peritoneo-venous shunting for ascites. Ann. Surg. 1974; 180: 580–591
195. **LeVeen, H.H., Ahmed, N., Hutto, R.B., Moon Ip, LeVeen, E.G.:** Coagulopathy post peritoneovenous shunt. Ann. Surg. 1987; 205: 305–311
196. **Lund, R.H., Moritz, M.W.:** Complications of Denver peritoneovenous shunting. Arch. Surg. 1982; 117: 924–928
197. **Markey, W., Payne, J.A., Straus, A.:** Hemorrhage from oesophageal varices after placement of the LeVeen shunt. Gastroenterology 1979; 77: 341–343
198. **Moskovitz, M.:** The peritoneovenous shunt: expectations and reality. Amer. J. Gastroenterol. 1990; 85: 917–929
199. **Prokesch, R.C., Rimland, D.:** Infectious complications of the peritoneovenous shunt. Amer. J. Gastroenterol. 1983; 78: 235–240
200. **Rubinstein, D., McInnes, I., Dudley, F.:** Morbidity and mortality after peritoneovenous shunt surgery for refractory ascites. Gut 1985; 26: 1070–1073
201. **Schumpelick, V., Riesener, K.-P.:** Peritoneo-venöser Shunt – Indikation, Grenzen, Ergebnisse. Chirurg 1993; 64: 11–15
202. **Smadja, C., Franco, D.:** The LeVeen shunt in the elective treatment of intractable ascites in cirrhosis. A prospective study on 140 patients. Ann. Surg. 1985; 201: 488–493
203. **Söderlund, C.:** Denver peritoneovenous shunting for malignant or cirrhotic ascites. A prospective consecutive series. Scand. J. Gastroenterol. 1986; 21: 1161–1172
204. **Tobe, S.W., Morali, G.A., Greig, P.D., Logan, A., Blendis, L.M.:** Peritoneovenous shunting restores atrial natriuretic factor responsiveness in refractory hepatic ascites. Gastroenterology 1993; 105: 202–207
205. **Unger, P., Moran, R.M.:** Ascitic pseudocyst obstructing superior vena cava as a complication of a peritoneo-venous shunt. Gastroenterology 1981; 81: 1137–1139

206. **Vaida, G.A., Laucius, J.R.:** LeVeen shunt dislodgement. J. Amer. Med. Ass. 1980; 243: 149–150
207. **Van Deventer, G.M., Snyder, N. III., Patterson, M.:** Superior vena cava syndrome. A complication of the LeVeen shunt. J. Amer. Med. Ass. 1979; 242: 1655–1656
208. **Warren, W.H., Altman, J.S., Gregory, St.A.:** Chylothorax secondary to obstruction of the superior vena cava: a complication of the LeVeen shunt. Thorax 1990; 45: 978–979
209. **Wormser, G.P., Hubbard, R.C.:** Peritonitis in cirrhotic patients with LeVeen shunts. Amer. J. Med. 1981; 71: 358–362

TIPS
210. **Boyer, T.D.:** Transjugular intrahepatic portosystemic shunt: Current status. Gastroenterology. 2003; 124: 1700–1710
211. **Degawa, M., Hamasaki, K., Yano, K., Kanao, K., Kato, Y., Sakamoto, I., Nakata, K., Eguchi, K.:** Refractory hepatic hydrothorax treated with transjugular intrahepatic portosystemic shunt. J. Gastroenterol. 1999; 34: 128–131
212. **Gerbes, A.L., Gülberg, V., Waggershauser, T., Holl, J., Reiser, M.:** Renal effects of transjugular intrahepatic portosystemic shunt in cirrhosis: comparison of patients with ascites, with refractory ascites, or without ascites. Hepatology 1998; 28: 683–688
213. **Rössle, M., Ochs, A., Gülberg, V., Siegerstetter, V., Holl, J., Deibert, P., Olschewski, M., Reiser, M., Gerbes, A.L.:** A comparison of paracentesis and transjugular intrahepatic portosystemic shunting in patients with ascites. New Engl. J. Med. 2000; 342: 1701–1707
214. **Thuluvath, P.J., Bal, J.S., Mitchell, S., Lund, G., Venbrux, A.:** TIPS for management of refractory ascites. Response and survival are both unpredictable. Dig. Dis. Sci. 2003; 48: 542–550
215. **Trotter, J.F., Suhocki, P.W., Rockey, D.C.:** Transjugular intrahepatic portosystemic shunt (TIPS) in patients with refractory ascites: effect on body weight and Child-Pugh score. Amer. J. Gastroenterol. 1998; 93: 1891–1894
216. **Younossi, Z.M., McHutchison, J.G., Broussard, C., Cloutier, D., Sedghi-Vaziri, A.:** Portal decompression by transjugular intrahepatic portosystemic shunt and changes in serum-ascites albumin gradient. J. Clin. Gastroenterol. 1998; 27: 149–151

Surgical treatment
217. **Baronofsky, I.D., Canter, J.W.:** The effect of endocrinectomy on ascites with especial reference to adrenalectomy and thyroidectomy. Amer. J. Surg. 1960; 99: 512–518
218. **Belli, L., Pisani, F., Forti, D., Parmeggiani, A.:** Une nouvelle technique de traitement chirurgical de l'ascite par sténose de la veine cave inférieure: l'hépatopexie par substances adhésives et plastifiantes. Lyon Chir. 1965; 61: 182–193
219. **Burchell, A.R., Rousselot, L.M., Panke, W.F.:** A seven-year experience with side-to-side portacaval shunt for cirrhotic ascites. Ann. Surg. 1968; 168: 655–668
220. **Canter, J.W., Kreel, I., Segal, R.L., Frankel, A., Baronofsky, I.D.:** Influence of thyroidectomy on experimental ascites. Proc. Soc. Exp. Biol. (N.Y.) 1959; 100: 771–774
221. **Coodley, E.L., Matsumoto:** Thoracic duct-subclavian vein anastomosis in management of cirrhotic ascites. Amer. J. Med. Sci. 1980; 279: 163–168
222. **Crosby, R.C., Cooney, E.A.:** Surgical treatment of ascites. New Engl. J. Med. 1946; 235: 581–585
223. **Drummond, D., Morison, R.:** A case of ascites due to cirrhosis of liver cured by operation. Brit. Med. J. 1896; 2: 728–729
224. **El-Toraei, I.:** Surgical treatment of cirrhotic ascites with a new operation (Pleuroperitoneostomy). J. Int. Coll. Surg. 1961; 35: 436–445
225. **Ferguson, C.:** Ureteroperitoneal anastomosis. Milit. Surg. 1948; 102: 178–179
226. **Gage, A.A.:** Hepatopexy for chronic cirrhotic ascites. Surgery 1966; 60: 1129–1136
227. **Gibbon, J.H., Flick, J.B.:** Present status of epiplopexy with report of ten cases. Ann. Surg. 1922; 75: 449–458
228. **Giuseffi, J., Werk, E.E.jr., Larson, P.U., Schiff, L., Elliott, D.W.:** Effect of bilateral adrenalectomy in a patient with massive ascites and postnecrotic cirrhosis. New Engl. J. Med. 1957; 257: 796–803
229. **Grinnell, R.:** Omentopexy in portal cirrhosis of the liver with ascites. A review of twenty-three cases. Ann. Surg.1935; 101: 891–901
230. **Leger, L., Prémont, M., Devissaguet, P.:** Le drainage ducanal thoracique dans les cirrhoses ascitiques. Etude dudébit lymphatique. Presse Méd. 1962; 70: 1643–1646
231. **Mallet-Guy, P., Devic, G., Feroldi, J., Desjacques, P.:** Etude expérimentale des ascites. Sténoses veineuses post-hépatiques et transposition du foie dans le thorax. Lyon Chir. 1954; 49: 143–172
232. **Marson, F.G.W.:** Total adrenalectomy in hepatic cirrhosis with ascites. Lancet 1954/II, 847–848
233. **Mulvany, D.:** Vesico-coelomic drainage for the relief of ascites. Lancet 1955/II, 748–749
234. **Neuhaus, P., Bechstein, W.O.:** Ascites und Lebertransplantation. Chirurg 1993; 64: 16–20
235. **Neumann, C.G., Adie, G.C., Hinton, J.W.:** The absorption of ascitic fluid by means of ileoentectropy in patients with advanced cirrhosis. Ann. Surg. 1957; 146: 700–705
236. **Ring-Larsen, H.:** Surgical treatment of ascites. Eur. J. Gastroenterol. Hepatol. 1991; 3: 735–740
237. **Ruotte, M.:** Abouchement de la veine saphène externe aupéritoine pour resorber les épanchements sciatiques. Lyon Med. 1907; 109: 574–577
238. **Stewart, J.:** Surgical treatment of cirrhotic ascites. Brit. Med. J. 1906; 2: 1298–1299
239. **Talma, S.:** Chirurgische Öffnung neuer Seitenbahnen für das Blut der Vena porta. Berlin. Klin. Wschr. 1898; 35: 833–836
240. **Welch, C.S., Welch, H.F., Carter, J.H.:** The treatment of ascites by side to side portacaval shunt. Ann. Surg. 1959; 150: 428–440

Symptoms and Syndromes
17 Hepatorenal syndrome

		Page:
1	*Definition*	330
2	***Pathogenesis***	330
2.1	Biochemical factors	330
2.2	Haemodynamic factors	331
3	***Clinical aspects***	331
3.1	Risks and predictive factors	331
3.2	Courses of disease	331
3.3	Diagnosis	332
3.4	Differential diagnosis	332
3.4.1	Pseudohepatorenal syndrome	333
3.4.2	Prerenal kidney insufficiency	333
3.4.3	Primary kidney diseases	333
3.4.4	Secondary kidney diseases	333
3.5	Prognosis	334
4	***Prophylaxis and therapy***	334
4.1	Maintaining homoeostasis	334
4.2	Improvement of liver function	334
4.3	Conservative treatment	334
4.4	Invasive therapy	335
	• References (1–58)	336
	(Figure 17.1; tables 17.1–17.6)	

17 Hepatorenal syndrome

▶ *Coexistence of liver and kidney disease is a frequent clinical event.* • Reports in the literature date back more than 100 years (F. Th. Frerichs, 1861; K.W.H. Nothnagel, 1874; P.J. Moebius, 1877; A. Weil, 1886). • In 1863 A. Flint noted the coexistence of cirrhosis with ascites and oliguria, although autopsy revealed the kidneys to be normal. • In animal experiments, M. Pawlow (1893) was able to show the occurrence of albuminuria after placement of a portacaval anastomosis. Jaundice mainly developed parallel to renal damage. Richardière (1890) coined the term "hépatonéphrite" to describe this clinical picture. (44) • In 1911 both P. Clairmont et al. and F. Steinthal reported for the first time on renal failure with fatal outcome following surgery on the bile ducts for obstructive jaundice. This renal failure in biliary obstruction was described by F.C. Helwig et al. in 1932 as *"liver-kidney syndrome"*. (25) • However, the coexistence of cirrhosis and the hepatorenal syndrome was first published by R. Hecker et al. in 1956. (24)

The term **"hepatorenal syndrome"** was introduced by P. Merklen in 1916 and taken up by W. Nonnenbruch in 1939. (39) The following description is still largely accepted today: *"A combination of anatomically defined liver disease with a sometimes severe restriction in the function of the kidneys, which display few, if any, morphological changes. Liver disease can be the outcome of hepatocellular damage of any type, i.e. it may be toxic or infectious and originate from cirrhosis or cancer."*

1 Definition

The hepatorenal syndrome (HRS) is a functional, oliguric, progressive and in principle reversible circulation-related kidney failure occurring in severe liver disease and portal hypertension as well as increasing liver insufficiency or in the setting of acute liver failure – assuming there are indeed no other causes of the renal insufficiency.

▶ This syndrome is, in fact, a prerenal kidney failure – *yet without response to an adjustment of the effective plasma volume*, i.e. expansion of the intravasal volume does not influence the renal function. • This functional renal failure is due to extreme intrarenal vasoconstriction and reduced perfusion in the area of the renal cortex, whereby the blood supply to the medullary parts of the kidney is largely normal. The extrarenal circulation is undisturbed (arterial vascular resistance and vascular filling as well as cardiac output are normal). • In cases of cirrhosis, systemic vasodilation becomes increasingly prevalent, together with hyperdynamic circulatory disturbance. • In clinical terms, the ultimate outcome is a reduced glomerular filtration rate, pronounced sodium and water retention with oliguria and excretion of practically sodium-free urine – without or with only slight (< 500 mg/dl) proteinuria.

2 Pathogenesis

The frequent **coexistence** of the *hepatorenal syndrome*, *ascites* and/or *hepatic encephalopathy* suggests that similar pathogenetic mechanisms are responsible for these three intricate developments in liver cirrhosis.

2.1 Biochemical factors

The numerous biochemical substances that may be considered regarding hepatic encephalopathy or ascites have been outlined in detail. (s. tabs. 15.2; 16.5) • Similarly, an extensive synopsis of pathogenetically effective biochemical factors can also be drawn up for HRS. All of them ultimately interfere – directly or indirectly – with the renal retention of sodium (= ascites) and water retention (= hyponatraemia) as well as the balance between vasodilation and vasoconstriction. RAAS and SNS are markedly activated; secretion of ADH is increased. (5, 26, 30, 36, 56, 58) (s. tab. 17.1) • Vasodilative factors under discussion include bilirubin, bile acids, nitric oxide (NO), false neurotransmitters, calcitonin peptide (23) and platelet-activating factor (PAF). In more recent studies, far higher plasma values of the vasoconstrictor leukotrienes (C4 and D4) (37) and endothelin 1 and 3 (36) were detected.

Biochemical factors	Liver	Plasma	Kidneys/Urine
Aldosterone breakdown	↓		
Angiotensin II breakdown	↓		
Angiotensinogen synthesis	↓		
Endotoxin breakdown	↓		
Kininogen synthesis	↓		
Renin breakdown	↓		
Vasopressin breakdown	↓		
Aldosterone		↑	
Angiotensin II		↑	
Antidiuretic hormone (ADH)		↑↑	
Calcitonin peptide (23)		↑↑	
Endothelin 2 and 3 (36)		↑↑	
Endotoxin		↑	
Leukotriene C_4 and D_4 (37)		↑↑	
Noradrenaline		↑	
Renin (56)		↑	
Vasopressin		↑	
Atrial natriuretic factor (ANF)		↓	
Bradykinin (56)		↓↓	
Kallikrein		↓	
Aldosterone			↑
Angiotensin II			↑
Bradykinin			↑
Endothelin			↑↑
Leukotriene E_4			↑↑
Prostacyclin			↑
Prostaglandin E_2 (58)			↑↑
Renin			↑
Thromboxane A_2 (58)			↑

Tab. 17.1: Synopsis of the activity of biochemical factors in the liver, plasma and kidneys or urine relating to the hepatorenal syndrome (with some references)

2.2 Haemodynamic factors

The hepatorenal syndrome is characterized by pronounced vasoconstriction of the renal cortex with tortuosity and narrowing of the interlobular and arcuate arteries. The blood supply to the renal cortex may be almost totally interrupted; at the same time, the blood flow is diverted into areas containing cortical vessels near the medulla. The renal medulla is, however, supplied with blood in a regular way, thus allowing the nephrons to function normally. The insufficient blood supply to the renal cortex is aggravated by intrarenal arteriovenous shunts, leading to rapid changes in haemodynamics. This instability in renal perfusion is possibly due to reduced synthesis of angiotensinogen in the liver. Disturbances in the renal blood supply can proceed continuously through the non-azotaemic and azotaemic stages to the oliguric final phase. • The **functional nature** of renal vasoconstriction was also shown by the fact that the ischaemia of the renal cortex, which had been ascertained by selective angiography in vivo, was not evident in the postmortem evaluation of the kidney. Indeed, the cortical vascular network had fully regained its normal structure. • Increased levels of *neuropeptide Y* were found in HRS. This is related to circulatory dysfunction as well as to stimulation of the sympathetic nervous system (SNS) and may contribute to renal vasoconstriction. • *The pathogenesis of renal vasoconstriction is thus multifactorial.* (5, 26, 30, 46, 48, 49)

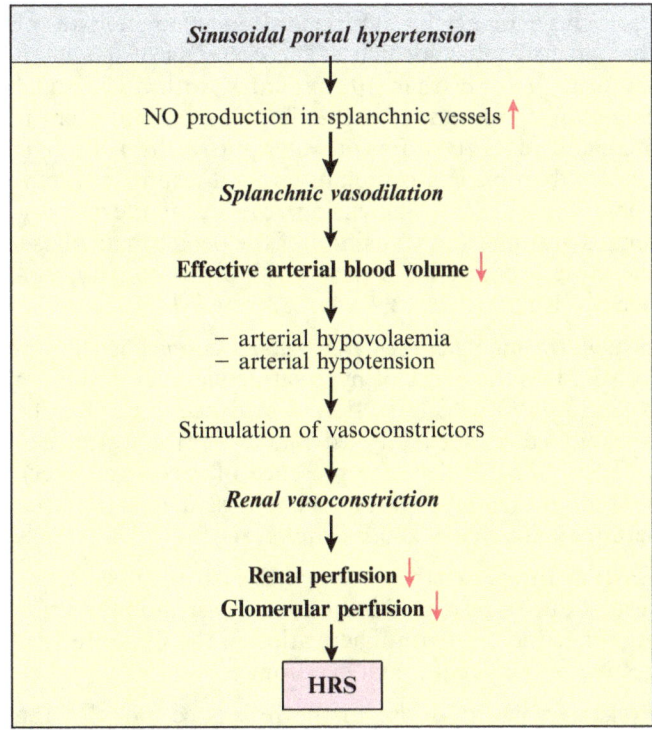

Fig. 17.1: Hypothetic pathogenesis of the hepatorenal syndrome in cirrhosis

3 Clinical aspects

In liver cirrhosis, the hepatorenal syndrome is nearly always (>80%) accompanied by ascites. HRS is most common in alcoholic cirrhosis. In some 75% of cases, hepatic encephalopathy is found at the same time, and jaundice is evident in about 40% of cases. HRS occurred in 18% of all cirrhotic patients with ascites within one year and in 32% within five years. (20, 47)

Histological findings are minimal in HRS. No constant or specific changes are known. In most cases, histology is either completely normal, or only minor degenerative changes of the tubuli and glomeruli are present. • Nevertheless, with a severe and protracted course of disease, the occurrence of acute tubular necroses can become more pronounced, resulting in end-stage renal failure.

3.1 Risks and predictive factors

Many risk situations trigger HRS, and various predictive factors make it possible to ascertain the development of HRS in non-azotaemic patients with cirrhosis and ascites. Often the cause is not directly recognizable (e.g. undisclosed alcohol abuse, environmental noxae). Typical liver function parameters do not help to anticipate the development of HRS. (11, 18, 49, 55) (s. tab. 17.2)

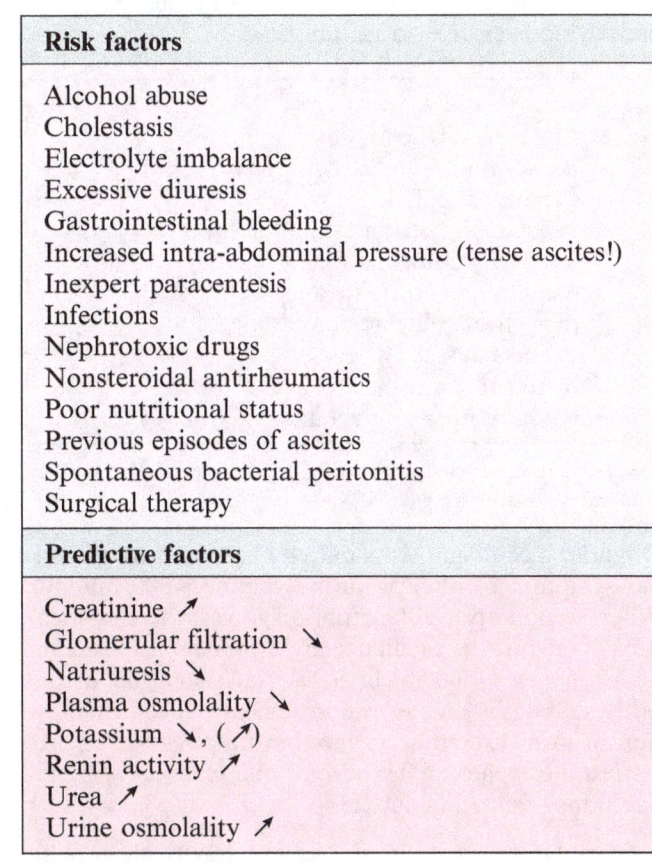

Tab. 17.2: Risk and predictive factors in patients with cirrhosis and ascites regarding the development of HRS

3.2 Courses of disease

There are **three ways** in which the hepatorenal syndrome can become manifest:

1. **Type I (acute HRS):** rapid elevation of creatinine (>2.5 mg/dl), reduction of 24-hour creatinine clearance (<20 ml/min), oliguria (<500 ml/day) and natriuria (<10 mmol/l) as well as jaundice, hypoprothrombinaemia,

hypalbuminaemia and encephalopathy — but no proteinuria. • All courses of disease which do not correspond to type I are assigned to one of the other two types;

2. **Type II (chronic HRS):** slow course of this complicated condition, renal function is more stable, reduction of 24-hour creatinine clearance (<40 ml/min). This (most frequent) form is often long-standing, although only slightly increased creatinine values in the serum (>1.5 mg/dl) and natriuria (<20 mmol/l) are clinically detectable. Type II is frequently accompanied by a diuretic-resistent ascites;

3. **Acutely exacerbated chronic HRS.**

3.3 Diagnosis

Subjective factors suggestive of HRS are unknown or uncharacteristic. The clinical picture is influenced by the underlying liver disease. (s. tab. 17.3)

1.	Liver cirrhosis, especially in
	– alcoholic cirrhosis
	– ascites and diuretic therapy
	– hepatic encephalopathy
	– oesophagogastrointestinal bleeding
2.	Acute liver failure
3.	Acute viral hepatitis (31, 40)
4.	Primary liver cell carcinoma (34)
5.	Liver metastases (45)
6.	Hemihepatectomy
7.	Acute fatty liver of pregnancy

Tab. 17.3: Severe liver diseases with the occurrence of a hepatorenal syndrome (with some references)

Oliguria: The diagnosis is initially based on the principal symptom of oliguria (urine volume <500 ml/day). When setting up a differential diagnosis, the classification of oliguria is facilitated by a *probationary volume replenishment* (1500 ml of 0.9% NaCl solution or 5% human albumin). A clear improvement in or normalization of urine excretion achieved in this way is evidence *against* the hepatorenal syndrome and *in favour of* prerenal kidney failure. (s. tab. 17.4)

Azotaemia: This condition develops progressively with increasing creatinine and urea, pointing to a drop in the glomerular filtration rate (GFR) and renal blood flow. The quotient of creatinine in the urine and plasma is high (>40) and that of urea-N in the urine and plasma is elevated (>8). There is a reduction in creatinine clearance within 24 hours to <40 ml/min. The serum value of urea displays a disproportionate increase (urea-N/creatinine ratio >20), since the tubular reabsorptive capacity with respect to urea depends on diuresis (maximum 2 ml/min). In the hepatorenal syndrome, the minimal urinary flow gives rise to a longer tubular period of contact with greater tubular reabsorption of urea.

Criteria	Hepato-renal syndrome	Acute kidney failure	Prerenal kidney insufficiency
Specific weight	>1,030	1,020	>1,030
Oliguria (<500 ml/day)	+	+	+
Azotaemia	+	+	+
Urine$_{osm}$ (mosm/kg)	>500	<350	>500
Urine$_{Na}$ (mmol/l)	<10	>30	<20
Urine$_{osm}$/P$_{osm}$	>1.3	<1.1	>1.3
Urine$_{urea}$/P$_{urea}$	>8	<3	>8
Urine$_{creat.}$/P$_{creat.}$	>30	<20	>30
Fe$_{Na}$ (%)	<1	>1.5	<1

Tab. 17.4: Urine findings for the differential diagnostic definition of the hepatorenal syndrome — provided that there has been no previous diuretic therapy. • Generally, however, this has proved necessary, which could be a reason for the considerable differences in the factors and figures reported in the literature

Urine: In general, the sediment in the urine is normal. Proteinuria or erythrocyturia are not characteristic of the hepatorenal syndrome. • The *excretion of sodium* in the urine is lower than 10 mmol/day, with a fractional excretion of sodium of <1%. For this reason, there is increased renal retention of water. • *Urine osmolality* is greater than plasma osmolality, which results in a quotient of >1.3. With increasing severity of the hepatorenal syndrome and transition of the penultimate phase, the urine becomes iso-osmotic with an osmolality quotient of 1 or <1. (18, 38, 48, 49, 55) (s. tab. 17.4)

Hyponatraemia: *Reduced free water clearance* is characteristic. It is the cause of hyponatraemia (serum sodium <130 mmol/l), which is often in evidence — this can be precipitated by an increased intake of free water (elevated sodium level in the presence of excessive water). This dilutional hyponatraemia is a sign of a reduced serum osmolality (<280 mosm/kg). (4)

Gastrin: In liver cirrhosis, elevated gastrin values in the serum, due to restricted excretion of gastrin in the urine and/or reduced gastrin inactivation in the liver, are suggestive of the hepatorenal syndrome.

Resistance index: A rise in the resistance index of the kidneys and a reduction in renal perfusion as shown by *Doppler sonography* provide an early diagnosis before renal dysfunction is clinically evident. (42) • *Colour-encoded sonography* has proved useful in determining renal haemodynamics (which deteriorates when the patient is in an upright position).

3.4 Differential diagnosis

The diagnosis of the hepatorenal syndrome calls for the exclusion of prerenal, renal or postrenal kidney insufficiency. (s. tabs. 17.4, 17.6) • *The presence of disease in the liver and kidney in the sense of a pseudohepatorenal syndrome must also be ruled out.* (s. tab. 17.5)

3.4.1 Pseudohepatorenal syndrome

Numerous diseases can impair both liver and kidneys at the same time. Each individual case reflects different levels of damage and severity, the liver and kidneys being affected to varying degrees. The prognosis is determined by this wide scope of variability. Simultaneously occurring diseases of the liver and kidneys are subsumed under the term **pseudohepatorenal syndrome** (H.O. Conn, 1973). (s. tab. 17.5)

1. **Circulatory disorders**
   - Cardiac insufficiency
   - Shock
2. **Congenital malformations**
   - Congenital liver fibrosis
   - Cystic liver and cystic kidney
3. **Experimental**
   - Choline deficiency
     etc.
4. **Infections**
   - Legionnaire's disease
   - Leptospirosis
   - Malaria
   - Sepsis
   - Viral hepatitis
   - Yellow fever
5. **Intoxications**
   - Burns
   - Chemicals
     - carbon tetrachloride
     - chrome, lead, arsenic, mercury
     - copper sulphate
     - trichloroethylene, methanol
   - Endotoxins
   - Hyperthermia
   - Mycotoxins
   - Snake venoms
   - Waterhouse-Friderichsen syndrome
6. **Medicaments**
   - Halothane
   - Iproniazid
   - Methoxyflurane
   - Paracetamol
   - Sulphonamide
   - Tetracycline
7. **Metabolic diseases**
   - Acute intermittent porphyria
   - Amyloidosis
   - Diabetes mellitus
   - Eclampsia
   - Glycogenosis I
   - Haemochromatosis
   - Reye's syndrome
   - Sickle-cell anaemia
   - Tyrosinaemia, oxalosis
   - Wilson's disease
8. **Systemic diseases**
   - Lupus erythematosus
   - Periarteritis nodosa
   - Rheumatoid arthritis
   - Sarcoidosis
9. **Tumours**
   - Hypernephroma
   - Metastases

Tab. 17.5: Coexistent disease of the liver and kidneys (comorbidity), so-called pseudohepatorenal syndrome (H.O. Conn, 1973)

3.4.2 Prerenal kidney insufficiency

Dehydration with diminished volume (bleeding, large water losses, diuretic therapy, paracentesis, intravasal volume shifting) can lead to prerenal azotaemia. Typically, renal function normalizes again when fluid intake is increased, *i.e. in contrast to the hepatorenal syndrome, the intravasal volume can be influenced by therapy.*

3.4.3 Primary kidney diseases

Initially, it is important to rule out primary kidney diseases, including all glomerular, interstitial and vascular forms, as well as acute tubular necrosis resulting, for example, from nephrotoxins, sepsis, hypoxia or shock. In severe or protracted kidney disease, various chemical findings can point to liver involvement (as suggested by a rise in GPT, GOT, GDH and AP or by impaired liver function). These pathological laboratory parameters are also reflected in cellular or canalicular forms of impairment. The treatment of primary kidney diseases (e. g. with immunosuppressives, cyclosporin) may give rise to liver damage, which can be ascertained morphologically and in laboratory investigations.

3.4.4 Secondary kidney diseases

In various diseases of the liver and biliary ducts, with or without jaundice, a wide range of secondary kidney diseases can occur. They differ greatly in their degree of severity and their prognosis and can cause considerable **difficulties** in the drawing up of a **differential diagnosis.** (49) (s. tab. 17.6)

Glomerular kidney diseases

1. Impaired renal function with acute viral hepatitis
2. Immune complex nephritis with chronic HBV and HCV infection
3. Glomerulosclerosis with cirrhosis
   - mesangial form
   - IgA nephropathy
   - membranous proliferative form

Tubular kidney diseases

1. Renal tubular acidosis
   - distal form (type I)
   - distal and proximal form (type II)
2. Acute tubular necrosis (acute kidney failure)
3. Biliary nephrosis

Tab. 17.6: Forms of secondary kidney damage in the course of hepatobiliary diseases

Mild renal dysfunction in the form of clinically non-significant proteinuria and erythrocyturia in acute viral hepatitis subsides once the acute viral hepatitis has been cured. Occasionally, serum creatinine levels may be slightly raised. Histologically, small deposits of immune complexes can be found in the glomeruli.

Immune complex nephritis is generally caused by the deposition of circulating immune complexes in the glomeruli, mostly in chronic viral hepatitis B and C (men are affected four times as often as women). Proteinuria and haematuria are in evidence, together with the retention of substances usually eliminated in the urine. A nephrotic syndrome possibly leading to renal insufficiency with hypertension may develop. Treatment of this perimembranous glomerulonephritis with interferon alpha has proved beneficial.

Glomerulosclerosis can be shown histologically in some 50—95% of patients with liver cirrhosis. The course of glomerulosclerosis may take *three different forms:* (*1.*) mesangial form with thickening of the mesangial matrix and basal membrane of the capillaries, (*2.*) glomerulosclerosis with glomerular deposition mainly of IgA (= IgA nephropathy), and (*3.*) membranous proliferous form with obvious cellular proliferation and additional glomerular deposition of IgA. As a rule, proteinuria and erythrocyturia are only minimal. Up to now, treatment has not been possible — and is usually not required. (s. tab. 17.6)

Renal tubular acidosis in liver cirrhosis is due to an inadequate concentration of sodium ions on the distal tubuli (type I). As a result, the secretion of hydrogen ions is reduced. This is attributed to cellular immune processes as well as to toxic effects such as copper or bile acids. (s. tab. 17.6)

Acute tubular necrosis can occur in the course of a hepatobiliary disease. In an aetiopathogenetical context, hypoxia, hypotension, nephrotoxins and so far undefined biochemical substances are deemed responsible. The outcome is a disruption in the reabsorption of sodium and water; the urine is less concentrated (isosthenuria). There is a greater excretion of sodium (>30 mEq/l) and of beta-2 microglobulin in the urine. Acute, yet in principle reversible renal failure can develop. Therapy thus consists of bridging the phase of insufficiency temporarily by dialysis.

Biliary nephrosis in its acute form reveals swellings of the tubular cells and bilirubin renal casts under histological investigation. This is due to elevated concentrations of bilirubin and bile acids in the serum. The kidneys show a marked sensitivity to oxygen deficiency, with the danger of acute kidney failure. That explains the relatively frequent occurrence of renal insufficiency in diseases of the extrahepatic bile ducts, in obstructive jaundice or following bile duct surgery. (s. tab. 17.6)

> **Hepatorenal syndrome:** After exclusion of these differential diagnostic possibilities in liver diseases with renal symptoms, the likely diagnosis is hepatorenal syndrome. In the case of a severe and protracted course, this functional impairment of the kidneys can progress to true, acute renal failure, even with tubular necrosis.

3.5 Prognosis

The prognosis of HRS, especially type 1, is poor with a **lethality rate** of 87—98%. The survival time amounts to 1.7—2.6 weeks. (19) Death results from acute renal failure or complications of cirrhosis, such as gastrointestinal bleeding or hepatic coma. Patients with HRS type II have a better prognosis (6—12 months). Spontaneous **reversibility** of the hepatorenal syndrome has been demonstrated following a decisive improvement in liver function — yet it can only be rarely expected (in 3—5% or 2—13% of cases). With the spontaneous regression of portal ascites, the impaired renal function is generally improved. Liver transplantation likewise led to a normalization of renal function (12, 28) — just as the kidneys of a patient with hepatorenal syndrome functioned normally again following transplantation into a patient with a healthy liver (M. H. KOPPEL et al., 1969). (5, 6, 11, 18, 19, 20, 39, 47, 55)

4 Prophylaxis and therapy

Prophylactic measures with regard to the hepatorenal syndrome are of decisive and vital importance. It must be borne in mind that the *water balance is extremely sensitive in cirrhotic patients*. The cause can almost always be found in an enormous iatrogenic intervention in the volumetric balance (aggressive diuresis, imbalance in the tapping of ascitic fluid, excessive restriction of fluid). For this reason, it is important to avoid all substances which could worsen renal function (e.g. nonsteroidal antirheumatics, aminoglycoside antibiotics) and all measures which could lead to a reduction in the effective plasma volume. Furthermore, care should be taken to apply the principles of prophylaxis and therapy for hepatic encephalopathy (s. p. 285) and ascites (s. p. 310). Spontaneous bacterial peritonitis should be treated at an early stage. (s. p. 309) • The most significant prophylaxis and therapy target is to decrease the tonus in the efferent vessel of the glomerule.

4.1 Maintaining homoeostasis

The *electrolyte balance* and *acid-base balance* should be restored in careful coordination with the renal function. In **hyponatraemia,** either the fluid intake should be reduced to 700—1,000 ml/day or a combination of a hypertonic salt solution (3%) and a loop diuretic should be administered intravenously. (s. p. 314) Likewise, an attempt can be made using a combination of diuretics and urea diuresis. Generally, sodium and water intake should be restricted. It is imperative to achieve an even volumetric balance, possibly supported by the cautious intake of fluid.

4.2 Improvement of liver function

To date, there is no effective therapy for the hepatorenal syndrome. Therapeutic possibilities are very limited due to the loss of function of two vital organs, liver and kidneys. The ideal goal would be to improve liver function, since clear improvement in the condition of the diseased liver has always preceded the reversibility of the hepatorenal syndrome. • Even if there is only a slight chance of improving liver function, certain biochemically justifiable and pharmacologically plausible procedures can indeed be implemented in serious cases of disease: (*1.*) *optimal nutrition*, (*2.*) *substitution measures* (e.g. multivitamins, trace elements, branched-chain amino acids, essential phospholipids), and (*3.*) *supportive therapy programme* (reducing endotoxinaemia by means of lactulose, influencing the synthesis of urea by means of ornithine aspartate, etc.). (5, 7, 9, 48, 57)

4.3 Conservative treatment

The overriding aim of therapy is to increase renal blood flow. This can be achieved either indirectly through splanchnic vasoconstriction or directly by encouraging renal vasodilation. Hereby, certain problems arise concerning substances which spill over into the splanchnic circulation, causing splanchnic vasoconstriction and at the same time exacerbating the renal vasoconstriction already present. (5–7, 10, 18, 20, 30, 38, 47, 55, 57)

Many investigations have focused on the efficacy of conservative treatment for improving both systemic and renal haemodynamics or for suppressing the activated hormone systems. • The complexity of the pathogenesis of the hepatorenal syndrome, which varies in each individual case, explains the differences in impact of the substances used. For this reason, there are pathogenetic grounds for the simultaneous application of the pharmacological possibilities mentioned.

Optimal **fluid management** is necessary. Fluid overload must be avoided. Measurement of the central venous pressure is important.

Attempts at treatment through **"head-out" water immersion** (M. Epstein et al., 1976) can be deemed relatively effective and, above all, low in risk, provided such a measure is feasible with a seriously ill patient. This simple method increases the central blood volume (= redirecting extracellular fluid to the vascular system). There is a significant rise in the volume of the urine and in natriuresis – although one must also reckon with a number of non-responders when applying this method.

A **lumbar blockade** of the sympathetic nervous system is a methodologically simple procedure, practically free from complications, which has proved to be effective in individual cases. (53)

Intravenous application of sodium-free **albumin** and/or 10% **mannitol** can be successful, possibly with the additional administration of low-dose *diuretics* (such as xipamide, torasemide), whereby due attention should be paid to renal function. Diuretics or aldosterone antagonists may only be used if the indication is precise and all risks have been considered.

Thought can be given to i.v. application of low-dosed **dopamine** (100 mg/12 hr or <5 μg/kg BW/hr). This vasodilator was able to improve the angiographic appearance of the renal cortical vasculature and the cortical blood flow. No change was seen in GFR or urine output. Dopamine alone cannot be recommended. (quot. 6, 21, 38)

Ornipressin is a vasopressin analogue that primarily leads to vasoconstriction of the splanchnic vasculature. The first report outlining its use was compiled in 1985 by K. Lenz et al. (33) Dosage was 25 IU/12 hr or 6 IU/4 hr. The outcome was a fall in renal vascular resistance and an improvement in the glomerular filtration rate.

(21; quot. 6, 10, 38) • The combined administration of *ornipressin* (2–6 IU/hr) and *albumin* (20–60 g/day) for a period of two weeks (with intensive care monitoring!) has led to remarkable therapeutic success. (22)

Terlipressin (2 mg/day, multiple doses) was likewise successfully administered over a temporary period. No side effects were reported. Terlipressin produced an improvement of renal function in 70–75% of cases and an increased survival in patients with type 1 HRS. (2, 11, 38, 52) • *Terlipressin* (0.5–2.0 mg/4 hr, i.v.) plus *albumin* (20–40 g/day) (18, 54) or plus *hydroxyethyl starch* (500 ml/day) appears to be an effective form of treatment for HRS. (15)

The combined application of **midodrine** and **octreotide** (i. e. an α-adrenergic agonist as a vasoconstrictor plus a substance inhibiting the release of endogenous vasodilators such as glucagon) led to an improvement in both GFR and natriuresis. (3)

Therapeutic attempts using **angiotensin II / noradrenalin** (first described by R. Ames et al. in 1965) or ACE inhibitors, sympathicomimetic agents and α- as well as β-receptor blockers yielded no (or only brief) success. • The combined i.v. application of noradrenalin (0.5–3.0 mg/day) plus albumin and furosemide shows a remarkable improvement in type 1 HRS. (13)

A therapeutic effect has been achieved by administering **N-acetylcysteine** (150 mg/kg BW for 2 hours and subsequently 100 mg/kg BW for 5 days). (27)

Likewise, reports have been published on the positive effect of **misoprostol**, a synthetic prostaglandin$_{E1}$, after oral administration (4 × 0.4 mg/day) (16) or with intra-arterial application.

A few isolated reports are available on the elimination of renal vasoconstriction, particularly using **ANP** (atrial natriuretic peptide) with its pronounced diuretic and natriuretic effects.

Treatment with **branched-chain amino acids** led to a reduction in azotaemia and creatinine as well as an increase in natriuresis. (9)

4.4 Invasive therapy

The infaust prognosis of the hepatorenal syndrome and the short space of time preceding its fatal outcome not only call for the swift and concurrent use of multiple conservative measures, but also make invasive therapy worth considering. Here, too, any decision with regard to therapy must initially focus on the clinical difficulties relating to the respective underlying disease.

Haemodialysis may be indicated after the condition has passed from functional renal failure to true renal insufficiency. Discussion should also centre on dialysis as a possible way to bridge the phase of renal insufficiency or to gain time for the liver function to improve and allow the hepatorenal syndrome to become reversible. (29) • **Peritoneal dialysis** achieved temporary success in treating azotaemia and hyponatraemia, but the lethality rate could not be reduced. Nevertheless, some cases of successful treatment were observed. (43)

PVS: There are many reports on experience made with peritoneovenous shunts (s. p. 317), the positive tenor of which justifies its incorporation when planning therapy for the hepatorenal syndrome with marked ascites. (14, 17, 29, 41)

TIPS: In its function as a portacaval side-to-side shunt (s. pp 267, 320, 899), TIPS has also proved to be successful in the treatment of HRS. The survival rate after 18 months was 35%, whereas only 10% of non-shunted patients survived 3 months. (8) However, patients with type I HRS and those with bilirubin levels of 15 mg/dl or higher as well as patients with a Child-Turcotte-Pugh score greater than 12 have a low response rate to TIPS and a high mortality rate.

MARS: A new therapeutic option that could improve renal function and prolong survival, especially in risk patients to TIPS, can be found in the molecular adsorbent recirculating system (MARS). It represents a cell-free liver dialysis technique and enables the selective removal of albumin-bound substances using an albumin-enriched dialysate fluid. Significant improvements for different biochemical and clinical parameters as well as a 30-day prolongation of survival were reported. (35) (s. p. 390)

Portacaval shunt: In some cases, the placement of a portacaval shunt (side-to-side) resulted in the restoration of normal renal function. (50, 51)

Liver transplantation: Where the hepatorenal syndrome occurs, consideration should understandably be given to liver transplantation in view of increasing liver insufficiency. (s. p. 903) With suitable cases, this intervention proved efficacious. (12, 20, 28, 32) In severe forms of HRS and with inadequate response to conservative therapy, the indication for liver transplantation should be reviewed without further delay. The feasibility of surgical intervention will largely depend on whether the phase of hepatic and renal insufficiency can be bridged — with as favourable clinical findings as possible and perhaps supported by suitable invasive measures — until transplantation is carried out. Three-year and four-year survival rates were both given as 65.7%. (20)

Support systems: Artificial renal and liver support systems may also be considered in order to bridge the period of time until liver transplantation is performed. (1)

References:

1. Alarabi, A.A., Danielson, B.G., Wikström, B., Kreuger, A., Tufveson, G.: Artificial renal and liver support in a severe hepatorenal syndrome of childhood. Acta Paediatr. 1992; 81: 75–78
2. Alessandra, C., Debernardi-Venon, W., Marzano, A., Barletti, C., Fadda, M., Rizzetto, M.: Renal failure in cirrhotic patients: role of terlipressin in clinical approach to hepatorenal syndrome type 2. Eur. J. Gastroenterol. Hepatol. 2002; 14: 1363–1368
3. Angeli, P., Volpin, R., Gerunda, G., Craighero, R., Roner, P., Merenda, R., Amodio, P., Sticca, A., Caregaro, L., Maffei-Faccioli, A., Gatta, A.: Reversal of type I hepatorenal syndrome with the administration of midodrine and octreotide. Hepatology 1999; 29: 1690–1697
4. Arroyo, V., Gines, P., Gerbes, A.L., Dudley, F.J., Gentilini, P., Laffi, G., Reynolds, T.B., Ring-Larsen, H., Schölmerich, J.: Definition and diagnostic criteria of refractory ascites and hepatorenal syndrome in cirrhosis. Hepatology 1996; 23: 164–176
5. Badalamenti, S., Graziani, G., Salerno, F., Ponticelli, C.: Hepatorenal syndrome. New perspectives in pathogenesis and treatment. Arch. Intern. Med. 1993; 153: 1957–1967
6. Bataller, R., Gines, P., Arroyo, V., Rodes, J.: Hepatorenal syndrome. Clin. Liver Dis. 2000; 4: 487–507
7. Biecker, E., Brensing, K.-A., Perz, J., Woitas, R., Sauerbruch, T.: Therapie des hepatorenalen Syndroms bei Leberzirrhose. Dtsch. Med. Wschr. 1999; 124: 1039–1042
8. Brensing, K.-A., Textor, J., Perz, J., Schiedermaier, P., Raab, P., Strunk, H., Klehr, H.U., Kramer, H.J., Spengler, U., Schild, H., Sauerbruch, T.: Long-term otcome after transjugular intrahepatic portosystemic stent-shunt in non-transplant cirrhotics with hepatorenal syndrome: a phase II study. Gut 2000; 47: 288–295
9. Cacciafesta, M., Bonavita, M.S., Ferri, C., Piccirillo, G., Ettorre, E., Marigliano, V., Santucci, A., Balsano, F.: A new therapeutic approach to hepatorenal syndrome. Curr. Therap. Res. 1991; 50: 888–895
10. Chutaputti, A.: Management of refractory ascites and hepatorenal syndrome (review). J. Gastroenterol. Hepatol. 2002; 17: 456–461
11. Colle, I., Durand, F., Pessione, F., Rassiat, E., Bernuau, E., Barriere, E., Lebrec, D., Valla, D.C., Moreau, R.: Clinical course, predictive factors and prognosis in patients with cirrhosis and type 1 hepatorenal syndrome treated with terlipressin: a retrospective analysis. J. Gastroenterol. Hepatol. 2002; 17: 882–888
12. Detroz, B., Honore, P., Monami, B., Meurisse, M., Canivet, J.L., Legrand, M., Damas, P., Jacquet, N.: Combined treatment of liver failure and hepatorenal snydrome with orthotopic liver transplantation. Acta Gastro-Enterol. Belg. 1992; 55: 350–357
13. Duvoux, C., Zanditenas, D., Hezode, C., Chauvat, A., Monin, J.L., Roudot-Thoraval, F., Mallat, A., Dhumeaux, D.: Effects of noradrenalin and albumin in patients with type 1 hepatorenal syndrome: a pilot study. Hepatology 2002; 36: 374–380
14. Epstein, M.: Peritoneovenous shunt in the management of ascites and the hepatorenal syndrome. Gastroenterology 1982; 82: 790–799
15. Fabrizi, F., Dixit, V., Martin, P.: Meta-analysis: Terlipressin therapy for the hepatorenal syndrome. Aliment Pharm. Ther. 2006; 24: 935–944
16. Fevery, J., van Cutsem, E., Nevens, F., van Steenbergen, W., Verberckmoes, R., de Groote, J.: Reversal of hepatorenal syndrome in four patients by peroral misoprostol (prostaglandin E1 analogue) and albumin administration. J. Hepatol. 1990; 11: 153–158
17. Fullen, W.D.: Hepatorenal syndrome: reversal by peritoneovenous shunt. Surgery 1977; 82: 337–341
18. Gentilini, P., Vizzutti, F., Gentilini, A., Zipoli, M., Foschi, M., Romanelli, R.G.: Update on ascites and hepatorenal syndrome. Dig. Liver Dis. 2002; 34: 592–605
19. Gines, A., Escorsell, A., Gines, P., Salo, J., Jimenez, W., Inglada, L., Navasa, M., Claria, J., Rimola, A., Arroyo, V., Rodes, J.: Incidence, predictive factors, and prognosis of the hepatorenal syndrome in cirrhosis with ascites. Gastroenterology 1993; 105: 229–236
20. Gonwa, T.A., Morris, C.A., Goldstein, R.M., Husberg, B.S., Klintmalm, G.B.: Long-term survival and renal function following liver transplantation in patients with and without hepatorenal syndrome – experience in 300 patients. Transplantation 1991; 51: 428–430
21. Gülberg, V., Bilzer, M., Gerbes, A.L.: Long-term therapy and retreatment of hepatorenal syndrome type I with ornipressin and dopamine. Hepatology 1999; 30: 870–875
22. Guevara, M., Gines, P.: Hepatorenal syndrome. Dig. Dis. 2005; 23: 47–55
23. Gupta, S., Morgan, T.R., Gordan, G.S.: Calcitonin generelated peptide in hepatorenal syndrome. A possible mediator of peripheral vasodilation? J. Clin. Gastroenterol. 1992; 14: 122–126
24. Hecker, R., Sherlock, S.: Electrolyte and circulatory changes in terminal liver failure. Lancet 1956; II/1221–1225
25. Helwig, F.C., Schutz, C.B.: A liver kidney syndrome. Clinical, pathological and experimental studies. Surg. Gynecol. Obstetr. 1932; 55: 570–580
26. Henriksen, J.H., Ring-Larsen, H.: Hepatorenal disorders: role of the sympathetic nervous system. Semin. Liver Dis. 1994; 14: 35–43
27. Holt, S., Goodier, D., Marley, R., Patch, D., Burroughs, A., Fernando, B., Harry, D., Moore, K.: Improvement in renal function in hepatorenal syndrome with N-acetylcysteine. Lancet 1999; 353: 294–295
28. Iwatsuki, S., Popovtzer, M.M., Corman, J.L., Ishikawa, M., Putnam, C.W., Katz, F.H., Starzl, T.E.: Recovery from "hepatorenal syndrome" after orthotopic liver transplantation. New Engl. J. Med. 1973; 289: 1155–1159

29. Kearns, P.J., Polhemus, R.J., Oakes, D., Rabkin, R.: Hepatorenal syndrome managed with hemodialysis, then reversed by peritoneovenous shunting. J. Clin. Gastroenterol. 1985; 7: 341–343
30. Lang, F., Gerok, W., Häussinger, D.: New clues to the pathophysiology of hepatorenal failure. Clin. Invest. 1993; 71: 93–97
31. Lazinik, H.: Das hepatorenale Syndrom bei Virushepatitis. Med. Welt 1980; 31: 1596–1598
32. Le Moine, O.: Hepatorenal syndrome-outcome after liver transplantation. Nephrol. Dialys. Transplant. 1998; 13: 20–22
33. Lenz, K., Hörtnagl, H., Druml, W., Reither, H., Schmid, R., Schneeweiss, B., Laggner, A., Grimm, G., Gerbes, A.L.: Ornipressin in the treatment of functional renal failure in decompensated liver cirrhosis. Effects on renal hemodynamics and atrial natriuretic factor. Gastroenterology 1991; 101: 1060–1067
34. Mas, A., Arroyo, V., Rodes, J., Bosch, J.: Ascites and renal failure in primary liver cell carcinoma. Brit. Med. J. 1975; 3: 629
35. Mitzner, St.R., Stange, R., Klammt, S., Risler, T., Erley, C.M., Bader, B.D., Berger, E.D., Lauchart, W., Peszynski, P., Freytag, J., Hickstein, H., Loock, J., Löhr, J.-M., Liebe, St., Emmerich, J., Korten, G., Schmidt, R.: Improvement of hepatorenal syndrome with extracorporeal albumin dialysis MARS: results of a prospective, randomized, controlled clinical trial. Liver Transplant. 2000; 6: 277–286
36. Moore, K., Wendon, J., Frazer, M., Karani, J., Williams, R., Badr, K.: Plasma endothelin immunoreactivity in liver disease and the hepatorenal syndrome. New Engl. J. Med. 1992; 327: 1774–1778
37. Moore, K.P., Taylor, G.W., Maltby, N.H., Siegers, D., Fuller, R.W., Dollery, C.T., Williams, R.: Increased production of cysteinyl leukotrienes in hepatorenal syndrome. J. Hepatol. 1990; 11: 263–271
38. Moreau, R.: Hepatorenal syndrome in patients with cirrhosis. J. Gastroenterol. Hepatol. 2002; 17: 739–747
39. Nonnenbruch, W.: Das hepatorenale Syndrom. Verh. Dtsch. Ges. Inn. Med. 1939; 51: 341–358
40. Phillips, A.O., Thomas, D.M., Coles, G.A.: Acute renal failure associated with non-fulminant hepatitis A. Clin. Nephrol. 1993; 39: 156–157
41. Pladson, T.R., Parrish, R.M.: Hepatorenal syndrome: recovery after peritoneovenous shunt. Arch. Intern. Med. 1977; 137: 1248–1249
42. Platt, J.F., Ellis, J.H., Rubin, J.M., Merion, R.M., Lucey, M.R.: Renal duplex Doppler ultrasonography: a noninvasive predictor of kidney dysfunction and hepatorenal failure in liver disease. Hepatology 1994; 20: 362–369
43. Poulos, A.M., Howard, L., Eisele, G., Rodgers, J.B.: Peritoneal dialysis therapy for patients with liver and renal failure with ascites. Amer. J. Gastroenterol. 1993; 88: 109–112
44. Richardière: Sur un cas d'ictère grave à forme rènale. Sem. Méd. 1890; 10: 401–402
45. Rosansky, S.J., Mullens, C.C.: The hepatorenal syndrome associated with metastatic angiosarcoma of the gallbladder. Ann. Intern. Med. 1982; 96: 191–192
46. Ruiz-del-Arbol, L., Monescillo, A., Arocena, C., Valer, P., Gines, P., Moreira, V., Milicua, J. M., Jimenez, W., Arroyo, V.: Circulatory function and hepatorenal syndrome in cirrhosis. Hepatology 2005; 42: 439–447
47. Sandhu, B. S., Sanyal, A. J.: Hepatorenal syndrome. Curr. Treat. Opin. Gastroenterol. 2005; 8: 443–450
48. Schelling, J.R., Linas, St.L.: Hepatorenal syndrome. Semin. Nephrol. 1990; 10: 565–570
49. Shear, L., Kleinerman, J., Gabuzda, G.J.: Renal failure in patients with cirrhosis of the liver. I. Clinical and pathological characteristics. Amer. J. Med. 1965; 39: 184–198
50. Schroeder, E.T., Anderson, G.H. jr., Smulyan, H.: Effects of a portocaval or peritoneovenous shunt on renin in the hepatorenal syndrome. Kidney Int. 1979; 15: 54–61
51. Schroeder, E.T., Numann, P.J., Chamberlain, B.E.: Functional renal failure in cirrhosis. Recovery after portocaval shunt. Ann. Intern. Med. 1970; 72: 923–928
52. Solanki, P., Chawla, A., Garg, R., Gupta, R., Jaim, M., Sarin, S.K.: Beneficial effects of terlipressin in hepatorenal syndrome: A prospective randomized placebo-controlled clinical trial. J. Gastroenterol. Hepatol. 2003; 18: 152–156
53. Solis-Herruzo, J.A., Duran, A., Favela, V., Castellano, G., Madrid, J.L., Munoz-Yague, M.T., Morillas, J.D., Estenoz, J.: Effects of lumbar sympathetic bloc on kidney function in cirrhotic patients with hepatorenal syndrome. J. Hepatol. 1987; 5: 167–173
54. Uriz, J., Gines, P., Cardenas, A., Sort, P., Jimenez, W., Salmeron, J.M., Bataller, R., Mas, A., Navasa, M., Arroyo, V., Rodes, J.: Terlipressin plus albumin infusion: an effective and safe therapy of hepatorenal syndrome. J. Hepatol. 2000; 33: 43–48
55. Watt, K., Uhanova, J., Minuk, G.Y.: Hepatorenal syndrome: diagnostic accuracy, clinical features, and outcome in a tertiary care center. Amer. J. Gastroenterol. 2002; 97: 2046–2050
56. Wong, P.Y., Talamo, R.C., Williams, G.H.: Kallikrein-kinin and renin-angiotensin systems in functional renal failure of cirrhosis of the liver. Gastroenterology 1977; 73: 1114–1118
57. Wong, F., Blendis, L.: New challenge of hepatorenal syndrome: prevention and treatment. Hepatology 2001; 34: 1242–1251
58. Zipser, R.D., Radvan, G.H., Kronborg, I.J., Duke, R., Little, T.E.: Urinary thromboxane B_2 and prostaglandin E_2 in the hepatorenal syndrome: evidence for increased vasoconstrictor and decreased vasodilator factors. Gastroenterology 1983; 84: 697–703

Symptoms and Syndromes
18 Hepatopulmonary syndrome

		Page:
1	*Definition*	340
2	*Epidemiology*	340
3	**Causes and pathogenesis**	340
3.1	Vasodilation	340
3.2	Shunt formations	341
3.3	Impairment in diffusion and perfusion	341
3.4	Ventilation-perfusion distribution disorder	342
4	**Clinical aspects**	342
5	*Hypertrophic osteoarthropathy*	342
6	**Therapy**	343
7	**Portopulmonary hypertension**	343
7.1	Definition, morphology and diagnosis	343
7.2	Endothelin and ET-receptor antagonist	344
7.3	Prognosis and therapy	344
	• References (1–77)	345
	(Figure 18.1; tables 18.1–18.3)	

18 Hepatopulmonary syndrome

▶ Recognition of a hepatopulmonary syndrome goes back over one hundred years (1884) to the detection of the **triad**: *cyanosis*, *clubbed fingers* and *liver cirrhosis*. (18). The same constellation of findings was described by A. GILBERT et al. in 1895 in juvenile patients suffering from hypertrophic biliary cirrhosis. • Reports on **hypertrophic osteoarthropathy** were published by A. A. HIJMANS VAN DEN BERGH in 1901. • A. M. SNELL detected **hypoxaemia** in chronic liver patients for the first time in 1935. (52) A right shift of the dissociation curve of oxyhaemoglobin was ascertained by A. KEYS et al. in 1938. In the course of acute progressive liver failure, R. RYDELL et al. (1956) also observed hypoxaemia; at autopsy, this patient showed intrapulmonary **arteriovenous shunts**. (45) Since then, there have been many reports on the detection of arteriovenous anastomoses in the lungs (further details in references 6, 7, 23). These arteriovenous shunts had already been attributed to vasoactive substances. The development of clubbed fingers was deemed to be the result of arteriovenous anastomoses in the tips of the fingers and the impact of reduced ferritin. (35, 53) • The term **hepatopulmonary syndrome** was used by T.C. KENNEDY et al. (1977) (26) and likewise by L.S. ERIKSON et al. (1989) to describe the correlation between hypoxaemia and liver cirrhosis.

1 Definition

The hepatopulmonary syndrome (HPS) is defined as a disorder in pulmonary gas exchange (= mismatch of ventilation and perfusion) due to intrapulmonary vasodilations (= reduction of pulmonary vascular resistance) in cases of chronic liver disease or acute liver failure. • Other criteria must also be met: (*1.*) ruling out of underlying pulmonary or cardiac disease, (*2.*) increase in the alveolar-capillary oxygen gradient (>20 mm Hg) without or with hypoxaemia (<70 mm Hg partial oxygen tension) with a clear drop of the O_2 value when changing from the supine to the upright body position, and (*3.*) detection of intrapulmonary vasodilations and/or a.-v. shunts.

2 Epidemiology

Hypoxaemia (p_aO_2 < 70 mm Hg) is found in 45–69% of patients suffering from cirrhosis or liver insufficiency. Only rarely has severe hypoxaemia been demonstrated (p_aO_2 < 50 mm Hg). (6, 31, 55, 58) • Intrapulmonary vasodilations could be ascertained in 13–47% of liver transplant candidates. (25) In about 50% of cirrhotic patients, a decline in the diffusion capacity for carbon monoxide was detected. (22) Some 30% of cases showed no (physiological) reduction in pulmonary vasoconstriction in hypoxia. The prevalence of HPS in cirrhosis varies between 4% and 19%. It occurs more frequently in patients with cirrhosis than with extrahepatic portal venous obstruction. (5, 20, 47)

3 Causes and pathogenesis

In theory, there are **three causes** of HPS (since hypoventilation is not deemed a possible cause): (*1.*) arteriovenous shunts, (*2.*) disturbed alveolocapillary oxygen diffusion in terms of impaired diffusion-perfusion, and (*3.*) mismatches between ventilation and perfusion. Consequently, there are numerous liver diseases which can be associated with HPS. (s. tab. 18.1)

Acute viral hepatitis (17, 40)	Liver cirrhosis
α_1-antitrypsin deficiency	Nodular regenerative
Biliary atresia	hyperplasia (9)
Budd-Chiari syndrome (13)	Peliosis hepatis (8)
Chronic active hepatitis (54)	Postsurgical shunt (21)
Chronic hepatic allograft rejection	Primary biliary cirrhosis
	Schistosomiasis
Congenital cystic fibrosis (19)	Tyrosinaemia
Fulminant liver failure (57)	Wilson's disease
Inf. vena cava obstruction (12)	

Tab. 18.1: Liver diseases associated with the hepatopulmonary syndrome (with some references). • Portal hypertension is considered to be an essential factor in the pathogenesis of HPS.

The existence of *portal hypertension* is probably the decisive factor in the development of HPS. The pathophysiological principles of HPS and the change in haemodynamics in cirrhotic patients were presented as a review in 1973. (6) A marked *pulmonary vasodilation* due to vasodilative substances is deemed to be the essential causative factor of HPS (K. R. REISMANN, 1956).

3.1 Vasodilation

Endotoxin is capable of inducing nitric oxide synthetases in the vascular endothelia of the liver and lung. *Nitric oxide* (NO) is a powerful **vasodilator** (through activation of guanylate cyclase) and is identical to the endothelium-derived relaxing factor (EDRF). An increase in NO in the vascular endothelia of cirrhotic patients is deemed to be one of the causative factors in the development of a hyperdynamic circulatory condition (= lower peripheral resistance), yet also of the hepatopulmonary syndrome (= lower pulmonary vascular resistance). NO concentration is increased in the expired air of patients with HPS. (5, 11) Animal experiments likewise suggested endothelial nitric oxide synthetase as being another causative factor. (16) In the same way, elevated values of glucagon, histamine, VIP, prostacyclin, calcitonin, substance P, atrial natriuretic factor and platelet-activating factor are considered to be vasodilators in the pulmonary vascular system. • Animal models of HPS showed that an increase of ET-1 production in

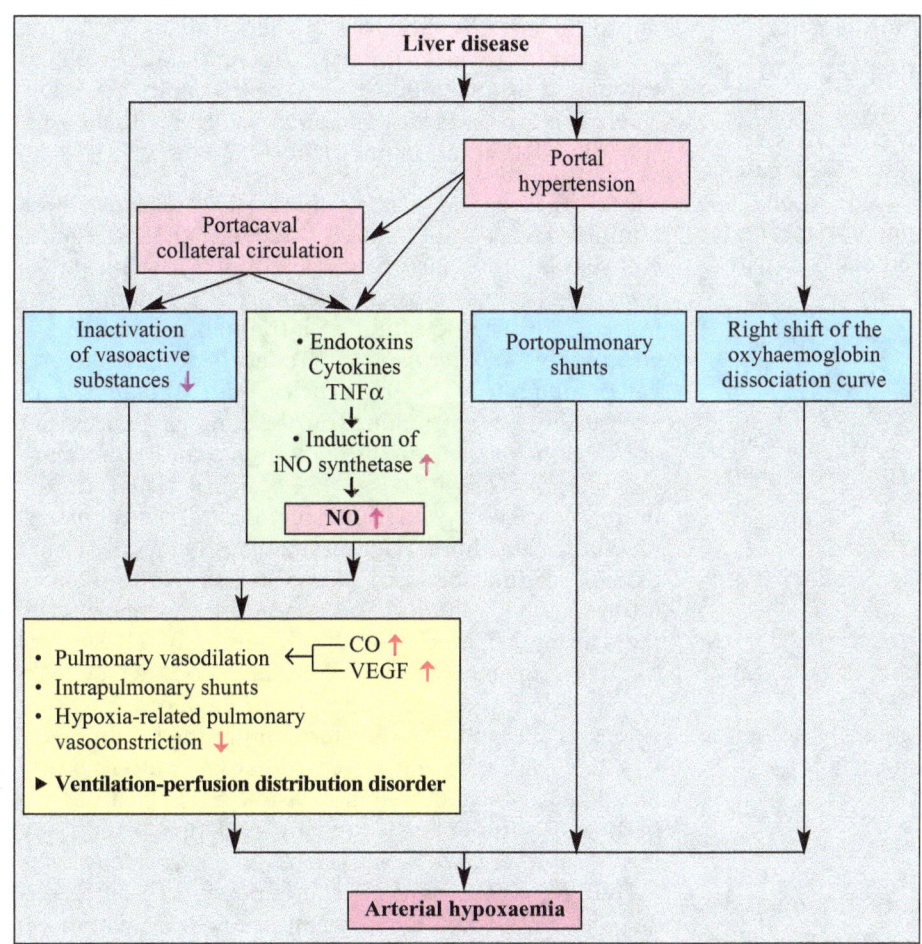

Fig. 18.1: Possible mechanisms in the pathogenesis of the hepatopulmonary syndrome. (VEGF = vascular endothelial growth factor, iNOS = inducible nitric oxide synthetase, TNF = tumour necrosis factor)

the liver correlates with both pulmonary nitric oxide synthase levels and pulmonary dysfunction. (5, 37, 59) In patients with liver cirrhosis, a markedly increased serum value of the vasoconstrictor ET-1 was demonstrated. Therefore it may be assumed that pronounced endothelinaemia leads to a modulation of NO production, which results in extensive intrapulmonary vasodilation.
• *In cirrhosis, a decrease in the pulmonary vascular resistance with formation of intrapulmonary shunts occurs more frequently than pulmonary hypertension; the reason for these different modes of reaction is unknown.*

3.2 Shunt formations

The assumption that **a.-v. shunts** play a causative role in HPS is founded on (*1.*) the presence of very small intrapulmonary a.-v. shunts in the lung parenchyma and on the pleura (= *pleural spider naevi*) at autopsy (7), (*2.*) dilation of the capillary and precapillary intrapulmonary vessels, particularly in the basal lung region, and (as a very rare finding) (*3.*) isolated links detected between the branches of the portal vein and the pulmonary vessels. • These a.-v. anastomoses are mainly **functional shunts.** They are found in about 50% of cirrhotic patients. Given a normal width of the lung capillaries (8–15 μm), precapillary vascular dilations can attain a diameter of 15–150 (–500) μm. This is reversible. HPS (probably only type 1) can therefore completely recede after liver transplantation – analogous to the hepatorenal syndrome. It remains uncertain, however, whether the vascular changes imply dilated capillaries or opened a.-v. anastomoses. • **Anatomic shunts,** which may be intrapulmonary and portopulmonary as well as pleural, are rare. In terms of haemodynamics, they have no noteworthy effect. (5, 9, 23, 24, 33, 44, 56, 57) (s. fig. 18.1)

3.3 Impairment in diffusion and perfusion

The pathogenesis of HPS has not yet been fully clarified. Presumably, however, substances with vasodilator activity can bypass the liver through collateral vessels, thus effecting vasodilation of the pulmonary vessels. There is oxygen desaturation of the erythrocytes flowing centrally through the dilated vessels (= increased distance from vessel wall to vessel centre). Moreover, insufficient oxygen saturation of the erythrocytes is induced by a hyperdynamic circulatory state (= reduced blood-oxygen contact time) – giving rise to a **diffusion-perfusion defect.** As a result, inadequately oxygenated or non-arterialized blood reaches the pulmonary veins, leading to hypoxaemia. (22, 58) (s. fig. 18.1)

3.4 Ventilation-perfusion distribution disorder

In poorly ventilated lung areas, perfusion is diminished (= *von Euler-Liljestrand reflex*). This reflex is impaired in liver cirrhosis. The decrease in or loss of hypoxia-induced pulmonary vasoconstriction leads to the greater perfusion of poorly ventilated lung areas; this results in an increase in the intrapulmonary shunt volume and thus in a ventilation-perfusion distribution disorder with hypoxaemia. (15, 22, 31, 33, 56, 58) (s. fig. 18.1)

A particular pathophysiological finding with HPS is a **right shift of the oxyhaemoglobin dissociation curve.** The cause of this diminished affinity of haemoglobin for oxygen is assumed to be the greater concentration of 2,3-diphosphoglycerate found in erythrocytes. This results in arterial hypoxaemia.

4 Clinical aspects

In most HPS patients, pulmonary discomfort or findings generally remain absent for a long period; the p_aO_2 is still within the normal range (>80 mm Hg). Some patients, however, display *dyspnoea* at an early stage.

HPS becomes manifest three to seven years after the development of portacaval and/or splenorenal collateral vessels. In a more or less rapidly progressing course of disease, *cyanosis* develops with even more pronounced *hypoxaemia* (p_aO_2 < 70 mm Hg). Both hypoxaemia and dyspnoea generally worsen in an upright position (see below) due to increased cardiac output with shortened pulmonary transit time. Patients with distinct *spider naevi* show more severe pulmonary disorders than those where this skin stigma of liver disease is absent or only developed to a minor degree. Frequently, signs of respiratory *alkalosis* due to hyperventilation are found. There is a decreased diffusing capacity for CO_2. • Some 85–90% of HPS patients show *platypnoea* (= clear improvement of dyspnoea when the body position is changed from the vertical to the horizontal) and/or *orthodeoxia* (= decrease in p_aO_2 of >3 mm Hg upon assuming an upright body position); it is usually accompanied by aggravated dyspnoea. (42) Orthodeoxia is diagnosed by blood gas analysis or pulse oximetry in both the recumbent and the standing position. The cause of platypnoea and orthodeoxia is the reinforced perfusion of the dilated pulmonary vessels in the poorly ventilated basal lung areas in an upright body position. This leads to a rise in shunt volume and hence to a deterioration of the ventilation-perfusion disorder. • *Hour-glass nails* and *drumstick fingers* are frequently observed. (s. fig. 4.19) • There might even be a connection with the formation of *oesophageal varices*. (10) • Patients with functional shunts and impaired diffusion and perfusion present significantly better values regarding the arterial O_2 partial pressure upon *inspiration of 100% O_2*; patients with anatomic shunts show no improvement. • Tachycardia, higher cardiac output and lower values of mean arterial pressure and peripheral vascular resistance point to a *hyperdynamic circulation*. There is always a risk of *bacterial infection* with a corresponding deterioration in prognosis. (6, 9, 20, 27, 33, 38, 47)

The *ECG* is regular. The *chest radiograph* usually shows reinforced basal, interstitial vascular markings (bilateral, basilar, nodular or reticulonodular opacities). (36) *Spirography* yields normal volumes and expiratory resistance. (32) • The detection of intrapulmonary shunts is effected by *scintigraphy* (^{99m}Tc-labelled macro-aggregated albumin). Tracer particles with a diameter of 20–60 μm are not retained in the lung capillaries, but are directly passed on through shunts and pulmonary vasodilations (positive = >3–6 heart beats) to the brain, liver, kidney and other organs. (2, 38) • By means of contrast-medium *echocardiography* (generally using oxypolygelatine solution), it is also possible to identify intrapulmonary shunts. This procedure is deemed to be the screening method for the diagnosis of HPS, prior to the occurrence of alterations in blood gas. (3, 38) • *Angiography* produces normal or reduced pressure values in the pulmonary artery, diminished pulmonary vascular resistance and increased cardiac output; a net-like dilated vascular system is visible. • The ventilation-perfusion status in the lung can be defined exactly by means of the *multiple inert gas elimination technique* (MIGET). At the same time, it is possible to differentiate between intrapulmonary shunts and vasodilations.

One can differentiate between **two distinct patterns** of HPS, whereby type 2 is only very rarely detectable (49):

Type 1: Using angiography, minor to pronounced vasodilations of speckled or sponge-like appearance may be demonstrated. Additionally, spider-like vascular ramifications are identifiable. Depending on the extent of the vasodilations, marked or only slight improvement in hypoxaemia is observed in patients following administration of 100% oxygen. Liver transplantation is the most successful approach in the treatment of type 1. With a good response to the administration of 100% oxygen, regression of HPS is to be expected after OLT.

Type 2: As a rule, only slight vascular changes resembling a.-v. shunts or vascular malformations are identified using angiography. No hypervascularization is found. There is no real improvement in hypoxaemia following administration of 100% oxygen. Liver transplantation is often unsuccessful regarding HPS. • In the individual case, embolization may be indicated.

5 Hypertrophic osteoarthropathy

Hypertrophic osteoarthropathy (hour-glass nails, clubbed fingers) (s. fig. 4.19), which has been known since 1884, is not caused by hypoxia, as has been assumed up to now. (18) The cause is to be found in the intrapulmonary arteriovenous shunts: from the venous limb of the pulmonary vessels, megakaryocytes and thrombocyte aggregates pass directly through the shunts into the arterial limb and hence (unfiltered, uncatabolized or not inactivated) into the circulation. These (and possibly other) substances are deposited in the acra; they effect the release of the platelet-derived growth factor. The PDGF induces nail bed oedema (= *hour-glass nails*) and an increase in collagen synthesis by activating the fibroblasts (= *drumstick fingers*). (14, 35, 53)

6 Therapy

Up to now, there is no satisfactory drug therapy for HPS available. Spontaneous improvement of HPS after recovery from an underlying liver disease has been reported. Often HPS has deteriorated despite stable liver function. Improvements in HPS with the help of various substances, for which a certain therapeutic effect was considered plausible, were only achieved in individual cases and for just a limited time. (27, 33, 38)

▶ By administering *100% oxygen* (as long-term oxygen therapy), a higher and nearly normal partial oxygen pressure can be achieved in the dilated pulmonary vessels (albeit only in some of the patients and just temporarily). • Intravenous application of *prostaglandin F_{2a}* has produced some improvement in hypoxaemia. With the help of *antibiotic therapy* (e.g. norfloxacin), which led to a reduction in bacterial endotoxins in the intestines, it was possible to improve the arterial hypoxaemia considerably. (4) *Indomethacin*, or a combination of indomethacin and PGF (51), has likewise been effective. By administering *allium sativum* (garlic) for a period of several months, a significant improvement in arterial O_2 saturation could be achieved. (1) Only isolated cases involving treatment with *methylene blue* (= inhibitor of NO-related guanylate cyclase) have been reported. (43, 46) In HPS due to multifocal nodular hyperplasia, *glucocorticoids* and *cyclophosphamides* have been successful. (9) *Somatostatin antagonist*, *NO antagonist* and *almitrine bimesylate* have proved ineffective.

▶ *Implantation of a TIPS* has brought about a clear improvement in cases of hypoxaemia, probably due to a decrease in endotoxinaemia and the resulting reduction in the formation of nitric oxide. There was a rise in pulmonary perfusion together with a marked decrease in pulmonary vascular resistance. Consequently, placement of a TIPS would serve to bridge the period of time until a liver transplantation can be carried out. (30, 33, 41, 50)

Liver transplantation: Like the hepatorenal syndrome (s. p. 336), HPS (probably only type 1) is, in principle, reversible after transplantation of the liver. The postoperative prognosis depends on the severity of hypoxaemia prior to transplantation (postoperative lethality is < 5% if preoperative hypoxaemia is > 50 mm Hg). An increase in arterial pO_2 when the patient is inhaling 100% O_2 in a horizontal position is a good prognostic sign for transplantation. It was possible to demonstrate improvement and normalization regarding arterial blood gas values and intrapulmonary shunt volumes as well as restoration of the responsive capacity of the von Euler-Liljestrand reflex. HPS may prove reversible within a few days of liver transplantation. However, other studies have shown that the process of recovery can last much longer (2–18 months). (5, 15, 28–30, 33, 34, 48) • *Embolization* may be indicated in the individual case of arteriovenous fistulas. (27, 33, 38)

7 Portopulmonary hypertension

This clinical picture was described for the first time in 1951 by F. MANTZ et al. (70) and confirmed in 1983 by P.J. McDONNELL et al. • Portopulmonary hypertension (PPH) is defined as a secondary form of pulmonary hypertension with portal hypertension (or as hypertension in combination with liver disease). Frequency in patients with cirrhosis is given as 2–4%, in patients in an advanced stage of cirrhosis (e.g. presenting for liver transplantation) as 5–10% of cases.

7.1 Definition, morphology and diagnosis

Definition: Characteristic criteria of PPH include (*1.*) elevated pulmonary artery pressure (>25 mm Hg), (*2.*) increased pulmonary vascular resistance (>120 dyne/sec/cm^{-5}), and (*3.*) normal pulmonary capillary wedge pressure (<15 mm Hg). An elevated transpulmonary gradient (mean pulmonary artery pressure/pulmonary capillary wedge pressure = >10 mm Hg) is likewise used as a diagnostic criterion. (67, 75) • *The presence of portal hypertension is considered as a prerequisite for the development of PPH.*

▶ The main difference between PPH and HPS is to be seen in the fact that the latter reveals an impaired gas exchange with hypoxaemia and a reduction in pulmonary vascular resistance due to vasodilation. The coexistence of these two pathological conditions (*vasodilation* on the one hand and *vasoconstriction* on the other hand) has recently become documented more often. Any illnesses which lead to pulmonary hypertension must be ruled out as part of the differential diagnosis.

Morphology: PPH is characterized by anatomically fixed pulmonary vasoconstriction. Vascular changes are brought about by (*1.*) vasoconstriction, (*2.*) structural remodelling of the pulmonary arteries (intimal fibroelastosis, hyperplasia of the media), and (*3.*) formation of microthrombi. Endothelial dysfunction may also arise due to shear stress, resulting from hypercirculation and/or autoimmune processes. In the further course of HPP, there is a proliferation of capillaries, followed by angioma-like changes with fibrinoid necroses of the arterial wall (= *plexogenic arteriopathy*). These findings are disseminated unevenly throughout the lungs. Thus the histological changes of PPH are similar to those of primary pulmonary hypertension. (73) • Remarkably, the combined occurrence of the primary antiphospholipid syndrome and PPH with anticardiolipin antibodies and microthrombi was observed. (61)

Diagnosis: Clinical symptoms of PPH can appear approximately five years after the diagnosis of portal hypertension. Initially, patients have no complaints regarding PPH. In the further course, however, effort dyspnoea, syncope and chest pains may occur. Occasionally, haemoptysis is observed. There is no cyanosis. Additional findings include a loud P_2 heart sound, systolic murmur (mostly right parasternal in the fifth ICS), prominent central pulmonary arteries on the chest roentgenogram and changes in the ECG (right ventricular hypertrophy, right axis deviation, right bundle branch block). • An initial diagnosis can be made using Doppler echocardiography. This proved to be an excellent screening test for identifying all patients with PPH before they presented for liver transplantation. (62) Respiratory alkalosis on room air arterial blood gas can be used as an adjunctive screening test, whereby exaggerated values are indicative of PPH. (68) The scintigraphy index with ^{99m}TMAA is <6%. Diagnosis is established using right heart catheterization, which is regarded as the "gold standard".

7.2 Endothelin and ET-receptor antagonist

Endothelin-1 was first isolated in 1988 by M. YANAGISAWA et al. from endothelial cells as a peptide comprising 21 amino acids linked through two sulphide bridges. In 1989 the same team discovered two further isoforms, endothelin-2 and endothelin-3, also in endothelial cells and smooth muscle cells. These endothelins closely resemble the cardiotoxic poison sarafotoxin, a potent vasoconstrictor toxin found in the Israeli mole viper. Endothelin-1 (ET) is the most important isoform in humans. The two ET receptors, ETA and ETB, can be detected on smooth muscle cells, in especially high densities in the pulmonary and coronary vessels, and produce intense vasoconstriction (T. SAKURAI et al., 1992). ETB receptors are likewise found in large numbers on endothelial cells. Activated under normal physiological conditions, they stimulate the release of vasodilatory substances (e.g. NO, prostacycline). Vasoconstriction is predominant under pathological conditions. Some results have shown that ETB receptors are upregulated in certain diseases, such as liver cirrhosis. (75). ET has a low plasma concentration and a short half-life of 4−7 minutes. It therefore acts as a local hormone rather than a circulating endocrine hormone. Apart from immediately producing vasoconstriction (ET is one of the strongest and slowest-acting endogenous vasoconstrictors), it stimulates numerous medium and long-term pathophysiological effects. (71, 76) (s. p. 300) (s. tab. 18.2)

Bosentan was first described as an ETA/ETB receptor antagonist by S.M. GARDINER et al. in 1994. These two receptors are features of the intense vasoconstrictory as well as the proliferative and profibrotic effects of ET. Pharmacological characterization was carried out in 1994 by M. CLOZEL et al. and in 1999 by S. ROUX et al.

The effects of bosentan have since been confirmed in numerous studies, and this substance was approved for use in the treatment of pulmonary arterial hypertension (WHO classes III and IV) in 2001. (63, 64, 72) • This dual ET receptor antagonist shows a number of important properties. (s. tab. 18.3)

Acute effects	• inflammation • platelet aggregation • stimulation of RAAS • stimulation of sympathetic nervous system • vasoconstriction • volume retention
Chronic effects	− cell proliferation − fibrosis − mitogenic effects − neuroendocrine activation − stimulation of growth factors

Tab. 18.2: Biological effects of endothelin

Antifibrotic effects
Antihypertrophic effects
Antiinflammatory effects
Buffering of other neurohormonal systems
Reduction in vascular resistance

Tab. 18.3: Main properties of bosentan

7.3 Prognosis and therapy

Prognosis: Prognosis is poor. The patients die as a result of liver insufficiency, right heart failure and/or various infectious diseases. The mean survival period after diagnosis was 15 months, with a six-month mortality of 50%. Mild forms can, however, exist without propression for several years.

Therapy: So far, no effective therapy is known. *Inhaled nitric oxide* as a specific pulmonary vasodilator may be useful perioperatively regarding liver transplantation. In several studies, the use of nitric oxide and *calcium channel blockers* only proved successful in single cases, and then just for a limited time. • *Epoprostenol* (prostacyclin) is a potent vasodilator with a short half-life (3–5 min), so that a permanent supply is required; this is made possible with the help of an indwelling i.v. catheter attached to a continuous pump. (66) A significant reduction in pulmonary hypertension could be achieved following a five-month period of application (8 ng/kg BW/min). (65) Further studies have also shown an improvement in haemodynamics and exercise tolerance as well as prolonged survival in patients with PPH. The application of *iloprost* (an inhaled analog of prostacyclin) was encouraging. It was also shown that long-term administration of epoprostenol led to a remodelling of the right ventricle. • Depending on the underlying liver disease, the use of *anticoagulants* may be indicated. The newly developed endothelin-receptor antagonist *bosentan* has also proved successful in the treatment of arterial pulmonary hypertension. (63, 64, 72) As a last resort, a combination of bosentan and epoprostenol (or other prostanoids) can be recommended. As yet, there have only been isolated cases involving the use of bosentan in PPH. The phosphodiesterase-5 inhibitor *sildenafil* improved the haemodynamics significantly. In the meantime, PPH is no longer considered to be an absolute contraindication for *liver transplantation*. The indication is given in cases involving a mild or moderate course of the disease. (60, 69, 74) A well-functioning right ventricle is a prerequisite for liver transplantation. In severe cases, liver-lung transplantation may be discussed.

References:

Hepatopulmonary syndrome

1. Abrams, G.A., Fallon, M.B.: Treatment of hepatopulmonary syndrome with Allium Sativum L. A pilot trial. J. Clin. Gastroenterol. 1998; 27: 232–235
2. Abrams, G.A., Nanda, N.C., Dubovsky, E.V., Krowka, M.J., Fallon, M.B.: Use of macroaggregated albumin lung perfusion scan to diagnose hepatopulmonary syndrome: a new approach. Gastroenterology 1998; 114: 305–310
3. Aller, R., Moreira, V., Boixeda, D., Moya, J.L., de Luis, D.A., Enriquez, J.L., Fogué, L.: Diagnosis of hepatopulmonary syndrome with contrast transthoracic echocardiography and histological confirmation. Liver 1998; 18: 285–287
4. Anel, R.M., Sheagren, J.N.: Novel presentation and approach to management of hepatopulmonary syndrome with the use of antimicrobial agents. Clin. Infect. Dis. 2001; 10: E 131–136
5. Arguedas, M.R., Fallon, M.B.: Hepatopulmonary syndrome. Curr. Treat. Opt. Gastroenterol. 2005; 8: 451–456
6. Baltzer, G., Arndt, H., Martini, G.A.: Sauerstoffuntersättigung und veränderte Hämodynamik bei Leberzirrhose. Klin. Wschr. 1973; 51: 1033–1042
7. Berthelot, P., Walker, J.G., Sherlock, S., Reid, L.: Arterial changes in the lungs in cirrhosis of the liver – lung spider nevi. New Engl. J. Med. 1966; 274: 291–298
8. Bindl, L., Wagner, N., Knöpfli, G., Gosseye, St., Lentze, M.J.: Peliosis hepatis with hepato-pulmonary syndrome. Klin. Paediatr. 1998; 210: 47–49
9. Cadranel, J.L., Milleron, B.J., Cadranel, J.F., Fermand, J.P., Andrivet, P., Brouet, J.C., Adnot, S., Akoun, G.M.: Severe hypoxemia-associated intrapulmonary shunt in a patient with chronic liver disease: improvement after medical treatment. Amer. Rev. Resp. Dis. 1992; 146: 526–527
10. Caruso, G., Catalano, D.: Esophageal varices and hepatopulmonary syndrome in liver cirrhosis. J. Hepatol. 1991; 12: 262–263
11. Cremona, G., Higenbottam, T.W., Mayoral, V., Alexander, G., Demoncheaux, E., Borland, C., Roe, J., Jones, G.J.: Elevated exhaled nitric oxide in patients with hepatopulmonary syndrome. Eur. Respir. J. 1995; 8: 1883–1885
12. De, B.K., Sen, S., Biswas, P.K., Sanyal, R., Majumdar, D., Biswas, J.: Hepatopulmonary syndrome in inferior vena cava obstruction responding to cavoplasty. Gastroenterology 2000; 118: 192–196
13. De, B.K., Sen, S., Biswas, P.K., Mandral, S.K., Das, D., Das, U., Guru, S., Bandyopadhyay, K.: Occurrence of hepatopulmonary syndrome in Budd-Chiari syndrome and the role of venous decompression. Gastroenterology 2002; 122: 897–903
14. Dickinson, C.J.: The aetiology of clubbing and hypertrophic osteoarthropathy. Eur. J. Clin. Invest. 1993; 23: 330–338
15. Eriksson, L.S., Söderman, C., Ericzon, B.-G., Eleborg, L., Wahren, J., Hedenstierna, G.: Normalization of ventilation perfusion relationship after liver transplantation in patients with decompensated cirrhosis: evidence for an hepatopulmonary syndrome. Hepatology 1990; 12: 1350–1357
16. Fallon, M.B., Abrams, G.A., Luo, B., Hou, Z., Dai, J.: The role of endothelial nitric oxide synthase in the pathogenesis of a rat model of hepatopulmonary syndrome. Gastroenterology 1997; 113: 606–614
17. Fiel, M.I., Schiaro, T.D., Suriawinata, A., Emre, S.: Portal hypertension and hepatopulmonary syndrome in a middle-aged man with hepatitis B infection. Semin. Liver Dis. 2000; 20: 391–395
18. Flückiger, M.: Vorkommen von trommelschlägelförmigen Fingerendphalangen ohne chronische Veränderungen an den Lungen oder am Herzen. Wien. Med. Wschr. 1884; 34: 1457–1458
19. Giniès, J.L., Couetil, J.P., Houssin, D., Guillemain, R., Champion, G., Bernard, O.: Hepatopulmonary syndrome in a child with cystic fibrosis. J. Pediatr. Gastroenterol. Nutr. 1996; 23: 497–500
20. Gupta, D., Vijaya, D.R., Gupta, R., Dhiman, R.K., Bhargava, M., Verma, D.M.J., Chawla, Y.K.: Prevalence of hepatopulmonary syndrome in cirrhosis and extrahepatic portal venous obstruction. Amer. J. Gastroenterol. 2001; 96: 3395–3399
21. Hannam, P.D., Sandokji, A.K.M., Machan, L.S., Erb, S.R., Champion, P., Buczkowski, A.K., Scudamore, C.H., Steinbrecher, U.P., Chung, S.W., Weiss, A.A., Yoshida, E.M.: Post-surgical shunt hepatopulmonary syndrome in a case of non-cirrhotic portal hypertension: lack of efficacy of shunt reversal. Eur. J. Gastroenterol. Hepatol. 1999; 11: 1425–1427
22. Hourani, J.M., Bellamy, P.E.B., Tashkin, D.P., Batra, P., Simmons, M.S.: Pulmonary dysfunction in advanced liver disease: frequent occurrence of an abnormal diffusing capacity. Amer. J. Med. 1991; 90: 693–700
23. Irle, U., Ohlms, F.B.: Leberzirrhose mit intrapulmonalen arteriovenösen Mikroanastomosen. Schweiz. Rundsch. Med. 1968; 57: 1720–1722
24. Jeffrey, G.P., Prince, R.L., van der Schaaf, A.: Fatal intrapulmonary arteriovenous shunting in cirrhosis; diagnosis by radionuclide lung perfusion scan. Med. J. Aust. 1990; 152: 549–553
25. Kaymakoglu, S., Kahraman, T., Kudat, H., Demir, K., Cakaloglu, Y., Adalet, I., Dincer, D., Besisik, F., Boztas, G., Sözen, A.B., Mungan, Z., Okten, A.: Hepatopulmonary syndrom in noncirrhotic portal hypertensive patients. Dig. Dis. Sci. 2003; 48: 556–560
26. Kennedy, T.C., Knudson, R.J.: Exercise-aggravated hypoxemia and orthodeoxia in cirrhosis. Chest 1977; 72: 305–309
27. Krowka, M.J., Cortese, D.A.: Hepatopulmonary syndrome – current concepts in diagnostic and therapeutic considerations. Chest 1994; 105: 1528–1537
28. Krowka, M.J., Porayko, M.K., Plevak, D.J., Pappas, S.C., Steers, J.L., Krom, R.A.F., Wiesner, R.H.: Hepatopulmonary syndrome with progressive hypoxemia as an indication for liver transplantation: case reports and literature review. Mayo Clin. Proc. 1997; 72: 44–53
29. Lange, P.A., Stoller, J.K.: The hepatopulmonary syndrome. Effect of liver transplantation. Clin. Chest Med. 1996; 17: 115–123
30. Lasch, H.M., Fried, M.W., Zacks, S.L., Odell, P., Johnson, M.W., Gerber, D.A., Sandhu, F.S., Fair, J.H., Shrestha, R.: Use of transjugular intrahepatic portosystemic shunt as a bridge to liver transplantation in a patient with severe hepatopulmonary syndrome. Liver Transplant. 2001; 7: 147–149
31. Lee, K.-N., Lee, H.-J., Shin, W.W., Webb, W.R.: Hypoxemia and liver cirrhosis (hepatopulmonary syndrome) in eight patients: comparison of the central and peripheral pulmonary vasculature. Radiology 1999; 211: 549–553
32. Lima, B.L.G., Franca, A.V.C., Pazin-Filho, A., Araujo, W.M., Martinez, J.A.B., Maciel, B.C., Simoes, M.V., Terra-Filho, J., Martinelli, A.L.C.: Frequency, clinical characteristics and respiratory parameters of hepatopulmonary syndrome. Mayo Clin. Proc. 2004; 79: 42–48
33. Mandel, M.S.: The diagnosis and treatment of hepatopulmonary syndrome. Clin. Liver Dis. 2006; 10: 387–405
34. Martinez, G.P., Barbera, J.A., Visa, J., Rimola, A., Pare, J.C., Roca, J., Navasa, M., Rodes, J., Rodriguez-Roisin, R.: Hepatopulmonary syndrome in candidates for liver transplantation. J. Hepatol. 2001; 34: 651–657
35. Martini, G.A., Hagemann, J.E.: Über Fingernagelveränderungen bei Leberzirrhose als Folge veränderter peripherer Durchblutung. Klin. Wschr. 1956; 34: 25–31
36. McAdams, H.P., Erasmus, J., Crockett, R., Mitchell, J., Godwin, J.D., McDermott, V.G.: The hepatopulmonary syndrome: radiologic findings in 10 patients. Amer. J. Roentgenol. 1996; 166: 1379–1385
37. Nunes, H., Lebrec, D., Mazmanian, M., Eapron, F., Heller, J., Tazi, K.A., Zerbib, E., Dulmet, E., Moreau, R., Dinh-Kuan, A., Simonneau, G.: Role of nitric oxide in hepatopulmonary syndrome in cirrhotic rats. Amer. J. Respir. Crit. Care Med. 2001; 164: 879–885
38. Palma, D.T., Fallon, M.B.: The hepatopulmonary syndrome. J. Hepatol. 2006; 45: 617–625
39. Poterucha, J.J., Krowka, M.J., Dickson, E.R., Cortese, D.A., Stanson, A.W., Krom, R.A.: Failure of hepatopulmonary syndrome to resolve after liver transplantation and successful treatment with embolotherapy. Hepatology 1995; 21: 96–100

40. **Regev, A., Yeshurun, M., Rodriguez, M., Sagie, A., Neff, G.W., Molina, E.G., Schiff, E.R.:** Transient hepatopulmonary syndrome in a patient with acute hepatitis A. J. Viral Hepat. 2001; 8: 83–86
41. **Riegler, J.L., Lang, K.A., Johnson, S.P., Westerman, J.H.:** Transjugular intrahepatic portosystemic shunt improves oxygenation in hepatopulmonary syndrome. Gastroenterology 1995; 109: 978–983
42. **Robin, E.D., Laman, D., Horn, B.R., Theodore, J.:** Platypnea related to orthodeoxia caused by true vascular lung shunts. New Engl. J. Med. 1976; 294: 941–943
43. **Rolla, G., Bucca, C., Brussino, L.:** Methylene blue in the hepatopulmonary syndrome. New Engl. J. Med. 1994; 331: 1098
44. **Rutishauser, M., Egli, F., Wyler, F.:** Juvenile Leberzirrhose mit multiplen arterio-venösen Aneurysmen der Lunge. Schweiz. Med. Wschr. 1972; 102: 514–517
45. **Rydell, R., Hoffbauer, F.W.:** Multiple pulmonary arteriovenous fistulas in juvenile cirrhosis. Amer. J. Med. 1956; 21: 450–460
46. **Schenk, P., Madl, C., Rezzaie-Majd, S., Lehr, St., Müller, C.:** Methylene blue improves the hepatopulmonary syndrome. Ann. Intern. Med. 2000; 133: 701–706
47. **Schenk, P., Schöniger-Hekele, M., Fuhrmann, V., Madl, C., Silberhumer, G., Müller, C.:** Prognostic significance of the hepatopulmonary syndrome in patients with cirrhosis. Gastroenterology 2003; 125: 1042–1052
48. **Scott, V., Miro, A., Kang, Y., DeWolf, A., Bellary, S., Martin, M., Kramer, A., Selby, R., Doyle, H., Paradis, I., Starzl, T.E.:** Reversibility of the hepatopulmonary syndrome by orthotopic liver transplantation. Transplant. Proc. 25 (1993), 1787–1788
49. **Scott, V.L., Dodson, S.F., Kang, Y.:** The hepatopulmonary syndrome. Surg. Clin. North Amer. 1999; 79: 23–41
50. **Selim, K.M., Akriviadis, E.A., Zuckerman, E., Chen, D., Reynolds, T.B.:** Transjugular intrahepatic portosystemic shunt: a successful treatment for hepatopulmonary syndrome. Amer. J. Gastroenterol. 1998; 93: 455–458
51. **Shijo, H., Sasaki, H., Miyajima, Y., Okumura, M.:** Prostaglandin $F_{2\alpha}$ and indomethacin in hepatogenic pulmonary angiodysplasia: effects on pulmonary hemodynamics and gas exchange. Chest 1991; 100: 873–875
52. **Snell, A.M.:** The effects of chronic disease of the liver on the composition and physicochemical properties of blood: changes in the serum proteins; reduction in the oxygen saturation of the arterial blood. Ann. Intern. Med. 1935; 9: 690–711
53. **Stein, H., Stein, S.:** Digital clubbing in cirrhosis of the liver. Lancet 1961/I: 999–1000
54. **Teuber, G., Teube, C., Dietrich, C.F., Caspary, W.F., Buhl, R., Zeuzem, St.:** Pulmonary dysfunction in non-cirrhotic patients with chronic viral hepatitis. Eur. J. Intern. Med. 2002; 13: 311–318
55. **Vachiéry, F., Mora, J, R., Hadengue, A., Gadano, A., Soupison, T., Valla, D., Lebrec, D.:** Hypoxemia in patients with cirrhosis: relationship with liver failure and hemodynamic alterations. J. Hepatol. 1997; 27: 492–495
56. **Whyte, M.K.B., Hughes, J.M.B., Peters, A.M., Ussow, W., Patel, S., Burroughs, A.K.:** Analysis of intrapulmonary right to left shunt in the hepatopulmonary syndrome. J. Hepatol. 1998; 29: 85–93
57. **Williams, A., Trewby, P., Williams, R., Reid, L.:** Structural alterations to the pulmonary circulation in fulminant hepatic failure. Thorax 1979; 34: 447–453
58. **Yao, E.H., Kong, B., Hsue, G., Zhou, A., Wang, H.:** Pulmonary function changes in cirrhosis of the liver. Amer. J. Gastroenterol. 1987; 82: 352–354
59. **Zhang, J.L., Ling, Y.Q., Luo, B., Tang, L.P., Ryter, S.W., Stockard, C.R., Grizzle, W.E., Fallon, M.B.:** Analysis of pulmonary heme oxygenase-1 and nitric oxide synthase alterations in experimental hepatopulmonary syndrome. Gastroenterology 2003; 125: 1441–1451

Portopulmonary hypertension

60. **Aucejo, F., Miller, C., Vogt, D., Eghtesad, B., Nakagawa, S., Stoller, J.K.:** Pulmonary hypertension after liver transplantation in patients with antecedent hepatopulmonary syndrome. A report of 2 cases and review of the literature. Liver Transplant. 2006; 12: 1278–1282
61. **Bayraktar, Y., Tanaci, N., Egesel, T., Gököz, A., Balkanci, F.:** Antiphospholipid syndrome presenting as portopulmonary hypertension. J. Clin. Gastroenterol. 2001; 32: 359–361
62. **Colle, I., Moreau, R., Godinho, E., Belghiti, J., Ertori, F., Cohen-Solai, A., Mal, H., Bernuau, J., Marty, J., Lebrec, D., Valla, D., Durand, F.:** Diagnosis of portopulmonary hypertension in candidates for liver transplantation: a prospective study. Hepatology 2003; 37: 401–409
63. **Halank, M., Ewert, R., Seyfarth, H.J., Hoeffken, G.:** Portopulmonary hypertension. J. Gastroenterol. 2006; 41: 837–847
64. **Hinterhuber, L., Graziadei, I.W., Kähler, E.M., Jaschke, W., Vogel, W.:** Endothelin – receptor antagonist treatment of portopulmonary hypertension. Clin. Gastroenterol. Hepatol. 2004; 2: 1039–1042
65. **Kähler, C.M., Graziadei, I., Wiedermann, C.J., Kneussl, M.P., Vogel, W.:** Successful use of continuous intravenous prostacyclin in a patient with severe portopulmonary hypertension. Wien. Klin. Wschr. 2000; 112: 637–640
66. **Krowka, M.J., Frantz, R.P., McGoon, M.D., Severson, C., Plevak, D.J., Wiesner, R.H.:** Improvement in pulmonary hemodynamics during intravenous epoprostenol (prostacyclin): a study of 15 patients with moderate to severe portopulmonary hypertension. Hepatology 1999; 30: 641–648
67. **Krowka, M.J.:** Evolving dilemmas and management of portopulmonary hypertension. Semin. Liver. Dis. 2006; 26: 265–272
68. **Kuo, P.C., Plotkin, J.S., Gaine, S., Schroeder, R.A., Rustgi, V.K., Rubin, L.R., Johnson, L.B.:** Portopulmonary hypertension and the liver transplant candidate. Transplantation 1999; 67: 1087–1093
69. **Levy, M.T., Torzillo, P., Bookallil, M., Sheil, A.G.R., McCaughan, G.W.:** Case report: Delayed resolution of severe pulmonary hypertension after isolated liver transplantation in a patient with cirrhosis. J. Gastroenterol. Hepatol. 1996; 11: 734–737
70. **Mantz, F., Craige, E.:** Portal axis thrombosis with spontaneous portocaval shunt and resultant cor pulmonale. AMA Arch. Pathol. 1951; 52: 91–97
71. **Masaki, T.:** The discovery of endothelins. Cardiovasc. Res. 1998; 39: 530–533
72. **Passarella, M., Fallon, M.B., Kawut, S.M.:** Portopulmonary hypertension. Clin. Liver Dis. 2006; 10: 653–663
73. **Rubin, L.J., Badesch, D.B., Barst, R.J., Galie, N., Black, C.M., Keogh, A., Pulido, T., Frost, A., Roux, S., Leconte, I., Landzberg, M., Simonneau, G.:** Bosentan therapy for pulmonary arterial hypertension. New Engl. J. Med. 2002; 346: 896–903
74. **Schraufnagel, D.E., Kay, J.M.:** Structural and pathologic changes in the lung vasculature in chronic liver disease. Clin. Chest Med. 1996; 17: 1–15
75. **Starkel, P., Vera, A., Gunson, B., Mutimer, D.:** Outcome of liver transplantation for patients with pulmonary hypertension. Liver Transplant. 2002; 8: 382–388
76. **Yang, Y.Y., Lin, H.C., Lee, W.C., Hou, M.C., Lee, F.Y., Chang, F.Y., Lee, S.D.:** Portopulmonary hypertension: distinctive hemodynamic and clinical manifestations. J. Gastroenterol. 2001; 36: 181–186
77. **Yokomori, H., Oda, M., Yasogawa, Y., Nishi, Y., Ogi, M., Takahashi, M., Ishii, H.:** Enhanced expression of endothelin B receptor at protein and gene levels in human cirrhotic liver. J. Pathol. 2001; 159: 1353–1362

Symptoms and Syndromes
19 Coagulopathy and haemorrhage

		Page:
1	***Coagulopathy***	348
1.1	Forms of haemostasis	348
1.2	Fibrinolysis	348
1.3	Vasopathies	348
1.4	Thrombocytopathies	348
1.5	*Plasmic coagulation disorders*	349
1.5.1	Synthesis disorders	350
1.5.2	Clearance function disorders	350
1.5.3	Increase in consumption	350
1.6	*Consumptive coagulopathy*	350
1.6.1	Definition	350
1.6.2	Clinical aspects	350
1.7	*Therapy of haemostatic disorders*	352
1.7.1	Prophylactic measures	352
1.7.2	Pharmacological therapy	352
2	**Upper gastrointestinal haemorrhage**	353
2.1	Definition	353
2.2	Forms	354
2.3	Causes	354
2.4	*Diagnostics*	354
2.5	Prognosis	356
2.6	*Therapy*	356
2.6.1	Basic therapy	356
2.6.2	Endoscopic haemostasis	357
2.6.3	Drug-controlled haemostasis	358
3	**Bleeding oesophageal varices**	358
3.1	Oesophageal varices as collateral circulation	358
3.2	Frequency and risks	359
3.3	Predictive haemorrhagic factors	359
3.3.1	Increase in pressure	359

		Page:
3.3.2	Endoscopic evaluation	359
3.3.3	Sonographic evaluation	360
3.3.4	Child-Pugh criteria	360
3.3.5	CT and MRI	361
3.4	*Clinical aspects*	361
3.5	*Conservative therapy*	361
3.5.1	Basic therapy	361
3.5.2	Sclerotherapy	361
3.5.3	Endoscopic variceal ligation	364
3.5.4	Balloon tamponade	365
3.5.5	Prevention of primary bleeding	366
3.5.6	Medicinal treatment	366
3.5.7	Bacteraemia	367
3.6	*Invasive treatment*	368
3.6.1	Transhepatic embolization	368
3.6.2	TIPS	368
3.7	*Surgical treatment*	369
3.7.1	Indications	369
3.7.2	Surgical methods	369
3.7.3	Timing of shunt operation	371
3.7.4	Prognosis	371
3.8	Liver transplantation	372
4	**Lower gastrointestinal haemorrhage**	372
4.1	Definition	372
4.2	Forms	372
4.3	*Diagnostics*	373
4.4	Aetiology	374
4.5	*Therapy*	374
	• References (1–209)	374
	(Figures 19.1–19.16; tables 19.1–19.7)	

19 Coagulopathy and haemorrhage

The leakage of blood from the blood vessels is referred to as **haemorrhage**. Its causes include: (*1.*) increased permeability of the vascular walls, (*2.*) pathological blood vessel condition, and (*3.*) injury to a blood vessel. • Generally, a haemorrhage may become considerably more severe in the presence of **coagulopathy**, i.e. clotting disorder. It is also possible for a coagulation defect to arise as a separate disorder even without existing tissue damage.

1 Coagulopathy

1.1 Forms of haemostasis

By means of the complex process of **haemostasis**, the organism seeks to protect itself directly from bleeding and the corresponding loss of blood. • **Three components** are available for achieving this end: (*1.*) blood vessels themselves (= vascular haemostasis), (*2.*) platelets and endothelial cells (= cellular haemostasis), and (*3.*) blood-clotting factors (= plasmic blood coagulation).

1. **Vascular haemostasis** comprises reflex contractions of the arteries, reinforced by the release of vasoconstrictor substances from the vessel walls (e.g. catecholamines, serotonin, thromboxane A_2).

2. **Cellular phases** of the arrest of bleeding commence as so-called **primary haemostasis,** during the course of which thrombocytes, with the aid of von Willebrand's factor, adhere to collagen fragments released from the injured vascular endothelium. The discharge of various factors from the thrombocytes then ensues. The prostaglandin-thromboxane system is directly involved in the subsequent aggregation of thrombocytes.

3. **Plasmic coagulation** is effected by a system of 15 coagulation factors. (s. p. 110) (s. tab. 5.12) So-called **secondary haemostasis** begins with the progressive activation of the plasmic coagulation system. All the coagulation factors involved are proteins and for the most part enzymatic. They are normally present in the plasma in their inactive form, and with the initiation of plasmic coagulation, they become successively activated. The clotting process (= **coagulation**) has the function of converting soluble fibrinogen into stable, insoluble fibrin. *Procoagulation and anticoagulation factors* regulate the process of coagulation.

Exogenous activation is initiated by tissue thromboplastin (= tissue factor) and the activated form of factor XII in the plasma. This complex is enlarged by ionic calcium and platelet factor 3. As a result, the activation of factors IX to IXa and X to Xa is triggered, thus forming a cross-connection between the endogenous and the exogenous system. (s. fig. 19.1)

Endogenous coagulation commences with the activation of factor XII. Factor XIIa then catalyzes the conversion of prokallikrein to kallikrein, plasminogen to plasmin and factor XI to XIa. The presence of factor XV is necessary for the activation of IX to IXa. This creates a complex comprising IXa, VIIIa, calcium and phospholipids, which then activates factor X to Xa. (s. fig. 19.1)

▶ Depending on the causative mechanism, either the exogenous or the endogenous coagulation system is activated. These progress differently until the activation of factor X, which then allows both pathways to merge into a common final phase of coagulation. • At this point, the activation of **prothrombin** II to thrombin by the Xa/Va/calcium/phospholipid complex represents the final step of both coagulation cascades. The prothrombin complex (factors II, VII, IX and X) does not exist as such – it refers to various proteins, the synthesis of which depends on vitamin K. • Soluble **fibrinogen** (I) is converted by thrombin into insoluble *fibrin*, which infiltrates and thereby solidifies the thrombocytic embolus. Thrombin simultaneously activates factor XIII to XIIIa and protein C to protein C_a. The fibrin network is further strengthened by factor XIIIa. • The most effective **inhibitors** of coagulation are antithrombin III, α_2-macroglobulin, C_1-inactivator and protein C_a as well as fibrinogen-fibrin degradation products.

1.2 Fibrinolysis

The minor coagulation processes constantly taking place in the vascular system (whereby fibrin is deposited) are counteracted by simultaneous fibrinolysis. *Coagulation and fibrinolysis are thus in continuous dynamic balance.* Plasminogen is converted to plasmin by activators such as urokinase PA (isolated from urine) and tissue PA (isolated from tissue). The effect of tissue PA is strongly enhanced by the presence of fibrin. Fibrinolysis is stimulated by protein C, while plasmin activity is maintained in balance by inhibitors (e.g. α_2-antiplasmin, α_2-macroglobulin). (s. fig. 19.1)

1.3 Vasopathies

Vasopathies may arise from direct injuries to the vessel wall, but also from pathological changes in the vessel wall or in the endothelium. It can be expected that vasopathies will occur or become more severe during the course of various liver diseases or with concomitant coagulopathy.

Osler-Rendu-Weber disease (*haemorrhagic telangiectasia*) is the most common congenital vasopathy. It is an autosomally inherited structural defect of the blood vessels with an accompanying decrease in muscular and elastic fibres in the capillaries and venules. Multiple telangiectases are most frequently found in the upper body and in the mucous membranes. Severe bleeding may occur from the nasal and pharyngeal passages as well as from the gastrointestinal tract.

Schoenlein-Henoch disease (*anaphylactoid purpura*) represents the most important acquired vasopathy. It is due to toxic or allergic inflammatory blood-vessel damage accompanied by immunological reactions. Bleeding may be present in the skin, in the form of petechiae or ecchymoses, or in the gastrointestinal mucosa.

1.4 Thrombocytopathies

Thrombocytopathies may arise in the course of a liver disease and during the measures taken to treat it as well

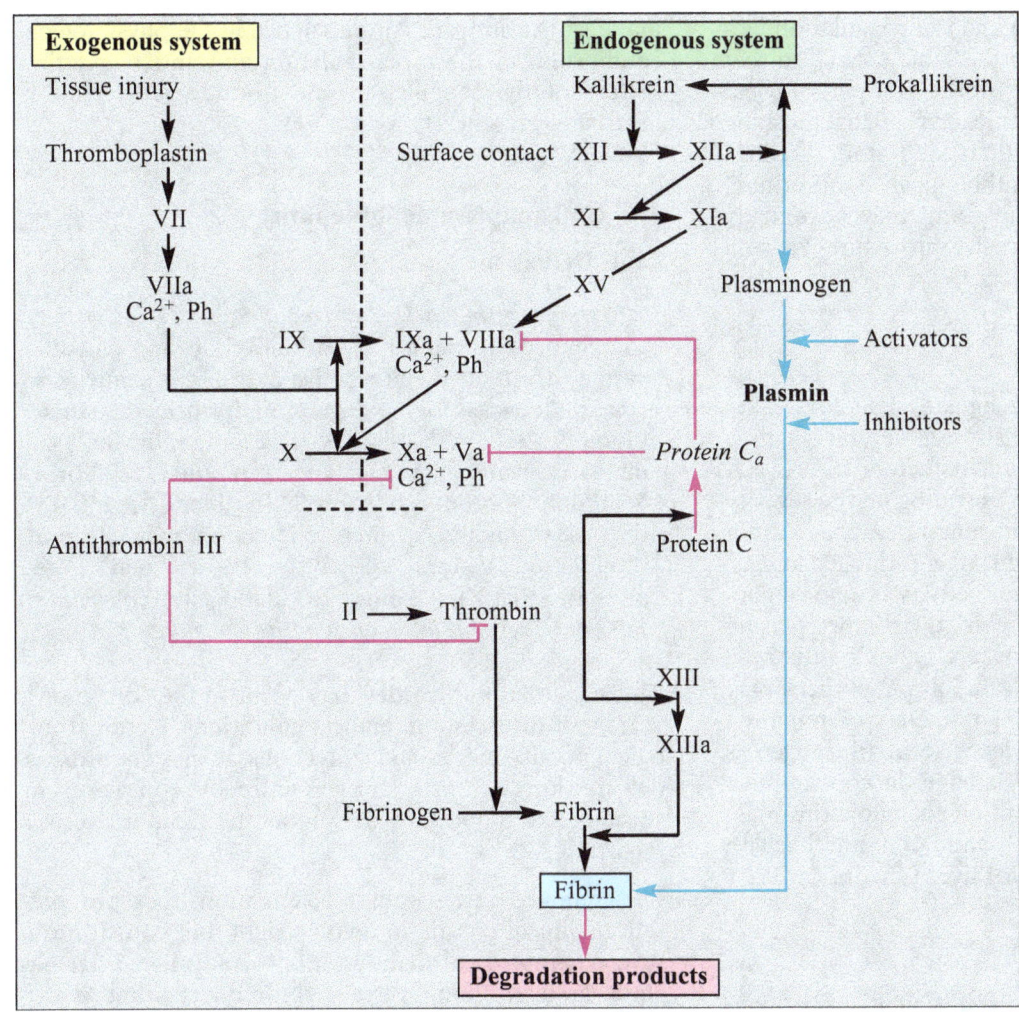

Fig. 19.1: Exogenous and endogenous plasmic coagulation cascade (with inhibition by antithrombin III and protein C_a) and the fibrinolysis pathway through plasminogen-plasmin. Proteolytic plasmin principally hydrolyzes the cross-linked fibrin clot into high molecular weight fragments and D fragment dimers (Ph = phospholipids) (s. tab. 5.12)

as from complications. This condition can lead to serious disturbances in haemostasis. Thrombocytic bleeding is typically observed as punctate or petechial haemorrhaging in mechanically stressed skin areas as well as in mucous membranes. Ecchymosis is found less frequently. • A *leftward shift* in the differential blood count may indicate thrombocytopathy. (17)

1. **Thrombocytopenia** may be caused by various metabolic disturbances: (*1.*) synthesis disorders (e.g. medicaments, alcohol, folic acid deficiency, thrombopoietin deficiency, increase in the platelet inhibitors prostacyclin and NO), (*2.*) replacement disorders (e.g. immunologically derived degradation, consumption coagulopathy, antiplatelet antibodies, loss of blood), and (*3.*) distribution disorders (e.g. increased sequestration in the enlarged spleen, involving up to 90% of the thrombocytes).

2. **Thrombocytosis** is a (generally temporary) rise in the thrombocyte count. Thromboembolic complications may arise. This disorder occurs in hepatocellular carcinoma, for example, following splenectomy or portosystemic anastomosis as well as after haemorrhage or cortisone therapy.

3. **Thrombocyte dysfunction** frequently emerges in the course of liver diseases and their complications, especially in the case of coagulation disorders and elevated fibrinolysis. Thus a decrease in both thrombocyte aggregation and the release of platelet factor 3 may occasionally be observed in cirrhosis. In most cases, this is caused by medication (acetylsalicylic acid, non-steroidal antirheumatic agents, dextran, antibiotics, etc.).

1.5 Plasmic coagulation disorders

Defects in liver function greatly affect the haemostatic system: (*1.*) most coagulation and fibrinolytic factors are synthesized in the liver; (*2.*) many procoagulation and anticoagulation factors must be metabolically converted into their functionally active forms in the liver, and (*3.*) various plasmic coagulation and fibrinolytic factors are removed from the bloodstream by clearance mechanisms in the liver. Thus liver diseases can disrupt the haemostatic system at various stages of coagulation or fibrinolysis and with varying degrees of intensity. It is the severity of the disease which is of decisive importance rather than its acute or chronic character or its aetiology (with the possible exception of liver carcinoma). Appropriate *diagnostic tests* are: thrombocyte count, Quick's value and AT III. Plasmic coagulation defects in liver disease are derived from acquired disorders in the synthesis of coagulation factors or from their accelerated breakdown. (1, 3, 6, 7, 10, 13–17)

In liver disease, procoagulation and anticoagulation factors are generally decreased to the same extent, so that haemostasis is kept in balance, albeit at a pathological level. Thus the clinical significance of haemostatic changes may be less serious than laboratory findings would seem to indicate. This pathological "equilibrium" is, however, extremely vulnerable and may be quickly destroyed by diagnostic or invasive procedures as well as by biochemical or toxic effects.

1.5.1 Synthesis disorders

The synthesis of almost all coagulation factors takes place in the liver. In liver disease, several factors, especially the vitamin K-dependent factors II, VII, IX and X, are affected differently, depending on the severity of the illness. Synthesis of non-functional coagulation factors, particularly fibrinogen (dysfibrinogenaemia), may also occur. Defects in factor activity become clinically manifest quite rapidly due to their short plasma half-life. (s. tab. 5.12) This is where Quick's value, the Colombi index and the AT III value, among others, play their part as accepted clinical parameters of impaired liver function. (s. p. 111) A decrease in fibrinogen is observed only in severe liver damage, in consumptive disease processes or in consumption coagulopathy. Plasminogen and factors XI, XII and XIII are likewise reduced in cases of severe loss of liver function.

1.5.2 Clearance function disorders

The liver has the unique ability to differentiate between inactive and active coagulation factors and to remove the latter, along with plasminogen activators, from the bloodstream. Cirrhosis greatly interferes with the clearance of t-PA. The fibrinogen-fibrin degradation products, which act as thrombin inhibitors, are likewise eliminated by a healthy liver. In severe liver disease, obstructive gall-bladder disorders, cholestasis or biliary cirrhosis, the clearance function of the liver (s. p. 69) as well as the elimination of coagulation factors (especially factor XIII) and fibrin degradation products can be seriously impaired. This disrupts the haemostasis system, and fibrinolysis increases.

1.5.3 Increase in consumption

An increased consumption of coagulation factors is found in extensive disseminated intravascular coagulopathy. Secondary hyperfibrinolysis evolves. Simultaneous activation of the coagulation cascade or fibrinolysis system leads to the consumption of coagulation factors and inhibitors. (17)

Haemostatic disturbances result in *hypocoagulopathy with a bleeding tendency* (= haemorrhagic diathesis) seen as manifest haemorrhage or in *hypercoagulopathy with a tendency to thrombosis* (= thrombophilia) seen as manifest thrombosis. An imbalance in the physiological equilibrium of the procoagulation and anticoagulation factors of the coagulation and fibrinolytic systems is invariably present. (17)

1.6 Consumptive coagulopathy

1.6.1 Definition

Disseminated intravascular coagulation (DIC) is due to enhanced formation of thrombi following an activation disorder in either the extrinsic or intrinsic coagulation cascades. Fibrin clots form in the small blood vessels and capillaries. In response, fibrinolysis increases, thus allowing large amounts of fibrin degradation products to reach the bloodstream. In the case of highly activated coagulation, platelets and coagulation factors are consumed in such large amounts that they cannot be adequately replaced. • DIC may develop into consumptive coagulopathy.

This coagulation disorder may occur in the course of a variety of diseases and clinical conditions. Aetiopathological possibilities include infections, toxins, endotoxins, dehydration, acidosis, antigen-antibody complexes or stasis of the blood flow as well as the tumour necrosis factor.

Disseminated intravascular coagulation does not present a clinical picture in its own right, but constitutes a severe pathological manifestation of an **altered haemostasis system.** Blood vessels, thrombocytes and endothelial cells, the coagulation system, fibrinolysis, inhibitors and activators as well as the kallikrein-kininogen system are all involved in this disorder. The haemostasis system is activated either exogenously by the release of tissue thromboplastin and its homologues or endogenously by direct proteolysis of one or several procoagulants. (1, 3, 4, 8, 14, 15, 17)

1.6.2 Clinical aspects

Clinical aspects and laboratory findings vary widely not only from patient to patient, but also during the course of DIC. Depending on the extent to which the coagulation system is activated, either an acute or chronic form develops. Furthermore, DIC may occur merely as an additional complication in an existing illness, without necessarily having serious consequences – or it may culminate in a life-threatening condition.

In the **initial stage** of DIC, the haemostasis system is activated via the exogenous and/or endogenous cascade. This stage is characterized by a state of hypercoagulability. There is consumption of thrombocytes and coagulation factors as well as of procoagulants and anticoagulants, with simultaneous intravascular release of thrombin. The fibrinolysis system undergoes secondary activation. (s. fig. 19.2) (s. tabs. 5.12, 5.13)

In the **second stage,** the intravascularly released thrombin begins to have an effect at various points in the pathological process. Thus (*1.*) fibrinogen and fibrin are converted into degradation products, (*2.*) factor XIII is activated, (*3.*) factors V and VIII are altered to more highly active forms with a fall in factor VIIIc, and (*4.*) aggregation of thrombin and thrombocytes occurs. The amount of monomeric fibrin rises, while the clearance capacity of the RES becomes progressively strained at the same time. Fibrin D fragments increase, as do fibrin-fibrinogen X, Y and E fragments. The monomers disintegrate into aggregates and, together with the thrombocytes, begin to form microthrombi and fibrin clots in the terminal vessels. Circulatory disorders arise with blood stasis, hypoxia and acidosis. These result in endothelial damage, involving cell destruction to the point of organ failure. Further consumption of coagulation factors leads to a state of *hypocoagulability* with a tendency towards bleeding, which is dramatically intensified by reactive *hyperfibrinolysis* and a growing AT III deficit – a consequence of the irreversible binding to thrombin as well as to factors IXa, Xa, XIa and XIIa. (2, 4, 5, 6, 9, 10, 11, 12–15, 17–19) (s. fig. 19.2) (s. tab. 5.13)

Latent and compensated forms of consumptive coagulopathy frequently occur in the course of severe acute or chronic liver disease. In 80–85% of cirrhosis patients, the values of at least one basic test (thrombocytes, Quick's value, fibrinogen, AT III, bleeding time) are pathological. In 15–30% of cases, clinically relevant haemorrhagic diathesis evolves.

Differential diagnosis, which is necessary for distinguishing consumptive coagulopathy from DIC in a short time, is often extremely difficult to draw up. It is only possible by implementing a closely woven series of laboratory tests. Plasma thrombin time or reptilase time (in the event of concurrent heparin therapy) are appropriate parameters to determine the transition into reactive hyperfibrinolysis. (s. tab. 19.1) • The diagnosis is complicated by the fact that laboratory values typical for disseminated intravascular coagulopathy might also be due to the reduced synthesis of blood-clotting factors. Likewise, evidence of fibrinogen-fibrin degradation products is not necessarily conclusive, since the diminished clearance capacity associated with the underlying liver malfunction often precludes an adequate elimination of these substances. *It may thus prove difficult in individual cases to distinguish between a synthesis disorder and the consumption of coagulation factors as possible causes of haemorrhagic diathesis or haemorrhage.*

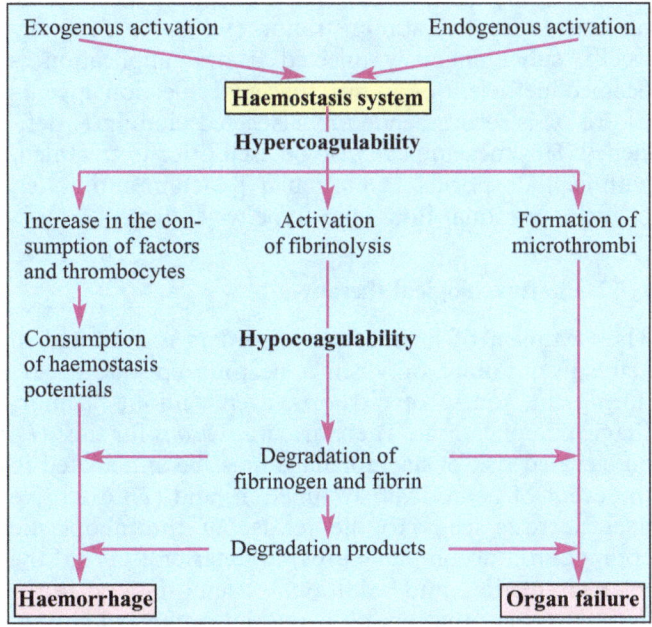

Fig. 19.2: Schematic course of consumptive coagulopathy

	Normal range	Compensated/de-compensated DIC
Thrombocytes Bleeding time	150,000–380,000 2–5 min	↓ – ↓↓ ↑ – ↑↑
Quick's value (% TPT) Fibrinogen (clottable) Antithrombin III (AT III) Partial thromboplastin time (PTT) Plasma thrombin time (TT) Factor XIII	70–120% 1.8–3.5 g/l 70–120% 28–40 sec 17–22 sec 70–120%	↓ – ↓↓↓ ↓ – ↓↓↓ ↓ – ↓↓↓ ↑ – ↑↑ ↑ – ↑↑ ↓ – ↓↓
Fibrin monomers (soluble) (= *hypercoagulability*)	< 15 mg/l	↑ – ↑↑
Fibrinogen degradation products (serum) D-dimer (= *hyperfibrinolysis*)	< 1 mg/l 20–400 µg/l	↑ – ↑↑ ↑ – ↑↑
Thrombin-antithrombin-III complex (TAT) (= *chronic DIC*)	1–4.1 µg/l	↑ – ↑↑

Tab. 19.1: Haemostasis parameters showing the normal range and corresponding changes in the course of hepatogenic consumption coagulopathy up to decompensation (s. tab. 5.12)

An accurate evaluation of the dynamics of clotting disorders or the development of disseminated intravascular coagulation as well as the further course of disease is only possible by monitoring the changes in the various laboratory parameters. Frequently repeated controls are far more important than determining each and every variable. (s. tab. 19.1)

The threshold between an inactive and an active coagulation system may be overcome abruptly at times by small stimuli, and haemostasis can then break down quite unexpectedly.

1.7 Therapy of haemostatic disorders

It is only possible to treat haemostatic disorders in liver disease *symptomatically*. In most cases, therapy also has to be adjusted to the individual patient. A causative effect on the haemostatic disorder can only be expected in the long term once liver function has begun to improve.

1.7.1 Prophylactic measures

Basic laboratory parameters concerning the haemostatic status should exceed a minimum level before any diagnostic or therapeutic procedure is initiated. The following values may be taken as a guideline (although in certain instances, some values may lie below those given): thrombocytes > 80,000, Quick's value > 40%, fibrinogen > 1.5 g/l, AT III > 40%, normal bleeding time.

Prevention of haemorrhage is always of particular importance. In view of the highly unstable nature of the haemostasis system, which – even though still in equilibrium – has a generally reduced factor level, the *insertion of catheters* (e.g. stomach probe, urinary bladder) is only carried out if particularly stringent indications are given. (7) Likewise, the administration of any medication which might affect the haemostatic system (e.g. acetylsalicylic acid, certain antibiotics, antihistamines, antirheumatic agents, clofibrate, dextran, diuretics, glucocorticoids, cardiac and psychotropic drugs, nitrofurantoin and radiological contrast medium) should be carefully evaluated. Even traces of acetylsalicylic acid, which may be "hidden" in some medicaments, can severely disrupt haemostasis and precipitate the collapse of the painstakingly maintained equilibrium. Application of H_2-*receptor antagonists* or *omeprazole* may prove to be a helpful preventive measure in controlling gastrointestinal haemorrhaging. *Infection-limiting measures* can also serve to prevent haemorrhage. *Intestinal cleansing* (purgation) using poorly absorbable antibiotics (e.g. neomycin, paromomycin) and/or lactulose to suppress gram-negative flora and diminish the danger from endotoxins is of vital importance. (s. pp 285, 286, 288)

If no haemorrhagic diathesis is present or when no invasive measures or techniques which might possibly distress the patient are planned, coagulation disorders generally **require no treatment.** *The equilibrium between haemostasis and fibrinolysis, which is based on lower clotting factor levels, is indeed somewhat unstable, yet it does not normally lead to spontaneous haemorrhaging.*

Should **substitution** of haemostatic factors be needed prior or subsequent to invasive procedures, *fresh plasma* is the agent of choice, since it contains not only a balanced mixture of procoagulant and anticoagulant factors, but also fibronectin, which serves to reinforce RES clearance. However, relatively large quantities of fresh plasma are required, and it is important that individual volume limits are adhered to for haemodynamic reasons. Preventive administration of *vitamin K* (10 mg/ week), subcutaneously injected if oral application is deemed inefficient or an intramuscular injection appears too risky, is recommended in suspected vitamin K deficiency. This measure can also be used prior to treatment with cephalosporins, in particular β-lactam antibiotics, or if the intestinal flora is in some way affected.

1.7.2 Pharmacological therapy

The **treatment** of haemostasis disorders is indicated in acute liver failure or when a necrotic episode occurs during the course of cirrhosis, even without haemorrhagic complications. There are *two reasons* for this: (*1.*) an elevated risk of haemorrhage must be anticipated in the event of acute liver dysfunction, and (*2.*) extensive liver necrosis leads to the release of thromboplastic compounds, accompanied by a deterioration in the microcirculation and additional haemostatic disturbances. In this situation, an early and optimized correction of coagulation and fibrinolysis parameters is thus essential. (1, 4, 10, 12, 16) (s. tab. 19.2)

Haemorrhage-related lethality of 20–30% (and more) has to be expected in the event that acute liver failure leads to **acute haemostasis disorders.** The following courses of treatment are recommended:

(*1.*) *Fresh frozen plasma* (FFP)*: 250 ml at six-hour intervals (10–20 ml/kg BW = 1,000–1,500 ml/day). Administration of 10 ml/kg BW (about 600–1,200 ml) serves to elevate the concentration of coagulation factors and inhibitors by 15–20%. The half-life of factor VII is only 6 hours, which is why dosage intervals of 6 to 12 hours must be maintained. IgA deficiency is a known contraindication. Adverse transfusion reactions may occur with a frequency of 1–5% of cases. Improvement in coagulopathy generally lasts one or two days. • Caution is called for, since accentuated coagulation entails the danger of thrombosis (if necessary, AT III replacement of up to 60–80%), and an overload of the intravascular volume must be avoided (monitoring of CVP!). (20) (s. tab. 19.2)

(2.) *Antithrombin III concentrate**: 1,000–2,000 U/day until the plasma AT III value exceeds 70%.

(3.) *Desmopressin acetate**: This vasopressin derivative (DDAVP) acts as an antidiuretic and antihaemorrhagic agent. It increases the turnover of factors VII, VIII, IX and XII and also shortens the bleeding time. The recommended dosage is 0.3–0.4 µg/kg BW as an i.v. infusion. This substance is contraindicated in the case of a thrombotic status. Further contraindications include ischaemic heart disease, cardiac arrhythmias and seizure disorders.

(4.) *Vitamin K**: 10 mg, subcutaneous administration, to be repeated for 3 to 7 days until the prothrombin time has been corrected. Be careful when using the intravenous route due to the risk of anaphylaxis and hypotension. Onset of action is within 6–12 hours, full impact is at 24 hours, subsequently lasting up to 7 days. An overdose should be avoided as it can cause a (sudden and dangerous) drop in Quick's value resulting from the formation of vitamin K oxide (s. tab. 19.2).

(5.) *PPSB**: Should Quick's value remain below 20% after treatment with fresh plasma, administration of 1,000–3,000 U/day is indicated (1 unit PPSB activates coagulation by 1–2%). This treatment should always be carried out in combination with fresh plasma and AT III concentrate to avoid the danger of thrombosis or the manifestation of DIC. It must also be borne in mind that PPSB (prothrombin [II]/proconvertin [VII]/Stuart-Prower factor [VIII]/antihaemophilic globulin B) may induce an increase in intravascular consumption in the presence of hypercoagulability, and indeed trigger haemorrhaging.

(6.) *Thrombocyte concentrates**: Administration of thrombocyte concentrates may be advisable when values lower than 30,000/µl are present, but this must be specifically indicated (e.g. thrombocyte deficit due to sequestration in the spleen, increase in consumptive coagulopathy, potential antibody formation).

(7.) *Fibrinogen**: Doses of 2–4 g (i.v.) at six to eight-hour intervals are recommended. Where haemorrhaging occurs, simultaneous administration of even small amounts of heparin is strongly contraindicated, particularly as the patient's heparin sensitivity may be highly elevated in this condition as well as after the administration of AT III. The use of heparin in such a situation thus involves very high risks. (s. tab. 19.2)

(8.) *Factor XIII**: The administration of *factor XIII* for fibrin stabilization (1,250 U, i.v. until cessation of bleeding) is worthy of consideration.

(9.) *Heparin**: Heparin was recommended as early as 1963 for the *prevention* of consumptive coagulopathy in cirrhosis patients. The interruption of intravascular thrombin coagulation by heparin has been confirmed in animal experiments. Soluble, circulating fibrin aggregates into microthrombi (within a few hours of the coagulation system being activated); heparin, however, cannot prevent this. The efficacy of heparin is dependent on normal AT III values. • *Heparin is no longer recommended as a prophylactic or therapeutic agent for DIC.*

*) The manufacturer's recommendations regarding application and dosage must be followed.

Treatment of **haemorrhagic complications** in acute or chronic liver disease initially focuses on the site of bleeding, i.e. in the upper or lower gastrointestinal tract. Mechanical, thermal and sclerotic measures are of prime importance. • Systemic clotting dysfunction is a potential contributory factor in more than 30% of cirrhotic patients with gastrointestinal bleeding. The seriousness of the haemorrhage depends to a great extent on the severity of the haemostatic disorder. Localized treatment must therefore be supplemented by additional corrective therapeutic measures, especially since a deterioration of the haemostatic potential in a haemorrhagic patient may occur rapidly and with serious consequences. The preparations listed above are also of value here, depending on the respective individual findings. (s. tab. 19.2)

1. **Local measures to arrest the bleeding**
2. **Correction of haemostasis disorders***   – antithrombin III concentrate   – desmopressin acetate   – factor XIII (factor rVII)   – fibrinogen   – fresh plasma/fresh blood   – PPSB   – thrombocyte or erythrocyte concentrate   – vitamin K

Tab. 19.2: Therapy of haemostasis disorders

It is not possible to draw up a "treatment schedule", since each individual case, including the financial status, calls for careful and critical evaluation of the respective measures. • The potentially deleterious countereffects produced by the haemostatic and fibrinolytic systems must be considered before any medication is administered.

2 Upper gastrointestinal haemorrhage

2.1 Definition

Upper (non-variceal) gastrointestinal (GI) haemorrhages comprise any bleeding occurring between the nasopharynx and the duodenojejunal fold (Treitz's arch), i.e. proximal to the duodenojejunal flexure. • *Such haemorrhages are especially problematic in cases where liver disease is also present.*

2.2 Forms

Acute gastrointestinal haemorrhage is the most frequent life-threatening emergency situation in gastroenterology. Incidence is as high as 50–100/100,000 population. In 85–90% of cases, upper gastrointestinal bleeding is involved. Differentiation can be made by applying various criteria relating to the haemorrhage, such as its course, extent, type and localization, as well as by classifying the bleeding activity. (s. tab. 19.3)

1. **Course of haemorrhage**
   - acute or chronic
2. **Extent of haemorrhage**
   - severe or slight bleeding
   - seeping bleeding
3. **Type of haemorrhage**
   - arterial, venous or capillary
4. **Source of haemorrhage**
   - petechiae, bleeding erosions, mucosal fissures, ulcer, variceal bleeding
5. **Classification of the bleeding activity of an ulcer**
   (J. A. H. Forrest et al., 1974)
   - I lesions with active bleeding
   - Ia spurting arterial bleeding
   - Ib seeping bleeding
   - II lesions with signs that bleeding has occurred
   - IIa visible vascular stump
   - IIb blood clot formation
   - IIc haematin at the bottom of the ulcer
   - III lesions without the above criteria, but with positive bleeding anamnesis

Tab. 19.3: Forms and classification of upper gastrointestinal haemorrhage, including the classification according to Forrest

2.3 Causes

Gastroduodenal ulcers account for 45–55% of cases of upper gastrointestinal bleeding, gastric or duodenal erosions for 25–35%, and oesophageal or fundus varices for the remaining 15–25%. Portal hypertensive gastropathy is frequently found together with portal hypertension. (22, 30, 37–39, 41, 46–48) Extensive haemorrhaging can often be observed in cases where a clotting dysfunction occurs simultaneously. • The spectrum of possible causes is exceptionally wide, particularly since manifest bleeding may originate from a combination of various (subthreshold) factors in individual cases. • Actually, approximately 5% of all cases of upper gastrointestinal haemorrhage remain aetiologically unresolved. (s. figs. 19.3–19.5) (s. tab. 19.4)

2.4 Diagnostics

Upper gastrointestinal bleeding may be either chronic or acute. It becomes manifest as severe or slight haemorrhages of arterial, venous or capillary origin. (s. tab. 19.3) Elimination of the blood is effected by vomiting or in the stool.

1. **Oesophageal, gastric and duodenal varices (18–25%)**
2. Angiodysplasia (1%) (s. fig. 19.5)
3. Boerhaave's syndrome
4. Bouveret's syndrome (31)
5. Clotting defects (s. fig. 19.4)
6. Dieulafoy's bleeding
7. Duodenal ulcer (25–30%)
8. Erosions (10–15%) (s. fig. 19.3)
9. Gastric ulcer (20–25%)
10. Haemobilia
11. Malignancies (3–5%)
12. Mallory-Weiss syndrome (5–8%)
13. Oesophagitis/reflux oesophagitis (8–10%)
14. Osler-Rendu-Weber's disease
15. Peptic jejunal ulcer
16. Portal hypertensive gastropathy or gastric antral vascular ectasia (GAVE) (22)
17. Watermelon stomach (36)

Tab. 19.4: Causes of upper gastrointestinal bleeding (with some references and frequencies)

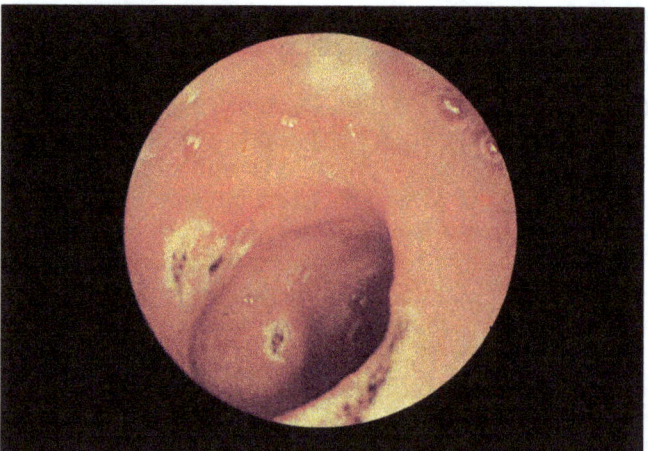

Fig. 19.3: Haemorrhagic erosions in the stomach as the cause of bleeding

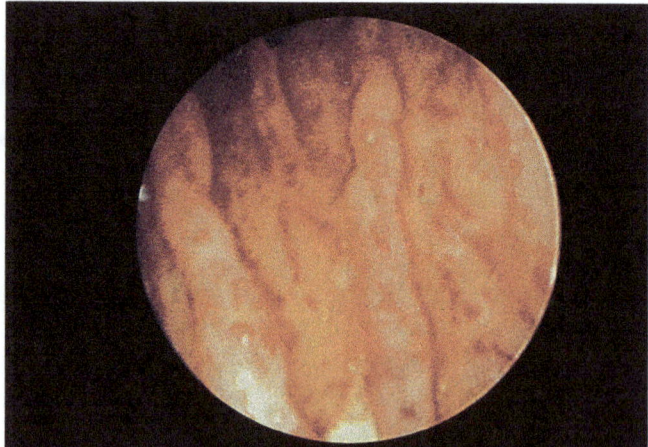

Fig. 19.4: Haemorrhagic gastritis in thrombopenia

Haematemesis: If bloody vomiting occurs immediately upon the onset of bleeding or if there is a deficiency of gastric hydrochloric acid or insufficient time for the formation of haematin, the vomited blood appears

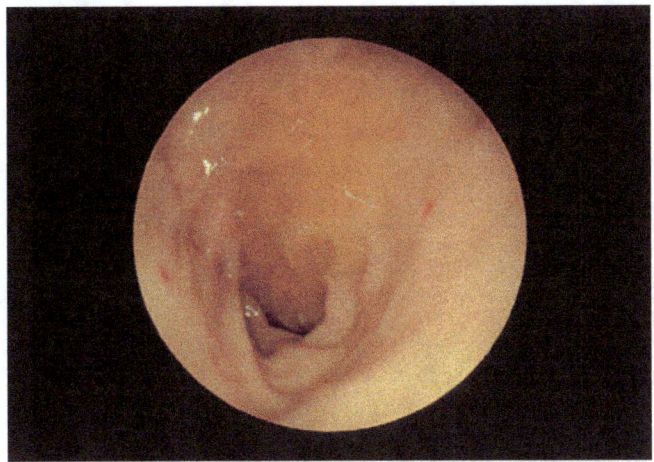

Fig. 19.5: Angiodysplasia in the duodenum

Allgoewer-Burri index
heart rate : *systolic RR = index*
index: 0.5 = normal; 1.0 to 1.5 = impending shock with circulating blood decreased by about 30%; exceeding 1.5 = circulating blood decreased by about 50%

bright red and is not foamy. After somewhat longer periods in the stomach, the blood becomes dark red to brown or black (= *coffee-ground vomiting*).

Melaena: A recognizable elimination of blood from the intestine normally takes place when more than 60–70 ml have accumulated in the lower intestine. As a result of bacterial and chemical action (lasting several hours), the stool becomes black in colour, so that a so-called *tarry stool* is observed. As a rule, the source of bleeding lies above the duodenojejunal flexure (ca. 90%). Melaena (s. p. 372) may, however, also arise from bleeding in the ileum or right colon – as could be demonstrated by the collection of blood in the caecum during appendectomy. The presence of larger amounts of blood in the intestine leads to an accelerated passage with diarrhoeal elimination.

Occult blood: Blood volumes of < 50 ml are not generally recognizable by discolouration of the stool, but must be demonstrated by special testing (e. g. test strips). (s. p. 372)

Diagnostic goals: The diagnostic procedure for upper gastrointestinal bleeding is largely standardized and has three main aims:

1. Estimation of the haemorrhagic activity
2. Quantification of the blood loss
3. Identification of the source of bleeding

Circulatory parameters: The determination of circulatory parameters allows a rough calculation of the amount of blood already lost as well as optimizing the subsequent diagnostic and therapeutic measures. Loss of more than 800–900 ml blood (or less in older patients and in cases of anaemia) causes *circulatory symptoms:* tachycardia, fall in blood pressure, decrease in both cardiac output and venous return to the heart. A central venous pressure (CVP) of < 5 cm H_2O suggests an unfavourable prognosis. The *Allgoewer-Burri index* has proved to be a useful, objective parameter:

Venous entries: Venous access points (one or possibly two) must be created as quickly as possible and kept open. Circulatory stabilization by means of *volume substitution*, at best with monitoring of the central venous pressure, is crucial. Diagnostic or therapeutic endoscopy is only possible once the circulation has been stabilized and any necessary *fresh blood* has been administered.

Loss of blood: Blood loss must be quantified by repeated determination of the *haemoglobin* and *haematocrit values*, because – depending on the severity of the bleeding – significant changes in these (and other) values only become evident after two to four hours due to the gradual flow of tissue fluid into the circulatory system.

Laboratory parameters: Once the initial blood sample has been taken to assess the blood loss, the following values must be determined immediately: *blood group, thrombocyte count, Quick's value, electrolyte profile* and *creatinine* as well as *fibrinogen* and *AT III levels*.

Endoscopy: It is essential that an endoscopic examination of the oesophagus, stomach and duodenum is carried out *as quickly as possible* under intensive care conditions with monitoring and pulsoximetry. The term "emergency endoscopy" is in fact misleading because upper gastrointestinal bleeding always constitutes an emergency and calls for immediate hospitalization and rapid diagnostic clarification.

▶ The **primary objectives** of initial endoscopy are: (*1.*) accurate identification of the location of the bleeding, (*2.*) evaluation of the bleeding activity, (*3.*) assessment of the danger of recurrent bleeding, and (*4.*) collection of coexisting findings. Endoscopy is 90–95% reliable in clarifying these questions (if necessary, repeated within a period of 12 to 24 hours). • The **secondary objective** is to decide on the therapeutic consequences, such as conservative and/or local treatment, or surgical intervention. To this end, the use of endoscopy with the possibility of simultaneous therapy is the method of choice, for which there is no viable alternative.

The grounds for the **primary use of endoscopy** to clarify upper (and lower) gastrointestinal bleeding are: (*1.*) endoscopy is acknowledged as the procedure which reveals the most conclusive information; (*2.*) this diagnostic procedure also provides the opportunity of using various endoscopic techniques to effect local haemostasis; (*3.*) endoscopic techniques are more likely to be readily available than scintigraphy or selective angiography; (*4.*) endoscopy is significantly more economical in terms of time and cost than scintigraphy or arteriography; (*5.*) endoscopy is less stressful for the patient and less invasive than angiography.

Complications cannot be attributed to endoscopy itself, but to the pre-existing conditions: localized perforations, risks associated with aspiration, cardiac problems, low blood pressure, etc. Premedication may be inappropriate in individual cases, and endotracheal intubation or endotracheal anaesthesia is then indicated.

Stomach tube: Use of a double-lumen stomach tube may be justified by several factors: (*1.*) detection of blood in the stomach, (*2.*) assessment of haemostasis, (*3.*) irrigation of the stomach to improve visibility during subsequent endoscopy, and (*4.*) permanent drip for clearing blood residues from the intestine to prevent the development of hepatic encephalopathy. (s. p. 285)

Scintillation scanning: In intermittent haemorrhagic lesions or subacute bleeding, valuable diagnostic data are yielded within a period of 24–36 hours by the use of scintillation scanning, employing ^{99m}technetium-labelled erythrocytes. The sensitivity of detection of bleeding is 93%, the specificity 95%, with an overall accuracy of 94%. Verification of bleeding is thus not only more reliable than arteriography, but is also far less invasive. (21)

Angiography: Selective angiography (coeliac artery, superior mesenteric artery) may be attempted if the haemorrhage site could not be localized by means of endoscopy and scintillation scanning. Angiography is also of intraoperative benefit. However, it is only possible to draw diagnostic conclusions with bleeding rates exceeding 0.5 ml/min. In individual cases, the administration of vasoconstrictor substances or an attempt at therapeutic embolization are rendered possible by using an in-situ angiography catheter.

2.5 Prognosis

Spontaneous haemostasis: Some 60–80% of all upper gastrointestinal haemorrhages cease spontaneously. Early diagnosis with simultaneous stabilization of the circulation facilitates such spontaneous haemostasis without further therapeutic measures being called for. In 10–15% of cases, the bleeding persists.

Risk factors: Several risk factors have a decisively negative influence on the prognosis. High-risk patients require particularly close observation. The necessity for surgical intervention may arise rapidly and often unexpectedly in such patients. Treatment is thus also directed at maintaining the patient in a permanent condition of operability. A new endoscopic index might possibly predict first bleeding from the upper gastrointestinal tract in patients with cirrhosis. (49) There is an almost linear correlation between the risk factors (s. tab. 19.5) and a negative prognosis or lethality. Larger vascular stumps at the base of ulcers (Forrest IIa, IIb) also show a tendency towards recurrent bleeding within 48 hours in 50% of cases. The risk remaining subsequent to the cessation of bleeding drops to less than 5% after three days and less than 1% after seven days. (28, 33, 42, 49)

Surgical measures: Surgical intervention is necessary in 5–25% of cases.

Lethality: Figures for lethality rates vary between 5–8% (and up to 30%). When no blood transfusion is necessary, the rate lies below 4%; when more than six units of blood have to be transfused, it can rise to 50%.

Prognosis: Decisive factors influencing the prognosis of acute GI bleeding include: (*1.*) immediate stabilization of circulation, (*2.*) prevention of aspiration, (*3.*) type of bleeding (varicose, arterial, diffuse), (*4.*) intensity of bleeding and blood loss, (*5.*) age and possible comorbidity of the patient, (*6.*) success of the treatment, and (*7.*) recurrent bleeding. (s. tab. 19.5)

1. State of shock in the hospitalized patient
2. Initial Hb value <7 g/dl or haematocrit <30%
3. Forrest state Ib/II
4. Insufficient circulatory stabilization despite optimal volume replacement
5. Consumption of >6 units of blood per 24 hours
6. Advanced age of patient, depending on biological aging
7. Concomitant illness: chronic liver, cardiac, pulmonary or kidney disease; diabetes mellitus; *etc.*
8. Short-term recurrence of bleeding
9. Ulcer patients after unsuccessful conservative therapy, possibly over an extensive period of time, and now requiring subsequent surgery

Tab. 19.5: Significant negative prognostic risk factors in upper gastrointestinal bleeding

In extensive bleeding from the larger arteries (e.g. gastroduodenal artery), surgery should be carried out immediately as opposed to losing valuable time with pointless endoscopic treatment.

2.6 Therapy

With coexisting liver disease, upper gastrointestinal bleeding poses special problems due to haemorrhagic complications or haemostatic disorders. Therapy is initially determined by the *form, location* and *classification* of the bleeding. (s. tab. 19.3) The *causes* of bleeding have a substantial influence on the therapy to be implemented – depending on the respective underlying disorder. (s. tab. 19.4) *Risk factors* that have a negative effect on the prognosis have to be considered in any decision regarding therapy, which is why the therapeutic procedures vary in individual cases. A bacterial infection is another important risk factor, so that the administration of antibiotics (e.g. norfloxacin) is recommended. (s. tab. 19.5) (s. fig. 19.12)

2.6.1 Basic therapy

Volume replacement: Adequate volume replacement, when possible through *two venous entry points*, is initially of utmost importance. A central vein entry point is strongly recommended to facilitate the constant monitoring of changes in CVP.

(*1.*) *Crystalloid i.v. solutions*, e.g. Ringer's solution, should only be used if the blood loss is relatively small (< 1 litre), since only 25–30% of the crystalloid i.v. solution has an effect on the volume. If administered in excessive amounts, this can lead to an undesired decrease in the colloidal pressure of the plasma. Crystalloid i.v. solutions, often with *glucose* as a principal energy source, also serve as carriers for any medicaments which have to be added to the drip infusion. HES is an acceptable plasma substitute. • *The use of fructose, xylose and lipid solutions, high concentration glucose (= rise in portal pressure) or dextran products (= inhibition of thrombocyte aggregation) is not advisable.*

(*2.*) **Human albumin solution** has proved extremely reliable, especially when used in conjunction with crystalloid infusions. (Synthetic iso-oncotic colloids should be avoided as far as possible because of their negative effects on coagulation and kidney function.)

(*3.*) *Packed red blood cells* are indicated when the blood loss is >25% (Hb < 7−8 g/dl). In this event, at least three or four units of blood should be readily available, and sufficient reserves must be on hand. An Hb value of 10−11 g/dl is seen as an adequate transfusion target. Degradation of the citrate normally present in conserved blood is delayed in the case of cirrhosis, so that a substitution of 10 ml calcium per four units of erythrocyte concentrate is advisable. In order to avoid transfusion acidosis (pH < 7.2), 40 mval bicarbonate are administered for every four or five transfusions.

(*4.*) *Frozen fresh plasma* is used in cases of high blood loss (> 50%), or even earlier if necessary (e. g. in the presence of concomitant coagulation defects). (s. p. 352)

Oxygen supply: Supplementary oxygen supply via a nasal tube is recommended. The air passages must be kept unobstructed, if necessary by intubation.

Gastrolavage using a double-lumen tube is of both diagnostic and therapeutic value in upper gastrointestinal haemorrhage. • Endobronchial intubation is recommended for disturbances of consciousness.

Bowel purgation: In gastrointestinal haemorrhage, large quantities of plasma proteins infiltrate the intestine. This results in an abundance of protein degradation products, which may cause **hepatic encephalopathy** in the presence of sustained failure regarding the detoxification function of the liver. In addition, the breakdown of intestinal blood releases a large amount of ammonia stored in the erythrocytes for systemic transport, thereby considerably accentuating the danger of HE. • *Any blood must therefore be removed as rapidly as possible from the gastrointestinal tract!* To this end, a gastric tube is used (during endoscopy) to aspirate blood from the stomach. A swift and thorough intestinal purge is achieved by administering a 10% *mannitol solution* or *Golytely solution* through nasal intubation until a state of haemostasis is assured. Residual blood may also be flushed from the lower colon by additional *high enemas* with 300 ml lactulose (plus 700 ml water). This intestinal purgation is followed by further treatment with lactulose. An additional infusion of *ornithine-aspartate concentrate* may be advisable for the prevention or treatment of HE. (s. p. 287)

In severe bleeding of portal hypertensive gastropathy, treatment with **thalidomide**, a potent inhibitor of angiogenesis, may be indicated. (32)

2.6.2 Endoscopic haemostasis

Spontaneous haemostasis, which is found without active therapy in about half the cases of upper gastrointestinal bleeding, should never encourage the assumption of a passive approach with the postponement of suitable therapeutic procedures. There is an enormous danger of massive renewed haemorrhage as well as of the development of complications within a few hours following spontaneous haemostasis. (s. fig. 19.15)

The development of effective procedures for endoscopic haemostasis − as well as the use of TIPS (45) − has significantly broadened the spectrum of treatment in cases of non-varicose, upper gastrointestinal bleeding. Endobronchial intubation is strongly recommended for disturbances of consciousness. In patients with acute upper GI bleeding, infusion of erythromycin (3 mg/kg BW over 30 minutes) before endoscopy improves the removal of blood and water from the stomach. Erythromycin is a motilin agonist and, as such, produces this favourable gastrokinetic effect. (27) These procedures have also improved the results achieved in differential therapy. In Forrest I and IIa, endoscopy is of prime importance. Three groups of **endoscopic methods** are available: (*1.*) topical procedures, (*2.*) thermal methods, and (*3.*) local injection techniques.

1. Topical procedures: Various compounds may be applied under endoscopic observation to the site of non-varicose bleeding or bleeding ulcerations following sclerotization. • The experience obtained with **adhesive fibrin** or **thrombin** is encouraging. This is also true of their application in *hypertensive gastropathy* and in *gastric antral vascular ectasia (GAVE)*. **Argon-plasma coagulation** (and possibly **laser** procedures) may also be used. Angiodysplasia is best managed using heat treatment, especially in the case of argon plasma coagulation.

2. Thermal methods: Various thermal methods may be employed successfully in clearly defined instances of non-varicose bleeding of the upper gastrointestinal tract:

(*1.*) The **heater technique** (R. L. PROTELL et al., 1978) involves the use of a plastic-coated metal probe, the tip of which is heated by means of a wire. Definitive haemostasis may be attained in 90−95% of cases. The heater probe has proved easy to operate and is free of complications. (25, 35)

Whereas the heat of the heater probe is directly transferred to the site of bleeding, in the following types of probes, the electrical energy is transferred by high frequency diathermy.

(*2.*) The **monopolar probe** (C. R. YOUMANS et al., 1970) has a small differential electrode inside a catheter, which may be routed to the site of bleeding through the endoscope. At the same time, the non-differential electrode surface is fastened to one of the patient's extremities. Highly concentrated electrical energy is emitted from the probe and effects deep tissue coagulation. Primary haemostasis was achieved in 79−91% of the reported cases; recurrent bleeding only occurred in 6−8%. (28)

(*3.*) The **bipolar probe** (D. C. AUTH et al., 1980) has no non-differential electrode, both electrodes being built into the tip. In the most widely used BICAP (= bipolar circumactive probe), a circular arrangement of several adjacent electrode pairs is incorporated into the probe tip. This limits the depth to which the electrical pulse penetrates the tissue. (28, 34, 43)

(4.) The **electrohydrothermoprobe** (EHT) (W. MATEK et al., 1983) is a refinement of the monopolar probe. It allows a stream of water to be directed through the probe: the site of bleeding can thus be irrigated and rendered more easily visible, and, at the same time, charring of the tissue in contact with the probe is prevented. In 92% of reported cases, definitive haemostasis was achieved, with recurrent bleeding in 11% of patients.

(5.) The high energy **neodymium YAG laser** (yttrium-aluminium garnet) has been used to treat bleeding gastrointestinal lesions (G. NATH et al., 1976). This method ensures deep tissue penetration of the energy, yet entails the disadvantage of a greater risk of perforation or ulceration. As with the monopolar probe, the tangential approach to the site of bleeding raises technical problems. On average, primary haemostasis was achieved in 90% (87–100%) of patients, and definitive haemostasis in 43–90%. Complication rates of up to 4% have been reported. (40, 43)

Analysis of the literature reveals no significant differences between electrocoagulation and (expensive) laser treatment procedures in terms of primary or definitive haemostasis. With laser therapy, the complication rate (0–4%) lies above that of electrocoagulation (0%). Heat and bipolar probes are regarded as the most "tissue-friendly", an inference supported by the results of animal experiments, while laser and monopolar probe methods are more "aggressive". The electrohydrothermal probe offers a compromise. In addition, electrocoagulation and EHT procedures are technically uncomplicated, locally applicable and lower in cost compared to laser methods.

3. **Local injection techniques:** Differentiation must be made between the use of local injections in the therapy of non-varicose bleeding in the upper gastrointestinal tract and the treatment of bleeding oesophageal varices. (24, 28, 40, 44)

Local injection treatment methods for non-varicose bleeding have proved uncomplicated, quick to carry out, independent of location, extremely reasonable in terms of cost and also very successful. • Absolute alcohol, adrenaline, polidocanol and hypertonic sodium solution are among the **active substances** used. A combination of suprarenin and polidocanol has meanwhile been established as first choice: adrenaline (0.005–0.01%) is injected into the mucous membrane surrounding the lesion in order to induce vasoconstriction. Directly afterwards, polidocanol (1%) or a hypertonic NaCl solution may be injected at the edges of the lesion, resulting in local oedema with vascular compression and thrombosis. The reported effectiveness of this method for primary haemostasis is 83–100%, and definitive haemostasis is attained in 91–94% of cases. The *complication rate* is <1%.

If a blood clot is found at the bleeding site, it should be removed straight away with the help of a probe or loop. This is followed by endoscopic therapy. In this way, the risk of rebleeding can be markedly reduced.

The spectrum of local injection treatment in gastrointestinal bleeding has been expanded and the results improved by the introduction of **N-butyl-2-cyanoacrylate** (J. P. GOTLIB et al., 1981). This "fluid tissue glue" polymerizes instantly on contact with blood and rapidly forms an embolus-like occlusion at the site of bleeding. (s. p. 362) • In addition, *fundus* and *stomach* as well as *duodenal varices* (K. OTA et al., 1998), which cannot be adequately assessed using standard sclerotization techniques, have become easier to treat. Tissue glue is still a possible therapy option.

4. **Haemoclips:** Using clips for bleeding ulcers can be problematic, since precise application is often unsuccessful in the presence of severe bleeding or when the ulcer has undergone deformation through scarring. Nevertheless, clips are nowadays regarded as the first-choice alternative if other forms of therapy fail. • Good results have meanwhile been achieved using haemoclips: recurrent bleeding was reduced to <10%. When this technique was combined with subcutaneous injection of hypertonic sodium solution or adrenaline, the rate of recurrent bleeding dropped to <3%. (29) The clips do not destroy the tissue, and the ulcer healing process is not impaired. If the ulcer base is too firm, it becomes more difficult to attach the clips and it may not be possible to use them at all. They are particularly suitable for dealing with Mallory-Weiss bleeding and Dieulafoy's ulcer. It should be mentioned that such clips are still relatively expensive. (24, 25, 29, 35)

2.6.3 Drug-controlled haemostasis

The use of particular substances may be considered in concordance with the existing haemorrhage situation. (s. tabs. 19.3–19.5) These may constitute either an adjuvant therapy to endoscopic haemostasis or be used when endoscopic or surgical measures are not indicated or not possible. (23, 26, 27, 38, 41, 48)

▶ Application of **pharmacological substances** in existing portal hypertension is aimed at reducing both the portal pressure and the hyperdynamic circulatory status as well as improving the microcirculation in the gastrointestinal mucosa. • Such substances are also used to correct the secretory and motor function status of the gastrointestinal tract, thus diminishing the overall vulnerability of the gastric mucosa. • The instability of the clotting system is controlled by the administration of fresh plasma. All these measures improve primary and definitive haemostasis as well as reducing the probability of any complications or recurrence of bleeding:

- Proton pump inhibitors
- H. pylori eradication

- Propranolol derivatives
- Vasopressin derivatives
- Somatostatin or octreotide
- Fresh plasma
- Thalidomide
- Sucralfate, antacids

3 Bleeding oesophageal varices

3.1 Oesophageal varices as collateral circulation

A serious **consequence of portal hypertension** is the formation of *collateral circulatory systems* with characteristic *haemodynamic circulation*. (s. p. 261) An awareness of these possibilities makes it easier to understand typical complications and provides grounds for the application of medicinal or invasive therapy for portal hypertension in the presence or absence of a haemorrhage. Enhanced inflow of blood from the splanchnic area into the portal vein or decreased resistance in the arterial splanchnic circulation (e.g. due to glucagon) increases portal hypertension. (s. tab. 14.8) (s. fig. 14.6)

▶ **Oesophageal varices,** like **cardia varices** and **fundus varices,** arise from a regional stasis of submucosal perioesophageal and paraoesophageal veins. • These varices are supplied by the left gastric vein and posterior gastric vein, while stomach varices are additionally served by the branches of the splenic vein and short gastric veins. Fundus varices may also receive a direct supply via a.v. shunts in the stomach wall. Neither the formation nor the presence of oesophageal varices shows any clinical signs. The development of Cruveilhier-von Baumgarten syndrome may protect cirrhotic patients from the risk of oesophageal varices forming and bleeding. (70) • *Elevated portal pressure is usually responsible for the formation of oesophageal varices.* (s. figs. 14.8 – 14.10)

3.2 Frequency and risks

Some 60 – 80% of all patients with portal hypertension develop oesophageal varices at some stage of their lives, half of them within two years and up to 90% within ten years of the initial diagnosis. Retrogression or spontaneous disappearance of oesophageal varices has been observed in less than 1% of patients within one year, mostly in the wake of extended and strict abstinence in cases of alcoholic cirrhosis. In 90 – 95% of cases, the varices are localized in the middle and lower third of the oesophagus (= "junction zone", i.e. in the area 2 – 6 cm above the oesophagogastric junction), and in 5 – 10% of cases, they are found in the area of the stomach fundus. Approximately 15% of patients have both oesophageal and stomach varices; these patients are particularly at risk with regard to haemorrhaging.

About 30 – 50% of oesophageal varix patients suffer from variceal bleeding during the course of their lives. • The risk of *initial haemorrhage* in a control group of untreated cirrhosis patients is approx. 20% per year (about 30% within three years). Most episodes of bleeding occur within the first year; altogether 70 – 90% occur within the first two years of observation. Some 20 – 30% cease spontaneously. The rate of *recurrent bleeding* (without prophylactic measures) is about 70% after the initial haemorrhage; the probability of a relapse is highest during the first week (75%), but is still relatively high after three months (30%). The prognosis is very poor in the event of early recurrent bleeding (more than twice within two days). (153)

Primary oesophageal bleeding proves fatal in 30 – 40% of cases despite adequate conservative treatment or emergency intervention. In general, 60 – 80% of patients survive longer than one year. Some 20 – 25% of all cirrhosis patients die as a direct result of bleeding oesophageal varices. • The lethality rate for each haemorrhage episode varies among the Child groups (A = 10%, B = 30 – 40%, C > 70%).

3.3 Predictive haemorrhagic factors

The *timing, degree of severity* and *frequency* of haemorrhage depend on numerous predisposing factors, which cannot, however, be used as sole criteria or in individual cases to predict the respective risk of bleeding. Full awareness of such established risk factors (s. tab. 19.6) is an important aid in defining previously non-haemorrhaging risk groups, giving the possibility of primary prophylactic measures. Severe splenomegaly and thrombopenia are also seen as risk factors. This aim has not become reality as yet. (125, 133, 134, 151)

Three pathogenetic mechanisms can trigger bleeding oesophageal varices: (*1.*) critical pressure increase in the varices, especially when it is sudden (= *explosion hypothesis*), (*2.*) flow turbulences with bidirectional blood flow in the varices (= *circulation hypothesis*), and (*3.*) inflammatory lesion at the varix surface with the formation of thin spots (= *erosion hypothesis*).

3.3.1 Increase in pressure

Oesophageal varices do not occur when the portal pressure lies below 10 – 12 mm Hg. It has been established that the risk of bleeding increases significantly in accordance with (*1.*) *size of the portohepatic pressure gradient,* (*2.*) *rise in the oesophageal varix pressure* (58, 135), and (*3.*) *subsequent growth in size of the varices.* The danger of recurrent bleeding also rises in relation to the variceal radius. A temporary elevation of the intravaricose pressure and the resulting increase in vessel wall tension may derive from one of several factors: the circadian rhythms (increase in nocturnal/early morning pressure), food intake, intra-abdominal pressure increase (from coughing, lifting heavy loads, choking, etc.) and even deep breathing as well as forceful respiratory movement. These may cause a sudden variceal rupture in isolated cases. (88, 131, 145, 149, 172) • An *upright posture* helps to limit the blood flow to oesophageal varices and hence reduces the risk of haemorrhage (101).

▶ The **pressure gradient** (HVPG) between the portal vein and the inferior vena cava (measured as the difference between WHVP and FHVP) is regarded as a more meaningful criterion than the simple portal pressure, which may be influenced by a variety of factors. (Portal vein pressure [P] = portal blood flow rate [F] x transhepatic vascular resistance [R]) (78) • Measurement of the blood flow in the **azygous vein** by means of thermodilution reveals a strong correlation between the oesophageal varix pressure and the varix size, but no correlation with the risk of bleeding. • The verification of a **hepatofugal blood flow** in the portal vein, splenic vein or superior mesenteric vein by duplex sonography predicts a limited risk of haemorrhage. The sonographic determination of a **hepatopetal blood flow** in the coronary veins correlates with a decreased tendency towards haemorrhaging. (192)

3.3.2 Endoscopic evaluation

In view of the methodological difficulties involved in the (direct or indirect) identification of relevant indicator levels, endoscopy is the only proven method available for identifying meaningful parameters concerning varices and hence for estimating the risk of haemorrhage. • The **various criteria** to be assessed in each endoscopy may also be of individual relevance for prognosis:

1. **Size of varices:** The determination of the size of varices is of fundamental significance in assessing the haemorrhage risk. This is done according to different criteria: *grade I* = 1–3 mm (small), visible or visible under strain; *grade II* = 3–5 mm (medium-sized), visible twisted, solitary or corkscrew-like; *grade III* = 6–10 mm (large), lumen-occluding; *grade IV* = >10 mm (very large), lumen-occluding, red patches, thin spots.

2. **Localization of varices:** The localization of varices may likewise be useful for evaluation purposes: those in the lower oesophagus and in the cardia area are more likely to rupture. The simultaneous presence of *oesophageal* and *fundus varices* (10–15%) carries an increased risk of haemorrhage.

3. **Surface of varices:** An assessment of the appearance of the variceal surface provides valuable criteria. The colour may be classified on a scale from (connective tissue-like) white to (blood clot-like) blue. Occasionally, there may be circumscribed red patches or stripes, corresponding to blocked and dilated vessels in the mucosa or submucosa. These are accompanied by an abnormal elevation of oesophageal varix pressure. They may be classified as small, *cherry-red spots* (A. E. DAGRADI et al., 1966), *red wall markings* in the form of stripes or *haemocystic spots* of over 4 mm in size resembling blood-filled blisters (K. BEPPU et al., 1981). *Diffuse red areas* may signify thin patches on the variceal wall. • *With elevated pressure in the varices, the growing increase in wall tension and decrease in wall thickness culminate in the formation of so-called* **thin spots,** *which are significant indicators of the risk of haemorrhage.* Varices with red-coloured signs are subject on average to about 40% more pressure than those without such signs, and haemorrhage occurs two or three times more frequently in such cases. (s. fig. 19.6)

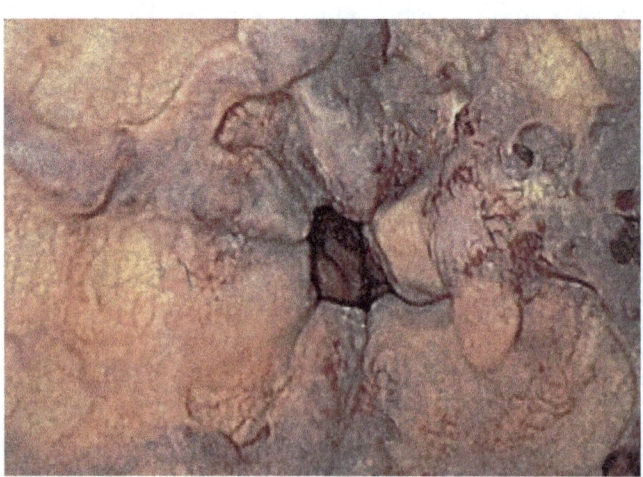

Fig. 19.6: Oesophageal varices with red wall signs

The **site of bleeding** can be located with precision in about 90% of cases. Haemorrhage may occur as seeping bleeding or as bright-red, spurting bleeding; there is often "pulsation", synchronous with respiration. An inactive haemorrhage site may occasionally be observed in the form of a coagulate or as a whitish thrombocytic embolus located at the point of rupture.

White nipple sign: No confirmation could be given of the findings reported by R. S. CHUNG et al. (1984) that a white nipple sign (= fibrin embolus) on a varicose node (= *Mount St. Helen's sign*) pointed to an unfavourable prognosis and recurrent haemorrhage. (171)

3.3.3 Sonographic evaluation

Endosonography may be regarded as a diagnostic improvement over sonography. (134, 139, 149, 162) (s. fig. 19.7) The recognition, diagnosis and sclerosing of varices is more reliably achieved by endosonography than by conventional endoscopy. (201) • A better evaluation of the risk of recurrent haemorrhage is also afforded by *duplex sonography.* (164)

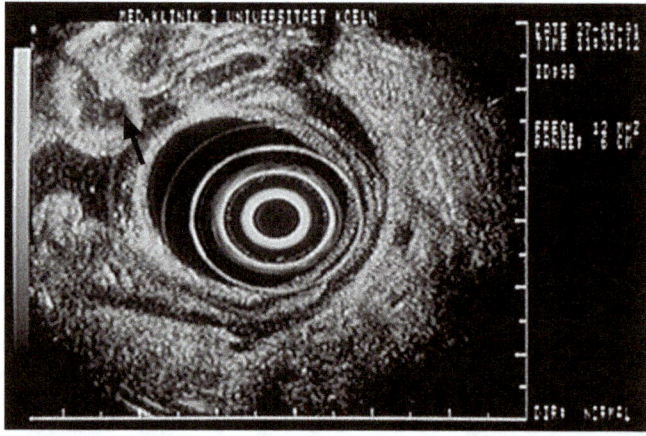

Fig. 19.7: Endosonographic detection of fundus varices (↑)

3.3.4 Child-Pugh criteria

Child-Pugh stage C (ascites, icterus, encephalopathy, albumin deficiency, drop in Quick's value) and regular alcohol abuse increase the frequency of haemorrhage and worsen the prognosis. *Coagulopathy* and *hyperfibrinolysis* are also considered to be additional risk factors, especially since higher fibrinolytic activity has been demonstrated in the mucosa of oesophageal varices. A correlation between the appearance of large *spider naevi* (>15 mm in diameter) on the skin surface and the onset of bleeding oesophageal varices was established by B. VARELA FUNTES et al. (1950). • A change in body position (e.g. bending over, lying down), cardia insufficiency, oesophagitis and gastro-oesophageal reflux have *no influence* on the tendency towards variceal bleeding.

3.3.5 CT and MRI

It is helpful to use CT with gastric varices (161, 197) and MRI with oesophageal varices (127), portal biliopathy (72) and bleeding of gall-bladder varices. (73)

3.4 Clinical aspects

Haematemesis: Oesophageal bleeding usually begins unexpectedly and without any characteristic preliminary signs. The onset is frequently in the evening, during the night or in the morning — possibly relating to the circadian rhythm of the portal pressure increase, vascular tone or clotting factors. (88, 131, 172) The haemorrhage often presents as surging haematemesis, and volumes of 500–1,000 ml of blood are vomited. The renewed accumulation of blood in the stomach may give rise to further surging haematemesis after a certain "pause in bleeding".

Endoscopic findings: An endoscopic diagnosis of the haemorrhaging should be undertaken as a matter of priority as quickly as possible after the circulation has been sufficiently stabilized. This has *three objectives*: (*1.*) exact localization of the source of bleeding, (*2.*) determination of the haemorrhage criteria, and (*3.*) assessment of coexistent findings. Additional, nonvariceal sources of haemorrhage occur in up to 30% of cases in the presence (and even absence) of varices. (s. fig. 19.8)

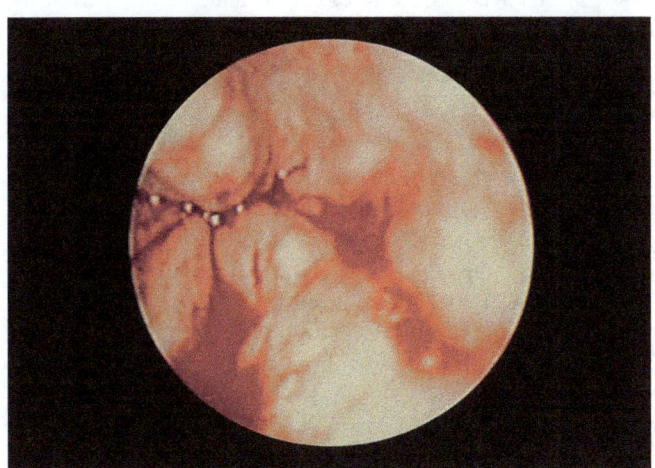

Fig. 19.8: Fresh bleeding of the oesophageal varices (first bleeding)

Circulatory disturbance: There is great variation in the effects of oesophageal bleeding on the circulation, depending on individual circumstances. Sometimes, only slight tachycardia and hypotension are presented despite extensive bleeding, whereas in other cases, a critical state of shock is rapidly induced, often leading to death. Sudden, unexpected transitions from an apparently compensated circulatory condition to a deleterious haemorrhagic shock must always be anticipated. The monitoring and evaluation of *circulatory parameters* are thus of utmost importance. (s. p. 355)

In the evaluation of the various **risk factors** hitherto discussed, which have also been expressed as quantifiable *scores* (NIEC score, München score), a simplified and practicable scheme may prove useful. (s. tab. 19.6)

Parameter	Low risk / I	High risk / III
1. Varix size	small (3–5 mm)	large (> 6 mm)
2. Fundus varices	absent	present
3. Red-coloured signs	slight	strong
4. Variceal pressure	< 15 mm Hg	> 16 mm Hg
5. Localization	mid-oesophagus	lower oesophagus
6. Alcohol	abstinent	habitual user
7. Hyperfibrinolysis	no	yes
8. Thrombopenia	no / slight	strong
9. Splenomegaly	slight	strong
10. Child-Pugh stage	A ⟶ B	C

Tab. 19.6: Relevant parameters as distinct risk factors for assessing the haemorrhagic tendency of oesophageal varices

Complications: The possible outcome of oesophageal haemorrhage can take the following forms: (*1.*) haemorrhagic shock, (*2.*) acute liver or kidney failure, (*3.*) hepatic encephalopathy (culminating in hepatic coma), (*4.*) consumptive coagulopathy, and (*5.*) aspiration pneumonia.

3.5 Conservative therapy

3.5.1 Basic therapy

Basic therapy of bleeding oesophageal varices is carried out under intensive care conditions. It essentially corresponds to the procedures for upper gastrointestinal haemorrhage (s. p. 356) and has **three main objectives:**

1. *Volume replacement* for circulatory stabilization
2. *Gastrointestinal irrigation* to prevent hepatic encephalopathy
3. *Monitoring of haemostasis* to prevent coagulopathy

Volume replacement should not increase CVP beyond 4–5 cm H_2O or the haematocrit beyond 35%, since there is a danger of recurrent bleeding from the oesophageal varices in the event of overcompensation. *Haemostasis parameters* (e.g. thrombocyte count, Quick's value, fibrinogen, AT III) must be continually monitored, so that any need for volume replacement is recognized immediately. • A *torsade de pointes* (special form of ventricular tachycardia) may arise in the case of an electrolyte imbalance combined with vasopressin and neuroleptics. (84) (s. fig. 19.9)

3.5.2 Sclerotherapy

▶ The sclerosing of bleeding oesophageal varices was first carried out by C. Crafoord et al. (1939). They injected the agent quinine-uretan (used at that time to sclerose haemorrhoids) into the varices via an oesophagoscope applying their own customized needle. This method was taken up by E. WODAK in 1958 and subsequently recommended for the periodic treatment of bleeding oesophageal varices. Positive clinical results employing a paravaricose sclerosing technique were likewise reported by H. DENK (1963).

Primary haemostasis: According to many publications, sclerotherapy has a success rate of 80—90% (60—100%) for establishing primary haemostasis.

Definitive haemostasis: Definitive haemostasis can only be considered as "certain" after the complete sclerosing of oesophageal varices carried out during four to six days of treatment in a period of six to eight weeks. • The sclerosing of oesophageal varices has meanwhile become standardized procedure.

Methods: Many technical modifications in the field of sclerotherapy have been reported and evaluated in a variety of publications. Variations in method include the range of instruments, injection technique, amount and concentration of the sclerosant per puncture as well as over the whole treatment period, needle gauge and time lapse between treatments. The results achieved are nonetheless largely identical. The method selected ultimately depends on the experience of the physician involved and, in individual cases, on the particular clinical picture. (174)

Rigid oesophagoscope: Endoscopic sclerosing is normally carried out under i.v. sedation, employing flexible instruments with a wide suction channel. General anaesthesia is recommended in difficult cases of severe bleeding. • The use of a rigid oesophagoscope may be advantageous for endotracheal anaesthesia in special circumstances (compression of strongly bleeding varices, localized focusing on varicose nodes within the endoscope aperture, improved aspiration of blood). Such a technique is, however, in itself more difficult. *Adequate experience in "rigid" methods is without doubt extremely advantageous in intensive care situations.*

Injection technique: Intravascular, paravascular (submucosal) or combined injection techniques may be employed. • An *intravaricose injection* results in immediate thrombosis and subsequent fibrosis of the varices. • The *paravaricose technique* facilitates first the compression of the haemorrhaging varices and then the (submucosal) formation of coarse scar tissue, which prevents variceal rupture and maintains the collateral integrity of the venous lumen at the same time. Replacement of the entire oesophageal mucosa by a connective tissue lining may be necessary to eradicate the varices completely. Paravascular injection often results in the sclerosing of varices. No significant differences between the efficacy of the two methods have been shown. Moreover, the "freehand" nature of clinical treatment renders any strict differentiation between intra- and paravascular methods difficult. • Preference is thus given to the *combined injection technique* (N. SOEHENDRA et al., 1981), since the sclerosing of varices is more rapidly achieved in this way and rebleedings or the appearance of new varices are more seldom. • It is important for successful treatment that sclerosing begins at the gastro-oesophageal junction and proceeds proximally.

Sclerosants: The following sclerosants are generally applied: polidocanol (0.5%—3.0%), ethanolamine oleate (5%), sodium morrhuate (2.5—5.0%), aqueous phenol solution (3%), sodium tetradecylsulphate (1—3%), ceplacolin (95%), phenolic almond oil (5%) and ethyl alcohol (45%). • **Polidocanol** (hydroxypolyethoxydodecane) is the most frequently used. The higher the concentration and the quantity of the sclerosing agent, the more common side effects are. However, the sclerosing impact is far more reliable, including the "desired" local inflammation with scar formation. • The most effective sclerosant (within ca. 20 seconds) is **N-butyl-2-cyanoacrylate** (0.5 ml + 0.7 ml lipiodol), which may only be injected into the varicose vein! It is already used widely as a method of choice. Technically speaking, an endoscopic operation is time-consuming and calls for perfect teamwork if tissue damage and clogging of the instrument are to be avoided. Risks for the patient include mediastinitis, local ulcerations and systemic embolisms. (81, 85, 122, 136, 179) • The combined use of butylcyanoacrylate and ethanolamine oleate has also been reported. (181)

Injection volumes of 1—2 ml per paravascular technique and 3—5 ml per intravascular technique are recommended, with a maximum of 30 ml per day. A total of ten injections may be required for each treatment session.

Injection interval: A one-week interval between treatment sessions (three to seven days for paravascular injection, at least seven days for intravascular injection) has proved to be effective for the obliteration of varices by means of repeated sclerosing (usually a total of five to six sessions).

Advantages: There are obvious advantages in using sclerotherapy: (*1.*) high effectiveness, (*2.*) low complication rate, (*3.*) no deleterious effects on haemodynamics or liver function, (*4.*) simplicity of use, (*5.*) patient acceptance, and (*6.*) well-balanced cost-benefit ratio.

Side effects: Side effects such as erosions, superficial ulceration or mucosal necrosis can be expected in >80% of cases. Sucralfate, cimetidine, ranitidine and omeprazole as well as fibrin adhesive have been used both for prevention and to promote healing. From a morphological viewpoint, these inflammatory tissue reactions are to a certain extent necessary to induce thrombosis and angiofibrosis. Fever, leucocytosis, chest pain and tension occur as frequent, yet usually insignificant concomitant reactions. Dysphagia or dysfunction of the oesophagus are of no clinical significance. The development of a gastro-oesophageal reflux is the subject of some controversy.

Complications: The frequency of complications fluctuates considerably, and thought must be given to the great differences between haemorrhage patients. Complicative developments can be anticipated in 10—20% of cases (when flexible instruments are used). Serious complications occur in 1—3% of cases. Lethality has been reduced to 1%. (56, 107) • Approximately *forty different types of complications* have been reported: radiologically demonstrable thoracic findings (80—85%) (166), oesophageal strictures (10—15%) (117), thrombosis of the subclavian vein, bleeding from sclerosing ulceration (5—10%) (165, 199), perforation of the oesophagus (1—2%), broncho-oesophageal fistula, mediastinitis, infection or bacteraemia (155) including pyogenic meningitis and cerebral abscess (195), formation of haematoma (159), gastro-oesophageal reflux (111), pleural effusion in 10—20% of cases (55, 109), chylothorax (68) and other pleuropulmonary complications (166), pericarditis or pericardial effusion (114), arrhythmias and myocardial ischaemia, peritonitis (178), ascites, thrombosis of the portal vein (119), development of squamous cell carcinoma (64, 91, 104, 118), etc. • The use of polidocanol can lead to considerable cardiodepressive effects. The potential danger of embolism, particularly of cerebral embolism, has been mentioned in connection with butylcyanoacrylate application. Disseminated coagulopathy has been described following repeated injections of ethanolamine oleate. • Life-threatening ventricular arrhythmias, so-called **torsade de pointes**, have been observed subsequent to the application of neuroleptics or vasopressin as well as in the case of electrolyte imbalances. (84) (s. fig. 19.9)

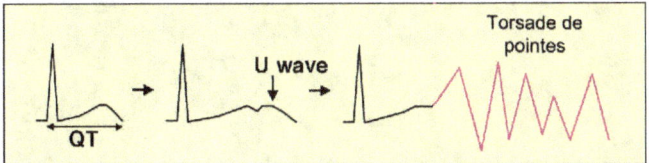

Fig. 19.9: Torsade de pointes: The QT interval represents the phase of myocardial spread of stimulus and repolarization. Excessive QT lengthening may be caused by certain drugs or electrolyte imbalance. In addition, a U wave can occur, whereby its amplitude exceeds the T wave in $V_4 - V_6$. Subsequently, a potential life-threatening arrhythmia of type torsade de pointes may develop. Clinical symptoms include vertigo and syncopes. This arrhythmia can spontaneously disappear, but also pass into ventricular fibrillation and thus end fatally

Indications: The use of sclerosing therapy – *which has been widely replaced by banding therapy!* – is based on three indications:

1. in acute bleeding of oesophageal varices
2. for preventing the recurrence of bleeding
3. as a preventive measure against primary haemorrhage

Primary haemostasis: *Acute sclerosing* is generally performed during the first endoscopic examination. The rate of haemostasis is 70–95(–100)%. Frequency of (early and late) recurrent bleeding has been reduced to 30–50%, most effectively after several months, when all varices have been obliterated. Nevertheless, an annual risk of recurrent bleeding of 10–20% remains due to newly formed varices, especially in the stomach fundus. Inpatient mortality is about 20%. However, more ways are being found to improve life expectancy. • If acute sclerosing is not possible or has failed due to massive haemorrhaging, the *balloon tamponade* may be used to provide temporary relief until the circulation has stabilized sufficiently. (s. p. 364) However, this is only effective for a limited period of time and in about 80% of patients. • Adjuvant *medicinal therapy* to reduce portal pressure is helpful. (s. p. 366) • At this stage, *elective sclerosing* can generally be performed with better visibility and circulatory conditions. In approx. 70% of cases, primary haemostasis can be achieved by means of acute or elective sclerosing. It is seldom necessary to perform portal vein surgery. (54, 57, 61, 73, 85, 86, 89, 90, 95, 106, 113, 126, 146, 168, 170, 174–176, 180, 181, 183, 184, 189, 190, 194)

The sclerosing of acutely bleeding fundus or stomach varices is more difficult from a technical point of view. (110, 161, 197) In this respect, the use of **butylcyanoacrylate** is a genuine step forward. (79, 81, 85, 122, 136) More effective haemostasis and a lower rate of late recurrent bleeding (about 8%) may also be achieved in sclerosing oesophageal varices using this substance, which is only administered intravascularly! Adverse effects include delayed rejection of the plastic-like plugs (after 6 to 8 weeks) and protracted healing of the defect. (s. p. 362) • *Pregnancy* does not preclude successful sclerotherapy. (102, 116) • *Nutrition* has no influence on the complication rate of sclerotherapy.

Interval sclerosing: There is *recurrence of bleeding* in 30–40% of patients within the first five or six days. Preventing a relapse is the most important consideration in the weeks following the successful treatment of primary haemorrhage. This *secondary prophylactic measure* helped to reduce the rate of potentially fatal recurrent bleeding from 70–80% to 30–40% over an observation period of one to four years as compared with a control group. The importance of acute sclerosing for primary haemostasis and of interval sclerosing for the prevention of relapses as well as in a long-term prophylactic strategy is undisputed. • The next sclerosing step is performed within the first three to seven days and repeated at weekly intervals until the varices are fully obliterated. Interval sclerosing, each time lasting one or two days, is undertaken during hospitalization. Endoscopic follow-up is carried out at two to three-month intervals, with further sclerosing in the event of any recurrence of varices. • During the **bleeding interval,** the following procedures are available: (*1.*) programmed *sclerosing* or *ligature treatment*, (*2.*) supplementary *drug therapy*, and (*3.*) portosystemic *shunting*. These procedures must be in accordance with the specific conditions of each case.

Prognosis: The *renewed formation* of collateral varicose lesions appears in 40–60% of patients within two years following the eradication of varices, although these patients tend to suffer fewer relapses of bleeding than those without new shunts. Fundus varices are found in 2–7% of cases. The question of a prognosis *quoad vitam* cannot be resolved simply in terms of the technical success of sclerosing, but is also substantially influenced by the prevailing liver function and by portal hypertension. In the first year, the survival rate in the Child A group proved to be significantly higher (80–95%) than in the Child C group (40%). Meta-analyses confirm the superiority of acute and interval sclerosing over non-endoscopic procedures not only with respect to primary haemostasis and the prevention of bleeding, but also regarding the improvement of survival time. Repeated sclerotherapy resulted in a five-year survival rate of 26%. (120) The prognosis for fundus varices, which are physically less accessible to therapeutic measures, is generally not so favourable. (71, 93, 120, 158, 176, 197)

Gastric varices are found in the fundus or in the region of the cardia. They have a lower rate of bleeding than oesophageal varices (5–10% of all acute variceal bleeding), but a higher lethality. Due to their deeper location in the submucosa in comparison to oesophageal varices, sclerotherapy or banding is generally ineffective and may even aggravate the bleeding. Isolated gastric varices are mainly found in splenic vein thrombosis. Therapy is based on direct injection of N-butyl-2-cyanoacrylate into the varices (52, 79, 81, 110, 112, 122, 136, 161, 167, 177), balloon tamponade (140) or balloon-occluded retrograde transvenous obliteration. (s. fig. 19.10)

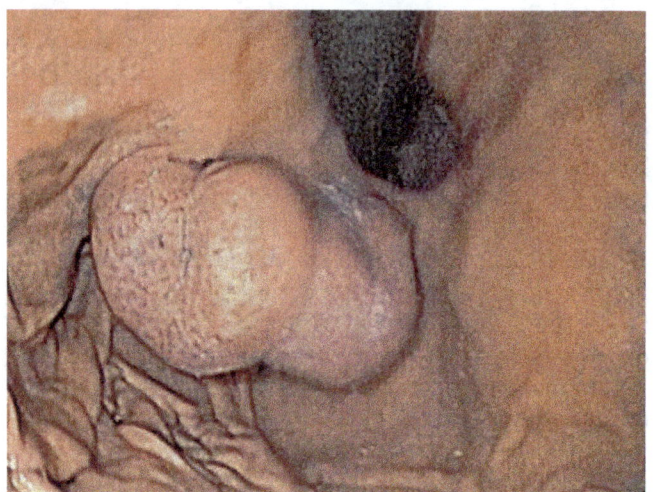

Fig. 19.10: Large varix in the gastric cardia

Duodenal varices are rare. Consequently, their frequency is poorly documented. They are present predominantly in patients with prehepatic portal hypertension. Therapy options include banding and medication (terlipressin, octreotide, later on β-blockers, etc.) or TIPS (provided there is no portal thrombosis). (59)

3.5.3 Endoscopic variceal ligation

▶ Following the propagation of rubber band ligation for haemorrhoids by J. BARRON (1963), oesophageal varix ligation was later introduced by G. VAN STIEGMANN et al. in 1986.

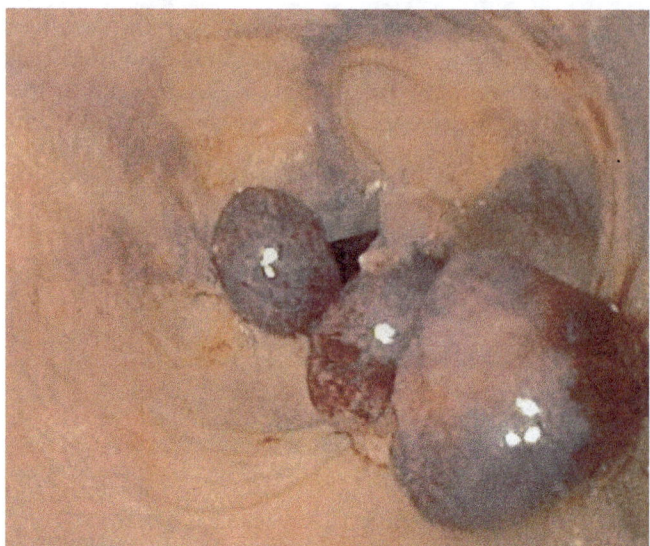

Fig. 19.11: Pronounced oesophageal varicosis: indication for ligation

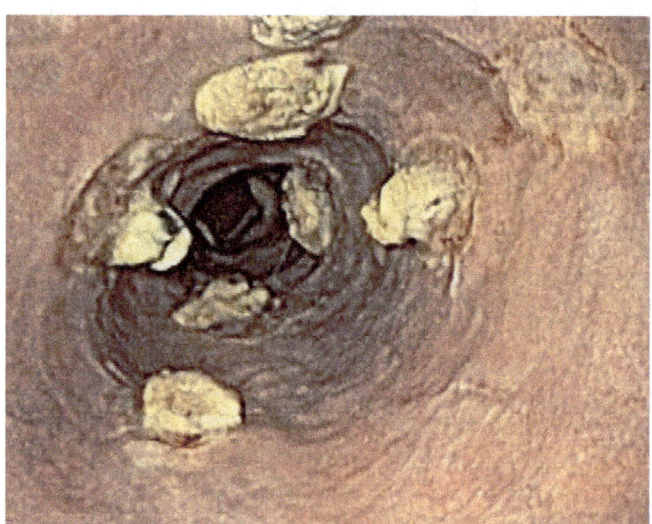

Fig. 19.12: Pronounced oesophageal varicosis: condition after ligation

Method: After sucking a varicose cord into a chamber at the tip of the endoscope, a rubber ring is applied around the respective varix in order to strangulate the bleeding varicose nodule. Between six and ten varices can be ligated during one session with the help of a speedband. Such an application set is available for clinical use. The multiligator top can carry as many as six to eight rings. As a rule, four or five sessions are held at weekly intervals. • A special *complication*, with lethal outcome in one case, is oesophageal perforation. This event can presumably be attributed to the entrapment of the oesophageal mucosa in the 6 mm aperture between endoscope and conductor, with subsequent rupturing upon further penetration of the piloting tube. Another rare complication is cerebral artery air embolism. (s. figs. 19.11, 19.12)

The reported **advantages** over sclerotherapy are (*1.*) lower rate of complications (2% vs. 22%), (*2.*) reduced occurrence of strictures or oesophageal dysphagia, (*3.*) swift and efficacious placement, (*4.*) lower frequency of recurrent bleeding (36% vs. 48%), (*5.*) ligation-related ulcerations are flatter and their healing is more rapid, (*6.*) fewer sessions are required, and (*7.*) mortality rate is lower (28% vs. 45%). The prerequisite is that the method is applied in such a way as to ensure precise placement. *This form of therapy has proved successful and even superior to sclerotherapy.* The ligation set, however, reduces the field of vision by about 30%, and aspiration of blood is hence rendered more difficult. At the Child A stage, this method is very efficient; in Child B, it is only indicated under certain conditions. This applies both to the treatment of acute variceal bleeding and secondary prophylactic strategy. In severe bleeding, a combination of ligation with somatostatin was more effective than sclerotherapy alone or drugs. • *After many years of experience, rubber-ring ligation has become the method of choice.* However, an initial rubber-ring ligature followed by sclerotherapy is also recommended. Mean success rate is 90−92%. (90, 122, 123, 126, 143, 145, 157, 160, 163, 170, 177, 179, 191, 198, 199)

3.5.4 Balloon tamponade

Massive bleeding can be effectively controlled by mechanical compression of bleeding oesophageal or fundus varices, yet only for a limited period of time. Unless the bleeding is life-threatening, it is necessary to carry out a preliminary endoscopic examination in order to localize the source of bleeding for ensuring accuracy in the selection and placement of the tube. (s. fig. 19.13)

The use of balloon tamponades in the form of the *Sengstaken-Blakemore tube* or *Linton-Nachlas tube* constitutes rapid and highly effective **emergency treatment**; this technique is initially necessary in some 10—15% of cases of acute bleeding. It guarantees primary haemostasis in about 80% (75—100%) of cases. Care should be taken in choosing a suitable balloon tube for each individual case. This method is indicated in cases of massive bleeding where no specific sclerotherapy or rubber-ring ligation is feasible because of greatly impaired visibility. The balloon tube may also be indicated in massive bleeding to bridge the time span until the circulation has been stabilized and the planned measures can be applied (even during transportation of the patient). It should also be possible to insert a balloon tamponade under intensive care conditions as and when required. As regards other causes of upper gastrointestinal bleeding, the balloon tamponade method is not appropriate, except under special circumstances. (87, 105, 140)

The **Sengstaken-Blakemore tube** (s. fig. 19.13) is the most widely used type. It comprises *four channels*: gastric tube, gastric balloon tube, oesophageal balloon tube, and tube for aspiration from the oesophagus via the tamponade. The tube is lubricated (using glycerine or liquid paraffin) and introduced through the nose (or, if necessary, through the mouth). The correct position of the tube in the stomach can be checked by auscultation (when air is blown through the lumen) or by X-ray. The gastric balloon is inflated with 150—250 ml air (secured with two clamps) and carefully fixed to the nose (or the mouth). It is not recommendable to weight down the tube. After the balloon has been positioned in the fundus, the oesophageal tube is inflated under manometric control to a pressure of about 40 mm Hg (generally, the oesophageal varix pressure does not exceed 30 mm Hg). At intervals of approximately two hours, the tube should be unblocked for 10 to 15 minutes to maintain the mucosal blood flow. It is imperative to keep the patient and the endoscopic technique under constant surveillance. Should the aspiration controls via the gastric and oesophageal tubes indicate a satisfactory degree of haemostasis, the oesophageal balloon is deflated, while leaving the gastric balloon inflated in the same position. After a further six to eight hours without recurrence of bleeding, the gastric balloon is likewise unblocked and the Sengstaken tube removed. The patient is kept in a head-up position throughout the whole procedure. • A different model, known as the **Minnesota tube**, is equipped with an additional feature to allow aspiration of the oesophageal contents above the balloon.

The **Linton-Nachlas tube** (s. fig. 19.14) has *three channels*: gastric tube with several lateral openings, tube for the pear-shaped gastric balloon, and oesophageal tube with lateral openings for aspiration. The gastric balloon is inflated with 350—500 ml air (depending on the physical stature of the patient) and drawn into the fundus and cardia area as well as into the lower oesophageal section by weight traction (500—750 g). This ensures good compression of the varices. As a rule, the tamponade can be maintained for 36 hours, with no intermittent unblocking. After this period of time, the

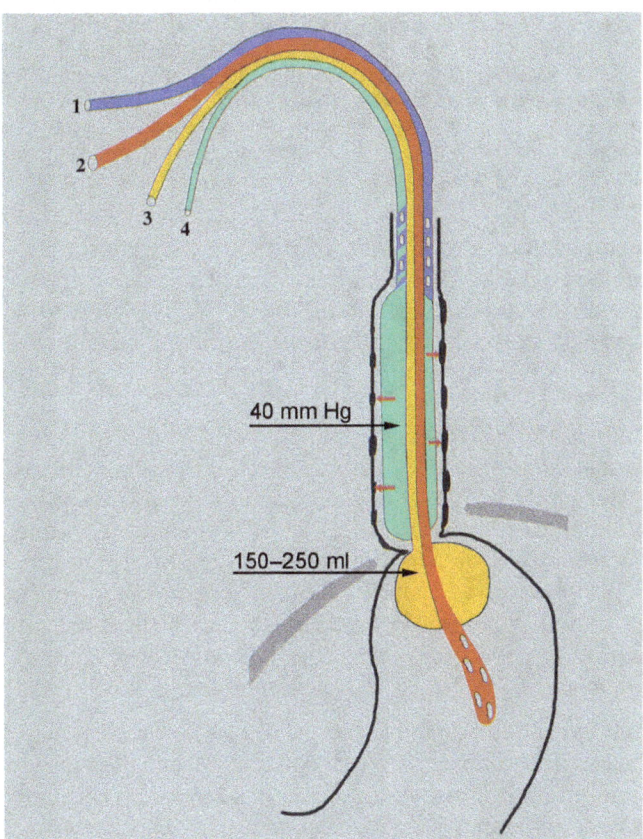

Fig. 19.13: Sengstaken-Blakemore tube (R.W. SENGSTAKEN, A.H. BLAKEMORE, 1950): 1. oesophageal tube, 2. gastric tube, 3. gastric balloon tube, 4. oesophageal balloon tube

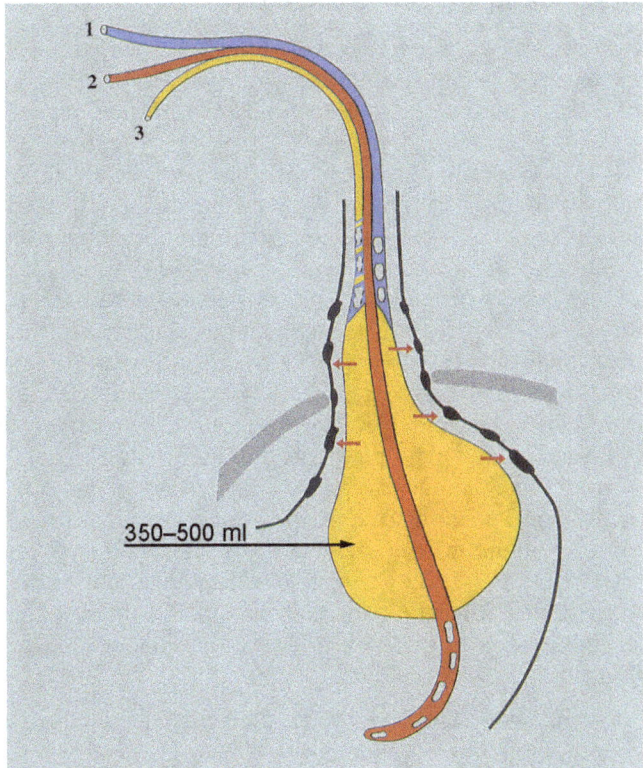

Fig. 19.14: Linton-Nachlas tube (R.R. LINTON, 1953; M.M. NACHLAS, 1955; L. BERTRAND, H. MICHEL, 1969): 1. oesophageal tube, 2. gastric tube, 3. balloon tube

weight for traction is removed, yet the position of the tube remains unchanged for a further period of 12 hours. Hourly lavage and aspiration yield reliable information on the therapeutic results. In order to prevent nasal ulcers, pressure and rubbing should be avoided as far as possible. It is imperative for the patient to maintain a supine position with the head raised and secured by means of sandbags. • *The tube currently in use was developed by L. BERTRAND and H. MICHEL (1969).*

Complications: In 15—20% of patients, aspiration pneumonia, ulceration, oesophageal rupture or asphyxia occur due to dislocation of the tube. Therefore, the *range of indications for endotracheal intubation* must be limited. Overall duration should not exceed 6 to 12 (to 24) hours. The use of the tube is in itself rather unpleasant. Care of the patient and medicotechnical measures are rendered difficult by the indwelling tubes. After the balloon tube has been removed, **recurrent bleeding** can be expected in 30—50% of cases. This may necessitate another tamponade; alternatively, endoscopic procedures or medication for haemostasis can be employed. • *In cases of inadequate therapeutic success, further measures for a definitive haemostasis of bleeding oesophageal varices must be initiated without delay.*

Self-expandable metal stent: A new type of stent with special introducers allowed correct placement without radiographic assistance in massive bleeding. Bleeding ceased immediately after implantation. The stent was left in position for 2—14 days. This method was safe and effictive. (97)

3.5.5 Prevention of primary bleeding

K. J. PAQUET (1982) suggested the **sclerosing of varices** as a preventive measure and put forward a system of grading to assess risk patients for primary prophylactic procedures. Even though the size of the varix (degrees III and IV) generally correlates with the risk of bleeding, the *compiling of a prognostic index* proved unreliable, since it is virtually impossible to estimate the danger of haemorrhaging in the individual. This applies especially to the risk associated with prophylactic sclerotherapy and shunt operations. The results made available in the meantime have proved variable and controversial, for which reason primary sclerosing is not recommended as a preventive measure. Nevertheless, according to a meta-analysis, primary prophylactic measures using polidocanol were far more effective in improving the survival time when compared to a reference group, particularly in patients with a greater risk of bleeding. (50, 124, 150, 156, 160, 187, 188) • Preventive **variceal ligation** is also effective and safe in Child-Pugh A and B, especially in combination with nadolol, and offers a greater chance of survival than do β-blockers. (99)

Prophylactic medication consists of *β-blocking agents* (propranolol, timolol, nadolol). (s. p. 267) The risk of primary bleeding could be reduced by about 50%. (65, 74, 132, 147, 156) • Parallel treatment with *isosorbide mononitrate, molsidomine* and *spironolactone* is recommendable from a pharmacological point of view. Portal venous pressure should be 20—30% lower. • Previous studies have shown that all patients with cirrhosis and oesophageal varices should be given primary prophylactic medication. • Alcohol, acetylsalicylic acid and NSAIDs should be avoided. There is no advantage to be gained from not consuming certain foods (such as spices) or from the long-term intake of H_2 blockers.

3.5.6 Medicinal treatment

In bleeding oesophageal varices, **adjuvant medication therapy** is advisable for reducing portal hypertension. This can be achieved by (*1.*) lowering vascular resistance with the help of vasodilators, (*2.*) cutting down the blood flow into the oesophageal collaterals with the help of substances which restrict the arterial splanchnic circulation, or (*3.*) applying a combination of these two therapeutic procedures. (57, 77, 92, 143)

In 1956 **vasopressin** was recommended for the first time to treat bleeding oesophageal varices (J. H. KEHNE et al.). Acute bleeding is temporarily arrested within a few hours in 50(—70)% of patients (0.4—0.8 U/min, i.v.). In addition to the pressure reduction in the splanchnic vascular bed (20—30%) and in the varices (ca. 15%), there are occurrences of coronary spasms, ventricular arrhythmia (84), hypertension, abdominal pain and ischaemic organ lesions. By combining vasopressin with **glyceryl trinitrate** (0.4 mg, sublingually or i.v.), the frequency of side effects can be reduced (31%) and the elevated portal pressure lowered. Vasopressin has largely been replaced by its synthetic derivative terlipressin.

Terlipressin has been used for bleeding oesophageal varices since 1975 (K. F. ARONSEN et al.). This "prodrug" is converted by enzymatic splitting off of the three glycine residues into active lysovasopressin, which results in an even distribution in the plasma and a prolonged effect (half-life of 3 or 4 hours). Terlipressin is administered at four- to six-hour intervals (1—2 mg in 10 ml isotonic NaCl solution). Following a bolus injection of 2 mg, the intravaricose pressure is reduced by about 30% within 2 minutes, and HVP is significantly reduced over a period of four hours. Haemostasis was achieved in 60—90% of cases. Terlipressin can be successfully combined with a **nitrovasodilator,** whereby the side effects of the vasoconstrictors are decreased. The combination of terlipressin and nitrates is the most beneficial drug regimen for bleeding oesophageal varices. Comparative studies on balloon tamponade, sclerotherapy and somatostatin have also demonstrated the efficacy of terlipressin. (53, 60, 86, 87, 100, 144, 169, 173) (s. p. 892)

Somatostatin has been recommended as medication for bleeding oesophageal varices since 1979 (L. THULIN et al.). It lowers the elevated portal pressure and reduces the blood flow in the azygous vein. The ideal dosage is 250 µg as an i.v. bolus administered immediately after emergency admission, followed by 250 (—500) µg/hour as i.v. infusion. The arterial splanchnic blood flow is decreased by 20—30% with unchanged systemic pressure. This facilitates sclerotherapy and improves therapeutic efficacy. In diabetes mellitus, it is advisable to check blood glucose levels repeatedly, since there may initially be a reduction and later an increase in blood glucose. Somatostatin probably antagonizes the effect of glucagon. The haemostatic effect of somatostatin is well documented (64% vs. 41%) (67); the drug has proved to be almost equivalent to terlipressin, and superior to vasopressin. Comparative studies with balloon tamponade or sclerotherapy also indicated that the results achieved with somatostatin were virtually identical in terms of primary haemostasis in 80% of cases. (54, 67, 105, 168) Somatostatin may also be indicated as concomitant treatment after sclerotherapy and ligation for five to seven days, since the danger of recurrent bleeding is particularly great during this period. (61, 106, 144) (s. p. 892) • The synthetic derivative **octreotide** shows good effects (reduction in mesenteric perfusion, HVWP, blood supply into the azygous vein and intravaricose pressure) in 80–85% of cases and has a much longer half-life than somatostatin (1–2 hours vs. 2 minutes). A dosage of 25–50 µg/hr is recommended as a continuous i.v. infusion. Octreotide has only few side effects. Recent results favour octreotide over vasopressin/terlipressin. (75)

	Initial bolus	Maintenance dose	Duration of therapy
Terlipressin*)	2 mg i.v.	1–2 mg/4 hr i.v.	2 days
Somatostatin	250 µg i.v.	250 µg/hr i.v.	5 days
Octreotide	50 µg i.v.	25–50 µg/hr i.v.	5 days
*) in combination with glyceryl trinitrate (20 mg/24 hr transdermally or 40–70 µg/min i.v.)			

Losartan is an antagonist of angiotensin-II receptor. With oral administration (25 mg/day), portal hypertension could be significantly reduced. Side effects were not observed.

Metoclopramide reduces the intravaricose pressure by restoring the normal tone to the lower oesophageal sphincter. The use of metoclopramide for the prevention and treatment of oesophageal varix bleeding is thus another pharmacological alternative. The haemodynamic effects of portal hypertension are not influenced.

Nitrates were used to produce a favourable effect on portal hypertension: isosorbide dinitrate, isosorbide mononitrate (51, 65, 123, 124, 132) and glyceryl trinitrate (87). *Glyceryl trinitrate* can easily be controlled owing to its short half-life of five minutes. It is also effective upon transdermal application (10 mg/day).

Molsidomine (L.R. DEL ARBOL et al., 1989) diminished the hepatic venous wedged pressure and the hepatic venous pressure gradient as an acute effect. Furthermore, in long-term oral treatment (3 to 6 months), the variceal pressure decreased by 28% and the hepatic venous pressure gradient by 25%, with a simultaneous reduction in the size of varices of about 17%. (98) A dose of 2 mg proved adequate. Orally applied molsidomine can thus be recommended for long-term prophylactic medication. •

In further studies, octreotide or the balloon tamponade were found to be superior to the combined application of nitroglycerin + terlipressin or nitroglycerin + vasopressin. (169) • The combination of *nitrates with β-blockers* has proved more effective than monotherapy in reducing portal hypertension. (190)

Propranolol was used for the first time as a *β-blocking agent* for prophylactic measures with regard to bleeding oesophageal varices (D. LEBREC et al., 1980). • By dilating the splanchnic vessels, it leads to a lower blood flow into the portal vein and thus a decrease in portal hypertension of 20–30%. This effect is only maintained when the intake is regular, although careful monitoring of the cardiac and circulatory function is still necessary, with particular attention being paid to a potential reduction in the cardiac output. In some patients, portal pressure cannot be diminished even with an adequate dosage of propranolol (non-responders). The frequency of *side effects* (such as hypotension, dizziness, Raynaud's syndrome, bradycardia, bronchoconstriction, impotence) is below 20%. • Propranolol can be used successfully as a prophylaxis for both oesophageal and fundus varices. The dosage (twice daily) should be continued until the pulse rate is reduced by approx. 25% of the initial value (generally down to 55–60/min); the blood pressure should not fall below 90 mm Hg. (92) • The risk of primary bleeding is lower when propranolol is applied as a primary prophylactic measure in patients with medium-sized or large varices and "red-coloured signs". (50, 74, 147) • *Long-term treatment* with propranolol may be successful in certain situations as a secondary prophylactic measure in order to prevent recurrent bleeding. (60, 124, 150, 189) This is particularly true of simultaneous interval sclerotherapy. (160, 163) The gastric mucosal blood flow was slowed down in portal hypertensive gastropathy; the serum gastrin level remained unaffected. • A combination of propranolol and molsidomine is considered to be efficient. • **Nadolol** has also been used with success as a β-blocking agent — in combination with nitrate — for the prevention of primary bleeding and relapses. It is only administered once daily; its elimination is predominantly renal. Side effects are markedly fewer (<5%) than with propranolol. (65, 123, 132, 190, 191)

3.5.7 Bacteraemia

Clinically relevant bacteraemia is seen in 5–15% of patients who undergo emergency sclerosing of oesophageal varices. Prophylactic treatment with poorly absorbable antibiotics led to a reduction in the frequency of bacteraemia and infections. The risk of rebleeding is increased by bacterial infection. *Thus it was possible to reduce cases of rebleeding significantly by administering an antibiotic prophylaxis for a period of three to seven days.* In this connection, the use of norfloxacin (2 × 400 mg/day for 1 week), ofloxacin or ceftriaxone proved beneficial. (63, 148, 155) (s. p. 310)

Synopsis

Primary prophylactic measures, such as administration of propranolol or nadolol (if necessary, combined with isosorbide mononitrate, molsidomine and spironolactone), sclerotherapy (50, 148, 187) or banding ligation (99, 124, 160), may be indicated in cirrhosis patients who present *major risk factors* for primary oesophageal bleeding. (s. tab. 19.6)

The various **conservative methods** used in the treatment of bleeding oesophageal varices have been investigated in a number of clinical studies. It might well be difficult to assess the results — often varying and occasionally controversial — since the individual findings within the frequently heterogeneous patient groups rarely permit any comparability between the studies. • Subsequent to the endoscopic confirmation of the diagnosis — which may only be omitted under exceptional circumstances — the decision must not only focus on the treatment procedures to be implemented, but on a flexible, sequentially structured process. This means using suitable, clinically well established procedures which have been selected from the entire scope of conservative treatment.

For **primary haemostasis,** *sclerotherapy* or *varix ligation* are considered to be the methods of choice. • Should sclerotherapy or ligation not be feasible (as yet) for primary haemostasis, *medication therapy* (first priority) with terlipressin and octreotide may be applied as an alternative — with the aim of carrying out subsequent sclerosing or ligation as soon as possible. • Should it be imperative to control massive bleeding without delay, the *balloon tamponade* method can be applied for a limited period of time. Here, too, the aim must be early sclerotherapy or ligation.

As a **secondary prophylactic step** against recurrent bleeding, eradicating sclerotherapy or ligation are the methods of choice. At the same time, β-blocking agents and nitrates may be given both as *adjuvant treatment* and subsequent *long-term therapy*. (200) Furthermore, spironolactone and/or molsidomine are also suitable in such cases.

The question concerning the use of **semi-invasive** or **surgical measures** arises once definitive haemostasis has been achieved. This depends on the liver function in each case and a careful review of the individual risk factors and behaviour as well as an assessment of the indications. • Variceal bleeding that has proved unresponsive to haemostatic efforts over a period of time exceeding two days (with a daily application of more than four units of packed red blood cells) in spite of all conservative measures must be subjected to semi-invasive or surgical therapy. This also applies to an early recurrence of bleeding.

3.6 Semi-invasive treatment

3.6.1 Transhepatic embolization

The transhepatic embolization of bleeding oesophageal varices, which was first used by A. LUNDERQUIST et al. (1974), is only of minor clinical importance today. With this procedure, a vascular catheter is introduced via the percutaneous transhepatic route into the portal system, and the convolute of varices is selectively thrombosed. (83)

3.6.2 TIPS

From a haemodynamic point of view, the transjugular intrahepatic portosystemic stent shunt (TIPS) constitutes a portacaval side-to-side anastomosis in the form of a nonsurgical link between the portal vein and the hepatic vein. The TIPS can be closely compared with the portacaval interposition shunt, because the pressure reduction also depends on the shunt lumen. Stent placement leads to a permanent *decrease in portal pressure*; in 60—70% of cases, it was possible to achieve the desired reduction in pressure to almost 12 mm Hg. In addition, the splanchnic blood pool decreased, the cardiac output increased, the RAAS was deactivated and renal function improved. (66, 128) (s. pp 267, 320, 336, 899) (s. figs. 16.15, 16.16)

This procedure, which is well documented in animal experiments, was introduced into clinical practice by R. F. COLAPINTO et al. in 1983. A self-expanding *Wall stent* with a width of 8 to 10 mm or a *Palmaz metal stent* (J. C. PALMAZ et al., 1985), which can be expanded up to a maximum of 16 mm, is applied. The latter was first used in clinical practice in 1989 (G. M. RICHTER et al.). • With this method, a catheter is inserted into a right liver vein through the internal jugular vein. The portal vein is punctured near the bifurcation by means of a needle inserted through the catheter, and a guide wire is introduced to an adequate extent into the portal branch. The liver tissue between the liver vein and the portal vein is predilated by means of a balloon catheter via the guide wire, and the Palmaz stent is subsequently inserted. • The problem of stenosis or restenosis of the stent can be largely prevented with the help of a newly developed stent type. (186)

Indications: The indications are: (*1.*) bleeding from oesophageal or gastric varices (acute, non-controllable bleeding, prophylactic measures against rebleeding, variceal embolization) (45, 59, 62, 89, 130, 163, 186), (*2.*) relapsing haemorrhage in hypertensive gastropathy, (*3.*) refractory ascites, (*4.*) Budd-Chiari syndrome, (*5.*) hepatogenic hydrothorax, (*6.*) hepatorenal syndrome, (*7.*) portal thrombosis, and (*8.*) bridging the period of time preceding liver transplantation. (153, 185)

Results: The results of this semi-invasive procedure are convincing: successful insertion of a TIPS by an experienced team could be achieved in 88—100% of cases, with a survival rate of 85% after one year and 78% after two years. The frequency of rebleeding was lowered to about 10%. The functionality of the TIPS could be maintained for 4 years. (130, 185, 196)

Mortality: Mortality during the application of TIPS is 1%, early mortality within the first four weeks amounts to approximately 2%, and in the case of an emergency TIPS, the rate is about 20%.

Complications: The application of a stent rapidly effects the formation of pseudointima. Through increased thrombosis development, this may even culminate in stent occlusion (4−22%), which could cause rebleeding. However, there is the possibility of placing a new stent. The reported frequency of hepatic encephalopathy is 20−30%. Haemobilia was observed in 4−5% and liver haematoma in 4% of cases. In view of such a high rate of hepatic encephalopathy, the subclinical stage should also be diagnosed (s. pp 211, 280) and systematically treated until the time is appropriate for the placement of a TIPS. During the following period, all possible dietary and medicinal measures should be taken to avert the frequent, albeit unexpected occurrence of serious hepatic encephalopathy.

The first **liver transplantations** after the positioning of a TIPS were performed by E. J. RING et al. (1992). (153) Meanwhile, other good results have been presented. (154) For transplantation purposes, a preceding TIPS is of decisive advantage as compared to a conventional shunt operation, since the extrahepatic vessels and the liver hilus remain intact. Therefore, TIPS is the method of choice when the time period preceding a transplantation has to be bridged for patients with stages Child B and C. (s. fig. 19.12)

3.7 Surgical treatment

As long ago as 1874, G. BANTI attempted for the first time to reduce the portal volume by means of splenectomy. In 1894 he developed this procedure further by carrying out the simultaneous resection of the short gastric veins in order to cut off the blood flow into the oesophageal collaterals. During the course of the past 100 years, countless surgical procedures and modifications for the treatment of portal hypertension and bleeding oesophageal varices have been published.

▶ The **tabular list** presented here consisting of more than 50 surgical procedures cannot be considered as complete or even totally accurate. • *These multiple and ingenious efforts undertaken by surgeons to control the most frequent and most life-threatening bleeding event − bleeding from oesophageal varices with portal hypertension − are worthy of admiration and respect.* • The diversity of the methods might, however, also reflect critical dissatisfaction on the part of the individual surgeon with the clinical results hitherto achieved.

> It is very interesting to compare a tabular overview of the surgical treatment of **bleeding oesophageal varices** (s. tab. 19.7) with a list of operative approaches for eliminating **refractory ascites.** (s. tab. 16.18)

3.7.1 Indications

Should it be necessary to consider surgical treatment for acute gastrointestinal bleeding, the decision depends on (*1.*) *cause of bleeding* in each case, (*2.*) *bleeding intensity*, and (*3.*) possibility of surgical elimination of the *source of bleeding*. The decision for operative intervention is taken in line with the following **criteria:**

1. Spurting arterial bleeding *(Forrest Ia)*
2. Volume replacement of >2 litres/day without definitive circulatory stabilization
3. Consumption of >5−6 units of blood/day without definitive haemostasis
4. Unfeasibility and inefficacy of conservative therapeutic measures in bleeding oesophageal varices or in hypertensive gastroenteropathy
5. Elective surgery for eliminating persistent recurrent bleeding from oesophageal and fundus varices (with strict adherence to selection criteria)
6. Ulcer patients with risk factors (initial Hb value <7 g/dl, *Forrest stages Ib/II*, signs of recurrent bleeding)
7. Secondary prophylactic measure at the request of the patient following objective presentation and discussion of the prevailing findings

3.7.2 Surgical methods

> Close cooperation with the surgeon is imperative for optimum treatment results in gastrointestinal bleeding. (s. fig. 19.12)

Of the many surgical methods used in the treatment of bleeding oesophageal varices, only two groups are of relevance: (*1.*) block surgery, and (*2.*) pressure-reducing shunt procedures. (76) (s. tab. 19.7)

I. Nonsurgical methods
1. **Local haemostatic methods** • Varicosclerosation (CRAFOORD, C., 1939) • Tamponade (gauze + thrombin) (BARNETT, C.B., 1949) • Sclerosing of the oesophageal wall (WODAK, E., 1956) • Transhepatic sclerosing (LUNDERQUIST, A., 1974)
II. Surgical methods
1. **Mediastinal tamponade** − upper and lower mediastinal tamponades (SOM, 1947) − gauze tamponade (HARLOCK, 1950) 2. **Varicotomy** − total oesophagogastrectomy (PHEMISTER, D.B., 1949) − subtotal oesophagogastrectomy (BARANOFSKY, I.D., 1949) − total small intestinal interposition (MEREDINO, K.A., 1950) − total prosthetic interposition (NACHLAS, M.M., 1956) − total colon interposition (KOOP, 1959) 3. **Purse-string ligation of varices** − abdom./thorac./subdiaphragmatic (HENSCHEL, C., 1938) − laparogastroscopic varicosclerosation (LUND, 1939)

- transthoracic/transoesophageal (Boerema, I., 1949)
- transabdominal (Welch, C.S., 1953)
- transthoracic/perioesophageal (Nissen, R., 1954)
- oesophageal dissection ligation (Vossschulte, K., 1957)
- transthoracic/oesophageal (Hartenbach, W., 1963)
- oesophageal dissection ligation (Boerema, I., 1967)

4. **Provocation of additional collaterals**
   - omentopexy (Talma, S., 1898)
   - displacement of the spleen into the abdominal wall (Holman, 1950)
   - splenopneumopexy (Nylander, E.E., 1950)
   - hepatopexy (Rousselot, L.M., 1959)
   - transthoracic displacement of the spleen and pole resection (Bourgeon, 1961)

5. **Reduction in portal venous volume**
   - splenectomy (Banti, G., 1874)
   - ligation of the left gastric artery and right gastroepiploic artery (Flerow, 1926)
   - ligation of the hepatic artery (Berman, E.J., 1950)
   - ligation of the splenic artery (Blain, A.W., 1950)
   - small intestine resection (Laufmann, 1954)
   - thoracic lymph fistula (Dumont, A.E., 1964)
   - laterolat. lymphoven. anastomosis (Defni, M., 1965)
   - terminolateral cervical lymphovenous anastomosis (Schreiber, H.W., 1968)

6. **Interruption of afferent collaterals**
   - resection of the short gastric veins by splenectomy (Banti, G., 1894)
   - ligation and resection of the coronary vein of the stomach (Rowntree, G., 1929)
   - subcardia gastric dissection (Tanner, N.C., 1950)
   - subtotal oesophageal resection (Cooley, D.H., 1954)
   - oesophageal transsection (Walker, R.M., 1960)
   - cardia reimplantation (Schmitt, W., 1963)
   - submucosal transsection (Stelzner, F., 1963)
   - circ. subcard. gastric dissection (Schreiber, H.W., 1964)
   - decongestion of the oesophagus and stomach (Hassab, M.A., 1967)
   - two-stage oesophageal dissection (Sugiura, M., 1973)
   - fundectomy (Hunt, H.A., 1964; Stelzner, F., 1975)
   - subcardia staple suture (Rinecker, H., 1975)

7. **Shunt operations**
   - Portacaval anastomosis
     - end-to-side (Vidal, M., 1903; Whipple, A.O., 1945)
     - side-to-side (Rosenstein, P., 1912)
     - crossed (double end-to-side) form (McDermott, W.V., 1960)
     - interposition shunt (Sarfeh, I.J., 1986)
   - Splenorenal anastomosis
     - mesentericocaval side-to-end anastomosis (Marion, P., 1953; Valdoni, P., 1954)
     - laterolateral form (Cooley, D.A., 1954)
     - distal form (Warren, W.D., 1967)
     - end-to-end anastomosis (Hivet, M., 1967)
     - proximal (central) form (Linton, R.R., 1974)
   - Coronariocaval anastomosis (Gütgemann, A., 1961)
   - Renomesent. renosplen. anastomosis (Erlick, D., 1964)
   - Saphenoumbilical anastomosis (Piccone, V.A., 1967)
   - Mesentericocaval side-to-side anastomosis (Maillard, J.N., 1970; Moreaux, J., 1972)
   - Mesentericocaval interposition shunt (Reynolds, T.B., 1951; Drapanas, T., 1972)
   - Splenocaval side-to-end shunt (Peiper, H.J., 1973)

Tab. 19.7: Overview of semi-invasive and surgical procedures for bleeding oesophageal varices and portal hypertension in chronological order (1874–1994). For reasons of simplification, only the first authors are named in each case. *(see also tab. 16.18!)*

1. **Block surgery:** This measure stops the venous flow to the bleeding oesophageal collaterals. The **disadvantage** is that portal hypertension is not influenced, so that there is a possibility of the collaterals and varices reforming and hence a danger of recurrent bleeding (40–60%). However, block surgery also has major **advantages:** (*1.*) it ensures rapid haemostasis, (*2.*) the duration of surgery is relatively short, (*3.*) the strain imposed on the patient by surgery is limited, (*4.*) the procedure is technically simple when using a stapler suture, (*5.*) liver perfusion is maintained, and (*6.*) there are no surgical problems with a subsequent shunt operation or liver transplantation. • Consequently, block surgery is performed as an emergency measure, particularly in cases of portal thrombosis. It is sometimes combined with splenectomy. (s. tab. 19.7)

Oesophageal transsection, as with the two-stage technique (Sugiura), and devascularization (Hassab, Paquet) have proved to be most valuable in cases of severe oesophageal bleeding which cannot be controlled by conservative measures. This is particularly true of high-risk patients. Haemostasis is guaranteed, recurrent bleeding is rare, and the frequency of encephalopathy is lower. Block surgery must be followed by systematic prophylactic measures against relapse. The indication for an elective shunt operation should be considered during the bleeding-free interval. Omeprazole and sucralfate have been used successfully in treating postoperative ulceration. (94, 129, 137, 184) (s. p. 900)

2. **Shunt operations:** Anastomoses are created in the portosystemic vascular area by way of this surgical method; they lead to a distinct and persistent reduction in pressure in the portal system. An operative shunt is the most effective method for attaining haemostasis and preventing recurrent bleeding. However, mortality is high: with the selective shunt, surgical lethality is 4–16% and late lethality 21–52%, whereas the respective rates for the total shunt are 4–13% and 18–69%. Before performing a shunt operation, indirect splenoportography and CT portography are the major examination methods. No shunt operation should be performed with a Quick's value of <40%. (108, 138, 141, 142) (s. p. 899)

> ▶ The classical form is the **portacaval end-to-side anastomosis** (laterolateral), applied for the first time in a dog by N.W. von Eck in 1877. Nevertheless, this was still a long way from clinical applicability. Not until 1901 was a clinical attempt made by R. Lenoir, yet without success. A renewed attempt to use this (end-to-side) shunt procedure undertaken by M. Vidal (1903) proved satisfactory. The first successful portacaval (side-to-side) anastomosis was reported by P. Rosenstein in 1912. Extensive clinical use of the portacaval shunt was encouraged by the studies of A.O. Whipple and A.H. Blakemore (1945). • The following years saw the development of a large number of varying shunt techniques and their modifications. (s. tab. 19.7)

The **complete shunt** involves a total bypassing of the portosystemic circulation. The liver blood flow is confined to the hepatic artery. This category includes the *portacaval end-to-side shunt*.

The **incomplete shunt** only effects a moderate reduction in pressure in the portal system, but residual mesentericoportal hepatic perfusion is generally maintained, which can be seen as a great advantage. This type of shunt includes: (*1.*) *portacaval side-to-side*, indicated particularly in ascites, (*2.*) *mesentericocaval interpo-*

sition, (3.) *portacaval interposition*, (4.) *laterolateral (proximal) splenorenal side-to-side*, and (5.) *proximal splenorenal end-to-side*, with splenic extirpation.

Deterioration of liver perfusion may possibly be prevented by **arterialization** of the portal vein stump (A. H. HUNT, 1952). Various arterialization techniques, including those which are pressure-adapted, have been tried out (D. BURLUI et al., 1968; J. N. MAILLARD et al., 1970; U. MATZANDER, 1974; and others). • The technical advantages of a **mesentericocaval anastomosis** can be seen in the simplified access to the superior mesenteric vein and the easier decompensation of the anastomosis in a liver transplantation later on. • **Disadvantages** include the twofold anastomosis and the use of a plastic vascular prosthesis with the associated higher rate of thrombosis of 15–30%.

A selective decrease in pressure coupled with the simultaneous maintenance of portal liver perfusion permits a **distal splenorenal anastomosis** (WARREN shunt). Decompression is then selectively limited to the gastrosplenic tract. Yet, this low-pressure area can only be maintained with an extensive surgical uncoupling of the circulation area of the splenic vein from the portal vein. Complete splenopancreatic disconnection comprising the left and right gastric veins as well as the epiploic veins is therefore necessary. Benefits include the much improved hepatic haemodynamics and the preserved clearance function. However, this shunt is technically more difficult and more time-consuming to implement, wide-lumen vessels are required and the rate of thrombosis can be as high as 50%. Moreover, due to the use of new venous links to the gastrosplenic area, the selectivity of the shunt is not guaranteed in the long term. **Splenoadrenal shunt** utilizing a left adrenal vein is deemed to be an excellent option in selected cases. (82, 96)

From a *haemodynamic point of view*, both complete and incomplete shunts are regarded as "complete shunts" because they lower portal pressure and decrease liver perfusion, albeit to varying degrees – depending on the technique and on subsequent structural changes to the liver or portal system. The portal perfusion rate in cirrhosis is reduced on average to approximately 30%, generally with arterial compensation and increased cardiac output. Cirrhosis patients show a stagnating or retrograde portal flow in 8–30% of cases. Shunt-associated *deficiency of the hepatic blood flow* would entail less serious consequences than total (or near total) failure of the liver as the major *clearance organ*.

3.7.3 Timing of shunt operation

When considering the ideal time point for a shunt operation, a distinction is made between (1.) emergency shunt, (2.) early elective shunt, and (3.) elective shunt.

▶ An **emergency shunt** is indicated in variceal bleeding that cannot be controlled by conservative measures. It is performed either as an **immediate shunt,** i.e. without previously attempted sclerosing, or as a **rescue shunt,** i.e. after unsuccessful sclerotherapy or ligation. Owing to the high rate of surgery-associated lethality (approx. 40%), the emergency shunt is generally used as a rescue shunt. In this respect, the *portacaval end-to-side shunt* is the most appropriate shunt form by virtue of its benefits: (1.) it is technically more simple to perform, (2.) the duration of the operation is relatively short (60–90 minutes), (3.) haemostasis is achieved rapidly, reliably and definitively, (4.) portal pressure is lowered swiftly and persistently, and (5.) with regard to the emergency situation, the surgical procedure is relatively well tolerated by the patient. Perioperative mortality is about 10% in Child A, 20–30% in Child B and over 50% in Child C. Moreover, this shunt entails the haemodynamic and functional late sequelae of a total shunt. The selective *distal splenorenal shunt* has also proved useful as an emergency measure, although the technique is more difficult and time-consuming, with greater operative lethality. If these emergency shunts are not feasible angiologically or for reasons pertaining to surgical techniques, a machine-performed block operation or oesophagogastric decongestion with splenectomy should be considered. (103, 108, 115, 152, 175, 180)

▶ An **early elective shunt** is created after initial haemostasis within one or two days if there are major grounds for immediate operative procedures. In principle, sclerotherapy or ligation should be continued for as long as possible, and thus such early elective shunts are rare.

▶ An **elective shunt** should be considered in situations where no definitive haemostasis was achieved (20–30% of cases) despite a sufficiently long sclerotherapy period and where there is still a danger of severe rebleeding. Choosing the most favourable shunt procedure should be done with due consideration of the individual case; there is no real answer to this issue, particularly as regards the decision in favour of a total or selective shunt, since the study data available can hardly be generalized (and are barely comparable). However, in most cases, preference is given to the distal renosplenic shunt and the mesentericocaval interposition shunt. (69, 121, 138, 141, 142, 182, 194)

3.7.4 Prognosis

The frequency of recurrent bleeding is 0–19% with elective shunts and 53–75% with sclerotherapy. Yet it is not possible to come to a universal decision in favour of a specific procedure. *In principle, all possibilities to prevent relapse that are afforded by conservative procedures should be fully exhausted.* (95, 113, 146, 175)

Operative lethality can be reduced to about 10% and the rate of recurrent bleeding to <10%. With careful internal treatment, the frequency of encephalopathy can be substantially diminished to 5–10% (from the previous rate of 20–30%). The *survival rate* (between 2 and 10 years) is 80–40% and can be decisively influenced by the patient's lifestyle, particularly as regards alcohol abstinence. Important *selective criteria* include: (1.) liver blood flow between 1,000 and 2,500 ml, (2.) selective portal blood flow of 15–40%, and (3.) timing of operation during the bleeding-free interval (elective) with careful pre- and aftertreatment.

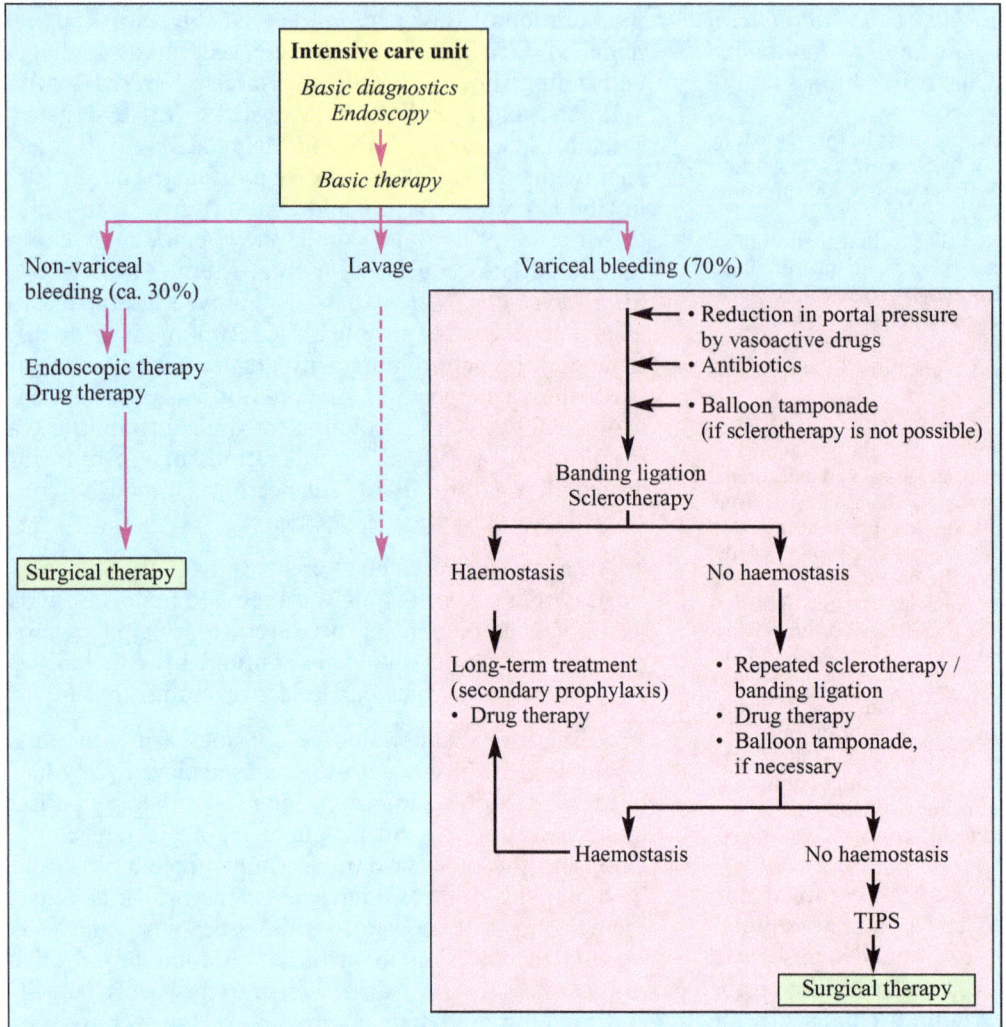

Fig. 19.15: Flow diagram: therapeutic spectrum for acute upper gastrointestinal bleeding, including bleeding oesophageal and gastric varices

3.8 Liver transplantation

Liver transplantation is the only way of ensuring elimination of the underlying liver disease with portal hypertension — and thus also eradication of the predominant and life-threatening complex of collateral circulation with its recurrent incidences of bleeding. A transplant operation is technically feasible both after TIPS and following block surgery. A mesentericocaval shunt is the surgical procedure of choice when a transplantation is planned at a later date. By contrast, the distal splenorenal shunt entails problems with operative techniques and haemodynamic difficulties. The four-year survival rate of patients who merely underwent sclerotherapy was 17%, whereas with an additional transplantation at a later date, a frequency of 73% was recorded. In appropriate cases, liver transplantation is a well-established therapeutic measure, equally suitable for the management of bleeding oesophageal varices. (108, 154)

4 Lower gastrointestinal haemorrhage

Lower gastrointestinal haemorrhage shows a frequency of 10—15%; some 3—5% of these cases develop in the small bowel. Intestinal bleeding as a result of liver disease is rare. The initial problem consists in the fact that (*1.*) numerous and varied causes of bleeding must be clarified by differential diagnosis and (*2.*) severe blood loss together with a concurrent liver disease is always particularly hazardous.

4.1 Definition

In lower gastrointestinal haemorrhage, the bleeding site is distal to the duodenojejunal ligament (Treitz's ligament) or the duodenojejunal recess (i.e. the passage of the duodenum retroperitoneally and its transition to the intraperitoneal jejunum).

4.2 Forms

Lower gastrointestinal bleeding is subdivided into the same *forms* as upper gastrointestinal bleeding: acute or chronic bleeding, minor or major bleeding, arterial or venous bleeding. (s. tab. 19.4) The *intensity of bleeding* may vary between acute or even life-threatening bleeding and chronic or occult loss of blood in the stools. Acute bleeding lasts less than three days. Occult bleeding is the most common form — in fact, the screening of symptom-free elderly people for occult blood in stools yielded positive results in 3% of cases. As regards the *nature of bleeding*, distinction must be made between melaena, reddish-brown stool, haemochezia and occult bleeding.

Melaena (= *tarry stool*) (s. p. 355) is defined as tarry, sticky stools resulting from the decomposition of blood by intestinal bacteria. The occurrence of melaena depends on the amount of blood and the time of gastrointestinal passage. Usually, melaena is only to be expected in lower gastrointestinal bleeding with a bleeding site in the upper part of the transverse colon. However, it may also be observed in the case of massive bleeding from the upper gastrointestinal area. • Melaena may be simulated by the intake of iron (iron preparations, black pudding), charcoal tablets, bismuth, liquorice, blueberries, etc.

Reddish-brown stool is generally encountered in chronic recurrent lower gastrointestinal bleeding, mostly below the right part of the colon.

Haemochezia (= bloody faeces) is defined as the discharge of fresh blood or small blood clots in the stools. This may be recognized as *blood on the surface* of a formed stool (especially with bleeding from the rectal or anal area) or *admixture of blood* in the stool (generally with a bleeding site in the upper sections of the colon). Major amounts of blood may greatly accelerate the gastrointestinal passage, which is why massive oesophageal or gastric bleeding can sometimes appear as a form of haemochezia.

Occult blood is defined as traces of blood in the stool which are not perceptible to the naked eye. Usually, the passage of blood into the intestinal contents is around 2 ml/day. Proof of occult blood is obtained by *chemical testing* (e.g. peroxidase reaction), although it is only possible to detect amounts of blood in excess of 1.5–2.0 ml/100 ml stool or to demonstrate them by means of an *immunological rapid diagnostic test* with a specificity of virtually 100%. The test usually comprises three specimens collected at different points in time. (s. p. 355)

4.3 Diagnostics

Lower gastrointestinal bleeding is less frequent than upper gastrointestinal bleeding (15–20% vs. 80–85%). Consequently, the presence of upper gastrointestinal bleeding has to be excluded first — even in the case of severe anal passage of blood and/or in cases of haemochezia. (202, 205, 209)

Inspection: Inspection of the stool facilitates an initial rough assessment of the nature of the gastrointestinal bleeding.

Laboratory parameters: Like in upper gastrointestinal bleeding, certain parameters are initially important, such as haemogram, haematocrit, blood group, coagulation values, electrolytes, plasma urea, creatinine, Allgöwer-Burri index. (s. p. 355)

Rectal examination: Rectal examination by inspection and palpation of the anus and rectum (especially after straining) is imperative. The presence of haemorrhoids must not be accepted as a potential source of bleeding without further diagnostic clarification.

Endoscopy: Basically, we consider intestinal endoscopy to be the method of choice. With a massive passage of blood, the examination is naturally very difficult; it requires optimum intestinal cleansing before and during the examination as well as expertise in managing the required techniques. Due to the multiplicity of the potential causes of bleeding, endoscopy should always be used as a primary diagnostic method (s. fig. 19.16).

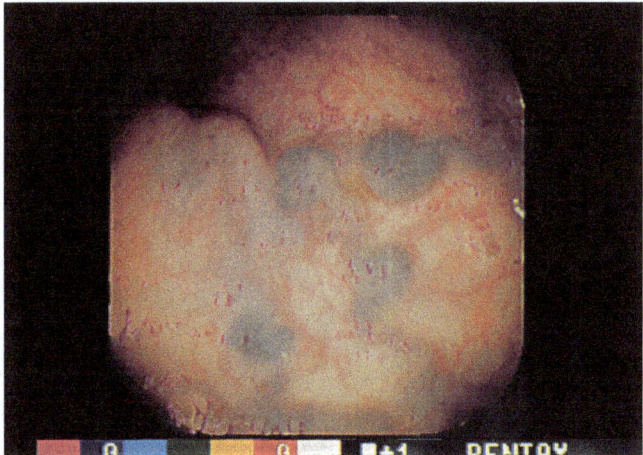

Fig. 19.16: Colonic varices in alcohol-toxic cirrhosis

With the help of **push enteroscopy,** it is possible to assess about 60 cm of the proximal jejunum. In this way, previously undetected sources of bleeding can be localized. (204) **Wireless capsule endoscopy** will improve endoscopic diagnosis of the small bowel considerably. The use of this capsule is currently limited to clarifying cases of intermittent bleeding. (203) Using this technique, mesenteric variceal bleeding could be identified.

Scintigraphy: Scintigraphy (e.g. with ^{99m}Tc-labelled erythrocytes) is the method of choice if endoscopy fails because of severe discharge of blood or due to technical difficulties, or if it yields no diagnosis. Amounts of blood exceeding 0.05–0.12 ml/min. are demonstrable. With an accuracy rate of 94%, overall reliability is higher than for angiography. One disadvantage is the imprecise localization of the bleeding source. (202, 205)

Angiography: Strong lower gastrointestinal bleeding can also be confirmed and possibly localized (in up to 70% of cases) by selective angiography of either the coeliac trunk or the (superior or inferior) mesenteric artery. A prerequisite condition for this is a bleeding rate in excess of 0.5 ml/min. By using anticoagulants to provoke bleeding, it was possible to raise the positive bleeding rate from 32% to 65%. Arteriography may also contribute to the differential diagnosis of lower gastrointestinal bleeding (e.g. diverticular bleeding, vascular anomaly, tumour). (202, 205)

All these diagnostic measures, when implemented specifically and step-by-step, yield a reliability of over 90% in lower gastrointestinal haemorrhage.

4.4 Aetiology

Numerous diseases of the lower gastrointestinal tract may be accompanied by bleeding. The **aetiological spectrum** is wide; the percentage frequency depends on the age distribution of the respective patients. Men are more frequently affected than women. At an advanced age, diverticulosis (overall frequency of bleedings about 50%, in old age about 40%) and angiodysplasia (overall frequency 1–3%, in old age about 30%) as well as haemorrhoids are the primary causes of bleeding. Furthermore, anal fissures, enterocolitis, polyps as well as benign and malignant tumours are worthy of mention. • Among the rare causes observed were proctitis, infections, parasitoses, endometriosis, collagenoses, congenital diseases (e.g. Meckel's diverticula, Osler-Rendu-Weber's disease) and mesenteric infarction. Some 80–85% of cases cease spontaneously. Lethality is 2–3%. (202, 209)

Lower gastrointestinal bleeding due to *liver disease* is very rare. The sources of bleeding develop in the course of portal hypertension. Intestinal erosions constitute the predominant mucosal changes in **portal hypertensive vasculopathy** in the gastrointestinal tract. They are usually responsible for the frequency of occult intestinal bleeding in cirrhosis patients.

During portal hypertension accompanied by the development of collaterals, **varices** also occur in the area of the duodenum, small intestine, colon and rectum. (205) Very severe, even life-threatening variceal bleeding may appear. (207)

4.5 Therapy

The therapeutic measures for lower gastrointestinal bleeding correlate with the **basic therapy** for upper gastrointestinal bleeding with respect to volume replacement, circulatory stabilization, restoration of the electrolyte balance and intestinal cleansing. • Depending on the respective findings, endoscopic **sclerotherapy**, the **banding ligation** of varices or the **clip technique** is carried out. (206, 209) The presence of portal hypertension is generally an indication for drug-induced **pressure reduction**. This may be necessary as a situation-related primary measure as well as in the form of adjuvant treatment with endoscopic techniques (208) or the placement of a **TIPS**. (207)

In the case of bleeding due to benign or malignant proliferation as well as in upper gastrointestinal bleeding, **thermic haemostatic procedures** are indicated.

Medicinal therapy is similar to that used for upper gastrointestinal bleeding, e.g. vasopressin, FFP, PPSB, fibrinogen (s. p. 358) and octreotide. • A novel therapeutic option in refractory bleeding from portal hypertensive gastropathy is given by the administration of thalidomide. (32)

If bleeding cannot be stopped endoscopically or conservatively, interventional radiology is indicated before any surgical measures can be taken. Exact localization of the source of bleeding is absolutely essential.

References:
Coagulopathy
1. **Amitrano, L., Guardascione, M.A., Brancaccio, V., Balzano, A.:** Coagulation disorders in liver disease. Semin. Liver Dis. 2002; 22: 83–96
2. **Bakker, C.M., Knot, E.A.R., Stibbe, J., Wilson, J.H.P.:** Disseminated intravascular coagulation in liver cirrhosis. J. Hepatol. 1992; 15: 330–335
3. **Boks, A.L., Brommer, E.J.P., Schalm, S.W., van Vliet, H.H.D.M.:** Hemostasis and fibrinolysis in severe liver failure and their relation to hemorrhage. Hepatology 1986; 6: 79–86
4. **Caldwell, S.H., Hoffman, M., Lisman, T., Macik, B.G. Northup, P.G. Reddy, K.R., Tripodi, A., Sanyal, A.J.:** Coagulation disorders and hemostasis in liver disease: Pathophysiology and critical assessment of current management. Hepatology 2006; 44: 1039–1046
5. **Carr, J.M.:** Disseminated intravascular coagulation in cirrhosis. Hepatology 1989; 10: 103–110
6. **DeCaterina., M., Tarantino, G., Farina, C., Arena, A., di Maro, G., Esposito, P., Scopacasa, F.:** Haemostasis unbalance in Pugh-scored liver cirrhosis: characteristic changes of plasma levels of protein C versus protein S. Haemostasis 1993; 23: 229–235
7. **Friedman, E.W., Sussman, I.I.:** Safety of invasive procedures in patients with the coagulopathy of liver disease. Clin. Lab. Haemat. 1989; 11: 199–204
8. **Gram, J., Duscha, H., Zurborn, K.-H., Bruhn, H.D.:** Increased levels of fibrinolysis reaction products (D-dimer) in patients with decompensated alcoholic liver cirrhosis. Scand. J. Gastroenterol. 1991; 26: 1173–1178
9. **Hersch, St.L., Kunelis, T., Francis, R.B.jr.:** The pathogenesis of accelerated fibrinolysis in liver cirrhosis: a critical role for tissue plasminogen activator inhibitor. Blood 1987; 69: 1315–1319
10. **Kaul, V., Munoz, S.J.:** Coagulopathy of liver disease. Curr. Treat. Opt. Gastroenterol. 2000; 3: 433–437
11. **Leebeek, F.W.G., Kluft, C., Knot, E.A.R., de Maat, M.P.M., Wilson, J.H.P.:** A shift in balance between profibrinolytic and antifibrinolytic factors causes enhanced fibrinolysis in cirrhosis. Gastroenterology 1991; 101: 1382–1390
12. **Mammen, E.F.:** Coagulopathies of liver disease. Clin. Lab. Med. 1994; 14: 769–780
13. **Paramo, J.A., Rocha, E.:** Hemostasis in advanced liver disease. Semin. Thromb. Hemost. 1993; 19: 184–190
14. **Plessier, A., Denninger, M.H., Consigny, Y., Pessione, F., Francoz, C., Durand, F., Francque, S., Bezeaud, A., Chauvelot-Moachon, L., Lebrec, D., Valla, D.C., Moreau, R.:** Coagulation disorders in patients with cirrhosis and severe sepsis. Liver Internat. 2003; 23: 440–448
15. **Porte, R.J.:** Coagulation and fibrinolysis in orthotopic liver transplantation: current views and insights. Semin. Thromb. Hemost. 1993; 19: 191–196
16. **Sallah, S., Bobzien, W.:** Bleeding problems in patients with liver disease. Ways to manage the many hepatic effects on coagulation. Postgrad. Med. 1999; 106: 187–195
17. **Trotter, J.F.:** Coagulation abnormalities in patients who have liver disease. Clin. Liver Dis. 2006; 10: 665–678
18. **Van Wersch, J.W.J., Russel, M.G.V.M., Lustermans, F.A.T.:** The extent of diffuse intravascular coagulation and fibrinolysis in patients with liver cirrhosis. Eur. J. Clin. Chem. Clin. Biochem. 1992; 30: 275–279
19. **Violi, F., Ferro, D., Basili, S., Cimminiello, C., Saliola, M., Vezza, E., Cordova, C.:** Prognostic value of clotting and fibrinolytic systems in a follow-up of 165 liver cirrhotic patients. Hepatology 1995; 22: 96–100
20. **Youssef, W.I., Salazar, F., Dasarathy, S., Beddow, T., Mullen, K.D.:** Role of fresh frozen plasma infusion in correction of coagulopathy of chronic liver disease: A dual phase study. Amer. J. Gastroenterol. 2003; 98: 1391–1394

Upper gastrointestinal (non variceal) haemorrhage

21. Bunker, S.R., Lull, R.J., Tanasecu, D.E., Redwine, M.D., Rigby, D., Landry, A.: Scintigraphy of gastrointestinal hemorrhage. Superiority of ^{99m}Tc red blood cells over ^{99m}Tc sulfur colloid. Amer. J. Roentgenol. 1984; 143: 543–548
22. Burak, K.W., Lee, S.S., Beck, P.L.: Portal hypertensive gastropathy and gastric antral vascular ectasia (GAVE) syndrome. Gut 2001; 49: 866–872
23. Carey, W.D.: Pharmacological management of portal hypertensive upper intestinal hemorrhage. Sem. Gastrointest. Dis. 1992; 3: 75–82
24. Chung, I.K., Ham, J.S., Kim, H.S., Park, S.H., Lee, M.H., Kim, S.J.: Comparison of the hemostatic efficacy of the endoscopic hemoclip method with hypertonic saline-epinephrine injection and a combination of the two for the management of bleeding peptic ulcers. Gastrointest. Endosc. 1999; 49: 13–18
25. Cipolletta, L., Bianco, M.A., Marmo, R., Rotondano, G., Piscopo, R., Vingiani, A.M., Meucci, C.: Endoclips versus heater probe in preventing early recurrent bleeding from peptic ulcer: a prospective and randomized trial. Gastrointest. Endosc. 2001; 53: 147–151
26. Cipolletta, L., Bianco, M.A., Rotondano, G., Marmo, R., Piscopo, R.: Outpatient management of low-risk nonvariceal upper GI bleeding: a randomized controlled trial. Gastrointest. Endosc. 2002; 55: 1–5
27. Coffin, B., Pocard, M., Panis, Y., Riche, F., Lainé, M.-L., Bitoun, A., Lémann, M., Bouhnik, Y., Valleur, P.: Erythromycin improves the quality of EGD in patients with acute upper GI bleeding: a randomized controlled study. Gastrointest. Endosc. 2002; 6: 174–179
28. Cook, D.J., Guyatt, G.H., Salena, B.J., Laine, L.A.: Endoscopic therapy for acute nonvariceal upper gastrointestinal hemorrhage: A metaanalysis. Gastroenterology 1992; 102: 139–148
29. Gevers, A.M., Goede, E.D., Momoens, M. Hiele, M., Rutgeerts, P.: A randomized trial comparing injection therapy with hemoclip and with injection combined with hemoclip for bleeding ulcers. Gastrointest. Endosc. 2002; 55: 466–469
30. Gostout, Ch.J., Viggiano, Th.R., Balm, R.K.: Acute gastrointestinal bleeding from portal hypertensive gastropathy: prevalence and clinical features. Amer. J. Gastroenterol. 1993; 88: 2030–2033
31. Heyd, R.L., Solinger, M.R., Howard, A.L., Rosser, J.C.: Acute upper gastrointestinal hemorrhage caused by gallstone impaction in the duodenal bulb. Dig. Dis. Sci. 1992; 37: 452–455
32. Karajeh, M.A., Huristone, D.P., Stephenson, T.J., Ray-Chaudhuri, D., Gleeson, D.C.: Refractory bleeding from portal hypertensive Gastropathy. A further novel role for thalidomide therapy? (case report). Eur. J. Gastroenterol. Hepatol. 2006; 18: 545–548
33. Kuntz, H.D., Burghof-Kozianka, G., May, B.: Upper gastrointestinal bleeding and prognosis. Retrospective analysis of clinical findings. Med. Welt 1986; 37: 970–972
34. Laine, L.: Multipolar electrocoagulation in the treatment of acute upper gastrointestinal tract hemorrhage. A prospective controlled trial. New Engl. J. Med. 1987; 316: 1613–1617
35. Lin, H.-J., Hsieh, Y.-H., Tseng, G.-Y., Perng, C.-L., Chang, F.-Y., Lee, S.-D.: A prospective, randomized trial of endoscopic hemoclip versus heater probe thermocoagulation for peptic ulcer bleeding. Amer. J. Gastroenterol. 2002; 97: 2250–2254
36. Ma, C.K., Rosenberg, B.F., Wong, D., Behrle, K.M., Zonca, M.C., Ansari, M.R.: Gastric antral vascular ectasia: the watermelon stomach. Surg. Pathol. 1988; 1: 231–239
37. Ohta, M., Yamaguchi, S., Gotoh, N., Tomikawa, M.: Pathogenesis of portal hypertensive gastropathy: a clinical and experimental review. Surgery 2002; 131 (Suppl.): 165–176
38. Panes, J., Piqué, J.M., Bordas, J.M., Llach, J., Bosch, J., Teres, J., Rodes, J.: Reduction of gastric hyperemia by glypressin and vasopressin administration in cirrhotic patitents with portal hypertensive gastropathy. Hepatology 1994; 19: 55–60
39. Primignani, M., Carpinelli, L., Preatoni, P., Battaglia, G., Carta, A., Prada, A., Cestari, R., Angeli, P., Gatta, A., Rossi, A., Spinzi, G., de Franchis, R.: Natural history of portal hypertensive gastropathy in patients with liver cirrhosis. Gastroenterology 2000; 119: 181–187
40. Pulanic, R., Vucelic, B., Rosandic, M., Opacic, M., Rustemovic, N., Krznaric, Z., Brkic, T., Jokic-Begic, N.: Comparison of injection sclerotherapy and laser photocoagulation for bleeding peptic ulcer. Endoscopy 1995; 27: 291–297
41. Quintero, E., Pique, J.M., Bombi, J.A., Bordas, J.M., Sentis, J., Elena, M., Bosch, J., Rodes, J.: Gastric mucosal vascular ectasias causing bleeding in cirrhosis. A distinct entity associated with hypergastrinemia and low serum levels of pepsinogen I. Gastroenterology 1987; 93: 1054–1061
42. Rockall, T.A., Logan, R.F., Devlin, H.B., Northfield, T.C.: Risk assessment after acute upper gastrointestinal haemorrhage. Gut 1996; 38: 316–321
43. Rutgeerts, P., Vantrappen, G., van Hootegem, P., Broeckaert, L., Janssens, J., Coremans, G., Geboes, K.: Neodymium-YAG laser photocoagulation versus multipolar electrocoagulation for the treatment of severely bleeding ulcers: a randomized comparison. Gastrointestin. Endosc. 1987; 33: 199–202
44. Savides, T.J., Jensen, D.M.: Therapeutic endoscopy for high risk nonvariceal gastrointestinal bleeding. Gastrointest. Clin. North Amer. 2000; 29: 465–488
45. Simpson, K.J., Chalmers, N., Redhead, D.N., Finlayson, N.D.C., Bouchier, I.A.D., Hayes, P.C.: Transjugular intrahepatic portasystemic stent shunting for control of acute and recurrent upper gastrointestinal haemorrhage related to portal hypertension. Gut 1993; 34: 968–973
46. Stewart, C.A., Sanyal, A.J.: Grading portal gastropathy: validation of a gastropathy scoring system. Amer. J. Gastroenterol. 2003; 98: 1758–1765
47. Yoo, H.Y., Eustace, J.A., Verma, S., Zhang, L., Harris, M., Kantsevoy, S., Lee, L.A., Kalloo, A.N., Ravich, W.J., Thuluvath, P.J.: Accuracy and reliability of the endoscopic classification of portal hypertensive gastropathy. Gastrointest. Endosc. 2002; 56: 675–680
48. Zhou, Y.N., Qiao, L., Wu, J., Hu, H.W., Xu, C.P.: Comparison of the efficacy of octreotide, vasopressin, and omeprazole in the control of acute bleeding in patients with portal hypertensive gastropathy: a controlled study. J. Gastroenterol. Hepatol. 2002; 17: 973–979
49. Zoli, M., Merkel, C., Magalotti, D., Marchesini, G., Gatta, A., Pisi, E.: Evaluation of a new endoscopic index to predict first bleeding from the upper gastrointestinal tract in patients with cirrhosis. Hepatology 1996; 24: 1047–1052

Bleeding oesophageal varices

50. Andreani, T., Poupon, R.E., Balkau, B.J., Trinchet, J.-C., Grange, J.-D., Peigney, N., Beaugrand, M., Poupon, R.: Preventive therapy of first gastrointestinal bleeding in patients with cirrhosis: results of a controlled trial comparing propranolol, endoscopic sclerotherapy and placebo. Hepatology 1990; 12: 1413–1419
51. Angelico, M., Carli, L., Piat, C., Gentile, S., Capocaccia, L.: Effects of isosorbide-5-mononitrate compared with propranolol on first bleeding and long-term survival in cirrhosis. Gastroenterology 1997; 113: 1632–1639
52. Arakawa, M., Masuzaki, T., Okuda, K.: Pathology of fundic varices of the stomach and rupture. J. Gastroenterol. Hepatol. 2002; 17: 1064–1069
53. Arcidiacono, R., Biraghi, M., Bonomo, G.M., Fiaccadori, F.: Randomized controlled trial with terlipressin in cirrhotic patients with bleeding esophageal varices: effects on precocious rebleeding and mortality rate. Curr. Ther. Res. 1992; 52: 186–195
54. Avgerinos, A., Nevens, S., Raptis, S., Fevery, J.: Early administration of somatostatin and efficacy of sclerotherapy in acute oesophageal variceal bleeding: the European acute bleeding oesophageal variceal episodes (ABOVE) randomized trial. Lancet 1997; 350: 1495–1499
55. Bacon, B.R., Bailey-Newton, R.S., Connors, A.F. jr.: Pleural effusions after endoscopic variceal sclerotherapy. Gastroenterology 1985; 88: 1910–1914
56. Baillie, J., Yudelman, P.: Complications of endoscopic sclerotherapy of esophageal varices. Endoscopy 1992; 24: 284–291
57. Banares, R., Albillos, A., Rincon, D., Alonso, S., Gonzales, M., Ruiz-del-Arbol, L., Salcedo, M., Molinero, L.-M.: Endoscopic treatment versus endoscopic plus pharmacological treatment for acute variceal bleeding. A meta-analysis. Hepatology 2002; 35: 609–615
58. Bandoh, T., Mitarai, Y., Kitano, S., Yoshida, T., Kobayashi, M.: Clinical significance of esophageal variceal pressure in patients with esophageal varices. J. Hepatol. 1994; 21: 326–331
59. Barange, K., Peron, J.M., Imani, K., Otal, P., Payen, J.L., Rousseau, H., Pascal, J.P., Joffre, F., Vinel, J.P.: Transjugular intrahepatic portosystemic shunt in the treatment of refractory bleeding from ruptured gastric varices. Hepatology 1999; 30: 1139–1143
60. Bernard, B., Lebrec, D., Mathurin, P., Poynard, T.: Betaadrenergic antagonists in the prevention of gastrointestinal rebleeding in patients with cirrhosis: a meta-analysis. Hepatology 1997; 25: 63–70
61. Besson, I., Ingrand, P., Person, B., Boutroux, D., Heresbach, D., Bernard, P., Hochain, P., Larricq, J., Gourlaouen, A., Ribard, D., Kara, N.M., Legoux, J.-L., Pillegand, B., Becker, M.-C., di Constanzo, J., Metreau, J.-M., Silvain, C., Beauchant, M.: Sclerotherapy with or without octreotide for acute variceal bleeding. New Engl. J. Med. 1995; 333: 555–560
62. Bilodeau, M., Rioux, L., Willems, B., Pomier-Layrargues, G.: Transjugular intrahepatic portocaval stent shunt as a rescue treatment for life-threatening variceal bleeding in a cirrhotic patient with severe liver failure. Amer. J. Gastroenterol. 1992; 87: 369–371
63. Blaise, M., Pateron, D., Trinchet, J.-C., Levacher, S., Beaugrand, M., Pourriat, J.-L.: Systemic antibiotic therapy prevents bacterial infection in cirrhotic patients with gastrointestinal hemorrhage. Hepatology 1994; 20: 34–38
64. Bochna, G.S., Harty, R.F., Harned, R.K., Markin, R.S.: Development of squamous cell carcinoma of the esophagus after endoscopic variceal sclerotherapy. Amer. J. Gastroenterol. 1988; 83: 564–568
65. Borroni, G., Salerno, F., Cazzaniga, M., Bissoli, F., Lorenzano, E., Maggi, A., Visentin, S., Panzeri, A., de Franchis, R.: Nadolol is superior to isosorbide mononitrate for the prevention of the first variceal bleeding in cirrhotic patients with ascites. J. Hepatol. 2002; 37: 315–321
66. Brensing, K.A., Hörsch, M., Textor, J., Schiedermaier, P., Raab, P., Schepke, M., Strunk, H., Schild, H., Sauerbruch, T.: Hemodynamic effects of propranolol and nitrates in cirrhotics with transjugular intrahepatic portosystemic stent-shunt. Scand. J. Gastroenterol. 2002; 37: 1070–1076
67. Burroughs, A.K., McCormick, P.A., Hughes, M.D., Sprengers, D., D'Heygere, F., McIntyre, N.: Randomized, double-blind, placebo-controlled trial of somatostatin for variceal bleeding. Emergency control and prevention of early variceal rebleeding. Gastroenterology 1990; 99: 1388–1395
68. Bury, T., Corhay, J.-L., Louis, R., Radermecker, M., Belaiche, J.: Chylothorax: a rare complication of endoscopic variceal sclerotherapy. Eur. J. Gastroenterol. Hepatol. 1993; 5: 293–294

69. Castells, A., Salo, J., Planas, R., Quer, J.C., Gines, A., Boix, J., Gines, P., Gassull, M.A., Teres, J., Arroyo, V., Rodes, J.: Impact of shunt surgery for variceal bleeding in the natural history of ascites in cirrhosis: a retrospective study. Hepatology 1994; 20: 584–591
70. Caturelli, E., Pompili, M., Squillante, M.M., Sperandeo, G., Carughi, S., Sperandeo, M., Perri, F., Andriulli, A., Cellerino, C., Rapaccini, G.L.: Cruveilhier-Baumgarten syndrome: An efficient spontaneous portosystemic collateral preventing oesophageal varices bleeding. J. Gastroenterol. Hepatol. 1994; 9: 236–241
71. Chalasani, N., Kalu, C., Francois, F., Pinto, A., Marathe, A., Bini, E.J., Pandya, P., Sitaraman, S., Shen, J.Z.: Improved patient survival after acute variceal bleeding: A multicenter, cohort study. Amer. J. Gastroenterol. 2003; 98: 653–659
72. Chandra, R., Kapoor, D., Tharakan, A., Chaudhary, A., Sarin, S.K.: Portal biliopathy. J. Gastroenterol. Hepatol. 2001; 16: 1086–1092
73. Chu, E.C., Chick, W., Hillebrand, D.J., Hu, K.Q.: Fatal spontaneous gallbladder variceal bleeding in a patient with alcoholic cirrhosis (case report). Dig. Dis. Sci. 2002; 47: 2682–2685
74. Conn, H.O., Grace, N.D., Bosch, J., Groszmann, R.J., Rodes, J., Wright, St.C., Matloff, D.S., Garcia-Tsao, G., Fisher, R.L., Navasa, M., Drewniak, St.J., Atterbury, C.E., Bordas, J.M., Lerner, E., Bramante, J.: Propranolol in the prevention of the first hemorrhage from esophagogastric varices: a multicenter, randomized clinical trial. Hepatology 1991; 13: 902–912
75. Corley, D.A., Cello, J.P., Adkisson, W., Ko, W.F., Kerlikowske, K.: Octreotide for acute esophageal variceal bleeding: a meta-analysis. Gastroenterology 2001; 120: 946–954
76. Crafoord, C., Frenckner, P.: New surgical treatment of varicous veins of the oesophagus. Acta Oto-laryngol. (Stockh.) 1939; 27: 422–429
77. D'Amico, G., Pietrosi, G., Tarantino, I., Pagliaro, L.: Emergency sclerotherapy versus vasoactive drugs for variceal bleeding in cirrhosis: a Cochrane meta-analysis. Gastroenterology 2003; 124: 1277–1291
78. D'Amico, G., Garcia-Pagan, J.C., Luca, A., Bosch, J.: Hepatic vein pressure gradient reduction and prevention of variceal bleeding in cirrhosis: A systematic review. Gastroenterology 2006; 131: 1611–1624
79. Datta, D., Vlavianos, P., Alisa, A., Westaby, D.: Use of fibrin glue (Beriplast) in the management of bleeding gastric varices. Endoscopy 2003; 35: 675–678
80. De Franchis, R., Arcidiacono, P.G., Carpinelli, L., Andreoni, B., Cestari, L., Brunati, S., Zambelli, A., Battaglia, G., Mannucci, P.M.: Randomized controlled trial of desmopressin plus terlipressin vs. terlipressin alone for the treatment of acute variceal hemorrhage in cirrhotic patients: a multicenter double-blind study. Hepatology 1993; 18: 1102–1107
81. Dhiman, R.K., Chawla, Y., Taneja, S., Biswas, R., Sharma, T.R., Dilawari, J.B.: Endoscopic sclerotherapy of gastric variceal bleeding with N-butyl-2-cyanoacrylate. J. Gastroenterol. Hepatol. 2002; 35: 222–227
82. Elwood, D.R., Pomposelli, J.J., Pomfret, E.A., Lewis, W.D., Jenkins, R.L.: Distal splenorenal shunt: preferred treatment for recurrent variceal hemorrhage in the patient with well-compensated cirrhosis. Arch. Surg. 2006; 141: 385–388
83. Evanson, E.J., McIvor, J., Murray-Lyon, I.M., Reynolds, K.W.: Survival after transhepatic embolization of gastro-oesophageal varices. Clin. Radiol. 1991; 44: 178–180
84. Faigel, D.O., Metz, D.C., Kochman, M.L.: Torsade de pointes complicating the treatment of bleeding esophageal varices: association with neuroleptics, vasopressin, and electrolyte imbalance. Amer. J. Gastroenterol. 1995; 90: 822–824
85. Feretis, C., Dimopoulos, C., Benakis, P., Kalliakmanis, B., Apostolidis, N.: N-butyl-2-cyanoacrylate (Histoacryl) plus sclerotherapy versus sclerotherapy alone in the treatment of bleeding esophageal varices: a randomized prospective study. Endoscopy 1995; 27: 355–357
86. Fiaccadori, F., Pedretti, G., Biraghi, M., Arcidiacono, R.: Terlipressin and endoscopic sclerotherapy control variceal bleeding and prevent early rebleeding in cirrhotic patients. Curr. Ther. Res. 1993; 54: 519–528
87. Fort, E., Sautereau, D., Silvain, Ch., Ingrand, P., Pillegand, B., Beauchant, M.: A randomized trial of terlipressin plus nitroglycerin vs. balloon tamponade in the control of acute variceal hemorrhage. Hepatology 1990; 11: 678–681
88. Garcia-Pagan, J.C., Feu, F., Castells, A., Luca, A., Hermida, R.C., Rivera, F., Bosch, J., Rodes, J.: Circadian variations of portal pressure and variceal hemorrhage in patients with cirrhosis. Hepatology 1994; 19: 595–601
89. Garcia-Villarreal, L., Martinez-Lagares, F., Sierra, A., Guevara, C., Marrero, J.M., Jimenez, E., Monescillo, A., Hernandez-Cabrero, T., Alonso, J.M., Fuéntes, R.: Transjugular intrahepatic portosystemic shunt versus endoscopic sclerotherapy for the prevention of variceal rebleeding after recent variceal hemorrhage. Hepatology 1999; 29: 27–32
90. Gimson, A.E.S., Ramage, J.K., Panos, M.Z., Hayllar, K., Harrison, P.M., Williams, R., Westaby, D.: Randomized trial of variceal banding ligation versus injection sclerotherapy for bleeding oesophageal varices. Lancet 1993; 342: 391–394
91. Gonzalez Bernal, A.C., de la Pena Garcia, J., Fernandez Marques, F., de las Heras Castano, G., Martin Ramos, L., Pons Romero, F.: Aparicion de cancer de esofago en paciente sometido a escleroterapia de varices esofagicas. Presentacion de un nuevo caso. Gastroenterol. Hepatol. 1994; 17: 373–375
92. Goulis, J., Burroughs, A.K.: Role of vasoactive drugs in the treatment of bleeding oesophageal varices. Digestion 1999; 60 (Suppl. 3): 25–34
93. Graffeo, M., Buffoli, F., Lanzani, G., Donato, F., Cesari, P., Benedini, D., Rolfi, F., Paterlini, A.: Survival after endoscopic sclerotherapy for esophageal varices in cirrhotics. Amer. J. Gastroenterol. 1994; 89: 1815–1822
94. Haciyanli, M., Genc, H., Halici, H., Kumkumoglu, Y., Gur. O.S., Ozturk, T.: Results of modified Sugiura operation in variceal bleeding in cirrhotic and noncirrhotic patients. Hepato-Gastroenterology 2003; 50: 784–788
95. Henderson, J.M., Kutner, M.H., Millikan, W.J. jr., Galambos, J.T., Riepe, St.P., Brooks, W.S., Bryan, F.C., Warren, W.D.: Endoscopic variceal sclerosis compared with distal splenorenal shunt to prevent recurrent variceal bleeding in cirrhosis. A prospective, randomized trial. Ann. Intern. Med. 1990; 112: 262–269
96. Henderson, J.M., Boyer, T.D., Kutner, M.H., Galloway, J.R., Rikkers, L.F., Jeffers, L.J., Abu-Elmagd, K., Connor, J.: Distal splenorenal shunt versus transjugular intrahepatic portal systematic shunt for variceal bleeding: A randomized trial. Gastroenterology 2006; 130: 1643–1651
97. Hubmann, R., Bodlaj, G., Czompo, M., Benkö, L., Pichler, P., Al-Kathib, S., Kiblböck, P., Shamyieh, A., Biesenbach, G.: The use of self-expanding metal stents to treat acute esophageal variceal bleeding. Endoscopy 2006; 38: 896–901
98. Hüppe, D., Jäger, D., Tromm, A., Barmeyer, J., May, B.: Dosisabhängige Akutwirkung und Langzeiteinfluß von Molsidomin auf die portale und kardiale Hämodynamik bei Patienten mit Leberzirrhose. Med. Klin. 1994; 89: 65–68
99. Imperiale, T.F., Chalasani, N.: A metaanalysis of endoscopic variceal ligation for primary prophylaxis of esophageal bleeding. Hepatology 2001; 33: 1003–1004
100. Ioannou, G.N., Doust, J., Rockey, D.C.: Terlipressin in acute oesophageal variceal haemorrhage (review). Alim. Pharm. Ther. 2003; 17: 53–64
101. Iwao, T., Oho, K., Sakai, T., Nakano, R., Yamawaki, M., Toyonaga, A., Tanikawa, K.: Upright posture decreases esophageal varices flow velocity in patients with cirrhosis. J. Hepatol. 1998; 28: 447–453
102. Iwase, H., Morise, K., Kawase, T., Horiuchi, Y.: Endoscopic injection sclerotherapy for esophageal varices during pregnancy. J. Clin. Gastroenterol. 1994; 18: 80–83
103. Jacobs, D.L., Rikkers, L.F.: Indications and results of shunt operations in the treatment of patients with recurrent variceal hemorrhage. Hepato-Gastroenterol. 1990; 37: 571–574
104. Jalan, R., Hayes, P.C., Morris, A.I., Jenkins, S., Krasner, N., Shields, R., Lombard, M., Walker, R.J.: Oesophageal variceal sclerotherapy: a risk factor for the development of oesophageal carcinoma. Dis. Esophagus 1993; 4: 51–53
105. Jaramillo, J.L., de la Mata, M., Mino, G., Costan, G., Gomez-Camacho, F.: Somatostatin versus Sengstaken balloon tamponade for primary haemostasia of bleeding esophageal varices. J. Hepatol. 1991; 12: 100–105
106. Jenkins, S.A., Shields, R., Davies, M., Elias, E., Turnbull, A.J., Bassendine, M.F., James, O.F.W., Iredale, J.P., Vyas, S.K., Arthur, M.J.P., Kingsnorth, A.N., Sutton, R.: A multicentre randomised trial comparing octreotide and injection sclerotherapy in the management and outcome of acute variceal haemorrhage. Gut 1997; 41: 526–533
107. Kahn, D., Jones, B., Bornman, P.C., Terblanche, J.: Incidence and management of complications after injection sclerotherapy: a ten-year prospective evaluation. Surgery 1989; 105: 160–165
108. Ka-Sic Ho, Lashner, B.A., Emond, J.C., Baker, A.L.: Prior esophageal variceal bleeding does not adversely affect survival after orthotopic liver transplantation. Hepatology 1993; 18: 66–72
109. Kayama, H., Inamori, M., Togawa, J., Shimamura, T., Tokita, Y., Umezawa, T., Sakaguchi, T., Naitoh, M., Nagare, H., Nakajima, A., Saito, T., Tominaga, S., Uenno, N., Tanaka, K., Sekihara, H.: Pleural effusions following endoscopic injection sclerotherapy for cirrhotic patients with esophageal varices. Hepato-Gastroenterol. 2006; 53: 376–380
110. Kim, T., Shijo, H., Kokawa, H., Tokumitsu, H., Kubara, K., Ota, K., Akiyoshi, N., Iida, T., Yokoyama, M., Okumura, M.: Risk factors for hemorrhage from gastric fundal varices. Hepatology 1997; 25: 307–312
111. Kinoshita, Y., Kitajima, N., Itoh, T., Ishido, S., Nishiyama, K., Kawanami, C., Kishi, K., Inatome, T., Fukuzaki, H., Chiba, T.: Gastroesophageal reflux after endoscopic injection sclerotherapy. Amer. J. Gastroenterol. 1992; 87: 282–286
112. Kitamoto, M., Imamura, M., Kamada, K., Aikata, M., Kawakanu, Y., Matsumoto, A., Kurihara, Y., Kono, H., Shirakawa, H., Nakanishi, T., Ito, K., Chayama, K.: Balloon-occluded retrograde transvenous obliteration of gastric fundal varices with hemorrhage. Amer. J. Gastroenterol. 2002; 178: 1167–1174
113. Kitano, S., Iso, Y., Hashizume, M., Yamaga, H., Koyanagi, N., Wada, H., Iwanaga, T., Ohta, M., Sugimachi, K.: Sclerotherapy vs. esophageal transection vs. distal splenorenal shunt for the clinical management of esophageal varices in patients with Child class A and B liver function: a prospective randomized trial. Hepatology 1992; 15: 63–68
114. Knauer, C.M., Fogel, M.R.: Pericarditis: complication of esophageal sclerotherapy. A report of three cases. Gastroenterology 1987; 93: 287–290
115. Knechtle, S.J., DπAlessandro, A.M., Armbrust, M.J., Musat, A., Kalayoglu, M.: Surgical portosystemic shunts for treatment of portal hypertensive bleeding: outcome and effect on liver function. Surgery 1999; 116: 708–711

116. Kochhar, R., Goenka, M.K., Mehta, S.K.: Endoscopic sclerotherapy during pregnancy. Amer. J. Gastroenterol. 1990; 85: 1132–1135
117. Kochhar, R., Goenka, M.K., Mehta, S.K.: Esophageal strictures following endoscopic variceal sclerotherapy. Antecedents, clinical profile, and management. Dig. Dis. Sci. 1992; 37: 347–352
118. Kokudo, N., Sanjo, K., Umekita, N., Harihara, Y., Tada, Y., Idezuki, Y.: Squamous cell carcinoma after endoscopic injection sclerotherapy for esophageal varices. Amer. J. Gastroenterol. 1990; 85: 861–864
119. Korula, J., Yellin, A., Kanel, G.C., Nichols, P.: Portal vein thrombosis complicating endoscopic variceal sclerotherapy. Convincing further evidence. Dig. Dis. Sci. 1991; 36: 1164–1167
120. Krige, J.E.J., Kotze, U.K., Bornman, P.C., Shaer, J.M., Klipin, M.: Variceal recurrence, rebleeding, and survival after endoscopic injection sclerotherapy in 287 alcoholic cirrhotic patients with bleeding esophageal varices. Ann. Surg. 2006; 244: 764–770
121. Lewis, W.D., Sanchez, H., Jenkins, R.L.: Indications and technique for the use of the porto-renal shunt in the treatment of variceal hemorrhage. Amer. J. Surg. 1993; 165: 336–340
122. Lo, G.H., Lai, K.H., Cheng, J.S., Chen, M.H., Chiang, H.T.: A prospective, randomized trial of butyl cyanoacrylate injection versus band ligation in the management of bleeding gastric varices. Hepatology 2001; 35: 1060–1064
123. Lo, G.H., Chen, W.C., Chen, M.H., Hsu, P.I., Lin, C.K., Tsai, W.L., Lai, K.H.: Banding ligation versus nadolol and isosorbide mononitrate for the prevention of esophageal variceal rebleeding. Gastroenterology 2002; 123: 728–734
124. Lui, H.F., Stanley, A.J., Forrest, E.H., Jalan, R., Hislop, W.S., Mills, P.R., Finlayson, N.D.C., MacGilchrist, A.J., Hayes, P.C.: Primary prophylaxis of variceal hemorrhage: a randomized controlled trial comparing band ligation, propranolol, and isosorbide mononitrate. Gastroenterology 2002; 123: 735–744
125. Madhotra, R., Mulcahy, H.E., Willner, I., Reuben, A.: Prediction of esophageal varices in patients with cirrhosis. J. Clin. Gastroenterol. 2002; 34: 81–85
126. Masci, E., Stigliano, R., Mariani, A., Bertoni, G., Baroncini, D., Cennamo, V., Micheletti, G., Casetti, T., Tansini, P., Buscarini, E., Ranzato, R., Norberto, L.: Prospective multicenter randomized trial comparing banding ligation with sclerotherapy of esophageal varices. Hepato-Gastroenterol. 1999; 46: 1769–1773
127. Matsuo, M., Kanematsu, M., Kim, T., Hori, M., Takamura, M., Murakami, T., Kondo, H., Moriyama, N., Nakamura, H., Hoshi, H.: Esophageal varices: Diagnosis with gadolinium-enhanced MR imaging of the liver for patients with chronic liver damage. Amer. J. Roentgenol. 2003; 180: 461–466
128. McAvoy, N.C., Hayes, P.C.: The use of transjugular intrahepatic portosystemic stent shunt in the management of acute oesophageal variceal haemorrhage. Eur. J. Gastroenterol. Hepatol. 2006; 18: 1135–1441
129. McCormick, P.A., Kaye, G.L., Greenslade, L., Cardin, F., Hobbs, K.E.F., McIntyre, N., Burroughs, A.K.: Esophageal staple transection as a salvage procedure after failure of acute injection sclerotherapy. Hepatology 1992; 15: 403–406
130. McCormick, P.A., Dick, R., Panagou, E.B., Chin, J.K.T., Greenslade, L., McIntyre, N., Burroughs, A.K.: Emergency transjugular intrahepatic portasystemic stent shunting as salvage treatment for uncontrolled variceal bleeding. Brit. J. Surg. 1994; 81: 1324–1327
131. Merican, I., Sprengers, D., McCormick, P.A., Minoli, G., McIntyre, N., Burroughs, A.K.: Diurnal pattern of variceal bleeding in cirrhotic patients. J. Hepatol. 1993; 19: 15–22
132. Merkel, C., Marin, R., Enzo, E., Donada, C., Cavallarin, G., Torboli, P., Amodio, P., Sebastianelli, G., Sacerdoti, D., Felder, M., Mazzaro, C., Beltrame, P., Gatta, A.: Randomised trial of nadolol or with isosorbide mononitrate for primary prophylaxis of variceal bleeding in cirrhosis. Lancet 1996; 348: 1677–1681
133. Merli, M., Nicolini, G., Angeloni, S., Rinaldi, V., de Santis, A., Merkel, C., Attili, A.F., Riggio, O.: Incidence and natural history of small esophageal varices in cirrhotic patients. J. Hepatol. 2003; 38: 266–272
134. Miller, L., Banson, F.L., Bazir, K., Korimilli, A., Liu, J.B., Dewan, R., Wolfson, M., Panganamamula, K.V., Carrasquillo, J., Schwartz, J., Chaker, A.E., Black, M.: Risk of esophageal variceal bleeding based on endoscopic ultrasound evaluation of the sum of esophageal variceal cross-sectional surface area. Amer. J. Gastroenterol. 2003; 98: 454–459
135. Nevens, F., Bustami, R., Scheys, I., Lesaffre, E., Fevery, J.: Variceal pressure is a factor predicting the risk of a first variceal bleeding: a prospective cohort study in cirrhotic patients. Hepatology 1998; 27: 15–19
136. Ogawa, K., Ishikawa, S., Naritaka, Y., Shimakawa, T., Wagatsuma, Y., Katsube, A., Kajiwara, T.: Clinical evaluation of endoscopic injection sclerotherapy using n-butyl-2-cyanoacrylate for gastric variceal bleeding. J. Gastroenterol. Hepatol. 1999; 14: 245–250
137. Orozco, H., Mercado, M.A., Takahashi, T., Hernandez-Ortiz, J., Capellan, J.F., Garcia-Tsao, G.: Elective treatment of bleeding varices with the Sugiura operation over 10 years. Amer. J. Surg. 1992; 163: 585–589
138. Orozco, H., Mercado, M.A., Takahashi, T., Capellan, F., Rojas, G., Chan, C.: Selective splenocaval shunt for bleeding portal hypertension: fifteen-year evaluation period. Surgery 1993; 113: 260–265
139. Palazzo, L., Hochain, P., Helmer, C., Cuillerier, E., Landi, B., Roseau, G., Cugnenc, P.H., Barbier, J.-P., Cellier, C.: Biliary varices on endoscopic ultrasonography: clinical presentation and outcome. Endoscopy 2000; 32: 520–524
140. Panes, J., Teres, J., Bosch, J., Rodes, J.: Efficacy of balloon tamponade in treatment of bleeding gastric and esophageal varices: results in 151 consecutive episodes. Dig. Dis. Sci. 1988; 33: 454–459
141. Paquet, K.-J., Mercado, M.A., Koussouris, P., Kalk, J.-F., Siemens, F., Cuan-Orozco, F.: Improved results with selective distal splenorenal shunt in a highly selected patient population. Ann. Surg. 1989; 210: 184–189
142. Paquet, K.-J.: Narrow-lumen mesocaval interposition shunt in liver cirrhosis and recurrent bleeding from oesophageal varices: standard method of the future for failure of sclerotherapyp? Dtsch. Med. Wschr. 1995; 120: 707–712
143. Patch, D., Sabin, C.A., Goulis, J., Gerunda, G., Greenslade, L., Merkel, C., Burroughs, A.K.: A randomized, controlled trial of medical therapy versus endoscopic ligation for the prevention of variceal rebleeding in patients with cirrhosis. Gastroenterology 2002; 123: 1013–1019
144. Pedretti, G., Elia, G., Calzetti, C., Magnani, G., Fiaccadori, F.: Octreotide versus terlipressin in acute variceal hemorrhage in liver cirrhosis. Emergency control and prevention of early rebleeding. Clin. Invest. 1994; 72: 653–659
145. Pereira-Lima, J.C., Zanette, M., Lopes, C.V., de Mattos, A.A.: The influence of endoscopic variceal ligation on the portal pressure gradient in cirrhotics. Hepato-Gastroenterol. 2003; 50: 102–106
146. Planas, R., Boix, J., Broggi, M., Cabré, E., Gomes-Vieira, M.C., Morillas, R., Armengol, M., de Leon, R., Humbert, P., Salva, J.A., Gassull, M.A.: Portocaval shunt versus endoscopic sclerotherapy in the elective treatment of variceal hemorrhage. Gastroenterology 1991; 100: 1078–1086
147. Plevris, J.N., Elliot, R., Mills, P.R., Hislop, W.S., Davies, J.M., Bouchier, I.A.D., Hayes, P.C.: Effect of propranolol on prevention of first variceal bleeding and survival in patients with chronic liver disease. Aliment. Pharmacol. Ther. 1994; 8: 63–70
148. Pohl, J., Pollmann, K., Sauer, P., Ring, A., Stremmel, W., Schlenker, T.: Antibiotic prophylaxis after variceal hemorrhage reduces incidence of early rebleeding. Hepato. Gastroenterol. 2004; 51: 541–546
149. Pontes, J.M., Leitao, M.C., Portela, F., Nunes, A., Freitas, D.: Endosonographic Doppler-guided manometry of esophageal varices: experimental validation and clinical feasibility. Endoscopy 2002; 34: 966–972
150. Psilopoulos, D., Galanis, P., Goulas, S., Papanikolaou, I.S., Elefsimiotis, I., Liatsos, C., Sparos, L., Marrogiannis, C.: Endoscopic variceal ligation vs. propranolol for prevention of first variceal bleeding: A randomized controlled trial. Eur. J. Gastroenterol. Hepatol. 2005; 17: 1111–1117
151. Rigo, G.P., Merighi, A., Chahin, N.J., Mastronardi, M., Codeluppi, P.L., Ferrari, A., Armocida, C., Zanasi, G., Cristani, A., Cioni, G., Manenti, F.: A prospective study of the ability of three endoscopic classifications to predict hemorrhage from esophageal varices. Gastrointest. Endosc. 1992; 38: 425–429
152. Rikkers, L.F., Jin, G.L., Langnas, A.N., Shaw, B.W.: Shunt surgery during the era of liver transplantation. Ann. Surg. 1997; 226: 51–57
153. Ring, E.J., Lake, J.R., Roberts, J.P., Gordon, R.L., LaBerge, J.M., Read, A.E., Sterneck, M.R., Ascher, N.L.: Using transjugular intrahepatic portosystemic shunts to control variceal bleeding before liver transplantation. Ann. Intern. Med. 1992; 116: 304–309
154. Ringe, B., Lang, H., Tusch, G., Pichlmayr, R.: Role of liver transplantation in management of esophageal variceal hemorrhage. World J. Surg. 1994; 18: 233–239
155. Rolando, N., Gimson, A., Philpott-Howard, J., Sahathevan, M., Casewell, M., Fagan, E., Westaby, D., Williams, R.: Infectious sequelae after endoscopic sclerotherapy of oesophageal varices: role of antibiotic prophylaxis. J. Hepatol. 1993; 18: 290–294
156. Saab, S., DeRosa, V., Nieto, J., Durazo, F., Han, S., Roth, B.: Costs and clinical outcomes of primary prophylaxis of variceal bleeding in patients with hepatic cirrhosis: A decision analytic model. Amer. J. Gastroenterol. 2003; 98: 763–770
157. Saeed, Z.A., Stiegmann, G.V., Ramirez, F.C., Reveille, R.M., Goff, J.S., Hepps, K.S., Cole, R.A.: Endoscopic variceal ligation is superior to combined ligation and sclerotherapy for esophageal varices: a multicenter prospective randomized trial. Hepatology 1997; 25: 71–74
158. Sakaki, M., Iwao, T., Oho, K., Toyonaga, A., Tanikawa, K.: Prognostic factors in cirrhotic patients receiving long-term sclerotherapy for the first bleeding from oesophageal varices. Eur. J. Gastroenterol. Hepatol. 1998; 10: 21–26
159. Salomez, D., Ponette, E., van Steenbergen, W.: Intramural hematoma of the esophagus after variceal sclerotherapy. Endoscopy 1991; 23: 299–301
160. Sarin, S.K., Lamba, G.S., Kumar, M., Misra, A., Murthy, N.: Comparison of endoscopic ligation and propranolol for the primary prevention of variceal bleeding. New Engl. J. Med. 1999; 340: 988–993
161. Sato, T., Yamazaki, K., Toyota, J., Karino, Y., Ohmura, T., Suga, T.: Color Doppler findings of gastric varices compared with findings on computed tomography. J. Gastroenterol. 2002; 37: 604–610
162. Sato, T., Yamazaki, K., Toyota, J., Karino, Y., Ohmura, T., Suga, T.: Evaluation of hemodynamics in esophageal varices. Value of endoscopic color Doppler ultrasonography with a galactose-based contrast agent. Hepatol. Res. 2003; 25: 55–61
163. Sauer, P., Hansmann, J., Richter, G.M., Stremmel, W., Stiehl, A.: Endoscopic variceal ligation plus propranolol vs. transjugular intrahepatic portosystemic stent shunt: a long-term randomized trial. Endoscopy 2002; 34: 690–697
164. Schmassmann, A., Zuber, M., Livers, M., Jäger, K., Jenzer, H.R., Fehr, H.F.: Recurrent bleeding after variceal hemorrhage: predictive value of portal venous duplex sonography. Amer. J. Roentgenol. 1993; 160: 41–47

165. **Schwaighofer, H., Koch, R., Vogel, W.:** Successful treatment of a bleeding esophageal sclerotheraphy ulcer with endoscopic injection of granulocyte-macrophage colony-stimulating factor. Gastrointest. Endosc. 2001; 54: 785–787
166. **Sethy, P.K., Kochhar, R., Behera, D., Bhasin, D.K., Raja, K., Singh, K.:** Pleuropulmonary complications of esophageal variceal sclerotherapy with absolute alcohol. J. Gastroenterol. Hepatol. 2003; 18: 910–914
167. **Shiba, M., Higuchi, K., Nakamura, K., Itani, A., Kuga, T., Okazaki, H., Fujiwara, Y., Arakawa, T.:** Efficacy and safety of balloon-occluded endoscopic injection sclerotherapy as a prophylactic treatment for high-risk gastric fundal varices: a prospective, randomized, comparativ clinical trial. Gastrointest. Endosc. 2002; 56: 522–528
168. **Shields, R., Jenkins, S.A., Baxter, J.N., Kingsnorth, A.N., Ellenbogen, S., Makin, C.A., Gilmore, I., Morris, A.I., Ashby, D., West, C.R.:** A prospective randomized controlled trial comparing the efficacy of somatostatin with injection sclerotherapy in the control of bleeding oesophageal varices. J. Hepatol. 1992; 16: 128–137
169. **Silvain, Ch., Carpentier, St., Sautereau, D., Czernichow, B., Metréau, J.-M., Fort, E., Ingrand, P., Boyer, J., Pillegand, B., Doffël, M., Dhumeaux, D., Beauchant, M.:** Terlipressin plus transdermal nitroglycerin vs. octreotide in the control of acute bleeding from esophageal varices: a multicenter randomized trial. Hepatology 1993; 18: 61–65
170. **Singh, P., Pooran, N., Indaram, A., Bank, S.:** Combined ligation and sclerotherapy versus ligation alone for secondary prophylaxis of esophageal variceal bleeding: a meta-analysis. Amer. J. Gastroenterol. 2002; 97: 623–629
171. **Siringo, S., McCormick, P.A., Mistry, P., Kaye, G., McIntyre, N., Burroughs, A.K.:** Prognostic significance of the white nipple sign in variceal bleeding. Gastrointest. Endosc. 1991; 37: 51–55
172. **Siringo, S., Bolondi, L., Sofia, S., Hermida, R.C., Gramantieri, L., Gaiani, S., Piscaglia, F., Carbone, C., Misitano, B., Corinaldesi, R.:** Circadian occurrence of variceal bleeding in patients with liver cirrhosis. J. Gastroenterol. Hepatol. 1996; 11: 1115–1120
173. **Söderlund, C., Magnusson, I., Törngren, S., Lundell, L.:** Terlipressin (Triglycyl-lysine-vasopressin) controls acute bleeding oesophageal varices. A double-blind, randomized, placebo-controlled trial. Scand. J. Gastroenterol. 1990; 25: 622–630
174. **Soehendra, N., Grimm, H., Maydeo, A., Nam, V.C., Eckmann, B., Brückner, M.:** Endoscopic sclerotherapy – personal experience. Hepato-Gastroenterol. 1991; 38: 220–223
175. **Spina, G.P., Santambrogio, R., Opocher, E., Cosentino, F., Zambelli, A., Passoni, G.A., Cucchiaro, G., Macri, M., Morandi, E., Bruno, S., Pezzuoli, G.:** Distal splenorenal shunt versus endoscopic sclerotherapy in the prevention of variceal rebleeding. First stage of a randomized, controlled trial. Ann. Surg. 1990; 211: 178–186
176. **Stringer, M.D., Howard, E.R.:** Longterm outcome after injection sclerotherapy for oesophageal varices in children with extrahepatic portal hypertension. Gut 1994; 35: 257–259
177. **Tait, I.S., Krige, J.E.J., Terblanche, J.:** Endoscopic band ligation of oesophageal varices. Brit. J. Surg. 1999; 86: 437–446
178. **Tam, F., Chow, H., Prindiville, T., Cornish, D., Haulk, T., Trudeau, W., Hoeprich, P.:** Bacterial peritonitis following esophageal injection sclerotherapy for variceal hemorrhage. Gastrointest. Endosc. 1990; 36: 131–133
179. **Tan, P.C., Hou, M.C., Lin, H.C., Liu, T.T., Chang, F.Y., Lee, F.Y., Lee, S.D.:** A randomized trial of endoscopic treatment of acute gastric variceal hemorrhage: N-butyl-2-cyanoacrylate injection versus band ligation. Hepatology 2006; 43: 690–697
180. **Terés, J., Bordas, J.M., Bravo, D., Visa, J., Grande, L., Garcia-Valdecasas, J.C., Pera, C., Rodes, J.:** Sclerotherapy vs. distal splenorenal shunt in the elective treatment of variceal hemorrhage: a randomized controlled trial. Hepatology 1987; 7: 430–436
181. **Thakeb, F., Salama, Z., Raouf, T.A., Kader, S.A., Hamid, H.A.:** The value of combined use of N-butyl-2-cyanoacrylate and ethanolamine oleate in the management of bleeding oesophagogastric varices. Endoscopy 1995; 27: 358–364
182. **Thomas, P.G., D'Cruz, A.J.:** Distal splenorenal shunting for bleeding gastric varices. Brit. J. Surg. 1994; 81: 241–244
183. **Tomikawa, M., Hashizume, M., Okita, K., Kitano, S., Ohta, M., Higashi, M., Akahoshi, T.:** Endoscopic injection sclerotherapy in the management of 2105 patients with esophageal varices. Surgery 2002; 131 (Suppl.): 171–175
184. **Triger, D.R., Johnson, A.G., Brazier, J.E., Johnston, G.W., Spencer, E.F.A., McKee, R., Anderson, J.R., Carter, D.C.:** A prospective trial of endoscopic sclerotherapy vs. oesophageal transection and gastric devascularisation in the long term management of bleeding oesophageal varices. Gut 1992; 33: 1553–1558
185. **Tripathi, D., Helmy, A., Macbeth, K., Balata, S., Lui, H.F., Stanley, A.J., Redhead, D.N., Hayes, P.C.:** Ten years' follow-up of 472 patients following transjugular intrahepatic portosystemic stent-shunt insertion at a single centre. Eur. J. Gastroenterol. Hepatol. 2004; 16: 9–18
186. **Tripathi, D., Ferguson, J., Barkell, H., Macbeth, K., Ireland, H., Redhead, D.N., Hayes, P.C.:** Improved clinical outcome with transjugular intrahepatic portosystemic stent-shunt utilizung polytetrafluoroethylene-covered stents. Eur. J. Gastroenterol. Hepatol. 2006; 18: 225–232
187. **Van Ruiswyk, J., Byrd, J.C.:** Efficacy of prophylactic sclerotherapy for prevention of a first variceal hemorrhage. Gastroenterology 1992; 102: 587–597
188. **Van Thiel, D.H., Dindzans, V.J., Schade, R.R., Rabinovitz, M., Gavaler, J.S.:** Prophylactic versus emergency sclerotherapy of large esophageal varices prior to liver transplantation. Dig. Dis. Sci. 1993; 38: 1505–1510
189. **Vickers, Ch., Rhodes, J., Chesner, I., Hillenbrand, P., Dawson, J., Cockel, R., Adams, D., O'Connor, H., Dykes, P., Bradby, H., Valori, R., Elias, E.:** Prevention of rebleeding from oesophageal varices: two-year follow up of a prospective controlled trial of propranolol in addition to sclerotherapy. J. Hepatol. 1994; 21: 81–87
190. **Villanueva, C., Balanzo, J., Novella, M.T., Soriano, G., Sainz, S., Torras, X., Cusso, X., Guarner, C., Vilardell, F.:** Nadolol plus isosorbide mononitrate compared with sclerotherapy for the prevention of variceal rebleeding. New Engl. J. Med. 1996; 334: 1625–1629
191. **Villanueva, C., Minana, J., Ortiz, J., Gallego, A., Soriano, G., Torras, X., Sainz, S., Boadas, J., Cusso, X., Guarner, C., Balanzo, J.:** Endoscopic ligation compared with combined treatment with nadolol and isosorbide mononitrate to prevent recurrent variceal bleeding. New Engl. J. Med. 2001; 345: 647–655
192. **Wachsberg, R.H., Simmons, M.Z.:** Coronary vein diameter and flow direction in patients with portal hypertension: evaluation with duplex sonography and correlation with variceal bleeding. Amer. J. Roentgenol. 1994; 162: 637–641
193. **Waked, I., Korula, J.:** Analysis of long-term endoscopic surveillance during follow-up after variceal sclerotherapy from a 13-year experience. Amer. J. Med. 1997; 102: 192–199
194. **Warren, D.W., Henderson, J.M., Millikan, W.J., Galambos, J.T., Brooks, W.S., Riepe, St.P., Salam, A.S., Kutner, M.H.:** Distal splenorenal shunt versus endoscopic sclerotherapy for long-term management of variceal bleeding. Preliminary report of a prospective, randomized trial. Ann. Surg. 1986; 203: 454–462
195. **Wen-Ming Wang, Chang-Yi Chen, Chang-Ming Jan, Li-Tzong Chen, Deng-Chyang Wu:** Central nervous system infection after endoscopic injection sclerotherapy. Amer. J. Gastroenterol. 1990; 85: 865–867
196. **Williams, D., Waugh, R., Gallagher, N., Perkins, K., Dilworth, P., Duggan, A., Selby, W.:** Mortality and rebleeding following transjugular intrahepatic portosystemic stent shunt for variceal haemorrhage. J. Gastroenterol. Hepatol. 1998; 13: 163–169
197. **Willmann, J.K., Weishaupt, D., Böhm, T., Pfammatter, T., Seifert, B., Marincek, B., Bauerfeind, P.:** Detection of submucosal gastric fundal varices with multi-detector row CT angiography. Gut 2003; 52: 886–892
198. **Yol, S., Belviranli, M., Toprak, S., Kartal, A.:** Endoscopic clipping vs band ligation in the management of bleeding esophageal varices. Surg. Endosc. 2003; 17: 38–42
199. **Young, M.F., Sanowski, R.A., Rasche, R.:** Comparison and characterization of ulcerations induced by endoscopic ligation of esophageal varices versus endoscopic sclerotherapy. Gastrointest. Endosc. 1993; 39: 119–122
200. **Zaman, A.:** Portal hypertension-related bleeding: management of difficult cases. Clin. Liver Dis. 2006; 10: 353–370
201. **Ziegler, K., Gregor, M., Zeitz, M., Zimmer, T., Habermann, F., Riecken, E.O.:** Evaluation of endosonography in sclerotherapy of esophageal varices. Endoscopy 1991; 23: 247–250

Lower gastrointestinal haemorrhage
202. **Enns, R.:** Acute lower gastrointestinal bleeding. Canad. J. Gastroenterol. 2001; 15: 509–521
203. **Fix, O.K., Simon, J.T., Farraye, F.A., Oviedo, J.A., Pratt, D.S., Chen, W.T., Cave, D.R.:** Obscure gastrointestinal hemorrhage from mesenteric varices diagnosed by video capsule endoscopy. Dig. Dis. Sci. 2006; 51: 1169–1174
204. **Hayat, M., Axon, A.T.R., O'Mahony, S.:** Diagnostic yield and effect on clinical outcomes of push enteroscopy in suspected small-bowel bleeding. Endoscopy 2000; 32: 369–372
205. **Kouraklis, G., Misiakos, E., Karatzas, G., Grogas, J., Skalkeas, G.:** Diagnostic approach and management of active lower gastrointestinal hemorrhage. Int. Surg. 1995; 80: 138–140
206. **Misra, S.P., Misra, V., Dwivedi, M.:** Effect of esophageal variceal band ligation on hemorrhoids, anorectal varices, and portal hypertensive colopathy. Endoscopy 2002; 34: 195–198
207. **Nayar, M., Saravanan, R., McWilliams, R.G., Evans, J., Sutton, R.J., Gilmore, I.T., Smart, M.L., Lombard, M.G.:** TIPSS in the treatment of ectopic variceal bleeding. Hepato-Gastroenterol. 2006; 53: 584–587
208. **Sato, T., Yamazaki, K., Toyota, J., Karino, Y., Ohmura, T., Suga, T.:** The value of the endoscopic therapies in the treatment of rectal varices. A retrospective comparison between injection sclerotherapy and band ligation. Hepatol. Res. 2006; 34: 250–255
209. **Zuckerman, G.R., Prakash, C.:** Acute lower gastrointestinal bleeding. Etiology, therapy, and outcomes. Gastrointest. Endosc. 1999; 49: 228–238

Symptoms and Syndromes

20 Acute and chronic liver insufficiency

		Page:
1	*Definition*	380
2	**Systematics**	380
2.1	Partial and global insufficiency	380
2.2	Compensation and decompensation	380
2.3	Acuteness and chronicity	380
2.4	Hepatic coma	380
3	**Acute liver insufficiency**	380
3.1	Definition	380
3.2	Morphology	381
3.3	Pathogenesis	381
3.4	Frequency and causes	381
3.5	Clinical findings	382
3.6	Laboratory parameters	383
3.7	Complications	384
3.8	Prognosis	385
3.9	Regeneration	385
4	**Chronic liver insufficiency**	385
4.1	Definition	385
4.2	Clinical findings	385
4.3	*Decompensation*	385
4.3.1	Impairment of liver functions	386
4.3.2	Hepatic encephalopathy	386
4.3.3	Ascites and oedema	386
4.3.4	Hepatorenal syndrome	386
4.3.5	Coagulopathy and haemorrhage	386
4.4	*Acute-on-chronic liver insufficiency*	386
5	**Therapy**	387
5.1	General therapeutic measures	387
5.2	Specific therapeutic measures	388
5.3	*Liver support systems*	389
5.3.1	Extracorporeal systems	389
5.3.2	Bioartificial systems	390
5.3.3	Extracorporeal liver perfusion	391
5.4	*Liver transplantation methods*	391
5.4.1	Orthotopic transplantation	391
5.4.2	Auxiliary partial orthotopic liver transplantation	392
5.4.3	Heterotopic transplantation	392
5.4.4	Xenotransplantation	392
5.5	*Transplantation of hepatocytes*	392
	• References (1–134)	393
	(Figures 20.1–20.5; tables 20.1–20.5)	

20 Acute and chronic liver insufficiency

1 Definition

The term "liver insufficiency" denotes a breakdown in the functions of the liver. The syndrome of functional liver failure covers a wide spectrum of clinical, biochemical and neurophysiological changes. In principle, liver insufficiency can occur without previous liver damage as well as with already-existing liver disease. It is characterized by a deterioration in the synthesizing, regulatory and detoxifying function of the liver. This final stage of liver disease terminates in hepatic coma.

2 Systematics

2.1 Partial and global insufficiency

Serious liver disease can affect the 12 main metabolic functions of the liver, with their 60—70 even more important partial functions, to widely differing degrees. (s. tab. 3.1) The result is either *global insufficiency* or *partial insufficiency*, each with very varied clinical and biochemical symptoms. The failure of certain metabolic functions is responsible to a greater or lesser extent for the development and intensity of liver insufficiency. Impairments in the functions of detoxification and protein metabolism are particularly significant in this respect.

2.2 Compensation and decompensation

The **compensated stage** does not usually display any signs of liver insufficiency (except possibly jaundice), nor are there any typical ailments. Functional parameters that can be quantified in routine laboratory tests (such as cholinesterase, albumin, Quick's value, bile acids) may still be normal or only minimally impaired in the individual instance. In contrast, liver function tests (galactose, indocyanine green, MEGX, etc.) demonstrate a reduction of liver function which is already quite considerable.

The **decompensated stage**, i.e. manifest liver insufficiency, can present as *cellular decompensation* (e.g. in the case of acute liver failure due to toxic or inflammatory mass necrosis) or be expressed only in the form of *portal decompensation* (e.g. in cases of postsinusoidal intrahepatic portal hypertension). • As a rule, chronic liver insufficiency is accompanied by a *combined decompensation* with a loss in function of the liver cells and, at the same time, the sequelae of portal decompensation (collateral varicosis, encephalopathy, ascites, hepatorenal syndrome, hepatopulmonary syndrome, variceal bleeding). *(see chapters 15—19 and 35)*

2.3 Acuteness and chronicity

Depending on the time period involved in the course of the disease, **acute liver failure** without pre-existing liver disease can initially be differentiated by massive liver cell disintegration due to a variety of causes. • In contrast, **chronic liver insufficiency** with pre-existing liver disease is mostly found in advanced liver cirrhosis with a progressive loss of function. • A *sudden necrotising episode* can also precipitate the change from chronic and still compensated liver insufficiency into acute liver failure (i.e. **"acute-on-chronic" insufficiency**) in the same way that acute liver failure which has been overcome may develop into chronic liver insufficiency. (60)

2.4 Hepatic coma

Hepatic coma can be subdivided according to its aetiology as follows: (*1.*) *hepatocyte disintegration coma* (= endogenous coma due to the loss of parenchyma), (*2.*) *liver cell failure coma* (= exogenous coma due to metabolic disorders, almost always in the presence of cirrhosis), (*3.*) *electrolyte coma* (= so-called "false" coma due to dyselectrolytaemia, almost always iatrogenic), and (*4.*) *mixed forms of coma*. (s. pp 281, 284, 386) (s. tab. 15.5)

3 Acute liver insufficiency

▶ J. W. Morgagni (1761) was probably the first to describe acute yellow atrophy of the liver, i.e. hepatic coma. Acute liver failure can be seen as identical to the "acute yellow atrophy" described by K. Rokitansky in 1842. This acute and severe clinical picture was subsequently termed "bilious dyscrasia" (P. J. Horaczek, 1844), "icterus gravis" (C. Ozanam, 1849), "acholia" (F. Th. Frerichs, 1858), "hepatolysis" (R. Ehrmann, 1922), "hepatodystrophy" (G. Herxheimer, 1935) or "liver dystrophy" (R. Böhmig, 1949). The terms "hepatargia" (H. I. Quincke, 1899) and "hepatic coma" were used to denote the final stage, which usually sets in at the end of acute or chronic liver failure. • Acute liver failure in the course of acute viral hepatitis was termed "fulminant hepatitis" by W. Lucké et al. (1946), who also defined a subacute form with a less severe course. (36)

3.1 Definition

Acute liver failure (ALF) is defined as an acute clinical picture with *jaundice* due to a most severe disorder in the liver function and/or massive liver cell necrosis which, without any pre-existing liver disease, culminates in *hepatic coma* (= endogenous coma) within 8 weeks. Potentially, the condition is fully reversible (C. Trey et al., 1970). • In addition, *coagulopathy* must also be present (D. F. Schafer et al., 1989).

Courses of disease

Clinically, there are three different courses of disease following the onset of **jaundice:** (*1.*) fulminant or *hyperacute liver failure* (= occurrence of hepatic encephalopathy in the 1st week), (*2.*) *acute liver failure* (= occurrence of hepatic encephalopathy between the 2nd and 4th week), and (*3.*) *subacute liver failure* (= occurrence of hepatic encephalopathy between the 5th and 8th week).
• Surprisingly, however, it could be shown that 30–40% of the hyperacute forms survived in spite of the development of hepatic coma and cerebral oedema. As opposed to this, the subacute forms displayed a survival rate of only 10–20% despite a lower frequency of cerebral oedema and better liver function. (s. tab. 20.1)

	Hyperacute liver failure	Acute liver failure	Subacute liver failure
Encephalopathy	++	++	++
Duration of icterus in days	0–7	8–28	29–72
Cerebral oedema	++	++	(+)
Quick's value	↓	↓↓	↓
Bilirubin	N-↑	↑↑	↑↑
Prognosis	favourable	poor	poor
Survival rate	30–40%	5–10%	10–20%

Tab. 20.1: Characteristics and prognosis of acute liver failure and its subtypes (modified according to J.G. O'Grady et al., 1993) (N = normal)

3.2 Morphology

In the **pathological-anatomical context,** *hepatomegaly* due to hyperaemia is often found at the outset. During the further course of disease, this can develop into *liver atrophy* as a result of parenchymal loss.

Histologically, acute liver failure shows a wide range of uncharacteristic changes. (*1.*) Depending on the underlying cause, the morphological picture of **acute necrotizing hepatitis** may develop, with extensive confluent cellular destruction. The extent of necrosis, measured by the morphologically evidenced hepatic volume fraction of the still functioning liver parenchyma, yields reliable information on the chance of survival (J. Scotto et al., 1973). Given a normal value of 85% **hepatic volume fraction** (HVF) of intact liver cells for each volume unit of the total liver, a decrease to <30% (threshold 28–35%) would possibly mean that the patient is unlikely to survive. (*2.*) In acute liver failure caused by toxins or hypoxia, **massive fatty degeneration** of the hepatocytes can vary substantially. In diffuse fatty degeneration featuring minute vacuoles and damage to the organelles, liver cell necrosis cannot, as a rule, be detected (e.g. acute fatty liver during pregnancy, Reye's syndrome, in association with tetracycline or valproic acid). (*3.*) Between these two "classical" morphological manifestations, there are also **compound forms,** i.e. courses of disease with a variety of histological changes of different intensities and combinations. On occasions, it is also possible to identify histological findings which point to a certain cause of the disease. (41, 59)

From a morphological point of view, acute liver failure is potentially reversible, so that even **complete regeneration** can be attained. Precursory cellular necrosis is hence less of a determinant than the capacity to regenerate.

There have been reports on the transition from virus-induced acute liver failure to **chronic hepatitis.** As the final stage of fulminant viral hepatitis (also known as acute liver dystrophy or submassive hepatitic necrosis), a **postdystrophic scarred liver** *("potato liver")* can develop. (s. fig. 35.14) Cicatricial distortions with a continuing effect, regenerative processes, intrahepatic vascular disorders and hypoxia-related damage lead to the conclusion that a *posthepatitic, postdystrophic scarred liver may well be a special form of cirrhosis.*

▶ Neither the functional state of liver insufficiency nor hepatic coma can be recognized histologically.

3.3 Pathogenesis

The common target structures for the various causes of acute liver failure are usually the cellular and subcellular biomembranes of the hepatocytes. Among other things, any damage to these biomembranes causes a massive inflow of calcium into the liver cells, which results in a severe disorder of the cell milieu and ultimately in cell death.

In **oxygen deficiency,** the oxidative stress is mainly localized in the extracellular spaces. This is where the Kupffer cells and neutrophils are involved in complex self-stimulating mechanisms, which can lead to the formation of inflammatory mediators and cytotoxic substances. • An important pathogenetic aspect is the "priming effect", which generally results in the increased production of oxygen radicals. The complex process of **lipid peroxidation** likewise effects massive liver cell damage in the form of self-perpetuation. • Excessive **immunological reactions,** which occur in acute liver failure due to viral hepatitis, halothane hepatitis, etc., are significant. There are also isolated cases in which **biotoxometabolites** are produced and may act as neo-antigens. (s. fig. 3.11)

Consequently, severe damage to liver cells and widespread necrosis are usually the result of a network of altered cellular and humoral reactions, which for their part are often the initial cause of acute liver failure due to their synergistic and interactive effects (H. Popper et al., 1986). Systemic reactions are responsible for the fact that other organs and functional sequences are equally affected, thus creating a wide spectrum of clinical findings and complications.

3.4 Frequency and causes

Acute liver failure is a rare occurrence. About five cases are found out of 6,000 hospital admissions (in the USA a total of ca. 2000 patients per year, in Germany ca. 150). However, there can be wide variations in frequency due to the effect of regional differences on individual aetiology. The causes of acute liver failure are numerous and varied. Diabetes mellitus and overweight (12) are extremely high risk factors. • Primary or secondary hepatitis viruses are deemed a frequent cause, although there are regional and individual variations (e. g. drug dependence, pregnancy) regarding the predominant virus type. • A further common cause (ca. 20%) are drugs (particularly paracetamol, often taken with suicidal intent, and halothane), followed by mycotoxins, alcohol and carbon tetrachloride (such as can be found in cleaning agents or solvents, and also with "glue sniffers"), heat-stroke (up to 10% of cases), Ecstasy, and vascular diseases. (12, 79) (s. tab. 20.2)

Paracetamol: The first report on acute liver failure due to paracetamol poisoning was published in 1966 (D. G. D. DAVIDSON et al.). Due to induced CYP II E2, paracetamol is metabolized to the extremely reactive molecule N-acetyl-p-benzoquinone-imine (NAPQI). This binds covalently to cellular proteins. A small amount of NAPQI is neutralized by glutathione; however, with a larger quantity of NAPQI (following an intake of >10 g paracetamol), the hepatic glutathione supplies are used up, so that the NAPQI becomes highly toxic. (s. fig. 20.3) There is hence a direct correlation between the degree of glutathione consumption and the severity of liver cell damage. The loss of glutathione can be compensated by i.v. administration of the glutathione precursor N-acetylcysteine. (s. p. 388)

Amanita phalloides: Mycotoxins, especially α-amatoxin, are extremely hepatotoxic as a result of the inhibition of mRNA polymerase B and the blocking of RNA synthesis. The lethal dose is approx. 0.1 mg amatoxin/kg BW (one to three fungi = 10–50 g), depending on the patient's age and state of health as well as the respective degree of intestinal absorption and diffusion in the tissue. The heat-resistant mycotoxins (amanitines) are capable of enterohepatic recirculation. (s. pp 388, 587)

1. **Primary hepatotropic viruses**
   HAV (0.2–0.3%) (6, 38, 68) • HBV (1–2%) (6, 40, 61, 67, 83) •
   HCV (ca. 1%) (29, 67, 69, 82) • HDV superinfection (ca. 20%) • HEV (10–20%) (6, 29) • HBV mutants • HCV + HAV (30–40%) (72)
2. **Secondary hepatotropic viruses**
   adenoviruses • Coxsackie (74) • cytomegaloviruses • dengue fever • Epstein-Barr (20) • herpes simplex (type 1,2) (71) • herpesvirus-6 (1) • influenza A (76) • parainfluenza virus • paramyxoviruses • parvovirus B 19 • varicella zoster virus • yellow fever (s. tab. 23.1)
3. **Bacteria and parasites**
   leptospira, listeria (70) • malaria • M. tuberculosis (24, 28), rickettsia, syphilis
4. **Chemical substances**
   carbon tetrachloride (53) • chloroform • nitropropane (25) • trinitrotoluene • yellow phosphorus (s. tab. 30.3)
5. **Fungal poisons**
   Amanita phalloides (26, 49, 111, 123) • lepiota (50)
6. **Toxins**
   B. cereus emetic toxin • microcystins of cyanobacteria
7. **Medicinal agents**
   allopurinol • amiodarone • antiretroviral agents • carbamazepine • cotrimoxazole (3) • cyproterone • dapsone • didanosine • disulfiram • Ecstasy (112, 116) • enflurane • flutamide • glitazone • gold • halothane • hydroxychloroquine • interferon • isoflurane • isoniazid • kava-kava • ketoconazole • lisinopril • methotrexate • methyldopa • mono-amine oxidase inhibitor • nilutamide • nimesulide • ofloxacin • omeprazole • paracetamol • phenhydane • phenothiazine • phenytoin • pirprofen • propylthiouracil • rifampicin • sulphasalazine • tetracycline • valproic acid (s. tab. 29.4)
8. **Alcohol**
9. **Metabolic causes**
   acute fatty liver in pregnancy (45) • $α_1$-antitrypsin deficiency • amyloidosis (31) • erythropoietic protoporphyria • hereditary fructose intolerance • galactosaemia • HELLP syndrome • Reye's syndrome, tyrosinaemia • Wilson's disease
10. **Ischaemia**
    Budd-Chiari syndrome • heatstroke • ligature of the hepatic artery • shock liver • veno-occlusive disease
11. **Malignant infiltration**
    hepatocellular carcinoma (37) • Hodgkin's disease (16) • leukaemia (4) • massive formation of metastases • melanoma • non-Hodgkin's lymphoma (5, 55, 80) • renal cell carcinoma (19)
12. **Autoimmune hepatitis** (44)
13. **Septic cholangitis**
14. **Heart failure** (77)
15. **Jejuno-ileal bypass** (11)

Tab. 20.2: Various causes of acute liver failure (with some references)

3.5 Clinical findings

The overall picture of acute liver failure is first and foremost determined by the clinical findings. The symptoms are dramatic and subject to swift change. The course of disease can advance within a matter of days or, in a subacute form, take several weeks. (12, 58, 62, 79)

General symptoms: The acute clinical picture develops swiftly with conspicuous symptoms, such as fatigability, loss of appetite, nausea, weakness, lassitude, meteorism, apathy and disruption of the circadian rhythm.

Encephalopathy: Rapidly, often within one or two days, there is evidence of dysarthria, muscle tremor, finger tremor, lack of concentration and asterixis. Restlessness, hyperkinesis and hallucinatory experiences occur. Even screaming attacks have been observed. These symptoms, which can still be classified under stages I and II, are fully reversible. Nevertheless, lethality of 30–35% must be anticipated in stage II. In contrast, stage III is clearly less reversible. Somnolence, stupor with confusion, deviant behaviour, hyperreflexia, Babinski's reflex, clonus and spasticity as well as nystagmus are now observed.

There is usually still a response to acoustic stimuli. The EEG shows a slowing down of basic activity (0.5–3.0/sec.) together with mainly biphasic and triphasic potentials. Lethality rises to over 50%. In stage IV, the patient is in a deep coma. There is evidence of areflexia, an absence of any corneal reflex and loss of tonicity; the brain waves flatten out to an isoelectric line. Irrespective of therapy, lethality is 80–90%. (s. tab. 15.5)

Cerebral oedema: As from coma stage III, cerebral pressure can increase (75–80% of cases) owing to water retention and/or vasodilation with hyperaemia, yet with a subsequent reduction in cerebral perfusion and hypoxia. Intracranial cerebral compression is > 20 mm Hg. Cerebral oedema is vasogenetic and/or cytotoxic, the latter feature appearing to predominate. Clinical symptoms include disorders in the respiratory rhythm (in particular tachypnoea), hypertension, bradycardia and increased muscular tonus. Singultus implies damage to and impending constriction of the brain stem. The pupils are dilated due to the pressure on the oculomotor nerve. Chemosis can develop, which is a fatal prognostic sign. (2) Intracranial blood circulation sinks rapidly. In 30–60% of cases, cerebral oedema is fatal. (9, 10, 39, 64, 66, 75, 78)

Jaundice: With the foudroyant disintegration of liver cells, a comatose condition can set in within a few hours, even before jaundice is identified. In most cases, however, jaundice is already present. The intensity and time of onset vary. Severe jaundice (> 20 mg/dl) is considered to be a poor prognostic sign.

Hepatic foetor: The sweet aromatic smell of the exhaled breath (mercaptan derivatives) is seen as a reliable sign of acute liver failure, but it is not always present. The administration of poorly absorbable antibiotics (e.g. paromomycin) improves the condition of hepatic foetor, and can even eliminate it temporarily. (s. pp 91, 275)

Fever: Fever often occurs; it mostly remains at 38 °C, but septic temperatures are possible. • In some cases, this may be a question of *aetiocholanolone fever*, whereby aetiocholanolone can also be quantified in the serum. • *Bacterial infections* likewise cause fever and require appropriate treatment. *Toxins* may also be responsible for the febrile condition (tissue toxins, endotoxins). (s. p. 761)

Liver size: The liver may have normal size or it can be enlarged due to hyperaemia or massive fatty infiltration. A rapid shrinking of the liver to less than 1000 ml in volume ("dystrophy", "acute atrophy") – requiring sonographic or CT monitoring at the bedside – is deemed to be a poor prognostic sign.

3.6 Laboratory parameters

At present, there is no specific laboratory investigation which facilitates the diagnosis of acute liver failure. In view of the severity of this clinical picture, there are, however, a number of laboratory parameters which show marked pathological changes and thus require full diagnostic clarification. Activin A serum levels were elevated, especially in patients with acute liver failure, due to a paracetamol overdose. This did not affect the final outcome, but was possibly a factor in the inhibition of liver regeneration. Serum follistatin was also increased in patients with fulminant liver disease. (27, 35) Furthermore, the laboratory values allow an assessment of the complications involved and an evaluation of the prognosis. (7, 13, 14, 58, 62, 79)

Various laboratory values are indicative of severe complications and thus considered to be **criteria** pointing to a poor prognosis. (s. tab. 20.3)

Decrease in cholinesterase	< 500 U/l
Decrease in factor V	< 20%
Fall in Quick's value	< 20%
Group-specific component protein	< 34 µg/ml
Hyperkalaemia	due to renal failure
Hypoalbuminaemia	< 2.5 g/dl
Hypocalcaemia	due to pancreatitis
Hyponatraemia	< 120 mval/l
Hyponatriuria	< 10 mmol/l
Lactatacidosis	> 3.5 mmol/l
Phosphataemia	> 2.5 mg/dl
Rapid drop in transaminases	subnormal values
Rise in bilirubin	over 20 mg/dl

Tab. 20.3: Criteria for a poor prognosis in acute liver insufficiency

1. **GPT, GOT, GDH, LDH:** These enzymes are greatly elevated in accordance with cell destruction (GOT ≫ GPT). A decrease in enzyme values during the further course of disease can be a sign of regressing cell necrosis, marked parenchymal loss or a disorder in enzyme synthesis. A rapid drop in the initially elevated enzyme values is considered to be an unfavourable prognostic sign.

2. **Bilirubin:** Serum bilirubin shows a pronounced and varied increase, although the conjugated bilirubin does not rise at all, or only minimally, since uptake and conjugation remain intact for a considerable period of time.

3. **Quick's value:** A drop in the coagulation factors II, V, VII, IX and X is a reliable indicator of the remaining liver function. Factor VIII increases. With massive liver cell destruction, a dangerous decrease in factors V and VII is observed within one or two days (corresponding to the half-life of the factors) together with a marked reduction in Quick's value and Colombi's index. (46, 48) (s. p. 111)

4. **Cholinesterase:** During the further course of disease, cholinesterase decreases in relation to its longer half-life and likewise allows a reliable assessment to be made of the remaining liver function. (s. p. 109)

5. **Electrolytes:** There is evidence of *hyponatraemia* (= dilutional hyponatraemia or reinforced natriuresis) as well as *hypokalaemia* (= inadequate supply, intensified kaliuresis, outflow of potassium into the body cells due

to i.v. glucose infusions). The serum values of *magnesium, phosphate* and *zinc* are also lower as a rule.

6. **Group-specific component protein:** This substance (= α_2-globulin) is synthesized in the liver and binds actin. GCP is released upon hepatocyte decay; its pronounced reduction in the serum results from the decrease in synthesis in acute liver failure. (57)

3.7 Complications

The course taken by acute liver failure varies in each case as a result of the respective complications, which also decidedly worsen the prognosis. Close-meshed and targeted laboratory investigations can usually identify complications early enough, so that successful therapy might still be possible.

Coagulation disorders: Some 35—55% of patients with acute liver failure are in danger of suffering from serious gastrointestinal bleeding. Extensive cutaneous haemorrhages also occur frequently. In addition, disseminated intravascular coagulation (DIC) sometimes develops. As a result, bleeding and coagulation disorders number among the most frequent causes of death (20—25%). Pathophysiology is based on the diminished synthesis of coagulation and fibrinolysis factors and inhibitors as well as a decrease in the breakdown of activated factors, a functional disorder of thrombocytes or thrombopenia, and latent consumptive coagulopathy. It is of great help to determine PTT and factor V. A high level of the thrombin-antithrombin III complex (TAT) points to a poor prognosis. The simultaneous development of portal hypertension in individual cases promotes a tendency towards nasopharyngeal and gastrointestinal bleeding. (33, 47, 48) (s. p. 349)

Renal failure: In about 50% of patients with acute liver failure, renal insufficiency develops. This can be expressed in three forms: (*1.*) *prerenal kidney failure* due to hypovolaemia, (*2.*) *acute tubular necrosis*, mainly secondary as a result of circulatory hypotension with cylindruria, a higher concentration of sodium in the urine (50—70 mmol/l) and a reduced urine creatinine/serum creatinine quotient (<20) or urine urea/serum urea quotient (<3), or (*3.*) *hepatorenal syndrome*. (42) (s. tab. 17.3)

Respiratory insufficiency: In general, respiratory alkalosis (pCO_2 < 30 mm Hg, pH > 7.5) is initially present, triggered by intensified respiration and tachypnoea. Despite this hyperventilation, there is evidence of hypoxia, which is largely due to a disorder in oxygen diffusion. The causes for this are microthromboses, interstitial formation of oedema and increased peripheral vasotonia. Central biochemical mechanisms together with an inadequate cerebral blood circulation as a result of a reduction in pCO_2 reinforce the respiratory insufficiency. Approximately 80% of patients in coma stages III and IV require artificial respiration. A total collapse of the pulmonary function can be occasioned by pneumonia (ca. 50% of cases) as well as by a leakage of fluid and/or bleeding in the lung area.

Acid-base disorders: Initial metabolic alkalosis (resulting from decreased urea synthesis with reduced bicarbonate consumption) may be superimposed by respiratory alkalosis as an outcome of disorders in lung function. During the further course, metabolic acidosis (with renal insufficiency) and respiratory acidosis (with pulmonary insufficiency) can be expected. In advanced or severe stages of the disease, lactate acidosis may develop in some 50% of all comatose patients owing to restricted gluconeogenesis.

Circulatory disorders: In general, acute liver failure is initially accompanied by hyperdynamic circulation. During the further course, approximately 80% of patients develop hypotension, which above all results in a considerable reduction in hepatic, cerebral and renal perfusion. At the same time, peripheral vasodilation is usually evident. Bradycardia, generally resulting from cerebral oedema, worsens the cardiovascular conditions and is considered to be a poor prognostic sign. Ultimately, the patient does not respond to volume expansion and catecholamines.

Hypoglycaemia: In 25—40% of cases, hypoglycaemia develops and can all too easily be overlooked. The cause is seen to be a reduction in liver glycogen content, diminished glycogen synthesis and gluconeogenesis as well as hyperinsulinaemia due to reduced degradation of insulin in the liver. (21) It is often difficult to eliminate such hypoglycaemia, even with i.v. glucose infusions. • Furthermore, there is a danger of **hypokalaemia** and even **hypophosphataemia,** necessitating phosphate substitution with continuous monitoring of the serum values of phosphate and calcium (reactive hypocalcaemia is dangerous).

Pancreatitis: The frequency of hyperamylasaemia is reported to be 55% of patients with acute liver failure; in 20—30% of cases, pancreatitis could be identified clinically and sonographically. The cause is multifactorial.

Infections: Because of their greater susceptibility, about 80% of patients with acute liver failure are subject to the threat of bacterial infection, which in 10% of cases is also the reason for their death. The typical signs of an infection, such as fever or leucocytosis, are often absent. Increased levels of *procalcitonin* (>0.58 ng/ml) are deemed to be a valid marker of bacterial infection. The respiratory tract and the urinary passages are most frequently affected. Regular bacteriological examinations (sputum or urine as well as catheter after removal) should therefore be carried out. Haemocultures have to be checked for both aerobians and anaerobians. Multiple serological tests may be necessary for aetiological clarification. There is also a certain risk of fungal infections. (51)

3.8 Prognosis

The survival rate in acute liver failure is 10–40%. This rate varies widely owing to a number of reasons. There is a *better prognosis* for poisoning from paracetamol or Amanita phalloides, since successful therapy procedures are already established for these forms of intoxication. Younger patients (10 to 40 years) have a better prognosis. This also applies to HAV infection. A *poor outcome* can be expected in obesity, Wilson's disease or the Budd-Chiari syndrome as well as in coma stages III and IV (lethality over 80%) due to various complications (e.g. bleeding, renal or respiratory insufficiency, infection) – especially with younger (<10 years) or older patients (>40 years). Acute liver failure which is due to halothane, the application of various medicaments or viral hepatitis (delta superinfection, HEV in pregnancy) likewise has a less favourable prognosis. • *Laboratory parameters* such as serum bilirubin, higher AFP values (especially during the first three hospital days), coagulation factors, galactose test and cholinesterase have proved helpful in assessing the course of disease, liver function and prognosis. (14, 18, 22, 43, 46, 59, 62, 79)

3.9 Regeneration

The regenerative ability of the liver is of utmost importance for overcoming such a severe disease. (40) After a regeneration period, an intact cell mass (hepatic volume fraction) of >45% is required for survival. (41) Various factors are indicative of good regeneration: rising values of α_1-foetoprotein (and also γGT), HGF, EGF, THFα, TNFα and interleukin-6 as well as a decline in serum phosphorous levels. (14) It was possible to improve *regeneration* by means of hepatotropic substances, such as *insulin* and *glucagon*, so that these substances are also referred to as "goodies" for the liver (S. SHERLOCK, 1976). Subsequent investigations proved to be contradictory. (23, 81) An increase in the regeneration rate of the liver cells can possibly be achieved either by hepatic arterial infusion of PGE_1 (56) or by *silymarin* through stimulation of RNA synthesis. (s. pp 44, 896) (s. fig. 3.5)

4 Chronic liver insufficiency

4.1 Definition

Chronic liver insufficiency is due to the progression of an already existing chronic liver disease. This generally tends to be advanced cirrhosis of varied aetiology. Basically, however, any liver disease can be a potential cause of chronic liver insufficiency. Alcohol, infections and certain medicaments are also deemed to be common causes. Thus a great number of substances and events can trigger liver insufficiency.

The clinical picture of chronic liver insufficiency comprises both a **compensated** and **decompensated** form. These two stages of manifest chronic liver insufficiency affect the hepatocellular area or the portal system either exclusively or predominantly (= **cellular** or **portal** compensation or decompensation); mostly they occur as a *combined form* of disease. The resulting spectrum of clinical and laboratory findings will reflect either a **global** or **partial** insufficiency of the liver. (s. p. 380)

4.2 Clinical findings

General manifestations of the disease: The clinical picture of chronic liver insufficiency is characterized by a number of symptoms such as fatigue, apathy, lack of appetite, lack of concentration, infirmity, sensation of repletion and meteorism.

Clinical findings: Organ-related so-called "minor signs" of liver insufficiency can be observed over a certain period of time. (s. tab. 20.4)

1. **Gastrointestinal tract** – meteorism
2. **Dermis and mucosa** – itching – skin stigmata of liver disease – tendency to "bruise" – nasal haemorrhage and ulorrhagia – tongue changes
3. **Stools** – intermittent acholic stool
4. **Urine** – intermittent dark urine
5. **Changes in the blood count** – anaemia   – thrombopenia – leucopenia   – macrocytosis
6. **Fever**
7. **Splenomegaly**
8. **Endocrine disorders**

Tab. 20.4: So-called "minor signs" of chronic liver insufficiency

Constant *meteorism* ("*first the wind and then the rain*") and intermittent changes in the colour of *stools* and *urine* are distinct signs of impending insufficiency. The "blossoming" of *spider naevi*, an intensification of *palmar erythema* and *tongue changes* (e.g. transition of the moist "scarlet tongue" into a dry "raspberry tongue") are common. Obvious features of the blood count are: *anaemia* (due to bleeding of the skin or mucosa, folic acid deficiency, reduced erythrocyte survival time) and *thrombopenia* (due to consumptive coagulopathy, dilutional thrombopenia with plasma dilution, immuno-thrombopenia, sequestration in splenomegaly and toxic inhibition of the bone marrow).

4.3 Decompensation

Decompensation in chronic liver insufficiency is characterized by the development of severe, life-threatening **complications**:

1. Ascites and oedema
2. Coagulopathy and bleeding
3. Hepatic encephalopathy
4. Hepatorenal syndrome
5. Hepatopulmonary syndrome
6. Impairment of liver functions

4.3.1 Impairment of liver functions

Of particular significance is the serious impairment of essential tasks performed by the liver such as the **detoxification function** (ammonia detoxification, biotransformation, radical scavenger function, clearance abilities of the RES, etc.), the **synthesis** of vital proteins and the **regulation** of biochemical systems and substances — these are considered to be precursors of complicative developments. Any insufficiency of bilirubin metabolism is reflected in increasing **jaundice**, likewise deemed to be an unfavourable sign with respect to prognosis.

4.3.2 Hepatic encephalopathy

The term **hepatic encephalopathy** (HE) describes the entire field of neuropsychiatric symptoms which can be found in patients suffering from acute or chronic liver disease. The term **portosystemic encephalopathy** (PSE) stresses the presence of portosystemic shunts, which are as a rule associated with liver cirrhosis. • **Hepatic coma** (in stages III and IV) is the ultimate and total loss of consciousness (coma = deep, sound sleep). In clinical terms, four or five stages can be defined, but the latent or subclinical stage as well as stages I and II may progress so rapidly that only the comatose final stage is actually determined. Generally, chronic liver insufficiency is seen as a liver failure coma, i.e. exogenous coma. Recurrent hepatic encephalopathy points to the existence of a chronic liver disease, particularly liver cirrhosis. The serum levels of TNF correlate positively with the severity of HE. *(see chapter 15)*

4.3.3 Ascites and oedema

Ascites and *oedema* are also found in severe hepatic diseases, pointing to serious disorders in the water and electrolyte metabolism. These complications are signs of decompensation in liver cirrhosis or chronic liver insufficiency. *Pleural effusion* may also be evident. Cirrhosis-related pleural effusion without concomitant ascites has been described as a rarity. *(see chapter 16)*

4.3.4 Hepatorenal syndrome

All liver diseases resulting in liver insufficiency can also give rise to the hepatorenal syndrome. This syndrome is most frequently found in decompensated liver cirrhosis ("renal insufficiency in the terminal stage of cirrhosis"). It involves massive vasoconstriction of the renal cortical vessels with a critical drop in the glomerular filtration rate (urine production < 500 ml/day, possibly developing into anuresis). At the same time, systemic vasodilation and hyperdynamic cardiac function are generally in evidence. The survival time is very short. Lethality is approx. 95%. *(see chapter 17)*

4.3.5 Coagulopathy and haemorrhage

In 15—30% of patients with liver cirrhosis, coagulopathy leads to clinically relevant haemorrhagic diathesis. Dangerous and considerable *bleeding* may occur (nasal, gingival), and there may well be pronounced cutaneous haemorrhages; the latter occasionally occur as sugillations, ecchymoses and petechial haemorrhages (s. fig. 20.1) or as disseminated petechiae, especially around postoperative scars. (s. fig. 20.2) Gastrointestinal bleeding can be assigned to the upper gastrointestinal area in 80—85% and to the lower intestinal area in 15—20% of cases. *(see chapter 19)*

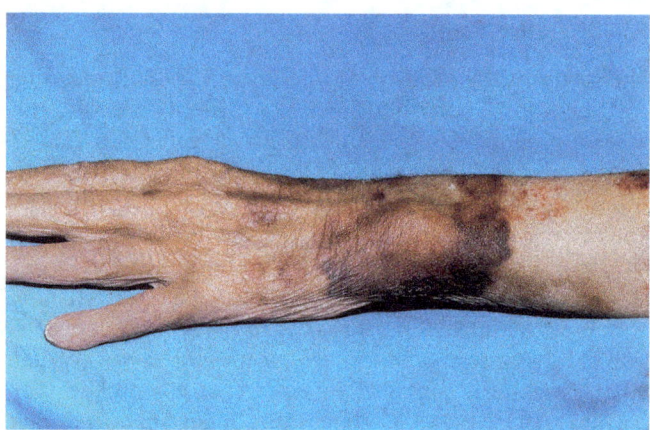

Fig. 20.1: Sugillations, ecchymoses and petechial haemorrhages in liver cirrhosis (with "paper money skin" and white nails) (s. figs. 4.8, 4.19)

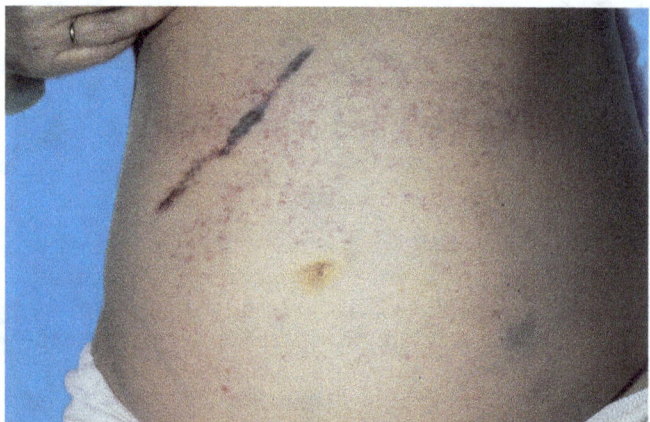

Fig. 20.2: Extensive purpura in the abdominal area with bleeding into the cholecystectomy scar

4.4 Acute-on-chronic liver insufficiency

This condition describes acute liver failure in cases of hitherto well-compensated liver disease. The result is a sudden deterioration in clinical status accompanied by jaundice as well as hepatic encephalopathy and/or the hepatorenal syndrome.

There are a number of *causes* including (*1.*) well-known hepatotoxic factors (e.g. superimposed viral infection, alcohol consumption, hepatotoxic drugs, intoxication) and (*2.*) endogenous factors (e.g. sepsis, variceal bleeding, gastrointestinal haemorrhage, diarrhoea, hypoxia). Acute liver failure is frequently the result of a chain of damaging events, like a vicious circle.

The clinical and laboratory *findings* of this sudden deterioration largely correspond to those of acute liver failure (see above). This also applies to potential *complications* such as coagulopathy, HE, ascites and/or HRS.

5 Therapy

Except for the treatment of, for example, paracetamol intoxication and Amanita phalloides poisoning, there is no causal therapy for liver insufficiency. All conservative treatment measures are based on **four principles:**

> 1. Prevention and treatment of complications
> 2. Substitution of substances which cannot be adequately produced in the liver as a result of hepatic synthesis disorders
> 3. Bridging the period of time until toxins have been eliminated, liver functions and regenerative processes have improved or liver transplantation can be carried out
> 4. Promotion of liver regeneration

▶ **Intensive care:** Patients with ALF or decompensated chronic liver insufficiency (e.g. coma stages II−IV, refractory ascites, hepatorenal syndrome, disseminated intravascular coagulation, gastrointestinal bleeding) require monitoring and treatment in an intensive care unit, preferably in a transplantation centre. (7, 13, 62, 79)

5.1 General therapeutic measures

Intensive care involves monitoring the *cardiovascular system* (blood pressure, pulse, ECG) and *respiratory frequency*. The patient's *temperature* and *urine excretion* have to be recorded every hour. The *body weight* is documented every day using a weighing bed. The water equilibrium should be carefully monitored. Consistent *preventive measures against infection* must be guaranteed for those patients who are particularly at risk. Regular physical measures for the *prevention of pneumonia* are a necessity. A moderate *head-up position* (30−40°) is recommended. • A *central venous catheter* (monitoring central venous pressure, parenteral feeding), a *nasogastral tube* and a *suprapubic bladder catheter* are positioned for supply and monitoring purposes. *Nasal oxygen supply* is advisable. The insertion of an epidural *intracranial pressure probe* is essential for early identification of cerebral oedema.

Feeding: Provided the patient does not have a paralytic ileus, *enteral feeding* via a nasogastral tube is advisable to prevent villous atrophy and thus reduce the risk of bacterial translocation. (s. p. 878) • **Parenteral feeding** (1,600−2,000 kcal/day) consists of a continuous intravenous supply of glucose and fat emulsions (MCT). Hypertriglyceridaemia may, in the case of lipid infusions, point to a lipid metabolism disorder, but it can also be due to increased glucose intake, which results in fatty degeneration of the hepatocytes and a corresponding reduction in liver function. Fructose, sorbitol and xylitol must be avoided! The supply of either liver-adapted amino acids or branched-chain amino acids is recommended for chronic liver insufficiency − but not advisable in cases of acute liver insufficiency, because almost all amino acids are elevated in the serum in endogenous hepatic coma. A high daily dosage of water-soluble vitamins (possibly divided into two doses) is important. Administration of zinc is recommended.

Electrolytes (Na, K, Ca, Mg) and **blood sugar** must be carefully monitored, and any deviation from the norm should be corrected immediately. The risk of **hypophosphataemia** must be eliminated by early parenteral substitution. During refractory episodes, such as those involving the acid-base equilibrium and **hyperhydration,** haemodialysis is usually indicated. In **hypoalbuminaemia,** substitution with salt-free albumin is necessary. • With about 75% of patients, **artificial respiration** is called for, the aim being controlled hyperventilation.

N-acetylcysteine is believed to promote the supply of oxygen to the tissues. (73) As a result, this substance, which is free from side effects, was also recommended for cases of CCl_4 intoxication (53) and is even considered helpful in acute liver failure with a different aetiology.

Prophylaxis: As a prophylaxis against bleeding in the upper gastrointestinal area, H_2 *antagonists* and omeprazole are recommended. • The timely and repeated administration of *fresh plasma* (FFB) as well as of antithrombin III has proved to be the most effective measure for balancing plasmatic coagulation disorders.

Bacterial infections are extremely common as a result of serious impairment of the cellular and humoral resistance (ca. 80%). Close-meshed bacteriological investigations are required in the frequent absence of clinical signs of infection. This leads to early antibiotic therapy based on an antibiotic sensitivity test. Although an antibiotic prophylaxis is not actually recommended, it should nevertheless be considered in the individual case, since the spreading of an infection has a decidedly negative impact on prognosis. • Administration of **selenite** (i.v.) may be advisable. Around 30% of patients develop a fungus infection, with a mortality rate of 50%. (s. p. 310) The administration of amphotericin B or fluconazol is an effective prophylactic measure. • Bacterial or fungal infection can also be effectively suppressed by *intestinal restimulating of the bacterial flora* or **intestinal sterilisation** by means of neomycin (or paromomycin), a combination of nystatin and gentamicin, or lactulose. (51, 54) (s. pp 285, 288, 310)

Essential phospholipids (EPL): In a pilot study, it was possible to achieve recompensation and lasting stabilization in nine out of ten patients suffering from severe liver insufficiency by i.v. administration of a new galenic form of polyenylphosphatidylcholine. (32) • This clinical result accords with other clinical studies and might be supported by the finding that a considerable deterioration in liver function was associated with a deficit of EPL. (15) (s. p. 894)

5.2 Specific therapeutic measures

Paracetamol intoxication: Liver damage due to paracetamol (>10 g) becomes manifest within ca. 48 hours after intake. (s. p. 382) For this reason, it is essential first of all to remove the non-absorbed fractions by *gastric lavage* and *intestinal cleansing*. As medicinal treatment, i.v. administration of the glutathione precursor *N-acetylcysteine* is the therapy of choice (L. F. Prescott et al., 1977). Dosage is 150 mg/kg BW with glucose as a rapid i.v. infusion (15—20 minutes), followed by 50 mg/kg BW over 4 hours and finally 100 mg/kg BW during the next 16 hours (= about 300 mg/kg BW within 20 hours). This therapy has to be commenced as soon as possible (no later than 12—15 hours after intoxication), even though a hepatoprotective effect can still be achieved up to 36 hours later. A serum concentration of <200 µg/ml within 4 hours or <60 µg/ml within 12 hours after intake can be considered prognostically favourable. (s. fig. 20.3)

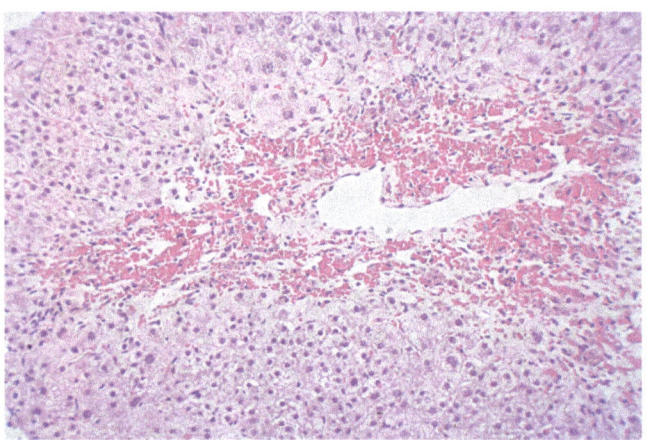

Fig. 20.3: Centrilobular, two-week-old liver cell necrosis resulting from paracetamol intoxication (HE)

Amanita phalloides poisoning: After a symptom-free latent period of about 12 hours, the gastroenteric phase sets in. (s. pp 382, 587) In this type of intoxication, it is imperative to carry out *gastric lavage* and *intestinal cleansing* as soon as possible with the help of saline agents using a nasogastral tube. The intestinal administration of medicinal charcoal is recommended. *Diuresis* must be enhanced by the administration of frusemide, if necessary with simultaneous volume substitution (CVP of about 10 cm H_2O). After another low-symptom period of about 1 day, the hepatorenal phase begins. The uptake of Amanita phalloides poison into the liver is inhibited by *penicillin* (1 mega unit/kg BW/day as i.v. solution over 3 days). The therapeutic efficacy of silymarin and *silibinin* was first detected in animal experiments in 1975 (G. Vogel et al.) and subsequently confirmed by further clinical studies. The recommended dose of silibinin is 30 (—50) mg/kg BW/day, administered in four separate doses in i.v. glucose infusions, each lasting two hours, over a period of three to four days. Penicillin and silibinin should be applied in combination. There is no specific antidote for Amanita toxins. Given timely and appropriate therapy, morbidity and mortality are surprisingly low. • In cases of therapy failure or a critical course of disease, liver transplantation may be indicated.

Cerebral oedema: *Mannitol* (0.5 g/kg BW or 100 ml, each as 20% solution) is used to treat the dreaded cerebral oedema. If renal function is sufficient, this course of therapy can be repeated every one to four hours, as required. Serum osmolality should not exceed 320 mosm/l, and intracranial pressure should not go above 20 mmHg. When renal function is restricted, dehydration must be effected by haemofiltration. *Artificial respiration* is required (often as PEEP ventilation). Continuous monitoring of the intracranial pressure using an epidural *intracerebral pressure probe* is extremely helpful. Frequently, there is increased susceptibility to cerebral convulsibility; therefore, phenytoin should be administered at an early stage. Therapeutic application of *thiopental* (A. Forbes et al., 1989) as i.v. solution (up to 150 mg/hour) calls for intracranial pressure probe monitoring. (22) Other means of lowering the intracerebral pressure include the use of aminophylline, ranitidine, luxus oxygenation and semirecumbent positioning. (8, 17, 34, 65) A prophylactic reduction in pCO_2 down to 25—35 mm Hg through **hyperventilation** can be advantageous in the initial stage of a brain oedema. (17, 65) Moderate **hypothermia** (core temperature down to 32—33 °C, for 10—12 hours) may be useful in reducing the intracerebral pressure and cerebral blood flow as well as the cerebral uptake of ammonia. (30)

Ornithine aspartate (40 g/8 hours as intravenous infusion) (52) and **flumazenil** are advisable for the treatment of hepatic precoma and coma.

Dopamine (2 to 4 µg/kg BW/hr) should be administered early on to stabilize the circulation and renal blood flow.

- **N-acetylcysteine** can be applied during oxygenation due to its positive effect on stabilizing the blood circulation and improving the serum coagulation factors. • **Indomethacine** reduces cerebral ammonia uptake.

Prostaglandin: The positive results achieved by the application of PGE_1 were reported in 1987 (M. ABACASSIS et al.). According to a subsequent prospective study, 71% of patients with fulminant and subfulminant hepatitis survived. (56, 63) The effect is attributed to improved arterial flow and regeneration of the liver (0.1 to 0.6 μg/kg BW/hr by means of perfusor for up to 18 hours, with the dosage gradually being phased out). • *Beware of hypotension!*

Glucocorticoids were first administered with some success in acute liver failure by H. DUCCI et al. in 1952. Good results were also achieved in the treatment of severe alcoholic hepatitis with liver insufficiency (R. A. HELMAN et al., 1971). The application of glucocorticoids in autoimmune hepatitis with acute liver failure did not prove successful. (44) • The first report containing good results after treating fulminant viral hepatitis B with **anti-HBs plasma** was published in 1971 (D. J. GOCKE). The treatment of fulminant hepatitis B with **interferon alpha** did not progress beyond initial attempts.

Lamivudine (100 mg/day) proved to be effective: it was possible to achieve a lasting improvement in liver function and to avoid liver transplantation. No side effects were observed.

In view of the loss of complex biochemical liver functions, drug intervention in the metabolic processes of the liver should be as varied as possible — even the use of therapeutic agents which are not clinically controlled may be biochemically or pharmacologically justified.

5.3 Liver support systems

The most important survival factor in acute liver failure is the **patient's age**. In the 15 to 25-year age group, 30−50% of patients survive, whereas those older than 30 years have hardly any chance of survival. It would appear that the good regenerative ability of the liver in young people is the best guarantee for survival. • An attempt must be made at **bridging the decompensatory phase** by means of optimum intensive care and monitoring of the cerebral pressure as well as by applying clinically proven or indeed new therapeutic procedures or medication until the liver has adequately regenerated or until liver transplantation can be carried out. • Basically, there are **three techniques** available for bridging the compensatory phase: (*1.*) extracorporeal systems (*2.*) biosynthetic artificial livers or hybrid organs, and (*3.*) transplantation of hepatocytes. (86, 87, 97, 98, 108)

5.3.1 Extracorporeal systems

1. **Exchange transfusion** (C. LEE et al., 1958): This method was used to fractionate and repeatedly exchange the entire circulatory blood of a patient. However, based on the results of subsequent studies, this procedure can no longer be recommended.

2. **Haemoperfusion:** The removal of both water-soluble and protein-bound substances from the plasma was first attempted by means of a haemoperfusion circuit, using a column filled with activated charcoal (D.C. SCHECHTER et al., 1958). Both the unwanted binding of corpuscular components and the danger of embolization from charcoal particles could largely be eliminated by coating the activated charcoal with a biocompatible membrane, i.e. microencapsulation (T.M.S. CHANG et al., 1964). Because of the greater aggregation of thrombocytes, however, thrombopenia often ensues. This event can generally be prevented by the administration of prostacyclin (C. A. E. GIMSON et al., 1980). Unfortunately, however, this procedure causes a loss of insulin and other hormones. (90)

3. **Cross-circulation:** *Homologous* cross-circulation with healthy volunteers was first attempted by J. M. BURNELL et al. in 1965. • Due to multiple problems, S. C. W. BOSMAN et al. introduced *heterologous* cross-circulation using a baboon in 1968; baboons are the only animal species which can tolerate human blood for five to seven days.

4. **Plasmapheresis:** This procedure is a further development of blood exchange (M. J. LEPORE et al., 1967). The patient's plasma is separated by centrifugation or other appropriate techniques and discarded, so that the protein-bound and fat-soluble toxins circulating in the plasma are removed. This plasma volume is replaced by fresh plasma. At the same time, the separated corpuscular components of the patient's blood are reinfused. Serious complications may arise from the transmission of viral hepatitis and the occurrence of transfusion-related lung disorders (ARDS). Nevertheless, the method involved is simple and has been carried out successfully in individual cases (89, 93, 104) even as plasma exchange with the administration of a high plasma volume (1.3 l/hr over 8 hours). • It has proved to be much more successful when the serum (ca. 3 l fresh frozen plasma/day) is infused into the femoral artery rather than into the vein.

5. **Plasma perfusion:** In 1974 patient plasma separated by plasmapheresis was for the first time passed through activated charcoal and artificial resin in order to absorb toxins. In this way, the patient's own purified plasma is reinfused together with the solid components of the blood. This procedure produces fewer side effects and is easy to carry out.

6. **Total body wash-out:** This technique is a modification of exchange transfusion. The circulatory system is washed out with electrolyte solutions and then refilled with donor blood whilst the patient is in a state of hypothermia (G. KLEBANOFF et al., 1972).

7. **Haemodialysis:** In 1968 temporary improvement could be achieved for the first time by means of haemodialysis in a patient presenting with fulminant hepatic failure (W. M. KEYNES). The procedure, however, is not generally recommended. It may be indicated in renal failure, acid-base disorders or with hyperhydration. Following haemodialysis, substitution of reduced amino acids is necessary.

8. **Haemofiltration:** This procedure turned out to be of more value than haemodialysis. No dialysate fluid is required. Instead, a solution containing buffered bicarbonate is used to replace the ultrafiltrate. In fulminant hepatic failure, continuous venovenous haemofiltration is recommended because of its advantages for the circulation and metabolism. Heparin or prostacyclin can be used as anticoagulants.

9. **Haemodiabsorption:** The BiologicDT system is a combination of haemodialysis and haemoadsorption (S. R. ASH et al. 1992). (84) Plasma separation was subsequently added to this system (S. R. ASH et al., 1998). (85) This newly developed BiologicDTPF facilitates direct plasma contact with the haemodiadsorber. The system, which makes use of both a charcoal and a cation exchanger, dialyzes blood across a parallel plate dialyzer with a cellulose mem-

brane. So far, results have been disappointing – only lactate, creatinine and bilirubin were reduced.

Albumin dialysis: The aim of albumin dialysis is to remove both soluble metabolites and albumin-bound substances (ABS) from the blood of patients with acute liver failure. (s. tab. 20.5)

benzodiazepines	fatty acids
bile acids	phenylalanin
bilirubin	several peptides
carbon hybrids	tryptophan
copper	*etc.*

Tab. 20.5: Albumin-bound substances (ABS) relevant in acute liver failure

SPAD: **S**ingle-**p**ass **a**lbumin **d**ialysis was the first method to be developed. The blood of the patient is extracporeally dialyzed through an albumin-impermeable membrane against albumin in the secondary circuit. The loaded albumin is discarded.

MARS: The SPAD method was further developed into a combination of dialysis, filtration and adsorption (= **m**olecular **a**dsorbent **r**ecycling **s**ystem). (105). The patient's blood is fed through a hollow-fibre filter and dialyzed against an albumin dialysate. The ABS (s. tab. 20.5) pass through the pores in the filter and become bonded. Plasma proteins, hormones and vitamins are not lost. The albumin dialysate is recirculated in a closed circuit where it is fed through a second dialyzer and two adsorber columns which bind the ABS. The albumin dialysate is returned to the hollow-fibre filter. It is dialyzed against a bicarbonate solution in order to remove the excess water and water-soluble substances (ammonia, creatinine, urea, iron, copper) as well as to stabilize the electrolyte and glucose levels and the pH value. The results obtained to date are promising. (95, 103, 106) (s. fig. 20.4)

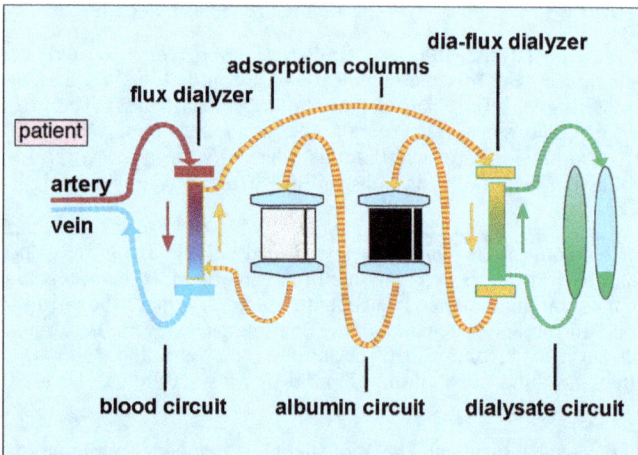

Fig. 20.4: Diagram showing the molecular adsorbent recirculating system (MARS)

FPSA: Fractioned **p**lasma **s**eparation and **a**dsorption is a very efficient and multifactorial method, employing membranes and adsorbants. (88) It is additionally characterized by the use of microparticles (2.0–3.5 μm), which are recirculated in suspension using high-speed flow (2–4 l/min) to optimize the in-line filtration process. In a further development, a special sulfone filter is applied.

Prometheus: In the meantime, the Prometheus method has been introduced. (99) Here, the plasma is separated out by an albumin-permeable filter and cleaned in a secondary circuit via an adsorber together with conventional high-flux haemodialysis. Direct contact between the albumin plasma and the adsorber helps to increase the efficiency of this method.

These liver support methods serve to detoxify the organism for a limited period of time. They are regarded as **supportive measures** in intensive care. Survival time has often been prolonged, yet only in isolated cases has the overall life-span of the patient been extended. These methods of treatment, which are costly and involve considerable resources, can only be carried out in medical units that are equipped with all the facilities of intensive care and thus in a position to effect epidural brain pressure measurement, blood purifying processes and liver perfusion methods. • Only young patients between the ages of 15 and 25 have a real chance of survival (40 to 50%), provided they receive optimum intensive care. With patients over 30 years, supportive techniques should only be applied to bridge the time period until a liver transplantation can be carried out.

However, **conservative treatment** may be attempted for four or five days under the following conditions irrespective of *age*: (*1.*) there is a chance of regeneration during this period that can be made use of; (*2.*) this period of time does not preclude the patient's chances of liver transplantation (which calls for two to four days' preparation time); (*3.*) should there be no signs of recovery or regeneration, not even in younger patients (<30 years), transplantation is nevertheless indicated. • After four or five days, however, severe *complications* develop, also in younger patients, which render transplantation difficult or even impossible. Especially older patients (>30 years) should undergo liver transplantation without delay.

5.3.2 Bioartificial systems

Temporary substitution of the liver function using hepatocytes (e.g. in haemofiltration systems or bioreactors) is conceivable in acute liver failure, possibly in conjunction with activated charcoal filtration or with plasma separation. The importance lies in bridging the phase of acute liver failure until compensation of the liver function or liver regeneration is achieved.

The bioreactor is filled with capillaries in which the patient's blood circulates; some of this blood has already been oxygenated extracorporeally. The efficacy of the system depends on an efficient exchange of the corresponding substances in both directions as well as stable hepatocyte functions. It is possible to use human (allogeneic) or animal (xenogeneic) hepatocytes as well as cell cultures (immortalized cells or tumour cell lines). If human cells are taken, 10^{10} hepatocytes per patient are required — as would be needed for a conventional liver transplant. Regarding the use of animal hepatocytes, there is a possible risk in that no solution has yet been found to the question of zoonosis transmission and there may be an immune reaction to foreign antigens. Bile flow also remains a problem. (92, 100, 101, 109, 110)

1. **Vital hepatocytes:** The so-called "artificial liver" system was developed by K. N. MATSUMURA et al. (1978). The procedure comprised haemodialysis across a suspension of vital hepatocytes. A semi-artificial liver was first used clinically in 1987 on a patient with bile-duct carcinoma and acute liver failure (K. N. MATSUMURA et al.).

2. **Liver enzymes:** The binding of microsomal liver enzymes to synthetic carriers is a promising method of temporarily compensating important liver functions (G. BRUNNER, 1981).

3. **Bioartificial liver (BAL):** Freshly isolated hepatocytes of pigs, immobilized on collagen-coated microcarriers, remained vital in-vivo and in-vitro over a longer period in a perfusion system; they were able to conjugate bilirubin and synthesize proteins. These results provided the basis for developing an extracorporeal bioartificial liver (A. A. DEMETRIOU et al., 1986). In more advanced systems, plasma was perfused through an activated charcoal column and a fibre system with cultured pig liver cells. (92, 97, 100, 110) • Using a BAL, the plasma is separated by centrifugation and directed into a reservoir in order to increase both the plasma and metabolite flow. By integrating an activated charcoal column, it is possible to effect a greater elimination of toxins. The separated plasma reaches the hollow-fibre bioreactor, where it is perfused through the previously inserted hepatocytes (7 ± 1 hours). • Such a system yielded increased production of coagulation factors in a patient with alcohol cirrhosis (D. F. NEUZIL et al., 1993). (s. fig. 20.5)

4. **Extracorporeal liver assistance device (ELAD):** Attention has recently focused on temporarily replacing the liver function with hepatocytes which have been cultured in the extracapillary space of a cellulose-acetate hollow-fibre unit. Each unit contains ca. 200 g C3A cells, an amount which is necessary for successful perfusion. ELAD has proved efficacious in clinical use. (108)

5. **BLSS:** The **b**ioartificial **l**iver **s**upport **s**ystem is made up of a blood pump, a heat exchanger to control the blood temperature, as well as an oxygenator and a bioreactor. The hollow-fibre bioreactor generally contains 70—100 g of porcine liver cells. Initial experience with BLSS is encouraging. (94)

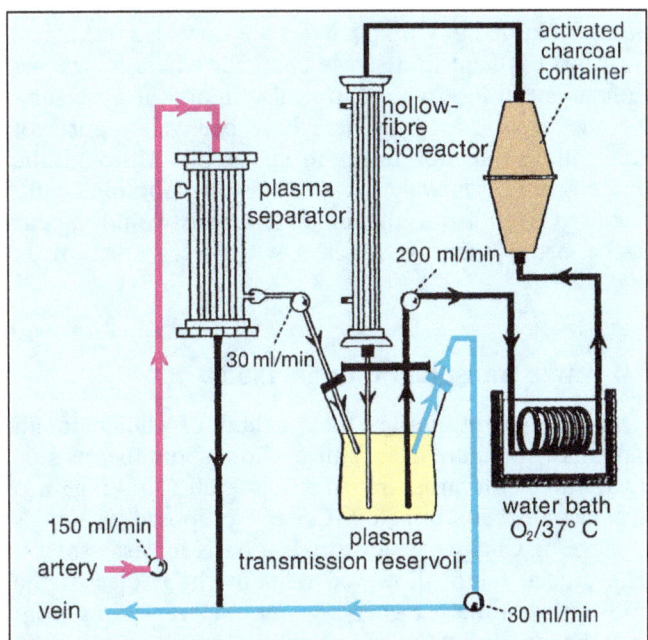

Fig. 20.5: Diagram showing a bioartifical liver (BAL) (98)

6. **BELS:** The **B**erlin **e**xtracorporeal **l**iver **s**upport system consists of a three-dimensional accumulation of approx. 500 g pig liver cells. These cells are linked by means of capillaries and provided with oxygen independently of the patient's blood, so that they function and stay vital for several weeks. (91)

MELS: The **m**odular **e**xtracorporeal **l**iver **s**upport system was developed from BELS. In contrast to BELS, however, it consists of three modules: (*1.*) a cell module with human hepatocytes, (*2.*) single-pass albumin dialysis, and (*3.*) a dialysis module for constant venovenous haemofiltration. (102)

The clinical significance of bioartificial systems largely depends upon whether it is possible (*1.*) to keep functional hepatocytes alive in extracorporeal systems for an adequate period of time and (*2.*) to make such systems available at short notice for use in emergencies.

5.3.3 Extracorporeal liver perfusion

The idea of extracorporeal liver perfusion (ECLP) for removing toxins by way of perfusion using an animal liver goes back to ANDREWS (1953), who used this technique for liver substitution in dogs. In 1958 J. J. OTTO et al. applied this method and demonstrated a clear reduction in pathologically elevated serum ammonia values in the dog. • In 1965 B. EISEMAN et al. first treated hepatic coma in humans by perfusion using a pig liver. • The use of baboon livers yielded further progress (S. SAUNDERS et al., 1968; T. S. LIE et al., 1976). Treatment was reported to be effective in isolated cases. This procedure has been successfully taken up again, using human livers which, for medical or organizational reasons, could not be transplanted. • Vital pig livers are now also used. The fresh liver is kept in a sterile chamber where it receives the patient's blood via the portal vein and, if necessary, via the hepatic artery. There have been no reports of xenogenous infection or rejection. (86, 107) Although the procedure is relatively safe, the results obtained with perfused livers from humans or baboons would appear to be better than is the case with livers taken from pigs. (96)

5.4 Liver transplantation methods

Liver transplantation is the method of choice in all patients with acute liver failure whose spontaneous survival rate without a transplant is <20%, taking into account all the parameters. Criteria proposed by King's College or Clichy provide a useful basis for assessment. The crucial factor, however, remains the choice of the appropriate time for carrying out the transplantation: (*1.*) the possibility of eliminating decompensation by means of regeneration should be exploited; (*2.*) delayed indications should not result in complications which would prevent a transplantation from being carried out (e. g. brain-stem herniation, sepsis). *(see chapter 40.7)*

5.4.1 Orthotopic transplantation

▶ The **survival rate** following orthotopic transplantation in acute liver failure is 50 to 80% after one year and about 60% after five years. When the **indication** for transplantation is given, it is impossible to foresee to what extent the patient's life might be lengthened. The decision as to whether and when a transplantation is indicated continues to be arbitrary. The question of which patients will benefit most from transplantation is still unresolved – particularly since liver diseases are, in general, potentially reversible. However, acute liver failure due to Wilson's disease or the Budd-Chiari syndrome is an indication for liver transplantation, because these conditions are always lethal otherwise. Of all liver transplantations in Europe, a constant 10–12% are carried out due to ALF. In patients under the age of 45, this figure is 20%. Meanwhile, OLT has already been carried out on four adolescents for Ecstasy-induced liver failure. • With an isoelectric line in the electroencephalograph and with irreversible cerebral oedema, transplantation is no longer possible. The prognosis is likewise poor for decompensated liver insufficiency as a result of "acute-on-chronic failure" (e. g. acute virus infection or intoxication in cirrhosis), even after conservative and invasive intensive care therapy or indeed after liver transplantation. (20, 45, 111–114, 122, 123, 126, 127) *(see chapter 40.7)*

Ultima ratio transplantation: The following *criteria* are indicators in those cases where the probability of survival without transplantation would be <20% (T. E. STARZL et al., 1989):

1. Foudroyant deterioration of the general state of health
2. Severe coagulation disorders
3. Coma stages III to IV
4. Metabolic acidosis
5. Liver atrophy
6. Circulatory insufficiency requiring catecholamines
7. Manifestation of septic multiple organ failure

SLT: Split **l**iver **t**ransplantation was developed as an alternative to OLT (121). The transplanted split should be around 1% of the body weight of the recipient. SLT has a higher complication rate than OLT.

LDLT: With regard to **l**iving **d**onor **l**iver **t**ransplantation, SLT has become particularly important in cases where no cadaver organ is readily available. Living donor liver transplantation was first carried out on children. The left lateral segment, usually segments II and III, of the donor's liver is used. Around 5% of OLT candidates are also suitable for LDLT. More than 2,500 living donor liver transplantations have been carried out worldwide. The donor mortality rate is 0.2–0.3%. (118, 119, 125)

5.4.2 Auxiliary partial orthotopic liver transplantation

In 1991 auxiliary partial orthotopic liver transplantation (APOLT) was successfully carried out for the first time in acute liver failure, with the subsequent possibility of dispensing with the transplant after regeneration of the patient's own liver. (115) The corresponding part of a donor liver is transplanted orthotopically as left lateral segments II and III into the acutely diseased liver. The requisite partial resection of the liver is considered difficult. (124) A European multicentre study (12 centres) achieved equally good results in 30 patients compared to orthotopic liver transplantation with the removal of the native liver (M.-P. CHENARD-NEU et al., 1996). APOLT is intended as a temporary measure in acute liver failure with the aim of discontinuing immunosuppressive therapy after the patient's own liver has regenerated. So far, results imply that more complications are experienced in APOLT than in OLT.

5.4.3 Heterotopic transplantation

The concept of heterotopic transplantation of a complete or even partial ("spliced") donor liver should also be pursued further. Heterotopic transplantation involves placing an auxilliary (additional) organ in the right upper abdomen (O. T. TERPSTRA et al., 1988). In surgical terms, this technique is considered to be demanding due to the application of the piggy-back method (= anastomosis of the donor liver with the appropriately prepared ostium of the hepatic veins to the infrahepatic caval vein, generally cranial to the opening of the renal vein). • These two methods (APOLT and auxiliary heterotopic liver transplantation) are particularly suitable for juveniles with acute liver failure because they bridge the critical time span preceding the regeneration of the diseased liver. Immunosuppression is thus only required for a restricted period of time. The transplant shrinks or is surgically removed. Acute liver failure induced by Ecstasy was successfully overcome using this technique. (116) It allows the liver function to be compensated and gives the diseased liver time to regenerate. (120)

5.4.4 Xenotransplantation

Pigs with human immune system genes are expected to facilitate the production of transgenic donor organs (D. WHITE, 1992). This is the basis of all endeavours to use transgenic pig liver for the purpose of xenotransplantation (J. PLATT, 1993). In the future, genetic engineering should make it possible to eliminate the immunobiological risk of complement-activated, hyperacute rejection. However, the problem regarding the transmission of zoonoses has not yet been resolved. To date, a survival period of 70 days has been achieved with three xenotransplants in ALF and chronic liver insufficiency (J. FUNG et al., 1997).

5.5 Transplantation of hepatocytes

Liver cells were successfully transplanted for the first time in experiments on rats (A.J. MATAS et al., 1976). The requirements for transplantation include absolute care in the production of an adequate quantity of **vital liver cells** of utmost purity as well as the possibility of cryopreservation and in-vitro culturing. The cells are injected locally into the implantation area or infused selectively into the organ through a vascular catheter. Special adhesive-supporting substances can be used in this process (agarose gel, micro-encapsulation into thin membranes, etc.). (128–134)

Among the experimentally tested **transplantation sites** are the spleen, kidneys, lungs, pancreas, peritoneum, greater omentum and fatty tissue. Up to now, the spleen has proved to be the most suitable site. The transplantation of foetal liver cells into the spleen may even culminate in a liver lobule-like formation with bile ducts and veins – however, the functional results have (so far) been no better than with normal hepatocytes.

The question of the required **number of hepatocytes** has still not been resolved: the collapse of a certain liver function (e.g. normalization of factor VIII values in serum) can be compensated by a far lower number of hepatocytes than is the case with total liver failure (e.g. acute liver failure). Calculations made up to now have claimed that there are at least 10^7–10^8 liver cells in partially resected liver parenchyma.

Indications for the transplantation of hepatocytes predominantly involve those liver diseases in which functional failures occur in the liver cells (not in the bile ducts). • Permanent transplantation would be indicated, for example, in order to eliminate *congenital metabolic disorders* of the liver cells. In this case, it is possible to use hepatocytes from the patient, with subsequent elimination of the defect by gene technology, as well as hepatocytes from healthy donors. A therapeutic effect lasting for over one year was achieved for the first time in a girl suffering from the Crigler-Najjar syndrome (I.J. FOX et al., 1998). • Human hepatocytes are most definitely more suitable than animal liver cells. The latter may well meet the requirements for a provisional substitute, but not for permanent transplantation.

Future prospects

▶ Looking into the future, it can be expected that the next few years will witness advances in gene technology (e.g. transgenic animal liver) and molecular biology (e.g. targeted blockade of the immune system against the liver transplant) or even produce new concepts of liver and hepatocyte transplantation.

▶ It is no longer too bold to pin legitimate hopes on the development of an artificial liver. The preliminary objective hereby must be to replace the most important liver functions for a longer period of time, thus affording the diseased liver of the patient a greater chance to regenerate.

References:

1. Aita, K., Jin, Y., Iris, H., Takahashi, I., Kobori, K., Nakasato, Y., Kodama, H., Yanagawa, Y., Yoshikawa, T., Shiga, J.: Are there histopathologic characteristics particular to fulminant hepatic failure caused by human herpesvirus-6 infection? A case report and discussion. Human Pathol. 2001; 32: 887–889
2. Akhtar, A.J.: Conjunctival edema. A marker of increased mortality in patients with advanced hepatic encephalopathy and hepatocellular failure. Dig. Dis. Sci. 2002; 47: 373–375
3. Alberti-Flor, J.J., Hernandez, M.E., Ferrer, J.P., Howell, S., Jeffers, L.: Fulminant liver failure and pancreatitis associated with the use of sulfamethoxazole-trimethoprim. Amer. J. Gastroenterol. 1989; 84: 1577–1579
4. Anderson, S.H.C., Richardson, P., Wendon, J., Pagliuca, A., Portmann, B.: Acute liver failure as the initial manifestation of acute leukaemia. Liver 2001; 21: 287–292
5. Ando, Y., Saito, A., Moriya, M., Okada, Y., Kawase, C., Hisamitsu, T., Obata, H.: Two cases of fulminant hepatic failure in malignant lymphoma. Acta Hepatol. Japon. 1993; 34: 819–824
6. Arora, N.K., Nanda, S.K., Gulati, S., Ansari, I.H., Chawla, M.K., Gupta, S.D., Panda, S.K.: Acute viral hepatitis types E, A, and B singly and in combination in acute liver failure in children in North India. J. Med. Virol. 1996, 48: 215–221
7. Bernal, W., Wendon, J.: Acute liver failure; clinical features and management. Eur. J. Gastroenterol. Hepatol. 1999; 11: 977–984
8. Blei, A.T.: Medical therapy of brain edema in fulminant hepatic failure. Hepatology 2000; 32: 666–669
9. Blei, A.T.: Pathophysiology of brain edema in fulminant hepatic failure, revisited. Metab. Brain Dis. 2001; 16: 85–94
10. Bosman, D.K., Deutz, N.E.P., de Graaf, A.A., van den Hulst, R.W.N., van Eijk, H.M.H., Bovée, W.M.M.J., Maas, M.A.W., Jörning, G.G.A., Chamuleau, R.A.F.M.: Changes in brain metabolism during hyperammonemia and acute liver failure: results of a comparative 1H-NMR spectroscopy and biochemical investigation. Hepatology 1990; 12: 281–290
11. Burkolter, D., Schär, B.: Acute liver failure with a history of morbid obesity. Schweiz. Med. Wschr. 2000; 130: 924–927
12. Canbay, A., Chen, S.Y., Gieseler, R.K., Malago, M., Karliova, M., Gerken, G., Broelsch, C.E., Treichel, U.: Overweight patients are more susceptible for acute liver failure. Hepato-Gastroenterol. 2005; 52: 1516–1520

13. **Capocaccia, L., Angelico, M.:** Fulminant hepatic failure. Clinical features, etiology, epidemiology, and current management. Dig. Dis. Sci. 1991; 36: 775–779
14. **Chung, P.Y., Sitrin, M.D., Te, H.S.:** Serum phosphorus levels predict clinical outcome in fulminant hepatic failure. Liver Transplant. 2003; 8: 248–253
15. **Clemmnesen, J.O., Hoy, C.E., Jeppesen, P.B., Ott, P.:** Plasma phospholipids fatty acid pattern in severe liver disease. J. Hepatol. 2000; 32: 481–487
16. **Dourakis, S.P., Tzemanakis, E., Deutsch, M., Kafiri, G., Hadziyannis, S.J.:** Fulminant hepatic failure as a presenting paraneoplastic manifestation of Hodgkin's disease. Eur. J. Gastroenterol. Hepatol. 1999; 11: 1055–1058
17. **Ede, R.J., Gimson, A.E., Bihari, D., Williams, R.:** Controlled hyperventilation in the prevention of cerebral oedema in fulminant hepatic failure. J. Hepatol. 1986; 2: 43–51
18. **Eisenhuber, E., Madl, C., Kramer, L., Steininger, R., Yeganehfar, W., Ratheiser, K., Gangl, A.:** Prognostic indicators in acute liver failure. Wien. Klin. Wschr. 1998; 110: 564–569
19. **Fang, J.W.S., Lau, J.Y.N., Wu, P.C., Lai, C.L.:** Fulminant hepatic failure in nonmetastatic renal cell carcinoma. Dig. Dis. Sci. 1992; 37: 474–477
20. **Feranchak, A.P., Tyson, R.W., Narkewicz, M.R., Karrer, F.M., Sokol, R.J.:** Fulminant Epstein-Barr viral hepatitis: orthotopic liver transplantation and review of the literature. Liver Transpl. Surg. 1998; 4: 469–476
21. **Fiaccadori, F., Pedretti, G., Ferrari, C., Pizzaferri, P., Riggio, O., Orlandi, N., Pezzarossa, A.:** Insulin and glucagon levels in fulminant hepatic failure in man. Dig. Dis. Sci. 1991; 36: 801–808
22. **Frohburg, E., Stölzel, U., Lenz, K., Schäfer, J.-H., Tung, L.G., Riecken, E.-O.:** Prognostic indicators in fulminant hepatic failure. Z. Gastroenterol. 1992; 30: 571–575
23. **Fujiwara, K., Ogata, I., Sato, Y., Tomiya, T., Ohta, Y., Oka, Y., Nagoshi, S., Yamada, S., Masaki, N., Takatsuki, K., Hayashi, S., Oka, H.:** Insulin and Glucagon therapy of acute hepatic failure. Dig. Dis. Sci. 1991; 36: 809–815
24. **Godwin, J.E., Coleman, A.A., Sahn, St.A.:** Miliary tuberculosis presenting as hepatic and renal failure. Chest 1991; 99: 752–754
25. **Harrison, R., Letz, G., Pasternak, G., Blanc, P.:** Fulminant hepatic failure after occupational exposure to 2-nitropropane. Ann. Intern. Med. 1987; 107: 466–468
26. **Hruby, K., Csomos, G., Fuhrmann, M., Thaler, H.:** Chemotherapy of Amanita phalloides poisoning with intravenous silibinin. Hum. Toxicol. 1983; 2: 183–195
27. **Hughes, R.D., Evans, L.W.:** Activin A and follistatin in acute liver failure. Eur. J. Gastroenterol. Hepatol. 2003; 15: 127–131
28. **Hussain, M., Mutimer, D., Harrison, R., Hubscher, S., Neuberger, J.:** Fulminant hepatic failure caused by tuberculosis. Gut 1995; 36: 792–794
29. **Jake Liang, T., Jeffers, L., Reddy, R.K., Silva, M.O., Cheinquer, H., Findor, A., de Medina, M., Yarbough, P.O., Reyes, G.R., Schiff, E.R.:** Fulminant or subfulminant non-A, non-B viral hepatitis: the role of hepatitis C and E viruses. Gastroenterology 1993; 104: 556–562
30. **Jalan, R., Olde Damink, S.W.M., Deutz, N.E.P., Hayes, P.C., Lee, A.:** Moderate hypothermia in patients with acute liver failure and uncontrolled intracranial hypertension. Gastroenterology 2004; 127: 1338–1346
31. **Köklü, S., Ödemis, B., Cengiz, C., Yüksel, O., Üscüdar, O., Turhan, N.:** Fulminant hepatic failure due to secondary amyloidosis. Dig. Liver Dis. 2006; 38: 208–216
32. **Kuntz, E.:** Pilot study with polyenylphosphatidylcholine in severe liver insufficiency. Med. Welt 1989; 40: 1327–1329
33. **Langley, P.G., Hughes, R.D., Forbes, A., Keays, R., Williams, R.:** Controlled trial of antithrombin III supplementation in fulminant hepatic failure. J. Hepatol. 1993; 17: 326–331
34. **Lidofsky, S.D., Bass, N.M., Prager, M.C., Washington, D.E., Read, A.E., Wright, T.L., Ascher, N.L., Roberts, J.P., Scharschmidt, B.F., Lake, J.R.:** Intracranial pressure monitoring and liver transplantation for fulminant hepatic failure. Hepatology 1992; 16: 1–7
35. **Lin, S.D., Kawakami, T., Ushio, A., Sato, A., Sato, S., Iwai, M., Endo, R., Takikawa, Y., Suzuki, K.:** Ratio of circulating follistatin and activin A reflects the severity of acute liver injury and prognosis in patients with acute liver failure. J. Gastroenterol. Hepatol. 2006; 21: 374–380
36. **Lucké, B., Mallory, T.:** The fulminant form of epidemic hepatitis. Amer. J. Pathol. 1946; 22: 867–945
37. **Mas, M.R., Simsek, I., Can, C., Ateskan, U., Erdem, H., Kocabalkan, F.:** Fulminant hepatic failure as the initial manifestation of primary hepatocellular carcinoma. Eur. J. Gastroenterol. Hepatol. 2000; 12: 575–578
38. **Masada, C.T., Shaw, B.W.jr., Zetterman, R.K., Kaufman, S.S., Markin, R.S.:** Fulminant hepatic failure with massive necrosis as a result of hepatitis A infection. J. Clin. Gastroenterol. 1993; 17: 158–162
39. **McClung, H.J., Sloan, H.R., Powers, P., Merola, A.J., Murray, R., Kerzner, B., Pollack, J.D.:** Early changes in the permeability of the blood-brain barrier produced by toxins associated with liver failure. Pediatr. Res. 1990; 28: 227–231
40. **Meyer, R.A., Duffy, M.C.:** Spontaneous reactivation of chronic hepatitis B infection leading to fulminant hepatic failure. Report of two cases and review of the literature. J. Clin. Gastroenterol. 1993; 17: 231–234
41. **Minuk, G.Y.:** Hepatic regeneration in fulminant hepatic failure. Can. J. Gastroenterol. 1993; 7: 545–546
42. **Moore, K.:** Renal failure in acute liver failure. Eur. J. Gastroenterol. Hepatol. 1999; 11: 967–975
43. **Nagel, R.A., Hayllar, K.M., Tredger, J.M., Williams, R.:** Caffeine clearance and galactose elimination capacity as prognostic indicators in fulminant hepatic failure. Eur. J. Gastroenterol. Hepatol. 1991; 3: 907–913
44. **Nakadate, I., Nakamura, A., Endo, R., Iwai, M., Kaneta, H., Shimotono, H., Sasaki, S., Takikawa, Y., Yamazaki, K., Madarame, T., Kashiwabara, T., Suzuki, K., Sato, S.:** Autoimmune hepatitis presenting with acute hepatic failure. Acta Hepatol. Japon. 1993; 34: 665–671
45. **Ockner, S.A., Brunt, E.M., Cohn, S.M., Krul, E.S., Hanto, D.W., Peters, M.G.:** Fulminant hepatic failure caused by acute fatty liver of pregnancy treated by orthotopic liver transplantation. Hepatology 1990; 11: 59–64
46. **Pereira, L.M.M.B., Langley, P.G., Hayllar, K.M., Tredger, J.M., Williams, R.:** Coagulation factor V and VIII/V ratio as predictors of outcome in paracetamol induced fulminant hepatic failure: relation to other prognostic indicators. Gut 1992; 33: 98–102
47. **Pereira, S.P., Langley, P.G., Williams, R.:** The management of abnormalities of hemostasis in acute liver failure. Semin. Liver Dis. 1996; 16: 403–414
48. **Pernambuco, J.R.B., Langley, P.G., Hughes, R.D., Izumi, S., Williams, R.:** Activation of the fibrinolytic system in patients with fulminant liver failure. Hepatology 1993; 18: 1350–1356
49. **Rabe, C., Scheurlen, C., Caselmann, W.H.:** Vorgehen bei Knollenblätterpilzvergiftung. Dtsch. Med. Wschr. 1999; 124: 1073–1076
50. **Ramirez, P., Parrilla, P., Sanchez Bueno, F., Robles, R., Antonio Pons, J., Bixquert, V., Nicolas, S., Nunez, R., Soledad Alegria, M., Miras, M., Manuel Rodriguez, J.:** Fulminant hepatic failure after Lepiota mushroom poisoning. J. Hepatol. 1993; 19: 51–54
51. **Rolando, N., Philpott-Howard, J., Williams, R.:** Bacterial and fungal infection in acute liver failure. Semin. Liver Dis. 1996; 16: 389–402
52. **Rose, C., Michalak, A., Rao, K.V., Quack, G., Kircheis, G., Butterworth, R.F.:** L-ornithine-L-aspartate lowers plasma and cerebrospinal fluid ammonia and prevents brain edema in rats with acute liver failure. Hepatology 1999; 30: 636–640
53. **Ruprah, M., Mant, T.G.K., Flanagan, R.J.:** Acute carbon tetrachloride poisoning in 19 patients: implications for diagnosis and treatment. Lancet 1985/I: 1027–1029
54. **Salmeron, J.M., Tito, L., Rimola, A., Mas, A., Navasa, M.A., Llach, J., Gines, A., Gines, P., Arroyo, V., Rodes, J.:** Selective intestinal decontamination in the prevention of bacterial infection in patients with acute liver failure. J. Hepatol. 1992; 14: 280–285
55. **Salo, J., Nomdedeu, B., Bruguera, M., Ordi, J., Gines, P., Castells, A., Vilella, A., Rodes, J.:** Acute liver failure due to non-Hodgkin's lymphoma. Amer. J. Gastroenterol. 1993; 88: 774–776
56. **Sato, T., Asanuma, Y., Hashimoto, M., Heianna, J., Kusano, T., Kurokawa, T., Yasui, O., Koyama, K.:** Efficacy of hepatic arterial infusion of prostaglandin E1 in the treatment of postoperative acute liver failure. – Report of a case. Hepato-Gastroenterol. 2000; 47: 846–850
57. **Schiodt, F.V., Rossaro, L., Stravitz, R.T., Shakil, A.O., Chung, R.T., Lee, W.M.:** Gc-globulin and prognosis in acute liver failure. Liver transplantation 2005; 11: 1223–1227
58. **Schneeweiss, B., Pammer, J., Ratheiser, K., Schneider, B., Madl, C., Kramer, L., Kranz, A., Ferenci, P., Druml, W., Grimm, G., Lenz, K., Gangl, A.:** Energy metabolism in acute hepatic failure. Gastroenterology 1993; 105: 1515–1521
59. **Sekiyama, K., Yoshiba, M., Inoue, K., Sugata, F.:** Prognostic value of hepatic volumetry in fulminant hepatic failure. Dig. Dis. Sci. 1994; 39: 240–244
60. **Sen, S., Williams, R., Jalan, R.:** The pathophysiological basis of acute-on-chronic liver failure. Liver 2002; 22 (Suppl. 2): 5–13
61. **Shafritz, D.A.:** Variants of hepatitis B virus associated with fulminant liver disease. New Engl. J. Med. 1991; 324: 1737–1738
62. **Shakil, A.O., Kramer, D., Mazariegos, G.V., Fung, J.J., Rakela, J.:** Acute liver failure: clinical features, outcome analysis, and applicability of prognostic criteria. Liver Transplant. 2000; 6: 163–169
63. **Sterling, R.K., Luketic, V.A., Sanyal, A.J., Shiffman, M.L.:** Treatment of fulminant hepatic failure with intravenous prostaglandin E1. Liver Transpl. Surg. 1998; 4: 424–431
64. **Stolze-Larsen, F., Wendon, J.:** Brain edema in liver failure: basic physiologic principles and management. Liver Transplant. 2002; 8: 983–989
65. **Strauss, G.I., Hansen, B.A., Knudsen, G.M., Stolze-Larsen, F.:** Hyperventilation restores cerebral blood flow autoregulation in patients with acute liver failure. J. Hepatol. 1998; 28: 199–203
66. **Strauss, G.I., Knudsen, G.M., Kondrup, J., Moller, K., Stolze-Larsen, F.:** Cerebral metabolism of ammonia and amino acids in patients with fulminant hepatic failure. Gastroenterology 2001; 121: 1109–1119
67. **Takano, S., Omata, M., Ohto, M., Satomura, Y.:** Prospective assessment of incidence of fulminant hepatitis in post-transfusion hepatitis: a study of 504 cases. Dig. Dis. Sci. 1994; 39: 28–32
68. **Taylor, R.M., Davern, T., Munoz, S., Han, S.H., McGuire, B., Larson, A.M., Hynan, L., Lee, W.M., Fontana, R.J.:** Fulminant hepatitis A virus infection in the United States: Incidence, prognosis, and outcomes. Hepatology 2006; 44: 1589–1597
69. **Theilmann, L., Solbach, C., Toex, U., Müller, H.M., Pfaff, E., Otto, G., Goeser, T.:** Role of hepatitis C virus in German patients with fulminant and subfulminant hepatic failure. Eur. J. Clin. Invest. 1992; 22: 569–571
70. **Tschumper, A., Streuli, H., Hottinger, S., Zimmermann, A., Müller, U.:** Fulminante Hepatitis bei Listeriensepsis. Schweiz. Med. Wschr. 1987; 117: 2010–2012

71. Velasco, M., Llamas, E., Guijarro-Rojas, M., Ruiz-Yagüe, M.: Fulminant herpes hepatitis in a healthy adult. A treatable disorder? J. Clin. Gastroenterol. 1999; 28: 386−389
72. Vento, S., Garofano, T., Renzini, C., Cainelli, F., Casali, F., Ghironzi, G., Ferraro, T., Concia, E.: Fulminant hepatitis associated with hepatitis A virus superinfection in patients with chronic hepatitis C. New Engl. J. Med. 1998; 338: 286−290
73. Walsh, T.S., Hopton, P., Philips, B.J., Mackenzie, S.J., Lee, A.: The effect of N-acetylcysteine on oxygen transport and uptake in patients with fulminant hepatic failure. Hepatology 1998; 27: 1332−1340
74. Wang, S.M., Liu, C.C., Yang, Y.J., Yang, H.B., Lin, C.H., Wang, J.R.: Fatal coxsackievirus B infection in early infancy characterized by fulminant hepatitis. J. Infect. 1998; 37: 270−273
75. Watanabe, A., Shiota, T., Tsuji, T.: Cerebral edema during hepatic encephalopathy in fulminant hepatic failure. J. Med. 1992; 23: 29−38
76. Whitworth, J.R., Mack, C.L., O'Connor, J.A., Narkewicz, M.R., Mengshol, S., Sokol, R.J.: Acute hepatitis and liver failure associated with influenza A infection in children (case report). J. Pediatr. Gastroenterol. Nutr. 2006; 43: 536−538
77. Wiesen, S., Reddy, K.R., Jeffers, L.J., Schiff, E.R.: Fulminant hepatic failure secondary to previously unrecognized cardiomyopathy. Dig. Dis. 1995; 13: 199−204
78. Wijdicks, E.F.M., Plevak, D.J., Rakela, J., Wiesner, R.H.: Clinical and radiologic features of cerebral oedema in fulminant failure. Mayo Clin. Proc. 1995; 70: 119−124
79. Williams, R.: Classification, etiology and considerations of outcome in acute liver failure. Semin. Liver Dis. 1996; 16: 343−348
80. Woolf, G.M., Petrovic, L.M., Rojter, S.E., Villamil, F.G., Makowka, L., Podesta, L.G., Sher, L.S., Memsic, L., Vierling, J.M.: Acute liver failure due to lymphoma. A diagnostic concern when considering liver transplantation. Dig. Dis. Sci. 1994; 39: 1351−1358
81. Woolf, G.M., Redeker, A.G.: Treatment of fulminant hepatic failure with insulin and glucagon. A randomized, controlled trial. Dig. Dis. Sci. 1991; 36: 92−96
82. Yanagi, M., Kaneko, S., Unoura, M., Murakami, S., Kobayashi, K.: Hepatitis C virus in fulminant hepatic failure. New Engl. J. Med. 1991; 324: 1895−1896
83. Yotsumoto, S., Kojima, M., Shoji, I., Yamamoto, K., Okamoto, H., Mishiro, S.: Fulminant hepatitis related to transmission of hepatitis B variants with precore mutations between spouses. Hepatology 1992; 16: 31−35

Liver support systems
84. Ash, S.R., Blake, D.E., Carr, D.J., Carter, C., Howard, T., Makowka, L.: Clinical effects of a sorbent suspension dialysis system in treatment of hepatic coma (the Biologic-DT). Intern. J. Artif. Org. 1992; 15: 151−161
85. Ash, S.R., Blake, D.E., Carr, D.J., Harker, K.D.: Push-pull sorbent based pheresis for treatment of acute hepatic failure: the Biologic-detoxifier/plasma filter system. ASAIO J. 1998; 44: 129−139
86. Butler, A.J., Rees, M.A., Wight, D.G.D., Casey, N.D., Alexander, G., White, D.J.G., Fried, P.J.: Successful extracorporeal porcine liver perfusion for 72 hr. Transplantation 2002; 73: 1212−1218
87. Dowling, D.J., Mutimer, D.J.: Artificial liver support in acute liver failure. Eur. J. Gastroenterol. Hepatol. 1999; 11: 991−996
88. Falkenhagen, D., Strobl, W., Vogt, G., Schrefl, A., Linsberger, I., Gerner, F.J., Schoenhofen, M.: Fractionated plasma separation and adsorption system: a novel system for blood purification to remove albumin bound substances. Artif. Organs 1999; 23: 81−86
89. Freeman, J.G., Matthewson, K., Record, C.D.: Plasmapheresis in acute liver failure. Int. J. Artif. Org. 1986; 9: 433−438
90. Gazzard, B.G., Weston, M.J., Murray-Lyon, I.M.: Charcoal hemoperfusion in the treatment of fulminant hepatic failure. Lancet 1974; I: 1301−1307
91. Gerlach, J.C., Encke, J., Hole, O., Muller, C., Ryan, C.J., Neuhaus, P.: Bioreactor for a larger scale hepatocyte in vitro perfusion. Transplantation 1994; 58: 984−988
92. Kim, S.S., Utsonomiya, H., Koski, J.A., Wu, B.M., Cima, M.J., Sohn, J., Mukai, K., Griffith, L.G., Vacanti, J.P.: Survival and function of hepatocytes on a novel three-dimensional synthetic biodegradable polymer scaffold with an intrinsic network of channels. Ann. Surg. 1998; 228: 8−13
93. Kondrup, J., Almdal, T., Vilstrup, H., Tygstrup, N.: High volume plasma exchange in fulminant hepatic failure. Internat. J. Artific. Org. 1992; 15: 669−676
94. Mazariegos, G.V., Patzer, J.F., Lopez, R.C., Giraldo, M., de Vera, M.E., Grogan, T.A., Zhu, Y., Fulmer, M.L., Amiot, B.P., Kramer, D.J.: First clinical use of a novel bioartificial liver support system (BLSS). Amer. J. Transplant. 2002; 2: 260−266
95. Novelli, G., Rossi, M., Pretagostini, R., Poli, L., Novelli, L., Bereoco, P., Ferretti, G., Iappelli, M., Cortesini, R.: MARS (molecular adsorbent recirculating system): experience in 34 cases of acute liver failure. Liver 2002; 22 (Suppl. 2): 43−47
96. Pascher, A., Sauer, I.M., Hammer, C., Gerlach, J.C., Neuhaus, P.: Extracorporeal liver perfusion as hepatic assist in acute liver failure: a review of world experience. Xenotransplantation 2002; 9: 309−324
97. Rahman, T.M., Hodgson, H.J.F.: Review article: liver support systems in acute hepatic failure. Aliment. Pharm. Ther. 1999; 13: 1255−1272
98. Rajvanshi, P., Larson, A.M., Kowdley, K.V.: Temporary support for acute liver failure (review). J. Clin. Gastroenterol. 2002; 35: 335−344
99. Rifai, K., Ernst, T., Kretschmer, U., Bahr, M.J., Schneider, A., Hafer, C., Haller, H., Manns, M.P., Fliser, D.: Prometheus (R) − a new extracorporeal system for the treatment of liver failure. J. Hepatol. 2003; 39: 984−990
100. Rozga, J., Holzman, M.D., Man-Soo Ro, Griffin, D.W., Neuzil, D.F., Giorgio, T., Moscioni, A.D., Demetriou, A.A.: Development of a hybrid bioartificial liver. Ann. Surg. 1993; 217: 502−511
101. Sanchez, E.Q., Goldstein, R.M., Klintmalm, G.B., Levy, M.F.: Porcine hepatocytes for use in bioartificial liver support. Verdauungskrankh. 2003; 21: 24−31
102. Sauer, I.M., Gerlach, J.C.: Modular extracorporeal liver support. Artif. Organs 2002; 26: 703−706
103. Shi, Y.F., He, J.L., Chen, S.B., Zhang, L.L., Yang, X.L., Wang, Z.H., Wang, M.M.: MARS: optimistic therapy method in fulminant hepatic failure secondary to cytotoxic mushroom poisoning. A case report. Liver 2002; 22 (Suppl. 2): 78−80
104. Singer, A.L., Olthoff, K.M., Kim, H., Rand, E., Zamir, G., Shaked, A.: Role of plasmapheresis in the management of acute hepatic failure in children. Ann. Surg. 2001; 234: 418−424
105. Stange, J., Mitzner, S., Ramlow, W., Gliesche, T., Hickstein, H., Schmidt, R.: A new procedure for the removal of protein bound drugs and toxins. ASAIO J. 1993; 39: M621−M625
106. Steiner, C., Mitzner, S.: Experiences with MARS liver support therapy in liver failure: analysis of 176 patients of the International MARS Registry. Liver 2002; 22 (Suppl. 2): 20−25
107. Stockmann, H.B., Hiemstra, C.A., Marquet, R.L., Jn, I.J.: Extracorporeal perfusion for the treatment of acute liver failure. Ann. Surg. 2000; 231: 460−470
108. Sussman, N.L., Chong, M.G., Koussayer, T., Da-ER He, Shang, T.A., Whisennand, H.H., Kelly, J.H.: Reversal of fulminant hepatic failure using an extracorporeal liver assist device. Hepatology 1992; 16: 60−65
109. Tsiaoussis, J., Newsome, P.N., Nelson, L.J., Hayes, P.C., Plevis, J.N.: Which hepatocyte will it be? Hepatocyte choice for bioartificial liver support systems. Liver Transplant. 2001; 7: 2−10
110. Van de Kerkhove, M.P., Hoekstra, R., Chamuleau, R.A.F.M., van Gulik, T.M.: Clinical application of bioartificial liver support systems (review). Ann. Surg. 2004; 240: 216−230

Transplantation
111. Beckurts, K.T., Holscher, A.H., Heidecke, C.D., Zilker, T.R., Natrath, W., Siewert, J.R.: The place of liver transplantation in the treatment of acute liver failure caused by Amanita phalloides poisoning. Dtsch. Med. Wschr. 1997; 122: 351−353
112. Brauer, R.B., Heidecke, C.D., Nathrath, W., Beckurts, K.T.E., Vorwald, P., Zilker, T.R., Schweigart, U., Hölscher, A.H., Siewert, J.R.: Liver transplantation for the treatment of fulminant hepatic failure induced by the ingestion of ecstasy. Transplant. Intern. 1997; 10: 229−233
113. Castaldo, E.T., Chari, R.S.: Liver transplantation for acute liver failure. HPB 2006; 8: 29−34
114. Fischer, L., Sterneck, M., Rogiers, X.: Liver transplantation for acute liver failure. Eur. J. Gastroenterol. Hepatol. 1999; 11: 985−990
115. Gubernatis, G., Pichlmayr, R., Kemnitz, J., Gratz, K.: Auxiliary partial orthotopic liver transplantation (APOLT) for fulminant hepatic failure: first successful case report. World J. Surg. 1991; 15: 660−666
116. Hellinger, A., Rauen, U., de Groot, H., Erhard, J.: Auxiliäre Lebertransplantation bei akutem Leberversagen nach Einnahme von 3,4-Methylendioxymetamphetamin („Ecstasy"). Dtsch. Med. Wschr. 1997; 122: 716−720
117. Kanazawa, A., Platt, J.L.: Prospects for xenotransplantation of the liver. Semin. Liver Dis. 2000; 20: 511−522
118. Liu, C.L., Fan, S.T., Lo, C.M., Yong, B.H., Fung, A.S.M., Wong, J.: Right-lobe live donor liver transplantation improves survival of patients with acute liver failure. Brit. J. Surg. 2002; 89: 317−322
119. Miwa, S., Hashikura, Y., Mita, A., Kubota, T., Chisuwa, H., Nakazawa, Y., Ikegami, T., Terada, M., Miyagawa, S., Kawasaki, S.: Living-related liver transplantation for patients with fulminant and subfulminant hepatic failure. Hepatology 1999; 30: 1521−1526
120. Moritz, M.J., Jarrell, B.E.: Heterotopic liver transplantation for fulminant hepatic failure: a bridge to recovery. Transplantation 1990; 50: 524−526
121. Neuhaus, P., Bechstein, W.O.: Split liver/auxiliary liver transplantation for fulminant hepatic failure. Liver Transpl. Surg. 1997; 3: 355−361
122. Pauwels, A., Mostefa-Kara, N., Florent, C., Levy, V.G.: Emergency liver transplantation for acute liver failure. Evaluation of London and Clichy criteria. J. Hepatol. 1993; 17: 124−127
123. Pouyet, M., Caillon, P., Ducerf, C., Berthaud, S., Bouffard, Y., Delafosse, B., Thomasson, A., Pignal, C., Pulce, C.: Transplantation orthotopique du foie pour intoxication grave par amanite phalloide. Presse Méd. 1991; 20: 2095−2098
124. Sudan, D.L., Shaw, B.W., Fox, I.J., Langnas, A.N.: Long-term follow-up of auxiliary orthotopic liver transplantation for the treatment of fulminant hepatic failure. Surgery 1997; 122: 771−777
125. Uemoto, S., Inomata, Y., Sakurai, T., Egawa, H., Fujita, S., Kiuchi, T., Hayashi, M., Yasutomi, M., Yamabe, H., Tanaka, K.: Living donor liver transplantation for fulminant hepatic failure. Transplantation 2000; 70: 152−157
126. Van Hoek, B., de Boer, J., Boudjema, K., Williams, J., Corsmit, O., Terpstra, O.T.: Auxiliary versus orthotopic liver transplantation for acute liver failure. J. Hepatol. 1999; 30: 699−705

127. **Van Thiel, D.H., Brems, J., Nadir, A., Idilman, R., Colantoni, A., Holt, D., Edelstein, S.:** Liver transplantation for fulminant hepatic failure. J. Gastroenterol. 2002; 37 (Suppl. 13): 78–81

Hepatocyte transplantation
128. **Bilir, B.M., Guinette, D., Karrer, F., Kumpe, D.A., Krysl, J., Stephens, J., McGavran, L., Ostrowska, A., Durham, J.:** Hepatocyte transplantation in acute liver failure. Liver Transplant. 2000; 6: 32–40
129. **Fereira Galvao, F.H., Ramos de Antrade Junior, D., Ramos de Antrade, D., Martins, B.C., Garms Marson, A., Bernard, C.V., Alves dos Santos, S., Bacchella, T., Cerqueira Cesar Machado, M.:** Hepatocyte transplantation: State of the art (review). Hepatol. Res. 2006; 36: 237–247
130. **Habibullah, C.M., Syed, I.H., Qamar, A., Taher-Uz, Z.:** Human fetal hepatocyte transplantation in patients with fulminant hepatic failure. Transplantation 1994; 58: 951–952
131. **Mito, M., Kusano, M., Kawaura, Y.:** Hepatocyte transplantation in man. Transplant. Proc. 1992; 24: 3052–3053
132. **Regimbeau, J.M., Mallet, V.O., Bralet, M.P., Gilgenkrantz, H., Houssin, D., Soubrane, O.:** Transplantation of isolated hepatocytes. Principles, mechanisms, animal models, clinical results. Gastroenterol. Clin. Biol. 2002; 26: 591–601
133. **Sundback, C.A. Vacanti, J.P.:** Alternatives to liver transplantation: From hepatocyte transplantation to tissue-engineered organs. Gastroenterology 2000; 118: 438–442
134. **Wang, X., Andersson, R.:** Hepatocyte transplantation: a potential treatment for acute liver failure. Scand. J. Gastroenterol. 1995; 30: 193–200

Clinical Aspects of Liver Diseases
21 Clinical and morphological principles

		Page:
1	***Attempt at a systematic approach***	398
1.1	Difficulties of systematization	398
1.2	Need for systematization	398
2	***Clinical forms of liver disease***	398
2.1	Primary and secondary liver diseases	398
2.2	Diffuse and focal liver diseases	399
2.3	Acute and chronic liver diseases	399
2.4	Aims of liver diagnostics	400
2.4.1	Rational and expedient diagnostics	400
2.4.2	Diagnostic and clinical issues	400
3	***Basic morphological processes of the liver***	400
3.1	*Cellular adaptation*	400
3.1.1	Membrane hyperplasia	400
3.1.2	Hyaline drops	401
3.1.3	Lipofuscinosis	401
3.2	*Hepatocellular degeneration*	401
3.2.1	Cellular changes	401
3.2.2	Nuclear changes	402
3.2.3	Cellular metabolic disorders	402
3.3	*Mesenchymal reactions*	403
3.3.1	Peliosis hepatis	404
3.3.2	Granulomas	405
3.4	*Cell death and necrosis*	406
3.4.1	Programmed cell death	406
3.4.2	Provoked cell death	406
3.4.3	Cell necrosis	407
3.5	*Regeneration*	408
3.6	*Fibrogenesis*	410
4	***Hepatitis and hepatosis***	411
4.1	Hepatitis	411
4.2	Hepatosis	411
5	***Fibrosis and cirrhosis***	412
5.1	*Fibrosis*	412
5.1.1	Scarred liver	412
5.1.2	Portal/periportal fibrosis	413
5.1.3	Perisinusoidal fibrosis	413
5.1.4	Perivenous fibrosis	414
5.1.5	Septal fibrosis	414
5.1.6	Liver collapse fibrosis	414
5.2	*Cirrhosis*	414
5.2.1	Basic criteria	414
5.2.2	Systematic approach	415
5.2.3	Morphological diagnosis	415
6	***Liver tumours***	416
6.1	Benign tumours	416
6.2	Malignant tumours	416
	• References (1–56)	417

(Figures 21.1–21.16; tables 21.1–21.6)

21 Clinical and morphological principles

1 Attempt at a systematic approach

Any attempt at setting up a systematic approach to liver disease has to incorporate the correlation between *morphological* and *functional* changes. At the same time, such an approach has to take account of *aetiological* and *pathogenic* factors. • However, any classification made is provisional by its very nature, since there is no uniform standpoint in this respect, and advances in medical knowledge can alter such classifications. (*see references* 2, 4, 9, 20)

1.1 Difficulties of systematization

It must be borne in mind that only relatively minor morphological changes might be evident in functional liver insufficiency. • Moreover, apparently normal hepatic functions may also prevail despite pronounced morphological changes in the liver.

Further consideration has to be given to the fact that different pathogenic factors can also trigger similar or even identical morphological changes as well as identical biochemical reactions.

▶ The term **hepatopathy** (G. v. Bergmann, 1936) (s. p. 78) — which cannot be defined precisely — must be viewed as a noble attempt to classify all liver diseases with their respective morphological and functional changes as one single entity. Above all, it should be noted that in those days there was little chance of making a detailed diagnosis of a liver disease during the patient's life.

1.2 Need for systematization

As early as 1947, H. Kalk strongly emphasized the need to systematize liver disease in line with morphological aspects. Initially, his approach was founded on laparoscopic criteria, i.e. size, colour and superficial structures of the liver. • Pathohistological examination, however, is indispensable in the classification of most liver diseases. Liver diagnostics is based on four essential pillars, of which histology is still the most important and, in cases of doubt, the decisive factor in determining the diagnosis. (s. pp 78, 79)

Even though it is still difficult today to systematize liver diseases, any such attempt can be of help, provided it takes due account of the aetiology, the clinical picture and the morphological changes. This facilitates an overview of the different liver diseases, including their variants and complications, and makes for a better understanding of certain individual forms of disease and the way in which the various forms are interrelated.

2 Clinical forms of liver disease

2.1 Primary and secondary liver diseases

All liver diseases can be classified into (*1.*) primary liver diseases and (*2.*) secondary liver diseases, with diverse clinical, therapeutic and prognostic relevance.

Primary liver diseases

The liver is primarily affected, and the involvement of the liver in the disease is paramount. A typical example would be acute viral hepatitis resulting from primary hepatotropic viruses. (s. tab. 5.16) • It is not possible to make a reliable *clinical* differentiation between the primary hepatotropic types of hepatitis; there are, however, certain distinctive hints derived from *histology* or *immunohistology* (e.g. HAV, HBV or HCV infection). Modern methods of *serology* and *immunology* render precise differentiation possible. • *Acute viral hepatitis does not exhibit any isolated specific morphological findings; it is the sum of the individual phenomena which results in the diagnosis.* (s. tab. 22.1)

Secondary liver diseases

The liver is secondarily affected by a systemic disease or shows a coreaction to extrahepatic organ processes. Involvement of the liver in the disease is not obvious. • Occasionally, the aetiology of the underlying disease can be diagnosed from liver biopsy material by means of characteristic morphological substrates or by the detection of pathogens. • In the majority of cases, these findings are ambiguous and are thus grouped together under the generic term "non-specific reactive hepatitis".

Non-specific reactive hepatitis

Concomitant hepatic lesions can occur as a consequence of a number of viral, bacterial, parasitic and mycotic infections as well as due to toxic effects. Owing to their ambiguity, however, these lesions do not allow closer aetiological specification. • *Therefore, the term "non-specific reactive hepatitis" is not actually considered to be a pathological entity in its own right.*

From the **pathohistological point of view,** the findings are (*1.*) degenerative liver cell changes with single focal liver cell necrosis, (*2.*) concomitant reaction of the Kupffer cells and formation of Kupffer cell nodules with a generalized reaction of the mononuclear phagocytosis system, usually inside dilated sinusoids, (*3.*) histiocytic and portal round-cell infiltration, and (*4.*) cholangitic reaction with sparse infiltrations of neutrophilic granulocytes around small bile ducts. (s. fig. 21.1)

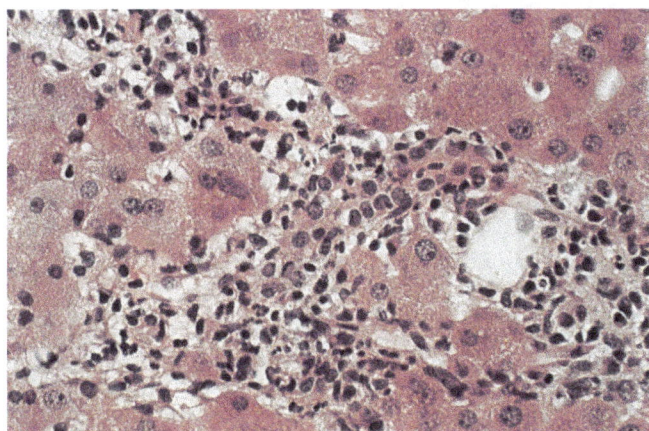

Fig. 21.1: Non-specific reactive hepatitis in sepsis due to cervical lymph node abscess: sparse single cell necrosis and periportal inflammation (HE)

The *pluriaetiological spectrum* involved in this condition already suggests the problematic nature of the generally accepted term non-specific reactive hepatitis. • The *confusion in terminology* is rendered all the more complex because the diagnosis of a non-specific reaction does not necessarily justify using the rather implicative term "hepatitis". • Moreover, an individual who is affected by non-specific reactive hepatitis cannot really be referred to as a "liver patient". We are also familiar with inflammatory secondary phenomena, such as leucocyte cellulations in alcoholic hepatitis or mesenchymal reactions due to drug abuse. In these cases, it can be equally problematic to apply terms like "non-specific", "hepatitis" or "liver disease".

That is why the **pathologist** will deliver a purely morphological description depending on the facts of the case, whereas it will be the task of the **clinician** to categorize these "non-specific" inflammatory secondary phenomena with respect to their aetiology and clinical significance.

2.2 Diffuse and focal liver diseases

In concordance with the morphological pattern associated with the liver condition, two further groups of diseases may be distinguished (s. tab. 4.1!):

1. **Diffuse liver diseases**
   The disease of the liver is largely diffuse; its occurrence can be either primary or secondary.
2. **Focal liver diseases**
   The liver only exhibits focal processes of disease, which may be primary or secondary and of non-specific or specific genesis.

Diffuse liver diseases: Certain *problems* with morphological definitions arise from the term diffuse liver disease. Individual cases present a genuine form of diffuse liver disease (e.g. in acute viral hepatitis), or portal-periportal lesions of different degrees of diffusion are evident (e.g. in bacterial cholangitis), or there are intraparenchymal diffusely localized changes (e.g. in listeriosis). • In diffuse liver diseases, the histological finding is representative in 80–100% of cases. (s. pp 165, 168)

Focal liver diseases: In contrast, it is frequently impossible to detect localized findings in the biopsy material, which is 1.5–2.0 cm in length and generally comprises up to 20 portal fields, especially since percutaneous biopsy only reaches a certain area of the right liver lobe. *Consequently, "negative" biopsy findings do not necessarily rule out the presence of localized hepatic changes!* (s. p. 160) • Larger focal lesions are detected by imaging procedures and can be assessed by guided biopsy, fine needle biopsy or laparoscopy.

2.3 Acute and chronic liver diseases

With regard to the time period involved in the course of a liver disease, distinction has to be made between two further groups, excluding the prodromal stage and the healing process (s. tab. 4.1) (s. p. 78):

1. **Acute liver diseases**
   In the individual case of acute liver disease, it is necessary to differentiate between *peracute* (i.e. *fulminant*), *subacute-necrotic* and *protracted* courses.
2. **Chronic liver diseases**
   Chronic liver diseases may show *protracted (subchronic)*, *"persistent"* or *"aggressive"* courses. The new classification of chronic hepatitis emphasizes its respective aetiology while at the same time categorizing the degree of inflammatory and necrotic activity as well as any fibrosis and additional changes in the hepatic architecture.

Chronic liver disease is characterized by inflammatory infiltrates and/or degenerative changes which have persisted for six to twelve months or longer; its prognosis is dubious. Chronic liver disease is thus defined by the following **triad:**

1. Prolonged course of disease (>6 months)
2. Inflammatory and/or degenerative morphological findings
3. Dubious prognosis
   - no general healing tendency
   - tendency towards progression
   - occurrence of complications

Chronic liver diseases (congenital or acquired) can be classified (schematically) into ten groups depending on their **aetiopathogenesis.** However, due to the close spatial intercalation of the mesenchymal and epithelial hepatic systems, the transition between the groups is fluent. As a result, chronic liver diseases can be classified according to their aetiopathogenesis as follows:

1. infectious	6. vascular
2. toxic	7. cardiac
3. autoimmune	8. malignant
4. metabolic	9. haematological
5. biliary	10. cryptogenic

2.4 Aims of liver diagnostics

2.4.1 Rational and expedient diagnostics

A diagnosis can only be regarded as expedient (i.e. thrifty and economical) if it has been reached by rational (i.e. logical and targeted) measures. Any irrational form of diagnostics will always be too expensive, even if it appears to be economically reasonable or is indeed presented as being cost-effective. (s. p. 77)

2.4.2 Diagnostic and clinical issues

In nearly every single case, the main diagnostic and clinical issues can be resolved, provided all the necessary (rational) diagnostic channels are pursued. (s. tab. 4.1) • This always includes the major differential diagnoses of **hepatomegaly** *(see chapter 11)*, **jaundice** *(see chapter 12)* and **cholestasis** *(see chapter 13)*. It is likewise of great clinical importance to establish the aetiopathogenesis of **portal hypertension** *(see chapter 14)*.

During the course of acute or chronic liver disease, it may be difficult for the liver to fulfill all biochemical tasks (s. p. 36) due to a profound impairment of its functional capacity. The result is inadequate functioning (= insufficiency) − this **liver insufficiency** is, however, still **compensated.** (s. p. 380) In the individual case, just a few liver functions may be affected to varying degrees (= *partial insufficiency*), or the functions of the liver can be extensively impaired in their entirety (= *global insufficiency*). The condition of compensated liver insufficiency may go unnoticed both subjectively and clinically − it is often revealed by laboratory analysis of the liver function. At this stage, the liver is still capable of maintaining the viability of the organism. • For this reason, the state of compensated liver insufficiency must be stabilized and maintained by the patient, on the one hand by preventing damage and on the other hand by establishing the best possible living conditions.

In the course of acute or chronic liver disease, the biochemical functions of the liver may be compromised indefinitely; the outcome is **decompensated liver insufficiency.** (s. p. 380) (s. tab. 20.4) The stage of decompensation is synonymous with the onset of life-threatening complications. These mainly take the form of *hepatic encephalopathy* with transition to hepatic coma *(see chapter 15)*, *oedema* and *ascites* with imbalance of the electrolytes and the acid-base equilibrium *(see chapter 16)* through to the *hepatorenal syndrome (see chapter 17)*, the hepatopulmonary syndrome *(see chapter 18)* and/or the development of *coagulopathy* as well as *bleeding oesophageal varices (see chapter 19)*.

The clarification of the diagnosis and the various clinical issues provides **statements** on (*1.*) course of disease (regressive, stationary, progressive), (*2.*) success of therapy, (*3.*) healing process, and (*4.*) prognosis. (s. p. 78)

3 Basic morphological processes of the liver

Despite the tremendous scope of morphological changes in liver diseases, the *pathomorphological reactions* of the liver are attributable to four main processes, which form the basis of **morphological diagnostics:**

1. Cell damage / degeneration (and sequelae)
2. Cell death / necrosis (and sequelae)
3. Fibrogenesis (and sequelae)
4. Regeneration

Pathobiochemical hepatic reactions can likewise be classified (schematically simplified) into four main disfunctional mechanisms, which form the basis of **biochemical diagnostics:**

1. Enzymopathies
2. Cholestasis / jaundice
3. Metabolic insufficiency
4. Immune reactions

3.1 Cellular adaptation

3.1.1 Membrane hyperplasia

During the course of biotransformation (s. p. 57), the need for *cell adaptation* often goes far beyond the normal scope of physiological activity as a result of excessive strain. This can lead to **membrane hyperplasia** (or agranuloreticular hypertrophy) of the smooth endoplasmic reticulum. (s. pp 59, 537, 559) The result is a considerable increase in liver cell volume, so that **hepatomegaly** is even clinically detectable. (s. p. 218) This in turn may cause increased glycogen deposition suppression of the mitochondria and of the granular reticulum in the cell periphery as well as an extremely fine-grain or net-like cytoplasm which is seen to be more eosinophilic and brighter. • This form of biotransformational proliferation of the smooth endoplasmic reticulum is easy to distinguish from the virus-induced (inflammatory) form − e.g. by aldehyde-thionine staining or through localization in the liver lobule. • *Membrane hyperplasia will persist as long as there is a surplus of substrate and will regress once the substrate pressure is relieved.* (s. fig. 21.2)

Clinical and morphological principles

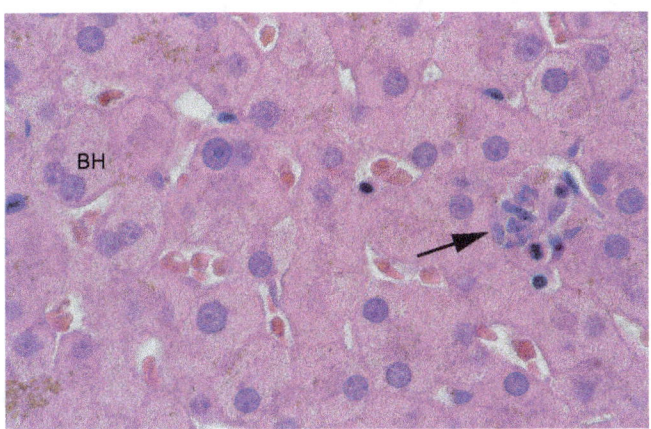

Fig. 21.2: Adaptive changes of hepatocytes due to hyperplasia of the smooth endoplasmic reticulum. Several binuclear hepatocytes (BH). Small Kupffer cell nodule following cell necrosis (↑) (HE)

3.1.2 Hyaline drops

In long-standing membrane hyperplasia, the affected membranes show regeneration and degradation. Electron microscopy reveals them to be cytoplasmic whorls, and light microscopy displays them as pale eosinophilic, occasionally layered homogeneous hyaline drops. • When persistent for a long time, this (physiological) cellular adaptation may gradually become cellular damage.

3.1.3 Lipofuscinosis

The peroxidation of unsaturated fatty acids from membrane hyperplasia remnants can cause lipofuscinosis. This consists of fine-grained, iron-free, yellowish-brown polymeric residual bodies (phospholipid protein complexes) within the lysosomes. These pigments are principally found in perivenular hepatocytes, in particular at the biliary pole. Due to their delayed breakdown, they are detectable for longer than membrane hyperplasia. • Lipofuscinosis is evident in older hepatocytes, at an advanced age ("wear-and-tear pigment"), in hepatic (brown) atrophy, malnutrition, cachexia, vitamin E deficiency, and with the Dubin-Johnson syndrome. In analgesic abuse, panlobular localization occurs. (s. figs. 21.3; 24.9)

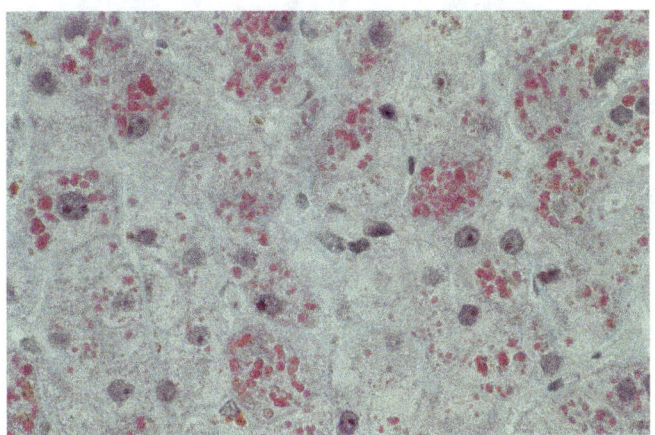

Fig. 21.3: Lipofuscinosis (metachromatic-red cytoplasmic pigments) following abuse of analgesics of the phenacetin type (Ladewig)

3.2 Hepatocellular degeneration

As a form of sublethal, yet generally reversible damage depending on the noxa, hepatocellular degeneration presents multiple changes in the cell and nucleus as well as cellular metabolic disorders.

3.2.1 Cellular changes

Hydropic-cell swelling: Disorders in the energy homeostasis in the hepatocyte biomembrane, with the associated failure of the ion pumps, leads to an increased influx of fluid from the extracellular space into the interior of the cell. This osmotic cellular oedema results in greater *cytoplasm transparency* and a reduction or even complete loss of cytoplasmic basophilia. The endoplasmic reticulum is dilated and the liver cell is enlarged. Collectively, a picture of *cellular hydrops* develops. • Later, a vacuolar swelling of the smooth ER is evident, and the organelles diminish. The cytoplasm is light-coloured, stringy or honeycombed, and in places optically "empty". There is a loss of glycogen as well as reduced chromatolysis, whereas protein accumulates. Such **ballooned hepatocytes** are seen as an early stage of a rapidly developing cellular lysis, as a result of which empty lattice fibres become visible. The ballooning is considered to be a severe, yet still reversible form of cell damage. (s. fig. 21.4)

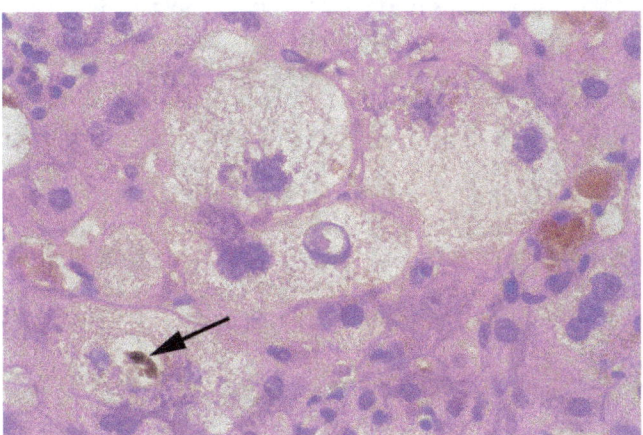

Fig. 21.4: Ballooned hepatocytes with intracellular bilirubinostasis (→) (HE)

Granular-cell swelling: In cases of turbid and/or granular swelling of the cell, usually toxin-related, the cell interior, which comprises numerous homogeneous eosinophilic granules, becomes lighter. This process is actually based on a swelling and proliferation of the mitochondria. At the same time, there is a substantial glycogen overload of the rough ER, which is subsequently displaced to the pole of the hepatocyte adjacent to the bile duct. • In some instances, this may lead to the development of **giant mitochondria**, which can reach a size comparable to that of the nucleus itself. These present as pale eosinophilic, well-defined, PAS-negative hyaline bodies. They appear in cases of chronic alcohol and/or medicament abuse, dermatosclerosis and local hypoxia. (s. fig. 28.4)

Feathery degeneration: Due to the detergent effect of retained bile acids, particularly in cases of long-term cholestasis, a net-like degeneration of the hepatocytic cytoplasm develops. The hepatocytes are hydropically swollen and appear foamy. They are also permeated with feather-like cytoplasmic filaments, which are often impregnated with bilirubin. Under an electron microscope, vorticose accumulations of membrane material can be seen. The smooth ER is dilated. Feathery degenerated cells are predominantly located in the periportal regions of the liver; being typically solitary, they are seldom found in groups. (s. figs. 13.4; 22.4)

Hyaline bodies are observed as round, eosinophilic, occasionally layered acidophilic corpuscles in the cytoplasm of degenerated hepatocytes. Diffusely distributed in the lobule, they are particularly evident in acute viral hepatitis A and B. • It was, in fact, in yellow fever that they were first described as **Councilman bodies** (W. T. Councilman) in 1890. • So-called **pin cells,** i.e. dehydrated, pin-shaped, compressed liver cells, may be regarded as precursors of the hyaline bodies. As a rule, they can be fully restored.

Ground-glass cells can be identified as enlarged liver cells with pale eosinophilic, turbid cytoplasm resulting from hyperplasia of the smooth ER. The nucleus is displaced to the cell margin. These cells are randomly distributed throughout the liver lobule. They are found in viral hepatitis B, glycogenosis (type IV) and hypofibrinogenaemia or can result from the impact of foreign substances. (s. figs. 5.7; 22.7) • From a differential diagnostic standpoint, they must be distinguished from **induced cells,** which may develop as a result of biotransformation stimuli. These cells are reversible, but can remain as hyaline droplets if noxic agents persist.

3.2.2 Nuclear changes

Nuclear changes are frequently observed in the form of **large nuclei** or **double nuclei** and reflect impaired reparatory nuclear division. The nucleoles are enlarged and basophilic. • This category likewise includes the so-called **glycogen vacuolation of the nuclei,** such as is found in diabetes mellitus, Wilson's disease and glycogenosis. (s. fig. 31.1) • It is often possible to observe cytoplasmic **intranuclear inclusions,** such as iron-containing inclusions (e. g. in haemochromatosis), protein-containing viral DNA (e. g. in cytomegaly), basophilic inclusions surrounded by a clear halo (e.g. in cytomegaly), eosinophilic *Cowdry type A* or basophilic *Cowdry type B* (e.g. herpes simplex virus) (s. fig. 23.2), herpes zoster virus, HB particles, and *Torres bodies* (e. g. in yellow fever). • **Sanded nuclei** (L. Bianchi, 1976) are finely granulated ("sand-like"), pale eosinophilic hepatocyte nuclei, stuffed with HB core particles, as found in chronic hepatitis B.

3.2.3 Cellular metabolic disorders

Lipid accumulation: The increased deposition of *triglycerides* in hepatocytes is deemed to be the most common morphological change in the liver. It begins within the endoplasmic reticulum, increasingly displacing the nucleus and organelles to the periphery of the cell. In lipid accumulation, fatty infiltration can be differentiated from fatty degeneration. The latter manifests as microvesicular or macrovesicular steatosis. (s. fig. 31.3) Fat deposits can both support and perpetuate liver cell damage. In addition, fatty liver cells are more vulnerable to damage from free radicals, endotoxins and hypoxia. • *Acute alcoholic foamy degeneration* of the liver is a particular form of microvesicular steatosis which diffusely affects the entire liver parenchyma. This rare and severe disorder was first described in 1983 by T. Uchida. (50) • *Labrea fever* is an equally uncommon and serious liver disease with microvesicular steatosis. It was first observed by B. Buitrago et al. in the Amazon River basin in 1986. Hepatitis D superinfection in chronic carriers of hepatitis B is considered to be the cause; the correspondingly modified hepatocytes are termed morula cells or spongiocytes. (7) • Cholesterol deposition mainly in the lysosomes is typical of *cholesteryl ester storage disease* (s. figs. 21.5; 31.15) and of *Wolman's disease*, while in *Tangier disease* (familiar HDL insufficiency), the cholesterol deposits are found free in the cytosol of these cells. • In *Gaucher's disease*, deposits of glucocerebroside are present. The pale cytoplasm contains PAS- and diastase-resistant material, which resembles folded paper. Such hepatocytes are called Gaucher cells. (s. fig. 31.17) • Similar cells are also encountered in chronic myeloid leukaemia, plasmacytomas and malignant lymphomas (= *pseudo-Gaucher cells*).

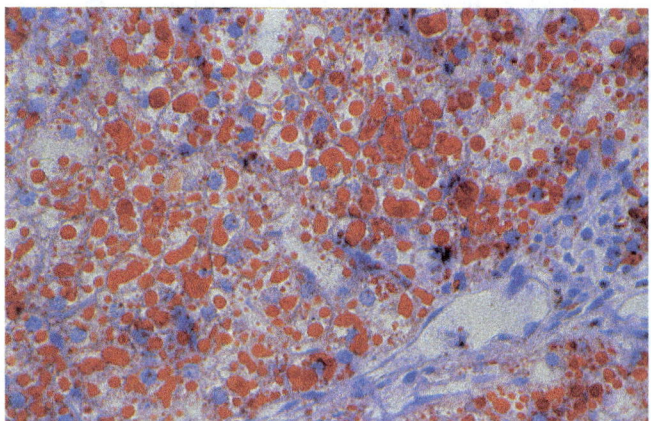

Fig. 21.5: Cholesterol ester storage disease (CESD). Micro-/macrovesicular fat droplets in hepatocytes and foam cells in a portal tract (Sudan III)

Cholestasis: The cytoplasm becomes brighter at the sinusoidal pole, and together with reinforced basophilia at the peribiliary pole, it points to toxic intrahepatic cholestasis. These changes often precede the deposition of bile. Histologically, bilirubin is normally not visible. Under pathological conditions, it appears yellowish-brown in the liver cells and greenish in the canaliculi. Bilirubin deposits are referred to as **bilirubinostasis**. (s. figs. 13.1; 21.4; 22.4; 29.4) • In a histological context, the term **cholestasis** is generally used. Thus the *morphological definition* of cholestasis (= bilirubin deposition) differs from the *clinical definition* of cholestasis (= increase in bile acids and alkaline phosphatase, yet without hyperbilirubinaemia). Depending on its location, the bilirubin stasis is classified as *hepatocellular* (= intracellular), *canalicular* (= inspissated bile plugs in dilated intercellular bile canaliculi, first appearing in acinar zone 3 and extending to zone 1) and *ductular* (= inspissated bile plugs in dilated bile ductules, especially in long-standing extrahepatic bile duct obliteration.) • In localized liver damage, **focal cholestasis** may also be detectable.

Glycogen accumulation: Large-scale deposition of glycogen gives hepatocytes a plant-like structure. The cells appear bright, are enlarged and have compressed sinusoids. These variations are found in glycogenosis IV (Anderson's disease), whereas in glycogenosis II, the cytoplasm contains fine, PAS-positive vacuoles. • *Lafora bodies* are characterized as round-to-oval-shaped, well-defined, slightly eosinophilic cell inclusions, which give the cytoplasm a fine-granular, homogeneous appearance. They are presumably composed of acidic mucopolysaccharides and mainly located in the periportal hepatocytes. Similar inclusions are found following the intake of disulfram and INH (= *pseudo-Lafora bodies*).

Pigment accumulation: Pigments are defined as coloured substances which are either produced in the body (endogenic) or introduced from the outside environment (exogenic). • Noteworthy here are *lipofuscine* (see above) and *ceroid pigment*. The latter is a coarse brown pigment found in hypertrophied Kupffer cells and macrophages. (s. fig. 21.6)

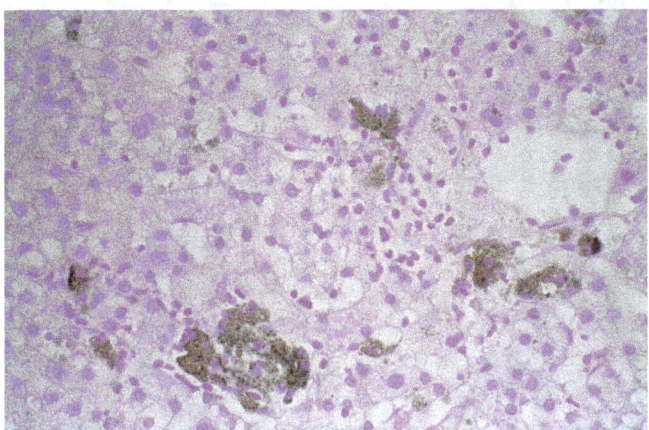

Fig. 21.6: Brownish ceroid ("decomposition pigment") in nested macrophages together with posthepatitic late-phase nodule (HE) (s. p. 424)

Ceroid pigment is both diastase-resistant as well as acid-fast. It derives from the phagocytosis of lipids released from dead hepatocytes (heterophagia). • In addition, *malarial pigment* (s. fig. 25.3), *schistosomatic pigment*, *melanotic pigment* and the *porphyrin pigments* are worthy of mention.

Inorganic substances: *Ferritin* represents the primary storage form of iron in hepatocytes. In the case of iron overload, ferritin is broken down into haemosiderin. It is a golden-brown, granular, iron-containing pigment which appears as blue granules when treated with Prussian blue stain. (s. fig. 31.28) • *Haemosiderin* is mainly located in lysosomes, but can also be found in the cytoplasm. In haemolysis, haemosiderin granules are chiefly stored in Kupffer cells and macrophages, where iron from necrotic liver cells is also present. • An increased storage of *copper* occurs in Wilson's disease, cholestasis and Indian childhood cirrhosis. The cytoplasmic copper granules can be displayed with rhodanine or orcein dyes. The periportal hepatocytes are mainly affected. (s. fig. 31.24) • In patients with pronounced anthracosis, *carbon* can also be detected in the liver cells. (s. fig. 21.7)

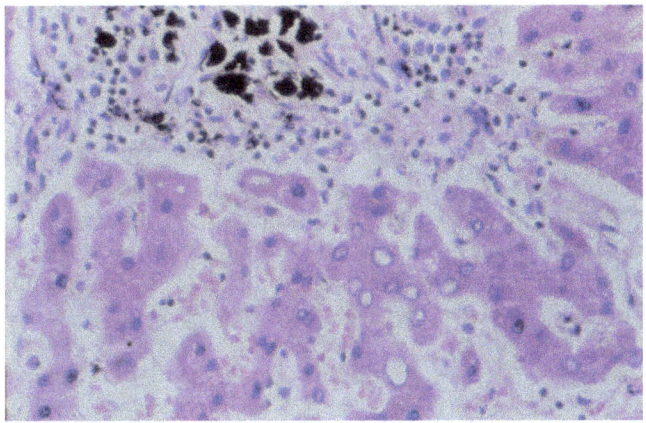

Fig. 21.7: Carbon pigment deposits in portal macrophages. Clinical diagnosis: pronounced anthracosis (HE)

Protein accumulation: The intracellular storage of protein can be an expression of both adaptive processes and metabolic disorders. While such deposits are often harmless, they may also facilitate or even directly cause damage to the cell. • *Fibrinogen* and *albumin* are examples of this. Proteinocholia reflects a hepatocellular metabolic disorder as well as a disturbance in bile acid excretion with marked feathery degeneration. (s. fig 22.4) • In α_1-*antitrypsine deficiency*, deposits of the altered proteinase inhibitor are found in hepatocytes, appearing as globular, eosinophilic, PAS-positive, diastase-resistant inclusions, mainly located in zone 1. (s. fig. 31.12) • *Mallory-Denk bodies* were first identified in alcoholic cirrhosis in 1911 by F. B. MALLORY, but they are not specific to alcohol abuse. These inclusions are also found in PBC, Wilson's disease, HCC, FNH, NASH, van Gierke's disease, abetalipoproteinaemia and chronic cholestasis as well as after intestinal bypass surgery and the use of certain medicaments (e.g. amidaron, diltiazem, nifidipin). Mallory-Denk bodies are aggregated, hyperphosphorylated cytoceratine filaments. They are irregularly shaped (branched, cord-like), thick, eosinophilic cytoplasmic inclusions, which can be detected immunohistochemically with antibodies to ubiquitin. Their pathogenesis is unclear. Up to now, no negative effects upon the existing liver disease are known. (11, 55!) (s. figs. 28.2, 28.3)

3.3 Mesenchymal reactions

As a result of degenerative changes, there may be mesenchymal reactions, such as the formation of *stellate cell nodules* (s. fig. 22.3), which reflect previous cellular decay, or a diffuse spread of *retothelial nodules* in toxic hepatosis. Portal *cellulations*, eosinophilic *pericholangitis* and *peliosis hepatis* as well as *granulomas* also belong to this group. • Eosinophilic depositions (antigen-AB precipitates) which accumulate in the immediate surroundings of fungi, parasites or bacterial colonies (i.e. perifocally) are classified under the term **Splendore-Hoeppli phenomenon** (E. Splendore, 1908; R. Hoeppli, 1932). (s. p. 509)

The occurrence of mesenchymal or even "inflammatory" lesions depends on the type of noxa and the respective exposure time. Turbid swelling, for example, can be an expression of enhanced cellular activity or a sign of impaired protein metabolism. Perhaps the deposits of minute fat droplets are a counter-regulatory mechanism. With degenerative changes, thought should therefore be given to the question of whether a finding is a compensatory mechanism or whether it constitutes damage and might, as such, evoke (secondary) mesenchymal reactions. Transitions may be fluid, just as epithelial and mesenchymal lesions of differing intensities can also combine. • *Histological terminology always depends on the respective findings at the various stages of change.*

In this context, it is reasonable to address the longstanding rejection of the term **hepatosis**. Even if the objections to the term hepatosis as defined by R. Rössle (1929) (s. p. 411) are absolutely justified, it is nevertheless true to say: *the primary degenerative lesions of the liver cell are of central significance – they can be considered as the key to the development of multiple functional and structural patterns of damage.*

3.3.1 Peliosis hepatis

When portal processes of varying aetiology spread, sinusoidal structures and cellular systems are damaged. (52, 54) Toxic effects or local increases in pressure in the sinusoids, for example, can lead to their dilation with concomitant epithelial lesions and the destruction of reticular fibres. The invasion of erythrocytes results in diffusely distributed cavities filled with blood ("globoid bleeding") of 0.5–2.0 mm, even up to 1.0 cm, in diameter. They were first described by E. Wagner in 1861 and termed peliosis hepatis by F. W. Schönlanck in 1916. Such cavities possess no endothelium. They are mostly disseminated, but sometimes arranged focally. All age groups and both sexes are affected equally. Peliosis hepatis is diagnosed with the help of ultrasound, CT or MRI. The diagnosis can be confirmed histologically with a liver biopsy. (s. figs. 21.8; 36.23)

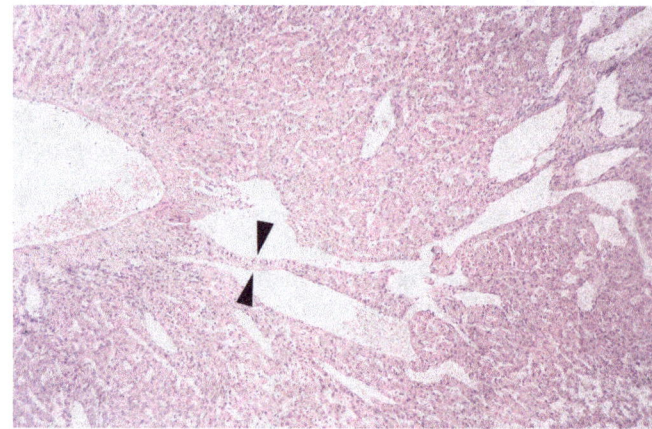

Fig. 21.8: Peliotic sinus dilatation in Osler's disease with small liver trabeculae (▶) (HE)

The blood-filled cavities of the **parenchymatous type** are linked with the sinusoids; their walls consist of trabeculae formed from flattened hepatocytes. In contrast, the blood-filled cavities of the **phlebosclerotic type** communicate with the sinusoids and the central veins. Indistinct sinusoidal dilations, so-called *hepatic spongiosis* (P. Bannasch et al., 1981), are a possible precursor of peliosis hepatis. • Peliosis can lead to bleeding into the parenchyma or abdominal cavity. It is nearly always found in adenomas and FNH. Secondary thrombi may appear at the centre of the peliotic foci. In the subsequent course of disease, fibrosis can develop. Despite elimination of the root cause, a regression is rarely possible. Intra-abdominal haemorrhages are often fatal. (s. p. 787)

The **causes** of peliosis hepatis are varied and include anabolic or androgenic steroids, oestrogens (52), azathioprine, arsenic, vinyl chloride, tamoxifen and danazol as well as tuberculosis, histiocytosis, leishmaniasis, leprosy, carcinoma, sprue, liver abscess, cytomegalovirus infection, glycogenosis (type I) (14) and marasmus. (46) • Congenital (angiomatous) abnormality of the vessels may also be a contributory factor. (5) The respective development of peliosis hepatis is still unclear.

▶ **Bacterial peliosis hepatis** has been determined in cases of HIV infection and cat-scratch fever, where it is caused by Rochalimaea quintana bacteria (Bartonella henselae). (s. p. 492) It presents as a proliferation of blood-filled cystic sinusoidal cavities, which are surrounded by fibromyxoid stroma (M. J. Dolan et al., 1993). Sometimes it is possible to identify the causative organism using PCR or staining with a silver dye (Warthin-Starry). Treatment can then follow with antibiotic agents, such as erythromycin, doxycyclin or clarithromycin.

3.3.2 Granulomas

Granulomas develop as a knot-like collection of macrophages, plasma cells, lymphocytes, histiocytes, fibroblasts and multinuclear giant cells of the Langhans' or foreign-body type. They are seen as a particular form of chronic inflammation. Two forms are differentiated: (*1.*) immune granulomas and (*2.*) foreign-body granulomas. • In *immune granulomas*, macrophages can, following antigen stimulation, transform into epithelioid cells, which produce large quantities of cytokines. The centre of these epithelioid granulomas are populated with $CD4^+$ cells, whereas the periphery is dominated by $CD8^+$ cells. Immune granulomas can also have a lymphohistiocytic structure. Due to the high turnover of their cells, immune granulomas are extremely dynamic entities, whose morphology can vary greatly. • *Foreign-body granulomas* typically contain the causative substance (e.g. starch, silicone, mineral oil, beryllium). Lipogranulomas are also included here. (13) Granulomas can sometimes completely degenerate, but in cases where the causative agent remains, they persist or scar over. Granulomas are generally distributed focally throughout the liver, mostly within the liver lobules and less frequently in the portal fields. As a rule, the normal lobular architecture is not affected. Granulomas located on the surface are visualized laparoscopically as small, greyish-white foci, which can be conveniently collected by forceps biopsy for histological examination. (s. figs. 21.9, 21.10; 24.3, 24.4, 24.8, 24.14; 29.6, 29.7) (s. p. 787)

In **genuine granulomas**, it is often possible to identify the underlying causative disease (e.g. tuberculosis, syphilis) as a specific form of reaction with typical tissue structures; one can sometimes demonstrate the presence of pathogenic organisms in the granuloma. • **Genuine, unspecific granulomas** constitute a largely uniform reaction of the liver to different causes. • **Lipogranulomas** result from the destruction of fatty liver cells. They are composed of phagocytizing and epithelioid cells and surrounded by ring-shaped histiocytes. In particular, they are found in alcoholic liver damage. (13) • With certain limitations, it is possible to distinguish **sarcoid-like granulomas,** which are considered to be a resorption phenomenon. They are made up of round cells and histiocytic epithelioid cellular tissue, occasionally with ceroid-containing macrophages or foreign-body giant cells; sometimes central necrosis or caseation is evident. Although the borders of the parenchyma are indistinct, they can still be identified. The healing process takes place with fine cicatrization. • **Eosinophilic granulomas** are seen as an expression of hyperergic immune reactions. They contain epithelioid cells and eosinophilic leucocytes. (8, 10, 12, 13, 18, 21, 25, 51, 53)

In over 80% of patients, tuberculosis, sarcoidosis and medicaments are the main **causal factors**. (51) In most cases, granulomas are discovered accidentally during liver biopsy. They cause no discomfort, and there are no clinical findings or any deviations from normal laboratory parameters. Granulomas may give valuable hints of the underlying disease. Therapy can only be directed at the underlying disease itself. (s. tab. 21.1)

Medicaments	**Parasites**
Acetylsalicylic acid	Amoebiasis
Allopurinol	Ankylostoma
Cephalexin	Ascaris lumbricoides
Clofibrate	Lambliasis
Diazepam	Larva migrans
Fluothane	Linguatula serrata
Halothane	Schistosomiasis
Hydralazine	Strongyloidiasis
Hydrochlorothiazide	Toxocara canis
Interferon-α	
Isoniazid	**Fungi**
Metahydrin	Aspergillosis
Methyldopa	Blastomycosis
Metolazone	Candidiasis
Penicillin	Coccidioidomycosis
Phenytoin	Cryptococcosis
Phenylbutazone	Histoplasmosis
Procainamide	Torulopsosis
Procarbazine	
Quinine	**Neoplasia**
Sulphonamide	Hodgkin's disease
Sulphonylurea	Intestinal adenocarcinoma
Bacteria	**Immunopathies**
Actinomycosis	Basedow hyperthyroidism
Brucellosis	BCG vaccine
Lepra	Erythematodes visceralis
Listeriosis	Granulomatosis infantisepticum
M. avium intracellulare	Hypogammaglobulinaemia
M. tuberculosis	Polymyalgia rheumatica
Melioidosis	Primary biliary cholangitis
Nocardiosis	Sarcoidosis
Salmonellosis	Vasculitis
Staphylococcal sepsis	Wegener's granulomatosis
Tularaemia	**Foreign bodies**
Yersiniosis	Berylliosis
Viruses	Drug abuse
Cytomegalovirus	Mineral oil
Felinosis	**Enteropathies**
Infectious mononucleosis	Crohn's disease
Influenza B	Eosinophilic gastroenteritis
Viral hepatitis A	Ulcerative colitis
Protozoiases	Whipple's disease
Rickettsiosis	
Toxoplasmosis	

Tab. 21.1: Possible causes of the formation of granulomas in the liver (s. figs. 21.9, 21.10; 24.3, 24.4, 24.8, 24.14; 29.6, 29.7)

Granulomatous hepatitis has been postulated as an independent diesease with fever of unknown origin, greater transaminase activity, lymphocytosis, splenomegaly, myalgia or arthralgia, weight loss, fatigue and malaise (M. Eliakim et al., 1968). • Yet, the concomitant increase in the blood sedimentation rate as well as the rise in alkaline phosphatase may well be assigned to rheumatic polymyalgia or autoimmune vasculitis (s. tab. 5.9!) — in the same way that the positive response to glucocorticoids points to an *immunopathy* which may really exist.

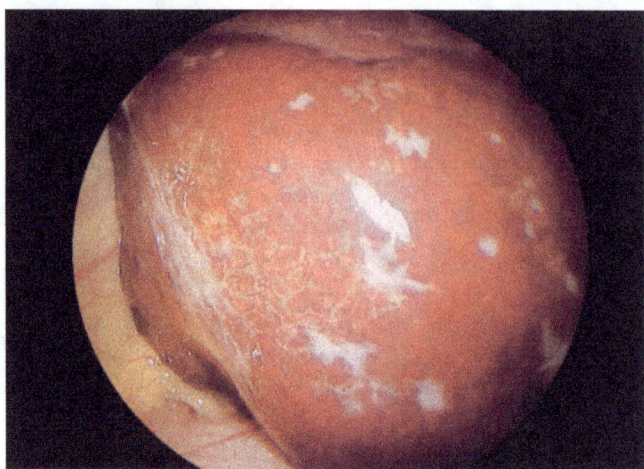

Fig. 21.9: Sarcoid granulomas (miliary type, up to the size of a lentil) on the liver surface (right liver lobe)

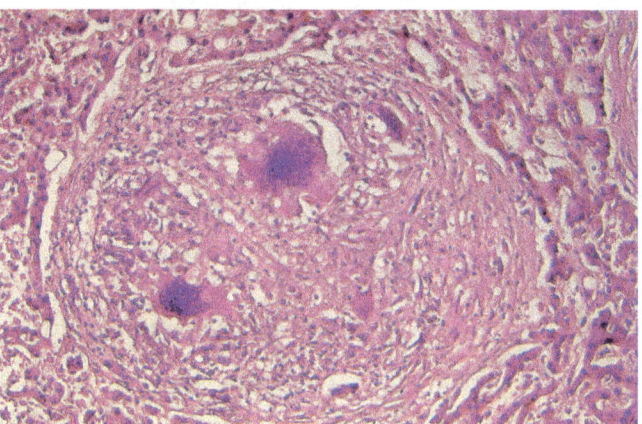

Fig. 21.10: Fibrosing epithelioid cell granuloma containing giant cells in sarcoidosis (HE)

From the pathologist's point of view, the term **granulomatous hepatitis** is incorrect: the detection of granulomas never represents a histomorphological picture of "hepatitis", even in cases where the granulomas are densely accumulated in the portal fields or indeed diffusely distributed in the parenchyma. Granulomas are considered to be harmless findings in the sense of a local mesenchymal or hyperergic concomitant reaction of the liver to toxic lesions as well as to extrahepatic causes — they do not actually constitute a liver disease, nor can they be seen as a liver disorder of any significance. (36)

3.4 Cell death and necrosis

3.4.1 Programmed cell death

Like practically all other tissue cells of the organism, hepatocytes are subject to **physiological ageing,** a process that is controlled by specific biochemical signal substances. The normal, genetically determined **life-span of hepatocytes** is 200 (150–400) days. This programmed cell death or death due to ageing (C. Vogt, 1842) is known as **apoptosis**, which in Greek means "falling of the leaves from the trees" (J. F. R. Kerr et al., 1972). (28) Apoptosis is of great significance for the homoeostasis of tissues and for the removal of old, injured or mutated cells. • It is a genetically programmed and regulated, active, energy-consuming process, whereby the liver cell controls its own death. Both physiological and pathological stimuli can initiate apoptosis. It is important that the integrity of the plasma membrane remains intact. Despite the death of individual liver cells, the tissue structure is not affected. The remaining apoptotic bodies are later phagocytized by macrophages. (4)

A cell surface receptor (CD 95/APO-1/Fas) that can trigger apoptosis was first described in 1989 (S. Yonehara et al.). Besides Fas, there are further receptors which mediate the apoptosis of hepatocytes, such as TNF-δ, TGF-β and TRAIL (= TNF-related apoptosis-inducing ligand). (16, 41) *Pro-apoptotic proteins* include Bcl-2, Bcl-w, Mcl-I and Brag-1; *anti-apoptotic proteins* include Bax, Bad, Bak and Bag. Only isolated cells are affected by apoptosis, usually 40–60 per 10^5 hepatocytes, mainly in the area of two cellular columns around the terminal liver vein. The process of apoptosis seems to be irreversible. At first, the cell disengages from the neighbouring cells, showing "wild movements" (= *boiling stage*). The stability of the cell membrane declines, and evaginations of the cell appear (= *zeiosis*). Finally, vesicles encompassed by membrane are discharged (= *blebbing stage*). The cell nucleus ruptures, and chromatin is condensed; the DNA is split. The organelles are unchanged, and no lysosomal enzymes are released. No inflammatory or fibrotic reactions occur. The remnants of the apoptotic hepatocytes form eosinophilic *acidophilic bodies,* which are then expelled from the cell aggregate and later phagocytized by Kupffer cells. These residual bodies are additionally found in viral hepatitis, drug-induced toxic liver damage and yellow fever; they are also called *Councilman bodies*. The shrunken cell or other cellular residues are likewise phagocytized. • The decomposed liver cells are replaced by new hepatocytes ("*moulting*"). It is assumed that the **normal values of liver enzymes** (with their low range of variation) are largely based upon this programmed cell death. (4, 32, 41)

> The genetically determined normal life-span of hepatocytes is, however, impaired by the negative effects of an unhealthy lifestyle, exogenous and endogenous noxae, or pathological processes. • *In such instances, the physiologically programmed death of cells due to ageing is prematurely triggered by provoked cell death.*

3.4.2 Provoked cell death

Provoked cell death is not genetically regulated, but is a passive, incidental process triggered by pathological stimuli. This is a non-energy-consuming process, whereby the integrity of the plasma membrane and of the organelles is destroyed, as is the overall tissue structure. The result is cellular disintegration with subsequent release of the cell contents into the extracellular space. This is followed by a concomitant inflammatory response, later progressing to tissue regeneration or fibrosis. Possible **causes** are: (*1.*) severe disorders of the mitochondrial energy metabolism with loss of ATP, (*2.*) loss of protective cellular substances, such as reduced glutathione, and (*3.*) release of lysosomal enzymes and toxic oxygen products (such as H_2O_2, hydroxyl radicals and singlet oxygen) by activated macrophages. (4) • These causal pathobiochemical factors affect hepatocytes in various modes and combinations as well as over different time sequences. The degenerative reactions are correspondingly variable and intensive. Provoked cell death always affects larger accumulations of liver cells. At the outset, the organelles are usually damaged, with a number of noxae initially causing harm to certain components of the cell (mitochondria, membranes, cytoskeleton, lysosomes, etc.). Lysosomal enzymes are released from the liver cells at an early stage. As a rule, inflammatory and scarring reactions are observed. • *Thus the degenerative changes, which are in themselves always reversible, can ultimately become irreversible and cause cell death.*

3.4.3 Cell necrosis

Cell necrosis in the form of coagulation necrosis or colliquation necrosis can be detected approximately 6 hours after the death of a liver cell. • **Coagulation necrosis** is characterized by a loss of water with subsequent concentration of the cytoplasm and shrinkage of the cell. This is also termed *acidophilic necrosis*. Shrinkage leads to eosinophilic, elongated and unevenly frayed hepatocytes, so-called *stift cells*. This breaks off its connection to adjacent cells. The nucleus becomes pyknotic and caryolytic. The remaining cytoplasm is strongly eosinophilic owing to the breakdown of RNA and denaturation of protein. • **Colliquation necrosis,** nowadays known as *lytic necrosis*, becomes evident in cases of water uptake and cell swelling (= ballooning). It is caused by the impact of hydrolytic enzymes (proteases, nucleotidases). Cytolysis, which is focused on the lobules, leads to patchy or string-like parenchymal loss. Inflammatory infiltrates occur as a reaction to lytic necroses. Various patterns of necrosis are differentiated according to the degree and distribution of cell destruction in the acinus. The liver cells disappear as a result of enzymatic lysis, and empty reticular fibre nets (s. p. 23) (s. fig. 2.7) or even collapsed fibre areas are the outcome. (3)

Programmed cell death (apoptosis) and cell necrosis can be differentiated by morphology. However, liver diseases are often accompanied by a combination of both processes, so that there is mostly no clear borderline. Therefore, the term **necrapoptosis** was introduced. (30) This coexistence of apoptosis and necrosis is often explained with the help of calcium-induced mitochondrial permeability transition (MPT).

A prerequisite for the development of cell necrosis is the loss of cellular ATP reserves. However, 15—20% of the normal ATP reservoir are sufficient to prevent cell lysis. In the same way, fructose (a glycolytic ATP donor) has been shown to inhibit cell necrosis in laboratory experiments. This could be an explanation for the fact that fructose infusion was formerly considered to be effective in liver diseases.

Single-cell necrosis: Necrotic hepatocytes are found both as groups and in isolation. Initially, they either form small patches or are disseminated throughout the liver. The reticular fibres at first remain, but are later removed.

Cell-group necrosis: Lytic necrosis comprising larger groups of hepatocytes can be located at certain positions within an acinus (= *zonal necrosis*) or throughout the entire lobule (= *panlobular necrosis*). • So-called *surgical necrosis* occurs mainly during abdominal operations and can manifest in single-cell or cell-group forms. It results from surgical trauma or hypoxia and is principally found in centroacinar areas.

Confluent necrosis: Cell-group necroses can merge within a lobule (= *submassive necrosis*) or connect affected areas in several different lobules (= *multilobular necrosis*).

Bridging necrosis: These are extensive types of confluent necroses lying within a single acinus or connecting neighbouring lobules (J. L. BOYER et al. 1970). The reticular fibre network collapses. Bridging necrosis can appear between the central veins (= *venovenous*) or the portal tracts (= *portoportal*) of neighbouring lobules. Once they have been removed, it is possible to identify a strand-like collapse of the reticular fibres of the sinusoids.

Piecemeal necrosis: This is the fundamental element of a progressive, chronic-inflammatory process. The necrosis is brought about by cytotoxic T lymphocytes, which may be located within a recess of the hepatocyte (= *peripolesis*) or inside the hepatocyte itself (= *emperipolesis*). (s. fig. 21.11) • The necrotic process takes place at the crossover between mesenchyma (portal tract, septa) and parenchyma, whereby mononuclear cells (primarily lymphocytes, plasma cells, macrophages) penetrate the boundary and infiltrate the acinus (= *interface hepatitis*). The interface between parenchyma and mesenchyma becomes blurred. Kupffer cells are hypertrophied and there is a proliferation of the ductuli. So-called *liver cell rosettes* are also occasionally found near piecemeal necroses. (31) These are light-coloured, hydropic hepatocytes which are arranged around a central lumen and often surrounded by fine connective-tissue fibres. Liver cell rosettes are deemed to be an expression of regenerative activity.

The progressive course of cell damage through to **cell death** is mainly characterized by *two biochemical meta-*

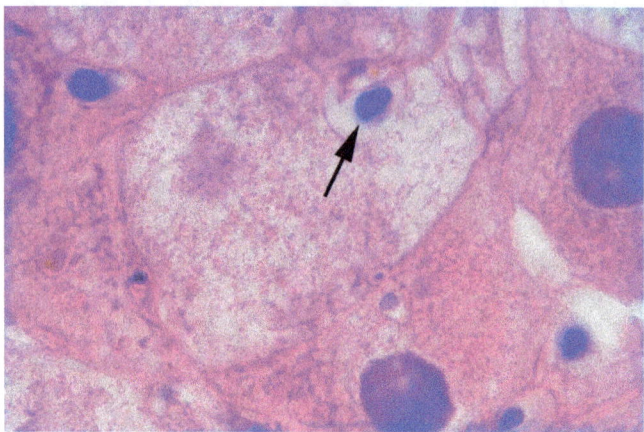

Fig. 21.11: Degenerated hepatocyte with either an intracellular lymphocyte, which is often surrounded by a narrow clear halo (= *emperipolesis*), or a lymphocyte invaginated in the cell membrane (= *peripolesis*) – it is perhaps a T lymphocyte. This condition points to immunologically induced liver damage in florid virus hepatitis B (HE)

bolic processes: (*1.*) oxidative stress and (*2.*) disruption of intracellular Ca^{2+} homoeostasis. These two processes interact, so that the oxidative stress induces the disruption of calcium homoeostasis; there are also, however, other reciprocal actions/effects involving further cellular metabolic processes. (27)

▶ **Oxidative stress** is caused by the dominance of pro-oxidants (= *reactive oxygen intermediates*) over anti-oxidants (= enzymatic or non-enzymatic anti-oxidants as well as auxiliary reactions supporting anti-oxidants). (s. p. 72) Several pro-oxidants have properties of radicals, rendering them reactive and unstable; some reactive oxygen intermediates (ROI) are not radicals. ROIs are indispensable to many metabolic processes – yet if they predominate, they precipitate severe damage to various biological substances. They can evoke the all-important oxidation of polyunsaturated fatty acids (= *lipid peroxidation*) (s. p. 73) or address target areas in carbohydrates and proteoglycans, proteins or enzymes, and nucleic acids. The disruption of different cellular substrates in various intensities and combinations can produce a multifaceted picture of biochemical damage and its outcome. In contrast, cell damage may not only be the upshot of oxidative stress, but also the cause of it, so that a *vicious circle* is set up, whereby the cellular damage is reinforced. An imbalance between pro-oxidants and anti-oxidants with a predominance of reactive oxygen intermediates or free radicals can therefore culminate in hepatocellular degeneration and provoke cell death. (15, 24, 44, 45) (s. fig. 21.12)

▶ **Disrupted calcium homoeostasis:** Normal concentrations of ionized calcium in the cytosol (0.05–0.2 µm), in the overall liver cell (0.5–2.0 µm) and in the extracellular space (1.0 µm) maintain the function of numerous Ca-dependent enzymes and structural elements of the liver cell. Calcium homoeostasis is maintained by the regulatory functioning of all Ca^{2+} transportation systems, energy supply in the form of ATP and intactness of the biomembranes. Defective calcium homoeostasis can cause an increase in calcium in the cytosol, which in turn activates calcium-dependent enzymes, alters the metabolic functions of the cell and disrupts the gap junctions and tight junctions. These biochemical changes result in various forms of hepatocellular degeneration and ultimately in cell death. (s. fig. 21.12)

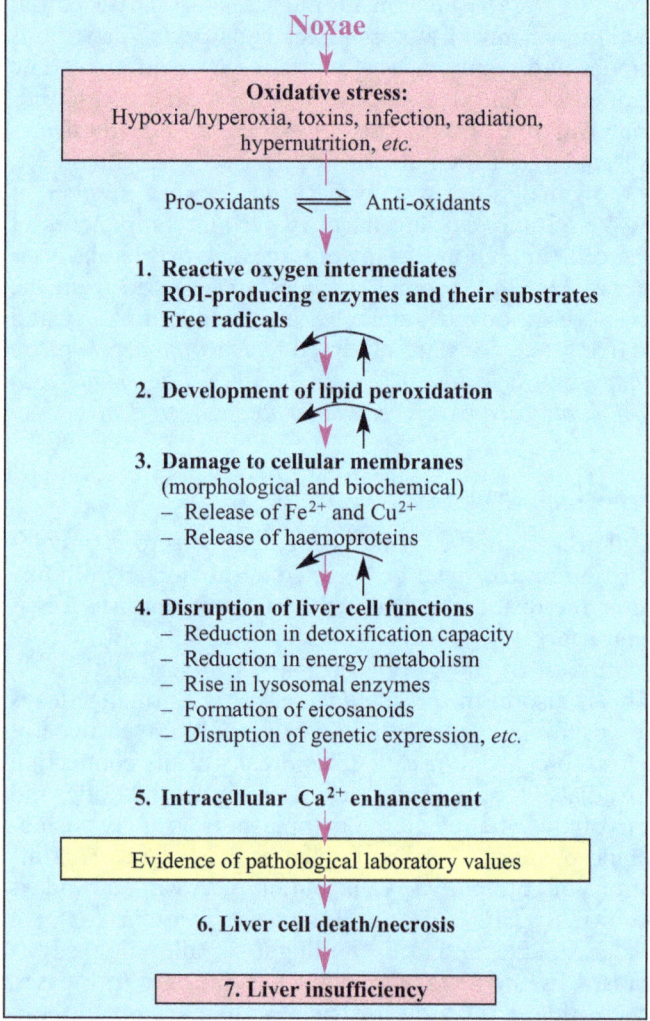

Fig. 21.12: Biochemical causative mechanisms of hepatocellular degeneration and cell death due to oxidative stress and disruptions of cellular calcium homoeostasis (similar to a vicious circle)

3.5 Regeneration

Our present knowledge concerning the extraordinarily complex process of liver regeneration stems almost exclusively from experiments on animals and isolated hepatocytes in culture. • *In principle, this exceedingly complicated concept depends on the close collaboration of hepatocytes, non-parenchymal cells and elements of the extracellular matrix as well as the fine coordination between proliferative and anti-proliferative factors.*

Physiological liver regeneration follows the physiological ageing of the liver cells (= programmed cell death). (s. p. 406) *Reparative liver regeneration* results from a loss of liver tissue or cell death caused by damage. *Complete regeneration* leads to normal histoarchitecture and return of all cell-specific functions. *Incomplete regeneration* is given if the defective area is filled with replacement tissue.

In the process of regeneration, irreversibly damaged or surgically removed liver tissue is replaced as far as possible by new growth. The *regeneration* of the liver (s. p. 5!) is a most important process in (*1.*) overcoming necrosis, (*2.*) determining the course of a liver disease, (*3.*) liver resection, (*4.*) partial liver transplantation, and (*5.*) liver cell transplantation. (29)

The morphological signs of liver regeneration include (*1.*) increase in cell proliferation (= bright cytoplasm of the hepatocytes) and mitoses, (*2.*) appearance of hepatocytes containing two to three nuclei with greater variability (= dyskaryostasis), (*3.*) formation of two to three rows of liver cell trabeculae, (*4.*) occurrence of liver cell rosettes around a central lumen, and (*5.*) proliferation of cholangiocytes. • The hepatocytes of a cirrhotic liver react to a much smaller extent to growth-stimulating factors than those of the normal liver (S. KISO et al., 1994).

The regenerative processes can largely be attributed to *enhanced cellular division,* i. e. compensating hyperplasia (= increase in the tissue volume through a rise in the number of cells), and to the differentiation and multiplication of *liver stem cells*, particularly in those cases where the remaining liver tissue is insufficient to induce adequately compensating hyperplasia. Thus a loss of <15% of liver tissue does not induce compensating hyperplasia, whereas a loss of >75% of liver tissue means that DNA synthesis does not suffice to compensate such extensive tissue damage. • With a loss ranging between 15 and 75%, DNA synthesis and the mitotic index are enhanced in the remaining liver in relation to the reduction in tissue volume. (39)

▶ **Liver regeneration** takes place in three phases: (*1.*) *pre-replicative phase*, with preparation for mitosis, (*2.*) *proliferative phase*, with wave-like mitoses at 6–8 hour intervals, and (*3.*) *restitution phase*, with reconstitution of the liver structure. • There are **two stages** to this whole process: (*1.*) *priming*, which is the transition of latent hepatocytes (G_0) into the mitotic cycle (G_1) – this reversible process is triggered by cytokines, hormones or other permissive substances, whereby the cells proliferate due to stimulation by the growth factor; (*2.*) *progression* is the transition from G_1 to DNA synthesis (S) – this transition point from G_1 to S is marked by the expression of cyclin D_1.

DNA synthesis begins just 10 to 12 hours after partial liver resection, and after another 10 to 20 hours, mitotic division reaches maximum activity. Replication in the endothelial cells and bile duct epithelia follows within one to three days. Some three or four weeks subsequent to a right-sided hemihepatectomy, the size, structure and function of the liver are largely restored, and six months later, regeneration is generally complete. • *After restoration of the normal organ size (with a fluctuation range of only 5–10%), the regenerative processes come to an end – there is no "overregeneration". Nor is there any formation of hepatomas or malignant transformations.* The best conditions for regeneration are found in young patients (10 to 45 years).

Regulation: The course taken by regenerative processes is regulated by **cyclins** and **CDK** (= cyclin-dependent kinases). The regenerative cycle is also controlled by cell-specific **regulator proteins.** They are designated by the letter "p" (protein) and their respective molecular weight (given in kD), e. g. p16, p21, p24, p27, p53, p107. • There are numerous **signal compounds** which are essential to the regeneration of the liver, acting in a stimulating or inhibiting capacity in accordance with the respective regeneration phase. They likewise consist of small protein particles which have a wide range of action. These signal substances act through receptors attached to the cell membrane. As a result, biochemical signals are directly transmitted to certain organelles in the cell and the nucleus, where the transcription of specific genes is controlled.

Stimulators such as *HGF* (= hepatocyte growth factor), *TGF-α* (= transforming growth factor), *EGF* (= epidermal growth factor), *FGF-1 and 2* (= fibroblast growth factor), *CT-1* (= cardiotrophin 1) and *HSS* (= hepatic stimulatory substance) affect DNA synthesis and the replication of hepatocytes. • The **permissive substances**, which are considered to be essential for the effectiveness of the growth factors, are glucagon, insulin, IGF-I and II, T_3 and T_4, calcitonin, ACTH, oestrogens, vasopressin and interleukins. • *HGF is regarded as the most effective mitogen, whereby this effect is enhanced by noradrenaline.* Merely one or two hours after a partial liver resection, the plasma levels of HGF increase to 15–17 times their normal value; 10 to 20 hours later, the rise in DNA synthesis commences. In fulminant liver failure, the HGF levels were found to be elevated, as they were in 80% of patients with CAH or cirrhosis; this is probably due to the insufficient hepatic clearance of HGF or to its increased formation in the extrahepatic cells. • *TGF is important in stimulating the proliferation and differentiation of hepatocytes. In contrast, FGF-2 and plasminogen are mainly responsible for the proliferation of non-parenchymal cells and for angiogenesis.*

Inhibitors of DNA synthesis and cell replication are *TGF-β* and *HPI* (= hepatic proliferation inhibitor). Their function is to block the growth-promoting factors once the nominal size of the liver has been reached. • The regeneration course is, however, also linked to a complex **network** of biochemical processes, including the polyamines (putrescine, spermidine and spermine) as well as the precursors of nucleic acids (orotate, thymidine and uridine). (17, 33, 47–49, 56)

> The coordinated and regulated **regeneration of the liver** can thus be regarded as one of the most outstanding features in human life — no other organ possesses this ability to regenerate, with the complete restoration of size, structure and function. • *Why* — one may ask — *was this ability attributed only to the liver as far back as antiquity, and not to any other organ?* Was this just a product of the imagination projected into this mantically meaningful organ, or had the repercussions of liver injury really been observed? *After all, the first two hints of the regenerative capacity of the liver go back almost 3,000 years! (s. p. 5)*

3.6 Fibrogenesis

The process of fibrogenesis results in an increase in the extracellular matrix, i.e. all insoluble organic constituents of the interstitial space. This represents an uniform, dynamic and potentially reversible reaction of the liver to chronic injury. Fibrosis is considered to be a possible forerunner of liver cirrhosis.

The **functions of the extracellular matrix** are manifold: *(1.)* stabilization of the tissue and organ structure, *(2.)* structural linkage of cells, *(3.)* transmission of information between the various types of cells within the tissue and the extracellular milieu, *(4.)* adhesion or migration of cells, and *(5.)* influence on the development and differentiation of cells and their polarity. • In fibrogenesis, collagen fibres build the framework in which the other components of the extracellular matrix are embedded. In line with this wide scope of functions, the extracellular matrix is not only organ-specific as regards its architecture, but it also displays variations at different locations within the liver, e.g. in Disse's space, in the periportal fields and within the acinus zones. • The extracellular matrix is a dynamic structure, i.e. there is a constant equilibrium between build-up (by matrix-metalloproteinases = **MMP**) and break-down (by tissue inhibitors of matrix metalloproteinases = **TIMP**).

The **main constituents of the extracellular matrix** are *(1.)* collagen, particularly the fibrillary types I (36%), III (36%) and V (16%) as well as the non-fibrillary types IV (9%), VI (0.2%) and to a minor degree also type VII, *(2.) glycoproteins* (fibronectin, tenascin, laminin, undulin, elastin, entactin), and *(3.) proteoglycans* of both the core protein and the glycosaminoglycan type (e.g. chondroitin, heparan sulphate, hyaluronic acid, dermatan sulphate).

Profibrogens: These matrix substances are produced in a variety of ways in the liver and sinusendothelial cells. The Ito cells, which are activated into myofibroblasts, are deemed the most important site of synthesis for virtually all types of matrix. Stellate cells take in apoptotic hepatocyte remnants. Thus, they produce ten times more collagen type I and eight times more $TGF_{\beta 1}$. The latter activates fibroblasts and keratinocytes. Perivenular myofibroblasts, portal fibroblasts, sinus endothelium and bile duct epithelium can also take over the synthesis of matrix proteins. Production of the matrix substances is stimulated by signal substances and controlled by regulatory factors. (s. tab. 21.2)

Profibrogens	Antifibrogens
Endothelin-1	HGF
FGF	Interferon-γ
ILGF	Interleukin-10
Interleukin-1, -4, -6	TNFα
Leptin (in ASH and NASH)	*etc.*
PDGF	
TGFα	
$TGF_{\beta 1}$	
Drug-related antifibrogenesis	
Canrenone	Baicalen
Captopril	Colchicine
Interferon-α	Glyzirrhicin
Pentoxyfilline	Halofuginone
Silymarin	PGE_2

Tab. 21.2: Some cytokines and peptides as well as chemical or herbal substances with profibrogenetic and antifibrogenetic effects

Antifibrogens: Some cytokines and peptides have an inhibitory effect on fibrogenesis. Formation and breakdown of the extracellular matrix are regulated by collagenases, stromelysin, proteases, endoglycosidases, etc. These *enzymes*, which are responsible for breaking down the components of the matrix, are mainly produced in Kupffer and endothelial cells as well as in fibroblasts. • A number of *substances* also have an antifibrogenic effect under clinical conditions. In this context, pentoxyfylline and silymarin are worth mentioning; of equal interest are halofuginon and baicalen extracted from the Chinese plant sho-saiko-to. (35) (s. tab. 21.2)

Pathologic fibrogenesis: As a rule, there are no abnormal matrix components in pathological fibrogenesis; the tendency is for the total mass to increase as much as eight to ten times the normal amount, albeit in varying proportions for each individual substance. There is an excess of collagen types I and IV as well as of hyaluronane, chondroitin sulphate and dermatan sulphate, with a relative reduction in heparan sulphate. The collagen content (with a normal level of 0.5%) may rise to 50% of the protein fraction of the liver, which is equivalent to three to six times the normal level of approximately 7 mg/g wet weight. Acetaldehyde produced during the metabolism of alcohol considerably stimulates fibrogenesis by enhancing the transcription of genes for matrix components, in particular collagen type I and fibronectin. Reactive oxygen intermediates as well as non-protein-bound iron in haemochromatosis also have a stimulating effect on fibrogenesis.

Standstill: It can be assumed that fibrogenesis will initially come to a standstill upon cessation of the causative factors or stimulating signals. When the extracellular matrix is only moderately increased, the lobular structure, the vascular supply and the bile flow from the periportal fields are undisturbed. A balance between the stimulation and inhibition of fibrogenesis can develop, stopping "liver fibrosis" at the point which has been reached.

Regression: It is of clinical relevance that an enzymatic breakdown occurs as well in order to cope with the augmented production of matrix components, thereby resulting in regression of fibrosis. Whether, on the other hand, pathological fibrogenesis progresses even after the causative factors cease to be present has not yet been clarified, even though this has been demonstrated in vitro. (6, 19, 23, 35, 37, 42)

4 Hepatitis and hepatosis

4.1 Hepatitis

▶ It was DIOGENES OF APPOLONIA who first used the term "hepatitis" when referring to the so-called "liver vessel". (s. p. 6) • In his "Historia hepatica" (1725), J. B. BIANCHI grouped the various types of diffuse inflammation of the liver under the term "hepatitis".

In histomorphological terms, **hepatitis** means "inflammation of the liver". The factor causing the disease may spread from the initially or predominantly affected **mesenchyma** to the liver cells (such as in kala-azar and malaria), or the primarily or mainly affected **liver cells** may subsequently incorporate the mesenchyma into the damaging process (as for example in yellow fever). • In leptospirosis and herpes virus infection, the morphological finding is determined almost exclusively by changes in the parenchyma, while mesenchymal reactions are hardly or not at all present.

As long as the interaction between the liver and the causative factor (viruses, toxins, noxae, etc.) is restricted to the *mesenchyma* or the connective tissue (particularly within the periportal field), i.e. if directly adjacent hepatocytes have not as yet been damaged, no rise in transaminase levels (GPT, GOT) is to be expected in laboratory examinations. These mesenchymal reactions range from signs of portal inflammation (cellulation, oedema, activation of fibroblasts) to Kupffer cell reactions (changes in shape, swelling, proliferation or pseudoproliferation) through to proliferation of the bile ducts and fibrotic processes.

The spread of the damaging processes to adjacent *hepatocytes* is signalled by an increase in transaminase activity; the liver cell membranes are also affected. The result is an enhanced release of cytoplasmic enzymes (GPT, to a lesser extent also GOT) into the serum. Ultimately, cell necrosis must be expected with a rise in mitochondrial enzymes in the serum (GDH, mGOT). From the point of view of biochemistry, the term hepatitis presupposes an increase in indicator enzymes once the hepatocytes have been damaged or destroyed. (s. pp. 101, 109) (s. tabs. 5.6, 5.7, 5.11)

The term hepatitis is frequently used with a variety of **differentiating attributes**, e.g. acute, necrotic, chronic, cholestatic, and with attributes which are not quite correct from a pathohistological viewpoint, e.g. diffuse, non-specifically reactive, granulomatous or focal. • Taking a histological and biochemical approach, the complex process of hepatitis can indeed be accepted as such and allocated to a larger group of clinical pictures. • This interpretation might make it easier to understand the terms *"serous inflammation"* (R. RÖSSLE, 1929) and *"acute interstitial serous hepatitis"* (H. EPPINGER, 1937).

The classical **inflammation criteria** such as *exudation*, *cellulation* and *proliferation* can only be applied to the liver with some reservations, since the emphasis in this instance is on the sinusoids, which already display maximum permeability under normal conditions. The increase in capillary permeability, required by the definition of inflammation, is really only applicable to the area of the vascularized portal fields, e.g. in purulent cholangitis. The definition of inflammation can only be applied to classic acute viral hepatitis. (s. p. 423)

It is to be expected that the current criteria of inflammation in hepatology will be reviewed and revised.

4.2 Hepatosis

▶ The term *hepatosis* was used for the first time (according to our research) by F. PIELSTICKER in 1921 (34) in analogy to the nephrosis-nephritis concept before being subsequently adopted by A. GÉRONNE. (22) It was then made known on a large scale and became the subject of controversial discussion as a result of the frequently quoted publication by R. RÖSSLE (1929). (38) Especially H. KALK (1957) showed a commitment to this concept. • Hepatosis can be defined as a *"metabolic disorder of the hepatocyte in the widest sense"* (L.-H. KETTLER, 1965), which is the focal point for the morphological approach during the entire course of disease (G. HOLLE, 1967; H. U. ZOLLINGER, 1968; W. DOERR, 1970; O. KLINGE, 1984).

Non-inflammatory, primary degenerative changes in the liver, which mostly affect only the parenchyma, are known under the term hepatosis. • The causative damage can be of an exogenous or endogenous nature. Electron microscopy has yielded a better understanding of the primary degenerative alterations of the liver parenchyma, which in turn has been the reason for a revival of the term hepatosis. (s. p. 404)

Endogenous hepatosis comprises endogenous metabolic disorders of the liver cell; the terminology used in this context refers to accumulated substances (e.g. glycogenosis), harmful substrate (e.g. fructose-1 phosphate) or enzyme defect (e.g. α_1-antitrypsin deficiency).

Exogenous hepatosis is caused by numerous and varying substances, which are taken up externally and transported to the liver cell, e.g. alcohol, medication, chemicals, toxins. Its pathogenesis is still unresolved, which is why the nomenclature remains subject to debate.

5 Fibrosis and cirrhosis

5.1 Fibrosis

Fibrosis is defined as local or diffuse augmentation of the extracellular matrix together with an additional disproportionate increase in its individual components. It is not possible to detect any structural or functional abnormality concerning the respective matrix substances, which are now being generated to a growing extent. The lobular structure remains intact. Fibrosis is a dynamic process which is potentially reversible.

Fibrosis is usually the consequence or concomitant symptom of a chronic hepatobiliary disease, the course of which can itself be unfavourably influenced by the fibrosis. The matrix substances, which are being produced in greater quantities, are increasingly deposited in Disse's space in the portal field and periportal area as well as around the terminal liver vein.

Morphological changes result from the increasing deposition of matrix components: more pronounced portal and periportal formation of connective tissue, constriction of lobular areas by connective tissue, narrowing or obstruction of small vessels, neovascularization within the connective tissue septa, and disorders in the lobular structure. • **Functional disorders** are also given: the haemodynamic system is increasingly impaired, resulting in portal hypertension with its own specific complications; the metabolic exchange of substrates, the oxygen supply and the clearance of toxic substances are greatly impeded; the bile flow from the portal fields is reduced. • Hepatic fibrosis can come to a *standstill* at any level, either temporarily or permanently, yet may even be *accelerated* by the activation of Ito cells. It is also possible for the fibrosis to *regress* due to enzymatic breakdown. (1, 6, 23, 35, 40)

▶ In line with the differences in aetiopathogenesis, there are various *mechanisms of fibrosis development:* (*1.*) fibrosis due to changes in preformed intralobular and portal fibres, (*2.*) fibrosis resulting from the destruction of liver cells (= *substitute fibrosis*), (*3.*) fibrosis as a consequence of the collapse of the reticulin-fibre scaffolding (yet without an increase in collagen fibres) with complete or partial lobular necrosis or bridging necrosis (= *collapse fibrosis*), (*4.*) enhanced neoformation or diminished breakdown of the extracellular matrix, and (*5.*) fibrosis resulting from the proliferation of bile ducts (= *periductal fibrosis*). (s. fig. 33.14)

Serum markers: The clinical validation of possible serum markers of fibrosis or fibrolysis causes great difficulties, since this condition generally shows only slow changes over a long period. Furthermore, the ubiquitous presence of molecules of the extracellular matrix in other organs can produce false values in liver fibrosis. • The propeptide of type III procollagen (**P-III-P**) is taken as a serum-related marker for assessing the metabolism of collagen. The P-III-P value is a criterion for measuring the turnover of extracellular matrix components. (s. p. 118) (26, 43) In the meantime, it is possible to measure several markers of matrix deposition (e.g. P-III-C, P-III-N, tenascin) or matrix removal (e.g. P-IV-C, P-IV-N, collagen IV, undulin) with the help of reproducible and relatively sensitive **sandwich ELISA tests**. Similarly, an elevated serum value of $TGF\beta_1$ can point to increased fibrogenesis. (1, 35) • A decrease in the **prothrombin index** less than or equal to 80% points to severe fibrosis. (8) The introduction of useful markers for connective-tissue metabolism would be of great importance for detecting progressive and regressive fibrosis as a result of antifibrotic therapy. (s. tab. 21.2)

Forms and courses: In line with the morphological **activity,** a distinction can be made between *progressive* and *stationary* fibroses, which appear either as mild or severe with regard to their intensity and can be reversible or irreversible in terms of their course. Depending on the extent of the inactive stationary fibrosis, the hepatic function is only slightly or not at all impaired. In contrast, active progressive fibrosis gives rise to portal hypertension, which can actually become reversible once the fibrosis is inactivated. • Fibrosis can be differentiated according to its **localization**: (*1.*) portal/periportal, (*2.*) perisinusoidal, and (*3.*) perivenous. In the case of (*4.*) diffuse fibrosis of the liver, all three areas are typically affected, but to varying degrees of intensity. Furthermore, there is (*5.*) periductal fibrosis. An exact discrimination of the various types is often impossible. • **Intralobular focal fibrosis** can be caused by minor losses of parenchyma, formation of granulomas, recovery of abscesses, obliteration of a cavernous haemangioma, reaction of parasites in the liver parenchyma, etc. • A **regression of fibrosis** is possible: this process could be demonstrated in successfully treated haemochromatosis, during abstinence following alcohol abuse, after IFN therapy in chronic hepatitis C, and in Indian childhood cirrhosis after penicillamine therapy.

5.1.1 Scarred liver

Scarred liver (H. KALK, 1957) develops following large-scale loss of parenchyma, which is replaced by scar tissue without bulbiform metaplasia. Outside this scar, the lobular architecture is retained. During laparoscopy, these multilobular necroses of the parenchyma are visible as concave greyish-white to greyish-red scars with deep retractions, depicting the so-called *funnel liver*. • The left liver lobe in particular can shrink to a slender scarred disc due to its poor blood supply. (s. figs. 21.13; 22.16; 35.1, 35.17!)

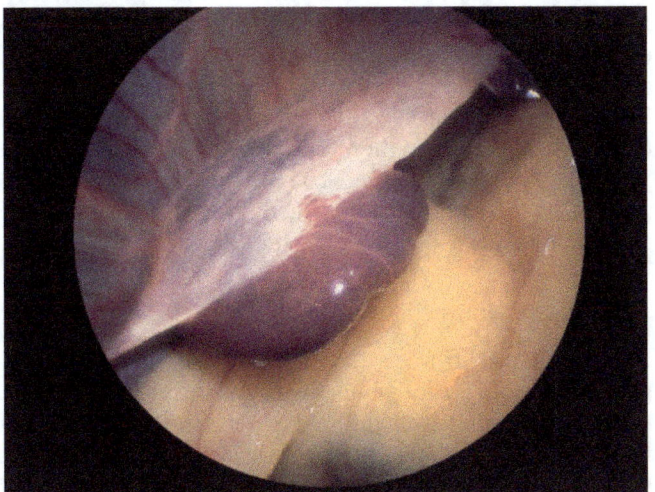

Fig. 21.13: Atrophy of left liver lobe due to acute viral hepatitis B

5.1.2 Portal/periportal fibrosis

A fibrotic widening of the portal fields (with differing intensity and often variable regional distribution) is a frequent finding in chronic hepatitis, and it plays an important role in staging. (s. p. 715) However, it may also be a remnant of previous hepatitis. In many cases, strands of connective tissue extend into the periportal parenchyma. Mostly, there is portal/periportal fibrosis with an irregular star-shaped pattern. (s. fig. 21.14)

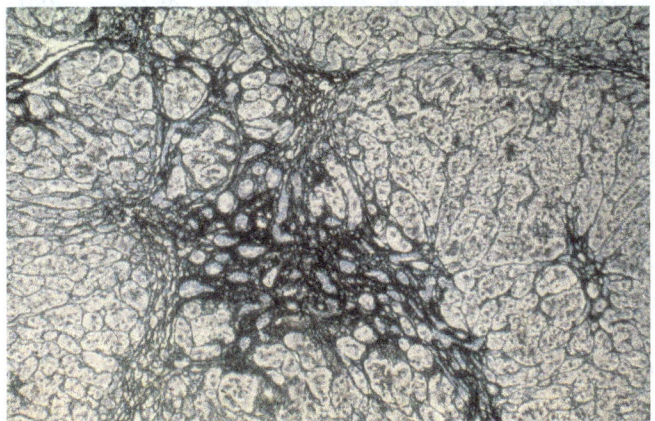

Fig. 21.14: Periportal and septal fibrosis following severe acute viral hepatitis B: clearly disrupted liver architecture; older collapse fields with condensed reticular fibres (Gomori's reticulin stain)

The reticular fibre structure of the sinusoids breaks apart, while liver cells try to remedy the parenchymatous defects in the area of the lobules. In chronic, alcohol-induced liver disease, *brushwood-like fibrosis* is often present. In hereditary haemochromatosis, there is usually evidence of a *holly-leaf fibrosis*: thickened portal fields and finger-like fibrosis with flat ends. Such a pattern is also seen in cholangitic processes with biliary portal fibrosis. The portal bile ducts become encircled by connective tissue in an onion-like manner, which is termed *periductular fibrosis*. Occasionally, *portal-centrolobular fibrosis* and *portal-perilobular fibrosis* can be detected. Particular mention should be made here of a special form in schistosomiasis, the so-called *pipe-stem fibrosis*. (s. fig. 25.14)

Portal/periportal fibrosis can be found in:	
α_1-AT deficiency	haemochromatosis
alcohol abuse	hepatoportal sclerosis
Byler's disease	methotrexate
chronic cholangitis	obstructive jaundice
congenital fibrosis	PBC, PSC
cystic fibrosis	schistosomiasis
galactosaemia	thorotrastosis
graft-versus-host	Wilson's disease, *etc.*

5.1.3 Perisinusoidal fibrosis

In perisinusoidal fibrosis (also called intermediate fibrosis), fibres develop along the sinusoids, or they encircle the individual hepatocyte in a pericellular manner. These forms either affect the whole lobule equally or they show a tendency to invade the periportal or central region of the lobule. Initially, the lobular structure is not affected, nor is the vascular supply restricted. • The progressive fibrogenesis leads to a **capillarization of sinusoids** (F. SCHAFFNER et al., 1963): the deposition of glygoproteins and collagen fibres in Disse's space causes the formation of a basal membrane below the endothelial cells. The sieve plate-like structure is lost, mainly due to alcohol and endotoxin. The endothelial cells express CD34, factor VIII, endothelin-1, etc. These factors induce the perisinusoidal cells to contract, supporting the development of portal hypertension. Such capillarization impedes the metabolic exchange of substrates, i.e. between plasma and the sinusoidal surface of the hepatocytes. • *Chicken-wire fibrosis* is a characteristic finding in chronic, alcohol-induced liver disease. (s. fig. 21.15) A particular example of a sinusoidal/pericellular fibrosis is connatal syphilis, which is termed *brimstone fibrosis*. (s. p. 489)

Perisinusoidal/pericellular fibrosis can be found in:	
• arsen intoxication	• myeloproliferative disease
• Budd-Chiari syndrome	• osteomyelosclerosis
• chronic alcohol abuse	• portal vein thrombosis
• chronic blood congestion	• Schönlein-Henoch
• connatal fibrosis	• vinyl chloride

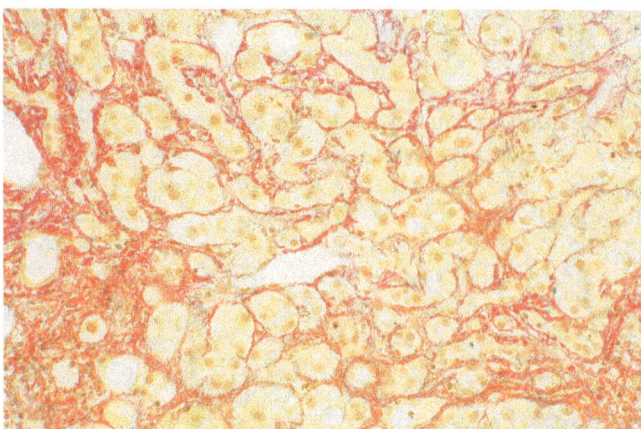

Fig. 21.15: Pericellular trabecular fibrosis with a wire mesh pattern (= *chicken-wire fibrosis*) due to chronic alcohol abuse (Sirius red)

5.1.4 Perivenous fibrosis

Central venules only contain a small amount of collagen, with the result that in this form of fibrosis, perivenous sinusoids are always involved. A typical example is perivenular fibrosis in chronic alcohol abuse. (s. fig. 21.16) Centrolobular fibrosis may also be detectable in healed viral hepatitis or following slight liver damage (e. g. Meulengracht's disease). *Central hyaline sclerosis*, which is due to chronic alcohol abuse with intermittently recurring alcohol hepatitis, is a particularly severe form of fibrosis.

Perivenous fibrosis can be found in:	
• Budd-Chiari syndrome	• healed hepatitis
• chronic alcohol abuse	• Meulengracht's disease
• chronic blood congestion	

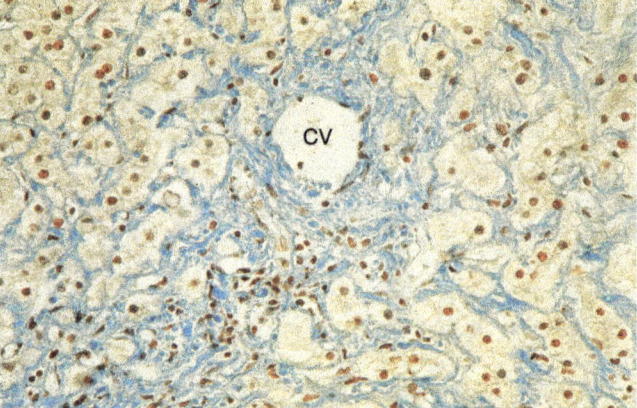

Fig. 21.16: Perivenular and perisinusoidal fine-meshed fibrosis and discreet cellular inflammatory reaction as a result of chronic alcohol abuse (ASH) (CV = central vein) (Ladewig)

5.1.5 Septal fibrosis

In persistent confluent and bridging necrosis, the development of correspondingly located **fibrotic septa** can be observed. • *Portoportal septa* connect neighbouring portal tracts, such as in progressive piecemeal necrosis and in chronic cholestasis with an extensive ductular reaction. • *Centrocentral septa* connect adjacent central veins as a result of confluent cell-group necrosis. • *Portocentral septa* join portal tracts with central veins following corresponding bridging necrosis. • *Active septa* display inflammatory infiltrates of mononuclear cells and are therefore difficult to differentiate from the neighbouring parenchyma. These inflammatory cells are able to stimulate further fibrogenesis. • *Passive septa* display no inflammatory infiltrates and are therefore easily differentiated from the adjacent parenchyma. They represent a cicatricial process in the healing of confluent necrosis. Septa older than six months can contain elastic fibres.

5.1.6 Liver collapse fibrosis

Liver collapse fibrosis must be differentiated from proper liver fibrosis, which displays increased deposition of a qualitatively altered extracellular matrix. It results from a collapse of the reticular fibres following liver cell necrosis. • A *primary collapse* arises subsequent to confluent cell-group necrosis in a previously normal parenchyma. • A *secondary collapse* develops as a result of extensive necrosis in previously damaged parenchyma (e. g. cirrhosis).

Inactive, stationary or even regressive liver fibrosis constitutes the healing of a pathological event by means of connective tissue. Such *partial (fibrous-defective) recovery through the formation of connective tissue* is regarded as a therapeutic success.

5.2 Cirrhosis

▶ *The elimination of the lobular structure is the essential component of all forms of cirrhosis.* • Pronounced necrosis or extensive proliferation of connective tissue do not serve as adequate criteria, nor are inflammatory processes a prerequisite in this respect. Neither aetiology nor the presence of regeneration nodes are criteria for liver cirrhosis. *(see chapter 35)*

5.2.1 Basic criteria

The criteria for the development and completion of liver cirrhosis can be assessed according to their importance:

1. Pronounced parenchymal necrosis, not balanced by reparative mechanisms
2. Diffuse increase in connective tissue
3. Varying degrees of nodular regeneration

4. *Elimination and metaplasia of the lobular structure, in principle covering the entire liver*
5. *Disruption of the intrahepatal (venous, portal and arterial) haemodynamic system*

5.2.2 Systematic approach

Aetiology: It would be beneficial to establish a systematic approach to cirrhosis based on the underlying aetiology, since this would allow both preventive and therapeutic measures to be initiated. Only some forms of cirrhosis allow aetiological identification from morphological criteria. Nevertheless, given the simultaneous application of all laboratory parameters, clinical findings and imaging procedures, it is possible to clarify the aetiology of cirrhosis − *the frequency of "cryptogenic" cirrhosis has been continually reduced in line with improvements made in detailed diagnostics. (see chapter 35)*

However, a systematic approach to cirrhosis can only be founded to a limited degree on aetiological principles, since (*1.*) it has not been possible to define the cause in many cases, (*2.*) one specific cause can trigger different morphological forms in different patients, (*3.*) several causes can result in the same form, and (*4.*) several causes often merge in a variety of combinations.

Morphology: A systematic approach to cirrhosis based on morphology has so far found the widest acceptance and consequently given rise to various principles regarding classification. (2, 20) Any such approach should, however, focus on the processes which are evident in each individual case:

1. *Formation of regeneration nodes*
   - macronodular (> 3 mm)
   - micronodular (< 3 mm)
   - mixed nodular
   - "smooth" surface cirrhosis
2. *Postdystrophic* (**monophasic**) *cirrhosis*
   (= incomplete postnecrotic cirrhosis)
3. *Pathogenic development*
   - regular forms of cirrhosis
   - irregular forms of cirrhosis
   - biliary cirrhosis
   - vascular cirrhosis
4. *Collapsed form and development of septa*

Experience shows that the course of cirrhosis can be reconstructed from the morphological findings although certain **mixed forms** are to be expected:

(*1.*) Atrophic, *finely nodular* cirrhosis, which is low in regenerative capacity and rich in connective tissue, generally develops if the underlying damage persists and its pronounced impact continues. (s. fig. 28.9)

(*2.*) Cirrhosis which is hypertrophic, *coarsely nodular*, rich in regenerative capacity and poor in fibrosis usually develops if the damage occurs in episodes with intermittent phases of respite. Consequently, the formation of regeneration nodes can be helpful in assessing the duration of the "recovery phases". (s. fig. 35.2)

(*3.*) *Mixed nodular* cirrhosis (i.e. fine and coarse nodules of varying site and number) (s. fig. 35.8)

(*4.*) *"Smooth"* cirrhosis (i.e. without recognizable nodules on the liver surface) (s. fig. 14.3)

Aetiopathogenetical and morphological criteria, are to be considered as separate, but complementary factors. In some cases, the aetiopathogenetic cause can be diagnosed by reliable morphological findings.

The **transformation of the lobular architecture** is initiated and maintained by at least two histomorphological processes: (*1.*) piecemeal necrosis and (*2.*) bridging necrosis, which provides string-like links between the central veins and the portal fields. Portocentral shunts, which are of significance for the "fate" of cirrhosis, make use of these bridges as routes for their development. During the course of time, these channels, which acquire solid basal membranes like capillaries, carry the portal blood directly to the venous flow-off. As a result, blood is withdrawn from the respective acini; these areas become more susceptible to disruption and damage and are forced to restructure anew. *(see chapter 35)*

▶ The **disruption of intrahepatic haemodynamics** due to *liver necrosis + shunts + formation of septa* ultimately constitutes self-perpetuating lobular transformation: *"This is the curse of every evil deed that, propagating still, it brings forth evil."* (F. VON SCHILLER in his tragedy "Wallenstein")

5.2.3 Morphological diagnosis

Morphological assessment of cirrhosis depends on whether the **liver material** was obtained by post-mortem autopsy (when lymphohistiocytic inflammatory reactions are hardly detectable) or biopsy using a Menghini needle (which rarely yields fully assessable cirrhotic material). In contrast, biopsies carried out with a Silverman needle produce an adequately sized biopsy cylinder.

Suspicion of cirrhosis is based on various **criteria:** (*1.*) fragments of the biopsy cylinder are surrounded by fibres, (*2.*) central veins have a non-eccentric arrangement, (*3.*) evidence of increased vascularization or vascular ectasia and possibly also of poor vascularization, (*4.*) variability of the nuclear pattern, (*5.*) different epithelial sizes with divergent glycogen content, and (*6.*) disordered, tubular or reticular epithelial areas.

It is possible that some of the **uncertainties in diagnosis** as well as any existing differences in the systematic approach to liver cirrhosis taken by pathologists and clinicians might simply be attributable to the fact that the material used for assessment has been considered as representative although it was, in fact, inadequate and obtained by faulty procurement techniques.

Clinical and scientific statements on the morphology of cirrhosis are based on certain **criteria** (s. pp. 165, 168):

> 1. in-vivo examination of tissue
> 2. tissue specimens obtained through laparoscopic biopsy (and not only by blind biopsy!)
> 3. sufficient compact hepatic tissue (best obtained using a Silverman needle)
> 4. additional documentation intended for the pathologist using colour photography of the liver surface (since the macroscopic images are frequently of greater relevance in postnecrotic, coarse-nodular transformation processes and it is obviously impossible to cover the entire process by way of biopsy)

6 Liver tumours

Both benign and malignant tumours may be found in the liver. They originate in (1.) liver cells, (2.) connective tissue, (3.) blood and lymph vessels, and (4.) bile ducts. An updated systematic classification and nomenclature for nodular hepatocellular lesions was set up in line with the agreement worked out in Los Angeles in 1994. (53) The classification is based on pathogenesis, aetiology and prognosis. A determinant factor for any systematization is the question of whether the cells prove to be regenerative or can be classified as dysplastic, or possibly even neoplastic, and which characteristics are displayed by the respective adjacent stroma of the liver.

6.1 Benign tumours

Benign liver tumours are no rarity. As a rule, they only give rise to symptoms or biochemical findings if they have reached a critical size or if they become noticeable due to the compression of blood vessels or bile ducts. Such tumours may be of clinical importance because of their potential precarcinogenicity in individual cases as well as their tendency to massive bleeding following traumatization. Benign liver tumours can be differentiated as (1.) *epithelial*, (2.) *cholangiolitic*, (3.) *vascular*, and (4.) *mesenchymal*. It is also possible to differentiate liver cysts (congenital or acquired). *(see chapter 36)*

(1) *Benign epithelioid tumours* include liver cell adenoma, biliary adenoma, biliary cystadenoma, biliary papillomatosis, *etc.*

(2) *Benign mesenchymal tumours* include angiomyolipoma, lymphangioma, haemangioma, infantile haemangioendothelioma, leiomyoma, *etc.*

(3) *Tumour-like lesions* include hamartoma, FNH, NRH, focal steatosis, peliosis hepatis, inflammatory pseudotumour, cysts, lobular hyperplasia, postnecrotic regenerative nodes, *etc.*

Regenerative lesions are the result of localized proliferation of liver cells and their stroma. They are seen as the main response to various types of liver damage. Generally, they are circumscribed and 0.5–3.0 cm (or more) in diameter. They can grow and build up daughter nodes ("nodule in nodule"). The parenchyma is regular; these lesions contain portal fields, bile ducts and blood vessels. The hyperplastic hepatocytes are arranged in enlarged liver cell columns consisting of two to three plates. Usually, there are no cell atypias. • Congenital or acquired vascular anomalies or irregularities of the arterial blood supply with focal hyperperfusion may cause the formation of regenerative lesions. A multitude of biochemical factors and hormones also play a key role. (53, 55) (s. p. 408) Regenerative lesions are classified in five main groups. (s. tab. 21.3)

> 1. Monoacinar regenerative nodes
>   - *diffuse nodular regenerative hyperplasia without fibrotic septa (NRH)*
>   - *diffuse nodular hyperplasia with fibrotic septa or within cirrhosis (DNH)*
> 2. Multiacinar regenerative nodes
> 3. Lobular or segmental hyperplasia
> 4. Cirrhotic nodule
>   - *monoacinar*
>   - *multiacinar*
> 5. Focal nodular hyperplasia (FNH)
>   - *solid type*
>   - *teleangiectatic type*
>   – *solitary*
>   – *multiple*

Tab. 21.3: Classification of regenerative lesions

Dysplastic lesions: Due to changes in the cytoplasm or the nucleus, dysplastic lesions exhibit histological features, such as irregular structure or growth. Genetic factors are probably involved (though appropriate criteria do not yet exist for all forms). (53) (s. tab. 21.4)

> 1. Hepatocellular adenoma
> 2. Dysplasia
> 3. Dysplastic focus
> 4. Dysplastic nodule
>   - low-grade (slightly dysplastic)
>   - high-grade (severely dysplastic)

Tab. 21.4: Classification of dysplastic lesions

6.2 Malignant tumours

In classifying malignant liver tumours, differentiation has to be made between primary and secondary liver tumours (J. B. GIBSON et al., 1978; K.G. ISHAK, et al., 1994). **Primary liver tumours** are differentiated in four groups. (s. tabs. 21.5; 37.1) *(see chapter 37)*

> 1. Epithelial tumours
> 2. Mesenchymal tumours
> 3. Neuroendocrine tumours
> 4. Mixed forms

Tab. 21.5: Classification of primary malignant liver tumours

Secondary malignant liver tumours can be divided into different groups. (s. tab. 21.6)

1. Liver metastases
2. Malignant infiltration (per continuitatem)
3. Myeloid metaplasia
4. Myeloproliferative disease
5. Lymphomatosis

Tab. 21.6: Classification of secondary malignant liver tumours

References:

1. **Afdahl, N.H., Nunes, D.:** Evaluation of liver fibrosis: A concise review. Amer. J. Gastroenterol. 2004; 99: 1160–1174
2. **Anthony, P.P., Ishak, K.G., Nayak, N.C., Poulsen, H.E., Scheuer, P.J., Sobin, L.H.:** The morphology of cirrhosis: definition, nomenclature, and classification. Bull. World Health Organ. 1977; 55: 521–540
3. **Bianchi, L.:** Necroinflammatory liver diseases. Semin. Liver Dis. 1986; 6: 185–198
4. **Bilodeau, M.:** Liver cell death: update on apoptosis. Canad. J. Gastroenterol. 2003; 17: 501–506
5. **Bracero, L.A., Gambon, T.B., Evans, R., Beneck, D.:** Ultrasonographic findings in a case of congenital peliosis hepatis. J. Ultrasound Med. 1995; 14: 483–486
6. **Brenner, D.A., Waterboer, T., Choi, S.K., Lindquist, J.N., Stefanovic, B., Burchardt, E., Yamauchi, M., Gillan, A., Rippe, R.A.:** New aspects of hepatic fibrosis. J. Hepatol. 2000; 32 (Suppl. 1): 32–38
7. **Buitrago, B., Popper, H., Hadler, S.C., Thung, S.N., Gerber, M.A., Purcell, R.H., Maynard, J.E.:** Specific histologic features of Santa Marta hepatitis: a severe form of hepatitis δ-virus infection in Northern South America. Hepatology 1986; 6: 1285–1291
8. **Croquet, V., Vuillemin, E., Ternisien, C., Pilette, C., Oberti, F., Gallois, Y., Trossaert, M., Rousselet, M.C., Chappard, D., Cales, P.:** Prothrombin index is an indirect marker of severe liver fibrosis. Eur. J. Gastroenterol. Hepatol. 2002; 14: 1133–1141
9. **De Groote, J., v. Desmet, J., Gedigk, P., Korb, G., Popper, H., Poulsen, H., Scheuer, P.J., Schmid, M., Thaler, H., Uehlinger, E., Wepler, W.:** A classification of chronic hepatitis. Lancet 1968/II: 626–628
10. **Denk, H., Scheuer, P.J., Baptista, A., Bianchi, L., Callea, F., de Groote, J., Desmet, V.J., Gudat, F., Ishak, K.G., Korb, G., Macsween, R.N.M., Phillips, M.J., Portmann, B., Poulsen, H., Schmid, M., Thaler, H.:** Guidelines for the diagnosis and interpretation of hepatic granulomas. Histopathology 1994; 25: 209–218
11. **Denk, H., Stumptner, C., Zatloukal, K.:** Mallory bodies revisited. J. Hepatol. 2000; 32: 689–702
12. **Devaney, K., Goodman, Z.D., Epstein, M.S., Zimmerman, H.J., Ishak, K.G.:** Hepatic sarcoidosis: clinicopathologic features in 100 patients. Amer. J. Surg. Path. 1993; 17: 1272–1280
13. **Dincsoy, H., Wessner, R.E., MacGee, J.:** Lipogranulomas in non-fatty human livers. A mineral oil induced environmental disease. Amer. J. Clin. Pathol. 1982; 78: 35–41
14. **Eising, E.G., Auffermann, W., Peters, P.E., Schmidt, H., Ullrich, K.:** Fokale Peliosis der Leber im Erwachsenenalter in Kombination mit einer Glykogenose Typ I (v. Gierke). Kasuistik und Übersicht über neuere Literatur. Radiologe 1990; 30: 428–432
15. **Elstner, E.F.:** Oxygen radicals-biochemical basis for their efficacy. Klin. Wschr. 1991; 69: 949–956
16. **Faubion, W.A., Gores, G.J.:** Death receptors in liver biology and pathobiology. Hepatology 1998; 29: 1–4
17. **Fausto, N.:** Liver regeneration. J. Hepatol. 2000; 32 (Suppl. 1): 19–31
18. **Ferrell, L.D.:** Hepatic granulomas: a morphologic approach to diagnosis. Surg. Path. 1990; 3: 87–106
19. **Friedman, S.I.:** Molecular regulation of hepatic fibrosis, an integrated cellular response to tissue injury. J. Biol. Chem. 2000; 275: 2247–2250
20. **Galambos, J.T.:** Classification of cirrhosis. Amer. J. Gastroenterol. 1979; 64: 437–451
21. **Gaya, D.R., Thorburn, D., Oien, K.A., Morris, A.J., Stanley, A.J.:** Hepatic granulomas: A 10 year single centre experience. J. Clin. Path. 2003; 56: 850–853
22. **Géronne, A.:** Zur Pathogenese einiger Formen des Ikterus. Klin. Wschr. 1922; 828–832
23. **Gressner, A.M.:** Mediators of hepatic fibrogenesis. Hepatogastroenterol. 1996; 43: 92–103
24. **Halliwell, B., Gutteridge, J.M.C., Cross, C.E.:** Free radicals, antioxidants, and human disease: where are we now? J. Lab. Clin. Med. 1992; 119: 598–620
25. **Harrington, P.T., Gutierrez, J.J., Ramirez-Ronda, C.H., Quinones-Soto, R., Bermudez, R.H., Chaffey, J.:** Granulomatous hepatitis. Rev. Inf. Dis. 1982; 4: 638–655
26. **Hayasaka, A., Saisho, H.:** Serum markers as tools to monitor liver fibrosis. Digestion 1998; 59: 381–384
27. **Kaplowitz, N.:** Mechanisms of liver cell injury. J. Hepatol. 2000; 32 (Suppl. 1): 39–47
28. **Kerr, J.F.R., Wyllie, A.H., Currie, A.R.:** Apoptosis: a basic biological phenomenon with wide-ranging implications in tissue kinetics. Brit. J. Cancer 1972; 26: 239–257
29. **Koniaris, L.G., McKillop, I.H., Schwartz, S.I., Zimmers, T.A.:** Liver regeneration. J. Amer. Coll. Surg. 2003; 197: 634–659
30. **Lemasters, J.J.:** Mechanisms of hepatic toxicity. V. Necrapoptosis and the mitochondrial permeability transition: shared pathways to necrosis and apoptosis. Amer. J. Physiol. 1999; 276: 1–6
31. **Nagore, N., Howe, S., Boxer, L., Scheuer, P.J.:** Liver rosettes: structural differences in cholestasis and hepatitis. Liver 1989; 9: 43–51
32. **Patel, T.:** Apoptosis in hepatic pathophysiology. Clin. Liver Dis. 2000; 4: 295–317
33. **Peters, M., Roeb, E., Pennica, D., Meyer zum Büschenfelde, K.-M., Rosejohn, S.:** A new hepatocyte stimulating factor: Cardiotrophin-1 (CT-1). FEBS Letters 1995; 372: 177–180
34. **Pielsticker, F.:** Die akute infektiöse stomatogene Hepatose. Dtsch. Med. Wschr. 1921; 289–290
35. **Pinzani, M., Rombouts, K.:** Liver fibrosis: From the bench to clinical targets (review). Dig. Liver Dis. 2004; 36: 231–242
36. **Rasenack, U.:** Die „granulomatöse Hepatitis". Dtsch. Med. Wschr. 1984; 109: 226–230
37. **Rockey, D.C.:** The cell and molecular biology of hepatic fibrogenesis: clinical and therapeutic implications. Clin. Liver Dis. 2000; 4: 319–355
38. **Rössle, R.:** Hepatose und Hepatitis. Schweiz. Med. Wschr. 1929; 59: 4–9
39. **Rubin, E.M., Martin, A.A., Thung, S.N., Gerber, M.A.:** Morphometric and immunhistochemical characterization of human liver regeneration. Amer. J. Path. 1995; 147: 397–404
40. **Sarin, S.K., Kapoor, D.:** Non-cirrhotic portal fibrosis: current concepts and management. (review) J. Gastroenterol. Hepatol. 2002; 17: 526–534
41. **Schattenberg, J.M., Galle, P.R., Schuchmann, M.:** Apoptosis in liver disease (review). Liver Internat. 2006; 26: 904–911
42. **Schuppan, D.:** Structure of the extracellular matrix in normal and fibrotic liver: collagens and glycoproteins. Semin. Liver Dis. 1990; 10: 1–10
43. **Schuppan, D., Jax, C., Hahn, E.G.:** Serum markers of liver fibrosis. Dtsch. Med. Wschr. 1999; 124: 1213–1218
44. **Sies, H.:** Biochemie des oxidativen Streß. Angew. Chem. 1986; 98: 1061–1075
45. **Sies, H.:** Strategies of antioxidant defense. Eur. J. Biochem. 1993; 215: 213–219
46. **Simon, D.M., Krause, R., Galambos, J.T.:** Peliosis hepatis in a patient with marasmus. Gastroenterology 1988; 95: 805–809
47. **Takiya, S., Tagaya, T., Takahashi, H., Kawashima, H., Kamiya, M., Fukuzawa, Y., Kobayashi, S., Fukatsu, A., Katoh, K., Kakumu, S.:** Role of transforming growth factor β1 on hepatic regeneration and apoptosis in liver diseases. J. Clin. Path. 1995; 48: 1093–1097
48. **Tomiya, T., Tani, M., Yamada, S., Hayashi, S., Umeda, N., Fujiwara, S.:** Serum hepatocyte growth factor levels in hepatectomized and non-hepatectomized surgical patients. Gastroenterology 1992; 103: 1621–1624
49. **Tsubouchi, H., Hirono, S., Gohda, E., Nakayama, H., Takahashi, K., Sakiyama, O., Kimoto, M., Kawakami, S., Miyoshi, H., Kubozono, O., Kawarada, Y., Mizumoto, R., Arakaki, N., Daikuhara, Y., Hashimoto, S.:** Human hepatocyte growth factor in blood of patients with fulminant hepatic failure. I. Clinical aspects. Dig. Dis. Sci., 1991; 36: 780–784
50. **Uchida, T., Kao, H., Quispe-Sjogren, M., Peters, R.L.:** Alcoholic foamy degeneration–a pattern of acute alcoholic injury of the liver. Gastroenterology 1983; 84: 683–692
51. **Valla, D.C., Benhamou, J.P.:** Hepatic granulomas and hepatic sarcoidosis. Clin. Liver Dis. 2000; 4: 269–285
52. **Van Erpecum, K.J., Janssens, A.R., Kreuning, J., Ruiter, D.J., Kroon, H.M.J.A., Grond, A.J.K.:** Generalized peliosis hepatis and cirrhosis after long-term use of oral contraceptives. Amer. J. Gastroenterol. 1988; 83: 572–575
53. **Wanless, I.R.:** Terminology of nodular hepatocellular lesions. Hepatology 1995; 22: 983–993
54. **Zafrani, E.S., Cazier, A., Baudelot, A.M., Feldmann, G.:** Ultrastructural lesions of the liver in human peliosis. A report of 12 cases. Amer. J. Pathol. 1984; 114: 349–359
55. **Zatloukal, K., French, S.W., Stumptner, C., Strnad, P., Harada, M., Toivola, D.M., Cadrin, M., Omary, M.B.:** From Mallory to Mallory-Denk bodies: What, how and why? Exper. Cell Res. 2007; 313: 2033–2049
56. **Zhang, B.H.:** Growth signals in liver regeneration. Hepatology 1997; 12: 44–46

Clinical Aspects of Liver Diseases
22 Acute viral hepatitis (A–SEN)

		Page:			Page:
1	*History of acute viral hepatitis*	421	4.8.3	Perinatal infection and antenatal care	436
2	*Morphology and aetiopathogenetic range*	422	4.8.4	Close physical contact	436
2.1	Histomorphological changes	423	4.9	Hepatitis B and medical personnel	437
2.2	Sonographic morphology	424	4.9.1	Medical personnel	437
2.3	*Specific courses of disease*	424	4.9.2	Hepatitis B and the dialysis unit	438
2.3.1	Minimal hepatitis	424	4.9.3	Hepatitis B and dentistry	438
2.3.2	Drug-induced hepatitis	424	4.9.4	Insurance questions	438
2.3.3	Cholestatic course of disease	424	4.10	Stages of disease	439
2.3.4	Anicteric course of disease	425	4.11	Extrahepatic manifestations	440
2.3.5	Fulminant course of disease	425	4.12	Specific clinical courses of disease	440
2.3.6	Giant-cell hepatitis	425	4.12.1	Subclinical course	440
2.4	*Aetiopathogenetic diversity*	425	4.12.2	Anicteric course	440
3	**Acute viral hepatitis A**	426	4.12.3	Protracted course	440
3.1	Definition	426	4.12.4	Recurrent course	441
3.2	Pathogen	427	4.12.5	Cholestatic course	441
3.2.1	Inactivation	427	4.12.6	Fulminant course	441
3.2.2	Detection	427	4.12.7	Subacute course	441
3.2.3	Replication	427	4.12.8	Chronic course	441
3.3	Transmission	427	4.13	Hepatitis B and pregnancy	442
3.4	Epidemiology	428	4.14	Hepatitis B and hepatocellular carcinoma	442
3.4.1	Frequency of disease	428	4.15	Prophylaxis	442
3.4.2	Obligation for notification	428	4.15.1	General hygiene measures	442
3.5	Pathogenesis	428	4.15.2	Passive immunoprophylactic measures	443
3.6	Serological diagnostics	429	4.15.3	Simultaneous vaccination	443
3.7	Stages of disease	429	4.15.4	Active protective vaccination	443
3.8	Extrahepatic manifestations	430	4.16	Therapy	445
3.9	Clinical courses of disease	430	4.16.1	Aims of treatment	445
3.10	Formation of granulomas	430	4.16.2	Methods of treatment	445
3.11	Prophylactic measures	430	4.17	Healing of hepatitis B	446
3.11.1	Passive immunization	430	4.17.1	Morphological healing process	446
3.11.2	Active vaccination	431	4.17.2	Biochemical healing process	447
3.11.3	Simultaneous vaccination	431	5	**Acute viral hepatitis C**	448
3.12	Therapy	431	5.1	Definition	448
4	**Acute viral hepatitis B**	431	5.2	Pathogen	448
4.1	Definition	431	5.2.1	Genotypes	448
4.2	Pathogen	431	5.2.2	Inactivation	449
4.2.1	Inactivation	432	5.3	Serological diagnostics	449
4.2.2	Pathogenesis	432	5.3.1	Anti-HCV test	449
4.3	Antigens and antibodies	432	5.3.2	RT-PCR test	449
4.4	HBV variants	433	5.4	Epidemiology	449
4.5	Specific serological courses of disease	434	5.5	Transmission	450
4.6	Chronic HBsAg carriers	434	5.6	Histological findings	451
4.7	Epidemiology	434	5.7	Stages of disease	451
4.7.1	Obligation for notification	435	5.8	Extrahepatic manifestations	452
4.8	Transmission	435	5.9	Hepatitis C and hepatocellular carcinoma	453
4.8.1	Parenteral infection	435	5.10	Prophylaxis and therapy	453
4.8.2	Sexual infection	436	6	**Acute viral hepatitis D**	454

Chapter 22

		Page:				Page:
6.1	Definition	454	7.2	Pathogen		457
6.2	Pathogen	454	7.3	Epidemiology		457
6.2.1	Mutants	454	7.4	Transmission		457
6.3	Transmission	454	7.5	Serological diagnostics		458
6.4	Epidemiology	455	7.6	Clinical aspects and courses of disease		458
6.5	Serological diagnostics	455	7.7	Prophylaxis and therapy		458
6.5.1	Coinfection	455	8	*Acute viral hepatitis NA-NE*		458
6.5.2	Superinfection	455	9	*HF virus*		458
6.6	Courses of disease	455	10	*HG virus*		458
6.6.1	Coinfection	455	11	*GB viruses*		459
6.6.2	Superinfection	456	12	*TT virus*		459
6.7	Special features of HDV infection	456	13	*SEN virus*		460
6.8	Prophylaxis	456	14	*Other viruses*		460
6.9	Therapy	456		● References (1–553)		461
7	*Acute viral hepatitis E*	456		(Figures 22.1–22.20; tables 22.1–22.9)		
7.1	Definition	457				

22 Acute viral hepatitis

1 History of acute viral hepatitis

> HIPPOCRATES described a potentially dangerous disease widely found in young people and accompanied by jaundice. • As early as 752, Pope ZACHARIAS wrote in a letter to St. Boniface, Bishop of Mainz (Germany), about "jaundice of a contagious nature" where those affected would have to be segregated.

▶ In 1629 HENRY DE BEER wrote about a **jaundice epidemic** in Spa (Belgium). In 1745 CLEGHORN described the clinical picture of jaundice prevalent during an epidemic in Menorca (Spain). In 1761 I. F. HERLITZ (14) observed many jaundice patients in Göttingen (Germany) and gave an impressive description of the clinical symptoms of this benign illness, which mainly occurred in winter; this was all the more interesting since he himself was suffering from it. The term **icterus epidemicus** in fact stems from him (and was also proposed by A. HENNIG in 1890). • Descriptions of jaundice epidemics were to follow from Bremen (Germany) (1760), Essen (Germany) (G. F. H. BRUENING, 1772), Genova (Italy) (1792), Lüdenscheid (Germany) (F. KERCKSIG, 1799), Greifswald (Germany) (L. MENDE, 1810), etc. In fact, more than 80 epidemics in Europe and 6 outside Europe were recorded by C. KÖHNHORN (1877) (16), C. FRÖHLICH (1879) (11) and A. HENNIG (1890). Numerous publications focused on the frequency of epidemic jaundice in garrisons and at theatres of war, so that the illness also became known as *"soldier's disease"*. • Its causal **origin** was deemed to be poor hygiene, vermin, overcrowding, climatic factors, monotonous and nauseating nutrition, mental trauma, physical strain and polluted water. (quot. in 4, 11, 16) H. EPPINGER (1908) believed that this apparently epidemic jaundice was, in fact, an accidental accumulation of non-infectious diseases. Almost all epidemics were accompanied by severe courses of disease and many deaths. As early as 1862, R. J. GRAVES pointed out that "the worst was to be feared if there were any signs of nervous symptoms during the course of jaundice" (hepatic encephalopathy?). He attributed the cause of jaundice to gastroenteritis and believed that it also affected the bile ducts. This opinion was so convincing for R. VIRCHOW (1864) (29) that he later adopted the term **icterus catarrhalis** for catarrhal jaundice, a term that had been introduced by H. QUINCKE (1903): the bile was thick and sticky with subsequent obstruction of the small bile ducts and development of jaundice. At a later date, he also assumed the cause to be an intercurrent mucous plug in the duodenal papilla. However, towards the end of the 19th century, it was increasingly thought to be an infectious disease (A. E. CH. CHAUFFARD, 1885; S. P. BOTKIN, 1888 [it was also known as **Botkin's disease** in Russia and the Baltic countries]; A. HENNIG, 1890; O. MINKOWSKI, 1904, etc.). The main localization of the disease was already considered to be in the liver parenchyma, but the source of the infection was unknown. Airborne transmission was also postulated. (6)

▶ Reports drawn up by LÜRMAN (20) and JEHN (15) on the epidemics in Bremen (Germany) and Merzig (Germany) following inoculation with smallpox vaccine are considered to be the first ever regarding the **parenteral route of infection** (i.e. HBV and HCV infections). In Bremen (Germany) 191 persons (out of 1,290 cases) and in Merzig (Germany) 144 persons (out of 510 cases) succumbed to the disease. Further reference to the parenteral transmissibility of infectious jaundice was made by A. FLAUM et al. (1926), G. M. FINDLAY et al. (1937), C. H. GROSSMAN et al. (1946), etc. After an inoculation campaign with a measles convalescent serum involving 109 children, A. S. MCNALTY (1937) observed the occurrence of jaundice in 47% of cases with a mortality rate of 22%. • W. SIEDE (1949) reported that 19% of 125 children developed jaundice after an infusion of insulin and dextrose. • In 1943 in the USA, the term *homologous serum jaundice* was introduced, but it was also known as *serum hepatitis*. Over the following years, the terms *haematogenous hepatitis*, *inoculation hepatitis, transfusion hepatitis* and **homologous serum hepatitis** were used as well. (21, 27)

▶ In 1919 F. LINDSTEDT introduced the term **hepatitis epidemica** for epidemic jaundice. In 1930, however, G. LEPEHNE proposed the term "hepatia" to avoid emphasizing its inflammatory character. The term **icterus simplex** can be attributed to G. V. BERGMANN (1931). Another term used was **infectious hepatitis,** proposed by G. M. FINDLAY et al. (1939). • Since the morphological studies carried out by H. EPPINGER et al. (1935) revealed "acute destructive hepatitis" and the characteristics of "serous inflammation" (R. RÖSSLE, 1929), icterus catarrhalis has also been considered morphologically as "hepatitis", and the term *"acute interstitial serous hepatitis"* is used. In 1937 H. EPPINGER distinguished the parenchymal from the periacinal or cholangiolitic form of hepatitis, an idea which is reflected by the present-day term of acute *viral hepatitis with cholestatic character*. H. EPPINGER was already familiar with the term *anicteric hepatitis*, which he called "icterus sine ictero" (1937). • In 1940 F. CORELLI claimed icterus catarrhalis to be an allergic inflammation which could possibly be improved by desensitization therapy. He reports on a number of interesting observations of icteric patients under a variety of conditions. (7)

First World War: The tremendous **jaundice epidemics** witnessed during the war in practically every army and those in the thirties among the civilian population called for a new definition. • An excellent monograph was drawn up by F. v. BORMANN (1940), critically evaluating the entire material available (406 publications quoted!). (4) The clinical picture was described in great detail, all theories and doctrines quoted and observations and experiments presented with the greatest of care. The viral nature of the pathogen was postulated on the basis of the findings. • The publication brought out in the same year (1940) by F. LAINER from Eppinger's hospital is an excellent supplement to the level of knowledge of that time — yet even in 1940, the opinion was still held that icterus catarrhalis occurred sporadically in the form of serous hepatitis, precipitated by endogenous or exogenous toxins and not by any specific icterogenic pathogen. (18) • T. TH. ANDERSEN et al. (1938) were the first to trigger jaundice in young swine by feeding them the **duodenal juice** of jaundice patients. This in turn could be transmitted in a second passage to other swine by feeding them the raw liver of the first icteric group. The administration of the blood of jaundice patients to swine also led to the occurrence of jaundice with microscopic liver changes. • *No pathogen was found and so it was generally assumed to be an invisible virus (1), as* MCDONALD *had already postulated in 1908.*

Second World War: Large-scale **epidemics**, even **pandemics**, of hepatitis were also rife during the Second World War. Entire military units were severely depleted by the illness. • *I was one of those affected in Russia in 1942.* • The number of cases of hepatitis in the Second World War has been estimated at approximately 16 million. In this period, the first transmission of an infectious agent was effected in a **self-experiment** by H. VOEGT (1941), *who was later to be my tutor in hepatology*. Within three or four weeks, the oral intake of duodenal juice from a hepatitis patient led to the contraction of hepatitis in both himself and in three medical student volunteers (who had not stayed in an epidemic area). Histological focus was on "capillaritis". Six other test persons, who were orally administered haemolyzed blood or urine taken from a jaundice patient (2 cases) or received serum or blood by s.c. or i.m. injection (4 cases), showed symptoms of hepatitis. • *The direct transmission path of an infectious virus was hence deemed proven (30) and the existence of "posthepatic residual damage" established (12).*

▶ In 1952 H. VOEGT told me personally at the university in Giessen (Germany) that he had changed the term **icterus infectiosus** (K. GUTZEIT, 1942) into **hepatitis contagiosa** (1942) — also used by A. DOHMEN in 1943. • The term **hepatitis infectiosa** was proposed by F. MAYTHALER in 1942. • In 1943 F.O. MACCALUM confirmed the transmissibility of an infectious agent. (22)

▶ In 1947 MACCALUM termed hepatitis epidemica as type A and inoculation hepatitis as type B. These results were validated by further studies. (13, 23, 24) S. KRUGMAN et al. (1967) introduced the terms MS1 and MS2 for these two types of virus, which at a later date were to correspond to HAV and HBV. (17) In 1970 virus B was detected by D. S. DANE et al. (8) — following the identification of the Australian antigen by B. S. BLUMBERG et al. (1965) (3) and A. M. PRINCE (1968). (25) In 1973 the hepatitis A virus was discovered by S. M. FEINSTONE et al. (9) In 1977 the delta virus was detected by M. RIZZETTO et al. (28) A pathogen termed hepatitis E virus was identified in 1983 in the stool of an infected volunteer (M.S. BALAYAN et al.). (2) It was assumed that another virus existed (10, 26), which was termed the hepatitis C virus after being identified by Q. L. CHOO et al. in 1989. (5) Detection of the hepatitis G virus (HGV) followed in 1996 (J. LINNEN et al.). (19)

Infectious jaundice is the most imposing clinical picture in hepatology and has occupied physicians for more than 2,500 years, caused epidemics and pandemics all over the world (thus significantly influencing the outcome of wars), led to innumerable experiments as well as controversial theories and culminated in absurd speculations including treatment by the oral administration of live sheep lice. • Today, hepatitis viruses have been (almost) fully explained down to the last molecular, biological and serological detail.

2 Morphology and aetiopathogenetic range

▶ Histologically, the suffix **"itis"** denotes inflammation, thus "hepatitis" can be defined as "inflammation of the liver". This term was coined by J. B. BIANCHI as early as 1725 in order to summarize various diffuse inflammations of the parenchyma.

The classical **criteria of inflammation** (*1.*) *exudation*, (*2.*) *cellulation* and (*3.*) *proliferation* can only partly be applied to the liver, since this organ is predominantly characterized by sinusoids rather than capillaries. An essential problem thus arises in the morphological context of the term "hepatitis". *Due to this specific vascular feature, the otherwise valid association between the terms "inflammation" and "infection" is only marginally true in the case of the liver. In fact, this association is only given with infectious changes within the vascularized fibrous tissue of the portal fields.* • *The problem concerning the definition of "hepatitis" has already been outlined in detail in the last chapter.* (s. p. 411)

Macroscopically, acute viral hepatitis presents as a **large red liver** (H. KALK, 1947). The *enlargement* is probably caused by hyperaemia and the oedematization of the portal area. The *reddening* is due to hyperaemia and the accumulation of large quantities of stagnating erythrocytes in the empty lattice fibre network.

2.1 Histomorphological changes

Histologically, the *parenchyma*, the *mesenchyma* and the *connective tissue* are affected in an almost identical manner. The combination of all lesions together with the onset of hepatocellular regeneration gives the typically **unsettled variegated picture** of acute viral hepatitis, which is more characteristic than any single finding on its own (H.-W. ALTMANN, 1971). • The liver lobules are affected as a whole and in all their components, whereby the hepatocytes at the centre of the lobule are most severely damaged. Therefore, acute viral hepatitis is seen to be **lobular hepatitis.** These changes are shown as constant or inconstant lesions. (31, 34, 36) (s. tab. 22.1)

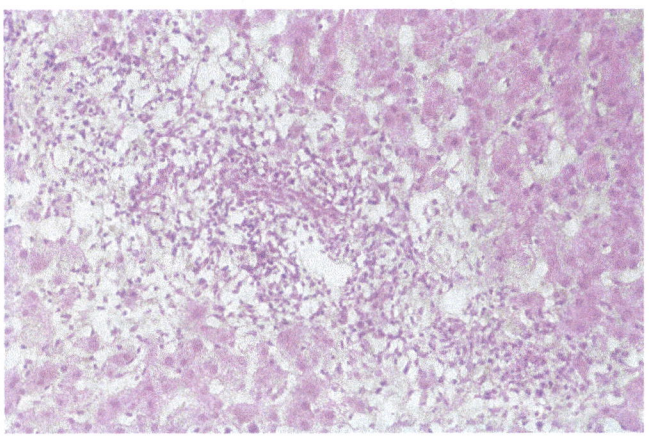

Fig. 22.1: Acute viral hepatitis A: Periportal inflammation and periportal cell loss (HE)

	Lobular	Portal and periportal
Con-stant	**Liver cell degenerations** (hydropic swelling, eosinophilic degeneration, pin cells, hyaline bodies); **cell polymorphy**; single cell **necrosis** (predominantly centrolobular, in the form of acidophilic Councilman bodies); **infiltration** (lymphocytes, macrophages and activated stellate cells, yet only few plasma cells and neutrophilic granulocytes); **proliferation** of sinusoidal cells.	**Lymphohistiocytic infiltration** (small lymphocytes, plasma cells and other mononuclear cells).
Incon-stant	Confluent liver cell necrosis, possibly developing into bridging necroses or multilobular (<3% of cases) or even massive necroses in B, B/D and C hepatitis, as well as in E hepatitis during pregnancy • Collapse of the lattice fibre network • Formation of passive septa, cholestasis, accumulation of ceroid and siderin in macrophages and stellate cells.	Flow of infiltrates into adjacent lobular areas, fibroblast activity • Damage to and proliferation of bile ducts • Accumulation of ceroid and siderin in macrophages.

Tab. 22.1: Morphological changes with acute viral hepatitis

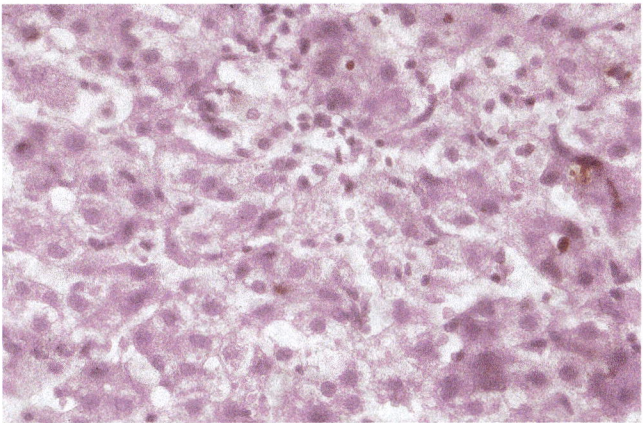

Fig. 22.2: Subsiding acute viral hepatitis A with lytic loss of hepatocytes and round-cell infiltrates (HE)

▶ **Mitoses:** Mitotic figures and binuclear hepatocytes with basophilic cytoplasm are found. The consumption of liver cells by necroses is considerable, as is the concurrent regeneration process, particularly at the onset of acute hepatitis and during the retrogressive phase. • This also explains the remarkable observation that patients with the *Dubin-Johnson syndrome* are found to have far fewer pigment-charged liver cells subsequent to acute viral hepatitis. (s. pp 231, 430)

Stellate cell activation: At the climax of acute viral hepatitis, the stellate cells are diffuse and highly activated.

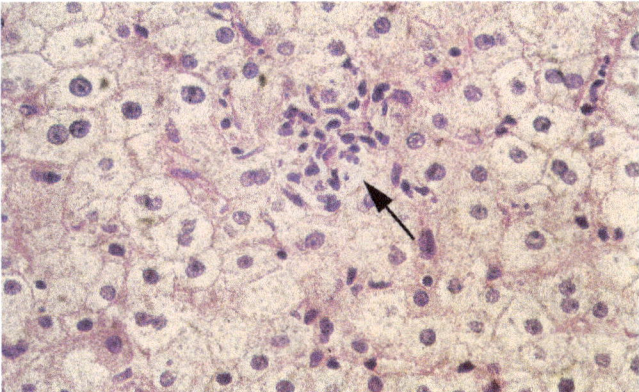

Fig. 22.3: Kupffer cell nodules (arrow) in subsiding acute viral hepatitis B; hydropic hepatocytes, often binuclear (HE)

Stellate cell nodules (s. fig. 22.3) are formed. The diffuse spread of the swelling and the proliferation of sinusoidal cells may recede during the retrogressive phase into localized proliferations. These indistinctly contoured stellate cell nodules are often detected in the necrotic area at an early stage. In this event, they generally contain the liver disintegration pigment **ceroid** (s. fig. 21.6), later also **lipofuscin** (s. fig. 21.3) and **siderin.** Such *resid-*

ual nodules (H. KALK et al., 1947) or *late-phase nodules* (W. WEPLER et al., 1968) are still found one to two months after the acute hepatitis is deemed to be clinically healed. The nodules remain diffusely distributed in the parenchyma until they gradually diminish, lose their pigment and ultimately disappear completely.

▶ **Regeneration:** Regenerative processes overlap with the slowly dwindling inflammation. They are characterized by a proliferation of the liver cell columns, an uneven pattern of cell nuclei, an increase in mitoses and the formation of liver cell rosettes. A modular − like pattern is visible in the trabecula architecture. • Minimal (but negligible) cholestasis is sometimes present. (s. p. 237) Acute viral hepatitis usually heals completely within a period of four to eight weeks.

Collagenation: The empty lattice fibre structure in a de-epithelialized area (with possible collapse of the lattice fibres) becomes increasingly collagenized, so that sclerosis appears at the centre of the lobules in place of lost liver cells. This process may be completely reversible if the regenerated liver cells succeed in respreading the fibres. Otherwise, central fibre scars persist for a longer time. This fibre production occurs far earlier and to a more pronounced extent at the periphery of the lobules. In delayed epithelial regeneration, the fibre layers or cicatrized changes remain as portal fibrosis. (s. p. 412)

2.2 Sonographic morphology

With the help of sonography, it is possible in acute viral hepatitis to obtain the following findings: (*1.*) hepatomegaly, (*2.*) slight increase in brightness, (*3.*) truncated lower liver margin, (*4.*) thickening of the gall-bladder wall (35), and (*5.*) increased blood flow (using duplex sonography).

2.3 Specific courses of disease

Various endogenous or exogenous factors can alter the histomorphological picture of acute viral hepatitis, so that specific courses of disease may become apparent.

2.3.1 Minimal hepatitis

The course of minimal hepatitis (O. KLINGE, 1976) is generally found in anicteric or subicteric patients and only shows minor histological lesions. It is even possible over a period of several years to detect the hyaline bodies, the activation of the sinusoidal cells and the moderate round-cell infiltration of the portal fields as well as single cell necrosis. These changes show no progression, so that histology largely corresponds to that of chronic persistent hepatitis.

2.3.2 Drug-induced hepatitis

Irrespective of the type of drug, acute hepatitis prevails in drug addicts. It is characterized by portal infiltration, often with many eosinophilic leucocytes. Cholestasis is common. The lobular borders may be difficult to define. In most cases, phagocytized exogenous pigments or waste substances are found in the macrophages. • The extent to which primary or secondary hepatotropic viruses are involved must be clarified. (s. tab. 5.16) • Histology, course of disease and prognosis are determined by the duration and intensity of drug intake, polytoxicomania or additional viral infections.

2.3.3 Cholestatic course of disease

▶ The "cholestatic course of disease" (W. SIEDE, 1942) is largely identical to the "periacinal form of icterus catarrhalis" (H. EPPINGER, 1937), "cholangiolitic hepatitis" (C.J. WATSON et al., 1946), "hepatitis with intrahepatic obstruction" (I. MAGYAR, 1953) and "hepatitis with a cholestatic element" (H. KALK, 1957).

Those forms of acute viral hepatitis that have a normal clinical course also present discrete quantities of bile to be found as intraepithelial drops and intercellular cylinders or deposits in the stellate cells. These findings cannot be confirmed biochemically. • A cholestatic course of disease is occasionally observed with a marked increase in alkaline phosphatase, particularly in older patients and in women. It is mostly accompanied by jaundice. The patient's general well-being is significantly compromised, and pruritus is pronounced in most cases.

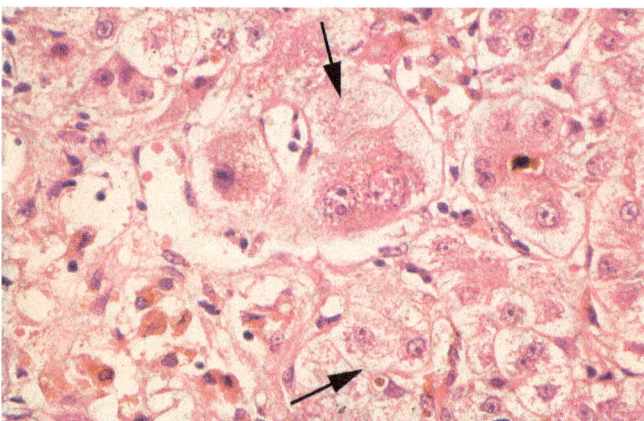

Fig. 22.4: Feathery degeneration (↑) of ballooned hepatocytes, massive liver cell oedema and canalicular bilirubinostasis. Clinically: cholestatic course of acute viral hepatitis B (HE) (s. fig. 13.4)

Histologically, changes linked to the respective stage of hepatitis can be observed together with an abundance of bile drops in the liver cells, above all in the centre of the lobule; in addition, there are bilirubin cylinders inside the canaliculi that are often dilated and tubular in shape. Sometimes, tubular reshaping of the liver cell plates is noticeable, with a bile canal in the centre. • **Cholestatic liver cell rosettes** develop in isolated surviving hepatocytes or small groups of hepatocytes within areas of collapse. These parenchymal islands of hepatocytes are arranged in a tubular pattern resembling that of the cholestatic liver cell rosettes. Evidence of bile retention is not always obvious, but copper and copper-associated protein are often demonstrable. Bile duct proliferation is usually inconspicuous. (s. p. 237) Bilirubin cylinders are detectable in the ductuli. In the portal fields, the picture of cholangiolitis is seen: small, round-cell infiltration with embedded leucocytes and degenerative changes of the portal bile ducts. (s. fig. 22.4)

2.3.4 Anicteric course of disease

As early as 1904, O. MINKOWSKI observed the anicteric form, and in 1937, H. EPPINGER described it using the term *"icterus sine ictero"*, i.e. the bilirubin values in the serum are not in excess of 1.5−1.8 mg/dl, with the result that no jaundice of the sclerae can develop. This is a clinical phenomenon and not a morphological one. There are reports of fatal acute liver necrosis without jaundice. Generally, the clinical findings are less pronounced than with the icteric course of disease. Bilirubinuria is only observed in isolated cases, whereas urobilinogenuria is usually detectable. (s. pp 430, 440)

2.3.5 Fulminant course of disease

Hepatitis fulminans (B. LUCKÉ et al., 1946) is the most severe course of viral hepatitis, and in 80−90% of cases, it is fatal. The term is used if signs of liver insufficiency emerge within 8 weeks following the onset of disease. (If this occurs later, preference is given to the term *"subacute necrotizing hepatitis"*.) • The clinical findings suddenly and swiftly multiply in intensity and acuity. In addition, fever, nausea, vomiting and hepatic foetor are present, and the sensorium becomes dulled. Cutaneous and mucosal bleeding occurs, and there may be evidence of oliguria and oedemas. Laboratory parameters show a considerable decrease in enzyme activity, serum iron (after an initial increase), Quick's value, albumin and cholinesterase. Leucocytosis is frequently observed. The morphological picture is characterized by extensive, confluent parenchymal necrosis (= *liver dystrophy*). There is virtually no sign of a mesenchymal reaction. Postdystrophic *scarred liver* is usually found in those surviving the disease. (s. figs. 21.13; 22.16; 35.1, 35.17)

2.3.6 Giant-cell hepatitis

Giant-cell hepatitis in children: During infancy, acute viral hepatitis can occur with the formation of syncytial, polynuclear balloon-like giant cells. Recessive autosomal *hereditary factors* are said to contribute to this hepatocyte reaction. In recurrent intrahepatic cholestasis of the Aagenaes type, giant-cell hepatitis may develop. The **pathogens** include cytomegaly, herpes, varicella, Coxsackie, ECHO, hepatitis B and rubella viruses as well as listeriosis, toxoplasmosis and syphilis. The pattern of epithelial damage largely corresponds to that of classic acute viral hepatitis − however, the histological picture is dominated by giant cells. (s. fig. 22.5) (s. p. 477)

Differentiation is made between **two types:** (*1.*) giant cells in a regular arrangement (with evenly placed giant cells around the former canaliculi) and (*2.*) giant cells in an irregular arrangement. Both types may appear simultaneously. • Their *development* is probably due to the confluence of liver cells following disintegration of the membrane − so-called confluent giant cells (O. KLINGE, 1970). This process is facilitated by the fact that in children up to the age of five, liver cells are usually still in a double epithelial plate-like arrangement. Following their cytolysis, the giant cells are replaced by regular epithelium. The prognosis is often good, but reports have also been received of severe courses of disease.

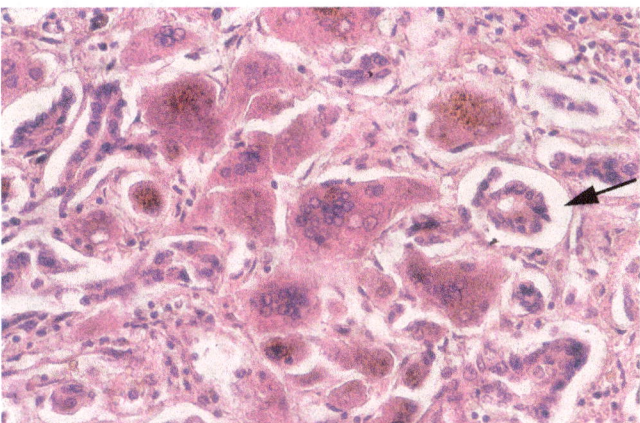

Fig. 22.5: Numerous multinuclear giant cells (centre of picture) with bile duct proliferation (arrow) in giant-cell hepatitis (HE)

Postinfantile giant-cell hepatitis: This term was introduced by H. THALER in 1982. The form itself is rare; about 70 cases have been reported so far. (33) It develops in a similar way to progressive cholestasis of unknown aetiology and mainly affects zone 3. The giant cells make up > 10% of the hepatocytes. They contain large numbers of nuclei (up to 40 per cell). Numerous luminae are found in the cytoplasm. Pathogenetically, this is a syncytial formation (and not amitotic cell regeneration as in the infantile form). The morphological spectrum extends from acute to chronic hepatitis and ultimately to cirrhosis. The giant cells are minimal and thus often undetectable in a biopsy specimen. The frequency of disease is possibly greater than has been assumed up to now. It may be caused by *infections, medication* (e.g. Plantago ovata) or *viruses* (e.g. Epstein-Barr, paramyxoviruses). The frequent evidence of autoantibodies (e.g. ANA) and significant increases in γ-globulin levels point to a close correlation between giant-cell hepatitis and autoimmune processes, such as PSC.

2.4 Aetiopathogenetic diversity

The problem of working in line with morphological classification is rendered more complicated by the aetiopathogenetic diversity of acute hepatitis. The tissue

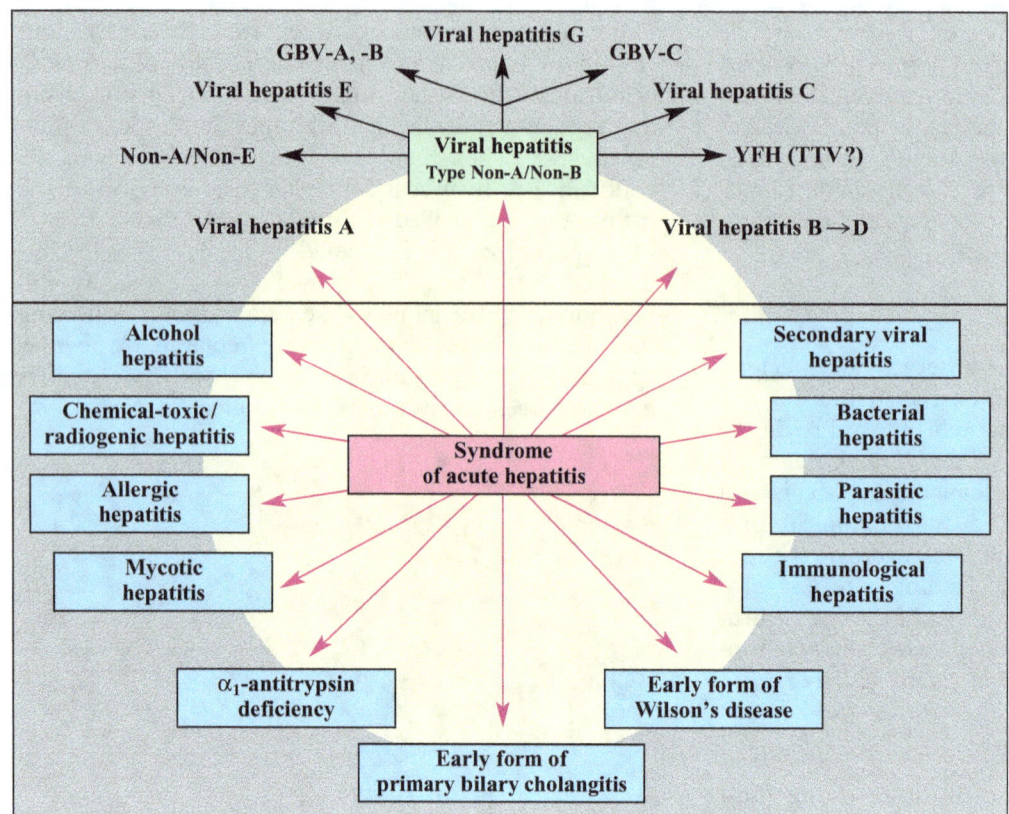

Fig. 22.6: Syndrome of acute hepatitis (s. tab. 5.16)

changes in acute hepatitis arise not only from primary hepatotropic viruses and secondary hepatotropic or exotic types of viruses, but also from bacterial or parasitic agents. • Changes identical to these can, however, also be caused by alcohol, chemical substances, toxins or allergic and immunological reactions as well as by reactions to radiation (*radiogenic hepatitis*), for example from cobalt — and even by the early forms of Wilson's disease or primary biliary cholangitis.

▶ A recently discovered form of acute hepatitis was attributed to a **deficiency of lipoamide dehydrogenase** (= catalytic subunit E3 of the pyruvate dehydrogenase complex). This LAD deficiency was allocated to chromosome 7 (q31-q32). So far, about ten well-documented cases have been reported. The patients all died during early childhood. (32)

▶ Recently, there were reports of **episodes of acute hepatitis**, each with significantly increased transaminases, slight jaundice and uncharacteristic symptomatology. Between the episodes, all the liver values were normal. Histological analyses only revealed minor findings in the form of non-specific reactive hepatitis. The aetiology could not be determined even though the entire range of clinical examinations was applied. This entity is considered to be identical to benign recurrent intrahepatic cholestasis. (37)

The respective lesions in the area of the lobules and portal fields and at the hepatocytes, the mesenchyma and connective tissue differ in intensity from case to case (also depending on the respective stage of the disease) — yet the picture of "acute hepatitis" predominates. • *In each case of liver disease which remains unresolved in terms of differential diagnosis, thought must be given to the possibility of acute hepatitis with its wide range of aetiological causes.* (s. fig. 22.6)

Acute hepatitis *is not an entity in itself, either clinically, aetiologically or morphologically — but indeed must be seen as a* **syndrome.**

3 Acute viral hepatitis A

3.1 Definition

Acute viral hepatitis A is caused by an enterally transmitted (+) RNA virus of 27 (−32) nm in diameter. It is self-limiting and usually self-healing, contracted by people lacking virus A antibodies — hence its preference for children. With good hygienic living standards, however, the tendency of infection shifts increasingly to adulthood. The disease seldom follows a biphasic or cholestatic course. A fulminant course of disease is very rare (ca. 0.01%). There is no causative correlation with primary liver cell carcinoma. Healthy HAV carriers are not known. The disease leaves the patient with life-long immunity. Transition into chronic hepatitis need not be feared. (s. p. 430!)

3.2 Pathogen

So far, **one serotype** has been identified. **Seven genotypes** of HAV are known to show serological cross-reactions. Three genotypes are deemed to be HAV strains, stemming from the *simian virus*. Recently, a new genotype 1 B variant was described. (43) By means of genotyping, it is possible to explain the geographic origin of the virus, the individual source of infection, etc. HAV have since been characterized in greater detail. (71, 115) (s. p. 118!) (s. fig. 5.4!)

> **Genotype:** More than 30% variability in the genome.
> **Quasispecies:** Less than 10% variability in the genome in the same individual.

3.2.1 Inactivation

HAV survives for up to three months in freshwater or sea water. It is completely inactivated by **heat** at 75 °C for 20 minutes or 85 °C for 1 minute, but only partly inactivated at 60 °C for 4 hours. Boiling water (< 15 minutes) is not enough to inactivate HAV completely, particularly if the instruments have not been mechanically cleaned with due care prior to heating. *Formalin* (diluted solution, 37 °C for 2 hours), *β-propriolactone, sodium hypochloride* and *glutaraldehyde* (2%) are suitable for inactivating HAV. • *Alcohol, ether or acids (up to pH 3) do not inactivate HAV; the virus also remains stable down to −70 °C.* (105)

3.2.2 Detection

Stools: With the aid of an electron microscope, HAV is detectable in the stools 7 to 11 days before the acute phase of disease begins. The rate of detection in the 1st week in no more than 50% of cases, in the 2nd week about 29% of cases and in the 3rd week merely 4% of cases. After the 4th week, HAV can generally no longer be found in the stools at all − by means of molecular hybridization or PCR, however, it may be possible to detect the viruses up to three months following the onset of the disease. In the event of clinical relapse, HAV is again apparent in the stools. (107) The presence of the virus (10^9−10^{11} particles/g stool) clearly means infectiosity − yet a negative test does not definitely rule out infectiousness. It has hitherto not been possible to validate either the replication of the virus in stools or its permanent excretion. Some two weeks after the initial occurrence of dark urine, intestinal excretion of the virus has generally ceased, and in addition, patients are no longer infectious with respect to their environment.

Serum: At the same time as viruses are excreted in the stools, viraemia is apparent. The highest concentrations are found shortly before the onset of the disease (> 10^7−10^9 particles/ml serum). Using PCR, it was possible to show that viraemia can exist for longer than three weeks, and even up to four months.

Cells: The HA antigen is detectable as granular fluorescence in the cytoplasm of the hepatocytes from the second week after infection, about one week prior to excretion in the stools. HAV could also be detected in the spleen and lymph nodes (P. KARAYIANNIS et al., 1986).

3.2.3 Replication

Replication of HAV is effected within the liver cell following its transportation into the interior via a "receptor": (*1.*) the capsid proteins are removed and the RNA is released; (*2.*) both are reproduced separately in the cytoplasm; (*3.*) new viruses are assembled from the RNA copies and the structural proteins; (*4.*) these viruses are packed into vesicles and released into the biliary pole; (*5.*) the viruses are excreted via the ductuli. The viruses enter the bile by way of the ductules and are subsequently excreted into the bile and stool as early as one to two weeks before onset of the disease.

3.3 Transmission

Transmission of HAV is effected by a **faecal-oral route.** The main danger, therefore, is *poor hygiene*, as is occasionally found in communal houses or flats, children's homes, prisons, shelters for the homeless and homes for the mentally handicapped as well as among injecting drug users, etc. (45, 57, 70, 82, 89, 108) A similar danger prevails for those who are constantly exposed to material that contains viruses, such as sewage and water purification plant workers (55), medical personnel (= *nosocomial infection*) (s. pp 437, 450) (68), dentists (53) and staff in neonatal intensive care units. (96, 118) • An additional hazard exists in infected drinking water and foodstuffs, such as ice cubes, ice-cream, frozen strawberries and raspberries, raw bilberries, salads, green onions, raw milk, hamburgers, cold meat, bread, cakes and pastries. (38, 43, 50, 64, 75, 76, 83, 88, 93, 99, 117) The warming up of food with microwave ovens (> 1 minute) has been shown to lower the risk of infection. (84) • Even chlorinated water in a swimming pool can serve as a vehicle for HAV infection. (78) Sexual transmission is rare, although an oral infection route may be responsible for infection in such cases, especially among homosexuals. (46, 110) The hands, in particular, are vehicles of HAV transmission to animate and inanimate surfaces. (81) HAV infection of an animal keeper at a zoo, transmitted for example by the apes he cares for, is accepted as an occupational disease. (100)

▶ **Oyster hepatitis:** The ingestion of oysters cultivated in pools or harbour basins has led to oyster hepatitis (B. ROOS, 1956). This is due to their mode of life: filtration of approx. 40 litres water/hr, whereby coliform bacteria are excreted again, leading to a 100-fold concentration of HAV. Usual boiling of oysters in water does not guarantee inactivation of such highly concentrated HAV. (52, 93) • The terrible epidemic in Shanghai in 1988 caused a sensation, with 292,301 cases of disease (4,083 per 100,000 inhabitants) being registered. The infection was brought on by the ingestion of inadequately boiled *Venus oysters* (Anadara subcrenata Lischke). (61, 112)

▶ **Posttransfusion transmission** was observed for the first time by T. Francis (1946) and A.G. Harden (1955). In isolated cases (e.g. collection of blood and blood plasma during viraemia), a haematogenic mode of transmission is conceivable (63, 103) (see observations of H. Voegt (30), S. Krugman et al. (17) on page 414). Infection of haemophiliacs from factor VIII preparations is likewise considered rare (59), as is infection in haemodialysis units. However, a total of more than 80 cases have actually been reported. • *There have been no reports of perinatal infection.*

3.4 Epidemiology

HAV is a ubiquitous virus, especially since it retains its stability in heat and cold under normal environmental conditions and is highly resistant to external influences. The risk of infection correlates with a low standard of hygiene. For this reason, a seven- to ten-fold increase in frequency of the disease must be anticipated when travelling to certain countries (some 20 cases of infection out of 1,000 travellers per month). The infection risk is even greater with so-called adventure trips (overland trekking, backpacking) in those countries. The same applies to persons engaged in humanitarian or development projects. Given these factors, prior active vaccination is a necessity, unless immunity already exists. (74, 87, 109)

▶ The **seasonal frequency** of infection in the late autumn and winter, which used to be most pronounced in the wake of dry summer months (at least in northern latitudes), is less evident today. It is possible that *closer physical contact* resulting from unfavourable weather conditions played a part here — especially since such seasonal fluctuations were not observed in southern regions.

▶ Recent decades have witnessed large-scale **epidemics** *in several countries*, generally caused by poor hygiene conditions and/or infected food or drinking water. • This is also true of the great epidemics and **pandemics** with their impact on the battle fronts and across the frontiers during the **Second World War:** from 1939–1945, between 5 to 6 million German soldiers and 3 to 4 million civilians (i.e. about 13% of the German population at that time) contracted an HAV infection. These figures do not include the undoubtedly large number of unidentified anicteric courses of disease. • A wide-scale regrouping of troops had to be carried out as a result of the losses in manpower due to HAV infection, as *I experienced myself when I likewise contracted the disease in Russia in 1942.* (s. p. 422)

The **infection rate** among the population of a country correlates with age, hygiene standards, socio-economic status and individual risk factors (drug addiction, homosexuality, close contact with infected persons, etc.). Men and women are subject to the same frequency of infection, irrespective of age or race and seasonal or regional factors. • In Germany, there has been a rapid decrease in natural immunity, because far fewer juveniles become infected with HAV today. Consequently, when people contract the infection at a more advanced age, there is a higher complication rate and greater mortality (2.7% vs. 0.004%).

3.4.1 Frequency of disease

The infection rate is established by determining anti-HAV IgG in the serum. Prevalence depends upon the epidemiological situation in a given country. At 40–50%, Germany ranks in the middle, with a clear dependence on age: some 5% of eighteen-year-olds and about 75% of seventy-year-olds are positive. Currently, 30–40% of those older than fifty are HAV-negative in Germany. The infection rate is about four to five times higher than the number of cases actually registered. (54)

3.4.2 Obligation for notification

Germany's fourth Federal Epidemic Control Act (1992) requires that all cases involving primary hepatotropic viruses (A, B, C and others) which result in disease or death are reported to the local Public Health Department. (s. tabs. 23.1, 23.2; 24.3; 25.1)

Frequency: There has been a continuously declining tendency in the number of HAV cases in numerous countries as a result of improved hygiene and active vaccination. However, there is in nearly all western countries an underreporting of up to 20% (74) • In *Germany*, the following frequencies of HAV disease were registered — although the actual figures were probably much higher (s. pp 435, 449):

1992 = 6,990	1997 = 4,596	2002 = 1,479
1993 = 5,839	1998 = 3,811	2003 = 1,365
1994 = 5,488	1999 = 3,131	2004 = 2,304
1995 = 6,639	2000 = 2,820	2005 = 1,507
1996 = 4,911	2001 = 2,274	2006 = 1,533

Mortality in the same period (1992–2006) was as follows:

1992 = 13	1997 = 15	2002 = 11
1993 = 14	1998 = 9	2003 = 4
1994 = 12	1999 = 13	2004 = 9
1995 = 12	2000 = 11	2005 = 7
1996 = 19	2001 = 17	2006 = 5

3.5 Pathogenesis

In principle, differentiation is made between **two phases:** (*1.*) initial *non-cytotoxic reaction* with a high HAV replication rate and (*2.*) *cytopathogenic reaction* with low virus production, histological signs of inflammation and development of immunity. • **Liver cell necrosis** is caused by T lymphocytes (CD^{8+}) specific to the virus, with T cell-induced cytolysis occurring in the course of the immunological response. The virus is subsequently neutralized by antibodies. • Given the right predisposition, HAV is deemed capable of triggering **autoimmune hepatitis** in a number of cases. (95, 116)

3.6 Serological diagnostics

Direct detection of **HAV** and **HAAg** in the blood or stools is only necessary for scientific purposes. • Serological diagnostics is based on the specific detection of **anti-HAV IgM,** the presence of which confirms acute viral hepatitis A. In differential diagnosis, it is necessary to rule out acute viral hepatitis E, with which anti-HAV IgM may likewise occur! Anti-HAV IgM rises in the serum during the first two weeks of the disease, i.e. three to four weeks after infection. It persists for two or three months, and in single cases for up to twelve months (69), with slowly diminishing titre values. A clinical relapse is usually accompanied by a renewed increase in anti-HA IgM; in protracted courses of disease, the drop in titre values is generally delayed. • A rise in **anti-HAV IgG** is observed four to six weeks after infection. This finding points to a subsiding HAV count or one which has long since run its course. The IgG specific to the virus persists for a lifetime and reflects the HAV immunity of the carrier (and the infection rate of the population or community). (74) (s. p. 118) (s. fig. 5.5!)

The mere detection of **anti-HAV** implies the presence of virus-specific IgG or IgM, but does not offer any information on acuity or immunity. For this purpose, it is necessary to determine the antibodies of the IgG or IgM. Maternal HA-antibodies pass to the foetus via the placenta and provide the infant with postnatal immunity for a certain period. The most sensitive method of detecting hepatitis A is by RT-PCR. HAV-RNA is also detected with high sensitivity using molecular hybridization (up to approx. 10^4 copies per ml).

3.7 Stages of disease

Incubation period
The period of time between HAV infection and the manifestation of symptoms ranges from 15 to 49 days, the mean period varying between 25 and 30 days. A shorter incubation period is often accompanied by a severe course of disease, i.e. fluctuations in the period of incubation depend on the respective quantity of the virus uptake and on the individual immune response.

Prodromal stage
Generally, the onset of the prodromal stage is characterized by nausea, vomiting, lack of appetite, a feeling of repletion and diarrhoea (or constipation), followed by weakness, fatigue, fever, headaches, itching, sore throat, painful joints, impaired sense of smell and taste, light sensitivity and coughing — in various degrees of intensity and frequency. These symptoms often take the form of a "febrile influenzal infection". In children and juveniles, "gastrointestinal" symptoms predominate, whereas adults more frequently present with jaundice as well as aching joints and muscles.

Clinical stage
In approximately 90% of all patients, acute viral hepatitis A is subclinical, i.e. it frequently goes undetected. The end of the prodromal and the beginning of the clinical phase is indicated by a *brown colouration of the urine*. Urobilinogenuria persists for a longer period of time than bilirubinuria. Mild proteinuria and microhaematuria can develop. *Stools are usually acholic.* • With the occurrence of *jaundice* (60−70% children, 80−90% adults), most of the subjective symptoms of the prodromal stage subside, whereas *fever* and *exanthema* often occur. *Hepatomegaly* is evident in 70−80% of cases (whereby the liver is sensitive to pressure due to capsular distension and has a soft consistency) and *splenomegaly* in 20−30%, more rarely *cervical lymphadenopathy* (10−20%). • **Children** show a moderate or asymptomatic course in >90% of cases.

From the end of the incubation period, **laboratory parameters** show a rise in *LDH* as an expression of virocyte duplication. They reach their maximum value in the prodromal stage and decline from the beginning of the icteric stage. • Already in the prodromal phase, the *indicator enzymes* GPT, GOT and GDH begin to rise, the increase in GPT being evident at an earlier point ("liver cell damage") and that of GOT somewhat later. The transaminase values (usually between 800−1,200 U/l GPT and 500−700 U/l GOT) do not necessarily correlate with the degree of severity. In approx. 95% of cases, the transaminases show one peak. Generally, the DeRitis quotient is <1 *("inflammation type")*. (s. p. 101) (s. tab. 5.6) (s. fig. 5.5) The *γ-GT* rises until the end of the icteric phase and then recedes to the normal range at a slower rate than the indicator enzymes − also reflecting regeneration of the liver cells. (s. p. 103) A rise in *serum iron* is an expression of liver cell damage. (s. p. 104) The *AP* and *LAP* only increase minimally. Conjugated *bilirubin* is elevated, where the bilirubin values − and to a far greater extent the duration of the jaundice − correlate with the degree of morphological severity. *IgM* in the serum is clearly higher. The *haemogram* initially reflects leucopenia and lymphopenia, the latter often developing into relative lymphocytosis with the production of *atypical lymphocytes*. All other parameters (electrophoresis, Quick's value, cholinesterase, autoantibodies, etc.) are normal. Zinc and selenium, which are important for the body's own defence, are often reduced; copper levels are elevated. (69) *Viraemia* may be longer-lasting than previously assumed: HAV RNA is detectable about 17 days before GPT increases and several days before HAV IgM appears. Viraemia persists for an average of 79 days after GPT increase, i.e. the main duration of viraemia is 95 days. (41)

Convalescence phase
The icteric phase lasts for two to six weeks. Laboratory parameters become normal after four to six months. Normalization of the *serum bile acid* is also deemed a

reliable parameter of recovery. The regression phase is often characterized by episodes of *fatigue* and pronounced *diuresis*. (54, 113)

3.8 Extrahepatic manifestations

Extrahepatic manifestations have repeatedly been described in viral hepatitis A. They can complicate the course of disease and cause considerable clinical difficulties. (s. tab. 22.2)

Acute renal failure (58, 91, 120)	Haemolysis (77)
Aplastic anaemia	Myalgia
Arthralgia (66)	Pancreatitis (49, 72, 104)
Ascites (47, 73)	Pleural effusion (106)
Cholecystitis (39, 85, 90)	Purpura (44)
Cryoglobulinaemia (65, 66)	Thrombocytopenia (44)
Encephalitis (62)	Urticaria (102)
Exanthemas	Vasculitis (48, 65, 66)
Guillain-Barré syndrome (42)	

Tab. 22.2: Extrahepatic manifestations with acute viral hepatitis A (with some references) (s. tabs. 22.6, 22.8)

3.9 Clinical courses of disease

Acute viral hepatitis A usually pursues an uncomplicated course (mild or asymptomatic in children) and heals without sequelae (90–99%). About 13% of elderly patients need clinical therapy. • Nevertheless, some particular courses of disease are worth mentioning:

Cholestatic course
Characteristic of this course of disease – mainly in elderly patients – are the greatly increased bilirubin values (15–30 mg/dl) lasting two to five months, accompanied by elevated AP (and LAP) values. Transaminase activity is relatively low (generally below 500 U/l). Clinical symptoms include itching, fever, malaise, bradycardia and weight loss. This complicated course of disease (up to 10%) finally heals without sequelae, often first after several months. (48, 60, 101, 119) (s. pp 424, 441) (s. fig. 22.4)

Fulminant course
Very rarely (0.01%), albeit more frequently in elderly patients and people with a compromised immune system (0.1–1.0%), viral hepatitis A takes a fulminant course. About 1.0% of all cases of fulminant viral hepatitis are caused by HAV. The mortality rate is >90%. (51, 80) (s. pp 425, 441)

Protracted course
Delayed or remittend courses of disease lasting 6 to 18 months (2–3%) have been observed repeatedly (also by us in three cases). The frequency is given at 5–15%. (101) (s. p. 440) • This protracted course of HAV infection can, however, be a sporadic, recurrent *HEV infection*, since HAV IgM also reacts positively here! • With both a protracted and a cholestatic course, thought must always be given to the combination of acute viral hepatitis with the *Dubin-Johnson syndrome* when drawing up a differential diagnosis. In one protracted and cholestatic case, we observed that it was ultimately the typical histological finding which produced the diagnosis. In such cases, percutaneous biopsy is essential for differential diagnosis. (s. pp 231, 423) (s. fig. 12.1) Generalized lymphadenopathy is considered to be a marker of ongoing inflammation. (86)

Anicteric (subclinical) course
The anicteric course is mainly found in children. However, it generally remains unidentified due to the multifarious complaints. For this reason, the condition can give rise to a chain of infections, particularly in nursery centres and schools. (92) (s. pp 424, 440)

Recurrent course
For reasons that cannot be explained (reinfection? reactivation?), relapse occurs in 5–15% of cases, especially in children. There may be renewed HAV excretion in the stools (with a danger of infection for the environment) and a more pronounced increase in anti-HAV IgM in the serum. The clinical course is usually milder than in the first phase of the disease, yet is more frequently accompanied by cholestasis and extrahepatic manifestations. Despite this relapse, the disease heals completely. (40, 107)

Chronic course

▶ A report on the (possibly) first case of acute hepatitis A developing into chronic active hepatitis (CAH) and cirrhosis has already been published. (67)

3.10 Formation of granulomas

As with various viral, bacterial or parasitic diseases, with Hodgkin's disease or after the intake of allopurinol, etc. (s. tab. 21.1), acute viral hepatitis A can be accompanied by intrahepatic fibrin-ring granulomas. (98)

3.11 Prophylactic measures

In principle, consideration has to be given to any measure that prevents faecal-oral HAV infection, e.g. correct **hygiene procedures** – particularly in risk situations. Generally, for water and food, is required: *"Cook it, peel it, boil it, or forget it!"* This includes the (worldwide) purification of drinking water and the operation of reliable sewage plants. (45, 46, 71, 74)

3.11.1 Passive immunization

Passive immunization using standard immunoglobulin (J. STOKES et al., 1945) requires an absence of HAV antibodies. The detection of anti-HAV renders immunization superfluous. Such protection is temporary, lasting two to four months. It is effective as both a **pre-exposure** measure (almost to 100%) and **postexposure** measure (in over 80% up to 14 days after exposure and possible infection). Passive immunization should also be given to pregnant women who have been exposed to infection. • Immunization is indicated to protect HAV-antibody-free persons in their contact with diseased persons or prior to a stay in high-risk regions. The immunization of antibody-free persons makes it possible to develop a temporary protective ring of immunity, preventing the infection from spreading when diseased persons are being cared for. This *vaccination seal* is recommended for families, schools and institutions where there is close physical contact. Such passive immunization should be extended to simultaneous vaccination as well. (45, 56, 76, 111)

Immunoglobulin A: The specific human immunoglobulin A is injected i.m. deeply at body temperature (0.02–0.06 ml/kg BW). With continued exposure, the injection must be repeated after six to eight weeks. Due to the known HAV IgG content, the effect is better and lasts longer than with standard immunoglobulin, in particular since batches of immunoglobulin can differ in antibody titre. Approximately 1% of vaccinated persons display side effects in the form of fever, rash, aching joints or local soreness at the site of injection. All of them are without consequence and disappear rapidly. There are no contraindications. • Should a **pregnant woman** be suffering from an acute HAV infection at the time of delivery, the newborn should be immunized simultaneously.

3.11.2 Active vaccination

Active vaccination (P.J. PROVOST et al., 1979) with an HAV live vaccine and an inactivated HAV vaccine has led to a higher antibody titre and longer efficacy than passive immunization. (94)

▶ The usual **commercially obtainable vaccine** is highly immunogenic and low in side effects. The former three-phase administration (i.m.) with a single dose of 720 IU can be replaced by a two-phase administration (i.m.) at zero and 6 (–12) months with a single dose of 1,440 IU. On average, an antibody titre of >4,000 IU/l is reached. Given an annual drop in the titre of 14%, a protection period of ten years can be expected. The vaccine protection expires at about 20 IU/l, which is why a booster inoculation ought to be carried out in due course. An **immunity** of almost 100% is achieved. By controlling the antibody titre, the time point for a **booster inoculation** can be established. The success rate is highest in younger people (under 40 years). • If protection has to be provided sooner, both injections may be administered within a period of two weeks, or a simultaneous injection of 5 ml HBV immunoglobulin can be used. **Side effects** are rare and without consequence, and disappear rapidly (tendency to diarrhoea, nausea, slightly increased transaminases, local soreness). (56, 76, 97)

The **indications** for active inoculation are (*1.*) people who are planning a stay in areas with a high HAV infection risk, (*2.*) those who are working in such areas or have close contact with HAV sufferers (e.g. cleaning and kitchen staff in medical facilities), (*3.*) homosexuals (46), (*4.*) homeless people (114), and (*5.*) patients with severe or chronic HAV-negative liver disease, since a superimposed HAV infection can result in a life-threatening situation.

In principle, hepatitis A inoculation should be a routine measure already carried out in childhood!

3.11.3 Simultaneous vaccination

Where rapid protection is required and at the same time long-term immunity is to be established as well, it is possible to carry out an active-passive vaccination with immunoglobulin A and active vaccine A. This is also indicated in the case of a newborn if the mother was suffering from acute viral hepatitis A during pregnancy. After the third inoculation with vaccine, all individuals displayed a good formation of antibodies to HAV.

3.12 Therapy

A *causal therapy* (with antiviral agents) is not yet possible. • *Bed rest* is usually kept in line with the situation of the patient and, as with other acute diseases, is recommended. • With inadequate oral intake, the *substitution* of fluid, calories (glucose infusions), electrolytes, trace elements and (water-soluble) vitamins is advisable. *Cholestyramine* may prove necessary for severe pruritus due to a cholestatic course of disease (4–8 g prior to breakfast) – if antihistamines were unsuccessful. With such a cholestatic course of disease, the application of *ursodeoxycholic acid* (2–3 × 250 mg) is most suitable. (166) In some cases with a fulminant course, *interferon alpha* has been successfully used. *"Special diets"*, *glucocorticoids* or other *medication* are not necessary.

4 Acute viral hepatitis B

4.1 Definition

A 42 nm DNA virus causes acute liver inflammation, which heals in the majority of cases; in 5–15% of patients, it becomes chronic or develops into a long-term virus carrier status. Occasionally, posthepatitic cirrhosis occurs, and there is a close correlation with the development of primary liver cell carcinoma.

4.2 Pathogen

The hepatitis B virus (**HBV**) belongs to the *hepadna virus* group. • This includes woodchuck hepatitis virus (**WHV**) and ground squirrel hepatitis virus (**GSHV**) (= orthohepadnaviruses) as well as Peking duck hepatitis virus (**DHBV**), heron hepatitis virus (**HHBV**) and crane hepatitis virus (**CHBV**) (= avihepadnaviruses). (196, 197, 209, 212, 216, 222, 252)

There are at least **eight genotypes** of HBV (A–H). Serologically, **nine subtypes** of HBsAg can be distinguished, all of which have component "a" in the main HBsAg. HBV only infects mature hepatocytes in humans and chimpanzees. • HBV DNA is a direct parameter of viral **replication** and infectivity, with a magnitude of 10^8 to 10^{13}/ml per day; replication of HBV is very high. It is possible to detect 10–100 viruses/ml using PCR. (129, 135, 161, 224) (s. p. 119!) (s. figs. 5.6, 5.9!) (s. tab. 22.3)

A	Central and East Africa, Japan, North-western Europe, Philippines, South Africa, USA
B	Brazil, China, Indonesia, Japan, Philippines, Taiwan, Vietnam
C	Australia, China, East Asia, Japan, Korea, Polynesia, Taiwan, Vietnam
D	Africa, Eastern Europe, India, Mediterranean area, Russia
E	Central and West Africa
F	Alaska, Central and South America, France, Polynesia
G	France, Germany, USA
H	Central America, Mexico

Tab. 22.3: Geographical distribution of HBV genotypes (areas of predominance)

4.2.1 Inactivation

Viruses are only deemed to be definitively inactivated once their nucleic acid has been irreversibly changed. This can be determined with electron microscopy or by a negative PCR. The individual types of virus may differ considerably in terms of morphology and biochemistry, so that the efficacy of disinfectants often varies greatly, both in mode and degree. Hepatitis B viruses number among the most resistant types of virus. This is why the hepatovirucide potential of a disinfectant is considered to be a criterion of its general effectiveness.

Hepatovirucidal substances such as aldehyde derivatives, chlorine preparations (as long as chlorine is released at a low pH), glyoxal, n-propanol and iodine have proved to be effective. • Virus destruction is also achieved by **heating** (e.g. 100°C >10 minutes, or hot air 180°C >2 hours, or steam 120°C >20 minutes at 1 bar). Just as effective in inactivating a virus is the boiling of instruments or equipment in a soda solution for 15 minutes. • As far as possible, linen should be disinfected by **boiling**, e.g. in an alkaline solution (pH 9–10 >30 minutes). • Linen which cannot be boiled should be decontaminated by **soaking** for 12 hours in a 16% aqueous solution of formalin or in a 1.5% chloramine-T solution. Crockery and cutlery should be boiled in a soda solution (>15 minutes) or soaked in either commercially available aldehyde compounds (2% >1 hour) or compounds of aldehyde glyoxal and ethylhexonal glyoxal (5% >15 minutes). • The careful **cleaning** of instruments prior to sterilization — any remaining blood must be removed — is of great importance. Instruments sensitive to heat are sanitized by **gas sterilization** using ethylene oxide or placed in a 3% formalin solution for 6 hours. • **Endoscopes** are sterilized by immersion in a commercially obtainable virucide disinfectant, by an ultrasound immersion method or in an endoscope disinfector. • Frequent **hand washing** with soap (ca. 3 minutes) and subsequent disinfection using an ordinary commercially obtainable preparation (approx. 2 minutes) is deemed adequate (yet not reliable). • *Reference should be made here to recognized disinfecting agents and procedures listed in the official guidelines of the individual countries.*

4.2.2 Pathogenesis

Virus docking: According to current knowledge on pathogenesis, virus docking with the liver cells ensues directly via specific receptors (e.g. pre-S1 domain). This capsid protein, which contains HBV DNA, is transported into the cell nucleus with the help of a nuclear localization signal. Now the development of the complete Dane particle starts, and the new viruses are secreted from the hepatocytes by the Golgi apparatus. About 5×10^{13} viruses are produced per day. It is possible that new therapeutic paths could be opened up by using specific peptides to prevent the virus from docking with the target cell or to stimulate the antibody response. The uptake of the virus is effected by endocytosis; the virus DNA reaches the cell nucleus.

Hepatocytolysis is caused by the cellular immune response to virus-coded or virus-induced antigens of the liver cell membrane. HBV itself is not directly cytopathogenic. The T lymphocytes are of prime importance for the cellular immune response to HBcAg (or HBeAg) at the liver cell membrane. The density of the virus determinants at the liver cell surface and the concentration of the antigens, determined by the human leucocyte antigen complex, are significant. Genetic factors and individual endogenous production of interferon also influence hepatocytolysis. The virus particles released by lysis are fixed by humoral antibodies and then phagocytized. (206, 214)

4.3 Antigens and antibodies

HBsAg is coded by the pre-S gene. Pre-S_1 and pre-S_2 antigens are detected in high concentrations in the serum. HBV expresses three forms of HBsAg: large (l), medium-sized (m) and small (s) proteins. Small HBsAg is the main component of mature HBV (approx. 90%). In a normal course, these surface antigens are eliminated well in advance of the decrease in the HBsAg titre. The elimination of HBsAg can be swift but also delayed and is usually effected within two to four months. Smooth endoplasmic reticulum containing HBsAg is histochemically detectable by orcein or aldehydethionine staining. However, this is only true for half of the hepatocytes. HBsAg is also detected in the liver cells by fluorescence microscopy. The affected hepatocytes have no preference for a particular site in the liver lobule. Nor is there any correlation with the respective HBsAg serum titre. Histologically, the HBsAg-containing hepatocytes resemble **ground glass cells** (S. Hadziyannis et al., 1973). (160) (s. figs. 5.7; 22.7, 22.8) (s. pp 120, 402)

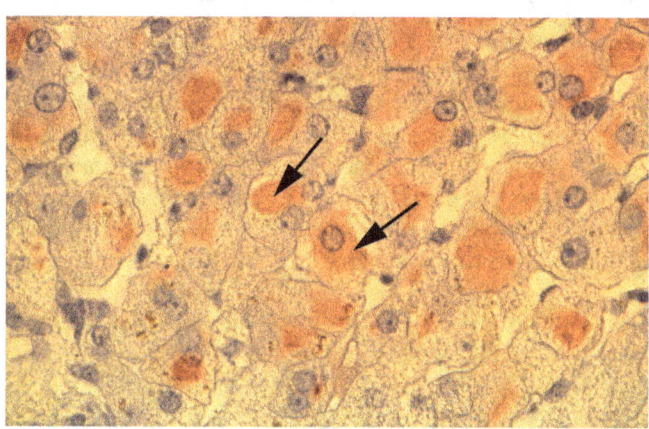

Fig. 22.7: HBsAg in the cytoplasm of hepatocytes (arrows). Clinically: HBsAg carrier (former drug abuse) with moderately increased transaminases (immunoperoxidase reaction). These findings correspond to the ground glass cells in HE (s. figs. 5.7; 22.8)

HBeAg is cleared from the serum in acute disease after several days or a few weeks. The significance of HBeAg is unclear (viral persistence?). It is not needed for HBV replication. HBeAg is seen as a breakdown product of HBcAg and, in conjunction with HBsAg and HBV DNA, determines the infectivity of the patient. Seroconversion of HBeAg to anti-HBe does not always guarantee active elimination of HBV, since viruses are still found by PCR in clinically healthy carriers of anti-HBe. In these cases, a decrease in the titre of anti-HBe is often accompanied by a reduction in the remaining virus load. Anti-HBe can persist for 10–20 years, even lifelong. Negativity of HBeAg may be a sign of mutants forming due to a stopcodon between the pre-core and core region, and thus HBeAg cannot be produced. Infections with HBeAg-negative mutants show a highly replicative course. (135, 177) (s. p. 434) (s. tab. 22.4)

HBcAg is not detectable in the serum, yet can be demonstrated by immunofluorescence in the nuclei of the hepatocytes. (s. fig. 22.8) The excessive formation of **intranuclear HBcAg** is occasionally expressed in the form of a microvesicular, eosinophilic brightening of the karyoplasm and a shift of chromatin to the core membrane. As a result of the metabolic strain on the liver cells due to the viral infection, functional core swelling occurs, subsequently leading to enlargement as well as basophilia of the nucleolus. HBcAg can be seen in the affected cores as an even, dense, finely granulated fluorescence. HBsAg and HBcAg are detectable in the liver cells both together and separate from one another. With serologically unresolved chronic hepatitis, the demonstration of HBsAg and HBcAg in the liver cells can bring clarity to the clinical picture.

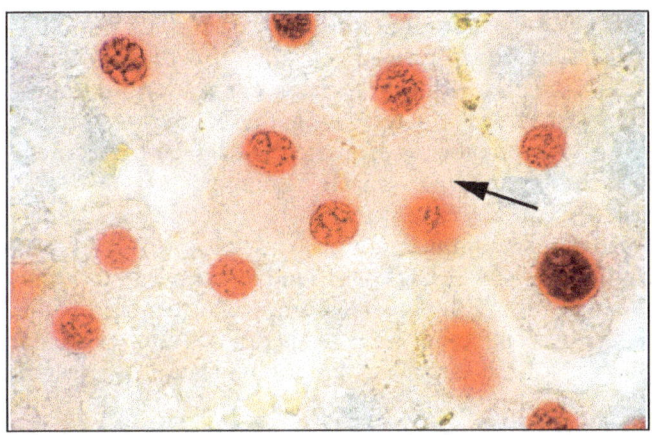

Fig. 22.8: Immunohistochemical detection of HBcAg in the nuclei of liver cells shown by monoclonal antibody. Hepatocytes with ground glass-like homogenization of the cytoplasm, so-called ground glass cells (arrow). HBsAg in the cytoplasm is not presented immunohistochemically in this case (s. figs. 5.7; 22.7)

Anti-HBs is found in the serum just two to three months after infection ("diagnostic window") and probably remains detectable for life (due to mild, continuous boosting from persistent hepatitis B viruses?). It guarantees immunity to HBV infection. Patients with anti-HBs titres are generally anti-HBc-positive. Some 10–15% of hepatitis B patients form no anti-HBs. In previous infections which date back a long time, titre levels can fall below the detection threshold. About 2% false-positive values are measured in the serum. (s. p. 121)

Anti-HBc IgM is the earliest immunological response of the body to HBV antigens. It is the most reliable marker, and once the disease is overcome, it can probably be demonstrated lifelong as **anti-HBc IgG.** In chronic hepatitis B carriers, low titre anti-HBc IgG may also be present. It is the most suitable marker for the HBV contamination rate of a population (more reliable than anti-HBs). The absence of HBsAg and anti-HBc IgM rules out acute HBV infection. In healthy patients who test positive for anti-HBc, latent viral replication is usually still found. This can be detected with the help of PCR. Active vaccination does not result in positive anti-HBc IgM. (s. p. 121)

HBxAg: The significance of the smallest coded region of the HBV genome (17 k Da) — as well as of its protein, which comprises 154 amino acids — is still unclear. It is deemed to be an early marker of acute hepatitis B. HBx reinforces the replication of HBV in the liver cell. It possibly has something to do with the development of liver cell carcinoma, especially since it is most prevalent in HBV-related liver cirrhosis and even in liver cell carcinoma. (143, 204)

▶ Serological markers of the HBV antigens and antibodies facilitate reliable diagnostic and prognostic statements as well as an evaluation of the existing infectivity of the patient. (s. pp 118–122) (s. tab. 5.17) (s. fig. 5.9)

4.4 HBV variants

Clinically relevant *mutations* at a relatively low rate (up to 10^{-5}) of about 1 nucleotide/10,000 bases/year can accumulate in cases of HBV infections which have existed for years. (s. tab. 22.4)

S gene:	loss of the "a" determinant (= absence of vaccine protection)
Pre-S gene:	loss of B and T cell epitopes or loss of the pre-S_2 promoter region or loss of the pre-S_2 start codon (= no neutralization of the virus by anti-HBs)
Pre-C/C gene:	inhibition of the "e" antigen synthesis (= severe course of disease)
C gene:	loss of T cell epitopes (= tendency to fulminant hepatitis) • so-called *escape mutant*
P gene:	loss of polymerase (= accelerated elimination of the virus, "unfit" mutant) • so-called *replication defect*

Tab. 22.4: Known HBV mutants and their possible biomolecular repercussions

Such mutations are found in all genes of the HBV. After the onset of acute hepatitis, they affect the course of disease in a variety of ways, resulting in fulminant development or rapid chronicity, or indeed latent virus persistence. The presence of mutations in the pre-C/C region prevents formation of the e-antigen. HBV mutants might be responsible for a situation which has long puzzled physicians, namely the occurrence of severe chronic hepatitis despite a complete immune response. It is likewise possible that the development of hepatocellular carcinoma is attributable to the integration of the viral genome (with its oncogenic domain) into that of the host cell or the mutants. Mutations in the "a" determinants can effect non-response to the administration of HBV vaccine. When using active vaccines composed of the S-gene product from wild type HBV sequences, mutated viruses are indeed capable of bringing about an infection in inoculated persons (= S-escape mutant). (131, 133, 177, 188, 234, 245, 253)

4.5 Specific serological courses of disease

(*1.*) **HBsAg-negative/anti-HBs-positive course:** This rare course of disease can occasionally be detected in fulminant hepatitis with rapid elimination of the virus, in cases of infection with HBV mutants, in HDV superinfection with suppression of the HBV infection and in non-apparent HBV infection in patients suffering from alcohol-related liver damage.

(*2.*) **HBsAg-positive/anti-HBs-positive course:** It is possible for this constellation to occur with vaccine *escape mutants*, with anti-HBs immune response to a subdeterminant rather than to the "a" antigen and with subsequent infection from another genotype with HBsAg positivity.

(*3.*) **Anti-HBc-positive course:** In negativity of HBsAg and anti-HBs, only anti-HBc can be identified. This constellation is found in approx. 1.5% of the population, in 0.9% of blood donors and in 15−25% of intravenous drug addicts. Anti-HBs in low titre, no longer measurable, may also be present, although positivity can occur in 35% of cases following a once-only "booster" and in 50% of cases after full vaccination. If a healthy individual shows anti-HBc positivity, there is the possibility of a latent infection with virus replication in hepatocytes. In order to verify this finding, it is necessary to use HBV-DNA determination or PCR.

(*4.*) **HBsAg-positive/anti-HBs-positive/anti-HBc-negative course:** The occurrence of this rare constellation may be attributable to a selective immune defect, HBcAg/anti-HBc immune complex formation and mutation in the core gene.

(*5.*) **HBe-minus-HBV mutant:** With fluctuating increases in transaminases, the reaction to HBV DNA can nevertheless be positive in the presence of anti-HBe. HBeAg formation is not induced. These patients are particularly endangered by a rapid development of CAH and cirrhosis. (s. tab. 22.3)

4.6 Chronic HBsAg carriers

A person is said to be an *HBsAg carrier* (*1.*) if HBsAg positivity has persisted for more than six months, (*2.*) if the clinical and chemical findings fail to show any signs of acute hepatitis, and (*3.*) if no (or only minimal) lesions are detectable histologically. • The *diagnosis* and differentiation of an HBV carrier can be established by PCR. Viral hepatitis B is only considered to be completely cured if HBV-DNA negativity is determined at least in the serum. Chronic hepatitis cannot be ruled out as long as HBV DNA is still detectable, even though HBsAg negativity as well as anti-HBs and anti-HBe positivity is given. • *Risk factors* involved in the development of a carrier state include youth, minimal quantity of inoculated viruses with a subclinical course, individual immune status, dialysis patients, etc. Only about 3% of carriers can recall having had acute hepatitis. • The *elimination rate* of HBsAg from the serum is about 2% per year. One case was recorded with almost 20 years of HBsAg persistence and infectivity!

Some 10% of patients with HBV infections develop a *carrier state* (men five or six times more than women). With regard to vertical infection, a carrier state is found in up to 90% of the affected children. • The long-standing existence of an HBsAg carrier state has the following *dangers*: (*1.*) superinfection with HAV and HCV, (*2.*) superinfection with HDV, (*3.*) chronic hepatitis culminating in cirrhosis (in 10−20% of cases), and (*4.*) two to four-fold risk of hepatocellular carcinoma (1 in ca. 250 carriers). • The *prognosis* is generally good for persons who become HBsAg carriers as adults. It is not possible, however, to make a long-term prediction regarding the course of a carrier state. If elevated transaminase values are detected at intervals of several months, the histological findings need to be clarified by liver biopsy. (121, 123, 140, 147, 164, 192)

HBsAg carriers are fundamentally deemed to be contagious, with the degree of *infectivity* fluctuating widely from viraemic, highly infectious carriers to non-infectious carriers. By determining the HBeAg and HBV DNA, it is possible to estimate the degree of infectivity, if necessary incorporating PCR findings. (193) Carriers can present a very real source of infection in interpersonal and intrafamilial contact (139, 147, 154, 193, 221, 244), particularly since HBsAg is found in various body secretions. (s. tab. 22.4) The newborn, too, is exposed to the danger of infection in the perinatal and postnatal phases, so that passive-active immunization is urgently recommended. (250)

> Chronic HBsAg carriers must be given detailed information on how they should behave. This is most important with respect to their occupation, especially for persons in the medical field. Care in complying with hygiene regulations, the wearing of gloves and avoiding procedures that may cause injury are matters of course.

4.7 Epidemiology

The HBV infection rate in Germany is 0.3−0.8% of the population (ca. 500,000 carriers), 0.1% of blood donors and 2−6% of i.v. drug addicts. In 5−8% of the population, anti-HBs and anti-HBc indicate a previous a HBV infection. • In Europe, 0.1−5.0% of the population are HBsAg-positive, with greater frequency in countries to the south (the highest values being found in southern

Italy and Greece). Among foreigners from endemic areas who are resident in Germany, the fraction of chronic HBV infected persons is ten times higher than in the general population. In the countries of Africa and East Asia as well as in some parts of South America, up to 30% of the population (sometimes even more) are HBsAg-positive. Very high infection rates are found in isolated population groups (such as the Alaskan Eskimo with 45% and the Australian aborigines with 85%). • The HBV reservoir is estimated at 350 million people worldwide. Some 250,000 patients die each year as a result of hepatitis B. (122, 199)

4.7.1 Obligation for notification

In Germany, **viral hepatitis** ranks second among infectious diseases that are subject to notification. After 1962 (passing of the Federal Epidemic Control Act), the number of cases ranged between 14,077 (minimum value, 1963) and 25,900 (maximum value, 1973), with a steady decline since that time. Nevertheless, the figures only relate to those cases which have been "registered". The actual number is probably more than five times higher, since anicteric cases are mostly not identified, the obligation to report the disease is possibly "forgotten" and the law can be subject to flexible interpretation. This has no doubt resulted in widespread "underreporting". The wording of the law does not differentiate between acute and chronic diseases. • A "healthy" chronic HBsAg carrier does *not* have to be reported – *nor* does a case of "suspected viral hepatitis".

▶ In *Germany*, the following **frequencies** of HBV disease were registered, whereby the actual figures are about five times higher. The continuously declining tendency is be found in numerous countries as a result of improved hygiene, optimized testing of blood as well as of blood constituents, and active vaccination (s. pp 428, 449):

1992 = 5,987	1997 = 6,133	2002 = 1,425
1993 = 5,497	1998 = 5,232	2003 = 1,304
1994 = 5,166	1999 = 4,570	2004 = 2,767
1995 = 6,152	2000 = 4,601	2005 = 2,474
1996 = 6,044	2001 = 2,427	2006 = 2,531

In the same period (1992–2006), **mortality** in Germany was as follows (males/females = 2 : 1):

1992 = 173	1997 = 190	2002 = 108
1993 = 175	1998 = 158	2003 = 119
1994 = 167	1999 = 96	2004 = 74
1995 = 148	2000 = 98	2005 = 78
1996 = 207	2001 = 93	2006 = 60

4.8 Transmission

Acute viral hepatitis B can present with up to 10^{13} viruses per millilitre of blood – indeed an inconceivably high figure. The typical maximum titre is about 10^8 viruses/ml serum. It is possible to detect $10^5 - 10^6$ particles by means of HBV DNA. A relatively small number of viruses suffices for an infection in the individual case. The PCR method identifies a very low number of HBV particles, although in practice the detection threshold of 100 to 1,000 HBV particles/ml is considered adequate. With such excessive viraemia, it must be assumed that B viruses pass into all body secretions and excretions – only their detection in the stools remains controversial. Sperm is considered to be particularly infectious. (s. tab. 22.5)

Amniotic fluid	Pancreatic juice
Articular effusion	Peritoneal dialysate
Ascites	Pleural effusion
Bile	Saliva (148, 173, 194, 244)
Breast milk (127)	Sperm (173)
Colostrum (186)	Stools
Gastric juice	Sweat
Lacrimal fluid (244)	Urine (173, 244)
Liquor (215, 246)	Vaginal secretion
Menstrual blood	

Tab. 22.5: HBsAg and HBV-DNA detection in body secretions and excretions (with some references)

4.8.1 Parenteral infection

In the past, the *infection route* was assumed to be solely *parenteral*, with blood transfusions being of paramount significance, followed by the parenteral administration of plasma preparations. Present-day extraction and processing techniques for blood and blood constituents have deprived this route of its significance (1 : 150,000 – 200,000). • Nevertheless, it must be borne in mind that the transfusion of HBsAg-negative, but anti-HBc-positive blood can lead to an HBV infection. (223) This diagnostic *risk gap* still exists when selecting blood donors (in the USA and France, for example, blood donors are already screened by means of anti-HBc). Every tenth to twentieth HBsAg-negative and anti-HBc-positive blood donor is considered infectious. This infection, which is for example caused by immune complexes (s. p. 440), has a longer period of incubation (> 120 days) and generally progresses without clinical symptoms.

A number of *unusual parenteral infection routes* have been observed as causing the onset of viral hepatitis B in individual instances (this can sometimes be of relevance when a medical expertise has to be drawn up): spring lancets for taking blood from the finger (219), infection from the interior of a syringe, tattooing (185, 233), acupuncture (175), mosquitoes, (207), bugs (198, 210), leeches that have been used several times, infection from skin diseases such as psoriasis or eczema, manicure or pedicure, shaving, infection from blood smears on thorn bushes, etc. Contagion from needles which have been improperly and carelessly discarded must be avoided. The frequent multiple use and sharing of needles and syringes explains the high rate of contamination and subsequent contraction of the hepatitis B virus among drug addicts (70–90% after >5 years).

4.8.2 Sexual infection

Infection via the sexual route is actually more frequent than has been assumed up to now (25–30% to 68%). *Infectious body fluids* include sperm, vaginal secretion, urine and menstrual blood. (s. tab. 22.4) Apart from the main inoculation route via mucosal lesions, discussion focuses on the cellular intake of the virus through lymphocytes (in which HBV latently exists and can also proliferate) or through mononuclear cells. • Hence, viral hepatitis B must be seen as a special form of *sexually transmitted disease* (STD), and any concomitant abuse of drugs succeeds in considerably heightening the risk of HBV infection. (154) • In 19%, 44% and 56% of documented cases, prostitutes proved to be HBsAg-positive, with a 75% concurrent drug dependence. (229) • *Homosexual males* are exposed to a high risk of infection (ca. 70%), especially since anal intercourse considerably increases the danger of HBV transmission. (158) • With these risk groups, *active immunization* is the safest and cheapest preventive measure in every case. In addition, it is important to encourage safer sex in order to contain the spread of hepatitis B.

4.8.3 Perinatal infection and antenatal care

Diaplacental infection from HBsAg-positive pregnant women to their unborn children (so-called **vertical infection**) is very infrequent in the first and second trimester, yet often prevails in the third trimester. With coexisting HBeAg positivity and in acute viral hepatitis B in the third trimester of pregnancy, the child is nearly always (>90%) infected. About 10% of HBV infections are acquired in utero. It is, however, difficult to decide whether the infection is diaplacental or perinatal. Of the foetuses examined, in fact only 8% showed signs of diaplacental infection. Consequently, diaplacental transmission of HBV is considered to be of minor importance. It is remarkable that HBsAg could be detected in the gastric juice in 96% of the newborns with HBsAg-positive mothers, thus pointing to the infectivity of the amniotic fluid. The most regular development of an HBsAg carrier state in children may be caused by intrauterine exposure to HBeAg: this antigen is transmitted via the placenta and can therefore induce immunologic tolerance in the foetus. (257)

Perinatal infection occurs during the course of delivery. The transmission mode is through skin injuries to the child, maternalfoetal microtransfusions due to placenta lesion or oral intake of HBsAg from maternal blood, amniotic fluid and vaginal secretion. There have been reports of fulminant hepatitis in newborns between the second and fourth month of life. Chronic hepatitis must be feared in >90% of cases, and the development of liver cirrhosis has also been observed. The probability of a perinatal infection correlates with the detection of HBeAg. Each HBsAg-positive pregnant woman must be considered infectious on principle, so that the newborn immediately receives a simultaneous vaccination. In this way, perinatal infection of the child is mostly averted before it can develop, and postnatal infection is prevented. Administration of lamivudine during pregnancy to reduce the risk of HBV infection is a further alternative. (124, 128, 132, 241, 247, 250, 254)

Postnatal infection also poses a danger for the non-vaccinated baby/infant in terms of breast milk (127), injury to the mamilla and close physical contact with regard to an HBsAg-positive mother. (128)

▶ **Statutory prenatal care:** Some 5,000 HBsAg-positive women become pregnant in Germany every year. In the past, just risk groups were tested for HBsAg. However, it became clear that only one third of the pregnant women who were HBsAg-positive could be assigned to

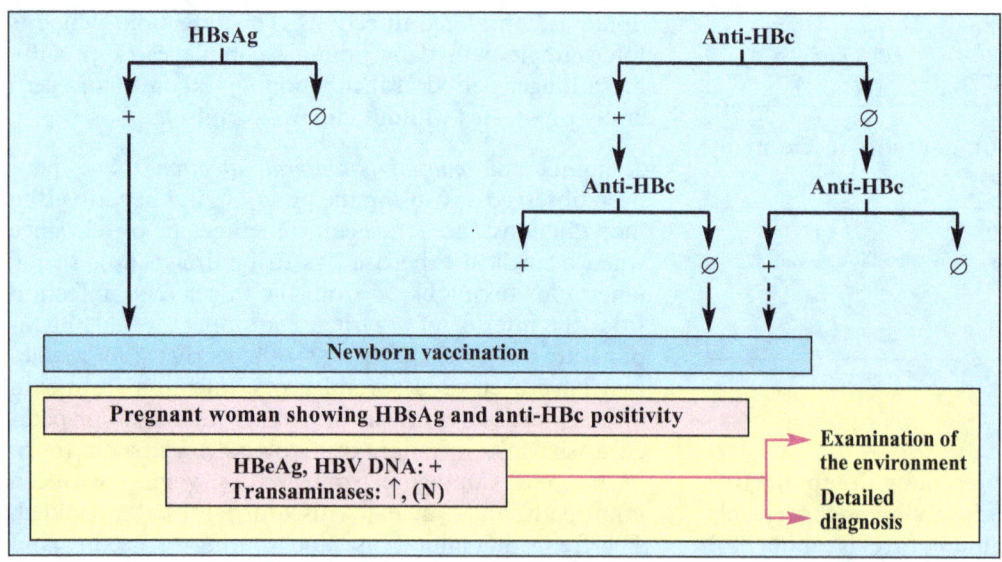

Fig. 22.9: Screening of pregnant women in the final trimester with indications for simultaneous vaccination of the neonate

a "classical" risk group, while two thirds remained unaccounted for. This explains why the guidelines applied throughout the respective countries did not lead to a decrease in the frequency of HBV infection in newborns. The cost of routine HBsAg testing and simultaneous prophylaxis for neonates with HBsAg-positive mothers amounted to a twentieth of the costs incurred annually for the treatment and care of those cases which were not protected from perinatally acquired hepatitis B infection. • In 1992 the respective **statutory maternal guideline** in Germany was changed accordingly, and now reads: "The blood shall be examined for HBsAg in all pregnant women after the thirty-second week of pregnancy and as near to the delivery date as possible." Thus general screening for hepatitis B in pregnancy has been anchored in law, and the costs, including those for simultaneous vaccination, are borne by the health insurance provider. (s. fig. 22.9)

4.8.4 Close physical contact

Infection during childhood can be related to close contact within the family or in day centres and schools (249), particularly those for mentally disabled children and adults. (142) The prevalence of HBV in child molesters is high. (155) Children normally maintain close physical contact, which may involve mutual skin injuries. (148, 211) Initial HBV infections sustained in childhood are generally associated with a very high carrier rate (20−30%), whereas with advancing age the predisposition to carrier state decreases to about 5%. An HBsAg-positive child can, therefore, be the source of *intrafamilial horizontal infection*. From this angle, too, the necessity of *preventive vaccination* is obvious. (171)

HBV infection in the home mainly affects the partner. Seromarkers were in evidence in about 50% of such cases, whereas only 17% of the other members of the household were affected. In 78% of partners who presented serological evidence of HBV infection, HBsAg, HBeAg and DNA polymerase were simultaneously detected, while HBsAg and anti-HBe were found in only 25% of cases. Without doubt, contact in the family or among people sharing a flat or a house constitutes a specific risk of HBV infection from HBsAg carriers. Each individual case must therefore be examined as to whether passive or active or simultaneous vaccination is indicated, and at what time. It should be noted that the infection rate in non-immune members of a household is about 30%. (139, 194, 221)

With *travellers to the tropics*, the rather high rate of HBV infection must be attributed to close physical contact in poor hygienic conditions and possibly to insect bites as well. An unusual report was published concerning an HBV infection in four employees (out of ten) in a *butcher's shop* within one year. (152) The 100 to 200-fold frequency of viral hepatitis in *prisons* as compared to that among the general population is striking (so-called *desmoteric infection*). (57)

Oral transmission of HBV (S. KRUGMAN et al., 1967) requires larger quantities of substrate (about 50-fold) than is the case with parenteral infection. Usually, oral HBV transmission has a longer incubation period and almost always takes an anicteric course.

4.9 Hepatitis B and medical personnel

4.9.1 Medical personnel

The term **nosocomial infection** (s. p. 427) should not only be applied to hospitals, but also to every *doctor's surgery*. At these locations, there are basically **three paths of transmission:**

1. HBV can be transmitted from one infectious inpatient to another (so-called cross infection).

2. Patients can be infected by contaminated blood and blood constituents as well as instruments or equipment. Here, too, cross infections are of considerable relevance. (174, 219, 225)

3. Infected physicians and nursing staff are frequently found to be hepatitis B carriers. (183, 213, 231, 236, 248) A considerable sensation was caused by the fact that in one report 41 patients had been infected by a single practitioner within four to five years. (157, 174)

▶ Compared with the general population, physicians (7.4-fold) and other medical personnel (16-fold) are exposed to a considerably **higher risk** (200 in 100,000) of contracting acute viral hepatitis from contact with HBV-infected patients. HBsAg positivity was detected in 1.5% and 1.6% of medical personnel as a whole, 16% of physicians, 22.4% of surgeons and 36.5% of laboratory staff. Likewise, physicians and medical staff of psychiatric hospitals (10−12%) and those engaged in pathology are risk groups. The greatest danger from hepatitis is found in dialysis centres. The so-called **Newcastle infection** clearly demonstrated the unfortunate chain of hepatitis disease when six members of the medical staff were infected by an HBV-positive patient who was admitted to hospital after having been injured in an accident. (226) • Of 133,000 **surgeons** in the USA, 1,900 proved to be chronically infected with HBV. In spite of this, the transmission of hepatitis B from surgeons to patients is considered unusual. Recently, however, a case was reported in which one HBV-infected surgeon had transmitted an acute HBV infection with positive HBc IgM to 19 patients who had been operated on by him (out of 144 assessable cases). (162) Similarly, a German thoracic surgeon, who had unknowingly become infected by HBV a long time before, was held responsible for the transmission of hepatitis B to 13 of his patients (1999). • The transmission of hepatitis B by **endoscopes** (provided they have been cleaned in compliance with the regulations) is considered improbable. (189)

The recommended **prophylactic vaccination** against HBV has led to a drastic drop in occupation-related HBV infections. Given an even greater acceptance of voluntary active immunization, it would be possible to prevent HBV infection almost completely in the medical sector. In accordance with the statutory regulations, non-immunized persons ought not to be engaged in HBV risk areas. With a genetically engineered vaccine available, all those whose occupations involve contact with blood, blood constituents, contaminated items or body secretions (s. tab. 22.5) should most definitely receive active hepatitis B inoculation. In conjunction with compliance to hygiene regulations, this measure would make it possible to eliminate the risk of nosocomial HBV infection almost completely (<1%). Vaccination against hepatitis B is soon to be compulsory for medical staff according to an EU directive. • In the case of **needlestick injury,** passive immunization should be effected within 6 hours if the following *infection constellation* is established (by means of a rapid test): donor = HBsAg-positive and recipient = anti-HBs-negative. At the same time, active immunization should be initiated. (179, 195, 225)

4.9.2 Hepatitis B and the dialysis unit

Physicians and medical staff at dialysis units, as well as the patients themselves, are exposed to a particularly high risk. At 15 American dialysis centres, the physicians presented an HBsAg frequency of 2.4%, which is five times higher than in the general population. In 1978 a total of 752 physicians and nursing staff contracted hepatitis B with five fatal cases in 350 European dialysis units. The number of lethal infections recorded in the field of dialysis totalled 65 between 1972 and 1978. However, the subsequently improved preventive measures, parallel to the separation of hepatitis-positive from hepatitis-negative units and, in particular, the employment of immunized staff have resulted in extensive elimination of HBV infection in the field of dialysis. (203)

Dialysis patients were found to be HBsAg-positive in 15−20% of cases. About two thirds of them were also HBeAg-positive and hence highly infectious. Chronic hepatitis can be expected to develop in about half such patients. HBsAg-negative dialysis patients must be vaccinated as soon as possible, perhaps initially with passive immunization, until they form their own antibodies. Unfortunately, however, a high percentage of such dialysis patients are *non-responders*. (144, 170) • **Our experience shows that it is in fact possible to achieve a response in some of these non-responders following adequate "substitution" of zinc, and in some cases selenium.** (s. p. 444)

Moreover, the **relatives of dialysis patients** are also exposed to the risk of an HBV infection. Altogether 26% of the contact persons examined presented serological signs of hepatitis B infection. The frequency rate rose to 35% in people assisting in home dialysis. Here, too, preventive measures are to be strictly observed; non-immune contact persons must be actively immunized.

4.9.3 Hepatitis B and dentistry

The first report that dentists (5.3%) were exposed to hepatitis more frequently than the general population was drawn up by A. Bernstein et al. (1953). • The **risk of contracting the disease** in a dental practice was calculated by G. Klavis et al. (1971) and by subsequent investigators as being 6−30 times higher than average. Some 80% of the hepatitis diseases contracted by dentists are considered to be related to their occupation. The number of dentists who have overcome viral hepatitis is given at approximately 14%. • Understandably, the question arises as to what extent an HBsAg-positive dentist poses a **risk** to his/her patients. The first report on this transmission mode, submitted to my knowledge by M. L. Levin et al. in 1974, focused on a dentist who had infected 12 patients as well as a dental nurse and a colleague. Other publications report on the infection of many patients, in one case up to 55 within a period of four years. (159)

Given the specific circumstances of this profession, dentistry is *ideal* for the transmission of HBV: (*1.*) to the attending dentist, the patients are a totally unknown group of persons with respect to hepatitis infectivity; (*2.*) dental treatment nearly always involves injuries in the oral cavity, where blood mixes with the saliva (which is deemed to be an infectious agent anyway) − the close contact of the dentist with blood and saliva predisposes him to HBV infection; (*3.*) the work of a dentist involves injuries to the skin from instruments as well as from nonvisible or unnoticed epithelial defects or rhagades (also caused by the frequent washing and brushing of hands); (*4.*) the application of high-speed turbine drills produces a spray of vapour comprising blood constituents, saliva and mucosal particles − in the case of an HBV carrier, this is highly infectious. It was demonstrated that the arm and hand of the dentist act as a "crash barrier", so that most of the spray is deflected and can easily be inhaled by the dentist (L. Winkler, 1970). • There are almost 40 publications available on the subject of the high occupational *risk of infection* to which dentists are exposed and on the transmission of hepatitis B from dentists to patients. (134, 159, 165, 178, 180, 181, 217, 218)

4.9.4 Insurance questions

The infection of dentists or physicians and their medical staff with HBV from infectious patients presents no particular problems in terms of accident insurance protection and recognition as an **occupational disease.** In the eyes of the law, it is of no importance whether hygiene regulations have been ignored, whether a situation can be attributed to negligence or whether use has been made of the opportunity for active immunization. Active immunization of dentists (physicians) and their personnel is, however, a top priority! In addition, care should be taken to comply with accident prevention regulations.

Nevertheless, the situation becomes more complex if patients appear to have been infected with viral hepatitis by a dentist or a doctor and claim compensation from the respective **personal liability insurance.** The decision taken here will be based on the general terms and conditions of the insurance policy itself. Likewise, the definition of "intent" and "gross negligence", as stipulated under German law, will have to be clarified once all relevant factors have been reviewed.

For the **legislator,** the question arises as to whether the (possible) infectivity of a dentist (physician) constitutes an exceptionally high risk and to what extent hygiene-related stipulations and other legal measures can provide a remedy. The legislator, however, reserves the right to "prohibit the practice of certain occupational activities in whole or in part". In some cases, this channel has already been pursued by the responsible authorities (even somewhat inappropriately).

> ▶ In 1978 we reported on a dentist who was given a two-year suspension. (180) The issues raised by this publication, in particular regarding the inadequacy of sometimes uncoordinated and unbalanced regulations, have still not been satisfactorily clarified by the discussions and statements that have meanwhile ensued. (181)

For chronic HBsAg carriers (s. p. 434), there are no comprehensive regulations to follow with respect to **professional conduct,** everyday routine and family life. Yet they must be well informed about their condition and should be fully aware of the danger they pose. Provided the respective hygiene measures are observed, restrictions in professional life are generally not necessary.

4.10 Stages of disease

Incubation period
The incubation period is (25−) 50−90 (−180) days. This wide range depends on (*1.*) route of transmission, (*2.*) quantity of virus transmitted, and (*3.*) immunity status of the infected person.

Prodromal stage
The prodromal stage can last from a few days up to two to four weeks. Non-specific prodromal symptoms (general, gastrointestinal, influenzal and arthritic/myalgic complaints as well as taste disorder) tend to develop more gradually, yet more severely, in hepatitis B than in hepatitis A. Otherwise, however, there are no great differences in terms of prodromal symptoms between the two types of hepatitis virus, so that it is not possible to differentiate hepatitis B from hepatitis A at the prodromal stage. (s. p. 429) Nor is this possible by establishing more pronounced enzyme activities or by means of initial histological findings. It is the presence of HBsAg (which is, however, absent from the serum in the early phase in about 5% of cases and thus usually remains unidentified) and above all of anti-HBc IgM as well as HBeAg and HBV DNA in the serum which makes differentiation possible. In the pre-icteric phase, there is as a rule evidence of leucopenia. Subsequently, lymphocytosis and monocytosis occur. (s. fig. 5.8)

Clinical stage
The clinical stage commences with the occurrence of jaundice. The level of bilirubin in the serum and especially the duration of the icteric phase correlate with the morphological degree of severity. Here, direct (conjugated) bilirubin mostly predominates. (s. tab. 22.6)

Depending on the degree of jaundice, pruritus usually occurs, the stools are light in colour (acholic) and the urine takes on a dark brown shade. Even prior to the

Parameters	Spectrum of values
GPT GOT DeRitis quotient	↑↑− ↑↑↑ ↑ − ↑↑ < 1
GDH γ-GT LDH	(↑)− ↑↑ ↑ − ↑↑ (↑)− ↑↑
Bilirubin (conjugated) − anicteric form	↑ − ↑↑ N −(↑)
AP LAP	(↑)− ↑↑ (↑)− ↑↑
Serum iron	↑ − ↑↑
Bile acids	↑ − ↑↑
Quick's value Colombi index Cholinesterase	N −(↓) N −(↓) N −(↓)
Immunoglobulins	↑ − ↑↑
Leucopenia Lymphocytosis, monocytosis	N − + N − +
γ-globulins	N − ↑

Tab. 22.6: Spectrum of laboratory parameters in acute viral hepatitis B, depending on the degree of severity and specific courses of disease (N = normal)

occurrence of jaundice, urobilinogen is excreted to a greater extent in the urine and remains detectable for the entire course of disease. The icteric phase lasts three to six weeks; 60−70% have an anicteric course. In most cases, the liver is enlarged so as to be palpable and is tender upon pressure; the spleen is frequently palpable, too, and, in 10−20% of patients, the lymph nodes are swollen. Arthritic pain, fever and skin eruptions are commonly experienced. In children, an anicteric form with lymphadenopathy as well as a non-pruritic, mostly populous exanthema, known as acrodermatitis papulosa infantum (= *Gianotti-Crosti syndrome*), can develop. (s. p. 88) The laboratory parameters show a wide spectrum, depending on the degree of severity and the course taken by the hepatitis. Microhaematuria and mild proteinuria are possible. The blood sugar is occasionally reduced, and isolated cases can present symptoms of hypoglycaemia. (s. tab. 22.7) (s. p. 429)

In the later course of disease, slight increases in IgA and IgG may be detected. (s. tab. 5.15). HBsAg is absent from the serum in approx. 90% of cases within two to four months. A lower Quick's value due to reduced absorption of vitamin K normalizes swiftly following the parenteral substitution of vitamin K (= Koller's test). The possible detection of antibodies (e.g. SMA, ANA, SLA, LMK) is of no significance. The return of bile acid values to normal constitutes a sensitive parameter for the regression and healing of the disease.

Convalescence phase

Given a natural course of disease, all laboratory values are normalized within four to six months. AFP and γ-GT may continue to be increased for a while as an expression of the regeneration of the liver cells. Weakness, fatigability, reduction in physical strength, etc. can also persist for a considerable period of time. (147)

4.11 Extrahepatic manifestations

The course of disease of viral hepatitis B can be changed or complicated by multiple extrahepatic manifestations. (78) They are probably caused by circulating *immune complexes* containing HBV antigens (U.E. NYDEGGER et al., 1980). Circulating antibodies are present in up to 80% of cases. It is assumed that virus antigens (HBs, HBe) constantly reach the blood from the liver cells, as do immune complexes formed in the liver. Antigenaemia triggers the production of circulating immune complexes in the blood. Inefficient clearance in the RES due to massive complement fixation then leads to the deposition of immune complexes in different organs. • Three forms of *glomerulonephritis* can be differentiated: (*1.*) membranous, (*2.*) membrano-proliferative, and (*3.*) endocapillary. (s. tabs. 22.2, 22.7; 34.7) (s. p. 719)

Ascites (130)
Colitis ulcerosa
Cryoglobulinaemia (144)
Diabetes mellitus
Encephalitis
Gianotti-Crosti syndrome (153, 202)
Glomerulonephritis (136, 182, 243, 251)
Guillain-Barré syndrome (215, 237)
Myelitis, myasthenia gravis
Myocarditis (240)
Nephrotic syndrome (128, 191)
Neuritis
Pancreatitis
Panmyelophthisis (200)
Peri-/polyarteriitis (156, 191, 201, 205, 235)
Pleural effusion
Polyarthritis (168)
Polymyalgia rheumatica
Polymyositis
Porphyria cutanea tarda
Psychosis (246)
Skin alterations (258)
Thrombopenic purpura (176)
Thyroiditis
Urticaria (145)

Tab. 22.7: Extrahepatic manifestations in viral hepatitis B (with some references) (s. tabs. 22.2, 22.9)

▶ D.J. GOCKE et al. (1970) reported on the first observation of HBsAg-associated vasculitis. Hepatitis B was initially associated with glomerulonephritis by B. COMBES et al. in 1971. Polymyositis was described by A.A. MIHAS et al. in 1978. Concomitant haematological reactions are relatively frequent, generally in the form of harmless haemolysis or thrombopenia. Severe complications include agranulocytosis and panmyelophthisis due to acute viral hepatitis, such as were described by E. LORENZ et al. in 1955 (at that time without the possibility of virus classification). Altogether, over 250 cases of panmyelophthisis or aplastic anaemia have been reported in the literature. (167, 176, 200)

4.12 Specific clinical courses of disease

As with HAV infection (s. p. 434), the clinical features of viral hepatitis B can be influenced by certain courses of disease. As a result, it often proves difficult to draw up a differential diagnosis, and further examination becomes necessary. Some of these initially unpredictable courses of disease are a considerable impediment to the self-limiting capacity of viral hepatitis B. (s. fig. 22.10)

4.12.1 Subclinical course

The term *"asymptomatic"* course should not be used. Even if no subjective symptoms or clinical findings exist and HBsAg is not detectable, at least the GPT is always elevated. The existence of an HBV infection is not to be dismissed unless the remaining HBV seromarkers, including HBV DNA, are negative as well. • In contrast, the term *"subclinical"* can be applied to a constellation comprising increased GPT (and GOT) values, HBsAg negativity (low-level carrier) and elevated HBV seromarkers. • Therefore, it is quite right for persons with elevated transaminase values (despite concurrent HBsAg negativity) to be excluded from being blood donors as a precautionary measure.

4.12.2 Anicteric course

In this course of disease (s. pp 424, 430), the immune reactions are weakened; consequently, liver cell lesions are less pronounced (= lower transaminase values as a rule) and virus elimination is delayed (= protracted course of disease in general), with the result that HBsAg persistence is also more common. Often, these patients are only identified by chance. Because of the frequent non-diagnosis, they continue to be exposed to the daily routine strain put on them at work and to chemical noxae, alcohol or medicaments, thus furthering the tendency towards chronicity of the disease.

4.12.3 Protracted course

This is characterized by a delayed normalization of the laboratory parameters and also by urobilinogenuria. By contrast, the serum bilirubin has mostly become normalized. Subjectively, there are no symptoms. Protracted hepatitis B can continue to be HBsAg-positive or become HBsAg-negative, or the HBsAg negativity, apparent from the very beginning, may remain unchanged the whole time. In these cases, however,

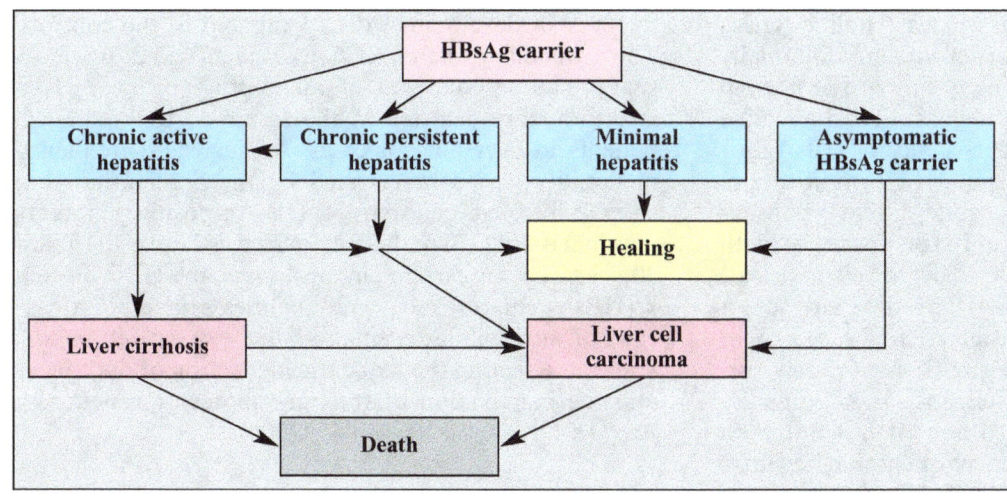

Fig. 22.10: Clinical courses of disease in the HBsAg carrier status (s. tabs. 5.17, 5.18) (s. p. 122)

HBV-DNA positivity still exists (by applying the PCR method, the sensitivity of HBV identification is increased 10 million-fold!). • Histologically, there are periportal residual infiltrates as well as late nodules and liver cell lesions with isolated cell necrosis. It is recommendable to establish morphological findings by means of percutaneous biopsy so as to have a basis for comparison with follow-up biopsies. Protracted hepatitis B is considered to be an important indicator for the further course, either towards the healing of the disease or its transition into chronic hepatitis.

4.12.4 Recurrent course

A renewed rise in the enzyme activities in the regular course of subsiding disease or during the posthepatitic phase of normal findings points to a relapse of hepatitis B (2–15% of cases). As a rule, the first occurrence of the disease and its relapse are only separated by an anicteric interval (H. THALER, 1982). The histological findings are generally more pronounced, since the disease has not yet morphologically healed. Routine everyday strain as already mentioned above (alcohol, chemical noxae, medication, etc.) may be a causative factor. Physical work, however, is not considered to induce a relapse. Activation of HBV replication by means of cytotoxic therapy has been described. (190) A relapse is understandably distressing to both patient and physician. In setting up the differential diagnosis, thought has to be given to secondary viral hepatitis (A, C, and especially D) as well as to an additional infection with secondary hepatotropic viruses (s. tab. 5.16) or indeed to a general virus infection. Superimposed hepatitis infections are greatly feared.

4.12.5 Cholestatic course

The frequency is given at 10–15%; including the minor cases of disease, however, it may even be as high as 30%. In the main, older persons are affected. When setting up the differential diagnosis, the numerous other causes of cholestasis have to be ruled out. (s. pp 424, 430) (s. tabs.

13.4–13.6, 13.8) (s. fig. 22.4) • *Explorative laparotomy is contraindicated!*

Fibrotic cholestatic hepatitis in HBV infection can be found in patients following liver transplantation and reinfection of the transplant as well as after bone marrow transplantation (S. E. DAVIES et al., 1991). The prognosis is poor. Therapy with lamivudine can be tried. (170) Usually, the transplant fails or the outcome is fatal within one year.

4.12.6 Fulminant course

The frequency of fulminant hepatitis B (s. pp 425, 430) is about 1%, yet it is clearly higher in an infection with HBV mutants and above all in a superinfection with HDV. Fulminant hepatitis B may be due to a combination of several unfavourable factors such as pre- or coexisting liver disease, coinfection with HDV (approx. 50%), virus load, virulence and route of infection (e.g. intravenous drug addicts), hormonal strain, additional infections, haemodialysis and inadequate (too fast, too pronounced) immune reactions. With rapid HBsAg negativity and anti-HBs positivity, the survival rate is clearly better at 47% than is the case with persistent HBsAg positivity at 17%. • Therapy with lamivudin can be recommended. (126, 131, 137, 169, 177, 184, 213, 232, 234, 238, 242, 253)

4.12.7 Subacute course

The subacute course is rare. It is found more frequently in women than in men. The onset is acute, the symptoms are more severe and the disease progresses for months. The prognosis is serious, since chronic liver insufficiency often develops. Mortality is high.

4.12.8 Chronic course

About 3–5 (–10)% of cases of acute hepatitis B become chronic. Chronicity occurs in 40% of 1- to 5-year-olds and in 90% of babies. (s. fig. 22.10) Enzyme activities (GPT, GOT, GDH) usually stabilize at moderately elevated levels, the liver function values (cholinesterase, Quick's value, albumin) are normal or only minimally reduced, while the gammaglobulins stay in the normal range or only display a modest increase. The IgG value shows a tendency to rise. The persistence of HBsAg for more than 10–12 weeks may point to chronification. Serological markers can present quite different constellations in individual cases, yet anti-HBc positivity (with distinctly and sometimes greatly elevated titre values) and HBV-DNA positivity always prevail. Evidence of HBsAg/IgM complexes is considered to be a sign of chronicity. (187) A defect in the pre-S1 region may further chronification. The risk of cirrhosis is 30% in a 20-year course of disease. • Up to now, it has not been possible to prevent the development of chronic hepatitis. The idea that earlier treatment with IFα might reduce the number of chronic courses is under discussion. *(see chapter 34.6.5)*

4.13 Hepatitis B and pregnancy

Some 40% of all liver diseases and some 50% of jaundice occurring during pregnancy are caused by acute viral hepatitis. • The **course** of acute hepatitis B is not influenced by pregnancy. More frequent development into chronic hepatitis or reactivation of chronic hepatitis need not be feared. • The **mortality rate** of 1.5% corresponds to that of acute viral hepatitis without pregnancy.

At 7.2%, the **miscarriage rate** in the event of pregnancy coinciding with acute hepatitis B is no greater than the frequency of spontaneous miscarriages. Only the **premature birth rate** at 15.7% is slightly higher than with normal pregnancies. The cause could be a greater sensitization of the uterus musculature to oxytocin as a result of higher bile acid values in the serum or an inadequate breakdown of placental hormones because of impaired liver function. • The **stillbirth rate** at 3.1% lies within the normal range. In the literature, however, there are reports of higher rates of premature birth (28.6%) and stillbirth (9.9%) if viral hepatitis occurs in the third trimester of pregnancy. • There is no increase in the frequency of **embryopathy** or *foetal deformity*. • As in acute viral hepatitis A, an **abortion** is not indicated. On the contrary, each termination must be seen as an abrupt intervention in the hormone system and the immune reaction status, which considerably endangers the pregnant woman. (124) • For *statutory antenatal care*, see page 436. (s. fig. 22.9)

4.14 Hepatitis B and hepatocellular carcinoma

There is a causal interrelation between the development of hepatocellular carcinoma (HCC) and an HBV infection. (s. fig. 22.10) This is also shown by the geographic correlation between the high HBsAg prevalence in Asian and African countries (up to 20%) and the higher HCC rate. HBsAg carriers have a 100 to 200-fold relative risk of developing HCC compared to the controls. The probability rate of HCC was calculated at 6% for 5 years. The seromarkers of an existing or past HBV infection were detected in the serum or liver of HCC patients in over 60% of cases. An increased frequency in families was demonstrated by the observation that several infected children of HBsAg-positive mothers developed HCC. The latency period is between 15 and 30 years. Under certain circumstances, the HBV protein x (HBx) acquires oncogenic qualities, triggering a cascade of intracellular events (= *step-wise carcinogenesis*) and thus effecting the sequential activation of oncogenes and the inactivation of tumour-suppressor genes. (123, 125, 143, 172, 220, 256) (s. pp 453, 800)

4.15 Prophylaxis

All preventive measures are facilitated by an awareness of the serological status of infected persons, individuals with suspected infection and those generally in need of protection. • *Prevention of acute viral hepatitis has the following aims:*

1. Inactivation of the pathogen
2. Interruption of the infection chain
3. Passive immunization
4. Active immunization

Inactivation of the hepatitis virus should be effected by suitable disinfection and sterilization measures. (s. p. 432) Interruption of the infection chain is easier with hepatitis A than with hepatitis B as a result of its faecal-oral mode of transmission and shorter period of infectivity. Because of the costs involved, it is difficult to build up a temporary immunization barrier around the B-infected patient. There is no legal obligation to have a patient with acute viral hepatitis hospitalized. When the patient is treated at home, however, the provisions of the Epidemic Control Act have to be adhered to, preferably with the involvement of the Public Health Department. Upon admission to an isolation unit, it is recommended to separate hepatitis A patients from B and C patients, since there is no cross immunity between the various hepatitis viruses, secondary infection is always possible, and thus constitutes a certain risk!

4.15.1 General hygiene measures

In order to *prevent* viral hepatitis and to *treat* hepatitis patients (in hospital and at home), strict compliance with **hygiene regulations** is a priority. Regular and thorough briefing of physicians and nursing staff is imperative. Eating and smoking should be prohibited in areas where a greater risk of hepatitis prevails. The sexual transmission of HBV is reliably prevented by using condoms. • *If all hygienic requirements are fulfilled, the risk of hepatitis infection can be reduced to <1%.*

4.15.2 Passive immunoprophylactic measures

Passive prevention is ensured by (*1.*) pre-exposure prophylaxis or (*2.*) postexposure prophylaxis. For this, *immunoglobulin (HBIG)* with an established anti-HBs content (generally 200 IU/ml) is available. The **efficacy** of passive immunoprophylactic measures depends on:

1. the existing hepatitis B virus load in the body
2. the amount of anti-HBs administered
3. the timing of the injection
4. the mode of application of the preparation

The **protective effect** of HBIG (0.06 ml/kg BW) sets in two to five hours following i.m. injection. It lasts for two to three months. If necessary, repeated vaccination may be advisable after one, three and possibly six months. The application of HBIG calls for critical assessment in view of the high costs involved.

Pre-exposure prophylactic measures with the cheaper traditional gammaglobulin are ineffective against hepatitis. In cases of non-immunity, **immunoglobulin B** (0.06 ml/kg BW) has to be administered without delay. Non-immune persons should know their own serological status, so that suitable preventive measures can be taken immediately after any probable contact. If necessary, a serological **rapid test** can be carried out first, although this involves a certain loss of time. • The protective effect of the immunization decreases with each hour, and just six hours after exposure, efficacy can no longer be guaranteed.

Postexposure prophylactic measures are, in contrast, of tremendous practical significance. This is true for the HBV infection of non-immune persons in the medical field as well as in everyday life (e.g. needlestick injury, swallowing infectious material, sexual contact, prevention of reinfection following liver transplantation). All preventive measures must be complemented by concurrent active vaccination in contralateral parts of the body (= *simultaneous vaccination*). • The mere detection of anti-HBc or anti-HBe in the suspect matter (e.g. blood) is suggestive of an infection and justifies vaccination of the exposed person (since HBV DNA may be present in a still unknown quantity). The demonstration of anti-HBe in the mother is an indication for the vaccination of the neonate. Newborns with HBsAg- and/or HBeAg-positive mothers are considered to be particularly at risk. For this reason, HBIG is administered immediately postpartum and repeated after one and three months. At the same time, active vaccination is initiated.

Side effects (e.g. local soreness, urticaria, exanthema, arthralgia) are rare, harmless and short-lived. The administration of HBIG in HBsAg positivity may lead to the formation of immune complexes, yet this complication has not been observed so far.

4.15.3 Simultaneous vaccination

In approximately 95% of cases, simultaneous vaccination affords protection against HBV infection. An **indication** is given for non-immune persons if their circumstances have led to HBV exposure and there is not enough time for active prophylactic immunization:

1. newborns with HBsAg-positive (and anti-HBc-positive, possibly even anti-HBe-positive) mothers
2. accidental inoculations (e.g. needlesticks, injuries, smear contacts)
3. sexual contact, particularly anal intercourse, with potentially infectious partners
4. dialysis patients and relatives caring for them (e.g. home dialysis)
5. current exposure through close physical contact (e.g. in institutionalized homes for the mentally disabled, in shelters for the homeless, among drug addicts)

In order to prevent infection with HAV or HBV, various **measures** are indicated. (s. fig. 22.11)

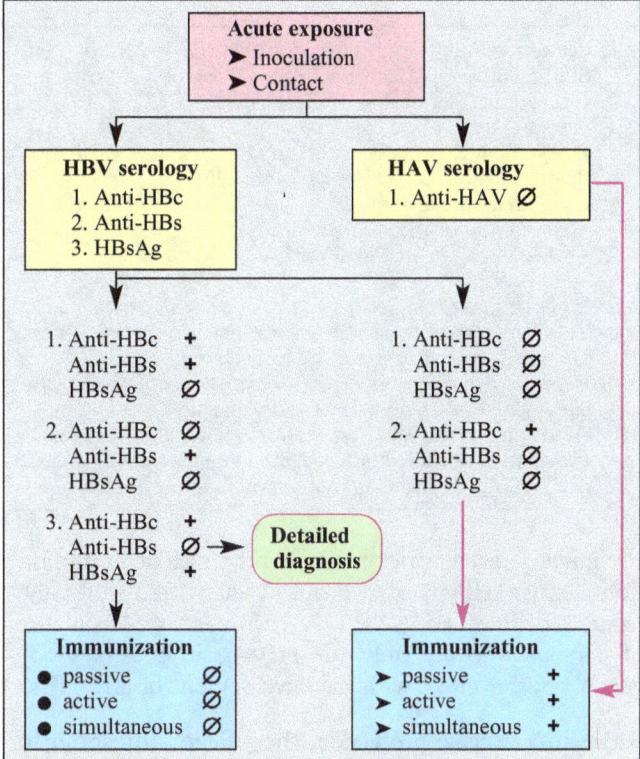

Fig. 22.11: Preliminary tests and measures in the event of exposure to or infection with HAV or HBV

4.15.4 Active protective vaccination

The **basic principle** for the development of a vaccine resulted from observations by S. KRUGMAN et al. (1970), according to which inoculation with heat-inactivated HBsAg prevented the outbreak of hepatitis B or lessened its severity in 80% of exposed persons as a result of the development of protective antibodies (anti-HBs). The first active immunization against HBV was carried out in 1973 (S. KRUGMAN et al.). • The **immunogenicity** of vaccines derived from plasma is comparable to that of gene-engineered vaccines: with 3 × 10 µg, anti-HBs is induced in 95–99% of children and adults (20–40 years); in older persons, the immune response is weaker.

A **vaccination schedule** involving injections (i.m. in the upper arm [!] or more effectively intradermal) at intervals of 1 and 6 months following the first injection (i.e. month

0, 1, 6) has proved successful. If an adequately high anti-HBs titre is to be attained as quickly as possible, the recommended intervals are 0, 1, 2 and 12 months.

Contraindications include acute infections and (possibly) certain allergies. **Side effects** are minimal (<5%) and harmless (e.g. fatigue, rise in temperature, local reddening of the skin). Rare reports have been received of thrombocytopenia, haemolysis or neuritis. Active vaccination can be carried out during **pregnancy**. (124) (s. fig. 22.9)

The **indication** for active vaccination is given for all non-immune persons (*1.*) who are most probably exposed to the danger of infection, (*2.*) for whom the necessary time for the development of a protective anti-HBs titre is available, (*3.*) who have not previously received active vaccination because of indicated simultaneous vaccination, and (*4.*) as a general rule all children (from infancy) and juveniles. These groups include:

1. Persons working in the health sector (179, 195, 226)
2. Staff members in contact with blood or blood constituents
3. Intimate partner of an HBsAg carrier
4. Homosexuals (158, 226)
5. Dialysis patients and, if necessary, the relatives caring for them (e.g. home dialysis) (141, 166, 226)
6. Care personnel or inmates
   – in homes for the mentally disabled
   – in shelters for the homeless
   – in prisons
7. Drug addicts (226)
8. Travellers to endemic areas, especially when these journeys are repeated or if hygienic conditions are poor
9. Patients with coexisting liver disease who would be greatly endangered by an additional HBV infection
10. According to the WHO report of 1995, hepatitis B vaccination is to be included in *vaccination programmes for infants and juveniles* – this is now common in many countries

Preliminary testing prior to active prophylactic immunization against HBV is carried out in line with a well established schedule. (s. figs. 22.11, 22.12) • Active vaccination of persons who are only anti-HBc-positive usually triggers a booster effect with the development of anti-HBs.

Regarding **vaccine protection,** the efficacy threshold for anti-HBs is deemed to be a titre of about 10 IU/l. The antibody titre is determined four to six weeks after the last vaccination. Depending on the titre attained, a *booster* may be required at various intervals. It is recommended to check the titre level some four weeks after the booster. It is thus possible to establish the effect of the previous vaccination and to fix a date for the next booster. About 25% of successfully vaccinated persons are no longer adequately protected after five years.

Anti-HBs titre (in IU/l)	Booster after
<10	immediately
10–100	3–6 months
100–1,000	1 year
1,000–10,000	3–5 years
>10,000	6–10 years

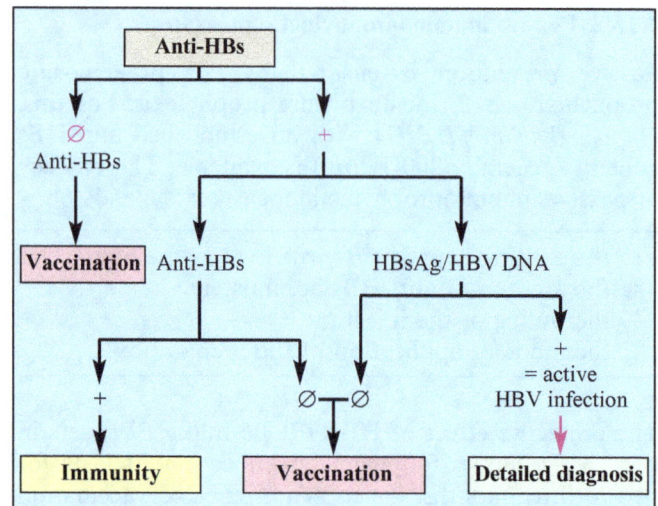

Fig. 22.12: Preliminary tests prior to active vaccination against hepatitis B (s. tab. 5.17)

▶ The **immune response** is mainly influenced by *age, gender* and *immune status*. Women usually show a better immune response than men. In almost every case, children form adequately high antibody titres (100% responders). Older people, starting at the age of about 50, show a slowly decreasing immune response. (149) Smokers, patients suffering from coeliac disease and overweight persons are more frequently non-responders, as are certain HLA types or those with IL-2 deficiency (e.g. dialysis patients). Dialysis patients or immunosuppressed persons are only capable of an immune response in about 50% of cases (or even less). • In 5–10% of cases, no antibodies are formed (non-responders). (227)

Relative non-responders only display a good immune response after an additional fourth, fifth or sixth injection. In alcoholics, a double vaccine dose is more effective. (230) Care must be taken to ensure that the ampoule is well shaken and the injection correctly placed (i.m.) in the upper arm. It must likewise be guaranteed that the vaccine storage directions are adhered to and the cooling chain is not interrupted prior to injection. • The trace elements **zinc** and **selenium**, which can be relatively or absolutely reduced under certain conditions, are also important for the functioning of the immune system. (s. p. 55) (s. tab. 3.15) In our experience, an adequately high "substitution" of zinc and selenium can prove beneficial prior to repeated injections (especially since the cost factor is low, and there are no known side effects). This measure is recommended for cirrhotic patients, in particular those with alcohol-induced cirrhosis, and indeed for all alcohol abusers. These persons, who generally display zinc deficiency, are hardly capable of an immune response, yet are very much exposed to the risk of HBV infection. • The experience we made after 1987 with additional zinc application in non-responders or in a reduced immune system could be confirmed in rats. (214)

Absolute non-responders are individuals who, in spite of all efforts, still show no immune response. Additional administration of interleukin-2 may open up new opportunities for treatment. (122, 230)

Measures for non-responders
1. Compliance with storage instructions and maintenance of the cooling chain for the vaccine
2. Shaking the ampoule
3. Injection in the upper arm (i.m., intradermal)
4. Additionally, 4th, 5th or 6th repeat injections, in general with double dose and at shorter intervals
5. Possibly pre-administration of zinc and selenium

▶ If there is a risk of HBV infection prior to the completion of vaccination and before anti-HBs values can give protection, the administration of HBIG is indicated. As a result, interim passive protection is provided and active vaccination can be completed. • *Active vaccination against hepatitis B is also considered to be the most effective prevention against the development of HBV-related hepatocellular carcinoma.* (256)

4.16 Therapy

Causal therapy (i.e. antiviral treatment) is not yet possible with viral hepatitis B. Both HAV and HBV are deemed to be self-restricting. • *HBV infection*, however, differs considerably from hepatitis A with regard to the following **criteria:**

1. Development of HBsAg carrier state
2. Progression to chronic hepatitis
3. Transmission mode
4. Penetration into body secretions and excretions
5. Correlation with HCC
6. Virus binding to the liver cell membrane
7. Mechanism of hepatocytolysis

4.16.1 Aims of treatment

The spontaneous recovery rate is 90−95%. The desired aims in treating viral hepatitis B can only be attained by means of therapeutic steps targeted at the pathogenesis of the HBV infection:

1. Shortening of the (acute and total) course of disease
2. Prevention of massive liver cell necrosis
3. Avoidance of chronic hepatitis

4.16.2 Methods of treatment

Symptomatic measures: The only forms of treatment available (at present) are those already used in general medicine or other reasonable symptomatic measures:

1. Avoidance of factors (possibly) damaging to the liver, such as alcohol, chemicals, medication, toxins, *etc.*
2. Avoidance of factors (possibly) straining the immune system, such as operations, vaccinations, special medication, mental stress, *etc.*
3. Treatment and stabilization of endocrine diseases, such as diabetes mellitus, hyperthyroidism, *etc.*
4. Avoidance of malnutrition
5. Avoidance of physical strain

Alcohol abstinence: Despite contradictory opinions, alcohol abstinence should be maintained during the acute course of disease as well as during the *posthepatitic vulnerable phase*. Even if just a minimal amount of alcohol is actually permitted, the patient is nevertheless likely to increase consumption at will.

Bed rest: Patients who feel ill and weak will keep to bed rest of their own accord and refrain from any unnecessary physical exertion. (s. p. 7) The fact that the hepatic blood flow is improved when the body is lying flat is an additional argument in favour of bed rest during the acute phase of disease.

Diet: The *diet* should be evenly balanced and in accordance with the principles of present-day dietetics; it must also be tolerated by the patient. There is no special diet for viral hepatitis patients. • The *water and electrolyte balance* is often disrupted in cases of acute viral hepatitis, possibly with the occurrence of oedemas and ascites (= *hepatitis oedematosa*) (47, 73, 130) (s. p. 303) or impaired renal function − as is recognizable from the diuresis which normally develops at the onset of the convalescence phase. An even balance of water and electrolytes should be maintained − this is supported by the patient lying flat. • In the event of inadequate nutrition or malnutrition, particularly when nausea and vomiting occur, substitution measures are advisable (e.g. vitamins, glucose and electrolyte infusions).

Moist warmth: The application of moist warmth in the region of the liver is one of the oldest modes of treatment of liver disease and dates back to CAELIUS AURELIANUS. (s. p. 7) This aims at an improved circulation in the liver, something which has not, however, been proved up to now. In the case of upper abdominal complaints, moist warmth is not only seen as beneficial, but it helps to avoid the use of splasmolytics and analgesics.

Cholestyramine may be advisable in cases of pronounced pruritus as a result of a cholestatic course of disease (4−8 g before breakfast).

Ursodeoxycholic acid was used to treat acute viral hepatitis B *without* cholestasis for the first time by our working group in 1988. (163) At the time, we attributed the markedly positive effect of treatment in 9 out of 10 patients to the potential immunomodulatory effect of UDCA. (146, 151, 208) In 1993 reports were also published by A.D. JORGE on the good results achieved in 22 patients suffering from acute viral hepatitis and cholestasis. • Administration in acute viral hepatitis is therefore recommended in controlled studies, since side effects are not to be expected and the current level of knowledge on the pharmacological effects of UDCA can be deepened. The beneficial effects of UDCA as reported so far in the cholestatic course of acute viral hepatitis are evidence of the success of this treatment.

Medicaments: *Glucocorticoids* are contraindicated. • Administration of *interferon* α is more dangerous than helpful. • *Other medicaments* should not be used unless this is absolutely necessary – it must be noted that the disturbed metabolism may alter in unforeseen ways. • In contrast, **misoprostol** (150) and **lamivudine** (138, 239, 241) showed remarkably positive effects. Especially in fulminant hepatitis B, administration of lamivudine (100–150 mg/day) proved to be effective. (238) • In patients with reactivation due to cytostatic therapy after liver transplantation, lamivudine was much more efficacious than famciclovir.

▶ The "treatment of jaundice with **sheep lice**" was first reported on by J.J. BECHER (1663). In a fascinating publication, K. QUECKE (1951) describes this topic in detail from the viewpoint of medical history. This procedure has long been common practice in folk medicine in the treatment of jaundice and involves the ingestion of a certain number of live sheep lice. There are inofficial reports that this absurd course of treatment is still practised in many regions of the world as well as in all social classes of the population, as I myself have experienced (cf. the German expression of *"eine Laus ist über die Leber gelaufen"* or the English exclamation of *"something is biting him"*). (s. p. 5)

4.17 Healing of hepatitis B

The term **healing** means the *complete restoration* of the previous normal condition. Such a *restitutio ad integrum* in morphological and biochemical terms often cannot be achieved in the case of acute viral hepatitis B. • The term **healing up** means *recovery*, although varying morphological or biochemical *residues* may remain – as is often the case with acute viral hepatitis B.

4.17.1 Morphological healing process

In simple terms, the morphological healing process comprises three steps: (*1.*) phase of remittent inflammation, (*2.*) phase of regeneration, and (*3.*) phase of residual defects. Even if the healing phases are fluid in their relation to one another, each individual stage is easy to identify in the "longitudinal histological pattern". (255) (s. figs. 22.13, 22.14)

(*1.*) The **phase of remittent inflammation** shows a *variegated histological picture*, which can be characterized as follows:

- increased deposition of glycogen in the hepatocytes
- accumulation of small liver cells with chromatin-rich nuclei and basophilic cytoplasm in the peripheral areas of the cleaned necrotic foci
- rise in acidophilic (and eosinophilic) single-cell coagulation necroses (= *Councilman bodies*), rejected from the cellular arrangement, whereby the histological picture is often dominated by condensed acidophilic hepatocytes with disintegrating nuclei
- rise in binuclear hepatocytes
- decrease in ballooned hepatocytes and histiocytic-lymphocytic cell elements in favour of plasmocytic forms as well as eosinophilic degeneration (= *dark liver cells*)
- reduced stellate cell reaction through to focal residues
- smoothing of the parenchymal portal field barrier, with inflammatory reactions receding to the portal fields; the liver cells grow in the direction of the central vein, making use of the intersinusoidal spaces as conveyance channels

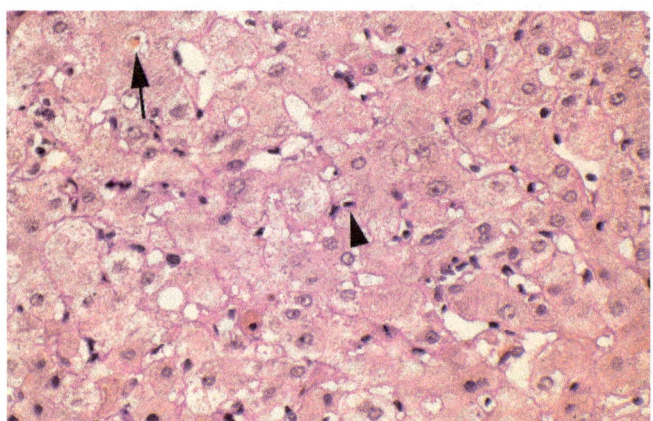

Fig. 22.13: Late stage of acute viral hepatitis B: moderate round-cell infiltration of the lobular parenchyma with small aggregates of Kupffer cells and Kupffer cell activation; slight disarray of liver cell trabeculae; minimal canalicular cholestasis (→); liver cell mitosis (▶) and binuclear hepatocytes (HE)

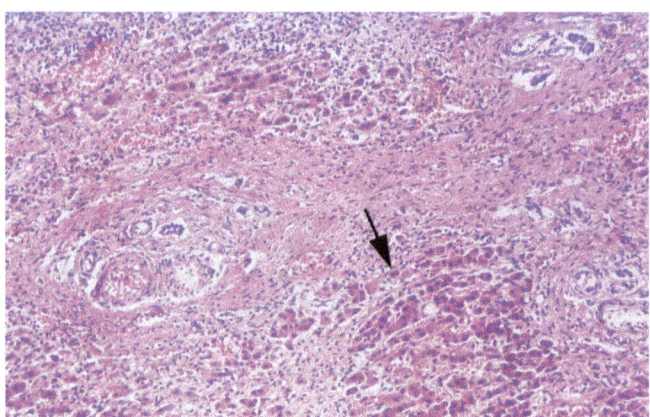

Fig. 22.14: Scarred area with fragmented parenchymal islets (→) after confluent necrosis in the wake of viral hepatitis B (HBsAg+). Localized round-cell infiltration in the remaining parenchymal areas (HE)

(*2.*) The **phase of regeneration** (s. p. 408) cannot be clearly delimited – the histological picture shows the superimposition of remittent inflammatory changes and signs of regeneration. Minor inflammatory reactions in the portal field may persist for some time after termination of the clinical course of disease. The liver cell degeneration pigment ceroid (s. fig. 21.6) is no longer present, the stored iron pigment is only gradually transported away and the intralobular late nodules (s. fig. 22.3) recede slowly. Fibrocytes and fibroblasts are produced and activated, apparently from the histiocytes.

(3.) The **phase of residual defects** continues to display so-called *late nodules* (even for several months). The portal fields are freed from inflammatory elements. Only occasionally is iron-positive pigment identified; this serves as the most reliable and longest detectable sign of a past acute viral hepatitis. Parallel fibrillar production of collagen is increasingly evident in the portal field. The portal field vein, initially still dilated, normalizes its lumen. Sometimes, there are minor fibrotic portal fields, with the fibres fringed at the corners. Condensation of the intralobular lattice fibre structure or fibrous sclerosis around the central vein may still be detectable. These connective tissue residues often prove to be reversible.

In severe hepatic necrosis with large losses of parenchyma, the regenerating epithelium is not always able to restore the affected area completely. There is a development of fibrous bundles, which are in some places connected with pronounced and partly fringed fibrotic tissue in the portal field. Moreover, extensive **cicatricial areas** are formed, occasionally embedded in small parenchymal islets. (s. fig. 22.14)

▶ After severe viral hepatitis had been overcome, we were often able to use photolaparoscopy to document extensive **parenchymal losses**, particularly in the area of the left liver lobe. We found not only (*1.*) diffusely distributed scarred retractions and defects in the connective tissue on the liver surface, but also (*2.*) circumscribed, relatively clearly defined grey-white and sunken scar plates, and even (*3.*) a largely dystrophic loss of the left liver lobe. (s. figs. 21.13; 22.15, 22.16)

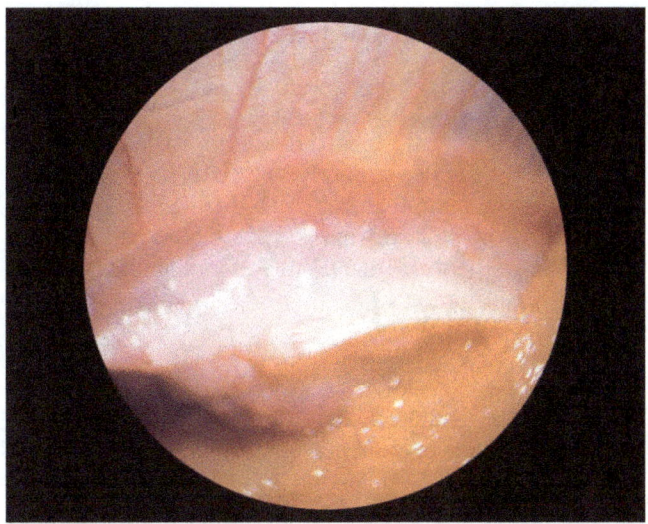

Fig. 22.16: Massive atrophy of the left liver lobe with pronounced capsular callosity following severe acute viral hepatitis B. This finding was completely misinterpreted when using sonography. (s. fig. 21.13; 35.1, 35.17)

Despite these often extensive fibrotic and scarred changes, sometimes with considerable parenchymal loss, liver function values are usually normal. The enzyme activities, likewise normalized, suggest the total disappearance of inflammatory reactions without any further liver cell damage. However, γ-GT can still be elevated, pointing to continued liver cell regeneration.

4.17.2 Biochemical healing process

Biochemical healing is demonstrated by the normalization of enzyme activities and liver function parameters. There are no obvious signs of any (possibly still) increased mesenchymal activity. Occasional posthepatitic (functional) hyperbilirubinaemia is of no significance; it disappears spontaneously. HBsAG elimination is 1—2% per year. Serologically, anti-HA IgG and anti-HBs IgG as well as anti-HBe (with the simultaneous disappearance of HBsAg and HBeAg) are considered to initiate a recovery phase with immunity. (255)

Nevertheless, these normalized laboratory parameters do not supply any information on the form of morphological healing; in individual cases, this can be either a *restitutio ad integrum* or a persistent *defect after healing* with pronounced parenchymal loss and fibrosis. (s. p. 412) With examinations using imaging procedures, thought should be given to the possibility of such posthepatitic defect healing processes – even on a large scale! (s. figs. 22.15, 22.16) – in cases where findings are difficult to interpret. It is necessary to use laparoscopy (and possibly targeted biopsy) in order to assess the type and severity of such morphological findings reliably and pinpoint their clinical significance in the light of laboratory tests.

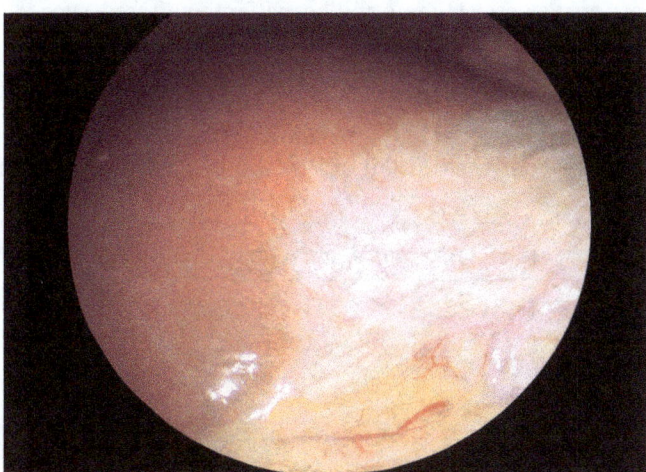

Fig. 22.15: Large sunken scar plate in the area of the left lobe of liver (about 6 × 4 cm) subsequent to massive dystrophic liver parenchymal necrosis due to severe viral hepatitis B

5 Acute viral hepatitis C

5.1 Definition

Acute viral hepatitis C is largely (about 90%) identical with the disease formerly known as acute **NANB** hepatitis. The main features of HCV infection are the persistence of the virus (in >80% of cases) and a high risk of chronification (in 60—80% of infected persons). *(see chapter 34.6.6!)*

5.2 Pathogen

As from 1981, cases of acute viral hepatitis not caused by HAV or HBV were known as non-A-non-B hepatitis (NANB) (H. Yoshizawa et al., 1981). • In 1989 Q.-L. Choo et al. succeeded in isolating another pathogen of acute viral hepatitis from the serum of an artificially infected chimpanzee suffering from chronic NANB hepatitis. (5) In the same year, the above mentioned working group presented a radioimmunoassay with which the antibodies to the C-virus were detectable. (307)

HCV is a (+) strand RNA virus with a total of some 9,400 nucleotides (9.4 kilobases). This virus has a diameter of 30—60 nm. Its nucleotide sequence displays homologies to the flaviviruses and pestiviruses of the flaviviridae family. HCV possesses a long open reading frame encoding a *polyprotein* precursor of about 3,000 amino acids. With the help of enzymatic degradation three **structural proteins** develop: nucleocapsid C (p21), envelope E1 (gp31) and envelope E2 (gp70). Region p7 forms the transition to the **non-structural proteins**. These include the regions NS2 (p23), NS3 (p70) (= protease/helicase), NS4A (p8), NS4B (p27), NS5A (p58) and NS5B (p68) (= replicase). The beginning of the structural proteins is denoted by 5'NCR, the end of the non-structural proteins by 3'NCR. (s. fig. 22.17)

The complete DNA sequence has meanwhile been clarified. HCV binds to the cell surface structure CD 81 via its envelope protein E2; for this reason, HCV can also infect other cell types (apart from hepatocytes). • Virus replication can be detected very early (within the first week after exposure). The viral particle load is $< 10^6$/ml serum, which is less than half of an HBV infection. The highest antibody titres are found in the pre-acute and early acute stages. • HCV can replicate extrahepatically, e.g. in leucocytes and B or T lymphocytes as well as, occasionally, in oral lichen tissue. (274) The spleen serves as a large extrahepatic reservoir for HCV. (270, 278, 307, 330, 341, 344) (s. p. 121)

5.2.1 Genotypes

HCV shows pronounced **genetic variability**. The cause lies in the fact that HCV mutates swiftly and continuously under immune pressure, so that several variants result (known as *quasi species*). The **mutation rate** is about 10 times higher than that of HBV. Worldwide, different virus isolates have been found and characterized in great detail. The genes for the envelope proteins E_1 and E_2 seem to be particularly variable. • Up to now, **6 genotypes** and up to **50 subtypes** have been distinguished. There are clear differences in their prevalence, depending on the geographic region. In Germany, for example, genotypes 1b (50—55%), 1a (18—23%) and 3a (15—18%) are most frequent, with i.v. drug dependence displaying an even higher prevalence of the HCV genotypes 2, 3a and 1a. Genotype 3a was particularly common in young patients. In cases of sporadic and posttransfusion hepatitis, there is greater correlation to type 1b, which could take a more severe course in liver transplant recipients due to the special circumstances involved. Type 1b was also frequently detected in patients with liver cell carcinoma in a non-cirrhotic liver. Furthermore, type 1b is more often associated with cirrhosis, and its response to interferon treatment is less marked, whereas types 2a and 3 display the highest responsiveness. Haemophiliac patients suffered successive infections with up to 3 HCV genotypes. • Types 4 and 5 are found mainly in Africa and type 6 in Asia. The assumption that certain genotypes are of significance for the course and prognosis of an HCV infection was not confirmed in an evaluation of 2,235 patients. •

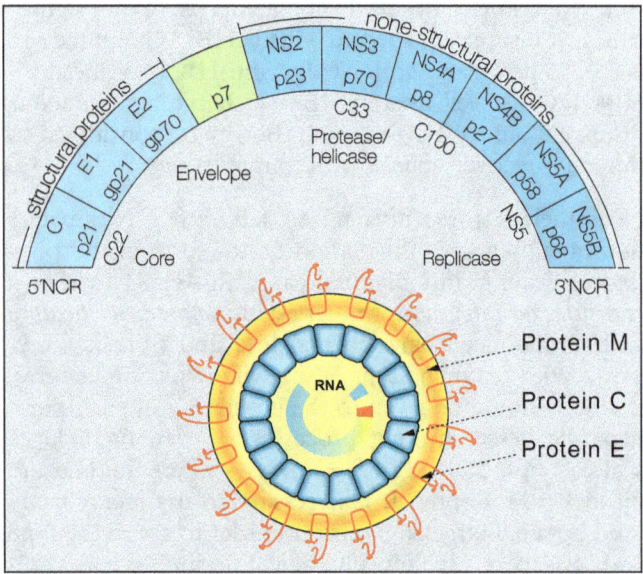

Fig. 22.17: Diagram of the genetic organization and structure of HCV.

Genotypes of HCV and their regional frequency	
Europe, USA	1, 2, 3
Australia	1, 2, 3
Far East	1, 2
Middle East	4
North Africa	4
South Africa	5
Southeast Africa	6

Tab. 22.8: Main geographical distribution of the HCV genotypes

It is most probable that the course of disease and the success of therapy largely depend on the genotype and the virus load. (272, 277, 329, 344, 370)

5.2.2 Inactivation

There are no particular measures for inactivating HCV, except for the same disinfecting procedures as applied for viral hepatitis B. Emphasis is thus placed on formalin, aldehyde derivatives and chlorine preparations as well as heating (e.g. 60 °C for 10 hours). (s. pp 427, 432)

5.3 Serological diagnostics

5.3.1 Anti-HCV test

▶ The anti-HCV test serves to identify chronic (and thus particularly infectious) HCV carriers and blood donors. The test does not identify any acute disease or HCV infection of a newborn with an HCV-positive mother, nor does it provide any information on specific immunity or infectivity. • *Although the term anti-HCV is generally used, antibodies to the intact C virus have not yet been detected.*

▶ The presence of anti-HCV affords no protection from another infection or reinfection. A reliable anti-HCV IgM test is not yet available. Experimental results, however, showed that the titre correlates with the activity of the disease and thus with the response to interferon therapy. A serum may contain HCV RNA, even though the anti-HCV test is negative. • *All sera testing positive for HCV RNA proved to be infectious.*

In acute viral hepatitis C, the HCV RNA usually clears from the serum once the infection is over – although the anti-HCV test remains positive for a longer time. However, the combination of increased GPT and a positive anti-HCV test nearly always points to infectious HCV. Subsequent to the EIA test, 95% of the positive sera demonstrated cRNA by PCR, so that infectivity was confirmed. For this reason, neither anti-HCV-positive blood donors nor blood units can be released for transfusion. • As a check for hepatitis B-negative patients with liver cell carcinoma, the EIA test displayed positivity in 83% of cases. In aetiologically unresolved cirrhosis, the EIA test was positive in 62% of patients, i.e. a large number of the cryptogenic chronic cases of hepatitis and cirrhosis were probably caused by HCV infection.

False-positive HCV tests are mainly found with autoimmunopathies, in particular autoimmune hepatitis type 2 (LMK-positive form). In cases of HCV infection which cannot be established serologically, the HCV RNA should be identified directly prior to commencement of INF therapy. In this way, the danger of deterioration in patients with autoimmune hepatitis is eliminated. (290, 320, 344)

5.3.2 RT-PCR test

Viraemia is best detected by determining the HCV RNA in the PCR test after prior reverse transcription (RT) (K. B. MÜLLIS, 1985). This also works in the incubation phase with patients who are still anti-HCV-negative with normal transaminase values as well as with serum that is still anti-HCV-negative in the acute phase. Thus the following **indications** are given for the PCR method:

(*1.*) identification of HCV infection during the incubation or acute phase, possibly after exposure

(*2.*) ascertainment of acute viral hepatitis C with negative anti-HCV test

(*3.*) detection of virus persistence and infectivity

(*4.*) measurement of the virus load as a follow-up, particularly prior to and after interferon therapy

(*5.*) testing newborns of mothers with a positive anti-HCV test

(*6.*) testing immunosuppressed patients for HCV infection

(*7.*) establishment of reinfection after organ transplantation

5.4 Epidemiology

The annual rate of new infections in Germany is estimated at 15,000–20,000. Generally, men are infected twice as often as women. The prevalence of HCV infection is 0.4 (−0.7)%, which equals approx. 500,000 chronic carriers of HCV. This includes both carriers with liver disease and people with an apparently healthy liver, since HCV RNA-positive persons show normal GPT values in 50–60% of cases, yet also display the histological signs of chronic hepatitis. • In the countries of south-eastern Europe, the prevalence is 1.5–4.0%. As with hepatitis B, there are regions with a particularly high rate of infection, such as the Pacific area with 75%. • Worldwide, the number of infectious HCV carriers is estimated at 200–300 million; the number of those infected with HCV is estimated at approx. 5 million in Europe and 4 million in the USA. (332, 337, 344, 345) *(see chapter 34.6.6)*

Obligation for notification: In Germany, since 2000, a differentiation has been made for notification purposes between HAV and HBV as well as HCV, HDV, HEV and "others". The following numbers for **NANB hepatitis** (including all hepatitis viruses except A and B) were registered (s. pp 428, 435):

1992 = 2,188	1995 = 4,272	1998 = 6,174
1993 = 2,498	1996 = 5,178	1999 = 5,987
1994 = 3,163	1997 = 6,272	

The following **frequencies of HCV** were registered, whereby the real figure is 8–10 times higher:

2000 = 6,274	2003 = 6,961	2006 = 7,558
2001 = 8,635	2004 = 9,081	
2002 = 6,745	2005 = 8,368	

The rate of **mortality** due to virus hepatitis excluding A and B (i.e. "other viruses") was as follows:

1992 = 62	1994 = 99	1996 = 156
1993 = 76	1995 = 98	1998 = 138

The rate of **mortality** due to virus hepatitis C was as follows:

1999 = 173	2002 = 127	2005 = 74
2000 = 168	2003 = 110	2006 = 99
2001 = 166	2004 = 87	

5.5 Transmission

The hepatitis C virus can be transmitted *parenterally* or *sporadically*. **Risk groups** with a high prevalence rate are haemophiliac patients (70–90%), i.v. drug addicts (50–90%), posttransfusion patients (60–80%), dialysis patients (5–30%) and liver transplant recipients. In 40–50% of patients with a positive anti-HCV test, the transmission route is still unknown. These cases are designated *"community-acquired"* or *"sporadic" hepatitis C*. The cause is rooted in poor hygienic conditions and close physical contact. (263) Fundamentally, the possibility of infection depends on the virus titre in the source person – it is considerably lower than with HBV infection. *Nosocomial infection* between patients has also been observed. (271, 318, 371)

Body secretions: HCV antibodies and HCV RNA could be detected in saliva, sweat, urine, ascites, ejaculate, breast milk, bile and lacrimal fluid. It can be assumed that (as with hepatitis B) the occurrence of HCV in various body fluids is directly correlated to the HCV concentration in the serum. (259, 280, 319, 326, 331)

Blood transfusion: Some 90% of cases of NANB posttransfusion hepatitis are caused by hepatitis C. The risk deriving from this greatly feared transmission route could be diminished by using the anti-HCV test to screen blood donors and blood units; this caused a reduction from 4.0% to 0.6% and to <1 for every 10,000 blood units (= residual risk if a so-called serological window is present). (285, 290, 293, 367, 376)

Blood products: The use of blood units or blood products with haemophiliac patients and the administration of immunoglobulin preparations in general (311, 335) were accompanied by high HCV positivity. Today, there is only a slight risk of HCV infection in this respect.

Haemodialysis: HCV prevalence (5–30%) depends on the duration of dialysis and hence on the number of blood units used. Transmission is also possible via the dialysis equipment itself. (286, 306, 323, 349, 360, 361)

Drug addicts: With i.v. drug abuse, above all due to the common practice of "needle sharing", HCV antibodies can be detected in 50–90% of cases. (289, 364)

Medical personnel: Infection can be caused by way of *needlestick injury* (264, 305, 312, 340, 369, 379) or percutaneously; sometimes the route of transmission is unknown. (386) The rate of contagion is 0.8 (–2.0)%. Medical personnel in transplantation units were particularly exposed to risk (300), as were those in dialysis and plasmapheresis centres. (284) Dentists, too, were infected 12 times more frequently with hepatitis C than a control group (1.7% vs. 0.14%). With dental surgeons, a contagion rate exceeding 9% was detected. (280, 295, 313) In emergency admission units, the frequency rates for positive anti-HCV tests were very high. An outbreak of acute hepatitis C was observed among volunteers participating in pharmacokinetic studies. (322) There was also a report regarding the risk of HCV transmission from patients to surgeons. (375) However, no serious risk of transmission emanating from an infected gynaecologist was demonstrated during a period of seven years. (357) In other studies, the risk of HCV infection in medical staff is largely identical to that found in the normal population; in cases of injury, no (not even short-term) IF therapy is indicated.

Transplantation: The transfer of an infected organ led to hepatitis C in about half the cases, which, because of the required immunosuppression, mainly took a fulminant or chronic course. As with HBV infection, reinfection can occur in up to 87% of cases within a 12-month period following the transplantation of a virus-free liver. This could be due to the duplication of the virus in extrahepatic cells. However, the transplanted liver only showed slight inflammatory reactions, so that HCV cirrhosis is deemed to be a clear indication for transplantation. (297, 317, 333, 363, 381, 383)

Skin injury: One report was received on the parenteral transmission of hepatitis C via a bite wound from an HCV-infected person (291) and another on transmission from shaving. (377) It is unclear whether mosquito bites also transmit hepatitis C. Large tattoos or acupuncture are considered to be another channel of infection. Worthy of mention is a report of an HCV-positive anaesthetist who infected 20 patients with hepatitis C. (282)

Endoscopy: There is no risk of infection provided the endoscope has been correctly cleaned. (353)

Intrafamilial infection: The frequency of intrafamilial infection, i.e. from close contact in the household and sexual contact between spouses, is clearly higher than with HCV-free families, yet it is still categorized as low. The notified rates of infection can vary considerably (3.2–23.0%). With children, positive anti-HCV tests were found in about 5% of cases. The sensitivity of the tests applied and the difference in the types of virus are probably responsible for the variations in the infection risk. (261, 279, 294, 310, 335, 346, 354)

Sexual transmission: In heterosexual partners, anti-HCV tests were positive in 5–23% of cases; a frequent change of partners seems to increase the risk of infection (some 10% of all HCV infections). Sexual transmission is more frequent from an infected male to a female than vice versa. Homosexuals show a low infection rate of 2–3% per year. In prostitutes, prevalence is 5–10%. In all, sexual transmission is of little significance, yet it has been validated in several studies. (268, 304, 331, 336, 354, 374, 378)

Vertical infection: In about 0.8% of pregnant women, the anti-HCV test is positive. The likelihood of transmission from the mother to the child is 5% (−10%), yet it increases in line with the titre value of the circulating HCV RNA. The chronicity rate may be as high as 90%! However, detection is only possible by means of PCR, since anti-HCV can also be transmitted passively to the newborn, irrespective of infection. Transmission of HCV has even been demonstrated over a number of generations. HCV-positive mothers should possibly refrain from breast-feeding their infants, since HCV RNA can be present in the breast milk. Nevertheless, a doctor's order against breast-feeding is unnecessary. So far, one fatal case of HCV infection in a child has been reported. Administration of immunoglobulin to the newborn is not indicated. Pregnancy is not contraindicated in HCV-infected women. HCV screening is not required in every case. (298, 316, 351, 352, 366, 385)

5.6 Histological findings

On the whole, the histological picture resembles that of toxic hepatitis. As a result, it can be difficult to make a differential diagnosis. In contrast to HAV and HBV infections, viral hepatitis C displays several *specific histological features* (301, 314, 315, 344, 365):

(*1.*) In 30−85% of cases, the liver cells show fatty degeneration.
(*2.*) Destruction of the bile ducts is frequently detectable.
(*3.*) Hyaline cytoplasm inclusions (Mallory-Denk bodies) are often detected.
(*4.*) Hyaline single cell necrosis (rather similar in appearance to Councilman bodies) is nearly always present. This condition is the result of cytotoxicity, mediated by T lymphocytes.
(*5.*) In the portal fields, plasmacellular and lymphocytic infiltrates prevail. However, they are also present in the liver parenchyma, arranged linearly inside the sinusoids, so that this finding is often mistaken for hepatitis mononucleosa. There are no granulocytic components.
(*6.*) Epithelioid cell granuloma and liver cell ballooning are found in rare cases.
(*7.*) With a chronic course of hepatitis C, the extent to which connective tissue is formed is far less than in chronic hepatitis B. In contrast, filigree bundles of fibre and small hyalinization foci are chiefly found.

▶ **Histological diagnosis** of chronic HCV positivity is *best guaranteed by means of targeted biopsy with laparoscopy if two or three bioptic specimens are taken, possibly from the right as well as from the left liver lobe.* Percutaneous biopsies, as a primary or follow-up measure, only reach a limited area of the right liver lobe (s. fig. 7.8). One single bioptic specimen is not necessarily representative of the total liver findings, as we have repeatedly discovered through our own experience. (s. pp 168, 713, 750)

Differential diagnosis: Such histological findings can lead to considerable difficulties in terms of diagnostic classification. Moreover, the course of hepatitis C can be uneventful; sometimes only minor fatty liver cell degeneration, often without any noteworthy inflammatory reactions, is found. Even in cases of validated HCV infection, percutaneous liver biopsy frequently shows "normal findings" (which, cannot in any way be seen as representative). Histological diagnosis is rendered very difficult by the occasional combination of an HBV infection with hepatitis C. The following *liver diseases* are important in terms of differential diagnosis:

> (*1.*) Exogenous toxic fatty liver cell degeneration with possible inflammatory reactions of fatty liver hepatitis. Especially *alcohol-toxic fatty liver* is the most frequent false diagnosis in hepatitis C.
> (*2.*) False diagnosis due to a certain similarity with *autoimmune hepatitis.*
> (*3.*) Histologically based suspicion of *primary biliary cholangitis.*
> (*4.*) Morphological similarity with *hepatitis mononucleosa.*

5.7 Stages of disease

The **incubation period** lasts for 15−150 days. Anti-HCV can only be demonstrated four to seven weeks after infection, whereas PCR is already positive within the first week. Current serological tests fail during the incubation phase, which is why those persons who are without clinical and biochemical symptoms can transmit HCV infection unnoticed (e.g. blood donors).

The **acute phase** is characterized by a continuous rise in the detection of anti-HCV. Only 5−10% still test negative for a certain period of time; in suspected infection, a serological check should therefore be carried out after four to six weeks. With individual patients, the immune response can be delayed by several months, although there are no signs of immunodeficiency. As with HAV or HBV infections, prodromal symptoms are milder or even absent. *The acute phase is clinically symptom-free in ca. 80% of cases!* Jaundice and/or hepatomegaly only occur in 15−30% of patients, whereby the jaundice is less pronounced. Enhanced fatigue may be evident. The mean transaminase activity is about half of that observed in hepatitis B, i.e. between 250−750 U/l. Often, an episodic fluctuating course ensues, alternating with transaminase values that may even be normal; therefore, normal values cannot be taken as a criterion for ruling out HCV infection. The clinical course frequently displays different episodes with monophasic (15%), biphasic (22%) or multiphasic transaminase levels as well as a plateau-like pattern of GPT values. The increase in transaminase activity can persist for a period of 12 months in half of the cases. The inflammatory changes correspond to the extent of viraemia, i.e.

the severity of the course of disease correlates with the anti-HCV titre. Often there is a significant increase in γ-GT (3 to 4 times the norm). This correlates with serious damage to the bile capillaries. • A *cholestatic course* is rare; generally, the disease progresses rapidly and can culminate in liver failure. Organ transplant patients are especially affected. • A *fulminant course* of disease is more frequent in Japan, yet is very rare in western countries (0.5−1.0%). (281, 302, 316, 372) This can be attributed to the higher HCV prevalence in Japan or to the divergence of HCV genotypes. • Superinfection with HAV has also been known to cause a fulminant course.

▶ In acute and chronic HCV infections, various **antibodies** such as ANA, SMA, LKM-1, anti-GOR, etc. (s. pp 123−127, 659) (up to 65% of cases) as well as a positive rheumatoid factor (approx. 20% of cases) were detected. The differentiation between "genuine" autoimmune hepatitis and HCV infection with autoimmune phenomena is of paramount clinical significance.

A **symptom-free course** is common with HCV infection. A subclinical course is often observed as well. It is therefore sometimes difficult to define the onset of the disease and the point when clinical healing begins. HAV infection can suppress HCV replication and therefore support the clearance of HCV. (288) Clarity is only obtained by reliable histology based on representative samples. (269)

The clinical course can be unfavourably affected by various **risk factors** (e.g. race, gender, advanced age, immune status, genetics) as well as by alcohol abuse (266, 325), toxins, coinfections and chemicals. Conversely, the course and prognosis of HBV, HDV and HIV infections as well as of metabolic diseases (e.g. porphyria cutanea tarda, α_1-antitrypsin deficiency) can deteriorate as a result of hepatitis C.

Course of disease: Some 15−30% of those infected with HCV recover spontaneously; another 25% are asymptomatic with consistently normal transaminase values and only minor histological lesions. About 25% of cases are icteric. In approx. 40% of patients, sonographically determinable abdominal lymphadenopathy develops. During the further course of disease, hepatitis C displays a high chronicity rate of 70−80%. In 20−30% of cases, liver cirrhosis can be expected to develop within 10−20 years. These figures apply both to posttransfusion and to sporadic HCV infections. In 5% of cases, death occurs within 5 years. (303, 359, 362, 373, 376)

The **diagnosis** of acute viral hepatitis C is based on the following parameters, whereby especially alcoholic liver damage must first be ruled out:

- moderate increase in GPT, GOT and GDH
- noticeably higher γ-GT value
- repeatedly positive anti-HCV test (plus titre determination in the blood)
- determination of the HCV genotype
- positive HCV RNA test
- histological criteria

HCV carrier state: A clinically asymptomatic carrier is demonstrated by the anti-HCV titre and HCV RNA (in serum and peripherical blood mononuclear cells) with normal transaminase values. This form is naturally found in immunodeficient patients, but also in cases of infection caused by genotype 3. Histology may be non-contributory (269, 349, 362, 365) − yet it can also reveal severe changes, in which case the GPT level is elevated.

5.8 Extrahepatic manifestations

As in acute viral hepatitis A and B, an HCV infection may induce extrahepatic manifestations and syndromes. (292, 343) Such associations with various diseases not only make differential diagnosis difficult, but can also have an unfavourable influence on the course of disease. The capability of the C virus to induce autoimmunity is of special significance. (s. tab. 22.9) (s. p. 719)

Agranulocytosis
Aplastic anaemia
Corneal ulceration (382)
Cryoglobulinaemia (260, 334, 339)
Diabetes mellitus (type 1)
Erythema exsudativum multiforme
Glomerulonephritis (283, 327, 347, 356)
Guillain-Barré syndrome (321)
Hyperlipasaemia (384)
Lichen ruber planus (348)
Non-Hodgkin lymphoma (287, 334)
Polyarteriitis nodosa (273, 275, 350)
Polyarthritis
Polyneuritis
Porphyria cutanea tarda (296, 342, 368)
Sialadenitis
Sjögren's syndrome (262)
Thrombocytopenia
Thyreoiditis

Tab. 22.9: Extrahepatic manifestations in viral hepatitis C (with some references) (s. tabs. 22.2, 22.7)

▶ Even during the acute course of disease, haematological manifestations in the form of **agranulocytosis** and transient **aplastic anaemia** have been observed. • Membranoproliferative **glomerulonephritis** is rare. HCV RNA, anti-HCV IgG antibodies and IgM rheumatoid factors are found in the immune complex deposits. At the same time, cryoglobulins and circulating immune complexes are often identified in the serum. No association of this manifestation with a particular HCV genotype is known. HCV replication in the renal epithelium has not been detected up to now. Treatment with interferon-α has been successful in producing a clear improvement of the renal function. • HCV RNA is detected in 42−95% of patients with essential compound **cryoglobulinaemia** of type II or III (in Germany, in about 25% of cases). These findings often coincide with the identification of the rheumatoid factor and/or a decrease in complement. This extrahepatic manifestation of an HCV infection also displayed a good response to interferon-α, whereas cessation of this therapy led to the reoccurrence of the clinical and biochemical symptoms. Long-term therapy might be helpful here, possibly with low-dose interferon-α. HCV RNA is a suitable follow-up parameter for the effectiveness of interferon therapy. In chronic HCV infection, a low-titre cryoglobulinaemia is often found without any signs of autoimmune disease typical for the condition. • **Polyarteriitis nodosa** is another extrahepatic manifestation of HCV infection. • In 70−80%

of cases, HCV infection could be associated with **porphyria cutanea tarda**, whereas in Germany and Ireland, the coexistence of an HCV infection with PCT could only be established in <10% of cases. A possible explanation for this variation in prevalence might be either regional differences in the frequency of congenital uroporphyrinogen-III decarboxylase deficiency or a specific genotype. • Moreover, some reports have focused on **dermatological** and **ophthalmological** associations. Histology has shown **lesions of the salivary gland** in up to 50% of cases.

5.9 Hepatitis C and hepatocellular carcinoma

The prevalence of anti-HCV antibodies in patients with HCC is 13−76%, i.e. there are considerable geographic differences. High rates of prevalence are found in Italy, Spain and Japan (55−76%). A combination with a concurrent HBV infection increases the risk of carcinoma. With posttransfusion NANB cirrhosis, the incidence of carcinoma is >5%. Given an appropriately long duration of HCV infection (20−30 years), primary liver cell carcinoma must be expected in up to 20% of cases, i.e. HCC occurs in 1−4% of patients with HCV cirrhosis every year. Likewise, in chronic hepatitis C, the frequency of HCC tends to be underestimated owing to the difficulty involved in making an early diagnosis. (267, 276, 287, 324, 358) (s. pp 442, 800)

HCC diagnostics: Priority is given to **sonography**, which should be carried out at intervals of six to nine months in cases of chronic HCV infection. • At the same time, the α_1 **foetoprotein** should be determined, since both results are complementary to each other. AFP values of <20 ng/ml do not give any cause for suspicion. Increasing values, however, should be checked at shorter intervals, since a continuous rise points to a high risk of carcinoma. The AFP values correlate well with the size of the tumour and the undifferentiation of HCC. • The next diagnostic step to be taken is a **CT** scan. It is important to mention that foci of 3−5 cm in diameter are still accessible for surgical resection. • *For the histological validation of a diagnosis of suspected HCC,* **laparoscopy** *is the first priority − there is no other real diagnostic alternative.* (s. p. 163) Such a technique facilitates targeted biopsies and, when using Robbers forceps, the targeted *removal of tissue* from various areas in an adequate quantity for possible specific pathological processing. *At the same time, it supports* **staging** *through inspection of the free abdominal cavity, which is generally required in any case and cannot be replaced by any other procedure.* • Percutaneous ("blind") or sonography-guided liver biopsy is not recommended, since it involves a considerably greater risk of bleeding in this situation than does laparoscopic forceps biopsy; moreover, percutaneous biopsy is only possible in a relatively small area of the right epigastric region (which does not always correspond to the localization of the focus). Further thought must be given to the fact that the obtained information is in itself limited, and usually the investigation has to be taken a step further by subsequent staging. *(see chapter 37.3)*

5.10 Prophylaxis and therapy

Prophylactic measures, as with HBV infection, include general hygiene measures and avoidance of exposure. Passive or active vaccination is not yet available. No therapy is required initially in a suspected infection with HCV due to needlestick injury. (All relevant findings and facts must be carefully documented!) However, GPT and GOT as well as PCR should be checked after two to three weeks and again after a further four to six weeks. If a virus infection is now detected, interferon therapy can be applied. In terms of behaviour on the part of the patient, the *treatment* of acute viral hepatitis C corresponds to that of acute viral hepatitis A or B. During antiviral therapy, HCV RNA should be monitored every three to six months. (265, 299, 338)

▶ Only an efficient **antiviral immune reaction** can eliminate the hepatitis C virus. In acute HCV infection, minimal (endogenous) interferon-α values are detectable in the serum, i.e. the virus effects a poor interferon induction in the organism. • The $CD8^+$ and $CD4^+$ T lymphocytes are mainly responsible for virus elimination. The problems of HCV infection lie in the fact that the patient has virtually no chance of spontaneous improvement or healing with a *chronic course* of disease, i.e. there is practically no self-limiting factor in a process that has become chronic.

Antiviral therapy

In 1992 **interferon-α** was used for the first time in acute HCV infection. The time at which therapy was commenced varied between three and four months after onset of the disease. Measured against the normalization of the transaminase values, success was attained in 60% of cases vs. 50% in the placebo group. After the end of therapy, the transaminase values may rise again. In the event of chronification, the course proved to be milder, and there was less histological activity. The long-term effect of interferon-α therapy in acute viral hepatitis C cannot be assessed as yet. Only in 20−25% of cases has it so far been possible to maintain remission of the disease. Patients with HCV genotypes 3 or 2 maintained remission in 30−40% of cases. • The recommended dosage of pegylated IFNα is 5 million U/day for 4 weeks and then 3×5 million U/week for 5 months, the aim being to achieve HCV RNA negativity and normalization of the transaminase levels as well as to avoid chronification (success rate 80−98%). (308, 380) With HCV RNA negativity and normalization of laboratory values, interferon therapy can be continued for another 6 months (3×3 million U/week). • In some 50% of patients suffering from hepatitis C, the immune reaction is sufficient to control the virus (i.e. its multiplication is suppressed); this is also the case in α superinfection with HAV. Presumably, complete elimination of the viruses cannot be achieved, even with an intact immune system. An increase in $CD4^+$ lymphocytes is indicative of an effective cellular immune response, so that the viral load is kept at a low level.

In 60–80% of people infected with HCV 2 or HCV 3, the virus load can be reduced below the detection threshold after six months of combination therapy with **interferon-α + ribavirin**; with interferon monotherapy, this is achieved merely in 30–40% of cases. • The question of improving the success rate by changing the dosage or period of application is still unresolved, yet worth considering in this special context. (309, 328, 355)

This is also true for the (pharmacologically plausible) adjuvant use of **antioxidants,** for example in the form of *silymarin* (2–3 × 140–170 mg/day) during treatment with interferon-α. • Moreover, not enough reliable data are available regarding treatment with **amantadine** (e.g. 2 × 100 mg/day for 3–6 months) subsequent to interferon therapy. *(see chapter 34.7.4)*

6 Acute viral hepatitis D

6.1 Definition

Acute viral hepatitis D/B is precipitated by an initially uncoated (incomplete, defective) human apathogenic viroid, which subsequently acquires HBsAg as its envelope protein. This hepatitis delta virus (HDV) becomes pathogenic as a result of two different infection modes: (*1*.) simultaneous infection of HBV and HDV (= coinfection) and (*2*.) infection of a chronic HBsAg carrier with HDV (= superinfection).

6.2 Pathogen

The **delta virus** was first detected in HBsAg carriers by M. RIZZETTO et al. in 1977. It was described as having a spherical form with a diameter of 36 nm. Subsequently, it was characterized as a causative agent of exceptional pathogenicity.

As a **viroid**, the delta particle comprises an uncoated, single-stranded RNA in closed (circular) chain form, with 1,758 bases (1.7 kilobases). Viroids are up to 100 times smaller than viruses. The delta RNA is similar in structure to the genome of viroids from the plant kingdom. The nucleoprotein of the delta viroid is made up of the actual delta antigen (HDAg), which is composed of two larger proteins (P24 = 24,000 kD, P27 = 27,000 kD). (s. fig. 22.18)

Because of its coating with "major" HBsAg (>95%), the delta viroid becomes a complete pathogenic virus (HDV), replicating in the host cells. In this form, it has also been shown to be transmissible in animal experiments (chimpanzees, marmosets). It has not been clarified whether coating material from other hepadna viruses is used to complete the virus – in any case, replication within the hepatocytes has been demonstrated in the absence of HBV. The infectivity of HDV is dependent on the presence of HBV. Pathogenic HDV also infects other body cells, such as renal cells and fibroblasts. HDV can be inactivated with formalin. (390, 393, 396, 399, 413, 414, 417)
• Only **three genotypes** (1–3) are known so far. These features of heterogeneity may all be found in a single patient. It can be assumed that mutants account for the difference in virulence of HDV and are also of significance for the clinical course, prognosis and therapy of the disease (e.g. genotype 1 is found mainly in fulminant hepatitis, cirrhosis and HCC). (400, 404, 406, 426)

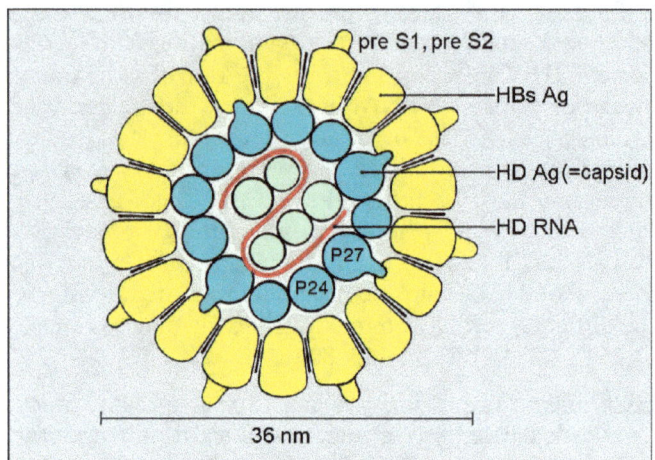

Fig. 22.18: Structure of the hepatitis D virus

6.2.1 Mutants

The presence of mutant forms has been postulated on the basis of certain observations that HDV infection can have a somewhat variable course of disease (*1*.) in animal experiments, (*2*.) in human disease, (*3*.) in various ethnic groups, and (*4*.) in different regions of the world.

6.3 Transmission

The transmission route of HDV corresponds to all the channels of infection of HBV, since its pathogenicity is coupled to the HBV as a helper virus. Thus HDV is mainly transmitted parenterally through blood and blood products as well as by sexual and even close physical contact. HDV infection cannot survive HBV infection. (395, 399, 412, 420, 421, 427, 428)

Vertical transmission from mother to child is rare. Nevertheless, newborns with HBsAg-positive and HDV-infected mothers are especially at risk. Today, examinations carried out in the final trimester of pregnancy regularly identify HBV-infected women by serological testing, so that perinatal infection should, in principle, no longer occur. (s. p. 436) (s. fig. 22.9)

Posttransfusion infection can be dangerous for the recipient (*1*.) if he/she is HBsAg-positive and if the donor blood, although proved to be HBsAg-negative in terms of the legal requirements, contains incomplete delta particles which can cause a superinfection and (2.) if the blood units have been obtained from an asymptomatic HDV carrier, where HBsAg synthesis in the donor is inhibited and his/her serological categorization proves to be false-HBsAg-negative. • *For this reason, blood units intended for HBsAg-positive recipients should be HDV-negative and also show normal transaminase values.*

6.4 Epidemiology

Retrospectively, the delta virus could be detected in Brazil in liver tissue dating back to the years after 1930 and also in blood specimens from the year 1947. Similar discoveries have been made in blood elsewhere since 1968. • HDV infection is actually present worldwide, yet there are considerable differences in frequency. The **highly endemic areas** with the greatest infection percentage are parts of Romania (80–85%), the Pacific Republic of Kiribati (ca. 70%) (424) and the Amazon region (ca. 60%). Other **endemic areas** include Egypt, Senegal, Gabon, Kenya, North India, Okinawa (Japan) and Tanzania as well as certain parts of Bolivia, Columbia and Venezuela. (391, 403) Significantly less endemic areas are to be found in the Balkans, southern Italy (25–30%) and countries of the Near and Middle East. There are estimated to be approx. 15 million HDV-infected people worldwide, i.e. some 5% of HBsAg-positive carriers. (417, 419, 423) • Outside the endemic regions, the highest figures are found among **risk groups:** haemophiliac patients (40–60%), i.v. drug addicts (up to 80%), dialysis patients and homosexuals (40–60%). (387, 392, 407, 418–420, 427) • In **Germany**, HDV infection is rare (0.5–3.0%), except in the above-mentioned risk groups (398):

Frequency		Mortality
2001 = 8	2004 = 26	2004 = 1
2002 = 12	2005 = 29	2005 = 1
2003 = 10	2006 = 26	2006 = 3

6.5 Serological diagnostics

Because of the different modes of infection with acute viral hepatitis D, as coinfection or superinfection, serology may also reveal special features. In this respect, HDAg as well as HDV RNA can be directly detected in the serum and liver cells by PCR. (388, 402, 405, 422) • An **indication** for an HDV check by means of the anti-HDV search test is given with (1.) an acute intermittent episode of chronic hepatitis B, (2.) an acute HBV infection in risk groups and patients from endemic areas, and (3.) a severe or fulminant course of acute viral hepatitis B. The persistence of anti-HDAg IgM can be considered as a *serological risk marker* for the development of a chronic form. A titre of >1:1,000 points to chronic hepatitis D. Generally, anti-HDV and HDV RNA are replication markers for an HDV infection. (s. p. 122)

6.5.1 Coinfection

HBsAg positivity is evident prior to the appearance of HDAg in the serum, just as HBcAg is found in the liver cell prior to the detection of HDAg. The other HBV seromarkers follow, as in viral hepatitis B when existing on its own. Anti-HBc IgM can be demonstrated at an early stage with a high titre. One or two months after an HDV infection, about 90% of the infected persons have antibodies (anti-HDV and anti-HDAg IgM), yet as a rule, the antibody titre is low. Anti-HDAg IgM can persist for 5–6 (–12) weeks. Anti-HDAg IgG is subsequently detectable – often within a serological "window". HDV IgG remains present for a number of years and points to a past HDV infection. With the occurrence of anti-HDV, the HDV RNA disappears. As the healing of the acute HDV coinfection progresses, the titre of anti-HDAg IgG gradually drops below the detection threshold. A past HDV infection can no longer be recognized retrospectively. HDAg and HDV RNA become negative in the hepatocytes as well. With the coinfection of HBV and HDV, the HBV RNA clears more rapidly from the serum than in the case of an HBV infection on its own. (s. fig. 22.19)

6.5.2 Superinfection

The HDV infection of a chronic HBsAg carrier leads to the suppression of HBV synthesis, so that HBsAg, HBcAg and HBeAg are no longer detectable. By contrast, anti-HDV can be identified earlier and at a higher titre. (s. fig. 22.19)

6.6 Courses of disease

The course of disease is determined equally by these two modes of infection. The incubation time is 20–70 days. Analogous to HBV infection, HDV infection can take on multiple forms. (388, 394, 405, 410, 418)

6.6.1 Coinfection

A healthy person is simultaneously infected with HBV and HDV. The pathogenic effect of HDV is usually restricted to the period of the generally self-limiting HBV infection, i.e. it can be expected to heal in approx. 90% of cases. For this reason, its clinical picture often cannot be distinguished from that of viral hepatitis B. In the event of a false-negative absence of HBV seromarkers, acute viral hepatitis D can be misinterpreted as HCV infection. Frequently (in some 30% of cases), a bimodal-like increase in the transaminase activity is registered at intervals of three to four weeks. This second rise in enzyme activity is probably caused by activation of HBV after synthesis was initially suppressed by HDV. (s. fig. 22.19) Such a biphasic course often correlates with the bilirubin level. The second phase of the disease is sometimes severe, developing into *fulminant hepatitis* in 2–20% of cases. (391) • In 2–7%

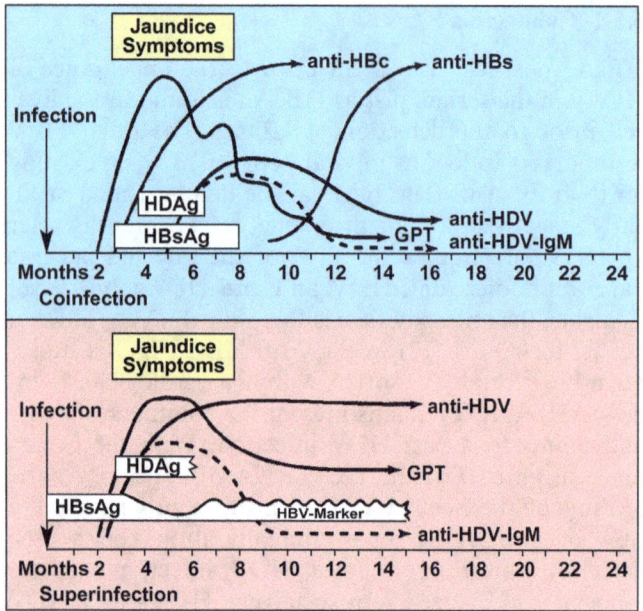

Fig. 22.19: Diagram of the immune status in the course of coinfection and superinfection with HDV

of patients, *chronic hepatitis D* may follow; 30–60% of these patients develop *cirrhosis*. A *hepatocellular carcinoma* might also appear after a 30 to 40-year latency period. (425)

6.6.2 Superinfection

A "healthy" or "diseased" HBsAg carrier is additionally infected with HDV. The incubation period is shorter than for coinfection. The transaminase values, hitherto normal or moderately increased, are now rapidly augmented, subsequently pursuing a plateau-like course. (s. fig. 22.19) As a result, superinfection normally takes a more severe course than coinfection. Consequently, transaminase values are generally higher than is usual in coinfection (approx. 300–400 U/l). The transaminase level is only insignificantly correlated with the extent of liver cell necrosis. A modest boost in bilirubin (3–6 mg/dl, higher values are rare) is observed after the rise in transaminase activity. Generally, alkaline phosphatase is elevated. • *Fulminant hepatitis* must be expected more often than in coinfection (10–25%). A rapid rise in transaminase values (>1,000 U/l) points to the onset of this severe clinical picture. No distinction can be made from the fulminant course of an HBV infection. (397, 411, 412) • *Chronic hepatitis D* occurs in 70–95% of cases of superinfection. Reactivation is frequent. Accordingly, the histological pattern of liver damage is more pronounced. (401) Chronic hepatitis D develops into *cirrhosis* at an increased rate and also at an (10–15 years) earlier stage. Likewise, there is a far higher danger of *hepatocellular carcinoma* following an appropriately long period of latency; the frequency is, however, no higher. • In single cases, reciprocal viral interference can effect the *healing* of HBV and HDV infections. (394, 408, 416, 429)

6.7 Special features of HDV infection

The occurrence of an asymptomatic **HDV carrier state** is possible, yet rare. With immunodeficiency, there is greater proneness to HDV infection and HDV replication. • Following **liver transplantation,** increased HDV replication can result from the use of immunosuppressives. There is a danger of reinfection of the transplant and development of chronic hepatitis D. Treatment with interferon-α had no influence on the replication of HBV, yet it reduced HDV replication. (415) • Disproportional to the absence or minimal presence of portal hypertension, distinct **splenomegaly** is found in approx. 20% of patients infected with chronic HDV. (410) • **Autoantibodies** of the LKM 3 type (liver kidney microsomes) are detectable in some 20% of patients. • The **extrahepatic manifestations** are similar to those found with HBV infection. (s. tab. 22.5) The special features of the serological and clinical course, as well as of the histological changes, can be attributed to the differing pathogenesis or degree of cytotoxicity. (389)

6.8 Prophylaxis

In terms of coinfection, prevention is only possible by means of passive or active immunization against HBV. It is imperative for chronic HBsAg carriers to avoid HDV endemic areas. However, should this not be possible, strict protective measures against HDV infection are called for.

6.9 Therapy

The treatment of acute viral hepatitis D is symptomatic; it is usually carried out in line with the same principles that apply to acute viral hepatitis A, B and C. • There is (not yet) any evidence for commencing antiviral therapy of the acute HDV infection. Recurrence of chronic hepatitis HDV after liver transplantation has also been observed. (409) *(see chapter 34.7.5)*

7 Acute viral hepatitis E

▶ The first thoroughly investigated epidemic of the disease known today as viral hepatitis E was in **New Delhi** in December 1955/January 1956. More than 29,000 cases of jaundice were reported. The three- to fourfold frequency among females and the prevalence in middle-aged people (30–40 years) were striking. Above all, pregnant women were affected, and the occurrence of the disease in the third trimester was accompanied by high mortality (15–25%). Everything pointed to contaminated drinking water as being the source of infection. (478) • At the time, serological tests were not available for the differentiation of acute hepatitis. Nevertheless, after the development of HAV seromarkers, deep-frozen sera from the 1955/56 epidemic were examined, and, amazingly, no HAV positivity was established. Thus this large-scale epidemic in New Delhi was − at least for the most part − not caused by HAV infection. There must have been a second type of (non-A) virus transmitted by the faecal-oral route. (463, 479)

In 1975 V.M. VILLAREJOS et al. likewise described an epidemic in **Costa Rica** with a faecal-oral transmission route which was not caused by HAV.

Evaluation of a hepatitis epidemic in **Kashmir** in November 1978 produced similar results to those found after the epidemic in New Delhi. HAV and HBV infections were not present. (452) Here, too, a faecal-oral transmission route via contaminated drinking water was found. • The greatest epidemic of all, registering about 120,000 diseased persons, was in **Xinjiang/China** (1986−1988).

7.1 Definition

Apart from HAV infection, acute viral hepatitis E is deemed to be a second enterally transmissible form of viral hepatitis. The incubation period and clinical picture are largely identical to those of an HAV infection, but HEV occurs more frequently in adults. Pregnant women are particularly susceptible, with a more severe course of disease, a higher abortion rate and increased mortality (15−25%).

7.2 Pathogen

The virus known as **HEV** was first identified in Moscow in 1983 after being recovered from the stools of a voluntarily infected person (M.S. BALAYAN et al.). In 1988 it was assigned to the *Caliciviridae* (D.W. BRADLEY et al.), to which it bears a similarity. It is also similar to that of the rubella virus, but because it lacks a protein coat, it cannot strictly be assigned to the Togaviridae. In all probability, it represents a new virus family. The genome was clarified in 1990. (465) HEV is a (+)-stranded, naked RNA virus, 27 to 34 nm in size, with a genome of 7,200 nucleotides in length and three open reading frames. Several isolates have already been cloned and sequenced. The processing of isolates from various geographical areas clearly demonstrated genetic heterogeneity. Up to now, **1 serotype** and **3 genotypes** have been identified. (431, 437, 443, 448, 454, 464−466)

7.3 Epidemiology

In all probability, HEV is a zoonosis which is transmitted to humans mainly by pigs (457), but possibly also by other animals, e.g. rodents. (445) HEV infection occurs *endemically* and *epidemically* as well as *sporadically* (because of travel). There have been many reports of epidemics and endemias of acute viral hepatitis E, such as in India (433, 438, 464, 471, 479), Pakistan (442, 474), Nepal (450), Afghanistan, China, Indonesia, Malaysia, Egypt (444), Israel (451), Somalia (459), Ethiopia (475), Turkey (473), Syria (431), Singapore (440), Venezuela (462) and Mexico (477). Sporadic diseases have been described in seroepidemiological studies in Europe (435), the USA, Korea, Australia (458), South Africa (446), Austria (447), Spain (449), Switzerland (455), Taiwan (456), Greece (472), Belgium (476) and Italy (481). • In view of travel and tourism, particularly adventure treks in countries with poor hygienic conditions, HEV infection must be considered when faced with the task of drawing up a differential diagnosis of acute viral hepatitis. • In **Germany**, up to 1% of the population are infected with HEV: 34 cases in 2001, 17 cases in 2002, 32 cases in 2003, 61 cases in 2004, 58 cases in 2005 and 62 cases in 2006.

The swine is considered to be the main reservoir of the virus; in the USA, the majority of pigs were found to be infected with HEV (genotype 3) within the first year of life. (457) This strain of HEV has been transmitted from swine to chimpanzee and from humans to swine. Such an HEV reservoir in swine has meanwhile been detected in several countries. Nevertheless, transmission from the animal reservoir to humans is extremely rare.

7.4 Transmission

HEV is transmitted by a **faecal-oral route.** (439, 441, 448, 467) Sources of infection are contaminated drinking water (particularly due to pigs) as well as food which is unboiled and contaminated by foul or waste water (463, 469, 479) as well as eating raw deer meat (e.g. in Japan). Only rarely is close intrafamilial contact deemed to be the route of infection. (430) In contrast, an epidemic of HEV infection has already occurred in schools. (434) At one school in India, 67 children and a great number of teachers contracted the disease. (433) The risk of the environment becoming infected by an HEV patient is only 1.5−2.5%, whereas in acute hepatitis A, an infection ensues in 10−20% of cases. HEV is excreted in the stools in considerably lower concentrations than HAV. (464) As a result of this, and because HEV is less stable than HAV, the danger of contagion by HEV is lower. Transmission of HEV from an infected mother to the newborn child is possible, resulting in significantly higher morbidity and mortality. (453) It is not known why pregnant women succumb to the disease more often, with a mortality rate of 15−25%. Possibly, a parenteral route of infection is involved. The i.v. transmission of HEV to primates led to higher transaminase values and evidence of virus particles in the blood as well as to the detection of HEV by PCR. Therefore, transmission by blood transfusion is assumed. In haemophiliacs, the i.v. risk of infection is low (480) or non-existent. Reinfection with the hepatitis E virus must be expected, since there is no lifelong immunity.

7.5 Serological diagnostics

The diagnosis of acute viral hepatitis E is possible through the detection of **HEV Ag** (482) and **anti-HEV IgM;** identification of **anti-HEV IgG** points to a past HEV infection. No results are available on the duration of anti-HEV IgG positivity and any possible immunity associated with it. *It is interesting to note that HAV IgM can be detected in acute HEV infection. This may lead to a false diagnosis of acute viral hepatitis A.* (s. p. 429) The specificity of positive anti-HEV IgG or IgM test results should always be validated by means of the corresponding Western blot test. In a self-infection experiment with HEV, the HEV RNA was detectable in the serum from the 22nd day after infection onwards; once the maximum GPT level had been reached (on the 46th day), the serum was no longer HEV-positive. Anti-HEV IgG could only be identified on the 41st day following infection (a short time after the occurrence of jaundice), and this persisted for more than 14 years. From the onset of the icteric phase, HEV could be demonstrated in the stools; this virus was also the cause of viral hepatitis E in related animal experiments. (439) In 10–20% of cases of HEV infection confirmed by PCR, neither anti-HEV IgM nor subsequently anti-HEV IgG could be detected. A negative anti-HEV IgM finding does not exclude acute HEV infection. (431, 441, 448)

7.6 Clinical aspects and courses of disease

The incubation period is 15–56 (mean period about 40) days. The symptomatic clinical picture which is given cannot be distinguished from that of acute viral hepatitis A — especially in cases where the HAV IgM is positive. (s. p. 429) The clinical findings and symptoms are regressive within a period of two or three weeks. The course is acute and self-limiting, especially in children moderate or asymptomatic. In individual cases, severe courses of disease occur with transaminase values above 2,000 U/l and a pronounced increase in bilirubin. (431, 435, 461) • Occasionally, there is a *cholestatic course* of disease with clearly elevated values of the cholestasis-indicating enzymes, bile acids and serum bilirubin. Although the disease lasts longer (as in acute viral hepatitis A), the prognosis is the same. • *Fulminant hepatitis* occurs in 2–3% of cases. This severe clinical picture is to be feared in children with HAV and HEV coinfection, in displaced peoples (436) as well as in pregnant women in the third trimester; mortality is high (10–25%). (438, 459, 460, 470) HEV superinfection produces severe decompensation in patients with chronic liver disease. • *Chronic courses* of HEV infection or HEV carrier state have not been observed. Nothing is known about a correlation between HEV infection and hepatocellular carcinoma. The *extrahepatic manifestations* seen in HAV infection can be anticipated in HEV infection as well. Mortality due to acute viral hepatitis E is 0.18–0.58% for a normal course of disease.

7.7 Prophylaxis and therapy

The hygienic and therapeutic measures correspond to those given for acute viral hepatitis A. • Recently, an active vaccination was introduced. (468)

8 Acute viral hepatitis NA-NE

▶ In the initial course of evaluating 17 epidemics from a total of 25 waterborne epidemics in India transmitted by faecal-oral route, it originally seemed that 16 epidemics had been caused by HEV. The seroepidemiological results showed, however, that the epidemic on the Andaman Islands, and possibly also several of the remaining 16 epidemics, might have been caused by a *third non-A-non-E virus* transmitted by faecal-oral route. This presumed *NA-NE* virus has not been conclusively identified so far. It has simply been assigned to the *flaviviruses*. (483) • Acute NA-NE hepatitis is found worldwide (20–60% of sporadic acute NANB hepatitis). Non-parenteral transmission is most common. There is no gender- or age-related preference. Usually, the disease is self-limiting; its course is often severe. Fulminant liver failure and the development of chronic hepatitis were observed. (484, 485)

9 HF virus

In 1994 N. Deka et al. detected virus-like particles of 27–37 nm in size in specimens of stools from French patients with virus hepatitis NANB. The authors provisionally named the infectious agent hepatitis French virus or HFV. (486) The patients tested seronegative for other hepatitis viruses, and no HAV or HEV was detectable in the stool specimens. Following i.v. application of such particles in rhesus monkeys, the hepatitis virus was produced and could be identified in the liver cells and stools of these primates. The genetic material was characterized as a double-stranded DNA of 20 kilobases in length. It was possible to reproduce the pathogens in cell culture. The existence of this pathogen and its epidemiological significance in relation to humans have not been confirmed up to now.

10 HG virus

In 1995 J.P. Kim et al. confirmed that they had identified another putative hepatitis agent in the serum of a patient with aetiologically unresolved chronic hepatitis by means of PCR. Because the letter F had already been used for the above mentioned unsubstantiated virus, the authors moved on to the next letter in the hepatitis alphabet and named this novel agent hepatitis G virus or HGV. The genomic structure of this enveloped RNA virus of the *flaviviridae* group (50–60 nm, plus strain) with its 9,125 and 9,392 nucleotides has already been clarified. (497) • In the meantime, anti-HGV (against the envelope protein E 2) has been developed as a serological marker. Up to now, 3 genotypes and 5 subtypes have been demonstrated, each with its own geographic distribution. (500) The virus seems to be spread worldwide and to have a prevalence of about 2%. HGV definitely has a long-term persistence rate (up to 16 years). (487, 491, 499) Studies using frozen blood specimens demonstrated that HGV has existed in Germany for at least 20 years. (489) Patients with chronic viral hepatitis B or C are coinfected with HGV in 10–20% of cases. HGV can be detected directly not only in the serum, but also in liver parenchyma and mononuclear cells. (503) In nearly all cases, infection occurs parenterally, e.g. blood transfusion (489, 498, 505), haemodialysis (491, 493, 504) and i.v. drug addicts (501, 502); more rarely it is due to plasma products (494) and sexual contact (490, 501). Vertical infection from mother to child is also possible. The clinical course is mostly asymptomatic. In patients showing an unclarified elevation of transaminases, hepatitis due to HGV should be considered. A rise in γGT and AP was associated with lesions of the small bile ducts as a result of HGV infection. (488) Overall, laboratory parameters and histology resembled HCV. (495, 496) The course of hepatitis with HAV, HBV or HCV is not influenced by an HGV infection. (487, 503) Examination of patients with cryptogenic chronic hepatitis did not point to HGV infection as being a causal factor. (492) Treatment of persistent HGV with interferon had only a limited effect. (495, 504) Liver transplants were not affected by this virus.

11 GB viruses

▶ In 1967 F. DEINHARDT et al. discovered an infectious agent in the serum of a 34-year-old surgeon in Chicago suffering from acute hepatitis. It was termed **GB virus** from the initials of the first and last names of the patient. The serum was taken on the third day of jaundice. This GBV was successfully transmitted to marmosets. Further serial passaging in marmosets and during filtration experiments strongly suggested a viral aetiology. (508) Subsequent studies showed that the GB agent was distinct from HAV, HBV, HCV and HEV. (518)

GBV A, GBV B: Almost 30 years later (1995), the GBV agent could be differentiated into two flavivirus-like genomes: GBV A (9,493 nucleotides) and GBV B (9,143 nucleotides). (520) Both virus types are simian viruses. Up to then, these two types had not been found in humans. However, GBV A antibodies have meanwhile been detected in 0.3% and GBV B antibodies in 1.2% of blood donors. Nevertheless, these two types of viruses are considered to be of no pathogenic significance for humans. It would, however, appear from animal experiments that GBV A potentiates GBV B infection. According to their genomic organization, the GB species A and B belong to the family of *flaviviridae*.

GBV C: Recently, another genome, GBV C (ca. 9,200 nucleotides), was identified by means of PCR. (512, 521) It is defined as a single-stranded (+) RNA virus and forms a separate species within the *flaviviridae* family. It seems that the original serum of GB contained no (or no more) GBV A, GBV B or GBV C RNA; thus the above mentioned surgeon's hepatitis remains unclarified with regard to the causative virus type. In the meantime, HCV could be differentiated into five subtypes: 1a, 1b, 2a, 2b and 3a.

It became evident that GBV-C and HGV are two isolates of the same virus, which is why the term **GBV C/HGV** is generally used. This virus can cause (mostly) asymptomatic as well as (rarely) acute hepatitis. Its RNA is detectable in the serum and saliva, but not in the urine, of infected patients. (519) There is a close correlation with the transmission of this virus from mother to child. (506) The incubation time is four to six months. The virus has no capability to replicate in liver cells and is considered to be an endosymbiont. In most cases, it is eliminated, but it can also remain in a latent state for some time. (511, 513, 514, 517, 523) It was possible to demonstrate the presence of GBV C/HGV RNA in 10–20% of patients with chronic hepatitis C. RNA was found in 1.2–16.0% of blood donors (507), in 3.0–20.0% of long term haemodialysis patients (515), in 17.3% among dental personnel (516) and in 30% of polytransfused patients. In Hungary, antibodies to GBV C/HGV were found in 28% of the population over the age of 60. (572) This virus is held responsible for (mild) chronic active hepatitis. Infection has also been reported due to sexual contact. (524) However, infection with GBV C/HGV does not always lead to liver disease. Aplastic anaemia was observed in the course of GBV C/HGV infection. (510) Even after liver transplantation in GBV C-positive patients, viraemia was still detectable in 75% of cases. In contrast, GBV C viraemia was found in 29% of HBV-positive patients and in 12% of HCV-positive patients following OLT. The occurrence of hepatitis in a liver transplant was not influenced by GBV C/HGV. There is no clear association with fulminant hepatitis.

12 TT virus

In 1997 another virus was detected in a Japanese patient with increased transaminases of unknown aetiology. The infectious agent was termed TT virus or TTV, based on the initials of the patient who had been infected as a result of a blood transfusion. (533) This genome is approx. 3,800 nucleotides in length. It is an antisense, circular, single-stranded DNA virus with no outer envelope. There are three conserved open reading frames. The size of the TTV is estimated to be 30—50 nm. It most probably belongs to the *circoviridae* family. (531)

TTV has not been shown by electron microscopy. Up to now, the virus could only be demonstrated in the serum due to the presence of TTV DNA. A total of 16 genotypes have now been differentiated. (536) Recently, a TTV isolate from non-human primates could be identified; the authors named it s-TTV. Overall, 10.5% of Japanese patients with liver disease were found to be infected with s-TTV, whereby two different genotypes were classified. (529) There have also been reports of TTV-like mini virus DNA, which are detectable in a large number of patients. (530) TTV replicates in various tissues, but changes in the liver are only mild. (537)

There is a high prevalence of TTV all over the world (41—93%), with striking differences in the various countries. Japan has a prevalence of 39—68%. (525) In Hungary, 18.5% of healthy persons and 50.4% of patients with hepatitis of unknown aetiology tested positive. (539) In Brazil, donated blood was shown to contain TTV in 62% of cases. In Germany, a TTV viraemia could be found in 14% of healthy donors and in 16—20% of the various risk groups. (535)

TTV can be transmitted by blood products and through common parenteral routes (532, 535, 536) as well as by haemodialysis. (520, 528) TTV could also be detected in umbilical cord blood, so that a neonatal (in utero) transmission is to be considered. (530) The likelihood of enteric transmission has been shown by the finding of TTV DNA in breast milk, saliva, duodenal fluid, bile juice and faeces. There is a higher viral load in saliva than in the corresponding serum. (527, 538) TTV displays ubiquitous diffusion in human tissue and is able to invade the central nervous system. (534) A high virus load has been demonstrated in patients with HCV-associated HHC. (540) Although TTV has been found in patients with a broad range of liver diseases, current evidence does not indicate a specific link with TTV infection in such cases.

13 SEN virus

In the year 2000, Italian scientists discovered a new virus isolated from an HIV-infected drug user. It was provisionally named SEN virus or SENV after the initials of the source patient, who showed elevated transaminases of unknown aetiology (D. PRIMI et al.).

This agent is also an antisense, circular, single-stranded DNA without an envelope. The genome is linear and contains ca. 3,900 nucleotides; it has at least three open reading frames. So far, eight genotypes have been reported (SENV-A to -H). There are remarkable parallels between SENV and various TTV subtypes, and it may be that both viruses share a common ancestor. (547)

Genotypes D and H are thought to be linked with non-A-non-E hepatitis. Therefore investigations have focused on these two strains. SENV-D and -H strains were detected in patients with fulminant hepatitis (32%), chronic hepatitis (27%), autoimmune hepatitis (33%), cirrhosis (31%) and primary biliary cirrhosis (46%). (546) The prevalence in the population is currently estimated to be 10—20%; in risk groups with parenteral exposure, the figures are remarkably high — up to 80% in transfused non-A to non-E hepatitis. (549) Coinfection with HBV or HCV is found in approx. 20% of patients. Perinatal transmission from mother to child has also been reported. (542) • SENV infection does not affect the course of a persistent HCV coinfection. (543) It was also shown that SENV has no influence on acute or chronic hepatitis A, B or C and is not the cause of cryptogenic hepatitis. (550) Genotypes D and H were more often present in patients with a high risk of parenterally acquired viral infection. (541, 552) SENV-H viraemia has been found mostly in patients with HIV. (545)

Infection with SENV-D and -H adversely affected the outcome of antiviral therapy for HCV (544), whereas in another study SENV did not influence the clinical or histological features of HCV at all. (549) SENV infection is not associated with increased evidence of liver disease or the risk of HCC. (548, 551) Likewise, this virus does not play any role in graft dysfunction after liver transplantation, although SENV was found in 35% of unselected liver transplant recipients. It is possible that SENV is a causative agent of posttransfusion-associated hepatitis, especially since specific DNA could be detected in liver tissue.

14 Other viruses

In 1994, using a total of 1,974 sera from patients with NANB hepatitis, the working group of G. BERENCSI (Budapest) was able to identify 133 cases of a positive cross-reaction with the **yellow fever antigen** *(YF IgG)*; in 19 instances, *YF-IgM positivity* was also demonstrated. The majority of the sera were HCV-negative. These patients had had no contact with yellow fever vaccines and they had never left Hungary. • Studies carried out so far suggest the existence of an independent, but not yet identified flavivirus in the Hungarian population which produces a positive cross-reaction with the YF antigen and is associated with posttransfusion hepatitis. (552)

The evolutionary distance of flaviviridae polyproteins was used to generate an **unrooted phylogenetic tree**. The GB viruses are considered to form a group of their own with a close relationship to HCV. (s. fig. 22.20)

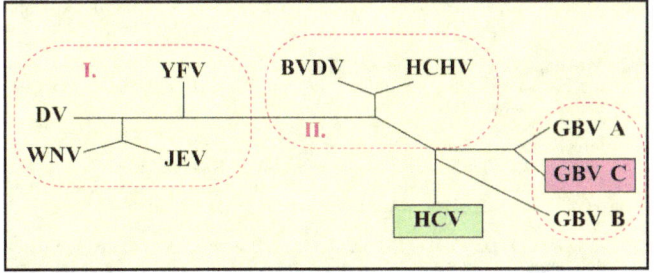

Fig. 22.20: Possible phylogenetic scheme of the HCV (*Hepaciviridae*) and GB viruses (especially GBV C/HGV) as well as other members of the *Flaviviridae* (I): DV = Dengue virus, WNV = West Nile virus, JEV = Japanese encephalitis virus, YFV = yellow fever virus, or *Pestiviruses* (II): BVDV = bovine viral diarrhoea virus, HCHV = hog cholera virus (mod. J. N. SIMONS et al., 2000)

References:

The history of acute viral hepatitis
1. Andersen, T.Th.: Untersuchungen über die Ätiologie der Hepatitis epidemica. (Dänisch) Ugeskr. Laeg. 1938: 777–778
2. Balayan, M.S., Andjaparidze, A.G., Savinskaya, S.S., Ketiladze, E.S., Braginsky, D.M., Savinov, A.P., Poleschuk, V.F.: Evidence for a virus in non-A, non-B hepatitis transmitted via the fecal-oral route. Intervirology 1983; 20: 23–31
3. Blumberg, B.S., Alter, H.J., Visnich, S.: A "new" antigen in leukemia sera. J. Amer. Med. Ass. 1965; 191: 541–546
4. Bormann, von, F.: Hepatitis epidemica. Ergebn. Inn. Med. 1940; 58: 201–284
5. Choo, Q.L., Kuo, G., Weiner, A.J., Overby, L.R., Bradley, D.W., Houghton, M.: Isolation of a cDNA clone derived from a blood-borne Non-A, Non-B viral hepatitis genome. Science 1989; 244: 359–361
6. Cockayne, E.A.: Catarrhal jaundice, sporadic and epidemic, and in relation to acute yellow atrophy of the liver. Quart. J. Med. 1912; 6: 1–29
7. Corelli, F.: Der Icterus catarrhalis als allergische Hepatitis. Die allergische Entzündung der Leber und der Gallenwege. Etiopathogenetisches Studium. Dtsch. Arch. Klin. Med. 1940; 185: 600–625
8. Dane, D.S., Cameron, C.H., Briggs, M.: Virus-like particles in serum of patients with Australia-antigen-associated hepatitis. Lancet 1970/I: 695–700
9. Feinstone, S.M., Kapikian, A.Z., Purcell, R.H.: Hepatitis A: detection by immune electron microscopy of a viruslike antigen associated with acute illness. Science 1973; 182: 1026–1028
10. Feinstone, S.M., Kapikian, A.Z., Purcell, R.H., Alter, H.J., Holland, P.V.: Transfusion-associated hepatitis not due to viral hepatitis type A or B. New Engl. J. Med. 1975; 292: 767–770
11. Fröhlich, C.: Ueber Icterusepidemien. Dtsch. Arch. Klin. Med. 1879; 24: 394–406
12. Gebhardt, F., Voegt, H.: Die verschiedenen Verlaufsformen der Hepatitis contagiosa. Dtsch. Med. Wschr. 1944; 70: 450–451
13. Havens, W.P.jr., Ward, R., Drill, V.A., Paul, J.R.: Experimental production of hepatitis by feeding icterogenic materials. Proc. Soc. Exp. Biol. Med. 1944; 57: 206–208
14. Herlitz, I.F.: De ictero speciatim epidemico Goettingae, grassante dissertatio Goettingae. Diss.-Inaug. 1761
15. Jehn: Eine Icterusepidemie in wahrscheinlichem Zusammenhang mit vorausgegangener Revaccination. Dtsch. Med. Wschr. 1885; 11: 354–356
16. Köhnhorn, C.: Ueber Gelbsucht-Epidemien. Berlin. Klin. Wschr. 1877: 89–90; 104–106; 132–134
17. Krugman, S., Giles, J.P., Hammond, J.: Infectious hepatitis. Evidence for two distinctive clinical, epidemiological, and immunological types of infection. J. Amer. Med. Ass. 1967; 200: 365–373
18. Lainer, F.: Zur Frage der Infektiosität des Ikterus. Wien. Klin. Wschr. 1940: 601–604
19. Linnen, J., Wages, J.jr., Zhang-Keck, Z.-Y., Fry, K.E., Krawczynski, K.Z., Alter, H., Koonin, E., Gallagher, M., Alter, M., Hadziyannis, St., Karayiannis, P. et al.: Molecular cloning and disease association of hepatitis G virus: a transfusion-transmissible agent. Science 1996; 271: 505–508
20. Lürman: Eine Icterusepidemie. Berlin. Klin. Wschr. 1885; 22: 20–23
21. Martini, G.A.: Die homologe Serum-Hepatitis. Dtsch. Med. Wschr. 1949; 18: 568–572
22. McCallum, F.O., Bradley, W.H.: Transmission of infective hepatitis to human volunteers. Lancet 1944/II: 228.
23. Neefe, J.R., Stokes, J.jr., Reinhold, J.G.: Oral administration to volunteers of feces from patients with homologous serum hepatitis and infectious (epidemic) hepatitis. Amer. J. Med. Sci. 1945; 210: 29–32
24. Paul, J.R., Havens, W.P.jr., Sabin, A.B., Philipp, C.B.: Transmission experiments in serum jaundice and infectious hepatitis. J. Amer. Med. Ass. 1945; 128: 911–915
25. Prince, A.M.: An antigen detected in the blood during the incubation period of serum hepatitis. Proc. Nat. Acad. Sci. USA 1968; 60: 814–821
26. Prince, A.M., Brotman, B., Grady, G.F., Kuhns, W.J., Hazzi, C., Levine, R.W., Millian, S.J.: Long-incubation post-transfusion hepatitis without serological evidence of exposure to hepatitis-B virus. Lancet 1974/II: 241–246
27. Purcell, R.H.: The discovery of the hepatitis viruses. Gastroenterology 1993; 104: 955–963
28. Rizzetto, M., Canese, M.G., Arico, S., Crivelli, O., Trepo, C., Bonino, F., Verme, G.: Immunofluorescence detection of new antigen-antibody system (δ/anti-δ) associated to hepatitis B virus in liver and in serum of HBsAg carriers. Gut 1977; 18: 997–1003
29. Virchow, R.: Über das Vorkommen und den Nachweis des hepatogenen, insbesondere des katarrhalischen Icterus. Virchow's Archiv 1864; 32: 117–125
30. Voegt, H.: Zur Aetiologie der Hepatitis epidemica. Münch. Med. Wschr. 1942; 89: 76–79

Morphological and aetiopathogenetic variety
31. Bianchi, L., de Groote, J., Desmet, V.J., Gedigk, P., Korb, G., Popper, H., Poulsen, H., Scheuer, P.J., Schmid, M., Thaler, H., Wepler, W.: Morphological criteria in viral hepatitis. Lancet 1971/I: 333–337
32. Barak, N., Huminer, D., Segal, T., Ben Ari, Z., Halevy, J., Tur Kaspa, R.: Lipoamide dehydrogenase deficiency: a newly discovered cause of acute hepatitis in adults. J. Hepatol. 1998; 29: 482–484
33. Fimmel, C.J., Guo, L., Compans, R.W., Brunt, E.M., Hickman, S., Perrillo, R.R., Mason, A.L.: A case of syncytial giant cell hepatitis with features of a paramyxoviral infection. Amer. J. Gastroenterol. 1998; 93: 1931–1937
34. Ishak, K.G.: Light microscopic morphology of viral hepatitis. Amer. J. Clin. Pathol. 1976; 65: 787–827
35. Kim, M.Y., Baik, S.K., Choi, Y.J., Park, D.H., Kim, H.S., Lee, D.K., Kwon, S.O.: Endoscopic sonographic evaluation of the thickened gallbladder wall in patients with acute hepatitis. J. Clin. Ultrasound 2003; 31: 245–249
36. Phillips, M., Purcell, S.: Modern aspects of the morphology of viral hepatitis. Hum. Pathol. 1981; 12: 1060–1084
37. Phillips, J.R., Angulo, P., Lindor, K.: Recurrent idiopathic hepatitis: a new entity? J. Clin. Gastroenterol. 2003; 37: 267–269

Acute viral hepatitis A
38. Becker, B., Prömse, B., Krämer, J., Exner, M.: Transmission of human pathogenic viruses via food: bakery products causing hepatitis A in Germany. Gesundheitswesen 1996; 58: 339–340
39. Black, M.M., Mann, N.P.: Gangrenous cholecystitis due to hepatitis A infection. J. Trop. Med. Hyg. 1992; 95: 73–74
40. Bornstein, J.D., Byrd, D.E., Trotter, J.F.: Relapsing hepatitis A. A case report and review of the literature. J. Clin. Gastroenterol. 1999; 28: 355–359
41. Bower, W.A., Nainan, O.V., Han, X., Margolis, H.S.: Duration of viremia in hepatitis A virus infection. J. Infect. Dis. 2000; 182: 12–17
42. Breuer, G.S., Morali, G., Finkelstein, Y., Halevy, J.: A pregnant woman with hepatitis A and Guillain-Barré. J. Clin. Gastroenterol. 2001; 32: 179–180
43. Chironna, M., Lopalco, P., Prato, R., Germinario, C., Barbuti, S., Quarto, M.: Outbreak of infection with hepatitis A virus (HAV) associated with a foodhandler and confirmed by sequence analysis reveals a new HAV genotype 1 B variant. J. Clin. Microbiol. 2004; 42: 2825–2828
44. Cohen, O., Mevorach, D., Ackerman, Z., Oren, R.: Thrombocytopenic purpura as a manifestation of acute hepatitis A. J. Clin. Gastroenterol. 1993; 17: 166–167
45. Conzelmann-Auer, C., Ackermann-Liebrich, U., Herzog, Ch., Bächlin, A.: An outbreak of hepatitis A in a kindergarden. Schweiz. Med. Wschr. 1992; 122: 1559–1566
46. Cotter, S.M., Sansom, S., Long, T., Koch, E., Kellerman, S., Smith, F., Averhoff, F., Bell, B.P.: Outbreak of hepatitis A among men who have sex with men: implications for hepatitis A vaccination strategies. J. Infect. Dis. 2003; 187: 1235–1240
47. Dagan, R., Yaqupsky, P., Barki, Y.: Acute ascites accompanying hepatitis A infection in a child. Infection 1988; 16: 360–361
48. Dan, M., Yaniv, R.: Cholestatic hepatitis, cutaneous vasculitis, and vascular deposits of immunoglobulin M and complement associated with hepatitis A virus infection. Amer. J. Med. 1990; 89: 103–104
49. Davis, T.V., Keeffe, E.B.: Acute pancreatitis associated with acute hepatitis A. Amer. J. Gastroenterol. 1992; 87: 1648–1650
50. Dentinger, C.M., Bower, W.A., Nainan, O.V., Cotter, S.M., Myers, G., Dubusky, L.M., Fowler, S., Salehi, E.D.P., Bell, B.P.: An outbreak of hepatitis A associated with green onions. J. Infect. Dis. 2001: 183: 1273–1276
51. Durst, R.Y., Goldsmidt, N., Namestnick, J., Safadi, R., Ilan, Y.: Familial cluster of fulminant hepatitis A infection. J. Clin. Gastroenterol. 2001; 32: 453–454
52. Enriquez, R., Frösner, G.G., Hochstein-Mintzel, V., Riedemann, St., Reinhardt, G.: Accumulation and persistence of hepatitis A virus in mussels. J. Med. Virol. 1992; 37: 174–179
53. Fagan, E.A., Partridge, M., Sowray, J.H., Williams, R.: Review of the herpes-viruses and hepatitis A: the potential hazards in dental care. Oral Surg. Oral Med. Oral Pathol. 1987; 64: 693–696

54. **Forbes, A., Williams, R.:** Changing epidemiology and clinical aspects of hepatitis A. Brit. Med. Bull. 1990; 46: 303–318
55. **Fröhlich, J., Zeller, I.:** Risk of HAV infection with employees of a sewage plant cooperative society. Arbeitsmed. Sozialmed. Präventivmed. 1993; 28: 503–505
56. **Fujiyama, S., Iino, S., Odoh, K., Kuzuhara, S., Watanabe, H., Tanaka, M., Mizuno, K., Sato, T.:** Time course of hepatitis A virus antibody titer after active and passive immunization. Hepatology 1992; 15: 983–988
57. **Gaube, J., Feucht, H.H., Laufs, R., Polywka, S., Fingscheidt, E., Müller, H.E.:** Hepatitis A, B, and C as desmoteric infections. Gesundheitswesen 1993; 55: 246–249
58. **Geltner, D., Naot, Y., Zimhoni, O., Gorbach, S., Bar-Khayim, Y.:** Acute oliguric renal failure complicating type A nonfulminant viral hepatitis. A case presentation and review of the literature. J. Clin. Gastroenterol. 1992; 14: 160–162
59. **Gerritzen, A., Schneweis, K.E., Brackmann, H.-H., Oldenburg, J., Hanfland, P., Gerlich, W.H., Caspari, G.:** Acute hepatitis A in haemophiliacs. Lancet 1992; 340: 1231–1232
60. **Gordon, S.C., Reddy, K.R., Schiff, L., Schiff, E.R.:** Prolonged intrahepatic cholestasis secondary to acute hepatitis A. Ann. Intern. Med. 1984; 101: 635–637
61. **Halliday, M.L., Kang, L.-Y., Zhou, T.-K., Hu, M.-D., Pan, Q.-C., Fu, T.-Y., Huang, Y.-S., Hu, S.-L.:** An epidemic of hepatitis A attributable to the ingestion of raw clams in Shanghai, China. J. Infect. Dis. 1991; 164: 852–859
62. **Hammond, G.W., MacDougall, B.K., Plummer, F., Sekla, L.H.:** Encephalitis during prodromal stage of acute hepatitis A. Can. Med. Ass. J. 1982; 126: 269–270
63. **Hollinger, F.B., Khan, N.C., Oefinger, P.E., Yawn, D.H., Schmulen, A.C., Dreesman, G.R., Melnick, J.L.:** Posttransfusion hepatitis A. J. Amer. Med. Ass. 1982; 250: 2313–2317
64. **Hutin, Y.J.F., Pool, V., Cramer, E.H., Nainan, O.V., Weth, J., Williams, I.T., Goldstein, S.T., Gensheimer, K.F., Bell, B.P., Shapiro, C.N., Alter, M.J., Margolis, H.S.:** A multistate foodborne outbreak of hepatitis A. New Engl. J. Med. 1999; 340: 595–602
65. **Ilan, Y., Hillman, M., Oren, R., Zlotogorski, A., Shouval, D.:** Vasculitis and cryoglobulinemia associated with persisting cholestatic hepatitis A virus infection. Amer. J. Gastroenterol. 1990; 85: 586–587
66. **Inman, R.D., Hodge, M., Johnston, M.E.A., Wright, J., Heathcote, J.:** Arthritis, vasculitis, and cryoglobulinemia associated with relapsing hepatitis A virus infection. Ann. Intern. Med. 1986; 105: 700–703
67. **Inoue, K., Yoshiba, M., Yotsuyanagi, H., Otsuka, T., Sekiyama, K., Fujita, R.:** Chronic hepatitis A with persistent viral replication. J. Med. Virol. 1996; 50: 322–324
68. **Jensenius, M., Ringertz, S.H., Berlid, D., Bell, H., Espinoza, R., Grinde, B.:** Prolonged nosocomial outbreak of hepatitis A arising from an alcoholic with pneumonia. Scand. J. Infect. Dis. 1998; 30: 119–123
69. **Kalkan, A., Bulut, V., Avci, S., Celik, I., Bingol, N.K.:** Trace elements in viral hepatitis. J. Trace Elem. Med. Biol. 2002; 16: 227–230
70. **Kern, G., Frisch-Niggemeyer, W., Wewalka, G., Bruns, C.:** An outbreak of hepatitis A in a homeless shelter in Vienna. Wien. Klin. Wschr. 1991; 23: 364–366
71. **Khanna, B., Spelbring, J.E., Innis, B.L., Robertson, B.H.:** Characterization of a genetic variant of human hepatitis A virus. J. Med. Virol. 1992; 36: 118–124
72. **Klar, A., Branski, D., Nadjari, M., Akerman, M.Y., Shoseyov, D., Hurvitz, H.:** Gallbladder and pancreatic involvement in hepatitis A. J. Clin. Gastroenterol. 1998; 27: 143–145
73. **Kuntz, E.:** Oedematous hepatitis: a special form of acute viral hepatitis due to secondary aldosteronism. Med. Klin. 1975; 70: 274–278
74. **Lemon, S.M.:** Type A viral hepatitis: epidemiology, diagnosis and prevention. Clin. Chemist. 1997; 43: 1494–1499
75. **Levy, B.S., Fontaine, R.E., Smith, C.A., Brinda, J., Hirman, G., Nelson, D.B., Johnson, P.M., Larson, O.:** A large food-borne outbreak of hepatitis. A. J. Amer. Med. Ass. 1975; 234: 289–294
76. **Levy, M.J., Herrera, J.L., di Palma, J.A.:** Immune globulin and vaccine therapy to prevent hepatitis A infection. Amer. J. Med. 1998; 105: 416–423
77. **Lyons, D.J., Gilvarry, J.M., Fielding, J.F.:** Severe haemolysis associated with hepatitis A and normal glucose-6-phosphate dehydrogenase status. Gut 1990; 31: 838–839
78. **Mahoney, F.J., Farley, T.A., Kelso, K.Y., Wilson, S.A., Horan, J.M., McFarland, L.M.:** An outbreak of hepatitis A associated with swimming in a public pool. J. Infect. Dis. 1992; 165: 613–618
79. **Matin, N., Grant, A., Granerod, J., Crowcroft, N.:** Hepatitis A surveillance in England. How many cases are not reported and does it really matter? Epidem. Infect. 2006; 134: 1299–1302
80. **Masada, C.T., Shaw, B.W.jr., Zetterman, R.K., Kaufman, S.S., Markin, R.S.:** Fulminant hepatic failure with massive necrosis as a result of hepatitis A infection. J. Clin. Gastroenterol. 1993; 17: 158–162
81. **Mbithi, J.N., Springthorpe, S., Boulet, J.R., Sattar, S.A.:** Survival of hepatitis A virus on human hands and its transfer on contact with animate and inanimate surfaces. J. Clin. Microbiol. 1992; 30: 757–763
82. **Meyerhoff, A.S., Jacobs, R.J.:** Transmission of hepatitis A through household contact. J. Viral Hepat. 2001; 8: 454–458
83. **Meyers, J.D., Romm, F.J., Tihen, W.S., Bryan, J.A.:** Food-borne hepatitis A in a general hospital. Epidemiologic study of an outbreak attributed to sandwiches. J. Amer. Med. Ass. 1975; 231: 1049–1053
84. **Mishu, B., Hadler, S.C., Boaz, V.A., Hutcheson, R.H., Horan, J.M., Schaffner, W.:** Foodborne hepatitis A: evidence that microwaving reduces risk? J. Infect. Dis. 1990; 162: 655–658
85. **Mourani, S., Dobbs, St.M., Genta, R.M., Tandon, A.K., Yoffe, B.:** Hepatitis A virus-associated cholecystitis. Ann. Intern. Med. 1994; 120: 398–400
86. **Mukhopadhya, A., Chandy, G.M.:** Generalized lymphadenopathy as a marker of ongoing inflammation in prolonged cholestatic hepatitis. Eur. J. Gastroenterol. Hepatol. 2002; 14: 877–878
87. **Nelson, K.E.:** Global changes in the epidemiology of hepatitis A virus infection. Clin. Infect. Dis. 2006; 42: 1151–1152
88. **Niu, M.T., Polish, L.B., Robertson, B.H., Khanna, B.K., Woodruff, B.A., Shapiro, C.N., Miller, M.A., Smith, J.D., Gedrose, J.K., Alter, M.J., Margolis, H.S.:** Multistate outbreak of hepatitis A associated with frozen strawberries. J. Inf. Dis. 1992; 166: 518–524
89. **O'Donovan, D., Cooke, R.P.D., Joce, R., Eastbury, A., Waite, J., Stene-Johansen, K.:** An outbreak of hepatitis A amongst injecting drug users. Epidem. Infect. 2001; 127: 469–473
90. **Ozaras, R., Mert, A., Yilmaz, M.H., Celik, A.D., Tabak, F., Bilir, M., Ozturk, R.:** Acute viral cholecystitis due to hepatitis A virus infection. (case report) J. Clin. Gastroenterol. 2003; 37: 79–81
91. **Phillips, A.O., Thomas, D.M., Coles, G.A.:** Acute renal failure associated with non-fulminant hepatitis A. Clin. Nephrol. 1993; 39: 156–157
92. **Pohl, Ö., Brojnas, J., Rusvai, E., Ördög, K., Siska, I., Faludi, G., Kapusinszky, B., Csohan, A., Lendvai, K., Lengyel, A., Mezey, I., Berencsi, G.:** Retrospective detection of a subclinical hepatitis A virus (HAV) epidemic affecting juvenile cohorts of the Hungarian population. FEMS Immun. Med. Microbiol. 2003; 1565: 1–7
93. **Portnoy, B.L., Mackowiak, P.A., Caraway, C.T., Walker, J.A., McKinley, T.W., Klein, C.A.jr.:** Oyster-associated hepatitis. Failure of shellfish certification programs to prevent outbreaks. J. Amer. Med. Ass. 1975; 233: 1065–1068
94. **Provost, P.J., Hillemann, M.R.:** Propagation of human hepatitis A virus in cell culture in vitro. Proc. Soc. Exp. Biol. Med. 1979; 160: 213–221
95. **Rahaman, S.M., Chira, P., Koff, R.S.:** Idiopathic autoimmune chronic hepatitis triggered by hepatitis A. Amer. J. Gastroenterol. 1994; 89: 106–108
96. **Rosenblum, L.S., Villarino, M.E., Nainan, O.V., Melish, M.E., Hadler, S.C., Pinsky, P.P., Jarvis, W.R., Ott, C.E., Margolis, H.S.:** Hepatitis A outbreak in a neonatal intensive care unit: risk factors for transmission and evidence of prolonged viral excretion among preterm infants. J. Infect. Dis. 1991; 164: 476–482
97. **Rosenthal, P.:** Cost-effectiveness of hepatitis A vaccination in children, adolescents, and adults. Hepatology 2003; 37: 44–51
98. **Ruel, M., Sevestre, H., Henry-Biabaud, E., Courouce, A.M., Capron, J.P., Erlinger, S.:** Fibrin ring granulomas in hepatitis A. Dig. Dis. Sci. 1992; 37: 1915–1917
99. **Schenkel, K., Bremer, V., Grabe, C., van Treeck, U., Schreier, E., Hohne, M., Ammon, A., Alpers, K.:** Outbreak of hepatitis A in two federal states of Germany: Bakery products as vehicle of infection. Epidem. Infect. 2006; 134: 1292–1298
100. **Schiller, W.-G., Ochs, A.:** Hepatitis A infection of a primate keeper as an occupational risk. Arbeitsmed. Sozialmed. Umweltmed. 1993; 28: 530–532
101. **Schiraldi, O., Modugno, A., Miglietta, A., Fera, G.:** Prolonged viral hepatitis type A with cholestasis: case report. Ital. J. Gastroenterol. 1991; 23: 364–366
102. **Scully, L.J., Ryan, A.E.:** Urticaria and acute hepatitis A infection. Amer. J. Gastroenterol. 1993; 88: 277–278
103. **Sheretz, R.J., Russell, B.A., Reuman, P.D.:** Transmission of hepatitis A by transfusion of blood products. Arch. Intern. Med. 1984; 144: 1579–1580
104. **Shrier, L.A., Karpen, S.J., McEvoy, C.:** Acute pancreatitis associated with acute hepatitis A in a young child. J. Pediatr. 1995; 126: 57–59
105. **Siegl, G., Weitz, M., Kronauer, G.:** Stability of hepatitis A virus. Intervirology 1984; 22: 218–226
106. **Simmons, W.W., Warren, R.E.:** Eosinophilic pleural effusion associated with recovery from viral hepatitis A. J. Clin. Gastroenterol. 1994; 19: 143–145
107. **Sjogren, M.H., Tanno, H., Fay, O., Sileoni, S., Cohen, B.D., Burke, D.S., Feighny, R.J.:** Hepatitis A virus in stool during clinical relapse. Ann. Intern. Med. 1987; 106: 221–226
108. **Staes, C.J., Schlenker, T.L., Risk, I., Cannon, K.G., Harris, H., Pavia, A.T., Shapiro, C.N., Bell, B.P.:** Sources of infection among persons with acute hepatitis A and no identified risk factors during a sustained community-wide outbreak. Pediatrics 2000; 106: 63–69
109. **Steffen, R., Kane, M.A., Shapiro, C.N., Billo, N., Schoellhorn, K.J., van Damme, P.:** Epidemiology and prevention of hepatitis A in travelers. J. Amer. Med. Ass. 1994; 272: 885–889
110. **Stene-Johansen, K., Jenum, P.A., Hoel, T., Blystad, H., Sunde, H., Skaug, K.:** An outbreak of hepatitis A among homosexuals linked to a family outbreak. Epidem. Infect. 2002; 129: 113–117
111. **Taliani, G., Gaeta, G.B.:** Hepatitis A: post-exposure prophylaxis. Vaccine 2003; 21: 2234–2237
112. **Tang, Y.W., Wang, J.X., Xu, Z.Y., Guo, Y.F., Qian, W.H., Xu, J.X.:** A serological confirmed, case-control study, of a large outbreak of hepatitis A in China, associated with consumption of clams. Epidemiol. Infect. 1991; 107: 651–657
113. **Texeira, M.R., Weller, I.V.D., Murray, A., Bamber, M., Thomas, H.C., Sherlock, S., Scheuer, P.J.:** The pathology of hepatitis A in man. Liver 1982; 2: 53–60
114. **Tjon, G.M., Gotz, H., Koek, A.G., de Zwart, O., Mertens, P.L., Coutinho, R.A., Bruisten, S.M.:** An outbreak of hepatitis A among home-

less drug users in Rotterdam, the Netherlands. J. Med. Virol. 2005; 77: 360–366
115. **Totsuka, A., Moritsugu, Y.:** Hepatitis A virus proteins. Intervirology 1999; 42: 63–68
116. **Vento, S., Garofano, T., Di Perri, G., Dolci, L., Concia, E., Bassetti, D.:** Identification of hepatitis A virus as a trigger for autoimmune chronic hepatitis type 1 in susceptible individuals. Lancet 1991; 337: 1183–1187
117. **Warburton, A.R.E., Wreghitt, T.G., Rampling, A., Buttery, R., Ward, K.N., Perry, K.R., Parry, J.V.:** Hepatitis A outbreak involving bread. Epidem. Infect. 1991; 106: 199–202
118. **Watson, J.C., Fleming, D.W., Borella, A.J., Olcott, E.S., Conrad, R.E., Baron, R.C.:** Vertical transmission of hepatitis A resulting in an outbreak in a neonatal intensive care unit. J. Infect. Dis. 1993; 167: 567–571
119. **Wolf, M., Oneta, C.M., Jornod, P., Seld, D., Wauters, J.P., Blum, A.L., Delarive, J.:** Cholestatic hepatitis A complicated by acute renal insufficiency. Zschr. Gastroenterol. 2001; 39: 519–522
120. **Zikos, D., Grewal, K.S., Craig, K., Jen-Chieh-Cheng, Peterson, D.R., Fisher, K.A.:** Nephrotic syndrome and acute renal failure associated with hepatitis A virus infection. Amer. J. Gastroenterol. 1995; 90: 295–298

Acute viral hepatitis B
121. **Akahane, Y., Okada, S., Sakamoto, M., Wakamiya, M., Kitamura, T., Tawara, A., Naitoh, S., Tsuda, F., Okamoto, H.:** Persistence of hepatitis B viremia after recovery from acute hepatitis B: correlation between anti-HBc titer and HBV DNA in serum. Hepatol. Res. 2002; 24: 8–17
122. **Alter, M.J.:** Epidemiology and prevention of hepatitis B. Semin. Liver Dis. 2003; 23: 39–46
123. **Alward, W.L.M., McMahon, B.J., Hall, D.B., Heyward, W.L., Francis, D.P., Bender, T.R.:** The long-term serological course of asymptomatic hepatitis B virus carriers and the development of primary hepatocellular carcinoma. J. Infect. Dis. 1985; 151: 604–609
124. **Ayoola, E.A., Johnson, A.O.K.:** Hepatitis B vaccine in pregnancy: immunogenicity, safety and transfer of antibodies to infants. Int. J. Gynaecol. Obstet. 1987; 25: 297–301
125. **Benvegnu, L., Fattovich, G., Noventa, F., Tremolada, F., Chemello, L., Cecchetto, A., Alberti, A.:** Concurrent hepatitis B and C virus infection and risk of hepatocellular carcinoma in cirrhosis. Cancer 1994; 74: 2442–2448
126. **Bianco, E., Stroffolini, T., Spada, E., Szklo, A., Marzolini, F., Ragni, P., Gallo, G., Balocchini, E., Parlato, A., Sangalli, M., Lopalco, P.L., Zotti, C., Mele, A.:** Case fatality rate of acute viral hepatitis in Italy: 1995–2000. An update. Dig. Liver Dis. 2003; 35: 404–408
127. **Boxall, E.H., Flewett, T.H., Dane, D.S., Cameron, C.H., MacCallum, F.O., Lee, T.W.:** Hepatitis-B surface antigen in breast milk. Lancet 1974/II: 1007–1008
128. **Broderick, A.L., Jonas, M.M.:** Hepatitis B in children. Semin. Liver Dis. 2003; 23: 59–68
129. **Brown, J.L., Carman, W.F., Thomas, H.C.:** The hepatitis B virus. Clin. Gastroenterol. 1990; 4: 721–746
130. **Calvet, X., Bruix, J., Bosch, J., Rodes, J.:** Portal pressure in patients with exudative ascites in the course of acute hepatitis B. Liver 1991; 11: 206–210
131. **Carman, W.F., Fagan, E.A., Hadziyannis, St., Karayiannis, P., Tassapoulos, N.C., Williams, R., Thomas, H.C.:** Association of a precore genomic variant of hepatitis B virus with fulminant hepatitis. Hepatology 1991; 14: 219–222
132. **Chang, M.-H., Hwang, L.-H., Hsu, H.-C., Lee, C.-Y., Beasley, R.P.:** Prospective study of asymptomatic HBsAg carrier children infected in the perinatal period: clinical and liver histologic studies. Hepatology 1988; 8: 374–377
133. **Chen, W.N., Oon, C.J.:** Hepatitis B virus mutants: An overview. J. Gastroenterol. Hepatol. 2002; 17 (Suppl.): 497–499
134. **Chobe, L.P., Chadha, M.S., Arankalle, V.A., Gogate, S.S., Banerjee, K.:** Hepatitis B infection among dental personnel in Pune and Bombay (India). Indian J. Med. Res. 1991; 93(A): 143–146
135. **Chu, C.J., Hussain, M., Lok, A.S.F.:** Hepatitis B virus genotype B is associated with earlier Hbe Ag seroconversion compared with hepatitis B virus genotype C. Gastroenterology 2002; 122: 1756–1762
136. **Combes, B., Shorey, J., Barrera, A., Stastny, P., Eigenbrodt, E.H., Hull, A.R., Carter, N.W.:** Glomerulonephritis with deposition of Australia antigen-antibody complexes in glomerular basement membrane. Lancet 1991/II: 234–237
137. **Comer, G.M., Mittal, M.K., Donelson, S.S., Lee, T.-P.:** Cluster of fulminant hepatitis B in crack users. Amer. J. Gastroenterol. 1991; 86: 331–334
138. **Connor, F.L., Rosenberg, A.R., Kennedy, S.E., Bohane, T.D.:** HBV associated nephrotic syndrome: resolution with oral lamivudine (case report). Arch. Dis. Childh. 2003; 88: 446–449
139. **Craxi, A., Tine, F., Vinci, M., Almasio, P., Camma, C., Garofalo, G., Pagliaro, L.:** Transmission of hepatitis B and hepatitis delta viruses in the households of chronic hepatitis B surface antigen carriers: A regression analysis of indicators of risk. Amer. J. Epidemiol. 1991; 134: 641–650
140. **De Franchis, R., Meucci, G., Vecchi, M., Tatarella, M., Colombo, M., del Ninno, E., Rumi, M.G., Donato, M.F., Ronchi, G.:** The natural history of asymptomatic hepatitis B surface antigen carriers. Ann. Intern. Med. 1993; 118: 191–194
141. **Dentico, P., Volpe, A., Buongiorno, R., Maracchione, N., Carbone, M., Manno, C., Proscia, F.:** Immunogenicity and efficacy of anti-hepatitis B vaccines in hemodialysis patients. Nephron 1992; 61: 324–325
142. **Devesa, F., Martinez, F., Moreno, M.J., Sanfrancisco, M., Ferrando, J., Rull, S.:** Marcadores de la hepatitis B en tres centros abiertos para disminuidos psiquicos. Rev. Esp. Enf. Digest. 1993; 84: 162–168
143. **Diamantis, I.D., McGandy, Ch.E., Cheng, T.-J., Liaw, Y.-F., Gudat, F., Bianchi, L.:** Hepatitis BX-gene expression in hepatocellular carcinoma. J. Hepatol. 1992; 15: 400–403
144. **Dienstag, J.L., Wands, J.R., Isselbacher, K.J.:** Hepatitis B and essential mixed cryoglobulinemia. New Engl. J. Med. 1977; 297: 946
145. **Dienstag, J.L., Rhodes, A.R., Bhan, A.K., Dvorak, A.M., Mihm, M.C.jr., Wands, J.R.:** Urticaria associated with acute viral hepatitis type B. Studies of pathogenesis. Ann. Intern. Med. 1978; 89: 34–40
146. **Fabris, P., Tositti, G., Mazzella, G., Zanetti, A.R., Nicolin, R., Pellizzer, G., Benedetti, P., de Lalla, F.:** Effect of ursodeoxycholic acid administration in patients with acute viral hepatitis: a pilot study. Aliment. Pharm. Ther. 1999; 13: 1187–1193
147. **Fattovich, G.:** Natural history and prognosis of hepatitis B. Semin. Liver Dis. 2003; 23: 47–58
148. **Fisker, N., Georgsen, J., Stolborg, T., Khalil, M.R., Christensen, P.B.:** Low hepatitis B prevalence among pre-school children in Denmark: saliva anti-HBc screening in day care centres. J. Med. Virol. 2002; 68: 500–504
149. **Fisman, D.N., Agrawal, D., Leder, K.:** The effect of age on immunologic response to recombinant hepatitis B vaccine: A meta-analysis. Clin. Infect. Dis. 2002; 35: 1368–1375
150. **Flisiak, R., Prokopowicz, D.:** Effect of misoprostol on serum beta(2)-microglobulin in the course of viral hepatitis B. Eur. J. Gastroenterol. Hepatol. 1999; 11: 1227–1230
151. **Galsky, J., Bansky, G., Holubova, T., König, J.:** Effect of ursodeoxycholic acid in acute viral hepatitis. J. Clin. Gastroenterol. 1999; 28: 249–253
152. **Gerlich, W.H., Thomssen, R.:** An outbreak of hepatitis B in a butchery. Dtsch. Med. Wschr. 1982; 107: 1627–1630
153. **Gianotti, F.:** Papular acrodermatitis of childhood: an australia antigen disease. Arch. Dis. Childh. 1973; 48: 794–799
154. **Gilson, R.J.C.:** Sexually transmitted hepatitis: a review. Genitourin. Med. 1992; 68: 123–129
155. **Giotakos, O., Bourtsoukli, P., Paraskeyopoulou, T., Spandoni, P., Stasinos, S., Boulougouri, D., Spirakou, E.:** Prevalence and risk factors of HIV, hepatitis B and hepatitis C in a forensic population of rapists and child molesters. Epidem. Infect. 2003; 130: 497–500
156. **Glück, T., Weber, P., Wiedmann, K.H.:** Hepatitis B-associated vasculitis. Dtsch. Med. Wschr. 1994; 119: 1388–1392
157. **Grob, P.J., Bischoff, B., Naeff, F.:** Cluster of hepatitis B transmitted by a physician. Lancet 1981/II: 1218–1220
158. **Hadler, S.C., Francis, D.P., Maynard, J.E., Thompson, S.E., Judson, F.N., Echenberg, D.F., Ostrow, D.G., O'Malley, P.M., Penley, K.A., Altman, N.L., Braff, E., Shipman, G.F., Coleman, P.J., Mandel, E.J.:** Long-term immunogenicity and efficacy of hepatitis B vaccine in homosexual men. New Engl. J. Med. 1986; 315: 211–214
159. **Hadler, S.C., Sorley, D.L., Acree, K.H., Webster, H.M., Schable, Ch.A., Francis, D.P., Maynard, J.E.:** An outbreak of hepatitis B in a dental practice. Ann. Intern. Med. 1981; 95: 133–138
160. **Hadziyannis, S., Gerber, M.A., Vissoulis, C., Popper, H.:** Cytoplasmic hepatitis B antigen in "ground-glass" hepatocytes of carriers. Arch. Pathol. 1973; 96: 327–330
161. **Halfon, P., Pol, S., Bourliere, M., Cacoub, P.:** Hepatitis B virus genotypes: clinical, epidemiological and therapeutic implications. Gastroenterol. Clin. Biol. 2002; 26: 1005–1012
162. **Harpaz, R., von Seidlein, L., Averhoff, F.M., Tormey, M.P., Sinha, S.D., Kotsopoulou, K., Lambert, S.B., Robertson, B.H., Cherry, J.D., Shapiro, C.N.:** Transmission of hepatitis B virus to multiple patients from a surgeon without evidence of inadequate infection control. New Engl. J. Med. 1996; 334: 549–554
163. **Homann, J., Petri, F., Deetjen, W., Kuntz, E., Matthes, K.J., Zellmer, R., Eimiller, A., Paul, F.:** Therapeutic effect of ursodeoxycholic acid in acute viral hepatitis? Z. Gastroenterol. 1988; 26: 623.
164. **Hoofnagle, J.H., Shafritz, D.A., Popper, H.:** Chronic type B hepatitis and the "healthy" HBsAg carrier state. Hepatology 1987; 7: 758–763
165. **Hurlen, B., Jonsen, J., Aas, E.:** Viral hepatitis in dentists in Norway. Acta Odont. Scand. 1980; 38: 321–324
166. **Hutin, Y.J.F., Goldstein, S.T., Varma, J.K., Odair, J.B., Mast, E.E., Shapiro, C.N., Alter, M.J.:** An outbreak of hospital-acquired hepatitis B virus infection among patients receiving chronic hemodialysis. Inf. Contr. Hosp. Epid. 1999; 20: 731–735
167. **Ide, T., Sata, M., Nouno, R., Yamashita, F., Nakano, H., Tanikawa, K.:** Clinical evaluation of four cases of acute viral hepatitis complicated by pure red cell aplasia. Amer. J. Gastroenterol. 1994; 89: 257–262
168. **Inman, R.D.:** Rheumatic manifestations of hepatitis B virus infection. Semin. Arthr. Rheum. 1982; 11: 406–420
169. **Joh, H., Hasegawa, K., Ogawa, M., Ishikawa, K., Iizuka, A., Naritomi, T., Kanai, N., Torii, N., Hashimoto, E., Hayashi, N.:** Genotypic analysis of hepatitis B virus from patients with fulminant hepatitis: comparison with acute self-limited hepatitis. Hepatol. Res. 2003; 26: 119–124
170. **Jung, S., Lee, H.C., Han, J.M., Lee, Y.L., Chung, Y.H., Lee, Y.S., Kwon, Y., Yu, E.S., Suh, D.J.:** Four cases of hepatitis B virus-related fibrosing cholestatic hepatitis treated with lamivudine (case report). J. Gastroenterol. Hepatol. 2002; 17: 345–350

171. **Kaganov, B.S., Nisevich, N.I., Uchaikin, V.F., Konev, V.A., Levina, E.I., Sizich, N.N., Chapligina, G.V.:** Acute viral hepatitis B in children: lack of chronicity. Lancet 1990; 336: 374–375
172. **Kalayci, C., Johnson, P.J., Davies, S.E., Williams, R.:** Hepatitis B virus related hepatocellular carcinoma in the non-cirrhotic liver. J. Hepatol. 1991; 12: 54–59
173. **Karayiannis, P., Novick, D.M., Lok, A.S.F., Fowler, M.J.F., Monjardino, J., Thomas, H.C.:** Hepatitis B virus DNA in saliva, urine, and seminal fluid of carriers of hepatitis Be antigen. Brit. Med. J. 1985; 290: 1853–1855
174. **Khan, A.J., Cotter, S.M., Schulz, B., Hu, Y.L., Rosenberg, J., Robertson, B.H., Fiore, A.E., Bell, B.R.:** Nosocomial transmission of hepatitis B virus infection among residents with diabetes in a skilled nursing facility. Inf. Contr. Hosp. Epidoma. 2002; 23: 313–318
175. **Kobler, E., Schmuziger, P., Hartmann, G.:** Hepatitis resulting from acupuncture. Schweiz. Med. Wschr. 1979; 109: 1828–1829
176. **Korman, S.H.:** Thrombocytopenic purpura during the incubation of hepatitis B. Acta Paediatr. Scand. 1991; 80: 975–976
177. **Kosaka, Y., Takase, K., Kojima, M., Shimizu, M., Inoue, K., Yoshiba, M., Tanaka, S., Akahane, Y., Okamoto, H., Tsuda, F., Miyakawa, Y., Mayumi, M.:** Fulminant hepatitis- B-induction by hepatitis-B virus mutants defective in the precore region and incapable of encoding e-antigen. Gastroenterology 1991; 100: 1087–1094
178. **Krebs, H.-J.:** Hepatitis B in dentists and dental staff. Münch. Med. Wschr. 1985; 127: 462–463
179. **Kunches, L.M., Craven, D.E., Werner, B.G., Jacobs, L.M.:** Hepatitis B exposure in emergency medical personnel. Prevalence of serologic markers and need for immunization. Amer. J. Med. 1983; 75: 269–272
180. **Kuntz, E., Kuntz, A.:** Prohibition to practice for dentists in the case of unfavourable hepatitis B serology. Münch. Med. Wschr. 1978; 120: 1407–1410; 1979; 121: 114–115
181. **Kuntz, E.:** Viral hepatitis and dental practice. Der Freie Zahnarzt 1982; 988–993
182. **Lai, F.M.-M., Lai, K.N., Tam, J.S.L., Lui, S.F., To, K.F., Li, P.K.T.:** Primary glomerulonephritis with detectable glomerular hepatitis B virus antigens. Amer. J. Surg. Path. 1994; 18: 175–186
183. **LeBrecque, D.R., Muhs, J.M., Lutwick, L.I., Woolson, R.F., Hierholzer, W.R.:** The risk of hepatitis B transmission from health care workers to patients in a hospital setting – a prospective study. Hepatology 1986; 6: 205–208
184. **Liang, T.J., Hasegawa, K., Rimon, N., Wands, J.R., Ben-Porath, E.:** A hepatitis B virus mutant associated with an epidemic of fulminant hepatitis. New Engl. J. Med. 1991; 324: 1705–1709
185. **Limentani, A.E., Elliot, L.M., Noah, N.D., Lamborn, J.K.:** An outbreak of hepatitis B from tattooing. Lancet 1979/II: 86–88
186. **Lin, H.-H., Hsu, H.-Y., Chang, M.-H., Chen, P.-J., Chen, P.-S.:** Hepatitis B virus in the colostra of HBeAg-positive carrier mothers. J. Pediatr. Gastroenterol. Nutr. 1993; 17: 207–210
187. **Ljunggren, K., Hanson, B.G., Nordenfelt, E.:** HBsAg/IgM complexes as a prognostic marker of chronicity in acute hepatitis B virus infection. Scand. J. Infect. Dis. 1991; 23: 529–534
188. **Locarnini, S.:** Molecular virology of hepatitis B virus. Semin. Liver Dis. 2004; 24 (Suppl.): 3–10
189. **Lok, A.S.F., Lai, C.L., Hui, W.M., Matthew, M.T., Wu, P.C., Lam, S.K., Leung, E.K.Y.:** Absence of transmission of hepatitis B by fibreoptic upper gastrointestinal endoscopy. J. Gastroenterol. Hepatol. 1987; 2: 175–180
190. **Lok, A.S.F., Liang, R.H.S., Chiu, E.K.W., Wong, K.-L., Chan, T.-K., Todd, D.:** Reactivation of hepatitis B virus replication in patients receiving cytotoxic therapy. Gastroenterology 1991; 100: 182–188
191. **Lortholary, O., Molinie, V., Jaccard, A., Amarenco, G., Boudes, P., Amouroux, J., Guillevin, L.:** Bladder neuropathy and gastric paralysis in polyarteritis nodosa associated with hepatitis B virus. Scand. J. Rheumat. 1990; 19: 442–443
192. **Luo, K.X., Zhou, R., He, C., Liang, Z.S., Jiang, S.:** Hepatitis B virus DNA in sera of virus carriers positive exclusively for antibodies to the hepatitis B core antigen. J. Med. Virol. 1991; 35: 55–59
193. **Marcellin, P., Martinot-Peignoux, M., Loriot, M.-A., Giostra, E., Boyer, N., Thiers, V., Benhamou, J.-P.:** Persistence of hepatitis B virus DNA demonstrated by polymerase chain reaction in serum and liver after loss of HBsAg induced by antiviral therapy. Ann. Intern. Med. 1990; 112: 227–228
194. **Marie-Cardine, A., Mouterde, O., Dubuisson, S., Buffet-Janvresse, C., Mallet, E.:** Salivary transmission in an intrafamilial cluster of hepatitis B. J. Pediatr. Gastroenterol. Nutrit. 2002; 34: 227–230
195. **Marinho, R.T., Moura, M.C., Pedro, M., Ramalho, F.J., Velosa, J.F.:** Hepatitis B vaccination in hospital personnel and medical students. J. Clin. Gastroenterol. 1999; 28: 317–322
196. **Marion, P.L., Oshiro, L.S., Regnery, D.C., Scullard, G.H., Robinson, W.S.:** A virus in beechey ground squirrels which is related to hepatitis B virus in man. Proc. Natl. Acad. Sci. USA 1980; 77: 2941–2945
197. **Mason, W.S., Seal, G., Summers, J.:** Virus of Peking ducks with structure and biological relatedness to human hepatitis B virus. J. Virol. 1980; 36: 829–836
198. **Mayans, M.V., Hall, A.J., Inskip, H.M., Lindsay, S.W., Chotard, J., Mendy, M., Whittle, H.C.:** Do bedbugs transmit hepatitis B? Lancet 1994; 343: 761–763
199. **McMahon, J.J.:** Epidemiology and natural history of hepatitis. B Glmin. Liver Dis. 2005; 25 (Suppl. 1): 3–8
200. **McSweeney, P.A., Carter, J.M., Green, G.J., Romeril, K.R.:** Fatal aplastic anemia associated with hepatitis B viral infection. Amer. J. Med. 1988; 85: 255–256
201. **Michalak, T.:** Immune complexes of hepatitis B surface antigen in the pathogenesis of periarteritis nodosa. A study of seven necropsy cases. Amer. J. Pathol. 1978; 90: 619–628
202. **Milbradt, R., Nasemann, T.:** The entity of the Gianotti-Crosti syndrome and its relationship to hepatitis B infection. Hautarzt 1975; 26: 471–479
203. **Moyer, L.A., Alter, M.J., Favero, M.S.:** Hemodialysis- associated hepatitis B: revised recommendations for serologic screening. Semin. Dialysis 1990; 3: 201–205
204. **Murakami, S.:** Hepatitis B virus X protein: structure, function and biology. Intervirology 1999; 42: 81–99
205. **Nakamura, H., Shimizu, T., Ohshiro, S., Aoki, H., Kaneko, M., Shioda, A., Saitoh, T., Moriyama, M., Tanaka, N., Arakawa, Y.:** An adult patient with acute hepatitis type B which was protracted and complicated by polyarteritis nodosa: A case report. Hepatol. Res. 2002; 24: 439–444
206. **Nassal, M.:** Hepatitis B virus replication: novel roles for virus-host interactions. Intervirology 1999; 42: 100–116
207. **Newkirk, M.M., Downe, A.E.R., Simon, J.B.:** Fate of ingested hepatitis B antigen in blood-sucking insects. Gastroenterology 1975; 69: 982–987
208. **Odeh, M., Oliven, A.:** Treatment of prolonged cholestasis of acute hepatitis B with ursodeoxycholic acid. Hepat. Res. 1998; 13: 37–41
209. **O'Gorman, M.A., Sharma, S., Groopman, J.D., Tennant, B.C., Tochkov, I.A., Schwarz, K.B.:** Decreased oxidative DNA damage and accelerated cell turnover in woodchuck hepatitis virus infected liver. Hepatol. Res. 2003; 25: 254–262
210. **Ogston, C.W., Wittenstein, F.S., London, W.T., Millman, I.:** Persistence of hepatitis B surface antigen in the bedbug Cimex hemipterus (Fabr.). J. Infect. Dis. 1979; 140: 411–414
211. **Oleske, J., Minnefor, A., Cooper, R.jr., Ross, J., Gocke, D.:** Transmission of hepatitis B in a classroom setting. J. Pediatr. 1980; 97: 770–772
212. **Omata, M., Uchiumi, K., Ito, Y., Yokosuka, O., Mori, J., Terao, K., Ye, W.-F., O'Connell, A.P., London, W.T., Okuda, K.:** Duck hepatitis B virus and liver diseases. Gastroenterology 1983; 85: 260–267
213. **Oren, I., Hershow, R.C., Ben-Porath, E., Krivoy, N., Goldstein, N., Rishpon, S., Shouval, D., Hadler, S.C., Alter, M.J., Maynard, J.E., Alroy, G.:** A common-source outbreak of fulminant hepatitis B in a hospital. Ann. Intern. Med. 1989; 110: 691–698
214. **Ozgenc, F., Aksu, G., Kirkpinar, F., Aituglu, I., Coker, I., Kutukculer, N., Yagci, R.V.:** The influence of marginal zinc deficient diet on postvaccination immune response against hepatitis B in rats. Hepatol. Res. 2006; 35: 26–30
215. **Penner, E., Maida, E., Mamoli, B., Gangl, A.:** Serum and cerebrospinal fluid immune complexes containing hepatitis B surface antigen in Guillain-Barre syndrome. Gastroenterology 1982; 82: 576–580
216. **Perlman, D., Hu, H.M.:** Duck hepatitis B virus virion secretion requires a double-stranded DNA genome. J. Virol. 2003; 77: 2287–2294
217. **Piazza, M., Guadagnino, V., Picciotto, L., Borgia, G., Nappa, S.:** Contamination by hepatitis B surface antigen in dental surgeries. Brit. Med. J. 1987; 295: 473–474
218. **Polakoff, S.:** Acute hepatitis B in patients in Britain related to previous operations and dental treatment. Brit. Med. J. 1986; 293: 33–36
219. **Polish, L.B., Shapiro, C.N., Bauer, F., Klotz, P., Ginier, P., Roberto, R.R., Margolis, H.S., Alter, M.J.:** Nosocomial transmission of hepatitis B virus associated with the use of a spring-loaded finger-stick device. New Engl. J. Med. 1992; 326: 721–725
220. **Pontisso, P., Morsica, G., Ruvoletto, M.G., Barzon, M., Perilongo, G., Basso, G., Cecchetto, G., Chemello, L., Alberti, A.:** Latent hepatitis B virus infection in childhood hepatocellular carcinoma. Analysis by polymerase chain reaction. Cancer 1992; 69: 2731–2735
221. **Porres, J.C., Carreno, V., Bartolome, J., Gutiez, J., Castillo, I.:** A dynamic study of the intrafamilial spread of hepatitis B virus infection. Relation with the viral replication. J. Med. Virol. 1989; 28: 237–242
222. **Prassolov, A., Hohenberg, H., Kalinina, T., Schneider, C., Cova, L., Krone, O., Frolich, K., Will, H., Sirma, H.:** New hepatitis B virus of cranes that has an unexpected broad host range. J. Virol. 2003; 77: 1964–1976
223. **Prati, D.:** Transmission of viral hepatitis by blood and blood derivatives: current risks, past heritage. Dig. Dis. Sci. 2002; 34: 812–817
224. **Pumpens, P., Grens, E., Nassal, M.:** Molecular epidemiology and immunology of hepatitis B virus infection. An update. Intervirology 2002; 45: 218–232
225. **Quale, J.M., Landman, D., Wallace, B., Atwood, E., Ditore, V., Fruchter, G.:** Déjà vu: Nosocomial hepatitis B virus transmission and fingerstick monitoring. Amer. J. Med. 1998; 105: 296–301
226. **Radvan, G.H., Hewson, E.G., Berenger, S., Brookman, D.J.:** The Newcastle hepatitis B outbreak. Observations on cause, management and prevention. Med. J. Aust. 1986; 144: 461–464
227. **Rehermann, B.:** Immune responses in hepatitis B virus infection. Semin. Liver Dis. 2003; 23: 21–37
228. **Rich, J.D., Ching, C.G., Lally, M.A., Gaitanis, M.M., Schwartzapfel, B., Charuvastra, A., Beckwith, C.G., Flanigan, T.P.:** A review of the case for hepatitis B vaccination of high-risk adults. Amer. J. Med. 2003; 114: 316–318
229. **Rosenblum, L., Darrow, W., Witte, J., Cohen, J., French, J., Gill, P.S., Potterat, J., Sikes, K., Reich, R., Hadler, S.:** Sexual practices in the transmission of hepatitis B virus and prevalence of hepatitis delta virus infection in female prostitutes in the United States. J. Amer. Med. Ass. 1992; 267: 2477–2481

230. Rosman, A.S., Basu, P., Galvin, K., Lieber, C.S.: Efficacy of a high and accelerated dose of hepatitis B vaccine in alcoholic patients: a randomized clinical trial. Amer. J. Med. 1997; 103: 217–222
231. Samandari, T., Malakmadze, N., Balter, S., Perz, J.E., Khristova, M., Swetnam, L., Bornschlegel, K., Philipps, M.S., Poshni, I.A., Nautiyal, P., Nainan, O.V., Bell, B.P., Williams, I.T.: A large outbreak of hepatitis B virus infections associated with frequent injections at a physician's office. Infect. Contr. Hosp. Epidem. 2005; 26: 745–750
232. Saracco, G., Macagno, S., Rosina, F., Caredda, F., Antinori, S., Rizzetto, M.: Serologic markers with fulminant hepatitis in persons positive for hepatitis B surface antigen. A worldwide epidemiologic and clinical survey. Ann. Intern. Med. 1988; 108: 380–383
233. Sebastian, V.J., Ray, S., Bhattacharya, S., Tin Maung, O., Md Saini, H.A., HJ Daud Jalani: Tattooing and hepatitis B infection. J. Gastroenterol. Hepatol. 1992; 7: 385–387
234. Shafritz, D.A.: Variants of hepatitis B virus associated with fulminant liver disease. New Engl. J. Med. 1991; 324: 1737–1738
235. Solis Herruzo, J.A., Munoz-Yague, T.: Polyarteritis nodosa and hepatitis B virus infection. Rev. Esp. Enferm. Dig. 2003; 95: 156.
236. Spijkerman, I.J.B., van Doorn, L.J., Janssen, M.H.W., Wijkmans, C.J., Bikert-Mooiman, M.A.J., Coutinho, R.A., Weers-Pothoff, G.: Transmission of hepatitis B virus from a surgeon to his patients during high-risk and low-risk surgical procedures during 4 years. Inf. Contr. Hosp. Epidem. 2002; 23: 306–312
237. Tabor, E.: Guillain-Barre syndrome and other neurologic syndromes in hepatitis A, B, non-A, non-B. J. Med. Virol. 1987; 21: 207–216
238. Tillmann, H.L., Hadem, J., Leifeld, L., Zachou, K., Canbay, A., Eisenbach, C., Graziadei, I., Encke, J., Schmidt, H., Vogel, W., Schneider, A., Spengler, U., Gerken, G., Dalekos, G.N., Wiedemeyer, H., Manns, M.P.: Safety and efficacy of lamirudine in patients with severe acute or fulminant hepatitis B, a multicenter experience. J. Vival Hepat. 2006; 13: 256–263
239. Torii, N., Hasegawa, K., Ogawa, M., Hashimo, E., Hayashi, N.: Effectiveness and long-term outcome of lamivudine therapy for acute hepatitis B. Hepatol. Res. 2002; 24: 34–41
240. Ursell, P.C., Habib, A., Sharma, P., Mesa-Tejada, R., Lefkowitch, J.H., Fenoglio, J.J.jr.: Hepatitis B virus and myocarditis. Hum. Pathol. 1984; 15: 481–484
241. Van Zonneveld, M., van Nunen, A.B., Niesters, H.G.M., de Man, R.A., Schalm, S.W., Janssen, H.L.A.: Lamivudine treatment during pregnancy to prevent perinatal transmission of hepatitis B virus infection. J. Viral Hepat. 2003; 10: 294–297
242. Vanclaire, J., Cornu, Ch., Sokal, E.M.: Fulminant hepatitis B as an infant born to a hepatitis Be antibody positive, DNA negative carrier. Arch. Dis. Childh. 1991; 66: 983–985
243. Venkataseshan, V.S., Lieberman, K., Kim, D.U., Thung, S.N., Dikman, S., D'Agati, V., Susin, M., Valderrama, E., Gauthier, B., Prakash, A., Churg, J.: Hepatitis-B- associated glomerulonephritis: pathology, pathogenesis, and clinical course. Medicine (Baltimore) 1990; 69: 200–216
244. Vittal, S.B.V., Dourdourekas, D., Steigmann, F.: Hepatitis-B antigen in saliva, urine and tears. Amer. J. Gastroenterol. 1974; 61: 133–135
245. Waters, J.A., Kennedy, M., Voet, P., Hauser, P., Petre, J., Carman, W., Thomas, H.C.: Loss of the common "a" determinant of hepatitis B surface antigen by a vaccine- induced escape mutant. J. Clin. Invest. 1992; 90: 2543–2547
246. Weber, H.C., Schoeman, J.F., Nowitz, A., Becker, M.L.B.: Case report: psychosis associated with hepatitis B. J. Med. Virol. 1994; 44: 5–8
247. Weizsäcker, von, F., Puet, I., Geiss, K., Wirth, St., Blum, H.E.: Selective transmission of variant genomes from mother to infant in neonatal fulminant hepatitis B. Hepatology 1995; 21: 8–13
248. Welch, J., Tilzey, A.J., Webster, M., Noah, N.D., Banatvala, J.E.: Hepatitis B infections after gynaecological surgery. Lancet 1989; 1: 205–206
249. Williams, I., Smith, M.G., Sinha, D., Kernan, D., Minor-Babin, G., Garcia, E., Robertson, B.H., Di Pentima, R., Shapiro, C.N.: Hepatitis B virus transmission in an elementary school setting. J. Amer. Med. Ass. 1997; 278: 2167–2169
250. Wong, V.C.W., Ip, H.M.H., Reesink, H.W., Lelie, P.N., Reerink-Brongers, E.E., Yeung, C.Y., Ma, H.K.: Prevention of the HBsAg carrier state in newborn infants of mothers who are chronic carriers of HBsAg and HBeAg by administration of hepatitis-B vaccine and hepatitis-B immunoglobulin. Lancet 1984/I: 921–926
251. Wrzolkowa, T., Zurowska, A., Uszycka-Karcz, M., Picken, M.M.: Hepatitis B virus-associated glomerulonephritis: electron microscopic studies in 98 children. Amer. J. Kidn. Dis. 1991; 18: 306–312
252. Yao, E.M., Tavis, J.E.: Kinetics of synthesis and turnover of the duck hepatitis B virus reverse transcriptase. J. Biol. Chem. 2003; 278: 1201–1205
253. Yotsumoto, S., Kojima, M., Shoji, I., Yamamoto, K., Okamoto, H., Mishiro, S.: Fulminant hepatitis related to transmission of hepatitis B variants with precore mutations between spouses. Hepatology 1992; 16: 31–35
254. Young, B.W.Y., Lee, S.S., Lim, W.L., Yeoh, E.K.: The long-term efficacy of plasma-derived hepatitis B vaccine in babies born to carrier mothers. J. Viral Hepat. 2003; 10: 23–30
255. Yuki, N., Nagaoka, T., Yamashiro, M., Mochizuki, K., Kaneko, A., Yamamoto, M., Omura, H., Hikiji, K., Kato, M.: Long-term histologic and virologic outcomes of acute self-limited hepatitis B. Hepatology 2003; 37: 1172–1179
256. Zanetti, A.: Hepatitis B vaccination: an important method of preventing HBV-related hepatocellular carcinoma. Ital. J. Gastroenterol. 1992; 24: 100–102
257. Zhu, Q.R., Yu, Q.J., Yu, H., Lu, Q., Gu, X.H., Dong, Z.Q., Zhang, X.Z.: A randomized control trial on interruption of HBV transmission in uterus. Chin. Med. J. 2003; 116: 685–687
258. Zurn, A., Schmied, E., Saurat, J.-H.: Les manifestations cutanees de l'infection par le virus de l'hepatite B. Schweiz. Rundsch. Med. 1990; 79: 1254–1257

Acute viral hepatitis C
259. Ackerman, Z., Paltiel, O., Glikberg, F., Ackerman, E.: Hepatitis C virus in various human body fluids: a systematic review. Hepatol. Res. 1998; 11: 26–40
260. Agnello, V.: Mixed cryoglobulinemia and hepatitis C virus. Hospital Pract. 1995; 30: 35–42
261. Akahane, Y., Aikawa, T., Sugai, Y., Tsuda, F., Okamoto, H., Mishiro, S.: Transmission of HCV between spouses. Lancet 1992; 339: 1059–1060
262. Almasio, P., Provenzano, G., Scimemi, M., Cascio, G., Craxi, A., Pagliaro, L.: Hepatitis C virus and Sjögren's syndrome. Lancet 1992; 339: 989–990
263. Alter, M.J., Margolis, H.S., Krawczynski, K., Judson, F.N., Mares, A., Alexander, J., Hu, P.Y., Miller, J.K., Gerber, M.A., Sampliner, R.E., Meeks, E.L., Beach, M.J.: The natural history of community-acquired hepatitis C in the United States. New Engl. J. Med. 1992; 327: 1899–1905
264. Arai, Y., Noda, K., Enomoto, N., Arai, K., Yamada, Y., Suzuki, K., Yoshihara, H.: A prospective study of hepatitis C virus infection after needlestick accidents. Liver 1996; 16: 331–334
265. Bekkering, F.C., Brouwer, J.T., Leroux-Roels, G., van Vlierberghe, H., Elewaut, A., Schalm, S.W.: Ultrarapid hepatitis C virus clearance by daily high-dose interferon in non-responders to standard therapy. J. Hepatol. 1998; 28: 960–964
266. Bhattacharya, R., Shuhart, M.C.: Hepatitis C and alcohol: interactions, outcomes, and implications. J. Clin. Gastroenterol. 2003; 36: 242–252
267. Bisceglie, di A.M.: Hepatitis C and hepatocellular carcinoma. Semin. Liver Dis. 1995; 15: 64–69
268. Bresters, D., Mauser, F.M., Bunschoten, E.P., Reesink, H.W., Roosendaal, G., van der Poel, C.L., Chamuleau, R.A.M., Jansen, P.L.M., Weegink, C.J., Cuypers, H.T.M., van den Berg, M.H.: Sexual transmission of hepatitis C virus. Lancet 1993; 342: 210–211
269. Brillanti, S., Foli, M., Gaiani, S., Masci, C., Miglioli, M., Barbara, L.: Persistent hepatitis C viraemia without liver disease. Lancet 1993; 341: 464–465
270. Brown, J.L.: Hepatitis C: the structure and biology of the virus and diagnostic tests. J. Infect. 1995; 30: 95–101
271. Bruguera, M., Saiz, J.C., Franco, S., Gimenez-Barcons, M., Sanchez-Tapias, J.M., Fabregas, S., Vega, R., Camps, N., Dominguez, A., Salleras, L.: Outbreak of nosocomial hepatitis C virus infection resolved by genetic analysis of HCV RNA. J. Clin. Microbiol. 2002; 40: 4363–4366
272. Bukh, J., Miller, R.H., Purcell, R.H.: Genetic heterogeneity of hepatitis C virus: quasispecies and genotypes. Semin. Liver Dis. 1995; 15: 41–63
273. Cacoub, P., Lunel-Fabiani, F., Huong Du, L.T.: Polyarteritis nodosa and hepatitis C virus infection. Ann. Intern. Med. 1992; 116: 605–606
274. Carrozzo, M., Quadri, R., Latorre, P., Pentenero, M., Paganin, S., Bertolusso, G., Gandolfo, S., Negro, F.: Molecular evidence that the hepatitis C virus replicates in the oral mucosa. J. Hepatol. 2002; 37: 364–369
275. Carson, C.W., Conn, D.L., Czaja, A.J., Wright, T.L., Brecher, M.E.: Frequency and significance of antibodies to hepatitis C virus in polyarteritis nodosa. J. Rheumatol. 1993; 20: 304–309
276. Castells, L., Vargas, V., Gonzalez, A., Esteban, J., Esteban, R., Guardia, J.: Long interval between HCV infection and development of hepatocellular carcinoma. Liver 1995; 15: 159–163
277. Chan, S.-W., McOmish, F., Holmes, E.C., Dow, B., Peutherer, J.F., Follett, E., Yap, P.-L., Simmonds, P.: Analysis of a new hepatitis C virus type and its phylogenetic relationship to existing variants. J. Gen. Virol. 1992; 73: 1131–1141
278. Chang, M., Williams, O., Mittler, J., Quintanilla, A., Carithers, R.L., Perkins, J., Corey, L., Gretch, D.R.: Dynamics of hepatitis C virus replication in human liver. Amer. J. Path. 2003; 163: 433–444
279. Chayama, K., Kobayashi, M., Tsubota, A., Koida, I., Arase, Y., Saitoh, S., Ikeda, K., Kumada, H.: Molecular analysis of intraspousal transmission of hepatitis C virus. J. Hepatol. 1995; 22: 431–439
280. Chen, M.; Yun, Z.-B., Sällberg, M., Schvarcz, R., Bergquist, I., Berglund, H.-B., Sönnerborg, A.: Detection of hepatitis C virus RNA in the cell fraction of saliva before and after oral surgery. J. Med. Virol. 1995; 43: 223–226
281. Chu, C.-M., Liaw, Y.-F.: Simultaneous acute hepatitis B virus and hepatitis C virus infection leading to fulminant hepatitis and subsequent chronic hepatitis C. Clin. Infect. Dis. 1995; 20: 703–705
282. Cody, S.H., Nainan, O.V., Garfein, R.S., Meyers, H., Bell, B.P., Shapiro, C.N., Meeks, E.L., Pitt, H., Mouzin, E., Alter, M.J., Margolis, H.S., Vugia, D.J.: Hepatitis C virus transmission from an anaesthesiologist to a patient. Arch. Intern. Med. 2002; 162: 345–350
283. Daghestani, L., Pomeroy, C.: Renal manifestations of hepatitis C infection. Amer. J. Med. 1999; 106: 347–354
284. Datz, C., Cramp, M., Haas, T., Dietze, O., Nitschko, H., Froesner, G., Muss, N., Sandhofer, F., Vogel, W.: The natural course of hepatitis C

virus infection 18 years after an epidemic outbreak of non-A, non-B hepatitis in a plasmapheresis centre. Gut 1999; 44: 563–567

285. Delage, G., Infante-Rivard, C., Chiavetta, J.A., Willems, B., Pi, D., Fast, M.: Risk factors for acquisition of hepatitis C virus infection in blood donors: results of a case-control study. Gastroenterology 1999; 116: 893–899

286. Delarocque-Astagneau, E., Baffoy, N., Thiers, V., Simon, N., de Valk, H., Laperche, S., Courouce, A.M., Astagneau, P., Buisson, C., Desencios, J.C.: Outbreak of hepatitis C virus infection in a hemodialysis unit: Potential transmission by the hemodialysis machine? Infect. Contr. Hosp. Epidem. 2002; 23: 328–334

287. Devita, S., Zagonel, V., Russo, A., Rupolo, M., Cannizzaro, R., Chiara, G., Boiocchi, M., Carbone, A., Franceschi, S.: Hepatitis C virus, non-Hodgkin's lymphomas and hepatocellular carcinoma. Brit. J. Canc. 1998; 77: 2032–2035

288. Deterding, K., Tegtmeyer, B., Cornberg, M., Hadern, J., Potthoff, A., Böker, K.H.N., Tillmann, H.L., Manns, M.P., Wedemeyer, H.: Hepatitis A virus infection suppresses hepatitis C virus replication and may lead to clearance of HCV. J. Hepatol. 2006; 45: 770–778

289. Dove, L., Phung, Y., Bzowej, N., Kim, M., Monto, A., Wright, T.L.: Vibal evolution of hepatitis C in injection drug users. J. Viral Hepat. 2005; 12: 574–583

290. Dow, B.C., Follett, E.A.C., Jordan, T., McOmish, F., Davidson, J., Gillon, J., Yap, P.L., Simmonds, P.: Testing of blood donations for hepatitis C virus. Lancet 1994; 343: 477–478

291. Dusheiko, G.M., Smith, M., Scheuer, P.J.: Hepatitis C virus transmitted by human bite. Lancet 1990; 336: 503–504

292. El-Serag, H.B., Hampel, H., Yeh, C., Rabeneck, L.: Extrahepatic manifestations of hepatitis C among United States male veterans. Hepatology 2002; 36: 1439–1445

293. Esteban, J.I., Lopez-Talavera, J.C., Genesca, J., Madoz, P., Viladomiu, L., Muniz, E., Martin-Vega, C., Rosell, M., Allende, H., Vidal, X., Gonzalez, A., Hernandez, J.M., Esteban, R., Guardia, J.: High rate of infectivity and liver disease in blood donors with antibodies to hepatitis C virus. Ann. Intern. Med. 1991; 115: 443–449

294. Everhart, J.E., Di Bisceglie, A.M., Murray, L.M., Alter, H.J., Melpolder, J.J., Kuo, G., Hoofnagle, J.H.: Risk for non-A, non-B (type C) hepatitis through sexual or household contact with chronic carriers. Ann. Intern. Med. 1990; 112: 544–545

295. Fagan, E.A., Partridge, M., Sowray, J.H., Williams, R.: Review of hepatitis non-A, non-B: the potential hazards in dental care. Oral Surg. 1988; 65: 167–171

296. Fargion, S., Piperno, A., Capellini, M.D., Sampietro, M., Fracanzani, A.L., Romano, R., Caldarelli, R., Marcelli, R., Vecchi, L., Fiorelli, G.: Hepatitis C virus and porphyria cutanea tarda: evidence of a strong association. Hepatology 1992; 16: 1322–1323

297. Feray, C., Gigou, M., Samuel, D., Paradis, V., Wilber, J., David, M.F., Urdea, M., Reynes, M., Brechot, C., Bismuth, H.: The course of hepatitis C virus infection after liver transplantation. Hepatology 1994; 20: 1137–1143

298. Fischler, B., Lindh, G., Lindgren, S., Forsgren, M., von Sydow, M., Sangfelt, P., Alaeus, A., Harland, L., Enockson, E., Nemeth, A.: Vertical transmission of hepatitis C virus infection. Scand. J. Infect. Dis. 1996; 28: 353–356

299. Gerlach, J.T., Diepolder, H.M., Zachoval, R., Gruener, N.H., Jung, M.C., Ulsenheimer, A., Schraut, W.W., Schirren, C.A., Waechtler, M., Backmund, M., Pape, G.R.: Acute hepatitis C: High rate of both spontaneous and treatment induced viral clearance. Gastroenterology 2003; 125: 80–88

300. Goetz, A.M., Ndimbie, O.K., Wagener, M.M., Muder, R.R.: Prevalence of hepatitis C infection in health care workers affiliated with a liver transplant center. Transplantation 1995; 59: 990–994

301. Goodman, Z.D., Ishak, K.G.: Histopathology of hepatitis C virus infection. Semin. Liver Dis. 1995; 15: 70–81

302. Gordon, F.D., Anastopoulos, H., Khettry, U., Loda, M., Jenkins, R.L., Lewis, W.D., Trey, C.: Hepatitis C infection: a rare cause of fulminant hepatic failure. Amer. J. Gastroenterol. 1995; 90: 117–120

303. Gordon, S.C., Bayati, N., Silverman, A.L.: Clinical outcome of hepatitis C as a function of mode of transmission. Hepatology 1998; 28: 562–567

304. Healey, C.J., Smith, D.B., Walker, J.L., Holmes, E.C., Fleming, K.A., Chapman, R.W.G., Simmonds, P.: Acute hepatitis C infection after sexual exposure. Gut 1995; 36: 148–150

305. Hernandez, M.E., Bruguera, M., Puyuelo, T., Barrera, J.M., Sanchez Tapias, J.M., Rodes, J.: Risk of needle-stick injuries in the transmission of hepatitis C virus in hospital personnel. J. Hepatol. 1992; 16: 56–58

306. Hinrichsen, H., Leimenstoll, G., Stegen, G., Schrader, H., Fölsch, U.R., Schmidt, W.E.: Prevalence and risk factors of hepatitis C virus infection in haemodialysis patients: a multicentre study in 2796 patients. Gut 2002; 51: 429–433

307. Houghton, M., Weiner, A.J., Han, J., Kuo, G., Choo, Q.-L.: Molecular biology of the hepatitis C viruses: Implications for diagnosis, development and control of viral disease. Hepatology 1991; 14: 382–388

308. Kamal, S.M., Ismail, A., Graham, C.S., He, Q., Rasenack, J.W., Peters, T., Tawill, A.A., Fehr, J., Khalifa, K.E, Madwar, M.M., Koziel, M.J.: Pegylated interferon alpha therapy in acute hepatitis C: Relation to hepatitis C virus-specific T cell response kinetics. Hepatology 2004; 39: 1721–1731

309. Kamal, S.M., Fouly, A.E., Kamel, R.R., Hockenjos, B., Al Tawil, A., Khalifa, K.E., He, Q., Koziel, M.J., El Naggar, K.M., Rasenack, J.: Peginterferon α-2b therapy in acute hepatitis C impact of onset of therapy on sustained vivologic response. Gastroenterology 2006; 130: 632–638

310. Kao, J.-H., Hwang, Y.-T., Chen, P.-J., Yang, P.-M., Lai, M.-Y., Wang, T.-H., Chen, D.-S.: Transmission of hepatitis C virus between spouses: the important role of exposure duration. Amer. J. Gastroenterol. 1996; 91: 2087–2090

311. Kenny-Walsh, E.: Clinical outcome after hepatitis C infection from contaminated anti-D immune globulin. New Engl. J. Med. 1999; 340: 1228–1233

312. Kiyosawa, K., Sodeyama, T., Tanaka, E., Nakano, Y., Furuta, S., Nishioka, K., Purcell, R.H., Alter, H.J.: Hepatitis C in hospital employees with needlestick injuries. Ann. Intern. Med. 1991; 115: 367–369

313. Klein, R.S., Freeman, K., Taylor, P.E., Stevens, C.E.: Occupational risk for hepatitis C virus infection among New York City dentists. Lancet 1991; 338: 1539–1542

314. Kobayashi, K., Hashimoto, E., Ludwig, J., Hisamitsu, T., Obata, H.: Liver biopsy features of acute hepatitis C compared with hepatitis A, B, and non-A, non-B, non-C. Liver 1993; 13: 69–72

315. Kodama, T., Tamaki, T., Katabami, S., Katamuma, A., Yamashita, K., Azuma, N., Kamijo, K., Kinoshita, H., Yachi, A.: Histological findings in asymptomatic hepatitis C virus carriers. J. Gastroenterol. Hepatol. 1993; 8: 403–405

316. Kong, M.-S., Chung, J.-L.: Fatal hepatitis C in an infant born to a hepatitis C positive mother. J. Pediatr. Gastroenterol. Nutrit. 1994; 19: 460–463

317. König, V., Bauditz, J., Lobeck, H., Lüsebrink, R., Neuhaus, P., Blumhardt, G., Bechstein, W.O., Neuhaus, R., Steffen, R., Hopf, U.: Hepatitis C virus reinfection in allografts after orthotopic liver transplantation. Hepatology 1992; 16: 1137–1143

318. Krause, G., Trepka, M.J., Whisenhunt, R.S., Katz, D., Nainan, O., Wiersma, S.T., Hopkins, R.S.: Nosocomial transmission of hepatitis C virus associated with the use of multidose saline vials. Infect. Contr. Hosp. Epidem. 2003; 24: 122–127

319. Kumar, R.M., Shahul, S.: Role of breast-feeding in transmission of hepatitis C virus to infants of HCV-infected mothers. J. Hepatol. 1998; 29: 191–197

320. Kuo, G., Choo, Q.L., Alter, H.J., Gitnick, G.L., Redeker, A.G., Purcell, R.H., Miyamura, T., Dienstag, J.L., Alter, M.J., Stevens, C.E., Tegtmeier, G.E., Bonino, F., Colombo, M., Lee, W.-S., Kuo, C., Berger, K., Shuster, J.R., Overby, L.R., Bradley, D.W., Houghton, M.: An assay for circulating antibodies to a major etiologic virus of human non-A, non-B hepatitis. Science 1989; 244: 362–364

321. Lacaille, F., Zylberberg, H., Hagège, H., Roualdés, B., Meyrignac, C., Chousterman, M., Girot, R.: Hepatitis C associated with Guillain-Barré syndrome. Liver 1998; 18: 49–51

322. Larglu, A., Zuin, M., Crosignani, A., Ribero, M.L., Pipia, C., Battezzati, P.M., Binelli, G., Donato, F., Zanetti, A.R., Podda, M., Tagger, A.: Outcome of an outbreak of acute hepatitis C among healthy volunteers participating in pharmacokinetic studies. Hepatology 2002; 36: 963–1000

323. Le Pogam, S., Le Chapois, D., Christen, R., Dubois, F., Barin, F., Goudeau, A.: Hepatitis C in a hemodialysis unit: molecular evidence for nosocomial transmission. J. Clin. Microbiol. 1998; 36: 3040–3043

324. Lee, H.-S., Han, C.J., Kim, C.Y.: Predominant etiologic association of hepatitis C virus with hepatocellular carcinoma compared with hepatitis B virus in elderly patients in a hepatitis B-endemic area. Cancer 1993; 72: 2564–2567

325. Lieber, C.S.: Hepatitis C and alcohol. J. Clin. Gastroenterol. 2003; 36: 100–102

326. Liou, T.C., Chang, T.T., Young, K.C., Lin, X.Z., Lin, C.Y., Wu, H.L.: Detection of HCV RNA in saliva, urine, seminal fluid, and ascites. J. Med. Virol. 1992; 37: 197–202

327. Loustaud-Ratti, V., Liozon, E., Karaaslan, H., Alain, S., le Meur, Y., Denis, F., Vidal, E.: Interferon alpha and ribavirin for membranoproliferative glomerulonephritis and hepatitis C infection. Amer. J. Med. 2002; 113: 516–519

328. Macedo, G., Correia, A., Ribeiro, T.: Antiviral treatment in acute hepatitis C. Hepato-Gastroenterol. 2003; 50: 1057–1059

329. Maggi, R., Vatteroni, M.L., Pistello, M., Avio, C.M., Cecconi, N., Panicucci, F., Bendinelli, M.: Serological reactivity and viral genotypes in hepatitis C virus infection. J. Clin. Microbiol. 1995; 33: 209–211

330. Major, M.E., Feinstone, S.M.: The molecular virology of hepatitis C. Hepatology 1997; 25: 1527–1538

331. Manavi, M., Baghestanian, M., Watkins-Riedel, T., Battistutti, W., Pischinger, K., Schatten, C., Witschko, E., Hudelist, G., Hofmann, H., Czerwenka, K.: Detection of hepatitis C virus (HCV) RNA in normal cervical smears of HCV-seropositive patients. Clin. Infect. Dis. 2002; 35: 966–973

332. Mansell, C.J., Locarnini, S.A.: Epidemiology of hepatitis C in the East. Semin. Liver Dis. 1995; 15: 15–32

333. Marzano, A., Smedile, A., Abate, M., Ottobrelli, A., Brunetto, M., Negro, F., Farci, P., Durazzo, M., David, E., Lagget, M., Verme, G., Bonino, F., Rizzetto, M.: Hepatitis type C after orthotopic liver transplantation: reinfection and disease recurrence. J. Hepatol. 1994; 21: 961–965

334. Mazzaro, C., Efremov, D.G., Burrone, O., Pozzato, G.: Hepatitis C virus; mixed cryoglobulinaemia and non-Hodgkin's lymphoma. Ital. J. Gastroenterol. Hepatol. 1998; 30: 428–434

335. Meisel, H., Reip, A., Faltus, B., Lu, M., Porst, H., Wiese, M., Roggendorf, M., Krüger, D.H.: Transmission of hepatitis C virus to children

and husbands by women infected with contaminated anti-D immunoglobulin. Lancet 1995; 345: 1209–1211
336. **Melbye, M., Biggar, R.J., Wantzin, P., Krogsgaard, K., Ebbesen, P., Becker, N.G.:** Sexual transmission of hepatitis C virus: cohort study (1981–9) among European homosexual men. Brit. Med. J. 1990; 301: 210–212
337. **Memon, M.I., Memon, M.A.:** Hepatitis C: An epidemiological review. J. Viral Hepat. 2002; 9: 84–100
338. **Micallef, J.M., Kaldor, J.M., Dore, G.J.:** Spontaneous vival clearance following acute hepatitis C infection: A systematic review of longitudinal studies. J. Vival. Hepat. 2006; 194: 53–60
339. **Misiani, R., Bellavita, P., Fenili, D., Vicari, O., Marchesi, D., Sironi, P.L., Zilio, P., Vernocchi, A., Massazza, M., Vendramin, G., Tanzi, E., Zanetti, A.:** Interferon alfa-2a therapy in cryoglobulinemia associated with hepatitis C virus. New Engl. J. Med. 1994; 330: 751–756
340. **Mitsui, T., Iwano, K., Masuko, K., Yamazaki, C., Okamoto, H., Tsuda, F., Tanaka, T., Mishiro, S.:** Hepatitis C virus infection in medical personnel after needlestick accident. Hepatology 1992; 16: 1109–1114
341. **Müller, H.M., Pfaff, E., Goeser, T., Kallinowski, B., Solbach, C., Theilmann, L.:** Peripher blood leukocytes serve as a possible extrahepatic site for hepatitis C virus replication. J. Gen. Virol. 1993; 74: 669–676
342. **Murphy, A., Dooly, S., Hillary, I.B., Murphy, G.M.:** HCV infection in porphyria cutanea tarda. Lancet 1993; 341: 1534–1535
343. **Nocente, R., Ceccanti, M., Bertazzoni, G., Cammarota, G., Gentiloni-Silveri, N., Gasbarrini, G.:** HCV infection and extrahepatic manifestations. Hepato-Gastroenterol. 2003; 50: 1149–1154
344. **Orland, J.R., Wright, T.L., Cooper, S.:** Acute hepatitis C. Hepatology 2001; 33: 321–327
345. **Palitzsch, K.-D., Hottenträger, B., Schlottmann, K., Frick, E., Holstege, A., Schölmerich, J., Jilg, W.:** Prevalence of antibodies against hepatitis C virus in the adult German population. Eur. J. Gastroenterol. Hepatol. 1999; 11: 1215–1220
346. **Peano, G.M., Fenoglio, L.M., Menardi, G., Balbo, R., Marenchino, D., Fenoglio, S.:** Heterosexual transmission of hepatitis C virus in family groups without risk factors. Brit. Med. J. 1992; 305: 1473–1474
347. **Perez-Calvo, J., Lasierra, P., Moros, M., Inigo, P.:** Role of ribavirin in membranoproliferative glomerulonephritis associated with hepatitis C virus infection refractory to alpha-interferon. Nephron 2002; 92: 459–462
348. **Pilli, M., Penna, A., Zerbini, A., Vescovi, P., Manfredi, M., Negro, F., Carrozzo, M., Mori, C., Giuberti, T., Ferrari, C., Missale, G.:** Oral lichen planus pathogenesis: A role for the HCV-specific cellular immune response. Hepatology 2002; 36: 1446–1452
349. **Puoti, C., Guido, M., Mangia, A., Persico, M., Prati, D.:** Clinical management of HCV carriers with normal aminotransferase levels. Dig. Liv. Dis. 2003; 35: 362–369
350. **Quint, L., Deny, P., Guillevin, L., Granger, B., Jarrousse, B., Lhote, F., Scavizzi, M.:** Hepatitis C virus in patients with polyarteritis nodosa. Prevalence in 38 patients. Clin. Experim. Rheumatol. 1991; 9: 253–257
351. **Resti, M., Azzari, C., Lega, L., Rossi, M.E., Zammarchi, E., Novembre, E., Vierucci, A.:** Mother-to-infant transmission of hepatitis C virus. Acta Paediatr. 1995; 84: 251–255
352. **Resti, M., Jara, P., Hierro, L., Azzari, C., Giacchino, R., Zuin, G., Zancan, L., Pedditzi, S., Bortolotti, F.:** Clinical features and progression of perinatally acquired hepatitis C virus infection. J. Med. Virol. 2003; 70: 373–377
353. **Rey, J.-F., Halfon, P., Feryn, J.-M., Khiri, H., Masseyeff, M.-F., Ouzan, D.:** Risque de transmission du virus de l'hepatite C par l'endoscopie digestive. Gastroenterol. Clin. Biol. 1995; 19: 346–349
354. **Rice, P.S., Smith, D.B., Simmonds, P., Holmes, E.:** Heterosexual transmission of hepatitis C virus. Lancet 1993; 342: 1052–1053
355. **Rocca, P., Bailly, F., Chevallier, M., Chevallier, P., Zoulim, F., Trepo, C.:** Early treatment of acute hepatitis C with interferon alpha-2b or interferon alpha-2b plus ribavirin: study of sixteen patients. Gastroenterol. Clin. Biol. 2003; 27: 294–299
356. **Rollino, C., Roccatello, D., Giachino, O., Basolo, B., Piccoli, G.:** Hepatitis C virus infection and membraneous glomerulonephritis. Nephron 1991; 59: 319–320
357. **Ross, R.S., Viazov, S., Thormahlen, M., Bartz, L., Tamm, J., Rautenberg, P., Roggendorf, M., Deisler, A.:** Risk of hepatitis C virus transmission from an infected gynecologist to patients. Results of a 7-year retrospective investigation. Arch. Intern. Med. 2002; 162: 805–810
358. **Saito, I., Miyamura, T., Ohbayashi, A., Harada, H., Katayama, T., Kikuchi, S., Watanabe, Y., Koi, S., Onji, M., Ohta, Y., Choo, Q.L., Houghton, M., Kuo, G.:** Hepatitis C virus infection is associated with the development of hepatocellular carcinoma. Proc. Nat. Acad. Sci. USA 1990; 87: 6547–6549
359. **Santantonio, T., Sinisi, E., Guastadisegni, A., Casalino, C., Mazzola, M., Gentile, A., Leandro, G., Pastore, G.:** Natural course of acute hepatitis C: A long-term prospective study. Dig. Liv. Dis. 2003; 35: 104–113
360. **Savey, A., Simon, F., Izopet, J., Lepoutre, A., Fabry, J., Desenclos, J.C.:** A large nosocomial outbreak of hepatitis C virus infections at a hemodialysis center. Infect. Contr. Hosp. Epidem. 2005; 26: 752–760
361. **Schlipkoter, U., Roggendorf, M., Cholmakow, K., Weise, A., Deinhardt, F.:** Transmission of hepatitis C virus (HCV) from a haemodialysis patient to a medical staff member. Scand. J. Infect. Dis. 1990; 22: 757–758
362. **Seeff, L.B., Miller, R.N., Rabkin, C.S., Buskell-Bales, Z., Straley-Eason, K.D., Smoak, B.L., Johnson, L.D., Lee, S.R., Kaplan, E.L.:** 45-year follow-up of hepatitis C virus infection in healthy young adults. Ann. Intern. Med. 2000; 132: 105–111
363. **Shiffman, M.L., Contos, M.J., Luketic, V.A., Sanyal, A.S., Purdum III, P.P., Mills, A.S., Fisher, R.A., Posner, M.P.:** Biochemical and histologic evaluation of recurrent hepatitis C following orthotopic liver transplantation. Transplantation 1994; 57: 526–532
364. **Silini, E., Bono, F., Cividini, A., Cerino, A., Maccabruni, A., Tinelli, C., Bruno, S., Bellobuono, A., Mondelli, M.U.:** Molecular epidemiology of hepatitis C virus infection among intravenous drug users. J. Hepatol. 1995; 22: 691–695
365. **Stanley, A.J., Haydon, G.H., Piris, J., Jarvis, L.M., Hayes, P.C.:** Assessment of liver histology in patients with hepatitis C and normal transaminase levels. Eur. J. Gastroenterol. Hepatol. 1996; 8: 869–872
366. **Steininger, C., Kundi, M., Jatzko, G., Kiss, H., Lischka, A., Holzmann, H.:** Increased risk of mother-to-infant transmission of hepatitis C virus by intrapartum infantile exposure to maternal blood. J. Infect. Dis. 2003; 187: 345–351
367. **Stevens, C.E., Taylor, P.E., Pindyck, J., Choo, Q.-L., Bradley, D.W., Kuo, G., Houghton, M.:** Epidemiology of hepatitis C virus. A preliminary study in volunteer blood donors. J. Amer. Med. Ass. 1990; 263: 49–53
368. **Stölzel, U., Köstler, E., Koszka, C., Stöffler-Meilicke, M., Schuppan, D., Somasundaram, R., Doss, M.O., Habermehl, K.O., Riecken, E.O.:** Low prevalence of hepatitis C virus infection in porphyria cutanea tarda in Germany. Hepatology 1995; 21: 1500–1503
369. **Sulkowski, M.S., Ray, S.C., Thomas, D.L.:** Needlestick transmission of hepatitis C. J. Amer. Med. Ass. 2002; 287: 2406–2413
370. **Takada, N., Takase, S., Takada, A., Date, T.:** Differences in the hepatitis C virus genotypes in different countries. J. Hepatol. 1993; 17: 277–283
371. **Tallis, G.F., Ryan, G.M., Lambert, S.B., Bowden, D.S., McCaw, R., Birch, C.J., Moloney, M., Carnie, J.A., Locarnini, S.A., Rouch, G.J., Catton, M.G.:** Evidence of patient-to-patient transmission of hepatitis C virus through contaminated intravenous anaesthetic ampoules. J. Viral Hepat. 2003; 10: 234–239
372. **Theilmann, L., Solbach, C., Toex, U., Müller, H.M., Pfaff, E., Otto, G., Goeser, T.:** Role of hepatitis C virus in German patients with fulminant and subfulminant hepatic failure. Eur. J. Clin. Invest. 1992; 22: 569–571
373. **Thimme, R., Oldach, D., Chang, K.-M., Steiger, C., Ray, S.C., Chisari, F.V.:** Determinants of viral clearance and persistence during acute hepatitis C virus infection. J. Exper. Med. 2001; 194: 1395–1406
374. **Thomas, D.L., Zenilman, J.M., Alter, H.J., Shih, J.W., Galai, N., Carella, A.V., Quinn, T.C.:** Sexual transmission of hepatitis C virus among patients attending Sexually Transmitted Diseases Clinics in Baltimore. An analysis of 309 sex partnerships. J. Infect. Dis. 1995; 171: 768–775
375. **Thorburn, D., Roy, K., Cameron, S.O., Johnston, J., Hutchinson, S., McCruden, E.A.B., Mills, P.R., Goldberg, D.J.:** Risk of hepatitis C virus transmission from patients to surgeons: Model based on an unlinked anonymous study of hepatitis C virus prevalence in hospital patients in Glasgow. Gut 2003; 52: 1333–1338
376. **Tong, M.J., El-Farra, N.S., Reikes, A.R., Co, R.L.:** Clinical outcomes after transfusion-associated hepatitis C. New Engl. J. Med. 1995; 332: 1463–1466
377. **Tumminelli, F., Marcellin, P., Rizzo, S., Barbera, S., Corvino, G., Furta, P., Benhamou, J.-P., Erlinger, S.:** Shaving as potential source of hepatitis C virus infection. Lancet 1995; 345: 658.
378. **Utsumi, T., Hashimoto, E., Okumura, Y., Takayanagi, M., Nishikawa, H., Kigawa, M., Kumakura, N., Toyokawa, H.:** Heterosexual activity as a risk factor for the transmission of hepatitis C virus. J. Med. Virol. 1995; 46: 122–125
379. **Vaglia, A., Nicolin, R., Puro, V., Ippolito, G., Bettini, C., de Lalla, F.:** Needlestick hepatitis C virus seroconversion in a surgeon. Lancet 1990; 336: 1315–1316
380. **Venezia, G., Licata, A., di Marco, V., Craxi, A., Almasio, P.L.:** Acute polymyositis during treatment of acute hepatitis C with pegylated interferon alpha-2b. Dig. Liver Dis. 2005; 37: 882–885
381. **Weinstein, J.S., Poterucha, J.J., Zein, N., Wiesner, R.H., Persing, D.H., Rakela, J.:** Epidemiology and natural history of hepatitis C infections in liver transplant recipients. J. Hepatol. 1995; 22 (Suppl. 1): 154–159
382. **Wilson, S.E., Lee, W.M., Murakami, C., Weng, J., Moninger, G.A.:** Mooren's corneal ulcers and hepatitis C virus infection. New Engl. J. Med. 1993; 329: 62.
383. **Wright, T.L., Donegan, E., Hsu, H.H., Ferrell, L., Lake, J.R., Kim, M., Combs, C., Fennessy, S., Roberts, J.P., Ascher, N.L., Greenberg, H.B.:** Recurrent and acquired hepatitis C viral infection in liver transplant recipients. Gastroenterology 1992; 103: 317–322
384. **Yoffe, B., Bagri, A.S., Tran, T., Dural, E.R., Shtenberg, K.M., Khaoustov, V.I.:** Hyperlipasemia associated with hepatitis C virus. Dig. Liv. Sci. 2003; 48: 1648–1653
385. **Zanetti, A.R., Tanzi, E., Romano, L., Zuin, G., Minola, E., Vecchi, L., Principi, N.:** A prospective study on mother-to-infant transmission of hepatitis C virus. Intervirology 1998; 41: 208–212
386. **Zuckerman, J., Clewley, G., Griffiths, P., Cockcroft, A.:** Prevalence of hepatitis C antibodies in clinical health-care workers. Lancet 1994; 343: 1618–1620

Acute viral hepatitis D
387. **Amarapurkar, D.N., Vishwanath, N., Kumar, A., Shankaran, S., Murti, P., Kalro, R.H., Desai, H.G.:** Prevalence of delta virus infection in high

risk population and hepatitis B virus related liver diseases. Ind. J. Gastroenterol. 1992; 11: 11–12
388. **Battegay, M., Simpson, L.H., Hoofnagle, J.H., Sallie, R., Di Bisceglie, A.M.:** Elimination of hepatitis delta virus infection after loss of hepatitis B surface antigen in patients with chronic delta hepatitis. J. Med. Virol. 1994; 44: 389–392
389. **Bichko, V., Netter, H.J., Wu, T.-T., Taylor, J.:** Pathogenesis associated with replication of hepatitis delta virus. Infect. Agents Dis. 1994; 3: 94–97
390. **Bordier, B.B., Marion, P.L., Ohashi, K., Kay, M.A., Greenberg, H.B., Casey, J.L., Glenn, J.S.:** A prenylation inhibitor prevents production of infectious hepatitis delta virus particles. J. Virol. 2002; 76: 10465–10472
391. **Buitrago, B., Popper, H., Hadler, S.C., Thung, S.N., Gerber, M.A., Purcell, R.H., Maynard, J.E.:** Specific histologic features of Santa Marta hepatitis: a severe form of hepatitis δ-virus infection in Northern South America. Hepatology 1986; 6: 1285–1291
392. **Caredda, F., Rossi, E., D'Arminio Monforte, A.:** An outbreak of delta agent among a group of drug addicts and their close contacts. J. Infect. Dis. 1984; 149: 286–287
393. **Carreno, V., Bartolome, J., Madejon, A.:** Hepatitis delta virus infection: molecular biology and treatment. Dig. Dis. 1994; 12: 265–275
394. **Colombo, P., Di Blasi, F., Magrin, S., Fabiano, C., Di Marco, V., D'Amelio, L., Lojacono, F., Spinelli, G., Craxi, A.:** Smouldering hepatitis B virus replication in patients with chronic liver disease and hepatitis delta virus superinfection. J. Hepatol. 1991; 12: 64–69
395. **Craxi, A., TinŁ, F., Vinci, M., Almasio, P., Camma, C., Garofalo, G., Pagliaro, L.:** Transmission of hepatitis B and hepatitis delta viruses in the households of chronic hepatitis B surface antigen carriers: a regression analysis of indicators of risk. Amer. J. Epidem. 1991; 134: 641–650
396. **Davies, S.E., Lau, J.Y.N., O'Grady, J.G., Portmann, B.C., Alexander, G.J.M., Williams, R.:** Evidence that hepatitis D virus needs hepatitis B virus to cause hepatocellular damage. Amer. J. Clin. Path. 1992; 98: 554–558
397. **Desai, P., Banker, D.D.:** Hepatitis B and delta viruses in fulminant hepatitis. Ind. J. Gastroenterol. 1990; 9: 209–210
398. **Erhardt, A., Knuth, R., Sagir, A., Kirschberg, O., Heintges, T., Häussinger, D.:** Socioepidemiological data on hepatitis delta in a German University Clinic-increase in patients from Eastern Europe and the Former Soviet Union. Zschr. Gastroenterol. 2003; 41: 523–526
399. **Farci, P.:** Delta hepatitis: an update. J. Hepatol. 2003; 39 (S): 212–219
400. **Foster, G.R., Carman, W.F., Thomas, H.C.:** Replication of hepatitis B and delta viruses: appearance of viral mutants. Semin. Liver Dis. 1991; 11: 121–127
401. **Govindarajan, S., De Cok, K.M., Redeker, A.G.:** Natural course of delta superinfection in chronic hepatitis B virus-infected patients: histopathological study with multiple liver biopsies. Hepatology 1986; 6: 640–644
402. **Gupta, S., Govindarajan, S., Cassidy, W.M., Valinluck, B., Redeker, A.G.:** Acute delta hepatitis: serological diagnosis with particular reference to hepatitis delta virus RNA. Amer. J. Gastroenterol. 1991; 86: 1227–1231
403. **Hadler, S.C., De Monzon, M., Ponzetto, A., Anzola, E., Rivero, D., Mondolfi, A., Bracho, A., Francis, D.P., Gerber, M.A., Thung, S., Gerin, J., Maynard, J.E., Popper, H., Purcell, R.H.:** Delta virus infection and severe hepatitis. An epidemic in the Yucpa Indians of Venezuela. Ann. Intern. Med. 1984; 100: 339–444
404. **Hsu, S.C., Syu, W.J., Sheen, I.J., Liu, H.T., Jeng, K.S., Wu, J.C.:** Varied assembly and RNA editing efficiencies between genotypes I and II hepatitis D virus and their implications. Hepatology 2002; 35: 665–672
405. **Jardi, R., Buti, M., Cotrina, M., Rodriguez, F., Allende, H., Esteban, R., Guardia, J.:** Determination of hepatitis delta virus RNA by polymerase chain reaction in acute and chronic delta infection. Hepatology 1995; 21: 25–29
406. **Lai, M.M.C., Lee, C.-M., Bih, F.-Y., Govindarajan, S.:** The molecular basis of heterogeneity of hepatitis delta virus. J. Hepatol. 1991; 13 (Suppl. 4): 121–124
407. **Lettau, L.A., McCarthy, J.G., Smith, M.H., Hadler, St.C., Morse, L.J., Ukena, T., Bessette, R., Gurwitz, A., Irvine, W.G., Fields, H.A., Grady, G.F., Maynard, J.E.:** Outbreak of severe hepatitis due to delta and hepatitis B viruses in parenteral drug abusers and their contacts. New Engl. J. Med. 1987; 317: 1256–1262
408. **Liaw, Y.-F., Chen, T.-J., Chu, C.-M., Lin, H.-H.:** Acute hepatitis delta virus superinfection in patients with liver cirrhosis. J. Hepatol. 1990; 10: 41–45
409. **Lucey, M.R., Graham, D.M., Martin, P., Di Bisceglie, A., Rosenthal, S., Waggoner, J.G., Merion, R.M., Campbell, D.A., Nostrant, T.T., Appelman, H.D.:** Recurrence of hepatitis B and delta hepatitis after orthotopic liver transplantation. Gut 1992; 33: 1390–1396
410. **Manesis, E., Zoumboulis, P., Georgiou, S., Vardaka, J., Hadziyannis, St.:** Splenomegaly in asymptomatic chronic carriers of hepatitis B and D viruses. Eur. J. Gastroenterol. Hepatol. 1994; 6: 793–796
411. **Mas, A., Buti, M., Esteban, R., Sanchez-Tapias, J.M., Costa, J., Jardi, R., Bruguera, M., Guardia, J., Rodes, J.:** Hepatitis B virus and hepatitis D virus replication in HBsAg-positive fulminant hepatitis. Hepatology 1990; 11: 1062–1065
412. **Mendez, L., Reddy, K.R., Di Prima, R.A., Jeffers, L.J., Schiff, E.R.:** Fulminant hepatic failure due to acute hepatitis B and delta co-infection: probable bloodborne transmission associated with a spring-loaded fingerstick device. Amer. J. Gastroenterol. 1991; 86: 895–897
413. **Moraleda, G., Bartolome, J., Martinez, M.G., Porres, J.C., Carreno, V.:** Influence of hepatitis delta virus replication in the presence of hepatitis B virus DNA in peripheral blood mononuclear cells. Hepatology 1990; 12: 1290–1294
414. **Negro, F., Rizzetto, M.:** Pathobiology of hepatitis delta virus. J. Hepatol. 1993; 17 (Suppl. 3) 149–153
415. **Ottobrelli, A., Marzano, A., Smedile, A., Recchia, S., Salizzoni, M., Cornu, C., Lamy, M.E., Otte, J.B., De Hemptinne, B., Geubel, A., Grendele, M., Colledan, M., Galmarini, D., Marinucci, G., Di Giacomo, C., Agnes, S., Bonino, F., Rizzetto, M.:** Patterns of hepatitis delta virus reinfection and disease in liver transplantation. Gastroenterology 1991; 101: 1649–1655
416. **Pastore, G., Monno, L., Santantonio, T., Angavano, G., Milella, M., Giannelli, A., Fiore, J.R.:** Hepatitis B virus clearance from serum and liver after acute hepatitis delta superinfection in chronic HBsAg carriers. J. Med. Virol. 1990; 31: 284–290
417. **Polish, L.B., Gallagher, M., Fields, H.A., Hadler, St.C.:** Delta hepatitis: molecular biology and clinical and epidemiological features. Clin. Microbiol. Rev. 1993; 6: 211–229
418. **Rizzetto, M.:** Hepatitis delta: the virus and the disease. J. Hepatol. 1990; 11: 145–148
419. **Rizzetto, M., Hadziyannis, S., Hansson, B.G., Toukan, A., Gust, I.:** Hepatitis delta virus infection in the world: epidemiological patterns and clinical expression. Gastroenterol. Internat. 1992; 5: 18–32
420. **Rosenblum, L., Darrow, W., Witte, J., Cohen, J., French, J., Gill, P.S., Potterat, J., Sikes, K., Reich, R., Hadler, S.:** Sexual practices in the transmission of hepatitis B virus and prevalence of hepatitis Delta virus infection in female prostitutes in the United States. J. Amer. Med. Assoc. 1992; 267: 2477–2481
421. **Rosina, F., Saracco, G., Rizzetto, M.:** Risk of transfusion infection with the hepatitis Delta virus. A multicenter study. New Engl. J. Med. 1985; 312: 1488–1491
422. **Salassa, B., Daziano, E., Bonino, F., Lavarini, C., Smedile, A., Chiaberge, E., Rosina, F., Brunetto, M.R., Pessione, E., Spezia, C., Bramato, C., Soranzo, M.L.:** Serological diagnosis of hepatitis B and delta virus (HBV/HDV) coinfection. J. Hepatol. 1991; 12: 10–13
423. **Stroffolini, T., Ferrigno, L., Cialdea, L., Catapano, R., Palumbo, F., Novaco, F., Moiraghi, A., Galanti, C., Bernacchia, R., Mele, A.:** Incidence and risk factors of acute Delta hepatitis in Italy: results from a national surveillance system. J. Hepatol. 1994; 21: 1123–1126
424. **Tibbs, C.J.:** Delta hepatitis in Kiribati: a pacific focus. J. Med. Virol. 1989; 29: 130–132
425. **Verme, G., Brunetto, M.R., Oliveri, F., Baldi, M., Forzani, B., Piantino, P., Ponzetto, A., Bonino, F.:** Role of hepatitis delta virus infection in hepatocellular carcinoma. Dig. Dis. Sci. 1991; 36: 1134–1136
426. **Wang, T.C., Chao, M.:** Molecular cloning and expression of the hepatitis delta virus genotype II b genome. Biochem. Biophys. Res. Comm. 2003; 303: 357–363
427. **Weisfuse, I.B., Hadler, S.C., Fields, H.A., Alter, M.J., O'Malley, P.M., Judson, F.N., Ostrow, D.G., Altmann, N.L.:** Delta hepatitis in homosexual men in the United States. Hepatology 1989; 9: 872–874
428. **Wu, J.-C., Lee, S.-D., Govindarajan, S., Lin, H.-C., Chou, P., Wang, Y.-J., Lee, S.-Y., Tsai, Y.-T., Lo, K.-J., Ting, L.-P.:** Sexual transmission of hepatitis D virus infection in Taiwan. Hepatology 1990; 11: 1057–1061
429. **Wu, J.-C., Chen, T.-Z., Huang, Y.-S., Yen, F.-S., Ting, L.-T., Sheng, W.-Y., Tsay, S.-H., Lee, S.-D.:** Natural history of hepatitis D viral superinfection: significance of viremia detected by polymerase chain reaction. Gastroenterology 1995; 108: 796–802

Acute viral hepatitis E
430. **Aggarwal, R., Naik, S.R.:** Hepatitis E: intrafamilial transmission versus waterborne spread. J. Hepatol. 1994; 21: 718–723
431. **Aggarwal, R., Krawczynski, K.:** Hepatitis E: an overview and recent advances in clinical and laboratory research. J. Gastroenterol. Hepatol. 2000; 15: 9 - 20
432. **Al-Azmeh, M., Frösner, G., Darwish, Z., Bashour, H., Monem, F.:** Hepatitis E in Damascus, Syria. Infection 1999; 27: 221–223
433. **Arankalle, V.A., Chadha, M.S., Mehendale, S.M., Banerjee, K:** Outbreak of enterically transmitted non-A, non-B hepatitis among schoolchildren. Lancet 1988; II: 1199–1200
434. **Arora, N.K., Panda, S.K., Nanda, S.K., Ansari, I.H., Joshi, S., Dixit, R., Bathia, R.:** Hepatitis E infection in children: study of an outbreak. J. Gastroenterol. Hepatol. 1999; 14: 572–577
435. **Balayan, M.S.:** Hepatitis E virus infection in Europe: regional situation regarding laboratory diagnosis and epidemiology. Clin. Diagn. Virol. 1993; 1: 1–9
436. **Boccia, D., Guthmann, J.P., Klovstad, H., Hamid, N., Tatay, M., Ciglenecki, I., Nizou, J.Y., Nicaud, E., Guerin, P.J.:** High mortality associated with an outbreak of hepatitis E among displaced persons in Darfur, Sudan. Clin. Infect. Dis. 2006; 42: 1679–1684
437. **Bradley, D.W.:** Hepatitis E virus: a brief review of the biology, molecular virology, and immunology of a novel virus. J. Hepatol. 1995; 22 (Suppl. 1): 140–145
438. **Chau, T.N., Lai, S.T., Tse, C., Ng, T.K., Leung, V.K.S., Lim, W., Ng, M.H.:** Epidemiology and clinical features of sporadic hepatitis E as compared with hepatitis A. Amer. J. Gastroenterol. 2006; 101: 292–296

439. Chauhan, A., Jameel, S., Dilawari, J.B., Chawla, Y.K., Kaur, U., Ganguly, N.K.: Hepatitis E virus transmission to a volunteer. Lancet 1993; 341: 149–150
440. Chow, W.C., Lee, A.S:G., Lim, G.K., Cheong, W.K., Chong, R., Tan, C.K., Yap, C.K., Oon, C.J., Ng, H.S.: Acute viral hepatitis E: clinical and serologic studies in Singapore. J. Clin. Gastroenterol. 1997; 24: 235–238
441. Clayson, E.T., Myint, K.S.A., Snitbhan, R., Vaughn, D.W., Innis, B.L., Chan. L., Cheung, P., Shrestha, M.P.: Viremia, fecal shedding, and IgM and IgG responses in patients with hepatitis E. J. Infect. Dis. 1995; 172: 927–933
442. De Cock, K.M., Bradley, D.W., Sandford, N.G., Govindarajan, S., Maynard, J.E., Redeker, A.G.: Epidemic non-A, non-B hepatitis in patients from Pakistan. Ann. Intern. Med. 1987; 106: 227–230
443. Derong, L., Rutong, H., Xing, T., Shurong, Y., Jun, W., Xiangrui, H., Baozhen, W., Ruixia, L., Yuchuan, L.: Morphology and morphogenesis of hepatitis E virus (strain 87 A). Chin. Med. J. 1995; 108: 126–131
444. El-Zimaity, D.M.T., Hyams, K.C., Imam, Z.E.T., Watts, D. M., Bassily, S., Naffea, E.K., Sultan, E., Emaru, K., Burans, J., Purdy, M.A., Bradley, D.W., Carl, M.: Acute sporadic hepatitis E in an Egyptian pediatric population. Amer. J. Trop. Med. Hyg. 1993; 48: 372–376
445. Favoro, M.O., Kosoy, M.Y., Tsarev, S.A., Childs, J.E., Margolis, H.S.: Prevalence of antibody to hepatitis E virus among rodents in the United States. J. Infect. Dis. 2000; 181: 449–455
446. Grabow, W.O.K., Favorov, M.O., Khudyakova, N.S., Taylor, M.B., Fields, H.A.: Hepatitis E seroprevalence in selected individuals in South Africa. J. Med. Virol. 1994; 44: 384–388
447. Hofmann, H., Holzmann, H.: Investigations regarding the occurrence of hepatitis E in Austria. Wien. Klin. Wschr. 1995; 107: 336–339
448. Irshad, M.: Hepatitis E virus: an update on its molecular, clinical and epidemiological characteristics. Intervirology 1999; 42: 252–262
449. Jardi, R., Buti, M., Rodriguez-Frias, F., Esteban, R.: Hepatitis E infection in acute sporadic hepatitis in Spain. Lancet 1993; 341: 1355–1356
450. Kane, M.A., Bradley, D.W., Shrestha, S.M., Maynard, J.E., Cook, E.H., Mishra, R.P., Joshi, D.D.: Epidemic non-A, non-B hepatitis in Nepal. J. Amer. Med. Assoc. 1984; 25: 3140–3145
451. Karetnyi, Y.V., Favorov, M.O., Khudyakova, N.S., Weiss, P., Bar-Shani, S., Handsher, R., Aboudy, Y., Varsono, N., Schwartz, E., Levin, E., Mendelson, E., Fields, H.A.: Serological evidence for hepatitis E virus infection in Israel. J. Med. Virol. 1995; 45: 316–320
452. Khuroo, M.S.: Study of an epidemic of non-A, non-B hepatitis. Possibility of another human hepatitis virus distinct from post-transfusion non-A, non-B type. Amer. J. Med. 1980; 68: 818–824
453. Khuroo, M.S., Kamili, S.: Aetiology, clinical course and outcome of sporadic acute viral hepatitis E in pregnancy. J. Viral Hepat. 2003; 10: 61–69
454. Lau, J.Y.N., Sallie, R., Fang, J.W.S., Yarbough, P.O., Reyes, G.R., Portmann, B.C., Mieli-Vergani, G., Williams, R.: Detection of hepatitis E virus genome and gene products in two patients with fulminant hepatitis E. J. Hepatol. 1995; 22: 605–610
455. Lavanchy, D.: Seroprevalence of hepatitis E virus in Switzerland. Lancet 1994; 344: 747–748
456. Lee, S-D., Wang, Y.-J., Lu, R.-H., Chan, C.-Y., Lo, K.-J., Moeckli, R.: Seroprevalence of antibody to hepatitis E virus among Chinese subjects in Taiwan. Hepatology 1994; 19: 866–870
457. Meng, X.J., Purcell, R.H., Halbur, P.G., Lehman, J.K., Webb, D.M., Tsareva, T.S., Haynes, J.S., Thacker, B.J., Emerson, S.U.: A novel virus in swine is closely related to the human hepatitis E virus. Proc. Natl. Acad. Sci. 1997; 94: 9860–9865
458. Moaven. L., van Asten, M., Crofts, N., Locarnini, St.A.: Seroepidemiology of hepatitis E in selected Australian populations. J. Med. Virol. 1995; 45: 326–330
459. Mushahwar, I.K., Dawson, G.J., Bile, K.M., Magnius, L.O.: Serological studies of an enterically transmitted non-A, non-B hepatitis in Somalia. J. Med. Virol. 1993; 40: 218–221
460. Nanda, S.K., Yalcinkaya, K., Panigrahi, A.K., Acharya, S.K., Jameel, S., Panda, S.K.: Etiological role of hepatitis E virus in sporadic fulminant hepatitis. J. Med. Virol. 1994; 42: 133–137
461. Nanda, S.K., Ansari, I.H., Acharya, S.K., Jameel, S., Panda, S.K.: Protracted viremia during acute sporadic hepatitis E virus infection. Gastroenterology 1995; 108: 225–230
462. Pujol, F.H., Favorov, M.O., Marcano, T., Este, J.A., Magris, M., Liprandi, F., Khudyakov, Y.E., Khudyakov, N.S., Fields, H.A.: Prevalence of antibodies against hepatitis E virus among urban and rural populations in Venezuela. J. Med. Virol. 1994; 42: 234–236
463. Ramalingaswami, V., Purcell, R.H.: Waterborne non-A, non-B hepatitis. Lancet 1988/II: 571–573
464. Ray, R., Aggarwal, R., Salunke, P.N., Mehrotra, N.N., Talwar, G.P., Naik, S.R.: Hepatitis E virus genome in stools of hepatitis patients during large epidemic in north India. Lancet 1991; 338: 783–784
465. Reyes, G.R., Purdy, M.A., Kim, J.P., Luk, K.-C., Young, L.M., Fry, K.E., Bradley, D.W.: Isolation of a cDNA from the virus reponsible for enterically transmitted non-A, non-B hepatitis. Science 1990; 247: 1335–1339
466. Schlauder, G.G., Mushahwar, I.K.: Genetic heterogeneity of hepatitis E virus. J. Med. Virol. 2001; 65: 282–292
467. Schwartz, E., Jenks, N.P., van Damme, P., Galun, E.: Hepatitis E virus infection in travellers. Clin. Inf. Dis. 1999; 29: 1312–1314
468. Shresta, M.P., Scott, R.M., Joshi, D.M., Mammen, M.P., Thapa, N., Myint, K.S.A., Fourneau, M., Kuschner, R.A., Shresta, S.K., David, M.P., Seriwatana, J., Vaughn, D.W., Safary, A., Endy, T.P., Innis, B.L.: Safety and efficacy of a recombinant hepatitis E vaccine. New Engl. J. Med. 2007; 356: 895–903
469. Skidmore, S.J., Yarbough, P.O., Gabor, K.A., Reyes, G.R.: Hepatitis E virus (HEV): the cause of a waterborne hepatitis outbreak. J. Med. Virol. 1992; 37: 58–60
470. Suzuki, K., Aikawa, T., Okamoto, H.: Fulminant Hepatitis E in Japan. New Engl. J. Med. 2002; 347: 1456.
471. Tandon, B.N., Joshi, Y.K., Jain, S.K., Gandhi, B.M., Mathiesen, L.R., Tandon, H.D.: An epidemic of non-A, non-B hepatitis in north India. Indian J. Med. Res. 1982; 75: 739–744
472. Tassopoulos, N.C., Krawczynski, K., Hatzakis, A., Katsoulidou, A., Delladepsima, I., Koutelou, M.G., Trichopoulos, D.: Role of hepatitis E virus in the etiology of community-acquired non-A, non-B hepatitis in Greece. J. Med. Virol. 1994; 42: 124–128
473. Thomas, D.L., Mahley, R.W., Badur, S., Palaoglu, K.E., Quinn, T.C.: Epidemiology of hepatitis E virus infection in Turkey. Lancet 1993; 341: 1561–1562
474. Ticehurst, J., Popkin, T.-J., Bryan, J.P., Innis, B.L., Duncan, J.F., Ahmed, A., Iübal, M., Malik, I., Kapikian, A.Z., Legters, L.J., Purcell, R.H.: Association of hepatitis E virus with an outbreak of hepatitis in Pakistan: serological responses and pattern of virus excretion. J. Med. Virol. 1992; 36: 84–92
475. Tsega, E., Krawczynski, K., Hansson, B.G., Nordenfelt, E., Negusse, Y., Alemu, W., Bahru, Y.: Outbreak of acute hepatitis E virus infection among military personel in northern Ethiopia. J. Med. Virol. 1991; 34: 232–236
476. Vandenvelde, C.: Hepatitis E virus infection in Belgian soldiers. Lancet 1994; 344: 747.
477. Velazquez, O., Stetler, H.C., Avila, C., Ornelas, G., Alvarez, C., Hadler, St. C., Bradley, D.W., Sepulveda, J.: Epidemic transmission of enterically transmitted non-A, non-B hepatitis in Mexico, 1986–1987. J. Amer. Med. Assoc. 1990; 263: 3281–3285
478. Viswanathan, R.: Infectious hepatitis in Delhi (1955–56): a critical study: epidemiology. Indian J. Med. Res.1957; 45 (Suppl.): 1–30
479. Wong, D.C., Purcell, R.H., Sreenivasan, M.A., Prasad, S.R., Pavri, K.M.: Epidemic and endemic hepatitis in India, evidence for a non-A, non-B hepatitis virus aetiology. Lancet 1980/II: 876–879
480. Zaaijer, H.L., Mauser-Bunschoten, E.P., ten Veen, J.H., Kapprell, H.P., Kok, M., von den Berg, M., Lelie, P.N.: Hepatitis E virus antibodies among patients with hemophilia, blood donors, and hepatitis patients. J. Med. Virol. 1995; 46: 244–246
481. Zanetti, A.R., Dawson, G.J.: Hepatitis type E in Italy: seroepidemiological survey. J. Med. Virol. 1994; 42: 318–320
482. Zhang, F., Li, X., Li, Z., Harrison, T.J., Chong, H., Qiao, S., Huang, W., Zhang, H., Zhuang, H., Wang, Y.: Detection of HEV antigen as a novel marker for the diagnosis of hepatitis E. J. Med. Vivol. 2006; 78: 1441–1448

Acute viral hepatitis NA-NE

483. Arankalle, V.A., Chadha, M.S., Tsarev. S.A., Emerson, S.U., Risbud, A.R., Banerjee, K., Purcell, R.H.: Seroepidemiology of water-borne hepatitis in India und evidence for a third enterically-transmitted hepatitis agent. Proc. Nat. Acad. Sci. (USA) 1994; 91: 3428–3432
484. Chu, C.M., Lin, D.Y., Yeh, C.T., Sheen, I.S., Liaw, Y.F.: Epidemiological characteristics, risk factors, and clinical manifestations of acute non-A-E hepatitis. J. Med. Virol. 2001; 65: 296–300
485. Rochling, F.A., Jones, W.F., Chau, K., DuCharme, L., Mimms, L.T., Moore, M., Scheffel, J., Cuthbert, J.A., Thiele, D.L.: Acute sporadic Non-A, Non-B, Non-C, Non-D, Non-E hepatitis. Hepatology 1997, 25: 478–483

F virus

486. Deka, N., Sharma, M.D., Mukerjee, R.: Isolation of the novel agent from human stool samples that is associated with sporadic non-A, non-B hepatitis. J. Virol. 1994; 68: 7810–7815

HG virus

487. Alter, M.J., Gallagher, M., Morris, T.T., Moyer, L.A., Meeks, E.L., Krawczynski, K., Kim, J.P., Margolis, H.S.: Acute non-A-E-hepatitis in the United States and the role of hepatitis G virus infection. New Engl. J. Med. 1997; 336: 741–746
488. Colombatto, P., Randone, A., Civitico, G., Monti Gorin, J., Dolci, L., Medaina, N., Oliveri, F., Verme, G., Marchiaro, G., Pagni, R., Karayiannis, P., Thomas, H.C., Hess, G., Bonino, F., Brunetto, M.R.: Hepatitis G virus RNA in the serum of patients with elevated gamma glutamyl transpeptidase and alkaline phosphatase: a specific liver disease. J. Viral Hepat. 1996; 3: 301–306
489. Feucht, H.H., Zollner, B., Polywka, S., Knodler, B., Schroter, M., Nolte, H., Laufs, R.: Prevalence of hepatitis G-viremia among healthy subjects, individuals with liver disease and persons at risk for parenteral transmission. J. Clin. Microbiol. 1997; 35: 767–768
490. Frey, S.E., Homan, S.M., Sokol-Anderson, M., Cayco, M.T., Cortorreal, P., Musial, C.E., di Bisceglie, A.: Evidence for probable sexual transmission of the hepatitis G virus. Clin. Infect. Dis. 2002; 34: 1033–1038
491. Hayashi, J., Furusyo, N., Sawayama, Y., Kishihara, Y., Kawakami, Y., Ariyama, I., Etoh, Y., Kashiwagi, S.: Hepatitis G virus in the general population and in patients as hemodialysis. Dig. Dis. Sci. 1998; 43: 2143–2148
492. Hollingsworth, R.C., Minton, E.J., Fraser-Moodie, C., Metivier, E., Rizzi, P.M., Irving, W.L., Jenkins, D., Ryder, S.D.: Hepatitis G infec-

tion: role in cryptogenic chronic liver disease and primary liver cell cancer in the UK. J. Vir. Hepat. 1998; 5: 165–169
493. Ideura, T., Tanaka, E., Nakatsuji, Y., Kobayashi, M., Kanno, Y., Oguchi, H., Hora, K.: Clinical significance of hepatitis G virus infection in patients on long-term haemodialysis. J. Gastroenterol. Hepatol. 1997; 12: 762–765
494. Jarvis, L.M., Davidson, F., Hanley, J.P., Yap, P.L., Ludlam, C.A., Simmonds, P.: Infection with hepatitis G virus among recipients of plasma products. Lancet 1996; 348: 1352–1355
495. Karayiannis, R., Hadziyannis, S.J., Kim, J., Pickering, J.M., Piatak, M., Hess, G., Yun, A., McGarvey, M.J., Wages, J., Thomas, H.C.: Hepatitits G virus infection: clinical characteristics and response to interferon. J. Viral Hepat. 1997; 4: 37–44
496. Kobayashi, M., Chayama, K., Fukuda, M., Tsubota, A., Suzuki, Y., Arase, Y., Koida, I., Saitoh, S., Murashima, N., Ikeda, K., Koike, H., Hashimoto, M., Miyano, Y., Kobayashi, M., Kumada, H.: Biochemical and histological features of hepatitis G virus infection. J. Gastroenterol. Hepatol. 1998; 13: 767–772
497. Linnen, J., Wages, J.jr., Zhang-Keck, Z.-Y., Fry, K.E., Krawczynski, K.Z., Alter, H., Koonin, E., Gallagher, M., Alter, M., Hadziyannis, St., Karayiannis, P. et al.: Molecular cloning and disease association of hepatitis G virus: a transfusion-transmissible agent. Science 1996; 271: 505–508
498. Moaven, L.D., Locarnini, S.A., Bowden, D.S., Kim, J.P., Breschkin, A., McCaw, R., Yun, A., Wages, J., Jones, B., Angus, P.: Hepatitis G virus and fulminant hepatic failure: evidence for transfusion-related infection. J. Hepatol. 1997; 27: 613–619
499. Nakatsuji, Y., Wai-Kuo Shih, J., Tanaka, E., Kiyosawa, K., Wages, J. jr., Kim, J.P., Alter, H.J.: Prevalence and disease association of hepatitis G virus infection in Japan. J. Viral Hepat. 1996; 3: 307–316
500. Saito, T., Shiino, T., Arakawa, Y., Hayashi, S., Abe, K.: Geographical characterization of hepatitis G virus genome: evidence for HGV genotypes based on phylogenetic analysis. Hepatol. Res. 1998; 10: 121–130
501. Stark, K., Bienzle, U., Hess, G., Engel, A.M., Hegenscheid, B., Schlüter, V.: Detection of the hepatitis G virus genome among injection drug abusers, homosexual and bisexual men, and blood donors. J. Infect. Dis. 1996; 174: 1320–1323
502. Thomas, D.L., Nakatsuji, Y., Shih, J.W., Alter, H.J., Nelson, K.E., Astemborski, J.A., Lyles, C.M., Vlahov, D.: Persistence and clinical significance of hepatitis G virus infection in injecting drug users. J. Infect. Dis. 1997; 176: 586–592
503. Torres, D., de Rueda, P.M., Ruiz-Extremera, A., Quintero, D., Palacios, A., Salmeron, J.: Genomic and antigenomic chains of hepatitis C virus and hepatitis G virus in serum, liver and peripheral blood mononuclear cells. Rev. Esp. Enferm. Dig. 2002; 94: 664–668
504. Umlauft, F., Wong, D.T., Underhill, P.A., Oefner, P.J., Jin, L., Urbanek, M., Gruewald, K., Greenberg, H.B.: Hepatitis G virus infection in hemodialysis patients and the effects of interferon treatment. Amer. J. Gastroenterol. 1997; 92: 1986–1991
505. Woelfle, J., Berg, T., Keller, K.M., Schreier, E., Lentze, M.J.: Persistent hepatitis G virus infection after neonatal transfusion. J. Pediat. Gastroenterol. Nutrit. 1998; 26: 402–407

GB viruses
506. Cheng, P.N., Chang, T.T., Jen, C.M., Ko, A.W., Young, K.C., Wu, H.L.: Molecular evidence for transmission of GB virus-C/hepatitis G virus infection within family: close relationship between mother and child. Hepato-Gastroenterol. 2003; 50: 151–156
507. Christensen, P.B., Fisker, N., Mygind, L.H., Krarup, H.B., Wedderkopp, N., Varming, K., Georgsen, J.: GB virus C epidemiology in Denmark: Different routes of transmission in children and low- and high-risk adults. J. Med. Virol. 2003; 70: 156–162
508. Deinhardt, F., Holmes, A.W., Capps, R.B., Popper, H: Studies on the transmission of human viral hepatitis to marmoset monkeys. Transmission of disease, serial passages, and description of liver lesions. J. Exper. Med. 1967; 125: 673–687
509. Heringlake, S., Ockenga, J., Tillmann, H.L., Trautwein, C., Meissner, D., Stoll, M., Hunt, J., Jou, C., Solomon, N., Schmidt, R.E., Manns, M.P.: GB virus-C / hepatitis G virus infection: a favorable prognostic factor in human immunodeficiency virus-infected patients? J. Infect. Dis. 1998; 177: 1723–1726
510. Kato, T., Mizokami, M., Nitta, M., Nakamura, M., Hiramatsu, H., Sugihara, K., Kato, A., Mukaide, M., Ueda, R.: Acute GB virus C / hepatitis G virus hepatitis preceding aplastic anemia. Hepatol. Res. 1997; 9: 164–171
511. Kiyosawa, K., Tanaka, E.: GB virus-C / hepatitis G virus. Intervirology 1999; 42: 185–195
512. Leary, T.P., Muerhoff, A.S., Simons, J.N., Pilot-Matias, T.J., Erker, J.C., Chalmers, M.L., Schlauder, G.G., Dawson, G.J., Desai, S.M., Mushahwar, I.K.: Sequence and genomic organization of GBV-C: a novel member of the flaviviridae associated with human Non-A-E hepatitis. J. Med. Virol. 1996; 48: 60–67
513. Meng, X.W., Komatsu, M., Ohshima, S., Nakane, K., Fujii, T., Goto, T., Yoneyama, K., Kuramitsu, T., Mukaide, M.: GB virus C virus infection: clinical significance. Can. J. Gastroenterol. 1999; 13: 814–818
514. Müller, C.: Pathogenicity of GBV-C / HGV infection. J. Vir. Hepat. 1999; 6 (Suppl. 1): 49–52
515. Okuda, K., Kanda, T., Yokosuka, O., Hayashi, H., Yokozeki, K., Ohtake, Y., Irie, Y.: GB-virus-C infection among chronic haemodialysis patients: clinical implications. J. Gastroenterol. Hepatol. 1997; 12: 766–770
516. Roy, K.M., Bagg, J., Kennedy, C., Cameron, S., Simmonds, P., Lycett, C., Hunter, I., Taylor, M.: Prevalence of GBV-C infection among dental personnel. J. Med. Virol. 2003; 70: 150–155
517. Sarrazin, C., Roth, W.K., Zeuzem, S.: Heterosexual transmission of GB virus-C / hepatitis G virus infection. Eur. J. Gastroenterol. Hepatol. 1997; 9: 1117–1120 • GB virus C / hepatitis G virus: discovery, epidemiology, diagnosis and clinical significance. Z. Gastroenterol. 1998; 36: 997–1008
518. Schlauder, G.G., Dawson, G.J., Simons, J.N., Pilot-Matias, T.J., Gutierrez, R.A., Heynene, C.A., Knigge, M.F., Kurpiewski, G.S., Buijk, S.L., Leary, T.P., Muerhoff, A.S., Desai, S.M., Mushahwar, I.K.: Molecular and serologic analysis in the transmission of the GB hepatitis agents. J. Med. Virol. 1995; 45: 81–90
519. Seemayer, C.A., Viazov, S., Philipp, T., Roggendorf, M.: Detection of GBV-C / HGV RNA in saliva and serum, but not in urine of infected patients. Infection 1998; 26: 39–41
520. Simons, J.N., Pilot-Matias, T.J., Leary, T.P., Dawson, G.J., Desai, S.M., Schlauder, G.G., Muerhoff, A.S., Erker, J.C., Buijk, S.L., Chalmers, M.L., van Sant, C.L., Mushahwar, I.K.: Identification of two flavivirus-like genomes in the GB hepatitis agent. Proc. Nat. Acad. Sci. 1995; 92: 3401–3405
521. Simons, J.N., Leary, T.P., Dawson, G.J., Pilot-Matias, T.J., Muerhoff, A.S., Schlauder, G.G., Desai, S.M., Mushawar, I.K.: Isolation of novel virus-like sequences associated with human hepatitis. Nature Med. 1995; 1: 564–569
522. Takacs, M., Szomor, K.N., Szendroi, A., Dencs, A., Brojnas, J., Rusvai, E., Berencsi, G.: Prevalence of GB virus C/hepatitis G virus in Hungary. FEMS Imm. Med. Microbiol. 2002; 34: 283–287
523. Stapleton, J.T.: GB virus type C/hepatitis G virus. Semin. Liver Dis. 2003; 23: 137–148
524. Tanaka, T., Takeuchi, T., Inoue, K., Tanaka, S., Kohara, M.: Acute hepatitis caused by sexual or household transmission of GBV-C. J. Hepatol. 1997; 27: 1110–1112

TT virus
525. Abe, K., Inami, T., Asano, K., Miyoski, C., Masaki, N., Hayaski, S., Ishikawa, K., Tokebe, Y., Win, K.M., El-Zayadi, A.R., Han, K.H., Zhang, D.Y.: TT virus infection is wide spread in the general populations from different geographical regions. J. Clin. Microbiol. 1999; 37: 2703–2705
526. Choi, M.S., Lee, J.H., Koh, K.C., Lee, J.H., Paik, S.W., Rhee, P.L., Rhee, J.C., Choi, K.W., Huh, W.S., Oh, H.Y.: TT virus infection in patients on maintenance hemodialysis in Korea. Hepato-Gastroenterol. 2003; 50: 170–173
527. Deng, X.W., Terunuma, H., Handema, R., Sakamoto, M., Kitamura, T., Ito, M., Akahane, Y.: Higher prevalence and viral load of TT virus in saliva than in the corresponding serum: Another possible transmission route and replication site of TT virus. J. Med. Virol. 2000; 62: 531–537
528. Gad, A., Tanaka, E., Orii, K., Rokuhara, A., Nooman, Z., El-Hamid-Serwah, A., El-Sherif, A., El-Essawy, M., Yoshizawa, K., Kiyosawa, K.: Clinical significance of TT virus infection in maintenance hemodialysis patients of an endemic area for hepatitis C infection. Hepatol. Res. 2002; 22: 13–19
529. Iwaki, Y., Aiba, N., Tran, H.T.T., Ding, X., Hayashi, S., Arakawa, Y., Sata, T., Abe, K.: Simian TT virus (S-TTV) infection in patients with liver diseases. Hepatol. Res. 2003; 25: 135–147
530. Matsubara, H., Michitaka, K., Horiike, N., Kihana, T., Yano, M., Mori, T., Onji, M.: Existence of TT virus DNA and TTV-like mini virus DNA in infant cord blood: mother-to-neonatal transmission. Hepatol. Res. 2001; 21: 280–287
531. Mushawar, I.K., Erker, J.C., Muerhoff, A.S., Leary, T.P., Simons, J.N., Birkenmeyer, L.G., Chalmers, M.L., Pilot-Matias, T.J., Dexai, S.M.: Molecular and biophysical characterization of TT virus: evidence for a new virus family infecting humans. Proc. Nat. Acad. Sci. 1999; 96: 3177–3182
532. Niel, C., de Oliveira, J.M., Ross, R.S., Gomes, S.A., Roggendorf, M., Viazov, S.: High prevalence of TT virus infection in Brazilian blood donors. J. Med. Virol. 1999; 57: 259–263
533. Nishizawa, T., Okamoto, H., Konishi, K., Yoshizawa, H., Miyakawa, Y., Mayumi, M.: A novel DNA virus (TTV) associated with elevated transaminase levels in posttransfusion hepatitis of unknown etiology. Biochem. Biophys. Res. Comm. 1997; 241: 92–97
534. Pollicino, T., Raffa, G., Squadrito, G., Constantino, L., Cacciola, I., Brancatelli, S., Alafaci, C., Florio, M.G., Raimondo, G.: TT virus has a ubiquitous diffusion in human body tissues: analyses of paired serum and tissue samples. J. Viral Hepat. 2003; 10: 95–102
535. Schröter, M., Feucht, H.-H., Zöllner, B., Knödler, B., Schäfer, P., Fischer, L., Laufs, R.: Prevalence of TTV viremia among healthy subjects and individuals at risk for parenterally transmitted diseases in Germany. Hepatol. Res. 1999; 13: 205–211
536. Simmonds, P., Davidson, F., Lycett, C., Prescott, L.E., MacDonald, D.M., Ellender, J., Yap, P.L., Ludiam, C.A., Haydon, G.H., Gillon, J., Jarvis, L.M.: Detection of a novel DNA virus (TTV) in blood donors and blood products. Lancet 1998; 352: 191–195
537. Suzuki, F., Chayama, K., Tsubota, A., Akuta, N., Someya, T., Kobayashi, M., Suzuki, Y., Saitoh, S., Arase, Y., Ikeda, K., Kumada, H.: Pathogenic significance and organic virus levels in patients infected with TT virus. Intervirology 2001; 44: 291–297

538. **Tajiri, H., Tanaka, T., Sawada, A., Etani, Y., Kozaiwa, K., Mushiake, S., Mishiro, S.:** Three cases TT virus infection and idiopathic neonatal hepatitis. Intervirology 2001; 44: 364–369
539. **Takacs, M., Balong, K., Toth, G., Balogh, Z., Szomor, K.N., Brojnas, J., Rusvai, E., Minarovits, J., Berencsi, G.:** TT virus in Hungary: sequence heterogeneity and mixed infections. FEMS Imm. Med. Microbiol. 2003; 35: 153–157
540. **Tokita, H., Murai, S., Kamitsukawa, H., Yagura, M., Harada, H., Takahashi, M., Okamoto, H.:** High TT virus load as an independence factor associated with the occurrence of hepatocellular carcinoma among patients with hepatitis C virus-related chronic liver disease. J. Med. Virol. 2002; 67: 501–509

SEN virus

541. **Kao, J.-H.H., Chen, W., Chen, P.-J., Lai, M.-Y., Chen, D.-S.:** Prevalence and implication of a newly identified infectious agent (SEN virus) in Taiwan. J. Infect. Dis. 2002; 185: 389–392
542. **Pirovano, S., Bellinzoni, M., Ballerini, C., Cariani, E., Duse, M., Altertini, A., Imberti, L.:** Transmission of SEN virus from mothers to their babies. J. Med. Virol. 2002; 66: 421–427
543. **Lin, J.G., Goto, T., Nakane, K., Miura, K., Mikami, K., Ohshima, S., Yoneyama, K., Watanabe, S.:** Clinical significance of SEN-virus on interferon response in chronic hepatitis C patients. J. Gastroenterol. Hepatol. 2003; 18: 1144–1149
544. **Rigas, B., Hasan, I., Rehman, R., Donahue, P., Wittkowski, K.M., Lebovics, E.:** Effect on treatment outcome of coinfection with SEN viruses in patients with hepatitis C. Lancet 2001; 358: 1961–1962
545. **Schröter, M., Laufs, R., Zöllner, B., Knödler, B., Schäfer, P., Sterneck, M., Fischer, L., Feucht, H.-H.:** Prevalence of SENV-H viremia among healthy subjects and individuals at risk for parenterally transmitted diseases in Germany. J. Viral Hepat. 2002; 9: 455–459
546. **Shibata, M., Wang, R.Y.-H., Yoshiba, M., Shih, J.W.-K., Alter, H.J., Mitamura, K.:** The presence of a newly identified infectious agent (SEN virus) in patients with liver diseases and in blood donors in Japan. J. Infect. Dis. 2001; 184: 400–404
547. **Tanaka, Y., Primi, D., Wang, R.Y.H., Umemura, T., Yeo, A.E.T., Mizokami, M., Alter, H.J., Shih, J.W.-K.:** Genomic and molecular evolutinonary analysis of a newly identified infectious agent (SEN virus) and its relationship to the TT virus family. J. Infect. Dis. 2001; 183: 359–367
548. **Tangkijvanich, P., Theambooniers, A., Sriponthong, M., Kullavanijaya, P., Poovorawan, Y.:** SEN virus infection and the risk of hepatocellular carcinoma: A case-control study. Amer. J. Gastroenterol. 2003; 98: 2500–2504
549. **Umemura, T., Yeo, A.E., Sottini, A., Moratto, D., Tanaka, Y., Wang, R.Y.-H., Shih, J.W.-K., Donahue, P., Primi, D., Alter, H.J.:** SEN virus infection and its relationship to transfusion-associated hepatitis. Hepatology 2001; 33: 1303–1311
550. **Umemura, T., Tanaka, E., Ostapowicz, G., Brown, K.E., Heringlake, S., Tassopoulos, N.C., Wang, R.Y.H., Yeo, A.E.T., Shih, J.W.K., Manns, M.P., Lee, W.M., Kiyosawa, K., Alter, H.J.:** Investigation of SEN virus infection in patients with cryptogenic acute liver failure, hepatitis-associated aplastic anemia, or acute and chronic non-A-E hepatitis. J. Infect. Dis. 2003; 188: 1545–1552
551. **Yoshida, H., Kato, N., Shiratori, Y., Shao, R.X., Wang, Y., Shiina, S., Omata, M.:** Weak association between SEN virus viremia and liver disease. J. Clin. Microbiol. 2002; 40: 3140–3145
552. **Wang, L.Y., Ho, T.Y., Chen, M.C., Yi, C.S., Hu, C.T., Lin, H.H.:** Prevalence and determinants of SENV viremia among adolescents in an endemic area of chronic liver disease. J. Gastroenterol. Hepatol. 2007; 22: 171–176

YF virus

553. **Takacs, M., Berencsi, G., Mezey, I., Brojnas, J., Barcsay, E., Garamvölgyi, E., Hütter, E., Ferenczi, E., Pipirasz, E., Hollos, I., Dömök, I.:** Detection of transfusion-associated hepatitis caused by non-A, non-B, non-C flavivirus. Acta Microbiol. Immunol. Hungar. 1994; 41: 83–89

Clinical Aspects of Liver Diseases
23 Acute concomitant viral hepatitis

		Page:
1	***Secondary hepatotropic viruses***	474
1.1	*Herpesviruses*	474
1.1.1	Infectious mononucleosis	474
1.1.2	Herpes simplex hepatitis	475
1.1.3	Herpesvirus hepatitis (HHV-6, HHV-8)	476
1.1.4	Varicella-zoster hepatitis	476
1.1.5	Cytomegalovirus	476
1.2	*Togaviruses*	477
1.2.1	Rubella hepatitis	477
1.2.2	Spring-summer encephalitis hepatitis	477
1.3	*Picornaviruses*	477
1.3.1	Coxsackie hepatitis	477
1.3.2	ECHO virus hepatitis	477
1.4	*Paramyxoviruses*	477
1.4.1	Measles hepatitis	477
1.4.2	Parotitis hepatitis	477
1.4.3	Giant-cell hepatitis	477
1.5	*Adenovirus hepatitis*	477
1.6	*Human parvovirus B19*	478
1.7	*HIV hepatitis*	478
2	***Exotic hepatotropic viruses***	478
2.1	Yellow fever	478
2.2	Dengue fever	479
2.3	Kyanasur Forest fever	479
2.4	Marburg virus disease	479
2.5	Ebola haemorrhagic fever	479
2.6	Lassa haemorrhagic fever	480
2.7	Rift Valley fever	480
	• References (1–116)	480
	(Figures 23.1–23.5; tables 23.1–23.2)	

23 Acute concomitant viral hepatitis

A multitude of viruses can affect the liver as a large, filtrating and reacting organ, and subsequently cause concomitant viral hepatitis in the course of an existing systemic viral infection. Laboratory and histological findings in this case are determined by the type of pathogen, including its particular hepatotropic character, and by the immune status or reactivity of the affected organism. Concomitant viral hepatitis does not generally cause symptoms, which is why it is often recognized purely by chance due to slight to moderate elevations in transaminases; minor increases in bilirubin or cholestasis-indicating enzymes are rarely detectable. Nevertheless, severe courses with vast hepatocellular necrosis can occur in patients with a weakened immune response. • In infancy, concomitant viral hepatitis is frequently accompanied by a predominant cholestasis syndrome. • On the one hand, an infant liver can be damaged by virus infections of a severe and even fatal course, yet on the other hand, it displays an astonishing capacity for regeneration and is indeed capable of restoring structures which have been destroyed.

1 Secondary hepatotropic viruses

The most important virus species with regard to their ability to cause concomitant inflammatory reactions of the liver are (1.) herpesviruses, (2.) rubella viruses, (3.) Coxsackie viruses, and (4.) paramyxoviruses. (s. tab. 23.1)

1. Herpesviruses		
– Epstein-Barr virus	D	E
– Herpes simplex virus 1, 2	D	E
– Human herpesvirus 6, 7, 8	D	E
– Varicella-zoster virus	(D)	
– Cytomegalovirus	D	E
2. Togaviruses		
– Rubella virus	D	E
– Spring-summer encephalitis virus	D	E
3. Picornaviruses		
– Coxsackie virus	D	E
– ECHO virus	D	E
4. Paramyxoviruses		
– Measles virus		E
– Parotitis virus	(D)	
– Giant-cell hepatitis virus	D	E
5. Adenoviruses	(S D	E)
6. Human parvovirus B 19		
7. HIV	laboratory test +	

Tab. 23.1: Secondary hepatotropic viruses causing viral hepatitis. • In Germany, **obligation for notification** is given in cases of suspicion (S), disease (D) or exitus (E). • But this varies from country to country. *If in doubt*, contact the Public Health Department!

1.1 Herpesviruses

Out of a group of approximately 40 herpesviruses (containing DNA, 100 nm in length), the following are classified as secondary hepatotropic: (1.) Epstein-Barr virus (types A, B), (2.) herpes simplex virus, (3.) herpesvirus-6, (4.) varicella-zoster virus, and (5.) cytomegalovirus.

1.1.1 Infectious mononucleosis

▶ "Pfeiffer's glandular fever" (E. Pfeiffer, 1889) or "infectious mononucleosis" (T.P. Sprungt et al., 1920) is caused by **human herpesvirus** 4 (= EB virus 4), which was discovered by M.A. Epstein, B.G. Achong and Y.M. Barr in 1964.

Infectious mononucleosis is a generalized reticuloendothelial infection, mainly found in adolescents and young adults. The total endemic infection rate in the more advanced age groups is 80–100%. • This condition is transmitted by close physical contact ("kissing disease"), sexual contact and blood transfusion. The incubation period of the orally transmitted virus is 8–21 days (up to 7 weeks). This is followed by a prodromal stage with headaches, tiredness and atypical fever. The clinical picture is defined by (chiefly cervical) swollen lymph nodes (95–100%), tonsillitis (>80%), splenomegaly (>50%), exanthema, mucosal petechiae in the oral cavity (30–50%) and leucocytosis with very large numbers of lymphomonocytoid cells. These "atypical lymphocytes" (W. Schultz, 1922) are activated T cells. Gallbladder wall thickening is detected by sonography. (17)

In about 50% of cases, **hepatitis mononucleosa** with hepatomegaly (10–25%) develops, displaying an increase in transaminases of 10–20 times the normal value. (15) Jaundice is found in 5–10% of cases, usually due to autoimmune-based haemolysis. (2, 4, 6, 7) There is a distinct elevation of LDH and alkaline phosphatase. (8) The following enzyme constellation can be evaluated as the *biochemical triad* of hepatitis mononucleosa:

LDH	↑↑↑	(90–95%)
AP	↑↑	(75–90%)
GPT, GOT	↑	(60–90%)

The *Paul-Bunnel test* (J.R. Paul, W.W. Bunnel, 1932) is positive from the 4th to 10th day in about 75% of cases. Serological proof of acute infection can be obtained by way of *anti-EB virus IgM*. The virus DNA is revealed by PCR. • *Hepatic lesions* are already found as from the 5th day and are most distinct between the 10th and 30th day of the disease. Portal/periportal and sinusoidal infiltrations of partially beaded lymphomonocytoid cells frequently appear in the form of small foci. Proliferations of Kupffer cells and bile capillaries as well as isolated focal hepatocellular necroses and granulomas are present. (2, 4, 9, 16) (s. fig. 23.1)

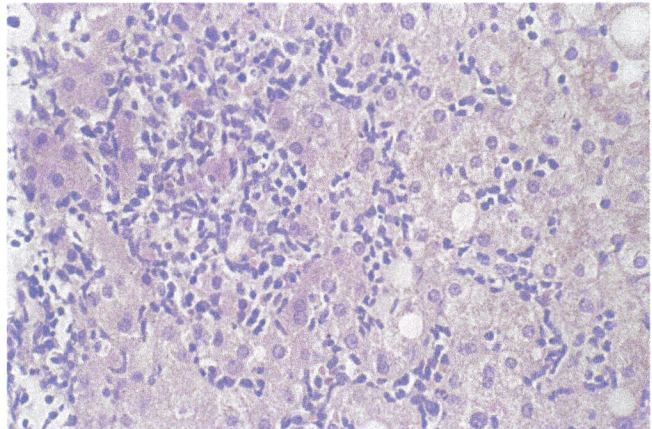

Fig. 23.1: Agglomeration of activated Kupffer cells (partially beaded), especially in the sinusoidal vessels, with single-cell necrosis. Clinical diagnosis: hepatitis mononucleosa (HE)

▶ *We observed a severe haemolytic course in a 23-year-old man, which took four months to subside: total bilirubin up to 34.8 mg/dl, haemoglobin decline to 7.7 g%, LDH up to 1,720 U/l, reticulocytosis 54‰, GPT 110 U/l, GOT 60 U/l, AP 308 U/l, γ-GT 148 U/l, increased erythropoiesis in bone marrow +, direct Coombs' test +, cold agglutinin +, and incomplete cold haemolysin +. (s. fig. 23.1)*

Some of the more *serious extrahepatic complications* include splenic rupture, thrombocytopenia, myocarditis or pericarditis, meningitis, pneumonia, nephritis and haemolytic anaemia; ascites was also reported in the course of severe hepatitis. (3) It should be noted that EBV sometimes triggers autoimmune hepatitis. (14) • Prognosis is good. Full recovery is generally achieved within 6—12 weeks. However, fatigue can persist for 8—9 months, which for athletes, for example, means an inability to train, resulting in a drop in performance. In this context, it has been suggested that the **fatigue syndrome** may be caused by a variant of EBV. • In rare cases, a *fulminant course*, possibly even with a fatal outcome, has been reported. (12) In sporadic fatal infection, the mortality rate is relatively high (40—45%). (1, 4, 7, 11—13) • A *chronic course* of EBV infection has been observed in some families, implying a genetic predisposition. Transition into chronic hepatitis or cirrhosis need not be feared, because it is extremely seldom. (4) In 50—70% of cases, an EBV infection developed following liver transplantation, and in 2% of these patients, *EBV hepatitis* occurred, sometimes with a lethal outcome. (10) • *Therapy* is symptomatic. Treatment with aciclovir or valacyclovir is reported to be encouraging. In complicated courses, erythromycin (*cave* ampicillin!) and glucocorticoids may be indicated.

1.1.2 Herpes simplex hepatitis

The herpesvirus hominis is a widespread virus affecting all tissues. Herpes simplex virus types 1 (mostly systemic) and 2 (genital herpes) are transmitted by droplet or smear infection. • In newborns, in patients with a weakened immune response or in immunosuppression (e. g. following liver transplantation or in AIDS) as well as in chronic diseases (e. g. colitis) and during pregnancy, the course of disease may be severe, even lethal. • The viraemia also causes *herpes hepatitis*. Clinical findings include fever, fatigue, abdominal discomfort (ca. 60%), hepatomegaly (ca. 35%), leucopenia and thrombopenia, marked increases in transaminases and distinct decreases in cholinesterase and albumin. Jaundice tends to be rare (with a value of < 5 mg/dl). Diagnosis can be established serologically by detecting herpesvirus antibodies of the IgM class or by demonstrating the presence of pathogens. Mucocutaneous changes are infrequent. (35) The liver surface usually displays variable, yellow-coloured focal necrosis with red borders. • *Histologically*, microvesicular fatty degeneration is detectable; focal hepatic necroses are surrounded by hepatocytes with intranuclear inclusion bodies of *Cowdry type A* (= surrounded by a bright area) (s. fig. 23.2) or *Cowdry type B* (= homogenous, ground glass-like).

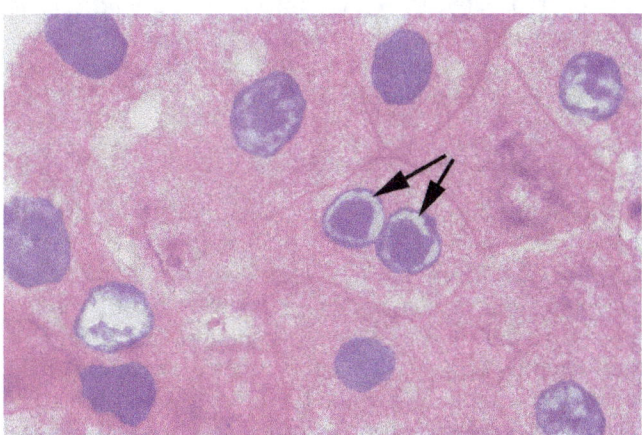

Fig. 23.2: Acute herpes simplex virus hepatitis with intranuclear bodies (Cowdry type A) (→) (HE)

The extent ranges from individual cell necroses to patchy confluent lobular necroses with irregular zoning. HSV are directly cytopathic; thus cellular necroses appear first, followed by inflammatory infiltrates. Herpesviruses are visible by electron microscopy; they can be cultured from the liver and rendered visible through staining by immunoperoxidase. • The *prognosis* is dubious in high-risk patients; mortality is 10—15%. In severe fibrosis following long-standing protracted HSV hepatitis, chronic cholestasis may develop (even with a lethal course). There have been reports of a fulminant course of disease. (25, 28, 31—34, 37, 38) • *Therapy* is effected, even during pregnancy, using aciclovir as the agent of choice with 5(—10) mg/kg BW/8 hours as i.v. infusion or, in severe and immunosuppressed cases, with 10 mg/kg BW. Ganciclovir has also proved effective with 2 mg/kg BW/12 hours as i.v. infusion. (19–22, 24, 26, 27, 29, 30)

1.1.3 Herpesvirus hepatitis

Human herpes virus-6: Infection with HHV-6 occurs in babies and infants of all races as well as in males and females in equal number - after maternal antibodies have waned. Primarily, T lymphocytes are affected, followed by monocytes and endothelial cells. Two variants (A and B) have been identified. This virus causes 3-day fever (= *exanthema subitum*) or a mononucleosis-like syndrome with chronic fatigue in older children or adults. A latent phase is also known and can be reactivated if the immune system is compromised. Diagnosis is made by serology or PCR. In immunodeficiency, there may be complications, such as pneumonia, encephalitis and *acute hepatitis*. There have also been reports of fulminant hepatitis. (18, 23, 36)

HHV-8 causes *Kaposi's sarcoma*. The liver is the most common site, with dark reddish-violet tumour nodes. Histological analysis reveals endothelial cell proliferations and growths of spindle-shaped fibroblast-like cells. The bile ducts may be altered. Transaminase levels are elevated, and jaundice occurs. There may be a causal relationship between HHV-8 infection and *multicentric Castleman's disease*. The latter usually implies the presence of peliosis hepatis, perisinusoidal fibrosis and nodular regenerative hyperplasia.

1.1.4 Varicella-zoster hepatitis

"Chickenpox" in infancy and "shingles" in adults are caused by the same varicella-zoster virus. Very rarely and almost exclusively in immunosuppressed patients, *concomitant hepatitis* occurs with pronounced (mainly focal) hepatocellular necrosis, sometimes even with a fatal course. (39, 43, 44) Leucocytic portal and periportal infiltration can spread to the blood vessels and bile capillaries. Intranuclear inclusion bodies are present (s. fig. 23.2). Diagnosis is based on increased GPT, GOT, GDH and γ-GT values as well as the presence of varicella IgM antibodies; alternatively, pathogens can also be demonstrated in cultures. In children, a differential diagnosis of Reye's syndrome must be considered. • As *therapy* in a severe course, aciclovir is indicated. (40–42, 45, 46)

Herpes zoster generally shows less severe concomitant viral hepatitis. In one particular case of zoster disease (s. fig. 23.3), we observed an unusually pronounced form of hepatitis. After recovery, the patient revealed normal laboratory values.

1.1.5 Cytomegalovirus

A cytomegalic infection is transmitted perinatally or postnatally (mainly unnoticed) by the cytomegalovirus (CMV) − a DNA herpesvirus − as well as by direct body contact (droplet-smear infection, breast milk, sexual intercourse) and blood transfusion. Some 60–80% of all adults in the USA and in Europe have overcome a cytomegalic infection and are now immune. (52)

In terms of liver involvement, a **pre-/perinatal infection** usually causes hepatosplenomegaly, moderate jaundice (ca. 60%), differing degrees of cholestasis (concomitant cholangitis) and mild *cytomegaly hepatitis*. In numerous cases, the characteristic intranuclear inclusion bodies (= *owl's eyes*) are found. The occurrence of *giant-cell hepatitis* (s. fig. 22.5) is considered to be an unusual event. Occasionally, *granulomatous hepatitis* with epithelioid cellular or histiocytic granulomas occurs. Histologically, the hepatic changes can persist for months or years. Therefore, non-cirrhotic portal hypertension may develop. (51) Mortality is about 20%.

Postnatal infection, providing it does not take a symptom-free course, displays the clinical picture of infectious mononucleosis with similar haematological findings and complicative developments (such as haemolytic anaemia, thrombopenic purpura, pneumonia) as well as retinitis, arthritis, acute portal vein thrombosis and colitis. In 25–35% of cases, *cytomegaly hepatitis* develops with moderate jaundice, hepatomegaly, a slight increase in transaminases and varying degrees of cholestasis. Cytomegaloviruses can persist in lymphocytes and other body cells and may be reactivated under conditions of diminished immunity or immunosuppression.

In **infancy,** cytomegalic infection is mainly symptom-free. Up to 40% of cases, however, show evidence of *cytomegaly hepatitis* with hepatomegaly. Virus excretion in the urine points to viraemia. • In **adulthood,** there is also evidence of *concomitant hepatitis* (55) and *granulomatous hepatitis* (48, 49) in addition to the generally pronounced cytomegalic infection, which is present to varying degrees during this phase of life. Moderately increased GPT, GOT, GDH and LDH activity is often evident; this is sometimes accompanied by a distinctly

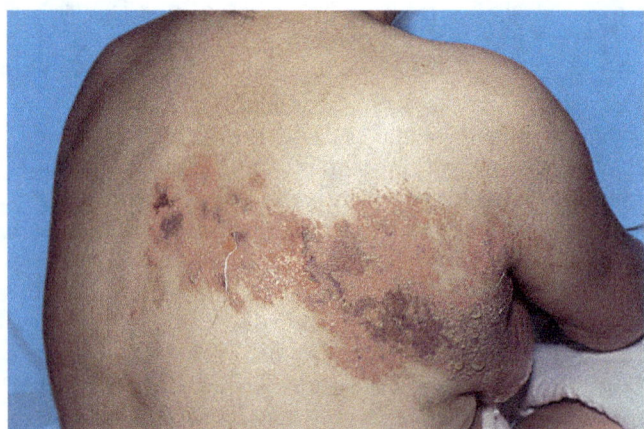

Fig. 23.3: Herpes zoster. Pronounced concomitant hepatitis: GPT 186 U/l, GOT 132 U/l, GDH 8.3 U/l, γ-GT 56 U/l, cholinesterase ↓; alkaline phosphatase and bilirubin normal

pronounced elevation of γ-GT (without an equivalent rise in AP) and decreased levels of serum iron. Occasionally, marked cholestasis occurs. In most cases, there is a reduction in serum iron. Bilirubin values are moderately elevated or completely normal. (54) • *Diagnosis* of cytomegalic infection is based on the antibody titer increase of CMV IgM (sometimes with reactivation), detection in the virus by PCR, virus excretion in urine or in situ hybridization. Histologically, the typical intranuclear inclusion bodies suggest a cytomegalic infection. (57–59) CMV infection is to be feared in the liver transplant; thus there is a danger of "vanishing bile-duct syndrome". (50, 53) Acute portal and mesenteric thrombosis is a rare complication. (47) • *Therapy* consists of ganciclovir (56) or foscarnet. CMV immunoglobulin is recommended for pre-exposure prophylaxis.

1.2 Togaviruses

1.2.1 Rubella hepatitis

Connatal infection due to the 60 nm RNA virus, which belongs to the togavirus group, is accompanied by a clearly enlarged liver and spleen as well as, on occasions, by jaundice. Histologically, cholestasis with bile pigmentation in the hepatic cells and with bile thrombi in the canaliculi is found. The portal fields are widened and irregular as a result of inflammatory infiltration, and the ductuli generally display pronounced proliferation. Occasionally, *giant-cell hepatitis* occurs. (s. fig. 22.5) • In adolescents and adults, *granulomatous hepatitis* is sometimes observed. In other cases, only slight histological changes are detectable, or the findings can be interpreted as insignificant *non-specific reactive hepatitis*. (s. fig. 21.1) In the later stages, fine calcification foci may develop (as in Ebola hepatitis). (60, 62–67)

1.2.2 Spring-summer encephalitis hepatitis

In spring and summer, ticks (especially Ixodes ricinus) can transmit meningo-encephalitic viruses of the togavirus family to human beings. During this disease, *concomitant hepatitis* may develop, with a moderate increase in transaminases. Histologically, pronounced focal hepatic cell lesions are found together with mesenchymal inflammatory reactions; all of these findings are attributable to non-specific reactive hepatitis. (61)

1.3 Picornaviruses

1.3.1 Coxsackie hepatitis

This virus species derived its name from the town of Coxsackie in New York State, where virological evidence was successfully obtained for the first time. Coxsackie viruses are assigned to the picornavirus group, consisting at present of 23 A and 6 B types. • *Coxsackie hepatitis* with mesenchymal reactions, portal infiltration and focal hepatocellular necrosis often occurs, especially in infants. Cholestatic, predominantly centrolobular forms of the disease, can develop in adults. Coxsackie hepatitis associated with myocaditis has also been observed. (70) A lethal course is extremely rare. (69–71) • An infection with the Coxsackie type B 4 or B 5 virus may give rise to the *Fitz-Hugh-Curtis syndrome* with the development of the typical violin string-like adhesive strands. (68) (s. fig. 24.2)

1.3.2 ECHO virus hepatitis

The widespread group of echoviruses, with its 31 known serotypes, has not yet been reliably categorized systematically or pathogenically. These viruses can also give rise to *concomitant hepatitis*, with type 4 and type 9 being held mainly responsible for this condition. (72)

1.4 Paramyxoviruses

1.4.1 Measles hepatitis

The measles virus, discovered in 1911, is a large (100–150 nm) paramyxovirus with a lipid envelope. Concomitant *measles hepatitis* occurs in 80% of all adults suffering from measles. It generally takes an anicteric, clinically bland course, and in most cases even goes unnoticed. Diagnosis is based on the elevation of transaminases and the detection of IgM antibodies. Cytologically, multinuclear giant cells are found in nasal secretion. The prognosis for measles hepatitis is good. Despite lifelong immunity, however, the measles virus is able to persist latently in cells, especially in lymphocytes (as in autoimmune hepatitis). (73, 75, 78)

1.4.2 Parotitis hepatitis

The parotitis virus, an RNA virus of the paramyxovirus group, can also cause *mumps hepatitis* with corresponding minimal histological and laboratory findings.

1.4.3 Giant-cell hepatitis

In 1991 in Canada, J. PHILLIPS et al. determined the presence of paramyxoviruses in patients with an infaust course of giant-cell hepatitis: out of ten patients, only five survived with the help of liver transplantation. Paramyxovirus nucleocapsid protein, with a diameter of 12–17 nm, was detected in the cytoplasm of the hepatocytes. (77) Until then, this paramyxovirus had been unknown. It can cause severe acute hepatitis, which might even be fatal. (74, 76, 79) (s. p. 425!)

1.5 Adenovirus hepatitis

Adenoviruses can be the cause of *hepatitis* in newborns or immunosuppressed persons, sometimes even with a *fulminant course*. They bring about the formation of inclusion bodies in the hepatocellular nuclei. Adenovirus infections are diagnosed either serologically or by virus isolation. (80–82)

1.6 Human parvovirus B19

HPV B19 causes infections erythema in children. It may also lead to acute hepatitis. Aplastic anaemia is found in adults with simultaneous, potentially massive liver cell necroses and fulminant liver failure. HPV B19 can be detected in the liver tissue using PCR. (83)

1.7 HIV hepatitis

By means of virological examination methods, it was possible to demonstrate HIV-1 RNA in hepatocytes, Kupffer cells and endothelial cells. The liver may be involved in systemic HIV disease both during primary infection and in the more advanced stages. The elevation, of GDH, γ-GT and the transaminases is highly significant. Hepatomegaly is occasionally detected and attributed to infection-related hyperplasia of the liver cells. *HIV-concomitant hepatitis* shows differing degrees of focal hepatocellular necrosis, inflammatory mesenchymal reactions, portal field infiltration, granulomas or peliosis hepatis. During the course of HIV infection, *HIV cholangiopathy*, frequently of the sclerogenic type, may also develop. Cryptosporidiosis of the bile ducts with cholangitis has only been observed in AIDS. (s. p. 671) • The most common opportunistic infective agents are Mycobacterium avium intracellulare (40–45%), cytomegalovirus (20–30%), cryptosporidium and various mycoses (histoplasmosis, cryptococcosis, coccidiomycosis). (84–90)

2 Exotic hepatotropic viruses

A large number of virus species found in tropical and subtropical countries are known to be hepatotropic pathogens. They can give rise to minor findings of *non-specific reactive hepatitis* (s. fig. 21.1) or fatty degeneration of the hepatocytes with cell necrosis.

1. Flaviviruses			
• yellow fever		D	E
• dengue fever		D	E
• Kyasanur Forest disease		D	E
• Semliki Forest disease (alphavirus)		D	E
2. Filoviruses			
• Marburg virus	S	D	E
• Ebola virus	S	D	E
3. Arenavirus			
• Lassa fever	S	D	E
• Bolivian haemorrhagic fever			
4. Bunyaviruses			
• Hantavirus		D	E
• Rift Valley fever (Phlebovirus)		D	E
• Crimea-Congo fever (Nairovirus)			

Tab. 23.2: Significant exotic hepatotropic viruses which can cause hepatic damage. • In Germany, the **obligation for notification** is given in cases of suspicion (S), disease (D) or exitus (E). • This can, however, vary from country to country. *If in doubt*, contact the Public Health Department!

Such viruses may also cause severe (even fatal) liver disease. All of them have been categorized under the generic term *exotic virus diseases*. (103, 105) They are pathogens from the family of flaviviruses, filoviruses, arenaviruses, and bunyaviruses. (s. tab. 23.2)

> **It should be noted, however:** The large number of people travelling all over the world on the one hand and the globalized economy on the other hand have overcome (nearly) all political barriers and geographical borders. Now to make matters worse, a warmer global climate is spreading to countries in the northern hemisphere. The annually increasing number of exotic hepatotropic virus diseases in Europe and North America is alarming! • *This is also a new challenge for hepatology!*

2.1 Yellow fever

The main epidemic regions are South America and equatorial Africa, i.e. the so-called *yellow fever belt* between the 15th northern latitude and the 15th southern latitude. The yellow fever virus is transmitted from human being to human being by infected mosquitoes, especially Aedes aegypti or Aedes simpsoni. There is a marked steatosis hepatis. Often a bacillary peliosis hepatis is found; it can be associated with the cutaneous bacillary angiomatosis. Rochalimaea henselae have been determined as a pathogen. In children with a coinfection of HIV and adenoviruses, fulminant hepatitis has been reported. An incubation period of 3–6 (–13) days is followed by fever with viraemia, jaundice, hepatosplenomegaly, arthralgia, myalgia, exanthema, bleeding and haematemesis ("vomito negro") as well as circulatory disorders and renal damage (largely in the form of fatty tubular degeneration). However, inapparent or bland courses of disease are equally possible.

Hepatic lesions in the case of yellow fever are more likely to correspond to those of hepatosis. (s. p. 411) There is also evidence of distinct acidophilic hepatocellular necrosis and microvesicular fatty degeneration of the hepatocytes. Hyaline, eosinophilic inclusions in the cytoplasm of degenerated hepatic cells (= *Councilman bodies*) are characteristic and were first identified by W. T. COUNCILMAN in 1890 in yellow fever (s. p. 402). Acidophilic inclusion bodies in the hepatocellular nuclei which are arranged concentrically around the nucleolus (= *Torres corpuscles*) correspond to the yellow fever virus (C. M. TORRES, 1928). The liver does not present any significant signs of inflammation. The reticular fibre structure is maintained, so that the liver architecture is usually completely restored, provided the outcome of the disease is favourable. (s. fig. 23.4)

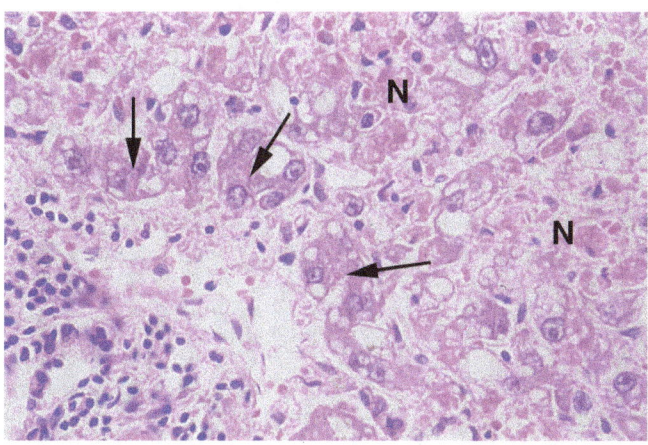

Fig. 23.4: Portal inflammation and acute parenchymal necrosis (N) due to shock (only periportal hepatocytes are intact). Clinical diagnosis: yellow fever (HE)

The *diagnosis* is established by determining the specific YF IgM antibodies and/or the virus RNA. Laboratory parameters reveal an elevation of the transaminases, GDH, γ-GT and LDH as well as a reduction in leucocytes, Quick's value and cholinesterase. Albuminuria is also present. *Mortality* (5–10%) is generally due to renal insufficiency. After *recovery*, immunity is lifelong. Chronic courses of disease are not known. When travelling to yellow fever regions, immunization (with live vaccine) is imperative; vaccine protection lasts for six to ten years. (s. p. 460) (96, 101, 115)

2.2 Dengue fever

The dengue virus is also related to the flavivirus species. It is transmitted by mosquitoes (of the Aedes type). The prognosis is relatively good – despite the fact that several hundred deaths have been recorded during epidemics (such as in Java and India in 1996). Altogether, some 55 million people contract the disease every year. The worldwide mortality rate is approx. 10%. In Germany, more than 1,500 cases of infection are registered annually. Following a five- to eight-day incubation period, the clinical picture comprises fever ("breakbone fever"), headache, nausea, haemorrhage (haematuria, melaena), myalgia and arthralgia, exanthema, lymphadenopathy, and even splenic rupture. • *Concomitant hepatitis* of different degrees of severity, often with centroacinar necrosis and microvesicular steatosis, can occur. Fulminant hepatitis is rare. Convalescence is protracted. Diffuse residual parenchymal calcifications may remain. No vaccine has been found so far. (95, 99, 104, 106)

2.3 Kyanasur Forest disease:

This disease was observed for the first time in 1959 in the Kyanasur forest of Karnataka on the southwest coast of India. The respective virus belongs to the family of flaviviruses. Especially monkeys and small mammals become infected. • It is transmitted to humans by forest ticks or direct contact with infected animals. The incubation period is two to seven days. Symptoms include fever, headaches, arthralgia, nausea and diarrhoea. Sometimes, haemorrhagies and *acute hepatitis* with elevated transaminases occur. In most cases, there is evidence of leukopenia. Diagnosis is generally made by serology and PCR. Lethality is 3–5 %. There is no known therapy at present Vaccines, however, are available. (91)

2.4 Marburg virus disease

In 1967 in Marburg (Germany), a total of 23 patients contracted a previously unknown infection caused by the "Marburg virus", which belongs to the filoviruses. Altogether, five outbreaks have been reported, with over 120 cases. It is a single-strand RNA virus, 790–970 nm in length and 80 nm in width. Infection resulted from direct, work-related contact with African apes (green guenons) as well as human transmission (partially due to sexual contact). After a five- to seven-day incubation period, the clinical picture became serious, with fever, vomiting, diarrhoea, exanthema, conjunctivitis, myalgia, haemorrhagic diathesis with thrombopenia, renal and hepatic damage as well as disorientation. • Laboratory parameters and histological examinations pointed to severe *hepatitis* with hepatosplenomegaly. Jaundice is extremely rare. Hyaline eosinophilic liver cell necrosis, microvesicular fatty degeneration and lymphomonocytic infiltration of the portal fields predominate. The patchy necroses tend to merge and form bridging necroses. Basophilic bodies can be found in the necrotic cells. The reticular fibre structure remains intact. • The prognosis is unfavourable: in the Marburg epidemic, mortality was 28%; in epidemics in the Sudan and in Zaire, it was 53% and 88%, respectively. (92, 102, 108, 109, 113, 114)

2.5 Ebola haemorrhagic fever

The Ebola virus disease was first observed in 1976 in southern Sudan (in the vicinity of the Ebola River) and northern Zaire. Altogether, 14 outbreaks have been reported. Apart from in Sudan, Ebola infections are frequent in the Congo and in Gabun. The incubation period is seven to ten days. Both the course of disease and the virus itself closely resemble the Marburg virus, although it is a virus in its own right and related to the filovirus species. Clinical findings include generalized pain, pharyngitis, conjunctivitis, bronchitis, exanthema and enanthema. Death usually occurs on the ninth day. The mortality rate of this haemorrhagic fever with pronounced hepatic damage (focal necrosis) was between 51% and 89%. (93, 98, 103, 105, 107) (s. fig. 23.5)

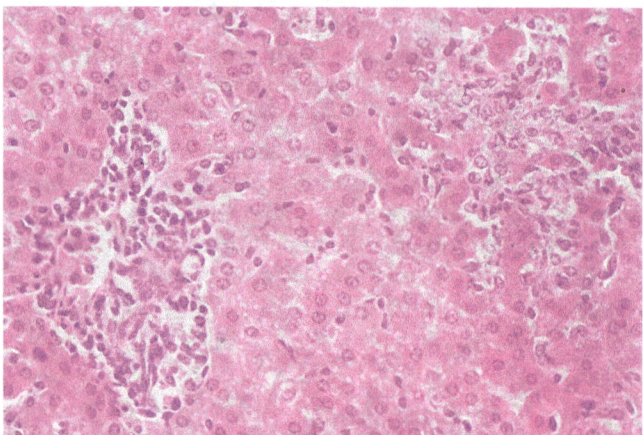

Fig. 23.5: Portal (left) and parenchymal (right) round-cell inflammation. Clinical diagnosis: Ebola fever (HE)

2.6 Lassa haemorrhagic fever

Lassa fever was first identified in 1969 in a missionary in Lassa (Nigeria). (94) The disease is also endemic in eastern Sierra Leone. Over 100,000 people worldwide contract the disease every year. A single-strand RNA virus of the arena group was isolated and characterized as the pathogen. (94) The disease is transmitted by rats. The incubation period is 3–16 days. • It manifests as haemorrhagic fever with ulcerous inflammation in the throat and mouth cavity, arthralgia, exanthema, alopecia, hearing impairment, lymphadenopathy as well as haemorrhages. In endemic areas, diagnosis is generally based (approx. 80% of cases) upon the *triad* (*1.*) fever and pharyngitis, (*2.*) proteinuria, and (*3.*) retrosternal pain. • The *liver* displays distinct acidophilic necrosis, frequently bridging necroses, and bleeding. Pronounced Kupffer-cell hyperplasia is evident. Deposits of lipofuscin are found. The transaminases and GDH are markedly increased; the blood count shows leucopenia and thrombopenia. The course is anicteric as a rule. Hepatosplenomegaly is present. The diagnosis is confirmed by the presence of IgM antibodies. Mortality is 35–40%. • Ribavirin has proved successful as therapy. There is still no vaccine available. (97, 100, 111, 116)

2.7 Rift Valley fever

This condition was first observed in the valley of the same name in Kenya in 1913. Since a wide-spread epidemic in 1931, this disease has spread across sub-Saharan Africa. The pathogen is a phlebovirus (single-strand RNS, 90–100 nm) and belongs to the family of Bunyaviridae. The virus infects ruminants and causes haemorrhagic fever with a lethality of 70–80%. • The disease is transmitted to humans by different species of mosquito, and by direct contact with infected animals; There is also an airborne path of transmission. The incubation period is 3 to 7 (to 12) days. As from the fourth day, diagnosis is possible by serology and PCR.

In most cases the course is moderate and influenza-like. However, patients also have a high temperature, headaches and myalgia. *Acute hepatitis* can occur, sometimes with pronounced liver cell necroses. Severe courses of the disease with meningitis, retinitis and haemorrhages as well as with *fulminant hepatitis* (110, 112) have been observed. Generally, prognosis is favourable. Treatment can be attempted with ribavirin. A well-tolerated vaccine is available.

References

Epstein-Barr virus
1. **Allen, U.R., Bass, B.H.:** Fatal hepatic necrosis in glandular fever. J. Clin. Path. 1963; 16: 337–341
2. **Bang, J., Wanscher, O.:** The histopathology of the liver in infectious mononucleosis complicated by jaundice, investigated by aspiration biopsy. Acta Med. Scand. 1945; 120: 437–446
3. **Devereaux, C.E., Bemiller, T., Brann, O.:** Ascites and severe hepatitis complicating Epstein-Barr infection. Amer. J. Gastroenterol. 1999; 94: 236–240
4. **Drebber, U., Kasper, H.U., Krupacz, J., Haferkamp, K., Kern, M.A., Steffen, H.M., Quasdorff, M., zur Hausen, A., Odenthal, M., Dienes, H.P.:** The role of Epstein-Barr virus in acute and chronic hepatitis. J. Hepatol. 2006; 44: 879–885
5. **Edoute, Y., Baruch, Y., Lachter, J., Furman, E., Bassan, L., Assy, N.:** Case report: Severe cholestatic jaundice induced by Epstein-Barr virus infection in the elderly. J. Gastroenterol. Hepatol. 1998; 13: 821–824
6. **Fuhrmann, S.A., Gill, R., Horwitz, C.A., Henle, W., Henle, G., Kravitz, G., Baldwin, J., Tombers, J.:** Marked hyperbilirubinemia in infectious mononucleosis. Arch. Intern. Med. 1987; 147: 850–853
7. **Harries, J.T., Ferguson, A.W.:** Fatal infectious mononucleosis with liver failure in two sisters. Arch. Dis. Child. 1968; 43: 480–485
8. **Hinedi, T.B., Koff, R.S.:** Cholestatic hepatitis induced by Epstein-Barr virus infection in an adult. Dig. Dis. Sci. 2003; 48: 539–541
9. **Jacobson, I.M., Gang, D.L., Schapiro, R.H.:** Epstein-Barr viral hepatitis: an unusual case and review of the literature. Amer. J. Gastroenterol. 1984; 79: 628–632
10. **Langnas, A.N., Markin, R.S., Inagaki, M., Stratta, R.J., Sorrell, M.F., Donovan, J.P., Shaw, B.W. jr.:** Epstein-Barr virus hepatitis after liver transplantation. Amer. J. Gastroenterol. 1994; 89: 1066–1070
11. **Markin, R.S.:** Manifestations of Epstein-Barr virus-associated disorders in liver. Liver 1994; 14: 1–13
12. **Papatheodoridis, G.V., Delladetsima, J.K., Kavallierou, L., Kapranos, N., Tassopoulos, N.C.:** Fulminant hepatitis due to Epstein-Barr virus infection. J. Hepatol. 1995; 23: 348–350
13. **Shaw, N.J., Evans, J.H.:** Liver failure and Epstein-Barr virus infection. Arch. Dis. Childh. 1988; 63: 432–433
14. **Vento, S., Guella, L., Murandola, F., Cainelli, F., Di Perri, G., Solbiati, M., Ferraro, T., Concia, E.:** Epstein-Barr virus as trigger for autoimmune hepatitis in susceptible individuals. Lancet 1995; 346: 608–609
15. **White, N.J., Juel-Jensen, B.E.:** Infectious mononucleosis hepatitis. Semin. Liver Dis. 1984; 4: 301–306
16. **Wills, E.J.:** Electron microscopy of the liver in infectious mononucleosis hepatitis and cytomegalovirus hepatitis. Amer. J. Dis. Childh. 1972; 123: 301–303
17. **Yamada, K., Yamada, H.:** Gallbladder wall thickening in mononucleosis syndromes. J. Clin. Ultrasound 2001; 29: 322–325

Herpes viruses
18. **Asano, Y., Yoshikawa, T., Suga, S., Yazaki, T., Kondo, K., Yamanishi, K.:** Fatal fulminant hepatitis in an infant with human herpesvirus-6 infection. Lancet 1990; 335: 862–863
19. **Dienes, H.P., Schirmacher, P., Weise, K., Falke, D.:** Herpes simplex virus hepatitis and related problems. Int. Rev. Exper. Path. 1994; 35: 2–38
20. **Fingeroth, J.D.:** Herpesvirus infection of the liver. Infect. Dis. North Amer. 2000; 14: 689–719
21. **Fink, C.G., Read, S.J., Hopkin, J., Peto, T., Gould, S., Kurtz, J.B.:** Acute herpes hepatitis in pregnancy. J. Clin. Pathol. 1993; 46: 968–971
22. **Goodman, Z.D., Ishak, K.G., Sesterhenn, I.A.:** Herpes simplex hepatitis in apparently immunocompetent adults. Amer. J. Clin. Path. 1986; 85: 694–699
23. **Härmä, M., Höckerstedt, K., Lautenschlager, I.:** Human herpesvirus-6 and acute liver failure. Transplantation 2003; 76: 536–539
24. **Hamory, B.H., Luger, A., Kobbermann, T.:** Herpesvirus hominis hepatitis of mother and newborn infant. South Med. J. 1981; 74: 992–995
25. **Ichai, P., Roque Alfonso, A.M., Gonzales, M.E. Codes, L., Azoulay, D., Saliba, F., Karam, V., Dussaix, E., Guettier, C., Castaing, D., Samuel, D.:** Herpes simplex virus-associated acute liver failure. A difficult diagnosis with a poor prognosis. Liver Transplant. 2005; 11: 1550–1555
26. **Kaufman, B., Gandhi, S.A., Louie, E., Rizzi, R., Illei, P.:** Herpes simplex virus hepatitis: case report and review. Clin. Infect. Dis. 1997; 24: 334–338

27. **Klein, N.A., Mabie, W.C., Shaver, D.C., Latham, P.S., Adamec, T.A., Pinstein, M.L., Riely, C.A.:** Herpes simplex virus hepatitis in pregnancy. Two patients successfully treated with acyclovir. Gastroenterology 1991; 100: 239–244
28. **Lüchtrath, H., Totovic, V., Deleon, F.:** A case of fulminant Herpes simplex hepatitis in an adult. Path. Res. Pract. 1984; 179: 235–241
29. **Markin, R.S., Langnas, A.N., Donovan, J.P., Zetterman, R.K., Stratta, R.J.:** Opportunistic viral hepatitis in liver transplant recipients. Transplant. Proc. 1991; 23: 1520–1512
30. **Marret, S., Buffet-Janvresse, C., Metayer, J., Fessard, C.:** Herpes simplex hepatitis with chronic cholestasis in a newborn. Acta Paed. 1993; 82: 321–323
31. **McCalmont, T.H., McLeod, D.L., Kerr, R.M., Hopkins, M.B., Geisinger, K.R.:** Fatal disseminated herpesvirus infection with hepatitis. Arch. Pathol. Labor. 1994; 118: 566–567
32. **Peters, D.J., Greene, W.H., Ruggiero, F., McGarrity, T.J.:** Herpes simplex-induced fulminant hepatitis in adults. A call for empiric therapy. Dig. Dis. Sci. 2000; 45: 2399–2404
33. **Pinna, A.D., Rakela, J., Demetris, A.J., Fung, J.J.:** Five cases of fulminant hepatitis due to herpes simplex virus in adults. Dig. Dis. Sci. 2002; 47: 750–754
34. **Rubin, M.H., Ward, D.M., Painter, J.:** Fulminant hepatic failure caused by genital herpes in a healthy person. J. Amer. Med. Ass. 1985; 253: 1299–1301
35. **Sharma, S., Mosunjac, M.:** Herpes simplex hepatitis in adults. A search for muco-cutaneous clues. J. Clin. Gastroenterol. 2004; 38: 697–704
36. **Tajiri, H., Nose, O., Baba, K., Okada, S.:** Human herpesvirus-6 infection with liver injury in neonatal hepatitis. Lancet 1990; 335: 863.
37. **Verma, A., Dhawan, A., Zuckerman, M., Hadzic, N., Baker, A.J., Mieli-Vergagni, G.:** Neonatal herpes simplex virus infection presenting as acute liver failure. Prevalent role of herpes simplex virus type I. J. Pediatr. Gastroenterol. Nutrit. 2006; 42: 282–286
38. **Wolfsen, H.C., Bolen, J.W., Bowen, J.L., Fenster, L.F.:** Fulminant herpes hepatitis mimicking hepatic abscesses. J. Clin. Gastroenterol. 1993; 16: 61–64

Varicella-zoster virus
39. **Anderson, D.R., Schwartz, J., Hunter, N.J., Cottrill, C., Bisaccia, E., Klainer, A.S.:** Varicella hepatitis: a fatal case in a previously healthy, immunocompetent adult. Arch. Intern. Med. 1994; 154: 2101–2106
40. **Eshchar, J., Reif, L., Waron, M., Alkan, W.J.:** Hepatic lesion in chickenpox. A case report. Gastroenterology 1973; 64: 462–466
41. **Ey, J.L., Smith, S.M., Fulginiti, V.A.:** Varicella hepatitis without neurologic symptoms or findings. Pediatrics 1981; 67: 285–287
42. **Myers, M.G.:** Hepatic cellular injury during varicella. Arch. Dis. Child. 1982; 57: 317–319
43. **Patti, M.E., Selvaggi, K.J., Kroboth, F.J.:** Varicella hepatitis in the immunocompromised adult: a case report and review of the literature. Amer. J. Med. 1990; 88: 77–80
44. **Pishvaian, A.C., Bahrain, M., Lewis, J.H.:** Fatal varizella-zoster hepatitis presenting with severe aldominal pain: A case report and review of the literature. Dig. Dis. Sci. 2006; 51: 1221–1225
45. **Pitel, P.A., McCormick, K.L., Fitzgerald, E., Orson, J.M.:** Subclinical hepatic changes in varicella infection. Pediatrics 1980; 65: 631–633
46. **Reinecke, P., Arning, M., Löhler, J., Bürrig, K.-F.:** Varizellenhepatitis. Pathologe 1990; 11: 208–214

Cytomegalovirus
47. **Amitrano, L., Guardascione, M.A., Scaglione, M., Menchise, A., Romano, L., Balzano, A.:** Acute portal and mesenteric thrombosis: unusual presentation of cytomegalovirus infection (case report) Eur. J. Gastroenterol. Hepatol. 2006; 18: 443–445
48. **Bonkowsky, H.C., Lee, R.V., Klatskin, G.:** Acute granulomatous hepatitis: occurrence in cytomegalovirus mononucleosis. J. Amer. Med. Ass. 1975; 233: 1284–1288
49. **Clarke, J., Craig, R.M., Saffro, R., Murphy, P., Yokoo, H.:** Cytomegalovirus granulomatous hepatitis. Amer. J. Med. 1979; 66: 264–269
50. **Finegold, M.J., Carpenter, R.J.:** Obliterative cholangitis due to cytomegalovirus: A possible precursor to paucity of intrahepatic bile ducts. Hum. Path. 1982; 13: 662–665
51. **Ghishan, F.K., Greene, H.L., Halter, S., Bernard, J.A., Moran, J.R.:** Non-cirrhotic portal hypertension in congenital cytomegalovirus infection. Hepatology 1984; 4: 684–686
52. **Griffiths, P.D.:** Cytomegalovirus and the liver. Semin. Liver Dis. 1984; 4: 307–313
53. **Kanji, S.S., Sharara, A.I., Clavien, P.A., Hamilton, J.D.:** Cytomegalovirus infection following liver transplantation: review of the literature. Clin. Infect. Dis. 1996; 22: 537–549
54. **Kanno, A., Abe, M., Yamada, M., Murakami, K.:** Clinical and histological features of cytomegalovirus hepatitis in previously healthy adults. Liver 1997; 17: 129–132
55. **Laskus, T., Lupa, E., Cianciara, J., Slusarczyk, J.:** Cytomegalovirus infection presenting as hepatitis. Digestion 1990; 47: 167–171
56. **Miguelez, M., Gonzalez, A., Perez, F.:** Severe cytomegalovirus hepatitis in a pregnant woman treated with ganciclovir. Scand. J. Gastroenterol. 1998; 30: 304–305
57. **Snover, D.C., Horwitz, C.A.:** Liver disease in cytomegalovirus mononucleosis: A light microscopical and immunoperoxidase study of six cases. Hepatology 1984; 4: 408–412
58. **Tanaka, S., Toh, Y., Minagawa, H., Mori, R., Sugimachi, K., Minamishima, Y.:** Reactivation of cytomegalovirus in patients with cirrhosis: analysis of 122 cases. Hepatology 1992; 16: 1409–1414
59. **Vanstapel, M.J., Desmet, V.J.:** Cytomegalovirus hepatitis: A histological and immunohistological study. Appl. Path. 1983; 1: 41–49

Togaviruses
60. **Arai, M., Wada, N., Maruyama, K., Nomiyama, T., Tanaka, S., Okazaki, I.:** Acute hepatitis in an adult with acquired rubella infection. J. Gastroenterol. 1995; 30: 539–542
61. **Hohenegger, M., Zeitlhofer, J.:** Clinical and morphological investigations regarding liver changes in early summer meningoencephalitis. Wien. Zschr. Inn. Med. 1965; 46: 486–492
62. **Kalo, T., Leport, C., Vilde, J.L.:** L'atteinte hépatique au cours de la rubéole acquise. Etude chez 10 malades. Med. Mal. Infect. 1991; 21: 241–243
63. **McLellan, R.K., Gleiner, R.A.:** Acute hepatitis in an adult with rubeola. J. Amer. Med. Ass. 1982; 247: 2000–2001
64. **Onji, M., Kumon, I., Kanaoka, M., Miyaoka, H., Ohta, Y.:** Intrahepatic lymphocyte subpopulations in acute hepatitis in an adult with rubella. Amer. J. Gastroenterol. 1988; 83: 320–322
65. **Strauss, L., Bernstein, J.:** Neonatal hepatitis in congenital rubella. A histopathological study. Arch. Pathol. 1968; 86: 317–327
66. **Tameda, Y., Kosaka, Y., Shiraki, K., Ohashi, Y., Hamada, M., Miyazaki, M., Ito, N., Takase, K., Nakano, T.:** Hepatitis in an adult with rubella. Intern. Med. 1993; 32: 580–583
67. **Zeldis, J.B., Miller, J.G., Dienstag, J.L.:** Hepatitis in an adult with rubella. Amer. J. Med. 1985; 79: 515–516

Coxsackie virus
68. **Brmbolic, B., Jevtovic, D., Zerjav, S., Surakovic, V.:** Fitz-Hugh Curtis syndrome. Presentation of a case. Gastroenterohepatol. Arh. 1990; 9: 137–139
69. **Morris, J.A., Elisberg, B.L., Pond, W.L., Webb, P.A.:** Hepatitis associated with Coxsackie virus group A, type 4. New Engl. J. Med. 1962; 267: 1230–1233
70. **Sun, N.C., Smith, V.N.:** Hepatitis associated with myocarditis: unusual manifestation of infection with coxsackie virus group B, type 3. New Engl. J. Med. 1966; 274: 190–193
71. **Wang, S.M., Liu, C.C., Yang, Y.J., Yang, H.B., Lin, C.H., Wang, J.R.:** Fatal coxsackievirus B infection in early infancy characterized by fulminant hepatitis. J. Infect. 1998; 37: 270–273

ECHO virus
72. **Schleissner, L.A., Portnoy, B.:** Hepatitis and pneumonia associated with ECHO virus, type 9 infection in two adult siblings. Ann. Intern. Med. 1968; 68: 1315–1319

Paramyxoviruses
73. **Berry, T.J.:** Hepatic damage associated with measles. Pen. Med. J. 1960; 63: 995–999
74. **Fimmel, C.J., Guo, L.S., Compans, R.W., Brunt, E.M., Hickman, S., Perrillo, R.R., Mason, A.L.:** A case of syncytial giant-cell hepatitis with features of a paramyxoviral infection. Amer. J. Gastroenterol. 1998; 93: 1931–1937
75. **Gavish, D., Kleinman, Y., Morag, A., Chajek-Shaul, T.:** Hepatitis and jaundice associated with measles in young adults. An analysis of 65 cases. Arch. Intern. Med. 1983; 143: 674–677
76. **Krech, R.H., Greenen, V., Maschek, H., Högemann, B.:** Adult giant cell hepatitis with fatal course. Clinical pathology case report and reflections on the pathogenesis. Pathologe 1998; 19: 221–225
77. **Phillips, M.J., Blendis, L.M., Poucel, S., Patterson, J., Petric, M., Roberts, E., Levy, G.A., Superina, R.A., Greig, P.D., Cameron, R., Langer, B., Purcell, R.H.:** Sporadic hepatitis with distinctive pathological features, a severe clinical course, and paramyxoviral features. New Engl. J. Med. 1991; 324: 455–466
78. **Siegel, D., Hirschman, S.Z.:** Hepatic dysfunction in acute measles infection of adults. Arch. Intern. Med. 1977; 137: 1178–1179
79. **Tordjmann, T., Grimbert, S., Genestie, C., Freymuth, F., Guettier, C., Callard, P., Trinchet, J.-C., Beaugrand, M.:** Hépatite à cellules multinucléées de l'adulte. Etude chez 17 malades. Gastroenterol. Clin. Biol. 1998; 22: 305–310

Adenovirus
80. **Carmichael, G.P., Zahradnik, J.M., Moyer, G.H., Porter, D.D.:** Adenovirus hepatitis in an immunosuppressed adult patient. Amer. J. Clin. Path. 1979; 71: 352–355
81. **Saad, R.S., Demetris, A.G., Lee, R.G., Kusne, S., Randhawa, P.S.:** Adenovirus hepatitis in the adult allograft liver. Transplantation 1997; 64: 1483–1485
82. **Varki, N.M., Bhuta, S., Drake, T., Porter, D.D.:** Adenovirus hepatitis in two successive liver transplants in a child. Arch. Path. Lab. Med. 1990; 114: 106–109

Human parvovirus B19
83. **Yoto, Y., Kudoh, T., Haseyama, K., Suzuki, N., Chiba, S.:** Human parvovirus B 19 infection associated with acute hepatitis. Lancet 1996; 347: 868–869

HIV hepatitis
84. **Bach, N., Theise, N.D., Schaffner, F.:** Hepatic histopathology in the acquired immunodeficiency syndrome. Semin. Liver Dis. 1992; 12: 205–212
85. **Cappell, M.S.:** Hepatobiliary manifestations of the acquired immune deficiency syndrome. Amer. J. Gastroenterol. 1991; 86: 1–15

86. Cello, J.P.: Human immunodeficiency virus-associated biliary tract disease. Semin. Liver Dis. 1992; 12: 213–218
87. Gordon, S.C., Reddy, K.R., Gould, E.E., McFadden, R., O'Brien, C., de Medina, M., Jeffers, L.J., Schiff, E.R.: The spectrum of liver disease in the acquired immunodeficiency syndrome. J. Hepatol. 1986; 2: 475–484
88. Lafon, M.-E., Kirn, A.: Human immunodeficiency virus infection of the liver. Semin. Liver Dis. 1992; 12: 197–204
89. Poles, M.A., Dieterich, D.T.: Infections of the liver in HIV-infected patients. Infect. Dis. Clin. North Amer. 2000; 14: 741–759
90. Trojan, A., Kreuzer, K.-A., Flury, R., Schmid, M., Schneider, J., Schröder, S.: Leberveränderungen bei AIDS. Retrospektive Analyse von 227 Sektionen HIV-positiver Patienten. Pathologe 1998; 19: 194–200

Exotic hepatotropic viruses
91. Adhikari-Prabha, M.R., Prabhu, M.G., Raghuveer, C.V., Bai, M., Mala, M.A.: Clinical study of 100 cases of Kyasanur Forest disease with clinicopathological correlation. Indian J. Med. 1993; 47: 124–130
92. Bechtelsheimer, H., Korb, G., Gedigk, P.: The morphology and pathogenesis of "Marburg Virus" Hepatitis. Human. Pathol. 1972; 3: 255–264
93. Bowen, E.T.W., Platt, G.S., Lloyd, G., Baskerville, A., Harris, W.J., Vella, E.E.: Viral haemorrhagic fever in southern Sudan and northern Zaire. Lancet 1977/II: 571–573
94. Buckley, S.M., Casals, J., Downs, W.G.: Isolation and antigenic characterization of Lassa virus. Nature 1970; 227: 174.
95. Couvelard, A., Marianneau, P., Bedel, C., Drouet, M.T., Vachon, F., Henin, D., Deubel, V.: Report of a fatal case of dengue infection with hepatitis: Demonstration of dengue antigens in hepatocytes and liver apoptosis. Hum. Pathol. 1999; 30: 1106–1110
96. De Filippis, A.M.B., Nogueira, R.M.R., Schatzmayr, H.G., Tavares, D.S., Jabor, A.V., Diniz, S.C.M., Oliveira, J.C., Moreira, E., Miagostovich, M.P., Costa, E.V., Galler, R.: Outbreak of jaundice and hemorrhagic fever in the Southeast of Brazil in 2001: detection and molecular characterization of yellow fever virus. J. Med. Virol. 2002; 68: 620–627
97. Edington, G.M., White, H.A.: The pathology of Lassa fever. Trans. R. Soc. Trop. Med. Hyg. 1972; 66: 381–389
98. Ellis, D.S., Simpson, D.I.H., Francis, D.P., Knobloch, J., Bowen, E.T.W., Lolik, P., Deng, I.M.: Ultrastructure of Ebola virus particles in human liver. J. Clin. Pathol. 1978; 31: 201–208
99. Fabre, A., Couvelard, A., Degott, C., Lagorce-Pages, C., Bruneel, F., Bouvet, E., Vachon, F.: Dengue virus induced hepatitis with chronic calcific changes (case report). Gut 2001; 49: 864–865
100. Frame, J.D., Baldwin, J.M., Gocke, D.J., Troup, J.M.: Lassa fever, a new virus disease of man from West Africa. I. Clinical descriptions and pathological findings. Amer. J. Trop. Med. Hyg. 1970; 19: 670–676
101. Francis, T.I., Moore, D.L., Edington, G.M., Smith, J.A.: A clinicopathological study of human yellow fever. Bull. WHO 1972; 46: 659–667
102. Gear, J.S.S., Cassel, G.A., Gear, A.J., Trappler, B., Clausen, L., Meyers, A.M., Kew, M.C., Bothwell, T.H., Sher, R., Miller, G.B., Schneider, J., Koornhoff, H.J., Gomperts, E.D., Isaäcson, M., Gear, J.H.S.: Outbreak of Marburg virus disease in Johannesburg. Brit. Med. J. 1975; 4: 489–493
103. Griffiths, P.D., Ellis, D.S., Zuckerman, A.J.: Other common types of viral hepatitis and exotic infections. Brit. Med. Bull. 1990; 46: 512–532
104. Hasler, C., Schorf, H., Enderlin, N., Gyr, K.: Imported dengue fever following a stay in the tropics. Schweiz. Med. Wschr. 1993; 123: 120–124
105. Howard, C.R., Ellis, D.S., Simpson, D.I.H.: Exotic viruses and the liver. Semin. Liver Dis. 1984; 4: 361–374
106. Huerre, M.R., Lan, N.T., Marianneau, P., Hue, N.B., Khun, H., Hung, N.T., Khen, N.T., Drouet, M.T., Huong, V.T.Q., Ha, DQ., Buisson, Y., Deubel, V.: Liver histopathology and biological correlates in five cases of fatal dengue fever in Vietnamese children. Virch. Arch. 2001; 438: 107–115
107. Johnson, K.M., Webb, P.A., Lange, J.V., Murphy, F.A.: Isolation and partial characterization of a new virus causing acute haemorrhagic fever in Zaire. Lancet 1977/II: 569–571
108. Korb, G., Slenczka, W., Bechtelsheimer, H., Gedigk, P.: Marburg virus hepatitis in animal experiments. Virch. Arch. A Path. Anat. 1971; 353: 169–184
109. Martini, G.A., Knauff, H.G., Schmidt, H.A., Mayer, G., Baetzer, G.: Über eine bisher unbekannte, von Affen eingeschleppte Infektionskrankheit: Marburg-Virus-Krankheit. Dtsch. Med. Wschr. 1968; 93: 559–571
110. McGarvan, M.H., Easterday, B.C.: Rift Valley fever virus hepatitis. Light and electron microscopic studies in the mouse. Amer. J. Path. 1963; 42: 587–607
111. McCormick, J.B., King, I.J., Webb, P.A., Scribner, C.L., Craven, R.B., Johnson, K.M., Elliot, L.H., Belmont-Williams, R.: Lassa fever. Effective therapy with Ribavirin. New Engl. J. Med. 1986; 314: 20–26
112. Mussgay, M.: Rift-valley fever. Dtsch. Med. Wschr. 1980; 105: 1265–1266
113. Rippey, J.J., Schepers, N.J., Gear, J.H.S.: The pathology of Marburg virus disease. S. Afr. Med. J. 1984; 66: 50–54
114. Smith, D.H., Johnson, B.K., Isaacson, M., Swanapoel, R., Johnson, K.M., Killey, M., Bagshawe, A., Siongok, T., Keruga, W.K.: Marburgvirus disease in Kenia. Lancet 1982: 816–820
115. Vieira, W.T., Gayotto, L.C., de Lima, C.P., de Brito, T.: Histopathology of the human liver in yellow fever with special emphasis on the diagnostic role of the Councilman body. Histopathology 1983; 7: 195–208
116. Winn, W.C.jr., Monath, T.P., Murphy, F.A., Whitfield, S.G.: Lassa virus hepatitis. Observations on a fatal case from the 1972 Sierra Leone epidemic. Arch. Path. 1975; 99: 599–604

Clinical Aspects of Liver Diseases
24 Bacterial infections and the liver

		Page:
1	*Pathogenesis*	484
2	*Types of lesion*	484
3	**Bacterial pathogens**	484
3.1	Pyogenic cocci	485
3.2	Neisseria gonorrhoea	485
3.3	Enterobacteriaceae	485
3.4	Mycobacteria	486
3.4.1	Mycobacterium tuberculosis	486
3.4.2	Mycobacterium scrofulaceum	487
3.4.3	Mycobacterium leprae	488
3.5	Spirochaetes	488
3.5.1	Leptospirosis	488
3.5.2	Syphilis	489
3.5.3	Borreliosis	490
3.6	Listeriosis	490
3.7	Brucellosis	490
3.8	Rickettsiosis	491
3.9	Tularaemia	491
3.10	Psittacosis	491
3.11	Clostridium welchii	491
3.12	Tropheryma whippeli	492
3.13	Campylobacter colitis	492
3.14	Rochalimaea	492
3.15	Actinomycosis	492
3.16	Burkholderia pseudomallei	492
	• References (1–148)	492
	(Figures 24.1–24.14; tables 24.1–24.3)	

24 Bacterial infections and the liver

A number of bacterial infections may affect the liver to varying degrees of intensity. The frequently observed liver involvement is attributed to a number of **causes:** (*1.*) size of this visceral parenchymatous organ, (*2.*) multiplicity and activity of the hepatic RES as a filtering system, (*3.*) double (portal and arterial) blood supply with transport of bacteria or their toxins, and (*4.*) lymphogenous spread of pathogenic organisms.

1 Pathogenesis

The pathogenesis of liver involvement in bacterial infections often remains unresolved. In this respect, **four pathomechanisms,** either alone or in combination, are assumed to play a role. (4, 9) (s. tab. 24.1)

1. Direct effects of pathogens • direct haematogenic spread • direct lymphogenous spread
2. Indirect effects of pathogens • toxins • endotoxins
3. Reactions due to the basic disease • hypoxaemia • fever, exsiccosis, acidosis • electrolyte imbalance, *etc.*
4. Therapy-induced liver damage

Tab. 24.1: Pathomechanisms of liver involvement in different bacterial diseases

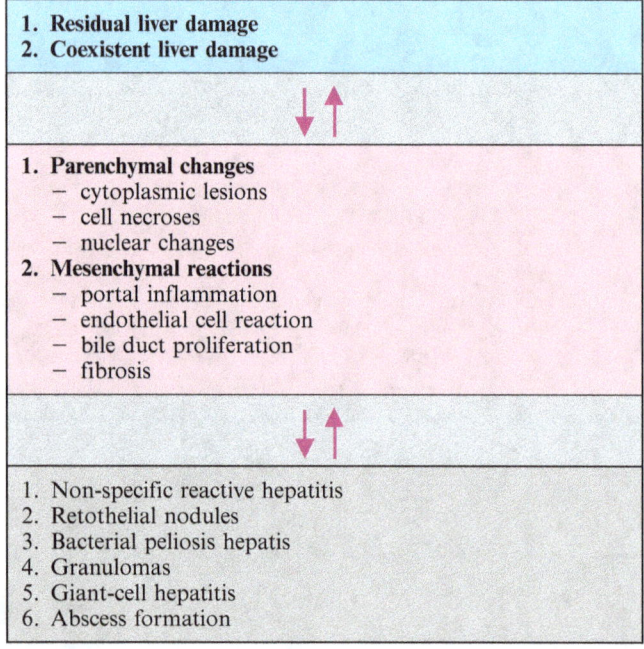

Tab. 24.2: Morphological reactions of the liver following various bacterial infections

2 Types of lesion

Liver involvement occurs in extrahepatically localized and generalized bacterial infections. Various **morphological reactions** depend on (*1.*) severity of infection, (*2.*) type of pathogen, (*3.*) respective morphological reaction of the liver, and (*4.*) possible previous liver damage – similar reactions also appear in viral hepatitis. Combined with the coexistence of scarred/fibrotic and chronic inflammatory liver changes, these acute infections may lead to morphological pictures that are difficult to interpret. The diversity of the morphological reactions may also be influenced by individual factors. (s. tab. 24.2)

3 Bacterial pathogens

The principal pathogenic agents causing liver damage are pyogenic cocci, gonococci, enteric bacteria, mycobacteria, spirochaetes, listeriae, brucellae, rickettsiae, chlamydiae and clostridiae. (4, 9) (s. tab. 24.3)

1. Pyogenic cocci – Pneumococci – Staphylococci – Streptococci				
2. Neisseria gonorrhoea		D		
3. Enterobacteriaceae – Escherichia coli – Shigella species – Salmonella species – Yersinia enterocolitica – Vibrio cholerae	(S) S S (S) S	D D D D D	E) E E E) E	
4. Mycobacteria – M. tuberculosis – M. scrofulaceum – M. leprae	 S	 D D D	 E E E	
5. Spirochaetes – Leptospira species – Treponema pallidum – Borrelia species	 P S	 D D D	 E E	
6. Listeriae	P	D	E	
7. Brucella species		D	E	
8. Rickettsia species	(S)	D	E	(R. prow.)
9. Francisella tularensis	S	D	E	
10. Chlamydia psittaci	S	D	E	
11. Clostridium species	(S)	D	E	(C. bot.)
12. Tropheryma whippeli				
13. Campylobacter jejuni	(S)	D	E)	
14. Rochalimaea species				
15. Actinomyces israelii				

Tab. 24.3: Various bacterial organisms causing liver damage. In Germany, **obligation for notification** is given in cases of suspicion (S), disease (D), exitus (E), or perinatal infection (P). But this varies from country to country. *If in doubt: contact the Public Health Department!*

3.1 Pyogenic cocci

Streptococcus pneumoniae: Infection with Streptococcus pneumoniae may cause toxic liver damage and pneumococcal hepatitis with focal necroses, leading to the corresponding laboratory findings. In lobar pneumonia, *jaundice (= biliary pneumonia)* frequently occurs in the so-called *grey hepatization stage*. In addition to predominantly bacterial haemolytic jaundice, increased transaminases (20%) and cholestasis (10%) are found. The condition always regresses completely. A *liver abscess* induced by pneumococci is a rare event. (5, 10)

Staphylococci, streptococci: In sepsis, toxic liver damage and portal granulocytic infiltration may be observed. Septic bacterial invasion of the liver mainly entails periportal, circumscribed and non-suppurative *septic foci* (s. fig. 24.1), and occasionally multiple microabscesses as well. (10) Cholestasis usually suggests a severe course of disease; likewise, prolonged jaundice generally points to a poor prognosis as far as the underlying disease is concerned. (1, 2, 6, 7, 11)

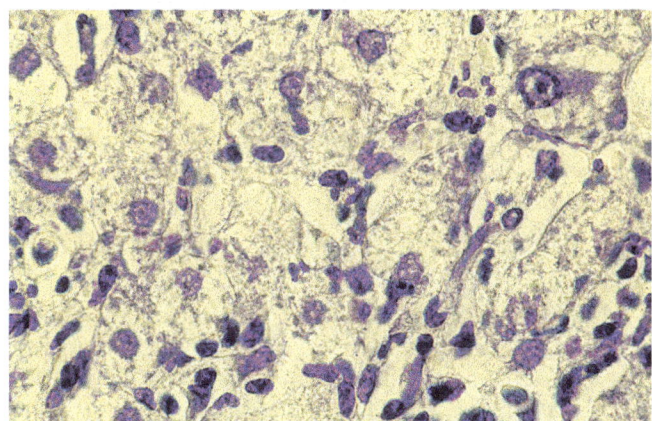

Fig. 24.1: Markedly altered, swollen hepatocytes. Focal intralobular accumulation of Kupffer cells, histiocytes and neutrophilic leucocytes. Clinical diagnosis: streptococcal sepsis (HE)

Myoplasma pneumoniae: This pathogen is classified between bacteria and viruses. It is a pleomorphic, immovable, and gram-negative germ, which is the cause of primary, atypical pneumonia. In rare cases, acute cholestatic hepatitis without lung involvement has been observed. (8)

3.2 Neisseria gonorrhoea

Gonococcal infection may lead to *toxic liver damage* or *concomitant hepatitis*, especially in the presence of gonococcal sepsis. Diagnosis of gonorrhoea is established by direct demonstration of pathogens (vaginal smear, liver tissue, liver capsule) or serologically by means of CFR (positive from the third week).

Acute gonorrhoeal perihepatitis: Of special relevance is a fibrinous inflammation of the subphrenic space without abscess formation, occurring as a sequel of gonorrhoeal adnexitis in women. It is also called the *Fitz-Hugh-Curtis syndrome* (A.H. Curtis, 1932; T. Fitz-Hugh, 1934), although it was first described by C. Stajano in Montevideo in 1920. Only two cases have so far been reported in men. Symptoms include severe epigastric pain (nearly always dextral), local peritonitis (dependent on respiration and movement), shoulder pain due to irritation of the phrenic nerve, and occasional friction rub. There are no other major subjective complaints or clinical findings. In the meantime, it has been demonstrated that, in addition to Neisseria gonorrhoeae, Chlamydiae and even Coxsackie virus B5 may also be responsible for this condition. (s. pp 477, 491) • A typical feature of the syndrome are the fine violin string-like adhesions between the liver surface and the abdominal wall, which are easily identified by means of laparoscopy. The syndrome can also be diagnosed retrospectively by laparoscopy through the detection of such lesions. (12–16)

▶ *In the one case that we observed, the patient was suffering from severe recurrent epigastric pain and had pathological, inflammation-related laboratory parameters. Following unsuccessful diagnostic efforts during an eight-month course, we were finally able to obtain a diagnosis by laparoscopy and confirm gonorrhoea as being the cause of the disease. (s. fig. 24.2)*

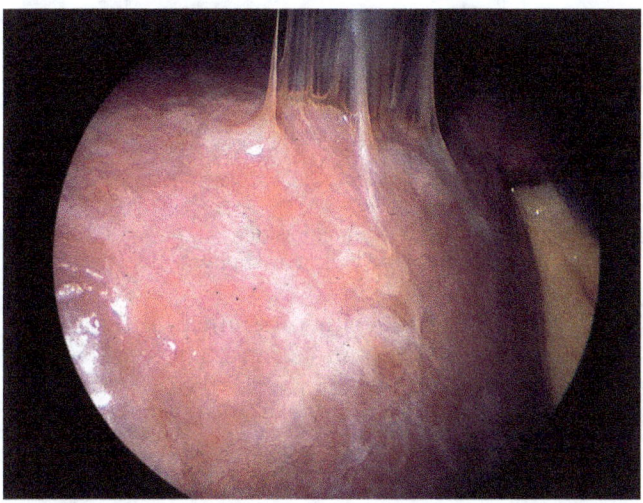

Fig. 24.2: Fitz-Hugh-Curtis syndrome: perihepatitis with violin string-like adhesions in gonorrhoeal infection

3.3 Enterobacteriaceae

Escherichia coli: In sepsis, occasionally massive endotoxinaemia may lead to major liver cell damage, accompanied by jaundice. Histologically, focal liver cell necrosis, giant-cell transformation, inflammatory infiltrations and signs of cholestasis are detectable. Escherichia coli is the most frequent cause of liver abscesses, followed by Friedländer's bacillus and Yersinia enterocolitica. In bacteraemia, a toxic shock syndrome can develop (2) with *cholangiolitis lenta* (M. Vyberg et al., 1984).

Salmonellosis: Infection with Salmonella paratyphi A, B or C can cause suppurative *cholangitis* with cholangiohepatitis, whereas Salmonella enteritidis mainly gives rise to *toxic hepatitis*. • In typhus abdominalis, hepatomegaly (20—30%) as well as an increase in transaminase and alkaline phosphatase activities are invariably observed from the second to third week after infection. Hyperbilirubinaemia is common, but manifest jaundice is rare. Histology may show signs of non-specific reactive hepatitis. Sometimes, submiliary nodules or *granulomas* (= *typhomas*) appear. Here, mainly intrasinusoidal proliferations of large plasma-rich cells with very small nuclei (so-called beef-like cells or typhoid cells) are found. These epithelioid cell clusters originating from reticular cells often contain multinuclear giant cells in their periphery. The toxic submiliary *typhoid nodules* (s. fig. 24.3), however, exhibit centroacinar necroses as well as proliferations of sinus endothelial cells and granulocytes with signs of regeneration. *Liver abscesses* have also been identified. (17, 18, 20, 21, 23, 25—27)

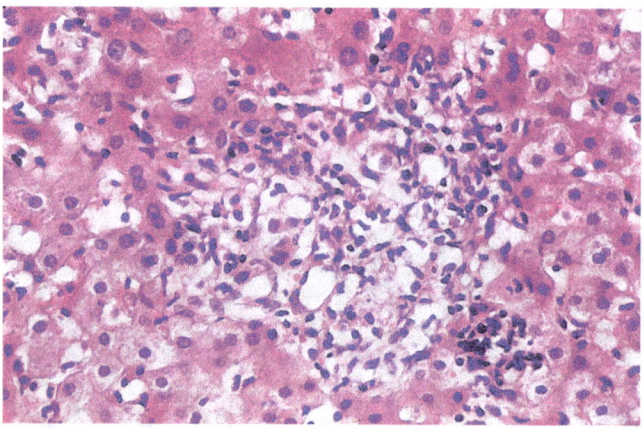

Fig. 24.3: Granuloma-like, lymphohistiocytic infiltrate in an area of parenchymal loss. Clinical diagnosis: typhus abdominalis (HE)

Ehrlichiosis: This infection is transmitted by the bite of a tick. The respective gram-negative, pleomorphic and intracellular organisms form inclusion bodies (= morula), in which they reproduce. They leave the cell by cytolysis. The incubation period is one week. Ehrlichiosis results in fever, chills, myalgia and panzytopenia. The transaminases are increased in 80—90% of cases. Histologically, it is possible to detect scattered lobular lymphohystiocytic foci, various diffuse infiltrations and Kupffer-cell hyperplasia with intense phagocytosis. Occasional injuries to the bile duct epithelium may also cause elevated AP activity. The development of liver abscesses can be observed. Laboratory findings and histology (which often vary in severity) suggest that host inflammatory or immune responses contribute to the liver injury. Therapy is based on doxycycline. (29)

Shigella: Infections with shigella are rarely accompanied by hepatitis. Direct involvement of the liver in the course of shigellosis is, however, to be feared, as first demonstrated by positive shigella identification from liver biopsy as early as 1910 (J. H. N. Knox Jr. et al.). Shigella-induced cholestatic hepatitis with jaundice and marked histological changes has likewise been reported. (22)

Yersinia enterocolitica: Infection with Y. enterocolitica or Y. pseudotuberculosis, together with haematogenous spread, may lead to a septic-typhoid course with hepatic and splenic abscess formation. Especially ulcerative colitis was frequently found to favour the formation of multiple *liver abscesses*. A genetic disposition is assumed in the presence of the HLA-B 27 gene. Patients with hepatic overload of iron are at special risk of Yersinia infection, since iron plays a major role in the metabolism of Yersinia. (19, 24, 28, 31, 32)

3.4 Mycobacteria

3.4.1 Mycobacterium tuberculosis

Tuberculous hepatic infections are transmitted **prenatally** and **perinatally** via the umbilical vein or the amniotic fluid; maternal placenta tuberculosa is a precondition for both infections. • The hepatic artery, portal vein and hepatopetal lymph vessels serve as **postnatal infection routes.**

1. The **tuberculous primary complex** in the liver with caseation of the associated hepatic hilar lymph nodes may become the source of spread causing early systemic generalization. Given the clinical picture of a coarse-nodular or a miliary tuberculosis, this may result in the death of the newborn child. (42, 51)

2. **Miliary tuberculosis** results in an attack on the liver by clustered miliary tubercles. They are visible on the liver surface using laparoscopy. (35, 40, 52, 56) GPT, GOT, GDH and AP are moderately increased. Clinical manifestations include severe malaise, hepato(spleno)megaly and fever — the cause of the latter often remain unclear for a long time. The haematogenous spread, occurring as intermittent episodes, provokes a number of small *tuberculous liver foci*. They show central caseation and fibrinoid necrosis. In the periphery, a corona of epithelioid cells of variable diameter is found, in which Langhans' giant cells are embedded. (s. fig. 24.4)

These granulomatous tubercles are surrounded by a loose rim of lymphocytes. Massive miliary spread to the liver may also cause acute liver failure (35, 46) as well as septic shock with multiorgan insufficiency. (56)

3. **Tuberculomas** can develop through enlargement and subsequent confluence of the miliary foci or tubercles as well as through nodular development of tuberculous foci in the tertiary stage. They appear as nodules with a diameter of 1—4 cm. Embedded calcifications are typical features of tuberculomas. They may penetrate bile ducts and cause *tuberculous cholangitis* with bile-duct stricture. (43, 44, 50, 52) These major tuberculous nodes become encapsulated in the course of time; the caseous

necrosis can still contain tubercle bacilli in its interior. The nodes are sometimes the source of haematogenic spread. They may also decompose as a result of caseous necrosis and thus lead to hepatic cavities such as *tuberculous abscesses* (47, 48, 52, 59, 64) or gravitation abscesses. Diagnosis of a liver abscess therefore includes differentiation from tuberculosis. Differential diagnosis from *pseudotumoural liver tuberculosis* is very difficult, even when using imaging techniques. (33, 34, 36−39, 41, 43, 45, 49, 53−55, 57, 58, 60−62, 67) (s. figs. 24.4, 24.5, 24.6)

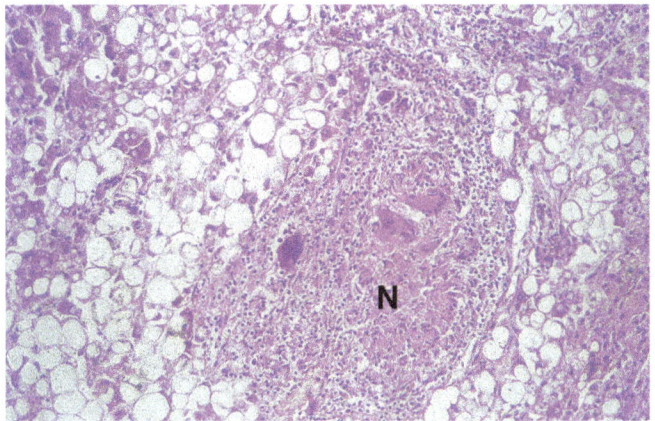

Fig. 24.4: Tuberculous epithelioid cell granuloma with Langhans' giant cells and small central necrosis (N); additional steatosis of hepatocytes (HE)

In the course of healing, miliary tuberculosis or small diffuse disseminated foci give rise to scarred transformation with the morphological picture of *tuberculous pseudocirrhosis* as a result of vascularization, fibroblasts and histiocytic connective tissue. As a rule, however, no major hepatic dysfunction results from the cicatrization of the healing process, which no longer (or barely) exhibits the specific character of granulation tissue.

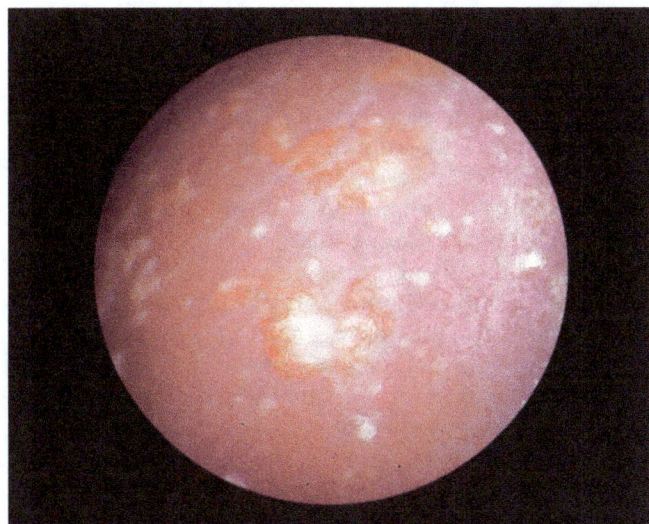

Fig. 24.5: Small nodular hepatic tuberculosis: foci, the size of a millet seed up to that of a lentil, in the right lobe of liver

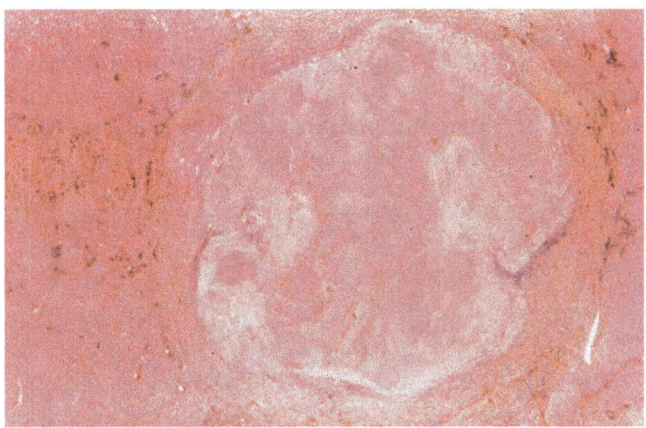

Fig. 24.6: Old intrahepatic tuberculoma. Encapsulated eosinophilic necrosis with marked caseation (HE)

4. Non-specific **toxic liver damage** may be evident; in this connection, possible tuberculostatic toxic effects must also be considered. With severe courses of tuberculosis, *peliosis hepatis* is often observed. Frequently, *retothelial nodules* are detectable, as demonstrated for the first time in tuberculosis patients by H. HAMPERL in 1953. (52) In the course of chronic pulmonary tuberculosis, *fatty infiltration of liver cells* was noted, as reported in several publications. (52) It was attributed to toxic effects and/or undernourishment or malnutrition. Secondary *hepatic amyloidosis*, developing in the course of chronic lung tuberculosis, has also been postulated. (52) A restriction of *hepatic function* in chronic tuberculosis, which was first observed by E. LEURET et al. in 1922, has been described in several studies. (53, 62, 65) Depending on the severity and duration of the disease as well as the tuberculostatic pretreatment, we found pathological laboratory parameters in 15−20% and 25−40% of cases respectively. (52)

If laboratory tests and imaging techniques have proved unsuccessful, it is only possible to obtain a reliable *diagnosis* and differentiation of the multiple manifestations of liver tuberculosis by means of laparoscopy and targeted biopsy. (64) (s. tab. 7.11) (s. figs. 7.11; 24.5, 24.6) Hepatic miliary tuberculosis is recognizable with the help of percutaneous biopsy in more than 90% of cases due to the dense arrangement of the foci. The aim should always be to demonstrate the presence of tubercle bacilli in the liver tissue, either directly or by culture (higher sensitivity can be obtained using PCR). (37) • *Treatment* consists of a fourfold combination: isoniazid (5 mg/kg BW/day), rifampicin (10 mg/kg BW/day), pyrazinamide (30 mg/kg BW/day), ethambutol (20 mg/kg BW/day) generally for 2−4 months, subsequently isoniazid + rifampicin for 6−12 months.

3.4.2 Mycobacterium scrofulaceum

Mycobacterium scrofulaceum may cause **granulomatous hepatitis**. Clinical findings include a clear increase in alkaline phosphatase as well as fever and general malaise. Diagnosis is confirmed by positive culture of the pathogen in liver biopsy specimens. (63) • Other **atypical mycobacteria** may also cause liver damage, possibly in the form of granulomatous hepatitis, above all in AIDS (20–50% of cases). (60) (s. fig. 24.7)

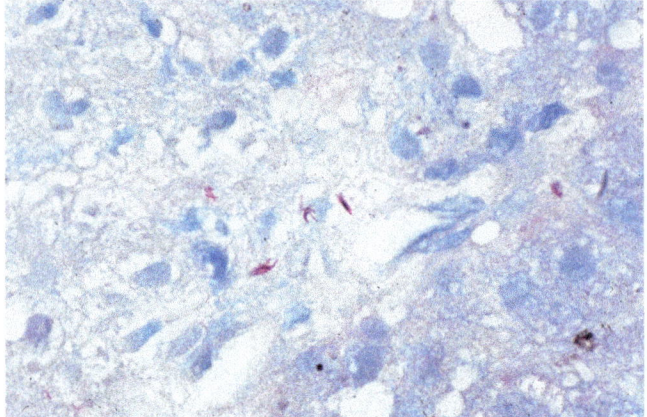

Fig. 24.7: Acid-fast bazilli of mycobacterium tuberculosis in the liver of an AIDS patient (Fite staining)

3.4.3 Mycobacterium leprae

Worldwide, about 500,000 people are suffering from leprosy; this number is steadily falling. The transmission route is via aerosolized drops emitted by nasal mucosa. Normal skin cannot be penetrated by the pathogen. The bacteria show tropism to macrophages and Schwann's cells. The incubation period is two to four years. A mere 5% of those who become contaminated are actually infected. Of these, no more than 25% develop the disease.

In lepromatous leprosy with a high germ count, the liver is affected in 50–90% of cases. Glisson's capsule is thickened and whitish. The number of *lepra granulomas* in the liver, which appear in the form of yellowish nodules, may be high enough to justify the term granulomatous hepatitis. Initially, these granulomas consist of histiocytic and lymphocytic infiltrates, which contain lepra bacteria in approximately 75% of cases. The lepra bacteria can be identified above all in Kupffer cells. Eventually, the characteristic bacteria-phagocytizing leprotic cells are formed (so-called *foam cells* or Virchow cells). These large-cell lepra granulomas are localized predominantly in the portal tract and show a tendency to central caseation. (s. fig. 24.8)

The *treatment regimen* consists of diphenylsulphone, clofazimine and rifampicin in combination for 6 to 24 months or longer (depending on the course of the disease). Thalidomide has also proved effective. • *BCG vaccination* is an effective prophylactic measure against infection induced by Mycobacterium leprae. (68–70)

3.5 Spirochaetes

3.5.1 Leptospirosis

▶ In 1886 A. WEIL reported four patients with an acute, highly feverish, infectious disease, accompanied by icterus and a high mortality rate. This disease was termed **icterus infectiosus Weil**. In 1915 R. INADA et al. in Japan and P. UHLENHUT et al. in Germany discovered virtually at the same time that the **Leptospira icterogenes** (or L. icterohaemorrhagica) were pathogenic agents (S. interrogans).

About 180 serotypes have been identified, all of which are generally pathogenic for humans and may provoke Weil's disease. • *Reservoir hosts* include rats, mice, hedgehogs, hamsters and various domesticated animals. Leptospirosis is therefore a globally distributed zoonosis. • *Transmission* to humans occurs via the oral or percutaneous route with small skin or mucosal lesions serving as portals of entry for the pathogens, which are excreted in the urine of infected animals.

Leptospirosis (Weil's disease) has an incubation period of 7 to 14 days. Subsequently, the septicaemic phase sets in with fever, chills, myalgia, arthralgia, headaches, haemorrhagic conjunctivitis, abdominal pain, vomiting and renal involvement (erythrocyturia, proteinuria). Histologically, interstitial nephritis with tubular necrosis is evident. • In a few days, icterus, hepatomegaly, increased transaminase activity and haemorrhagic diathesis occur, especially in severe cases. Histology reveals focal centrilobular lesions (acidophilic degeneration, turbid swelling), lymphocytic infiltration of the portal tract, stellate cell proliferation, bile thrombi in the canaliculi and active hepatocyte mitosis. The histological picture corresponds to that of *cholestatic hepatitis* (cholestasis is usually not verifiable by laboratory tests). • Identification of pathogens is performed in blood and CSF (first week) and in the urine (second week); increasing antibody titres (up to four times the norm) are detectable in the serum as from the second week. Proof of specific IgM is possible. • As the disease advances, a typical iridocyclitis as well as meningitis or encephalomyelitis with brain oedema can appear. Convalescence, which may take a long time, is characterized

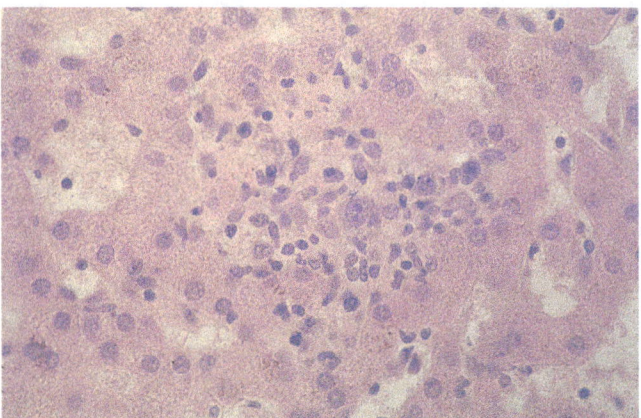

Fig. 24.8: Lepra: granuloma-like, lymphohistiocytic infiltration in the liver parenchyma (HE)

by adynamia and loss of hair. Mortality ranges from 4 to 50%, depending on the course — anicteric or icteric — and is mostly due to renal insufficiency. The recommended *therapy* consists of penicillin (10—20 million U/day) or doxycycline (2 × 100 mg/day). (71—75)

▶ We observed a lethal case (treatment with doxycycline was unsuccesful) showing massive amounts of leptospirae in the serum and in the centrifuged urine under dark-field examination. Maximum values were: GPT 4,200 U/l, GOT 2,290 U/l, GDH 1,080 U/l, serum bilirubin 11 mg/dl and Quick's value 17%, but with normal AP (!); such pathological levels have repeatedly been reported in the literature. Autopsy revealed severe interstitial nephritis, tubular necrosis (laboratory findings corresponding to severe renal insufficiency), brain oedema (680 g), severe hepatic dystrophy with marked centrozonal necroses and diffuse small-droplet fatty degeneration of the liver cells as well as haemorrhagic organ lesions. (s. fig. 24.9)

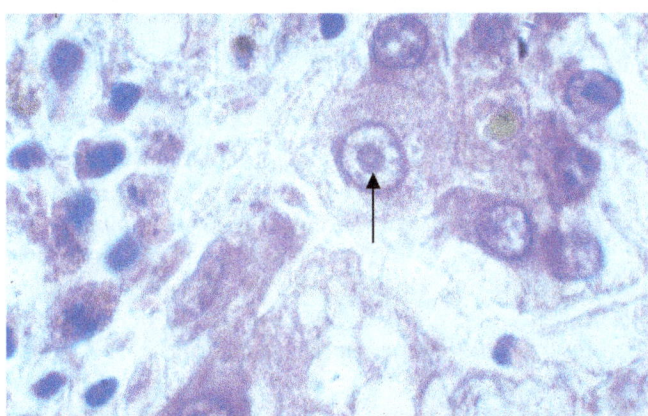

Fig. 24.9: Enlargement of hepatocytes with large nucleoles (arrow), distinct icterus with (green) bile thrombi in the biliary capillaries and hepatocytes. Multivacuolar steatosis of isolated liver cells. Groups of histiocytes (left) with phagocytized nuclear material and lipofuscin. Clinical diagnosis: Weil's disease (HE)

3.5.2 Syphilis

The coexistence of jaundice and syphilis was described by PARACELSUS as early as 1585. • In all stages of congenital or acquired syphilis, liver involvement is possible. The **pathogen** (anaerobic, gram-negative) is very sensitive to environmental factors and perishes rapidly. The period of cellular fission is 36 hours. Treponema pallidum is occasionally verifiable in histological preparations as corkscrew-shaped structures, 6—10 µm in length and 0.2 µm in diameter.

Lues connata (congenital syphilis) is a form of syphilis transmitted to the foetus after the fourth month of pregnancy. If neither foetal death nor abortion occurs (approx. 30%), hepatosplenomegaly, "capillaritis" and *interstitial syphilitic hepatitis* develop. The liver cell plates are split into small epithelial groups. Subsequent swift interstitial fibrosis leads to microgranular intralobular cirrhosis. Focal cell necrosis in the liver of the neonate causes the formation of miliary *syphilomas*, which contain giant cells, epithelioid cells, lymphocytes and macrophages. (s. fig. 24.10) • Obliterative endarteritis, fine-spot bleeding and large siderin deposits lead to the so-called **brimstone liver.** (s. p. 413)

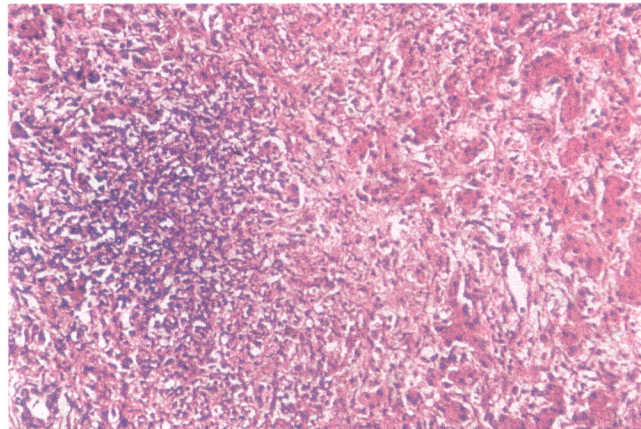

Fig. 24.10: Lues connata: Severe inflammatory infiltration (especially left of picture); sinusoidal fibrosis; irregular liver cell plates (far right of picture). Also called "interstitial syphilitic hepatitis" (HE)

▶ A 38-year-old patient had been suffering from subfebrile temperatures, general malaise, moderately increased GPT, GOT, GDH and γ-GT, markedly augmented alkaline phosphatase (430 U/l), reduced ChE and albumins as well as moderately elevated γ-globulins for a period of several weeks. All the other laboratory values and examinations with imaging techniques were within the normal range. Syphilis was originally not considered in the differential diagnosis. However, percutaneous biopsy provided evidence of corkscrew-shaped pathogens within lesions, now interpreted as syphilitic hepatitis. Subsequent serological tests for specific antibodies were positive. (s. fig. 24.11)

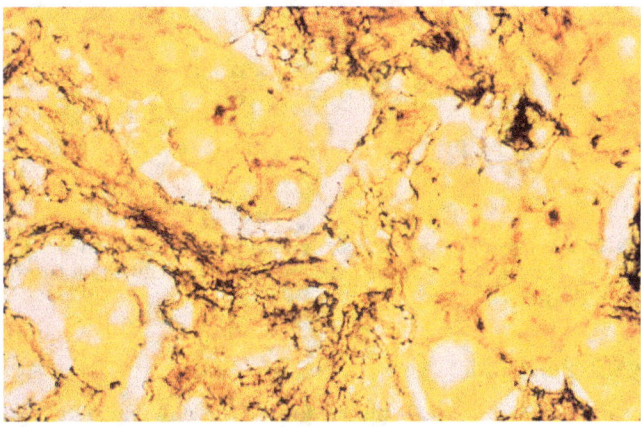

Fig. 24.11: Syphilis, secondary stage: hepatitis syphilitica. In the liver parenchyma, massive amounts of corkscrew-shaped syphilis pathogens, 6—10 µm in length, are visible (= treponema pallidum) (silver impregnation)

Lues acquisita progresses as (*1.*) *early syphilis* throughout the primary and secondary stages, lues latens seropositiva (= early latent form) and (*2.*) *late syphilis* in the tertiary stage, lues latens seronegativa (= late latent form) and stage IV. (81, 83, 88, 90) • From the primary complex, haematogenous dissemination of the pathogen in the body takes place, with development of the primary and secondary stages. *Syphilitic hepatitis* is found in 10% of cases, with focal liver cell necrosis, infiltrates of lymphocytes, eosinophils and granulocytes, focal activation of the stellate cells and portal infiltrations. (78, 79, 81, 84–86, 89) (s. fig. 24.11) Epithelioid cell granulomas are mostly localized in the central lobule. The portal bile ducts are narrowed by infiltrations, resulting in pronounced cholestasis. The portal vessels show signs of vasculitis. Hepatomegaly of hard consistency is present. About 50% of patients exhibit elevated transaminases. Usually, the antimitochondrial antibody M_1 is positive. (76) Healing is accompanied by fibrosis. Cirrhosis may also develop. • In the *tertiary stage*, occurring in 30–40% of cases after years of latency, *gumma syphiliticum* may be observed in the liver, where it is either solitary or multiple and mostly localized in the right lobe. Gummas are large, closely circumscribed, nodular structures with a diameter of a few millimetres up to several centimetres. They consist of central caseation, which is surrounded by vascularized granulation tissue resembling a capsule and by plasma and giant cells. (77, 80, 82, 87) (s. fig. 24.12) The hepatic architecture is not affected. Usually, endarteritis develops. Treponemas are rarely found in the gumma. • In the case of multiple occurrence with associated deep grooves and scar formation, the striking picture of *hepar lobatum* appears.

Relapsing fever: The epidemic (European) form of fever is induced by the spirochaete Borrelia recurrentis (obermeyeri), which is transmitted by lice. After an incubation period of 3 to 15 days, there are sudden repeated (up to ten) attacks of fever separated by fever-free intervals together with parallel hepatomegaly and splenomegaly, cutaneous and mucosal bleeding (e.g. colon, nose), myalgia, arthralgia, iridocyclitis, facial paresis and meningism.

Jaundice is often observed. Histologically, signs of non-specific *reactive hepatitis* with spotty liver cell necrosis are detectable in most cases.

3.6 Listeriosis

Listeria monocytogenes is most common in animals. **Transmission** to humans is effected through the secretions of infected animals or contaminated food (e.g. milk and dairy products, raw meat). An increased proneness to listeriosis is found in drug-related immunosuppression, pregnancy, liver cirrhosis, diabetes mellitus and AIDS. In connatal (diaplacental) transmission *(= granulomatosis infantiseptica)*, listeriosis leads to abortion or premature delivery with meningoencephalitis and multiple organ abscesses, so that the neonate dies within a few days. • The **disease course** varies from uncharacteristic "flu-like" manifestations to (*1.*) septic, (*2.*) central nervous, (*3.*) glandular or cutaneous, and (*4.*) chronic septic forms with isolated organic affection. • **Treatment:** ampicillin and amoxicillin at high dosage are the remedies of choice, but only in the first four days. (98, 99, 103)

Liver involvement is reflected in elevated transaminases, histologically detected monohistiocytic *granulomas* and miliary *microabscesses* (frequently with gram-positive rods). (96, 100, 101) There is occasional evidence of *non-specific reactive hepatitis*. (95, 97) Fulminant hepatitis has been reported in listeria sepsis. (102) (s. fig. 24.13)

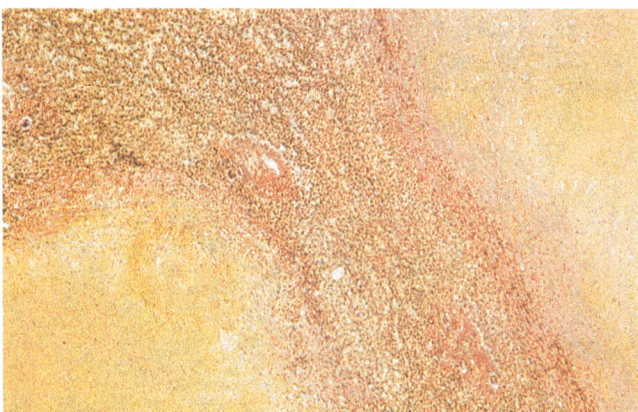

Fig. 24.12: Hepatic gumma from syphilitic hepar lobatum. Intrahepatic necrotic zones surrounded by a thin layer of granulation tissue (Sirius red)

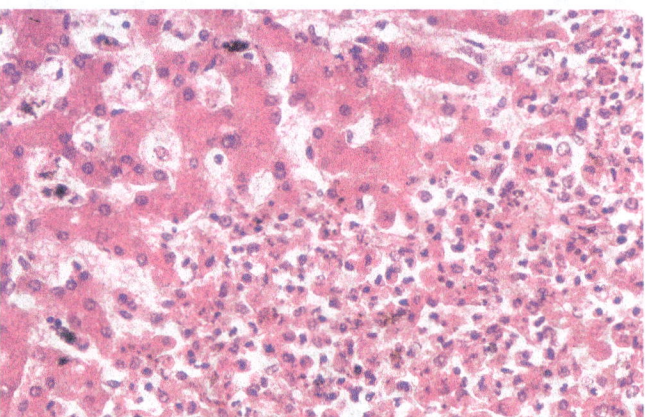

Fig. 24.13: Dense, granulocytic infiltration in the environment of fresh hepatocellular necrosis (right lower half of the picture). Clinical diagnosis: listeriosis (HE)

3.5.3 Borreliosis

Lyme borreliosis was first observed in Lyme (USA) in 1976. It is caused by Borrelia burgdorferi and transmitted by insects, especially ticks. The multisystemic clinical picture initially includes erythema chronicum migrans with non-specific manifestations. During the following weeks and months, cardiac involvement, polymeningoradiculoneuritis and arthritis may be seen.

In some cases, severe *Lyme hepatitis* develops. The pathogen is often found in liver cells and sinusoids. *Therapy* consists of doxycycline or erythromycin. (91–94)

3.7 Brucellosis

Brucellae are gram-negative, aerobic, non-motile, rod-shaped bacteria, with a natural **reservoir** in some mammals: B. abortus in cattle (Bang's disease), B. melitensis (in goats and sheep, the "Malta fever" is a special form), B. suis (especially in pigs, the natural host of the Brucellae), B. ovis (in sheep) and B. canis (in dogs). The pathogens enter the host via skin lesions or mucosa (conjunctiva, respiratory tract, gastrointestinal tract).

Brucellosis is the generic term for diseases induced by the various Brucella species in animals and humans. Following an incubation period of approximately 14 days, headaches, pronounced fatigue, myalgia, arthralgia, swollen lymph nodes and especially undulant fever occur. Frequently, organ manifestations (cholecystitis, endocarditis, meningoencephalitis, nephritis, prostatitis, pneumonia, etc.) are in evidence. • Hepatosplenomegaly and moderate increases in transaminases and in alkaline phosphatase are found. Histologically, histiocytic *granulomas* are present (in 90—95% of cases), often with central necrosis, portal and peripheral infiltration and hyperplasia of the Kupffer cells. (104, 109) Up to now, about 30 cases of *hepatic brucelloma* have been reported in the literature. (105, 107) They result from the caseation of a granulomatous reaction by persistent brucellae in macrophages. The imaging methods show central calcification and peripheral necrotic areas, which imitate malignant tumours or pyogenic liver abscesses. In many patients, fatty infiltration of liver cells, lipofuscinosis and siderosis are found. Extensive focal necrosis may occur in infections with B. melitensis and B. suis. Severe courses, possibly with acute liver failure, are rarely observed. Ascites can appear. Hepatic *abscesses* are seldom. Fewer than 50 cases have been described in the literature. (105, 106, 108) • The *diagnosis* is confirmed by serological tests, culture of pathogens or animal experiments. As *treatment*, the combination of rifampicin (900 mg/day) + doxycycline (200 mg/day) for three months or doxycycline + gentamycin, possibly also tetracycline + streptomycin, has proved effective. In chronic brucellosis, treatment with tetracycline must be repeated.

3.8 Rickettsiosis

Rickettsiae are gram-negative pathogens living as cellular parasites in the gastrointestinal tract of arthropods (especially lice, fleas, ticks and mites). They may be transmitted to human beings and cause endemic and epidemic rickettsioses, generally showing a typhoid-like clinical picture. Major rickettsioses include *classic spotted fever* (R. prowazeki), *Rocky Mountain spotted fever* (R. rickettsii), *Q fever* (R. burneti), *Boutonneuse fever* (R. conori) and *murine endemic spotted fever* (R. typhi). Following infection, the pathogens may spread haematogenously to all organs and colonize the endothelial cells of the small arteries and capillaries, so that partial or complete vascular obstruction ensues.

Each of the ten Rickettsia species pathogenic to humans may cause *concomitant hepatitis*. Clinical findings include hepatomegaly with an increase in the transaminases as well as (occasionally) in alkaline phosphatase and bilirubin. Histology reveals *granulomas* of round cells, granulocytes, proliferated stellate cells and polynuclear giant cells as well as spotty infiltrations with single-cell necrosis and portal infiltrates. (s. fig. 24.14) Chronic Q-fever hepatitis has been reported. Typical fatty granulomas (often surrounded by a fibrin ring) are frequently found in the liver lobules or in the portal tracts. *Treatment* consists of doxycycline, chloramphenicol or tetracycline. (110—117)

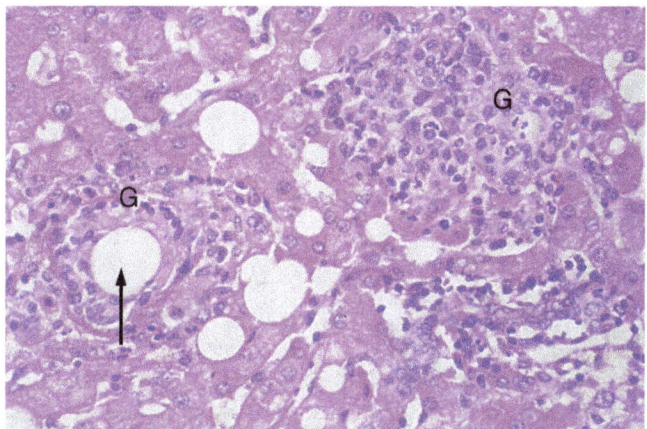

Fig. 24.14: Two intraparenchymal granulomas, one of which has the appearance of a lipogranuloma (→). Clinical diagnosis: Q fever (HE)

3.9 Tularaemia

This clinical picture was observed for the first time in Tulare, California in 1911 (G. W. McCoy). The causative pathogen was identified as Bacterium tularense by G. W. McCoy et al. (1912) and W. B. Wheery et al. (1914). The gram-negative, aerobic and non-motile **Francisella tularense** is transmitted to humans by arthropods infected by sick rodents, directly by the rodents themselves or through contaminated water.

After a short incubation period, lasting one to three days, a clinical picture develops comprising high fever, chills, lymphadenitis and local ulceration, sometimes also meningitis, pneumonia or pulmonary abscesses and mediastinitis. • In the course of this severe disease, *liver granulomas* up to 2 mm in diameter may occur with central necrosis, epithelioid cells and giant cells. The portal fields show inflammatory infiltration. *Liver abscesses* and the clinical picture of *cholangitis* or obstructive jaundice have also been observed; ascites is rarely seen. There is evidence of hepatomegaly together with the corresponding pathological laboratory parameters. *Diagnosis* is confirmed by serology or skin tests. *Treatment* consists of antibiotics (e.g. tetracycline, streptomycin, gentamycin, ampicillin). (118, 119)

3.10 Psittacosis

Chlamydia psittaci is the causative pathogen of **ornithosis** (psittacosis or parrot disease). It is transmitted to humans by birds via their droppings. The incubation period is 4 to 28 days. In the course of the occasionally severe pneumonia, *concomitant hepatitis* may be in evidence. (120, 122, 123) The *Fitz-Hugh-Curtis syndrome* rarely develops. (121, 124) (s. fig. 24.2) Clinical findings generally include hepatomegaly and slightly increased transaminases. *Diagnosis* of this infectious disease is confirmed by CFR. *Treatment* consists of tetracycline.

3.11 Clostridium welchii

In the course of the rare systemic gas gangrene caused by Clostridium perfringens (gram-positive, anaerobic, rod-shaped, spore-forming bacterium, formerly known as Clostridium welchii), severe *clostridial hepatitis* may ensue. Necrotic foci, abscesses and aerogenesis develop. The pathogens can be cultivated from biopsy material and PCR. A major harmful factor is the respective exotoxin, which sometimes causes pronounced haemolytic icterus. (125)

3.12 Tropheryma whippeli

Whipple's disease (G.H. WHIPPLE, 1907) with feverish, sprue-like symptoms is generally accompanied by polyadenopathy, arthritis, polyserositis and endocarditis or pericarditis. Men are affected eight times more often than women. • Liver involvement occurs in the form of *granulomas*, in which macrophages loaded with bacteria are present. The gram-positive bacterium Tropheryma whippeli has been identified as the causative pathogen. It is assigned to the group of Actinomyces. (126, 127)

3.13 Campylobacter colitis

The intestinal disease with fever and arthralgia caused by Campylobacter colitis may show findings corresponding to *non-specific reactive hepatitis* in terms of laboratory parameters and histology. (128, 129)

3.14 Rochalimaea

The gram-negative Rochalimaea species (R. quintana, R. henselae, R. vinsonii, R. bacilliformis) are responsible for **four clinical syndromes:** (*1.*) cat-scratch disease, (*2.*) bacterial angiomatosis, (*3.*) bacterial peliosis hepatis, and (*4.*) relapsing fever with bacteriaemia (= trench fever). • The *cat-scratch disease* (R. DEBRÉ et al., 1950) was first attributed to a new pathogen, named Afipia felis; more recent studies point to a species of Rochalimaea (Bartonella henselae) as the causative pathogen. The incubation period ranges from 3 to 20 days. Thereafter, feverish lymphadenitis with a morbilliform rash appears. Painful hepatomegaly is experienced. The transaminases are elevated. Diagnosis involves specific serological tests, PCR or liver biopsy. • Liver involvement is manifested by *granulomas* with occasional central star-shaped microabscesses, in which pathogens can be demonstrated, and by *focal infiltrates*, possibly also with *single-cell necrosis*. Adaequate *therapy* with erythromycine is recommended. (130–135)

3.15 Actinomycosis

The abdominal form of the so-called ray-fungus disease (actinomycosis) is a non-contagious, mostly chronic infectious disease induced through the gram-positive, anaerobic rod-shaped bacterium **Actinomyces israelii**. It is a pseudomycosis. Under favourable conditions, this human saprophyte can cause enterocolitis.

Pronounced formation of *granulomas* or *microabscesses* and major (hyperdense) liver abscesses with cauliflower-like *druses* may be due to haematogenous spread of the pathogen to the liver (portal vein, systemic circulation) or, occasionally, to direct encroachment on the liver. The pus of the abscess typically contains so-called *sulphur granules*. • *Treatment* consists of penicillin G (e.g. 2 × 10 million U/day i.v. for approximately 4 weeks), ampicillin, tetracycline, clindamycin or metronidazole. (136–147)

3.16 Burkholderia pseudomallei

Burkholderia pseudomallei is an aerobic, motile and rod-shaped bacterium, causing *melioidosis*, which is endemic in the different subtropical and tropical countries. Patients with diabetes mellitus are particularly susceptible to infection. Acute melioidosis displays large numbers of both localized and disseminated necrotic foci, which produce confluent abscesses, sometimes with a diameter of 2–3 mm. The presence of pathogens can be confirmed using Giemsa staining. Chronic melioidosis is characterized by epithelioid cell granuloma with giant cells and central necrosis. Pathogens (previously known as pseudomonas) are only rarely found in the foci themselves. • *Therapy* is based on ceftadizine, which is the antibiotic of first choice. (148)

References:

Pyogenic cocci
1. **Girisch, M., Heininger, U.:** Scarlet fever associated with hepatitis. A report of two cases. Infection 2000; 28: 251–253
2. **Gourley, G.R., Chesney, P.J., Davis, J.P., Odell, G.B.:** Acute cholestasis in patients with toxic-shock syndrome. Gastroenterology 1981; 81: 928–931
3. **Grüllich, C., Baumert, T.F., Blum, H.E.:** Acute Mycoplasma pneumoniae infection presenting as cholestatic hepatitis. J. Clin. Microbiol. 2003; 41: 514–515
4. **Larrey, D.:** Bacterial hepatitis. Gastroenterol. Clin. Biol. 2003; 27 (Suppl.): 27–31
5. **Lund-Tonnesen, St.:** Liver abscess: an unusual manifestation of pneumococcal infection. Scand. J. Infect. Dis. 1995; 27: 397–398
6. **Pieron, R.:** Miliary abscess of the liver during septicaemia caused by staphylococcus. Peritoneoscopic diagnosis. Sem. Hop. Paris 1977; 53: 383–388
7. **Quale, J.M., Mandel, L.J., Bergasa, N.V., Straus, E.W.:** Clinical significance and pathogenesis of hyperbilirubinemia associated with staphylococcus aureus septicemia. Amer. J. Med. 1988; 85: 615–618
8. **Romero-Gomez, M., Otero, M.A., Sanchez-Munoz, D., Ramirez-Arcos, M., Larraona, J.L., Suarez Garcia, E., Vargas-Romero, J.:** Acute hepatitis due to Mycoplasma pneumoniqe infection without lung involvement in adues patients (case report). J. Hepatol. 2006; 44: 827–828
9. **Sikuler, E., Guetta, V., Keynan, A., Neumann, L., Schlaeffer, F.:** Abnormalities in bilirubin and liver enzyme levels in adult patients with bacteremia. A prospective study. Arch. Intern. Med. 1989; 149: 2246–2248
10. **Tugwell, P., Williams, A.O.:** Jaundice associated with lobar pneumonia. Quart. J. Med. 1977; 46: 97–118
11. **Verbanck, J., Ponette, J., Verbanck, M., Vanderwiele, I., Segaert, M.:** Sonographic detection of multiple Staphyococcus aureus hepatic microabscesses mimicking Candida abscess. J. Clin. Ultrasound 1999; 27: 478–481

Neisseria gonorrhoea
12. **Amman, R., Zehender, O., Jenny, S., Bass, G.:** Die Perihepatitis acuta gonorrhoica (Fitz-Hugh-Curtis-Syndrom). Dtsch. Med. Wschr. 1971, 96: 1515–1519
13. **Hauk, G., Mall, K., Ebel, J.:** Perihepatitis acuta gonorrhoica (Fitz-Hugh-Curtis-Syndrom). Med. Klin. 1974; 61: 338–340
14. **Kimball, M.W., Knee, S.:** Gonococcal perihepatitis in a male. New Engl. J. Med. 1970; 282: 1082–1083
15. **Lopez-Zeno, J.A., Keith, L.G., Berger, G.S.:** The Fitz-Hugh-Curtis syndrome revisited. Changing perspectives after half a century. J. Reprod. Med. 1985; 30: 567–582

16. McLain, L.G., Decker, M., Nye, D.: Gonococcal perihepatitis. J. Amer. Med. Ass. 1978; 239: 339–341

Enterobacteriaceae
17. Ayhan, A., Cokoz, A., Karacadac, S., Telatar, H.: The liver in typhoid fever. Amer. J. Gastroenterol. 1973; 59: 141–146
18. Calva, J.J., Ruiz-Palacios, G.M.: Salmonella hepatitis: detection of Salmonella antigens in the liver of patients with typhoid fever. J. Infect. Dis. 1986; 154: 373–374
19. Colizza, F., LePage, S., LaJoie, J.-F., Duperval, R., Marcoux, A., Mongeau, J., Bergeron, D.: Multiple hepatic abscesses following Yersinia enterocolitica septicemia. Canad. J. Gastroenterol. 1990; 4: 179–183
20. Diem, L.V., My, T.Q., Chi, N.V., Nhon, N.T., Thuc, T.K.: Typhoid fever with hepatitis. J. Trop. Med. Hyg. 1976; 79: 25–27
21. El-Newihi, H., Alamy, M.E., Reynolds, T.B.: Salmonella hepatitis: analysis of 27 cases and comparison with acute viral hepatitis. Hepatology 1996; 24: 516–519
22. Horney, J.T., Schwarzmann, St.W., Galambos, J.T.: Shigella hepatitis. Amer. J. Gastroenterol. 1976; 66: 146–149
23. Khan, M., Coovadia, Y.M., Karas, J.A., Connolly, C., Sturm, A.W.: Clinical significance of hepatic dysfunction jaundice in typhoid fever. Dig. Dis. Sci. 1999; 44: 590–594
24. Khanna, R., Levendoglu, H.: Liver abscess due to Yersinia enterocolitica: case report and review of the literature. Dig. Dis. Sci. 1989; 34: 636–639
25. Morgenstern, R., Hayes, P.C.: The liver in typhoid fever: always affected, not just a complication. Amer. J. Gastroenterol. 1991; 86: 1235–1239
26. Pramoolsinsap, C., Viranuvatti, V.: Salmonella hepatitis. J. Gastroenterol. Hepatol. 1998; 13: 745–750
27. Ramachandran, S., Godfrey, J.J., Perera, M.V.F.: Typhoid hepatitis. J. Amer. Med. Ass. 1974; 230: 236–240
28. Saebo, A., Lassen, J.: Acute and chronic liver disease associated with Yersinia enterocolitica infection: a Norwegian 10-year follow-up study of 458 hospitalized patients. J. Intern. Med. 1992; 231: 531–535
29. Sehdev, A.E.S., Dumler, J.S.: Hepatic pathology in human monocytic ehrlichiosis. Ehrlichia chaffeensis infection. Amer. J. Clin. Path. 2003; 119: 859–865
30. Soni, P.N., Hoosen, A.A., Pillay, D.G.: Hepatic abscess caused by Salmonella typhi. A case report and review of the literature. Dig. Dis. Sci. 1994; 39: 1694–1696
31. Stjernberg, U., Silseth, C., Ritland, S.: Granulomatous hepatitis in Yersinia enterocolitica infection. Hepatogastroenterol. 1987; 34: 56–57
32. Vadillo, M., Corbella, X., Pac, V., Fernandez-Viladrich, P., Pujol, R.: Multiple liver abscesses due to Yersinia enterocolitica discloses primary hemochromatosis: three case reports and review. Clin. Infect. Dis. 1994; 18: 938–941

Tuberculosis
33. Alcantara-Payawal, D.E., Matsumura, M., Shiratori, Y., Okudaira, T., Gonzalez, R., Lopez, R.A., Sollano, J.D., Omata, M.: Direct detection of Mycobacterium tuberculosis using polymerase chain reaction assay among patients with hepatic granuloma. J. Hepatol. 1997; 27: 620–627
34. Alvarez, S.Z.: Hepatobiliary tuberculosis. J. Gastroenterol. Hepatol. 1998; 13: 833–839
35. Asada, Y., Hayashi, T., Sumiyoshi, A., Aburaya, M., Shishime, E.: Miliary tuberculosis presenting as fever and jaundice with hepatic failure. Hum. Pathol. 1991; 22: 92–94
36. Bengoa Hernandez, R., Lopez Barbarin, J.M., Galdos Ayala, J., Alvarez Rubio, M., Delgado Fontaneda, E., Garcia Campos, F.: Tuberculosis hepatica pseudotumoral. Rev. Esp. Enf. Digest. 1994; 86: 687–689
37. Blangy, S., Cornud, F., Sibert, A., Vissuzaine, C., Saraux, J.L., Benacerraf, R.: Hepatitis tuberculosis presenting as tumoral disease on ultrasonography. Gastrointest. Radiol. 1988; 13: 52–54
38. Caroli-Bosc, F.-X., Conio, M., Maes, B., Chevallier, P., Hastier, P., Delmont, J.-P.: Abdominal tuberculosis involving hepatic hilar lymph nodes. J. Clin. Gastroenterol. 1997; 25: 541–543
39. Cherki, S., Cotte, E., Boibieux, A., Baulieux, J., Adham, M.: Hepatic tuberculosis: Case report pseudotumoral form. Gastroenterol. Clin. Biol. 2006; 30: 1317–1320
40. Chien, R.-N., Lin, P.-Y., Liaw, Y.-F.: Hepatic tuberculosis: comparison of miliary and local form. Infection 1995; 23: 5–8
41. Desai, C.S., Josh, A.G., Abraham, P., Desai, D.C., Deshpande, R.B., Bhaduri, S., Shah, S.R.: Hepatic tuberculosis in absence of disseminated abdominal tuberculosis. Ann. Hepatol. 2006; 5: 41–43
42. Emre, A., Akpinar, E., Acarli, K., Alper, A., Cevikbas, V., Ariogul, O.: Primary solitary tuberculosis of the liver. HPB Surgery 1992; 5: 261–265
43. Essop, A.R., Posen, J.A., Hodkinson, J.H., Segal, I.: Tuberkulosis hepatitis: A clinical review of 96 cases. Quart. J. Med. 1984; 53: 465–477
44. Fan, S.T., Ng, J.O.L., Choi, T.K., Lai, E.C.S.: Tuberculosis of the bile duct: a rare cause of biliary stricture. Amer. J. Gastroenterol. 1989; 84: 413–414
45. Huang, W.T., Wang, C.C., Chen, W.J., Cheng, Y.F., Eng, H.L.: The nodular form of hepatic tuberculosis: a review with five additional new cases. J. Clin. Pathol. 2003; 56: 835–839
46. Hussain, W., Mutimer, D., Harrison, R., Hubscher, S., Neuberger, J.: Fulminant hepatic failure caused by tuberculosis. Gut 1995; 36: 792–794
47. Ismail, R., Larabi, K., Alyoune, M., Nadir, S., Jamil, D., Cherkaoui, A.: Abcès tuberculeux du foie. A propos de deux observations. Ann. Gastroenterol. Hepatol. 1994; 30: 212–214
48. Jain, R., Sawhney, S., Gupta, R.G., Acharya, S.K.: Sonographic appearances and percutaneous management of primary tuberculous liver abscess. J. Clin. Ultrasound 1999; 27: 159–163
49. Kawamori, Y., Matsui, O., Kitagawa, K., Kadoya, M., Takashima, T., Yamahana, T.: Macronodular tuberculoma of the liver: CT and MR findings. Amer. J. Radiol. 1992; 158: 311–313
50. Kok, K.Y.Y., Yapp, S.K.S.: Tuberculosis of the bile duct – A rare cause of obstructive jaundice. J. Clin. Gastroenterol. 1999; 29: 161–164
51. Krami, H., Fadli, F., Benzzoubeir, N., Marzouk, N., Ouazzani, L., Ouzzani, H., Dafiri, N., Bennani, A.: La tuberculose hépatique primitive. Ann. Gastroenterol. Hepatol. 1998; 34: 71–74
52. Kuntz, E.: Über Leberveränderungen durch Tuberkulose. Beitr. Klin. Tuberk. 1960; 123: 26–40
53. Lamache, A., Bourel, M., Chevrel, M.L., Richier, J.L.: Foie et tuberculose. Sem. Hop. (Paris) 1961; 37: 803–813
54. Levine, C.: Primary macronodular hepatic tuberculosis: US and CT appearances. Gastrointestin. Radiol. 1990; 15: 307–309
55. Maharaj, B., Leary, W.P., Pudifin, D.J.: A prospective study of hepatic tuberculosis in 41 black patients. Quart. J. Med. 1987; 63: 517–522
56. Mandak, M., Kerbl, U., Kleinert, R., Höfler, G., Zeichen, R., Denk, H.: Miliare Tuberkulose der Leber als Ursache eines septischen Schocks mit Multiorganversagen. Wien. Klin. Wschr. 1994; 106: 111–114
57. Mitlehner, W., Dissmann, W.: Pseudotumoröse Lebertuberkulose mit multiplen Organabszessen. Dtsch. Med. Wschr. 1987; 112: 760–763
58. Moumen, M., Jamil, D., Cherkaoui, A., El Fares, F.: Tuberculose hépatique à forme pseudo-tumorale. A propos de trois cas. Sem. Hop. (Paris) 1993; 69: 358–361
59. Nampoory, M.R.N., Halim, M.M.A., Sreedharan, R., Al-Sweih, N.A.S., Gupta, R.K., Constandi, J.N., Johny, K.V.: Liver abscess and disseminated intravascular coagulation in tuberculosis. Postgrad. Med. J. 1995; 71: 490–492
60. Navarro, V., Guix, J., Ferrer, C., Bernacer, B., Nieto, A., Borras, R., Sabater, V.: Tuberculosis hepatica y virus de la immunodeficiencia humana. Gastroenterol. Hepatol. 1992; 15: 351–356
61. Oliva, A., Duarte, B., Jonasson, O., Nadimpalli, V.: The nodular form of local hepatic tuberculosis. A review. J. Clin. Gastroenterol. 1990; 12: 166–173
62. Pariente, R., Etienne, J.P., Chrétien, J.: Etude de 22 cas de tuberculose du foie anatomiquement démontrée. (Considérations étiologiques, cliniques, laparoscopiques et histologiques). Rev. Tuberc. Pneumol. 1963; 27: 1177–1192
63. Patel, K.M.: Granulomatous hepatitis due to Mycobacterium scrofulaceum: report of a case. Gastroenterology 1981; 81: 156–158
64. Rahmatulla, R.H., Al-Mofleh, I.A., Al-Rashed, R.S., Al-Hedaithy, M.A., Mayet, I.Y.: Tuberculous liver abscess: a case report and review of literature. Eur. J. Gastroenterol. Hepatol. 2001; 13: 437–440
65. Thomas, M.R., Goldin, R.D.: Tuberculosis presenting as jaundice. Brit. J. Clin. Pract. 1990; 44: 161–163
66. Troschel, P., Clemens, G., von Düsterlho, J., Homann, J.: Kasuistik einer durch Laparoskopie gesicherten Peritoneal-Tuberkulose. Med. Welt 1999; 50: 433–435
67. Varela, M., Fernandez, J., Navasa, M., Bruix, J.: Pseudotumoral hepatic tuberculosa. J. Hepatol. 2003; 39: 654

M. leprae
68. Chen, T.S.N., Drutz, D.J., Whelan, G.E.: Hepatic granulomas in leprosy. Arch. Path. Labor. Med. 1976; 100: 182–185
69. Karat, A.B.A., Job, C.K., Rao, P.S.S.: Liver in leprosy: histological and biochemical findings. Brit. Med. J. 1971/I 307–310
70. Sehgal, V.N., Tygai, S.P., Kumar, S., Gupta, M.C.: Microscopic pathology of the liver in leprosy patients. Int. J. Dermatol. 1972; 11: 168–172

Leptospirosis
71. Den Haan, P.J., van Vliet, A.C.M., Hazenberg, B.P.: Weil's disease as a cause of jaundice. Nederl. J. Med. 1993; 42: 171–174
72. Gordon, M.E.: Clinical problem-solving: Leptospirosis. New Engl. J. Med. 1993; 329: 2040–2041
73. Notheis, W.F., Krämer, B.K., Leser, H.-G., Rüschoff, J., Kromer, E.P., Riegger, A.J.G.: Schwerer Verlauf einer Leptospirose mit akutem Nierenversagen und ausgeprägtem Ikterus (Morbus Weil). Dtsch. Med. Wschr. 1993; 118: 1437–1441
74. Thurner, J., Haas, P.: Leberveränderungen bei Leptospiren-Infektionen (Leptospira icterohaemorrhagia und Leptospira pomona). Münch. Med. Wschr. 1973; 115: 147–150
75. Vinetz, J.M., Glass, G.E., Flexner, C.E., Mueller, P., Kaslow, D.C.: Sporadic urban leptospirosis. Ann. Intern. Med. 1996; 125: 794–798

Syphilis
76. Comer, G.M., Mukherjee, S., Sachdev, R.K., Clain, D.J.: Cardiolipin-fluorescent (M1) antimitochondrial antibody and cholestatic hepatitis in secondary syphilis. Dig. Dis. Sci. 1989; 34: 1298–1302
77. Fischbach, W., Mössner, J., Dämmrich, J., Jenett, M.: Tertiäre Lues mit Lebergummen. Dtsch. Med. Wschr. 1991; 116: 1013–1017
78. Gschwantler, M., Gulz, W., Schrutka-Kölbi, C., Kogelbauer, G., Schober, G., Bibus, B., Weiss, W.: Acute hepatitis as the only symptom of secondary syphilis. Dtsch. Med. Wschr. 1996; 121: 1457–1461
79. Jozsa, L., Timmer, M., Somogyi, T., Feher, J.: Hepatitis syphilitica. A clinico-pathological study of 25 cases. Acta Hepatogastroenterol. 1977; 24: 344–347
80. Maincent, G., Labadie, H., Fabre, M., Novello, P., Derghal, K., Patriarche, C., Licht, H.: Tertiary hepatic syphilis. A treatable cause of multinodular liver. Dig. Dis. Sci. 1997; 42: 447–450

81. **Mandache, G., Coca, C., Caro-Sampara, F., Haberstezer, F., Coumaros, D., Blickle, F., Andres, E.:** A forgotten aetiology of acute hepatitis in immunocompetent patient: Syphilitic infection. J. Intern. Med. 2006; 259: 214–215
82. **Peeters, L., van Vaerenbergh, W., van der Perre, C., Lagrange, W., Verbeke, M.:** Tertiary syphilis presenting as hepatic bull's eye lesions (case report). Acto Gastro-Enterol. Belg. 2005; 68: 435–439
83. **Rampal, P., Veyres, B., Agrati, D., Saint-Paul, M.C., Rampal, A., Francois, E., Lafon, J., Delmont, J.:** Les atteintes hépatiques de la syphilis. Ann. Gastroent. Hepatol. 1986; 22: 77–81
84. **Schlossberg, D.:** Syphilitic hepatitis: a case report and review of the literature. Amer. J. Gastroenterol. 1987; 82: 552–553
85. **Seeberger, U., Aksü, T., Linke, J., Hengstmann, J.:** Granulomatous hepatitis in secondary syphilis. Internist 2002; 43: 541–547
86. **Sehgal, V.N., Rege, V.L.:** Malignant syphilis and hepatitis. Case report. Brit. J. Vener. Dis. 1974; 50: 237–238
87. **Shapiro, M.P., Gale, M.E.:** Tertiary syphilis of the liver: CT appearance. J. Comput. Assist. Tomogr. 1987; 11: 546–547
88. **Sobel, H.J., Wolf, E.H., Passaic, N.J.:** Liver involvement in early syphilis. Arch. Path. 1972; 93: 565–568
89. **Tiliakos, N., Shamma'a, J.M., Nasrallat, S.M.:** Syphilitic hepatitis. Amer. J. Gastroenterol. 1980; 73: 60–61
90. **Weiss, H., Weiss, A., Wehner, H.:** Syphilis der Leber–ein selten gewordenes Krankheitsbild. Inn. Med. 1987; 14: 21–25

Borreliosis
91. **Chavanet, P., Pillon, D., Lancon, J.P., Waldner-Combernoux, A., Maringe, E., Portier, H.:** Granulomatous hepatitis associated with Lyme disease. Lancet 1987; II: 623–624
92. **Goellner, M.H., Agger, W.A., Burgess, J.H., Duray, P.H.:** Hepatitis due to recurrent Lyme disease. Ann. Intern. Med. 1988; 108: 707–708
93. **Horowitz, H.W., Dworkin, B., Forseter, G., Nadelman, R.B., Connolly, C., Luciano, B.B., Nowakowski, J., O'Brien, T.A., Calmann, M., Wormser, G.P.:** Liver function in early Lyme disease. Hepatology 1996; 23: 1412–1417
94. **Killmann, H., Lind, P., Stanek, G.:** Akute Hepatitis bei Lyme–Borreliose. Wien. Med. Wschr. 1987; 14: 343–346

Listeriosis
95. **Bourgeois, N., Jacobs, F., Lourdes Tavares, M., Rickaert, F., Deprez, C., Liesnard, C., Moonens, F., van de Stadt, J., Gelin, M., Adler, M.:** Listeria monocytogenes hepatitis in a liver transplant recipient: a case report and review of the literature. J. Hepatol. 1993; 14: 284–289
96. **Brönnimann, S., Baer, H.U., Malinverni, R., Büchler, M.W.:** Listeria monocytogenes causing solitary liver abscess. Dig. Surg. 1998; 15: 364–368
97. **Desprez, D., Blanc, P., Larrey, D., Galindo, G., Ramos, J., Feldmann, G., Michel, H.:** Hépatite aiguë due à une infection par Listeria monocytogenes. Gastroenterol. Clin. Biol. 1994; 18: 516–519
98. **De Vega, T., Echevarria, S., Crespo, J., Artinano, E., San Miguel, G., Pons Romero, F.:** Acute hepatitis by Listeria monocytogenes in an HIV patient with chronic HBV hepatitis. J. Clin. Gastroenterol. 1992; 15: 251–255
99. **Hardie, R., Roberts, W.:** Adult listeriosis presenting as acute hepatitis. J. Infect. 1984; 8: 256–258
100. **Jenkins, D., Richards, J.E., Rees, Y., Wicks, A.C.B.:** Multiple listerial liver abscesses. Gut 1987; 28: 1661–1662
101. **Marino, P., Maggioni, M., Preatoni, A., Cantoni, A., Invernizzi, F.:** Liver abscesses due to Listeria monocytogenes. Liver 1996; 16: 67–69
102. **Tschumper, A., Streuli, H., Hottinger, S., Zimmermann, A., Müller, U.:** Fulminante Hepatitis bei Listeriensepsis. Schweiz. Med. Wschr. 1987; 117: 2010–2012
103. **Yu, V.L., Miller, W.P., Wing, E.J., Romano, J.M., Ruiz, C.A., Burns, F.J.:** Disseminated listeriosis presenting as acute hepatitis. Case reports and review of hepatic involvement in listeriosis. Amer. J. Med. 1982; 73: 773–777

Brucellosis
104. **Aygen, B., Sümerkan, B., Doganay, M., Sehmen, E.:** Prostatitis and hepatitis due to Brucella melitensis: a case report. J. Infect. 1998; 36: 111–112
105. **Carazo, E.R., Parra, F.M., Villares, M.P.J., Garcia, M.D.C., Calvente, S.L.M., Benitez, A.M.:** Hepatosplenic brucelloma: Clinical presentation and imaging features in six cases. Abdom. Imag. 2005; 30: 291–296
106. **Cosme, A., Barrio, J., Ojeda, E., Ortega, J., Tejada, A.:** Sonographic findings in brucellar hepatic abscess. J. Clin. ultrasound 2001; 29: 109–111
107. **Halimi, C., Bringard, N., Boyer, N., Vilgrain, V., Panis, Y., Degott, C., Brouland, J.-P., Boudiaf, M., Valleur, P., Henry-Biabaud, E., Valla, D.:** Brucellome hépatique: deux nouveaux cas et revue de la literature. Gastroenterol. Clin. Biol. 1999; 23: 513–517
108. **Vaquero Gajate, G.J., Costo Campoamor, A., Santos Santos, J.M., Del Amo Olea, E., Murillo Diez, J.:** Absceso hepatico brucelar: presentacion de un caso y revision de la literatura. Rev. Esp. Enf. Ap. Digest. 1989; 76: 409–412
109. **Williams, R.K., Crossley, K.:** Acute and chronic hepatic involvement of brucellosis. Gastroenterology 1982; 83: 455–458

Rickettsiosis
110. **Abril Lopez de Medrano, V., Ortega Gonzales, E., Ruiz Cavanilles, C., Soler Ros, J.J., Fraile Farinas, T., Monzo Ingles, V., Herrera Ballester, A.:** Afectacion hepatica en la fiebre Q y la fiebre botonosa del Mediterraneo. Estudio comparativo. Rev. Esp. Enf. Digest. 1994; 86: 891–893
111. **Adams, J.S., Walker, D.H.:** The liver in rocky mountain spotted fever. Amer. J. Clin. Pathol. 1981; 75: 156–161
112. **Dupont, H.L., Hornick, R.B., Levin, H.S., Rapaport, M.I., Woodward, T.E.:** Q fever hepatitis. Ann. Intern. Med. 1971; 74: 198–206
113. **Guardia, J., Martinez-Vazquez, J.M., Moragas, A., Rey, C., Vilaseca, J., Tornos, J., Beltran, M., Bacardi, R.:** The liver in boutonneuse fever. Gut 1974; 15: 549–551
114. **Hofmann, C.E., Heaton, J.W.jr.:** Q fever hepatitis. Clinical manifestations and pathological findings. Gastroenterology 1982; 83: 474–479
115. **Picchi, J., Nelson, A.R., Waller, E.E., Razavi, M., Clizer, E.E:** Q-fever associated with granulomatous hepatitis. Ann. Intern. Med. 1960; 53: 1065–1074
116. **Westlake, P., Price, L.M., Russel, M., Kelly, J.K:** The pathology of Q fever hepatitis. A case diagnosed by liver biopsy. J. Clin. Gastroenterol. 1987; 9: 257–363
117. **Yale, St.H., de Groen, P.C., Tooson, J.D., Kurtin, P.J.:** Unusual aspects of acute Q fever-associated hepatitis. Mayo Clin. Proc. 1994; 69: 769–773

Tularaemia
118. **Cortez, J.C., Shapiro, M., Awe, R.J.:** Case report: Pasteurella multocida liver abscess. Amer. J. Med. Sci. 1986; 292: 107–109
119. **Ortego, T.J., Hutchins, L.F., Rice, J., Davis, G.R.:** Tularemic hepatitis presenting as obstructive jaundice. Gastroenterology 1986; 91: 461–463

Chlamydia
120. **Dan, M., Tyrrell, L.D.J., Goldsand, G.:** Isolation of Chlamydia trachomatis from the liver of a patient with prolonged fever. Gut 1987; 28: 1514–1516
121. **Haight, K.B., Ockner, S.A.:** Chlamydia trachomatis perihepatitis with ascites. Amer. J. Gastroenterol. 1988; 83: 323–325
122. **Manesis, E.K., Kittou, N., Kolokotronis, P., Hatziantoniou, P., Papadimitriou, K., Hadziyannis, S.:** Biochemical acute hepatitis in Chlamydia psittaci infection. Hellen. J. Gastroenterol. 1985; 8: 155–160
123. **Schmid, H.J.:** Ornithose mit hepatitischem Bild. Gastroenterologia 1962; 98: 15–18
124. **Simson, J.N.L.:** Chlamydial perihepatitis (Curtis-Fitz-Hugh-syndrome) after hydrotubation. Brit. Med. J. 1984; 289: 544–545

Clostridium
125. **Ashley, D.J.B.:** Two cases of clostridial hepatitis. J. Clin. Pathol. 1965; 18: 170–174

Tropheryma whippeli
126. **Ehrbar, H.U., Bauerfeind, P., Dutly, F., Koelz, H.R., Altwegg, M.:** PCR-positive tests for Tropheryma whippelii in patients without Whipple's disease. Lancet 1999; 353: 2214
127. **Raoult, D., Birg, M.L., La Scola, B., Fournier, P.E., Enea, M., Lepidi, H., Roux, V., Piette, J.-C., Vandenesch, F., Vital-Durand, D., Marrie, T.J.:** Cultivation of the bacillus of Whipple's disease. New Engl. J. Med. 2000; 342: 620–625

Campylobacter
128. **Brmbolic, B.:** Multiple abscesses of the liver caused by Campylobacter jejuni. J. Clin. Gastroenterol. 1995; 20: 307–309
129. **Reddy, K.R., Farnum, J.B., Thomas, E.:** Acute hepatitis associated with Campylobacter colitis. J. Clin. Gastroenterol. 1983; 5: 259–262

Rochalimaea
130. **Danon, O., Duval-Arnould, M., Osman, Z., Boukobza, B., Kazerouni, F., Cadranel, J.F., Neuenschwander, S., Nocton, F.:** Hepatic and splenic involvement in cat-scratch disease: imaging features. Abdom. Imag. 2000; 25: 102–183
131. **Lenoir, A.A., Storch, G.A., de Schryver-Kecskemeti, K., Shakelford, G.D., Rothbaum, R.J., Wear, D.J., Rosenblum, J.L.:** Granulomatous hepatitis associated with cat scratch disease. Lancet 1988/I: 1132–1136
132. **Le Tallec, W., Abgueguen, P., Pichard, E., Chennebault, J.M., Bellec, W., Delbos, V., Rousselet, M.C., Dib, N., Boyer, J.:** Hepatosplenic localization of cat scratch disease in immunocompetent adults. Two cases. Gastroenterol. Clin. Biol. 2003; 27: 225–229
133. **Rocco, V.K., Roman, R.J., Eigenbrodt, E.H:** Cat scratch disease. Report of a case with hepatic lesions and a brief review of the literature. Gastroenterology 1985; 89: 1400–1406
134. **Schwartzman, W.A.:** Infections due to Rochalimaea: the expanding clinical spectrum. Clin. Infect. Dis. 1992; 15: 893–902
135. **Vukelic, D., Benic, B., Bozinovic, D., Vukovic, B., Dakovic Rode, O., Culig, Z., Vukovic, J., Batinica, S., Visnjic, S., Puljiz, I.:** An unusual outcome in a child with hepatosplenic cat-scratch disease (case report). Wien. Klin. Wschr. 2006; 118: 615–618

Actinomycosis
136. **Bhatt, B.D., Zuckerman, M.J., Ho, H., Polly, S.M.:** Multiple actinomycotic abscesses of the liver. Amer. J. Gastroenterol. 1990; 85: 309–310
137. **Cheng, Y.F., Hung, C.F., Liu, Y.H., Ng, K.K., Tsai, C.C.:** Hepatic actinomycosis with portal vein occlusion. Gastrointest. Radiol. 1989; 14: 268–270

138. **Deivert, D.E., Potteiger, C.E., Komar, M. Dubagunta, S., Meschter, S.:** Primary hepatic actinomycosis: Case report and literature review. Pract. Gastroenterol. 2007; 31: 92–100
139. **Kasano, Y., Tanimura, H., Yamaue, H., Hayashido, M., Umano, Y.:** Hepatic actinomycosis infiltrating the diaphragm and right lung. Amer. I. Gastroenterol. 1996; 91: 2418–2420
140. **Kazmi, K.A., Rab, S.M.:** Primary hepatic actinomycosis. Amer. J. Trop. Med. Hyg. 1989; 40: 310–311
141. **Meade, R.H.:** Primary hepatic actinomycosis. Gastroenterology 1980; 78: 355–359
142. **Mongiardo, N., de Rienzo, B., Zanchetta, G., Lami, G., Pellegrino, F., Squadrini, F.:** Primary hepatic actinomycosis. J. Infect. 1986; 12: 65–69
143. **Nazarian, L.N., Spencer, J.A., Mitchell, D.G.:** Multiple actinomycotic liver abscesses: MRI appearances with etiology suggested by abdominal radiography. Case report. Clin. Imag. 1994; 18: 119–122
144. **Roesler, P.J., Wills, J.S.:** Hepatic actinomycosis: CT feature. J. Comput. Assist. Tomogr. 1986; 10: 335–337
145. **Sharma, M., Briski, L.E., Khatib, R.:** Hepatic actinomycosis: an overview of salient features and outcome of therapy. Scand. J. Infect. Dis. 2002; 34: 386–391
146. **Sugano, S., Matuda, T., Suzuki, T., Makino, H., Iinuma, M., Ishii, K., Ohe, K., Mogami, K.:** Hepatic actinomycosis: case report and review of the literature in Japan. J. Gastroenterol. 1997; 32: 672–676
147. **Tambay, R., Cote, J., Bourgault, A.M., Villeneuve, J.P.:** An unusual case of hepatic abscess (case report). Canad. J. Gastroenterol. 2001; 15: 615–617

Burkholderia pseudomallei
148. **Piggot, J.A., Hochholzner, L.:** Human melioidosis. A histopathologic study of acute and chronic melioidosis. Arch. Pathol. Labor. Med. 1970; 90: 101–111

Clinical Aspects of Liver Diseases
25 Parasitic infections and the liver

		Page:
1	***Protozoiases***	498
1.1	*Amoebiasis*	498
1.1.1	Definition	498
1.1.2	Epidemiology and pathogens	498
1.1.3	Courses of disease	499
1.1.4	Hepatic amoebiasis	499
1.1.5	Therapy	500
1.2	*Lambliasis*	500
1.3	*Cryptosporidiosis*	501
1.4	*Leishmaniasis*	501
1.5	*Malaria*	501
1.5.1	Pathogens	501
1.5.2	Malarial cycle	502
1.5.3	Clinical findings	502
1.5.4	Prophylactic measures	502
1.5.5	Therapy	503
1.6	*Toxoplasmosis*	503
1.6.1	Congenital toxoplasmosis	503
1.6.2	Acquired toxoplasmosis	503
1.6.3	Therapy	504
1.7	*Trypanosomiasis*	504
2	***Helminthiases***	504
2.1	*Nematodes*	504
2.1.1	Ascaris lumbricoides	504
2.1.2	Capillaria hepatica	506
2.1.3	Pentastomum denticulatum	506
2.1.4	Strongyloides stercoralis	506
2.1.5	Toxocariasis	506
2.1.6	Trichinella spiralis	507
2.2	*Trematodes*	507
2.2.1	Clonorchis sinensis	507
2.2.2	Dicrocoelium dentriciticum	507
2.2.3	Fasciola hepatica	507
2.2.4	Fasciolopsis buski	508
2.2.5	Opisthorchiasis	508
2.2.6	Schistosomiasis	509
2.3	*Cestodes*	510
2.3.1	Echinococcus cysticus	510
2.3.2	Echinococcus alveolaris	512
	• References (1–161)	514
	(Figures 25.1–25.22; tables 25.1–25.2)	

25 Parasitic infections and the liver

A number of parasitic diseases result in a **coexisting liver reaction** or even lead to **coexisting liver disease.** However, most of these parasitoses are rarely encountered in the temperate zones, and if at all, they occur only sporadically in the wake of immigration and tourist travel to endemic regions.

▶ In recent times, an great number of people (9–10 million) have immigrated to Europe from the Near East and from African and Asian countries. Moreover, hundreds of thousands of people travel every year to remote regions of the earth in search of adventure and new experiences, often living in unhygienic conditions such as those common to backpacking and trekking. In addition, some parasitic diseases that are barely known up to now nevertheless have to be constantly considered for differential diagnosis when unresolved symptoms of disease are present.

Protozoiases	
1. Amoebiasis	(S D E)
2. Lambliasis	
3. Cryptosporidiosis	
4. Leishmaniasis	
5. Malaria	D E
6. Toxoplasmosis (congenital)	P D E
7. Trypanosomiasis	
Helminthiases	
1. Nematodes	
1. Ascaris lumbricoides	
2. Capillaria hepatica	
3. Pentastomum dentriculatum	
4. Strongyloides stercoralis	
5. Toxacara canis	
6. Trichinella spiralis	D E
2. Trematodes	
1. Clonorchis sinensis	
2. Dicrocoelium dentriticum	
3. Fasciola hepatica	
4. Fasciolopsis buski	
5. Opisthorchis felineus	
6. Opisthorchis viverrini	
7. Schistosomiasis	
3. Cestodes	
1. Echinococcus	

Tab. 25.1: Parasitic diseases caused by protozoiases and helminthiases which may lead to liver involvement or concomitant liver disease. The **obligation for notification** in Germany is given in cases of suspicion (S), disease (D), exitus (E) or perinatal infection (P). But this varies from country to country. *If in doubt, contact the Public Health Department*

Generally, the clinical manifestations of the respective parasitosis predominate, and the involvement of the liver may even go unnoticed, especially in the early stages. In individual cases, the laboratory parameters indicative of liver damage are only slightly changed. The various parasites mainly affect either the biliary tract or the liver cells. Consequently, inflammatory infiltration, liver cell necrosis, granulomas, abscesses, fibrosis, vascular occlusion and biliary obstruction as well as the deposition of eggs or larvae in the liver may be observed. Thus there are multiform morphological findings. Parasitoses with potential liver involvement belong to the group of protozoiases and helminthiases. (s. tab. 25.1)

1 Protozoiases

Protozoa are unicellular organisms with a well-defined cell nucleus. Some species are capable of sexual reproduction, while others reproduce asexually. In addition to their vegetative (usually motile) forms, most protozoa also develop cysts as a permanent state under unfavourable external conditions. They move with the aid of flagella or cilia, by amoeboid locomotion or in a winding and gliding manner.

1.1 Amoebiasis

1.1.1 Definition

Amoebiasis is defined as the invasion of the human body by the protozoal organism Entamoeba histolytica, with or without ensuing symptoms of disease or clinical manifestations.

1.1.2 Epidemiology and pathogens

Entamoeba histolytica is an obligate pathogen. It has worldwide distribution and is the third most common parasitic pathogen, with a prevalence of 20–90% among the populations of tropical and subtropical countries. However, given unfavourable hygiene conditions, Ent. histolytica can also be encountered in the temperate zones, particularly when imported by individuals after a stay in the tropics. The frequency of infection is less than 1% in Germany and other European countries, whereby the disease/infection ratio ranges between 1:300 and 4:10. Homosexual males showed a higher incidence of amoebic abscesses.

Cysts: The resistant quadrinucleate (in the immature stage, mononuclear or binuclear) cysts are the permanent forms of Ent. histolytica. The organisms, 10–16 μm in diameter, are round with a monoplastic cytoplasm, in which chromidium bodies may be embedded. They develop from the vegetative minuta form in the lower intestine as a result of increasing dehydration in this area. Both the cysts and the vegetative minuta forms are excreted in semi-solid stools. The minuta form is rapidly destroyed in the external environment. • *For this reason, it is the cysts which are the mode of transmission of Ent. histolytica.*

Minuta form: Following oral ingestion of the cyst, four trophozoites (= minuta form) are generated from each cyst in the intestine. This form, which inhabits the intestinal lumen, has an asymmetric structure, 12–20 μm in diameter, and displays one or two nuclei in its cytoplasm, occasionally with ingested bacteria in the vacuoles. It is capable of amoeboid movement. • *The minuta form is probably a primarily non-pathogenic amoeba, i.e. it is sometimes the cause of mild dysenteric symptoms.*

Magna form: The minuta form reaches the intestinal wall and is converted into the magna form. This is an asymmetric organism, 20–30 (–60) μm in size, with delicate, honeycomb-like cytoplasm and phagocytized erythrocytes (= haematophagous trophozoites), which produce proteolytic enzymes. • Magna forms are excreted from intestinal ulcers or transported to the liver in the portal blood. Very rarely, they can be directly transmitted through small skin or mucosal lesions. *Detection of the magna form is the only reliable criterion of manifest (invasive) intestinal amoebiasis.*

The minuta and magna forms excreted in the faeces in intestinal amoebiasis are usually not infectious, as they perish rapidly in the stools once they have been excreted. Differentiation can be made between the two forms using molecular biology techniques. Only the **cysts** are responsible for transmission, but they are not present in the stool in the acute phase: infection from the cysts is transmitted by the faecal-oral route and hence only in the symptom-free, chronic stage of the disease. An exact incubation period has not been defined. The latent period may last for several years.

1.1.3 Courses of disease

▶ **Intestinal amoebiasis:** Initially, clinical differentiation must be made between diffuse colonic amoebiasis and the (rare) circumscribed involvement of the colon. *Diffuse amoebiasis* of the colon may take different courses: (*1.*) asymptomatic, (*2.*) symptomatic, and (*3.*) symptomatic, but non-dysenteric. (11)

1. **Asymptomatic intestinal amoebiasis** may be found both with and without excretion of cysts or the minuta form of the pathogen. The tissue may, however, also be invaded without the appearance of symptoms, so that patients with extraintestinal amoebiasis do not complain of diarrhoea either during consultation or in the anamnesis. This is obviously of clinical and therapeutic relevance.

2. **Symptomatic intestinal amoebiasis** may, in rare instances, follow a *fulminant course*, whereby the entire colon is affected with clinical symptoms resembling severe shigellosis. Usually, the symptomatic intestinal form is either *acute* or *chronic recurrent*. The cardinal symptoms are: diarrhoea of gradual, sometimes also sudden onset (evacuation frequency 6–8 [–20]/day), small stools of semi-solid or watery consistency with bloody raspberry jelly-like mucous contents as well as lower abdominal spasms, tender abdominal walls and an episodic course of disease. Laboratory tests reveal changes in the blood count (anaemia, leucocytosis, eosinophilia) and inflammation-related parameters. Endoscopic examination of the rectum, sigmoid and colon reveals mucosal ulceration resembling ulcerative colitis or Crohn's disease. The diagnosis can only be confirmed by the identification of the magna forms (mucosal smear, smear preparation of fresh stool specimens, mucosal biopsy or culture method).

3. **Symptomatic, non-dysenteric courses** of disease elicit minor symptoms in the form of loss of appetite, nausea, meteorism, rectal tenesmus, slight diarrhoea alternating with constipation, and diffuse abdominal pain of varying intensity. In patients whose physical defence response is weakened, exacerbation may occur at any moment. • In most cases, amoebic dysentery affects only isolated colonic sections, leaving intermediate regions largely free from lesions. • In the rare instance of **circumscribed intestinal amoebiasis**, the rectum and coecum or sigmoid are primarily and predominantly affected. **Amoebic appendicitis** and **perianal cutaneous amoebiasis** are seen as particular forms of manifestation. • Focal inflammatory infiltration of the abscessed intestinal wall is called **amoeboma**. This consists of granulation tissue with a bleeding tendency. It is mainly localized in the coecum and rectosigmoid. In the case of amoeboma, it can be rather difficult to set up a differential diagnosis to distinguish it from carcinoma, especially in the presence of a symptom complex of stenosis.

Complications: Potential complications include the perforation of the intestinal wall (covered or open), stenosis and stricture as well as intussusception or haemorrhage.

▶ **Extraintestinal amoebiasis:** In the event of an imbalance between the pathogen and the host organism due to various factors (s. tab. 26.1), the minuta form becomes pathogenic. Although it normally inhabits the intestinal mucosa, the minuta form infiltrates the intestinal wall with the aid of a cytolytic enzyme and is converted into the magna form. These magna forms then pass via the portal vein to the *liver*, where they are partially destroyed. Moreover, the liver may now become involved in the amoebiasis. • Extraintestinal dissemination of amoebiasis is effected haematogenically; after passing the hepatic sinusoids, it reaches the lung and brain, rarely also the spleen and kidney. Intestinal amoebiasis may encroach on the neighbouring areas (e.g. peritoneum, pericardium, pleura, female pelvic organs) through direct contact (per continuitatem).

1.1.4 Hepatic amoebiasis

1. **Non-specific mesenchymal reactions:** The reaction to acute intestinal affection from Ent. histolytica consists of moderate diffuse swelling and multiplication of the stellate cells. Other morphological lesions are generally not detectable. The liver may be enlarged and sensitive to pressure.

2. **Liver amoebiasis:** The propagation of amoebae in the liver leads to focal cell necrosis, which regresses spontaneously. Further episodes of focal necrosis may follow. Occasionally, *granulomas* are formed as well. The liver is generally enlarged and sensitive to pressure. The transaminases are slightly elevated. This involvement is called *non-suppurative amoebiasis of the liver*. Liver amoebiasis does not lead to cirrhosis. • There is no evidence of "hepatitis", "chronic non-suppurative hepatitis" or "chronic amoebic hepatitis".

3. **Liver abscess:** In 5—10% of patients with acute invasive intestinal amoebiasis, liver abscesses are formed, which are either solitary (50—70%) or multiple (30—50%). The right lobe of liver is affected five times as often as the left lobe (80—90%). Strictly speaking, the term "abscess" is not correct in this context, since there is actually no leucocytic abscess formation but a pathogen-free cytolytic necrosis. This consists of a viscous, creamy, yellowish-green to chocolate-brown mass, which does not contain any amoebae. Trophozoites are only found in the viable, cell-infiltrated tissues of marginal areas. Secondary infections of the amoebic abscesses are possible. • *Clinical observations* include fever (occasionally with chills), tachycardia, sweats, pain in the right epigastrium radiating to the right shoulder and back, an enlarged liver that is sensitive to pressure, a right costal arch that is sensitive to percussion and a tickling sensation in the throat. Men are affected significantly more often by an abscess than women. • *Laboratory findings* reveal severe bacterial inflammation, a slight increase in the transaminases and a distinct rise in alkaline phosphatase. Hyperbilirubinaemia is a rare occurrence. IgM antibodies against Ent. histolytica can be detected in 90—100% of patients. These antibody titres persist for months or even years. Apart from ELISA, the highly sensitive EIA test and the indirect haemagglutination test are available. Evidence of amoebae is rarely obtained (<10% of cases) by stool examination. • *Imaging techniques* facilitate the diagnosis. In ultrasonography, an amoebic liver abscess appears as a vaguely delineated, hypoechoic (yet not echo-free) space-occupying lesion. (s. fig. 25.1) CT yields the same information. With scintigraphy, "cold" areas are visible. (s. fig. 9.2) Radiological evaluation often shows an elevation or restricted movement of the right diaphragm, atelectasis or infiltration in the right lower area of the lung as well as a marginal angular effusion. Diagnostic puncture is not necessary as a rule; however, PCR may provide proof of Ent. histolytica DNA in the abscess content.

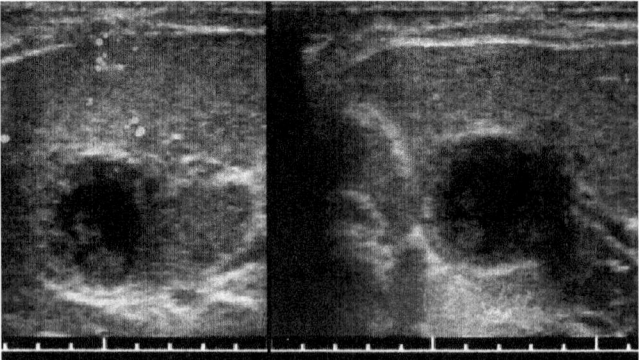

Fig. 25.1: Ultrasonographic visualization of an amoebic abscess in the right lobe of liver (s. fig. 9.2)

Complications: One of the major complications is the confluence of abscesses with subsequent necrosis of large areas of the liver. Furthermore, there is a risk of a covered perforation or rupture into the free abdominal cavity or the adjacent organs, e.g. pleura, pericardium (possibly with the formation of a hepatobronchial fistula) (3), stomach, lung, intestine, gall bladder, bile ducts. Rupture occurs more frequently (20—25%) than in pyogenic liver abscess. Moreover, thrombosis of the inferior vena cava (6) or the portal vein as well as obstructive jaundice may be observed. Arrosion of blood vessels sometimes leads to considerable bleeding. Metastatic spread (e.g. brain) has been observed. (2, 4, 5, 7—12) • With early diagnosis and appropriate treatment, **lethality** is well below 1%, yet ranges between 6.2% (thorax) and 29.6% (pericardium) in cases of abscess perforation. (16)

1.1.5 Therapy

Treatment consists of metronidazole (4 × 500 or 3 × 750 mg/day, orally) for about 10 to 14 days. As an alternative approach, tinidazole (3 × 800 mg/day, orally) for 7 to 10 days or ornidazole (2 × 0.5—1.0 g/day) for 10 to 12 days may be administered. Satranidazole seems to be a new and better alternative. Additional administration of chloroquine (600 mg) for 2 days followed by 300 mg for approx. 2 weeks may be advisable. For decontamination of the intestinal lumen, this regimen should be combined with diloxanide furoate (3 × 500 mg) for 10 to 12 days or paromomycin (3 × 500 mg) for approx. 1 week or iodoquinol (3 × 650 mg) for approx. 3 weeks. Therapeutic progress is monitored by ultrasound (possibly also by CT). If therapy is not entirely successful, the course of treatment is prolonged. • Regression following medication may take several months (even >6). With large abscesses (>6 cm in diameter), impending rupture or lack of impact of the treatment within 5 to 7 days, the abscess should be emptied by means of puncture or drainage. (1) Surgical procedures are only necessary in very severe and/or therapy-resistant cases, especially in necrosis of the left lobe of liver. (2, 10)

1.2 Lambliasis

A pear-shaped, 10—20 μm sized parasite of the small intestine, **Lamblia intestinalis** (or *Giardia lamblia*), is the causative pathogen of lambliasis (or giardiasis). (13) This semipathogenic organism shows a high prevalence in tropical and subtropical regions, but is also repeatedly found in Central European countries — particularly following a stay in the tropics by travellers. • It causes an **infection of the small intestine**. The lambliae attach themselves to the cryptic epithelium of the small intestinal mucosa with the aid of sucking disks. Here, they can form such an extensive and dense lamblia covering that steatorrhoea sometimes results from the disrupted absorption.

Liver involvement can occasionally be recognized by the occurrence of *granulomas*. (14) Laboratory findings reveal a slight increase in γ-GT and AP, pointing to the involvement of the small bile ducts, possibly in the form of *lamblia-induced cholangiopathy*. (14) After parasitization of the gall bladder, *cholecystitis* may occur. • Evidence of highly motile lambliae is readily obtained by examining A, B or C bile procured with the help of a nasoduodenal tube, secretion taken from the small intestine, or suspended and centrifuged stool specimens. In the meantime, tests for the detection of giardia antigens in the stool are available as well. • *Treatment* is effected with iodoquinol (3 × 650 mg), ornidazole, tinidazole (1.5 g) or metronidazole (2 × 250 mg) for a period of five to ten days.

1.3 Cryptosporidiosis

Cryptosporidiosis is classed as traveller's diarrhoea, particularly endemic on the Caribbean islands. The pathogen, an opportunistic protozoon (2−4 µm), is transmitted through contaminated water or food. Clinical findings include watery faeces (5−22 days) with subsequent exsiccation and acetonaemia, headaches and limb pain, vomiting and severe general malaise. The disease persists for up to six weeks. • This infection is also observed in AIDS patients (in 6% of all patients and in 21% of patients with diarrhoea). • The biliary system and the gall bladder are especially affected: epigastric pain and anicteric cholestasis are present. Sonography and CT show dilated bile ducts with mural thickening. ERC may reveal findings similar to those found in primary sclerosing *cholangitis*, while papillary stenosis is also observed on occasions. Frequently, a coexisting cytomegalovirus infection has been found. (15−17)

1.4 Leishmaniasis

▶ Leishmania (W. B. Leishman, 1900) is a parasite with host exchange between humans and female sandflies (Phlebotomus sp.). Leishmaniasis occurs as a zoonosis, usually found in dogs and rodents. Of pathological relevance to humans is **Leishmania donovani** (India, East Africa), an oval, gram-negative, basophilic organism, 3 µm in length. It is the causative pathogen of *visceral leishmaniasis* (kala-azar = black fever, dumdum fever, tropical splenomegaly). These organisms multiply in the RES and macrophages (spleen, liver, small intestine, lymph nodes). L. infantum (Mediterranean region) and L. chagasi (South America) are less frequently found. • *Evidence* is based on cultural or microscopic examination of biopsy specimens (liver, spleen, sternum, tibia or lymph node) and on immunological methods (ELISA, indirect fluorescence test). The leishmaniae penetrate the skin and multiply there, causing an ulcer at the site of entry. • The **infection** may be self-limiting (the pathogens are eliminated in the skin or the liver), or it may become systemic in patients with a weakened immune system and develop into visceral leishmaniasis. The incubation period lasts two to three weeks, and even up to eight months.

The disease runs a course similar to that of an insidious infection with remittent fever (often with a dromedary curve during the day), tickling of the throat, diarrhoea and lymphadenopathy. Hepatosplenomegaly develops as a result of affected sinus endothelia and the subsequent neoformation and multiplication of these cells (a process which is also found in the lymph nodes). A blackish hyperpigmentation (face, hands, feet and abdomen) is a characteristic symptom of visceral leishmaniasis. • *Laboratory tests* reveal a marked increase in IgM

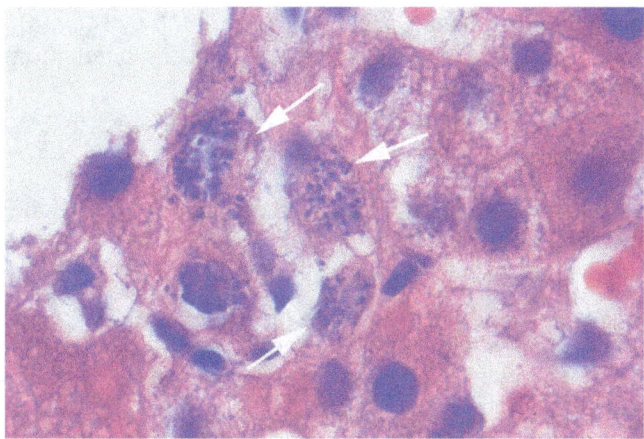

Fig. 25.2: Amastigotes of Leishmania Donovani in swollen Kupffer cells (→) (HE)

and γ-globulins as well as anaemia, leucopenia, thrombopenia and slightly elevated transaminases. Leucosis is a common tentative, albeit incorrect, diagnosis. Liver biopsy is a useful diagnostic tool. (18) • The *liver* is enlarged, the hepatocytes are free of pathogens. The Kupffer cells are severely affected; the basophilic Leishman bodies (2−5 µm in length) can be detected in their interior. (s. fig. 25.2) Non-specific reactive *hepatitis* is present: the portal tracts show dense, small and round-cell infiltrations; lobular peripheral single-cell necrosis and centrolobular fatty degeneration of the liver cells are found. (20) Occasionally, *granulomas* (21) and periportal *fibrosis* develop, in some cases with portal hypertension. (19) • *Treatment* consists of sodium stibogluconate (10−20 mg/kg BW for approx. 20 days) and meglumine antimoniate. Recurrence is possible (even after several years). Combined treatment with γ-interferon or aminosidin is thought to be promising. As alternative regimens, amphotericin B and pentamidine may also be used. With the new drug miltefosin, oral therapy has proved very successful and represents a true breakthrough in the treatment of visceral leishmaniasis. (23) If untreated, the disease is fatal in over 80% of cases as a result of cachexia and/or superinfection. (22, 24)

1.5 Malaria

With 300−500 million new infections annually, malaria is one of the most common infectious diseases in the world. The mortality rate is about two million/year. • In Germany, approximately 1,000 cases are reported each year, and the tendency is rising. About half of them are due to tropical malaria.

1.5.1 Pathogens

Quartan malaria is caused by Plasmodium malariae (incubation period of 18−40 days), *tertian malaria* by Plasmodium vivax and Plasmodium ovale (incubation period of 10 to 18 days), and *tropical malaria* by Plasmodium falciparum (incubation period of 7 to 14 days); administering malaria drugs can extend the incubation period by up to six weeks.

1.5.2 Malarial cycle

The **sexual cycle** (sporogony) takes place in the female anopheline mosquito, while the **asexual cycle** (schizogony) takes place in humans.

Following the bite of an infected female mosquito, the **sporozoites** injected from her salivary gland are rapidly conducted through the bloodstream to the liver cells, where either the pre-erythrocytic or exoerythrocytic phase commences. The sporozoites turn into **schizonts**, which rupture and release massive numbers of **merozoites** into the blood (after 6 to 16 days of maturation), invading the erythrocytes within 20–30 seconds. The erythrocytic phase produces trophozoites and schizonts (which, in turn, discharge large amounts of merozoites into the blood) as well as male and female **gametocytes**, which also reach the blood, possibly to be ingested by another Anopheles mosquito while biting. Sporozoites are formed in intermediary stages in the mosquito stomach, completing the malarial infection cycle. • A certain number of Pl. vivax and Pl. ovale may persist in the liver cells (perhaps even for several years) and provoke late relapses of tertian or tropical malaria. • **Evidence of plasmodias** is obtained in the peripheral blood using the "thin-film method" or the "thick-film method" with the help of Giemsa stain. A **quick test** is now available. Such tests are helpful, but are not considered to be an alternative to stained blood smears.

1.5.3 Clinical findings

The typical bouts of fever (in tertian malaria, every three days with a tendency to recur for up to one year; in quartan malaria, every four days with relapses over a period of up to four years; in tropical malaria, at irregular intervals without late relapses) and chills are caused by the release of merozoites from the erythrocytes. Interestingly, "influenza" is the most common incorrect diagnosis in malaria. Symptoms include headaches and limb pain, severe malaise and hepatosplenomegaly. A reduced HDL cholesterol level is a reliable (and early) indicator of malarial infection. The generally mild jaundice is mainly caused by haemolysis – which correlates with the increased LDH. A moderate rise in the transaminases, possibly also in alkaline phosphatase, and a marked increase in IgG and IgM with a reduction in cholinesterase are observed in some cases, particularly when the course of disease is severe. (28) Leucocytosis suggests a poor prognosis. Especially with Pl. vivax, marked splenomegaly is present (= hyperreactive malaria splenomegaly syndrome) with a danger of splenic rupture. This can also lead to a lymphoproliferative disease. (27) In severe cases and with high pathogen counts, consumptive coagulopathy may develop from microthrombi. • The so-called *airport malaria* is clinically significant. In the vicinity of European airports, anopheles mosquitoes brought inadvertently into the country in summertime can result in unexpected cases of malaria. • During pregnancy, this infection may be passed on to the child by transplacental or perinatal transmission, resulting in initially unexplained fever. • *Liver* histology shows isolated hepatocytes with phagocytized erythrocytes and finely grained siderin. The generally distended sinusoidal cells contain large amounts of haemozoin: small brownish-black balls, 1–2 μm in diameter, of an iron-porphyrin-protein complex, exhibiting a characteristic double refraction under the polarizing microscope. This *malarial pigment* is abundant in quartan malaria. (26, 30, 31) (s. fig. 25.3)

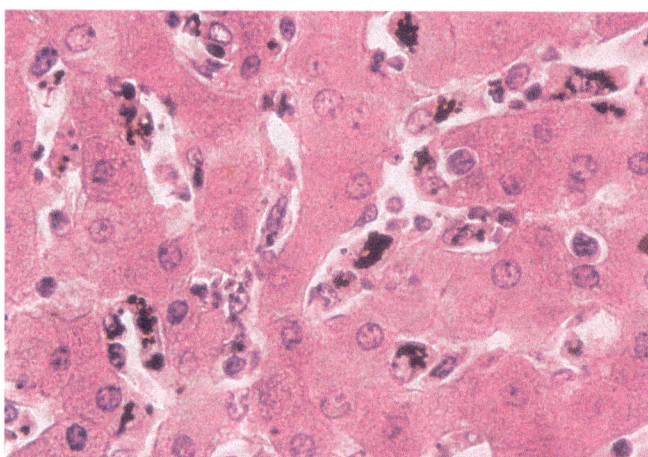

Fig. 25.3: Malarial pigment: marked haemozoin deposition in the hepatic macrophages (HE)

With the augmented deposition of haemozoin, the grey discolouration of the malaria liver develops. In the acute stage, single-cell necrosis may also be detected; chronic malaria generally shows blocks of malarial pigment in the portal field, lobular central sclerosis and occasionally non-specific *granulomas* consisting of histiocytes. Findings of non-specific reactive hepatitis or centroacinar liver cell necrosis might be due to a disrupted microcirculation or hypoxia. Cirrhosis does not occur as a sequela of malaria. • The *lethality* of severe malaria tropica is still >10% despite intensive medical care.

1.5.4 Prophylactic measures

Prevention of malaria comprises exposure prophylaxis and chemoprophylaxis.

1. **Exposure prophylaxis,** i.e. avoiding mosquito bites, may considerably reduce the risk of malaria when carried out systematically. This means applying mosquito repellants to uncovered skin areas, wearing sufficient clothing to protect as much of the skin surface as possible, staying in rooms kept free of mosquitoes (air-conditioning, insect screens) and using insecticide-impregnated mosquito nets. The additional use of insecticides (spray, aerosol) in rooms and vaporizers or smoke spirals outdoors (e.g. on the patio) may be very effective. Preventing exposure is imperative, particularly at dawn and dusk and during the night, since these are the times when Anopheles mosquitoes are active.

2. **Chemoprophylactic measures** have become extremely complex and more difficult to apply due to increasing resistance. Varying degrees of resistance to virtually every **antimalarial agent** can be expected, depending on the geographic region. Multiresistance is also on the rise. According to a WHO classification, the malaria areas are defined as **zone A** (areas without chloroquine resistance or without Pl. falciparum), **zone B** (areas with resistance to chloroquine) and **zone C** (areas with extreme resistance to chloroquine or multiresistance). • In the light of this zone definition, chemoprophylaxis based on *chloroquine* (300–450 mg/week), *proguanil* (200 mg/day) or *mefloquine* (250 mg/week) is recommended. *Tafenoquine* (250 mg/day for 3 days) may be a new drug for the prevention of malaria; the prophylactic effect is given as 7 weeks. • *Preventive inoculation* is still in the experimental stage.

1.5.5 Therapy

In suspected malaria, *self-treatment* with halofantrine (3 × 500 mg = 3 × 2 tablets at intervals of 6 hours) on day 1 and day 8 should commence if immediate diagnosis and treatment are not possible. Alternatively, mefloquine can also be given (1,000 mg = 4 tablets or 15 mg/kg BW as a single dose; with a body weight of >60 kg, another 250 mg may have to be given after 6 hours and 12 hours). • In non-immune patients, malaria tropica must be treated in a hospital as an emergency. Treatment consists of quinine (3 × daily, approx. 10 mg/kg BW, orally) for a period of 8 days, and in complicated cases as i.v. infusion, possibly with simultaneous administration of doxycycline. Other regimens include mefloquine or halofantrine. • In tertian and quartan malaria, chloroquine, mefloquine or halofantine are used. Additionally, primaquine (15 mg = 1 tablet for 14 days) is imperative for eliminating persistent (proerythrocytic) hypnozoites; if necessary, treatment is repeated with a maximum total dosage of 280–420 mg. • New drug combinations for combating tropical malaria are proguanil plus atovaquone (29) and arthemether plus lumefantrin. In cerebral malaria, artemisinin has been used successfully. (25)

1.6 Toxoplasmosis

Toxoplasmosis is caused by **Toxoplasma gondii** (2–7 μm in size). There is a secondary exchange of hosts with a developmental cycle (coccidian cycle) in cats (and possibly other Felidae) as specific hosts with excretion of oocysts in the faeces. Such an acyclic development is found in all mammals, various birds (= non-specific hosts) and humans. The **infection** is transmitted through exposure to cat faeces, by consumption of raw meat infected with oocysts, in the breast milk or via the placenta. The exact incubation period is unknown. Toxoplasma is one of the most widespread parasites, especially in humid and warm climates. The frequency of toxoplasma infection in the population is extremely high, although there are considerable regional and individual differences. Both the acute and the chronic stages of disease are asymptomatic. Consequently, toxoplasmosis presents a mild pathological picture, since the virulence of the pathogen is balanced by the undisturbed immunological response of the organism; in this case, an infection with Toxoplasma gondii is of no consequence. Occasionally observed concomitant symptoms (fatigue, basophilia in the blood, lymphadenopathy, etc.) are signs of an immunization process. Swollen lymph nodes may therefore persist for some months before the condition regresses spontaneously. • Toxoplasmosis will only lead to a serious clinical picture in the presence of an **impaired immune response.** Most cysts are found in the CNS, the myocardium and the liver, where the parasite can multiply longest. In these tissues, late sensitization leads to the destruction of the parasite with simultaneous development of varying degress of tissue necrosis.

1.6.1 Congenital toxoplasmosis

Toxoplasma infections occurring before pregnancy have no effect on the child: the parasite is not transmitted to the foetus. • During pregnancy, the infection is transmitted in approx. 50% of cases; the later the maternal infection is acquired, the greater the frequency (approx. 15% in the first, approx. 25% in the second and approx. 65% in the third trimenon). Massive parasitization leads to stillbirth or premature delivery, usually with severe defects. Besides generalized invasion, the parasites are localized in the CNS, whereby chorioretinitis is also in evidence. • From the hepatological viewpoint, marked jaundice and hepatosplenomegaly as well as anasarca and ascites are worth mentioning. The endothelial cells of the liver are distended, and this is where the slightly falcate pathogens are also detectable. Isolated cases present liver cell degeneration and necrosis; later on there may be evidence of microcalcification.

1.6.2 Acquired toxoplasmosis

In early infancy, liver involvement manifests as *giant-cell hepatitis* (s. fig. 22.5) or *non-specific reactive hepatitis.* (s. fig. 21.1) Furthermore, granulomas (s. p. 398) may develop, sometimes with marked density. The transaminases are elevated; cholestasis is also frequently detectable. (32, 33, 35, 37)

In children and adults, signs of *non-specific reactive hepatitis* have also been observed. (36) Acidophilic liver cell necrosis occasionally develops, depending on the type of red corpuscles. The endothelial cells are distended, the portal zones show inflammatory infiltration, and *granulomas* or retothelial nodules are frequently found. (s. fig. 25.4) The pathogens can be demonstrated in the liver. *Cirrhosis* may develop, especially after the destruction of the lobular architecture as a sequela of extensive parenchymal necrosis. • There are various *serological tests* available, including the Sabin-Feldmann dye test, the indirect immunofluorescence test (IFT), the indirect haemagglutination test (IHA) and the ELISA test. Evidence of IgM antibodies is obtained as early as five days after infection. Direct identification of the pathogen is achieved by means of the PCR technique. (34)

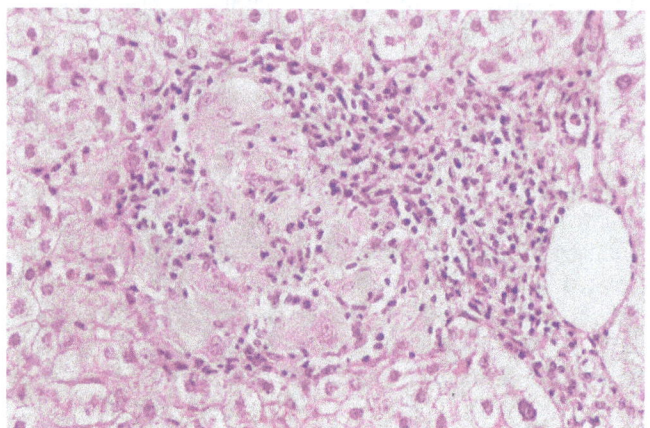

Fig. 25.4: Granuloma close to a portal field. Clinical diagnosis: Toxoplasmosis (HE)

1.6.3 Therapy

Asymptomatic or uncomplicated primary infection does not require treatment. Severe courses of disease are treated with pyrimethamine (50 mg/day for approx. 2 weeks, followed by 25 mg/day for approx. 2 weeks) or sulphamethoxydiazine (50 mg for day 1, 25 mg as from day 2 or 3) + pyrimethamine (100 mg/kg BW/day) or clindamycin + pyrimethamine. As an alternative approach (e. g. in the first trimester of pregnancy), spiramycin may be given. In order to reduce the myelotoxicity of pyrimethamine, the administration of folic acid (10–15 mg/day) is recommended.

1.7 Trypanosomiasis

Trypanosomes belong to the genus of flagellates with a spindle-shaped thin body, large central nucleus, small kinetoplasts and a highly motile flagellum. The cycle of development requires both vertebrate and insect hosts. • **Diagnosis** of the blood parasite is obtained by dark-field and phase-contrast microscopy, Giemsa stain, culture and tissue biopsy. Serological evidence is based on the FTA test as well as on CFR and IgM antibodies in the liquor. • **Treatment** in early stages (also as a preventive measure) consists of suraminum natricum or pentamidine; in the tertiary stage, tryparsamide or melarsoprol are recommended.

The **transmission** of **Tryp. gambiense** and **Tryp. rhodesiense** (*"African sleeping sickness"*) is caused by tsetse flies. Outside the body, these pathogens only survive for a brief period. Multiplication takes place in the peripheral blood, possibly also in the lymph nodes, CSF and bone marrow. The incubation period is one to three weeks (= primary stage with headaches, limb pain and fever). Pathogenic invasion of the blood and lymph vessels (= secondary stage) causes swelling of the lymph nodes, splenomegaly and bouts of fever. When the CNS is affected, a serious clinical picture appears, which can culminate in death after a few weeks or months if untreated. • The **liver** shows centroacinar cell necrosis and inflammatory infiltration, especially in the portal fields.

The **transmission** of **Tryp. cruzi** is caused by reduviid bugs, which excrete infectious trypanosomes in their faeces. These enter the body through small skin or mucosal lesions. They cause the "South American sleeping sickness", also called *Chagas' disease* (C. CHAGAS, 1908). • In the **liver** only portal round-cell infiltrates are found.

2 Helminthiases

Infections caused by helminths often lead to liver involvement. The parasites or their immature forms may reach the **liver** (*1.*) via the *portal vein* (e. g. eggs of schistosomes), (*2.*) via the *hepatic artery* (e. g. scolices of echinococci), (*3.*) transperitoneally through *Glisson's capsule* (e. g. larvae of Fasciola hepatica), and (*4.*) ascending through the *bile ducts* (e. g. larvae of the Clonorchis sinensis). • *Histological signs* of the parasitization of the liver often include granuloma formation, fibroblast activation and an eosinophilic cellular reaction. • *Laboratory parameters* frequently reveal eosinophilia and an increase in IgE. • Under certain circumstances, three different **helminth species** can appear: (*1.*) nematodes (roundworms or eelworms), (*2.*) trematodes (flukes), and (*3.*) cestodes (tapeworms). (s. tab. 25.1)

2.1 Nematodes

2.1.1 Ascaris lumbricoides

Ascariasis is one of the most common parasitoses: approx. 800 million people are infected. The **ascarid** is cream-coloured, generally 4–6 mm in diameter and 15–25 cm (males) or 20–40 cm (females) in length, the latter showing an involuted posterior part. The worm lives mainly in the jejunum. The female lays nearly 200,000 eggs daily during her life span of about one year, so that faecal evidence is relatively easy to obtain. • The compact oval **ascaris eggs** (up to 60 μm in diameter) show a peculiarly structured surface, yellowish-brown in colour. (s. fig. 25.5)

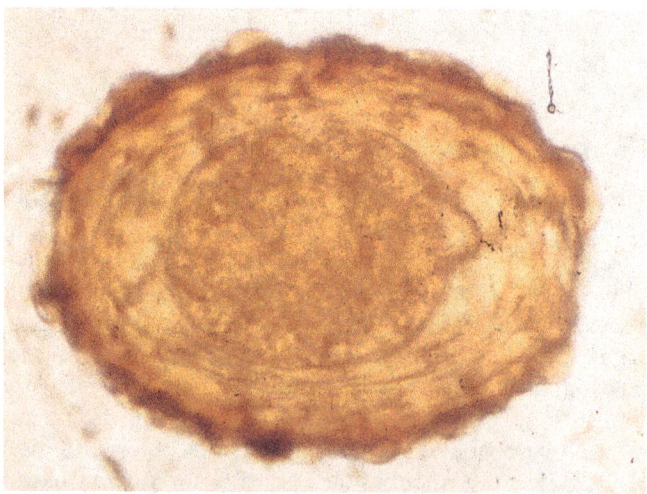

Fig. 25.5: Egg of Ascaris lumbricoides in bile fluid (obtained by means of a nasogastroduodenal probe)

After fertilization, the larvae in the eggs mature in about 2 (−8) weeks at the appropriate temperature (= **larval stages 1 and 2**). The route of infection is faecal-oral. After oral ingestion, the eggs reach the small intestine, where the **larvae** shed the egg membrane. They penetrate the intestinal mucosa and enter the lymph vessels and bloodstream before migrating to the liver (= **larval stage 3**), where a major part of the larvae is destroyed. The rest travel to the lung, where they leave the capillaries and reach the alveoli (= **larval stage 4**). The larvae are transported via the bronchial tract to the trachea and larynx. The pulmonary larval migration may be accompanied by transitory, often multiple eosinophilic lung infiltrates, sometimes with asthmatic symptoms for the individual and, in the case of secondary infection, by bronchopneumonia. When swallowed, the larvae reach the small intestine a second time (= **larval stage 5**). Here, in roughly 3 months, they mature to become ascarids of separate sexes. Their life span as intestinal parasites is 12 to 18 months.

Diagnosis: The diagnosis is confirmed by the presence of Ascaris eggs in the stool or bile. (s. fig. 25.5) With X-ray examination, the ascarids are shown to form a recess in the contrast medium in the bowl (s. figs. 25.6, 25.7); alternatively, they are detectable one day later due to their intestinal resorption of the CM. The ascarids sometimes travel to the common bile duct, so that they can be confirmed by ultrasound (40, 46, 50) (s. fig. 25.8), ERC, CT or MRT. (43, 47) (s. tab. 25.2).

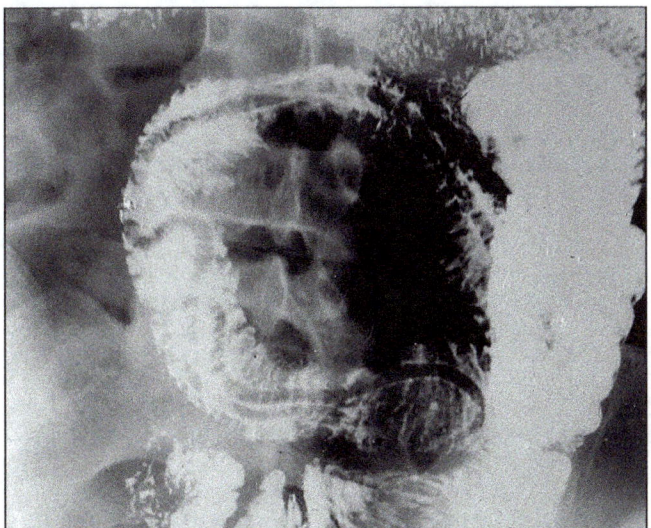

Fig. 25.6: X-ray with contrast medium showing two ascarids in the duodenum

The **clinical picture** is characterized by different symptoms; in some cases, the ascarid leads to diffuse abdominal pain of varying severity. By entering the bile ducts, it causes recurrent biliary colics and fever, sometimes also haemobilia, and the symptom complex of obstructive cholestasis, cholangitis or cholecystitis. (39, 42, 43, 45, 50) Residues of a dead ascarid in the bile duct may

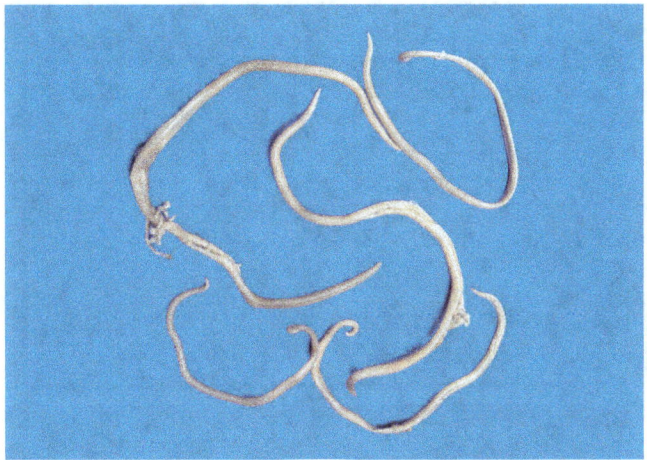

Fig. 25.7: Passage of the ascaris pair and three young ascarids (not shown by the X-ray above) through the intestine following antihelminthic treatment

Sonography

1. Single, long-linear or curved echogenic nonshadowing structure
  – without an inner tube *(= stripe sign)*
  – containing either a central anechogenic tube or tubular structure *(= inner tube sign)*
2. Multiple, long linear overlapping echogenic structure *(= spaghetti sign)*

ERC
1. Smooth, long-linear filling defects with tapering ends; mostly dilated common bile duct
CT
1. Bull's eye appearance in postcontrast scans
MRT
1. Linear, hyperintense tubular structure with central hypointense area 2. Linear, hypointense filling defects in massive biliary ascariasis

Tab. 25.2: Key features of imaging techniques for the diagnosis of biliary ascariasis

calcify or trigger the formation of bile concrement. The abdominal complaints are not relieved by spasmolytics, especially since the parasite can now penetrate even further into the bile ducts. (s. fig. 25.8) • The ascarids may migrate from the biliary system to the liver parenchyma and can even reach below Glisson's capsule. This may entail vascular thrombosis and abscesses, mainly in the left lobe of liver. The colonization by larvae or eggs provokes granulomas with giant cells and eosinophilic margins as well as portal infiltration. (41, 44)

Various **complications** are known: pneumonia, asthmatic attacks *(= asthma verminosum)*, parasitization of the biliary tract (= cholangitis) (38, 45, 48), liver (= hepatic lesions), pancreatic duct (= pancreatitis), appendix (= appendicitis) and entanglement of worms (= ileus).

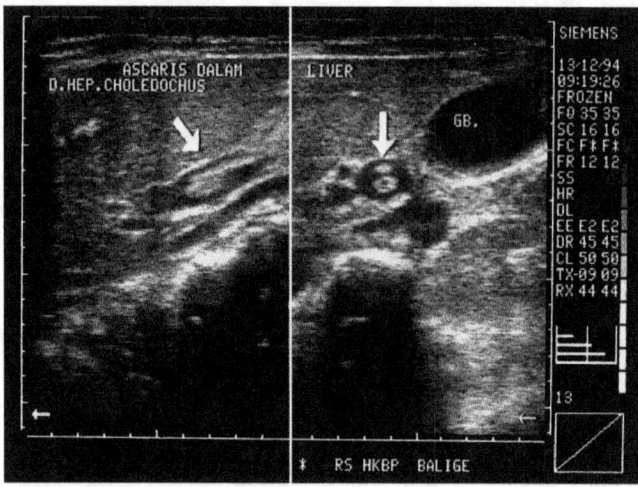

Fig. 25.8: Sonographic visualization of an Ascaris lumbricoides in the common bile duct (longitudinal/transverse imaging). Clinical findings: colicky pain, cholestasis and slight jaundice

Therapy: The treatment regimen consists of levamisole (1 × 150 mg) or albendazole (400–800 mg), flubendazole (1 × 200 mg), pyrantel pamoate (1 × 10 mg/kg BW), piperazine (1 × 75 mg/kg BW, up to a maximum total dosage of 4 g) as well as mebendazole (2 × 100 mg/day for 3 days). • Endoscopic measures for the removal of an ascarid from the common bile duct, possibly after sphincterotomy, are sometimes necessary. (38, 43, 48–51) If endoscopic extraction has failed, surgical intervention becomes necessary.

2.1.2 Capillaria hepatica

Capillaria hepatica is encountered in the livers of vertebrates such as rats, squirrels, dogs, beavers and pigs. The worm measures 35–50 (–60) mm in length. Humans are infected through the ingestion of worm eggs excreted in the faeces of these host animals, occasionally also through the consumption of the liver of infected animals. The worm eggs are transported to the coecum, where the larvae hatch. They penetrate the coecal wall and reach the liver via the portal system. This is where the maturation of the adult worms takes place. The females die after some weeks, and a large number of eggs are released into the liver. The infection with Capillaria hepatica may be mild or asymptomatic or lead to weight loss, general malaise, fever, oedema and eosinophilia as well as hepatomegaly, with an increase in the transaminases and alkaline phosphatase. Histiocytic granulomas develop in the liver, with an abundance of eosinophilic granulocytes. Their identification by liver biopsy yields the diagnosis. • No *treatment* for this worm disease is yet known.

2.1.3 Pentastomum denticulatum

Pentastomum denticulatum is the final larva of the nasal worm Linguatula serrata. The adult parasites (4–5 mm long) live in the nasal cavities and respiratory tracts of carnivorous animals and snakes. Infection is transmitted through oral ingestion of the eggs, with subsequent development of the larvae in the small intestine. They travel via the portal vein to the *liver*, where they encyst and form hard, yellow nodules of ca. 3 mm in diameter. Histology reveals fibrous alterations as well as granulomatous infiltrates; fine calcifications can occasionally be detected. • No *therapy* is known.

2.1.4 Strongyloides stercoralis

The **dwarf threadworm** has two separate developmental phases: a *strongyloid type* with a parthenogenetic, parasitic cycle and a free-living *saprozoic type* of both sexes. The filariform larvae penetrate the skin and reach the lungs via the bloodstream; then they migrate through the trachea to the oesophagus, where they are swallowed, and subsequently make their way to the upper section of the small intestine. Here the female parasites mature and lay eggs (no eggs are found in the liver). The larvae hatch and are either excreted in the stool or re-enter the body in the bloodstream after penetrating the intestinal wall (= *endoautoinvasion*) or perianal skin (= *exoautoinvasion*), so that a new developmental phase begins via the lung. The two types of autoinfection and the additional free-living cycle account for the extreme obstinacy of strongyloidosis. Sometimes, major gastrointestinal disorders with bloody diarrhoea, pulmonary infiltrates and asthma verminosum occur.

Liver: In the liver, the larvae cause portal infiltration and granulomas. The parasites can also invade the bile ducts, giving rise to cholestasis or cholangitis, even obstructive jaundice or cholecystitis. *Diagnosis* is based on finding motile larvae (ca. 300 μm) in the stool or duodenal juice (perhaps after enrichment) and by an indirect immunofluorescence test or ELISA. *Treatment* consists of thiabendazole (2 × 25 mg/kg BW for 5 days), mebendazole (2 × 200 mg for 3 days), albendazole (400–800 mg for 3 days) or ivermectin (100 μg/kg BM/day for 2 days). • In Germany, the infection is seen as an *occupational disease* among miners and tunnel workers with obligation for notification. (52) (s. p. 583)

2.1.5 Toxocariasis

Toxocariasis is transmitted to humans by dogs (T. canis) and more rarely by cats (T. cati) through oral infection with eggs. The adult worms measure 4–12 cm in length. The larvae mature in the eggs and after hatching in the intestinal tract, pass into various organs, including the liver and lungs.

Liver: In the liver, the larvae cause local inflammatory infiltrates, eosinophilic portal infiltration, small abscesses and granulomas. The latter, which often contain Charcot-Leyden crystals, may become confluent and form conglomerates. Many of the larvae die in the liver, the rest encyst in the granulomas. (55) Fibrous alterations can occur. This liver infestation is also known as *visceral larva migrans disease*. (54, 55, 57) • *Diagnosis* is obtained using ELISA and liver biopsy. (53, 55, 56) Clinically, there is evidence of fever, nausea, eosinophilia, hepato(-spleno)megaly, bronchopulmonary disorders and an increase in γ-globulins, AP and γ-GT. Migration of the larvae to the eyes (chorioretinitis, iridocyclitis) (57), the lungs and the myocardium may lead to severe complications. The disease is mostly self-limiting, no *therapy* being required. In severe cases, treatment consists of diethylcarbamazine (9 mg/kg BW/day), given in three single doses per day for a period of three weeks. As an alternative regimen, thiabendazole (50 mg/kg BW/day) may be administered, possibly combined with steroids, mebendazole or ivermectine.

2.1.6 Trichinella spiralis

Infection with *Trichinella spiralis* is caused by consumption of raw meat from pigs or wild boars containing encysted larvae. The larvae are released in the stomach or duodenum and grow within five to seven days to sexually mature parasites. Following fertilization, the female trichinae burrow into the intestinal wall and discharge living larvae into the bloodstream and lymph vessels. They are deposited as trichina cysts in muscles, with involuted trichinae. The diagnosis is established by antibody detection (unfortunately, not until the third or fourth week). It may also be possible to establish the presence of nucleinic acids using PCR.

Liver: The trichinae also reach the liver, where they invade the sinusoids and may cause an inflammatory mesenchymal reaction. There is likewise an abundance of liver granulomas. (58, 59) • *Treatment* for trichinosis during the motile phase consists of mebendazole and possibly thiabendazole (in a gradually increasing dosage, with additional administration of glucocorticoids, if necessary).

2.2 Trematodes

2.2.1 Clonorchis sinensis

The **Chinese liver fluke** measures 1.0–2.5 cm in length. It is most common in China, Japan and South East Asia. Transmission is via consumption of raw or undercooked freshwater fish. The main hosts are pigs, dogs, cats and humans. The yellowish-brown eggs are approx. 30 µm in size and have an "operculum". (s. fig. 25.9)

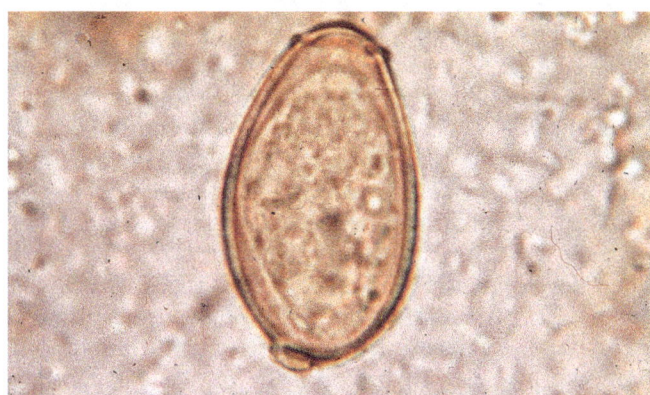

Fig. 25.9: Egg of Clonorchis sinensis in bile fluid (obtained by a nasogastroduodenal probe)

The eggs, which contain a miracidium, are excreted in the faeces. They are eaten by water snails. The latter excrete cercarias, which penetrate fish as metacercarias and encyst in their muscles. After these fish have been ingested, the cercarias are released in the duodenum and migrate to the bile ducts, where they mature into parasitic worms within the space of one month. The worms can live in the bile ducts for several years. (s. fig. 25.10)

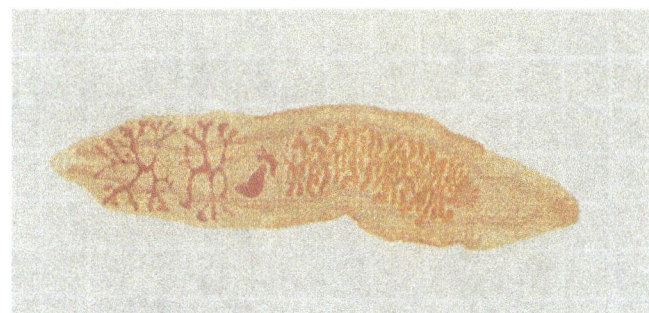

Fig. 25.10: Chinese liver fluke (Clonorchis sinensis)

The *clinical picture* of clonorchiasis is characterized by epigastric pain and fever, sometimes with chills, diarrhoea, weight loss, hepatomegaly, eosinophilia, slight jaundice and an increase in enzymatic markers of cholestasis. The blood-sucking liver flukes cause proliferation and adenoma-like growth with periductal fibrosis in the area of the affected *bile ducts*. Potential late sequelae of chronic cholangitis are miliary liver abscesses, intrahepatic gallstones and biliary cirrhosis. Cholangiocarcinoma and carcinoma of the gall bladder may also develop. (60–66, 68–70) • *Diagnosis* is confirmed by the presence of eggs in stool specimens, but more reliably in the bile after nasoduodenal probing (especially in the so-called B bile after choleretic stimulation). Sonographically, widened bile ducts with inhomogeneous reflexes are detectable. (62, 67, 69) ERC shows filling defects and mural irregularities of the bile ducts. • *Treatment* is with praziquantel (3×25 mg/kg BW/day) for about two days.

2.2.2 Dicrocoelium dentriciticum

This **small liver fluke** (5–12 mm long) evolves in two intermediate hosts. A special snail species excreting metacercarias is necessary as the first host. They are ingested by cattle and sheep. Human infection is rare. • The cercarias travel through the duodenum to the bile ducts, where they grow into mature liver flukes. Dicrocoeliasis is characterized by biliary ailments and respective findings.

2.2.3 Fasciola hepatica

The **large liver fluke** (length: 2–3 cm, diameter: 0.8–1.5 cm) is a leaf-shaped biliary parasite. It is found worldwide, its main natural reservoirs being in sheep and cattle. Human infection is accidental. (72, 84) The eggs are excreted in the faeces. The larvae (miracidia) emerge from the eggs and penetrate freshwater snails (Lymnaea species), which, in turn, release cercarias. As metacercarias, they attach themselves to water plants, especially watercress. (89) When infected plants are ingested, the metacercarias are released in the upper intestinal tract. They penetrate the intestinal wall, reach the free abdominal cavity and invade other organs, particularly the liver parenchyma via Glisson's capsule. It takes them several weeks to reach the biliary system, where the parasite then develops in a hermaphroditic fashion. (s. fig. 25.11)

During their migration through the *liver parenchyma*, the young parasites cause major lesions, cell necroses, haemorrhages and inflammatory infiltration. (74, 82, 89) The eggs deposited in the liver tissue lead to the forma-

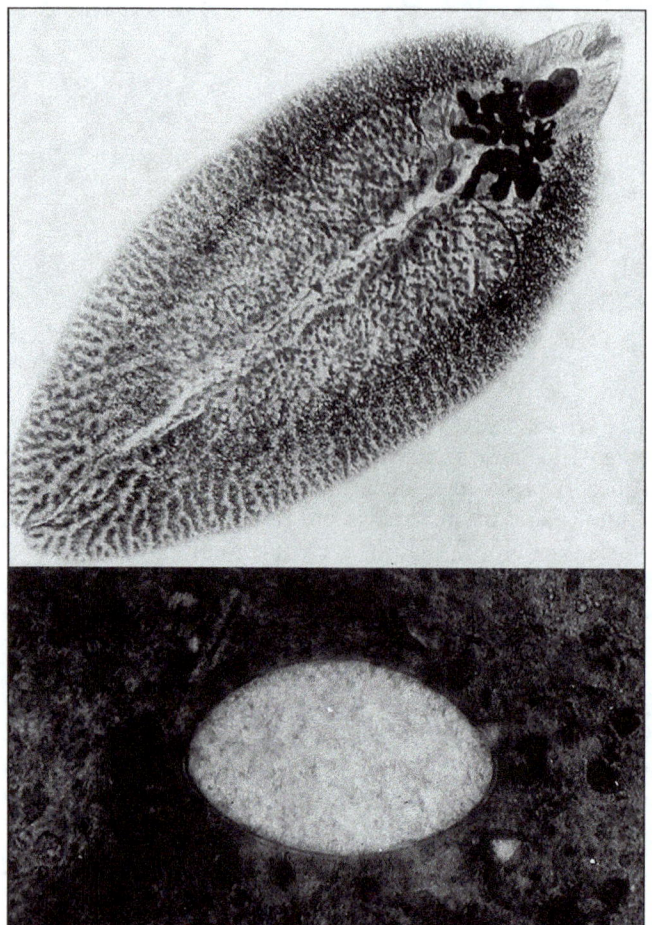

Fig. 25.11: Fasciola hepatica (large liver fluke), 2.9 × 1.1 cm (× 3). • Ovum of Fasciola hepatica, approx. 0.13 × 0.07 mm, in bile fluid (obtained by means of a nasogastroduodenal probe) (× 400)

tel. (83, 87) If oral therapy proves unsuccessful, an endoscopic rinsing of the biliary system using a povidone-iodine solution is recommended. Invasive methods (sphincterotomy, insertion of endoprostheses) and surgical intervention are necessary in some cases. (74, 75, 79)

2.2.4 Fasciolopsis buski

This **large intestinal fluke** is a common parasite in East Asia. It is the largest trematode (5–7 cm by 1.2–1.5 cm) to infect humans. (s. fig. 25.12) Infection occurs through consumption of freshwater plants, especially raw water-nuts, infected with metacercarias. Water snails serve as intermediate hosts. • Infection leads to fever, weight loss, vomiting, abdominal pain, bloody diarrhoea (later greyish-yellow stool), anaemia and ascites as well as cholangitis and liver abscesses, with corresponding laboratory findings.

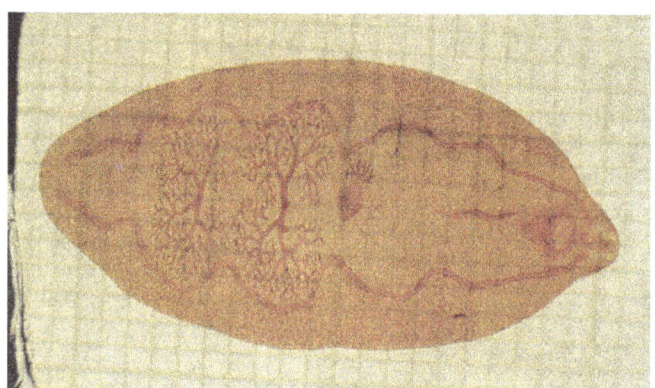

Fig. 25.12: Large intestinal fluke (Fasciolopsis buski)

tion of granulomas. The bile ducts display epithelial proliferation, budding processes and proliferation of the connective tissue with the associated circumscribed inflammatory narrowing of the affected bile ducts. Cholangitis can occur, possibly with abscess formation. (78, 81, 88) The bile ducts may be obstructed by the liver flukes and their eggs. • *Clinical findings* during the liver invasion and migration phase (5 or 6 days after ingestion) feature pain in the right epigastrium, hepato(spleno)megaly, fever, vomiting, diarrhoea, loss of appetite, urticaria, meteorism as well as leucocytosis, eosinophilia, increased ESR, slight jaundice and elevated liver enzymes. (75) Over a period of years, chronic cholangitis and biliary cirrhosis may develop. (74) • *Diagnosis* is based on the presence of eggs (0.14 × 0.08 mm in size) in the stool or bile fluid. (s. fig. 25.11) Serological tests are also available. Nodular changes (4–10 mm), small liver abscesses and bile-duct irregularities may be identified by ultrasound (71, 73, 76, 79, 81), CT (73, 74, 78, 79, 81, 85) (s. tab. 8.2) or cholangiography. (86) • *Treatment* is based on bithionol (30–50 mg/kg BW, in three single doses, every second day for 2–3 weeks), or alternatively triclabendazole (1–2 × 10 mg/kg BW) and nitazoxanide (80), possibly also with (the less potent) praziquan-

2.2.5 Opisthorchiasis

Opisthorchis felineus: This fluke, also called *Siberian liver fluke* (K.N. VINOGRADOV, 1891), is found mainly in Asia, but to an increasing extent in Europe as well. It measures 0.7–1.2 cm in length by 2–3 mm in diameter and is of a light reddish colour. The pale brown eggs, with a length of 20–30 μm and a diameter of 10–14 μm, are somewhat smaller than the eggs of Clonorchis sinensis; they also have an "operculum". (s. fig. 25.9) Their development is similar to that of the Chinese liver fluke. • This fluke infection of the *biliary tract* likewise leads to severe reactive cholangitis with proliferation, adenoma-like growth and fibrosis as well as chronic cholangitis, liver abscesses, haemobilia and cholelithiasis. Biliary cirrhosis and cholangiolar carcinoma may develop. (90–93) • *Treatment* is with praziquantel (40–75 mg/kg BW in three doses).

Opisthorchis viverrini: This fluke is also encountered in East Asia, mainly in Thailand, Laos and Cambodia, and has the same course of development as Clonorchis sinensis. It causes similar alterations in the biliary tract and liver. (92, 93)

2.2.6 Schistosomiasis

▶ Some 200–250 million people in over 70 countries are suffering from schistosomiasis (bilharziosis). This parasitosis is found in large areas of Africa, South America, Asia and Puerto Rico. • The eggs (approx. 150 μm long with a **characteristic side "thorn"**) reach the water in the environment with the stools and are ingested by freshwater snails; subsequently, cercarians develop in these intermediate hosts. Humans are exposed to **infection** when coming into contact with contaminated water; the larvae penetrate the skin by way of borer glands or, alternatively, infection occurs via mucous membranes. During this process, the larvae discard their tails before making their way through the venous system into the right heart and the pulmonary capillaries, subsequently passing through the left heart into the arterial circulation and hence to the **liver**. Here, within a space of four to six weeks, the larvae develop into worms, 10–20 mm in length and 1–2 mm in diameter, each with two sucking disks on the head and another two on the posterior part of the body. The worms migrate hepatofugally in pairs into the **portal system,** mainly into the superior mesenteric vein (and through anastomoses also into the pelvic veins). The worms can reside here for years, living either in sexual segregation or as pairs, the females laying up to 350 eggs daily. Some eggs are excreted in the stool, others reach the liver via the portal system and embolize into the perisinusoidal venoles. (96, 97, 103)

Four of the five species infecting humans may cause liver disease: S. mansoni. S. japonicum, S. intercalatum and S. mekongi. The disease has an incubation period of four to six weeks. It manifests as fever ("Katayama fever"), chills, headaches, arthralgia, pain in the right epigastrium, blood-flocked mucous diarrhoea, loss of weight, lymphadenopathy and urticarial skin reactions. The liver and the spleen are moderately enlarged, especially in the case of S. japonicum and S. mansoni (= hepatolienal bilharziosis). Chronic schistosomiasis develops (in about 10% of infected persons) after years or even decades. Laboratory values reveal eosinophilia, thrombopenia (as a predictor of portal hypertension) (101) and anaemia, markedly increased inflammatory parameters (e.g. ESR, α- and γ-globulins, CRP) as well as a moderate rise in the transaminases, γ-GT and alkaline phosphatase. Jaundice is rare. (97, 103, 104, 107)

During the early stages of larval and worm migration and at the outset of egg-laying, the *liver* often shows signs of non-specific reactive *hepatitis*. The Kupffer cells frequently contain an iron-free pigment. The deposited eggs lead to the formation of *granulomas* with lamellar wall structures and perigranulomatous inflammatory reactions. (98, 99, 103, 107, 112) (s. fig. 25.13) • The eggs are detectable inside the granulomas and may occasionally calcify. Especially in cases of infection (e.g. Staphylococcus pyogenes aureus, Streptococcus intermedius), conglomerates of bacteria in the form of granules can develop. (110) Because of their grape-like shape, they are termed bothryomycosis (but they are not fungi!). They form eosinophilic antigen-antibody precipitates, which surround fungal foci, parasites or abscesses and appear as radiating eosinophilic spokes or thick eosinophilic rings. This condition is known as the **Splendore-Hoeppli phenomenon**. (110) (s. p. 404) • There is subsequent formation of marked portal and perilobular *fibrosis*, which

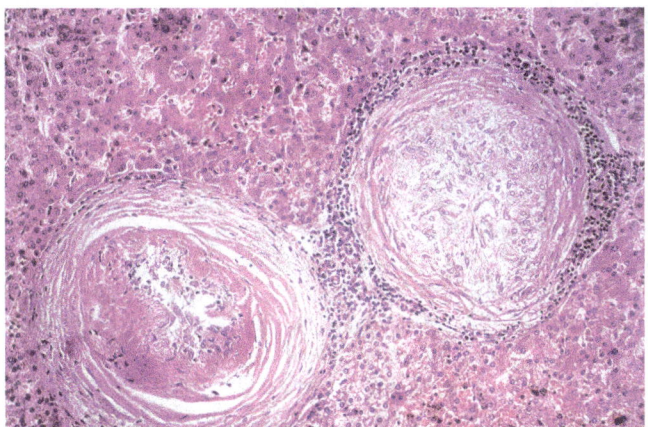

Fig. 25.13: Schistosomiasis: cicatricial granulomas with lamellar walls; perifocal lymphohistiocytic inflammatory rim (HE)

is most pronounced with S. mansoni and S. japonicum. (s. fig. 25.14) Especially in the case of S. mansoni, white *clay pipe-stem fibrosis* is characteristically present (W. S. C. SYMMERS, 1904). The lobular structure is retained. The portal branches reveal a thickening of the walls, with clot formation and rarefaction, resulting in the picture of *endophlebitis obliterans*. • Portal hypertension occurs as a sequela of presinusoidal block formation. (s. p. 255) As a result of compression of the small liver veins by granulomas, postsinusoidal block formation can arise as an additional feature. Splenic infarcts with perisplenitis are frequently detectable. Isolated bilharzia eggs are also found in the spleen. Even in the early stage of the disease, oesophageal and fundus varices are formed as a result of *portal hypertension*, and there is a danger of bleeding. (100, 102, 109, 111) Oedemas and ascites are often observed. Hepatic encephalopathy need not be feared owing to the intact liver function; nor does cirrhosis occur. In the course of time, however, the liver (especially the left lobe) shows signs of shrinkage.

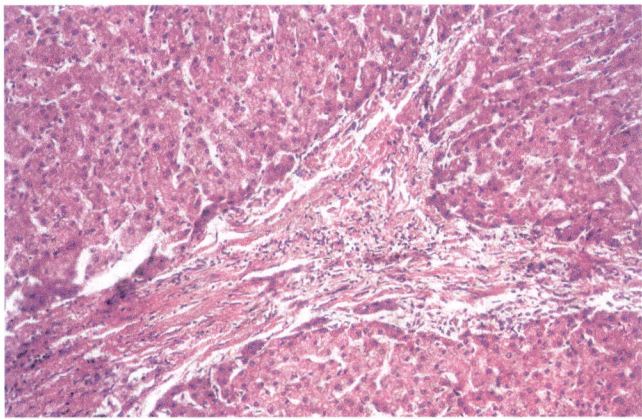

Fig. 25.14: Schistosomiasis: portal fibrosis (so-called clay pipe-stem fibrosis) (HE)

▶ Schistosomiasis is frequently accompanied by an additional *HBV* or *HCV infection*, corresponding to the respective regional infection rate. As a result, the course of disease is generally more severe, portal hypertension becomes progressive more rapidly, and there is a greater disposition towards hepatobiliary carcinoma. (95, 108)

The *diagnosis* can be established by identification of eggs in the stool as well as by rectal and/or sigmoidal mucosa biopsy or liver biopsy. Serological tests (e.g. ELISA) may be useful. The PCR technique can also be applied. Imaging techniques (ultrasound, CT) are of diagnostic value. (94, 97, 102, 105–107, 111, 114) Early oesophagogastroscopy and follow-ups are necessary. In advanced stages, the laboratory parameters usually show only moderate cholestasis and γ-globulinaemia. (99)

The *treatment* for all forms of schistosomiasis consists of praziquantel (30–45 mg/kg BW as a single dose). In severe courses of the disease or with an S. japonicum infection, 60 mg/kg BW daily, in three single doses, should be administered. A six-day course of therapy with 30 mg/kg BW/day is likewise recommended. S. mansoni is also effectively treated with oxamniquine (20 mg/kg BW/day for 3 days). (97, 104, 107)

2.3 Cestodes

Infections with Taenia, a genus belonging to the family of tapeworms, is of no consequence for the human liver and bile ducts. • In contrast, **echinococcosis** is a helminthic infection of major clinical significance.

▶ Hepatic hydatids were reported for the first time by F. RUYSCH in 1691. • The pathogens responsible for echinococcosis are found worldwide and comprise four different species: (*1.*) **Echinococcus cysticus** (E. granulosus, E. hydatidosus), (*2.*) **Echinococcus alveolaris** (E. multilocularis), (*3.*) **Echinococcus oligarthrus**, and (*4.*) **Echinococcus vogeli**. All forms of echinococcosis differ greatly with respect to epidemiology, pathomorphology and clinical findings. • E. oligarthrus and E. vogeli have been identified in isolated cases in Africa and South America. So far, only a few instances of parasite diseases have been reported in humans. E. vogeli is the cause of polycystic echinococcosis.

2.3.1 Echinococcus cysticus

With a frequency rate of over 90%, E. cysticus (E. granulosus) is the major causative pathogen of echinococcosis and is encountered frequently in countries where intensive cattle breeding is common. (124, 134, 150) • The *principal hosts* (final hosts) of the dog tapeworm are various canine species such as dogs, wolves, jackals and hyenas. Sheep, pigs, cattle, horses and deer serve as *intermediate hosts*. Humans infected by the principal host serve as *false intermediate hosts* (secondary host), since the developmental process of the dog tapeworm cannot be brought to an end in humans. • Echinococcus cysticus is 3–6 mm long and is generally made up of 3 (–7) proglottids. The eggs are discharged into the intestinal lumen in each case from the last proglottid. The head (scolex) is equipped with four suckers and a double-hooked crown. Humans are infected by oral ingestion of Echinococcus eggs (embryophores), 30–40 μm in diameter, which are present in the stool and sputum of infected dogs. The larvae (oncospheres) are released in the intestine, where they penetrate the intestinal wall and gain access to the portal system. Within three to four hours, they reach the liver. About 70% stay in the liver, while the remaining 30% are transported into the lungs and via the arterial circulation into the brain, spleen, bone, kidney and other organs. • The larvae encyst and form fluid-filled cysts or **hydatids** (cysticercus) with a three-layered wall. The outer, milky-white lamellar layer, about 1 mm thick, is a PAS-positive chitin membrane; the middle layer is a hyaline membrane, and the inner wall constitutes the germinal layer, 10–15 μm thick, where internal brood capsules are formed, initially without, but later with scolices. These capsules may rupture and release protoscolices as "hydatid sand" into the hydatids. Other brood capsules are formed which grow outwards through the hydatid wall and later become "free" daughter cysts. (s. figs. 25.15)

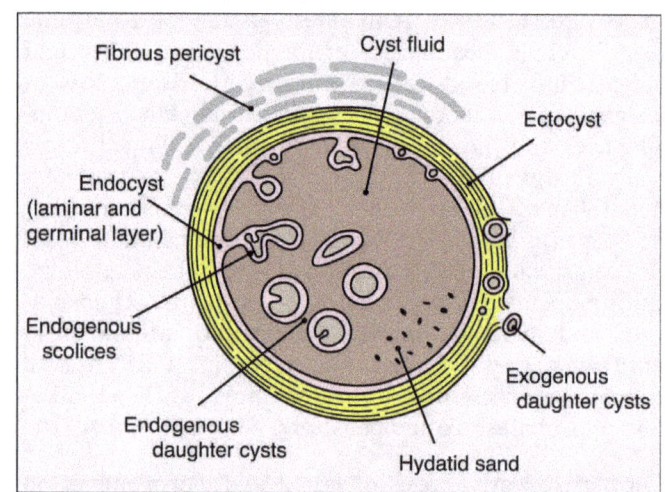

Fig. 25.15: Morphology of a hydatid cyst (E. cysticus) in the liver

Through hydatid rupture (e.g. surgery, puncture), the partly free-floating scolices are disseminated, resulting in the formation of secondary cysts (E. multicysticus). The release of allergenic hydatid fluid may cause a strong anaphylactic reaction. • The hydatids grow ca. 0.5–1.0 (–5.0) cm/year and only lead to clinical symptoms after a number of years. In 7–10% of cases, the cysts may disappear spontaneously or remain unchanged. The secondary cysts frequently perish in human beings, remaining only in a sterile and calcified form. (s. fig. 25.18, 25.19) • If the main hosts ingest organs containing hydatids with mature head structures, the developmental course will be completed, i.e. tapeworms are again formed in the intestine of the final host, and eggs are excreted. (128, 145)

Clinical symptoms appear after three to five years at the earliest, the peak of their manifestation being in the third decade. Some patients complain of fatigue, food intolerance, pruritus, loss of weight and episodes of fever. Further symptoms depend on the localization, size and growth of the hydatids. The liver is nearly always affected, most frequently the right lobe. With increasing hydatid growth, the right epigastrium or costal arch may show protrusion; in cranial localization, the right diaphragm is elevated. When the left lobe is affected, the increase in hydatid size leads to epigastric protrusion. Depending on the mechanical situation, a sensation of pressure and repletion as well as pain is felt by the patient. With the exception of eosinophilia (30–40% of cases) and an occasional increase in γ-GT and the transaminases, laboratory parameters are not particularly striking. When the bile ducts are compressed, there is an increase in the enzymatic markers of cholestasis, and mild jaundice may be seen. (119, 150)

Diagnosis is based on sonography, possibly with four or six-stage classification. (s. fig. 25.16) (124, 128, 145, 150, 156) Additional information is yielded by CT (s. fig. 25.17), MRT (126, 142, 147, 148) and by routine X-ray of the chest and abdomen (elevated right diaphragm, reduced respiration-related movement of the diaphragm, pleural effusion, pulmonary foci, evidence of calcification). (s. fig. 25.18) Hydatids can be identified in the large bile ducts by ERC. Angiography (only indicated in individual cases) shows a poorly vascularized area with a discolouration of the capsule. F-18-fluorodeoxyglucose (FDG) positron-emission tomography shows a sensitivity of 81% and a specificity of 92% versus Echinococcus cysticus. This technique also allows follow-up during benzimidazole therapy. (157)

Laparoscopically, the cyst appears on the liver surface with an irregularly thickened capsule and moderately diffuse vascular irritation (but no "breaks"). Slight fibrinous exudates may be seen at the adjacent peritoneum. (s. fig. 25.19) Palpation by probe reveals a distended elastic consistency. Although puncture is con-

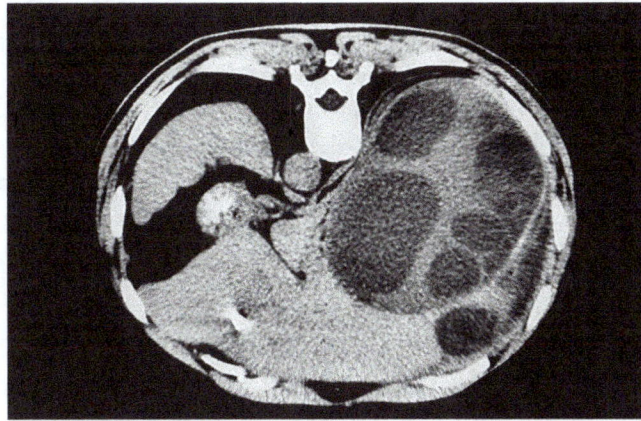

Fig. 25.17: CT showing Echinococcus cysticus in the liver

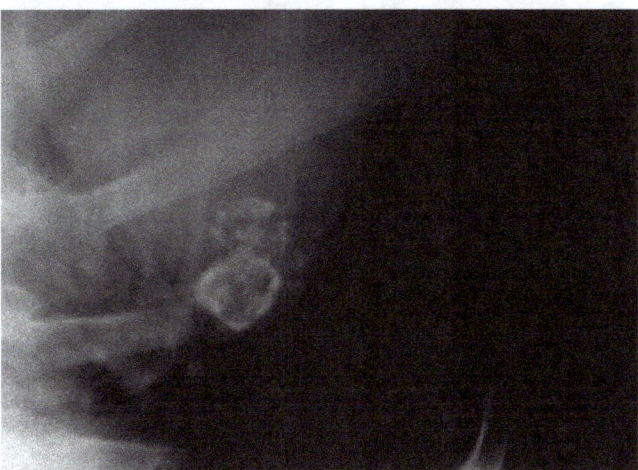

Fig. 25.18: Calcified Echinococcus cysticus in the liver

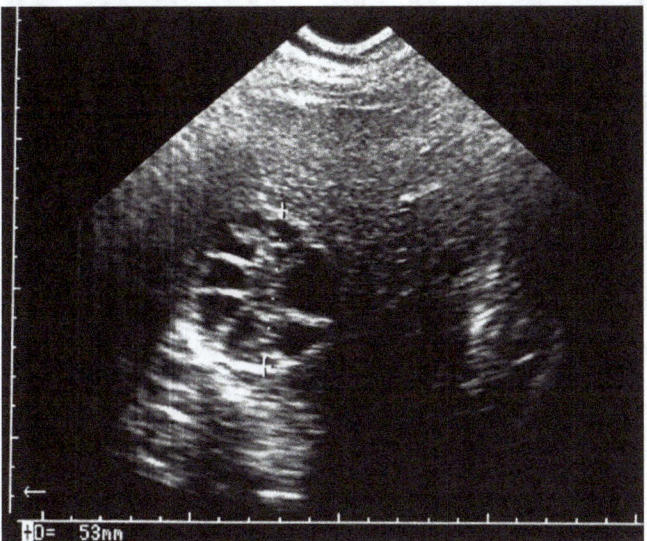

Fig. 25.16: Echinoccus cysticus (stage II B): bizarre conglomerate with peripheral daughter cysts

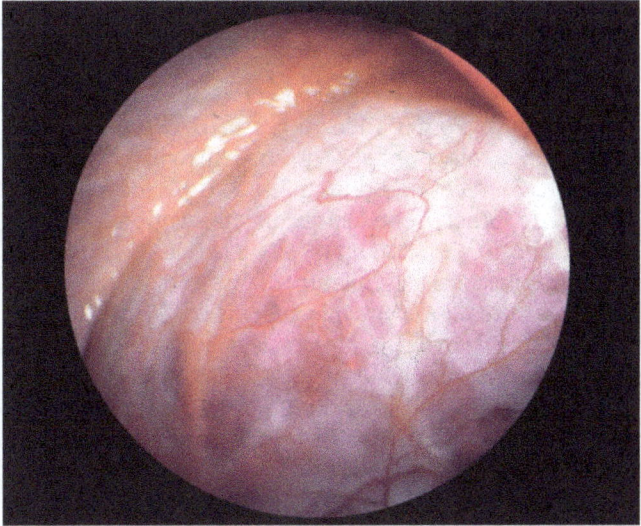

Fig. 25.19: Laparoscopic view of a large Echinococcus cysticus hydatid in the right lobe of liver: irregularly thickened hypervascular capsule. Fibrin deposition at the adjacent peritoneum. Distended elastic consistency

sidered to be dangerous, it is often performed for diagnostic and therapeutic reasons; it is less dangerous when carried out under laparoscopic surveillance. (156)

Serological tests (Em-2-ELISA, indirect haemagglutination, indirect immunofluorescence) are positive in some 85%–95% of cases. All tests may yield false-positive or false-negative results. The tests are negative if the hydatid shows no leak or contains no or only dead scolices. Differentiation of the species is effected successfully by Western blot. (134)

Complications in the form of a rupture into the free abdominal cavity (with anaphylactic shock) (143, 144, 147), bile ducts (159, 160), duodenum, large intestine, pleura and lungs have been reported, as has the Budd-Chiari syndrome after rupture into the liver veins and bronchobiliary fistulas. (149, 154) Secondary infection may appear following damage to the cystic wall, presenting the clinical picture of a liver abscess. Rare manifestations comprise formation of gallstones in the cysts, obstructive jaundice (135), obstruction of the inferior vena cava (141) or glomerulonephritis as an immunological reaction. Complications may also occur as a result of localization and growth in other organs (brain, lung, kidney, bones, etc.). (s. fig. 25.20) (122, 128, 140, 158)

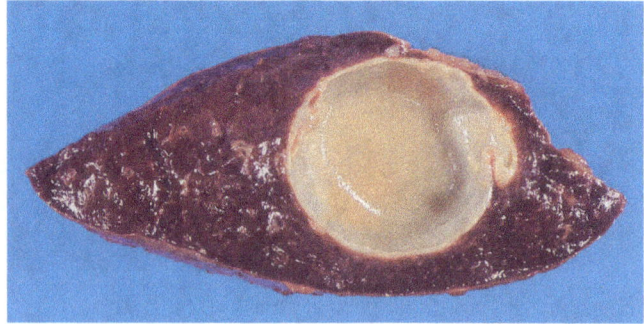

Fig. 25.20: Hydatid cyst of Echinococcus cysticus in the spleen

Treatment of choice is surgical removal of the hydatid cyst (pericystectomy) following systemic pretreatment with albendazole, possibly with concurrent partial liver resection. Surgical deroofing is easy to perform and, in contrast to other minor surgical interventions, universally applicable. (114, 115, 118, 123, 127, 129, 139, 150, 155) For intraoperative destruction of the scolices, the cyst may, before resection, be injected with a 10–30% common salt solution, a highly concentrated glucose solution, hydrogen peroxide, alcohol (90%), PVD iodine (10%), cetrimide (0.5%) or even mebendazole. • Percutaneous aspiration or drainage treatment was reported to be successful. (113, 117, 120, 130, 133, 138, 150, 152, 155) The PAIR procedure (**p**uncture/**a**spiration/**i**njection/**r**easpiration) (M. GARGOURI et al., 1990) has proved generally effective when using a sodium chloride solution (20%, 10 min) and ethanol (95%, 10 min). The two solutions can also be administered successively. These therapeutic measures are performed with a higher degree of reliability under laparoscopic control (M. ERTEM et al., 1998). • Medicamentous treatment consists of mebendazole (40–100 mg/kg BW daily in three single doses) together with meals of a high fat content, initially for a period of four to six months, but in most cases for life. It is essential to have a guaranteed serum level of >10 ng/ml or a plasma level of >200 mmol/l for about four hours after the morning intake; a higher plasma level is attained by additional administration of cimetidine. The dose is adjusted daily in accordance with the control values in the serum. Albendazole (2×400 mg/day for 4 weeks, followed by a therapy-free period of 2 weeks and a new treatment cycle) and fenbendazole as well as a combination of chemotherapy with albendazole and praziquantel (50 mg/kg BW) have also proved effective. (114, 116, 125, 131, 132, 136, 138, 146, 150, 151, 153)

2.3.2 Echinococcus alveolaris

The *principal host* of E. alveolaris (E. multilocularis) is the fox; more rarely, the dog and the cat are infected as well. *Intermediate hosts* include the common field mouse and other wild animals. Humans can also be infected as intermediate hosts. (124, 134) • This tapeworm inhabiting the small intestine has a length of 1.0–3.5 mm and possesses five proglottids. *Infection* with eggs results from consuming contaminated food (wild berries, windfall fruit, vegetables) and from contact with fox pelts. E. alveolaris is found worldwide, particularly in the various endemic areas. Apart from these endemic areas, there are "hyperendemic" regions, where the prevalence is 1:1000. (s. fig. 25.21)

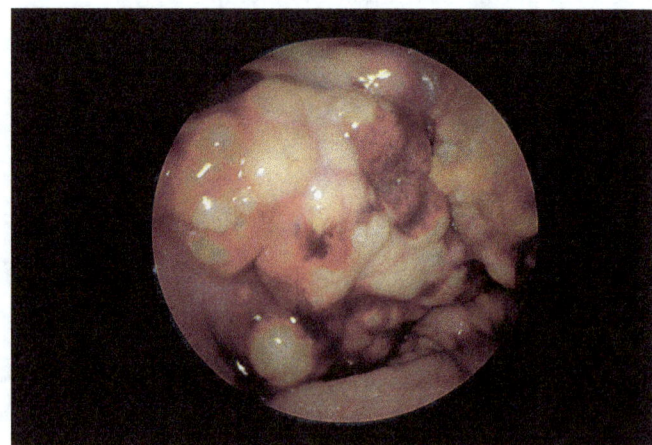

Fig. 25.21: Laparoscopic view of multiple Echinococcus alveolaris hydatids in the right lobe of liver

The *development cycle* is identical to that of E. cysticus. In 90% of cases, only the liver is affected. The cysticercus, however, grows in an infiltrative, destructive manner from organ to organ, i.e. the growth pattern shows tumour-like aggression. Metastatic spread is systemic (e.g. lungs, brain, bones) and lymphogenic. Many daughter cysts, up to the size of a hazelnut and coarse in structure, are formed on the surface of the small primary cyst, producing a crunching noise when cut. These cystoid proliferations have no proper capsules. Their interiors display necrotic cavities and colloidal, jelly-like contents. (s. fig. 25.22)

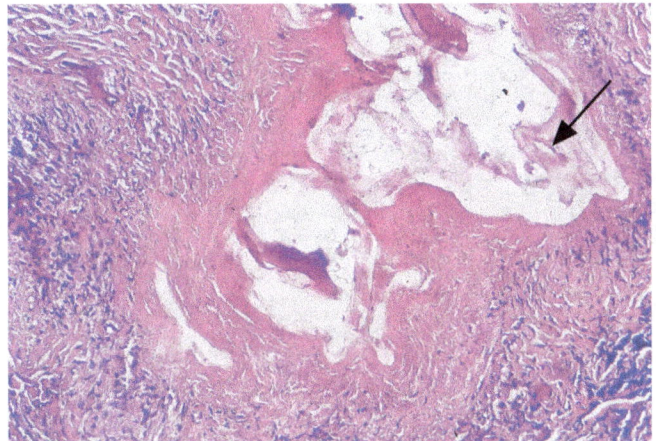

Fig. 25.22: Echinococcus alveolaris hydatid: pseudocyst surrounded by a rim of radially arranged histiocytes. Markedly damaged adjacent liver parenchyma. Small parasitic membranes in the bright lumen of the pseudocyst (arrow) (HE)

Macroscopy: In terms of macroscopy, alveolar echinococcosis presents in two different forms, whereby the latter is more common:

(*1.*) *pseudometastatic multinodular form* (= generally isolated, white, hard nodules on the liver surface without the central retractions found in metastases)

(*2.*) *confluent form* (= irregular, yellowish-white plaques on the liver surface)

Diagnosis: Alveolar echinococcosis is a rare, but severe disease. Diagnostics and therapy resemble that of carcinoma. The incubation period is unknown. The latency period before clinical symptoms appear is 5—15 years. As with E. cysticus, an early diagnosis is not possible. However, uncharacteristic ailments can occur earlier and with greater intensity. From the clinical viewpoint, there is a discrepancy between the good general state of health of the patient and the increasingly severe organic destruction. The outbreak of disease possibly depends upon the individual immunogenetic predisposition or resistance. • Over the years, hepatomegaly develops. Fever, growing malaise and epigastric pain with occasional radiation to the right shoulder are in evidence. In some cases, right-side pleural effusion, transitory erythema, tingling in the nose and sweats are observed. Tuberous resistance, as hard as cartilage, may be palpable in the area of the liver. • Laboratory examinations reveal eosinophilia in ca. 40% of cases; inflammatory parameters (ESR, CRP, leucocytes, α- and γ-globulins) and enzymatic activities (GPT, GOT, γ-GT, AP) are generally elevated. Slight jaundice is sometimes detectable. The diagnosis is obtained by confirmation of specific antibodies (e.g. using Em1-/Em2-antigen). Thus a differentiation can be made between the cystic and the alveolar type of echinococcus. Direct identification of the pathogen is achieved by means of PCR. • In ultrasonography, E. alveolaris is seen as irregularly delineated, with an echogenic and hypoechoic, inhomogeneous internal structure, so that it is often indistinguishable from a malignant tumour. (126) (s. p. 144) In angiography, E. alveolaris also resembles a malignant tumour, showing a constricting, stretching or corkscrew-shaped arrangement, irregularities in the walls and convolutions of the arteries. CT and MRT provide a better basis for differential diagnosis. MRT shows the areas of necrosis and the periportal or perihepatic spread on T_1. (142) (s. p. 182) • In laparoscopy, white or grey, hard nodular proliferations up to the size of a hazelnut are visible on the surface. Sufficient material can be obtained by forceps biopsy (there is no danger of anaphylactic shock).

Complications: The following complications have been reported: (*1.*) cholangitis, (*2.*) obstructive jaundice, (*3.*) intrahepatic cholelithiasis, (*4.*) sepsis, (*5.*) portal hypertension (oesophageal varices, portal vein thrombosis, chronic Budd-Chiari syndrome, etc.), (*6.*) thrombosis of the inferior vena cava, (*7.*) amyloidosis, (*8.*) immune complex-associated glomerulonephritis, (*9.*) metastases, (*10.*) "acute on chronic" liver insufficiency or acute liver failure, and (*11.*) bronchobiliary fistula.

Treatment: Treatment of E. alveolaris has no influence on the generally poor prognosis. In isolated cases with an early diagnosis, some improvement has been attained by extensive surgical procedures (e.g. en bloc resection of the liver with lymphadenectomy). At best, this method is applicable in 20—40% of patients. As a rule, however, no successful surgical intervention is possible because of the advanced hepatic infiltration. (161) • Orthotopic liver transplantation, already reported in more than 40 incurable cases, would, therefore, seem to be the last resort. An indication is given if the lesions are inaccessible and cannot be removed by partial resection of the liver, in cases of chronic Budd-Chiari syndrome or in secondary biliary cirrhosis, and if no metastases are present. The survival rate after liver transplantation is about 65% after five years. Late mortality may be attributed to relapses in the transplant or the formation of metastases. (121) • Medicamentous therapy (mebendazole) starts some four weeks before surgery and is continued until the normalization of serologic parameters, if necessary in adequate dosage life-long. • The ten-year survival rate of inoperable patients could be improved with the aid of consistent and continuous chemotherapy (mebendazole, albendazole, benzimidazole) by up to 85% (as compared to 10% without this therapy). (113, 127, 137)

References:

Amoebiasis
1. **Agarwal, D.K., Baijal, S.S., Roy, S., Mittal, B.R., Gupta, R., Choudhuri, G.:** Percutaneous catheter drainage of amebic liver abscesses with and without intrahepatic biliary communication: a comparative study. Europ. J. Radiol. 1995; 20: 61–64
2. **Badalamenti, S., Jameson, J.E., Reddy, K.R.:** Amebiasis. Curr. Treat. Opin. Gastroenterol. 1999; 1: 97–103
3. **Birgelen, von, C., von Schönefeld, J., Görge. G-. Fabry, W., Layer, P.:** Amoebic liver abscess with hepatobronchial fistula. Dtsch. Med. Wschr. 1994; 119: 1034–1038
4. **Bloch, S., Ustianowski, A., Pasvol, G.:** Amoebic abscess in the left lobe of the liver masquerading as pyelonephritis (case report). J. Infect. 2003; 46: 249–250
5. **Chuah, S.Y., Chang-Chien, C.S., Sheen, I.S., Lin, H.H., Chiou, S.-S., Chiu, C.-T., Kuo, C.-H., Chen, J.-J., Chiu, K.W.:** The prognostic factors of severe amebic liver abscess: a retrospective study of 125 cases. Amer. J. Trop. Med. Hyg. 1992; 46: 398–402
6. **Hodkinson, J., Couper-Smith, J., Kew, M.C.:** Inferior vena cava and right atrial thrombosis complicating an amebic hepatic abscess. Amer. J. Gastroenterol. 1988; 83: 786–788
7. **Maltz, G., Knauer, C.M.:** Amebic liver abscess: a 15-year experience. Amer. J. Gastroenterol. 1991; 86: 704–710
8. **Meng, X.Y., Wu, J.X.:** Perforated amebic liver abscess: clinical analysis of 110 cases. South Med. J. 1994; 87: 985–990
9. **Mondragon-Sanchez, R., Cortes-Espinoza, T., Alonzo-Fierro, Y., Labra-Villalobos, M.I., Maldonado, R.B.:** Amebic liver abscess "a 5-year Mexican experience with a multimodality approach". Hepato-Gastroenterol. 1995; 42: 473–477
10. **Petri, W.J.:** Recent advances in amebiasis. Crit. Rev. Clin. Lab. Sci. 1996; 33: 1–37
11. **Reed, S.L.:** New concepts regarding the pathogenesis of amebiasis. Clin. Infect. Dis. 1995; 21 (Suppl. 2): 182–185
12. **Sharma, M.P., Dasarathy, S., Verma, N., Saksena, S., Shukla, D.K.:** Prognostic markers in amebic liver abscess: a prospective study. Amer. J. Gastroenterol. 1996; 91: 2584–2588

Lambliasis
13. **Osterholm, M.T., Forfang, J.C., Ristinen, T.L., Dean, A.G., Washburn, J.W., Godes, J.R., Rude, R.A., McCullough, J.G.:** An outbreak of foodborne giardiasis. New Engl. J. Med. 1981; 304: 24–28
14. **Roberts-Thomas, I.C., Anders, R.F., Bhathal, P.S.:** Granulomatous hepatitis and cholangitis associated with giardiasis. Gastroenterology 1982; 83: 480–483

Cryptosporidiosis
15. **Margulis, S.J., Honig, C.L., Soave, R., Govoni, A.F., Mouradian, J.A., Jacobson, I.M.:** Biliary tract obstruction in the acquired immunodeficiency syndrome. Ann. Intern. Med. 1986; 105: 207–210
16. **Teixidor, H.S., Godwin, T.A., Ramirez, E.A.:** Cryptosporidiosis of the biliary tract in AIDS. Radiology 1991; 180: 51–56
17. **Wolfson, J.S., Richter, J.M., Waldbron, M.A., Weber, D.J., McCarthy, D.M., Hopkins, C.C.:** Cryptosporidiosis in immunocompetent patients. New Engl. J. Med. 1985; 312: 1278–1282

Leishmaniasis
18. **Artan, R., Yilmaz, A., Alecam, M., Aksoy, N.H.:** Liver biopsy in the Diagnosis of visceral leisemaniasis. J. Gastroenterol. Hepatol. 2006; 21: 299–302
19. **Bukte, Y., Nazaroglu, H., Mete, A., Yilmaz, F.:** Visceral leishmaniasis with multiple nodular lesions of the liver and spleen: CT and sonographic findings. Abdom. Imag. 2004; 29: 82–84
20. **Koshy, A., Al-Azmi, W.M., Narayanan, S., Grover, S., Hira, P.R., Idris, M., Madda, J.P.:** Leishmaniasis diagnosed by liver biopsy. Management of two atypical cases. J. Clin. Gastroenterol. 2001; 32: 266–267
21. **Moreno, A., Marazuela, M., Yerba, M., Hernandez, M.J., Hellin, T., Montalban, C., Vargas, J.A.:** Hepatic fibrin-ring granulomas in visceral leishmaniasis. Gastroenterology 1988; 95: 1123–1126
22. **Murray, H.W., Berman, J.D., Davies, C., Saravia, N.:** Advances in leishmaniasis. Lancet 2005; 366: 1561–1577
23. **Sundar, S., Iha, T.K., Thakur, C.P., Engel, J., Sindermann, H., Fischer, C., Junge, K., Bryceson, A., Berman, J.:** Oral miltefosine for Indian visceral leishmaniasis. New Engl. J. Med. 2002; 347: 1739–1746
24. **Wilson, M.E.:** Leishmaniasis. Curr. Opin. Infect. Dis. 1993; 6: 331–341

Malaria
25. **Adjuik, M., Agnamey, P., Babiker, A., Borrmann, S., Brasseur, P., Cisse, M., Cobelens, F., Diallo, S., Faucher, J.F., Garner, P., Gikunda, S., Kremsner, P.G., Krishna, S., Lell, B., Loolpapit, M., Matsiegui, P.-B., Missinou, M.A., Mwanza, J., Ntoumi, F., Olliaro, P., Osimbo, P., Rezbach, P., Some, E., Taylor, W.R.J.:** Amodiaquine-artesunate versus amodiaquine for uncomplicated Plasmodium falciparum malaria in African children: a randomized, multicentre trial. Lancet 2002; 359: 1365–1372
26. **Cook, G.C.:** Malaria in the liver. Postgrad. Med. J. 1994; 70: 780–784
27. **Crane, G.G.:** Hyperreactive malarious splenomegaly (tropical splenomegaly syndrome). Parasit. Today 1986; 2: 4–9
28. **Joshi, Y.K., Tandon, S.K., Acharya, S.K., Babu, S., Tandon, M.:** Acute hepatic failure due to Plasmodium falciparum liver injury. Liver 1986; 6: 357–360
29. **Lundgren, J.D., Gragsted, U.B.:** Atovaquone / proguanil. Prophylaxis and treatment of malaria. Ugesker. Laeger. 2000; 162: 4177–4181
30. **Planche, T., Krishna, S.:** The relevance of malaria pathophysiology to strategies of clinical management. Curr. Opin. Infect. Dis. 2005; 18: 369–375
31. **Rosen, S., Roycroft, D.W., Hano, J.E., Barry, K.G.:** The liver in malaria. Electron microscopic observations on a hepatic biopsy obtained 15 minutes post mortem. Arch. Pathol. 1967; 83: 271–277

Toxoplasmosis
32. **Marazuela, M., Moreno, A., Yebra, M., Cerezo, E., Gomez-Gesto, C., Vargas, J.A.:** Hepatic fibrin-ring granulomas: a clinicopathologic study on 23 patients. Hum. Pathol. 1991; 22: 607–613
33. **Ortego, T.J., Robbey, B., Morrison, D., Chan, C.:** Toxoplasmic chorioretinitis and hepatic granulomas. Amer. J. Gastroenterol. 1990; 85: 1418–1420
34. **Sijpkens, Y.W.J., DeKnegt, R.J., van der Werf, S.D.J.:** Unusual presentation of acquired toxoplasmosis in an immuncompetent adult. Neth. J. Med. 1994; 45: 174–176
35. **Tiwari, I., Rolland, C.F., Popple, A.W.:** Cholestatic jaundice due to toxoplasma hepatitis. Postgrad. Med. J. 1982; 58: 299–300
36. **Vethanyagam, A., Pryceson, A.D.M.:** Acquired toxoplasmosis presenting as hepatitis. Trans. Roy. Soc. Trop. Med. Hyg. 1976; 70: 524–525
37. **Weitberg, A.B., Alper, J.C., Diamond, I., Fligiel, Z.:** Acute granulomatous hepatitis in the course of acquired toxoplasmosis. New Engl. J. Med. 1979; 300: 1093–1096

Ascaridiasis
38. **Al-Karawi, M., Sanai, F.M., Yasawy, M.I., Mohammed, A.E.:** Biliary strictures and cholangitis secondary to ascaris: endoscopic management. Gastrointest. Endosc. 1999; 50: 695–697
39. **Cremin, B.J., Fisher, R.M.:** Biliary ascariasis in children. Amer. J. Radiol. 1976; 126: 352–357
40. **Ferreyra, N.P., Cerri, G.G.:** Ascariasis of the alimentary tract, liver, pancreas and biliary system: its diagnosis by ultrasonography. Hepatogastroenterol. 1998; 45: 932–937
41. **Fogaca, H.S., Oliveira, C.S., Barbosa, H.T., Lanfredi, R.M., Chagas, V.:** Liver pseudotumor: a rare manifestation of hepatic granulomata caused by Ascaris lumbricoides ova. Amer. J. Gastroenterol. 2000; 95: 2099–2101
42. **Hsu, F.-H.:** Clinical observation on 110 cases of ascaris invasion into the biliary tract. Nagoya J. Med. Sci. 1962; 24: 215–233
43. **Kamath, P.S., Joseph, D.C., Chandran, R., Rao, S.R., Prakasch, M.L.S., D'Cruz, A.J.:** Biliary ascariasis: ultrasonography, endoscopic retrograde cholangiopancreatography, and biliary drainage. Gastroenterology 1986; 91: 730–732
44. **Kim, S.R., Maekawa, Y., Matsuoka, T., Imoto, S., Ando, K., Muta, K., Kim, H.B., Nakajima, T., Ku, K.S., Koterazawa, T., Fukuda, K., Yano, Y., Nakaji, M., Kudo, M., Kim, K.I., Hirai, M., Hayashi, Y.:** Eosinophilic pseudotumor of the liver due to Ascaris suum infection (case report) Hepatol. Res. 2002; 23: 306–314
45. **Lloyd, D.A.:** Massive hepatobiliary ascariasis in childhood. Brit. J. Surg. 1981; 68: 468–473
46. **Mani, S., Merchant, H., Sachdev, R., Rananavare, P., Cunha, N.:** Sonographic evaluation of biliary ascariasis. Austral. Radiol. 1997; 41: 204–206
47. **Pereira-Lima, J.C., Jacobs, R., da Silva, C.P., Coral, G.P., da Silveira, L.L., Rynkowski, C.B., Riemann, J.F.:** Endoscopic removal of Ascaris lumbricoides from the biliary tract as emergency treatment for acute suppurative cholangitis. Z. Gastroenterol. 2001; 39: 793–796
48. **Sandouk, F., Haffar, S., Zada, M.M., Graham, D.Y., Anand, B.S.:** Pancreatic-biliary ascariasis: experiences of 300 cases. Amer. J. Gastroenterol. 1997; 92: 2264–2267
49. **Shah, O.J., Robanni, I., Khan, F., Zargar, S.A., Javid, G.:** Management of biliary ascariasis in pregnancy. World J. Surg. 2005; 29: 1294–1998
50. **Shah, O.J., Zargar, S.A., Robbani, I.:** Biliary ascariasis: a review. World J. Surg. 2006; 30: 1500–1506
51. **Zargar, S.A., Khan, B.A., Javid, G., Yattoo, G.N., Shah, A.H., Gulzar, G.M., Singh, J., Khan, M.A., Shah, N.A.:** Endoscopic management of early postoperative biliary ascariasis in patients with biliary tract surgery. World J. Surg. 2004; 28: 712–715

Strongyloidiasis
52. **Concha, R., Harrington, W., Rogers, A.I.:** Intestinal strongyloidiasis: recoquition, management, and determinants of outcome. J. Clin. Gastroenterol. 2005; 39: 203–211

Toxocariasis
53. **Bhatia, V., Sarin, S.K.:** Hepatic visceral larva migrans evolution of the lesion, diagnosis, and role of high-dose albendazole therapy. Amer. J. Gastroenterol. 1994; 89: 624–627
54. **Hartleb, M., Januszewski, K.:** Severe hepatic involvement in visceral larva migrans. Eur. J. Gastroenterol. Hepatol. 2001; 13: 1245–1249
55. **Kaplan, K.J., Goodman, Z.D., Ishak, K.G.:** Eosinophilic granuloma of the liver. A characteristic lesion with relationship to visceral larva migrans. Amer. J. Surg. Path. 2001; 25: 1316–1321
56. **Leone, N., Baronio, M., Todros, L., David, E., Brunello, F., Artioli, S., Rizzetto, M.:** Hepatic involvement in larva migrans of Toxocara canis: Report of a case with pathological and radiological findings. Dig. Liver Dis. 2006; 38: 511–514

57. **Zinkham, W.H.:** Visceral larva migrans. A review and reassessment indicating two forms of clinical expression: visceral and ocular. Amer. J. Dis. Child. 1978; 132: 627–633

Trichinosis
58. **Burg, H.:** Serumtransaminasen und Plasmaproteine bei Trichinose. Med. Klin. 1968; 63: 534–535
59. **Guattery, J.M., Milne, J., House, R.K.:** Observations on hepatic and renal dysfunction in trichinosis. Anatomic changes in these organs occurring in cases of trichinosis. Amer. J. Med. 1956; 21: 567–582

Clonorchiasis
60. **Chan, H.H., Lai, K.H., Lo, G.H., Cheng, J.S., Huang, J.S., Hsu, P.I., Lin, C.K., Wang, E.M.:** The clinical and cholangiographic picture of hepatic clonorchiasis. J. Clin. Gastroenterol. 2002; 34: 183–186
61. **Choi, B.I., Kim, H.J., Han, M.C., Do, Y.S., Han, M.H., Lee, S.H.:** CT findings in clonorchiasis. Amer. J. Radiol. 1989; 152: 281–284
62. **Choi, D., Hong, S.T., Lim, J.H., Cho, S.Y., Rim, H.J., Ji, Z., Yuan, R., Wang, S.Y.:** Sonographic findings of active Clonorchis sinensis infection (case report). J. Clin. Ultrasound 2004; 22: 17–23
63. **Choi, D., Lim, J.H., Lee, K.T., Lee, J.K., Choi, S.H., Heo, J.S., Jang, K.T., Lee, N.Y., Kim, S., Hong, S.T.:** Cholangiocarcinoma and Clonorchis sinensis infection. A case-control study in Korea. J. Hepatol. 2006; 44: 1066–1073
64. **Chow, C.W., Allen, P.W.:** Clonorchis sinensis infestation of liver associated with cholangiocarcinoma. Pathology 1978; 10: 174–175
65. **Kim, K.H., Kim, C.D., Lee, H.S., Lee, S.J., Jeen, Y.T., Chun, H.J., Song, C.W., Lee, S.W., Um, S.H., Choi, J.H., Ryu, H.S., Hyun, J.H.:** Biliary papillary hyperplasia with clonorchiasis resembling cholangiocarcinoma. Amer. J. Gastroenterol. 1999; 94: 514–517
66. **Kim, S.H., Park, Y.N., Yoon, D.S., Lee, S.J., Yu, J.S., Noh, T.W.:** Composite neuroendocrine and adenocarcinoma of the common bile duct associated with Clonorchis sinensis: a case report. Hepato-Gastroenterol. 2000; 47: 942–944
67. **Lim, J.H.:** Radiologic findings in clonorchiasis. Amer. J. Radiol. 1990; 155: 1001–1008
68. **Ona, F.V., Dytoc, J.N.T.:** Clonorchis-associated cholangiocarcinoma: a report of two cases with unusual manifestations. Gastroenterology 1991; 101: 831–839
69. **Rinn, H.-J.:** Clonorchiasis: an update. J. Helminthol. 2005; 79: 269–281
70. **Schwartz, D.A.:** Cholangiocarcinoma associated with liver fluke infection: a preventable source of morbidity in Asian immigrants. Amer. J. Gastroenterol. 1986; 81: 76–79

Fascioliasis
71. **Bassily, S., Iskander, M., Youssef, F.G., El-Masry, N., Bawden, M.:** Sonography in diagnosis of fascioliasis. Lancet 1989/I: 1270–1271
72. **Bechtel, U., Feucht, H.E., Held, E., Vogl, T., Nothdurft, H.D.:** Fasciola hepatica. Infection of a family. Dtsch. Med. Wschr. 1992; 117: 978–982
73. **Beers, van, B., Pringot, J., Geubel, A., Trigaux, J.-P., Bigaignon, G., Dooms, G.:** Hepatobiliary fascioliasis: non-invasive imaging findings. Radiology 1990; 174: 809–810
74. **Chen, M.G., Mott, K.E.:** Progress in assessment of morbidity due to Fasciola hepatica infection: a review of recent literature. Trop. Dis. Bull. 1990; 87: 1–37
75. **Christmann, M., Henrich, R., Mayer, G., Ell, C.:** Infection with Fasciola hepatica causing elevated liver-enzyme results and eosinophilia – serologic and endoscopic diagnosis and therapy. Z. Gastroenterol. 2002; 40: 801–806
76. **Cosme, A., Ojeda, E., Poch, M., Bujanda, L., Castiella, A., Fernandez, J.:** Sonographic findings of hepatic lesions in human fascioliasis. J. Clin. Ultrasound 2003; 31: 358–363
77. **Dowidar, N., El-Sayad, M., Osman, M., Salem, A.:** Endoscopic therapy of fascioliasis resistants to oral therapy. Gastrointest. Endosc. 1999; 50: 345–351
78. **Gulsen, M., Savas, M.C., Koruk, M., Kadayifci, A., Demirci, F.:** Fascioliasis: A report of five cases presenting with common bile duct obstruction. Netherl. J. Med. 2006; 64: 17–19
79. **Kabaalioglu, A., Cubuk, M., Senol, U., Cevikol, C., Karaali, K., Apaydin, A., Sindel, T., Luleci, E.:** Fascioliasis: US, CT, and MRT findings with new observations. Abdom. Imag. 2000; 25: 400–404
80. **Kabil, S.M., El-Ashry, E., Ashraf, N.K.:** An open-label clinical study of nitazoxanide in the treatment of human fascioliasis. Curr. Ther. Res. 2000; 61: 339–345
81. **Kim, J.C., Lee, S.K., Sco, D.W., Lee, S.S., Kim, M.H.:** Fasciola hepatica in the common bile duct. Gastrointest. Endosc. 2006; 63: 501
82. **Liu, L.X., Harinasuta, K.T.:** Liver and intestinal flukes. Gastroenterol. Clin. North Amer. 1996; 25: 627–636
83. **Mannstadt, M., Sing, A., Leitritz, L., Brenner-Maucher, K., Bogner, J.:** Conservative management of biliary obstruction due to Fasciola hepatica. Clin. Inf. Dis. 2000; 31: 1301–1303
84. **Mas-Coma, S.:** Epidemiology of fascioliasis in human endemic areas. J. Helminthol. 2005; 79: 207–216
85. **Pagola Serrano, M.A., Vega, A., Ortega, E., Gonzales, A.:** Computed tomography of hepatic fascioliasis. J. Comput. Assist. Tomogr. 1987; 11: 269–272
86. **Roses, L.L., Alonso, D., Iniguez, F., Mateos, A., Bal, M., Agüero, J.:** Hepatic fascioliasis of long-term evolution: diagnosis by ERCP. Amer. J. Gastroenterol. 1993; 88: 2118–2119
87. **Schiappacasse, R.H., Mohammadi, D., Christie, A.J.:** Successful treatment of severe infection with Fasciola hepatica with praziquantel. Trop. Med. Parasit. 1985; 36: 88–90
88. **Teichmann, D., Grobusch, M. P. Gobels, K., Müller, H. P., Koehler, W., Suttorp, N.:** Acute fascioliasis with multiple liver abscesses. Scand. J. Gastroenterol. 2000; 32: 558–560
89. **Wood, I.J., Stephens, W.B., Porter, D.D.:** Fascioliasis causing hepatitis in two eaters of water cress. Med. J. Austr. 1975; 2: 829–831

Opisthorchiasis
90. **Berger, B., Vierbuchen, M.:** Opisthorchiasis simultaning malignoma. Zschr. Gastroenterol. 2001; 39: 173–175
91. **Cherdron, A., Fiegel, P.:** Opisthorchis felineus – der kleine Kaztenleberegel. Differentialdiagnose des rechtsseitigen Oberbauchschmerzes. Dtsch. Med. Wschr. 1992; 117: 328–331
92. **Kurathong, S., Lerdverasirikul, P., Wongpaitoon, V., Pramoolsinsap, C., Kanjanapitak, A., Varavithya, W., Phuapradit, P., Bunyaratvej, S., Upatham, E.S., Brockelman, W.Y.:** Opisthorchis viverrini infection and cholangiocarcinoma. A prospective, case-controlled study. Gastroenterology 1985; 89: 151–156
93. **Schwartz, D.A.:** Helminths in the induction of cancer: Opisthorchis viverrini, Clonorchis sinensis and cholangiocarcinoma. Trop. Geogr. Med. 1980; 32: 95–100

Schistosomiasis
94. **Abdel-Wahab, M.F., Esmat, G., Farrag, A., El-Boraey, Y.A., Strickland, G.T.:** Grading of hepatic schistosomiasis by the use of ultrasonography. Amer. J. Trop. Med. Hyg. 1992; 46: 403–408
95. **Andoh, H., Yasui, O., Kurokawa, T., Sato, T.:** Cholangiocarcinoma coincident with schistosomiasis japonica (case report). J. Gastroenterol. 2004; 39: 64–68
96. **Andrade, Z.A., Peixoto, E., Guerret, S., Grimaud, J.-A.:** Hepatic connective tissue changes in hepatosplenic schistosomiasis. Hum. Pathol. 1992; 23: 566–573
97. **Bica, I., Hamer, D.H., Stadecker, M.J.:** Hepatic schistosomiasis. Infect. Clin. North Amer. 2000; 14: 583–604
98. **Bonard, P., Kalach, N., Cadranel, J.F., Remoué, F., Riveau, G., Capron, A.:** Digestive and hepatic signs of schistosomiasis. Gastroenterol. Clin. Biol. 2000; 24: 409–419
99. **Camacho-Lobato, L., Borges, D.R.:** Early liver dysfunction in schistosomiasis. J. Hepatol. 1998; 29: 233–240
100. **Cordeiro, F.:** Variceal sclerosis in schistosomic patients: a five year follow-up study. Gastrointest. Endosc. 1990; 36: 475–478
101. **De Araujo-Souza, M.R., Fischer-de-Toledo, C., Borges, D.R.:** Thrombocytemia as a predictor of portal hypertension in schistosomiasis. Dig. Dis. Sci. 2000; 45: 1964–1970
102. **De Cleva, R., Herman, P., Pugliese, V., Zilberstein, B., Abrao-Saad, W., Gama-Rodrigues, J.J., Atilio-Laudanna, A.:** Prevalence of pulmonary hypertension in patients with hepatosplenic mansonic schistosomiasis. Prospective study. Hepato-Gastroenterol. 2003; 50: 2028–2030
103. **Domingues, A.L.C., Lima, A.R.F., Dias, H.S., Leao, G.C., Coutinho, A.:** An ultrasonographic study of liver fibrosis in patients infected with Schistosoma mansoni in north-east Brazil. Trans. R. Soc. Trop. Med. Hyg. 1993; 87: 555–558
104. **Elliott, D.E.:** Schistosomiasis. Pathophysiology, diagnosis and treatment. Gastroenterol. Clin. North. Amer. 1996; 25: 599–625
105. **Fataar, S., Bassiony, H., Satyanath, S., Rudwan, M.A., Kaffaji, S., El Magdy, W., Al-Ansari, A.G., Hanna, R.:** CT of hepatic schistosomiasis mansoni. Amer. J. Radiol. 1985; 145: 63–66
106. **Monzawa, S., Uchiyama, G., Ohtomo, K., Araki, T.:** Schistosomiasis japonica of the liver: contrast-enhanced CT findings in 113 patients. Amer. J. Roentgenol. 1993; 161: 323–327
107. **Nompleggi, D.J., Farraye, F.A., Singer, A., Edelman, R.R., Chopra, S.:** Hepatic schistosomiasis: report of two cases and literature review. Amer. J. Gastroenterol. 1991; 86: 1658–1664
108. **Pereira, L.M.M.B., Melo, M.C.V., Lacerda, C., Spinelli, V., Domingues, A.L.C., Massarolo, P., Mies, S., Saleh, M.G., McFarlane, I.G., Williams, R.:** Hepatitis B virus infection in schistosomiasis mansoni. J. Med. Virol. 1994; 42: 203–207
109. **Raja, S., da Silva, L.C., Gayotto, L.C.C., Forster, S.C., Fukushima, J., Strauss, B.:** Portal hypertension in schistosomiasis: a long-term follow-up of a randomized trial comparing three types of surgery. Hepatology 1994; 20: 398–403
110. **Schlossberg, D., Pandey, M., Reddy, R.:** The Splendore – Hoeppli phenomenon in hepatic botryomycosis. J. Clin. Pathol. 1998; 51: 399–400
111. **Shet, N.P.:** Schistosomal portal hypertension. J. Amer. Coll. Surg. 2006; 202: 201
112. **Widman, A., Souza-de-Oliveira, I.R., Speranzini, M.B., Cerri, G.G., Saad, W.A., Gama-Rodrigues, J.:** Portal thrombosis: late postoperative prevalence in Mansoni's schistosomiasis. Hepato-Gastroenterol. 2003; 50: 1463–1466

Echinococcosis
113. **Akhan, O., Özmen, M.N., Dincer, A., Sayek, I., Göcmen, A.:** Liver hydatid disease: long-term results of percutaneous treatment. Radiology 1996; 198: 259–264
114. **Ammann, R.W.:** Chemotherapy alone or as adjuvant treatment to surgery for alveolar and cystic echinococcosis. Chirurg 2000; 71: 9–15
115. **Avgerinos, E.D., Pavlakis, N., Stathoulopoulos, A., Manoukas, E., Skarpas, G., Tsatsoulis, P.:** Clinical presentations and surgical management of liver hydatidosis: Our 20 year experience. HPB 2006; 8: 189–193

116. **Bartolini, C., Tricerri, A., Guidi, L., Gambassi, G.:** The efficacy of chemotherapy with mebendazole in human cystic echinococcis. Long-term follow-up of 52 patients. Ann. Trop. Med. Parasitol. 1992; 86: 249–256
117. **Bastid, C., Azar, C., Doyer, M., Sahel, J.:** Percutaneous treatment of hydatid cysts under sonographic guidance. Dig. Dis. Sci. 1994; 39: 1576–1580
118. **Bektas, H., Lehner, F., Werner, U., Bartels, M., Piso, P., Tusch, G., Schrem, H., Klempnauer, J.:** Surgical therapy of cystic echinococcis of the liver. Zbl. Chir. 2001; 126: 369–373
119. **Biava, M.F., Dao, A., Fortier, B.:** Laboratory diagnosis of cystic hydatic disease. World J. Surg. 2001; 25: 10–14
120. **Bosanac, Z. B., Lisanin, L.:** Percutaneous drainage of hydatid cyst in the liver as a primary treatment: Review of 52 consecutive cases with long-term follow-up. Clin. Radiol. 2000; 55: 839–848
121. **Bresson-Hadni, S., Koch, S., Miguet, J.P., Gillet, M., Mantion, G.A., Heyd, B., Vuitton, D.A.:** Indications and results of liver transplantation for Echinococcus alveolar infection: An overview. Langenbecks Arch. Surg. 2003; 388: 231–238
122. **Cebollero, M.P., Cordoba, E., Escartin, J., Cantin, S.:** Hydatid cyst of the spleen. J. Clin. Gastroenterol. 2001; 33: 89–90
123. **Cirenei, A., Bertoldi, I.:** Evolution of surgery for liver hydatidosis from 1950 to today: analysis of a personal experience. World J. Surg. 2001; 25: 87–92
124. **Cook, G.C.:** Echinococcus granulosus and E. multilocularis in Europe. Eur. J. Gastroenterol. Hepatol. 1992; 10: 778–783
125. **Crippa, F.G., Bruno, R., Brunetti, E., Filice, C.:** Echinococcal liver cysts: treatment with echo-guided percutaneous puncture PAIR for echinococcal liver cysts. Ital. J. Gastroenterol. 1999; 31: 884–892
126. **Davolio Marani, S.A., Canossi, G.C., Nicoli, F.A., Alberti, G.P., Monni, S.G., Casolo, P.M.:** Hydatid disease: MR imaging study. Radiology 1990; 175: 701–706
127. **Dhaliwal, R.S., Kalkat, M.S.:** One-stage surgical procedure for bilateral lung and liver hytatid cysts. Ann. Thor. Surg. 1997; 64: 338–341
128. **Eckert, J., Deplazes, P.:** Biological, epidemiological, and clinical aspects of edinococcosis, a zoonosis of increasing concerning. Microbiol. Clin. Prev. 2004; 17: 107–135
129. **Ertem, M., Karahasanoglu, T., Yavuz, N., Erguney, S.:** Laparoscopically treated liver hydatid cysts. Arch. Surg. 2002; 137: 1170–1173
130. **Filice, C., Brunetti, E., Bruno, R., Crippa, F.G.:** Percutaneous drainage of echinococcal cysts (PAIR-puncture, aspiration, injection, reaspiration): results of a worldwide survey for assessment of its safety and efficacy. Gut 2000; 47: 156–157
131. **Frider, B., Larrieu, E., Odriozola, M.:** Long-term outcome of asymptomatic liver hydatidosis. J. Hepatol. 1999; 30: 228–231
132. **Gil-Grande, L.A., Rodriguez-Caabeiro, F., Prieto, J.G., Sanchez-Ruano, J.J., Brasa, C., Aguilar, L., Garcia-Hoz, F., Casado, N., Barcena, R., Alvarez, A.I., Dal-Re, R.:** Randomised controlled trial of efficacy of albendazole in intra-abdominal hydatid disease. Lancet 1993; 342: 1269–1272
133. **Giorgio, A., Tarantino, L., de Stefano, G., Francica, G., Mariniello, N., Farella, N., Perrotta, A., Aloisio, V., Esposito, F.:** Hydatid liver cyst. An 11-year experience of treatment with percutaneous aspiration and ethanol injection. J. Ultrasound Med. 2001; 20: 729–738
134. **Gottstein, B.:** Epidemiology and systematik of cystic and alveolar hydatid disease. Chirurg 2000; 71: 1–8
135. **Greulich, T., Kohler, B.:** Obstruction jaundice caused by rupture of cystic echinococcosis into the biliary tract. Zschr. Gastroenterol. 2000; 38: 301–306
136. **Ishizu, H., Uchino, J., Sato, N., Aoki, S., Suzuki, K., Kuribayashi, H.:** Effect of albendazole on recurrent and residual alveolar echinococcosis of the liver after surgery. Hepatology 1997; 25: 528–531
137. **Kadry, Z., Renner, E.C., Bachmann, L.M., Attigah, N., Renner, E.L., Ammann, R.W., Clavien, P.A.:** Evaluation of treatment and long-term follow-up in patients with hepatic alveolas echinococcosis. Brit. J. Nurg. 2005; 92: 1110–1116
138. **Kern, A.:** Echinococcus granulosus infection: Clinical presentation, medical treatment and outcome. Langenbecks Arch. Surg. 2003; 388: 413–420
139. **Khuroo, M.S., Wani, N.A., Javid, G., Khan, B.A., Yattoo, G.N., Shah, A.H., Jeelani, S.G.:** Percutaneous drainage compared with surgery for hepatic hytatid cysts. New Engl. J. Med. 1997; 337: 881–887
140. **Kilani, T., El-Hammami, S., Horchani, H., Ben-Miled-Mrad, K., Hantous, S., Mestiri, I., Sellami, M.:** Hydatid disease of the liver with thoracic involvement. World J. Surg. 2001; 25: 40–45
141. **Kocak, F.S., Bumin, C., Erdem, E., Dolapci, M., Erden, I., Imamoglu, K.:** Unusual complication of hydatid cysts: Acute inferior vena caval thrombosis. Dig. Surg. 1993; 10: 114–115
142. **Kodama, Y., Fujita, N., Shimizu, T., Endo, H., Nambu, T., Sato, N., Todo, S., Miyasaka, K.:** Alveolar echinococcosis: MR findings in the liver. Radiology 2003; 228: 172–177
143. **Kök, A.N., Yurtman, T., Aydin, N.E.:** Sudden death due to ruptured hydatid cyst of the liver. J. Forens. Sci. 1993; 38: 978–980
144. **Kurt, N., Oncel, M., Gulmez, S., Ozkan, Z., Uzun, H.:** Spontaneous and traumatic intra-peritoneal perforation of hepatic hydatid cysts: a case series. J. Gastrointest. Surg. 2003; 7: 635–641
145. **Lewall, D.B.:** Hydatid disease: biology, pathology, imaging and classification. Clin. Radiol. 1998; 53: 863–874
146. **Liu, Y.H., Wang, X.G., Wu, J.Q.:** Continuous long-term albendazole therapy in intraabdominal cystic echinococcosis. Chin. Med. J. 2000; 113: 827–832
147. **Losanoff, J.E., Richman, B.W., Jones, J.W.:** Organ-sparing surgical treatment of giant hepatic hydatid cysts. Amer. J. Surg. 2004; 187: 288–290
148. **Marani, S.A.D., Canossi, G.C., Nicoli, F.A., Alberti, G.P., Monni, S.G., Casolo, P.M.:** Hydatid disease: MR imaging study. Radiology 1990; 175: 701–706
149. **Mazziotti, S., Gaeta, M., Blandino, A., Barone, M., Salamone, I.:** Hepatobronchial fistula due to transphenic migration of hepatic echinococcosis: MR demonstration. Abdom. Imag. 2000; 25: 497–499
150. **McManus, D.P., Zhang, W.B., Li, J., Bartley, P.B.:** Echinococcosis: Lancet 2003; 362: 1295–1304
151. **Nahmias, J., Goldsmith, R., Soibelman, M., El-On, J.:** Three-to 7-year follow-up after albendazole treatment of 68 patients with cystic echinococcosis (hydatid disease). Ann. Trop. Med. Parasitol. 1994; 88: 295–304
152. **Paksoy, Y., Odev, K., Salin, M., Arslan, A., Koc, O.:** Percutaneous treatment of liver hydatid cysts. Comparison of direct injection of albendazole and hypertonic saline solution. Amer. J. Roentgenol. 2005; 185: 727–734
153. **Saimot, A.G.:** Medical treatment of liver hydatidosis. World J. Surg. 2001; 25: 15–20
154. **Senturk, H., Mert, A., Ersavasti, G., Tabak, F., Akdogan, M., Ulualp, K.:** Bronchobiliary fistula due to alveolar hydatid disease. Report of three cases. Amer. J. Gastroenterol. 1998; 93: 2248–2253
155. **Smego, R.A., Bhatti, S., Khaliq, A.A., Beg, M.A.:** Percutaneous aspiration-injection-respiration drainage plus albendazole or mebendazole for hepatic cystic echinococcosis: a meta-analysis. Clin. Infect. Dis. 2003; 37: 1073–1083
156. **Stefaniak, J., Lemke, A.:** Clinical aspects of the hepatic cystic echinococcosis. Differential diagnosis of echinococcus cysts in the liver by ultrasonography and fine needle aspiration biopsy. Hepatol. Polska 1995; 2: 33–38
157. **Stumpe, K.D., Renner-Schneiter, E.C., Kuenzle, A.K., Grimm, F., Kadry, Z., Clavien, P.A., Deplaces, P., von Schulthess, G.K., Muellhaupt, B., Ammann, R.W., Renner, E.L.:** F-18-fluorodeoxyglucose (FDG) positron-emission tomography of Echinococcus multilocularis liver lesions. Prospective evaluation of its value for diagnosis and follow-up during benzimidazole therapy. Infection 2007; 35: 11–18
158. **Thameur, H., Abdelmoula, S., Chenik, S., Bey, M., Ziadi, M., Mestiri, T., Mechmeche, R., Chaouch, H.:** Cardiopericardial hydatid cysts. World J. Surg. 2001; 25: 58–67
159. **Ulualp, K.M., Aydemir, I., Senturk, H., Eyuboglu, E., Cebeci, H., Unal, G., Unal, H.:** Management of intrabiliary rupture of hydatid cyst of the liver. World J. Surg. 1995; 19: 720–724
160. **Vargas-Serrano, B., Rodriguez-Romero, R., Coarasa-Cerdan, A.:** Hepatic hydatid cyst communicating with the biliary tract. J. Clin. Ultrasound 1995; 23: 259–262
161. **Wilson, J.F., Rausch, R.L., Wilson, F.R.:** Alveolar hydatid disease. Review of the surgical experience in 42 cases of active disease among Alaskan Eskimos. Ann. Surg. 1995; 221: 315–323

Clinical Aspects of Liver Diseases

26 Mycotic infections and the liver

		Page:
1	*Predisposing factors*	518
2	*Pathogens*	518
3	*Diagnostics*	518
4	*Morphological findings*	519
5	**Hepatobiliary organ mycoses**	519
5.1	Candidosis	519
5.2	Aspergillosis	519
5.3	Blastomycosis	520
5.4	Trichosporosis	520
5.5	Cryptococcosis	520
5.6	Coccidioidomycosis	520
5.7	Histoplasmosis	520
5.8	Torulopsosis	520
5.9	Mucormycosis	520
5.10	Prototothecosis	521
5.11	Coniothyrium mycosis	521
6	*Therapy*	521
	• References (1–65)	521
	(Tables 26.1–26.3)	

26 Mycotic infections and the liver

▶ *The clinical diagnosis of any mycosis requires proof of the pathogenic fungus and, as far as possible, additional differentiation by fungal culture.* • **Endogenous mycosis** is a fungal infection caused by saprophytic fungi, i.e. normal inhabitants of the gastrointestinal tract, especially as secondary mycosis following other immunocompromising diseases. • **Exogenous mycosis** is caused by primary pathogenic fungi: it may be localized or generalized, and it may have a preference for certain tissues or systems. • **Systemic mycosis** shows widespread dissemination, predominantly affecting particular organs and tissues; it may originate from endogenous or exogenous mycosis. • *Thus, a mycotic disease of the liver and biliary tract is always systemic.*

1 Predisposing factors

Hepatic or biliary mycosis is only likely to occur with a deficiency of the endogenic defence response. However, in isolated cases, discussion has also centred on locally impaired defence mechanisms (e.g. after ERCP (17), choledocholithiasis, papillotomy) which cause or exacerbate an existing mycotic focus. There have been several cases without any noticeable immunosuppression (e.g. aspergillosis and candidosis). Both systemic and organ mycosis are causally related to factors or events leading to a reduced immune response, especially the clearance function of the hepatic RES. Saprophytic fungi thus become opportunistic pathogens, which, like exogenous primary pathogenic fungi, gain the upper hand over the body's defence system. (s. tab. 26.1)

2 Pathogens

Hepatobiliary organ mycosis may be caused by several fungal forms, whereby the Candida species by far outnumber the others. With the exception of the Candida and Mucor species, all hepatotoxic fungi have an airborne route of infection. (s. tab. 26.2)

3 Diagnostics

Even though hepatobiliary mycosis is rare in terms of numbers, the possibility of mycotic infection should always be considered in the presence of predisposing factors or respective events. • Signs of such a complication include additional **complaints**, e.g. loss of appetite, increasing malaise, tenderness in the right epigastrium, and **clinical symptoms**, e.g. fever of unknown origin – especially in nonresponse to antibiotics – and hepato(spleno)megaly.

1. Medicaments
   - immunosuppressants
   - glucocorticoids
   - cytostatics
   - antibiotics
2. Immunological diseases
   - e.g. AIDS, collagenosis
3. Haematological diseases
   - e.g. leukaemia, aplastic anaemia
4. Malignant diseases
5. Organ transplantation
6. Severe hepatic dysfunction
7. Serious acute diseases
   - e.g. pancreatitis, endocarditis, peritonitis
8. Chronic renal diseases
   - e.g. glomerulonephritis, dialysis
9. Intensive care
   - e.g. artificial respiration, parenteral feeding
10. Infectious diseases
    - e.g. salmonellosis, tuberculosis
11. Diabetes mellitus
12. Burns
13. Major surgery
14. Prepartal and postpartal complications
15. Chronic alcoholism
16. Malnutrition
17. Ileus
18. Tooth extraction
19. ERCP, papillotomy

Tab. 26.1: Predisposing factors for mycosis of the liver and biliary tract

1. Candida species
   - C. albicans, C. glabrata, C. krusei
     C. parapsilosis, C. tropicalis
2. Aspergillus species
   - A. flavus, A. fumigatus, A. niger
3. Blastomyces species
   - B. brasiliensis, B. dermatitidis
4. Trichosporon species
   - T. beigelii, T. capitatum
5. Cryptococcus neoformans
6. Coccidioides immitis
   Paracoccidioides brasiliensis
7. Histoplasma capsulatum
8. Torulopsis glabrata
9. Mucor indicus
10. Prototheca wickerhamii
    Prototheca zopfii
11. Coniothyrium fuckelii

Tab. 26.2: Fungal species causing hepatobiliary organ mycosis in the presence of predisposing factors

Several **laboratory parameters**, e.g. increase in the transaminases, alkaline phosphatase, bilirubin, ESR, CRP, decrease in ChE, are important. (s. tab. 27.4) • **Ultrasound** and **CT** only reveal hepato(spleno)megaly or suggest multiple foci similar to small abscesses, possibly in the form of a "snowstorm" – and occasionally biliary congestion as a result of obstruction due to fungal masses. (1, 2, 13, 15, 25, 26, 28, 29) • **MRI** is a better diagnostic tool (85–100%) – equally reliable information was also obtained with MRI when monitoring the treatment and follow-up of hepatolienal mycoses. (7)

These hints of hepatolienal mycosis can be confirmed by **liver biopsy** or **fine needle biopsy.** (9, 18, 20, 51, 52) In this respect, however, only a small area is examined by the puncture technique, with the result that negative histological findings are not always representative of the liver as a whole. Diagnostic reliability is, of course, increased by taking two or three biopsy samples from the two lobes of liver during laparoscopy. (s. pp 157, 161) • Conclusive proof of **mycosis** is obtained by (*1.*) microscopic examination, (*2.*) serological tests or immunoassays, and (*3.*) fungal culture.

4 Morphological findings

Systemic organ mycosis is characterized by different manifestations in the area of the liver or biliary tract. The manifestations vary depending on the type of mycosis, and indeed some of them have only been seen in certain mycosis forms. Various morphological findings have been reported. (s. tab. 26.3)

1. Granulomas
   Granulomatous suppurative or caseating foci
2. Microabscesses and small abscesses
3. Cholangitis
4. Hepatitis
   – portal, often eosinophilic cellular infiltration
   – focal inflammatory lesions
   – single-cell necrosis
5. Mesenchymal reactions
6. Splendore-Hoeppli phenomenon (s. p. 404, 509)
7. Biliary obstruction by fungal conglomerates
8. Perihepatic adhesions

Tab. 26.3: Morphological findings in mycosis of the liver and biliary tract

5 Hepatobiliary organ mycoses

5.1 Candidosis

Some facultative pathogenic Candida species are common pathogens responsible for mycosis of the hepatobiliary system. (s. tab. 26.2) This candida mycosis, also called thrush or moniliasis, is a typical **opportunistic mycosis,** generally known more than 140 years ago as the *"disease of the sick"*. The human intestinal tract serves as a reservoir for pathogens in the body. As a rule, thrush initially manifests in the area of the oral and pharyngeal mucosa. Depending on the degree of impairment of the body's own defence mechanisms, the candida infection can disseminate further into the tracheobronchial system and gastrointestinal tract, where it penetrates the intestinal wall and, via the vascular system, affects most of the other organs (liver, lungs, spleen, bone marrow, eyes, CNS, endocardium) as well; it may also spread systematically, possibly as septicaemic candidosis. (11)

Hepatolienal candidosis: In most cases, the liver and spleen are concurrently and similarly affected, especially in the form of microabscesses. A greater risk of candidosis exists for patients with severe hepatic dysfunction, in particular cirrhosis or acute liver failure (5, 19, 32), after marrow or liver transplantation (3, 6, 8) and with leukaemia or carcinoma. (1, 4, 31) Fever of unknown origin and non-response to antibiotics are suggestive of systemic candidosis. Alkaline phosphatase is always elevated. (14, 21, 24, 25) • *Morphological findings* include granulomas (12, 20, 21, 30), hepatitis-like lesions (18), microabscesses (1, 2, 4, 28), cholangitis (16), biliary obstruction by fungal conglomerates (10, 22, 23) and perihepatic adhesions. (12) • *Sonography* shows multiple small abscesses (> 5 mm in diameter), which are detectable as hypoechoic areas and target zones; however, aetiological clarification is not possible. "Wheels within wheels" is considered to be more characteristic: a round, hypoechoic (fibrosis-related) focus shows an inner hyperechoic (inflammation-related) zone, which, in turn, exhibits an inner hypoechoic (caseation-related) area. (26) Sonographic clues to candidosis of the (generally enlarged) liver and spleen (9, 13, 15, 24–28) are further underpinned by *CT* and *MRI*, using gadolinium as a contrast medium. Cytological or histological clarification and cultural or serological tests as well as DNA analysis (PCR) are now indicated. Lethality is 40–50%.

5.2 Aspergillosis

▶ **Environmental reservoirs** for the Aspergillus species (s. tab. 26.2) include damp cellars and old stone walls, soil in flowerpots (thus possibly in hospital rooms!) and mouldy food. The aflatoxins of the mould Aspergillus flavus (e.g. in mouldy nuts) are deemed to have a high *carcinogenic potential*.

The aspergillus spores enter the body by *airborne transmission*, usually via the respiratory tract. Under normal conditions (good defence response, no excessively high germ count), aspergillus is eliminated. In cases of reduced body-own defence (s. tab. 26.1), the mucosa is affected more severely, and after vascular invasion, generalized aspergillosis also occurs. The lungs are mainly impaired by bronchopulmonary aspergillosis, aspergilloma or pneumonia. Generalization may also involve other organs.

Liver and *spleen* are often affected. Focal lesions can be detected by imaging techniques. (35, 37) Disseminated aspergillosis has also been reported in acute liver failure. (36, 38) Following liver transplantation, aspergillosis is a feared and relatively frequent complication (6—10% of cases). (3, 8, 33, 34, 37)

5.3 Blastomycosis

Blastomyces species cause South American (B. brasiliensis) and North American (B. dermatitidis) blastomycosis (s. tab. 26.2), the budding forms of which are also found in body tissue. The pathogens are mainly transmitted via the respiratory tract, which explains why bronchopulmonary infections clearly predominate. Yet, multiple organ involvement, particularly with Blastomyces dermatitidis, is also known.

Hepatobiliary system: An interesting case report of blastomycosis with liver involvement describes the following conditions: the development of chronic cholangitis in the area of the left hepatic duct with encroachment of the mycotic inflammation to the left lobe of liver in cases of predisposing and/or pre-existing choledocholithiasis, histological evidence of liver granulomas and periportal fibrosis, and a marked increase in alkaline phosphatase and γ-GT. (39, 40)

5.4 Trichosporosis

Systemic infection induced by the Trichosporon species (s. tab. 26.2) sometimes leads to sepsis and, in the liver, to distinct hepatitis-like findings, granulomas and microabsesses. Several laboratory tests revealed an increase in the transaminases, alkaline phosphatase and bilirubin. Diagnosis was confirmed by liver biopsy and fungal culture. (41, 42)

5.5 Cryptococcosis

Mycosis caused by *Cryptococcus neoformans*, also termed European blastomycosis, is airborne and reaches the organism via the respiratory tract. The source of infection is mostly bird excrement, especially pigeon droppings. The pathogen consists of large round yeast cells, 10 μm in diameter, surrounded by gelatinous capsules. It can be selectively demonstrated by mucicarmine staining or Chinese ink.

Liver: In generalized cryptococcosis, hepatitis-like findings, simulating a surgical emergency (47) or causing peritonitis (44) and cholangitis (43), were reported; in a further case, the clinical picture of primary sclerosing cholangitis was imitated. (45) Cryptococcosis is mainly found in AIDS patients. Both acute liver failure and liver cirrhosis have also been provoked by cryptococcosis. (46, 48) Proof is obtained by histological and microscopic examination as well as by fungal culture, and, if necessary, by serological tests.

5.6 Coccidioidomycosis

The mycelial fungus *Coccidioides immitis*, affecting both humans and animals, is rarely encountered in Europe, whereas endemic areas are known in America. • In this context, coccidioidomycosis (*Paracoccidioides brasiliensis*) should also be mentioned.

Liver: In disseminated coccidioidomycosis (A. POSADA, 1894), lung involvement is predominant; however, in 45—60% of cases, autopsy findings showed the liver to be affected as well. The principal manifestations are granulomas and small abscess-like foci. Clinical findings include fever, hepatomegaly and eosinophilia as well as a rise in the transaminases and serum bilirubin. Liver biopsy provided the diagnosis in most cases. (49—54)

5.7 Histoplasmosis

▶ Disseminated infection with *Histoplasma capsulatum* is a form of mycosis frequently found in North and South America, but rarely in Europe. It affects both animals and humans. Henhouses and caves inhabited by bats are ideal breeding grounds. Infection is usually by inhalation of dust, which is why the lungs are primarily affected. In body tissue, the pathogen is demonstrable as yeast cells, 3—5 μm in diameter, mainly localized intracellularly. The course of pulmonary infection is mild with a good healing tendency.

Lymphogenous dissemination from the primary pulmonary focus leads to serious generalized disease in the form of chronic, slowly progressive reticuloendotheliosis with fever, lymphadenopathy and splenomegaly.

Liver: In cases involving the liver, there is evidence of hepatomegaly with many epithelioid cell granulomas, some with central necrosis. These granulomas may subsequently become fibrous and even calcify. The fungus can be demonstrated in the RES cells and in the granulomas by PAS staining or silver impregnation. Histoplasmosis can remain latent in the body for decades before being reactivated. (55—58)

5.8 Torulopsosis

Of the approximately 36 Torulopsis species known so far, *T. glabrata*, also classified as a Candida species, is a human pathogen. Dissemination leads to colonization of the fungus in many organs and the development of liver abscesses. Severe hepatobiliary torulopsosis was also diagnosed in one patient with diabetes and bile duct stricture, secondary to chronic pancreatitis. (59)

5.9 Mucormycosis

Mucormycosis of the liver is a rare condition. In one reported case, widespread dissemination of *Mucor indicus*, resulting from isolated ileocoecal mucormycosis with markedly reduced body-own defence, led to liver infection with multiple abscesses. A serious clinical picture with fever, hepatomegaly and icterus developed. The multiple abscesses could be identified by CT and the fungal infection confirmed by microscopic examination or cultures of biopsy specimens. (60–62)

5.10 Protothecosis

Of the many Protheca species, only *P. wickerhamii* and *P. zopfii* cause disease in humans. Infection occurs when the body's defence system is seriously impaired. Liver involvement is rare. In one noteworthy case, a severe feverish hepatobiliary disease simulating sclerosing cholangitis, as demonstrated by ERC, was reported. Liver biopsy showed portal infiltration with eosinophilic cells and granulomas as well as fibrosis. (63, 64)

5.11 Coniothyrium mycosis

Liver infection with *Coniothyrium fuckelii* in a female patient with leukaemia was reported for the first time in 1987. (65) The acute clinical picture consisting of fever, arthralgia and myalgia, nightly sweats, increased inflammatory parameters and enhanced alkaline phosphatase could be identified, after extensive examination, as a fungal infection of the liver. Histology revealed focal, partly granulomatous inflammatory lesions, from which *C. fuckelii* was demonstrated by culture.

6 Therapy

The fungistatic therapy, which has been used so far, includes (liposomal) amphotericin B, also in combination with 5-fluorocytosine, fluconazole, ketoconazole and itraconazole. Side effects occur often.

▶ The possibility of **mycosis** should be considered in all those patients with liver disease and reduced body-own defence who are experiencing growing malaise and fever!

References:

1. Bartley, D.L., Hughes, W.T., Parvey, L.S., Parham, D.: Computed tomography of hepatic and splenic fungal abscesses in leukemic children. Pediatr. Infect. Dis. 1982; 1: 317–321
2. Berlow, M.E., Spirt, B.A., Weil, L.: CT follow-up of hepatic and splenic fungal microabscesses. J. Comput. Assist. Tomogr. 1984; 8: 42–45
3. Castaldo, P., Stratta, R.J., Wood, R.P., Markin, R.S., Patil, K.D., Shaefer, M.S., Langnas, A.N., Reed, E.C., Li, S., Pillen, T.J., Shaw, B.W.jr.: Clinical spectrum of fungal infections after orthotopic liver transplantation. Arch. Surg. 1991; 126: 149–156
4. Maxwell, A.J., Mamtora, H.: Fungal liver abscesses in acute leukaemia – a report of two cases. Clin. Radiol. 1988; 39: 197–201
5. Rolando, N., Harvey, F., Brahm, J., Philpott-Howard, J., Alexander, G., Casewell, M., Fagan, E., Williams, R.: Fungal infection: a common unrecognised complication of acute liver failure. J. Hepatol. 1991; 12: 1–9
6. Rossetti, F., Brawner, D.L., Bowden, R., Meyer, W.G., Schoch, H.G., Fisher, L., Myerson, D., Hackman, R.C., Shulman, H.M., Sale, G.E.,
Meyers, J.D., McDonald, G.B.: Fungal liver infection in marrow transplant recipients: prevalence at autopsy, predisposing factors, and clinical features. Clin. Infect. Dis. 1995; 20: 801–811
7. Semelka, R.C., Kelekis, N.L., Sallah, S., Worawattanakul, S., Ascher, S.M.: Hepatosplenic fungal disease: diagnostic accuracy and spectrum of appearances on MR imaging. Amer. J. Roentgenol. 1997; 169: 1311–1316
8. Wade, J.J., Rolando, N., Hayllar, K., Philpott-Howard, J., Casewell, M.W., Williams, R.: Bacterial and fungal infections after liver transplantation: an analysis of 284 patients. Hepatology 1995; 21: 1328–1336

Candidosis
9. Bondestam, S., Jansson, S.-E., Kivisaari, L., Elonen, E., Ruutu, T., Anttinen, I.: Liver and spleen candidiasis: imaging and verification by fine-needle aspiration biopsy. Brit. Med. J. 1981; 282: 1514–1515
10. Carstensen, H., Nilsson, K.O., Nettleblad, S.-C., Cederlund, C.-G., Hildell, J.: Common bile duct obstruction due to an intraluminal mass of candidiasis in a previously healthy child. Pediatrics 1986; 77: 858–861
11. Eiff, von M., Essink, M., Roos, N., Hiddemann, W., Büchner, T., van de Loo, J.: Hepatosplenic candidiasis, a late manifestation of Candida septicaemia in neutropenic patients with haematologic malignancies. Blut 1990; 60: 242–248
12. Gordon, S.C., Watts, J.C., Veneri, R.J., Chandler, F.W.: Focal hepatic candidiasis with perihepatic adhesions: laparoscopic and immunhistologic diagnosis. Gastroenterology 1990; 98: 214–217
13. Grünebaum, M., Ziv, N., Kaplinsky, C., Kornreich, L., Horev, G., Mor, C.: Liver candidiasis. The various sonographic patterns in the immunocompromised child. Pediatr. Radiol. 1991; 21: 497–500
14. Haron, E., Feld, R., Tuffnell, F., Patterson, B., Hasselback, R., Matlow, A.: Hepatic candidiasis: an increasing problem in immunocompromised patients. Amer. J. Med. 1987; 83: 17–26
15. Ho, B., Cooperberg, P.L., Li, D.K.B., Mack, L., Naiman, S.C., Grossman, L.: Ultrasonography and computer tomography of hepatic candidiasis in immunosuppressed patients. J. Ultrasound Med. 1982; 1: 157–159
16. Irani, M., Truong, L.D.: Candidiasis of the extrahepatic biliary tract. Arch. Pathol. Lab. Med. 1986; 110: 1087–1090
17. Ito, M., Kato, T., Sano, K., Hotchi, M.: Disseminated Candida tropicalis infection following endoscopic retrograde cholangiopancreatography. J. Infect. 1991; 23: 77–80
18. Johnson, T.L., Barnett, J.L., Appelman, H.D., Nostrant, T.: Candida hepatitis. Histopathologic diagnosis. Amer. J. Surg. Pathol. 1988; 12: 716–720
19. Nair, S., Kumar, K.S., Sachan, P., Corpuz, M.: Spontaneous fungal peritonitis (Candida glabrata) in a patient with cirrhosis. J. Clin. Gastroenterol. 2001; 32: 362–364
20. Jones, J.M.: Granulomatous hepatitis due to Candida albicans in patients with acute leukemia. Ann. Intern. Med. 1981; 94: 475–477
21. Lewis, J.H., Patel, H.R., Zimmerman, H.J.: The spectrum of hepatic candidiasis. Hepatology 1982; 2: 479–487
22. Magnussen, C.R., Olson, J.P., Ona, F.V., Graziani, A.J.: Candida fungus balls in the common bile duct. Arch. Intern. Med. 1979; 139: 821–822
23. Marcucci, R.A., Whitely, H., Armstrong, D.: Common bile duct obstruction secondary to infection with Candida. J. Clin. Microbiol. 1978; 7: 490–492
24. Miller, J.H., Greenfield, L.D., Wald, B.R.: Candidiasis of the liver and spleen in childhood. Radiology 1982; 142: 375–380
25. Müller, D., Kopka, L., Grabbe, E.: Imaging of hepatosplenic candidosis. Fortschr. Röntgenstr. 1999; 170: 587–590
26. Pastakia, B., Shawker, T.H., Thaler, M., O'Leary, T., Pizzo, P.A.: Hepatosplenic Candidiasis: wheels within wheels. Radiology 1988; 166: 417–421
27. Pines, E., Malbec, D., Lepennec, M.P., Hilpert, F., Boudon, P.: Candidose hépatique à Candida glabrata. Ann. Gastroenterol. Hepatol. 1994; 30: 208–211
28. Schmidt, H., Fischedick, A.-R., Peters, P.E., Lengerke, H.-J.: Candida-Abszesse in Leber und Milz. Sonographische und computertomographische Morphologie. Dtsch. Med. Wschr. 1986; 111: 816–820
29. Shirkhoda, A.: CT findings in hepatosplenic and renal candidiasis. J. Comput. Assist. Tomogr. 1987; 11: 795–798
30. Tashjian, L.S., Abramson, J.S., Peacock, J.E.jr.: Focal hepatic candidiasis: a distinct clinical variant of candidiasis in immunocompromised patients. Rev. Infect. Dis. 1984; 6: 689–703
31. Thaler, M., Pastakia, B., Shawker, T.H., O'Leary, T., Pizzo, P.A.: Hepatic candidiasis in cancer patients: the involving picture of the syndrome. Ann. Intern. Med. 1988; 108: 88–100
32. Triger, D.R., Goepel, J.R., Slater, D.N.: Systemic candidiasis complicating acute hepatic failure in patients treated with cimetidine. Lancet 1981/II: 837–838

Aspergillosis
33. Green, M., Wald, E.R., Tzakis, A., Todo, S., Starzl, T.E.: Aspergillosis of the CNS in a pediatric liver transplant recipient: case report and review. Rev. Infect. Dis. 1991; 13: 653–657
34. Lie, T.S., Höfer, M., Höhnke, C., Krizek, L., Kühnen, E., Iwantscheff, A., Köster, O., Overlack, A., Vogel, J., Rommelsheim, K.: Aspergillose nach Lebertransplantation als Hospitalismusinfektion. Dtsch. Med. Wschr. 1987; 112: 297–301
35. Ow, C., Maldjian, C., Shires, G.T., Markisz, J., Kazam, E.: CT, US and MR imaging of hepatic aspergilloma. J. Comput. Assist. Tomogr. 1991; 15: 852–854

36. **Park, G.R., Drummond, G.B., Lamb, D., Durie, T.B.M., Milne, L.J.R., Lambie, A.T., Cameron, E.W.J.:** Disseminated aspergillosis occurring in patients with respiratory, renal, and hepatic failure. Lancet 1982/I: 179–183
37. **Varkey, B.:** Liver disease and aspergillosis. J. Amer. Med. Ass. 1983; 249: 2020
38. **Walsh, T.J., Hamilton, S.R.:** Disseminated aspergillosis complicating hepatic failure. Arch. Intern. Med. 1983; 143: 1189–1191

Blastomycosis
39. **Ryan, M.E., Kirchner, J.P., Sell, T., Swanson, M.:** Cholangitis due to Blastomyces dermatitidis. Gastroenterology 1989; 96: 1346–1349
40. **Witorsch, P., Utz, J.P.:** North American blastomycosis: a study of 40 patients. Medicine 1968; 47: 169–200

Trichosporosis
41. **Korinek, J.K., Guarda, L.A., Bolivar, R., Stroehlein, J.R.:** Trichosporon hepatitis. Gastroenterology 1983; 85: 732–734
42. **Rivera, R., Cangir, A.:** Trichosporon sepsis and leukemia. Cancer 1975; 36: 1106–1110

Cryptococcosis
43. **Bucuvalas, J.C., Bove, K.E., Kaufman, R.A., Gilchrist, M.J.R., Oldham, K.T., Balistreri, W.F.:** Cholangitis associated with Cryptococcus neoformans. Gastroenterology 1985; 88: 1055–1059
44. **Cleophas, V., George, V., Mathew, M., Samal, S.C., Chandry, G.M.:** Spontaneous fungal peritonitis in patients with hepatitis B virus-related liver disease. J. Clin. Gastroenterol. 2000; 31: 77–79
45. **Lefton, H.B., Farmer, R.G., Buchwald, R., Haselby, R.:** Cryptococcal hepatitis mimicking primary sclerosing cholangitis. Gastroenterology 1974; 67: 511–515
46. **Lin, J.I., Kabir, M.A., Tseng, H.C., Hillman, N., Moezzi, J., Gopalswarmy, N.:** Hepatobiliary dysfunction as the initial manifestation of disseminated cryptococcosis. J. Clin. Gastroenterol. 1999; 28: 273–275
47. **Procknow, J.J., Benfield, J.R., Rippon, J.W., Diener, C.R., Archer, F.L.:** Cryptococcal hepatitis presenting as a surgical emergency. J. Amer. Med. Ass. 1965; 191: 93–98
48. **Sabesin, S.M., Fallon, H.J., Andriole, V.T.:** Hepatic failure as a manifestation of cryptococcosis. Arch. Intern. Med. 1963; 11: 661–669

Coccidioidomycosis
49. **Bayer, A.S., Yoshikawa, T.T., Glabin, J.E., Guze, L.B.:** Unusual syndromes of coccidioidomycosis: diagnostic and therapeutic considerations. A report of 10 cases and a review of the English literature. Medicine 1976; 55: 131–152
50. **Coodley, E.L.:** Disseminated coccidioidomycosis: diagnosis by liver biopsy. Gastroenterology 1967; 53: 947–952
51. **Dodd, L.G., Nelson, S.D.:** Disseminated coccidioidomycosis detected by percutaneous liver biopsy in a liver transplant recipient. Amer. J. Clin. Pathol. 1990; 93: 141–144
52. **Howard, P.F., Smith, J.W.:** Diagnosis of disseminated coccidioidomycosis by liver biopsy. Arch. Intern. Med. 1983; 143: 1335–1338
53. **Ward, J.R., Hunter, R.C.:** Disseminated coccidioidomycosis demonstrated by needle biopsy of the liver. Ann. Intern. Med. 1958; 48: 157–163
54. **Zangerl, B., Edel, G., von Manitius, J., Schmidt-Wilcke, H.A.:** Coccidioidomycosis causing granulomatous hepatitis. Med. Klinik 1998; 93: 170–173

Histoplasmosis
55. **Jain, R., McLaren, B., Bejarano, P., Sherman, K.E.:** Diagnostic problem in clinical hepatology. A 69-year-old man with cholestatic liver disease. Semin. Liver Dis. 1996; 16: 445–449
56. **Lamps, L.W., Molina, C.P., West, A.B., Haggitt, R.C., Scott, M.A.:** The pathologic spectrum of gastrointestinal and hepatic histoplasmosis. Amer. J. Clin. Path. 2000; 113: 64–72
57. **Lanza, F.L., Nelson, R.S., Somayayi, B.N.:** Acute granulomatous hepatitis due to histoplasmosis. Gastroenterology 1970; 58: 392–396
58. **Okudaira, M., Straub, M., Schwarz, J.:** The etiology of discrete splenic und hepatic calcifications in an endemic area of histoplasmosis. Amer. J. Pathol. 1961; 39: 599–611

Torulopsosis
59. **Friedman, E., Blahut, R.J., Bender, M.D.:** Hepatic abscesses and fungemia from Torulopsis glabrata. Successful treatment with percutaneous drainage and amphotericin B. J. Clin. Gastroenterol. 1987; 9: 711–715

Mucormycosis
60. **Borg, ter, F., Kuijper, E.J., van der Lelie, H.:** Fatal mucormycosis presenting as an appendiceal mass with metastatic spread to the liver during chemotherapy-induced granulocytopenia. Scand. J. Infect. Dis. 1990; 22: 499–501
61. **Clark, R.M.:** A case of mucormycosis of the duodenum, liver and cecum. Gastroenterology 1957; 33: 985–990
62. **Tsaousis, G., Koutsouri, A., Gatsiou, C., Paniara, O., Peppas, C., Chalevelakis, G.:** Liver and brain mucormycosis in a diabetic patient type II successfully treated with liposomial amphotericin B. Scand. J. Inf. Dis. 2000; 32: 335–337

Protothecosis
63. **Chan, J.C., Jeffers, L.J., Gould, E.W., Hutson, D., Martinez, O.V., Reddy, K.R., Hassan, F., Schiff, E.R.:** Visceral protothecosis mimicking sclerosing cholangitis in an immunocompetent host: successful antifungal therapy. Rev. Infect. Dis. 1990; 12: 802–807
64. **Cox, G.E., Wilson, J.D., Brown, P.:** Protothecosis: a case of disseminated algal infection. Lancet 1974/II: 379–382

Coniothyrium
65. **Kiehn, T.E., Polsky, B., Punithalingam, E., Edwards, F.F., Brown, A.E., Armstrong, D.:** Liver infection caused by Coniothyrium fuckelii in a patient with acute myelogenous leukemia. J. Clin. Microbiol. 1987; 25: 2410–2412

Clinical Aspects of Liver Diseases
27 Liver abscess

		Page:
1	*Definition*	524
2	*Pathogenesis*	524
3	*Pathogens*	524
4	**Causes**	525
5	**Clinical picture and diagnosis**	525
5.1	Clinical findings	525
5.2	Imaging procedures	525
5.3	Aspiration material	526
5.4	Laboratory parameters	527
6	**Localization**	527
7	**Complications**	527
8	**Therapy**	527
8.1	Conservative treatment	527
8.2	Aspiration treatment	528
8.3	Percutaneous drainage	528
8.4	Surgical drainage	528
8.5	Liver resection	528
9	*Prognosis*	528
	• References (1–104)	529
	(Figures 27.1–27.2; tables 27.1–27.4)	

27 Liver abscess

1 Definition

The term liver abscess describes a circumscribed, often encapsulated, purulent inflammation with necrosis of the local parenchyma which is caused by a multitude of pathogens (bacteria, protozoa, helminths) and fungi. Liver abscesses can be detected as either a solitary or a multiple occurrence. Microabscesses are also observed, diffusely affecting the entire liver, sometimes as the outcome of purulent, suppurative cholangitis.

2 Pathogenesis

Infection can develop in five different ways, whereby a weakening of the body's defence system enormously heightens susceptibility. (13, 38, 80) (s. tab. 27.1)

1. **haematogenic:** via the *proper hepatic artery* in severe septic processes (e.g. furunculosis, osteomyelitis) as a metastatic-pyaemic liver abscess, or via the *portal vein* as a pylephlebitic liver abscess (such as in appendicitis, colitis, diverticulitis), and occasionally via the *umbilical vein* as omphalophlebitis
2. **biliary:** via the bile ducts, arising from cholecystitis or cholangitis as well as from the invasion of parasites or foreign bodies
3. **in continuity:** spread of inflammatory processes to the adjacent areas (e.g. gall-bladder empyema, subphrenic or perinephritic abscess)
4. **posttraumatic:** following injuries to the liver or as a result of intrahepatic haematoma
5. **postoperative**

Tab. 27.1: Various access routes leading to the development of liver abscesses

3 Pathogens

Fundamental differentiation may be made between four types of liver abscess, depending on their **aetiology:**

1. bacterial abscess
2. protozoal abscess
3. helminthic abscess
4. fungal abscess

The causative **pathogen** can be detected directly from the abscess or by cultures set up from the blood or bile, sometimes even from the urine or stool. It is also detectable by microscopy (e.g. evidence of parasites or their eggs and larvae) and sometimes by serology or sonography (e.g. Ascaris lumbricoides, see figs. 25.5−25.8) as well as by other imaging techniques. For diagnosis, it is necessary to select the examination method which is most suitable for the detection of the respective pathogen. When applying suitable bacteriological techniques, anaerobes are found in 30−40% of cases. Solitary liver abscesses (63%) displayed a polymicrobial pathogenic spectrum in twice as many cases as did multiple abscesses (30%). (13) Streptococcus milleri is a very common cause. (63) It can be cultured in a medium enriched with carbon dioxide. (s. tab. 27.2)

Gram-negative aerobes
Acinetobacter
Brucella species (76, 96)
Campylobacter jejuni (14)
Citrobacter freundii
Edwardsiella tarda (104)
Ehrlichiosis (43)
Eikenella corrodens
Escherichia coli
Klebsiella species (20)
Proteus species
Pseudomonas species (97)
Salmonella species (33, 85)
Yersinia species (1, 6, 28, 45, 52, 94)

Gram-positive aerobes
Listeria monocytogenes (56, 74)
Mycobacterium tuberculosis (18, 39)
Pediococcus acidilactici (82)
Staphylococcus (35, 98)
Streptococcus pneumoniae (54)
Streptococcus species (63)

Gram-negative anaerobes
Aeromonas hydrophilia (86)
Bacteroides species
Fusobacterium nucleatum (79)

Gram-positive anaerobes
Actinomyces (9, 61)
Clostridium species (48)
Diphtheria species
Lactobacillus (11)
Peptostreptococcus
Streptococcus anaerobius

Protozoa
Amoebiasis

Helminths
Ascaris lumbricoides
Fasciola hepatica

Fungi
Aspergillosis
Candida species (81)
Mucormycosis
Torulopsis glabrata
Trichosporon species

Tab. 27.2: Main pathogens (bacteria, protozoa, helminths, fungi) of liver abscesses and microabscesses (with some references) *(see chapters 24, 25 and 26)*

4 Causes

The frequency of **cryptogenic liver abscesses** (at one time 30–40%) has been reduced to 10–15% due to modern contrast-medium imaging procedures and improved or more advanced serological, bacteriological and parasitological methods. Improved diagnostic clarification of the clinical picture in terms of the respective pathogens and other causes has led to better treatment results and a clear drop in mortality. (80, 101)

1. Biliary diseases
   – cholecystitis
   – cholangitis
   – cholelithiasis, choledocholithiasis (5, 32)
   – biliary tract surgery (16, 57)
   – parasitosis
   – malignant tumours (102)
   – strictures
   – Sump syndrome following choledochoduodenostomia
2. Intestinal diseases
   – appendicitis with perityphlitic abscess
   – diverticulitis (70, 99)
   – colitis
   – Crohn's disease (7, 30, 46, 55, 60, 64, 91, 95)
   – malignant tumours (93, 102)
   – intestinal surgery
3. Gastric diseases
   – perforation of an ulcer
   – gastric surgery
4. Pancreatic diseases
   – pancreatitis (3, 72)
   – pancreatic carcinoma (102)
   – pancreatic surgery
5. Trauma, abdominal injuries
6. Abscesses of adjacent organs
   – perinephritic abscess
   – subphrenic abscess
   – retrocaecal abscess
   – gall-bladder empyema
   – gall-bladder carcinoma (102)
7. Parasitoses
   – amoebiasis
   – Fasciola hepatica
   – Ascaris lumbricoides
8. Thrombophlebitis
   – portal vein (pylephlebitis)
   – umbilical vein (omphalophlebitis)
9. Alcohol injections for HCC (29, 40, 66, 83)
10. Leukaemia
11. Chronic granulomatosis (34, 37)
12. Arterial embolization (78)
13. Ligature of the hepatic artery (42, 90)
14. Haemosiderosis and yersiniosis (6, 94)
15. Haemorrhoidectomy (67)
16. Infected liver cysts and echinococcus cysts
17. Passage of a swallowed toothpick (2, 44) or fish bone through the stomach into the liver
18. Cryptogenic diseases

Tab. 27.3: Underlying diseases and other causes relating to the development of liver abscesses (with some references)

The **spectrum** of causative diseases in the development of a liver abscess has changed significantly over the past ten years, as have the respective frequency rates. The perityphlitic abscess, once predominant in appendicitis, is now relatively rare; in contrast, traumatic injuries to the liver or adjacent organs as a result of accidents have increased in frequency (by 10%); the biliary infection route has acquired much greater significance (35–40%). Of note is the rising number of liver abscesses caused by the Yersinia species in patients suffering from haemosiderosis or haemochromatosis, or following long-term substitution of iron, since the metabolism of the Yersiniae is iron-dependent. • With regard to all these causative factors, a *weakening of the body's own defence system* (s. tab. 26.1), such as in diabetes mellitus and alcoholism or during a course of treatment with immunosuppressants, glucocorticoids and chemotherapeutic agents, increases the risk of infection. (13, 15, 27, 51, 79) The causes of abscesses hitherto reported have been numerous and diverse. (s. tab. 27.3)

5 Clinical picture and diagnosis

5.1 Clinical findings

In **clinical** terms, continuous or intermittent *fever* predominates. (47) In children with fever of unknown aetiology, a liver abscess should always be considered when setting up the differential diagnosis. Additional signs of febrile infection include bursts of perspiration, night sweats, lack of appetite, loss of weight, nausea, weakness and a general malaise. *Local symptoms* are abdominal pain in the right upper quadrant, radiation of pain to the right shoulder, occasional respiratory pain on the right side and irritable (dry) cough. The liver is often enlarged and tender on pressure; guarding of abdominal muscles is usually in evidence. (47) The clinical course can proceed gradually, yet may also show dramatic symptoms (e.g. shivers, sepsis, jaundice, shock), especially in the case of purulent cholangitis.

5.2 Imaging procedures

Sonography is the method of choice for identifying a liver abscess (sensitivity 71–92% for foci > 1.5 cm). Frequently, especially with small and multiple foci, the liver structure is initially inhomogeneous; clearly definable focal lesions only develop during the further course of disease. As a rule, sonographic morphology shows circular foci which are hypoechoic to anechoic. The echogenic focus usually appears as fluid-filled with several internal echoes. Sometimes, however, a fluid level can actually be detected. Multiple small abscesses aggregate, suggesting the beginning of coalescence into a single larger abscess (= *cluster sign*). (41) Should no gas be present in the abscess, a dorsal reduction in sound waves (= *comet tail*) is observed. Splenomegaly is frequently found. In addition, particularly with mycotic abscesses, an anechoic focus is visible with a centre that is rich in echoes (= *target phenomenon*); such an abscess occasionally presents an anechoic centre inside the echo-rich area (= *double wheel structure*). (15, 17, 18, 52, 98) (s. p. 141) (s. figs. 6.14; 25.1)

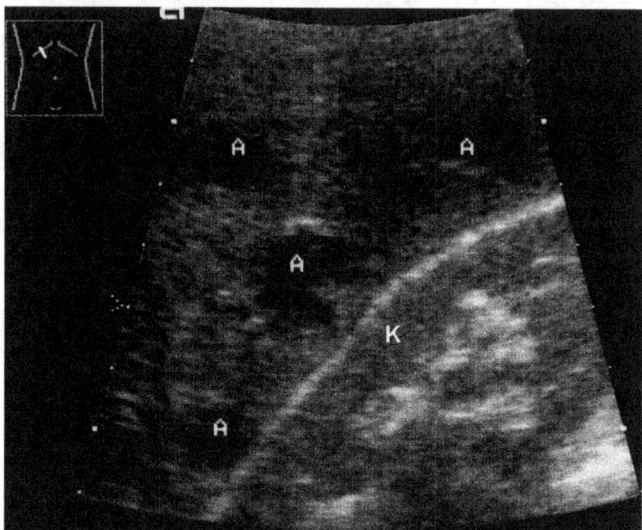

Fig. 27.1: Multiple hypoechoic microabscesses (A) in the right liver lobe (K = kidney)

Computer tomography, besides establishing the diagnosis (in 86—93% of cases with foci >0.5 cm), also makes it possible to locate the abscess exactly. (s. fig. 27.2)

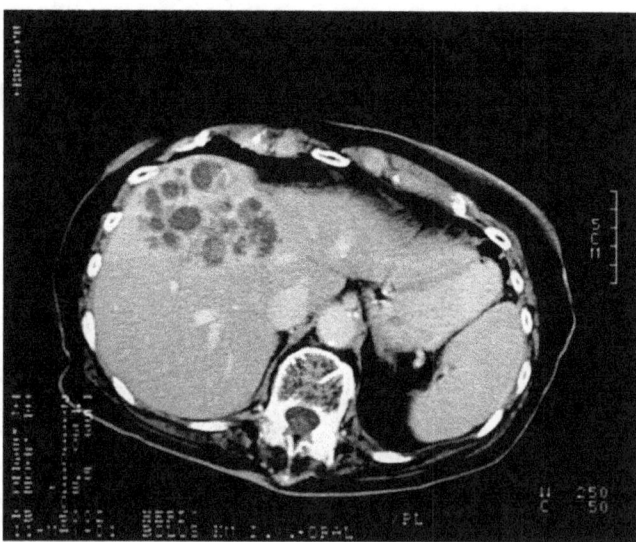

Fig. 27.2: CT scan shows multiple pyogenic liver abscesses in segment 4 (a and b) following perforation in diverticulitis (E. coli). Full recovery

When enhanced with a contrast medium, CT can differentiate an abscess from an intrahepatic metastasis. Pyogenic and mycotic abscesses are visible as hypodense areas both in their natural state as well as after administration of a contrast medium; occasionally, the contrast medium is visible as a ring-shaped enhancement.

A small amount of ascites may be detectable. With the help of ultrasonography and computer tomography, it is possible to carry out guided aspiration or drainage of an abscess reliably. (15, 52) (s. p. 183)

X-ray examination of the chest and abdomen is still imperative, despite the paramount importance of ultrasonography. These standardized routine techniques are usually applied prior to computer tomography because of the wide spectrum of findings acquired as well as the considerably lower costs involved. (13) • In the case of liver abscess, the following findings can be detected in the area of the *thorax*: (*1.*) lack of diaphragmatic motion or right-sided diaphragmatic elevation (40—65%), (*2.*) masking of the right-sided phrenicocostal angle, (*3.*) pleural effusion on the right (40—50%), (*4.*) hypoventilation and atelectasis of the right lower pulmonary lobe, (*5.*) subdiaphragmatic air-fluid level, (*6.*) free air in the subdiaphragmatic area, and (*7.*) infiltration of the lungs. • In the *abdominal area*, the following findings are occasionally observed: (*1.*) evidence of intrahepatic air, (*2.*) intrahepatic air-fluid level, (*3.*) free air in the biliary tract, and (*4.*) foreign bodies.

Cholangiography: If a biliary cause is suspected, cholangiography (i.v., ERC, PTC) may be indicated. With PTC, multiple abscesses mimic the picture of sclerosing cholangitis. (49, 88)

Angiography is deemed indispensable during the course of preoperative preparations for an extensive partial resection of the liver in order to demonstrate atypical arteries. It can also be helpful in detecting multiple small abscesses, where vessels as well as hypervascular zones surrounding small avascular areas are typically pushed aside or displaced.

Scintigraphy, preferably using ^{99m}Tc sulphur colloid or ^{67}Ga-citrate, detects a focal lesion with an abscess of >1.5 cm in approximately 80% of cases. (s. fig. 9.2) • However, the rate of false-negative findings is quite high, and differentiation cannot be made between abscess, tumour, cyst or haemangioma. For this reason, scintigraphy is of no clinical relevance for diagnosing an abscess.

Magnetic resonance imaging produces different elevations of the signal intensity in the T_2-weighted image in 70—75% and hypointensity in the T_1-weighted image in approx. 60% of cases. A perifocal oedema (pointing to an inflammatory process), which receded rapidly after good response to therapy, was detected in 30—40% of cases. After administration of a contrast medium, over 80% of cases displayed wheelspoke-like enhancement. (59)

5.3 Aspiration material

Diagnosis is reached by means of needle aspiration of the abscess guided by ultrasonography or computer tomography and subsequent examination of the abscess contents. In pyogenic abscesses, it is possible to detect one or several pathogens in 62—95% of cases. (quot. 62, 75) Gram-negative aerobic bacteria are found in approx. 60% and gram-positive aerobic pathogens in 15—20% of cases. In order to detect anaerobic bacteria (approx. 20% of cases), utmost care is required when collecting the anaerobic cultures; so-called sterile cultures are often due to mistakes made during the process of collection or are attributable to preceding antibiotic therapy.

(36, 77) The aspiration material should also be tested by selective culture, since mixed infections resulting from both bacteria and fungi may be present. Microscopic examination sometimes makes it possible to differentiate between tumorous and mycotic material. The respective results determine therapy requirements; with targeted treatment, greater efficacy can be achieved.

5.4 Laboratory parameters

Laboratory investigation reveals signs of infection and liver disease based on the degree of severity, course of disease and extent of involvement of the bile ducts. (10, 13, 26, 58, 65, 80, 87, 101) (s. tab. 27.4)

1. *Signs of infection*
   - changes in the blood count (leucocytosis, left shift, anaemia)
   - BSR ↑, CRP reaction +, serum iron ↓
   - fibrinogen, LDH ↑
   - changes in electrophoresis (α_2- and γ-globulins ↑, albumin ↓)

2. *Signs of liver disease*
   - GPT, GOT, GDH ↑
   - γ-GT, alkaline phosphatase ↑
   - serum bilirubin ↑
   - cholinesterase, Quick's value ↓
   - bile acids ↑

Tab. 27.4: Laboratory parameters in liver abscess(es) depending on the degree of severity, course of disease and involvement of the biliary tract

6 Localization

The right lobe of liver, especially the dorsal segments, is most frequently involved (60–70%). In 20–30% of cases, both lobes are affected. Solitary abscesses are localized in the right lobe of liver in 80–90% of cases. Multiple abscesses can be observed in approx. 40% of cases. Subhepatic localization of an abscess was observed following the perforation of a gastric ulcer (11) and conventional cholecystectomy.

7 Complications

With pyogenic abscesses, the most frequent complication is septicaemia and its deleterious sequelae. The abscess can also penetrate the biliary tract and the intrahepatic vascular system (19, 53), or rupture into the abdominal cavity and subphrenic space. (23) Sometimes, thrombosis of the portal and/or hepatic vein develops. Contrast-enhanced CT shows the thrombosis to have non-enhancing linear structures, which, however, do not expand the lumen of the vein. Penetration through the diaphragm into the pleural cavity and the pulmonary parenchyma is likewise to be feared. Pyogenic or mycotic sepsis can give rise to endophthalmitis, particularly in patients suffering from diabetes mellitus. (24, 89) Initial signs of eye symptoms in cases of liver abscess call for immediate examination by the ophthalmologist and, if necessary, appropriate treatment. • *Gas-forming pyogenic abscess:* Many pathogens are capable of gas formation, especially klebsiella pneumoniae. There are four major constituents: nitrogen, oxygen, carbon dioxide and hydrogen. This composition implicates mixed acid fermentation of glucose as the mechanism of gas formation. (22)

8 Therapy

8.1 Conservative treatment

1. Multiple, small and minute abscesses are not accessible to invasive or surgical treatment. Hence it is important to sanitize any focus of infection to prevent it from spreading and to combat the infectious toxic process by suitable therapeutic measures. A bacteriological analysis must be obtained as early as possible by aspiration of the abscess area using a thin needle. Until the pathogenic result is available, a combination of antibiotics should be administered which covers the aerobic as well as the anaerobic spectrum of the most frequent pathogens (e. g. E. coli, Proteus, Klebsiella, Bacteroides fragilis, aerobic and anaerobic streptococci, staphylococci). A suitable combination is cephalosporin + metronidazole + aminoglycoside, but aminoglycoside + clindamycine has also proved helpful. Once the bacteriological result is available, the antibiotic combination is altered in line with the antibiogram, possibly supplemented by a fungistatic agent. The duration of parenteral administration is 10–14 (–21) days with subsequent oral treatment for about 3 to 4 weeks. Prior to cessation of the antibiotic therapy, a check-up should be carried out by ultrasonography and/or computer tomography. In the case of successful treatment, the abscess is either obliterated or at least significantly reduced.

2. It is probable that antibiotics will reach the interior of those abscesses which are still relatively small and have only existed for a short period of time. In these cases, too, the spectrum of aerobic and anaerobic bacteria should initially be covered non-specifically by the above-mentioned combination of antibiotics. At the same time, the presence of an amoebic abscess or echinococcosis should be ruled out serologically (as quickly as possible) and aspirated material collected for bacterial and mycotic testing. Depending on the results, the respective antibiotic (and possibly fungistatic) therapy is effected. After two to four days, the efficacy of this targeted treatment is reviewed clinically, biochemically and ultrasonographically. If the treatment is considered to have been effective, it is continued until obliteration of the abscess foci is achieved. (12, 30, 65, 80, 87, 101)

8.2 Aspiration treatment

1. Should initial antibiotic therapy fail to show any success within the limited period of two to four days (persistence of fever, leucocytosis, bacteriaemia), percutaneous aspiration of the abscess contents, if necessary repeated several times during the next few days, usually proves successful. Antibiotic therapy is continued during the course of percutaneous aspiration treatment.

2. In an extremely large abscess, percutaneous aspiration of the focus with evacuation of the pus is carried out as an initial measure. Generally, several punctures have to be performed with respective aspiration of the focal contents until the abscess cavity is gradually obliterated under the impact of specific antibiotics. The outcome of such treatment is thought to be more favourable, and the concomitant complications (e. g. intraperitoneal contamination, bleeding) are less numerous than with percutaneous drainage. (4, 12, 13, 26, 33, 38, 71, 75, 81, 87, 101, 103)

8.3 Percutaneous drainage

▶ Percutaneous drainage was initially attempted by A. F. S MacFadzen et al. in 1953. It was later introduced into clinical routine by J.R. Haaga et al. (1976) (s. tab. 7.2) using the CT-guided method. An improved technique was subsequently applied by S.G. Gerzof et al. (1981). This led to successful results in the treatment of liver abscesses.

Puncture is effected using a teflon-coated 18 (or 20) gauge needle. After aspiration of the contents, a pigtail catheter (7 or 8 Charrière scale) is placed in the cavity of the abscess by means of a guidewire. Subsequently, the **position of the catheter** and the abscess cavity itself are checked by computer tomography to ensure that there is no septation and that the abscess cavity is completely drained. Once the catheter has been placed in an optimal position, the pus is totally evacuated and the cavity rinsed clean with a physiological NaCl solution. The original catheter may be replaced later, if necessary, by one with a wider lumen (14–16 Charrière scale). • Simultaneous **antibiotic therapy** is readjusted according to the bacteriological results and the antibiogram. Additional injection of antibiotics into the abscess cavity can further improve the efficacy of the parenteral and subsequent oral antibiotic treatment.

It is possible to remove the drainage if ultrasonography or computer tomography show the abscess cavity to be completely (or extensively) obliterated, if no more fluid can be detected and if the white blood cell count has dropped to below $10,000/mm^3$. This method of treatment of liver abscesses has proved its worth; success rates are of 70–90%. (8, 26, 27, 31, 38, 47, 50, 58, 63, 68, 71, 73, 75, 84, 100, 101)

8.4 Surgical drainage

Percutaneous drainage may be limited by antelocated intestinal loops or by abscesses that are difficult to reach. Similarly, surgery is indicated following unsuccessful percutaneous drainage, in extensive cavernous or multifocal abscesses, in tissue sequestration, after formation of enteral fistula and viscous abscess contents as well as in the case of local recurrences. • With abscess perforation or the existence of other purulent foci in the abdomen, surgical intervention is called for immediately.

The **surgical approach** depends on the location of the abscess, any abdominal investigation that may be required, and possible sanitization of a focus. • The respective **access routes** are: (1.) transperitoneal, (2.) extraperitoneal, (3.) in special cases also retroperitoneal or infrapleural, and (4.) transpleural as well as transdiaphragmatic. Evidence of biliary genesis calls for operative or endoscopic sanitization of the biliary tracts and safeguarding of the biliary flow, possibly via a T drain in the choledochus. (8, 26, 38, 47, 63, 69, 75, 101)

Laparoscopic drainage: An alternative to the open surgical drainage of abscesses can be found in laparoscopic drainage. This method is deemed to be safe and successful. In a group of 20 patients, there were no intraoperative or postoperative complications. (92) Consequently, before deciding on open surgery, the possibility of laparoscopic abscess drainage should be considered.

8.5 Liver resection

Resection of a liver abscess is reserved for exceptional circumstances. The **advantages** of this method are definitive sanitization of the abscess, an insignificant degree or indeed absence of peritoneal contamination, short-term postoperative antibiotic therapy and the possibility of histological clarification in the event of suspected superinfected malignant tumours. Moreover, the quality of life is nowhere near as limited as with the various operative drainage procedures, nor is the treatment as drawn-out and burdensome. A prerequisite for resection is the fundamental operability of the patient and a residual liver parenchyma that is still intact. • **Indications** for liver resection are as follows: large abscess cavities without any tendency to regression but possibly with rigid walls and septation, multifocal abscess systems, abscesses of unresolved status of benignancy/malignancy as well as necrotized and superinfected malignant tumours. Usually, low-complication postoperative courses without mortality have been reported. (25, 69) In some cases, the liver parenchyma completely regenerates along the edge of the abscission scar.

9 Prognosis

Prior to the introduction of liver scintigraphy, a mere 20% of liver abscesses were diagnosed antemortem; the mortality rate was correspondingly 80–100%. Following the introduction of scintigraphy in 1965, approx.

80% of all liver abscesses could be diagnosed, and the mortality rate dropped to 28%. • Early diagnosis and the correct choice of aspiration or drainage treatment procedures have further reduced the mortality rate to below 20%; the rate for solitary abscesses is now below 10%, sometimes as low as 3%. • **Risk factors** include: advanced age, impairment of the body's defence system, sepsis, diabetes mellitus, alcoholism, considerable prior liver damage, increasing hepatic and renal insufficiency, multiple and/or cavernous abscesses, biliary causes of infection, gas-forming abscesses – all depending on the situation in the respective case. (19, 21, 80, 101)

> *In view of such risk factors, each liver abscess calls for individual therapy planning discussed at an interdisciplinary level!*

References:

1. Albrecht, H., Stellbrink, H.-J., Nägele, H.-H., Guthoff, A., Greten, H.: Leberabszesse durch Yersinia enterocolitica. Dtsch. Med. Wschr. 1991; 116: 331–334
2. Allimant, P., Rosburger, C., Zeyer, B., Frey, G., Morel, E., Bietiger, M., Dalcher, G.: Une cause insolite d'abces hepatique. Ann. Gastroenterol. Hepatol. 1990; 26; 5–6
3. Ammann, R., Münch, R., Largiader, F., Akovbiantz, A., Marincek, B.: Pancreatic and hepatic abscesses: a late complication in 10 patients with chronic pancreatitis. Gastroenterology 1992; 103: 560–565
4. Baek, S.Y., Lee, M.-G., Cho, K.S., Lee, S.C., Sung, K.-B., Auh, Y.H.: Therapeutic percutaneous aspiration of hepatic abscesses: effectiveness in 25 patients. Amer. J. Roentgenol. 1993; 160: 799–802
5. Barek, L., Orron, D.E., Behar, D.J.: Hepatic abscesses due to occult biliary stones. J. Comput. Assist. Tomogr. 1987; 11: 31–34
6. Beeching, J.B., Hart, H.H., Synek, B.J., Bremner, D.A.: A patient with hemosiderosis and multiple liver abscesses due to Yersinia enterocolitica. Pathology 1985; 17: 530–532
7. Benhidjeb, T., Ridwelski, K., Wolff, H., Gellert, K., Lüning, M., Pertschy, J.: Liver abscess as a first manifestation of Crohn's disease. Dig. Surg. 1992; 9: 288–292
8. Bertel, C.K., van Heerden, J.A., Sheedy, P.F.: Treatment of pyogenic hepatic abscesses, surgical vs percutaneous drainage. Arch. Surg. 1986; 121: 554–558
9. Bhatt, B.D., Zuckerman, M.J., Ho, H., Polly, St.M.: Multiple actinomycotic abscesses of the liver. Amer. J. Gastroenterol. 1990; 85: 309–310
10. Bissada, A.A., Bateman, J.: Pyogenic liver abscess: a 7-year experience in a large community hospital. Hepatogastroenterology 1991; 38: 317–320
11. Bouaziz, M., Hammami, A., Beyrouti, I., Zouari, R., Jeddi, H.M.: Abces sous-hépatique à Lactobacillus. Sem. Hop. 1992; 68: 594–595
12. Bowers, E.D., Robison, D.J., Doberneck, R.C.: Pyogenic liver abscess. World J. Surg. 1990; 14: 128–132
13. Branum, G.D., Tyson, G.S., Branum, M.A., Myers, W.C.: Hepatic abscess. Changes in etiology, diagnosis and management. Ann. Surg. 1990; 212: 655–662
14. Brmbolic, B.: Multiple abscesses of the liver caused by Campylobacter jejuni. J. Clin. Gastroenterol. 1995; 20: 307–309
15. Callen, P.W., Filly, R.A., Marcus, F.S.: Ultrasonography and computed tomography in the evaluation of hepatic microabscesses in the immunosuppressed patient. Radiology 1980; 136: 433–434
16. Carrel, T., Lerut, J., Baer, H., Blumgart, L.H.: Hepatic abscess following biliary tract surgery. Acta Chir. Europ. J. Surg. 1991; 157: 209–213
17. Catalano, O., Sandomenico, F., Raso, M.M., Siani, A.: Low mechanical index contrast-enhanced sonographic findings of pyogenic hepatic abscesses. Amer. J. Roentgenol. 2004; 182: 447–450
18. Chen, H.C., Chao, Y.C., Shyu, R.Y., Hsieh, T.Y.: Isolated tuberculous liver abscesses with multiple hyperechoic masses on ultrasound: A case report and review of the literature. Liver Internat. 2003; 23: 346–350
19. Chen, S.C., Lee, Y.T., Lai, K.C., Cheng, K.S., Jeng, L.B., Wu, W.Y., Chen, C.C., Lee, M.-C.: Risk factors for developing metastatic infection from pyogenic liver abscesses. Swiss. Med. Week. 2006; 136: 119–126
20. Cheng, D.-L., Liu, Y.-C., Yen, M.-Y., Liu, C.-Y., Wang, R.-S.: Septic metastatic lesions of pyogenic liver abscess. Their association with Klebsiella pneumoniae bacteremia in diabetic patients. Arch. Intern. Med. 1991; 151: 1557–1559
21. Chou, F.-F., Sheen-Chen, S.-M., Chen, Y.-S., Chen, M.-C., Chen, F.-C., Tai, D.-I.: Prognostic factors for pyogenic abscess of the liver. J. Amer. Coll. Surg. 1994; 179: 727–732
22. Chou, F.-F., Sheen-Chen, S.-M., Chen, Y.-S., Lee, T.-Y.: The comparison of clinical course and results of treatment between gas-forming and non-gas-forming pyogenic liver abscess. Arch. Surg. 1995; 130: 401–405
23. Chou, F.-F., Sheen-Chen, S.-M., Lee, T.-Y.: Rupture of pyogenic liver abscess. Amer. J. Gastroenterol. 1995; 90: 767–770
24. Chou, F.-F., Kou, H.-K.: Endogenous endophthalmitis associated with pyogenic hepatic abscess. J. Amer. Coll. Surg. 1996; 182: 33–36
25. Christein, J.-D., Kendrick, M.-L., Qua, F.G.: What affects mortality after the operative management of hepatic abscen? (review) HPB 2006; 8: 175–178
26. Chu, K.-M., Fan, S.-T., Lai, E.C.S., Lo, C.-M., Wong, J.: Pyogenic liver abscess. An audit of experience over the past decade. Arch. Surg. 1996; 131: 148–152
27. Civardi, G., Filice, C., Caremani, M., Giorgio, A.: Hepatic abscesses in immunocompromised patients: ultrasonically guided percutaneous drainage. Gastrointest. Radiol. 1992; 17: 175–178
28. Colizza, F., LePage, S., LaJoie, J.-F., Duperval, R., Marcoux, A., Mongeau, J., Bergeron, D.: Multiple hepatic abscesses following Yersinia enterocolitica septicemia. Can. J. Gastroenterol. 1990; 4: 179–183
29. De Baère, T., Roche, A., Amenabar, J.M., Lagrange, C., Ducreux, M., Rougier, P., Ellias, D., Lasser, P., Patriarche, C.: Liver abscess formation after local treatment of liver tumors. Hepatology 1996; 23: 1436–1440
30. De Ronde, T., Melange, M., Trigaux, J.P., van Beers, B., Pouthier, F., Dive, C.: Abcès hépatiques compliquant une maladie de Crohn iléale en rémission. Efficacité de l'antibiothérapie. Gastroenterol. Clin. Biol. 1990; 14: 175–177
31. Donderlinger, R.F., Kurdziel, J.-C., Gathy, C.: Percutaneous treatment of pyogenic liver abscess: a critical analysis of results. Cardiovasc. Intervent. Radiol. 1990; 13: 174–182
32. Edelman, K.: Multiple pyogenic liver abscesses communicating with the biliary tree: treatment by endoscopic stenting and stone removal. Amer. J. Gastroenterol. 1994; 89: 2070–2072
33. Giorgio, A., Tarantino, L., de Stefano, G.: Hepatic abscess caused by Salmonella typhi: diagnosis and management by percutaneous echo-guided needle aspiration. Ital. J. Gastroenterol. 1996; 28: 31–33
34. Grund, K.E., Klotter, H.-J., Lemmel, E.-M.: Chronische Granulomatose als seltene Ursache rezidivierender Leberabszesse. Med. Welt. 1982; 33: 202–203
35. Guillois, B., Guillemin, M.G., Thoma, M., Sizun, J., Monnery, J.L., Alix, D.: Staphylococcie pleuro-pulmonaire néonatale avec abcès hépatiques multiples. Ann. Pediatr. 1989; 36: 681–684
36. Gupta, U., Sharma, M.P.: Etiology of liver abscess with special reference to anaerobic bacteria. Ind. J. Med. Res. 1991; 91: 21–23
37. Hague, R.A., Eastham, E.J., Lee, R.E.J., Cant, A.J.: Resolution of hepatic abscess after interferon gamma in chronic granulomatous disease. Arch. Dis. Childh. 1993; 69: 443–445
38. Huang, C.-J., Pitt, H.A., Lipsett, P.A., Ostermann, F.A., Lillemoe, K.D., Cameron, J.L., Zuidema, G.D.: Pyogenic hepatic abscesses. Changing trends over 42 years. Ann. Surg. 1996; 223: 600–607
39. Ismail, R., Larabi, K., Alyoune, M., Nadir, S., Alaoui, R., Jamil, D., Cherkaoui, A.: Abcès tuberculeux du foie. A propos de deux observations. Ann. Gastroenterol. Hepatol. 1994; 30: 212–214
40. Isobe, H., Fukai, T., Iwamoto, H., Satoh, M., Tokumatsu, M., Sakai, H., Andoh, B., Sakamoto, S., Nawata, H.: Liver abscess complicating intratumoral ethanol injection therapy for HCC. Amer. J. Gastroenterol. 1990; 85: 1646–1648
41. Jeffrey, R.B.jr., Tolentino, C.S., Chang, F.C., Federle, M.P.: CT of small pyogenic hepatic abscesses: the cluster sign. Amer. J. Roentgenol. 1988; 151: 487–489
42. Jochimsen, P.R., Zike, W.L., Shirazi, S.S., Pearlman, N.W.: Iatrogenic liver abscesses. A complication of hepatic artery ligation for tumor. Arch. Surg. 1978; 118: 141–144
43. Kager, L., Kostner, U., Gadner, H., Stanek, G.: Pyogenic liver abscess caused by human granulocytic ehrlichiosis in a 15^1/$_2$-years-old child. Infection 2001; 29 (Suppl.): 86
44. Kanazawa, S., Ishigaki, K., Miyake, T., Ishida, A., Tabuchi, A., Tanemoto, K., Tsunoda, T.: A granulomatous liver abscess which developed after a toothpick penetrated the gastrointestinal tract: report of a case. Surg. Today 2003; 33: 312–314
45. Khanna, R., Levendoglu, H.: Liver abscess due to Yersinia enterocolitica: case report and review of the literature. Dig. Dis. Sci. 1989; 34: 636–639
46. Kotanagi, H., Sone, S., Fukuoka, T., Narisawa, T., Koyama, K., Yagisawa, H., Chiba, M., Masamune, O.: Liver abscess as the initial manifestation of colonic Crohn's disease: report of a case. Japan. J. Surg. 1991; 21: 348–351
47. Kuntz, H.-D.: Status febrilis mit Oberbauchbeschwerden. Zur Klinik, Differentialdiagnose und Therapie des Leberabszesses. Münch. Med. Wschr. 1987; 129: 91–94
48. Kurtz, J.E., Claudel, L., Collard, O., Limacher, J.M., Bergerat, J.P., Dufour, P.: Liver abscess due to Clostridium septicum. A case report and review of the literature. Heptogastroenterol. 2005; 52: 1557–1558
49. Lam, Y.H., Wong, S.K.H., Lee, D.W.H., Lau, J.Y.W., Chan, A.C.W., Yiu, R.Y.C., Sung, J.J.Y., Chung, S.S.C.: ERCP and pyogenic liver abscess. Gastrointest. Endosc. 1999; 50: 340–344

50. **Lambiase, R.E., Deyoe, L., Cronan, J.J., Dorfman, G.S.:** Percutaneous drainage of 335 consecutive abscesses: results of primary drainage with 1-year follow-up. Radiology 1992; 184: 167–179
51. **Lee, K.-T., Sheen, P.-C., Chen, J.-S., Ker, C.-G.:** Pyogenic liver abscess: multivariate analysis of risk factors. World J. Surg. 1991; 15: 372–377
52. **Leyman, P., Baert, A.L., Marchal, G., Fevery, J.:** Ultrasound and CT of multifocal liver abscesses caused by Yersinia enterocolitica. J. Comput. Assist. Tomogr. 1989; 13: 913–915
53. **Liou, T.-C., Ling, C.-C., Pang, K.-K.:** Liver abscess concomitant with hemobilia due to rupture of hepatic artery aneurysm: a case report. Hepato-Gastroenterol. 1996; 43: 241–244
54. **Lund-Tonnesen, St.:** Liver abscess: an unusual manifestation of pneumococcal infection. Scand. J. Infect. Dis. 1995; 27: 397–398
55. **Macpherson, D.S., Scott, D.J.A.:** Liver abscess and Crohn's disease. Amer. J. Gastroenterol. 1985; 80: 399–402
56. **Marino, P., Maggioni, M., Preatoni, A., Cantoni, A., Invernizzi, F.:** Liver abscesses due to Listeria monocytogenes. Liver 1996, 16: 67–69
57. **Matthews, J.B., Gertsch, P., Baer, H.U., Blumgart, L.H.:** Hepatic abscess after biliary tract procedures. Surg. Gynec. Obstetr. 1990; 170: 469–475
58. **McDonald, M.I., Corey, G.R., Gallis, H.A., Durack, D.T.:** Single and multiple pyogenic liver abscesses. Natural history, diagnosis and treatment, with emphasis on percutaneous drainage. Medicine (Baltimore) 1984; 63: 291–302
59. **Mendez, R.J., Schiebler, M.L., Outwater, E.K., Kressel, H.Y.:** Hepatic abscesses: MR imaging findings. Radiology 1994; 190: 431–436
60. **Mir-Madjlessi, S.H., McHenry, M.C., Farmer, R.G.:** Liver abscess in Crohn's disease. Report of four cases and review of the literature. Gastroenterology 1986; 91: 987–993
61. **Miyamoto, M.I., Fang. F.C.:** Pyogenic liver abscess involving Actinomyces: case report and review. Clin. Infect. Dis. 1993; 16: 303–309
62. **Moore-Gillon, J.C., Eykyn, S.J., Philips, I.:** Microbiology of pyogenic liver abscess. Brit. Med. J. 1981; 283: 819–821
63. **Naef, M., Frei, E., Soucek, M., Berthold, M., Schweizer, W., Czerniak, A.:** Die chirurgisch-radiologisch-interventionelle Behandlungstaktik bei Leberabszessen mit Streptococcus anginosus Milleri. Helvet. Chir. 1993; 60: 121–125
64. **Nelson, A., Frank, H.D., Taubin, H.L.:** Liver abscess. A complication of regional enteritis. Amer. J. Gastroenterol. 1979; 72: 282–284
65. **Northover, J.M.A., Jones, B.J.M., Dawson, J.L., Williams, R.:** Difficulties in the diagnosis and management of pyogenic liver abscess. Brit. J. Surg. 1982; 69: 48–51
66. **Okada, S., Aoki, K., Okazaki, N., Nose, H., Yoshimori, M., Shimada, K., Yamamoto, J., Takayama, T., Kosuge, T., Yamasaki, S., Takayasu, K., Moriyama, N.:** Liver abscess after percutaneous ethanol injection (PEI) therapy for hepatocellular carcinoma. A case report. Hepato-Gastroenterol. 1993; 40: 496–498
67. **Parikh, S.R., Molinelli, B., Dailey, T.H.:** Liver abscess after hemorrhoidectomy. Report of two cases. Dis. Colon Rectum 1994; 37: 185–189
68. **Peer, A., Strauss, S., Pik, A.:** Percutaneous catheter drainage of multiple pyogenic liver abscess: a case report. Europ. J. Radiol. 1990; 10: 35–37
69. **Pitt, H.A.:** Surgical management of hepatic abscesses. World J. Surg. 1990; 14: 498–504
70. **Posthuma, E.F.M., Bieger, R., Kuypers, T.J.A.:** A rare case of a hepatic abscess: diverticulitis of the ileum. Nederl. J. Med. 1993; 42: 69–72
71. **Rajak, C.L., Gupta, S., Jain, S., Chawla, Y., Gulati, M., Suri, S.:** Percutaneous treatment of liver abscesses: needle aspiration versus catheter drainage. Amer. J. Roentgenol. 1998; 170: 1035–1039
72. **Reddy, K.R., Jeffers, L., Livingstone, A.S., Gluck, C.A., Schiff, E.R.:** Pyogenic liver abscess complicating common bile duct stenosis secondary to chronic calcific pancreatitis. A rare presentation. Gastroenterology 1984; 86: 953–957
73. **Rendon Unceta, P., Soria de la Cruz, M.J., Rodriguez Pardo, M.J., Diaz Garcia, J., Ruiz Guinaldo, A., Martin Herrera, L.:** Drenaje percutaneo guiado por ecografia de los abscesos hepaticos. Resultados y complicaciones. Rev. Esp. Enf. Digest. 1994; 85: 103–106
74. **Ribière, O., Coutarel, P., Jarlier, V., Bousquet, O., Balderacchi, U.:** Abcès du foie à Listeria monocytogenes. Chez une malade diabétique. Presse Méd. 1990; 19: 1538–1540
75. **Robert, J.H., Mirescu, D., Ambrosetti, P., Khoury, G., Greenstein, A.J., Rohner, A.:** Critical review of the treatment of pyogenic hepatic abscess. Surg. Gynec. Obstetr. 1992; 174: 97–102
76. **Rovery, C., Rolain, J.M., Raoult, D., Brouqui, P.:** Shell vial culture as a tool for isolation of Brucella melitensis in chronic hepatic abscess. J. Clin. Microbiol. 2003; 41: 4460–4461
77. **Sabbaj, J., Sutter, V.L., Finegold, S.M.:** Anaerobic pyogenic liver abscess. Ann. Intern. Med. 1972; 77: 629–638
78. **Satoh, H., Takeda, T., Takashima, M., Sumiyoshi, K., Imaizumi, N.:** Gas-forming liver abscess following transcatheter hepatic arterial embolization for an iatrogenic intrahepatic pseudoaneurysm: report of a case. Jpn. J. Surg. 1995; 25: 361–364
79. **Scoular, A., Corcoran, G.D., Malin, A., Evans, B.A., Davies, A., Miller, R.F.:** Fusobacterium nucleatum bacteraemia with multiple liver abscesses in an HIV-1 antibody-positive man with IgG_2 deficiency. J. Infect 1992; 24: 321–325
80. **Seeto, R.K., Rockey, D.C.:** Pyogenic liver abscess. Changes in etiology, management, and outcome. Medicine 1996; 75: 99–113
81. **Singh, S., Gupta, S., Mirdha, B., Hak, S., Singh, Y.N.:** Large single candidal liver abscess treated with aspiration and antifungal drugs. Ind. J. Gastroenterol. 1992; 11: 176–177
82. **Sire, J.M., Donnio, P.Y., Mesnard, R., Pouedras, P., Avril, J.L:** Septicemia and hepatic abscess caused by Pediococcus acidilactici. Europ. J. Clin. Microbiol. Inf. Dis. 1992; 11: 623–625
83. **Solinas, A., Erbella, G.S., Distrutti, E., Malaspina, C., Fiorucci, St., Clerici, C., Bassotti, G., Morelli, A.:** Abscess formation in hepatocellular carcinoma: complications of percutaneous ultrasound-guided ethanol injection. J. Clin. Ultrasound 1993; 21: 531–533
84. **Sommariva, A., Donisi, P.M., Leoni, G., Ardit, S., Renier, M., Gnocato, B., Tremolada, C.:** Pyogenic liver abscess: is drainage always possible ? (case report). Eur. J. Gastroenterol. Hepatol. 2006; 18: 435–436
85. **Soni, P.N., Hoosen, A.A., Pillay, D.G.:** Hepatic abscess caused by Salmonella typhi. A case report and review of the literature. Dig. Dis. Sci. 1994; 39: 1694–1696
86. **Spencker, F.B., Greiner, C., Tischer, W., Herrmann, E., Handrick, W.:** Leberabszeß durch Aeromonas hydrophila. Kinderärztl. Praxis 1991; 59: 123–125
87. **Srivastava, E.D., Mayberry, J.F.:** Pyogenic liver abscess: a review of aetiology, diagnosis and intervention. Dig. Dis. 1990; 8: 287–293
88. **Steinhart, A.H., Simons, M., Stone, R., Heathcote, J.:** Multiple hepatic abscesses: cholangiographic changes simulating sclerosing cholangitis and resolution after percutaneous drainage. Amer. J. Gastroenterol. 1990; 85: 306–308
89. **Tan, Y.M., Chee, S.P., Soo, K.C., Chow, P.:** Ocular manifestations and complications of pyogenic liver abscess. World J. Surg. 2004; 28: 38–42
90. **Tanaka, K., Nishimura, A., Hombo, K., Furoi, A., Ikoma, A., Yamauchi, T., Taira, A.:** The development of a pyogenic liver abscess following radical resection of cholangiocellular carcinoma with ligation of the right hepatic artery: report of a case. Jpn. J. Surg. 1994; 24: 659–662
91. **Tavarela Veloso, F., Araujo Teixeira, A., Saraiva, C., Carvalho, J., Maia, J., Fraga, J.:** Hepatic abscess in Crohn's disease. Hepato-Gastroenterol. 1990; 37: 215–216
92. **Tay, K.H., Ravintharan, T., Hoe, M.N.Y., Sec, A.C.H., Chng, H.C.:** Laparoscopic drainage of liver abscesses. Brit. J. Surg. 1998; 85: 330–332
93. **Teitz, S., Guidetti-Sharon, A., Manor, H.:** Pyogenic liver abscess: warning indicator of silent colonic cancer. Dis. Colon Rectum 1995; 38: 1220–1223
94. **Vadillo, M., Corbella, X., Pac, V., Fernandez-Viladrich, P., Pujol, R.:** Multiple liver abscesses due to Yersinia enterocolitica discloses primary hemochromatosis: three case reports and review. Clin. Infect. Dis. 1994; 18: 938–941
95. **Vakil, N., Hayne, G., Sharma, A., Hardy, D.J., Slutsky, A.:** Liver abscess in Crohn's disease. Amer. J. Gastroenterol. 1994; 89: 1090–1095
96. **Vaquero Gajate, G.J., Costo Campoamor, A., Santos Santos, J.M., del Amo Olea, E., Murillo Diez, J.:** Absceso hepatico brucelar: presentacion de un caso y revision de la literatura. Rev. Esp. Enf. Ap. Digest. 1989; 76: 409–412
97. **Vatcharapreechasakul, T., Suputtamongkol, Y., Dance, D.A.B., Chaowagul, W., White, N.J.:** Pseudomonas pseudomallei liver abscesses: a clinical, laboratory, and ultrasonographic study. Clin. Inf. Dis. 1992; 14: 412–417
98. **Verbanck, J., Ponette, J., Verbanck, M., Vandewiele, I., Segaert, M.:** Sonographic detection of multiple staphylococcus aureus hepatic microabscesses mimicking candida abscesses. J. Clin. Ultrasound 1999; 27: 478–481
99. **Wallack, M.K, Brown, A.S., Austrian, R., Fitts, W.jr.:** Pyogenic liver abscess secondary to asymptomatic sigmoid diverticulitis. Ann. Surg. 1976; 184: 241–243
100. **Wong, K.-P.:** Percutaneous drainage of pyogenic liver abscesses. World J. Surg. 1990; 14: 492–497
101. **Wong, W.M., Wong, B.C.Y., Hui, C.K., Ng, M., Lai, K.C., Two, W.K., Lam, S.K., Lai, C.L.:** Pyogenic liver abscess: Retrospective analysis of 80 cases over a 10-year period. J. Gastroenterol. Hepatol. 2002; 17: 1001–1007
102. **Yeh, T.-S., Jan, Y.-Y., Jeng, L.-B., Hwang, T.-L., Chao, T.-C., Chien, R.-N., Chen, M.-F.:** Pyogenic liver abscesses in patients with malignant disease. A report of 52 cases treated at a single institution. Arch. Surg. 1998; 133: 242–245
103. **Yu, S.C., Ho, S.S., Lau, W.Y., Yeung, D.T., Yuen, E.H., Lee, P.S., Metreweli, C.:** Treatment of pyogenic liver abscess: prospective randomized comparison of catheter drainage and needle aspiration. Hepatology 2004; 39: 932–938
104. **Zighelboim, J., Williams, T.W.jr., Bradshaw, M.W., Harris, R.L.:** Successful medical management of a patient with multiple hepatic abscesses due to Edwardsiella tarda. Clin. Inf. Dis. 1992; 14: 117–120

Clinical Aspects of Liver Diseases
28 Alcohol-induced liver damage

		Page:			Page:
1	*The "alcohol" factor*	532	4.6	Chemical additives in alcoholic drinks	542
1.1	Use of alcohol	532	4.7	Coexistent hepatotoxic agents	543
1.2	Abuse of alcohol	532	4.8	Malnutrition and undernourishment	543
1.3	Addiction to alcohol	533	5	*Clinical features of alcoholic liver damage*	543
1.4	Alcohol as a cause of disease	533	5.1	Types of disease	543
1.5	Costs for the economy	533	5.1.1	Alcoholic fatty liver	543
2	*Biochemical effects of alcohol*	534	5.1.2	Alcoholic hepatitis	544
2.1	Alcoholic hypoglycaemia	534	5.1.3	Alcoholic cirrhosis	546
2.2	Alcoholic hyperglycaemia	534	6	*Complications*	547
2.3	Alcoholic hyperlipidaemia	534	6.1	Alcoholic ketoacidosis	547
2.4	Alcoholic hyperuricaemia	535	6.2	Zieve's syndrome	547
2.5	Alcoholic porphyria	535	6.3	Cholestasis	547
2.6	Haematological disturbances	535	6.4	Fat embolism	547
2.7	Formation of addictive substances	536	6.5	Portal hypertension	547
2.8	Effects of disulfiram	536	6.6	Primary liver cell carcinoma	548
2.9	Alcohol-related interactions	536	7	*Diagnostic alcohol markers*	548
2.10	Lipid peroxidation	537	7.1	Questionnaire	548
2.11	Immune reactions	537	7.2	Laboratory findings as markers	548
3	*Morphological effects of alcohol*	537	8	*Prognosis*	550
3.1	Adaptation	537	9	*Therapy*	550
3.2	Types of damage	537	9.1	Alcohol abstinence	550
3.3	Steatosis hepatis and fatty liver	539	9.2	Nutrition	550
3.4	Hepatic fibrosis	540	9.3	Substitution	550
3.5	Liver cirrhosis	541	9.4	Physical exercise	551
4	*Pathogenesis*	541	9.5	Drug therapy	551
4.1	Genetic predisposition	542	9.6	Liver support system	552
4.2	Gender	542	9.7	Liver transplantation	552
4.3	Age	542	•	References (1–151)	552
4.4	Previous liver damage	542		(Figures 28.1–28.19; tables 28.1–28.7)	
4.5	Alcohol consumption	542			

28 Alcohol-induced liver damage

1 The "alcohol" factor

1.1 Use of alcohol

We do not know when and where drinkable grape juice was originally pressed from wild vines, nor when and where wine was produced and enjoyed for the first time following fermentation and purification. • The oldest find is probably a grape squeezer containing grape seeds found in the region south of Damascus, dating back to the time around 6000 BC. • Wine consumption and drunkenness are described in the EPIC OF GILGAMESH, which goes back to 4000–3000 BC. God told Noah, who is called Utnapishtim in the epic, to grow grapevines following the Flood (around 4000 BC). This he did: *"And he drank of the wine, and was drunken"* (Genesis, 9.21). • About 2700 BC, Chinese writings mention the benefits as well as the dangers of consuming wine. • Many descriptions pertaining to the consumption of wine (and also beer) as well as to drunkenness can be found in the rock tombs at El Kab in Upper Egypt (around 2500 BC), in the EBER'S Papyrus (around 1550 BC) and in various other discoveries. • A Babylonian clay tablet from the year 2230 BC shows a prescription written by a Sumerian physician regarding the use of wine for medical purposes. The TALMUD defines the correct way to drink wine and praises its medical applications. However, in the Old Testament, (ISAIAH, 5.11) expresses his anger saying: *"Woe unto them that rise up early in the morning, that they may follow strong drink; that continue until night, till wine inflame them!"* HOMER was aware of the early onset of drunkenness due to a rapid intake of alcohol and complained: *"Often times did you wet my garment, infront, at my bosom, spilling wine from your mouth, in clumsy childishness"* (s. p. 64), *"The wine must have been doing you a mischief, as it does with all those who drink immoderately"* (Odyssey, 21.293). OVID also admonished: *"When drinking, I will set you a limit: Head and feet must never fail."* The wild drunken orgies of the unleashed bacchantes, priestesses of Dionysus, were dreaded events. PLUTARCH, however, wrote on the moderate consumption of wine: *"The most exquisite amongst all beverages, the most pleasant amongst all foodstuffs, the most appetizing amongst all remedies."* • In the 11th century, pure alcohol was made from strong old wine for the first time in Southern Italy. From ca. 1250, this new substance was offered in Italian chemist's shops as a panacea and acclaimed as **aqua vitae** ("water of life"), aqua ardens ("burning water"), spiritus vini ("spirit of wine") or quinta essentia ("fifth essence" = filling the space between the cosmic bodies). The term **"alcohol"** was most probably introduced by PARACELSUS about 1530, from the Arabic word al-kuhl, meaning "the finest part of something".

As far as is known, the time around 6000 BC marks the beginning of a development in which man became more and more familiar with the manifold **use and effect** of wine or other alcoholic beverages, e.g. as roborant, tonic, sedative, narcotic, appetizer, aphrodisiac, disinfectant or an externally applied antiphlogistic. Apart from that, alcohol was an essential part of festive banquets or religious rituals, but was also identified as a cause of drunkenness, physical dysfunction, disease and liver damage when consumed to excess.

1.2 Abuse of alcohol

▶ Alcohol abuse is defined as overindulgence, i.e. **abnormal** or **pathological drinking behaviour** (according to quantity and modality). However, there are no generally accepted threshold values regarding this definition, since intake and metabolism of alcohol are influenced by many factors varying from individual to individual. Apart from that, alcohol metabolism and tolerance mainly depend on whether the intake is a *singular, intermittent* or *continuous event*. (s. p. 65) **Lethal alcohol poisoning** generally occurs at blood alcohol concentrations ranging between 3.1 and 5.6‰ (2.0–3.5 g/kg BW). (84) However, there have been reports of isolated cases in which considerably higher concentrations did not lead to death. In this context, reduced tolerance (e.g. caused by coexistent hepatic disease, organopathies, hypothermia, age, drinking speed, drinking habits and type of drink) plays an important role. (4) (s. p. 65) • Excessive alcohol intake to the point of abuse (with the alcohol dose varying from person to person) is characterized by the occurrence of **somatic damage.** • Alcohol abuse bears a certain relationship to the average intake per capita (in litres). In Germany, **annual consumption** increased from 3.1 l (1950) to 12.5 l (1980) and has remained at a level of about 12.0 l ever since. These statistics, however, do not take into account the large amounts of home-made cider or spirits, which cannot be recorded. Other countries, such as Denmark, Spain, Italy, France and Portugal, also sadly feature in this "top group" with 12–13 l per capita and year. At 7–8 l, consumption is, however, considerably lower in the Netherlands and the U.K., and lowest of all in Norway at 4 l. Worldwide, alcohol consumption has almost tripled since 1970. (67) • Alcohol abuse is found in **all social strata,** with people drinking at social occasions and parties, due to worry or poverty, when doing business and because of stress as well as success. • *Any of the above mentioned circumstances can easily pave the way to abuse.* (s. tab. 28.1)

1.3 Addiction to alcohol

▶ A kind of (low-dose) dependence may also develop when alcohol is consumed daily, albeit in minor quantities. *As a rule of thumb, alcohol always makes people dependent when consumed on a regular basis − no matter what the dose may be.* • Alcohol addiction comprises (*1.*) **physical dependence** including increased tolerance as well as the withdrawal syndrome and (*2.*) **psychological dependence** with an uncontrollable desire for permanent or intermittent alcohol consumption, reduced self-control as well as changes in behaviour. (s. tab. 28.1) Alcohol abuse includes addiction without actually being identical to it. • Neither the **brain's reward system** (A. HERZ et al., 1989) nor the **addiction memory** (J. BÖNING, 1992) are stimulated by *occasional alcohol consumption*. Another explanation for this phenomenon could be that there are no alcohol-specific receptors in the brain and that the effects of alcohol are initiated "on loan" mainly via the GABAergic and glutamergic systems.

Alpha alcoholism
− Conflict- or relief-related drinking, no loss of control
− Certain degree of psychological dependence

Beta alcoholism
− Periodic and occasional drinking
− No psychological dependence

Gamma alcoholism
− Drinking in association with psychological dependence, including loss of control
− Later also signs of physical dependence

Delta alcoholism
− Habitual drinker (continued drinking: with abstinence of more than 24 hours being impossible), no loss of control
− Physical dependence

Epsilon alcoholism
− Episodic excessive heavy drinking with respective episodic loss of control *("quarterly drinker")*

Tab. 28.1: Types of alcoholism (E. M. JELLINEK)

The term **alcoholism** (M. HUSS, 1852) should only be used when there are signs of dependence. In Germany, the concept of alcoholism as a disease (C. TROTTER, 1780; E. M. JELLINEK, 1960) was given official recognition as early as 1968.

1.4 Alcohol as a cause of disease

▶ An individual's **susceptibility to disease** and the average **duration of disease** are greatly increased by alcohol abuse. • A central feature here is alcohol-induced *liver damage*. • In the area of the *upper intestinal tract*, alcohol abuse is assumed to have various sequelae: stomatitis, carcinoma of the oral cavity and oesophagus, parotitis, reflux oesophagitis and gastritis. *Pancreatic diseases* occur about 20 times more often in alcoholics than in the rest of the population. In 30−50% of chronic alcoholics, *dilatative cardiomyopathy* is observed. In addition, *essential hypertension* and *cerebral infarct* seem to be associated with alcohol abuse. *Bronchopulmonary diseases* occur more frequently. In the course of chronic alcohol abuse, *cerebral damage*, psychic disorders and polyneuropathy appear. Any therapeutic approach is thus limited or proves unsuccessful, since alcoholics displaying such cerebral damage are no longer willing to understand their condition and take an active part in any treatment. Damage to the *immune system* is accompanied by endogenous immune deficiency. Alcoholism is often correlated with *malnutrition* or *undernourishment*. Moreover, *obesity, gout, latent or manifest diabetes, hyperlipidaemia, endocrinological disorders, myopathy* and *osteoporosis* may be anticipated. • Chronic alcohol abuse shortens **life expectancy** by 10 to 12 years, i.e. 9−12% in men and 13−15% in women, compared to the normal population. Every year, 30,000−40,000 people in Germany die due to **alcohol consumption.** These are grouped as follows: (*1.*) direct cause of death (acute alcohol poisoning, alcohol withdrawal syndrome (M. VICTOR et al., 1953), (*2.*) typical fatal sequelae (hepatic, pancreatic, and heart diseases), (*3.*) frequently fatal sequelae (hypertension, cerebral complications, pneumonia, hypoglycaemia, carcinoma, tuberculosis), and (*4.*) fatal incidents (accidents, suicide). (67)

1.5 Costs for the economy

It is impossible to approximate the economic and social costs arising from alcohol abuse, as these are said to be "inestimable" or "enormous." They may, however, be grouped in (*1.*) quantifiable, material costs and (*2.*) nonquantifiable, non-material costs, which vary in form and degree in the individual case. • **Quantifiable costs** comprise (*1.*) *social costs* pertaining to disease and therapy (i.e. about 10−11 million days of hospitalization/year, with each fourth to fifth bed occupied due to alcohol sequelae), rehabilitation measures, costs associated with loss of working hours including any additional costs (e. g. about 25% of wages), 3.5 times as many industrial accidents, about 16 times higher absentee rate, causing losses to employers of ca. 1.6 billion US dollars, costs due to accidents (workplace, traffic, leisure time, skiing, fights, etc.), costs arising from an increase in criminal offences (estimated figure 30−50%), legal costs, general living costs, administrative expenses and (*2.*) *private costs* pertaining to individual persons and/or their family.

Today, there are an estimated 2.5 million alcoholics in Germany − while some 4 million people are believed to be suffering extensively from the consequences of alcohol abuse, and about 10 million more are thought to be at risk. Each alcoholic is legally entitled to rehabilitation measures. However, no more than 30,000 people are treated as inpatients per year; for this small figure alone, the costs already amount to ca. 250 million US dollars. If the claims for inpatient rehabilitation measures were calculated for the total number of 2 million alcoholics (assuming this was at all possible in terms of bed and personnel capacity), the costs would amount to ca. 22.5 billion US dollars − a sum that would overtax any state or society. In the outpatient sector, costs are estimated at ca. 1,000 US dollars annually for each alcoholic. A person retiring early at the age of 45 due to alcoholism costs the state ca. 200,000 US dollars. The total average costs for an alcoholic amount to ca. 30,000 US dollars per year. In the time from early invalidity retirement to a usually premature death, the overall costs for the 2 million alcoholics amount to ca. 400 billion US dollars. All in all, the aggregate quantifiable material costs arising from alcoholism and alcohol abuse range between 24—26 billion US dollars per year, including all measures for inpatient treatment. (67) • In Germany, ca. 17.5 billion US dollars are spent annually on alcoholic drinks. This results in approx. 4 billion US dollars revenue from taxation.

Realistic prevention programmes have been repeatedly suggested from all sides. Apart from that, recommendations have also been made on how to cope (at least partially) with the enormous secondary costs caused by alcoholism, such as appropriating the tax revenue from alcohol sales with a simultaneous increase in duty on alcohol, particularly wine and beer, as well as introducing a law requiring the (considerable!) private production of alcohol to be declared. (67) • *All the above mentioned figures for Germany apply equally to most other comparable societies.*

▶ Although alcohol is considered to be the **number one civilisation drug,** it is also an integral part of human existence, unless its use is prohibited by strict religious laws or a fundamental attitude to life. A moderate and careful approach towards alcohol is thus called for. • As a **rule of thumb** for the use of alcohol, one could say: *"Drink moderately, but not on a daily basis."* During abstinence, the liver enjoys the possibility of full recovery; daily alcohol intake inhibits protein synthesis in the liver cells as well as cell recovery. Furthermore, any risk of addiction is avoided if alcohol is only consumed in an irregular manner, i.e. **interposed days of abstention.**

2 Biochemical effects of alcohol

As soon as alcohol reaches the liver cells, alcohol catabolism is initiated immediately and swiftly. Some 90% of the alcohol are metabolized by **ADH** and **MEOS,** whereby the intermediary metabolism of the liver cell is changed markedly. This is true for both the cytosolic and mitochondrial redox systems. • Alcohol breakdown via the MEOS involves the consumption of oxygen and NADPH. In contrast, its catabolism by ADH results in the production of NADH and formation of ATP, which, because of the rise in the **NADH/NAD ratio,** affects numerous redox reactions in the liver cell. Of special importance in this context is a reduced activity of the citric acid cycle as well as of both pyruvate and fatty acid oxidation. • Some 75% (up to 85%) of the oxygen intake into the liver cell are used for alcohol oxidation, i.e. the cellular metabolic reactions which depend on sufficient O_2 supply are compromised during alcohol catabolism by **cellular hypoxia,** particularly in the perivenous areas. If this process is a singular one, of short duration or intermittent, the hepatocellular reactions will quickly normalize. However, due to its high O_2 consumption, **continued alcohol catabolism** will result in all NAD-dependent redox systems being compromised, so that subsequent disorders in the liver cell metabolism can occur. (s. p. 66) • Research has shown that vitamins, hormones and trace elements play both a regulatory and a dysregulatory role in cellular metabolic processes in a far more varied manner than previously assumed. This may explain the persistent effects of alcohol-induced disturbances on numerous hepatocellular biochemical reactions with regard to the metabolic processes of vitamins, hormones and trace elements. (14, 17, 24, 36, 40, 54, 60, 70, 72, 76, 127, 138) *(see chapter 3.14)*

A rise in the NADH/NAD ratio and the associated increase in the redox potential as well as the formation of acetaldehyde result in a variety of **metabolic disturbances** in the hepatocellular oxidation processes, so that pathophysiological consequences are observed. • This large variety of alcohol-induced metabolic disturbances is responsible for many situations of clinical importance, and thus acute and chronic alcohol abuse will eventually result in additional **metabolic complications.** (s. tab. 28.2)

2.1 Alcoholic hypoglycaemia

In 10—20% of cases, hypoglycaemia is the cause of sudden, unexpected death following alcohol intoxication. When the person has been fasting before alcohol intake, the mortality rate is significantly higher. • Careful **monitoring of the blood sugar values** in patients with alcohol intoxication is required in order to treat them in time with i.v. glucose infusions. (s. tab. 28.2)

2.2 Alcoholic hyperglycaemia

In patients with a normal nutritional status, alcohol often results in hyperglycaemia. Apart from an alcohol-induced increase in catecholamines and cortisol (or ACTH), the reason for this also seems to be a reduced sensitivity of insulin receptors (e.g. due to zinc deficiency) (s. p. 55) and/or a lower glucose tolerance factor. (s. p. 56) (s. tab. 28.2)

2.3 Alcoholic hyperlipidaemia

Hypertriglyceridaemia is predominant in about 80% of all cases, whereby this condition is aggravated and potentiated by the simultaneous intake of dietary fat. • **Beware of the often recommended postprandial "small brandy" allegedly for better digestion after a fatty meal!** • The various metabolic disturbances (s. tab. 28.2, no. 13) ultimately lead to alcoholic fatty liver. • Alcohol-induced hyperlipidaemia and fatty liver thus have **four causes:** (*1.*) increased lipid transport due to nutrition and lipolysis, (*2.*) hypertriglyceridaemia, (*3.*) reduction in fatty acid oxidation, and (*4.*) limited removal of fat from the liver cell. (24) (s. tab. 28.2)

1. **Disturbances in hormone metabolism** (s. p. 49)
   - Hypogonadism
     (gonadotropins ↓, testosterone ↓, oestrogen ↑, zinc ↓)
   - Disturbance in T_3-T_4 conversion, TSH ↓
     5-deiodase ↓ (hyperthyroid state of liver)
   - ACTH ↑, cortisol ↑
   - Renin ↑, aldosterone ↑
   - Catecholamines ↑
2. **Disturbances in vitamin metabolism** (s. p. 51)
   - Folic acid, B_1, B_2, B_6, B_{12}, C ↓
   - A, D, E, K, F ↓
   - Conversion disorders of retinol
   - Occurrence of toxic retinol intermediary products
3. **Disturbances in trace elements** (s. p. 53)
   - Zinc, selenium, copper ↓
   - Manganese ↓ (later, manganese ↑)
4. **Loss of electrolytes**
   - Potassium ↓, magnesium ↓
5. **Disturbances in cellular energy metabolism** (s. p. 48)
   - Hyperthyroid state of hepatocytes (see above)
   - Uncoupling of the respiratory chain due to stimulation of the sodium/potassium ATPase
   - Microsomal hypermetabolism
     (O_2 consumption ↑, basal metabolism ↑, thermogenesis ↑)
6. **Increase in lipid peroxidation** (s. p. 73)
   - Glutathione ↓
   - Zinc, selenium, transferrin, ceruloplasmine/copper, cysteine, methionine, vitamins C, A, E ↓
   - Malondialdehyde equivalents ↑
7. **Alcoholic sympatheticotonia**
   - Catecholamines ↑
     (lipolysis ↑, glycogenolysis ↑, vascular reactions ↑)
8. **Alcoholic hypoglycaemia**
   - Glycogen reserves in liver cells ↓ (s. p. 45)
   - Gluconeogenesis ↓ (s. p. 45)
     (inhibition of the citric acid cycle with a decrease in oxalacetate, alanine deficiency)
9. **Alcoholic hyperglycaemia**
   - Release of catecholamine ↑
   - Release of cortisol ↑
   - Inadequate insulin secretion
10. **Alcoholic hyperuricaemia**
    - Breakdown of purine nucleotides ↑
    - Acidosis/ketoacidosis
11. **Inhibition of pyruvate oxidation**
    - Hyperlactataemia → acidosis
    - Fatty acid synthesis ↓
12. **Increase in ketogenesis** (s. p. 46)
    - Ketoacidosis
13. **Disturbances in lipid metabolism** (s. p. 46)
    - Sympathicotonic lipolysis ↑ →, fatty acids ↑
    - VLDL production ↑ →, triglycerides ↑
      (pre-β-lipoproteins ↓)
    - α-glycerophosphate ↑ →, triglycerides ↑
    - LCAT activity ↓ →, cholesterol ↑
    - Pyruvate ↓ →, fatty acid synthesis ↑
    - Cholinphospholipids ↓
    - Fatty acid oxidation ↓
14. **Disturbances in collagen metabolism**
    - Acetaldehyde ↑ →, collagen synthesis ↑
    - Proliferation of myoblasts, fibromyoblasts, monocytes, lymphocytes ↑ →, collagen synthesis ↑
    - Hyperlactataemia →, collagen synthesis ↑
    - Proline oxidase ↓ →, proline ↑
    - Collagenase ↓ →, collagen degradation ↓
15. **Disturbances in amino acid metabolism** (s. p. 42)
    - Consumption of cysteine ↑
    - Consumption of methionine ↑ →, α-aminobutyrate ↑
    - Consumption of glutathione ↑
    - Glutamic acid ↑ →, α-aminobutyrate ↑
    - Glutamic acid ↑ →, proline synthesis ↑
    - Reduction in BCAA
16. **Disturbances in protein metabolism** (s. p. 44)
    - Albumin synthesis ↓
    - Carrier proteins ↓ (e.g. transferrin)
    - Protein accumulation in the liver ↑
17. **Disturbances in porphyrin metabolism** (s. p. 38)
    - δ-aminolaevulinic acid synthetase ↑
    - δ-aminolaevulinic acid dehydratase ↓
    - Coproporphyrinogen oxidase ↓
    - Ferrochelatase ↓
    - Uroporphyrinogen synthase ↑
    - Uroporphyrin decarboxilase ↓
18. **Disturbances in neurotransmitter metabolism**
    - Disturbances in decarboxylation of biogenic amines
19. **Formation of addictive substances**
    - Salsolinol, tetrahydropapaveroline, β-carbolines

Tab. 28.2: Significant alcohol-induced metabolic disturbances and changes in biochemical reactions in the liver

2.4 Alcoholic hyperuricaemia

A rise in uric acid values up to an acute gout attack can only be attributed to a minor extent to diminished uric acid excretion from the kidneys, since decreased uricosuria due to hyperlactacidaemia is not observed unless the lactate value is >2 mmol. Excessive production of uric acid due to increased catabolism of preformed purine nucleotides is seen as an essential cause. This is also supported by the observation that the purine nucleotide content in liver cells is reduced after prolonged alcohol consumption. (36) (s. tab. 28.2)

2.5 Alcoholic porphyria

Alcohol may cause hepatic porphyria. This is true of both porphyria cutanea tarda, including latent phases of chronic hepatic porphyria, and the acute form. Given a genetic predisposition, alcohol inhibits uroporphyrin decarboxylase and induces δ-aminolaevulinic acid synthetase. This causes a rise in uroporphyrinogen, which is discharged to a greater extent in the urine. Consequently, in cases of porphyria cutanea tarda, it is not only imperative to avoid sunlight, but also alcohol. (s. p. 36) (s. figs. 4.13; 7.10)

2.6 Haematological disturbances

Alcohol has a dose-related toxic effect on erythropoiesis. In this context, vacuolization of the nuclei and plasma of the proerythroblasts (= *McCurdy cells*) can mostly be observed. The mean corpuscular volume of erythrocytes (MCV) increases with rising alcohol consumption in 50–60% of patients, particularly when consuming high-proof alcoholic drinks. Megaloblastic anaemia may occur due to vitamin deficiency (folic acid, B_1, B_2, B_6, B_{12}). Haemolytic anaemia can be found with or without Zieve's syndrome. Sideroblastic anaemia may be present when the iron metabolism is disturbed (as happens in 30—40% of cases). In 15—20% of cases, thrombopenia may be seen, and in 10—20% leucopenia can arise. The reason for an additional dysfunction in the leucocytes seems to be an increase in intracellular cyclic adenosine monophosphate, since alcohol activates the membrane-bound adenyl cyclase. (s. tab. 28.2)

2.7 Formation of addictive substances

Acetaldehyde, which is about 15 times more toxic than alcohol, enters into so-called condensation reactions with endogenous biogenic amines to form **opioid peptides**: acetaldehyde together with dopamine leads to the formation of *salsolinol* as well as *tetrahydropapaveroline* and *β-carbolines*. The development of these (and similar) substances may explain why addiction results from alcohol abuse. • However, alcoholic drinks also contain **methanol** in different quantities, e.g. beer <7mg/l, whisky 100—300 mg/l, spirits made from fruit juice 1,000—5,000 mg/l. (!) Its metabolite is a toxic agent called formaldehyde. Methanol (or the toxic substance formaldehyde) probably plays a much more crucial role in the pathophysiology of alcoholic liver damage and in the development of alcoholism than does ethanol. Moreover, formaldehyde is considered a more suitable partner for the synthesis of habit-forming substances than acetaldehyde. (117, 129) Thus the (high or low) methanol content in alcoholic drinks might also be important in the development of liver damage or alcohol addiction of varying intensities (E. V. Dunn et al., 1985).

2.8 Effects of disulfiram

Competitive inhibitors of acetaldehyde dehydrogenase block the breakdown of acetaldehyde. Especially **disulfiram** acts as an inhibitor, which is why the simultaneous intake of alcohol and disulfiram leads to increased acetaldehyde levels in the blood. This results in a *flush syndrome*, including perspiration, tachycardia, nausea, vomiting and even severe circulatory failure. • **A similar effect to that of disulfiram** is achieved by *medicaments* such as chloramphenicol, metronidazole, tolbutamide, chlorpropamide, griseofulvin, tolazoline, nitrofurantoin and quinacrine. The simultaneous intake of alcohol and inhaled *nitrogen*, e.g. from fertilizers, which has a disulfiram-like effect, is also of toxicological relevance. The combination of alcohol and a mushroom called *Coprinus atramentarius* (which is usually well-tolerated) may also cause a severe reaction resembling that of disulfiram. Such effects result from contact with *chemical agents* at the workplace (e.g. carbon disulphide, calcium cyanamide, dimethylformamide, butylaldoxim).

2.9 Alcohol-related interactions

Interactions between alcohol and various xenobiotics, particularly medicaments, are of considerable clinical importance. However, this depends upon the question of whether alcohol consumption is acute or chronic and whether these interactions are caused by gastric or hepatic ADH, MEOS or aldehyde dehydrogenase. The causes of such interactions are manifold. (s. tab. 28.3) • Gastric **ADH**, for example, is inhibited by pyrazole, cimetidine and ranitidine (but not by omeprazole or famotidine), which results in an increase in the blood alcohol concentration. A gastric isoenzyme of ADH (δ-ADH) causes the detoxification of a procarcinogen called nitrobenzaldehyde, occasionally found in foodstuffs. Similar ADH isoenzymes, which are equally capable of detoxifying procarcinogens, are also found in the colonic and rectal mucosa. Moreover, ADH is inhibited by agents such as chloralhydrate and metamizole. (40, 123, 127) The **MEOS** depends on the cytochrome P 450 (2E1, 4A1). (34) • **Acute alcohol consumption** leads to an **inhibition** of microsomal metabolization and thus a prolongation of the half-life of xenobiotics, e.g. pentobarbital, lorazepam, tolbutamide, phenytoin, diazepam, warfarin, paracetamol, caffeine, methadone (considerable increase in concentration in the liver and brain!) as well as the procarcinogen dimethylnitrosamine. • **Chronic alcohol consumption** causes an **induction** of the alcohol-specific cytochrome P 450 (2E1, 4A1). Thus numerous xenobiotics or pharmacons are metabolized much more rapidly, i.e. their half-life is clearly shorter; this is especially true in situations where no alcohol is found in the organism at the time of drug intake. This rapid breakdown of medicinal preparations may either shorten the period of therapeutic effect or result in intermediary products of a higher or even toxic concentration (e.g. isoniazid, paracetamol, vinyl chloride, dimethylnitrosamine, carbon tetrachloride, acetone, cocaine, halothane and butanol). Usually, this (primarily) metabolic drug tolerance then leads to higher redosing due to diminished, or a lack of, therapeutic effects. This may result in the intermediary products being present in dangerously toxic quantities. The induction of the alcohol-specific cytochrome continues for several weeks, even if no more alcohol is consumed. Furthermore, the original situation is re-established as soon as alcohol is consumed again. • Inhibition of **ALDH** may also be caused by numerous xenobiotics, which is why a *disulfiram effect* (see above) may be expected. (44) (s. p. 68)

2.10 Lipid peroxidation

Molecular oxygen is not always completely reduced in the metabolism of xenobiotics, so that partially decreased oxygen intermediates may be formed, such as H_2O_2, O_2^- and OH^-. Due to its extreme chemical reactivity, OH^- can attack every macromolecule. (s. p. 73) Consumption of alcohol causes both enhanced formation of toxic oxygen intermediates catalyzed by iron and antioxidant deficiency (e.g. zinc, selenium, glutathione, cysteine, and vitamins A, C, E). This creates an oxidative stress situation for the liver cells, with damage to the biomembranes (s. p. 408) and stimulation of the collagen-gene expression (= alcoholic hepatic fibrosis). Furthermore, lipid peroxidations are responsible for the inactivation of enzymes and the oxidative modification of lipoproteins, proteins, free amino acids and nucleic acids. (51, 99, 138, 141) (s. fig. 21.12)

1. Effects on enteral resorption
2. Changes in gastric or intestinal mucosal metabolism
3. Additive or supra-additive effects on receptors
4. Effects on microsomal enzyme systems
5. Effects on non-microsomal cellular metabolic processes
6. Effects of disulfiram

Tab. 28.3: Causes of interaction between alcohol and xenobiotics, particularly medicinal preparations

2.11 Immune reactions

Immunologically, an alcoholic fatty liver is seen as indifferent, while pronounced alcohol-induced cirrhosis mainly shows hyporeactivity. By contrast, alcoholic hepatitis displays obvious immunological activity. It was possible to show the existence of lymphocytes with cytotoxic activity as well as antibodies against cytokeratin filaments, nucleic components and cell membranes. Sometimes, the **IgA value** in the serum is elevated and IgA deposits are observed along the sinusoids. The cell-mediated immunity may be impaired, so that intracutaneous tests and vaccinations (e.g. against HBV) show negative results (= alcohol-related non-responders). Following alcohol intake, endotoxins and other agents are also transported from the intestinal tract to the liver, which leads to the **release of cytokines** (e.g. interleukins, tumour necrosis factor), since endotoxins are potent cytokine stimulators. Among other things, cytokines are thought to cause the stimulation of fibrogenesis, just as they are held responsible for various clinical symptoms (e.g. fever, catabolism, hypermetabolism, hypoalbuminaemia). LSP and protein aldehyde adducts are seen as target antigens for the formation of antibodies. Verification of a **histon 2B antibody** (anti-H2B) is of particular clinical importance. (s. p. 127) (s. tabs. 5.19, 5.20; 32.1) • It is uncertain whether we are dealing with individual epiphenomena or whether these findings are of pathogenic relevance. (10, 59, 68, 142)

3 Morphological effects of alcohol

Both acute alcohol consumption (in high doses and with toxic effects) and chronic alcohol intake result in manifold biochemical changes to the liver metabolism, which can be of varying intensity in the individual case in line with the respective influencing factors. (s. tab. 28.2) • Apart from these alcohol-induced changes to the hepatic metabolism, morphological modifications can also be observed at the subcellular and cellular levels, depending on the quantity and duration of alcohol consumption. This leads to an aggravation of liver damage and ultimately to extensive transformation processes. Structural changes in the organelles can be seen as an expression of an adaptation process triggered by pronounced acute or chronic strain on liver cells, but they may also constitute alcohol-induced damage. (145)

> There is a fluid transition between adaptation and alteration, with complete reversibility being possible if the damage does not exceed a certain limit.

3.1 Adaptation

As far as laboratory findings are concerned, the adaptation of metabolically active cell organelles or microsomal enzyme systems is generally reflected by an increase in **γ-GT activity** following a certain period of alcohol intake. In this context, an increase in γ-GT alone is an adaptive, physiological phenomenon as well as a sign that γ-GT has been released from its membrane binding. (s. pp 58, 103)

Adaptation to an alcohol intake of sufficient duration and quantity becomes morphologically visible when **proliferation** of the smooth endoplasmic reticulum as well as the Golgi complex is observed. This kind of induction can, for a certain period of time, only be detected with the aid of an electron microscope, but subsequently becomes visible under a light microscope as well. (s. pp 400, 559) (s. fig. 21.2)

3.2 Types of damage

With dose- and time-dependent alcohol intake, signs of morphological damage are found in important cellular components, irrespective of the catabolic path of the alcohol, when (*1.*) the cholesterol content of biomembranes increases, which leads to a rise in membrane fluidity and permeability, (*2.*) storage of lipids and proteins in the cytosol causes an enlargement of liver cells, (*3.*) mitochondria show a swelling and structural change in their cristae, (*4.*) the Golgi complex undergoes hyperplasia, (*5.*) ribosomes are released and diminish in number, (*6.*) multivesicular lysosomes can be seen, and (*7.*) cytoskeletal structures are damaged. The morphological changes, which are mainly caused by hypoxia, usually originate in the lobular centre (zone 3), from where they gradually progress to the periphery. (5, 50, 55, 64, 100)

Changes in the phospholipid composition and metabolism of hepatic biomembranes are now seen as one of

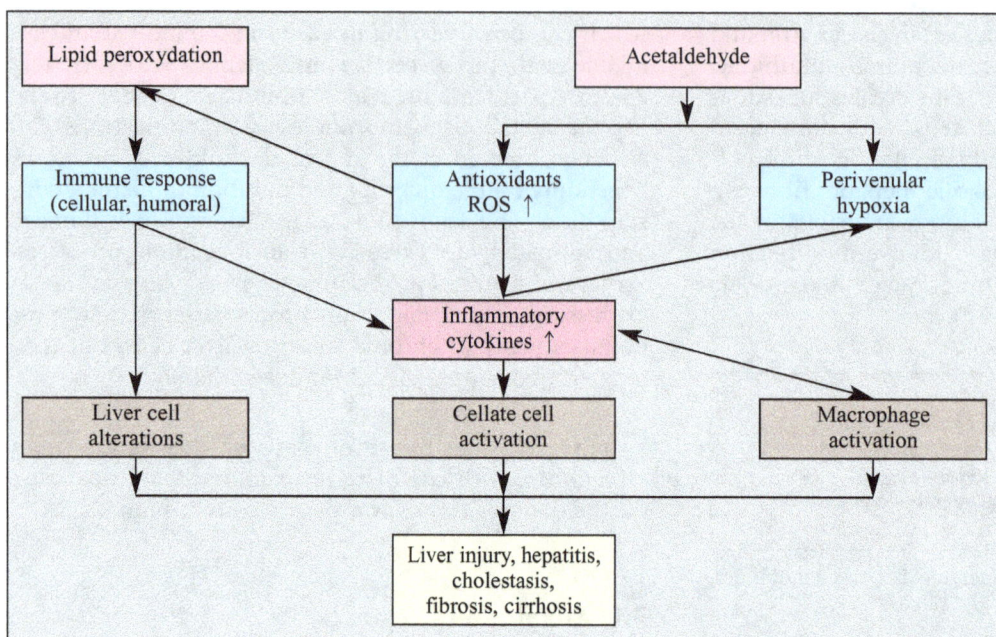

Fig. 28.1: Important alcohol-related effects via lipid peroxydation and acetaldehyde leading to the development of different forms of ALD

the most important mechanisms of alcoholic liver disease. This was recently confirmed by proton magnetic resonance spectroscopy (122)

An early (and specific) biochemical sign of hepatocellular damage is an increase in **GPT activity**. (86) It can be demonstrated once the damage rate is >1 g hepatocytes (>170 million liver cells). (s. p. 102) • In pronounced vitamin B_6 deficiency due to alcohol abuse, GPT formation may be inhibited, so that GPT activities appear misleadingly low.

Alcoholic hyalin: Alcoholic hyalin is seen as a characteristic maldevelopment in cellular protein synthesis and can be found in enlarged and bloated hepatocytes. Although these cells may recover, they are often subject to cytolysis and removed by leucocytes. Alcoholic hyalin, which contains a cellular stress protein called *ubiquitine*, is (more appropriately) referred to as a **Mallory-Denk body**, since it can also be found in liver diseases not related to alcohol. Mallory-Denk bodies present as string-like or lumpy, sometimes granular-branched, light-refracting and acidophilic structures, which take on a bright red colour when coming into contact with aniline blue or Masson stain. They consist of an abnormal accumulation of microfilaments. Ubiquitination of damaged intermediary filaments already occurs at an early stage of alcoholic hepatocellular damage before any Mallory-Denk bodies are observed. Thus, moderate and early forms of hepatocellular damage due to alcohol can be detected via *ubiquitin-specific antibodies* displaying high sensitivity and specificity (J. Lowe et al., 1988). (31) (s. p. 403!) (s. figs. 28.2, 28.3)

Granular swelling: Granular swelling is due to the swelling and multiplication of mitochondria as well as the formation of **giant mitochondria**. (s. fig. 28.4) (s. pp 401,

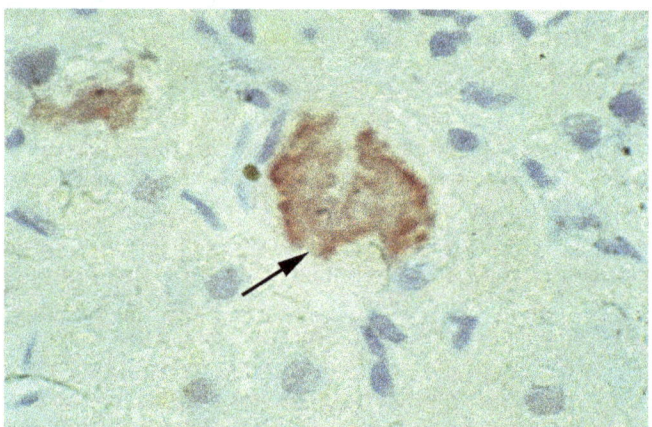

Fig. 28.2: Mallory-Denk bodies: immunohistochemical reaction with an antibody against ubiquitin (arrow)

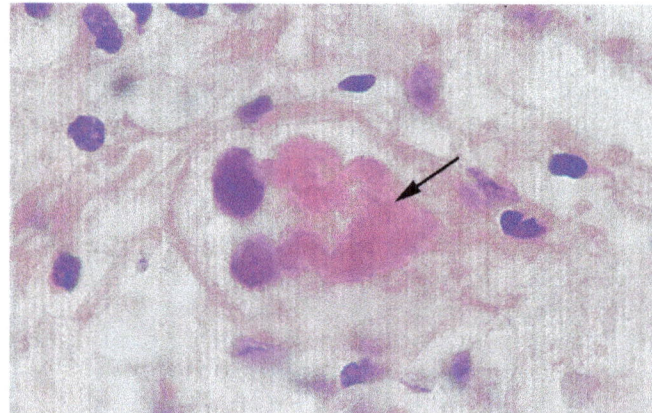

Fig. 28.3: Hydropic-degenerated hepatocyte with Mallory-Denk body (→) (HE)

559) These are eosinophilic, homogeneous, well-defined protein droplets of 10–20 μm in size within the cytoplasm of the mostly enlarged granular liver cells. (21)

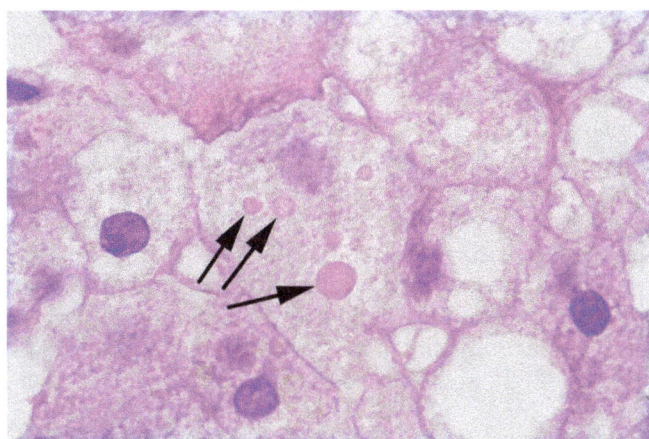

Fig. 28.4: Hepatocyte with megamitochondria (→) in alcoholic fatty liver (HE)

Liver cell hydrops: Liver cell hydrops is characterized by swollen hepatocytes, which contain a lot of liquid, but are mostly free of fat. Hydropic liver cells may be two to four and even ten times the size of normal hepatocytes. Cell hydrops is fully reversible when abstention is maintained. These cells usually die when alcohol intake is continued and are subsequently removed by macrophages and leucocytes. This leads to an alteration in the cytoskeleton. Hydropically degenerated liver cells and hyaline liberated from Mallory bodies produce a leucocytic inflammatory reaction. Unless it is compensated by regenerative processes, this cellular deficit results in defective healing by fine-fibred, cell-poor fibrils.

Protein storage: Protein storage in the cytoplasm of the liver cell is caused by antisecretory action, probably in the area of the microtubular system and the Golgi complex. This results in a **ballooning** of the hepatocytes. (s. p. 403) • Alcohol-induced *hepatomegaly* is therefore due to the concurrence of hepatocellular protein and lipid storage and liver cell hydropsy; this can indeed lead to a 50—100% weight increase (without cellular multiplication) of the liver, i.e. up to 3,000—4,000 g (or more). (s. fig. 28.6)

Single-cell necrosis: Single-cell necrosis (s. pp 407, 560) becomes manifest as the destruction of fatty liver cells and as hyaline necrosis. The latter is either drained haematogenically or removed by stellate cells, which may generate stellate cell nodules. When disposing of fatty liver cells, the stellate cells take in lipoid from the necrotic epithelium and become foam-like. This may result in the formation of **lipophagic granulomas.** (s. p. 405) However, leucocytes also participate, sometimes even exclusively, in the removal of fatty hepatocytes.

Cholestasis: Cholestasis is often identifiable by way of laboratory findings (*see chapter 13*) and becomes manifest in a pericanalicular arrangement of the rough endoplasmic reticulum. The final result is the impaired intracellular secretion of bile with yellowish guttate cell occlusions as well as excretory disorders with the formation of biliary casts. (100) (s. pp 402, 560) (s. figs. 13.2, 13.4; 28.17—28.19)

Siderosis: Siderosis, especially in the form of granular *stellate cell siderosis*, can often be observed in cases of alcohol abuse and is caused by enhanced phagocytosis of erythrocytes. For this reason, it is particularly prevalent in cases of Zieve's syndrome, which means that granular stellate cell siderosis may be a hint of past stages of this syndrome or of its "formes frustes". General activation of stellate cells does not fit into the histological picture of alcoholic liver damage.

Liver cell siderosis mainly becomes manifest in the periphery of the hepatic lobules and is most likely to appear due to both an increase in iron supply or resorption and parenchymal lesions. Iron overload with varying degrees of severity is often found in the liver and other organs during the end-stage of alcoholism, whereby HFE-1 is absent. (s. fig. 28.5)

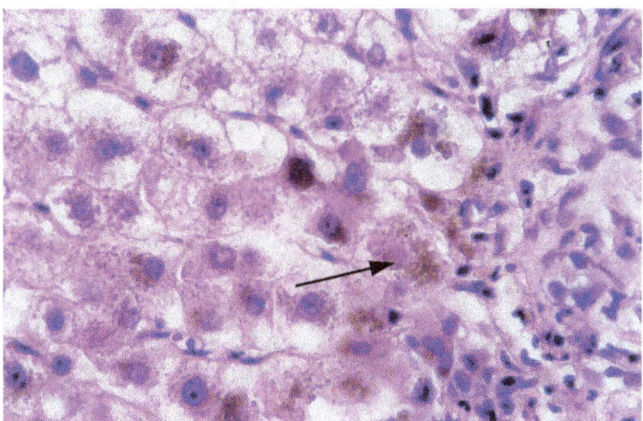

Fig. 28.5: Siderogranular deposits (↑) in hepatocytes (siderosis) in chronic alcohol abuse (HE)

3.3 Steatosis hepatis and fatty liver

Steatosis of hepatocytes is considered to be the most common form of alcohol-induced liver damage and constitutes a complex hepatocellular metabolic disorder. (s. tab. 28.2, no. 13) There is an imbalance between the storage of fat in the liver cell and its removal. (12, 29) (s. tab. 31.1) • **Peripheral** fatty changes in liver cells are mainly caused by infectious or toxic damage which directly and haematogenically affects the peripheral areas most involved in lipid metabolism. (s. fig. 31.4) • **Centroacinar** fatty changes in liver cells are mostly found in oxygen deficiency, nutritional damage, diabetes mellitus and alcohol abuse; in general, this is considered to be the more serious form of damage. (s. fig. 31.5) • **Zonal** fatty changes in liver cells occur when only certain areas of a lobule are affected. Finally, a **diffuse** fatty change of the whole lobule can be observed. (s. fig. 31.3)

A further increase in size of the stored lipid droplets will ultimately fill the liver cell completely, enlarge it and press the cytoplasm as well as the pitted nucleus towards the cell membrane. This impairs or even stops the division of the nucleus. At the same time, the liver cell undergoes glycogen depletion. Removal of the nucleic glycogen, so-called **glycogen vacuolation of the nuclei** develops (s. fig. 31.1). This may be present in various diseases, particularly in the area of the portal zones. The large-droplet fatty changes result in **fat cysts** of various sizes due to the cell membrane being torn. (s. fig. 31.2) • Fatty changes in liver cells constitute a **fatty liver** when *more than 50%* of the liver cells show the form of *medium* and *large fatty droplets*, and when *diffuse dissemination* occurs. (s. tab. 31.2) (s. fig. 31.3) A fatty liver may regress without any consequences. However, it may occur in an excessive form (up to 100% fatty liver cell changes have been observed) with a high fatality rate, e. g. in acute alcohol intoxication. (s. fig. 28.6)

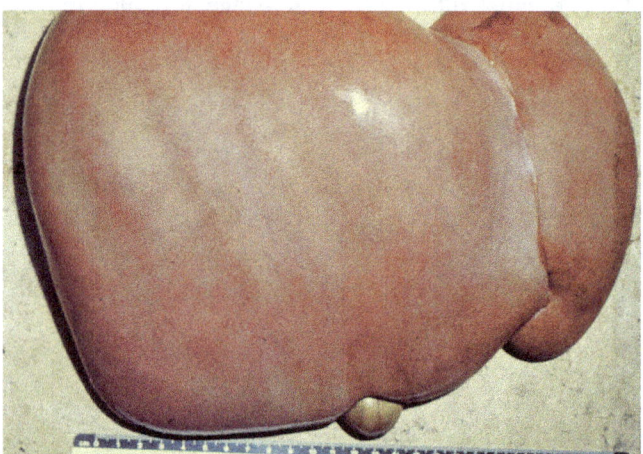

Fig. 28.6: Massive fatty liver (4,750 g hepatic wet weight) after acute alcohol intoxication ("brandy drinking bet"); exitus four days later

3.4 Hepatic fibrosis

Fibrogenesis, which occurs in the course of alcohol-induced toxic liver disease, is of decisive clinical and prognostic importance. The increase in fibres is not dependent on the degree and duration of the fatty changes. Hepatic fibrosis can be observed in some 40% of all patients suffering from a fatty liver. *Determination of P-III-P* and *apolipoprotein I* is a reliable **biochemical indicator** of progressive fibrosis. (77) (s. p. 410)

In alcohol-induced liver disease, fibre growth originates in the central veins. During this process, the delicate reticular fibres of collagen III are transformed into dense double-refracting collagen I. Elastic fibres are also found in increasing numbers. This **centrilobular perivenular fibrosis** (s. fig. 21.16) consists of a coat of collagenous fibres running mainly in a longitudinal direction around the central vein (H. A. EDMONDSON et al., 1967) and is a precursory stage of alcoholic liver cirrhosis (C. S. LIEBER, 1979). Collagenation of Disse's space occurs, mostly at the centre of the lobules, with the sinusoids being coated in a basal membrane-like manner and the sinusendothelium fenestration (= *capillarization of sinusoids*) being neutralized. (24, 55) (s. p. 413) This results in **perisinusoidal fibrosis.** (63, 83, 120, 146) • **Sclerosing hyaline fibrosis** can develop when larger centrilobular cell groups, which had been loaded with alcoholic hyalin, perish and are replaced by scarred, cell-poor, fine-fibred fibrils. In persistent alcohol abuse, such fibrosis may quickly lead to portal hypertension due to sinusoidal blockage. In most cases, it swiftly initiates transformation processes in the liver. (s. pp 255, 413) Peripheral sclerosis proceeds from the portal tracts and continues towards the centre as **periportal fibrosis** in a periacinar and intraacinar direction. (92) (s. figs. 21.14; 28.7) Hereby, single liver cells or small cell groups are drawn in from all sides and detached from their neighbouring structures. This spider-like fibrotic network continues to infiltrate the lobules until it connects with the central fibrosis, thus resulting in a picture which resembles so-called **chicken-wire fibrosis** (W. WEPLER et al., 1968). (s. figs. 21.15, 28.8) • It is via **proliferation of the ductules** that portal-periportal fibrosis assumes its characteristic features. Round-celled leucocytic infiltrates and periductular fibres may develop during this process, mimicking chronic cholangitis. • In up to 80% of patients suffering from hepatic fibrosis associated with a fatty liver, alcoholic hepatitis occurs if alcohol consumption is continued.

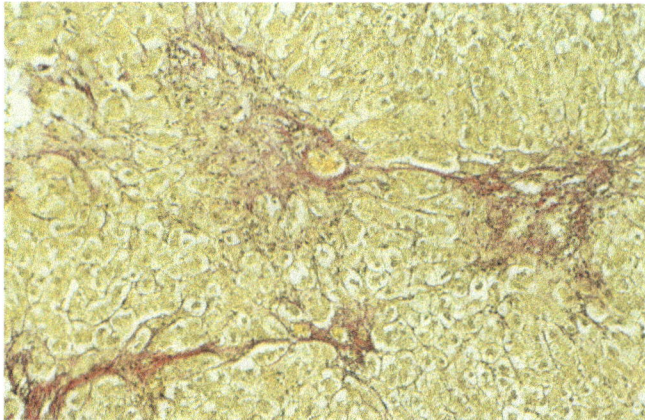

Fig. 28.7: Alcohol-induced periportal and centrilobular fibrosis, partially spider leg-like (Sirius red) (s. fig. 21.14)

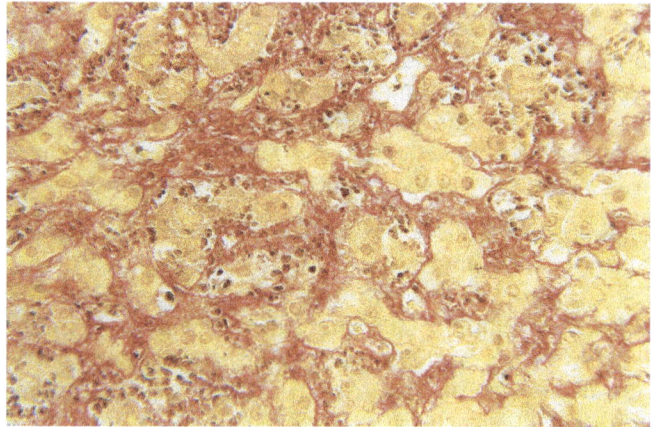

Fig. 28.8: Meshwire fibrosis in alcoholic steatohepatitis (Sirius red)

3.5 Liver cirrhosis

▶ *From a morphological perspective, alcohol-induced fatty liver or alcoholic hepatitis can always develop into cirrhosis.* • The fibrous ramifications of the various portal fields make contact with one another and with other centrilobular fibre formations. This ultimately causes pronounced fibrosis of the liver, which leads to a cirrhotic transformation if alcohol consumption continues. • In general, cirrhosis occurs as an insidious process characterized by permanent liver cell necrosis and fibrillogenetic stimulation. Pseudoacini and vascular shunts with impaired microcirculation develop, as do fibre paths, which show increasing signs of capillarization in the lobular structures. Finally, alcoholic cirrhosis presents as a uniform, micronodular condition. (s. fig. 28.9) • Histologically, it is often difficult to distinguish micronodular, postnecrotic alcoholic cirrhosis from posthepatitic/postnecrotic cirrhosis (although this is generally possible by laparoscopy). (s. figs. 28.10, 28.11) Alcoholic cirrhosis may even appear macroscopically as "smooth cirrhosis", which is rich in interstitial fibres, but has a poor capacity to regenerate. (s. fig. 14.3) (s. p. 415)

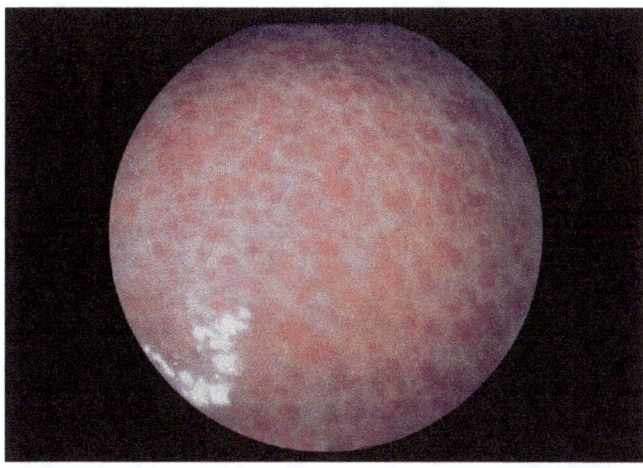

Fig. 28.11: Septate liver fibrosis without cirrhotic transformation in chronic alcohol abuse (misinterpreted, however, as cirrhosis in sonographic examination)

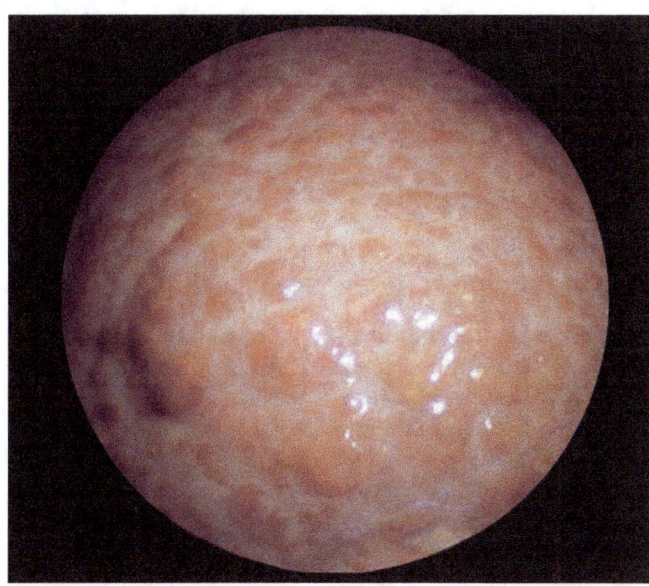

Fig. 28.9: Micronodular alcohol-induced liver cirrhosis

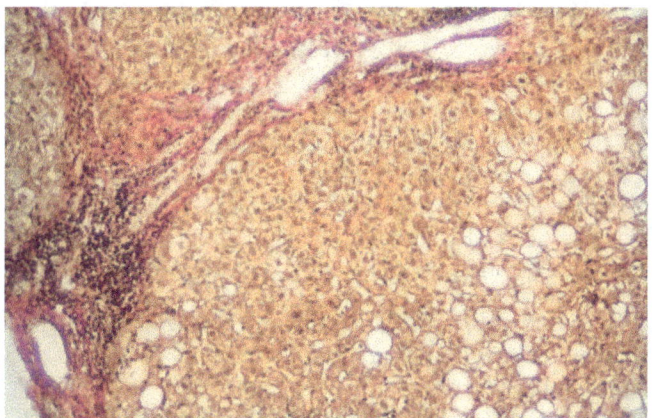

Fig. 28.10: Chronic moderate periportal and portal inflammatory reaction with septal fibrosis and centrilobular steatosis in chronic alcoholic liver damage (DD: mild chronic viral hepatitis C!) (van Gieson)

4 Pathogenesis

The various metabolic, morphological and clinical aspects of alcoholic liver disease can only be explained by the concurrence of a variety of exogenous and endogenous factors typical for the individual. Acetaldehyde, reactive O_2 species, free radicals and endotoxins are particularly important in *pathogenesis*. Consequently, there is evidence of GSH depletion, lipid peroxidation and antigen-antibody reactions. Alcohol consumption supports the growth of endotoxin-forming, gram-negative bacteria in the small intestine. The endotoxins stimulate especially the Kupffer cells, whereby principally cytokines (IL 1, 6 and 8, TNF_α) are produced. As a result, the microcirculation is impeded, T lymphocytes are stimulated and leucocytic inflammation can occur. Such pathogenesis is complex and differs in the individual case; this explains the various degrees of severity and the phenomenon of progession despite abstinence. (5, 39, 45, 48, 59, 61, 66, 74, 75, 107, 120, 141, 145, 147) (s. tab. 28.4)

Endogenous factors	
1. Genetic predisposition	4. Previous liver damage
2. Gender	5. Coexistent diseases
3. Age	6. Immunopathies
Exogenous factors	
1. Amount of alcohol intake per day	
2. Duration of alcohol consumption	
3. Continuity of alcohol consumption	
4. Chemical additives	
5. Coexistent hepatotoxic agents	
6. Malnutrition or undernourishment	

Tab. 28.4: Pathogenetic factors responsible for alcoholic liver disease

4.1 Genetic predisposition

Evidence of ethnic differences and family frequency, studies concerning twins and adopted children as well as animal experiments suggest a genetic disposition *towards* — as well as protection *against*! — alcoholism and a higher (or lower) incidence of alcoholic liver diseases. This is also seen in the different distribution of *ADH* and *ALDH* subtypes (e.g. ADH_2, ADH_3, $ALDH_2$) in various races and populations. • Even though findings concerning an *HLA association* have not yet been substantiated, the increases in frequency reported to date reveal interesting aspects, e.g. B8 (United Kingdom), BW40 (Scandinavia), B13 (Chile), B28 (Australia), A2, DR3 and DR2. • Apart from that, there is also genetic polymorphism of *cytochrome P450* (e.g. 2E1, 2D6, 4A1). (2, 8, 13, 32, 44, 79, 151) (s. pp 57, 67)

4.2 Gender

Liver disease progresses more rapidly in women, with the incidence of cirrhosis being two or three times higher than in men. Gender-specific differences in the gastric and hepatic alcohol metabolism are thought to be the factors responsible for this.

4.3 Age

ADH is not present before the age of three; alcohol should therefore not be given to infants. • With advancing age, the capacity to catabolize alcohol decreases, the prevalence of alcohol-induced liver and CNS disease rises, and blood alcohol concentrations are higher because the distribution volume is smaller in older people. Gastric δ-ADH diminishes in older men, so that there is no longer a difference between men and women in later life as far as gastric ADH is concerned. Moreover, the function of the smooth endoplasmic reticulum deteriorates with advancing age, a fact which is of particular importance when older people consume medicaments and alcohol at the same time! The decrease in the antioxidant glutathione in older people is also crucial. With advancing age, concentrations of the toxic agent acetaldehyde rise.

4.4 Previous liver damage

Previous liver damage resulting in limited hepatic function and/or accompanied by considerable loss of tissue affects hepatic alcohol catabolism in a negative way. **Coexistent diseases** may then prove to be extremely detrimental if they compromise the cellular reactions of alcohol catabolism. Generally, this applies to obesity, hyperlipidaemia, diabetes mellitus, gout, endocrinopathies, etc. **Immunopathies** may cause further immunological disturbances due to alcohol-induced immune responses. A striking feature in this context is the frequent presence of **HCV** antibodies as well as their close connection to portal and/or lobular inflammations. (16, 18, 38, 106, 118, 124, 136)

4.5 Alcohol consumption

The **daily quantity** of alcohol consumed is the decisive factor in the development of alcoholic liver disease. Following the intake of about 300 g alcohol, severe fatty infiltration of hepatocytes occurs within 2 to 4 days, whereas ingestion of 150 g alcohol leads to steatosis hepatis after about 21 days. • *The critical amount for the development of liver cirrhosis is a daily alcohol intake of >40 g for men and >20 g for women over a period of 5 years.* • Another important factor for alcohol-induced liver disease is the **duration of alcohol intake.** In this context, a single alcohol dose of >400 g, particularly as a result of *rapid drinking* ("drinking bet"!), will usually have fatal consequences. (s. fig. 28.4) The alcohol quantity and the duration of alcohol intake are thus closely related to the manifestation of liver damage. • The **regularity** of alcohol consumption is also important, namely whether alcohol consumption is continuous or irregular, i.e. three or four days of abstention between alcohol intake. During such abstention, the liver usually has enough time for metabolic and morphological restitution. With irregular ("sporadic") drinking, there is practically no chance for biochemical *addiction potential* to develop. (4, 12, 69, 101, 108)

> Single postprandial doses of 28 g or 71 g of alcohol resulted in blocked albumin synthesis or albumin and fibrinogen synthesis respectively. (143)

4.6 Chemical additives in alcoholic drinks

▶ Little is known about the content of additives in alcoholic beverages (either in *"standardized" industrial production* or in *"individual" home production*!) or their respective metabolism in the liver and potential toxicity. On the other hand, reliable information is available regarding the greatly varying amounts of **methanol** (ca. 5−5,000 mg/l!) and its metabolic effects (or those of its metabolite formaldehyde). The present level of knowledge regarding methanol is remarkable, but more research is required. (117, 129) (s. p. 536) • Apart from methanol, **butanol** and **propanol** or their derivatives are found in alcoholic beverages, likewise in varying quantities. Further chemical **constituents**, which are only mentioned in very general terms, include: fusel oil, ester, acids, aromatic compounds, essential oils, sulphur, phenols, histamine-like substances, artificial colouring, preservatives and so-called stabilizers − possibly also residues of insecticides. Moreover, too little is known about different components of wooden barrels in which various alcoholic beverages are stored for longer periods. • By contrast, certain additives (such as flavonoids) are thought to have an antioxidant effect.

> Considering our (still) insufficient knowledge of *chemical constituents* in individual alcoholic drinks, it is problematic *merely* to take the known ethanol content as a basic value for measurement and comparison or as a basic factor for prognosis. A critical approach is called for as long as the data are incomplete!

4.7 Coexistent hepatotoxic agents

It is with good reason that alcohol should be avoided when taking **medication** at the same time — however, this rule of thumb should always be complied with and not only heeded in specific cases or in advanced age. Predictions as to whether, when and what kind of biotoxometabolites will form due to biotransformatory interactions are difficult to make. (s. pp 59, 536) (s. fig. 3.11) With an estimated number of 400,000 to 500,000 persons addicted to pharmacons in Germany, this factor is of considerable importance in all statements concerning epidemiologic statistics. *(see chapter 29)* • **Chemical agents** encountered at work, at home, during leisure time and in connection with do-it-yourself activities may have a hepatotoxic effect and cause additive or even potentiated toxicity, given the individual peculiarities of ethanol metabolism. The most important reason for this development is alcohol-induced glutathione deficiency. *(see chapter 30)*

4.8 Malnutrition and undernourishment

Both malnutrition and undernourishment can be a cause or a result of alcoholic liver disease; indeed, the well-founded assumption of a vicious circle seems most likely. There is often evidence of secondary malnutrition due to alcohol-related disturbances affecting the intermediary metabolism. Malnutrition is brought about by the fact that each gram of alcohol supplies 7.1 kcal, so that the organism's basic need for calories can be satisfied predominantly by *"empty" alcohol calories*; on the other hand, alcohol-induced pancreatic insufficiency or damaged mucosa in the small intestine might result in maldigestion or malabsorption of various nutrients. Chronic alcoholics are able to satisfy more than half their daily calorie requirement with alcohol. A bottle of wine contains about 700 alcohol calories. Usually, a *deficiency in lipotropic substances* is observed (e. g. choline, methionine); therapeutic administration in cases of alcoholic liver disease has, however, proved unsuccessful. In addition, there is a deficiency in cysteine and glutathione, vitamins, electrolytes and trace elements. (s. tab. 28.2, nos. 2–4) • Alcohol causes a *deficiency in phospholipids* and *phosphatidylcholine* in the cellular biomembranes, particularly in the membrane of the mitochondria. (122) This can be corrected by substitution. Both substances also proved successful in preventing alcohol-induced fibroses. • *For this reason, "essential" phospholipids and S-adenosylmethionine can be used in therapy as "supernutrients".* (1, 61, 73–75, 95, 143)

Alcohol abuse may be considered as the biggest mass experiment for developing liver disease voluntarily carried out by mankind to date. About 50–60% of all liver diseases in Germany are caused by alcohol.

5 Clinical features of alcoholic liver damage

5.1 Types of disease

The total range of alcoholic liver diseases can be divided into three basic forms: (*1.*) fatty liver, (*2.*) alcoholic hepatitis, and (*3.*) cirrhosis. (7) With continued alcohol consumption, the forms may indeed develop in this given sequence; the transitions are smooth, and particular courses can be observed in individual cases. • Alcoholic fatty liver, for example, may regress completely or develop into fatty liver hepatitis, or it may take the form of liver fibrosis and remain in this state of partial recovery, or progress into cirrhosis if alcohol consumption is not brought to a halt. Any acute, severe alcohol intoxication will usually be fatal within a few (1–3) days. (84) (s. fig. 28.5) Acute alcoholic hepatitis is characterized by an upregulated inflammatory system. (97) It can turn (in about 40% of all cases) into a chronic form and finally into cirrhosis; in 10–20% of cases, it is accompanied by cholestasis and heals completely albeit with certain tissue defects (in about 50% of patients). Unfortunately, a lethal outcome must be anticipated in 10 to 15% of cases, and in fulminant courses even in about 90%. Occasionally, alcoholic hepatitis develops in addition to the existing alcoholic cirrhosis.

Exact differentiation is only possible morphologically. In this respect, the most reliable tool is laparoscopy, since a biopsy sample can only be taken from the strictly limited area of the right hepatic lobe using percutaneous biopsy. (s. fig. 7.8) *However, the biopsy specimen might not be sufficiently representative of the liver as a whole in advanced forms, e. g. chronic inflammation or fibrosis.* (s. fig. 28.10)

5.1.1 Alcoholic fatty liver

Fatty infiltrations of liver cells or fatty liver (s. pp 539, 595) are the most common morphological findings (up to 90% of all cases) in alcohol abuse. Both may develop within a short period of time (three or four weeks), but may also regress completely within a few weeks or months, depending on the degree of severity. (5, 12, 29, 33) • **Subjective complaints** are often absent, or there is unspecific or dyspeptic discomfort such as bloating, meteorism, flatulence, inappetence, fatigue, drop in performance, intolerance of food and drink, impotence and a sensation of pressure in the right upper abdomen (= hepatomegaly). These complaints are reported in 30–50% of cases. • **Clinical findings** are consistent with severity and duration. The most common symptom is *hepatomegaly* (60–80%) caused by infiltration of fat, water and protein as well as by proliferation of the SER. An enlarged liver has a blunt edge generally tender on pressure and weighs 2.0–2.5 kg or more. Liver weight can be as much as 6 kg. The various skin stigmata of liver diseases (s. pp 83–91) are observed with varying frequency (10–30%). Jaundice or scleral icterus are rare. • **Laboratory parameters** generally show an increase in γ-GT and CRP as well as, in more severe cases, an elevation of cholinesterase (60–70%). The transaminases are slightly elevated and GPT synthesis is often reduced owing to alcohol-induced B_6 deficiency, while the alcohol-induced release of GOT from the extrahepatic tissues is enhanced, with the result that GOT activity is occasionally higher than that of GPT. In several cases, GDH is likewise moderately elevated. An increase in alkaline phosphatase is a sign of a cholestatic form. Impaired liver function can easily be determined, particularly by means of i.v. galactose elimination capacity and the indocyanine green test. • **Sonography** shows a typical "large, white liver" with diffusely pronounced echogenicity; single reflexes are coarsened, and sound transmission is reduced. By contrast, milder forms of fatty infiltration of liver cells are not, or only unreliably, identifiable. • The degree of steatosis hepatis can only be demonstrated by **histology.** (s. figs. 31.1–31.5) In this way, it is also possible to detect inflammatory reactions and activities resulting in fibrosis, both of which are relevant for prognosis. In steatosis hepatis, the result of percutaneous biopsy is considered representative of the liver as a whole. • **CT** shows a reduction in density in relation to the degree of severity of the fatty liver. The vessels and bile ducts appear "brighter" (so-called reversal of contrast). (s. p. 180) More pronounced regional or segmental areas of fatty infiltration can be detected in individual cases. (s. figs. 8.2–8.4)

Pseudotumoural areas are often found in alcoholic liver disease, mainly in heavy drinkers. Multiple hypervascular nodules are visible in CT. (25) Sometimes they also appear in ultrasound in the form of ring-shaped foci (similar to those seen in porphyria cutanea tarda) (s. fig. 31.21)

Alcoholic foamy degeneration is seen as a variant of alcoholic fatty liver (T. UCHIDA et al., 1983). There is evidence of microvesicular steatosis, giant mitochondria, focal cell necrosis (with elevation of GPT, GOT and GDH) and cholestasis (with increase of AP and sometimes of bilirubin), whereas inflammatory alterations are rare and Mallory-Denk bodies totally absent. Likewise, there is no sign of fever or leucocytosis. (135)

5.1.2 Alcoholic hepatitis

Morphologically, this form is characterized by fatty infiltration (especially perivenular), liver cell damage to the point of necrosis, presence of inflammatory reactions with polymorphonuclear leucocytes (occasionally also macrophages and lymphocytes) as well as formation of fibrosis (perivenular and pericellular). (s. figs. 21.15, 21.16) The hepatocytes are swollen (= ballooned degeneration). Mallory-Denk bodies (s. figs. 28.2, 28.3) and giant mitochondria (s. fig. 28.4) can be found. There is proliferation of the bile ducts. Kupffer cells are activated. The cytokeratic skeleton of hepatocytes is damaged or destroyed. (120) (s. fig. 28.12)

Laparoscopy shows a brick-red liver surface, reticulated fibrosis, enhanced vascularization of the capsule with perivascular fibrosis, reddish speckles and an irregular liver surface with scattered light reflection. (s. fig. 28.13) • The **clinical spectrum** of alcoholic hepatitis covers various forms: (*1.*) asymptomatic, (*2.*) chronic persistent, (*3.*) chronic aggressive, and (*4.*) fulminant. These forms include anicteric, icteric and cholestatic courses. • A variant of alcoholic hepatitis is **alcoholic steatohepatitis** with fat deposition in the hepatocytes and inflammatory changes. Necroses are rare. This course is more common than alcoholic hepatitis, where cell necroses and inflammations are predominant.

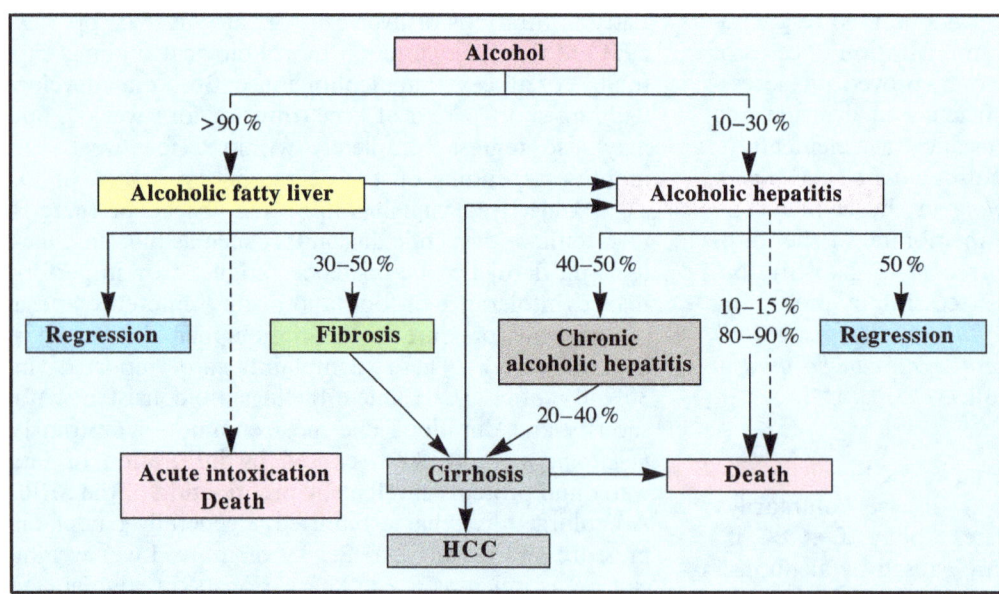

Fig. 28.12: Spectrum and course of alcoholic liver diseases (---▶ fulminant course)

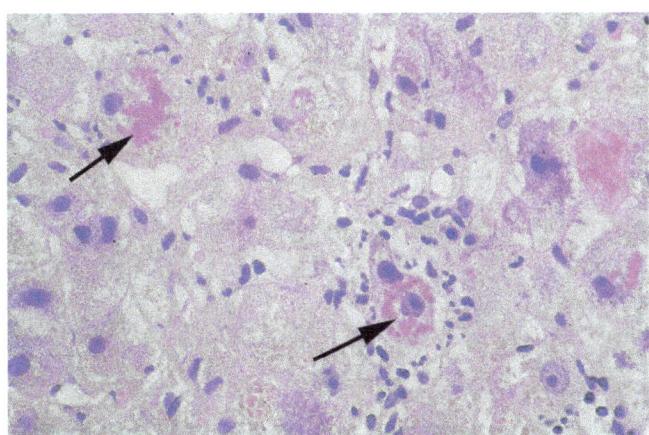

Fig. 28.13: Alcoholic steatohepatitis. Satellitosis of neutrophilic granulocytes surrounding hydropic-degenerated hepatocytes with Mallory hyalin (→) (HE)

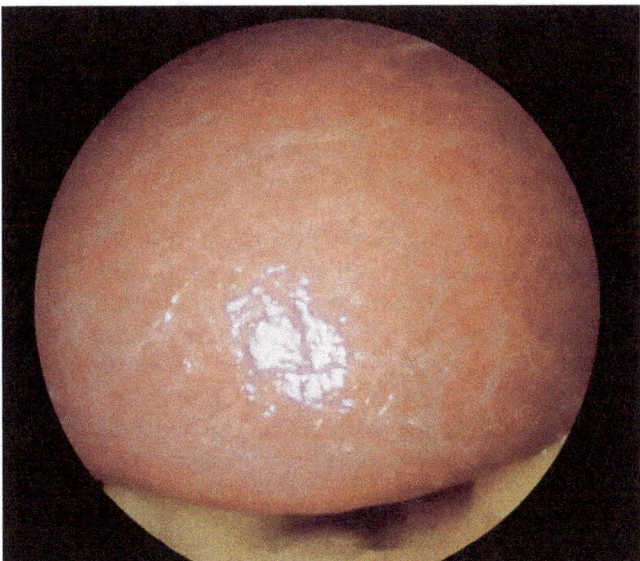

Fig. 28.14: Chronic alcohol-induced fatty liver hepatitis: scattered light reflection due to irregular surface; brick-red colour with reddish-speckled pattern; reticular fibrosing process with enhanced vascularization of the capsule

Symptoms include nausea, fever, vomiting, inappetence, meteorism, weight loss and a sensation of pressure in the right upper abdomen. The symptoms may vary in intensity and frequency depending upon severity and the respective alcohol consumption (30−80%). • **Clinical findings** present in the form of hepatomegaly and mild splenomegaly, possibly with icterus, skin stigmata of liver diseases, or oedema/ascites (30−60%), or hepatic encephalopathy. As in cases of severe fatty liver, symptoms of latent hepatic encephalopathy are also found in alcoholic hepatitis. Gastric colonization by *Helicobacter pylori*, which reduces gastric ADH activity, is considered to be a risk factor (47). (s. pp 61, 274) • **Laboratory findings** are characterized by the different types of course and their severity. In general, *GDH* is increased. *Leucocytosis* (often considerable), reduced *albumin synthesis* and *fever* are presumably caused by endotoxinaemia. The laboratory parameters may be changed to varying degrees − depending upon the clinical forms described above. (5, 9, 10, 72, 80, 85, 119, 126, 129, 145) (s. tab. 28.5) • The *Maddrey risk index* is a useful tool for assessing the degree of severity in acute alcoholic hepatitis. It is based on the *formula*: serum bilirubin value (mg/dl) plus (extension of prothrombin time in sec. × 4.6). A value of >90 indicates a severe course, a value of 30−90 a moderate course and <30 a mild course. (81) • **Sonographically**, there is often evidence of a dilation of the hepatic artery (= *pseudoparallel channel sign*). (49, 134) • **Morphological findings** are decisive for diagnostic classification and prognostic evaluation. Thus liver biopsy is indispensable, and especially reliable during laparoscopy (including simultaneous photographic documentation). (s. figs. 28.9, 28.11, 28.14, 28.18, 28.19) It was (unexpectedly) possible to find evidence of non-alcoholic liver disease in 20% of alcoholics using morphological findings. • Explorative laparotomy is contraindicated due to high mortality following surgical intervention (about 50%). (26, 50, 64, 76)

Continued alcohol abuse, which results in chronic alcoholic hepatitis in 60−70% of cases, can have a course of several years and may ultimately pass into cirrhosis. This final stage of cirrhosis will develop rapidly and in a relatively short period of time in about 40% of cases. A healing process is not expected. • In acute alcoholic hepatitis, the mortality rate is about 10%. A fulminant form is often observed after acute alcohol excess, with a fatal outcome in 90−100% of cases. (10, 33, 47, 81, 85, 89, 105) (s. fig. 28.6!)

γ-GT	↑ − ↑↑↑	γ-globulins	N − ↑↑
CDT: total transferrin	↑	Leucocytes	N − ↑↑
GDH	(↑) − ↑↑	Hyperchromia	N − ↑↑
GOT	(↑) − ↑↑	P III P	N − ↑
GPT	N − ↑	Galactose test	↓ − ↓↓
GOT : GPT	>1 − (>2)	Cholinesterase	N − ↓↓
Urea	↓	Quick	N − ↓
Alkaline phosphatase	N − ↑↑	Albumin	N − ↓
IgA	N − ↑↑↑	Magnesium	N − ↓
Triglycerides	↑ − ↑↑↑	Zinc	N − ↓

Tab. 28.5: Laboratory parameters in chronic alcohol-induced liver disease (N = normal)

Total abstinence from alcohol renders the prognosis considerably more favourable: some 30% of patients enjoy a return to full health; a further 50–60% develop a chronic course lasting several years, whereby about half of this latter group finally enjoy complete recovery. Cirrhosis is found in some 20% of all patients.

Treatment can be tried with pentoxifylline (3, 82) or, under strict indications, together with prednisolone. (11, 19, 23, 57, 82, 114) • A combination of steroids with infliximab cannot be recommended. (130) In serious cases, liver transplantation may be indicated for non-responders. In order to bridge the time gap until a liver is available, it is advisable to use MARS, which also leads to a reduction in portal pressure.

The **healing process** is based on regression of the inflammatory and degenerative reactions, and lasts several months. The state of fibrosis present in the individual case remains as diffuse organ damage. This fibrosis may recede to a certain extent. • Despite total abstinence, the disease may worsen due to **self-perpetuation** until the stage of cirrhosis is reached. Immunological phenomena (possibly antigen-antibody reactions, such as antihistone 2B) (s. tabs. 5.20; 32.1) may be responsible for this deterioration.

5.1.3 Alcoholic cirrhosis

There is a close relationship between alcohol consumption and the development of cirrhosis. Nevertheless, only 20–30% of all chronic alcoholics actually reach this final stage. It should, however, be mentioned that in up to 40% of cases, the presence of cirrhosis was only discovered at autopsy. The reason for this is that alcoholic cirrhosis is characterized by a wide clinical spectrum, ranging from mostly symptom-free forms through to severe disease, sometimes with high rates of mortality. In Europe, alcohol is considered to be the most common cause of cirrhosis (50–70%). (5, 12, 69, 74, 89, 101–103, 108, 126)

To a large extent, *subjective complaints, clinical findings* and *laboratory values* correspond to those present in more severe forms of chronic alcoholic hepatitis. • It is often the respective *complications* which point to the full picture of cirrhosis: portal hypertension, splenomegaly, oedema and ascites, coagulopathies, bleeding tendency, hepatic encephalopathy, jaundice, more pronounced skin stigmata of liver diseases, feminization, VOD and oesophageal varices. Osteoporosis in alcoholic cirrhosis is poorly understood. Circulating osteoprotegerin was recently identified as an inhibiting factor in osteoclastogenesis. This may cause a negative balance in bone remodelling. (35) Spontaneous bacterial peritonitis and the hepatorenal syndrome seem to be frequent in patients suffering from alcoholic cirrhosis. (15, 33, 46, 50, 64, 70, 76, 80, 102, 111)

Sonographic scanning and other *imaging techniques* can be helpful in further substantiating the existing form of alcoholic liver cirrhosis and in differentiating it more closely as far as portal hypertension or ascites formation are concerned. (s. figs. 28.15, 28.16)

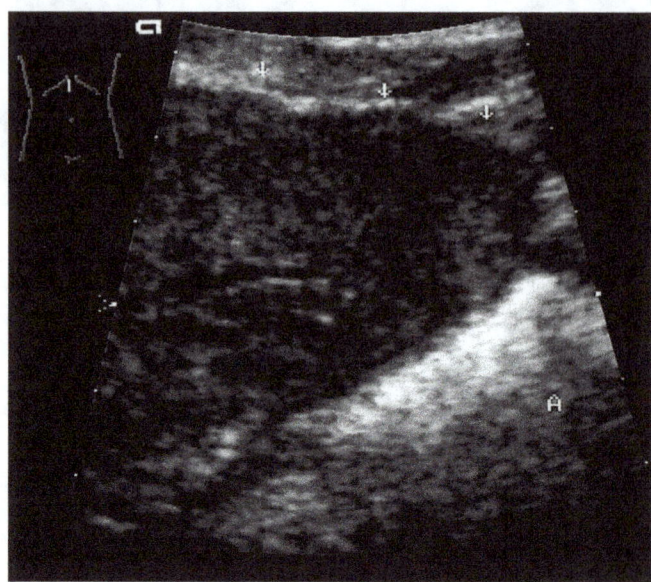

Fig. 28.15: Alcohol-related complete liver cirrhosis: sonographically spotted coarsening of the structure with a distinctly wavy edge (arrows) (A = ascites)

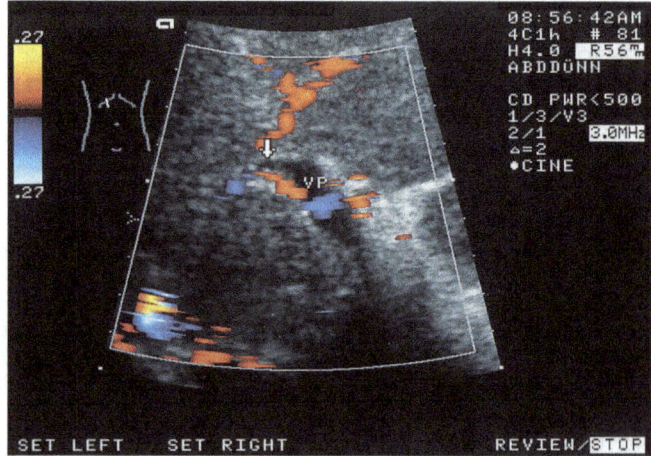

Fig. 28.16: Alcoholic cirrhosis with portal hypertension: stenosis of the portal vein (see arrow) with stagnation of blood flow in the portal vein (VP) and portal flow reversal (blue = hepatofugal) as well as enhanced arterial flow (red). Arterial signals are visible in the flow profile. Inhomogeneous liver structure

The final morphological diagnosis is reached by means of *laparoscopy* with photographic documentation (s. figs. 28.8, 28.9, 28.11, 28.14, 28.18, 28.19) and targeted biopsies. (s. figs. 28.7, 28.8, 28.10, 28.13, 28.16, 28.17) Laparoscopy is indicated in suspected hepatocellular carcinoma due to an increase in the α_1-foetoprotein value and/or sonographic peculiarities.

6 Complications

6.1 Alcoholic ketoacidosis

Alcohol-induced ketoacidosis must be differentiated from a similar metabolic complication in diabetes mellitus (E.S. DILLON et al., 1940). With chronic alcohol consumption and concurrent malnutrition, metabolic acidosis is caused by a still unclear multifaceted pathogenesis (hypoinsulinaemia, lipolysis, extreme increase in free fatty acids, rise in ketone bodies). The clinical picture shows nausea, vomiting, dehydration, hyperventilation, fruity odour on breath, acetonuria and acetonaemia as well as a moderate form of hyperglycaemia. This syndrome probably occurs more often than has been hitherto assumed. (54)

6.2 Zieve's syndrome

The syndrome described by L. ZIEVE (1958) (150) consists of the **triad** (1.) *jaundice*, (2.) *hyperlipidaemia*, and (3.) *haemolysis*. Hyperlipidaemia involves all fractions. The rapidly developing anaemia results in reticulocytosis; it is also responsible for enhanced erythropoiesis and an increase in lipid-storing reticular cells (= *foam cells*) in the bone marrow. This syndrome can occur in all forms of alcoholic liver disease. It nearly always affects men, mostly around the age of forty. Abortive forms only rudimentarily show this triad of symptoms at a subthreshold level, or any one of the other symptoms is missing altogether. The syndrome, mostly evident after acute alcohol consumption, becomes manifest in the form of lack of appetite, nausea, vomiting, diarrhoea, and often severe colic-like abdominal pain, possibly mimicking an acute abdomen (explorative laparotomy is absolutely contraindicated!). The pathogenesis is still unresolved. This syndrome is usually reversible within a few weeks of abstaining from alcohol.

6.3 Cholestasis

In 15–25% of all patients with alcoholic liver disease, **cholestasis** can be detected both histologically and in laboratory findings. There is a correlation between malnutrition and cholestasis. (*see chapter 13*)

Histological analysis reveals deposits of bile pigments in the hepatic cells and bile casts. With increasing severity, the laparoscopic picture of the liver becomes more and more striking. (s. figs. 28.17, 28.18)

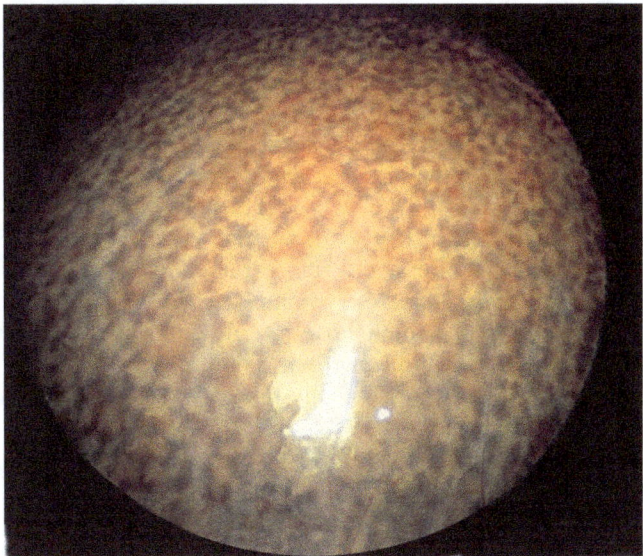

Fig. 28.18: Alcohol-induced cholestasis in a fatty liver

A severe **cholestatic syndrome** (H. BALLARD et al., 1961) can be observed in patients suffering from alcoholic fatty liver. The clinical picture may correspond to that of obstructive jaundice and cause great problems in dif-

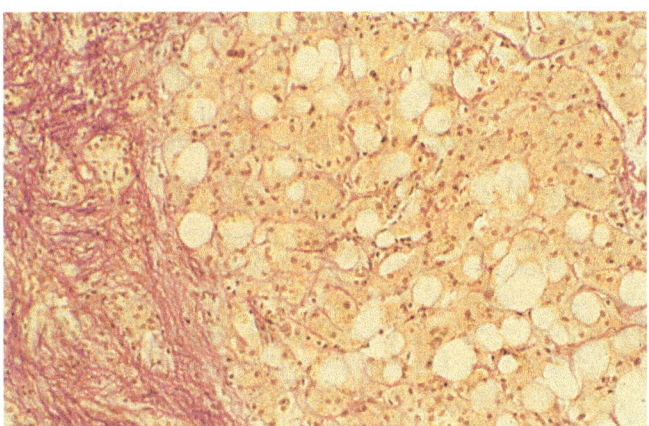

Fig. 28.17: Alcoholic cirrhosis with parenchymal steatosis and slight cholestasis (Sirius red)

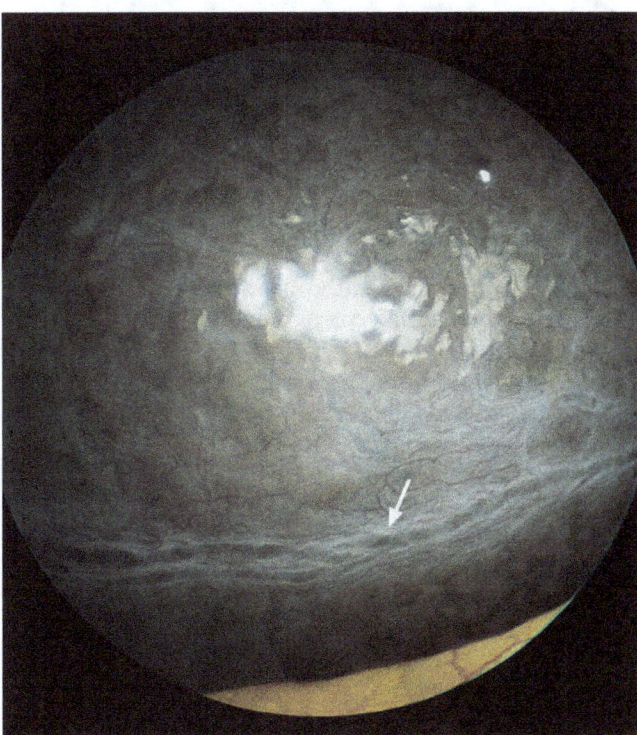

Fig. 28.19: Severe alcohol-induced cholestasis syndrome in alcoholic hepatitis. Dilated lymph vessel due to lymphostasis (↓)

ferential diagnosis, mainly because such patients may not have been known before to be suffering from alcohol-induced liver disease. Extreme forms to the point of acute liver failure have been observed. (s. fig. 28.19)

6.4 Fat embolism

In severe fatty liver, there is a risk of fat embolism occurring in the lungs, brain and kidneys. In view of the considerable fat masses stored in the hepatic parenchyma due to this condition, R. VIRCHOW suspected the manifestation of fat embolism as early as 1886. Blunt traumatism of the (enlarged) liver with subsequent mobilization of fat is thought to be the cause of this condition. It is not clear at present whether this so-called *inundation theory* offers sufficient explanation or whether it needs to be amended or even replaced by the so-called *segregation theory* (high lipaemia, de-emulsification of blood fats, etc.). While hepatic fat embolism may be rare, it is nevertheless clinically relevant.

6.5 Portal hypertension

Portal hypertension may occasionally develop in the course of severe fatty liver, since the sinusoids and hepatic veins are compressed by massive fat deposits. Even oesophageal varices, including bleeding, have been observed. Fibrosing processes have not (yet) occurred in the liver, so that portal hypertension is completely reversible once the fatty liver has been cured.

6.6 Primary liver cell carcinoma

Hepatocellular carcinoma (HCC) is found more often in alcoholics predominantly suffering from irregular, mixed nodular cirrhosis. The incidence is reported as being 10–20% (3–4/100,000 inhabitants). In patients with alcoholic cirrhosis, HCC is found two to six times more often than in cirrhosis of a different genesis. Additional deterioration of the individual's general state, loss of weight, pain in the right upper abdomen, slight fever or (pronounced) jaundice may point to the development of HCC in alcoholic cirrhosis. There is a substantial increase in α-fetoprotein (slightly elevated and mainly constant values can also be found as a result of regenerative processes in the liver or in cholestasis). Alpha fetoprotein is a valuable marker in the follow-up of a cirrhosis. • Neoangiogenesis is another important factor in the development of HCC. The major mediators are VEGF, b-FGF, a-FGF, EGF, angiogenin, etc. (132) • With the help of sonography, it is usually possible to detect HCC in alcoholic cirrhosis if the diameter is >1 cm; in cases of suspicion, CT is recommended. Alcohol itself is not carcinogenic, but is considered to be a cofactor. A case of spontaneous regression of histologically proven HCC in a patient suffering from cirrhosis following total abstinence attracted great attention (E. B. GOTTFEIER et al.,

1982). • Apart from hepatic hyperregeneration, other factors feature prominently in the pathogenesis of HCC, e.g. alcohol-induced changes in membrane properties with respect to the cellular absorption of carcinogenic agents, disturbances in the biotransformation, enhanced activities of carcinogenic agents due to alcohol. There is a close connection between HCC and HBV or HCV infection. (137) (s. pp 442, 453, 799) *(see chapter 37)*

7 Diagnostic alcohol markers

▶ Special questionnaires and laboratory tests have been developed for the early diagnosis or differential diagnosis of alcohol-induced liver disease, but also with respect to an assessment of therapeutic success and thus prognosis.

7.1 Questionnaire

The Michigan Alcoholism Screening Test (**MAST**) (M. L. SELZER, 1971), which is probably more common than any other test, has been simplified as brief MAST (**BMAST**) (A. D. POKORNY et al., 1972) and short MAST (**SMAST**) (M. L. SELZER, 1975). • The Munich Alcoholism Test (**MALT**) (W. FEUERLEIN et al., 1977) has also proved successful. • A test which is often used and easy to carry out is the **CAGE Test** (D. MAYFIELD et al., 1974). (88) It consists of *four brief questions*: (*1.*) Have you ever had the feeling you should cut down on your alcohol consumption? (= **C**ut down); (*2.*) Have you ever felt annoyed when your drinking behaviour was criticized? (= **A**nnoyed about criticism); (*3.*) Have you ever felt guilty about your drinking habits? (= **G**uilty feelings); (*4.*) Have you ever needed an "eye-opener" in the morning? (= **E**ye-opener). If you answer one or two of these questions in the affirmative, you have an alcohol problem.

7.2 Laboratory findings as markers

The markers currently available still do not fulfil the criteria of an ideal marker, particularly with respect to sensitivity and specificity. However, when several tests are combined, it is possible to gain some useful knowledge. • The most simple and most specific test is, of course, the detection of **ethanol**, e.g. in the blood, which means that acute alcohol intake can be determined in a "non-alcoholic". In chronic alcohol consumption, however, the problem arises that an "alcoholic" possesses a higher catabolic rate, i.e. alcohol is more rapidly broken down. • The use of **two biological marker types** would be of considerable clinical importance: a kind of marker that reacts to alcohol consumption over a few days only (e.g. in order to recognize relapses) and another kind of marker which only reacts to long-lasting alcohol abuse (e.g. for long-term control). However, it has not actually been possible to meet these requirements up to now. (9, 20, 28, 29, 37, 86, 112, 117, 119, 120, 125, 126, 129, 144) (s. tabs. 28.6, 28.7)

Acute intake of alcohol		
Ethanol	↑	= immediately
Acetate	↑	= 1– 6 hours
Methanol	↑	= 10–12 hours
5-HTOL	↑	= 20–30 hours
5-HIES	↓	= 20–30 hours
Ethylglucuronide	↑	= 1–80 hours
Blood sugar	↓	
Triglycerides	↑	
Potassium	↓	
Magnesium	↓	

Tab. 28.6: Biomarkers (plus detectability time) and laboratory parameters giving evidence of a single intake of alcohol (5-HTOL = 5-hydroxytryptophol; 5-HIES = 5-hydroxyindolacetic acid)

Chronic consumption of alcohol			
CDT	↑ = 2–3 weeks		
γ-GT	↑ = 4–6 weeks		
MCV	↑ = 4–8 weeks		
mGOT	↑	IgA	↑
mGOT	↑	Apo-A1, -A2	↑
GOT/GPT	↑	Triglycerides	↑
GTH	↑		

Tab. 28.7: Laboratory parameters (some of them with detectability time) giving evidence of long-term alcohol consumption

Ethylglucuronide develops through esterification of alcohol with UDP-glucuronic acid in the hepatocytes. It is a specific and extremely sensitive parameter, which is still detectable up to three days after alcohol consumption. Due to the fact that it is only present following the intake of alcohol, ethylglucuronide is an important clinical and forensic tool.

Gamma-GT is the most commonly used biological alcohol marker. Any increase is an expression of microsomal enzyme induction and solubilisation of biomembranes. But this enzyme is not alcohol-specific. It is found in increased concentrations in numerous hepatobiliary diseases as well as in many extrahepatic conditions. Figures regarding γ-GT positivity in alcoholic patients thus range from 30–90%. In general, positivity can only be observed in *regular* and *considerable* alcohol consumption; the γ-GT value usually remains normal in long-term, low-level alcohol intake. Intermittent alcohol consumption (with several days of abstention in between) does not result in an increase in γ-GT. Even an epsilon drinker (s. tab. 28.1) has normal γ-GT values. Alcohol-induced cholestasis results in enhanced neosynthesis of γ-GT and is also responsible for the rise in the serum value. Sensitivity is ca. 55%, specificity ca. 85%. The half-life of the positivity is 26 days. (58, 96) (s. p. 103)

Carbohydrate-deficient transferrin (CDT) is among the best markers of alcohol abuse. The carbohydrate content of this protein was found to be abnormal in alcoholics (H. STIBLER et al., 1978), due to a deficiency in sialic acid, neutral galactose and N-acetylglucosamine. Sensitivity ranges between 39–94%, while specificity reaches almost 100%. These values are considerably lower in women. A reaction occurs with an alcohol dose of 50–80 g/day over a period of at least seven days. A positive result is obtained at >26 U/l in women and >20 U/l in men. It is only primary biliary cholangitis/cirrhosis which gives false-positive results, while false-negative values occur in alcoholics suffering from liver insufficiency. The half-life of increased CDT is about two weeks. (30, 42, 96, 131) • The **CDT/total transferrin quotient** becomes elevated to >1.3% (sensitivity 81%, specificity 97%) (L. M. FLETCHER et al., 1991).

An increase in **mitochondrial GOT** displays relatively good specificity and sensitivity. It can be detected in the serum by immunological methods (B. NALPAS et al., 1986). The positive prognostic value of the increased mGOT/cGOT ratio was around 90%. (6)

The **GOT/GPT ratio** increases in many cases to >1.5. A rise to >2.0 is considered to be a reliable indicator of alcohol-induced liver disease. (s. p. 101)

A rise in **GDH** may be interpreted as an alcohol marker since, as an intramitochondrial enzyme, it is mainly localized in the perivenous area of the acinus. It is here that most of the alcohol-induced liver cell damage occurs. GDH is of minor importance as a marker on its own and is only of relevance in combination with other marker values. (93) (s. p. 102)

A connection between macrocytosis and alcoholism was discovered in 1938 (A. BIANCO et al.). The **mean corpuscular volume** of erythrocytes (MCV value) has been used as a marker of alcohol since 1974 (K. W. UNGER et al.). The pathogenesis of alcohol-induced macrocytosis is still unresolved (potentially toxic effect of alcohol, folic acid deficiency). However, an elevated MCV value (>95 fl) is a clear sign of heavy drinking, in particular the consumption of high-proof spirits. Due to the longevity of erythrocytes of about 120 days, elevated MCV values take several months to fall during abstention. Determination of MCV is part of modern blood analysis and this value is therefore regarded as a routine test. Sensitivity is 34–89%, specificity is 26–91%.

Immunoglobulin A is often increased in alcoholics. An increase of IgA/transferrin ratio the IgA_2/IgA_1 ratio can also be helpful in differential diagnosis. However, IgA is not elevated directly by alcohol, but by the underlying alcoholic liver disease. (142)

HDL cholesterol rises at an alcohol intake of >75 g/day over a period of five weeks; however, the underlying mechanism remains uncertain. This value may also be influenced by medication or smoking, for example, just as a decrease in HDL cholesterol may be caused by alcohol-induced liver damage. • The rise in **apolipoprotein A II** (based on >60 g alcohol/day over 3 weeks) seems to be more specific in this context. This value, however, normalizes very quickly during abstention.

Detection of **β-hexosaminidase** in the blood and urine is sensitive enough (69−86%) and indeed suitable for routine testing. The result is, however, greatly influenced by extrahepatic and hepatic factors or diseases. (56)

A rise in urinary **dolichol** proved to be promisingly sensitive, particularly because a positive value was already observed after just one to three days of alcohol intake, with a half-life of only three days; however, positive values may also be observed under numerous other conditions, and thus the specificity is reduced considerably. (116)

Progressive fibrosis under continued alcohol consumption can, if deemed necessary, be evaluated by determination of **P-III-P** (s. p. 118) (77, 98, 140) or **apolipoprotein** A1 and A2.

Previous experience has shown that some markers are important, while others are only of minor value. Sensitivity may be improved to over 80% with certain combinations of single tests, in particular when the principle of discriminant functional analysis is applied (D.M. CHALMERS el al., 1981). • In order to examine **chronic alcohol consumption,** a triple test combination would be of advantage, which, in the individual case, could be supported by additional values derived from the set of four tests. (s. tab. 28.7) • When determining and differentiating **acute alcohol consumption,** the values of the triple test combination can be upgraded by additional tests for better clinical reliability. This would also help to determine important, so-called *alcohol-typical emergency situations*, including Zieve's syndrome. (s. tab. 28.6, 28.7)

8 Prognosis

Several factors are decisive in achieving a favourable prognosis for alcoholic liver disease: (*1.*) total *abstention from alcohol*, (*2.*) extent of irreversible *loss of liver parenchyma*, (*3.*) exclusion of other *risk factors* (e.g. obesity, diabetes mellitus, malnutrition), (*4.*) additional effects of *hepatotoxic substances* (e.g. medication, chemical agents), and (*5.*) coexistence of further alcohol-induced *organ damage*. (5, 22, 37, 79, 80, 85, 100, 103, 109)

The prognosis for *alcoholic fatty liver* is good when abstention is strictly maintained, and complete reversibility can be expected within a few weeks or months. • In contrast, *alcoholic hepatitis* has a fatal outcome in 10−20% of cases. When alcohol consumption is continued, about 40% of patients develop cirrhosis, while some 60% persist for several years. However, when alcohol abstention is maintained, only 15−20% of cases develop cirrhosis, some 50−60% persist for up to three years, and 20−30% recover completely. Half of the persistent cases normalize again. There is a five-year survival rate in 50−70% of patients (depending on severity), with the mortality rate remaining almost constant after the third year. • In *alcoholic cirrhosis*, the two-year mortality rate can reach 85% with continued alcohol consumption, but falls to 10% with strict abstention. (2)

Risk factors
1. Non-compliance with alcohol abstinence
2. Severity of existing liver damage
3. Existing metabolic disorders
4. Additional toxic substances
5. Further alcohol-induced organ damage

9 Therapy

9.1 Alcohol abstinence

Complete and life-long abstention is an absolute necessity − this is the decisive factor for any prognosis. • The initiation and stabilization of abstinence from alcohol is made easier by a new antiethylic substance called **acamprosat,** which is water-soluble and permeates the blood-brain barrier. Above all, it has almost no side effects. • *Optimally, an addict must aim at total abstinence, i.e. "remaining dry". This happens in 35−50% of cases. Every individual relapses on renewed consumption of alcohol.*

9.2 Nutrition

Nutrition should provide a balance between carbohydrates, proteins and fats. Preference should be given to lactovegetarian proteins (0.9−1.1 [−1.3] g/kg BW). Lipid intake should contain a certain percentage of unsaturated fatty acids; however, in digestive insufficiency for example, the administration of medium-chain triglycerides is required. Great importance should be attached to ensuring a sufficient supply of vitamins and trace elements. • Calorie intake needs to be adjusted to the patient's nutritional status. Obesity should be reduced. Enteral feeding is better than parenteral feeding. Malnutrition requires parenteral feeding, as do severe courses of disease. In a catabolic state, as is often found in chronic alcoholics, it is important to achieve a positive nitrogen balance, which is obtainable by amino acid infusions, in particular branched-chain amino acids (0.3 g/kg BW). • Nutrition should be in accordance with the individual state of the patients and their metabolic condition. As a general rule, three normal meals and two additional snacks are recommended. (5, 61, 65, 90, 121, 128, 133) (s. pp 765, 878)

9.3 Substitution

Among other things, chronic alcohol intake results in **vitamin deficiency,** particularly of B_1, B_6 and folic acid as well as vitamins A and E. (91, 138) The reasons for this include (*1.*) insufficient food intake, (*2.*) reduced intestinal resorption, or (*3.*) intrahepatic disorder of the vitamin metabolism. Apart from that, (*4.*) intestinal vitamin resorption becomes diminished in later life. As a result, the necessary amount and diversity of vitamins cannot be obtained through normal nutrition. Apart from a diet "rich in vitamins", a daily dose of multivitamin preparations is advisable. Here, too, resorption losses need to be taken into account. When parenteral feeding is necessary, multivitamins are also added. • Alcoholics often suffer from a considerable B_1 deficiency, with the risk of developing polyneuropathy and Wernicke's encephalopathy. Administration of the fat-soluble B_1 prodrug **benfotiamine** is therefore recommended. • With chronic alcohol intake, **zinc** and **selenium** deficiency is often in evidence. (138, 148) Owing to their important biological functions, especially as antioxidants, daily substitution (i.v. if necessary) is advisable. Zinc can also be administered intravenously. (s. pp 55, 886)

9.4 Physical exercise

In severe forms of alcoholic liver disease, **bed rest,** either in strict or semistrict form, is called for. • Once the disease has reached a phase in which **muscular activity** seems to be desirable, non-strenuous sport, gymnastics or swimming might be helpful. Physical exercises that can be carried out at home have proved successful in such cases (and also in latent HE): 2 or 3 times a day 10 to 15 slow knee-bends, 10 to 15 toe-stands, 10 to 15 arm-bends, and 10 to 15 back-bends, so that some 60% of the musculature are regularly used. (s. pp 551, 683, 765)

9.5 Drug therapy

When treating alcoholic liver diseases, it should be taken into account that one is generally dealing with chronic alcoholics. Therefore, one should be aware of the fact that a **withrawal syndrome** might occur, possibly requiring the application of clomethiazole, haloperidol or clonidine. • In this complicated phase, the administration of *zinc* is likewise recommended. (140)

Reviewing treatment strategies in alcoholic liver diseases is difficult. On the one hand, individual (exogenous and endogenous) pecularities in the alcoholic play an important role and are not easy to assess, and on the other hand, it is difficult to determine respective severity or current stage of disease. (s. tab. 28.4) (s. fig. 28.8) In all treatment groups, numerous uncertainties remain. This may be the reason for the frequently controversial results which arise even in well-designed clinical studies. (5, 48, 71, 73, 80, 82) (s. pp 60, 878)

Antioxidants: Combined application of the antioxidants zinc, selenium and tocopherol yielded better treatment results and a reduced mortality rate in alcoholic hepatitis. Alcohol-induced liver diseases are considered to be diseases associated with "free radicals": oxidative stress is thought to be a contributory factor of disease. (51)

Silymarin: Its main active ingredient silibinin, used in treating amanita poisoning, has been tested in almost 100 experimental and more than 120 clinical studies. The *effects* are: (*1.*) protection of biological membranes against noxious agents, (*2.*) antioxidant effect (= radical scavenger), (*3.*) inhibition of fibrosis, and (*4.*) stimulation of protein synthesis. Recommended *dosage*: 300 – 500 mg/day in two or three single doses. (s. p. 896)

EPL: The substance known as "essential" phospholipid is the highly purified fraction of phosphatidylcholine with polyunsaturated fatty acids in positions C_1 and C_2 (= PPC), whereby 1,2 dilinoleylphosphatidylcholine is the main active ingredient. This exact biochemical definition is important, since *similar substances* do not display the effects of EPL as far as cell protection against toxic substances and inhibition of fibrosis are concerned – as was shown in many experimental and clinical studies. • Recommended *dosage*: 3×300 mg/day over a longer period of time. (71, 73) (s. p. 894!)

Glucocorticoids: In florid alcoholic hepatitis, particularly in acute intermittent attacks, administration of glucocorticoids in the form of prednisolone has beneficial effects, for example in reducing early mortality. A sign of a good prognosis is the decrease in bilirubin by >25% of the initial value after six to nine days of therapy. (94) Diagnosis of acute alcoholic hepatitis should be made using liver biopsy prior to commencement of prednisolone therapy. Treatment was given over a period of four to six weeks, with subsequent step-by-step dose reduction. A long-term course of treatment is not recommended. In alcoholic cirrhosis, the prognosis is more likely to worsen. (11, 19, 23, 57, 110, 114)

Colchicine: Since its first administration by M. ROJKIND et al. in 1973, the good results could not be repeated. Today colchicine is no longer recommended. (27)

Pentoxifylline: Increasing levels of the tumour necrosis factor are associated with an increase in the mortality rate in severe acute alcoholic hepatitis. (10) Recently, it was reported that pentoxifylline (an inhibitor of TNF) can improve short-term survival due to a decrease in the risk of developing the hepatorenal syndrome. Dosage was 3×400 mg orally/day.

Anabolic steroids: In order to improve anabolism and to stimulate hepatic regeneration, application of *oxandrolone* (80 mg/day over four to five weeks) may be considered. Good results have been achieved in alcoholic hepatitis following initial treatment.

Propylthiouracil: The therapeutic aim is the inhibition of a hypermetabolic status and the prevention of pericentral necrotizing processes. Dosage: 300 mg/day. So far, no efficacy could be proved.

S-adenosylmethionine: In animal experiments, S-adenosylmethionine (SAMe) protected the liver against alcohol-induced damage. SAMe is an important donor of methyl groups. The alcohol-related lack of glutathione in the liver and the erythrocytes can be compensated with SAMe. Good results could also be achieved in alcoholic cirrhosis. SAMe is without side effects and relatively inexpensive. It can be administered orally or intravenously. (87) The effectiveness of this substance is seen in its alleged capacity to stabilize the biological membranes. (s. p. 893)

Anti-TNF$_\alpha$ (infliximab at 5 mg/kg BW) has proved effective in alcoholic hepatitis. (53, 130)

Zinc supplementation successfully prevents alcohol-related liver injury by inhibiting the generation of free-radicals and enhancing the activity of antioxidant pathways. (149) (s. p. 55)

9.6 Liver support system

MARS: A new therapy option is the use of a macromolecular adsorbed recirculating system. (52, 62) (s. p. 390)

9.7 Liver transplantation

Patients suffering from alcoholic liver cirrhosis in the Child-Pugh C stage may well benefit from liver transplantation. However, **prerequisites** are: (*1*.) a minimum period of six months and (predictable) continued abstention, (*2*.) emotional stability, (*3*.) stable socio-economic situation, (*4*.) no other alcohol-induced organ damage, and (*5*.) subsequent psychotherapeutic support. • *Treatment results* are no worse than in non-alcoholic patients: the five-year survival rate is about 70% in both groups, the alcohol relapse rate is about 10%. • Without liver transplantation, the survival rate with continued alcohol consumption was 40% after five years, but when abstinence was maintained, it was 63%. (41, 78, 104, 113, 115)

References:

1. **Achord, J.L.:** Malnutrition and the role of nutritional support in alcoholic liver disease. Amer. J. Gastroenterol. 1987; 82: 1–7
2. **Agarwal, D.P. Goedde, H.W.:** Medicobiological and genetic studies on alcoholism. Role of metabolic variation and ethnicity on drinking habits, alcohol abuse and alcohol-related mortality. Clin. Invest. 1992; 70: 465–477
3. **Akriviadis, E., Botla, R., Briggs, W., Han, S., Reynolds, T., Shakil, O.:** Pentoxifylline improves short-term survival in severe acute alcoholic hepatitis: a double-blind, placebo-controlled trial. Gastroenterology 2000; 119: 1637–1648
4. **Arico, S., Galatola, G., Tabone, M., Corrao, G.:** Amount and duration of alcoholic intake in patients with chronic liver disease: an Italian multicentre study. Ital. J. Gastroenterol. 1994; 26: 59–65
5. **Arteel, G., Marsano, l., Mendez, C., Bentley, F., McClain, C.J.:** Advances in alcoholic liver disease. Best Pract. Clin. Gastroenterol. 2003; 17: 625–647
6. **Baldi, E., Burra, P., Plebani, M., Salvagnini, M.:** Serum malondialdehyde and mitochondrial aspartate aminotransferase activity as markers of chronic alcohol intake and alcoholic liver disease. Ital. J. Gastroenterol. 1993; 25: 429–432
7. **Baptista, A., Bianchi, L., de Groote, J., Desmet, V.J., Gedigk, P., Korb, G., MacSween, R.N.M., Popper, H., Poulsen, H., Scheuer, P.J., Schmid, M., Thaler, H., Wepler, W.:** Alcoholic liver disease: morphological manifestations. Review by an International Group. Lancet 1981/I: 707–711
8. **Bassendine, M.F., Day, C.P.:** The inheritance of alcoholic liver disease. Baill. Clin. Gastroenterol. 1998; 12: 317–335
9. **Bell, H., Skinningsrud, A., Raknerud, N., Try, K.:** Serum ferritin and transferrin saturation in patients with chronic alcoholic and non-alcoholic liver diseases. J. Intern. Med. 1994; 236: 315–322
10. **Bird, G.L.A., Sheron, N., Goka, A.K.J., Alexander, G.J., Williams, R.:** Increased plasma tumor necrosis factor in severe alcoholic hepatitis. Ann. Intern. Med. 1990; 112: 917–920
11. **Black, M., Tavill, A.S.:** Corticosteroids in severe alcoholic hepatitis. Ann. Intern. Med. 1989; 110: 677–680
12. **Bode, J.C., Kruse, G., Mexas, P., Martini, G.A.:** Alkoholfettleber, Alkoholhepatitis und Alkoholzirrhose. Trinkverhalten und Häufigkeit klinischer, klinisch-chemischer und histologischer Befunde bei 282 Patienten. Dtsch. Med. Wschr. 1984; 109: 1516–1521
13. **Bosron, W.F., Ehrig, T., Li, T.-K.:** Genetic factors in alcohol metabolism and alcoholism. Semin. Liver Dis. 1993; 13: 126–135
14. **Bradford, B.U., Enomoto, N., Ikejima, K., Rose, M.L., Bojes, H.K., Forman, D.T., Thurman, R.G.:** Peroxisomes are involved in the swift increase in alcohol metabolism. J. Pharm. Exper. Ther. 1999; 288: 254–259
15. **Bradlow, A., Mowat, A.G.:** Dupuytren's contracture and alcohol. Ann. Rheum. 1986; 45: 304–309
16. **Brillanti, S., Masci, C., Siringo, S., di Febo, G., Miglioli, M., Barbara, L.:** Serological and histological aspects of hepatitis C virus infection in alcoholic patients. J. Hepatol. 1991; 13: 347–350
17. **Caballeria, J.:** First-pass metabolism of ethanol: its role as determinant of blood alcohol levels after drinking. Hepato-Gastroenterol. 1992; 39: 62–66
18. **Caldwell, St.H., Jeffers, L.J., Ditomaso, A., Millar, A., Clark, R.M., Rabassa, A., Reddy, R., de Medina, M., Schiff, E.R.:** Antibody to hepatitis C is common among patients with alcoholic liver disease with and without risk factors. Amer. J. Gastroenterol. 1991; 86: 1219–1223
19. **Carithers, R.L.jr., Herlong, H.F., Diehl, A.M., Shaw, E.W., Combes, B., Fallon, H.J., Maddrey, W.C.:** Methylprednisolone therapy in patients with severe alcoholic hepatitis. A randomized multicenter trial. Ann. Intern. Med. 1989; 110: 685–690
20. **Chan, A.W.K., Welte, F.W., Whitney, R.B.:** Identification of alcoholism in young adults by blood chemistries. Alcohol 1987; 4: 175–179
21. **Chedid, A., Mendenhall, C.L., Tosch, T., Chen, T., Rabin, L., Garcia-Pont, P., Goldberg, S.J., Kiernan, T., Seeff, L.B., Sorrell, M., Tamburro, C., Weesner, R.E., Zetterman, R.:** Significance of megamitochondria in alcoholic liver disease. Gastroenterology 1986; 90: 1858–1864
22. **Chedid, A., Mendenhall, C.L., Gartside, P., French, S.W., Chen, T., Rabin, L.:** Prognostic factors in alcoholic liver disease. Amer. J. Gastroenterol. 1991; 86: 210–216
23. **Christensen, E.:** Alcoholic hepatitis – glucocorticosteroids or not? J. Hepatol. 2002; 36: 547–612
24. **Clark, S.A., Angus, H.B., Cook, H.B., George, P.M., Oxner, R.B.G., Fraser, R.:** Defenestration of hepatic sinusoids as a cause of hyperlipoproteinaemia in alcoholics. Lancet 1988/II: 1225–1227
25. **Colli, A., Massironi, S., Faccioli, P., Conte, D.:** "Pseudotumoral" hepatic areas in acute alhoholic hepatitis. A computed tomography and histological study. Amer. J. hastroenterol. 2005; 100: 831–836
26. **Colombat, M., Charlotte, F., Ratzin, V., Poynard, T.:** Portal lymphocytic infiltrate in alcoholic liver disease. Hum. Path. 2002; 33: 1170–1174
27. **Cortez-Pinto, H., Alexandrino, P., Camilo, M.E., Gouveia-Oliveira, A., Santos, P.M., Alves, M.M., Moura, M.C.:** Lack of effect of colchicine in alcoholic cirrhosis: Final results of a double blind randomized trial. Eur. J. Gastroenterol. Hepatol. 2002; 14: 377–381
28. **Crabb, D.W.:** Biological markers for increased risk of alcoholism and for quantitation of alcohol consumption. J. Clin. Invest. 1990; 85: 311–315
29. **Day, C.P., Yeaman, S.J.:** The biochemistry of alcohol-induced fatty liver. Biochem. Biophys. Acta 1994; 1215: 33–48
30. **De Feo, T.M., Fargion, S., Duca, L., Mattioli, M., Cappellini, M.D., Sampietro, M., Cesana, B.M., Fiorelli, G.:** Carbohydrate-deficient transferrin, a sensitive marker of chronic alcohol abuse, is highly influenced by body iron. Hepatology 1999; 29: 658–663
31. **Denk, H., Stumptner, C., Zatloukal, K.:** Mallory bodies revisited. J. Hepatol. 2000; 32: 689–702
32. **Dick, M.M., Foroud, T.:** Candidate genes for alcohol dependence. A review of genetic evidence from human studies. Alcoh. Clin. Exper. Res. 2003; 27: 868–879
33. **Diehl, A.M.:** Alcoholic liver disease. Med. Clin. North. Amer. 1989; 73: 815–830
34. **Dilger, K., Metzler, J., Bode, J.C., Klotz, U.:** CYP 2 E1 activity in patients with alcoholic liver disease. J. Hepatol. 1997; 27: 1009–1014
35. **Fabrega, E., Orive, A., Garcia-Suarez, C., Garcia-Unzuela, M., Amado, J.A., Pons-Romero, F.:** Osteoprotegerin and RANKL in alcoholic liver cirrhosis. Liver Internat. 2005; 25: 305–310
36. **Faller, J., Fox, I.H.:** Ethanol-induced hyperuricemia. New Engl. J. Med. 1982; 307: 1598–1602

37. **Fantozzi, R., Caramelli, L., Ledda, F., Moroni, F., Masini, E., Blandina, P., Botti, P., Peruzzi, S., Zorn, A.M., Mannaioni, P.F.:** Biological markers and therapeutic outcome in alcoholic disease: a twelve-year survey. Klin. Wschr. 1987; 65: 27–33
38. **Fong, T.-L., Kanel, G.C., Conrad, A., Valinluck, B., Charboneau, F., Adkins, R.H.:** Clinical significance of concomitant hepatitis C infection in patients with alcoholic liver disease. Hepatology 1994; 19: 554–557
39. **French, S.W.:** Mechanisms of alcoholic liver injury. Canad. J. Gastroenterol. 2000; 14: 327–332
40. **Frezza, M., di Padova, C., Pozzato, G., Terpin, M., Baraona, E., Lieber, C.S.:** High blood alcohol levels in women. The role of decreased gastric alcohol dehydrogenase activity and first-pass metabolism. New Engl. J. Med. 1990; 322: 95–99
41. **Gertsch, P.:** Transplantation hépatique chez le cirrhotique alcoolique: arguments pour. Schweiz. Med. Wschr. 1992; 122: 631–633
42. **Gjerde, H., Johnsen, J., Bjorneboe, A., Bjorneboe, G.-E.A.A., Morland, J.:** A comparison of serum carbohydrate-deficient transferrin with other biological markers of excessive drinking. Scand. J. Lab. Invest. 1988; 48: 1–6
43. **Godart, B., Mennetrey, L., Schellenberg, F., Pages, J.C., Bacq, Y.:** Carbohydrate – deficient transferrin and gamma-glutamyl transpeptidase in the evaluation of alcohol consumption. A five-year retrospective study of 633 outpatients in a single center. Gastroenterol. Clin. Biol. 2005; 29: 113–116
44. **Goedde, H.W., Agarwal, D.P., Fritze, G.:** Frequency of $ALDH_2$ and $ALDH_5$ genotypes in different populations and implications for alcohol sensitivity and alcohol drinking habits. Hum. Genet. 1992; 88: 344–346
45. **Goldin, R.:** The pathogenesis of alcoholic liver disease. Int. J. Exp. Path. 1994; 75: 71–78
46. **Goodman, Z.D., Ishak, K.G.:** Occlusive venous lesions in alcoholic liver disease. A study of 200 cases. Gastroenterology 1982; 83: 786–796
47. **Gubbins, G.P., Moritz, T.E., Marsano, L.S., Talwalkar, R., McClain, C.J., Mendenhall, C.L., VA-Group:** Helicobacter pylori is a risk factor for hepatitic encephalopathy in acute alcoholic hepatitis: the ammonia hypothesis revisited. Amer. J. Gastroenterol. 1993; 88: 1906–1910
48. **Haber, P.S., Warner, R., Seth, D., Gorrell, M.D., McCaughan, G.W.:** Pathogenesis and management of alcoholic hepatitis (review). J. Gastroenterol. Hepatol. 2003; 18: 1332–1344
49. **Han, S.H.B., Rice, S., Cohen, S.M., Reynolds, T.B., Fong, T.L.:** Duplex Doppler ultrasound of the hepatic artery in patients with acute alcoholic hepatitis. J. Clin. Gastroenterol. 2002; 34: 573–577
50. **Hall, P.M. de la:** The pathological spectrum of alcoholic liver disease. Pathology 1985; 17: 209–218
51. **Hayes, P.C., Bell, D., Plevris, J.N., Dawes, J., Bouchier, I.A.D.:** Free radical production and neutrophil activation in the pathogenesis of alcoholic liver disease. Eur. J. Gastroenterol. 1989; 1: 101–105
52. **Hessel, F.P., Mitzner, S.R., Rief, J., Guellstorff, B., Steiner, S., Wasem, J.:** Economic evaluation and 1-year survival analysis of MARS in patients with alcoholic liver disease. Liver Internat. 2003; 23: 66–72
53. **Hill, D.B., McClain, C.J.:** Anti-TNF therapy in alcoholic hepatitis (editorial). Amer. J. Gastroenterol. 2004; 99: 261–263
54. **Hintze, G., Cüppers, H.J., Mokry, H., Hein, D., Köbberling, J.:** Die alkoholische Ketoacidose. Eine wichtige Differentialdiagnose zur diabetischen Ketoacidose. Dtsch. Med. Wschr. 1988; 113: 725–727
55. **Horn, T., Christoffersen, P., Henriksen, J.H.:** Alcoholic liver injury: Defenestration in noncirrhotic livers – a scanning electron microscopic study. Hepatology 1987; 7: 77–82
56. **Hultberg, B., Isaksson, A., Berglund, M., Moberg, A.-L.:** Serum β-hexosaminidase isoenzymze: a sensitive marker for alcohol abuse. Alcohol. Clin. Exp. Res. 1991; 15: 549–552
57. **Imperiale, T.F., McCullough, M.:** Do corticosteroids reduce mortality from alcoholic hepatitis? A meta-analysis of the randomized trials. Ann. Intern. Med. 1990; 113: 299–307
58. **Ishii, H., Ebihara, Y., Okuno, F., Munakata, Y., Takagi, T., Arai, M., Shigeta, S., Tsuchiya, M.:** γ-Glutamyl transpeptidase activity in liver of alcoholics and its histochemical localization. Alcohol. Clin. Exper. Res. 1986; 10: 81–85
59. **Israel, Y., Orrego, H., Niemelae, O.:** Immune responses to alcohol metabolites: pathogenic and diagnostic implications. Semin. Liver Dis. 1988; 8: 81–90
60. **Isselbacher, K.J.:** Metabolic and hepatic effects of alcohol. New. Engl. J. Med. 1977; 296: 612–616
61. **Jacobs, R.M., Sorrell, M.F.:** The role of nutrition in the pathogenesis of alcoholic liver disease. Semin. Liver Dis. 1981; 1: 244–253
62. **Jalan, R., Sen, S., Steiner, C., Kapoor, D., Alisa, A., Williams, R.:** Extracorporeal liver support with molecular adsorbent recirculating system in patients with severe acute alcoholic hepatitis. J. Hepatol. 2003; 38: 24–31
63. **Junge, J., Horn, T., Vyberg, M., Christoffersen, P., Svendsen, L.B.:** The pattern of fibrosis in the acinar zone 3 areas in early alcoholic liver disease. J. Hepatol. 1991; 12: 83–86
64. **Kagata, Y., Okudaira, M., Uchikoshi, T., Nakano, M.:** Histological study on alcoholic liver disease. Acta Hepatol. Japon. 1993; 34: 710–717
65. **Kearns, P.J., Young, H., Garcia, G., Blaschke, T., O'Hanlon, G., Rinki, M., Sucher, K., Gregory, J.:** Accelerated improvement of alcoholic liver disease with enteral nutrition. Gastroenterology 1992; 102: 200–205
66. **Keshavarzian, A., Holmes, E.W., Patel, M., Iber, F., Fields, J.Z., Pethkar, S.:** Leaky gut in alcoholic cirrhosis: a possible mechanism for alcohol-induced liver damage. Amer. J. Gastroenterol. 1999; 94: 200–207
67. **Kuntz, E.:** Alkohol als soziale und ökonomische Belastung. Münch. Med. Wschr. 1984; 126: 549–552
68. **Laskin, C.A., Vidins, E., Blendis, L.M., Soloninka, C.A.:** Autoantibodies in alcoholic liver disease. Amer. J. Med. 1990; 89: 129–133
69. **Lelbach, W.K.:** Cirrhosis in the alcoholic and its relation to the volume of alcohol abuse. Ann. NY Acad. Sci. 1975; 252: 85–105
70. **Lester, R., Eagon, P.K., van Thiel, D.H.:** Feminization of the alcoholic: the estrogen/testosterone ratio (E/T). Gastroenterology 1979; 76: 415–417
71. **Li, J., Kim, C., Leo, A.M., Mak, K.M., Rojkind, M., Lieber, C.S.:** Polyunsaturated lecithin prevents acetaldehyde-mediated hepatic collagen accumulation by stimulating collagenase activity in cultured lipocytes. Hepatology 1992; 15: 373–381
72. **Lieber, C.S.:** Biochemical factors in alcoholic liver disease. Semin. Liver Dis. 1993; 3: 136–153
73. **Lieber, C.S., Robins, S.J., Li, J.J., DeCarli, L.M., Mak, K.M., Fasulo, J.M., Leo, M.A.:** Phosphatidylcholine protects against fibrosis and cirrhosis in the baboon. Gastroenterology 1994; 106: 152–159
74. **Lieber, C.S.:** Hepatic and metabolic effects of ethanol: pathogenesis and prevention. Ann. Med. 1994; 26: 325–330 • Ethanol metabolism, cirrhosis and alcoholism. Clin. Chim. Acta 1997; 257: 59–84 • Role of oxidative stress and antioxidant therapy in alcoholic and non-alcoholic liver diseases. Adv. Pharmacol. 1997; 38: 601–628
75. **Lieber, C.S.:** Alcoholic liver disease: new insights in pathogenesis lead to new treatments. J. Hepatol. 2000; 32 (Suppl. 1): 113–128
76. **Lindros, K.O.:** Alcoholic liver disease: pathobiological aspects. J. Hepatol. 1995; 23 (Suppl. 1): 7–15
77. **Lotterer, E., Gressner, A.M., Kropf, J., Grobe, E., von Knebel, D., Bircher, J.:** Higher levels of serum aminoterminal type III procollagen peptide, and laminin in alcoholic than in nonalcoholic cirrhosis of equal severity. J. Hepatol. 1992; 14: 71–77
78. **Lucey, M.R., Beresford, T.P.:** Alcoholic liver disease: to transplant or not to transplant? Alcohol Alcoholism 1992; 27: 103–108
79. **Lumeng, L., Crabb, D.W.:** Genetic aspects and risk factors in alcoholism and alcoholic liver disease. Gastroenterology 1994; 107: 572–578
80. **Lumeng, L., Crabb, D.W.:** Alcoholic liver disease. Curr. Opin. Gastroenterol. 2001; 17: 211–220
81. **Maddrey, W.C.:** Alcoholic hepatitis: clinicopathologic features and therapy. Semin. Liver. Dis. 1988; 8: 91–102
82. **Madhotra, R., Gilmore, I.T.:** Recent developments in the treatment of alcoholic hepatitis. Quart. J. Med. 2003; 96: 391–400
83. **Maher, J.J.:** Hepatic fibrosis caused by alcohol. Semin. Liver Dis. 1990; 10: 66–74
84. **Mallach, H.J., Pedal, I., Völz, T.:** Über tödliche Alkoholvergiftungen. Med. Welt 1980; 31: 1657–1661
85. **Mathurin, P., Abdelnour, M., Ramond, M.J., Carbonell, N., Fartoux, L., Serfaty, L., Valla, D., Poupon, R., Chaput, J.C., Naveau, S.:** Early change in bilirubin levels is an important prognostic factor in severe alcoholic hepatitis treated with prednisolone. Hepatology 2003; 36: 1363–1369
86. **Matloff, D.S., Selinger, M.J., Kaplan, M.M.:** Hepatic transaminase activity in alcoholic liver disease. Gastroenterology 1989; 78: 1389–1392
87. **Mato, J.M., Camara, J., Fernandez-de-Paz, J., Caballeria, L., Coll, S., Caballero, A., Garcia-Buey, L., Beltran, J., Benita, V., Caballeria, J., Sola, R., Moreno-Otero, R., Barrao, F., Martin-Duce, A., Correa, J.A., Pares, A., Barrao, E., Garcia-Magaz, I., Puerta, J.L., Moreno, J., Boissard, E., Ortiz, P., Rodes, J.:** S-adenosylmethionine in alcoholic liver cirrhosis: a randomized, placebo-controlled, double-blind, multicenter clinical trial. J. Hepatol. 1999; 30: 1081–1089
88. **Mayfield, D., McLeod, G., Hall, P.:** The CAGE questionnaire: validation of a new alcoholism screening instrument. Amer. J. Psychiat. 1974; 131: 1121–1123
89. **McCullogh, A.J., O'Connor, J.F.B.:** Alcoholic liver disease: proposed recommendations for the American College of Gastroenterology. Amer. J. Gastroenterol. 1998; 93: 2022–2036
90. **Mezey, E., Caballeria, J., Mitchell, M.C., Pares, A., Herlong, H.F., Rodes, J.:** Effect of parenteral amino acid supplementation on short-term and long-term outcomes in severe alcoholic hepatitis: a randomized controlled trial. Hepatology 1991; 14: 1090–1096
91. **Mezey, E., Potter, J.J., Rennie-Tankersley, L., Caballeria, J., Pares, A.:** A randomized placebo controlled trial of vitamin E for alcoholic hepatitis. J. Hepatol. 2004; 40: 40–46
92. **Michalak, S., Rousselet, M.C., Bedossa, P., Pilette, C., Chappard, D., Oberti, F., Gallois, Y., Cales, P.:** Respective roles of porto-septal fibrosis and centrilobular fibrosis in alcoholic liver disease. J. Path. 2003; 201: 55–62
93. **Mills, P.R., Spooner, R.J., Russell, R.I., Boyle, P., MacSween, R.N.M.:** Serum glutamate dehydrogenase as a marker of hepatocyte necrosis in alcoholic liver disease. Brit. Med. J. 1981; 283: 754–755
94. **Morris, J.M., Forrest, E.H.:** Bilirubin response to corticosteroids in severe alcoholic hepatitis. Eur. Gastroenterol. Hepatol. 2005; 17: 759–762
95. **Müller, M.J.:** Alcohol and body weight. Z. Gastroenterol. 1999; 37: 33–43
96. **Nalpas, B., Hispard, E., Thépot, V., Pot, St., Dally, S., Berthelot, P.:** A comparative study between carbohydrate-deficient transferrin and gamma-glutamyltransferase for the diagnosis of excessive drinking in a liver unit. J. Hepatol. 1997; 27: 1003–1008

97. Naveau, S., Balian, A., Capron, F., Raynard, B.R., Fallik, D., Agostini, H., Grangeot-Keros, L., Portier, A., Galanaud, P., Chaput, J.C., Emilie, D.: Balance between pro- and antiinflammatory cytokines in patients with acute alcoholic hepatitis. Gastroenterol. Clin. Biol. 2005; 29: 269–274
98. Naveau, S., Chollet-Martin, S., Dharancy, S., Mathurin, P., Jouet, P., Piquet, M.A., Davion, T., Oberti, F., Broet, P., Emilie, D.: A double-blind randomized controlled trial of infliximab associated with prednisolon in acute alcoholic hepatitis. Hepatology 2004; 39: 1390–1397
99. Niemelä, O., Risteli, J., Blake, J.E., Risteli, L., Compton, K.V., Orrego, H.: Markers of fibrogenesis and basement membrane formation in alcoholic liver disease. Relation to severity, presence of hepatitis, and alcohol intake. Gastroenterology 1990; 98: 1612–1619
100. Niemelä, O., Parkilla, S., Britton, R.S., Brunt, E., Bacon, B.: Hepatic lipid peroxidation in hereditary hemochromatosis and alcoholic liver injury. J. Lab. Clin. Med. 1999; 133: 451–460
101. Nissenbaum, M., Chedid, A., Mendenhall, C., Gartside, P.: Prognostic significance of cholestatic alcoholic hepatitis. Dig. Dis. Sci. 1990; 35: 891–896
102. Norton, R., Batey, R., Dwyer, T., MacMahon, St.: Alcohol consumption and the risk of alcohol-related cirrhosis in women. Brit. Med. J. 1987; 295: 80–82
103. Ohtomo, K., Baron, R.L., Dodd III, G.D., Federle M.P., Miller, W.J., Campbell, W.L., Cofner, S.R., Weber, K.M.: Confluent fibrosis in advanced cirrhosis: appearance at CT. Radiology 1993; 188: 31–35
104. Orrego, H., Blake, J.E., Blendis, L.M., Medline, A.: Prognosis of alcoholic cirrhosis in the presence and absence of alcoholic hepatitis. Gastroenterology 1987; 92: 208–214
105. Osorio, R.W., Ascher, N.L., Avery, M., Bacchetti, P., Roberts, J.P., Lake, J.R.: Predicting recidivism after orthotopic liver transplantation for alcoholic liver disease. Hepatology 1994; 20: 105–110
106. Pares, A., Caballeria, J., Bruguera, M., Torres, M., Rode, J.: Histological course of alcoholic hepatitis. Influence of abstinence, sex and extent of hepatic damage. J. Hepatol. 1986; 2: 33–42
107. Parés, A., Barrera, J.M., Caballeria, J., Ercilla, G., Bruguera, M., Caballeria, L., Castillo, R., Rodes, J.: Hepatitis C virus antibodies in chronic alcoholic patients: association with severity of liver injury. Hepatology 1990; 12: 1295–1299
108. Parlesak, A., Schäfer, C., Schütz, T., Bode, J.C., Bode, C.: Increased intestinal permeability to macromolecules and endotoxemia in patients with chronic alcohol abuse in different stages of alcohol-induced liver disease. J. Hepatol. 2000; 32: 742–747
109. Pequignot, G., Chabet, C., Eydoux, H., Courcoul, M.A.: Augmentation du risque de cirrhose en fonction de la ration d'alcool. Rev. Alcool. 1974; 20: 192–201
110. Pessione, F., Ramond, M.C., Peters, L., Pham, B.N., Batel, P., Rueff, B., Valla, D.C.: Five-year survival predictive factors in patients with excessive alcohol intake and cirrhosis. Effect of alcoholic hepatitis, smoking and abstinence. Liver Internat. 2003; 23: 45–53
111. Phillips, M., Curtis, H., Portmann, B., Donaldson, N., Bomford, A., O'Grady, J.: Antioxidants versus corticosteroids in the treatment of severe alcoholic hepatitis. A randomised clinical trial. J. Hepatol. 2006; 44: 784–790
112. Plevris, J.N., Hauer, J.L., Hayes, P.C., Bouchier, I.A.D.: The hands in alcoholic liver disease. Amer. J. Gastroenterol. 1991; 86: 467–471
113. Poynard, T., Aubert, A., Bedossa, P., Abella, A., Naveau, S., Paraf, F., Chaput, J.C.: A simple biological index for detection of alcoholic liver disease in drinkers. Gastroenterology 1991; 100: 1397–1402
114. Poynard, T., Barthelemy, P., Fratte, S., Boudjema, K., Doffoel, M., Vanlemmens, C., Miguet, J.P., Mantion, G., Messner, M., Launois, B., Naveau, S., Chaput, J.C.: Evaluation of efficacy of liver transplantation in alcoholic cirrhosis by a case-control study and simulated controls. Lancet 1994; 344: 502–507
115. Ramond, M.-J., Poynard, T., Rueff, B., Mathurin, P., Théodore, C., Chaput, J.-C, Benhamou, J.-P.: A randomized trial of prednisolone in patients with severe alcoholic hepatitis. New Engl. J. Med. 1992; 326: 507–512
116. Rohner, A.: La transplantation hépatique dans la cirrhose alcoolique est-elle légitime? Schweiz. Med. Wschr. 1992; 122: 628–630
117. Roine, R.P., Turpeinen, U., Ylikahri, R., Salaspuro, M.: Urinary dolichol – a new marker of alcoholism. Alcohol. Clin. Exp. Res. 1987; 11: 525–527
118. Roine, R.P., Erikson, C.J.P., Ylikahri, R., Penttilä, A., Salaspuro, M.: Methanol as a marker of alcohol abuse. Alcohol. Clin. Exp. Res. 1989; 13: 172–175
119. Rosman, A.S., Paronetto, F., Galvin, K., Williams, R.J., Lieber, C.S.: Hepatitis C virus antibody in alcoholic patients. Arch. Intern. Med. 1993; 153: 965–969
120. Sass, D.A., Shaikh, O.S.: Alcoholic hepatitis. Clin. Liver Dis. 2006; 10: 219–237
121. Savolainen, V., Perola, M., Lalu, K., Penttilä, A., Virtanen, I., Karhunen, P.J.: Early perivenular fibrogenesis – precirrhotic lesions among moderate alcohol consumers and chronic alcoholics. J. Hepatol. 1995; 23: 524–531
122. Schenker, S., Halff, G.A.: Nutritional therapy in alcoholic liver disease. Semin. Liver Dis. 1993; 13: 196–209
123. Schlemmer, H.-P.W., Sawatzki, T., Sammet, S., Dornacher, I., Bachert, P., van Kaick, G., Waldherr, R., Seitz, H.K.: Hepatic phospholipids in alcoholic liver disease assessed by proton-decoupled (31) P magnetic resonance spectroscopy. J. Hepatol. 2005; 42: 752–759
124. Seitz, H.K., Egerer, G., Simanowski, U.A., Waldherr, R., Ecky, R., Agarwal, D.P., Goedde, H.W., v. Wartburg, J.-P.: Human gastric alcohol dehydrogenase activity: effect of age, sex, and alcoholism. Gut 1993; 34: 1433–1437
125. Serra, M.A., Escudero, A., Rodriguez, F., del Olmo, J.A., Rodrigo, J.M.: Effect of hepatitis C virus infection and abstinence from alcohol on survival in patients with alcoholic cirrhosis. J. Clin. Gastroenterol. 2003; 36: 170–174
126. Sharpe, P.C., McBride, R., Archbold, G.P.R.: Biochemical markers of alcohol abuse. Quart. J. Med. 1996; 89: 137–144
127. Sillanaukee, P.: The diagnostic value of a discriminant score in the detection of alcohol abuse. Arch. Path. Lab. Med. 1992; 116: 924–929
128. Simanowski, U.A., Egerer, G., Oneta, C., Keil, T., Pares, X., Conradt, C., Arce, L., Waldherr, R., Stickel, F., Russell, R.M., Aderjan, R., Klee, F., Seitz, H.K.: Helicobacter pylori infection decreases gastric alcohol dehydrogenase activity and first-pass metabolism of ethanol in man. Digestion 1998; 59: 314–320
129. Simon, D., Galambos, J.T.: A randomized controlled study of peripheral parenteral nutrition in moderate and severe alcoholic hepatitis. J. Hepatol. 1988; 7: 200–207
130. Soyka, M., Gilg, T., von Meyer, L., Ora, I.: Methanolstoffwechsel bei chronischem Alkoholismus. Wien. Klin. Wschr. 1991; 103: 684–689
131. Stibler, H.: Carbohydrate-deficient transferrin in serum: a new marker of potentially harmful alcohol consumption reviewed. Clin. Chem. 1991; 37: 2029–2037
132. Stickel, F., Schuppan, D., Hahn, E.G., Seitz, H.K.: Cocarcinogenic effects of alcohol in hepatocarcinogenesis (review). Gut 2002; 51: 132–139
133. Stickel, F., Hoehn, B., Schuppan, D., Seitz, H.K.: Review article: Nutritional therapy in alcoholic liver disease. Alim. Pharm. Ther. 2003; 18: 357–373
134. Sumino, Y., Kravetz, D., Kanel, G.C., McHutchinson, J.G., Reynolds, T.B.: Ultrasonographic diagnosis of acute alcoholic hepatitis "pseudoparallel channel sign" of intrahepatic artery dilation. Gastroenterology 1993; 105: 1477–1488
135. Suri, S., Mitros, F.A., Ahluwalia, J.P.: Alcoholic foamy degeneration and a markedly elevated GGT. A case report and literature review. Dig. Dis. Sci. 2003; 48: 1142–1146
136. Takase, S., Tsutsumi, M., Kawahara, H., Takada, N., Takada, A.: The alcohol-altered liver membrane antibody and hepatitis C virus infection in the progression of alcoholic liver disease. Hepatology 1993; 17: 9–19
137. Tamburro, C.H., Lee, H.M.: Primary hepatic cancer in alcoholics. Clin. Gastroenterol. 1981; 10: 457–477
138. Tanner, A.R., Bantock, I., Hinks, L., Lloyd, B., Turner, N.R., Wright, R.: Depressed selenium and vitamin E levels in an alcoholic population: possible relationship to hepatic injury through increased lipid peroxidation. Dig. Dis. Sci. 1986; 31: 1307–1312
139. Thabut, D., Naveau, S., Charlotte, F., Massard, J., Ratzin, V., Imbert-Bismut, F., Cazals-Hatem, D., Abella, A., Messous, D., Beuzen, F., Munteanu, M., Taieb, J., Moreau, R., Lebrec, D., Poynard, T.: The diagnostic value of biomarkers (AshTest) for the prediction of alcoholic steato-hepatitis in patients wit chronic alcoholic liver disease. J. Hepatol.2006; 44: 1175–1185
140. Tome, S., Lucey, M.R.: Review article: Current management of alcoholic liver disease. Aliment. Pharm. Ther. 2004; 19: 707–714
141. Van de Casteele, M., Zaman, Z., Zeegers, M., Servaes, R., Fevery, J., Nevens, F.: Blood antioxidant levels in patients with alcoholic liver disease correlate with the degree of liver impairment and are not specific to alcoholic liver injury itself. Alim. Pharm. Ther. 2002; 16: 985–992
142. Van de Wiel, A., van Hattum, J., Schuurman, H.-J., Kater, L.: Immunoglobulin A in the diagnosis of alcoholic liver disease. Gastroenterology 1988; 94: 457–462
143. Volpi, E., Lucidi, P., Cruciani, G., Monacchia, F., Santoni, S., Reboldi, G., Brunetti, P., Bolli, G.B., de Feo, P.: Moderate and large doses of ethanol differentially affect hepatic protein metabolism in humans. J. Nutr. 1998; 128: 198–203
144. Watson, R.R., Mohs, M.E., Eskelson, C., Sampliner, R.E., Hartmann, B.: Identification of alcohol abuse and alcoholism with biological parameters. Alcohol. Clin. Exp. Res. 1986; 10: 364–385
145. Willner, I.R., Reuben, A.: Alcohol and the liver (review) Curr. Opin. Gastroenterol. 2005; 21: 323–330
146. Worner, T.M., Lieber C.S.: Perivenular fibrosis as precursor lesion of cirrhosis. J. Amer. Med. Ass. 1985; 254: 627–630
147. Xiong, S., She, H., Sung, C.K., Tsukamoto, H.: Iron-dependent activation of NF-kappa B in kupffer cells: a priming mechanism for alcoholic liver disease. Alcohol 2003; 30: 107–113
148. Zachara, B.A., Borowska, K., Koper, J., Rybakowski, J., Pilaczynska, E.: Selen- und Zinkgehalte im Serum bei chronischen Alkoholikern. Z. Ges. Hygiene 1988; 34: 187–189
149. Zhou, Z.X., Wang, L.P., Song, Z.Y., Saari, J.T., McClain, C.J., Kang, Y.J.: Zurc supplementation prevents alcoholic liver injury in mice through attenuation of oxidative stress. Amer. J. Pathol. 2005; 166: 1681–1690
150. Zieve, L.: Jaundice, hyperlipidemia and hemolytic anemia: a heretofore unrecognized syndrome associated with alcoholic fatty liver and cirrhosis. Ann. Intern. Med. 1958; 48: 471–496
151. Zintzaras, E., Stefanidis, I., Santos, M., Vidal, F.: Do alcohol-metabolizing enzyme gene polymorplusms increase the risk of alcoholism and alcoholic liver disease? Hepatology 2006; 43: 352–361

Clinical Aspects of Liver Diseases
29 Drug-induced liver damage

		Page:
1	*Drugs as foreign substances*	556
2	*Frequency*	556
3	***Pathogenesis***	557
3.1	Obligate hepatotoxins	558
3.2	Facultative hepatotoxins	558
4	***Morphological reactions***	559
4.1	Adaptive changes	559
4.2	Morphological changes	559
4.2.1	Steatosis	560
4.2.2	Necrosis	560
4.2.3	Cholestasis	560
4.2.4	Inflammatory reactions	561
4.2.5	Vascular reactions	562
4.2.6	Liver tumours	563
4.2.7	Fulminant liver failure	564
5	***Clinical aspects***	565
5.1	Clinical courses	565
5.2	Anamnesis	566
5.3	Clinical findings	566
5.4	Laboratory findings	566
5.5	Search for causes	567
5.6	Herbal remedies	567
5.7	Test procedures	568
5.7.1	Withdrawal trial	568
5.7.2	Re-exposure trial	569
6	*Prognosis*	569
7	*Therapy*	569
8	***Hepatotoxic remedies (selection)***	570
	• References (1–162)	569
	(Figures 29.1–29.15; tables 29.1–29.11)	

29 Drug-induced liver damage

1 Drugs as foreign substances

Xenobiotics: Xenobiotics are defined as exogenously administered or endogenously produced foreign substances that impair and ultimately damage the ecology and homoeostasis of cellular systems. This definition also includes medicinal preparations. (s. p. 56)

All orally or parenterally administered drugs enter the liver and from here, after passing through **biotransformation systems,** are released into the cardiovascular system in an unconverted or a metabolically converted state. In addition, systemic effects have to be anticipated in cases of topical administration (cutaneous, inhalant). • Metabolic processes generate **metabolites,** more specifically *catabolites* (= degradation products) and *anabolites* (= synthesis products). These biochemical processes are catalyzed or controlled inside and outside the cell by enzymes, hormones and the neurovegetative system. • Exogenous substances may also be metabolized and excreted without enzymatic processing by spontaneous chemical conversion (= **metabonates**).

▶ Of the many different xenobiotics, only a small fraction are sufficiently water-soluble to be excreted in an unchanged state via the kidneys or the bile. These are strongly polar groups such as penicillin, cephalosporin, tetracycline, thiazide, amiloride and cromoglycic acid; so far, no metabolites of these substances have been found. The phase-I reaction comprises non-synthetic processes such as the oxidation, reduction or hydrolysis of medicinal products. This largely takes place in the endoplasmic reticulum via the cytochrome P-450 isoenzyme system. Concerning the metabolism of foreign substances, CYP3A4 is quantitatively important. • The mainly lipophilic foreign substances can only be eliminated by **biotransformation,** i.e. by the metabolic production of water-soluble compounds. Phase-II reactions also occur due to specific transferases. The medicinal preparation as well as its metabolites are conjugated by various substances; this mainly takes place in the cytosol of the hepatocytes. These conjugation processes develop slowly during the first weeks of life. The metabolization of drugs via the kidneys, intestinal mucosa, muscles, lungs and skin is of minor importance in this context. (s. pp 56–60) **Biotoxometabolites** (or biotoxometabonates) may occur as a result of faulty biochemical reactions. (s. fig. 3.11) • The metabolization of medicaments also involves *antioxidants* (s. p. 72) as well as some functions of the *hepatic RES*. (s. pp 69–70) • The biochemical mechanisms related to the metabolism of xenobiotics may be affected by **non-variable factors,** such as genetics, gender and age, or by **variable factors.** In individual cases, these factors are of crucial importance. (s. tab. 3.18) (s. fig. 3.11) • The pharmacokinetic characteristics of a certain drug can be largely determined by the *pharmacogenetics* of the single patient. The enzymes responsible for biotransformation are also influenced by *genetics*; this affects mainly the phase-II reactions (and occasionally the oxidation process in phase I). *Genetic polymorphism* prevails if a certain enzyme variant is found in ≥ 1% of the population. (10, 37, 80, 121)

Medicaments that have a hepatic clearance of >60% when passing through the liver (bioavailability = 30–40%) are termed "high clearance substances". The rate of clearance depends on the hepatic circulation. • Medicaments with a hepatic clearance rate of <30% (bioavailability = 70–80%) are termed "low clearance substances". The clearance process itself largely depends on the metabolic function of the liver. • With increasing age and/or with the existence of liver disease, hepatic clearance and the biotransformation of medicaments decline, whereby phase I is mostly affected. Thus medicinal products that are mainly metabolized during phase II are not impaired. *(see chapter 3.12).*

The recognition that a system which metabolizes drug products can also produce highly reactive **toxic metabolites** has proved crucial. As the liver has the highest number of enzyme biotransformation systems, it is the main site of production of such reactive metabolites and is thus more susceptible to damage. • Medicaments must therefore be regarded as **potentially hepatotoxic substances.** Basically, they can trigger a vast range of functional and morphological changes in the liver. The resulting hepatic damage can mimic almost any acute or chronic liver disease. • *This means that in terms of function, morphology and clinical presentation, it is virtually impossible to differentiate between drug-induced liver diseases and the non-iatrogenic liver diseases they mimic.*

Drugs always have to be considered in the differential diagnosis of any case of liver disease lacking unequivocal clarification. The diagnosis of a pharmacon-related liver disease depends on the reliable exclusion of other potential causes of the existing disease as well as on the so-called withdrawal trial.

2 Frequency

Quantification: With regard to their frequency, adverse side effects are classified as (*1.*) *frequent* (>10%), (*2.*) *occasional* (1–10%), (*3.*) *rare* (<1%), (*4.*) *very rare* (<0.1%), and (*5.*) *isolated cases* (not yet quantifiable).

Surprisingly — but also understandably, given the great difficulties related to any reliable quantification — very little information is available regarding the **frequency** of adverse side effects in patients taking medication. A total of 2.3% or 1.9–6.2%, sometimes even up to 20%, of all hospitalizations have been attributed to drug-related diseases; 2–5% of all hospitalized types of jaundice and 25% of all cases with acute necrotizing hepatitis have been diagnosed as medication-induced toxicosis.
• A ten-year study carried out in Sweden between 1966 and 1975 listed 274 deaths due to pharmaceutical preparations, 23 (9%) of them with toxic liver damage. (12) In Denmark, the incidence of drug-induced side effects doubled within the space of ten years (1978–1987). (42) In Japan, there was an eleven-fold rise in such side effects during a period of 30 years. One French study gives the incidence of drug-induced liver damage as 13.9%. (130) • Various types of liver damage have been identified as resulting from some 1,000 medicinal preparations produced worldwide. Acute liver failure may be caused by approximately 40 medicaments. The fatality rate was reported at 11.9%, whereby the risk of death did not differ significantly between hepatocellular and cholestatic patterns. (63) Over the past fifteen years, the incidence of drug-induced chronic hepatitis or cirrhosis has dropped to <10% due to the fact that "dubious drugs" are not administered so frequently and that there is greater care and prudence in drug usage. This also applies to certain other forms of damage, e.g. malignancy, VOD, adenoma, FNH. (6, 12, 31, 108)

Survey: A comprehensive survey carried out in 1988 in a total of 2,008 medical practices in Germany found drug toxicity in 12.4% of the 7,095 patients suffering from liver disease (75): on average, the patients had been taking medication for approximately four years, with a maximum period of regular intake of up to 30 years (!). In 32.4% of patients, the liver had been exposed to a "double burden" as a result of the concomitant and regular daily ingestion of alcohol. The combination of two or more hepatotoxic drugs increased the risk considerably! This finding is of remarkable practical relevance. • In 1989 we conducted a **renewed survey** in an additional 2,990 medical practices (2,650 in Germany and 340 in Austria) and found that 17.7% of cases of acute liver disease in Germany and 14.3% of cases in Austria had been caused by drug toxicity, while 25.1% of cases of chronic hepatic disease in Germany and 22.1% of cases in Austria were attributable to the intake of different medicaments. (76)

3 Pathogenesis

The pathogenesis of drug-induced liver damage is an individual, albeit multifactorial process. (84) The main **mechanisms** known to date include:

(1) *Lipid peroxidation:* Free radicals induce peroxidation of the unsaturated fatty acids of the ER. As a result, there is fatty degeneration of the liver, whereby the mitochondria and biomembranes are damaged (possibly leading even to cell death).

(2) *Oxidative stress:* This process causes a depletion of glutathione in the hepatocytes with subsequent disturbance of calcium homoeostasis and damage to (and even death of) liver cells.

(3) *Inhibition of β-oxidation:* The enhanced formation of mitochondrial oxygen radicals in the presence of fatty degeneration of the liver causes lipid peroxidation, which can lead to steatohepatitis and fibrosis or cirrhosis.

(4) *Inhibition of protein synthesis:* Some substances can inhibit RNA polymerase II and III (s. fig. 3.5). This in turn impairs the synthesis of enzymes, structural proteins and apolipoproteins. The result is fatty degeneration of the liver and cell necrosis.

(5) *Disorder of haem synthesis:* Inhibition of hepatic coproporphyrinogen oxidase and uroporphyrinogen decarboxylase can give rise to secondary coproporphyrinuria and uroporphyrinuria or porphyria cutanea tarda.

(6) *Inhibition of bile acid transport:* More than 100 medicaments can cause intrahepatic cholestasis. In this case, the canalicular transport mechanisms are impaired. The retained bile acids damage the cells.

(7) *Immunoallergenic reactions:* Chemically generated neoantigens trigger a cytotoxic immune response to those hepatocytes that have such neoantigens on their surface.

(8) *Carcinogenesis:* Highly active or metabolically activated foreign substances may form DNA adducts, which culminate in mutations, above all in the p 53 gene.

Drug metabolism in the liver is subject to numerous endogenic and exogenic **influences**. They interfere with various biotransformational reactions, alter the sensitivity of the liver to drug products and determine the pattern of damage (see above):

(1) *Non-variable factors* are genetics, gender and age.
(2) *Variable factors* are coexisting diseases (diabetes, liver or renal disease, endocrinopathies), overweight, malnutrition (e.g. lack of protein), alcohol, additional medication, tobacco smoke particles, heavy metals and pregnancy as well as the long-term intake or even overdose of drugs and the respective administration techniques. (s. tab. 3.18)

Foreign substances, including medicinal products, are classified as *obligate* (directly effective) or as *facultative* (indirectly effective) hepatotoxins, depending on their degree of hepatic toxicity. Hepatotoxins are therefore grouped as either directly toxic or indirectly toxic according to the pathogenetic mechanisms of liver damage. Indirect hepatotoxins may, however, also cause an idiosyncratic type of liver impairment through immunological or metabolic mechanisms. (69, 80, 82, 88, 106, 112, 121, 141) (s. tab. 29.1) (s. fig. 29.1)

3.1 Obligate hepatotoxins

Direct hepatotoxins cause liver damage in all exposed persons (i.e. it is predictable). They cause **toxic damage.** This direct toxic response occurs either because the hepatotoxic foreign substance cannot be detoxified at all or because detoxification by biotransformation does not proceed rapidly enough. Following a relatively short and usually stable latent period, the hepatotoxin directly effects the destruction of cellular structures, e.g. by inactivating enzymes of the intermediary metabolism, by denaturation of cellular proteins or by lipid peroxidation. (s. fig. 21.12) This leads to *fatty infiltration* or *necrosis* of the liver cells. Obligate hepatotoxic medicaments are rarely clinically tested, since their hepatic toxicity is normally recognized at an early stage in animal testing. However, negative results from tests carried out on animals cannot guarantee absolute safety. This has been demonstrated with the preparations benoxaprofen and ticrynafen, in which the respective hepatic toxicity was only recognized after they had been administered to "thousands of patients". (82) Obligate hepatotoxic pharmacons are only likely to be tested clinically if their therapeutic benefit substantially outweighs their hepatic toxicity (e.g. as an effective cytostatic agent). • Some medicinal preparations that were shown initially to be non-hepatotoxic may, however, become obligate (directly) hepatotoxic substances in overdoses (= intoxification), as is the case with isoniazid, mercaptopurine, methotrexate, paracetamol, tetracycline, etc.

3.2 Facultative hepatotoxins

In contrast, indirect hepatotoxins only cause liver damage in a small number of exposed persons (i.e. it is not predictable). There is an individual, situation-related propensity towards the biotransformational production of indirect hepatotoxins or a manifestation of individual hypersensitivity (= idiosyncrasy). • **Indirect toxic hepatic damage** results from the interference of foreign substance metabolites (which are, strictly speaking, biotoxometabolites) with specific reactions of the intermediary metabolism. Such primary metabolic disorders include, for example, the alkylation or acylation of proteins, a lack of ATP or UTP, the blocking of receptors as well as of SH groups, or the binding to nucleoproteins. Only at a subsequent stage do these disorders result in structural damage: *steatosis* or *necrosis* of liver cells, *cholestasis* and also *tumour formation*. This type of impairment displays the features of facultative hepatotoxins. • **Idiosyncratic liver damage** is caused by facultative hepatotoxins. It only occurs in persons with a specific hypersensitivity to the ingested foreign substance or to one of its metabolites. Idiosyncratic liver damage may take an immunological or a metabolic course.

In the **immunological type** of hepatotoxicity, the foreign substance or one of its metabolites is bound to a liver cell protein. This leads to the production of a hapten (antigen), which in turn triggers a humoral or cell-mediated immune reaction and helps to detect autoantibodies, especially LKM-2 and LKM-3. Immunology-related liver damage is often accompanied by allergic symptoms (e.g. fever, exanthema, pruritus, arthralgia, eosinophilia) and by correspondingly identifiable histological findings (granulomas, eosinophilic infiltrations). • The **metabolic type** is reflected in an abnormal metabolic reaction, which occurs in a small number of

Criteria	Hepatotoxic xenobiotics	
	• obligate (= direct)	• facultative (= indirect)
	Liver damage	

	• directly toxic	• indirectly toxic
		• idiosyncratic
		  – immunological
		  – metabolic

1. Predictable toxicity 2. Latent period 3. Dose dependency 4. Reproducibility 5. Evidence from animal experiments	+ short, relatively stable + + +	∅ long, varied (weeks → months) ∅ ∅ ∅

Tab. 29.1: Pathogenetic criteria of hepatotoxic xenobiotics and the basic types of liver damage induced by foreign substances

exposed persons who are highly sensitive to the xenobiotic or to one of its metabolites. In general, this abnormal type of metabolism is primarily a genetic disorder. It results in the production of biotoxometabolites. This mechanism is thought to come into play with isoniazid and iproniazid, to name two examples. Symptoms of cholestasis are present, and AMA-M_6 positivity is frequently observed. (59) Idiosyncratic damage is also characterized by *steatosis* or *necrosis* of the liver cells as well as by a *hepatitic reaction*. (s. fig. 29.1)

▶ However, these two types of damage resulting from facultative hepatotoxins do not explain all pathological metabolic effects, such as the occasional occurrence of allergens, mutagens, procarcinogens, antivitamins and "new" toxins. (s. fig. 3.11) • In this context, **two hypotheses** are conceivable: on the one hand, these pathological "end products" may develop in combined toxic/idiosyncratic liver impairment and on the other hand, the "end products" may develop as a result of biotoxometabolites binding to specific cellular proteins or, in a certain number of cases, to "altered" cellular proteins after the occurrence of toxic liver damage.

substances, but they may be evident as an unspecific finding in chronic hepatitis B. The cytoplasm is fine-grained or fine-alveolate and looks pallidly eosinophilic. The nucleus, as well as the rough endoplasmic reticulum, move to the clearly contoured cell membrane. Anisokaryosis and binuclear liver cells point to an **accelerated cell metabolism.** In addition, **giant mitochondria** are often present. (s. fig. 28.3) (s. pp 401, 538)

If a sufficient level of adaptation cannot be achieved, **regressive alterations** occur; homogeneous cytoplasm droplets are produced, which are then transformed into pigment granules of the lipofuscin type. It is a characteristic of *lipofuscinosis* that, after the xenobiotically induced adaptation of the smooth reticulum (s. p. 401), it appears in enlarged, hypertrophied liver cells − unlike lipofuscinosis in brown atrophy. (s. fig. 21.3) • There is no sharp distinction between adaptive and alterative hepatic changes. **Single-cell necrosis** may already be present in this border area, possibly activating the local stellate cell system. • In addition, there could be a vast range of morphological changes, depending on the individual manifestation, the pathogenetic mechanisms and the administered dosage of a drug as well as the duration of its intake.

4 Morphological reactions

4.1 Adaptive changes

The xenobiotic-related induction of the biotransformation system usually leads to an initial adaptive response: **hyperplasia of the SER** (= smooth endoplasmic reticulum) occurs. (s. pp 58, 400, 537) (s. fig. 21.2) The cytoplasm takes on the turbid appearance of opalescent glass. These **ground glass hepatocytes** (s. pp 120, 402, 432) (s. figs. 5.7; 22.8) are not produced by all foreign

4.2 Morphological changes

Alterations in the liver parenchyma as a result of foreign substances are characterized by several parenchymal, mesenchymal and vascular basic reactions as well as by benign or malignant neoplasia. It seems reasonable to classify the morphological findings in accordance with the acuteness and chronicity of their occurrence − bearing in mind all fundamental and individual reservations with regard to their systematization. (s. tab. 29.2).

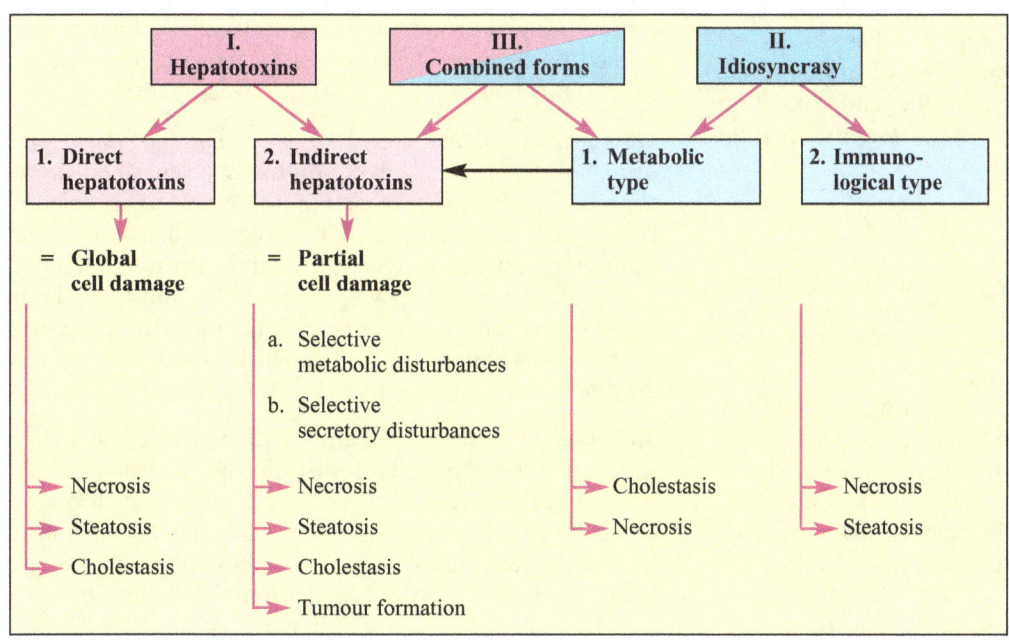

Fig. 29.1: Diagram illustrating potential pathogenetic mechanisms related to drug-induced toxic liver damage

Acute liver damage	Chronic liver damage

1. **Parenchymal findings**
 • Steatosis
  – microvesicular
  – macrovesicular
  – phospholipidosis
 • Necrosis
  – single
  – focal
  – diffuse
  – group necroses
 • Cholestasis
  – canalicular
  – hepatocanalicular
 • Jaundice
2. **Vascular changes**
 • Intimal hyperplasia
 • Dilation of sinusoids
 • Peliosis hepatis
 • Portal vein thrombosis
3. **Inflammatory reactions**
 • Infiltrations
	1. **Parenchymal findings**
	 • Chronic hepatitis
	 • Cirrhosis
	 • Primary biliary cholangitis
	2. **Inflammatory reactions**
	 • Granulomas
	3. **Vascular changes**
	 • Veno-occlusive disease
	 • Budd-Chiari syndrome
	4. **Fibrosis**
	5. **Tumours**
	 • Adenomas
	  – adenoma
	  – focal nodular hyperplasia
	 • Carcinomas
	  – hepatocellular
	  – cholangiolar
	 • Sarcoma
	 • Angiosarcoma

4. **Combined forms**	6. **Combined forms**

Tab. 29.2: Xenobiotic-induced acute and chronic types of morphological liver damage (with fundamental and individual reservations) (s. tab. 29.11)

4.2.1 Steatosis

Microvesicular steatosis (s. p. 598) presents as deposits of tiny lipid particles in the cisterns of the endoplasmic reticulum. The lipid particles are thus surrounded by a membrane. The nucleus remains at the centre of the cell.
• **Macrovesicular steatosis** (s. p. 596) often develops further into necrosis if the intake of a foreign substance is continued. (s. tab. 29.11) • **Phospholipidosis** is regarded as a special type of steatosis. The hepatocytes are enlarged and display a foamy cytoplasm resulting from a marked increase in phospholipids. Electron microscopy shows crystalline inclusions. Such an idiosyncratic hepatic lesion of the metabolic type has been observed for example during the administration of amiodarone. This substance has a long half-life and therefore remains in the liver for several months. Potentially fatal cirrhosis may occur. (s. p. 598)

4.2.2 Necrosis

Hepatocellular necrosis usually presents as coagulation necrosis. It is aetiologically unspecific and has various causes, but it constitutes the most significant type of xenobiotic-induced hepatic damage. Cellular necrosis may affect either single cells or cell groups. (s. p. 407) A characteristic feature of drug-induced toxicity are group necroses that are usually perivenously localized, sometimes sector-like and accentuated, always clearly demarcated and often confluent. Idiosyncratic liver damage induced by *halothane* leads to necrosis affecting the entire liver lobule diffusely. (s. fig. 29.2) • Cellular necrosis is frequently preceded by **cell ballooning** (s. p. 401)

(s. fig. 21.4), which may appear as (*1.*) *toxic swelling of cells*, or (*2.*) *cellular hydrops*. The hydropic cells are enlarged; they do not store any glycogen and look pallid. Cytoplasmic basophilia is reduced. The cisterns of the smooth endoplasmic reticulum are greatly enlarged as a result of fluid storage. The hyperchromatic nucleus perishes due to karyolysis; cell death follows. (s. tab. 29.11)

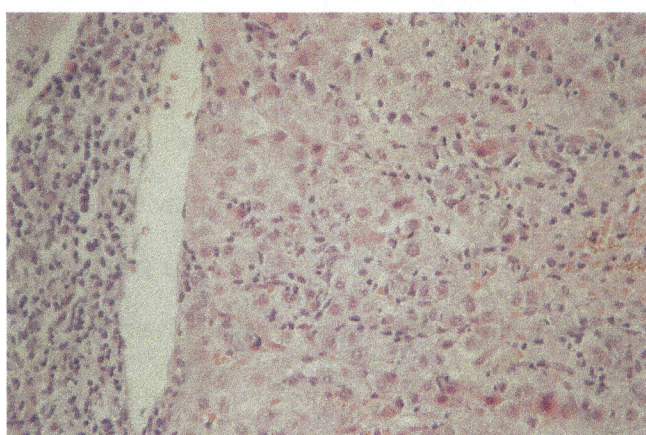

Fig. 29.2: Necroinflammatoric ("toxic") hepatitis after halothane intoxication (HE) (s. tab. 29.11)

4.2.3 Cholestasis

Xenobiotic-induced cholestasis is detected in three morphological types: (*1.*) intercellular in the form of **biliary thrombi,** which are found in the dilated canaliculi, with adjacent hepatic cells usually displaying pericanalicular condensation of the rough endoplasmic reticulum as well as frequent manifestation of cellular hydrops; (*2.*) intracellular in the form of **bile droplets,** which can be demonstrated as bile deposits of varying sizes or as small bile-imbibed protein particles – this type points to severe cell damage; (*3.*) mixed form of **intercellular and intracellular cholestasis.** (s. p. 237) (s. figs. 13.2, 13.5; 29.3, 29.4) Disturbed bile acid excretion is often accompanied by **feathery degeneration** of hepatic cells. (51, 78, 85, 115, 141) (s. figs. 13.4; 22.4) (s. tab. 29.11)

Ductopenia: Occasionally the *vanishing bile duct syndrome* is observed. This condition is given when more than half of the portal fields in a large biopsy specimen fail to feature a bile duct. The irregular distribution of the lesions can make it very difficult to form a diagnosis based on just one biopsy specimen. The safest way is to carry out several biopsies (e. g. with the help of laparoscopy) and to make an assessment based on more than 20 portal areas. (9, 40, 117, 145, 157) (s. tabs. 29.3; 29.11)

Jaundice: Hyperbilirubinaemia may be caused by drug-induced haemolysis. This disorder is regarded as an undesired drug action rather than liver damage brought about by foreign substances, since the bilirubin metabolism of the hepatic cells is not affected. Differential diagnosis must first rule out this haemolytic aetiology. (s. tab. 12.3) Jaundice (icterus) may be ascribed to various

Ajmaline	Flucloxacillin
Amitryptyline	Gold salts
Amoxycillin	Haloperidol
Ampicillin	Imipramine
Azathioprine	Methyltestosterone
Barbiturates	Norandrostenolone
Carbamazepin	Perchlorperazin
Carbutamide	Phenytoin
Chlorothiazide	Promethazine
Chlorpromazine	Tenoxicam
Cimetidine	Tetrazycline
Clindamycin	Tiabendazole
Cyclohexylproprionat	Tiopronin
Cyproheptadin	Tolbutamide
Erythromycin	Trimethoprim
Estradiol	Trioleandomycin

Tab. 29.3: Some medicaments that may provoke ductopenia (= vanishing-bile duct syndrome) in isolated cases. (s. tab. 29.11)

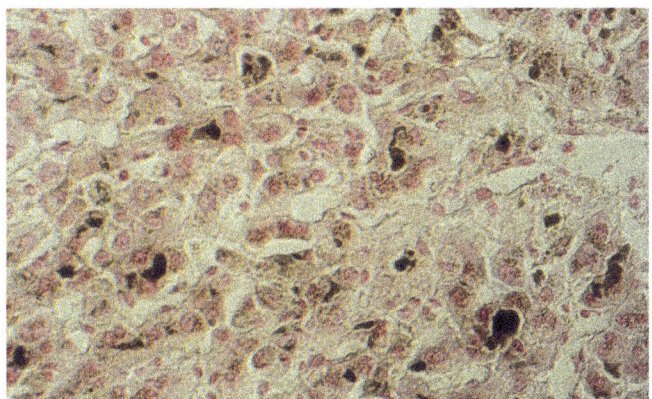

Fig. 29.3: Mixed (intracellular and canalicular) cholestasis following the use of dextropropoxyphene hydrochloride (HE) (s. tab. 29.11)

causes. Laboratory examinations and light microscopy have shown that several medicaments can (initially) cause a specific *jaundice type*, which continues in this same form until it disappears completely. If the effect of the substance and the course of the jaundice persist, this drug-induced disorder can lead to cholestasis and morphological changes. (32, 53, 61, 162)

▶ In a study of our own, we were able to demonstrate thiamazole-induced jaundice (maximum serum bilirubin 8.2 mg/dl with constantly normal values of AP, LAP and the transaminases) over a period of more than five months. (s. fig. 29.4)

4.2.4 Inflammatory reactions

The pattern of damage is as follows: steatosis, necrosis and cholestasis. These conditions occur either as defined individual phenomena or (more frequently) in combination. Depending on the severity and extent of these morphological findings, *two forms* of inflammatory reaction are possible: (*1.*) mesenchymal reaction and (*2.*) cellular infiltration.

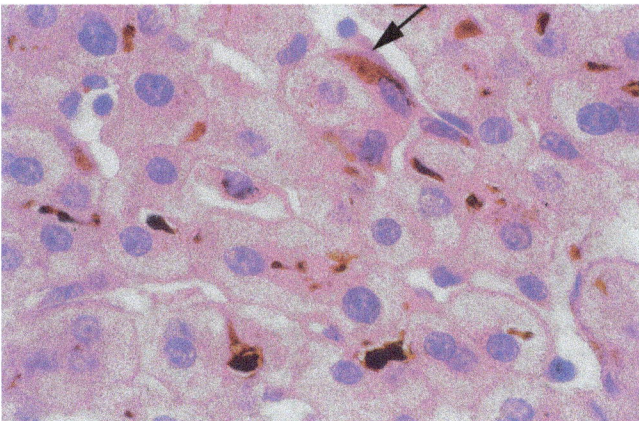

Fig. 29.4: Pronounced bilirubinostasis and cholate stasis as well as Kupffer cell cholestasis (see arrow) following administration of thiamazole (HE) (s. tab. 29.11)

Mesenchymal reaction shows an activated stellate cell system; the stellate cells and the mononuclear phagocytosis system proliferate. (s. p. 403) *Stellate cell nodules* form. (s. fig. 22.3) This process spreads from the sinusoids at the site of the lesion to include neighbouring parenchymal cells. The reticular lattice fibre is damaged or even destroyed. • In a more massive lesion, the inflammatory process spreads to the portal zone; histiocytes, lymphocytes and eosinophilic leucocytes lead to *portal zone cellulations* with oedematous dilations, sometimes subsequent to *portal fibrosis* (s. fig. 21.14) or *cholangitis* of the PBC type (s. fig. 29.5) and PSC type.

Granulomas: The hepatic mesenchyma may also respond with the formation of granulomas. (13, 72) (s. p. 405) This is often the only morphological reaction provoked by foreign substances, although the formation of granulomas can sometimes be accompanied by the phenomena of steatosis, necrosis or cholestasis. From the pathogenetic perspective, granulomas can be caused by direct toxic or idiosyncratic lesions. The formation of granulomas has been observed during the administration of numerous pharmacons, e.g. sulphonyl urea. (s. fig. 29.6) • *Collidon* (polyvinylpyrrolidon) is used in plasma sub-

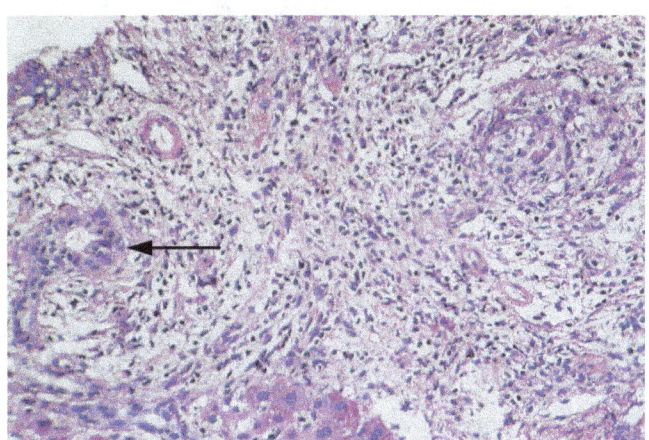

Fig. 29.5: Slightly florid, destructive cholangitis (see arrow) resulting from an ACE inhibitor (HE) (s. tab. 29.11)

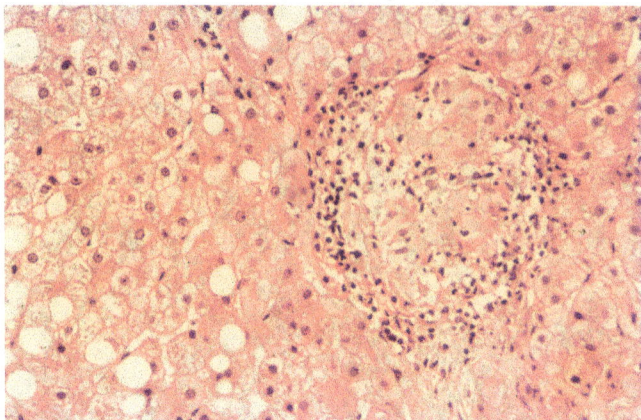

Fig. 29.6: Epithelioid cell granuloma resulting from sulphonyl urea therapy (HE) (s. tab. 29.11)

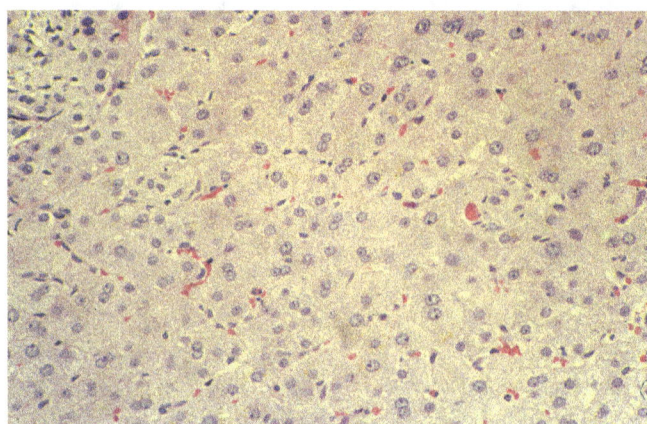

Fig. 29.8: Hepatic impairment with monocellular infiltration following administration of carbamazepine (HE) (s. tab. 29.11)

stitutes. It is stored in Kupffer cells if the molecular weight is > 80,000. The substance has a yellowish-brown colour, which with HE staining presents as greyish-blue, coarse-grained pigment. Collidon is PAS-positive. Generally, it can only be detected six months after administration. (s. fig. 29.7)

Cellular infiltration may vary in its degree, depending on the extent of the parenchymal lesion as well as on the type and duration of the toxic effect. A more severe inflammatory reaction corresponds to *non-specific reactive hepatitis.* (s. p. 398) (s. figs. 21.1; 29.8)

In this context, cell infiltrates consisting of leucocytes and lymphocytes can be found within the acinus and/or in the portal field; in contrast, in immunological-allergic impairment mechanisms, it is primarily lymphocytic and eosinophilic-leucocytic infiltrations that become manifest. This cellular reaction is reversible.

4.2.5 Vascular reactions

Medicinal agents (such as contraceptives) may result in proliferations of the intima in the hepatic artery and its branches. In some cases, these **arterial alterations** were associated with thrombosis in the hepatic veins. • Pharmacons can trigger three different forms of damage to the sinusoids: (*1.*) **dilation of the sinusoids** (e. g. by contraceptives), (*2.*) **perisinusoidal fibrosis** (e. g. by azathioprine, vitamin A and cytostatic agents), and (*3.*) **peliosis hepatis** (e. g. by contraceptives, anabolic and androgenic steroids, azathioprine, chenodesoxycholic acid). (15, 36, 159) (s. p. 404) (s. fig. 21.8)

The hepatic veins may be affected by xenobiotic-induced occlusion resulting from thrombosis or from proliferation starting in the intima and subsequently producing (secondary) thrombosis. An occlusion of the large hepatic veins is known as the **Budd-Chiari syndrome.** There are two distinct types, the truncular and the radicular form, the latter corresponding to veno-occlusive disease. (s. p. 257) Contraceptives (J.A. Ecker et al., 1966) and cytostatic agents are held responsible. Women develop this type of hepatic disease more than twice as often as men. (s. fig. 29.9)

Occlusion of the small hepatic veins is called **veno-occlusive disease** (VOD) (G. Bras et al., 1954; K.L. Stuart et al., 1957). It is identical to the radicular type of the Budd-Chiari syndrome. (s. p. 257) Cytostatics and azathio-

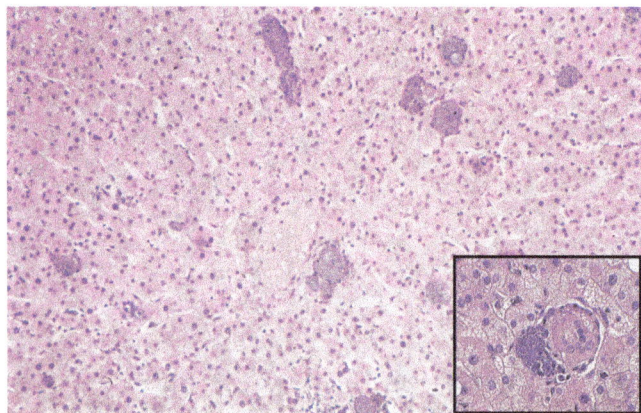

Fig. 29.7: Collidon storage: resorptive reaction of Kupffer cells and multinuclear macrophages to collidon deposits ten months after administration of plasma expander volume. *Insert:* Collidon granuloma (HE)

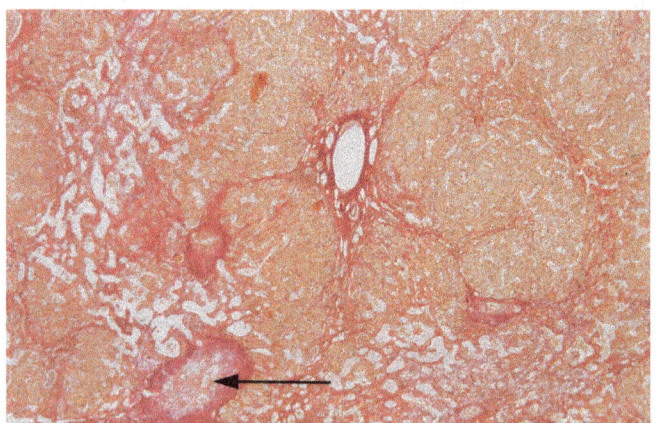

Fig. 29.9: Budd-Chiari syndrome with obliterated radicular vein (see arrow) after administration of contraceptives (van Gieson) (s. tab. 29.11)

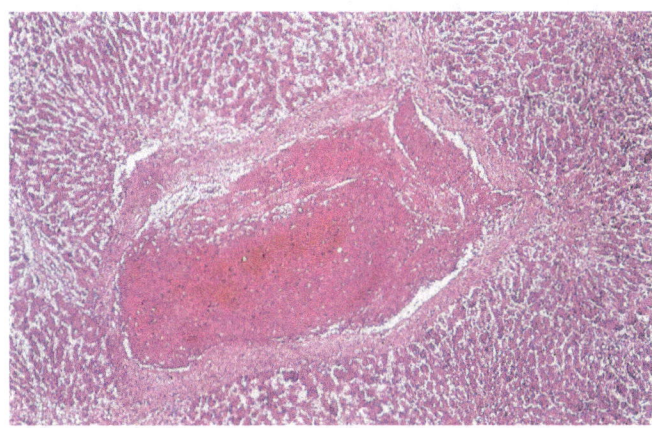

Fig. 29.10: Intima proliferation and thrombosis of a (radicular) hepatic vein resulting from Senecio alkaloids (HE) (s. tab. 29.11)

prine are among the alleged causal agents. (149, 159) Diagnosis is based on various imaging techniques (ultrasound, CEDS, CT) and, in individual cases on liver biopsy. (s. fig. 29.10) *(see chapter 39)*

4.2.6 Liver tumours

Benign tumours
With regard the neoformation of benign tumours, distinction is made between nodular adenoma and focal nodular hyperplasia (FNH). Because there are several transitional types between these two forms, they are generally considered to be variants of the same basic type of tumour (H.-W. ALTMANN, 1980). Both of these types may be multiple. (s. tab. 29.11)

Diagnosis: Benign hepatic tumours triggered by medicaments are generally diagnosed at a late stage or coincidentally during abdominal sonography. The tumour develops asymptomatically over an extended period of time. • **Symptoms**, which include upper abdominal pressure and occasional pain radiating to the back or to the right shoulder, only appear when the tumour has grown to a certain size. This may point to tumoural bleeding, the formation of subcapsular haematoma or impending rupture. A rupture is accompanied by the obvious signs of acute abdomen and the symptoms of haemorrhagic shock (possibly with simultaneous abdominal trauma, straining or retching). • Diagnosis is possible by **ultrasound** and other **imaging techniques** (if necessary, with contrast medium). **Laparoscopy** also provides a reliable diagnosis. If at all, biopsy is only indicated by laparoscopy and using a fine needle or Robbers forceps (there is a possible danger of bleeding due to the high degree of vascularization). • Values beyond the normal **laboratory parameters** (bilirubin, AP, LAP, GPT, cholinesterase, etc.) are only evident once the tumour has reached a certain size. We have found *subnormal* or *very low GGT values* in almost all women taking oestrogen. Increased γ-GT values were accompanied by the onset of cholestasis. *(see chapter 36)*

Adenoma: The potential association of hepatic adenoma with the long-term use of oral contraceptives was first suggested by I. K. BAUM et al. in 1973. Although the detection of adenoma was extremely rare before 1954, more than 400 cases were published by 1985. This figure has probably risen even further, but such findings have seldom been published since that time, as the diagnosis was often deemed not worth reporting. Thanks to the ultrasound technique, which is now used on a routine basis, hepatocellular adenomas rarely escape detection today. Most of them are located close to the surface. (98) (s. p. 776) *(We have extensive data on eight unpublished cases)* (s. fig. 29.11)

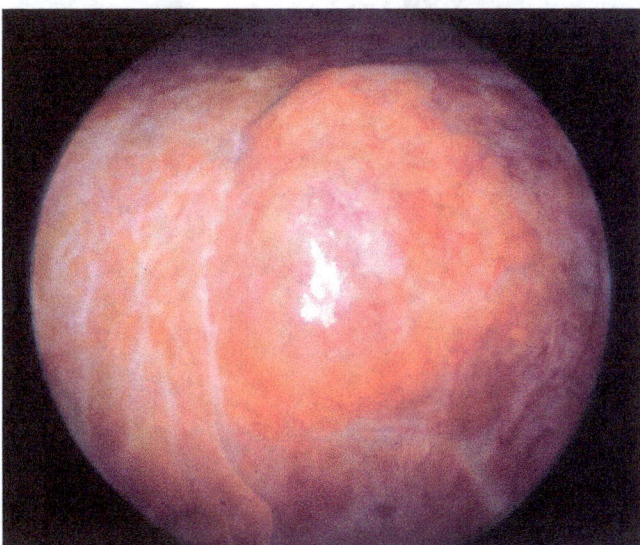

Fig. 29.11: Adenoma (approximately 5 cm in diameter) following long-term use of oral contraceptives (s. tab. 29.11)

Focal nodular hyperplasia: FNH is the most common benign hepatic neoplasia. As with adenoma, it may develop after the patient has taken oestrogens for a longer period (usually more than 4 or 5 years). In some cases, the lesion develops within 6 to 12 months after intake begins. (15) When the oral contraceptives are discontinued, the tumour regresses or disappears completely. The rate of both oestrogen-induced hepatocellular adenoma and FNH was considerably reduced after the introduction of low-dose oral contraceptives.

A genetic predisposition is assumed on the basis of frequency within families. The liver-damaging effect seems to be closely connected to the C_{18} and C_{19} steroid ring and alkylation in the 17α-position. Even the simultaneous occurrence of an adenoma and FNH under oestrogen administration has been described.

While there is a clear connection between adenoma formation and the intake of oestrogens, the association between FNH and oestrogens, albeit plausible, still lacks confirmation. *However, our own observations strongly suggest a causal relationship.* (s. figs. 29.12,

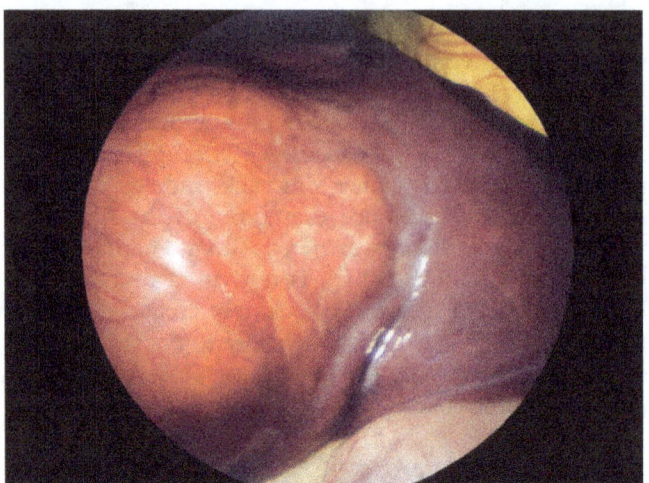

Fig. 29.12: Focal nodular hyperplasia in the left liver lobe following seven years' use of oestrogen (same patient as in fig. 29.13)

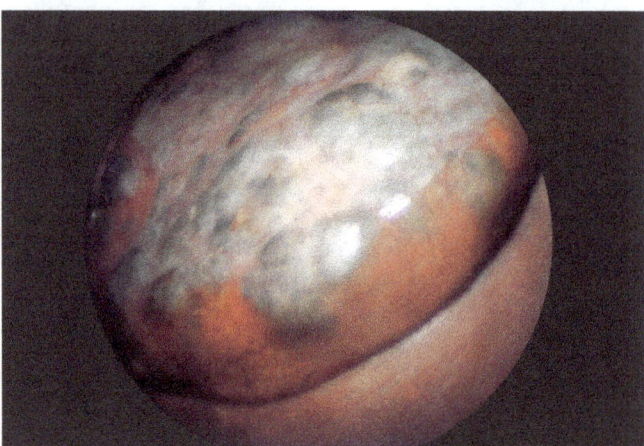

Fig. 29.14: Liver cell adenoma after 21 years' use of oestrogens, with subcapsular focal bleedings and malignant degeneration (hepatocellular carcinoma) (s. tab. 29.10)

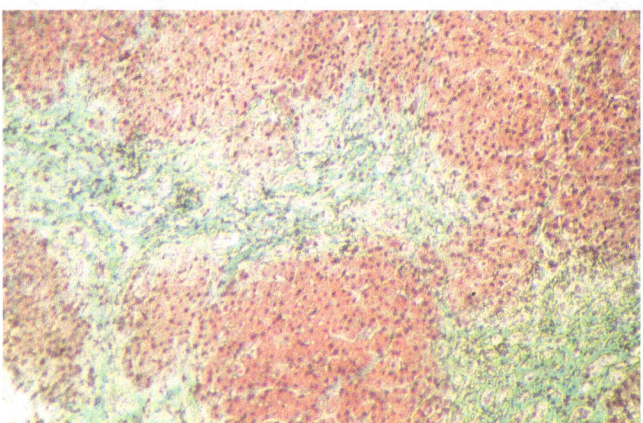

Fig. 29.13: Focal nodular hyperplasia with parenchymal nodules between fibrotic areas resembling portal zones (Goldner) (same patient as in fig. 29.12)

29.13) FNH may also be caused by various substances, e. g. azathioprine, clofibrate, nitrofurantoin.

Malignant tumours
Evidence that *focal nodular hyperplasia* tends to degenerate into malignant tumours is still lacking. • *Hepatocellular adenomas* pose the (rare) risk of developing into hepatocellular carcinoma (M. Davis et al., 1975). Several cases have been published in recent years. (57, 110, 146) We can add our own observation here. (s. fig. 29.14)

▶ *A 60-year-old female patient was referred to us for differential diagnosis of cholestasis after having taken oestrogen for about 21 years (substitution following bilateral removal of polycystic ovaries): AP 206 U/l, LAP 52 U/l, γ-GT 7 U/l (!), GPT 42 U/l, GOT 32 U/l, GDH 12 U/l, copper 192 μg/dl, cholinesterase 2,150 U/l. Repeated measurements gave normal values for $α_1$-foetoprotein; haemogram, LDH, iron, etc. were normal; demonstration of adenoma by ultrasound and CT, but with additional "unclear structures." Laparoscopy confirmed the adenoma, together with several subcapsular bleeding foci and hepatocellular carcinoma (identified by forceps biopsy).*

In contrast to primary hepatocellular carcinoma, the $α_1$-*foetoprotein values* are normal (G. Klatskin, 1977), which is also true of the case we presented above. However, a rapid increase and significant rise in AFP values have also been reported. *Metastasis* formation is rare and always relatively late. • It has been observed that *hepatocellular carcinoma* can follow the intake of hormone-based contraceptives as well as long-term administration (several years) of 17α-alkylated androgenic, anabolic steroids and methotrexate. *Cholangiocarcinoma* may also be caused by the long-term intake (several years) of hormone-based contraceptives, androgenic agents and α-methyldopa. The formation of *angiosarcoma* has likewise been attributed to the long-term use of oral contraceptives, oestrogens, androgenic and anabolic drugs. (s. tab. 29.11)

Diagnosis: Malignant tumour formation is accompanied by inappetence and weight loss, pain in the upper right abdominal quadrant, fever, specific laboratory findings and paraneoplastic symptoms. *(see chapter 37)*

4.2.7 Fulminant liver failure

Fulminant or protracted liver failure is caused by medicaments in 10−15% of cases. A reduction in the functional liver mass to <20−35% is deemed to be a critical stage. However, the death of the patient may already occur due to secondary metabolic disorders *(= exogenous hepatic coma)* before the extent of the parenchymal loss has fallen below the critical threshold *(= endogenous hepatocellular disintegration coma)*. (s. tab. 29.11)

Three forms of drug-induced liver failure are distinguished: (*1.*) obligate, dose-dependent toxicity (e. g. *paracetamol*, (s. fig. 20.3), (*2.*) unpredictable, idiosyncratic liver insufficiency (e. g. *isoniazid*), and (*3.*) immunoallergic idiosyncrasy (e. g. *halothane*) (s. fig. 29.2).

Initially, unspecific **complaints** frequently include nausea, inappetence and fatigue. • In some patients, idiosyncratic hepatocellular damage may be accompanied by **hypersensitive reactions** (e.g. fever, exanthema, eosinophilia, lymphocytosis, arthralgia).

Obligate, dose-dependent drug-induced toxicity need not be feared, since substances which predictably cause severe toxicity are not usually applied as medical remedies. It is only in cases where the therapeutic effect clearly outweighs the known type of damage that an obligate toxic substance is administered as a therapeutic agent — but in accordance with strict criteria!

It should be mentioned that almost all cases of fulminant or protracted liver failure caused by a certain substance are isolated occurrences that cannot be foreseen. They develop as a result of individual idiosyncrasy despite correct dosage and observation of all possible interactions. (s. tab. 29.4)

Acarbose	Ketoconazole
Allopurinol	Labetalol
Amiodarone	Levofloxacin (28)
Amoxicillin (39)	Leflunomide
Amphotericin B	Lisinopril
Antirheumatics	MAO inhibitor
Benoxaprofen	Methotrexate
Bromfenac (52, 105)	Methyldopa
Carbamazepine	Minocyclin
Carbimazol	Minocycline
Chlorpromazine	Nefadozone
Clozapine (91)	Nibutamid
Cotrimoxazole	Nimesulide (95)
Cyproterone	Niperotidine
Cytostatics	Ofloxacin
Diapsone	Omeprazole
Dicoumarol (18)	Paracetamol (81, 96)
Didanosine	Pemoline
Dideoxyinosine	Phenhydrane
Disulfiram (160)	Phenprocoumon (102)
Duloxetine (55)	Phenytoin
Ebrotidine (4)	Piroxicam
Ecstasy (7, 55, 122)	Pirprofen
Enflurane	Probenecid
Etoposide	Prophylthiouracil (64, 123)
Exifon	Pyrazinamide
Fluconazole	Rifampicin
Flutamide	Rosiglitazone
Gemcitabine (119)	Sulphonamide
Halothane	Tetrabamate
Hydroxychloroquine	Tetracycline
Ibuprofen	Triazolam (67)
Imatinib	Tolcapone
Imipramine	Troglitazone (47)
Interferon-α	Usnic acid (35)
Isoflurane	Valproic acid
Isoniazid	Zoxazolamine

Tab. 29.4: Some medicaments that may provoke idiosyncratic fulminant or protracted liver failure in isolated cases (with some references) (s. tab. 29.11)

The **mortality rate** depends on the cause of disease, the patient's age as well as the intensity and duration of encephalopathy. Since the introduction of liver transplantation (65) and temporary liver-support systems, the mortality rate in ALF has fallen markedly. (62, 83)

The initial **diagnosis** is based mainly on the determination of *laboratory values*, which can be used as a starting point for assessing the further course of disease. • The same applies to *sonography* as regards the determination of liver size and echo structure. Liver size may also be determined exactly by means of *CT*. (s. tab. 29.5)

GC protein (group-specific component) is an α_2-globulin which is synthesized in the liver and which binds actin released due to hepatocyte decay. Decreased GC-protein values in the plasma are thus attributable both to its reduced synthesis in acute liver failure and its increased binding to actin as a result of hepatocellular disintegration. A value of < 34 µg/ml was associated with a lethal outcome in some 70% of cases.

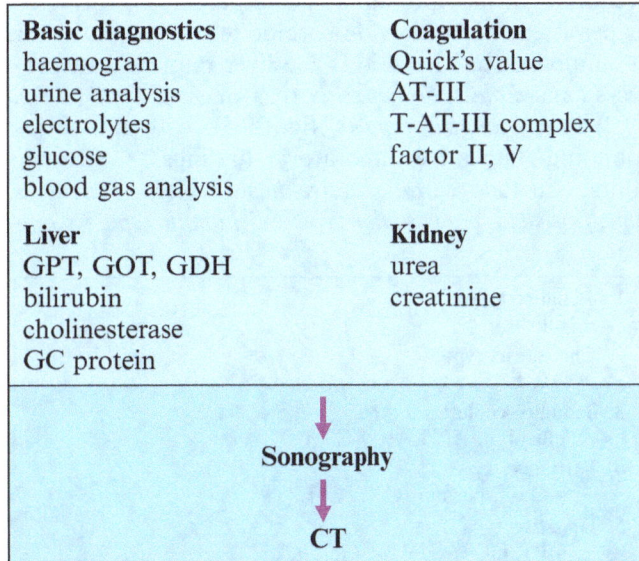

Tab. 29.5: Diagnostic measures in suspected fulminant liver failure

5 Clinical aspects

Liver damage caused by drug-induced toxicity, more specifically the intrahepatic obstructive type of jaundice resulting from the intake of arsphenamine, was first described by F.M. Hanger et al. in 1940. (53)

5.1 Clinical courses

Toxic liver damage does not produce a characteristic clinical picture. It is determined by the underlying lesion pattern. Clinical courses range from asymptomatic to symptomatic and from acute to chronic. (1, 10, 35, 63, 69, 79, 88, 89, 93, 104, 106, 108, 109, 128, 141)

• asymptomatic
• symptomatic
1. acute → normalized
2. acute → chronic
3. chronic → chronic
4. chronic → normalized
→ healed with residual fibrosis

Differential diagnosis: Drug-related hepatic damage can mimic almost any liver disease and must, therefore, always be included in the differential diagnosis. (s. tab. 29.6) • Thus a pure *jaundice type* can occur with unconjugated hyperbilirubinaemia, or a *cholestasis type* is observed, which may or may not be accompanied by simultaneous jaundice. (s. figs. 29.3, 29.4) The *fatty liver type* often starts out uneventfully with no abnormal laboratory values until increased levels of γ-GT and, in several cases, an additional rise in GPT and ChE occur. The *hepatitis type* with greatly varying laboratory values also produces a clinical picture with multiple interpretations: it may present as acute hepatitis, protracted or persistent hepatitis, non-specific reactive hepatitis or "granulomatous" hepatitis. The liver damage can progress as a *cholestatic hepatitis type, necrotic type* (s. fig. 29.2) or *cholangitis type* (s. fig. 29.5), with the corresponding indicative laboratory findings. • Chronic courses include *chronic active hepatitis type, cirrhosis type, fibrosis type, vascular type* and *tumour type*. • Combined forms of damage are also frequent. Their diagnostic categorization presents considerable difficulties. (s. tab. 29.6)

5.2 Anamnesis

Sometimes, there are no complaints at all. Mostly, however, patients have atypical complaints, which are possibly suggestive of toxic liver damage:

common cold	lack of appetite	nausea
diarrhoea	lacrimation	pruritus
fever	malaise	

5.3 Clinical findings

The following clinical findings are considered as additional symptoms for the detection of liver damage caused by drug-induced toxicity:

abdominal pain	leucocytosis/leucopenia
arthralgia	lymphadenopathy
conjunctivitis	myalgia
eosinophilia	pruritus
exanthema	rhinitis

5.4 Laboratory findings

The focus is on determining **γ-GT** as an indicator of long-term (several weeks) intensive activation of the biotransformation system due to drug intake − after excluding other causes of elevated γ-GT. (s. p. 103) Generally, the γ-GT level remains normal during intake of oral contraceptives or long-term contact with halothane (values are even subnormal in patients taking oestrogen). • A rise in **GPT** (usually also in GOT) suggests the development of drug-induced hepatocellular damage. Generally, a so-called inflammatory type (DeRitis quotient < 1) can be identified. (s. p. 101) In this context, γ-GT is regarded as the screening enzyme for drug-related activation of the biotransformation system, and GPT is seen as the screening enzyme for the resulting liver damage. • Decreased levels of **cholinesterase** point to a reduction in ChE synthesis in the area of the rough endoplasmic reticulum due to drug-related toxicity. Intake of hormone-based contraceptives likewise diminishes ChE activity. (s. p. 109) • The increase in **AP** suggests a toxic hepatic lesion of the cholestasis type (with or without jaundice), possibly with simultaneously augmented or normal GPT (and GOT). (s. p. 107) • This **threefold pattern** (γ-GT, GPT, ChE) is an efficient and rational test to demonstrate hepatic damage with a sensitivity of approx. 95%. Cholestasis is detected by the **fourfold pattern** (γ-GT, GPT, ChE, AP) with a sensitivity of approx. 96%. (s. p. 109) (s. tab. 5.11) More diagnostic findings can be generated from the **enzyme ratios.** (s. p. 101) (s. tabs. 5.6, 5.7; 29.5, 29.6)

1. **Jaundice type**
− bilirubin ↑
2. **Cholestasis type**
− AP, LAP, γ-GT ↑
3. **Jaundice-cholestasis type**
− bilirubin, AP, LAP, γ-GT ↑
4. **Fatty liver type**
− γ-GT ↑, perhaps GPT, ChE ↑
5. **Hepatitis type**
− GPT, GOT, GDH, γ-GT ↑
DeRitis quotient < 1
6. **Cholestatic hepatitis type**
− GPT, GOT, GDH, γ-GT, AP ↑
7. **Necrosis type**
− GPT, GOT, GDH ↑
DeRitis quotient > 1
generally bilirubin, AP, γ-GT ↑; ChE, Quick ↓
8. **Cholangitis type**
− GPT, GOT, GDH, γ-GT, AP ↑
possibly bilirubin ↑, ChE ↓
possibly autoantibodies +
9. **Chronic hepatitis type**
10. **Cirrhosis type**
11. **Fibrosis type**
12. **Vascular type**
13. **Tumour type**
14. **Combined forms**

Tab. 29.6: Morphological reactions or laboratory findings resulting from hepatic damage caused by drug-induced toxicity (s. tab. 29.11)

Evidence of **autoantibodies,** such as *ANA, AMA* and *SMA,* points to the immuno-allergic pathogenesis of drug-induced liver damage. These autoantibodies can be detected both singly and in a combined form. Usually, they occur in low titres. As a rule, they have been found with clometazine, fenofibrate, oxyphenisatin, papaverine, etc. *Anti-LKM 2* was detected after the administration of ticrynafene, and *anti-LM* after dihydralazine. (The subgroup *AMA anti-M_6* was identified as a specific antibody following the intake of iproniazid (59); it has not been found since iproniazid was taken off the market). However, autoantibodies are of no diagnostic value in medication-induced liver damage.

5.5 Search for causes

In most cases, the search for the causal toxin must be carried out meticulously. However, neither in the physician's practice nor in the hospital can this search be conducted with the required precision, since the time available is not sufficient to establish the individual medication history in depth, or the patient is generally agitated and cannot answer detailed and direct questions satisfactorily. Drug- and/or chemical-related anamneses are often incomplete or unreliable, because the patient was not given sufficient time at the doctor's surgery and was not able to take a close look at the medicines kept at home in order to provide more precise answers. • For these reasons, our **check-list**, which is given to the patient in the form of a *questionnaire*, has proved to be of great assistance over many years. (s. tab. 29.7)

Very few terms in this questionnaire require further explanation, and we also include some brief instructions about how to answer the questions. The patient has sufficient time to think about the individual questions either at home or in the hospital, is able to consult family members and may even have several days to complete the questionnaire. While discussing the responses with the doctor, further information can be added. This often requires repeated and sometimes outright *"inquisitory questioning"*, as the patient (*1.*) may have forgotten to mention certain medicaments or may not consider them as such (e.g. laxatives), (*2.*) may be ashamed to admit taking or abusing certain agents (e.g. aphrodisiacs – sometimes of rather obscure composition), (*3.*) may fear detection or may not wish anyone to know (e.g. abuse of drugs, alcohol, analgesics or soporifics), or (*4.*) may consciously (or subconsciously) repress the problems connected with toxic liver damage in line with a generally increasing tendency towards self-medication and a firm belief in tablets.

However, it must be considered that it is often only the **combined intake** of medicaments, alcohol and other chemical substances or the **age** of the patient that gives rise to such biotoxometabolites, which do not form when the respective substance is taken on its own. (75, 76) (s. tab. 29.8)

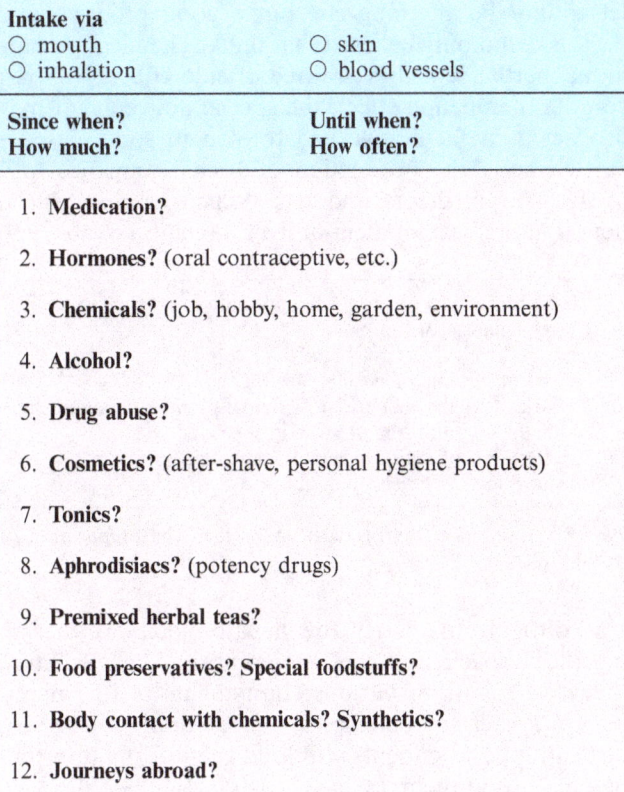

Tab. 29.7: Check-list for the detection of possible hepatotoxic xenobiotics

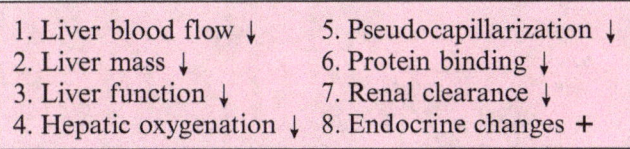

Tab. 29.8: Factors causing reduced drug metabolism in increasing age (>55 years)

▶ **Discrepancies** between pathologically altered laboratory parameters and minor or uncharacteristic histological changes, or even normal findings in the biopsy specimen, are regarded as almost typical for liver damage resulting from drug-induced toxicity. • In individual cases, however, the histological findings can be attributed to a specific chemical substance once the toxin has been identified. • As a rule, laboratory and morphological findings are all the more distinctive when the hepatic detoxification mechanisms have been constantly used and are ultimately exhausted.

5.6 Herbal remedies

Remedies prepared from herbal extracts have been used by all peoples since ancient times. • In recent years, herbal remedies have enjoyed growing popularity in modern societies. This trend can be explained by the following factors: (*1.*) ecological movements in industrialized states call for a return to natural products, (*2.*) there is a widespread naive opinion that a natural product cannot be anything else but a good product, and (3.) it is commonly believed that unlike chemical preparations, herbal remedies are free of side effects. • Apart from its therapeutic effect, the special active agent may also act as a facultative hepatotoxin in some cases. • Furthermore, the production of herbal remedies may involve certain errors and risks which can be crucial factors in the development of liver damage. (s. tab. 29.9)

1. Misidentification of the medicinal plant
2. Contamination of the plant
   – e.g. chemicals, heavy metals, microorganisms
3. Use of unsuitable or wrong parts of the plant
4. Variations in the formation of active plant substances due to changed conditions of growth
5. Adulteration of active agents during conditioning
6. Mislabelling of the end product

Tab. 29.9: Certain errors or risks involved in the preparation of herbal remedies

It is difficult to clarify the hepatotoxicity of herbal remedies, especially if they are comprised of a mixture of several plants or various components of one plant. Moreover, herbal remedies are often applied as automedication, and patients withhold the information that they have used them. (s. tab. 29.10) (s. fig. 29.15)

Plants containing pyrrolizidine alkaloids			
– Crotalaria			
– Heliotropium			
– Senecio			
– Symphytum officinale			
• These alkaloids are the main cause of VOD			
Reported hepatotoxicity	**Hepatitis**	**Necrosis**	**ALF**
Atractylis gummifera	+	+	(R)
Callilepsis laureola	+	+	(R)
Cascara sagrada	+		
Cassia angustifolia (Senna)	+		
Chinese herbs	+	+	(R)
Larrea tridentata (Chaparral) (46, 71, 131)	+	(R)	
Lycopodium serratum (Jin Bu Huan) (113)	+		(R)
Pennyroyal (Hedeoma pulegioides)	+	+	(R)
Piper methysticum (Kava) (124, 142)	+	+	+
Teucrium chamaedrys (Germander) (34, 115)	+	+	(R)
Viscum album	+	+	
Suspected hepatotoxicity			
Azadirachza indica	Scutellaria lacteriflora		
Berberis vulgaris	Teucrium polium (133)		
Borage officinalis	Valeriana officinalis etc.		

Tab. 29.10: Medicinal plants with reported or suspected facultative hepatotoxicity (ALF = acute liver failure, R = rare) (with some references)

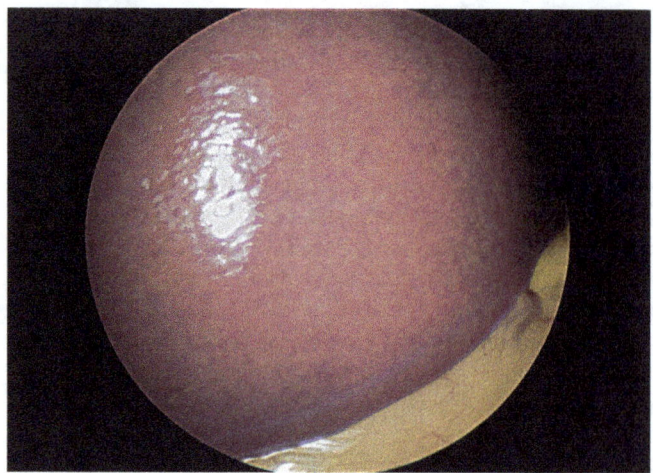

Fig. 29.15: Chronic toxic hepatitis after ten months chaparral ("creosote bush") automedication. • Laparoscopy: marked acinar structure, irregular chagreen-like surface (splintered light reflex) and extremely fine fibrosis. Histology: single cell necrosis, slight inflammatory infiltrations and moderate steatosis

Information about the effectiveness or safety of herbal remedies is based on experience transmitted over centuries rather than on controlled trials or toxicity studies. Numerous medicinal plants have been reported to possess facultative hepatotoxicity, or there is suspicion thereof. (16, 44, 63, 86, 90, 92, 97, 114, 118, 134, 135)

Kava extracts can, if overdosed (>60–120 mg kavapyrones/day) and/or taken over a longer period (>3 months), cause hepatotoxicity in the form of hepatic reactions and liver cell necrosis; in rare cases, they may even cause cholestasis and acute liver failure (possibly leading to liver transplantation). Risk factors include the concomitant intake of medicaments (especially St. John's Wort) and alcohol as well as a genetically based deficiency of cytochrome P 450 2 D6. (124, 142)

5.7 Test procedures

5.7.1 Withdrawal trial

The elimination of the causal noxa leads to an improvement in the pathological laboratory values, which represents an important diagnostic finding. This procedure constitutes the most significant therapeutic measure. • If various medicaments or substances are suspected to have caused the damage, one noxa after the other should be discontinued, and the effect of discontinuation on laboratory parameters should be tested after four to six weeks. The causal noxa normally "reveals itself" during this test. The drugs shown to be non-toxic can then be administered again, although laboratory parameters should be tested continuously to rule out any "false diagnosis". If a false diagnosis is established, the procedure (i.e. diagnostic and therapeutic withdrawal trial) will have to be repeated. • When hepatotoxicity due to home- or workplace-related exposure is suspected, laboratory parameters should be tested just *before* the patient goes on holiday as well as *immediately* after his/her return. This is of special significance if the patient is absent from work and/or home for at least two or three weeks. • Alcohol intake, in any form or quantity, must be prohibited during the withdrawal trial. This also applies to holiday trips that are intended to be used for such a test. • *Reliable results can only be achieved if the patient complies fully with the stringent requirements of a withdrawal trial and cooperates well!*

5.7.2 Re-exposure trial

▶ Re-exposure trials are regarded as *unacceptable* because dangerous exacerbations may occur. In addition, negative re-exposure trial results would not suffice to rule out drug-related liver damage completely.

> At present, there are no biochemical methods that facilitate early and reliable identification of the drug-induced toxicity causing the liver damage.

6 Prognosis

Patients with liver damage resulting from drug-induced toxicity mostly have a good prognosis. Changes regress completely after discontinuation of the implicated drug. However, it may take several weeks or months for the laboratory values and morphological findings to normalize. • Changes in the connective tissue remain (unless there is spontaneous reversal). These alterations appear histologically as fine periportal or periacinous fibroses (15), and laparoscopically as delicate, partly reticular fibroses, perivascular connective tissue or as a finely pimpled hepatic surface. (s. figs. 28.7, 28.10) • Vessels affected by thrombosis generally remain closed unless spontaneous thrombolysis or recanalization occurs. • Mortality is high for acute necrosing types of damage (e. g. 30–50% of halothane-induced cases). Prognosis is often poor when various toxins take effect at the same time. The disease can progress even though the causal toxin is eliminated. An autoimmune process may have been triggered, or another chemical substance may have taken over the function of the eliminated causal noxa.

7 Therapy

> ▶ Liver damage may not only be caused by a certain substance, but also by an interaction of a combination of substances (e.g. multidrug therapy, numerous constituents in plants) — moreover, this can happen in different individual ways.

The treatment of drug-induced liver damage comprises various measures: (*1.*) *Discontinuation* of the implicated noxa is regarded as the most effective therapy. • (*2.*) In cases of acute intoxication, *elimination* of the noxa from the body is essential (e.g. gastrointestinal lavage, forced diuresis) • (*3.*) In certain intoxications, the application of an *antidote* is required (e.g. N-acetylcysteine, silibinin, deferoxamine) (s. pp 387, 587, 644). • (*4.*) In lipid peroxidations, it is not known precisely to what extent a therapeutic effect is achieved by adjuvant treatment with *antioxidants*. (s. p. 72) • (*5.*) This also applies to adjuvant efforts to treat drug-induced *cholestasis* by reducing toxic-hydrophobic bile acids (e.g. lithocholic acid) with the help of ursodeoxycholic acid. The use of S-adenosyl-L-methionine has been considered in this context. (s. p. 249) EPL effectively inhibited the development of cyclosporine-induced cholestasis as well as liver damage due to antituberculous agents and cancer chemotherapy. (s. p. 587) • (*6.*) In rare cases, the use of glucocorticoids may be indicated. • (*7.*) *Symptomatic measures* can be undertaken in individual cases. They include increased intake of fluids and vitamins as well as electrolytes (if required). • (*8.*) In those patients who experience severe courses, the therapeutic measures are the same as in acute liver failure.

8 Hepatotoxic remedies (selection)

Medicaments	Jaundice	Cholestasis (with/without jaundice)	Cholestatic hepatitis	Hepatitis	Necrosis	Steatosis	Granuloma	Chronic hepatitis, Cirrhosis	Peliosis hepatis	Budd-Chiari syndrome, VOD	Adenoma	Focal nodular hyperplasia	Cholangitis	Ductopenia	Malignant tumours
Acarbose[+] (17, 60)			+												
Acenocoumarol (32)	+														
Acetohexamide			+					+							
Acetylsalicylic acid	+	+	+		+	+	+								
Acyclovir		+	+	+											
Acipimox		+													

Medicaments	Jaundice	Cholestasis (with/without jaundice)	Cholestatic hepatitis	Hepatitis	Necrosis	Steatosis	Granuloma	Chronic hepatitis, Cirrhosis	Peliosis hepatis	Budd-Chiari syndrome, VOD	Adenoma	Focal nodular hyperplasia	Cholangitis	Ductopenia	Malignant tumours
Adriamycine										+					
Ajmaline	+	+	+					+					+	+	
Albendazole				+											
Alendronate (30)				+		+									
Allopurinol[+]			+		+		+						+	+	
Alosetron (147)				+	+										
Amiodarone[+] (87)				+	+	+		+							
Amitriptyline		+	+	+	+								+	+	
Amoxicillin[+] (8, 48, 117)	+		+	+	+			+					+	+	
Amphotericin B[+]				+	+	+								+	
Aprindine				+	+										
Asparaginase (126)					+	+									
Azathioprine (120)		+	+	+			+	+	+	+		+	+	+	
Azithromycine (21)		+	+												
Barbiturates		+		+	+								+	+	
Bendazac				+											
Benosilate				+											
Benoxaprofen[+]				+	+										
Bromfenac[+] (62, 105)	+			+	+										
Buprobin	+		+												
Busulphan (41)	+	+								+		+			
Camustine										+					
Candesartan		+													
Captopril	+	+	+												
Carbamazepine[+] (40)		+	+	+	+			+					+	+	
Carbason				+											
Carbenicillin				+											
Carbenoxolone				+											
Carbimazole[+]			+	+	+	+	+								
Carbromal[+]					+										
Carbutamide	+			+										+	
Carisoprodol				+											
Carmustine					+					+					
Celecoxib (20)				+	+										
Cephalosporin		+	+					+							
Cetirizine (38)		+													
Chlorambucil	+	+	+	+				+		+					
Chloramphenicol	+	+		+	+										
Chlordiazepoxide				+	+										
Chlormezanone		+	+												
Chloroquine			+												
Chlorothiazide	+	+	+	+	+		+	+					+	+	
Chlorpromazine[+]	+	+	+	+	+			+	+				+	+	
Chlorpropamide	+	+	+	+				+							
Chlortetracycline			+		+	+									
Chlortalidone		+	+												
Chlorzotocin			+												
Cimetidine			+	+	+									+	
Ciprofloxacin (78, 161)		+	+	+	+										
Cisplatin			+		+										
Clofibrate				+			+					+			
Clomethiazole[+]				+	+			+							
Clopidogrel				+											
Clorazepat				+											
Cloxacillin (45)				+											
Clozapine[+] (91)	+		+	+	+			+							
Colchicine				+											
Contraceptives (36, 57, 98, 110, 149)	+	+	+		+			+	+	+	+	+		+	+
Cotrimoxazole[+]	+	+	+												
Cromoglicic acid													+		

Medicaments	Jaundice	Cholestasis (with/without jaundice)	Cholestatic hepatitis	Hepatitis	Necrosis	Steatosis	Granuloma	Chronic hepatitis, Cirrhosis	Peliosis hepatis	Budd-Chiari syndrome, VOD	Adenoma	Focal nodular hyperplasia	Cholangitis	Ductopenia	Malignant tumours
Cryoteron		+		+											
Cyclophosphamide				+	+					+					
Cyclosporine			+												
Cyproterone[+]				+	+										
Cytarabine		+								+	+				
Dacarbazine[+]										+	+				
Dactinomycin[+]		+		+	+					+	+				
Danazol[+]				+	+				+	+					
Dantrolene[+]			+	+	+	+		+							
Dapsone[+]	+		+												
Daunorubicin									+	+	+				
Desipramine[+]				+	+										
Dextropropoxyphene		+													
Diazepam	+			+	+		+						+		
Diclofenac (52)			+	+			+								
Dicoumarol[+] (18)		+	+												
Didanosine[+]		+	+												
Diethystilboestrol				+	+				+		+			+	+
Dihydralazine[+]	+	+		+	+			+					+		
Diltiazem				+	+			+							
Disopyramide			+	+											
Disulfiram[+] (160)	+		+	+	+										
Doxorubicin		+	+	+	+					+					
Duloxetine[+] (55)				+	+										
Ebrotidine[+] (4)	+			+	+										
Ecstacy[+] (58, 122)				+	+										
Enalapril			+	+	+										
Enflurane[+]				+	+										
Erythromycin[+]	+	+	+	+									+	+	
Etacrynic acid	+		+	+	+										
Ethambutol			+												
Ethinylestradiol			+	+	+										
Ethionamid (74)	+	+	+												
Etofoside				+	+										
Etretinate			+	+	+	+		+							
Exifon			+	+	+										
Ezetimibe (136)				+	+										
Famotidin				+											
Fenbufen				+	+										
Fenofibrate (43)				+	+			+				+			
Flavaspidic acid	+														
Floxuridine													+		
Flucloxacilline				+									+		
Fluconazole[+]				+	+										
Fluoxymesterone		+	+						+						+
Fluphenazine		+	+												
Flupirtin				+											
Flurazepam				+		+									
Flutamide[+] (25, 116)	+	+		+	+				+						
Furadantin			+	+	+		+		+						
Gabapentin		+													
Gatifloxacin	+			+	+										
Gemcitabine[+] (119)			+												
Glafenine				+	+										
Glibenclamide	+	+	+	+	+										
Gliclazide (23)				+	+										
Glimepiride (24)		+													
Glucocorticosteroids						+	+		+	+					

Medicaments	Jaundice	Cholestasis (with/without jaundice)	Cholestatic hepatitis	Hepatitis	Necrosis	Steatosis	Granuloma	Chronic hepatitis, Cirrhosis	Peliosis hepatis	Budd-Chiari syndrome, VOD	Adenoma	Focal nodular hyperplasia	Cholangitis	Ductopenia	Malignant tumours
Gold salts+) (9, 27)		+	+		+	+								+	
Griseofulvin	+	+	+												
Haloperidol		+	+					+							
Halothane+) (37, 50, 101)	+		+	+	+		+	+					+	+	
Heparin			+		+	+									
Hycanthon			+		+	+									
Hydralazine			+				+								
Hydrochlorothiazide				+	+		+								
Ibuprofen+)				+	+	+									
Idoxuridine		+													
Imatinib				+	+										
Imipramine+)		+	+	+	+										
Indomethacin+)			+	+	+	+									
Indinavir (162)	+												+	+	
Infliximab			+												
Interferone (14)								+							
Iprindol		+													
Iproclozide+)				+	+										
Iproniazid+) (59)		+	+	+	+										
Irbesartan (5)			+			+									
Iron sulphate				+	+		+								
Isocarboxazid+)				+	+										
Isoflurane+)				+	+										
Isoniazid+) (103, 152)	+		+	+	+	+	+	+							
Itraconazole (139)		+		+	+										
Ketoconazole+)			+	+	+										
Ketoprofen				+	+										
Labetolol		+		+											
Lamivudine				+											
Leflunomide (129)				+	+										
Levofloxacin+) (28)				+	+										
Lisinopril+)			+		+										
Losartan				+											
Lovastatin	+		+												
Mebendazol				+											
Mefloquine						+									
Megestrol acetate	+	+													
Mepacrine			+												
Meprobamate		+	+												
Mercaptopurine+)	+	+	+	+	+			+	+	+					
Mesalamine (13)							+								
Mesalazine (137)		+					+								
Mesantoin				+	+										
Mestranol				+											
Metformin		+		+											
Methamizol				+											
Methandienone	+	+													
Methandrostenolone		+		+		+									+
Methotrexate+) (140, 144, 150, 158)				+		+		+			+				+
Methoxyflurane				+	+	+									
Methyldopa+)				+	+	+	+	+							+
Methylpentinol		+													
Methyltestosterone		+		+	+			+	+	+	+	+	+	+	
Metolazone							+		+						
Metronidazol			+												
Mianserin			+	+											
Midecamycin (143)			+	+	+										
Minocycline+)			+	+	+										

Drug-induced liver damage

Medicaments	Jaundice	Cholestasis (with/without jaundice)	Cholestatic hepatitis	Hepatitis	Necrosis	Steatosis	Granuloma	Chronic hepatitis, Cirrhosis	Peliosis hepatis	Budd-Chiari syndrome, VOD	Adenoma	Focal nodular hyperplasia	Cholangitis	Ductopenia	Malignant tumours
Mirtazapine (61)	+														
Mithramycin				+	+	+									
Mitomycine			+	+	+										
Naproxen				+		+									
Natriumperchlorat			+		+										
Nefadozone[+)]		+	+												
Nevirapine[+)]				+											
Nicotinic acid			+	+	+					+					
Nifedipine	+	+	+			+									
Nimesulide[+)] (95, 151)				+	+										
Niperotidine[+)]				+											
Nitrofurantoin		+	+	+	+		+	+	+			+			
Nizatidine				+											
Nomifensine	+						+		+	+					
Norethandrolone	+		+						+						
Norethylnodrel		+		+	+			+							
Norfloxacin			+				+								
Nortriptyline[+)]		+	+	+											
Novobiocin	+		+	+									+		
Nystatin		+	+	+											
Obidoxime chloride	+	+													
Oleandomycin	+	+	+												
Omeprazol[+)]				+											
Ornidazole (138)			+												
Oxacillin		+	+	+		+	+								
Oxymetholone (146)		+	+						+		+				+
Oxyphenbutazone				+				+							
Oxyphenisatine				+	+			+	+						
Pamaquine				+											
Pantoprazole				+											
Papaverine		+	+				+								
Paracetamol[+)] (66, 81, 94, 96, 148)			+	+	+	+		+					+		
Paramethadione			+												
Paroxetin			+												
PAS		+	+	+	+			+							
Pemoline[+)]				+											
Penicillamine			+												
Penicillin			+	+	+		+	+							
Peracine				+											
Perhexiline			+	+		+		+						+	
Perphenazine			+	+	+										
Phenacetin	+	+	+												
Phenazone				+											
Phenazopyridine				+											
Phenelzin														+	
Phenformin		+													
Phenobarbital			+	+	+										
Phenprocoumon[+)] (102, 127)	+		+	+	+										
Phenylbutazone[+)]	+		+	+	+		+	+					+		
Phenyramidol (73)		+	+												
Phenytoin[+)]			+	+			+							+	
Pioglitazon			+												
Piperazine			+												
Piroxicam			+		+								+		
Polythiazide				+	+			+							
Prajmalium bitartrate		+	+				+								
Practolol													+		
Pravastatin (56)			+	+											

Medicaments	Jaundice	Cholestasis (with/without jaundice)	Cholestatic hepatitis	Hepatitis	Necrosis	Steatosis	Granuloma	Chronic hepatitis, Cirrhosis	Peliosis hepatis	Budd-Chiari syndrome, VOD	Adenoma	Focal nodular hyperplasia	Cholangitis	Ductopenia	Malignant tumours
Probenecid[+]				+	+										
Procainamide			+					+							
Procarbazine		+	+					+							
Prochlorperazine		+													
Promazine	+	+	+											+	
Promethazine			+											+	
Propafenone (29)			+												
Propylthiouracil[+] (64, 123, 154)	+	+		+	+	+	+								
Protionamide				+											
Pyrazinamide[+] (2, 70)	+			+	+	+									
Pyridylmethanol			+												
Pyrimethamine[+]				+	+										
Pyritinol				+											
Quinethazone		+	+												
Quinidine		+		+	+										
Rafecoxib			+												
Ramipril		+	+												
Ranitidine			+												
Reserpine		+													
Rifampicin[+] (77, 103)	+	+	+	+	+	+									
Risedronate				+	+										
Ritodrine (19)				+											
Rofecoxib (156)			+												
Rosiglitazone[+] (33, 99)	+		+		+		+								
Roxatidin				+											
Roxithromycine		+	+	+											
Sertraline (111)				+											
Sodium perchlorate[+]				+	+										
Spironolactone			+				+								
Stanozolol (51)	+	+		+											+
Stavudine				+	+										
Sulfasalazine[+]			+	+	+		+	+							
Sulfonamide[+]	+	+	+	+	+		+	+							
Sulindac			+	+	+	+									
Suloctidil			+	+											
Tacrine				+	+										
Tamoxifen	+	+								+					
Telithromycin (26)				+	+										
Tenoxicam (70, 145)														+	
Terbinafine			+												
Terfenadine (125)		+		+											
Testosterone		+		+	+										+
Tetrabamate[+]	+			+	+										+
Tetracycline[+]	+		+	+	+	+								+	
Thalidomide (54)				+	+										
Thiamazole	+	+		+		+									
Thioguanin		+								+					
Thiopental				+											
Thioridazine	+	+													
Tiabendazole[+]			+	+	+									+	
Ticlopidine (3, 49, 85, 100, 132)	+		+	+											
Tidozone					+										
Tolazamide		+	+	+											
Tolbutamide[+]		+	+				+	+					+	+	
Tolcapone[+] (11)															
Tolterodine		+		+		+									
Tranylcypromine					+	+									
Triaziquone		+													
Triazolam (67)			+	+	+										

Medicaments	Jaundice	Cholestasis (with/without jaundice)	Cholestatic hepatitis	Hepatitis	Necrosis	Steatosis	Granuloma	Chronic hepatitis, Cirrhosis	Peliosis hepatis	Budd-Chiari syndrome, VOD	Adenoma	Focal nodular hyperplasia	Cholangitis	Ductopenia	Malignant tumours
Trichlormethiazide							+								
Trifluoperazine		+													
Trimethadione		+	+	+	+										
Trimethoprim (157)				+	+									+	
Troglitazone⁺⁾ (47)				+	+										
Usnic acid (35)				+	+										
Valproic acid⁺⁾ (156)	+		+	+	+	+	+			+		+			
Verapamil	+	+	+	+	+										
Vinblastine										+					
Vincristine										+					
Vitamin A (107)			+	+					+	+					
Vitamin K	+			+											
Warfarin	+	+	+												
Zidovudin (22)	+			+	+	+									
Zonisamide (153)														+	
Zoxazolamine				+	+										

Table 29.11: Table of 314 (selected) medicaments potentially causing liver damage. (6, 84, 89, 108, 141) • ⁺⁾ Drugs which may cause acute liver failure or lethal liver damage. *(We would be grateful for any suggestions, corrections or additions)*

References:

1. **Aithal, P.G., Day, C.P.:** The natural history of histologically proved drug-induced liver disease. Gut 1999; 44: 731–735
2. **Al Sarraf, K.A.A., Michielsen, P.P., Hauben, E.I., Lefebure, A., Ramon, A.M., van Marck, E.A., Pelckmans, P.A.:** Hepatotoxicity after a short course of low-dose pyrazinamide. Acta Gastro-Enterol. Belg. 1996; 59: 251–253
3. **Amaro, P., Nunes, A., Macoas, F., Ministro, P., Baranda, J., Cipriano, A., Martins, I., Rosa, A., Pimenta, I., Donato, A., Freitas, D.:** Ticlopidine-induced prolonged cholestasis: a case report. Eur. J. Gastroenterol. Hepatol. 1999; 11: 673–676
4. **Andrade, R.J., Lucena, M.I., Martin-Vivaldi, R., Fernandez, M.C., Nogueras, F., Pelaez, G., Gomez-Outes, A., Garcia-Escano, M.D., Bellot, V., Hervas, A., Cardenas, F., Bermudez, F., Romero, M., Salmeron, J.:** Acute liver injury associated with the use of ebrotidine, a new H-2 receptor antagonist. J. Hepatol. 1999; 31: 641–646
5. **Andrade, R.J., Lucena, M.I., Fernandez, M.C., Vega, J.L., Garcia-Cortes, M., Casado, M., Guerrero-Sanchez, E., Pulido-Fernandez, F.:** Cholestatic hepatitis related to use of irbesartan: a case report and a literature review of antiotensin II antagonist-associated hepatotoxicity. Eur. J. Gastroenterol. Hepatol. 2002; 14: 887–890
6. **Andrade, R.J., Lucena, M.I., Fernandez, M.C.:** Drug-induced liver injury: an analysis of 461 incidences submitted to the spanish registry over a 10-year period. Gastroenterology 2005; 129: 512–521
7. **Andreu, V., Mas, A., Bruguera, M., Salmeron, J.M., Moreno, V., Nogue, S., Rodes, J.:** Ecstasy: a common cause of severe acute hepatotoxicity. J. Hepatol. 1998; 29: 394–397
8. **Barrio, J., Castiella, A., Lobo, C., Indart, A., Lopez, P., Garcia-Bengoechea, M., Cosme, A., Arenas, J.I.:** Hepatitis colestasica aguda secundaria a amoxicillina-acido clavulanico. Papel del acido ursodesoxicolico en la colestasis inducida por drogas. Rev. Esp. Enferm. Dig. 1998; 90: 523–526
9. **Basset, C., Vadrot, J., Denis, J., Poupon, J., Zafrani, E.S.:** Prolonged cholestasis and ductopenia following gold salt therapy (case report). Liver Internat. 2003; 23: 89–93
10. **Berson, A., Fréneaux, E., Larrey, D., Lepage, V., Douay, C., Mallet, C., Fromenty, B., Benhamou, J.-P., Pessayre, D.:** Possible role of HLA in hepatotoxicity. An exploratory study in 71 patients with drug-induced idiosyncratic hepatitis. J. Hepatol. 1994; 20: 336–342
11. **Borges, N.:** Tolcapone-related liver dysfunction. Implications for use in Parkinson′s disease therapy. Drug Saf. 2003; 26: 743–747
12. **Böttiger, L.E., Furhoff, A.K., Holmberg, L.:** Fatal reactions to drugs. A 10-year material from the Swedish Adverse Drug Reaction Committee. Acta Med. Scand. 1979; 205: 451–456
13. **Braun, M., Fraser, G.M., Kunin, M., Salamon, F., Kaspa, R.T.:** Mesalamine-induced granulomatous hepatitis. Amer. J. Gastroenterol. 1999; 94: 1973–1974
14. **Byrnes, V., Afdahl, N., Challies, T., Greenstein, P.E.:** Drug-induced liver injury secondary to interferon-beta (IFN-beta) in multiple sclerosis (case report). Ann. Hepatol. 2006; 5: 56–59
15. **Cadranel, J.-F., Cadranel, J., Buffet, C., Fabre, M., Pelletier, G., d'Agay, M.-F., Ink, O., Roche, A., Milleron, B., Etienne, J.-P.:** Nodular regenerative hyperplasia of the liver, peliosis hepatis, and perisinusoidal fibrosis. Gastroenterology 1990; 99: 268–273
16. **Cardenas, A., Restrepo, J.C., Sierra, F., Correa, G.:** Acute hepatitis due to Shen-Min. A herbal product derived from Polygonum multiflorum. J. Clin. Gastroenterol. 2006; 40: 629–632
17. **Carrascosa, M., Pascual, F., Aresti, S.:** Acarbose-induced acute severe hepatotoxicity. Lancet 1997; 349: 698–699
18. **Castedal, M., Aldenborg, F., Olsson, R.:** Fulminant hepatic failure associated with dicoumarol therapy. Liver 1998; 18: 67–69
19. **Ceriani, R., Borroni, G., Bissoli, F.:** Ritodrine-related liver injury. Case report and review of the literature. Ital. J. Gastroenterol. Hepatol. 1998; 30: 315–317
20. **Chamouard, P., Walter, P., Baumann, R., Poupon, R.:** Prolonged cholestasis associated with short-term use of celecoxib (case report). Gastroenterol. Clin. Biol. 2005; 29: 1286–1288
21. **Chandrupatla, S., Demetris, A.J., Rabinovitz, M.:** Azithromycin-induced intrahepatic cholestasis (case report). Dis. Dis. Sci. 2002; 47: 2186–2188
22. **Chariot, P., Drogou, I., de Lacroix-Szmania, I., Eliezer-Vanerot, M.C., Chazaud, B., Lombès, A., Schaeffer, A., Zafrani, E.S.:** Zidovudine-induced mitochondrial disorder with massive liver steatosis, myopathy, lactic acidosis, and mitochondrial DNA depletion. J. Hepatol. 1999; 30: 156–160
23. **Chitturi, S., Le, V., Kench, J., Loh, C., George, J.:** Gliclazide-induced acute hepatitis with hypersensitivity features. Dig. Dis. Sci. 2002; 47: 1107–1110
24. **Chounta, A., Zouridakis, S., Ellinas, C., Tsiodras, S., Zoumpouli, C., Kopanakis, S., Giamarellou, H.:** Cholestatic liver injury after glimepiridine therapy (case report). J. Hepatol. 2005; 42: 944–946
25. **Cicognani, C., Malavolti, M., Morselli-Labate, A.M., Sama, C., Barbara, L.:** Flutamide-induced toxic hepatitis. Potential utility of ursodeoxycholic acid administration in toxic hepatitis. Dig. Dis. Sci. 1996; 41: 2219–2221
26. **Clay, K.D., Hanson, J.S., Pope, S.D., Rissmiller, R.W., Purdum, P.P., Banks, P.M.:** Brief communication: Severe hepatotoxicity of telithromycin: Three case reports and literature review. Ann. Intern. Med. 2006; 144: 415–420

27. Closa, A.S., Rovira, E.C., Lopez, J.V.A., Gispert, J.S.: Necrosis hepatica submassiva asociada a tratamiento con salos de oro. Gastroenterol. Hepatol. 1983; 6: 468–470
28. Coban, S., Ceydilek, B., Ekiz, F., Erden, E., Soykan, I.: Levofloxacin-induced acute fulminant hepatic failure in a patient with chronic hepatitis B infection (case report). Ann. Pharmacol. 2005; 39: 1737–1740
29. Cocozella, D., Curciarello, J., Corallini, O., Olivera, A., Alburquerque, M.M., Fraquelli, E., Zamagna, L., Olenchuck, A., Cremona, A.: Propafenone hepatotoxicity – report of two new cases. Dig. Dis. Sci. 2003; 48: 354–357
30. Daifotis, A.G., Yates, A.J.: Liver damage due to alendronate. New Engl. J. Med. 2000; 343: 365–366
31. De Abajo, F.J., Montero, D., Madurga, M., Garcia Rodriguez, L.A.: Acute and clinically relevant drug-induced liver injury: a population based case-control study. Brit. J. Clin. Pharmacol. 2004; 58: 71–80
32. De Bruyne, E.L.E., Bac, D.J., de Man, R.A., Dees, A.: Jaundice associated with acenocoumarol exposure. Neth. J. Med. 1998; 52: 187–189
33. Dhawan, M., Agrawal, R., Ravi, J., Gulati, S., Silverman, J., Nathan, G., Raab, S., Brodmerkel, G.: Rosiglitazone-induced granulomatous hepatitis (case report). J. Clin. Gastroenterol. 2002; 34: 582–584
34. Dourakis, S.P., Papanikolaou, I.S., Tzemanakis, E.N., Hadziyannis, S.J.: Acute hepatitis associated with herb (Teucrium capitatum L.) administration (case report). Eur. J. Gastroenterol. Hepatol. 14: 693–695
35. Durazo, F.A., Lassman, C., Han, S.H.B., Saab, S., Lee, N.P., Kawano, M., Saggi, B., Gordon, S., Farmer, D.G., Yersiz, H., Goldstein, R.L.I., Ghobrial, M., Busuttil, R.W.: Fulminant liver failure due to usnic acid for weight loss (case report). Amer. J. Gastroenterol. 2004; 99: 950–952
36. Erpecum, van, K.J., Janssens, A.R., Ruiter, D.J., Kroon, H.M.J.A., Grond, A.J.K.: Generalized peliosis hepatis and cirrhosis after long-term use of oral contraceptives. J. Amer. Gastroenterol. 1988; 83: 572–575
37. Farrell, G., Prendergast, D., Murray, M.: Halothane hepatitis. Detection of a constitutional susceptibility factor. New Engl. J. Med. 1985; 313: 1310–1314
38. Fong, D.G., Angulo, P., Burgart, L.J., Lindor, K.D.: Cetirizine-induced cholestasis. J. Clin. Gastroenterol. 2000; 31: 250–253
39. Fontana, R.J., Obaid Shakil, A., Greenson, J.K., Boyd, I., Lee, W.M.: Acute liver failure due to amoxicillin and amoxicillin/clavulanate. Dig. Dis. Sci. 2005; 50: 1785–1790
40. Forbes, G.M., Jeffrey, G.P., Shilkin, K.B., Reed, W.D.: Carbamazepine hepatotoxicity: another cause of vanishing bile duct syndrome. Gastroenterology 1992; 102: 1385–1388
41. Foschi, F.G., Savini, P., Marano, G., Musardo, G., Bedeschi, E., Girelli, F., Emiliani, F., Aldi, M., D'Errico, A., Bernardi, M., Stefanini, G.F.: Focal nodular hyperplasia after busulfan treatment (case report). Dig. Liver Dis. 2005; 37: 619–621
42. Friis, H., Andreasen, P.B.: Drug-induced hepatic injury: an analysis of 1100 cases reported to the Danish Committee on Adverse Drug Reactions between 1978 and 1987. J. Intern. Med. 1992; 232: 133–138
43. Ganne-Carié, N., de Leusse, A., Guettier, C., Castera, L., Levecq, H., Bertrand, H.-J., Plumet, Y., Trinchet, J.-C., Beaugrand, M.: Hépatites d'allure auto-immune induites par les fibrates. Gastroenterol. Clin. Biol. 1998; 22: 525–529
44. Gioro, R., Hourmand-Ollivier, I., Mosquet, L., Rousselot, P., Salame, E., Piquet, M.A., Dao, T.: Fulminant hepatitis during self-medication with hydroalcoholic extract of green tea (case report). Eur. J. Gastroenterol. Hepatol. 2005; 17: 1135–1137
45. Goland, S., Malnick, St., D.H., Gratz, R., Feldberg, E., Geltner, D., Sthoeger, Z.M.: Severe cholestatic hepatitis following cloxacillin treatment. Postgrad. Med. J. 1998; 74: 59–60
46. Gordon, D.F., Rosenthal, G., Hart, J., Sirota, R., Baker, A.L.: Chaparral ingestion: the broadening spectrum of liver injury caused by herbal medications. J. Amer. Med. Ass. 1995; 273: 489–490
47. Graham, D.J., Green, L., Senior, J.R., Nourjah, P.: Troglitazone-induced liver failure: a case study. Amer. J. Med. 2003; 114: 299–306
48. Gresser, U.: Amoxicillin-clavulanic acid therapy may be associated with severe side effects – review of the literature. Eur. J. Med. Res. 2001; 6: 139–149
49. Grieco, A., Vecchio, F.M., Greco, A.V., Gasbarrini, G.: Cholestatic hepatitis due to ticlopidine: clinical and histological recovery after drug withdrawal. Case report and review of the literature. Europ. J. Gastroenterol. Hepatol. 1998; 10: 713–715
50. Gut, J., Christen, U., Huwyler, J.: Mechanisms of halothane toxicity: novel insights. Pharmacol. Ther. 1993; 58: 133–155
51. Habscheid, W., Abele, U., Dahm, H.H.: Anabolic steroids as a cause of severe cholestasis and renal failure in a bodybuilder. Dtsch. Med. Wschr. 1999; 124: 1029–1032
52. Hackstein, H., Mohl, W., Püschel, W., Stallmach, A., Zeitz, M.: Acute cholestatic hepatitis associated with diclofenac. Z. Gastroenterol. 1998; 36: 385–389
53. Hanger, F.M., Gutman, A.B.: Post-arsphenamine jaundice. Apparently due to obstruction of intrahepatic biliary tract. J. Amer. Med. Ass. 1940; 115: 263–271
54. Hanje, A.J., Shamp, J.L., Thomas, F.B., Meis, G.M.: Thalidomide-induced severe hepatotoxicity. Pharmacotherapy 2006; 26: 1018–1022
55. Hanje, A.J., Pell, L.J., Votolato, N.A., Frankel, W.L., Kirkpatrick, R.B.: Case report: Fulminant hepatic failure involving duloxetine hydrochloride. Clin. Gastroenterol. Hepatol. 2006; 4: 912–917
56. Hartleb, M., Rymarczyk, G., Januszewski, K.: Acute cholestatic hepatitis associated with pravastatin. Amer. J. Gastroenterol. 1999; 94: 1388–1390
57. Helling, T.S., Wood, W.G.: Oral contraceptives and cancer of the liver: a review with two additional cases. Amer. J. Gastroenterol. 1982; 77: 504–508
58. Henry, J.A., Jeffreys, K.J., Dawling, S.: Toxicity and deaths from 3,4-methylenedioxymethamphetamine ("ecstasy"). Lancet 1992; 340: 384–387
59. Homberg, J.C., Stelly, N., Andreis, I., Abuaf, N., Saadoun, F.: A new antimitochondrial antibody (anti-M6) in iproniazid-induced hepatitis. Clin. Exp. Immunol. 1982; 47: 93–102
60. Hsiao, S.H., Liao, L.H., Cheng, P.N., Wu, T.J.: Hepatotoxicity associated with acarbose therapy (case report). Ann. Pharmacother. 2006; 40: 151–154
61. Hui, C.K., Yuen, M.F., Wong, W.M., Lam, S.K., Lai, C.L.: Mirtazapine-induced hepatotoxicity (case report). J. Clin. Gastroenterol. 2002; 35: 270–271
62. Hunter, E.B., Johnston, P.E., Tanner, G., Pinson, C.W., Awad, J.A.: Bromfenac (Duract)-associated hepatic failure requiring liver transplantation. Amer. J. Gastroenterol. 1999; 94: 2299–2301
63. Ibanez, L., Perez, E., Vidal, X., Laporte, J.-R.: Prospective surveillance of acute serious liver disease unrelated to infectious, obstructive, or metabolic disease: epidemiological and clinical features, and exposure to drugs. J. Hepatol. 2002; 37: 572–580
64. Ichiki, Y., Akahoshi, M., Yamashita, N., Morita, C., Maruyama, T., Horiuchi, T., Hayashida, K., Ishibashi, H., Niho, Y.: Propylthiouracil-induced severe hepatitis: a case report and review of the literature. J. Gastroenterol. 1998; 33: 747–750
65. Idilman, R., Ersoz, S., Coban, S., Kumbasar, O., Bozkaya, H.: Antituberculous therapy-induced fulminant hepatic failure: successful treatment wit liver transplantation and nonstandard antituberculous therapy. Liver Transpl. 2006; 12: 1427–1430
66. James, L.P., Mayeux, P.R., Hinson, J.A.: Acetaminophen-induced hepatotoxicity. Drug Metab. Disp. 2003; 31: 1499–1506
67. Kanda, T., Yokosuka, O., Fujiwara, K., Saisho, H., Shiga, H., Oda, S., Okuda, K., Sugawara, Y., Makuuchi, M., Hirasawa, H.: Fulminant hepatic failure associated with triazolam. Dig. Dis. Sci. 2002; 47: 1111–1114
68. Kaplowitz, N.: Hepatotoxicity of herbal remedies: insights into the intricacies of plant-animal warfare and cell death. Gastroenterology 1997; 113: 1408–1412
69. Kaplowitz, N.: Biochemical and cellular mechanisms of toxic liver injury. Semin. Liver Dis. 2002; 22: 137–144
70. Katsinelos, P., Katsos, I., Patsiaoura, K., Xiarchos, P., Goulis, I., Eugenidis, N.: Tenoxicam-associated hepatic injury: a case report and review. Europ. J. Gastroenterol. Hepatol. 1997; 9: 403–406
71. Katz, M., Saibil, F.: Herbal hepatitis: subacute hepatic necrosis secondary to chaparral leaf. J. Clin. Gastroenterol. 1990; 12: 203–206
72. Knobel, B., Buyanowsky, G., Dan, M., Zaidel, L.: Pyrazinamide-induced granulomatous hepatitis. J. Clin. Gastroenterol. 1997; 24: 264–266
73. Köksal, A.S., Köklü, S., Filik, L., Sasmaz, N., Sahin, B.: Phenyramidol-associated liver toxicity. Ann. Pharmacol. 2003; 37: 1244–1246
74. Kuntz, E., Liehr, H., Pfingst, W.: Toxische Leberschäden durch Äthionamid. Dtsch. Med. Wschr. 1967; 92: 1718–1722
75. Kuntz, E., Ordnung, W., Schmidt, U., Wildhirt, E., Engels, Ch.: Leber und Umwelt. Eine anamnestische Praxisstudie. Kassenarzt 1988; 7: 32–40
76. Kuntz, E.: Lebererkrankungen aus der Sicht der niedergelassenen Ärzte. (Befragung von 2990 Ärzten). Notabene medici 1989; 19: 243–246
77. Kuntz, H.-D., Rausch, V.: Hepatotoxische Nebenwirkungen von Rifampicin – eine vergleichende Studie. Prax. Pneumol. 1977; 31: 925–932
78. Labowitz, J.K., Silverman, W.B.: Cholestatic jaundice induced by ciprofloxacin. Dig. Dis. Sci. 1997; 42: 192–194
79. Lammert, F., Matern, S.: Hepatopathien durch Medikamente. Schweiz. Rundsch. Med. 1997; 86: 1167–1171
80. Larrey, D., Pageaux, G.P.: Genetic predisposition to drug-induced hepatotoxicity. J. Hepatol. 1997; 26: 12–21
81. Larson, A.M., Polson, J., Fontana, R.J., Davern, T.J., Lalani, E., Hynan, L.S., Reisch, J.S., Schiodt, F.V., Ostapowicz, G., Shakil, A.O., Lee, W.M.: Acetaminophen-induced acute liver failure: Results of a United States multicenter, prospective study. Hepatology 2006; 42: 1364–1372
82. Lauterburg, B.H.: Arzneimittelschäden der Leber: Rolle von reaktiven Metaboliten und Pharmakokinetik. Schweiz. Med. Wschr. 1985; 115: 1306–1312
83. Lee, K.H., Lee, M.K., Sutedja, D.S., Lim, S.G.: Outcome from molecular adsorbent recycling system (MARS) (TM) liver dialysis following drug-induced liver failure. Liver Internat. 2005; 25: 973–977
84. Lee, W.M.: Drug-induced hepatotoxicity. New Engl. J. Med. 2003; 349: 474–485
85. Leone, N., Giordanino, C., Baronio, M., Morgando, A., David, E., Rizzetto, M.: Ticlopidine-induced cholestatic hepatitis successfully treated with corticosteroids: A case report. Hepatol. Res. 2004; 28: 109–112
86. Levitsky, J., Alli, T.A., Wisecarver, J., Sorell, M.F.: Fulminant liver failure associated with the use of black whosh (case report). Dig. Dis. Sci. 2005; 50: 538–539
87. Lewis, J.H., Mullick, F., Ishak, K.G., Ranard, R.C., Ragsdale, B., Perse, R.M., Rusnock, E.J., Wolke, A., Benjamin, S.B., Seeff, L.B., Zimmerman, H.J.: Histopathologic analysis of suspected amiodarone hepatotoxicity. Hum. Pathol. 1990; 21: 59–67

88. **Lewis, J.H., Ahmed, M., Shobassy, A., Palese, C.:** Drug-induced liver disease. Curr. Opin. Gastrornterol. 2006; 22: 223–233
89. **Ludwig, J., Axelsen, R.:** Drug effects on the liver. An updated tabular compilation of drugs and drug-related hepatic diseases. Dig. Dis. Sci. 1983; 28: 651–666
90. **Lynch, C.R., Folkers, M.E., Hutson, W.R.:** Fulminant hepatic failure associated with the use of black cohosh: A case report. Liver Transplant. 2006; 12: 989–992
91. **Macfarlane, B., Davies, S., Mannan, K., Sarsam, R., Pariente, D., Dooley, J.:** Fatal acute fulminant liver failure due to clozapine: a case report and review of clozapine-induced hepatotoxicity. Gastroenterology 1997; 112: 1707–1709
92. **MacGregor, F.B., Abernethy, V.E., Dahabra, S., Cobden, I., Hayes, P.C.:** Hepatotoxicity of herbal remedies. Brit. Med. J. 1989; 299: 1156–1157
93. **Maddrey, W.C.:** Drug-induced hepatotoxicity. J. Clin. Gastroenterol. 2005; 39: 83–89
94. **Mahadevau, S.B., McKiernan, P.J., Davies, P., Kelly, D.A.:** Paracetamol induced hepatotoxicity. Arch. Dis. Cildh. 2006; 91: 598–603
95. **McCormick, P.A., Kennedy, F., Curry, M., Taylor, O.:** Cox 2 inhibitor and fulminant hepatic failure. Lancet 1999; 353: 40–41
96. **McCormick, P.A., Treanor, D., McCormack, G., Farrell, M.:** Early death from paracetamol (acetaminophen) induced fulminant hepatic failure without cerebral oedema. J. Hepatol. 2003; 39: 547–551
97. **McRae, C.A., Agarwal, K., Mutimer, D., Bassendine, M.F.:** Hepatitis associated with Chinese herbs. Eur. J. Gastroenterol. Hepatol. 2002; 14: 559–562
98. **Meissner, K.:** Hemorrhage caused by ruptured liver cell adenoma following long-term oral contraceptives; a case report. Hepato-Gastroenterol. 1998; 45: 224–225
99. **Menees, S.B., Anderson, M.A., Chensue, S.W., Moseley, R.H.:** Hepatic injury in a patient taking rosiglitazone (case report). J. Clin. Gastroenterol. 2005; 39: 638–640
100. **Meyer, M.I., Kuhn, M., Bühler, H., Bertschinger, P.:** Ticlopidine-induced cholestasis. Schweiz. Med. Wschr. 1999; 129: 1405–1409
101. **Minoda, Y., Kharasch, E.D.:** Halothane-dependent lipid peroxidation in human liver microsomes is catalized by cytochrome P 450 2A6 (CYP 2A6). Anesthesiology 2001; 95: 509–514
102. **Mix, H., Wagner, S., Böker, K., Gloger, S., Oldhafer, K.J., Behrend, M., Flemming, P., Manns, M.P.:** Subacute liver failure induced by phenprocoumon treatment. Digestion 1999; 60: 579–582
103. **Moitinho, E., Salmeron, J.M., Mas, A., Bruguera, M., Rodes, J.:** Hepatotoxicidad grave por tuberculostaticos. Incremento de la incidencia. Gastroenterol. Hepatol. 1996; 19: 448–451
104. **Montessori, V., Harris, M., Montaner, J.S.G.:** Hepatotoxicity of nucleoside reverse transcriptase inhibitors. Semin. Liver Dis. 2003; 23: 167–171
105. **Moses, P.L., Schroeder, B., Alkhatib, O., Ferrentino, N., Suppan, T., Lidofsky, S.D.:** Severe hepatotoxicity associated with bromfenac sodium. Amer. J. Gastroenterol. 1999; 94: 1393–1396
106. **Navarro, V.J., Senior, J.R.:** Drug-related hepatotoxicity. New Engl. J. Med. 2006; 354: 731–739
107. **Nollevaux, M.C., Guiot, Y., Horsmans, Y., Leclercq, I., Rahier, J., Geubel, A.P., Sempoux, C.:** Hypervitaminosis A-induced liver fibrosis: Stellate cell activation and daily dose consumption. Liver Internat. 2006; 26: 182–186
108. **Novak, D., Lewis, J.H.:** Drug-induced liver disease. Curr. Opin. Gastroenterol. 2003; 19: 203–215
109. **O'Connor, N., Dargan, P.I., Jones, A.L.:** Hepatocellular damage from non-steroidal anti-inflammatory drugs. Quart. M. Med. 2003; 96: 787–791
110. **Palmer, J.R., Rosenberg, L., Kaufman, D.W., Warshauer, M.E., Stolley, P., Shapiro, S.:** Oral contraceptive use and liver cancer. Amer. J. Epidemiol. 1989; 130: 878–882
111. **Persky, S., Reinus, J.F.:** Sertraline hepatotoxicity – a case report and review of the literature on selective serotonin reuptake inhibitor hepatotoxicity (case report). Dis. Dis. Sci. 2003; 48: 939–944
112. **Pessayre, D.:** Role of reactive metabolites in drug-induced hepatitis. J. Hepatol. 1995; 23 (Suppl. 1) 16–24
113. **Picciotto, A., Campo, N., Brizzolara, R., Giusto, R., Guido, G., Sinelli, N., Lapertosa, G., Celle, G.:** Chronic hepatitis induced by Jin Bu Huan. J. Hepatol. 1998; 28: 165–167
114. **Pittler, M.H., Ernst, E.:** Systematic review: Hepatotoxic events associated with herbal medicinal products. Alim. Pharm. Ther. 2003; 18: 451–471
115. **Polymeros, D., Kamberoglou, D., Tzias, V.:** Acute cholestatic hepatitis caused by Teucrium polium (Golden germander) with transient appearance of antimitochondrial antibody. J. Clin. Gastroenterol. 2002; 34: 100–101
116. **Pontiroli, L., Sartori, M., Pittau, S., Morelli, S., Boldorini, R., Albano, E.:** Flutamide-induced acute hepatitis: investigations on the role of immunoallergic mechanisms. Ital. J. Gastroenterol. Hepatol. 1998; 30: 310–314
117. **Richardet, J.P., Mallat, A., Zafrani, E.S., Blazquez, M., Bognel, J.C., Campillo, B.:** Prolonged cholestasis with ductopenia after administration of amoxicillin/clavulanic acid. Dig. Dis. Sci. 1999; 44: 1997–2000
118. **Rifai, K., Flemming, P., Manns, M.P., Trautwein, C.:** Severe drug hepatitis caused by Chelidonium (case report). Internist 2006; 47: 496–751
119. **Robinson, K., Lambiase, L., Li, J.J., Monteiro, C., Schiff, M.:** Fatal cholestatic liver failure associated with gemcitabine therapy (case report). Dig. Dis. Sci. 2003; 48: 1804–1808
120. **Romagnuolo, J., Sadowski, D.C., Lalor, E., Jewell, L., Thomson, A.B.R.:** Cholestatic hepatocellular injury with azathioprine: A case report and review of the mechanisms of hepatotoxicity. Can. J. Gastroenterol. 1998; 12: 479–483
121. **Roots, I.:** Genetische Ursachen für die Variabilität der Wirkungen und Nebenwirkungen von Arzneimitteln. Internist 1982; 23: 601–609
122. **Roques, V., Perney, P., Beaufort, P., Hanslick, B., Ramos, J., Durand, L., Le Bricquir, Y., Blanc, F.:** Hépatite aiguë à l'ecstasy. Presse Med. 1998; 27: 468–470
123. **Ruiz, J.K., Rossi, G.V., Vallejos, H.A., Brenet, R.W., Lopez, I.B., Escribano, A.A.:** Fulminant hepatic failure associated with propylthiouracil. Ann. Pharmacother. 2003; 37: 224–228
124. **Russmann, S., Barguil, Y., Cabalion, P., Kritsanida, M., Duhet, D., Lauterburg, B.H.:** Hepatic injury due to traditional aqueous extracts of kava root in New Caledonia (case report). Eur. J. Gastroenterol. 2003; 15: 1033–1036
125. **Sahai, A., Villeneuve, J.:** Terfenadine-induced cholestatic hepatitis. Lancet 1996; 348: 552–553
126. **Sahoo, S., Hart, J.:** Histopathological features of L-asparaginase-induced liver disease. Semin. Liver Dis. 2003; 23: 295–299
127. **Seidl, C., Thomsen, R., Lohse, A., Grouls, V.:** Phenprocoumon-associated hepatitis. A rare complication of oral anticoagulation. Leber Magen Darm 1998; 28: 178–182
128. **Selim, K., Kaplowitz, N.:** Hepatotoxicity of psychotropic drugs. Hepatology 1999; 29: 1347–1351
129. **Sevilla-Mantilla, C., Ortega, L., Agundez, J.A.G., Fernandez-Gutierrez, B., Ladero, J.M., Diaz-Rubio, M.:** Leflunomide-induced acute hepatitis. Dis. Dis. 2004; 36: 82–84
130. **Sgro, C., Clinard, F., Ouazir, K., Chanay, H., Allard, C., Guilleminet, C., Lenoir, C., Lemoine, A., Hillon, P.:** Incidence of drug-induced hepatic injuries: a French population-based study. Hepatology 2002; 36: 451–455
131. **Sheikh, N.M., Philen, R.M., Love, L.A.:** Chaparral-associated hepatotoxicity. Arch. Intern. Med. 1997; 157: 913–919
132. **Skurnik, Y.D., Tchemiak, A., Edlan, K., Sthoeger, Z.:** Ticlopidine-induced cholestatic hepatitis. Ann. Pharmacother. 2003; 37: 371–375
133. **Starakis, I., Siagris, D., Leonidou, L., Mazokopakis, E., Tsamandas, A., Karatza, C.:** Hepatitis caused by the herbal remedy reucrium polium L. (case report). Eur. J. Gastroenterol. Hepatol. 2006; 18: 681–683
134. **Stickel, F., Pöschl, G., Seitz, H.K., Waldherr, R., Hahn, E.G., Schuppan, D.:** Acute hepatitis induced by Greater Celandine (Chelidonium majus). Scand. J. Gastroenterol. 2003; 38: 565–568
135. **Stickel, F., Egerer, G., Seitz, K.H.:** Hepatotoxicity of botanicals. Public Health Nutr. 2000; 3: 113–124
136. **Stolk, M.F.J., Becx, M.C.J.M., Kuypers, K.C., Seldenrijk, C.A.:** Severe hepatic side effects of ezetimibe. Clin. Gastroenterol. Hepatol. 2006; 4: 908–911
137. **Stoschus, B., Meybehm, M., Spengler, U., Scheurlen, C., Sauerbruch, T.:** Cholestasis associated with mesalazine therapy in a patient with Crohn's disease. J. Hepatol. 1997; 26: 425–428
138. **Tabak, F., Ozaras, R., Erzin, Y., Celik, A.F., Ozbay, G., Senturk, H.:** Ornidazole-induced liver damage: report of three cases and review of the literature. Liver Internat. 2003; 23: 351–354
139. **Talwakar, J.A., Soetikno, R.E., Carr-Locke, D.L., Berg, C.L.:** Severe cholestasis related to itraconazole for the treatment of onychomycosis. Amer. J. Gastroenterol. 1999; 94: 3632–3633
140. **ter Borg, E.J., Seldenrijk, C.A., Timmer, R.:** Liver cirrhosis due to methotrexate in a patient with rheumatoid arthritis. Nederl. J. Med. 1996; 49: 244–246
141. **Teschke, R.:** Drug-induced liver diseases. Z. Gastroenterol. 2002; 40: 305–326
142. **Teschke, R.:** Kava, kavapyrones and toxic liver injury. Z. Gastroenterol. 2003; 41: 395–404
143. **Thevenot, T., Mathurin, P., Martinez, F., Moussalli, J., Poynard, T., Opolon, P., Chosidow, O.:** Acute hepatitis during hypersensitivity syndrome due to midecamycin. Europ. J. Gastroenterol. Hepatol. 1997; 9: 1249–1250
144. **Tilling, L., Townsend, S., David, J.:** Methotrexate and hepatic toxicity in rheumatoid arthritis and psoriatic arthritis. Clin. Drug Invest. 2006; 26: 55–62
145. **Trak-Smayra, V., Cazals-Hatem, D., Asselah, T., Duchatelle, V., Degott, C.:** Prolonged cholestasis and ductopenia associated with tenoxicam (case report). J. Hepatol. 2003; 39: 125–128
146. **Treuner, J., Niethammer, D., Flach, A., Fischbach, H., Schenck, W.:** Hepatozelluläres Karzinom nach Oxymetholonbehandlung. Med. Welt 1980; 31: 952–955
147. **Turgeon, D.K., Tayeh, N., Fontana, R.J.:** Acute hepatitis associated with alosetron (Lotrones®) (case report). J. Clin. Gastroenterol. 2005; 39: 641–642
148. **Vale, J.A., Proudfoot, A.T.:** Paracetamol (acetaminophen) poisoning. Lancet 1995; 346: 547–552
149. **Valla, D., Le, M.G., Poynard, T., Zucman, N., Rueff, B., Benhamou, J.-P.:** Risk of hepatic vein thrombosis in relation to recent use of oral contraceptives. A case-control study. Gastroenterology 1986; 90: 807–811
150. **van Outryve, S., Schrijvers, D., van den Brande, J., Wilmes, P., Bogers, J., van Marck, E., Vermorken, J.B.:** Methotrexate-associated liver toxicity in a patient with breast cancer: case report and literature review. Netherl. J. Med. 2002; 60: 216–222
151. **Van Steenbergen, W., Peeters, P., de Bondt, J., Staessen, D., Büscher, H., Laporta, T., Roskams, T., Desmet, V.:** Nimesulide-induced acute hepatitis: evidence from six cases. J. Hepatol. 1998; 29: 135–141

152. **Vasudeva, R., Woods, B.:** Isoniazid-related hepatitis. Dig. Dis. 1997; 15: 357–367
153. **Vuppalanchi, R., Chalasani, N., Saxena, R.:** Restoration of bile ducts in drug-induced vanishing bile duct syndrome due to zonisamide (case report). Amer. J. Surg. Pathol. 2006; 30: 1619–1623
154. **Williams, K.V., Nayak, S., Becker, D., Reyes, J., Burmeister, L.A.:** Fifty years of experience with propylthiouracil-associated hepatotoxicity: what have we learned? J. Clin. Endocrin. Metabol. 1997; 82: 1727–1733
155. **Willmore, L.J., Triggs, W.J., Pellock, J.M.:** Valproate toxicity: risk-screening strategies. J. Child. Neurol. 1991; 6: 3–6
156. **Yan, B., Leung, Y., Urbanski, S.J., Myers, R.P.:** Rofecoxib-induced hepatotoxicity: A forgotten complication of te coxiber. (case report). Canad. J. Gastroenterol. 2006; 20: 351–355
157. **Yao, F., Behling, C.A., Saab, S., Li, S., Hart, M., Lyche, K.D.:** Trimethoprim-sulfamethoxazole-induced vanishing-bile duct syndrome. Amer. J. Gastroenterol. 1997; 92: 167–169
158. **Zachariae, H., Kragballe, K., Sogaard, H.:** Methotrexate induced cirrhosis: studies including serial liver biopsies during continued treatment. Brit. J. Dermatol. 1980; 102: 407–412
159. **Zafrani, E.S., Pinaudeau, Y., Dhumeaux, D.:** Drug-induced vascular lesions of the liver. Arch. Intern. Med. 1983; 143: 495–502
160. **Zala, G., Schmidt, M., Bühler, H.:** Fulminant hepatitis caused by disulfiram. Dtsch. Med. Wschr. 1993; 118: 1355–1360
161. **Zimpfer, A., Propst, G., Mikuz, G., Vogel, W., Terracciano, L., Stadlmann, S.:** Ciprofloxacin-induced acute liver injury: case report and review of literature. Virch. Arch. 2004; 444: 87–89
162. **Zucker, S.D., Qin, X.F., Rouster, S.D., Yu, F., Green, R.M., Keshavan, P., Feinberg, J., Sherman, K.E.:** Mechanism of indinavir-induced hyperbilirubinemia. Proc. Nat. Acad. Sci. USA 2001; 98: 12671–12676

Clinical Aspects of Liver Diseases

30 Liver damage due to toxic substances

		Page:
1	*Historical review*	580
2	*Detoxification of toxic substances*	581
3	*Pathophysiology*	582
4	*Morphology*	582
5	**Toxic substances**	582
5.1	Regulations governing occupational diseases	583
5.2	*Industrial toxins*	584
5.2.1	Halogenated hydrocarbons	584
5.2.2	Hydrocarbon derivatives	585
5.2.3	Aromatic amines	585
5.2.4	Inorganic substances	586
5.2.5	Thorotrast	586
5.3	*Mycotoxins*	586
5.4	*Phytotoxins*	587
5.4.1	3,4-benzpyrene	587
5.4.2	Pyrrolizidine alkaloids	587
5.4.3	Amanita phalloides	587
5.4.4	Helvella esculenta	588
5.5	*Endotoxins*	588
5.6	*Drugs*	588
6	**Diagnostics**	588
6.1	Chronic intoxication	588
6.2	Acute poisoning	589
7	*Therapeutic aspects*	589
8	**Industrial hepatotoxic agents**	590
	• References (1–78)	591
	(Figures 30.1–30.3; tables 30.1–30.3)	

30 Liver damage due to toxic substances

The *"chemicalization" of the environment* in the course of the last 100 years has proceeded virtually without restraint, on the one hand as a result of ever-advancing technologies and on the other hand because of the continuously rising demands of society and increased industrial productivity. • The liver, however, which is at the centre of the detoxification mechanisms (s. pp 56–61), is not in a position to adapt to new demands on the detoxification process within three to four generations. Adaptations of this kind by an organ or an organism to harmful or life-threatening influences can only take place over a much longer period of time, if at all (as has indeed been shown on numerous occasions in the animal and plant kingdoms).

The *"chemicalization" of the workplace* can be kept almost completely under control by compliance with industrial hygiene regulations. In this way, it is generally possible to avoid toxic liver damage. Specific **exposure** can, however, be expected in *occupational medicine* in the following situations: (*1.*) inadequate protective measures at work, (*2.*) the appearance of new, hitherto unforeseen or (as yet) unknown toxic compounds following a particular incident or due to a change in working techniques, and (*3.*) the combined impact of various toxic substances, especially in conjunction with alcohol and/or drugs. • In *agriculture*, the increasing use of fertilizers, animal feed additives, preservatives and pesticides has become a considerable problem. The occurrence of disulfiram-like effects has also been observed. • Generally, insufficient attention is paid to the risks of toxic liver damage encountered in *hobbies* or *do-it-yourself activities*. Handling chemical substances — frequently in small, poorly ventilated rooms over lengthy periods of time — can easily increase the danger of liver damage although under normal circumstances there is basically nothing to fear if the manufacturer's instructions are strictly adhered to. Nevertheless, it could happen that the risk of damaging one's own health is unconsciously suppressed or indeed goes unnoticed.

For every liver disease that cannot be clarified with certainty, each differential diagnosis should always include toxic substances in food, at work, in the house or garden and in those places where people pursue leisure activities. It is extremely difficult to identify the causal noxa. In the individual case, however, identification can be of considerable importance for general assessment purposes and possibly when an expertise is required.

1 Historical review

▶ In the nineteenth century, cases were observed of workers in the match industry who suffered liver damage due to **phosphorus** contamination leading to acute hepatic dystrophy. • *Since then, the relationship between exogenous noxae and liver disease has been considered unequivocal.*

Arsenic: Liver damage due to arsenic was first described in 1774 by F. L. Bang. In 1888 E. Ziegler et al. reported on damage caused by arsenic to the hepatocytes and sinusoids with subsequent scarring. The occurrence of melanosis, hyperkeratosis and liver fibrosis or cirrhosis was described as *"Reichenstein's disease"* (L. Geyer, 1898). It was observed in Reichenstein (Silesia) and Freiberg (Saxony) and traced back to chronic arsenic poisoning through contaminated drinking water (containing up to 25 mg arsenic per litre). Toxic liver damage, even culminating in cirrhosis, due to the presence of arsenic in beer was observed in 1900. Over the following years, there were further reports of arsenic poisoning from drinking water, e.g. in Argentina (A. Ayerza, 1918), Mexico and Taiwan. In 1974 a comprehensive study was published on chronic arsenic poisoning caused by contamination of the river Tononce in Antofagasta (Chile): several hundred people became ill between 1955 and 1972; arsenic was even found in fruit juice, beer and cola as well as in milk and food. (77) • Arsenic was officially introduced as a pesticide in viniculture in 1925 (after being used for this purpose for some time!). Since 1942 its use as a pesticide has been banned. Consumption of the so-called *wine-grower's house drink* led to severe liver damage, liver fibrosis with portal hypertension and even oesophageal varix bleeding, carcinoma and haemangioendothelioma of the liver. This homemade wine, which was produced by watering down the wine obtained from a second pressing of the grape skins and which had a low alcohol (3–5 vol. %) but high arsenic content, was consumed in large quantities (3–5 litres per day). • The severe arsenic poisoning of an aircraft pilot who had been spraying arsenic calcium carbonate dust as a pesticide was reported in 1930. • Extensive liver damage was also observed during the long-term treatment of psoriasis with Fowler's solution. • Cases of well-water poisoning due to arsenic pesticides were registered as late as 1984 in the USA (2) (s. p. 586) and again in 1998 to an incredible extent in Bangladesh.

Thorotrast: Thorotrast was introduced into radiology by K. Frik et al. in 1928 on the grounds of its excellent opaque properties and good tolerance. As early as 1933, the carcinogenic effect of ThO_2 was pointed out by

C. OBERLING et al. The occurrence of an angiosarcoma 12 years after the administration of thorotrast was reported by H. E. McMahon et al. in 1947. Production was stopped in 1950, but thorotrast was still occasionally used up to 1958. All in all, about one million patients using thorotrast between 1928 and 1958 were examined. ^{232}ThO$_2$ is a 90% α-emitter with a half-life of approximately 400 years. It is never excreted from the body. Most of it (70−75 %) is stored in the liver, although the highest relative concentration per gram tissue is found in the spleen. In total, more than 125 thorotrast-induced cases of malignancy have been reported in the literature − even 36, 39 and 44 years after administration. (23, 72) (s. figs. 30.2, 30.3) (s. p. 586)

Thioacetamide: In 1942 thioacetamide was introduced in the USA as a citrus fruit preservative. Shortly after ingestion of this fruit, liver damage (cell necrosis, steatosis) and cirrhosis occurred. There were even reports of fatalities. • Animal experiments showed that the liver damage was caused with such rapidity and reliability by thioacetamide that this substance came to be used as the most potent poison (apart from CCl$_4$) for producing liver damage in animal experiments.

Vinyl chloride: Hepatolienal diseases caused by vinyl chloride (VC) were first reported in Russia in 1949 (S. L. TRIBUKH et al.). Severe changes to the liver were observed by J. M. CORDIER et al. in France in 1960 and by J. SUCIU et al. in Romania in 1963. The carcinogenic effect of VC was demonstrated by P. L. VIOLA in animal experiments in 1970. Vinyl chloride can induce two different types of liver tumour: haemangiosarcoma and hepatocellular carcinoma (C. MALTONI et al., 1974). J. B. BLOCK reported on haemangiosarcoma in more detail in 1974, and in 1976 J. M. GOKEL et al. described hepatocellular carcinoma in persons exposed to VC. The two forms of carcinoma may also occur simultaneously. (s. p. 584)

Hexachlorobenzene: Between 1955 and 1959, more than 3,000 people in Turkey contracted porphyria cutanea tarda after hexachlorobenzene had been used as a preservative for cereals. (53)

Aflatoxin: Fatal liver necrosis was reported in about 100,000 turkeys and ducks in England by A. J. STEVENS et al. in 1960. The causative agent was found to be aflatoxin from mouldy peanut meal derived from animal feed. (s. p. 587)

Methylene dianiline: In 1965 at least 84 people in the English town of Epping contracted toxic hepatitis with jaundice and cholestasis (= **Epping disease**) after eating bread which contained flour that had been contaminated by a hardening agent for synthetic resin: methylene dianiline (4.4′-diaminodiphenyl methane). Histology showed signs of portal infiltrations, manifestations of cholangitis and centrilobular cholestasis. Pronounced hepatomegaly was also reported. (33, 34, 49) (s. p. 585)

Polybrominated diphenylene: In 1973 in the USA, about 30,000 cattle and some 1.6 million chickens died or had to be slaughtered (so-called "Michigan catastrophe") after being given feed to which a flame retardant containing polybrominated diphenylene had been mistakenly added in place of a fattening additive. Fortunately, however, none of the exposed persons showed any signs of poisoning. (1)

Dioxin: The first (8-fold chlorinated) dioxin was prepared as early as 1872 by the German chemists MERZ and WEITH. Tetrachlorodiphenyl-p-dioxin ("dioxin") was synthesized in 1957 (W. SANDERMANN et al.). The first large-scale case of intoxication was reported in Virginia/USA in 1949. Following the accident at the BASF chemical plant in Germany in 1953, 6 of the affected 53 persons developed liver damage. In the period leading up to the chemical disaster in Seveso/Italy on 10th July in 1976, there had been 21(!) such incidents reported in various countries, 6 of them in Germany (B. HOLMSTEDT, 1980). Following Seveso, some 27 years after the first chemical accident with dioxin in 1949, the irresponsible underestimation and ignorance of "chloracne" poisoning − known for nearly three decades − finally became public knowledge. (s. p. 585) Only then was it evident that dioxin was *"the most toxic carcinogenic and teratogenic chemical substance ever made by man"*.

Salad oil: Since 1981 more than 24,000 persons have become ill (with 357 fatalities up to 1985) in Spain due to the consumption of salad oil. The suspected cause was poisoning by oil which had been adulterated by being mixed with cheap industrial oil containing, among other things, aniline, acetanilide and quinoline. The patients showed generalized damage to the capillaries, including those of the liver. (65, 73)

2 Detoxification of toxic substances

Like medicaments, toxic substances can also enter the body by the oral, percutaneous, parenteral and respiratory routes. The detoxification and elimination of toxic substances essentially takes place via the same **biotransformation** mechanisms that are responsible for the metabolism of drugs. (s. p. 558) Overall, the capacity of the liver to eliminate foreign substances is dependent both on microsomal enzyme activity (which is affected by a number of factors) and on the blood flow through the liver. (s. tab. 3.18) Biotransformation can, however, lead to the production of **biotoxometabolites** (or biotoxometabonates), which are sometimes considerably more toxic than the original substance taken up by the body or which (by reacting with cellular proteins) can lead to the development of new hazardous substances such as mutagens, carcinogens or antigens. (s. pp 56−61) (s. fig. 3.11) For the elimination of various toxic substances including cadmium, manganese, lead, etc., the **functions of the RES** are also utilized. (s. p. 69) In addition, the

antioxidant systems may sometimes be necessary for the elimination of other toxic substances. (s. p. 72)

3 Pathophysiology

While medicaments (with few exceptions) can be regarded as facultative (indirect) hepatotoxins, almost all toxic chemicals act as obligate (direct) hepatotoxins. (s. tab. 29.1; s. fig. 29.1) • The extent and type of hepatic damage caused by toxic substances is determined by a number of influencing **factors.** (s. tab. 30.1)

1. Amount of noxious substance
2. Concentration
3. Duration of action
4. Method of uptake
5. Extent of protein binding
6. Degree of distribution or accumulation of the noxa within the liver or other organs
7. Radioactivity of the substance
8. Excretability of the noxa
9. Previous liver damage or coexisting liver disease
10. Coexistent strain caused by alcohol and drugs
11. Age, gender
12. Nutritional status

Tab. 30.1: Factors influencing the extent and type of liver damage caused by toxic substances

A variety of cellular sites of attack, sometimes very difficult to differentiate and often in combination with one another, have to be considered with regard to the **pathomechanisms** of liver damage. (s. tab. 30.2)

1. Direct toxic damage to membranes and organelles
2. Occurrence of biotoxometabolites
3. Formation of free radicals
4. Interactions with DNA
5. Interference with bilirubin metabolism
6. Interference with bile acid metabolism
7. Inhibition of protein synthesis
8. Inhibition of lipoprotein synthesis

Tab. 30.2: Pathogenic and pathophysiological mechanisms of liver damage caused by toxic substances

Liver damage due to toxic substances sometimes only appears and becomes recognizable after a latent period of several years. This applies especially to radioactive substances (e.g. thorotrast, with a latent period of up to 40 years). Exogenous factors (alcohol, medicaments and chemicals) can substantially impair the course and prognosis of intoxication. This may be due to (*1.*) acute multiple intoxication by simultaneous exposure to various toxic substances or (*2.*) the fact that the noxa is administered during the "deficiency period" of a biotransformative induction, since toxic substances cause greater hepatic lesions in this phase.

In the individual case, the personal reaction to exposure to toxic substances can vary greatly. Long-term exposure to toxins, even in low concentrations, often leads to liver damage. (66)

4 Morphology

Upon the intake of direct toxic noxae, the detoxification systems of the liver are only able to react with adaptive processes in isolated cases. The "force of the respective toxicity" leads to cell damage so rapidly that there is generally no chance for time-consuming adaptation to take place.

Morphological changes due to toxic substances are characterized by **four parenchymal alterations,** which also occur in alcohol-mediated or drug-induced liver damage: (*1.*) enlargement of cells, (*2.*) steatosis, (*3.*) cholestasis, and (*4.*) necrosis. These changes are not specific to particular noxae, even though a certain pattern of damage may predominate. There are frequent reports concerning fulminant liver failure. • In addition to these parenchymal changes, there may also be **mesenchymal reactions** with stellate cell activation, portal infiltration, reticular fibre sclerosis, fibrosis and vascular changes. Parenchymal and mesenchymal alterations of varying degrees often occur in combination. • After **long-term exposure,** the occurrence of liver fibrosis, cirrhosis or even malignant tumours can be expected.

5 Toxic substances

Toxically relevant substances have been recognized as such either as a result of animal experiments or casuistic observations. Here, too, it has been seen that findings from animal experiments can only be applied to humans to a certain extent. The dosage and duration of exposure are extremely relevant: the lesion pattern after acute, high exposure (e.g. in an accident or attempted suicide) can differ considerably from that after chronic exposure (to both high and low quantities). • A clear differentiation must be made from *naturally occurring liver noxae and carcinogens*. These can be present in plants, particularly in fungi (e.g. 3.4′-benzpyrene) and in bacteria (e.g. ethionine, endotoxins, 3.4′-benzpyrene). As a result, beverages and foodstuffs sometimes contain toxic substances, which were present naturally in the original raw material, derive from intentionally added pesticides, preservatives and animal feed, or have been inadvertently introduced into the final product in some way. (s. tab. 30.3)

▶ **Survey:** In 1988 we carried out a survey in 2,008 doctor's practices (37): liver damage was ascertained in 7,095 patients and confirmed morphologically in one third of cases. Long-term exposure to commercially available chemicals was found in 9.3% of those questioned, whereby the liver damage was ascribed to such chemical noxae in 7.4% of cases. Regular simultaneous alcohol consumption was confirmed by 34.1% of these patients. The following (in order of frequency) were found to be long-term contact noxae probably responsible for liver damage: hydrocarbons, carbon tetrachloride, lead, phenols, trichloroethylene, methyl alcohol, aniline, vinyl chloride, chloroform, heavy metals, pesticides and herbicides, lyes, carbides, glue, nitrosamines, inorganic acids and dioxins. (s. tab. 30.3)

▶ **Survey:** In a further survey in 2,650 doctor's practices in Germany (G) and 340 in Austria (A) carried out by us in 1989, the following statistics were obtained (38): existing *acute liver disease* was ascribed to household chemicals in 11.2% (G) and 9.3% (A) of patients. The most common cause of existing *chronic liver disease* was thought to be job-related noxae in 23.4% (G) and 21.8% (A) of cases; household chemicals were held to be responsible in 8.3% (G) and 7.2% (A) of patients. Sectors associated with the development of job-related toxic liver damage were found to be as follows: painting and varnishing trades in 46.0% (G) and 41.8% (A), mineral oil processing industries (including the production of solvents, dyes and adhesives) in 35.0% (G) and 30.8% (A), dry cleaning in 28.4% (G) and 38.8% (A), pesticide production in 27.6% (G) and 24.8% (A), and food preservation in 2.5% (G) and 3.3% (A) of cases. • Genuine proof that the respective noxa is the real and sole cause of the disease can naturally only be provided in a small number of cases. However, the high patient figures in Austria and former West Germany considerably increase the validity of these findings. (s. tab. 30.3)

5.1 Regulations governing occupational diseases

In the current German regulations on *occupational diseases due to industrial toxins*, the respective substances are divided into six classes and assigned specific numbers. *Occupational disease* is a legal term defined under German accident insurance law; *occupation-related disease* is a medical diagnosis. In individual cases, diseases are recognized as occupation-related and appropriate compensation is awarded, provided that they meet the pertinent legal requirements based on the most recent level of medical knowledge (so-called *opening clause*). The following are of importance in hepatology:

Arsenic and its compounds
Benzene and its homologues
Dimethylformamide
Halogenated alkyl, aryl or alkylaryl oxides
Halogenated hydrocarbons
Methyl alcohol (methanol)
Nitrobenzene or amino-benzene compounds (with their homologues or derivatives)
Phosphorus and its inorganic compounds

▶ When there are *good reasons for suspecting* the existence of an *occupation-related disease*, this must be reported immediately to the regional medical officer responsible for workplace health and safety, the respective governmental department for industrial medicine or directly to the appropriate industrial accident insurance provider. • Notification is mandatory for every registered doctor and dentist. No declaration of consent by the insured person is necessary, nor is there any right of objection. Notification does not constitute a breach of doctor-patient confidentiality. Insured persons or the employer can also report a suspected occupation-related disease themselves. In 1995 a total of 86,705 suspected cases were reported in Germany, of which about one fifth were accepted as occupational diseases.

▶ The doctor's obligation to report cases or suspected cases of poisoning is laid down in the German regulations on notification concerning toxic substances. This notification must be made in accordance with the *German chemicals law* using an appropriate form.

▶ *Food poisoning* does not have to be reported to the authorities unless it involves a disease covered by the German Epidemic Control Act. It is, however, strongly advisable to inform the appropriate authorities when food poisoning occurs or is suspected (see, for example, regulations relating to aflatoxin).

As regards **clarification by a medical expert,** four points are of great importance: (*1.*) gathering information for compiling a comprehensive job-history (specific job characteristics, exposure pattern, materials used, presence of additional chemical substances at the workplace), (*2.*) objectifying and quantifying the suspected liver noxa in the air (i. e. maximum allowable concentration) and in the biological material used for the job, (*3.*) assessment of the hepatotoxic potency of the working materials on humans, and (*4.*) exclusion of other possible causal factors (previous or present liver disease, alcohol, metabolic diseases, medicaments). In individual cases, discussion will focus on the extent or deterioration of already existing damage. Possible interference from potentially injurious factors must be taken into account. • The **measures for combating** such occupation-related diseases are based on the principles of the respective employers' liability insurance:

1. **Prophylactic medical measures**   – recruitment criteria   – monitoring criteria
2. **Technical measures**   – informing staff members   – ventilation, monitoring the air in rooms (industrial threshold values), protective clothing, masks   – technical modifications
3. **Medical and social measures**   – acceptance as an occupational disease, *etc.*

An individual's **reduction in earning capacity** is assessed in accordance with the usual criteria for evaluating liver diseases: (*1.*) fatty liver (20–40%), (*2.*) toxic hepatitis

(20–40%), (3.) chronic hepatitis (40–60%), (4.) liver cirrhosis (40–100%), (5.) acute intoxication (100%), and (6.) malignant tumours (100%).

5.2 Industrial toxins

A tabular compilation of all important known toxins can be useful for recording suspected cases of liver damage by toxic agents. (s. tab. 30.3) • Some substances are described separately below. (3, 7, 13, 14, 22, 24, 28, 39, 40, 48, 56–59, 63, 66–68, 71)

Cirrhosis/fibrosis: The following substances may cause cirrhosis or fibrosis of the liver:

Arsenic	Iron
Cadmium	Phosphorus
Carbon tetrachloride	Tetrachloroethane
Chloronaphthalene	Tetranitromethylaniline
Copper	Thioacetamide
Dichlorobenzene	Trinitrotoluene
Dimethylnitrosamine	Vinyl chloride
Dinitrotoluene	

Malignant tumours: Some toxic substances can induce the formation of malignant tumours. This has been demonstrated in humans for some substances, whereas for others it has so far only been confirmed in animal experiments. Protein deficiency increases the frequency of carcinoma considerably. Such substances include:

Acrylonitrile	Tetrachlorodiphenyl-p-dioxin
Arsenic	Thioacetamide
Butter yellow	Thorium dioxide
Carbon tetrachloride	Vinyl chloride
Dimethylnitrosamine	

5.2.1 Halogenated hydrocarbons

Aliphatic and aromatic halogenated hydrocarbons are widely used as industrial reagents, cleaning agents and solvents. The toxicity of the individual substances is very varied, e.g. relative to trichloroethane (nominal toxicity = 1), trichloroethylene, chloroform and carbon tetrachloride have a toxicity of 8, 60 and 190, respectively. (s. tab. 30.3)

Chlorinated halogenated hydrocarbons are taken up via the respiratory tract and the skin (even perorally in suicide attempts). In addition, they are also dangerous in their solid form. The so-called **perna disease** is named after an insulating material mainly consisting of "**per**chloro**na**phthalene". This substance, which is commonly used in the electrical industry, produces toxic vapour during soldering; that may cause severe liver cell necrosis and acute liver dystrophy.

Acute and high-dosage intoxication by **trichloroethylene** leads to severe symptoms associated with the central nervous system, but **not** to (noteworthy) liver damage.

▶ *We were able to confirm this condition in a 29-year-old female patient with severe acute trichloroethylene poisoning after taking 80–90 ml trichloroethylene perorally with suicidal intent. Despite a six-day comatose state, intensive care produced a complete recovery. Throughout the three-week period of treatment, all of the liver enzymes remained normal, and percutaneous liver biopsy yielded normal histology.*

In contrast, *chronic exposure to trichloroethylene* may lead to severe liver damage or even cirrhosis. (69)

Dichlorodiphenyl trichloroethane (DDT) was introduced as an insecticide in 1941. Its use in Germany has been prohibited since 1971. Toxic liver damage (steatosis, necrosis) and fatalities following liver dystrophy have been described. The strongly lipophilic properties of DDT, its accumulation in fatty tissue over many years and its resistance to all forms of inactivation or degradation are indicative of its long-term toxic potential. It can also be detected in high concentrations in breast milk. DDT greatly increased induction of the cytochrome P-450 system: Japanese workers in the plastics industry were found to have reduced bilirubin values due to continuous and strong enzyme induction with subsequent accelerated coupling of glucuronic acid and increased excretion of bilirubin. Peroral intake of 3–6 g DDT (e.g. with suicidal intent) causes fatal poisoning.

Carbon tetrachloride: Chronic intoxication due to year-long inhalation of even small quantities of hydrocarbons, including carbon tetrachloride, can lead to the development of cirrhosis. An already existing fatty liver promotes the toxicity of CCl_4 through the elevated affinity of the adipose tissue. The presence of trichloroethylene, vitamin A and alcohol likewise increases the hepatotoxicity of even small quantities of CCl_4. When there is a decrease in the activity of CCl_4-metabolizing enzymes (e.g. in cases of protein deficiency), a decrease in the toxicity of CCl_4 can also be expected. CCl_4 itself is atoxic; the high toxicity is produced by hepatic formation of the toxic radicals CCl_3, Cl and $CHCl_3$ due to CYP 2E1, CYP 2B1 and CYP 2B2. Severe impairment of the membranes of the liver cells and their organelles produces massive and diffuse liver damage with steatosis and necrosis, which finally results in the collapse of liver functions, particularly haemostasis. The degree of damage to the liver and kidneys by CCl_4 can apparently be reduced by high intravenous doses of acetylcysteine. (4, 27, 60, 62, 76)

Vinyl chloride: The gaseous, pleasantly sweet-smelling vinyl chloride (VC), which also has a slight anaesthetic effect, was formerly used in the production of polyvinyl chloride (PVC). Hepatolienal damage by VC was recognized in 1949 and 1960. (s. p. 581) As far as such cases could be recorded, a total of 109 fatalities occurred worldwide up to 1985. Symptoms included elevations of GPT, GOT, GDH, γ-GT and AP together with a decrease in ChE (60–70%), splenomegaly (40–50%), portal hypertension with oesophageal varices sometimes with bleeding (10–15%), as well as liver fibrosis and malignant tumours (haemangiosarcoma and/or hepatocellular carcinoma). (s. fig. 30.1) Laparoscopy shows striking Glisson's capsule fibrosis (initially linear like a *"star-filled sky"*). Histology reveals severe pre-/intrasinusoidal fibrosis, often with cavernoma-like enlarged sinusoids. It was found that it is not the inhaled VC that is toxic, but rather the highly reactive epoxide chloroethylene oxide produced by biotransformation. Considerably improved regulations for protection have in the meantime prevented any new cases of the disease occurring, as far as we know. However, in view of the long latency period of about 20 years, further manifestations of the disease must be expected. (10–12, 43–45, 70)

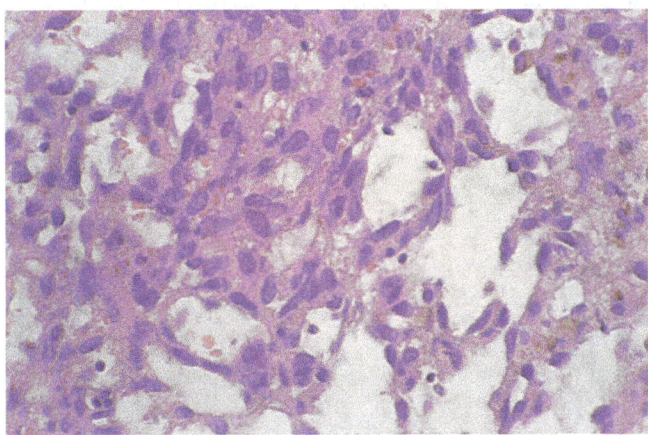

Fig. 30.1: Haemangiosarcoma in a case of disease induced by vinyl chloride. Tumorous endothelial proliferation with blood cavities and vascular fissures containing erythrocytes (HE)

Dioxin: Of the approx. 200 isomers of dioxin, tetrachlorodiphenyl-p-dioxin (TCDD) is seen as the most toxic: its half-life in the soil is about ten years, whereas in humans and animals, the half-life is up to one year (due to its lipophilic properties). In the region of the liver, dioxin causes steatosis, cell necrosis, haemofuscin deposits and fibrosis with portal hypertension and oesophageal varices. In Missouri (USA) in 1971 marked fibrosis was observed in poisoned animals following contact with contaminated oil. (s. p. 581) The long-term damage caused by this highly carcinogenic substance is serious; this effect may be exacerbated by the simultaneous action of other chlorinated hydrocarbons, dibenzofurans or hexachlorocyclohexane. Following the use of dioxin as a defoliant in the Vietnam war ("agent orange"), a fourfold increase in the frequency of liver cancer was recorded. The number of malformations due to VC-induced foetotoxicity was described as enormous.

5.2.2 Hydrocarbon derivatives

Pentachlorophenol: Because of its good fungicidal, pesticidal and preservative properties, pentachlorophenol (PCP) is frequently used for industrial and domestic purposes. Numerous cases of intoxication, even via bath water, with considerable liver damage are known. Infant fatalities have been reported after nappies were washed with PCP. (78)

Polychlorinated biphenyls are still used in large quantities in electrical and condenser technology. One of the main members of this group of substances is perchlorobiphenyl (PCB). In fires involving polychlorinated biphenyls, toxic dioxins can be released. Biphenyls lead to a powerful induction of the cytochrome P-450 system. Following exposure, biphenyls can be detected in adipose tissue and breast milk. Severe cases of liver damage, including fatalities, have been reported.

Hexachlorocyclohexane: During the production of this substance from chlorine and benzene under the influence of light, various isomers are also formed, particularly the toxic substance lindane. Isomers of hexachlorocyclohexane (HCH) are found in air, soil, water, food and even breast milk. Lindane is used in large quantities in agriculture and forestry as a wood preservative as well as in veterinary medicine. Provided that the required safety measures are adhered to, no liver damage occurs during the production of lindane. On the other hand, liver cell necrosis was observed in animal experiments after HCH isomers were added to the feed; a carcinogenic effect was seen after long-term administration. An increased toxic potential is to be expected when there is simultaneous exposure to DDT, PCB, contraceptives, etc.

Paints and varnishes: On the basis of our experience and data in the literature (13, 41), working as a *painter, spray-varnisher* or *floor layer* must be regarded as more hazardous in comparison to non-exposed groups with respect to toxic liver damage. Even though dispersion pigments are mainly (i.e. not exclusively) used, paints and sprays nevertheless contain a broad range of organic solvents and substances, including fungicides and pesticides. Despite observance of the specified industrial threshold values, so-called combination effects can never be totally ruled out. The risk of illness is hence greater in single cases, and it may be further aggravated by additional individual factors. Elevated transaminases are found, while steatosis and focal necrosis have been demonstrated histologically.

▶ It is always open to question as to what extent the risk threshold for chemical noxae may be exceeded due to altered technical working procedures and individual conditions despite compliance with the legal regulations. *The recruitment and monitoring criteria prescribed by the employers' liability insurance association are of great importance in this respect.*

5.2.3 Aromatic amines

Methylene dianiline (4,4-diaminodiphenylmethane) is used as a liquid hardening agent for epoxy resins. Its high hepatotoxicity was clearly seen in **Epping disease** in 1965. (s. p. 581) In the following decades (1974, 1985), severe toxic liver damage with liver cell necrosis, cholestasis and hepatomegaly was also found in workers who had been poisoned by percutaneous uptake of this substance (through carelessness). (33, 34, 49) • Other aromatic amines or nitrocompounds (e. g. dinitrobenzene: dye and paint industry; dinitrotoluene: explosives; dimethyl nitrosamine: anticorrosive agents) can likewise lead to steatosis and cell necrosis if there has been sufficient exposure. (s. tab. 30.3)

5.2.4 Inorganic substances

Phosphorus: Poisoning by phosphorus and its inorganic compounds is rare. While insoluble red phosphorus is only slightly toxic, yellow and (above all) white forms of phosphorus show considerable hepatotoxicity. Occasional instances of toxicosis occur through rat poison containing phosphorus. Phosphorus poisoning causes a loss of glycogen in the liver cells, subsequently leading to marked steatosis and cell necrosis with portal infiltration. Jaundice appears at an early stage. The transaminases are considerably elevated, whereas ChE and Quick's value generally fall. Signs of increasing liver insufficiency and azotaemia are prognostically unfavourable symptoms. Postnecrotic cirrhosis (or scarred liver) can develop in survivors. (18)

Arsenic: Arsenic poisoning is of great medicohistorical interest. (s. p. 580) Chronic arsenic intoxication can be caused by inhalation or, more frequently, by oral uptake. Hepatomegaly is found in the majority of cases. Steatosis and cell necrosis occur in the liver; fibrosis or cirrhosis with portal hypertension and oesophageal varices develop. The presence of liver adenoma and VOD as well as liver carcinoma or haemangioendothelioma has been described. (16, 42, 51, 54, 61, 77) In an animal experiment, trivalent arsenic stimulated endothelial cell capillarization and vessel remodelling, portal fibrosis and vascularization of the peribiliary vascular plexus, and constriction of hepatic arterioles. This may well explain portal hypertension. (68)

Lead: Lead poisoning (= *saturnism*) results in mild, rapidly regressive toxic hepatitis in about 30% of cases. Occasionally, eosinophilic, acid-resistant inclusions are found in the nuclei of the liver cells (so-called lead protein complexes). Steatosis and liver-cell necrosis have also been observed. Although there is a correlation between exposure to lead and severity of damage, individual sensitivity to lead nevertheless varies. In addition, lead intoxication causes an inhibition of erythrocyte δ-aminolaevulinic acid dehydratase and an induction of δ-aminolaevulinic acid synthase. This brings about the manifestation of acute intermittent porphyria. (8)

5.2.5 Thorotrast

The introduction of thorotrast into radiological diagnostics (1928) despite foreseeable radiation damage is one of the less positive aspects of twentieth century medicine. Thirty years passed before the use of thorotrast was stopped (after numerous reports of severe organ damage and the development of malignancies). (s. p. 580) • The term **thorotrastosis** subsumed (*1.*) aplastic anaemia, leukaemia and osteomyelofibrosis, (*2.*) atrophy of lymphatic organs with scarring obliteration, (*3.*) fibrosis of the liver and spleen with scarred areas (= *dystrophia lenta*, H. F. BRUNNER, 1955), (*4.*) development of scarred areas in the form of granulomas around thorotrast extravasations (H. F. BRUNNER, 1960), and (*5.*) occurrence of malignancies. (30, 32, 50) • The development of FNH due to thorotrast was first reported in 1998. (6) In the liver, thorotrast is initially stored in the Kupffer cells; after their destruction, it is deposited in the periportal areas. From here, periportal and periacinar fibrosis as well as Glisson's capsule fibrosis develop. (s. figs. 30.2, 30.3)

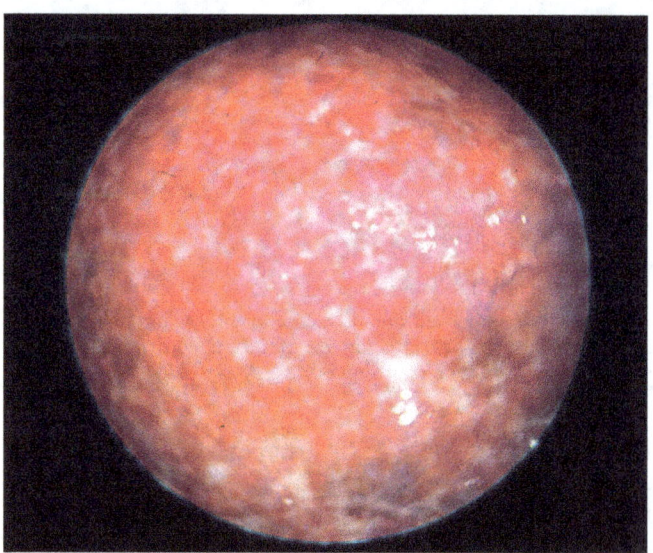

Fig. 30.2: Thorotrast liver: dark brown colouring of the liver surface with reticular bright white fibrosis

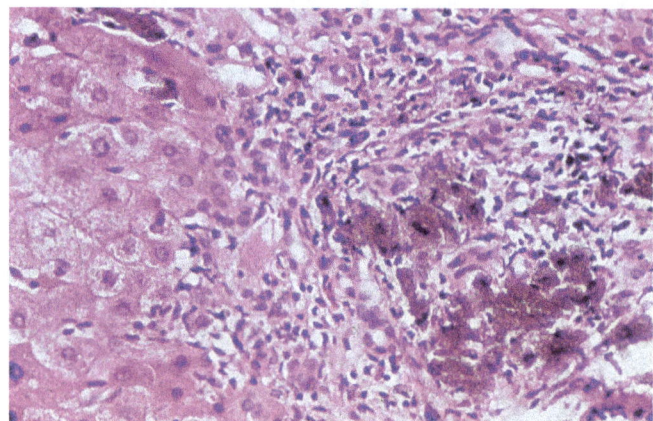

Fig. 30.3: Thorotrastosis: deposits of thorotrast in portal and perisinusoidal macrophages; periportal fibrosis and inflammation (HE)

5.3 Mycotoxins

▶ The following hepatotoxic mycotoxins are worthy of note: *aflatoxin* (Aspergillus flavus), *griseofulvin* (Penicillium griseofulvum), *ochratoxin A* (Aspergillus ochraceus), *maltrozyne* (from the fermentation of rice wine) and *luteoskyrin* (Penicillium islandicum). Their toxicity is increased by protein deficiency in the organism.

A disease of epidemic proportions affected more than 1,000 persons in India in 1974. The patients suffered from jaundice and ascites. Histological examination revealed centroacinar necrosis, inflammatory mesenchymal reactions and bile-duct proliferation; fibrosis and septal formation, sometimes ultimately cirrhosis, were determined. Mortality was 10%. The cause was thought to be the additive effect of several unidentified mycotoxins (B. N. TANDON et al., 1977).

Aflatoxins: So far, 13 types of aflatoxin (B, G, M) have been identified in various Aspergillus fungi. Their great toxicity is due to their alkylating effect with blocking of the DNA-dependent RNA polymerase. The highest toxicity to date has been ascribed to aflatoxin B_1. Under warm and humid conditions, certain agricultural products (rice, soybeans, peanuts, almonds, pistachios, hazelnuts, cereals, etc.) are attacked by Aspergillus fungi. (s. p. 581) Aflatoxins may be present in peanuts in vending machines. Some types (B, M) have also been detected in dairy products. Aflatoxins can be neither seen, smelt nor tasted. • Acute poisoning leads to jaundice, steatosis and liver cell necrosis; ascites and fulminant liver failure have likewise been observed. In cases of chronic intoxication, it is possible that cholestasis, bile-duct proliferation, fibrosis and the clinical picture of biliary cirrhosis will occur. Since 1968, aflatoxin has been regarded as the most potent hepatocarcinogenic substance; it can act alone as a carcinogen or, in the case of HBV infection, as a co-carcinogen. (15, 35, 46, 52) (s. p. 519)

5.4 Phytotoxins

The plant kingdom contains numerous phytotoxins. Their number is, however, far higher than has been realized so far. They are also of great significance as direct hepatotoxins. • A list of the most important phytotoxins includes *fungal poisons* (e.g. amanitin, phalloidin, gyromitrin), *pyrrolizidine alkaloids, cycasin* from the sago palm, *safrol* from the gassafras tree, *tannins* and *3.4'-benzpyrene*.

Carcinogenic phytotoxins	
Cycasin	Pyrrolizidine alkaloids
Luteoskyrin	Safrol
Maltrozyn	Tannins
Ochratoxin A	

There have been repeated reports of intoxication by still largely unknown phytotoxins: liver cell necrosis and cholestasis following the consumption of herbal medicine made from *mulberry tree bark* (S. TOZUKA et al., 1983); liver cell necrosis (even fatal) following the intake of a root extract from the *distaff thistle* (G. LEMAIGRE et al., 1975); poisoning by a decoction from *Callilepsis laureola* (J. WAINWRIGHT et al., 1977) and due to *mint oil* (J. B. SULLIVAN et al., 1979).

5.4.1 3.4'-benzpyrene

This polycyclic, aromatic hydrocarbon is produced continuously by almost all plants, irrespective of their habitat, and remains qualitatively and quantitatively constant. The normal content of the carcinogenic 3.4'-benzpyrene equals 1 µg/100 g dried plant material. The assumed quantity of carcinogenic polycyclic hydrocarbons ingested daily with food and drinking water is calculated at 10 µg/day. Food of animal origin, even in roasted, smoked or grilled form, contains substantially less benzpyrene than that derived from plants.

5.4.2 Pyrrolizidine alkaloids

Pyrrolizidine alkaloids are found in more than 200 crotalaria, senecio and heliotrope plants, but only about 100 types are toxic. Even honey may contain such pyrrolizidine alkaloids collected in pollen by bees from these plants. These alkaloids were held responsible for **veno-occlusive disease** in reports simultaneously published in South Africa (K. B. MOKHOBO) and Jamaica (K. R. HILL) in 1951. As early as 1920, however, F. C. WILLMOT et al. had described the development of cirrhosis due to senecio poisoning. Generally, intake was in the form of "bush tea", such as an Indian herbal tea for psoriasis (P. S. GUPTA et al., 1963), a dubious form of maté tea (J. D. MCGEE et al., 1976), an antirheumatic tea (C. L. LYFORD et al., 1976) and a Mexican antitussive tea (A. E. STILLMAN et al., 1977). Likewise in Europe, various types of herbal tea may contain senecio alkaloids. • Liver damage manifests as hepatomegaly, epigastric pain, a rise in liver enzymes and an occasional ascites. Hepatomegaly is due to the 10−20 fold enlargement of hepatocytes, which is a result of the anti-mitotic effect of pyrrolizidine alkaloids. Centrolobular necrosis, steatosis and obliterative hepatic endophlebitis as well as an acute or chronic **Budd-Chiari syndrome** may appear. Diagnosis is established with the aid of imaging techniques. In cases of acute poisoning, death often occurs within a few days. About half the affected persons survive. Chronic intoxications sometimes lead to the development of cirrhosis and possibly malignant liver tumours. (s. p. 856)

5.4.3 Amanita phalloides

The highly poisonous Amanita phalloides is easily confused with the field mushroom and yellow knight fungus. About 15−25% of all fungal poisonings and 50−60% of all fatalities are due to the ingestion of Amanita phalloides. Four **Amanita species** can be distinguished: (*1.*) *Amanita phalloides* (green type), (*2.*) *Amanita virosa* (white type), (*3.*) *Amanita citrina mappa* (yellowish type), and (*4.*) *Amanita verna* (spring amanita mushroom). The fungal toxins α-*amanitin* and *phalloidin* are not destroyed by drying or heating. Some 25 g of fungus contain about 4.0−4.5 mg α-amanitin, i.e. one mushroom (approx. 50 g) is sufficient for the fatal poisoning of one or two persons. • The maximum serum value is reached within 3 hours of ingesting the fungal poison. As a result of the enterohepatic circulation, the serum concentration remains virtually constant for about 18 hours before beginning to fall steadily. The latency period (5−24 h) is asymptomatic. In the gastrointestinal phase (24−48 h), vomiting, gastric spasms, diarrhoea and dehydration occur, with loss of electrolytes and zinc. Metabolic alkalosis can abruptly change into metabolic acidosis. This phase is caused by the rapid onset of phallotoxic action. The hepatorenal phase sets in from about the third day onwards, with hepatic encephalopathy, cerebral oedema, a rise in transaminases, jaundice, a drop in the clotting factors, and hypoglycaemia. Death due to haemorrhagic diathesis in coma and/or uraemia occurs within five days; later deaths are unknown (or very rare).

▶ **Wieland test:** The section plane of the fungus, which is cut open, is rubbed on a newspaper. One drop of 6 NHCl is then added to the dried sap, which takes on a blue colour in the presence of amanitin.

Supporting measures include gastric lavage, nasogastral intestinal lavage, for example with 100 g lactulose + active charcoal + Ringer's solution, and a high cleansing enema; haemoperfusion or forced diuresis can be carried out if necessary. Therapy consists of silibinin (30 mg/kg BW in 500 ml glucose solution, four times daily) and penicillin G (1 mega/kg BW, i.v.); both of these substances have proved their therapeutic value. N-acetylcysteine, fresh plasma, glucose, AT III and vitamins can be administered as supportive measures. The therapeutic success achieved with silibinin is good; it should be administered as soon as there is suspicion of amanita poisoning without waiting for the mushroom to be identified in the urine (RIA, HPCL). It is important to keep samples of the fungi, stomach contents, blood, urine, etc. (5, 9, 17, 19, 20, 31, 55) (s. pp 382, 388)

▶ *Our own experience with the immediate use of silibinin in three validated cases of poisoning showed almost reaction-free survival.*

5.4.4 Helvella esculenta

The toxins in Helvella esculenta (Gyromitra esculenta) can be completely removed by boiling, but this boiled water must not be re-used as it contains the fungal poison. The toxin was found to be *gyromitrin*, a hydrazine derivative. Liver damage manifests as extensive cell necrosis. With a rapid rise in the transaminases and serum bilirubin, the illness progresses to liver insufficiency followed by hepatic coma and death. • No *antidote* is known. • *Therapy* consists of thorough gastrointestinal lavage with the addition of active charcoal and, where applicable, haemoperfusion. It is also advisable to use supportive measures (see above). Where appropriate, thioctic acid (5 × 200 mg i.v.), zinc and selenium can be applied.

5.5 Endotoxins

Endotoxins are fragments of long-chain lipopolysaccharides. They pass from the cell membrane − mainly from gram-negative bacteria in the intestine − into the circulation and, as potential hepatotoxins, subsequently lead to liver damage. In the liver cells, they bring about a decrease in the activity of tryptophan pyrrolase as well as an increase in the activity of tyrosine-α-ketoglutarate transaminase. It is therefore understandable that a continuous flow of intestinal endotoxins via the portal vein may well exacerbate an existing liver disease, in particular liver cirrhosis. At the same time, these endotoxins cause fever, leucopenia, blood-clotting disorders and kinin activation. The burden on the RES leads to a rise in γ-globulins with a simultaneous depressor effect on albumin synthesis.

5.6 Drugs

Elevated transaminases are found in more than 60% of anicteric drug addicts. It is, however, difficult to relate the respective liver damage to a particular drug as there is usually abuse of several addictive substances, including alcohol (= polytoxicomania). It is likewise extremely difficult to obtain an accurate medical history from drug addicts. Examinations by liver biopsy have presented a picture of chronic non-specific, chronic persistent or active chronic hepatitis. • Recently, there have been increasing reports of Ecstasy intoxications (and even acute liver failure requiring liver transplantation) as well as the development of liver fibrosis following Ecstasy abuse. (21, 25, 26, 29, 75)

6 Diagnostics

6.1 Chronic intoxication

The diagnosis of liver damage due to toxic substances is based on a detailed **medical history.** In addition to general anamnesis, precise information on alcohol intake and medication is of primary importance. Alcohol and medication are regarded as substantial uncertainty factors in the differential diagnosis and assessment of liver damage due to chemical toxins. Knowledge of existing metabolic diseases and special aspects in the person's lifestyle is also important. Even though subjective symptoms are generally uncharacteristic, observations concerning the commencement of the illness, its intensity and, of course, any striking factors can nevertheless simplify diagnostic clarification. The attempt to compile a comprehensive occupational history can then begin. A certain flair for detective work may sometimes be necessary in this connection. • *It is important to obtain documentation of certain workplace-related chemicals and working materials!*

Objective **clinical findings** are obtained by *physical examination*, determination of *laboratory parameters* (γ-GT, GPT, GOT, GDH, AP, ChE) and *sonography*. Clarification of hepatitis serology is necessary. Additional laboratory parameters for differential diagnosis or long-term monitoring (e. g. immunoglobulins, P-III-P, electrophoresis) are helpful in some cases. Although these findings mainly serve to determine the hepatological status, the possibility or even probability of toxically induced liver damage can often be assessed as well. In the individual case, the constellation of *histological changes* also facilitates an aetiological assessment. • Definitive elucidation is only achieved once the respective occupational physician and industrial toxicologist have clarified the relevant conditions at the workplace. When there is any suspicion that the working environment has caused liver damage, it is necessary to notify the authorities, who will then instigate all requisite diagnostic measures and draw up expertises.

Objectification and quantification of the suspected liver noxa(e) at the workplace and in the respective industrial materials are carried out in accordance with the current state of knowledge concerning toxicology in occupational medicine. *Even in cases where the chemically induced liver damage is not obviously related to the patient's place of work, it is nevertheless recommended to seek advice from institutions dealing with occupational medicine and toxicology.*

6.2 Acute poisoning

In cases of acute poisoning (e. g. after suicide attempts or industrial accidents), it is generally possible to connect the poisoning to a specific chemical noxa. Numerous **poison information centres** are accessible − round the clock (!) − for rapid toxicological and therapeutic consultation. The prognosis for poisoning depends on the early commencement of therapeutic measures. • For the initial care of patients with acute poisoning, the **five-finger rule** should be observed:

1. removal of the toxin
2. antidote therapy (if possible)
3. elementary assistance (respiration, circulation)
4. transport to the hospital
5. collecting evidence of the intoxication

It should be noted, that medical confidentiality applies in all cases.

7 Therapeutic aspects

Acute poisoning is the result of **three parameters:** *toxin + toxin uptake + toxin action*. **Three corresponding therapeutic equivalents** should be applied: *antidote therapy + detoxification + first-aid treatment*. Detoxification and first-aid treatment are at the fore until an antidote (provided one exists) can be used (information obtainable from special **emergency centres for poisons** or from an antidote list). Depending upon the type of toxin involved, detoxification can be effected by gastrointestinal lavage, diuretic therapy, blood exchange, peritoneal dialysis, haemodialysis, ultrafiltration or haemoperfusion. In severe intoxication with acute liver failure, **liver transplantation** is indicated. (20, 25, 67) In this context, a report has been published about the successful treatment of acute potassium dichromate poisoning by means of liver transplantation. (67)

In **chronic intoxication,** the objective is removal of the patient from the site of exposure and elimination of the noxa from the body (detoxification measures, infusions of calcium-disodium EDTA in cases of lead poisoning, etc.). There is no justification for therapeutic nihilism. • With the aid of *dietetic measures* and *adjuvant therapy* (e. g. N-acetylcysteine, antioxidants, UDCA, S-adenosyl-methionine, BCAA, vitamins B and C, ornithine-aspartate, zinc), both clinical course and prognosis can be favourably influenced. EPL was shown to correct hepatotoxicity in patients chronically exposed to toxic chemical substances (e. g. organic solvents, uranium, lead, mercury compounds). (s. p. 894) • Insufficient regression or inadequate normalization of laboratory parameters and histological changes despite removal of the patient from the area of exposure arouse suspicion of *still existing noxae* (alcohol, drugs, other chemicals).

Despite the presence of numerous potential hepatotoxic substances at the workplace, the frequency of industrial toxic liver damage is nevertheless low. This is no doubt due to the success of screening programmes in occupational medicine, tolerance limits for toxic substances at the workplace as laid down by law and careful compliance with all preventive measures. • However, experience has shown that one must always reckon with new, potentially hepatotoxic substances. Indeed, far more attention must be paid to those chemicals belonging to the category of "recreational and hobby noxae", which are often handled with an irresponsible disregard of all risks.

8 Industrial hepatotoxic agents

1. **Aliphatic halogenated hydrocarbons**
   +Chloroform (= trichloromethane)
   Chloroprene (= 2-chloro-1,3-butadiene)
   +1,1-dichloroethane, 1,2-dichloroethane
   1,1-dichloroethene, 1,2-dichloroethene
   Dichloromethane
   Fluorchloromethane
   Methyl bromide (= monobromomethane)
   Methyl chloride (= monochloromethane)
   Methylene chloride (= dichloromethane)
   Methyliodide (= monoiodomethane)
   +Pentachloroethane
   Propylene dichloride (= dichloropropane)
   +Tetrachloroethane
   Tetrachloroethene (PER)
   +Tetrachloromethane (= carbon tetrachloride)
   1,1,1-trichloroethane, 1,1,2-trichloroethane
   +Trichloroethen (TRI)
   Vinyl chloride

2. **Aromatic halogenated hydrocarbons**
   Benzyl chloride (= monochlorobenzene)
   Chlorinated benzene derivatives
   Chlorinated naphthalenes
   +Chlorobiphenyl
   Dichlorodiphenyltrichloro-ethane (DDT)
   +Perchlorobiphenyl (PCB)

3. **Aliphatic hydrocarbons and cycloalcans**
   Cyclohexane
   Cyclopropane
   N-heptane
   N-hexane

4. **Aromatic hydrocarbons**
   Benzene
   Diphenyl
   +Naphthalene
   Styrene (= ethyl benzene)
   Toluene (= methyl benzene)
   Xylene (= dimethyl benzene)

5. **Aliphatic amines**
   2-acetylaminofluorene
   Ethanolamine (= aminoethanole)
   Ethylenediamine (= 1,2-diaminoethane)

6. **Aromatic amines**
   4,4-diaminodiphenyl methane
   3,3-dichlorobenzidine and its salts
   4-dimethylamino-azobenzene (= "butter yellow")
   4,4-methylene-bis(2-chloroaniline)

7. **Nitro compounds**
   +Dinitrobenzene
   4,6-dinitro-o-cresol (DNOC)
   +Dinitrophenole
   2,4-dinitrotoluene
   Nitrobenzenel
   Nitroparaffins (nitroalkanes)
   Nitrophenol
   Nitropropane
   N,N-dimethylnitrosamine
   +Picric acid (= 2,4,6-trinitrophenol)
   Tetryl (= nitramine)
   +Toluene diamine (= neutral red)
   +2,4,6-trinitrotoluene (TNT)

8. **Nitriles**
   Acetonitrile
   Acrylonitrile

9. **Acetates and silicates**
   Amyl, N-butyl, ethyl, isopropyl, methyl and N-propyl acetates
   Ethyl silicate

10. **Halogens and halogenides**
    Bromine
    Bromide
    Hydrobromic acid

11. **Ethers and epoxides**
    Diethyl ether
    +Dioxane (= 1,4-dioxane)
    Epichlorohydrin
    Ethylene oxide
    Ethylglycol ether and derivatives

12. **Alcohols and derivatives**
    Allyl alcohol
    Dichloropropanol (= 1,3-dichloro-2-propanol)
    Ethanol (= ethyl alcohol)
    Ethylene chlorhydrin (= 2-chloroethanol)
    Methanol (= methyl alcohol)

13. **Carboxylic acids and anhydrides**
    Phthalic acid anhydride

14. **Phenols and derivatives**
    Cresol (= methyl phenol)
    Pentachlorophenol (PCP)
    Phenol

15. **Cyanides and Cyanates**
    Cyanhydric acid (= prussic acid)
    +Isocyanate

16. **Pesticides**
    Dipyridyl (= 2,2-bipyridine)
    +Paraquat (= paraquat dichloride)
    +Thallium sulphate

17. **Other organic compounds**
    Aldehydes
    Betapropiolactone
    Carbon disulfide
    Dimethyl sulphate
    +Hydrazine and derivatives
    Mercaptans
    N,N-dimethylacetamide
    +N,N-dimethylformamide
    N-nitrosodimethylamine
    Pyridine
    Tetrachlorodiphenyl-p-dioxin (TCDD)
    Tetramethylthiuram disulphide (= thiram)
    Turpentine

18. **Metal and inorganic compounds**
    +Arsenic
    +Arsines
    Beryllium
    Bismuth and bismuth compounds
    Boron and boron compounds
    Cadmium and cadmium compounds
    Carbonyle
    Chromium and chromium compounds
    Germanium
    Iron
    Copper
    Lead
    Manganese
    Mercury and mercury compounds
    Nickel and nickel compounds
    Phosphine (= hydrogen phosphide)
    +Phosphorus and phosphorus compounds
    Selenium and selenium compounds
    Stibium (= antimony hydrogen)
    +Thallium and thallium compounds
    Thorium dioxide
    Tin and tin compounds
    Uranium and uranium compounds

Tab. 30.3: Table of important, mainly industrially used, toxic substances (selection). ($^+$ = causes very severe liver damage, severe toxic hepatitis and acute liver failure) • *We would appreciate any corrections, supplements or additions.*

References:

1. **Anderson, H.A., Wolff, M.S., Lilis, R., Holstein, E.C., Valciukas, J.A., Anderson, K.E., Petrocci, M., Sarkozzi, L., Selikoff, I.J.:** Symptoms and clinical abnormalities following ingestion of polybrominated-biphenyl-contaminated food products. Ann. N. Y. Acad. Sci. 1979; 320: 684–702
2. **Armstrong, C.W., Stroube, R.B., Rubio, T., Siudyla, E.A., Miller, G.B.:** Outbreak of fatal arsenic poisoning caused by contaminated drinking water. Arch. Environ. Hlth. 1984; 39: 276–279
3. **Babany, G., Bernuau, J., Cailleux, A., Cadranel, J.-F., Degott, C., Erlinger, S., Benhamou, J.-P.:** Severe monochlorobenzene-induced liver cell necrosis. Gastroenterology 1991; 101: 1734–1736
4. **Bagnell, P.C., Ellenberger, H.A.:** Obstructive jaundice due to a chlorinated hydrocarbon in breast milk. Canad. Med. Ass. J. 1977; 117: 1047–1048
5. **Bartoloni, S., Omer, F., Giannini, A., Botti, P., Caramelli, L., Ledda, F., Peruzzi, S., Zorn, M.:** Amanita poisoning: a clinical-histopathological study of 64 cases of intoxication. Hepato-Gastroenterol. 1985; 32: 229–231
6. **Beer, T.W., Carr, N.J., Buxton, P.J.:** Thorotrast-associated nodular regenerative hyperplasia of the liver. J. Clin. Pathol. 1998; 51: 941–942
7. **Boewer, C., Enderlein, G., Wollgast, U., Nawka, S., Palowski, H., Bleiber, R.:** Epidemiological study on the hepatotoxicity of occupational toluene exposure. Int. Arch. Occup. Environ. Health 1988; 60: 181–186
8. **Carton, J.A., Diaz, J., Vallina, E., Arribas, J.M.:** Hepatitis bei Saturnismus. Dtsch. Med. Wschr. 1984; 109: 195–196
9. **Covic, A., Goldsmith, D.J.A., Gusbeth-Tatomir, P., Volovat, C., Dimitriu, A.G., Cristogel, F., Bizo, A.:** Successful use of molecular adsorbent regenerating system (MARS) dialysis for the treatment of fulminant hepatic failure in children accidentally poisoned by toxic mushroom ingestion. Liver Internat. 2003; 23 (Suppl. 3): 21–27
10. **Creech, J.L., Johnson, M.N.:** Angiosarcoma of liver in the manifacture of polyvinylchloride. J. Occup. Med. 1974; 16: 150–151
11. **Dietz, A., Langbein, G., Permanetter, W.:** Das Vinylchloridinduzierte hepatozelluläre Karzinom. Klin. Wschr. 1985; 63: 325–331
12. **Doss, M., Lange, C.E., Vellman, G.:** Vinylchloride-induced hepatic coproporphyrinuria with transition to chronic hepatic porphyria. Klin. Wschr. 1984; 62: 175–178
13. **Dossing, M., Arlien-Soborg, P., Petersen, L.M., Ranek, L.:** Liver damage associated with occupational exposure to organic solvents in house painters. Eur. J. Clin. Invest. 1983; 13: 151–157
14. **Dossing, M.:** Occupational toxic liver damage. J. Hepatol. 1986; 3: 131–135
15. **Enwonwu, C.O.:** The role of dietary aflatoxin in the genesis of hepatocellular cancer in developing countries. Lancet 1984/II; 956–958
16. **Falk, H., Caldwell, G.G., Ishak, K.G., Thomas, L.B., Popper, H.:** Arsenic-related hepatic angiosarcoma. Amer. J. Indust. Med. 1981; 2: 43–50
17. **Faybik, P., Hetz, H., Baker, A., Bittermann, C., Berlakovich, G., Werba, A., Krenn, C.G., Steltzer, H.:** Extracorporeal albumin dialysis in patients with Amanita phalloides poisoning. Liver Internat. 2003; 23 (Suppl. 3): 28–33
18. **Fernandez, O.U.B., Canizares, L.L.:** Acute hepatotoxicity from ingestion of yellow phosphorus-containing fireworks. J. Clin. Gastroenterol. 1995; 21: 139–142
19. **Floersheim, G.L.:** Treatment of human amatoxin mushroom poisoning: myths and advances in therapy. Med. Toxicol. Adv. Drug Exp. 1987; 2: 1–9
20. **Galler, G.W., Weisenberg, E., Brasitus, T.A.:** Mushroom poisoning: the role of orthotopic liver transplantation. J. Clin. Gastroenterol. 1992; 15: 229–232
21. **Gilbert, H.S., Stimmel, B.:** Abnormal liver function and elevated hemoglobins in heroin addicts. Amer. J. Gastroenterol. 1975; 64: 49–54
22. **Haratake, J., Furuta, A., Icasa, T., Wakasugi, C., Imazu, K.:** Submassive hepatic necrosis induced by dichloropropanol. Liver 1993; 13: 123–129
23. **Hardt, M., Geisthövel, W.:** Malignes Hämangioendotheliom der Leber 39 Jahre nach einmaliger Thorotrast-Applikation. Med. Klin. 1988; 83: 151–153
24. **Harrison, R., Letz, G., Pasternak, G., Blanc, P.:** Fulminant hepatic failure after occupational exposure to 2-nitropropane. Ann. Intern. Med. 1987; 107: 466–468
25. **Hellinger, A., Rauen, U., De Groot, H., Erhard, J.:** Auxiliäre Lebertransplantation bei akutem Leberversagen nach Einnahme von 3,4-Methylendioxymetamphetamin ("Ecstasy"). Dtsch. Med. Wschr. 1997; 122: 716–720
26. **Henry, J.A., Jeffreys, K.J., Dawling, S.:** Toxicity and death from 3,4-methylenedioxymetamphetamine ("ecstasy"). Lancet 1992; 340: 384–387
27. **Hoshino, H., Komatsu, M., Ono, A., Funaoka, M., Kato, J., Ishii, T., Kuramitsu, T., Miura, K., Masamune, O., Hojo, H.:** A case of acute carbon tetrachloride poisoning. Acta Hepatol. Japon. 1994; 35: 882–886
28. **Kaufmann, L., Höpker, W.W., Deutsch-Diescher, O.G., Seitz, H.K., Götz, R., Kommerell, B.:** Leberschädigung durch chronische Cadmiumintoxikation. Leber Magen Darm 1984; 14: 103–106
29. **Khakoo, S.I., Coles, C.J., Armstrong, J.S., Barry, R.E.:** Hepatotoxicity and accelerated fibrosis following 3,4-methylenedioxymetamphetamine ("Ecstasy") usage. J. Clin. Gastroenterol. 1995; 20: 244–247
30. **Khan, A.A.:** Thorotrast-associated liver cancer. Amer. J. Gastroenterol. 1985; 80: 699–703
31. **Kleist-Retzow, von, J.-C., Vierzig, A., Fuchshuber, A., Roth, B., Michalk, D.V.:** Klinik und Therapie der Knollenblätterpilzvergiftung im Kindesalter. Mschr. Kinderheilk. 1995; 143: 1118–1127
32. **Kojiro, M., Kawano, Y., Kawasaki, H., Nakashima, T., Ikezani, H.:** Thorotrast-induced hepatic angiosarcoma, and combined hepatocellular and cholangiocarcinoma in a single patient. Cancer 1982; 49: 2161–2164
33. **Kopelman, H., Robertson, M.H., Sanders, P.G., Esch, I.:** The Epping jaundice. Brit. Med. J. 1966/I: 514–516
34. **Kopelman, H.:** Epping jaundice after two years. Postgrad. Med. J. 1968; 44: 78–81
35. **Krishnamachari, K.A.V.R., Nagarajan, V., Bhat, R.V., Tilak, T.B.G.:** Hepatitis due to aflatoxicosis. An outbreak in Western India. Lancet 1975/I: 1061–1063
36. **Kuntz, E., Neumann-Mangold, P.:** Die akute perorale Trichloraethylen-Vergiftung. Med. Welt 1965: 2872–2874
37. **Kuntz, E., Ordnung, W., Schmidt, U., Wildhirt, E., Engels, Ch.:** Leber und Umwelt. Eine anamnestische Praxisstudie. Kassenarzt 1988; 7: 32–40
38. **Kuntz, E.:** Lebererkrankungen aus der Sicht der niedergelassenen Ärzte. (Befragung von 2990 Ärzten). notabene medici 1989; 19: 243–246
39. **Kuntz, H.D., May, B.:** Berufsbedingte Lebererkrankungen. Münch. Med. Wschr. 1980; 122: 1059–1062
40. **Kuntz, H.D., May, B.:** Gewerblich-bedingte toxische Leberschäden. Atemw.-Lungenkrankh. 1984; 10: 477–483
41. **Kurrpa, K., Husman, K.:** Car painters exposure to a mixture of organic solvents: serum activities of liver enzymes. Scand. J. Work Environ. Health 1982; 8: 137–140
42. **Labadie, H., Stoessel, P., Callard, P., Beaugrand, M.:** Hepatic venoocclusive disease and perisinusoidal fibrosis secondary to arsenic poisoning. Gastroenterology 1990; 99: 1140–1143
43. **Langbein, G., Permanetter, W., Dietz, A.:** Hepatozelluläres Karzinom nach Vinylchlorid-Exposition. Dtsch. Med. Wschr. 1983; 108: 741–745
44. **Lange, C.E., Jühe, S., Veltmann, G.:** Über das Auftreten von Angiosarkomen bei zwei Arbeitern in der PVC-herstellenden Industrie. Dtsch. Med. Wschr. 1974; 99: 1598–1599
45. **Lelbach, W.K.:** Leber und Umweltgifte. Klin. Wschr. 1985; 63: 1139–1151
46. **Linsell, A.:** Incidence of hepato-carcinoma in relation to aflatoxin intake. Arch. Toxicol. 1980; 3: 13–18
47. **Mazumder, D.N.G.:** Effect of chronic intake of arsenic-contaminated water on liver. Tox. Appl. Pharm. 2005; 206: 169–175
48. **Matsumoto, T., Matsumori, H., Kuwabara, N., Fukuda, Y., Ariwa, R.A.:** A histopathological study of the liver in paraquat poisoning. An analysis of fourteen autopsy cases with emphasis on bile duct injury. Acta Path. Japon. 1980; 30: 859–870
49. **McGill, D.B., Motto, J.D.:** An industrial outbreak of toxic hepatitis due to methylenedianiline. New Engl. J. Med. 1974; 291: 278–282
50. **Morant, R., Rüttner, J.R.:** Thorotrast-Spätschäden. Schweiz. Med. Wschr. 1987; 117: 952–957
51. **Nevens, F., Fevery, J., van Steenbergen, W., Sciot, R., Desmet, V., de Groote, J.:** Arsenic and non-cirrhotic portal hypertension. A report of eight cases. J. Hepatol. 1990; 11: 80–85
52. **Olsen, J.H., Dragstedt, L., Autrup, H.:** Cancer risk and occupational exposure to aflatoxins in Denmark. Brit. J. Canc. 1988; 58: 392–396
53. **Peters, H.A.:** Hexachlorbenzene poisoning in Turkey. Fed. Proc. 1976; 35: 2400–2403
54. **Piontek, M., Hengels, K.J., Borchard, F., Strohmeyer, G.:** Nicht-zirrhotische Leberfibrose nach chronischer Arsenintoxikation. Dtsch. Med. Wschr. 1989; 114: 1653–1657
55. **Piqueras, J.:** Hepatotoxic mushroom poisoning: diagnosis and management. Mycopathologia 1989; 105: 99–110
56. **Pond, S.M.:** Effects on the liver of chemicals encountered in the workplace. West J. Med. 1982; 137: 506–514
57. **Pond, S.M.:** Manifestations and management of paraquat poisoning. Med. J. Aust. 1990; 152: 256–259
58. **Raithel, H.-J., Zober, A., Valentin, H.:** Berufsbedingte toxische Leberschäden. Inn. Med. 1983; 24: 16–24
59. **Redlich, C.A., West, A.B., Fleming, L., True, L.D., Cullen, M.R., Riely, C.A.:** Clinical and pathological characteristics of hepatotoxicity associated with occupational exposure to dimethylformamide. Gastroenterology 1990; 99: 748–757
60. **Reuber, M.D., Glover, E.L.:** Carbon tetrachloride-induced cirrhosis. Effect of age and sex. Arch. Path. 1968; 85: 275–279
61. **Roat, J.W., Wald, A., Mendelow, H., Pataki, K.J.:** Hepatic angiosarcoma associated with short-term arsenic ingestion. Amer. J. Med. 1982; 73: 933–936
62. **Ruprah, M., Mant, T.G.K., Flanagan, R.J.:** Acute carbon tetrachloride poisoning in 19 patients: implications for diagnosis und treatment. Lancet 1985/I: 1027–1029
63. **Scailteur, V., Lauwerys, R.R.:** Dimethylformamide (DMF) hepatotoxicity. Toxicology 1987; 43: 231–238
64. **Sinniah, D., Baskaran, G., Looi, L.M., Leong, K.L.:** Reye-like syndrome due to Margosa oil poisoning: report of a case with post mortem findings. Amer. J. Gastroenterol. 1989; 87: 158–161
65. **Solis-Herruzo, J.A., Vidal, J.V., Colina, F., Castellano, G., Munoz-Yagüe, M.T., Morillas, J.D.:** Clinico-biochemical evolution and late hepatic lesions in the toxic oil syndrome. Gastroenterology 1987; 93: 558–568
66. **Sotaniemi, E.A., Sutinen, S., Sutinen, S., Arranto, A.J., Pelkonen, R.O.:** Liver injury in subjects occupationally exposed to chemicals in low doses. Acta Med. Scand. 1982; 212: 207–215

67. **Stift, A., Friedl, J., Längle, F., Berlakovich, G., Steininger, R., Mühlbacher, F.:** Successful treatment of a patient suffering from severe acute potassium dichromate poisoning with liver transplantation. Transplantation 2000; 69: 2454–2455
68. **Straub, A.C., Stolz, D.B., Ross, M.A., Hernandez-Zavala, A., Soucy, N.V., Klei, L.R., Barchowsky, A.:** Arsenic stimulates sinusoidal endothelial cell capillarization and vessel remodeling in mouse liver. Hepatology 2007; 45: 205–212
69. **Texter, E.C., Grunow, W.A., Zimmermann, H.J.:** Massive centrizonal necrosis of the liver due to inhalation of 1,1,1-trichloroethane. Gastroenterology 1979; 76: 1260–1268
70. **Thiele, D.L., Eigenbrodt, E.H., Ware, A.J.:** Cirrhosis after repeated trichloroethylene and 1,1,1-trichloroethane exposure. Gastroenterology 1982; 83: 926–929
71. **Thomas, L.B., Popper, H., Berk, P.D., Selikoff, I., Falk, H.:** Vinyl-chloride-induced liver disease. From idiopathic portal hypertension (Banti's syndrome) to angiosarcomas. New Engl. J. Med. 1975; 292: 17–22
72. **Triebig, G., Weltle, D., Schaller, K.-H., Valentin, H.:** Chronische Lösemittel-Expositionen und Leberenzyme. Fortschr. Med. 1985; 103: 271–275
73. **Underwood, J.C.E., Huck, P.:** Thorotrast-associated hepatic angiosarcoma with 36 years latency. Cancer 1978; 2610–2612
74. **Velicia, R., Sanz, C., Martinez-Barredo, F., Sanchez-Tapias, J.M., Bruguera, M., Rodes, J.:** Hepatic disease in the Spanish Toxic Oil Syndrome. A thirty months follow-up study. J. Hepatol. 1986; 3: 59–65
75. **Ward, E., Boffetta, P., Andersen, A.:** Update of the follow-up of mortality and cancer incidence among European workers employed in the vinyl chloride industry. Epidemiology 2001; 12: 710–718
76. **Williams, A.T., Burk, R.F.:** Carbon tetrachloride hepatotoxicity: an example of free radical-mediated injury. Semin. Liver Dis. 1990; 10: 279–284
77. **Zaldivar, R.:** Arsenic contamination of drinking water and foodstuffs causing endemic chronic poisoning. Beitr. Path. Anat. 1974; 151: 384–400
78. **Zober, A., Schaller, K.-H., Gossler, K., Krekeler, H.-J.:** Pentachlorphenol und Leberfunktion: Eine Untersuchung an beruflich belasteten Kollektiven. Int. Arch. Occup. Environ. Health 1981; 48: 347–356

Clinical Aspects of Liver Diseases
31 Metabolic disorders and storage diseases

		Page:			Page:
1	*Definition*	595	9.2	Disturbances of the urea cycle	611
2	*Pathogenesis*	595	9.3	Cystinosis	611
3	**Non-alcoholic fatty liver disease**	595	9.4	Homocystinuria	612
3.1	Physiological aspects	595	10	**Carbohydrate storage diseases**	612
3.2	Definition	596	10.1	Glycogenoses	612
3.3	Pathogenesis	596	10.2	Galactosaemia	614
3.4	Morphology	596	10.3	Hereditary fructose intolerance	614
3.4.1	Fatty infiltration	596	10.4	Fructose-biphosphatase deficiency	615
3.4.2	Fatty degeneration	598	11	**Lipid storage diseases**	615
3.4.3	Phospholipidosis	598	11.1	Wolman's disease	615
3.5	Causes	599	11.2	Cholesterol ester storage disease	615
3.6	*Non-alcoholic steatohepatitis*	599	11.3	Cerebrotendinous xanthomatosis	616
3.6.1	Definition	599	11.4	Abetalipoproteinaemia	616
3.6.2	Epidemiology	600	11.5	Hypoalphalipoproteinaemia	617
3.6.3	Pathogenesis	600	11.6	Debré's syndrome	617
3.6.4	Morphology	600	12	**Sphingolipid storage diseases**	617
3.7	Diagnostics	601	12.1	Gaucher's disease	617
3.8	Prognosis	602	12.2	Fabry's disease	618
3.9	Complications	602	12.3	Gangliosidoses	618
3.10	Therapy	603	12.4	Niemann-Pick disease	619
4	**Faulty nutrition**	604	12.5	Mucopolysaccharidoses	619
4.1	Malnutrition	604	12.6	Mucolipidoses	620
4.2	Kwashiorkor	604	13	**Mucoviscidosis**	620
4.3	Tropical juvenile cirrhosis	605	14	**Zellweger's syndrome**	620
4.4	Infantile sclerosis	605	15	**Porphyrias**	621
4.5	Obesity	605	15.1	Definition	621
4.5.1	Diabetes mellitus	605	15.2	Classification	621
4.5.2	Hyperlipidaemia	605	15.3	Biochemistry	621
5	**Reye's syndrome**	606	15.4	Genetics	622
5.1	Causes	606	15.5	Clinical aspects	623
5.2	Clinical picture	606	15.6	Erythropoietic porphyrias	623
6	**Acute fatty liver of pregnancy**	606	15.6.1	Congenital erythropoietic porphyria	623
6.1	Clinical picture	606	15.6.2	Erythropoietic protoporphyria	623
6.2	Prognosis	607	15.7	Hepatic porphyrias	623
6.3	Treatment	607	15.7.1	Acute intermittent porphyria	624
7	**Mauriac's syndrome**	607	15.7.2	Variegate porphyria	625
8	**Protein storage diseases**	607	15.7.3	Hereditary coproporphyria	625
8.1	α_1-antitrypsin deficiency	607	15.7.4	Doss porphyria	626
8.1.1	Pathogenesis	607	15.7.5	Porphobilinogen synthase defect	626
8.1.2	Clinical picture	608	15.7.6	Porphyria cutanea tarda	626
8.1.3	Diagnostics and treatment	608	15.8	Hepatoerythropoietic porphyria	628
8.2	Amyloidosis	609	16	**Wilson's disease**	628
8.2.1	Clinical picture and diagnostics	609	16.1	Definition	629
8.2.2	Prognosis and treatment	610	16.2	Frequency	629
8.3	α_1-antichymotrypsin deficiency	610	16.3	Pathogenesis	629
9	**Amino acid storage diseases**	610	16.4	Pathophysiology	630
9.1	Hereditary tyrosinaemia	610	16.5	Morphological changes	630
9.1.1	Clinical picture	610	16.5.1	Hepatic manifestation	630
9.1.2	Treatment	611	16.5.2	Extrahepatic manifestations	631

		Page:
16.6	Clinical picture	632
16.7	Laboratory findings	633
16.8	Diagnostic measures	633
16.9	Prognosis	634
16.10	Treatment	634
16.10.1	Dietary measures	634
16.10.2	Drug therapy	634
16.10.3	Dialysis therapy	635
16.10.4	Liver transplantation	635
16.11	Indian childhood cirrhosis	635
17	***Haemochromatosis***	635
17.1	Definition	635
17.2	Classification	636
17.2.1	HFE-related haemochromatosis	636
17.2.2	Non-HFE-related haemochromatosis	636
17.2.3	Aceruloplasminaemia	637
17.2.4	Atransferrinaemia	637
17.2.5	Neonatal haemochromatosis	637
17.3	*Hereditary haemochromatosis*	637

		Page:
17.3.1	Frequency	637
17.3.2	Pathogenesis	637
17.3.3	Iron toxicity	638
17.3.4	Morphology	639
17.3.5	Early diagnosis	640
17.3.6	Preventive diagnostics	640
17.3.7	Manifestation	640
17.3.8	Prognosis	642
17.3.9	Treatment	643
18	***Haemosiderosis***	645
18.1	Alcohol abuse	645
18.2	Porphyria cutanea tarda	645
18.3	Blood transfusion	645
18.4	Haemolytic anaemia	645
18.5	Chronic liver disease	646
18.6	African iron overload	646
	• References (1–473)	646
	(Figures 31.1–31.30; tables 31.1–31.18)	

31 Metabolic disorders and storage diseases

1 Definition

Primary metabolic disorders and storage diseases are caused by endogenous factors, usually a gene mutation. Since the congenital defect is predominantly or exclusively located in the liver, the resulting diseases also become manifest in this organ.

Secondary metabolic disorders and storage diseases are present in almost all liver diseases and occur with more or less pronounced intensity. • They are, however, also caused by faulty nutrition as well as by many exogenous factors or noxae — just as latent metabolic disorders may generally become manifest due to such factors.

Thesaurismoses are storage diseases caused by the accumulation of metabolic products or substances in body fluids, organs or cells as a result of metabolic disorders.

2 Pathogenesis

▶ The pathogenic processes leading to the development of **primary** metabolic disorders or storage diseases are essentially caused by *two mechanisms*: (*1.*) formation of atypical macromolecules and (*2.*) extensive or complete blockage of a metabolic pathway. • These pathologically formed macromolecules cannot be broken down or secreted, with the result that they accumulate in the cells, including hepatocytes, or in the extracellular spaces. • Blockage of a metabolic pathway leads to (*1.*) insufficient production of certain metabolites, (*2.*) metabolite accumulation at the point of blockage, or (*3.*) formation of abnormal metabolites. This gives rise to the respective primary metabolic disorder or storage disease. It is, however, largely unclear what kind of mechanisms are actually responsible for liver cell damage.

▶ The pathogenesis of **secondary** metabolic disorders or storage diseases depends on the specific metabolic influence resulting from the character of the existing liver disease as well as other individual factors (e. g. malnutrition, alcohol abuse, chemicals, toxins). • Either a severe deficiency or an excessive supply of nutrients can cause persistent disorders in the hepatic metabolism and possibly result in morphological changes. That may also trigger a latent metabolic disorder which leads to further hepatocellular damage. This is especially true when the hepatic metabolism is compromised by a combination of stress factors, such as are present with diabetes mellitus, obesity, alcoholism or hyperlipidaemia.

▶ In primary or secondary metabolic disorders or storage diseases, almost all **metabolic functions** of the liver may be affected.

Bilirubin metabolism (= jaundice)	
Bile acid metabolism (= cholestasis)	
Amino acid metabolism	Lipid metabolism
Carbohydrate metabolism	Lipoprotein metabolism
Copper metabolism	Mucopolysaccharide metabolism
Glycolipid metabolism	Porphyrin metabolism
Iron metabolism	Protein metabolism

Genetically induced disorders of **bilirubin metabolism** affect (*1.*) bilirubin conjugation or (*2.*) bilirubin excretion through the canalicular membrane. This results in *functional hyperbilirubinaemia*. (s. tabs. 12.1, 12.4) (*see chapter 12*)

Genetically induced disorders of **bile acid metabolism** cause non-obstructive intrahepatic *cholestasis*. Cholestasis due to primary storage diseases also belongs to this group of disorders. (s. tab. 13.4) (*see chapter 13*)

3 Non-alcoholic fatty liver disease

3.1 Physiological aspects

Usually, the liver contains 0.8−1.5% of its wet weight in the form of extractable, finely dispersed structural fats, which cannot be detected by normal histological techniques. Under the light microscope, the liver fat, which is mainly made up of small droplets of triglycerides, only becomes visible when an increase up to 2−3% occurs. Above this value, hepatocytes "register" this event as a pathological process per se.

Triglycerides: Triglycerides are formed by the esterification of fatty acids, with glycerophosphate being produced by glycolysis. • Short- and medium-chain fatty acids from foodstuffs as well as fatty acids derived from lipolysis within adipose tissue are bound to albumin and transported to the liver cells through the portal vein. Long-chain fatty acids from foodstuffs become inserted as triglycerides in the chylomicrons within the mucosal cells of the small intestine. After having been broken down by endothelial lipoprotein lipase, the chylomicrons reach the hepatocytes in the form of remnants together with fatty acids. There, the fatty acids are beta-oxidized (to acetate and ketone bodies) in order to release energy or to synthesize phospholipids, cholesterol ester and triglycerides. The liver cell is also capable of de-novo synthesis of fatty acids from acetyl coenzyme A. Triglycerides are synthesized rapidly, particularly when there is a sufficient supply of α-glycerophosphate and acetyl coenzyme A. This also explains the influence of glucose and insulin on the regulation of the hepatocellular metabolism. High carbohydrate (and alcohol) levels increase the esterification of fatty acids to form glycerides. Partial conjugation of lipids and apoproteins takes place at the contact surfaces (i.e. membranes) of the smooth and rough endoplasmic reticulum, while the carbohydrate component is subsequently added within the Golgi complex, so that a complete VLDL particle is formed. It is only in this form, and together with cellular membrane lipids, that triglycerides can be actively exported from the liver cell by way of exocytosis. Otherwise, both retention and thus storage occur in the liver cell. • VLDL particles secreted from the hepatocyte are once more broken down in the capillaries by lipoprotein lipase to form LDL and fatty acids. In this way, the fatty acids can be reused as an energy source, stored in fat depots or remetabolized in the hepatocytes. • The lipids stored in fat depots are likewise broken down by triglyceride lipase into fatty acids (and glycerin) and reach the liver cells again via the blood stream, where the same possibilities of metabolization exist. • The liver cell is capable of either synthesizing or metabolizing lipid substances separately within itself, both in terms of time and place. *It should be noted that these metabolic processes can occur parallel to and independently of each other.* (s. p. 47) (s. fig. 3.8)

3.2 Definition

Liver steatosis is defined as a condition when there are small or medium-sized fat droplets in singular, disseminated liver cells and when the fat content is 3–10% of liver wet weight. • **Fatty liver** is defined as a condition when the fat storage is >10% of liver wet weight, when >50% of the hepatocytes contain fat droplets in different sizes (small to large) and when fat deposition shows a diffuse pattern in the parenchyma. • *Storage of fat in the liver cell is the most common form of morphological hepatocellular damage.*

▶ **Symptom:** Low-grade fat storage in liver cells, ranging from the deposition of tiny to medium-sized droplets, is deemed to be a mere symptom (or "metabolic siding") and therefore a harmless phenomenon. • Such a finding can be seen as a "dynamic" (short-term) liver steatosis after a high-fat meal, particularly together with alcohol.

▶ **Disease:** A diffuse fatty liver showing medium and large-sized droplets is regarded as a disease when the severity increases to a point where >50% of hepatocytes are involved (= *"from symptom to disease"*). Occasionally, excessive fat storage occurs (up to 100% of hepatocytes involved) with a high mortality rate, e.g. in acute alcohol intoxication (s. fig. 28.6) and acute poisoning due to chemicals or toxins. A maximum fat storage rate of 24% of liver wet weight has been observed.

3.3 Pathogenesis

When the hepatocytes are continuously inundated by fatty acids, from either the intestines or fat depots, their oxidative degradation or synthesis capacity may be reduced and triglyceride binding to lipoproteins can be depleted. This is most likely to happen whenever apoprotein synthesis or lipoprotein formation is compromised by noxae (e.g. alcohol). • Fat storage in hepatocytes is a *question of equilibrium* since accelerated or increased formation of triglycerides in the liver cell is *not* compensated by sufficient synthesis of lipoproteins and adequate secretion of VLDL from the liver cell. • Therefore, both exogenous and endogenous pathogenic factors may be responsible for the development of liver steatosis. In this process, additive as well as potentiating metabolic disorders sometimes occur, resulting in a biochemical/morphological *vicious circle*. (s. tab. 31.1)

Exogenous
1. Increase in lipid uptake from the intestine
2. Enhanced supply of glyceride precursors (glucose, fructose, galactose)
Endogenous
1. Increase in peripheral lipid mobilization   • Lipolysis ↑ (= triglyceride lipase activity ↑) (by ACTH, cortisol, catecholamines, prostaglandins, caffeine, alcohol, nicotine)
2. Inhibition of lipid utilization in hepatocytes   • β-oxidation ↓   • Fatty acid-binding protein ↓
3. Increase in lipid synthesis in hepatocytes   • Formation of fatty acids ↑   • Formation of triglycerides ↑
4. Reduction in lipid export   • Secretion of VLDL ↓   • Synthesis of apoproteins B, C_1–C_3, E ↓   • Disturbance in gluconeogenesis

Tab. 31.1: Pathogenesis of liver steatosis and fatty liver

3.4 Morphology

▶ The earliest histological criteria of **fatty liver** were described by W. Bowman in 1842. • As early as 1861, F. T. Frerichs demonstrated the development of hepatic steatosis and its reversibility in dogs. He gave a detailed description of minute fat droplets in liver cells and their continuous growth. Even at that time, he differentiated between **fatty infiltration** and **fatty degeneration.** Indeed, he considered fatty degeneration to be more "pernicious" than fatty infiltration. (1861, volume I, pp 285–324; figs. 41, 42) • (see below: W. S. Hartroft et al., 1968)

3.4.1 Fatty infiltration

Fat storage in liver cells starts with tiny droplets being deposited inside the endoplasmic reticulum and cytoplasm. This fatty deposition in the form of **small droplets** without a surrounding membrane is also called *fatty infiltration* (type A) (W. S. Hartroft et al., 1968). (14) Ini-

Formation of fat droplets
1. Deposits of tiny fat droplets
   Formation of small fat droplets
   = **small-droplet liver steatosis**

   ↓

2. Increase in size of fat droplets
   = **medium-droplet liver steatosis**

   ↓

3. Further increase in size of fat droplets
   Confluence of fat droplets
   Impairment of nuclear functions
   = **large-droplet liver steatosis**

   ↓

   = mixed-droplet liver steatosis
   = formation of fat cysts

Localization of liver steatosis
1. peripheral   3. zonal
2. centroacinar   4. diffuse

Liver steatosis
1. *Low-grade liver steatosis*
   = ca. 5% of WW
   = 10–15% of hepatocytes
2. *Medium-grade liver steatosis*
   = 6–8% of WW
   = 15–30% of hepatocytes
3. *Pronounced liver steatosis*
   = 8–9% of WW
   = 30–50% of hepatocytes

Fatty liver
4. *Severe fatty changes in liver cells*
   = 10–12% of WW
   = >50% of hepatocytes
     (medium-sized and large droplets, diffuse)
5. *High-grade fatty changes in liver cells*
   = 12–17% of WW (300–500 mg/g)
   = >70% of hepatocytes

Tab. 31.2: Formation, localization and various courses of liver steatosis resulting in the development of fatty liver (WW = wet weight of liver)

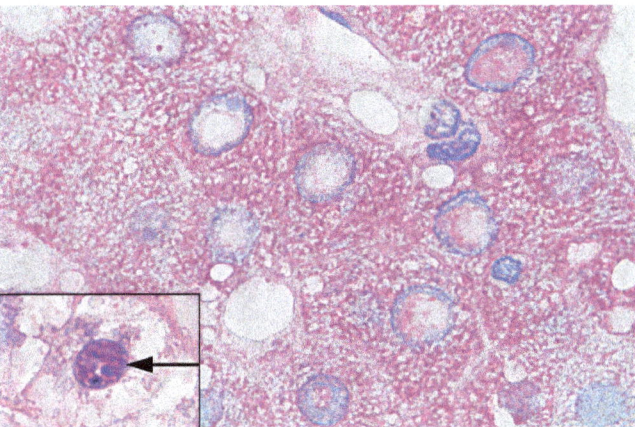

Fig. 31.1: Glycogenated nuclei (so-called glycogen vacuolations of the nuclei) in diabetes mellitus. *Insert:* nucleus strongly laden with glycogen (↑) (PAS) (s. pp 402, 540, 605, 613, 630, 639)

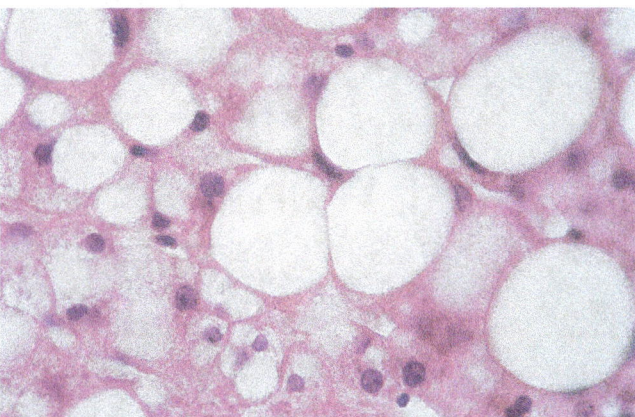

Fig. 31.2: Large-droplet (coarse-vacuolar) fatty liver in diabetes mellitus (preliminary stage of fat cyst formation) (HE)

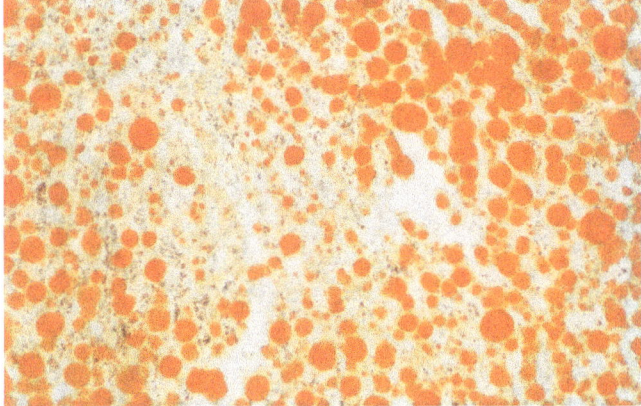

Fig. 31.3: Pronounced mixed-droplet fatty liver (Sudan red)

tially, only a few hepatocytes are affected by small-droplet deposits, whereas later on whole clusters are grouped together, mainly at the periphery of the lobules or in the centroacinar area. • Slowly but steadily, the droplets become larger, resulting in **medium-droplet steatosis**. The stored fatty droplets increase further in size and eventually fill the hepatocytes completely (= *macrovesicular steatosis*). (19, 23, 39, 48) (s. tab. 31.2)

As a result of **large-droplet steatosis,** the hepatocytes become enlarged, the fine cytoplasmatic structures are destroyed and the nucleus is pushed towards the cellular membrane. The functions of the nucleus are impaired or even halted. This also results in a strong tendency of the fatty cells to develop necrosis even under mildly toxic conditions. At the same time, the hepatocyte loses more and more glycogen. **Glycogen vacuolations of the nuclei** form when nuclear glycogen is removed. (s. fig. 31.1) They are observed in various diseases (e.g. diabetes mellitus), mostly in the area of the portal fields. • So-called **fat cysts** of various sizes are the result of large-droplet steatosis due to the cellular membrane being torn apart. (s. fig. 31.2) This fat-storing process results ultimately in a diffuse **mixed-droplet** fatty liver. (s. fig. 31.3) • **Peripheral** fat deposits (zone 1) are mainly caused by infectious or toxic damage directly affecting the

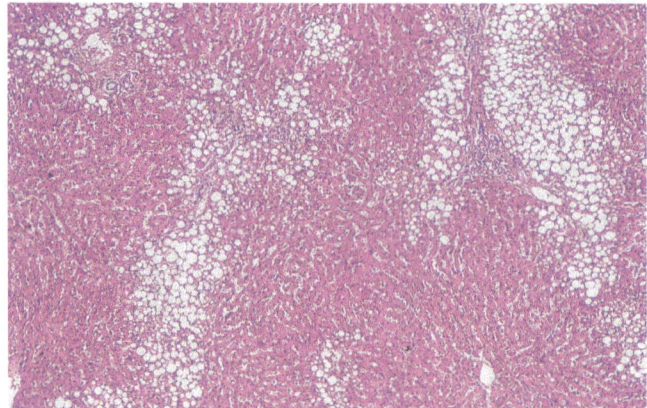

Fig. 31.4: Steatosis in periportal liver parenchyma. Clinical diagnosis: chronic phosporus poisoning (HE)

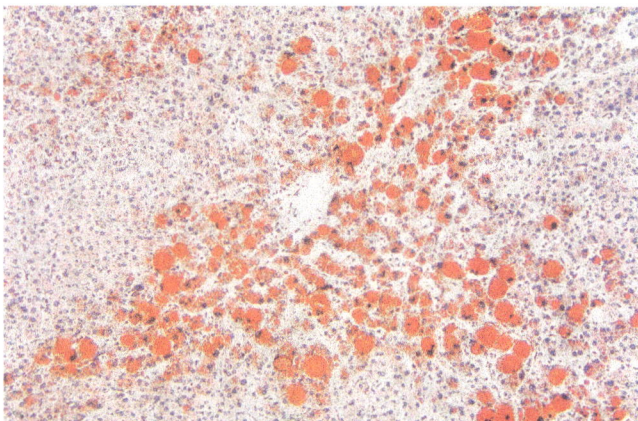

Fig. 31.5: Centroacinar steatosis. Clinical diagnosis: chronic alcohol abuse (Sudan red)

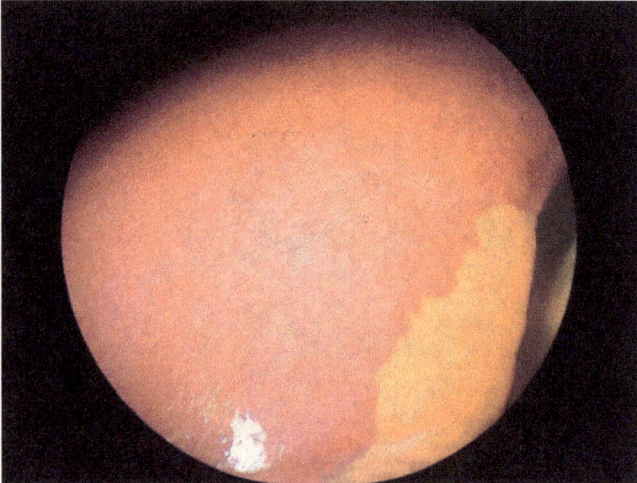

Fig. 31.6: Fatty liver with pronounced, thumb-sized fatty changes at the periphery of the left lobe (so-called "yellow spot")

periphery, where the liver cells are more involved in lipid metabolism via the blood stream. (s. fig. 31.4) • **Centroacinar** steatosis (zone 3) is often found in O₂ deficiency, nutrition-related damage, diabetes mellitus and alcohol abuse. It is seen as the more severe form of damage. (s. fig. 31.5) • **Zonal** steatosis occurs when only certain zones or areas of a lobule are affected. • This eventually results in **diffuse** steatosis of the whole lobule. (s. fig. 31.3)

In general, the left lobe shows less homogeneous steatosis than the right lobe. Regionally more pronounced fatty changes — which were formerly known laparoscopically as "yellow spots" (s. fig. 31.6), can be clearly detected as **focal** (s. fig. 8.3) or **segmental** fatty infiltration (s. fig. 8.4) by means of CT. (8, 12, 17, 25, 39)

3.4.2 Fatty degeneration

This form of microvesicular fat storage in hepatocytes, which is also termed type B (W.S. HARTROFT et al., 1968) (14), is a rare but prognostically serious condition. The cytoplasm is filled with small non-confluent fat particles which are surrounded by a delicate membrane. This may give the hepatocytes a foamy appearance. The nucleus remains largely unmodified in the centre of the cell.

Such *microvesicular degeneration* can be found in various thesaurismoses, different liver conditions and numerous drug-induced diseases. (15) (s. tab. 31.3)

1. **Acute fatty liver of pregnancy**
2. **Alcoholic foamy fat syndrome**
3. **Jamaican vomiting sickness** (33)
4. **Kwashiorkor** (29, 37)
5. **Reye's syndrome**
6. **Thesaurismoses**
– cholesterol ester storage disease
– disturbance of the urea cycle
– HDV hepatitis in northern South America
– Wolman's disease
7. **Drugs**
– acetylsalicylic acid   – pirprofen
– amineptin   – tetracycline
– fialuridine   – valproic acid
– ibuprofen   – warfarin
– ketoprofen   *etc.*

Tab. 31.3: Causes of microvesicular fatty degeneration (with some references)

3.4.3 Phospholipidosis

Enhanced lysosomal storage of phospholipids due to the inhibition of phospholipases is another special form of hepatic steatosis. The hepatocytes are enlarged and exhibit a distinctive foamy lucency of the cytoplasm. Crystalline inclusions and an agglomeration of myelin structures are visible in the lysosomes using electron microscopy. Mallory-Denk bodies may also be found. This idiosyncratic metabolic liver damage can even develop into cirrhosis. (s. tabs. 29.2; 31.4)

1. **Amiodarone**	4. **Chlorpromazine**
2. **Amitriptyline**	5. **Imipramine**
3. **Chloroquine**	6. **Perhexiline maleate**

Tab. 31.4: Some drugs causing phospholipidosis

3.5 Causes

Causes of fatty liver are manifold, and combinations of causes quite common. **Acquired causes** are by far the most frequent, but there are also rare causes, e. g. coeliac disease (9, 24), parenteral nutrition. (27, 28) • **Congenital metabolic disorders** can also lead to the development of a fatty liver, as in the case of a rare thesaurismosis. • It is of considerable therapeutic and prognostic importance to differentiate between an alcoholic fatty liver (AFL) and alcoholic steatohepatitis (ASH) (s. pp 529, 531) as well as between non-alcoholic fatty liver (NAFLD) and non-alcoholic steatohepatitis (NASH). (2, 19, 23, 34) (s. tabs. 31.5–31.7)

The frequency of NAFLD in the general population is given as 3–58%, whereby the great variability is due to socio-economic factors (average value is 20–23%). The development of NAFLD is more closely correlated with obesity than with alcohol abuse. In combined obesity and alcohol abuse, the frequency of fatty liver is estimated to be 50–60%. About one third of overweight patients suffer from type II diabetes, which in turn is responsible for NAFLD. Obesity can also lead to the formation of ASH and NASH. Consequently, if several causal factors of NAFLD coincide, the frequency and severity of fatty liver increases.

1. **Nutritional causes**
   Gastric bypass
   Hyperalimentation/obesity (1, 4, 5, 18, 32, 49, 73)
   Jejunoileostomy
   Malnutrition (11)
   – malabsorption, starvation, kwashiorkor (29, 37)
   Parenteral feeding (27, 28)
2. **Metabolic disorders**
   Diabetes mellitus (21, 32, 38)
   Gout
   Hyperlipidaemia (54)
   Thesaurismoses (s. tab. 31.6)
3. **Alcohol**
4. **Drugs** (s. tabs. 29.11; 31.3, 31.4, 31.7)
5. **Chemical substances** (47)
6. **Phytotoxins, mycotoxins**
7. **Infections**
   Bronchiectasis
   Chronic osteomyelitis
   Chronic tuberculosis
   Hepatitis C
   HIV infection
   Sprue
   Ulcerative colitis/Crohn's disease (9, 24)
   Yellow fever
8. **Oxygen deficiency**
   – anaemic – respiratory – cardiac
9. **Endocrinopathies**
   Acromegaly
   Cushing's syndrome
   Myxoedema (56)
10. **Liver surgery**
    Liver resection, jejuno-ileal bypass
    Primary dysfunction of a transplanted liver (44, 59)
11. **Cryptogenic fatty liver** (10)

Tab. 31.5: Acquired causes of liver steatosis or fatty liver (including some references)

Abetalipoproteinaemia	Mucoviscidosis
Cholesterol ester storage	Niemann-Pick disease
Fructose intolerance	Refsum's disease
Galactosaemia	Sphingolipidosis
Glycogenoses	Tyrosinaemia
Homocystinuria	Weber-Christian disease
Hypoalphalipoproteinaemia	Wilson's disease
Mauriac syndrome	Wolman's disease
Mucolipidosis	*etc.*

Tab. 31.6: Congenital causes of liver steatosis or fatty liver (so-called thesaurismoses)

1. **Medication** Flurazepam Glucocorticosteroids Hydrazine Mercaptopurine Methotrexate Naproxen Nifedipine Phenylbutazone Probenecid Rifampicin STH Tamoxifen, *etc.* 2. **Chemical substances** Antimony Arsenic Chloronaphthalene	Carbon tetrachloride Chloroform Chromium DDT Dinitrobenzene Dioxins Hexachlorocyclohexane Lead Pentachloroethane Phosphorus Tetrachloroethane Toluilendiamine, *etc.* 3. **Phytotoxins and mycotoxins** Aflatoxins Amanitins Gyromitrin, *etc.*

Tab. 31.7: Liver steatosis or fatty liver due to medication, chemical substances or toxins (s. tab. 29.11!)

3.6 Non-alcoholic steatohepatitis

▶ In 1980 the term non-alcoholic steatohepatitis (NASH) was introduced by J. LUDWIG et al. to denote chronic liver disease with increased enzymatic activity and the histological picture of alcohol-induced hepatitis. (57) • *The histological feature itself was described by H. THALER as early as 1962 in his paper "Fatty liver and its relationship to cirrhosis".* (72) • Over the following years, transition from a diabetic fatty liver into cirrhosis (S. ITOH et al., 1979) and from an obesity-induced fatty liver into cirrhosis (M. ADLER et al., 1979) were reported.

3.6.1 Definition

Histologically, non-alcoholic steatohepatitis shows moderate to high-grade, mainly macrovesicular fatty degeneration of the liver cells with inflammatory infiltrates and formation of fibrosis. Cirrhosis often develops. • Despite the morphological similarity to alcohol-induced fatty liver hepatitis, no (noteworthy) alcohol consumption is involved in NASH. Viral or autoimmune hepatitis are not detectable either. • There are no or only moderate subjective complaints. The transaminases are normal or slightly elevated. NASH is mostly associated with obesity and/or type II diabetes. • *Thus NASH is regarded as the hepatic manifestation of a metabolic syndrome.*

3.6.2 Epidemiology

Once alcohol consumption, viral hepatitis or autoimmune hepatitis have been ruled out, NASH is deemed the most common cause of a long-term increase in the transaminases. • The information available on prevalence and general frequency is not yet sufficient. In 2−6% of the US population, however, an increase in GPT (ALT) was detected without chronic liver disease being diagnosed. (53) Based on liver biopsies, a prevalence of 1.2−9.0% was determined. NASH is frequently associated with obesity (ca. 40%), non-insulin-dependent diabetes mellitus (ca. 20%) and hyperlipidaemia (ca. 20%). Women (particularly in middle age) are more often affected than men. (49, 53, 73, 74) • NASH may indeed also be found in children. (58, 64, 69). In this context, it was associated with obesity in 83% and with a disorder of the lipid metabolism in 50% of cases, while diabetes mellitus could only be detected in 5% of patients (but with increasing frequency during the further course of life, as was shown in the follow-up). (64)

3.6.3 Pathogenesis

The development of **liver steatosis** is attributable to various exogenous and endogenous mechanisms, which may combine with and/or potentiate each other. Numerous causal factors must be considered in the pathogenesis of fatty liver. (s. tab. 31.1) • With the increasing storage of fat, the liver cells also become more and more vulnerable to **noxae.** Thus oxidative stress may cause augmented oxidation of free fatty acids in the peroxisomes as well as enhanced activity of cytochrome P450 2E1. The biotoxometabolites (e. g. malonyldialdehyde, 4-hydroxynonenal) arising during this process provoke inflammatory infiltrations and fibrosis.

Second-hit hypothesis: The *first hit* is considered to be the development of *fatty liver*, particularly due to hyperalimentation and obesity resulting in insulin resistance. *However, the presence of a fatty liver is no prerequisite for the development of NASH!* • As *second hit* follows the mobilization of free fatty acids from fat depots, especially in cases of central obesity, and their transport to the liver cells. This leads to a massive increase of *free radicals* due to *oxidative stress* with *lipid peroxidation* and induction of *cytokines* (TNFα, TGFβ, IL8, IL1). (s. pp 71−73, 408) As a result, there is a reactive formation of uncoupling protein (UCP2) with a subsequent decrease in hepatocyte ATP and a disturbance of macrophage function with higher sensitivity to endotoxin. This leads to an inflammatory reaction, cell death and the formation of fibrosis. (43, 62)

A *genetic basis* seems to be necessary as a predisposition of NASH; however, such mechanisms are still unknown. It is discussed that genes can influence the degree of oxidative stress, the severity of steatosis, the regulation of immune reactions and apoptosis.

The pathogenesis of NASH is multifactorial, i.e. in the presence of steatosis, it is attributed to the additional (even combined) influence of different noxae (e. g. oxygen deficiency, endotoxins, medicaments, chemicals, iron, biotoxometabolites). • There should be no laboratory findings pointing to alcohol abuse; chronic hepatitis B and C as well as autoimmune hepatitis (71) must also be ruled out.

▶ From present knowledge, it can be assumed that numerous cases of cryptogenic chronic hepatitis or cryptogenic cirrhosis are attributable to the presence of NASH in terms of aetiopathogenesis.

3.6.4 Morphology

The diagnosis of NASH and the assessment of its prognosis are most reliably derived from liver histology. • In the lobule, *steatosis* is distributed mainly in a macrovesicular and diffuse manner, but sometimes it is concentrated microvesicularly and perivenously. Glycogen vacuolation of nuclei is common. • The *inflammatory reaction* consists of granulocytic and lymphocytic infiltrates, which are more frequently found in the portal and perivenous area than intralobular, with or without focal necrosis. Cell ballooning, Mallory's hyaline and ubiquitin (60) are generally present, while megamitochondria are also found occasionally. Steatosis and mild lobular chronic inflammation alone are insufficient for diagnosing NASH. The histological alterations are mainly localized in zone 3. • First of all, *fibrosis* appears within the perisinusoidal area, then additionally within the portal field (41); subsequently, it develops as bridging fibrosis giving rise to architectural remodelling, and eventually results in *cirrhosis* with portal hypertension. The histological picture of NASH can be mistaken for chronic hepatitis C, steroid-treated AIH, drug-induced hepatitis or the early stage of Wilson's disease. It is even more difficult for the pathologist to differentiate between a cirrhosis as a result of NASH, chronic hepatitis C and AIH. Often a diagnosis of cryptogenic cirrhosis has to be made. (10, 39, 42, 43, 50, 52, 58, 60, 63, 67, 69) (s. fig. 31.7)

▶ There are no morphological differences between alcoholic steatohepatitis and NASH. • In some 30(−50)% of patients with NASH, predominantly micronodular cirrhosis develops within five years.

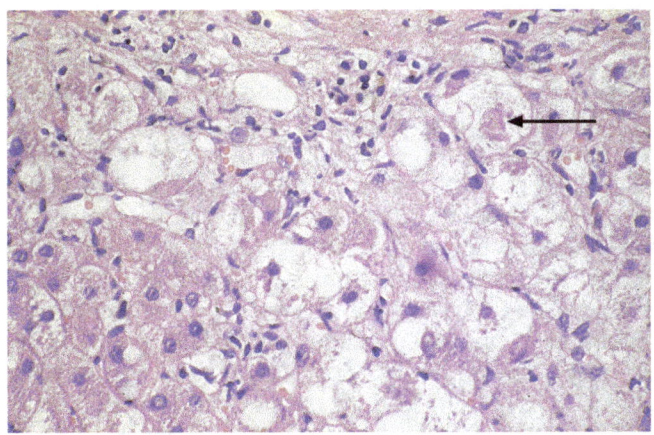

Fig. 31.7: Non-alcoholic steatohepatitis: Hydropic degenerated hepatocytes with Mallory's hyaline (←); lymphocytic and granulocytic infiltration as well as activated Kupffer cells (HE)

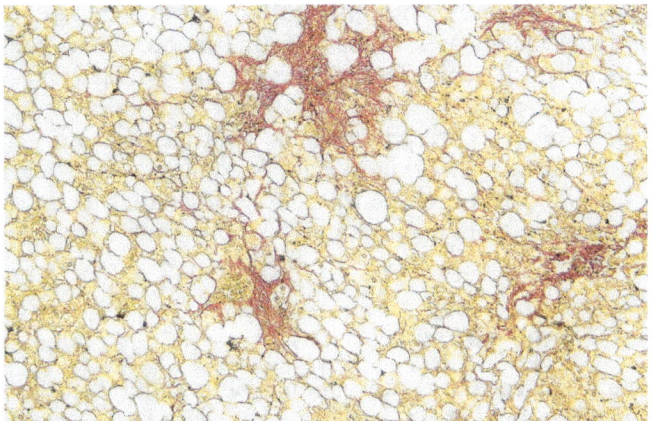

Fig. 31.8: Non-alcoholic steatohepatitis with massive steatosis and fibrosis. A 10-year-old boy with diabetes mellitus type 2

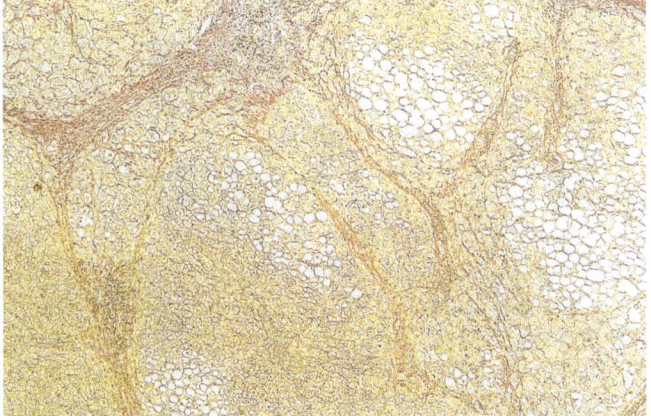

Fig. 31.9: Liver cirrhosis in non-alcoholic steatohepatitis. A 24-year-old adipose woman with insufficiently treated diabetes mellitus type 2 (Sirius red)

3.7 Diagnosis

Clinical findings: Steatosis does not generally cause any subjective complaints or clinical symptoms; it remains undetected or is discovered incidentally when diagnostic screening is being carried out for another disease. The presence of *risk factors* (overweight, diabetes, gout, hyperlipidaemia, medication, malnutrition, etc.) is of considerable diagnostic importance. • *Subjective complaints* include fatigue, repletion, malaise or loss of appetite. In hepatomegaly, right upper quadrant abdominal discomfort may occur, especially when stooping or lying on the right side. In obesity, which is present in most cases, hepatomegaly is often not palpable, so that the actual size of the liver can only be demonstrated by sonography (or CT). *Hepatomegaly* correlates with the severity of the fatty liver, allowing determination of the course. *Splenomegaly* is found in 20–25% of patients. (36) • In advanced cases, *skin stigmata* of liver disease and signs pointing to portal hypertension might be in evidence. Left ventricular diastolic dysfunction can be shown in ECG. (13) (s. tab. 31.8)

Laboratory diagnostics: With increasing severity of a fatty liver or NASH, some laboratory parameters are pathological in 80–90% of cases, i.e. 10–20% of patients show normal values. There is an initial rise in *γ-GT*, and subsequently in *GPT* and *GOT*. As a rule, the mildly to moderately increased values are detected purely by chance during a medical check-up. The DeRitis quotient is <1 (cf. alcoholic hepatitis with >1). While this constellation in itself is a useful hint of liver cell damage induced by toxins or metabolic processes, an increase in *cholinesterase* actually suggests the presence of disturbed lipid metabolism or a fatty liver. Decreased functioning of the liver, detectable at an early stage, can be determined by measuring the *galactose elimination capacity* (s. p. 114) or by applying the *indocyanine green test* (s. p. 114); these tests may also be used in long-term follow-up. • Other important laboratory parameters include alkaline phosphatase, bilirubin, electrophoresis, ferritin, leptin (46, 65), thioredoxin (70) and parameters connected with lipid metabolism. Progressive and severe courses correlate closely with laboratory values well outside the normal range. Sonographic signs of liver steatosis indicate screening for *diabetes mellitus*, if necessary with the help of the oral glucose tolerance test. (6, 34, 50, 52, 53, 68, 70) (s. tab. 31.8)

Sonography: Hepatomegaly can be confirmed by sonography (vertical diameter liver enlargement in MCL > 11–12 cm), with the liver mostly showing a plump form. Echogenicity is increased due to the high number of water/fat boundary layers, and the single reflexes are coarsened (unlike the renal parenchyma). The hepatic veins are difficult to visualize. In pronounced fatty liver, sonographic signs of portal hypertension may appear (= sinusoidal block). There is a positive correlation between the degree of fatty changes and the rise in echogenicity (= *large, white liver*). Fatty changes below 10–20% cannot be reliably detected by US. (s. p. 138) • Often, it is difficult to differentiate *focal fatty changes* (circumscribed density of the echo pattern) from malignant foci, so that further clarification using scintigraphy or CT is required. *Fibrosis* shows an inhomogeneous parenchymal structure in relation to the degree of severity. (7, 8, 12, 22) (s. tab. 31.8)

CT: In a fatty liver, CT scanning shows diffuse density reduction with a corresponding decrease in Hounsfield units (HU). (26) A fatty liver is markedly darker than the spleen (= *large, grey liver*). The vessels and bile ducts are hyperdense as compared to the parenchyma. There is a linear relationship between the extent of fat deposition and the reduction in density. The diagnostic reliability of a fatty liver determined by CT is 85–95%. *Focal fatty changes* or segmental fatty changes are easy to differentiate since, in contrast to metastases, they do not have any vascular branching. A 10% increase in the relative fat content results in a density reduction of 17–20 HU; i.e. in fatty changes of 80%, a density decrease to about −50 HU occurs. (s. p. 180) • Investigations have also been carried out to determine whether it is possible to quantify the fat content of the liver by **MRT**. (17, 20, 26) (s. tab. 31.8)

1. **Determination of potential risk factors** (obesity, alcohol, diabetes, gout, malnutrition, chemicals, hyperlipidaemia, medication, *etc.*)
2. **Hepatomegaly**   **Splenomegaly**
3. **Laboratory parameters**   • γ-GT ↑, GPT ↑, GOT ↑   • cholinesterase ↑, ferritin ↑   − galactose elimination capacity +   − indocyanine green test +   − alkaline phosphatase ↑   − triglycerides ↑, cholesterol ↑, glucose ↑   − lipid electrophoresis +, leptin ↑, thioredoxin ↑
4. **Sonography**   **CT**
5. **Morphology**   • percutaneous biopsy   • laparoscopy + biopsy

Tab. 31.8: Diagnosis of fatty liver or NASH, involving determination of the degree of severity, differential diagnosis and course

Liver biopsy: Only morphology provides a definitive diagnosis of fatty changes in the liver cells or a fatty liver. Apart from revealing *fatty changes*, it is even more important histologically to detect *inflammatory reactions* and to determine whether there is any sign of *progressive fibrosis* (e.g. due to iron overload). (6) The result of grading and staging (42) is decisive for the prognosis. (s. tabs. 34.2, 34.3) • Laparoscopic evaluation of the liver surface is of considerable diagnostic importance, as is the targeted biopsy of hepatic areas which are suspected of being pathological.

3.8 Prognosis

A fatty liver has a good prognosis, since complete reversibility can be achieved if the causes are fully eliminated. However, existing fibrotic processes generally remain. • A fatty liver should in no way be underestimated, since it involves many **dangers:** (*1.*) the manifold liver cell functions may be distinctly compromised, causing unfavourable effects on the liver or the organism as a whole; (*2.*) fatty changes in the liver cells make them susceptible to noxae or toxins, so that there is an increased tendency towards steatonecrosis and an impaired regeneration capacity; (*3.*) a fatty liver responds strongly to inflammatory processes with mesenchymal reactions; (*4.*) a severe fatty liver sometimes results in a narrowing of the intrahepatic vessels with ensuing impairment of biliary flow and haemodynamics, or it may even lead to the development of portal hypertension. Prognosis is essentially dependent on whether the causes of fatty liver as well as any additional risk factors can be eliminated. NASH develops into fibrosis or cirrhosis within five to ten years in 10–40% of cases. Some 10–15% of these patients die within 10 years as a result of complications associated with cirrhosis. • Risk factors showing that NASH is progressing include: age > 50 years, body mass index > 30, type II diabetes, hyperlipidaemia, DeRitis quotient > 1, thrombopenia, and the presence of Mallory-Denk bodies. (16, 34, 52, 63, 67) • *Metastases* originating from a colorectal carcinoma are rarely found in fatty liver.

3.9 Complications

The occurrence of complications points to the fact that fatty liver should not generally be regarded as a harmless disorder. A fatty liver and the various risk factors may give rise to complications which occasionally manifest as a separate disease. (19, 34, 63) (s. tab. 31.9)

1. Development of fatty liver hepatitis progressing to fatty fibrosis (50%) or cirrhosis (15%) (e.g. via *non-alcoholic steatohepatitis*)
2. Formation of intrahepatic cholestasis with or without jaundice, possibly even similar to obstructive jaundice (3)
3. Fat embolism (R. Virchow, 1886) (30)
4. Compression and narrowing of sinusoids (31) with potentially reversible portal hypertension – but also with formation of collaterals and ascites
5. Intrahepatic narrowing of the inferior vena cava, with occurrence of leg oedema
6. Hepatic insufficiency (3%)

Tab. 31.9: Possible complications of fatty liver

Such complications must be reckoned with in fatty liver if (*1.*) the cause or any additional risk factors have not been eliminated and continue to have an effect, (*2.*) the underlying cause has not been identified despite all efforts (= *cryptogenic fatty liver*) and thus no real starting point for therapeutic measures is given, and (*3.*) specific causes of fatty liver, and the occurrence of NASH in particular, already have a tendency towards progression. • In such patients, there is evidence of *liver cell necrosis* and inflammatory *infiltration*, both of which are reversible. However, in some cases, particularly with simultaneous *lipid peroxidation*, a vicious circle can develop with subsequent mesenchymal reactions. The outcome is increasing *fibrosis* or, in some cases, even *cirrhosis*.

3.10 Therapy

The search continues for a medicament that can normalize the disturbed hepatocellular lipid metabolism or bring about the release of the fat stored in liver cells.

▶ Fatty liver has no specific therapy. Exclusion of the *cause* and elimination of additional *risk factors* – in as far as these two basic therapeutic requirements can be accomplished – usually result in complete regression of steatosis. • Should these measures fail to bring about a regression within a period of three to six months, it is assumed that *either* exclusion of the cause and elimination of risk factors have not been successful *or* the real underlying cause was not identified, so that no effective treatment measures were actually applied. • A lack of regression thus necessitates (*1.*) renewed investigation of the cause and risk factors as well as (*2.*) consistent implementation of the therapy that results from this!

Strict *alcohol abstinence* is called for – even in cases where alcohol is not the cause of fatty liver. The same applies to the adjustment of the *blood-sugar levels* in diabetes mellitus or the *uric acid values* in gout. *Hyperlipidaemia* may likewise necessitate a specific drug therapy depending on the respective type and course. • In *obesity* due to overeating, it is imperative to lose weight (gradually!) by means of reduced caloric intake, especially a low-carbohydrate ketogenic diet (35), based on the principles of the physiology of nutrition. Proteins and water-soluble vitamins should be administered at a higher daily dosage than is usually required. The effect of dietary measures can generally be supported by *orlistat*. Regression of a fatty liver is best achieved by constant weight reduction (200–250 g/day). Given a normal body weight, reducing the intake of fat in the diet (below the level that is usually needed) does not influence the regression of hepatic steatosis. (11, 26)

Although the therapeutical principles described above are generally accepted knowledge, pharmacological possibilities for facilitating the release of fat from the liver cells by administering **specific medication** have been repeatedly sought in the past. This process is ongoing, but first results have been relatively promising.

Adjuvant therapy: In view of the fact that it has hitherto proved difficult to restore a fatty liver by means of medication, attention has focused on the possibility of averting the pathomorphological forms of damage described above (and thus the development of a complicative progression) with the help of medicaments as an adjuvant therapy.

Prevention of fibrosis is of great importance. Three substances have already proved their worth in the **inhibition of fibrosis:** *essential phospholipids* (EPL or PPC), *silymarin* and *UDCA*. • The antifibrogenic effect of EPL has been demonstrated repeatedly in experiments; it is mainly based on the stimulation of collagenase. (s. fig. 40.3) • The antifibrogenic efficacy of silymarin is attributed to the proven inhibition and transformation of Ito cells as well as the reduction in gene expression of ECM and TGF-β. (s. tab. 40.13) • An antifibrogenic effect of UDCA in alcoholic liver disease has also been reported.

The occurrence of **lipid peroxidation** normally results in inflammatory tissue reactions and progression of the morphological process. Under experimental conditions, elimination of the free radicals responsible for lipid peroxidation has proved useful in therapy. The administration of antioxidants may thus be advisable as adjuvant therapy. Effective active agents include *essential phospholipids* (s. fig. 40.3), *silymarin* (s. tab. 40.13) and *N-acetylcysteine*. In this connection, it was possible to observe stimulation of superoxide dismutase, inhibition of lipoxygenase, reduction in malonyl dialdehyde, decreased consumption of glutathione, etc. Administration of *vitamin C* and *vitamin E* as antioxidants led to the regression of fibrosis. (51) Likewise, *probucol*, an agent with antioxidant properties, caused a significant decrease in GPT and GOT. The use of *pentoxifylline* (1600 mg/day) led to a decrease in liver enzymes.

Lipotropic substances show a particular affinity to fats and have counteracted hepatic steatosis in animal experiments. • In a 12-month course of therapy involving patients with a fatty liver, *EPL* led to a significant and lasting improvement and even to normalization of the increased transaminases and γ-GT within four weeks. (61) • *Choline* is substantially involved in the mobilization of triglycerides from the liver cell, because it uses these neutral fats to form transportable phospholipids. • However, choline needs *betaine* for demethylation. Thus betaine has an important function in transmethylation processes of lipid metabolism. Resynthesis of methionine likewise requires the assistance of betaine (increase of SAMe concentration in the liver). A dosage of 20 g/day (over 1 year) led to a reduction of the transaminases, liver steatosis and inflammatory activity. (40) • *Atorvastatin* (10 mg/day) was effective in patients with hyperlipidaemia. *Clofibrat* proved ineffective in patients with NASH. *Gemfibrozil* (600 mg/day), which reduces the mobilization of free fatty acids from the fat depots, brought about a decrease in the transaminases. • By contrast, the use of *pioglitazone* or *rosiglitazone*, a peroxisome proliferator-activated receptor (PPAR), led to an improvement in the histological and biochemical findings. This could imply that insulin resistance is significant in the pathogenesis of NASH. (60) *Metformin*, an insulin-sensitizing drug, led to positive changes in the histological pattern.

The use of *ursodeoxycholic* acid is advisable in cases involving a cholestatic course of NAFLD or NASH. It has a cytoprotective and anti-apoptotic effect. With a dosage of 13–15 mg/kg BW/day, it was possible to achieve an improvement in the transaminase values and the fat content of the liver. An increase in dosage to 20–25 mg/kg BW/day might be advisable. (55) A combination of UDCA and vitamin E (over two years) showed good results. • In animal experiments, *taurine* led to a restorative effect of NASH (inhibition of lipid peroxidation, improvement in lipid and glucose metabolism, decreased synthesis of TFNα and TFNβ, enhanced synthesis of adiponectin. (45)

A *phlebotomy* reduces transaminase levels and increases iron parameters in patients with NASH. This is understandable, since intrahepatic iron storage correlates with the severity of fibrosis.

Liver transplantation may be indicated in patients with considerable cirrhosis-related complications. However, NASH can also reoccur in the transplanted liver. (44, 60) This observation points to a systemic disorder of the lipid metabolism.

4 Faulty nutrition

A **healthy liver** is capable over a longer time of tolerating considerable changes in the pattern of food intake (irregular meals) or with respect to the quantity and quality of the food itself. • However, even a healthy liver reacts with functional disturbances or morphological changes to long-term **malnutrition.** During a state of hunger or a period of low protein intake, for example, almost all toxic substances have more severe effects, while the ability of the immune system to fight infections is compromised. • General **hyperalimentation** results in surplus calorie supply. The excess in carbohydrates and fat usually goes together with simultaneous protein deficiency. In this context, both the kind of fat or carbohydrate and any imbalance between lipogenic and lipotropic substances are important.

Animal experiments have shown that **faulty nutrition**, i.e. > 90% fat, < 10% protein and < 2 mg choline per day, leads to pronounced fatty liver and even fatty cirrhosis within a few weeks. The same changes could be observed when the protein intake remained more or less normal, while extremely little methionine and choline was offered. • With a **partial surplus** of certain foodstuffs, the special nature of the excessive nutritional components is also of considerable importance. • The term **partial malnutrition** may, for example, be associated with a pronounced protein deficiency (and thus possibly inadequate production of lipoproteins) or a lack of lipotropic substances (such as methionine, choline, cystine, glycocollbetaine, pyridoxine, casein and various N- or S-methylated substances). *Protein deficiency has particularly severe consequences when toxic substances are absorbed at the same time or when the organism has to fight bacterial or parasitic infections.* • A **diseased liver** reacts to both a serious deficiency in and an excessive supply of different nutrients (e.g. proteins, certain kinds of amino acids, various lipids, trace elements) with unfavourable or even complicative developments during the course of disease.

4.1 Malnutrition

Functional disturbances and morphological cell damage of the liver can be observed after prolonged general malnutrition. They are fully reversible using nutritional therapy. In *anorexia nervosa*, there may also be an increase in the transaminases or a pathological tendency shown in liver function tests.

Lipofuscin: The presence of lipofuscin is without pathological relevance and can be observed when medication is taken (e.g. phenacetin, chlorpromazine) (s. fig. 21.3), with advancing age and during prolonged malnutrition. The yellowish-brown pigment granules, some 1 μ in size, are PAS-positive, orcein-negative and acid-proof. They are produced from cell-own material and stored in the centroacinar hepatocytes, i.e. between the nucleus and bile canaliculi (= *centroaxial pigment pathways*).

Ceroid: The presence of ceroid is occasionally seen in both malnutrition and in acute viral hepatitis. It is PAS-positive, orcein-positive and acid-proof. This orange-brown granular pigment is mainly stored centroacinarly. (s. fig. 21.6)

Brown atrophy: In malnutrition, the liver shows a decrease in cell and nucleus size, glycogen depletion, pigment deposits, occasional siderosis and proliferation of Kupffer cells. The liver as a whole becomes smaller (by as much as two thirds of its normal weight). Due to its pigment deposits, particularly siderin, the liver takes on a brown colour. These changes have been subsumed under the term brown atrophy (H. POPPER, 1948).

4.2 Kwashiorkor

Kwashiorkor (meaning in the Ghanaian language "a disease which develops in a baby when it is replaced by a new baby and is weaned from the breast onto starch paps") was first described by C. WILLIAMS in 1933. It is caused by a diet which is poor in protein, particularly animal protein, whereas the supply of carbohydrates and fat calories is too high. Two new hypotheses of aetiology emerged suggesting that the disease stems from (*1.*) the action of excess free radicals (M.N.H. GOLDEN et al., 1987) or (*2.*) the action of dietary toxins, e. g. cyanogens, aflatoxins (R.G. HENDRICKSE, 1991). Manifestation is attributable to intercurrent intestinal infections. In both children and adults, the symptoms include dermatosis, muscle atrophy, oedema due to hypoalbuminaemia, diarrhoea and growth retardation. The hair shows typical depigmentation (red hair), at the same time becoming straight, thin and soft. There is severe fatty liver (mainly in zone 1), often with enormous hepatomegaly. Striking dark red skin patches appear, mostly in the periumbilical and/or inguinal areas as well as in the nuchal region. This skin discoloration together with the red hair gave the illness the name "red boy". When animal protein is supplied, e. g. skimmed milk, complete restitution can be achieved. • Kwashiorkor as such does not result in liver fibrosis or cirrhosis. However, lymphocytic infiltration of the portal fields and progressive periportal/perilobular fibrosis (as well as pancreatic fibrosis and endocardial sclerosis) are often observed; there is also evidence of necrosis and collapse areas as well as signs of cirrhosis. Such changes are due to the high susceptibility of kwashiorkor patients to infections and toxic effects (e. g. aflatoxin). (29, 37) • A remarkable histological effect of EPL was seen in African children with a fatty liver due to nutritional imbalance as well as protein and vitamin deficiency. (s. p. 894)

4.3 Tropical juvenile cirrhosis

This clinical picture is also caused by animal protein deficiency. However, it was common practice in the affected regions to use beaver oil as a laxative, and this is known to be extremely toxic to the liver. Fatty liver, hepatomegaly and jaundice were observed; ultimately, cirrhosis of a more biliary type developed.

4.4 Infantile sclerosis

This disease has mainly been encountered in Jamaica. Severe fatty liver with hepatomegaly developed together with early ascites (but no jaundice) and an increasing deterioration in liver synthesis performance. Death occurs in liver coma. Morphologically, there was evidence of fibrosis as well as veno-occlusive disease, features which suggested a combination of protein-deficient nutrition and phytotoxins.

4.5 Obesity

In 30—50% of cases of obesity, *fatty liver* is detected. A statistical evaluation of available data (1996) revealed that 15—17% of the German population displayed a **body mass index** of > 30; BMI = *body weight (in kg): body size (in m^2)*. Another 40% are overweight, with a BMI of 25—30. (4) Thus the German population occupies a leading position in the world with regard to the percentage of persons who are considerably overweight. The degree of obesity correlates with the severity of fatty liver. Adipose people suffering from android distribution of fat (i. e. bulk of the fat in the abdominal area) also develop more pronounced fatty liver. (18) Steatosis is predominantly macrovesicular and localized in zone 3. The increased release of fatty acids is responsible for diminished glucose utilization, whereby blood sugar rises and insulin secretion is stimulated, with simultaneous insulin resistance. Apart from that, any excessive carbohydrates are used for liponeogenesis. The outcome is a *metabolic disorder similar to diabetes* with increasing fatty changes in the liver; this condition is further aggravated by an enhanced production of endogenous cortisol due to adiposity, with the result that a vicious circle is established. (1, 2, 5, 32, 49, 58, 73, 74)

Leptin, an anti-obesity hormone, can prevent "lipotoxicity" from damaging hepatocytes by limiting triglyceride accumulation. A deficiency of leptin could be a risk factor for NASH. (65) Hyperleptinaemia correlates with the severity of fatty liver, but not with inflammation or fibrosis. • *Thioredoxin* is a stress-inducible, thiol-containing protein. It is elevated in NASH compared to patients with simple fatty liver. There is a correlation with increasing iron accumulation in the liver cells. Therefore, the pathogenesis of NASH may be associated with iron-related oxidative stress.

4.5.1 Diabetes mellitus

In type II diabetes, *fatty liver* is detectable with a frequency of 30—40%, principally due to adiposity and insulin resistance. The course is generally more aggressive with rapid progression to cirrhosis; mortality is also higher. (39) In diabetics, fatty acid oxidation in the liver cell remains undisturbed as far as coenzyme A acetate; glucose deficiency then stops any further oxidation within the citric-acid cycle. The additional energy required has to be supplied through increased degradation of fatty acids in the fat depots (= lipolysis) or reduced storage (= lipogenesis). This inevitably results in *hyperlipidaemia*, fatty liver and ketosis. Often, so-called *glycogen vacuolization of the nuclei* is found, mainly in the vicinity of the portal fields. Ketoacidosis increases lipolysis, causing steatosis to progress. • In a type I diabetes, however, fatty liver is less common and is indeed only to be expected in a ketotic metabolic situation, e.g. if the diabetes is not well-regulated. The course is more favourable; the mortality rate is not influenced. (2, 21, 32, 38, 61, 74) (s. fig. 31.1)

4.5.2 Hyperlipidaemia

Disorders of lipid metabolism, particularly type IV (endogenous hypertriglyceridaemia), cause fatty liver to develop. Hyperlipidaemia is present in approximately 50% of patients with sonographically determined fatty liver. (2, 54) • In a similar way, patients suffering from **gout** are very often found to have a fatty liver. Both these metabolic disorders frequently appear in combination with obesity.

5 Reye's syndrome

▶ This syndrome was described by W.R. Brain et al. in 1929. (77) In 1963 it was differentiated as a clinical pathological entity by R.D.K. Reye et al. and defined as a feverish disease of unclear aetiology in infancy. Almost half the children who were found to be suffering from this syndrome died of various cerebral manifestations, including brain oedema. (87)

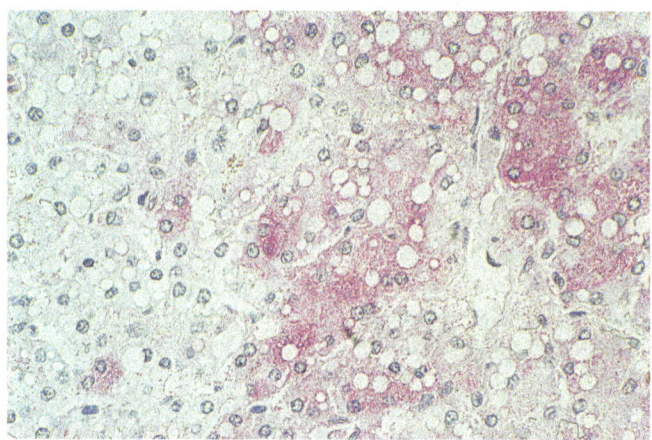

Fig. 31.10: Reye's syndrome (newborn): fine-droplet fatty changes of hepatocytes as well as glycogen depletion; no signs of inflammation (PAS)

5.1 Causes

Causes, which are generally linked to a genetic *disposition*, include *viral infection* (e.g. influenza, varicella) and the administration of *salicylates* (involved in some 95% of cases). (86) • In the USA, as many as 2,900 cases were observed in 1973 alone, with more than 800 fatalities; a further 1,207 cases were reported between 1980 and 1997. (76) About 98% of these patients were younger than 20 years of age. The frequency peak was 1978 to 1980; the disease appeared predominantly in December to April, i.e. during the influenza peak. It only occurs rarely nowadays: from 1994 to 1997 only two cases were observed. It should be mentioned that during administration of *Azadirachza indica* (= Margosa oil) toxic liver damage of the Reye type was reported. (75, 78, 80, 81, 83) (s. p. 279)

5.2 Clinical picture

The onset of the disease is an influenza-like, feverish syndrome. Uncontrollable vomiting results in severe hypoglycaemia. Progressive CNS disturbances develop along with convulsions, clouding of consciousness and brain oedema. Laboratory values show a pronounced increase in the transaminases, distinct hyperammoniaemia and moderate cholestasis (without jaundice). Striking features are elevated serum levels of alanine, glutamine and lysine. There are severe blood coagulation disorders. • The tumour-necrosis factor is increased. Hepatomegaly and microvesicular fatty changes in the liver cells predominate. The hepatocytes are swollen and depleted of glycogen. Cell necrosis is found at the periphery of the lobules. The smooth endoplasmic reticulum and peroxisomes are clearly increased, while the mitochondria are swollen and deformed; no signs of inflammation are present. (s. fig. 31.10) Development of chronic liver disease has not been observed as yet. The mortality rate is 30–50%. (78, 79, 82, 85, 88)

6 Acute fatty liver of pregnancy

▶ The first descriptions of acute fatty liver of pregnancy were given by H.J. Stander et al. (1934) (102); H.L. Sheehan (1940) later defined this disease as a separate syndrome. (100)

6.1 Clinical picture

This severe clinical picture occurs more often than has previously been assumed; nowadays, however, the survival rate is higher. Incidence is about 1 in 13,000 births. (91, 98, 99, 107) • The cause is still unknown. Up to now, a correlation with high-dosage intravenous tetracycline has been assumed. (92) An analogy to Reye's syndrome is also under discussion, as this clinical picture is considered to be part of the spectrum of pre-eclampsia. Primigravidas and multigravidas are equally affected. There is evidence of an already existing genetic enzyme defect (3-hydroxyacyl-CoA dehydrogenase?). (96, 104) Acute fatty liver of pregnancy occurs in the third trimester, particularly in the $34^{th}-36^{th}$ week. The disease begins in a state of complete well-being and a hitherto uncomplicated pregnancy. It comprises nausea and vomiting (often coffee-ground-like), polydipsia, right-sided abdominal pain, headaches and jaundice. Pruritus is rare. Sometimes, gastrointestinal bleeding, oedema and ascites occur. Encephalopathy develops with neurological symptoms similar to eclampsia. Hypertension, tachycardia, proteinuria and oliguria as well as signs of acute pancreatitis are frequently observed. The whole clinical picture is characterized by multiple organ insufficiency with haemorrhagic diathesis and fulminant hepatic failure. However, relatively asymptomatic and moderate courses with jaundice are also known.

Laboratory values show progressive hyperbilirubinaemia up to 15 mg/dl, an increase in alkaline phosphatase (3 to 5 times the normal range) and triglycerides as well as a rise in the transaminases up to 500 U/l. Usually, γ-GT is normal. Uric acid, which is mostly elevated, is seen as an early laboratory marker. Severe hypoglycaemias are evident. A striking feature is pronounced leucocytosis (> 50,000/µl), with neutrophils predominating. The differential blood count shows giant thrombocytes, target cells and normoblasts. There is a tendency towards bleeding due to thrombopenia as well as to a decrease in Quick's value, fibrinogen and AT III; disseminated intravascular coagulopathy is usually present. (93, 99)

Computer tomography provides evidence of massive fatty deposits in the liver. (94, 105) • *Sonography*, however, does not generally demonstrate such steatosis. There is pronounced hepatomegaly. (90)

Liver biopsy may be required for diagnosis — unless there are any contraindications. (s. tab. 7.4) In order to detect the characteristic microvesicular (mainly centroacinar) fatty changes, fixation without alcohol and examination of the biopsy material in the form of a frozen section are necessary. (101) The hepatocytes are swollen and resemble so-called foam cells. The nucleus is pyknotic. The mitochondria are deformed. (s. fig. 31.11)

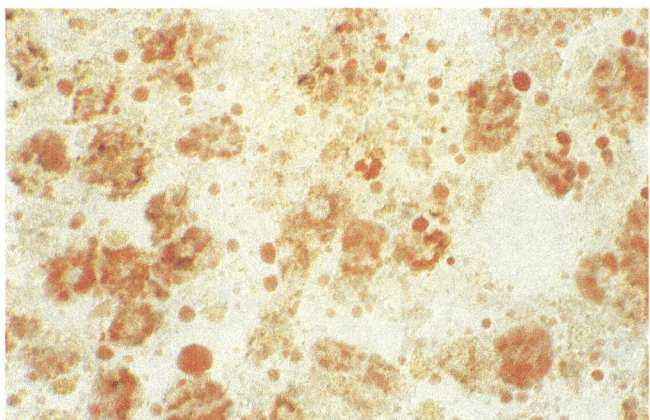

Fig. 31.11: Microvesicular fatty changes of liver cells in acute fatty liver of pregnancy (Sudan red)

Complications: Additional complications were observed during the course of disease, including pronounced cholestasis (106), portal hypertension and liver rupture (95).

6.2 Prognosis

The prognosis depends on early diagnosis and subsequent early (even premature) delivery. When a pregnant woman in the third trimester suddenly suffers from complaints and/or when the laboratory liver values are pathological, acute fatty liver of pregnancy should be suspected and other hepatobiliary diseases excluded as soon as possible. • The previous mortality rates for mother (ca. 90%) and child (ca. 70%) have been reduced to 10−35% and 7−50% respectively. The duration of the disease up to the death of the mother was on average 11 days (3 days up to 6 weeks), and in cases of survival from 2 to 8 weeks. (91, 93, 98, 103) • After acute fatty liver of pregnancy has been overcome, the liver values

normalize within a few days. There is no danger of chronic liver damage. In subsequent pregnancies, there is no tendency to relapse, and there are no contraindications against further pregnancies. (89, 107) However, a certain risk remains, so that the women affected should be given the relevant information. Usually, the patient prefers not to risk a further pregnancy.

6.3 Treatment

Immediate delivery (per section or vaginally) is the most important treatment. Further therapy consists of intensive medical care. (106) In individual cases, liver transplantation may be indicated. (97)

7 Mauriac's syndrome

This clinical picture was described by P. Mauriac in 1930. Pathogenesis is attributed to pluriglandular dysregulation. In combination with difficult-to-control infantile or juvenile diabetes mellitus, secondary glycogenosis may develop due to large deposits of glycogen and fat in the hepatocytes, resulting in *hepatomegaly*. • In addition to considerable fluctuations between hyperglycaemia and hypoglycaemia, there is evidence of hypercholesterolaemia, hyperlipidaemia and acetonuria. The clinical picture is characterized by repeated abdominal colic, meteorism, venectasias of the abdominal wall, buffalo obesity, moon face, retarded growth and osteoporosis. Careful monitoring and stabilization of diabetes mellitus are the most essential aspects of the treatment. (108)

8 Protein storage diseases

Numerous proteins are produced in the liver. *Genetically induced disorders* of protein metabolism may cause proteins to be stored in the hepatocytes or even deposited in the intestinal tract. Primary storage diseases in this context include: (*1*.) α_1-antitrypsin deficiency, (*2*.) amyloidosis, and (*3*.) α_1-antichymotrypsin deficiency.

8.1 α_1-antitrypsin deficiency

▶ The association between lung emphysema and α_1-antitrypsin (α_1AT) deficiency was recognized by C. B. Laurell et al. in 1963. The development of liver cirrhosis due to α_1AT deficiency was first observed in children by E. Freier et al. in 1968 and in adults by N. O. Berg et al. in 1972.

8.1.1 Pathogenesis

This disease is biochemically more correctly termed α_1-**protease inhibition deficiency** since the protein acts against trypsin and numerous serine proteases, in particular chymotrypsin and leucocyte elastase. In the pulmonary alveoli, for example, elastase inhibits the breakdown of elastin. • Serum α_1AT is a glycoprotein with 394 amino acids and 3 carbohydrate chains. It is generally synthesized in the Golgi apparatus of the hepatocytes, although small amounts are also formed in the gastrointestinal tract and in macrophages. Due to gene mutation, the transport of α_1AT from the endoplasmic reticulum (high-mannose type) to the Golgi apparatus is inhibited, so that the "secretion-competent complex" cannot be produced (= α_1AT deficiency). (118) Thus α_1AT is not transferred to the blood by way of exocytosis, but remains stored in the endoplasmic reticulum in the form of **globular deposits** and is subsequently broken down. • The α_1AT gene is localized on chromosome 14 q 32 and possesses about 100 allelic variants, which are named according to the **Pi nomenclature** (= *protease inhibitor*). In homozygosity, *normal allele PiM* regulates the formation of the normal phenotype PiMM, which is present in >90% of the population. • Alpha$_1$-antitrypsin deficiency is caused by an autosomal recessive mutation of two alleles. • **Homozygous defective alleles** are: PiZZ, PiSS, PiZnull, PiPP, PiWW, Pinull, PiMmalton. They show plasma concentrations between 0% and 15% of the normal α_1-AT value. *These homozygous combinations of defective alleles are accompanied by a high risk of pulmonary emphysema, newborn cholestasis, infantile hepatitis, cirrhosis and hepatocellular carcinoma.* • PiMS, PiMZ, PiSZ, PiFZ and PiMnull are deemed to be **heterozygous defective alleles.** In Europe, the allele type PiMZ is found in 3%, PiMS in 7%, and PiSZ as well as PiZZ in 1% of the population. Plasma values range between 42% and 60% of the normal α_1AT value. Heterozygosity thus causes only moderate and/or intermediary α_1-AT deficiency, but is nevertheless seen as a *predisposing factor of liver disease*. (110, 111, 113, 119, 124, 126)

8.1.2 Clinical picture

The great variability of this clinical picture depends upon allele type, age at initial manifestation and individual progression. • About 0.02−0.06% (1 : 1,500−3,500) of all newborns are **homozygous** carriers of defective alleles. In 10−12% of these, conjugated hyperbilirubinaemia with intrahepatic cholestasis and pruritus develops within the first months of life. A lethal course is possible; in most cases, the cholestasis present in the newborn disappears by the age of six or seven years. Hepatosplenomegaly generally persists. In 10−15% of the patients, cirrhosis is most likely to develop. Additional genetic or exogenous factors, especially indomethacine (123), are held responsible for manifestation and progression. An α_1-antitrypsin deficiency of the PiZZ type caused *cirrhosis* in 45−50% (as shown after autopsy) and *liver carcinoma* in 25−30% of adults. In some 50% of homozygous patients, nothing more than an increase in the transaminases was observed. Uninhibited neutrophilic elastase results in a loss of elasticity in the lung, so that emphysema and obstructive pulmonary disease develop. However, a combined hepato-pulmonary disease is rarely found. Extrahepatic manifestations include pancreas fibrosis, panniculitis, glomerulonephritis and arterial aneurysm. (s. fig. 31.12)
• **Heterozygous** α_1-antitrypsin deficiency does not cause any manifest hepatic or pulmonary diseases, but it is considered to be a predisposing factor. Heterozygotes of type PiZ have a higher risk of HCC, both in a non-cirrhotic liver and in the absence of liver disease. Heterozygous carriers are in any case overrepresented in patients suffering from cryptogenic or viral chronic hepatitis and cirrhosis. A higher prevalence of PiMZ was found in idiopathic haemochromatosis; greater frequency was likewise observed in pregnancies and twin births. There was a higher prevalence of PiZ in polyarthritis rheumatica. (109, 113, 115, 117, 119, 120, 125−127)

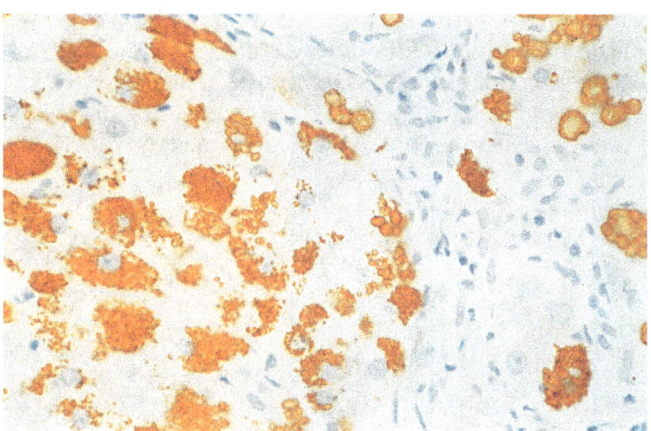

Fig. 31.12: Serologically confirmed α_1-antitrypsin deficiency type PiZ in a juvenile patient (homozygosity). Globular α_1-antitrypsin deposits in the hepatocytes; PiZ immunohistochemistry with PiZ antibody ATZ11

8.1.3 Diagnostics and treatment

Diagnosis: Evidence of conjugated jaundice in neonates and frequent bronchopulmonary infections in infants arouse suspicion of α_1-antitrypsin deficiency. In later life, this genetic cause needs to be ruled out in cryptogenic chronic hepatitis or cirrhosis. • Reduction in the α_1-globulin fraction in electrophoresis to <2 rel.% is an important indicator of α_1-antitrypsin deficiency, because α_1AT is the main component of α_1-globulins (90%). Diagnosis is confirmed by determination of α_1AT in the serum. *Normal values* range between 190−330 mg/dl or 80−147 IU/ml. Half-life is about five days. Values <20% of the normal level suggest a homozygous type, while a 40−70% reduction below normal points to a heterozygous type. Identification of the phenotype of α_1AT is possible. Alpha$_1$-AT is also found in tears, rhinal secretion, saliva, duodenal juice, bronchial secretion, cerebrospinal fluid and breast milk.

Liver histology points to cholestasis or changes in the biliary ductules. PAS-positive, diastasis-resistent, 1−40 µm sized globular deposits of α_1AT in the hepatocytes are typical features, mainly found in the periportal area (zone 1), but only in homozygosity. (112, 113, 119, 125) (s. fig. 31.12) Inflammatory and fibrotic reactions are detectable in the vicinity, although α_1AT is not considered to be a toxic agent. Copper content in the liver is increased. In progressive fibrosis, there is generally a rise in P-III-P in the serum. The prognosis for α_1-antitrypsin cirrhosis is much poorer than for other types of cirrhosis; the mean survival rate is reported to be two years after a diagnosis has been established. In 10−30% of cases, hepatic carcinoma can be expected. (122, 128)

Causal treatment is not yet possible, but *gene therapy* may prove feasible, i.e. integration of a normal allele M into the genome of the patient's somatic cells. *Substitution* with α_1AT (e.g. infusion or aerosol inhalation of α_1AT) is less promising. An increase in α_1AT synthesis has been attempted by means of androgens and oestrogen antagonists (e.g. tamoxifen). • Smoking is strictly forbidden! In progressive cirrhosis and imminent liver failure, *liver transplantation* is indicated. (116, 121) The five-year survival rate in children was 83%. (114) Transplantation generally allows a phenotypical healing process to take place.

8.2 Amyloidosis

Amyloid is an insoluble protein-polysaccharide complex consisting of fibrillary protein, AP component and glycosaminoglycan; this AP protein is identical with the regular serum amyloid P (= SAP). Amyloid is mainly stored in the extracellular spaces. The substance shows a strong affinity to iodine (R. VIRCHOW, 1854: "amyloid" = "starch-like") and Congo red (H. PUCHTLER et al., 1962). Under a polarizing microscope, amyloid shows a green staining with double refraction. Electron microscopy reveals a fibrillary structure with 7−10 μm fibres. Various amyloid types can be distinguished, depending on the different kinds of protein in the fibrils. Secondary amyloidosis is the most common form. • Autosomal dominant hereditary amyloidosis is transmitted by means of structurally altered transthyretin (TTR). Meanwhile, more than 60 mutations of TTR have been detected. The gene responsible is located on chromosome 18; a gene test is already available. (130, 133)

AA amyloid appears in a generalized form and is mainly stored perireticularly in the kidney, spleen and liver. This kind of amyloidosis occurs as (*1.*) a **congenital** form in cases of familial Mediterranean fever, (*2.*) an **idiopathic** (= primary) form without any associated basic disease, and (*3.*) a **reactive** (= secondary) form in chronic inflammations or tumours (e.g. Hodgkin's disease) as well as in drug abuse and AIDS.

AL amyloid possesses fibrils composed of fragments from Ig light chains of the *kappa* or *lambda* type. This amyloid is stored pericollagenically both in a generalized and organ-localized form. Deposits in organs, including the liver, may take the form of nodules (= amyloid tumour or paramyloid). AL amyloidosis may be: (*1.*) **idiopathic** (= primary) without any associated basic disease or (*2.*) **reactive** (= secondary) in cases of multiple myeloma, Waldenström's syndrome, Bence-Jones plasmocytoma and various type B cell tumours.

Further differentiation distinguishes between **AF amyloid** (ATTR) (amyloid types in familial amyloidosis), endocrine **EA amyloid**, **AS amyloid** (occasionally detected in old age in its isolated form in the heart and brain) and **AB amyloid** (Aβ_2m) (often observed in the osseous system during long-term dialysis).

8.2.1 Clinical picture and diagnosis

Clinically, pronounced *hepatomegaly* predominates; later on, splenomegaly usually develops as well. An increase in *alkaline phosphatase* is observed at an early stage. Severe courses of intrahepatic cholestasis have been observed. (129, 136, 138, 139, 143, 146, 147) These mostly involve obstructive cholestasis due to deposits of fibrils between the sinusoidal wall and hepatocytes, so that the canaliculi and the ductules are compressed. Hepatic enzymes and liver function tests are normal or deviate slightly from normal values. *Jaundice*, which appears in the late phases, is indicative of a poor prognosis. A decrease in *cholinesterase* is seen as a sign of increasing amyloid deposition with subsequent compromising of de novo synthesis. Factor X is often decreased. • In *CT scanning*, a reduced contrast medium enhancement in the area of amyloid storage may be detected. (141, 142). *Scintigraphy* using ^{99m}Tc-sulphocolloid shows markedly decreased uptake in the spleen as compared to the liver, and also metastasis-like storage defects. (148) • The tracers ^{123}I-SAP or ^{99m}Tc-SAP show abnormal uptake into amyloid deposits. (135) In some cases, *involvement of other organs* − kidney (129, 132), heart, spleen (142, 144, 147), intestines, CNS, carpal tunnel syndrome − suggests the existence of amyloidosis. Sometimes, there is reddish-brown dyschromia. (133) • Rectum biopsy, when carried out expertly, provides diagnostic accuracy in 80−85% of cases. Aspiration biopsy from bone marrow or subcutaneous abdominal fat tissue only has an accuracy of 40−50%. (s. fig. 31.13)

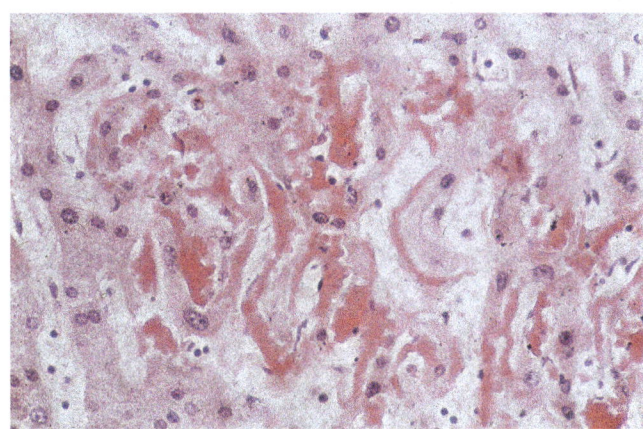

Fig. 31.13: Liver amyloidosis: Perisinusoidal amyloidosis with atrophic hepatocyte trabeculae (HE)

Morphology: Amyloid is also stored in the small portal vein branches of the liver. Depending on the guiding fibres used by amyloid, it is possible to differentiate between perireticular and pericollagenous amyloidosis. The vascular amyloid involvement together with the solidity and fragility of the liver are the cause of occasional excessive *haemorrhagic tendency* (134); this condition is also given after liver biopsy. Therefore, **percutaneous liver biopsy** must be considered as a *contraindication*. (s. tab. 7.4) If liver histology is required, the sample should be obtained by **laparoscopic liver biopsy,** so that targeted treatment measures can be applied "with visual control" if complicative bleeding occurs. The biopsy specimen is pale pink. The liver surface appears pale and wax-like with coarse reddish marbling. (s. fig. 31.13)

8.2.2 Prognosis and treatment

The **prognosis** for amyloidosis is poor. In AL amyloidosis, fewer than 20% of patients had a five-year survival rate. A course of one to two years is regarded as a mean survival period. The outcome depends mainly upon renal and cardiac amyloidosis; the prognosis regarding the liver is determined by the development of portal hypertension or acute liver failure. (131, 149) Cytostatics are recommended for the **treatment** of benign or malignant B cell tumours in type AL amyloidosis, while melphalan and prednisolone are used for concomitant amyloidosis. However, therapeutic measures are generally limited. The mobilization of amyloid deposits can be attempted by administering dimethyl sulphoxide (1.5–10.0 g/day). • In secondary amyloidosis, treatment of the underlying disease is important; individual cases have been reported in which amyloidosis disappeared due to successful therapy. • In hereditary amyloidosis, the indication for *liver transplantation* is given, since the liver is the main site of transthyretin synthesis. Mutant transthyretin is no longer detectable in the serum after transplantation. (137, 140, 145, 147) Regression of extrahepatic amyloid deposits has also been reported.

8.3 α₁-antichymotrypsin deficiency

In genetically (autosomal dominant) induced α_1-antichymotrypsin deficiency, this inhibitor of serine proteases is not secreted in sufficient quantities from the hepatocytes or alveolar macrophages. Therefore α_1-antichymotrypsin is stored in these cells. The deposits can be detected as cellular inclusions by light microscopy. Patients suffering from this condition may develop chronic hepatitis and cirrhosis. (150–152)

9 Amino acid storage diseases

9.1 Hereditary tyrosinaemia

▶ This clinical picture was described for the first time by M. D. BABER in 1956; it was identified as an enzyme deficiency by B. LINDBLAD et al. in 1977.

Tyrosinaemia type I is very rare (incidence 1 : 100,000 births). It is caused by an autosomal recessive defect of fumarylacetoacetate hydrolase (localized on chromosome 15 q 23–25), which impairs tyrosine degradation. Tyrosine metabolites accumulate at the point where the metabolic process is compromised. This results in either an **acute** clinical course initiated immediately after birth and usually leading to a quick death or a **chronic** course in which patients reach adult age. (153, 154, 156, 157)

Tyrosinaemia type II is caused by reduced activity of tyrosine aminotransferase, resulting in greater concentration in the serum. This may develop into an independent **congenital-hereditary** clinical picture or physiological hypertyrosinaemia, which occurs in about 10% of newborns as a **neonatal-transitory** event.

9.1.1 Clinical picture

The gene mutation inhibits hydrolytic cleavage of fumarylacetoacetate into fumarate and acetoacetate. Consequently, the toxic precursors maleylacetoacetate and fumarylacetoacetate accumulate in the liver and kidneys. They possess a reactive double bond and can therefore react with macromolecules to assume the properties of alkylating substances. In addition, intracellular glutathione deficiency develops due to the stable complex formation with glutathione, favouring *lipid peroxidations*. Enhanced formation of δ-aminolaevulinic acid can also be observed during occasional attacks of acute intermittent porphyria (G. MITCHEL et al., 1990).

The **acute course** in newborns is characterized by vomiting and diarrhoea as well as growth disturbances. Hepatosplenomegaly, hypoalbuminaemia, hypercholesterinaemia and hypoglycaemia as well as oedema/ascites and coagulopathy develop rapidly. A striking feature is the early and marked rise in the α_1-foetoprotein value in the serum. Excretion of succinylacetone (> 50 nmol/l) and delta-aminolaevulinic acid in the urine is noticeably increased. Methionine, phenylalanine and tyrosine are elevated in the serum. A slight rise in the transaminases and serum bilirubin occurs. Death is due to acute liver failure. There is histologic evidence of extensive necrosis, fatty infiltration, cholestasis and regenerative nodes in the liver. • If the newborn survives the first few months, the proximal renal tubule suffers complex damage, resulting in the clinical picture of **Fanconi's syndrome**: glucosuria, aminoaciduria, phosphaturia including osteomalacia, and renal tubular acidosis with polyuria.

The **chronic course** is characterized by a milder form. The general symptoms are less pronounced, and often they do not appear before the patient reaches school age. Hepatosplenomegaly is present. Laboratory findings include hypoalbuminaemia, coagulopathy and markedly elevated serum values of α_1-foetoprotein, methionine, tyrosine and phenylalanine. Activity of the fumarylacetoacetate hydrolase in leucocytes, fibroblasts and hepatocytes is increased. • The *liver* is granular and firm with a yellowish colour. Histologically, the picture is similar to that of galactosaemia (fatty changes, tubular transformation, cholestasis, periportal fibrosis, central sclerosis). Within a few months, micronodular cirrhosis is detectable with early multifocal liver cell carcinoma. (153, 156, 159) • *Fanconi's syndrome* (see above) also develops in the chronic course. Occasionally, there are symptoms of peripheral neuropathy.

9.1.2 Treatment

The *prognosis* is determined by the early onset of acute liver failure in the newborn and, in the following months or years, by the development of hepatocellular carcinoma. (156, 160) • A *liver transplantation* is thus recommended as from the second or third year of life. (155) Dietary measures (avoidance of methionine, tyrosine and phenylalanine as nutritional components) have not proved particularly successful. • Good therapeutic results were achieved when *nitisinone* (2 mg/kg BW/day) was applied. This substance is an inhibitor of 4-hydroxyphenylpyruvate dioxygenase, which prevents the accumulation of succinylacetone. (158) Even the risk of HCC development was reduced by this substance.

9.2 Disturbances of the urea cycle

Six enzymes are involved in the urea cycle: (*1.*) carbamoylphosphate synthetase (CPS), (*2.*) ornithine transcarbamylase (OTC), (*3.*) argininosuccinate synthetase, (*4.*) argininosuccinate lyase, (*5.*) arginase, and (*6.*) N-acetyl glutamate synthetase − as well as enzymes involved in supply reactions. They may be compromised by a genetic defect. Up to now, six congenital disorders of the urea cycle are known. The cumulative frequency is estimated at 1 : 8,000. • The genetic disorder is autosomal recessive; only the ornithine transcarbamylase disorder (= OTC deficiency) shows a dominant chromosomal pattern of transmission (chromosome p 21.1). This is the most frequently detected intramitochondrial defect to date (1 : 14,000). (165) • Following preliminary detoxification of ammonia at the site of formation by reaction with glutamate (whereby glutamine is formed), definitive detoxification takes place in the urea cycle and by hepatic glutamine synthesis. • The **urea cycle** has two other functions: (*1.*) denovo synthesis of arginine and (*2.*) regulation of the acid-base balance by consumption of bicarbonate. (s. pp 62, 63) (s. figs. 3.12, 3.15)

The **clinical symptomatology,** which is almost the same in all enzymatic disturbances of the urea cycle, is caused by hyperammonaemia. • An *arginase defect* results in enhanced excretion of lysine, ornithine and cystine. Neurological symptoms such as athetosis and hyperreactivity followed by paresis and tetraplegia predominate.

In neonatal manifestation of *OTC deficiency*, lethargy, vomiting, refusal to take food, hyperventilation and hypothermia develop quickly. Death ensues in coma within a few days. Manifestation in infants or adolescents is based upon the residual activity of the defective enzyme. This course is also characterized by vomiting and lethargy. The clinical picture is aggravated by a protein-rich diet, whereas protein reduction improves the clinical situation. Without treatment, death occurs in a hepatic coma.

A defect in *argininosuccinate synthetase* coincides with markedly elevated citrulline values in the blood. Neither citrullinaemia nor a carbamylphosphate synthetase defect cause liver damage. • By contrast, an *argininosuccinase defect* leads to microvesicular steatosis and megamitochondria with dilatation of the ER. (s. p. 279)

Diagnosis is based upon hyperammonaemia, which is detectable either spontaneously or after the oral intake of proteins − or, most obviously, following intravenous infusion of amino acids. The respective amino acids are increased in the serum prior to the disturbed metabolic reaction. Argininosuccinate is only detectable in the urine. A striking feature in these patients is their thin, brittle hair. With defective ornithine transcarbamylase, there is an increase in orotic acid, uridine and uric acid in the urine, while the respective citrulline concentration is decreased. Determination of OTC activity in liver tissue verifies the diagnosis and facilitates a genomic analysis. The allopurinol test can be applied for the identification of heterozygosity (or the mild form of OTC deficiency). The liver shows steatosis, portal inflammation and portal fibrosis.

Treatment involves a low-protein diet (0.5−0.7 g/kg BW/day) with sufficient calories. Substitution of essential amino acids (in about the same quantity) is required. • Administration of benzoate (0.1−0.25 g/kg BW/day), arginine hydrochloride (1 mmol/kg BW/day) or sodium phenylacetate (0.3−0.5 g/kg BW/day) (phenylbutyrate may be more effective) facilitates nitrogen excretion via other metabolic pathways. (161−164) • With enhanced excretion of orotate or other metabolites of pyrimidine synthesis, administration of allopurinol leads to an increase in the excretion of nitrogen via metabolites from pyrimidine synthesis. Ammonia and urea precursors are eliminated by haemodialysis. In some cases, liver transplantation is indicated. (161−163)

9.3 Cystinosis

Autosomal recessive cystinosis is caused by an enzyme-induced blockage of cystine degradation, particularly in the RES lysosomes of the bone marrow, liver, spleen and kidneys. Especially in the stellate cells of the spleen and to a lesser extent of the hepatic lobule centres, hexagonal and rectangular cystine crystals are found, pointing at an early stage to cystinosis. There is evidence of hepatosplenomegaly and microvesicular steatosis. The clinical picture of the infantile type presents as a *Fanconi syndrome*. (s. pp 610, 611) The children affected die in the first five years of life.

9.4 Homocystinuria

This rare disease has an autosomal recessive inheritance pattern. It is based on a deficiency of cystathion-β synthase, so that homocystein and other metabolites (e.g. methionine) accumulate and are eliminated in increased quantities in the urine. There is evidence of disturbed mental development and a marked tendency to thrombosis in the arterial system. Liver steatosis (mainly in zone 1) and hepatomegaly with subsequent portal fibrosis can be seen.

10 Carbohydrate storage diseases

Carbohydrate storage diseases generally include: (*1.*) glycogenoses, (*2.*) galactosaemia, (*3.*) hereditary fructose intolerance, and (*4.*) fructose-1,6-biphosphatase deficiency.

10.1 Glycogenoses

Glycogenoses are congenital metabolic diseases with enzyme defects in which glycogen cannot be broken down to glucose. This results in normal or structurally changed glycogen being stored in the organs in ever-increasing quantities. To date, **ten types** (types I–X) have been defined. Types VIII–X are very rare and partly present as subgroups of the other types. • The **incidence** of types I–VII ranges between 1:20,000 and 1:40,000 births with geographic differences. A relative frequency was determined from 1,192 cases: type I (23%), type II (15%), type III (21%), type IV (2.5%), type V (6%), type VI (30%) and type VII (2.5%). • Transmission is **autosomal recessive.** With regard to the extent of the enzymatic disturbance or the involvement of regulatory enzymes, pronounced heterogeneity can be observed within the individual types. • **Liver disease** only develops in types I, III, IV and VI. *Hepatomegaly* is also found in type II and in the rare types IX and X. • Differential diagnosis of glycogenoses and their subtypes is not possible simply using liver histology. However, it can be achieved by means of additional *histochemistry*, quantitative determination of *glycogen* and *enzyme analysis.* (167, 172, 180, 181)

Gierke's disease (type I)

Hepatorenal glycogenosis was described by S. VAN CREVELD in 1928 and resolved in terms of pathological morphology by E.O.E. VON GIERKE in 1929. This genetic defect (localized on chromosome 17) causes the complete or partial absence of **glucose-6-phosphatase** activity **(subtype Ia).** (173) • Enzymatic activity is only detectable after the application of detergents. There is a defect in the translocase of glucose-6-phosphatase at the endoplasmic reticulum membrane. This defect is also found in adults **(subtype Ib).** • Disturbance of the microsomal phosphate/pyrophosphate translocase may occur **(subtype Ic).** • Glucose-6-phosphatase is needed for the discharge of glucose from the liver when glucose-1-phosphate is supplied by glycogenolysis. This leads to an accumulation of **glucose-1-phosphate,** which in turn stimulates the neosynthesis of glycogen. However, glucose-1-phosphate is also broken down by glycolysis, with increased formation of lactate, acetyl-coenzyme A and glycerol-3-phosphate. The last two are basic products for the hepatic synthesis of fatty acids and triglycerides.

The **clinical picture** is characterized by hepatomegaly due to deposits of glycogen and triglycerides and by marked kidney enlargement (no splenomegaly as occurs in lipoidosis or cirrhosis). • Severe metabolic disorders such as hypoglycaemia and hyperlipidaemia (triglycerides, free fatty acids, cholesterol) as well as increased VLDL and LDL values are found, leading to the development of skin and tendon xanthomas, lactate acidosis, a slight increase in the transaminases, a tendency towards infection (due to leucopenia related to abnormal glucose-6-phosphatase transport), weakened skeletal muscles, bleeding tendency (due to abnormal platelet function), hyperuricaemia (with possible manifestations of gout, nephrocalcinosis, kidney stones) and osteoporosis. Hyposomia with fat pads, particularly in the buccal area, is often found. Diagnosis is additionally confirmed by a glucagon test (no or inadequate rise in the blood sugar level) as well as fructose or galactose tests and liver biopsy. (s. fig. 31.14)

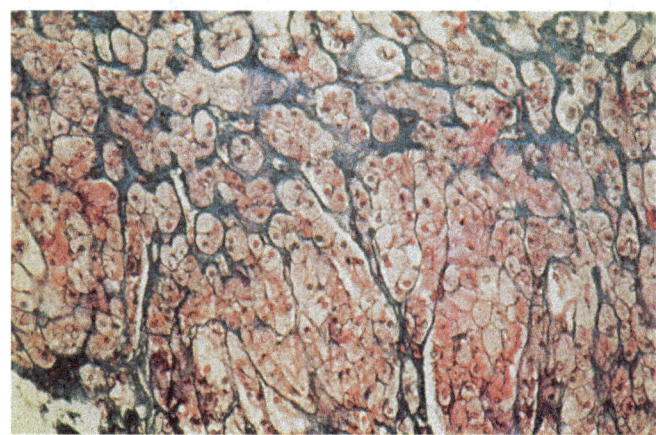

Fig. 31.14: Gierke's disease: phytocyte-like hepatocytes surrounded by a delicate network of fibrosis (Ladewig)

The occurrence of adenoma or HCC is associated with an increase in fatty acid synthesis. Subtype Ib is characterized above all by susceptibility to infection with leucopenia. Recurrent oral ulcers are often a cardinal symptom. The *liver* shows evidence of enlarged, polygonal hepatocytes with bright cytoplasm and centrally located small nuclei due to glycogen storage. Occasionally, Mallory-Denk bodies and glycogen vacuolation of the nuclei are seen. The hepatocytes have a pronounced (phytocell-like) cellular membrane. (168, 170, 171, 173–178)

Treatment consists of prevention or elimination of hypoglycaemia. In newborns and infants, this can be achieved by the continuous application of formula diets, if required via nasogastric tube feeding. The administration of allopurinol may also be advisable. A starch diet (e.g. uncooked corn starch) is then used to ensure that glucose is released and resorbed slowly in the intestinal tract. (166, 171) After puberty, the course of disease is usually less pronounced. In the long term, especially in adenoma-related complications, liver transplantation may be indicated. (179)

Pompe's disease (type II)

Generalized glycogenosis type II, also called Pompe's disease (J.C. POMPE, 1932), is caused by a deficiency of lysosomal acidic **α1,4 glucosidase.** This enzyme is responsible for the degradation of glycogen and maltose within the lysosomes. Glycogen is accumulated in all organs, particularly in the heart, but also in the liver. The disease mostly appears in the newborn (death due to heart failure, often within the first 12 months of life), but may also become manifest in infants and adults. • **Clinical symptoms** include weakened skeletal muscles, hyperlipidaemia, increased values of the muscle enzymes aldolase and CK, macroglossia as well as pronounced cardiomegaly and *moderate hepatomegaly.* Mental development is not impaired. The glucagon test is normal; hypoglycaemia does not occur. Diagnosis is confirmed by the detection of reduced enzyme activity in biopsy material obtained from the liver or muscle. Vacuoles can be demonstrated in the liver cells. • **Therapy** is based on the genetic engineering of alpha glucosidase (30 mg/kg BW every 14 days). In the later stages of life, the prognosis quoad vitam is determined by heart failure, pneumonia and respiratory insufficiency.

Cori's disease (type III)

Hepatomuscular glycogenosis (G.B. FORBES, 1952; G.H. HERS, 1959) is caused by a deficiency of **amylo-1,6-glucosidase** (debranching enzyme). Consequently, degradation of the glycogenic branched chains is impaired, yielding an abnormal residual molecule (limit dextrinosis). Gluconeogenesis from lactate is possible. In **Forbes subtype,** deposits of the markedly branched glycogen (with short external chains) are observed in the heart, liver and musculature; in **Forbes-Hers subtype,** they are found in the hepatocytes only. Further subtypes (up to III F) have been described.

Clinical symptoms include hepatomegaly, increased transaminases, hypoglycaemia (glucose may be released from glycogen when the terminal glucose fragments split off), hyperlipidaemia and moderate lactate acidosis. The glucagon tolerance test is positive (= no increase in blood sugar); the galactose test and the fructose test are normal. Liver histology shows numerous *glycogen vacuolizations of the nuclei* (s. fig. 31.1), slight steatosis and periportal fibrosis (also transition to cirrhosis and HCC) (169). Adenomas frequently appear. • The **treatment** consists of frequent small meals rich in carbohydrates and proteins plus additional dietary corn starch preparations.

Andersen's disease (type IV)

Liver-cirrhotic, reticulo-endothelial glycogenosis type IV (D.A. ANDERSEN, 1956) is a defect of the branching enzyme **amylo-1,4-1,6-transglucosidase.** There is a disturbance in the formation of glycogen side-chains, which results in the production of a low-branched glycogen with long side-chains (amylopectinosis). This abnormal structure causes low solubility, resulting in the **deposition** of the malstructured glycogen in the hepatocytes at the periphery of the lobule in the form of eosinophilic or colourless, granular, PAS-positive substances. This abnormal glycogen has a cellulotoxic effect. It is also deposited in the spleen, lymph nodes and RES.

Clinical symptoms include hepatosplenomegaly and increased transaminases as well as an occasional rise in cholestasis-indicating enzymes. Histologically, the liver specimen shows a number of giant cells, cell necrosis and cholestasis. The abnormal glycogen stored in the hepatocytes can to a certain extent be removed by diastasis digestion, and it takes on a violet stain when in contact with iodine (in contrast to the usual reddish-brown colour); PAS staining is positive. Diagnosis can also be reached using rectal biopsy: macrophages with globular inclusions containing amylopectin are found. The further course is determined by portal hypertension with the formation of ascites and a haemorrhagic tendency. In addition, diminished reflexes, muscular atrophy and motor dysfunctions as well as dilative cardiomyopathy may be observed. The disease can also take a protracted course, so that the patient even reaches adolescence. • There is no specific course of **treatment**. Liver transplantation is indicated, whereby a surprisingly positive effect on extrahepatic complications and growth retardation can be expected. (179)

Hers' disease (type VI)

Hepatic glycogenosis (type VI) (G.H. HERS, 1959) is due to hepatic phosphorylase deficiency. Subtype VIa is caused by a lack of **phosphorylase-B kinase,** and it is transmitted by the x-chromosomal recessive route. Subtype VIb generally shows a deficiency in **glycogen phosphorylase,** and its transmission is autosomal recessive. In the musculature, the analogous enzyme is, however, intact. Nevertheless, there is pronounced genetic and phenotypical heterogeneity in most cases.

The **clinical picture** shows moderate hepatomegaly. The normal glycogen is stored in a focal form at the periphery of the lobules. There is a mixed pattern of small and large hepatocytes, giving the picture of an irregular mosaic. Hypoglycaemia occurs only during fasting. No other biochemical deviations are observed. The prognosis is relatively good when dietary instructions are adhered to. Mental functions are normal.

Type IX and type X

These benign glycogenoses are due to a defect in hepatic phosphorylase kinase or cAMP-dependent phosphorylase kinase. Glycogen is deposited unevenly in the hepatocytes; there is evidence of hepatomegaly with fine-droplet steatosis and occasional fibrosis. Hyperlipidaemia and elevated GPT values are present. In the course of time, the patient is able to catch up on physical growth, and hepatomegaly recedes.

10.2 Galactosaemia

Hereditary galactose intolerance (A. v. Reuss, 1908; F. Göppert, 1917) is caused by an autosomal recessive disorder in the galactose metabolism. • Type II is characterized by an enzyme defect in **galactose-1-phosphate uridyltransferase.** (Type I, caused by a defect of galactokinase, only affects the eyes and is therefore not discussed here.) Transferase deficiency affects several organs, particularly the liver, and results in severe damage. Galactonate and galactite develop as **toxic metabolites,** which are deposited in the tissues; galactite is also detectable in the urine. (182, 185)

The **prevalence** of the disease is 1:35,000 to 1:70,000 births. With the help of neonate screening, the defect can be discovered and treated at an early stage. • The enzyme coding for transferase is on **chromosome 9 p 13**; there are various mutations and pronounced polymorphisms. Accordingly, several **variants** displaying different kinds of enzymatic activities have been described in many different places (the Duarre, Rennes, Los Angeles and Chicago variants as well as the Caucasian and Negroid variants). Usually, the defect can only be detected by means of the **galactose tolerance test.** A healthy person oxidizes 30–50% of orally administered galactose to CO_2 in five hours, whereas in transferase deficiency, only 0–8% is oxidized. • Galactonate causes synthesis disorders of glycoproteins and glycolipids in the liver cell by the consumption of UDP. Due to the accumulation of **galactose-1-phosphate,** the consumption of phosphate is increased with a subsequent decrease in ATP and gluconeogenesis. • The deposits of galactose-1-phosphate in the proximal renal tubular cells lead to the development of *Fanconi's syndrome* (glucosuria, aminoaciduria, phosphaturia, acidosis). (s. pp 610, 611)

The **clinical picture** sets in immediately after birth, as soon as milk (including breast milk) is given. The symptoms are vomiting, diarrhoea, no weight gain and galactosuria. As early as the second week, pronounced hepatomegaly (or hepatosplenomegaly) is observed, often accompanied by jaundice and cholestasis. The findings correspond to those in haemolysis. Transaminases are elevated, liver functions are increasingly compromised, and metabolic acidosis is generally in evidence. Cataracts develop. • The diagnosis is confirmed by galactosuria and a rise in galactose and galactose-1-phosphate concentrations in the blood as well as reduced transferase activity in the erythrocytes. • Histologically, the *liver* shows mixed-droplet fatty changes, cholestasis with ductular proliferations, liver cell necrosis, collapse of reticular fibre structures as well as pseudoglandular and/or tubular transformation processes of the liver cell plates around the canaliculi. Within a period of three to six months, micronodular cirrhosis develops, followed by ascites and increasing liver insufficiency. (183, 184, 186)

Treatment is successful when the disease is recognized early enough and when nutrition is free of galactose and lactose, so that the prognosis is generally considered to be favourable. Organ damage can be halted or indeed prevented completely; occasionally, there is (partial) recession. The UDP galactose required for cell metabolism is supplied from UDP glucose. (186)

10.3 Hereditary fructose intolerance

Hereditary fructose intolerance is caused by an autosomal recessive hereditary defect of the enzyme **fructose-1-phosphate aldolase.** Whenever fructose is supplied, severe hypoglycaemia and functional disorders occur in the liver, kidneys and CNS. • The **prevalence** is estimated at 1:20,000 births. As with galactose intolerance, the gene which codes aldolase B is also localized on **chromosome 9.** This enzyme defect causes fructose-1-phosphate to accumulate in the liver and tissue. The cleavage of fructose-1,6-biphosphate is only slightly compromised since the enzymes aldolase A and C are available for this process. • The consumption of phosphate and ATP in the tissue results in various **functional disorders:** (*1.*) inhibition of gluconeogenesis in the liver and kidneys, (*2.*) increase in lactate in the serum with metabolic acidosis, (*3.*) decrease in protein synthesis in the liver, and (*4.*) functional disorders of the proximal tubular cells with development of **Fanconi's syndrome.** (s. pp 610, 611) (187, 189, 191)

The **clinical picture** is characterized by nausea, vomiting, diarrhoea, abdominal pain, dizziness and hypoglycaemia, not only following the intake of fructose (oral, intravenous), but also after sorbitol infusions (sorbitol is converted to fructose in the organism). Growth failure is observed in babies and infants. • During adolescence and in adults, a chronic course may develop, characterized by hepatomegaly, hypophosphataemia, hypoglycaemia, blood coagulation disorders and an increase in the transaminases as well as jaundice and moderate cholestasis. Phosphaturia results in osteomalacia. Hypermagnesaemia is a striking feature. • *Histological findings* include a fatty liver with liver cell necrosis and increasing fibrosis; the liver cell plates show tubular transformation. Giant cells are often found. At a later stage, cirrhosis develops. (187–190) • When the intake of fructose (or sorbitol) is avoided, even patients with a homozygous genotype are symptom-free. The diagnosis is based upon the determination of liver aldolase B or on the *fructose tolerance test*.

> **Method:** Oral administration of 200 mg/kg BW fructose in a 20% solution over a period of 30 minutes. After establishing the initial values, both glucose and phosphate are determined every 10 minutes; after 1 hour, the intervals are extended to 30 minutes. The test findings are pathological when serum glucose decreases to <40 mg/dl and phosphate to <1.5 mg/dl. Hypoglycaemia requires an immediate i.v. glucose infusion.

Treatment consists of completely avoiding fructose and commercially available cane sugar as well as excluding sorbitol from i.v. infusions. If this regime is strictly adhered to, prognosis is good and life expectancy unaffected in most cases.

10.4 Fructose-1,6-biphosphatase deficiency

Due to the autosomal recessively inherited reduction in fructose-1,6-biphosphatase activity in the liver, the gluconeogenesis of lactate, glycerine and glucogenic amino acids is inhibited. If fructose or glycerine are supplied, phosphate and bicarbonate are consumed in higher quantities and lactate production is increased. This results in metabolic acidosis.

The **clinical picture** is much less pronounced than in hereditary fructose intolerance (type aldolase B). When fructose is supplied or when infections develop, the affected children may suffer from metabolic disorders, such as hypoglycaemia, nausea, vomiting, diarrhoea, hyperventilation, convulsions, lactate acidosis and ketosis. The glucagon tolerance test is pathological (= no increase in blood sugar). • Histology shows a fatty liver. Diagnosis can be confirmed by measuring the fructose-1,6-biphosphatase activity in the liver tissue.

Treatment consists of completely avoiding fructose and, if necessary, in correcting metabolic acidosis, electrolytes and blood sugar values.

11 Lipid storage diseases

11.1 Wolman's disease

Xanthomatosis, an autosomal recessive inherited disorder, was described by A. ABRAMOV, S. SCHORR and M. WOLMAN in 1956. Probably, this rare clinical picture (about 40 cases have been reported to date) was already published by H. DIENST and H. HAMPERL as early as 1927. Some cases may have been attributed erroneously to Niemann-Pick disease. • Wolman's disease is caused by a considerable reduction or complete absence of **intralysosomal lipase activity.** In acid pH, the lipase catalyzes the hydrolytic cleavage of cholesterol esters and triglycerides in the lysosomes. This enzyme defect results in an excessive storage of cholesterol esters and triglycerides in the abdominal organs, skin and nervous system. The mutant gene for isoenzyme A of acidic lysosomal lipase is located on **chromosome 10.** In homozygotes, lipase activity in the liver is reduced to less than 10% of the normal value, in heterozygotes to around 50%. • The **enzyme defect** is responsible for (*1.*) storage of cholesterol esters and triglycerides in the hepatocytes, Kupffer cells, macrophages and various other body cells, and (*2.*) disturbance of cholesterol homoeostasis in the blood, since the lysosomes release an insufficient quantity of free cholesterol into the cytosol. For this reason, the regulation of the cholesterol metabolism in the cytosol is considerably impaired: (*1.*) inadequate or no inhibition of the synthesis of cholesterol and the LDL receptor, and (*2.*) inadequate or no stimulation of cholesterol esterification with saturated fatty acids.

The **clinical picture,** which appears in early infancy, comprises vomiting, diarrhoea, growth failure and meteorism. Hepatosplenomegaly and anaemia develop rapidly. Multiple xanthomas of the skin appear. CT scanning shows enlarged adrenal glands (due to xanthomatous redifferentiation), often with finely spotted calcifications. Deposits of cholesterol esters, triglycerides and, to a certain extent, phospholipids are found in the spleen, liver, small intestine, lymph nodes, lungs, skin and nervous system. The foam cells detectable in the bone marrow differ from Pick cells in that they lack sphingomyelin. The transaminases are increased; liver function is markedly compromised. Death usually ensues within the first year of life. (192–194)

11.2 Cholesterol ester storage disease

> ▶ Cholesterol ester storage disease (CESD) was first described by D. S. FREDRICKSON in 1966. No more than 20 cases of this **very rare disease** have been reported to date, with twice as many girls being affected as boys. • Just like *Wolman's disease*, it is transmitted as an autosomal recessive mutation with the gene localization on **chromosome 10.** Due to this defect, degradation of cholesterol esters and triglycerides in the lysosomes is inhibited. Therefore, these lipids are stored in the hepatocytes, Kupffer cells and macrophages as well as in other somatic cells. Although CESD displays the same biochemical and metabolic disorders as Wolman's disease, it is less severe. It does not become evident until adulthood.

▶ *It was possible for us to describe this clinical picture in detail from our own observations of a 13-year-old girl. We detected a very high content of cholesterol ester in the biopsy sample and a deficiency of lysosomal α-naphthyl-acetate esterase in the fibroblast culture. (198) (s. figs. 21.5; 31.15, 31.16)*

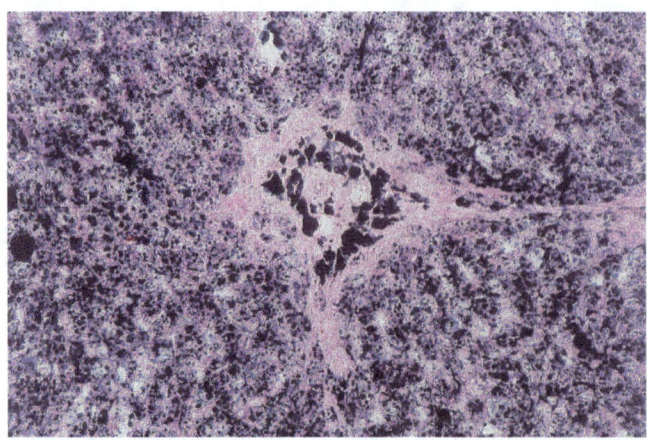

Fig. 31.15: Cholesterol ester storage disease. Fine-droplet fatty changes in the hepatocytes. Widely extensive small and larger lipid vacuoles in the liver cells and foam cells of the portal field (Sudan black) (s. fig. 21.5). Same patient as in fig. 31.16

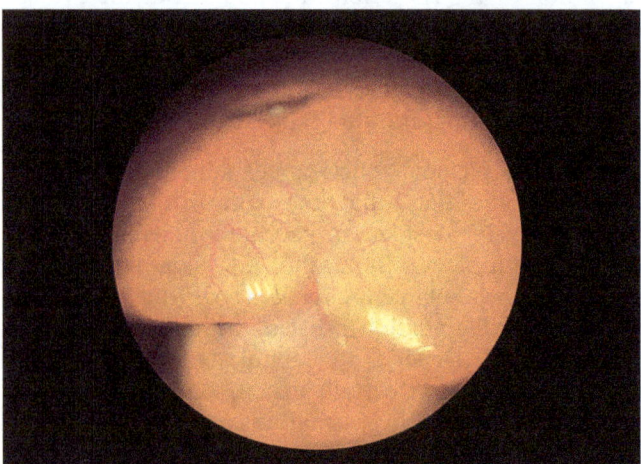

Fig. 31.16: Light yellowish-red, smooth surface in fatty liver due to cholesterol ester storage (13-year-old girl). Same patient as in fig. 31.15

Initially, the **clinical picture** is largely asymptomatic. The average age of the patients reported to date was 6.5 years at the time of diagnosis. Striking features are hepatomegaly and, occasionally, splenomegaly. (199) The cholesterol ester content of the liver can be up to 10% of the liver wet weight, while the total lipid content of the liver ranges between 22% and 28%. • *Laboratory findings* show a slight increase in the transaminases and bile acids as well as reduced liver function. In most cases, jaundice is observed. Markedly augmented concentrations of cholesterol, triglycerides and LDH are characteristic. (197) Foam cells can be found in the bone marrow. Diagnosis is confirmed by determination of lysosomal acidic lipase in the leucocytes and skin fibroblasts. • Corresponding to the high lipid content, the *liver surface* has an orange-yellowish colour, as does the liver specimen. (198) The lipid drops found in the hepatocytes and Kupffer cells are surrounded by a lysosomal membrane; they replace the cytoplasm and nucleus. In polarized light, the hepatocellular lipids show birefringence of the Maltese Cross type. The hepatocytes contain finely floccular, PAS-positive glycogen deposits. On the whole, the prevalent picture is that of mixed-droplet fatty changes. (198) In the further course, hepatic fibrosis or micronodular cirrhosis develop. Both the course and prognosis depend to a great extent on whether cirrhosis develops as well as what its concomitant complications are. (195, 196)

11.3 Cerebrotendinous xanthomatosis

This disease is caused by an autosomal recessive gene mutation (localization on chromosome 2) and leads to an enzyme defect in mitochondrial **steroid-27 hydroxylase.** The enzyme itself is responsible for the breakdown of cholesterol side-chains in bile acid synthesis. Such a defect results in the formation of **cholestanol,** a reduction product of cholesterol. It is deposited in various organs, particularly in the tendons and in the nervous system, because the substance cannot be broken down adequately. **Deposition** takes place conjointly with cholesterol. (202)

The **clinical picture** is characterized by xanthomas, particularly on the tendons (especially the Achilles tendon). Xanthomas consist of cholesterol and cholestanol. The enzyme defect also results in disturbed vitamin D metabolism. Osteoporosis is thus observed quite often, with a tendency towards spontaneous fractures. (201) Striking clinical features are cerebral functional disorders (from deviant behaviour to severe dementia, motor disturbances and convulsions) as well as peripheral neurological symptoms caused by cholestanol deposits. (203) High concentrations of apolipoprotein B and cholestanol are found in the CSF. (205) • **Treatment** is based on the administration of chenodeoxycholic acid (750 mg/day). Effectiveness is generally improved if HMG-CoA reductase inhibitors (e. g. pravastatin) are used concomitantly. (200, 204)

11.4 Abetalipoproteinaemia

In this autosomal recessive disease, the disorder does not involve the gene on chromosome 2, which is responsible for apoprotein assembly, but the **MTP gene** (microsomal triglyceride transfer protein), which is localized on chromosome 4 q 22−24. In the endoplasmic reticulum, MTP transfers cholesterol esters, triglycerides and phospholipids to the nascent apoprotein B. This process is a prerequisite for the transport of the complete **lipoproteins** (e. g. chylomicrons, VLDL) to the Golgi complex and their secretion into the blood via subsequent exocytosis. In the case of MTP deficiency, lipoprotein particles are not secreted, with the result that any superfluous **apoprotein B** is broken down in the endoplasmic reticulum. (206, 208, 211, 212)

Even in infants fed with high-fat milk, the **clinical picture** is characterized by malabsorption leading to fatty

stools and diarrhoea. This results in a deficiency of fat-soluble vitamins with all the respective complications.
• Reduced elimination of lipids from the *liver* leads to hepatomegaly with large-droplet fatty changes, possibly causing the formation of fat cysts and larger fat pools. (s. fig. 31.2) Splenomegaly often occurs due to fat storage in the macrophages of the spleen as well as to portal hypertension, which may be caused by an increased resistance in the sinusoids in cases of fatty liver. (207, 209) Development of cirrhosis has also been reported. •
As far as *laboratory findings* are concerned, a marked decrease in cholesterol (usually < 40 mg/dl) and triglycerides (usually < 10 mg/dl) is relevant for the diagnosis; VLDL (= pre-beta lipoproteins) are not found. The haemogram shows deformed (e.g. crenated) erythrocytes due to their altered membrane lipids. (210) • **Treatment** is based on the administration of triglycerides with medium-chain fatty acids (MTC diet) with strict avoidance of other fats. Fat-soluble vitamins have to be substituted (if necessary, orally in high doses).

11.5 Hypoalphalipoproteinaemia

▶ In 1961 D.S. FREDRICKSON et al. described an autosomal recessive disease called hypo- or analphalipoproteinaemia. This lipid storage disease is also known as **Tangier disease** — named after the small Tangier Island in Chesapeake Bay/Maryland — where it was first observed in two siblings. The cause is a gene mutation on chromosome 9q31 (= deficiency of the cholesterol-efflue regulatory protein). (213)

The most important **clinical feature** is the storage of cholesterol esters in the RES. The noticeably enlarged tonsils are of a distinctive yellowish or orange colour. There is evidence of lymphadenopathy and hepatosplenomegaly as well as polyneuropathy. PAS-positive foam cells or foamy Kupffer cells are found in the bone marrow, lymph nodes and liver. • *Laboratory findings* show an increase in triglyceride and a decrease in cholesterol and HDL. α_1-lipoprotein deficiency and moderate jaundice; occasionally, thrombopenia and leucopenia are observed. • The **prognosis** is generally good. Therefore, the disease is often diagnosed for the first time in adulthood. (213–215)

11.6 Debré's syndrome

This metabolic disorder with simultaneous storage of fat and glycogen in the liver was described by A.R. DEBRÉ et al. in 1934. Within a few weeks of birth, infants suffer from considerable hepatomegaly (without splenomegaly). There is evidence of hyperlipidaemia with hypercholesterolaemia, a tendency towards fasting hypoglycaemia, and disturbed glucose mobilization following exposure to insulin or adrenaline. • *It should be noted, however, that this form of glycolipidosis has still not been reliably classified.*

12 Sphingolipid storage diseases

The biochemical group of sphingolipids comprises: sphingomyelin, cerebroside, sulphatide, gangliosides, ceramide trihexosides, etc. Depending on the substance stored, differentiation is made between (*1.*) glucosyl ceramidoses (e.g. gangliosidoses, ceramide trihexosidosis, cerebrosidoses, sulphatidosis), (*2.*) phosphoryl ceramidoses (e.g. sphingomyelinosis), and (*3.*) mucopolysaccharidoses.

12.1 Gaucher's disease

▶ This form of glucosyl ceramidosis is the longest known lipid storage disease. It was described by P.C.E. GAUCHER as early as 1882 and recognized as a separate entity with systemic character by F. SCHLAGENHAUFER in 1907.

The condition is an autosomal recessive disease with reduced activity of the lysosomal **β-glucocerebrosidase**. (Instead of an enzyme defect, the cause may be the absence of cofactor **saposin C**.) The relevant gene is localized on **chromosome 1**. There is considerable genetic **heterogeneity**. While some gene mutations are responsible for more frequent neurologic and severe courses, others have been recognized, particularly in older patients, as causing a late onset and more moderate course of disease. The gene mutations are detectable with varying frequency in different ethnic groups. Due to the enzyme defect, sphingolipids are only broken down to the level of the glucocerebroside, whereby this glycolipid is subsequently stored. **Prevalence** is 1 : 30,000 – 1 : 50,000

Glucocerebroside is stored predominantly in the RES cells, but also in the spleen, hepatocytes, bone marrow and lymph nodes; rod-like tubules (20–40 nm) develop. • The storage of glucocerebroside leads to the formation of so-called **Gaucher cells**. These oval or polygonal cells are characterized by their light, striated ("crumpled") cytoplasm and a swollen cell body with a decentralized nucleus; occasionally, there are two or more hyperchromatic nuclei at the periphery. Apart from glucocerebroside, Gaucher cells also contain lysosomal acidic phosphatase. They are PAS-positive, 20–100 µm in size and grouped within the hepatic lobule; in some areas, the cells fill the sinusoids and are likewise found in the portal fields, where they originate from histiocytes.

Type I *(chronic visceral type)*: This is the most common course and may manifest at any time in life; most often, however, it occurs between the ages of 20 and 40. The patients are able to lead relatively normal lives. Clinical features include pronounced *hepatosplenomegaly*, *ostealgia* with spontaneous fractures, backache and pain in the extremities, fever and *haematopoetic disorders* (microcytic anaemia, leucopenia, thrombopenia with haemorrhagic diathesis). The transaminases and the liver function values are usually normal; alkaline phosphatase is increased. Portal hypertension and ascites can occur due to obstruction or compression of the sinusoidal pathway. (224) After a course of several years, yellowish brown, patchy pigmentations (containing melanin) appear in the face, particularly at the root of the nose, and on the legs. Yellowish grey pingueculae may be present around the eyes (nasal or bilateral). Diagnosis is confirmed by the detection of acidic phosphatase in the cells and a reduced activity of glucocerebrosidase in leucocyte suspensions or fibroblast cultures. Meanwhile, the various types of Gaucher's disease can be identified by PCR. There are no neurologic symptoms. The cholesterol level is normal. (221, 223, 226) • Prognosis is determined by haematological complications, an increased susceptibility to infections and a higher rate of lymphoproliferative diseases. Transition to cirrhosis has often been observed, as have bleeding oesophageal varices. (216, 224, 228, 230, 232)

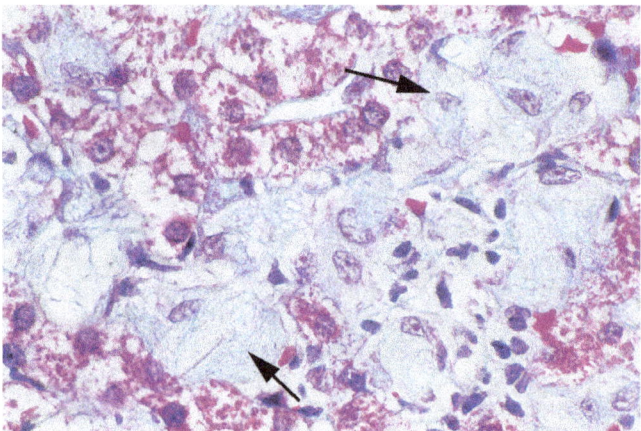

Fig. 31.17: Gaucher's disease. Gaucher cells (sphingolipid-storing macrophages) within the liver parenchyma (arrow), shown here as pale-blue cells with an internal structure similar to cigarette paper (PAS)

▶ *We were able to observe a family with 6 children, 4 of whom (3 boys and 1 girl) suffered from Gaucher's disease. I examined one of the children laparoscopically. All 4 children showed pronounced hepatosplenomegaly with symptoms of abdominal organ displacement; splenectomy was carried out in good time. (231) (s. fig. 31.17)*

For successful **treatment**, *β-glucocerebrosidase* gained from the placenta or recombinant imiglucerase can be used as an intravenous infusion every second week. (217–219, 222, 225, 227) • A novel form of oral treatment with N-butyldeoxynojirimycin over a period of up to 12 months produced good results. Further trials with this substance, which inhibits the synthesis of glucocerebrosides, are justified. Diarrhoea was a frequent side effect (79%). (220) • Following *liver transplantation*, there was a regression in glucosylceramide deposition in the extrahepatic organs – the metabolic defect was not corrected however. (236) Long-term follow-up showed good results after *bone-marrow transplantation*. (229)

Type II *(acute infantile neurological type):* Type II becomes manifest within the first few months of life. Splenomegaly followed by hepatomegaly can be observed at a very early stage. A striking feature is the cerebral and neurological symptomatology. The affected child usually dies within the first year of life due to bronchopulmonary infection.

Type III *(chronic juvenile neurological type):* At the onset of the disease, splenomegaly and, subsequently, hepatomegaly are observed. Gaucher cells are found in the bone marrow at an early stage. There are severe cerebral and neurological disorders.

12.2 Fabry's disease

The enzymatic defect in glycoprotein and lipid metabolism in this disease, which is based on X-chromosomal transmission, is most likely to be **α-galactosidase-A deficiency.** Storage products consist of sphingolipids, mainly GL-3. They are principally stored in the kidneys, vascular walls and smooth musculature, but also in the **liver** (stellate cells, portal macrophages, vascular endothelium). These affected cells take on a yellowish-brown colour. The hepatocytes are finely vacuolated; the Kupffer cells and macrophages are hypertrophic and contain cholesterol and lipofuscin. • The clinical picture, which usually begins with swelling of and burning pains in the limbs as well as skin changes and corneal opacity, was simultaneously described by J. Fabry and by W. Anderson in 1898. • *Treatment* with recombinant agalsidase beta has proved successful.

12.3 Gangliosidosis

Among other things, gangliosidosis may also affect the liver. The deposition of gangliosides (particularly of the G_{M1} and G_{M2} type) in the liver causes hepatomegaly to develop. In 1964 B.H. Landing et al. described *familial neurovisceral lipidosis* as a disease in its own right, although this entity had probably been observed by J. Caffey as early as 1951. The type of metabolic disorder was defined by J.S. O'Brien et al. in 1965. It is in fact an autosomal recessive G_{M1} **gangliosidosis** of the infantile generalized type I. The disease is caused by **β-galactosidase A, B and C deficiency**, so that the cleavage of the terminal galactose of both the ganglioside G_{M1} and the mucopolysaccharides is inhibited. These abnormal products are then stored. Foam cells with PAS-positive substances develop, which in turn involves the total RES and hence the stellate cells and portal histiocytes as well. Progressive hepatomegaly is present. Familial neurovisceral lipidosis causes the death of the child in the first or second year of life. (Type II G_{M1} gangliosidosis is considered to be a juvenile type without visceral involvement.)

G_{M2} **gangliosidosis** is caused by a deficiency of **hexosamidase A** and **B**. It was described for the first time by K. Sandhoff et al. as *Sandhoff's disease* in 1968. This biochemical variant (type II) largely corresponds to Tay-Sachs disease, which is also autosomal recessive. Renal globoside (ceramide trihexoside) is stored in the visceral organs, particularly in the liver and spleen. Hepatomegaly is present, occasionally with splenomegaly. The lysosomes within the hepatocytes become considerably larger until they are as big as the nucleus and show lamellar structures.

12.4 Niemann-Pick disease

▶ In 1914 A. NIEMANN described a type of storage disease which, however, he did not recognize. In 1926 L. PICK differentiated this clinical picture from Gaucher's disease and called it "lipid cellular splenomegaly". The substance predominantly stored was identified as sphingomyelin by E. KLENK in 1934. Thus, this condition is a kind of phosphoryl ceramidosis.

The disease is based upon a deficiency of the lysosomal enzyme **sphingomyelinase,** mainly in the RES cells. This autosomal recessive enzyme defect results in **sphingomyelin** being stored in the liver (hepatocytes, Kupffer cells, portal macrophages), spleen, bone marrow and lungs. These pale storage cells, the so-called **Pick cells** (20–40 μm) display a mulberry-like, alveolate structure, and, in addition to sphingomyelin, contain cholesterol and triglycerides as well as pigment ceroid (s. fig. 21.6). The cell inclusions are granular and double-refractory. Due to vacuolation, the Pick cells look like foam cells. (234)
• Meanwhile, five biochemical and **clinical types** have been differentiated (types A–E); type A is equivalent to the classical Niemann-Pick disease observed in infants. To date, some 200 cases have been reported.

Type A is already present in infancy. The following symptoms rapidly develop: anorexia, vomiting, weight loss, growth retardation, hepatosplenomegaly, lymphadenopathy, profuse sweating, a brownish-yellow waxy complexion and a pronounced cerebral and neurological symptomatology (muscular hypotonia, areflexia, deafness, loss of sight). In about 5 % of cases, cherry-red spots with yellowish prominence can be found on the fundus of the eye. Liver cell damage and cell necrosis as well as cholestasis develop. The affected child dies before reaching the age of 2 years. (236, 240)

Type B is often characterized by neonatal cholestasis, which disappears in the later course of disease. The condition becomes manifest in childhood and progresses slowly. Hepatosplenomegaly develops, as does cirrhosis with portal hypertension. (237) The lungs occasionally display a miliary picture due to the interstitial storage of sphingomyelin; chronic bronchitis is often observed. No neurological or cerebral symptoms are in evidence. The haemogram shows anaemia and thrombopenia. • *Treatment* with allogeneic bone marrow transplantation has been reported. (238)

Type C is characterized by a slow course with neurological symptoms and gradual mental deterioration. A rare event is the development of neonatal cholestasis (235, 239) or HCC (233).

Type E is also known as the **sea-blue histiocytes syndrome** and is considered to be a special form of Niemann-Pick disease found in adults. The stored, ceroid-like, acid-proof and PAS-positive pigment shows a sea-blue colour on Giemsa staining. Hepatosplenomegaly is present; thrombopenia is likewise in evidence due to bone marrow involvement. Cirrhosis may develop. The prognosis is considered to be good. (235)

12.5 Mucopolysaccharidoses

These are congenital disturbances in the enzymatic degradation of acidic mucopolysaccharides (MPS) by the lysosomes. *Four types of mucopolysaccharides* (glycosaminoglycam, dermatan sulfate, heparan sulfate, chondroitin-6 sulfate) are stored, ultimately compromising all organs and tissues. In addition, ganglioside is stored in the CNS. Depending on the respective disease, varying distribution patterns can be found, with storage forms occurring individually or in combination. To date, **ten individual forms** have been identified; others, however, have remained unclassified. In all forms, there is increased elimination of the above-mentioned MPS in the urine.

Six out of a total of ten forms are accompanied by **liver involvement** *(storage in the hepatocytes, Kupffer cells and portal macrophages as well as vacuolization of the cytoplasm)* and **hepatomegaly**. The liver is firm and has a bluish-yellow or greyish-yellow colour. The stored mucopolysaccharides are PAS-positive, but not diastasis-resistant. During a longer course, *fibrosis* develops and *cirrhosis* may occur.

Some forms overlap in symptomatology and cannot be distinguished by enzyme or urinary assays. • A **new therapy** for α-L-iduronidase deficiency using enzyme replacement (= *laronidase*) as i.v. infusion has proved safe and efficacious (J. WRAITH et al., 2004).

Pfaundler-Hurler syndrome *(type I):* This syndrome is caused by an α-L-iduronidase deficiency (M. v. PFAUNDLER, 1920; G. HURLER, 1920). It is autosomal recessive and panethnic, with an incidence of approx. 1:100,000 live births. A major cause of morbidity and mortality is respiratory insufficiency together with cardiac compromise (valvular dysfunction).

Ullrich-Scheie's syndrome *(type V):* This is also characterized by an α-L-iduronidase deficiency, but it does not appear before school age (O. ULLRICH et al., 1943; H. G. SCHEIE et al., 1962). Further symptoms are above-normal growth and head size, chronic otitis, chronic rhinitis, hepatosplenomegaly, corneal clouding, ankylosis and mental retardation.

Hunter's syndrome *(type II):* Initially, this disease was erroneously classified as type I. Its nosological independence and X-chromosomal recessive transmission were recognized in 1964 (A. NJA). The disease is based on a deficiency of L-iduron-sulphate sulphatase and sulphoiduronate sulphatase. The syndrome may appear in a moderate or severe form.

Sanfilippo's syndrome *(type III):* This syndrome exhibits a similar clinical picture as described above with at least two different enzyme defects: heparan-sulphamidase deficiency (type A) and N-acetyl-α-D-glucosamidase deficiency (type B) and possibly types C or D as well (S. J. SANFILIPPO et al., 1963).

Morquio's syndrome *(type IV):* This syndrome is a result of a galactosamine-6-sulphatase deficiency (type A) or a beta-galactosidase deficiency (type B) (L. MORQUIO, 1929; J. F. BRAILSFORD, 1929).

Maroteaux-Lamy syndrome *(type VI):* This syndrome is due to an arylsulphatase B deficiency. It appears in a severe or moderate form (P. MAROTEAUX et al., 1965).

12.6 Mucolipidoses

Mucolipidoses are characterized by a **combined metabolic disorder** of mucopolysaccharides, lipids, and glycoproteins. Lysosomal storage and foamy swollen Kupffer cells with hepatomegaly may be seen. In some of the numerous types, the underlying enzymatic defects have not yet been detected. • Type II is also called **Leroy syndrome** (J.G. LEROY et al., 1967). Due to distinctive cytoplasmic inclusions in fibroblast cultures, this disorder is also known as **"inclusion cell disease"** (J.G. LEROY et al., 1971). Foamy altered stellate cells, macrophages and also epithelioid foam cell granulomas are found.

Fucosidosis, being a so-called mucolipidosis, can be grouped among the mucopolysaccharidoses. It is due to α-fucosidase deficiency (localized on chromosome 1p 34). The storage products are deposited in the form of granular or lamellar inclusions in the lysosomes. This autosomal recessive disorder was first observed by P. DURAND et al. in 1967 and clarified by F. VAN HOOF et al. in 1968. Besides hepatomegaly, splenomegaly also sometimes occurs.

Mannosidosis, first observed by P.-A. ÖCKERMAN in 1967, is caused by α-mannosidase deficiency. The gene defect (autosomal recessive) is localized on chromosome 19p, 13, 2-q12. Hepatosplenomegaly, steatosis and perisinusoidal fibrosis are in evidence. PAS-positive vacuoles, consisting of lysosomally stored substances, are found in the cytoplasm of the hepatocytes.

Mucosulphatidosis is caused by arylsulphatase deficiency (types A, B and C). Metachromatic granules are found mostly in portal macrophages and less frequently in hepatocytes or Kupffer cells.

Lafora's disease (H. UNVERRICHT et al., 1891) is seen as an autosomal recessive enzyme defect. A striking feature are the severe CNS disorders. The myocardium, liver and musculature are also involved. The affected hepatocytes are similar to *ground glass cells* and mostly found at the periphery of the lobules. The coarse granular and lamellar cytoplasmic inclusions are PAS-positive glycoprotein-mucopolysaccharide particles, also known as *Lafora bodies* (C.R. LAFORA, 1911). Liver biopsy shows signs of unspecific reactive hepatitis and fibrosis. Death occurs in infancy.

13 Mucoviscidosis

Mucoviscidosis or **cystic fibrosis (CF)** is indeed one of the most common autosomal recessive diseases. It is characterized by the production of a viscous secretion in the excretory glands. Accordingly, pancreatic cystic fibrosis can be observed in the pancreatic area and cylindrical bronchiectases in the pulmonary area. The inspissation of bile and mucus leads to obstruction of the bile canaliculi and subsequently to cholestasis. The gene product is characterized as cystic fibrosis transmembrane regulator (CFTR). (246) The gene defect, which is located on chromosome 7, causes a disorder of the intracellular transport of chloride ions (probably also of chloride ion secretion) and thus triggers the occurrence of CF. The incidence of mucoviscidosis is about $1:2,000-4,500$.

Liver involvement: In protracted disease, the liver becomes involved in 20−25% of cases. Rarely, a symptomatic hepatobiliary disease, mostly in the form of fatty liver but also as focal biliary cirrhosis, occurs in the first few weeks of life. Proliferation of the ductuli and dilatation of the intralobular bile ducts can be detected. (241, 242) As a result of this, crumbly products are deposited and the lumina are completely sealed off. These retained crumbly products have not yet been differentiated specifically; they are, however, PAS-positive and mucin-negative and consist mainly of precipitated protein. Hepatomegaly is due to macrovesicular steatosis. Inflammatory changes in the bile canaliculi and the small bile ducts with cholestasis and infiltration of the portal fields are often observed. (244, 248) With progressive proliferation of the ductules and liver fibrosis, there is a rise in γ-GT, AP and 5' NU. In the further course, a slight increase in the transaminases as a sign of hepatocellular damage is detectable. A score can be used for the sonographic diagnosis of liver involvement in CF. (252) Scintigraphy may be applied for the quantification of impaired secretion. (250) Liver function is assessed using ChE, Quick's value, GEC (s. p. 114) and ICG tests (s. p. 114). Gene mutation is easily confirmed by direct genetic screening with allele-specific oligonucleotides. The inflammatory and reactive-fibrosing processes may ultimately result in necrotizing cholangitis and multilobular biliary cirrhosis, possibly with bleeding oesophageal varices; frequency is reported to be 5−20%. (244, 248, 249)

Treatment: The only effective therapy is gene replacement. (247, 253) Symptomatically, liver damage and cholestasis can be reduced by UDCA. (243) It is also advisable to achieve an optimum nutritional status and to use essential phospholipids as long-term therapy. (251) In severe cases, there may possibly be an indication for liver transplantation or indeed combined liver-lung transplantation. (245)

14 Zellweger's syndrome

This **cerebro-hepatorenal syndrome** was described by P. BOWEN, C.S. LEE, H. ZELLWEGER and R. LINDENBERG in 1964 on the basis of observations originally made by Zellweger. It is an autosomal recessive disease, with a lack of peroxisomes due to a mutation of the mRNA peroxisome-assembly factor 1. In this complex syndrome, there are various malformations with *disturbances in the amino-acid balance and β-oxidation of long chain fatty acids as well as iron metabolism resulting from a disorder* *of bile acid synthesis* at the side chain. The blood shows hypersideraemia, and there are increases of different intensity regarding alanine, lysine, isoleucine, methionine, phenylalanine and serine. Signs of substantial cholestatic liver damage, siderosis, portal inflammation, fibrosis and the potential development of cirrhosis are evident. (254–258) (s. p. 242)

15 Porphyrias

15.1 Definition

> Porphyrias are metabolic disorders caused by hereditary enzyme defects or acquired disorders of haem synthesis. These result in the increased formation of porphyrins and porphyrinogens and their precursors, which are either stored in the tissue or excreted in the urine or faeces. The term porphyria is derived from the Greek word "porphuros", which means purple and describes the purple-red crystalline porphyrins. Depending on the underlying enzyme defect or the respective aetiopathogenesis, porphyrias can become clinically manifest with neurological, photocutaneous, cerebral, cardiovascular, abdominal or hepatic symptomatology.

15.2 Classification

▶ **Primary porphyrias** are caused by hereditary enzyme defects in haem synthesis. They can be differentiated clinically into **acute** and **chronic** porphyrias as well as pathogenetically into **hepatic** and **erythropoietic** porphyrias. • **Secondary porphyrias** are symptomatic porphyrias present in various diseases or caused by poisoning or chemical substances, particularly alcohol. • Depending on the preferred **manifestation site** of the enzyme defect, either in the hepatocytes or in the erythrocytes (bone marrow), the porphyrias are subdivided into hepatic, erythropoietic and hepatoerythropoietic forms. However, this classification is not always strictly applicable. • Based on the **course of disease**, acute and chronic forms may be differentiated in primary hepatic porphyrias. The acute form is characterized by a congenital regulatory disturbance of porphyrin and haem synthesis together with the induction of ALA synthase within the hepatocyte. The acute forms are less frequent, but associated with a higher risk. Only acute hepatic porphyrias show convulsive gastrointestinal and neuropsychiatric symptoms. Chronic hepatic porphyrias are due to congenital or acquired enzyme defects; they are the most frequent forms and always involve liver damage. • Only the erythropoietic forms are accompanied by acute phototoxic reactions. Skin changes have been observed in variegate porphyria and porphyria cutanea tarda. (s. tab. 31.10)

Primary porphyrias may arise from a *hereditary defect* in any of the **eight enzymes** involved in haem synthesis: (*1.*) δ-aminolaevulinic acid synthase (which causes a sideroblastic anaemia), (*2.*) porphobilinogen synthase, (*3.*) porphobilinogen deaminase, (*4.*) uroporphyrinogen III synthase, (*5.*) uroporphyrinogen decarboxylase, (*6.*) coproporphyrinogen oxidase, (*7.*) protoporphyrinogen oxidase, and (*8.*) ferrochelatase. • A most important **branching point** in haem synthesis is the transformation of porphobilinogen (by PBG deaminase) into pre-uroporphyrinogen. The latter is transformed by uroporphyrinogen III synthase into uroporphyrinogen III; in the case of reduced enzyme activity, uroporphyrinogen I is spontaneously formed and subsequently eliminated in the urine. (300) (s. fig. 3.2)

▶ **Secondary porphyrias** are symptomatic and hepatic porphyrias. (300) They are coproporphyrinurias with simultaneously increased protoporphyrin concentrations in blood plasma. For prophylactic, prognostic and therapeutic reasons, it is important to differentiate between primary porphyria and secondary coproporphyrinuria. • Only in coproporphyrinuria caused by lead intoxication and in tyrosinaemia can δ-aminolaevulinaciduria be found at the same time. The alcohol-liver-porphyrinuria syndrome is the most important form of secondary porphyrinuria. In chronic alcohol abuse, secondary coproporphyrinuria may develop into chronic hepatic porphyria. (272) • *Some 30% of patients suffering from chronic liver disease later develop pathological coproporphyrinuria.* (s. tab. 31.11)

15.3 Biochemistry

Glycine and **succinyl coenzyme A** are the *initial substrates* for porphyrin synthesis, from which δ-aminolaevulinic acid (ALA) is formed with the help of ALA synthase. This initial biosynthetic step takes place in the mitochondria. Porphobilinogen (PBG) develops in the cellular cytosol due to the connection of 2 mol ALA. Uroporphyrinogen is then formed from 4 mol PBG and subsequently decarboxylated, thus producing coproporphyrinogen. Further decarboxylation occurs within the mitochondria, leading to the production of protoporphyrin. Due to its lipophilic qualities, the latter is not filtered by the kidneys and is therefore subject to enterohepatic circulation. With the help of ferrochelatase, iron is stored and haem is formed. • **Haem** is the *final product* of porphyrin synthesis, which may take place in all cells. It is required as a prosthetic group by enzymes or pigments (catalase, cytochrome, haemoglobin, myoglobin, etc.). Via feedback, haem regulates the limiting enzyme *ALA synthase* and thus the whole porphyrin synthesis. The activity of ALA synthase is increased by various drugs (s. tab. 31.13), chemical agents and endogenous metabolic products. • Induction of ALA synthase can be suppressed by glucose. Due to the short half-life of

Primary porphyrias	Abbreviations	Enzyme defect	Hereditary transmission
Erythropoietic porphyrias			
1. *Congenital erythropoietic porphyria* (Günther's disease)	CEP	Uroporphyrinogen III synthase	autosomal recessive
2. *Erythropoietic protoporphyria*	EPP	Ferrochelatase	autosomal dominant
Hepatic porphyrias			
1. *Acute hepatic porphyrias*			
• Acute intermittent porphyria	AIP	Uroporphyrinogen I synthase	autosomal dominant
• Variegate porphyria	VP	Protoporphyrinogen oxidase	autosomal dominant
• Hereditary coproporphyria	HCP	Coproporphyrinogen oxidase	autosomal dominant
• Doss porphyria	DP	Aminolaevulinic acid dehydratase	autosomal recessive
• Porphobilinogen synthase defect	PS	Porphobilinogen synthase	autosomal recessive
2. *Chronic hepatic porphyrias*			
• Porphyria cutanea tarda	PCT	Uroporphyrinogen III decarboxylase	autosomal dominant
• Hepatoerythropoietic porphyria	HEP	Uroporphyrinogen III decarboxylase	autosomal recessive

Tab. 31.10: Primary (erythropoietic, hepatic, hepatoerythropoietic) porphyrias

ALA synthase of 70−80 minutes, inhibition or induction of this enzyme quickly affects haem synthesis. Haem deficiency due to an enzyme defect causes an increase in δ-aminolaevulinic acid. Free haem is either integrated into various apoproteins or intervenes as a haem repressor with the nuclear gene chain, which leads to the formation of specific mRNA for ALA synthase.
• Synthesis and consumption of haem are synchronized precisely. The organism produces some 300 mg haem per day, with only 1% being excreted unused in the urine or faeces. (264, 266, 291, 300) (s. p. 38) (s. tab. 3.3)

Secondary coproporphyrinurias and protoporphyrinaemias
1. **Poisoning**
• Alcohol
• Heavy metals
– lead, arsenic, iron, gold
• Chemical agents
– benzenes, hydrocarbons, *etc.*
2. **Liver diseases**
• Acute and chronic hepatitis, alcohol-induced fatty liver, cirrhosis, cholestasis, haemochromatosis
3. **Blood diseases**
• Haemolytic anaemia, sideroachrestic anaemia, aplastic anaemia, pernicious anaemia, leukaemia, Hodgkin's disease, *etc.*
4. **Infectious diseases**
5. **Diabetes mellitus**
6. **Hereditary metabolic defects**
• Benign recurrent cholestasis
• Dubin-Johnson syndrome
• Rotor's syndrome
• Tyrosinaemia type I
7. **Neoplastic diseases**
8. **Cardiac infarction**
9. **Pregnancy**
10. **Starvation**
11. **Iron metabolism disturbances**
12. **Medication** (s. tab. 31.13)

Tab. 31.11: Secondary (symptomatic, acquired) disorders of porphyrin metabolism

▶ The colourless porphyrinogens easily convert to coloured *red-fluorescent uroporphyrins* at 366 nm when there is sufficient oxygen. This gives the urine a red colour, which becomes darker (burgundy red) when left in contact with air. The *red-fluorescent specimen* obtained by liver biopsy in chronic hepatic porphyria is impressive. (s. pp 153, 166) (s. fig. 7.10)

15.4 Genetics

Primary porphyrias are genetically determined, whereby their expression varies in intensity, i.e. there is either a reduction in or instability of the enzyme affected by gene mutation. A total loss of enzyme activity or a lack of enzyme protein is inconsistent with the viability of the organism. Transmission is autosomal dominant in five forms of porphyrias, but autosomal recessive in congenital erythropoietic porphyria (CEP), hepatoerythropoietic porphyria (HEP) and the so-called Doss porphyria. (s. tab. 31.10) • Any type of porphyria may be caused by various gene mutations, which results in pronounced genetic heterogeneity. Two different types of porphyria may even become manifest within one family. The penetrance of the relevant gene mutation is low, so that about 80% of the persons involved are without clinical or laboratory findings. The probability of the enzyme defect being passed on to a child is about 50%. (267, 275, 281, 299, 300)

Not only genetic factors figure in the manifestation of porphyria, but also endogenous and exogenous causes such as alcohol (272), medicaments, stress situations, fasting, intoxication, metabolic products, effects of light and chemical agents (e.g. polyhalogenized biphenyls, dioxin). • In a well-known case in Turkey, about 4,000 people contracted hepatocutaneous porphyria after eating wheat contaminated with the fungicide hexachlorobenzene. (s. p. 581)

15.5 Clinical aspects

In cases of suspected hepatic porphyria, **instant orientation** is gained by examining the urine for evidence of δ-aminolaevulinic acid and porphobilinogen – using the *Watson-Schwartz test* (C.J. Watson et al., 1941) or *Hoesch test* (K. Hoesch, 1947) – as well as for the presence of porphyrins. (Hoesch test: 2 ml Ehrlich's reagent + 3 drops of urine = pinkish-red discoloration after shaking, revealing positive evidence of porphobilinogen.) • Further **differentiation** of porphyrins excreted in the urine and faeces or present in plasma and erythrocytes as well as of the distribution pattern of porphyrin metabolites is necessary; for this purpose, thin-layer chromatography, ion-exchange chromatography and HPLC are available. • Identification of asymptomatic **gene carriers,** which is important for preventive measures, can be achieved by determining the enzymes involved in porphyrin synthesis.

The **symptomatology** of porphyrias is of such complexity and variability that there is always a danger of misinterpretation. Wrongly indicated laparotomy due to suspected acute abdomen entails a high risk! The initiation of incorrect treatment measures may also have grave consequences. Owing to the extremely complex interdisciplinary symptomatology, an emergency due to porphyria must be interpreted in terms of surgery, internal medicine or neurology, and depending on the results obtained, the patient is referred to the corresponding department. • *Porphyria can imitate numerous diseases.*

15.6 Erythropoietic porphyrias

The enzymatic metabolic defect is mainly restricted to the erythrocytes or bone marrow. Two distinct clinical pictures can be differentiated: *congenital erythropoietic porphyria (CEP)* and *erythropoietic protoporphyria (EPP)* (W. Kosenow et al., 1953; I.A. Magnus et al., 1961). From a hepatological point of view, only EPP is important. (s. tab. 31.12)

15.6.1 Congenital erythropoietic porphyria

This clinical picture is also termed *Günther's disease* (H. Günther, 1911). About 200 cases have been described so far. An autosomal recessive deficiency of uroporphyrinogen III synthase (chromosome 10q25) results in augmented accumulation of porphyrin isomers of type I, which cannot be used biologically. This causes an increase in uroporphyrin with the occurrence of fluorocytes (mostly erythrocytes, but sometimes also hepatocytes). A red discolouration of urine has already been observed in infants. Exposure to the sun leads to severe burns with the formation of blisters (the content of which may fluoresce) and necroses. Pronounced mutilations on the face and hands develop in the course of time.

	CEP	EPP
Urine		
Total porphyrins	+++	N/v
Uroporphyrin	++	N/v
Coproporphyrin	+	N/v
Porphobilinogen	N	N
ALA	N	N
Faeces		
Total porphyrins	++	+
Uroporphyrin	+	N/v
Coproporphyrin	+	v
Protoporphyrin	+	++
Erythrocytes		
Total porphyrins	+++	+++
Uroporphyrinogen I	+++	N/v
Coproporphyrin	++	N/v
Protoporphyrin	++	+++
Plasma		
Total porphyrins	++	+

Tab. 31.12: Constellation of findings in erythropoietic porphyrias (v = variable, N = normal)

The teeth are discoloured reddish-brown due to the deposition of porphyrins in dentine. Haemolytic anaemia with splenomegaly may develop. • *CEP causes neither neurologic disorders nor (substantial) liver damage.*

15.6.2 Erythropoietic protoporphyria

An autosomal dominant ferrochelatase deficiency causes enhanced accumulation of protoporphyrin within the erythrocytes. The gene for ferrochelatase has been detected on chromosome 18q21. EPP is considered to be the third most frequent porphyria (1:100,000). (306) Red-fluorescing erythrocytes form as a result of the high porphyrin content. EPP becomes manifest already in childhood, but the course of disease may be latent for a long time. Exposure to the sun causes skin reactions, such as painful erubescence, oedema and blisters. After long-term insolation, permanent skin infiltrations are observed. Prognosis is generally good. • The liver is damaged by increasing deposits of porphyrins. Cholestasis as well as liver fibrosis and cirrhosis may become manifest. Pigment gallstones can occur. Acute liver failure with a fatal outcome has also been reported. (265, 284, 298) • **Treatment** consists of the administration of β-carotene and vitamin E in order to capture the oxygen radicals which are present in greatly increased numbers in the skin following exposure to sunlight and thus to prevent the triggering of phototoxic reactions. Administration of chenodeoxycholic acid, cholestyramine and glucose (>300 g/day) is likewise recommended. Liver transplantation may be indicated. (263, 267, 269, 271, 282, 287, 289, 294, 295, 297, 300, 308, 310)

15.7 Hepatic porphyrias

Hepatic porphyrias show the following *characteristics:* (*1.*) intermittent course, (*2.*) increased ALA synthase activity, and (3.) acute attacks induced or manifesting during the latency period due to numerous causes such as alcohol (272), hunger, carbohydrate deficiency, hormones, stress, intoxication, metabolic products and medicaments. (s. tab. 31.13)

Alcohol	Lofepramine
Allopurinol	Medrogestone
Amiodarone	Meprobamate
Barbexaclon	Mesuximide
Barbiturates	Methyldopa
Benegrid	Metoclopramide
Carbamazepine	Metronidazole
Carbromal	Nalidixic acid
Chloramphenicol	Nicethamide
Chlordiazepoxides	Nifedipine
Chlormezanone	Nitrofurantoin
Chloroquine	Oral contraceptives
Chlorpropamide	Oestrogens
Clonazepam	Oxazepam
Clonidine	Paramethadione
Cyclophosphamide	Pentazocines
Danazol	Pentetrazol
Dapsone	Phenacetin
Diazepam	Phenoxybenzamine
Dichloralphenazone	Phensuximide
Diclofenac	Phenylbutazone
Dimenhydrinate	Phenytoin
Ergotamine preparations	Piroxicam
Ethosuximide	Primidone
Eucalyptus oil	Progesterone
Fern extract	Pyrazinamide
Flufenamic acid	Pyrazolone derivatives
Frusemides	Pyrimethamine
Gestagens	Ranitidine
Glibenclamide	Rifampicin
Gliquidone	Spironolactone
Glutethimide	Steroids
Griseofulvin	Sulphonamides
Halothane	Sulthiame
Hydralazine	Theophyllines
Ibuprofen	Tolbutamide
Imipramines	Trimethadione
Ketoconazole	Valproic acid
Lidocaine	etc.

Tab. 31.13: Drugs which are able to trigger acute hepatic porphyria (AIP, VP, HCP) with differing degrees of risk (s. tab. 31.10)

	AIP	VP	HCP	PCT
Urine				
Total porphyrins	++	++	++	+++
Uroporphyrins	++	+	+	++
Coproporphyrins	++	++	++	+
Porphobilinogen	+→+++	+→+++	+→+++	N
β-ALA	+→+++	+→+++	+→+++	N
Faeces				
Coproporphyrin	N/v	+	+++	N/v
Protoporphyrin	+	++	+	N/v
Uroporphyrin	N/v	+/v	N/v	+
Plasma				
Total porphyrins	N/v	N/v	+→++	+→++

Tab. 31.14: Porphyrin and porphyrin precursor content in urine and faeces for the differentiation of hepatic porphyrias (v = variable, N = normal) (s. tab. 31.10)

The *diagnosis* is based upon the clinical symptomatology and the excretion pattern of the porphyrins or their precursors in the urine and faeces as well as their concentrations in the erythrocytes and plasma. (s. tab. 31.14)

▶ Patients suffering from hepatic porphyria receive a **porphyria pass** as well as all important **information** referring to the disease; in particular, they must be informed about risk factors leading to manifestation, e. g. avoidance of porphyria-inducing drugs (s. tab. 31.13) and xenobiotics, alcohol abstinence. A diet rich in carbohydrates is important as a preventive measure, because this reduces ALA activity in the liver. • It is essential to examine other **family members** in order to recognize any potential genetic carriers or to identify a relative afflicted by porphyria which is still in the latency phase. Such persons are likewise informed about the disease, particularly with respect to potential manifestation factors, and they also receive a porphyria pass.

Acute hepatic porphyrias

There are pathophysiological and clinical transitions between all forms of acute hepatic porphyrias. Due to the complex clinical symptomatology, including abdominal, neurological and cardiovascular findings, misinterpretations are possible, and often the diagnosis is made too late. Skin symptoms are observed when porphyrins have accumulated in the tissue, causing reactive oxygen intermediates to form following exposure to sunlight. *In all acute hepatic porphyrias, the excretion of δ-aminolaevulinic acid, porphobilinogen and porphyrins is increased in the urine.* However, no augmentation in the excretion of PBG is observed in defective PBG synthase. Even genetically identified acute hepatic porphyrias may remain latent for a considerable period of time. Their frequency is given at about 5:100,000, with remarkable geographic variations. There are four (or five) different forms of acute hepatic porphyria. (300, 303) (s. tab. 31.10)

15.7.1 Acute intermittent porphyria

Acute intermittent porphyria (AIP) is the second most frequent form of porphyria; it occurs three to four times more often in women than in men. The peak rate is between the ages of 20 and 40 years. This autosomal dominant form is responsible for a deficiency in porphobilinogen deaminase (uroporphyrinogen I synthase). The genetic defect of this enzyme is localized on chromosome 11q24. Several genetic variants (>4) exist. The frequency of gene defects shows geographic variations. **Manifestation** of AIP is also caused by numerous exogenous or endogenous factors (see above). In women, the first clinical manifestation is often associated with the premenstrual phase. Some women suffer from cycle-related episodes of the disease. The overall frequency of AIP is 5−10: 100,000. • There are **five cardinal symptoms,** which may appear with widely differing intensity: (*1.*) cardiovascular findings such as tachycardia, hypertension and changes in the ECG, (*2.*) intermittent and diffuse abdominal pain, often localized in the lower abdomen, which may take the form of colic, including vomiting and ileus-like features, (*3.*) severe obstipation, largely unresponsive to treatment (onset mostly during puberty), (*4.*) peripheral neurological and muscular disorders, which may result in pareses or paralyses, and (*5.*) neurotic or psychotic behaviour (confusion, depression, anxiety, hallucinations, delirium and coma). In cases of hyponatraemia (insufficient ADH secretion), encephalopathy may become manifest. If cardiovascular and psychiatric symptoms coincide, the picture may be misinterpreted as a thyrotoxic crisis, particularly because the serum values of T_3 and T_4 are increased in approximately 20% of patients suffering from AIP. The causes of the clinical symptoms are thought to be abnormal biochemical stimuli, triggering dysregulations in peripheral and autonomic innervation. However, there are no skin changes in AIP, and there is no photosensitivity. (261)

Occasionally, the **liver** is also involved: slight increases in the transaminases and bilirubin, and possibly impaired excretory functions as well. Initially the hepatocytes reveal ultrastructural changes, and later slight steatosis and siderosis. The liver bioptate shows no signs of red fluorescence. In AIP, there is a high risk of *cirrhosis* and *liver cell carcinoma* developing. (259, 262, 268, 285) In some patients suffering from such conditions, liver transplantation has proved successful.

Acute attacks often coincide with oliguria and hyponatraemia. It is relatively simple to demonstrate the enhanced excretion of porphobilinogen in the urine using the Watson-Schwartz test or Hoesch test. Urinary excretion of ALA is increased. In about 60% of cases, the urine takes on a burgundy-red colour as a result of uro- and coproporphyrin when allowed to stand (due to the action of light and O_2). For evaluating prognosis and preventive measures, it is important to consider the different **AIP disease phases:** (*1.*) enzymatic defect, (*2.*) compensated latency period with moderate excretion of porphyrins, (*3.*) decompensated latency period with stronger excretion of porphyrins and discrete clinical symptomatology, and (*4.*) resultant clinical period with acute porphyria syndrome. When PBG is discharged in small amounts during remission, no acute episodes need to be feared. • **Misdiagnoses** include: acute abdomen, ileus, pancreatitis and peritonitis (= *beware of laparotomy!*), poliomyelitis, psychosis, hysteria, hypertonic crisis, thyrotoxic crisis, heart attack, etc. • A **prognosis** is difficult to make regarding an acute attack, which may be life-threatening. An acute sporadic attack has to be treated immediately. Morphological damage to nerves and also demyelination can develop after a long period of paralysis following an acute attack. The regression of these forms of damage often takes many months. Residual defects may remain, mostly in the hands and feet. If corresponding preventive measures are carried out to curtail the factors triggering the disease, the prognosis is quite favourable.

Treatment consists of i.v. glucose infusions ($2 \times 2,000$ ml, 20% per day) plus administration of **haemarginate** (3 mg/kg BW/day on four consecutive days and at varying sites of injection) (s. p. 893), possibly with simultaneous administration of metalloporphyrin (for the inhibition of haemoxygenase) (292) as well as intensive care measures and administration of cimetidine (283) or iron. In cases with peripheral or CNS symptoms, prednisolone (100 mg/day) may be administered in addition. (260, 280, 286, 287, 303, 304, 309)

15.7.2 Variegate porphyria

Variegate porphyria is caused by protoporphyrinogen oxidase deficiency. Transmission is autosomal dominant (chromosome 1 q 23). The frequency is 1 : 100,000. • The **clinical picture** is characterized by skin changes similar to PCT (men > women), abdominal pain and internal as well as neurological symptoms similar to AIP (women > men). Therefore, VP is also called "mixed porphyria". Skin symptoms (increased photosensitivity, vulnerability, formation of blisters, pigmentation, hypertrichosis) are observed in 85% of patients, beginning mostly between the ages of 20 and 30 years. Constipation, vomiting and hypertension are even more common in PV than in AIP. Growth is retarded. • **Laboratory findings** show relatively high increases in total porphyrins, porphobilinogen and ALA, particularly in acute attacks. Enhanced excretion of coproporphyrin in the urine and faeces is observed, even in the preclinical period. The following are considered to be characteristic features of VP: (*1.*) increased excretion of porphyrin-peptide (x-porphyrin) in faeces and (*2.*) maximum absorption of porphyrins in the plasma at 626 nm, while the maximum is 619 nm in all other porphyrias. • The liver biopsy sample shows no red fluorescence. No significant or even characteristic histological liver changes are in evidence. • Factors triggering an acute attack correspond to those found in AIP. The prognosis is quite good when such noxae are avoided. (270, 288)

15.7.3 Hereditary coproporphyria

This is an autosomal dominant coproporphyrinogen oxidase deficiency (chromosome 3 q 12). The frequency is 1 : 100,000. An increase in porphyrins, coproporphyrin and porphobilinogen is found in the urine. This form of acute hepatic porphyria is very rare. Its clinical course is largely identical to that of AIP, whereby acute gastrointestinal and neuropsychiatric symptoms predominate. However, they are less pronounced and cannot be detected with the same frequency as in AIP and VP. Skin symptoms (in about 30% of cases) include photosensitivity, pigmentation and hypertrichosis. The liver displays red fluorescence due to the accumulation of porphyrin (s. fig. 7.10), but no morphological damage. Coexistence with PCT has been described. (273)

15.7.4 Doss porphyria

This rare, autosomal recessive form of porphyria is based on 5'-aminolaevulinic acid dehydratase deficiency (chromosome 9q34). A symptomatic disease only occurs in homozygotes or double heterozygotes. No more than seven cases have been described to date. Urinary excretion of ALA and coproporphyrin is increased; greater amounts of protoporphyrin accumulate in the erythrocytes. Neuropathy develops, as in AIP. Repeated severe neurological crises may necessitate liver transplantation. Heterozygotes are considerably endangered by lead, because lead inhibits ALA and thus triggers the manifestation of porphyria (= *plumboporphyria*).

15.7.5 Porphobilinogen synthase defect

This rare form shows a very varied symptomatology. The disease may become manifest during puberty with severe pain or it may present later in life (beyond the fifth decade) with the clinical picture of moderate polyneuritis. ALA as well as uroporphyrins and coproporphyrins are augmented in the urine, whereas no abnormalities are evident in faeces or plasma.

Chronic hepatic porphyrias

Chronic hepatic porphyrias appear in two variants: (*1.*) porphyria cutanea tarda and (*2.*) hepatoerythropoietic porphyria. Chronic hepatic porphyria develops in about 10% of patients suffering from chronic liver disease. (s. tabs. 31.10, 31.11)

15.7.6 Porphyria cutanea tarda

This is the most common form of porphyria (prevalence 20–50 : 100,000). The primary enzyme defect is a *uroporphyrinogen III decarboxylase* deficiency. The coded gene for the enzyme defect is on chromosome 1q34. Porphyria cutanea tarda (PCT) is characterized by pronounced genetic heterogeneity. • As far as its transmission is concerned, two forms can be differentiated: (*1.*) **familial form** (type 2), which is characterized by an autosomal dominant transmission route with heterozygote enzyme deficiency (about 50% enzyme activity) in all tissues (e. g. erythrocytes, liver, fibroblasts) – other family members are frequently affected as well; (*2.*) **acquired form** (type 1), which is also autosomal dominant, displays a uroporphyrinogen decarboxylase deficiency, but only in the liver (normal enzymatic activity in erythrocytes). This "sporadic" type occurs about four to six times as often as the familial form. • Probably, there is also a third form of PCT, namely another familial form, in which, however, the inheritance is not confirmed. The URO-D in the hepatocytes is normal (100%) in these patients. The enzyme defect seems to be limited to the liver. (275) It is (not yet) possible to differentiate clinically between these forms.

▶ As is the case with all hepatic porphyrias except HEP, additional **realization factors** such as (*1.*) alcohol, (*2.*) oestrogens, and (*3.*) haemodialysis (together with a genetically induced enzyme defect) are required for the clinical manifestation of PCT. Alcohol may cause the manifestation of PCT due to the induction of MEOS and an alcohol-related increase in iron in the liver. However, (*4.*) pharmacons (particularly lipophilic medicaments) may also be responsible for PCT, e. g. barbiturates, diazepam, hydantoin, rifampicin, antipyrin, cyclophosphamide (290), hexachlorobenzene. (s. p. 581) These substances also trigger induction of the cytochrome P 450 system, but no regulatory disorder of haem synthesis, so there is no compensatory increase in ALA synthase. A rise in PBG and ALA is therefore not detectable in the urine; this means that no neuropsychiatric symptoms appear in PCT. • Apart from that, there are substances which act as **provocation factors**, e. g. xenobiotics, steroids, lead, iron and mercury. Iron interferes with porphyrin metabolism by inhibiting uroporphyrinogen decarboxylase and probably the subsequent ferrochelatase as well, so that PCT becomes manifest. While these factors trigger an acute life-threatening porphyric process in acute hepatic porphyrias, they are generally well tolerated in PCT (e. g. all drugs), at least for a short period of time. (274, 276, 300)

While PCT was formerly observed with greater **frequency** in men (peak rate between the third and fifth decade), the ratio between the sexes nowadays is assumed to be 1:1, with women occasionally being even more prone to the disease. This situation is possibly attributable to oestrogen intake (e. g. contraceptives) and increased alcohol consumption among women. Obviously, hepatic siderosis is a prerequisite for the expression of the "sporadic" form. The frequency of PCT is estimated to be 1% of the population in the age groups 30–70 years.

Predisposition: The additional liver damage caused by the accumulation of urocarboxyporphyrins (UCP) and heptacarboxyporphyrins (HCP) in hepatic tissue is a prerequisite for clinically manifest PCT. Several forms of **liver disease** increase susceptibility to PCT, e. g. viral hepatitis B, and more particularly type C (277, 278, 293, 300), fibrosis, siderosis, cirrhosis, alcohol-induced liver disease and liver cell carcinoma. Chronic liver disease is found in 30–40% of patients with PCT. (276, 296)

The **pathogenesis** of PCT is thus caused by a combination of *four factors:*

---
1. Defective uroporphyrinogen decarboxylase
2. Realization and provocation factors
3. Accumulation of UCP and HCP in the liver
4. Liver disease

Clinical picture: The clinical picture is characterized by skin lesions and liver damage. • The **skin changes** usually begin between the ages of 40 and 70 years. Photosensitivity is due to porphyrin deposits in the skin, where their distribution pattern resembles that in the urine and serum. The lesions are so typical that there are hardly any misinterpretations. They are found at locations exposed to light such as the dorsal surface of the hands and fingers, face, neck, auricle and hairless areas of the head. The following forms are evident: (*1.*) vesiculated erosive blisters of 2 mm to 3 cm in size, which "migrate" when subjected to pressure (= *Nikolsky's phenomenon*), (*2.*) bloody scabs after the blisters have ruptured, with a poor tendency to heal, but only a slight inclination to secondary bacterial infection, (*3.*) healed vesiculated erosive blisters with atrophic scar formation and blotchy hyperpigmentation or depigmentation as well as whitish epithelial cysts, the size of a pinhead, filled with pearly bodies, (*4.*) hypertrichosis and facial cyanosis as well as melanotic hyperpigmentation, (*5.*) chronic actinic skin changes (premature skin ageing, cutis rhomboidalis, elastosis), and (*6.*) pseudosclerodermia on skin areas exposed to sunlight. (s. figs. 4.13; 31.18)

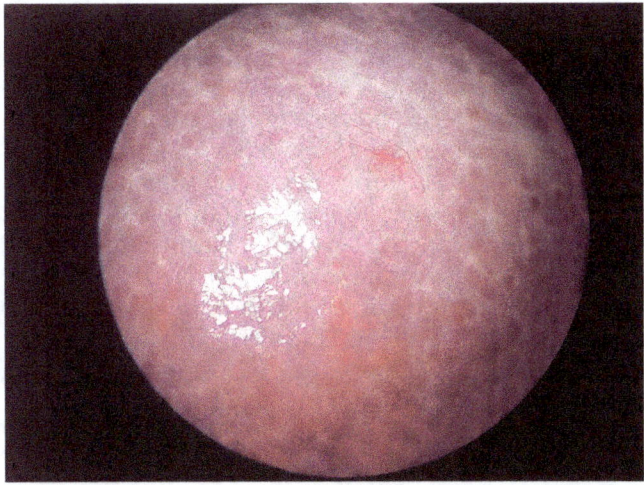

Fig. 31.19: Chronic active hepatitis in PCT: dispersed light reflection, capsular fibrosis with pronounced net-like fibrosis. Spider-like subcapsular neovascularization (s. fig. 33.13)

Histology shows deposits of needle-like porphyrins and large-droplet fatty changes in the hepatocytes, moderate iron deposits in the hepatocytes and Kupffer cells, and signs of non-specific reactive hepatitis. (s. fig. 31.20)

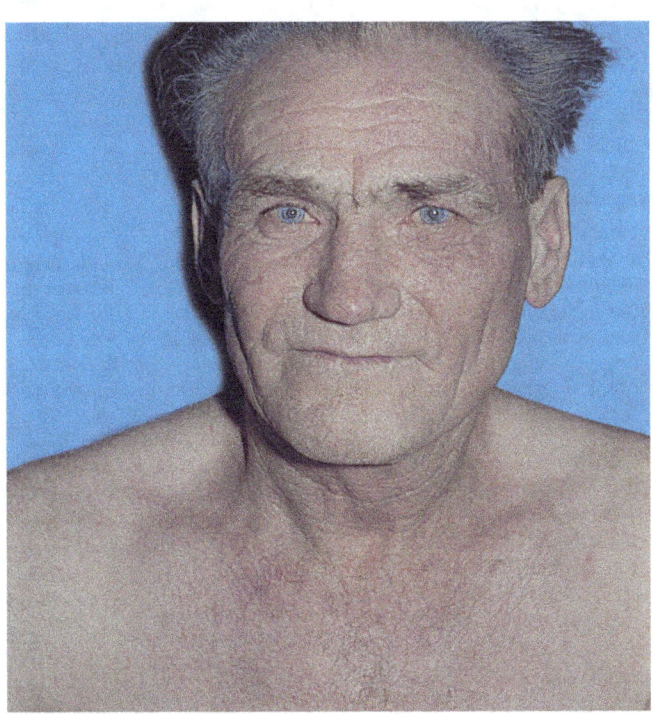

Fig. 31.18: Skin changes (face, front part of the neck) in porphyria cutanea tarda (s. fig. 4.13)

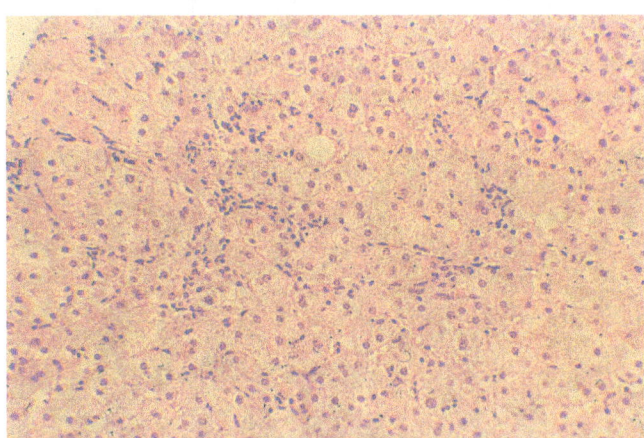

Fig. 31.20: Chronic porphyria: uncharacteristic lobular hepatitis histologically correlating to increased liver enzyme levels (HE)

Liver damage is clinically recognizable as hepatomegaly. There is a rise in the transaminases, GDH, γ-GT, serum iron (increased saturation of transferrin) with secondary polycythaemia, and occasionally alkaline phosphatase. Reduced liver function results from decreased cholinesterase. • Depending on the duration and progression of PCT, changes in the *liver surface* range from a faded lobular pattern on a reddish-brown coloured liver to finely granulated areas with fine whitish fibrosis on a diffuse blue-grey surface colour (due to porphyrin deposits) and brownish speckled areas as well as flat tuberous surfaces with scar formation. (s. fig. 31.19)

In the bluish-grey areas, the porphyrin content is three to four times higher than in the lighter liver sections. In *UV examinations* (366 nm), to which every liver bioptate should be subjected, the red fluorescence has different intensities, facilitating classification into *PCT groups A–D*: types A and B (no clinical symptoms) show dot-like fluorescence, type C (latent PCT) has mostly reticular fluorescence, and type D (manifest PCT) is characterized by homogeneous red fluorescence. (s. fig. 7.10!) (s. pp 153, 166) • In the further course, scar tissue or micronodular cirrhosis develop. There is a greater risk of hepatocellular carcinoma (15–25%) (due to concomitant HBV or HCV infection as well as haemochromatosis?). (296, 300–302)

Diagnosis of PCT is based upon *skin changes* with characteristic anamnesis and *detection of porphyrins* in the urine and faeces. (s. tab. 31.14) There is evidence of increased uroporphyrins, particularly heptacarboxyporphyrin and coproporphyrin in the urine as well as elevated uroporphyrin in the faeces and plasma. Dark red discolouration of the urine resulting from enhanced release of porphyrin (>15 μmol/day) has often been observed. Subclinical forms can be detected three times more frequently using targeted diagnostics! • In most cases, *HLA-A3* and *HLA-B7* (as in haemochromatosis) are present in the serum. *Serum iron* is elevated. The undoubtedly important role of **iron** in the pathogenesis of PCT has still not been clarified. Mutations of the HFE gene in haemochromatosis (C 282 Y, H 63 D) are also much more numerous in PCT. Probably, these (and other?) mutations cause an enhanced resorption of iron from the intestine. (275, 301) • There is a close coincidence of PCT and **HCV** infection (mainly genotype I b). A great geographical variation in frequency has been reported, from which an average of HCV positivity in PCT patients of about 45% can be determined. Interactions between the two diseases have not been clarified as yet; however, it is striking that both conditions generally show siderosis as well as being influenced to a particularly unfavourable degree by alcohol. (275, 278, 279, 293)

Sonography: Even at an early stage of porphyria, ring-shaped foci with marginal hyperechoic ring and central hypoechoic reflexes can be detected. (s. fig. 31.21)

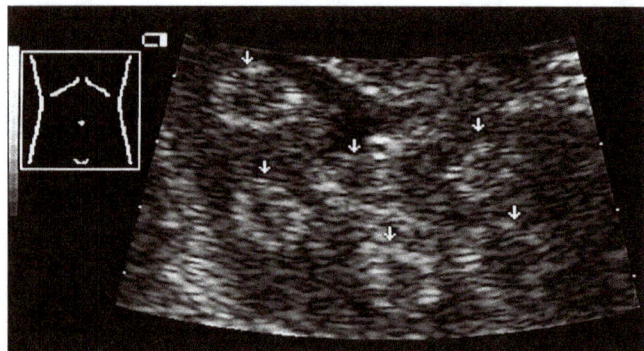

Fig. 31.21: Chronic hepatic porphyria: Sonographically, multiple, ring-shaped foci with marginal hyperechoic ring and central hypoechoic reflexes. (Completely reversible after alcohol abstinence)

These foci result from porphyrin deposition and are often discovered by chance since there is no evidence of a chronic porphyria. They can be mistaken for tumours or metastases; neither the foci nor their neighbouring parenchyma are hypervascularized. With abstinence of alcohol and avoidance of oestrogens, they are completely reversible. In a chronic porphyria, there may be a uniform increase in density due to diffuse porphyrin storage. (s. p. 544)

Treatment comprises avoidance of *trigger factors* (alcohol, oestrogens, sunlight, etc.) and application of sunblocks. *Venesection* with its withdrawal of iron results in inhibition of ALA synthetase, while uroporphyrinogen III decarboxylase activity is increased. This blood-letting therapy is based on 500 ml per week, after 4–6 weeks at monthly intervals. As an alternative, plasmapheresis has also been applied. *Chloroquine* (2 x 50 mg/day or 2 x 125 mg/week) is administered every second day for 6–12 months; it combines biochemically with porphyrins in the hepatocytes, thus improving the elimination of porphyrins from the liver. Venesection and chloroquine therapy may be carried out jointly. *Alkalization* of the renal metabolism enhances the elimination of porphyrins via the kidneys. (287)

15.8 Hepatoerythropoietic porphyria

This is a very rare form of chronic hepatic porphyria. As with PCT, the enzymatic defect is a deficiency of uroporphyrinogen decarboxylase. But the genetic defect is homozygous. It may also be caused by exogenous factors. Hepatoerythropoietic porphyria manifests in early childhood with high photosensitivity, sclerodermia, hypertrichosis and anaemia. • The *liver* shows red fluorescence. Histologically, siderosis and non-specific hepatitis are found. Development of cirrhosis is possible. • No effective *therapy* is known. (305, 307)

16 Wilson's disease

▶ The first clinical and morphological description of the disease was published by S.A.K. Wilson in 1912. (383) This article did not mention the previous reports by K.F.O. Westphal (1883) and A. von Strümpell (1898); they distinguished between the neuropsychiatric picture of the disease, assigning to it the rather unfortunate term *"pseudosclerosis"*, derived from multiple sclerosis, which was already clearly defined at that time. • In 1921 H.C. Hall maintained that Wilson's disease and pseudosclerosis were actually one and the same thing and that it was even hereditary; he coined the term *"hepatolenticular degeneration"*. • The *storage of copper* in the liver and brain was postulated by A. Rumpel in 1913 and confirmed by F. Haurowitz in 1930. The brown-green colour of the corneal ring described by B. Kayser (1902) (339) and B. Fleischer (1902) (320, 321) is due to copper deposits, as was confirmed by W. Gerlach in 1934. J.N. Cumings (1948) identified copper as the cause of disease. *Hypercupriuria* was first described by B.M. Mantelbrote et al. (1948) and *hypocupraemia* by A.G. Bearn et al. (1952). This abnormality in copper metabolism was clarified by the detection of *hypoceruloplasminaemia* (I.H. Scheinberg et al., 1952). In 1960 A.G. Bearn demonstrated the recessive autosomal transmission.

The *first therapeutic attempts* to eliminate the increased copper content of the tissue by way of chelating agents go back to J.N. Cumings (1948) and D. Denny-Brown et al. (1951). For this purpose, *dimercaprol* and *ethylenediaminetetraacetic acid* (EDTA) were used. Treatment with *potassium sulphide* was recommended by M.M. Wintrobe et al. in 1954. The final breakthrough came with examinations carried out by J.M. Walshe (1956), who recognized the copper-binding properties of β,β-dimethylcysteine (penicillamine). Another copper-chelating substance, *trientin-dihydrochloride*, was introduced by J.M. Walshe in 1969. (379) The therapeutic effectiveness of zinc in patients suffering from Wilson's disease had been reported as early as 1961 (G. SCHOUWINK), while the therapeutic principle itself was described later on by T. U. HOOGENRAAD et al. (1978). (325)

16.1 Definition

Wilson's disease is a genetically determined, autosomal recessive copper storage disease with a reduced discharge of copper into the bile. Due to pathological copper deposits in the liver and brain as well as various other organs, sequelae develop above all in the liver and CNS. The other affected organs are generally involved in the disease as late manifestation. The chromosomal defect is still not fully clarified.

16.2 Frequency

The incidence rate is 1:100,000 inhabitants/year. The prevalence of this disease in patients with manifestation is estimated at 1:30,000 and in heterozygote symptom carriers at 1:100 to 1:200 of the population, i.e. 5–30 patients/1 million inhabitants. • Wilson's disease appears in childhood, adolescence and early adulthood. Initial occurrence before the 5th or after the 35th year of life is considered to be an exception. However, mild courses of disease have also been diagnosed beyond the age of 50. (314, 316) Most patients develop the first clinical symptoms around the age of 15. Geographical or race-related differences in frequency have not been reported. However, a higher incidence is found in regions with strong consanguinity (e.g. Sardinia, Israel).

16.3 Pathogenesis

The metabolic defect in Wilson's disease is located in the liver on chromosome 13 (M. FRYDMAN et al., 1985), close to the esterase-D locus (ATP 7B). (312, 318, 329, 338, 352) Apparently, this is a genetically determined disturbance of **hepatobiliary copper** discharge due to a *defect in lysosomal copper-transporting ATPase*, which is localized in the trans-Golgi network. As a result, apoceruloplasmin cannot be loaded with copper, and is therefore degraded. The reduced secretion of ceruloplasmin explains the low copper level in the serum (D. J. FROMMER, 1974). So far, more than 250 different mutations of Wilson's gene have been described. (320, 351) This disorder may be located (*1.*) in the area of the sinusoidal membrane (transfer into the blood via ceruloplasmin) or (*2.*) in the area of the canalicular membrane (transfer into the bile via copper-binding ATPase). About 80% of the copper absorbed enterally is excreted via the bile, while in Wilson's disease, the biliary excretion is reduced to 10–20%. Neither reabsorption of copper excreted via the bile nor intestinal copper resorption are increased. (325, 340, 363, 376, 384)

In the first three to four months of life, the **newborn** usually shows findings concerning copper metabolism which correspond to those found in Wilson's disease. It is therefore assumed that the conversion of foetal copper metabolism to that normally found later on in life is effected by a control gene. From birth onwards, 10–20 mg copper are accumulated every year. It usually takes 6–15 years before clinical symptoms become apparent as a result of the cumulative copper deposition. • In **siblings,** there may be considerable differences regarding clinical and laboratory findings. It can therefore be concluded that *exogenous* or *endogenous factors* modify the genetically determined process or alter the gene expression within the families involved. In other words, there is *genetic heterogeneity.*

Copper: The daily intake from food is 0.8–2.0 mg; it is released into the portal vein via copper-transporting ATPase. The transport of copper, which is toxic in its free form, is effected by the binding to ceruloplasmin, albumin and transcuprin. • Copper is bound to reduced glutathione and metallothionein in the hepatocytes and distributed to various organelles or incorporated into enzymes. The biological effects of copper are manifold and essential for some cellular functions. (s. p. 54) Copper is toxic not only in its free form, but also in cases of overload (e.g. cirrhosis in childhood due to the consumption of water from copper pipes). Copper homoeostasis is regulated via biliary excretion (normal value: about 1.2–2.0 mg/day), so that the **normal value** in serum is 75–130 µg/dl. (314, 316, 363, 374, 377) (s. p. 108)

Ceruloplasmin binds eight copper atoms per molecule and is of an intense blue colour. The coding gene is localized on chromosome 3. (385) Ceruloplasmin is the most important transport protein for copper in circulating blood (about 75–95% binding capacity). Another important function of this protein is the catalysis of oxidative metabolic reactions; it also possesses antioxidative features for the elimination of reactive oxygen intermediates. (s. tab. 3.25) The **normal value** in serum is 20–35 mg/dl.

The **reduction** in the serum value of ceruloplasmin led to the assumption that a primary synthesis disturbance was of particular pathogenic importance. There are several observations which contradict this hypothesis, suggesting that the *disturbance in ceruloplasmin synthesis* is probably a secondary consequence of the underlying metabolic defect. The introduction of copper into ceruloplasmin is possibly inhibited as a result of a dysfunctional apoprotein of ceruloplasmin.

Transcuprin is another transport protein for copper in circulating blood (about 7% binding capacity). • Apart from being bound to glutathione and metallothionein, copper may also be bound intracellularly to *another protein* that has only recently been detected.

16.4 Pathophysiology

The **toxicity of copper** is due to (*1.*) its binding to SH groups of cysteine, which is converted into an irreversible form by oxidation, and (*2.*) the fact that it is responsible for the formation of reactive oxygen intermediates (e. g. hydroxyl radicals), resulting in lipid peroxidation, which, in turn, is responsible for functional and structural disturbances of biomembranes. (334) In addition, a reduction in vitamin E likewise encourages the occurrence of lipid peroxidations. • Initially, copper is diffusely distributed in the cytosol and then stored in the hepatocellular lysosomes. At this point, it can also be demonstrated histochemically. Rapid transfer from the cytosol to the lysosomes may lead to increased lipid peroxidation with cell necrosis. (363, 374) • *Abrupt discharge of copper from the lysosomes into the bloodstream results in intravasal haemolysis and widespread liver cell necroses with fulminant hepatitis.*

16.5 Morphological changes

16.5.1 Hepatic manifestation

Electron-microscopically, the *mitochondria* – an essential target of toxic copper – show swelling and altered morphology, separation of external and internal membranes, greater density of the matrix, and granular or vacuolic inclusions. The *peroxisomes* are characterized by their increase in size and altered form as well as a granular matrix. Secretion of lipids is reduced. These structural changes result in discernible steatosis of the hepatocytes. • The *lysosomes* grow in number and size; finally, they decay and release lysosomal enzymes. (341) Apart from that, structural changes in the endoplasmic *reticulum* and *cytoskeleton* can be observed (= **stage I**).

Histologically, fine-droplet, ultimately also large-droplet, *steatosis* in the peripheral lobules and the occasional formation of *Mallory-Denk bodies* can be found. There are no signs of fat cysts. Steatosis subsides with increasing duration of disease. The lysosomes, meanwhile overloaded with copper, are deposited mainly at the bile pole of the hepatocytes and resemble lipofuscin-like pigment bodies. Degenerative changes in the hepatocytes, hypertrophy of Kupffer cells and an accumulation of glycogen in the nuclei with formation of *glycogen vacuolations* can be observed. (s. fig. 31.1) • Rapid intracellular redistribution of copper causes extensive cell necrosis. In this intermediate stage (= **stage II**), inflammatory reactions (very probably of an autoimmune nature) and proliferations of the bile ducts are evident. The histological picture – as well as the laparoscopic image of the liver surface – may at this point correspond to that of chronic hepatitis. (s. fig. 31.22) • The late stage shows increased fibrogenesis with variable fibre contents, and micronodular cirrhosis develops (= **stage III**). (s. figs. 31.23 – 31.25)

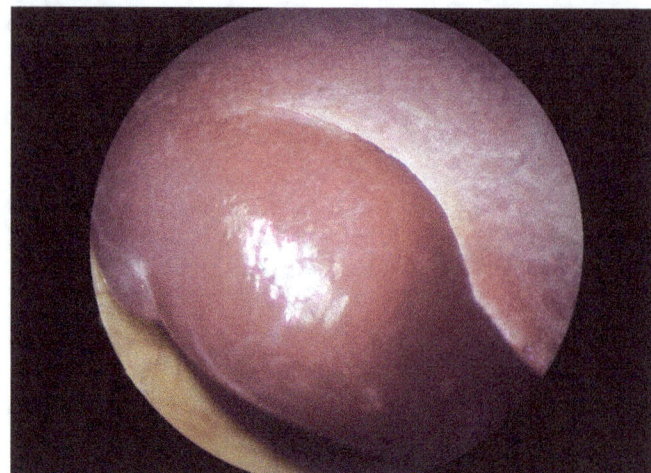

Fig. 31.22: Chronic hepatitis in Wilson's disease. Pronounced "simian cleft" with barely recognizable hepar succenturatum (s. p. 19)

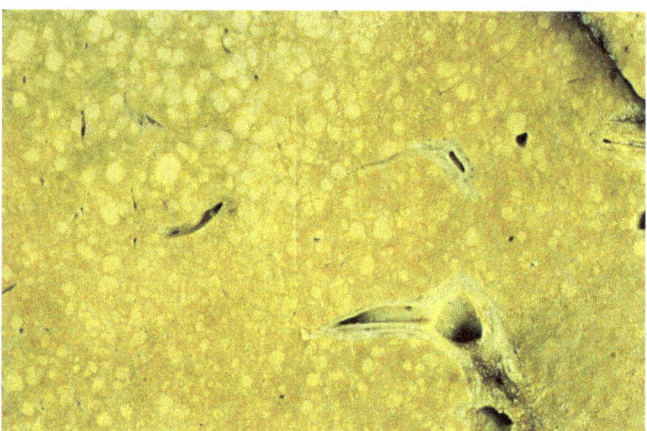

Fig. 31.23: Explanted liver with micronodular (regenerative-weak) cirrhosis in Wilson's disease (18-year-old woman presenting with acute liver failure) (Sirius red)

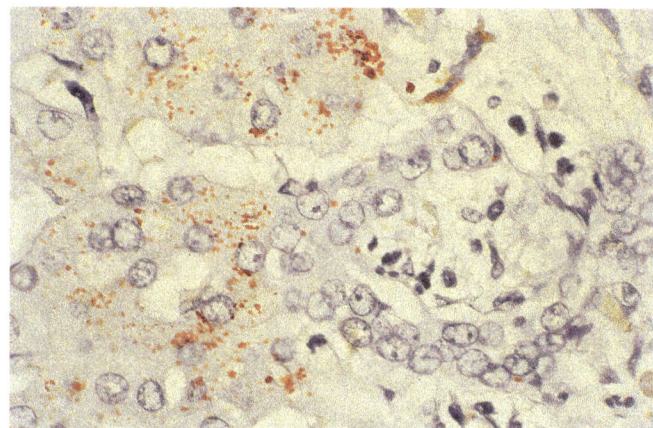

Fig. 31.24: Cirrhosis in Wilson's disease. Numerous copper deposits in periportal liver epithelia (Rhodanine)

The *distribution of copper* in the liver is concentrated in the peripheral lobules, but its pattern is irregular (even in advanced stages): there may be areas with very high copper concentrations adjacent to regions which are almost copper-free; this can give rise to false-negative findings during histochemical examination of the liver

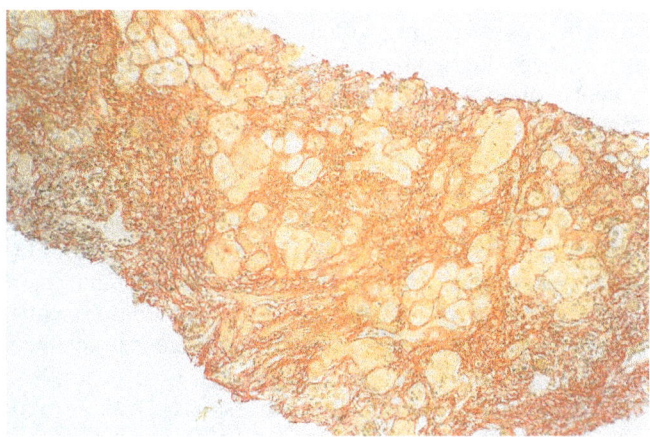

Fig. 31.25: Active progredient liver cirrhosis in Wilson's disease

bioptate. The *detection of copper* is possible using (unreliable) rhodanine staining, while the copper bound to metallothionein in the lysosomes is demonstrable by orcein staining (likewise not reliable). The copper content of the liver (normal 15–55 µg/g dry weight) may rise to 3,000 µg/g. If untreated, Wilson's disease shows rapid progression, also in the liver. (332, 340, 347, 373) With an effective therapeutic reversal of copper deposition, the copper balance can be restored. The patient returns to an asymptomatic course of Wilson's disease. However, the organ damage that has hitherto occurred is irreversible (= **stage IV**).

The **morphological spectrum** may therefore range from steatosis, acute hepatitis, fulminant course, chronic hepatitis, aggressive episodes in chronic hepatitis and liver fibrosis through to micronodular cirrhosis. Complete cirrhosis can exist in children aged four to five years. (312) • The development of *hepatocellular carcinoma* is extremely rare (353); it is assumed that copper has a protective effect against malignant transformation. (380, 382)

16.5.2 Extrahepatic manifestations

After complete saturation of the copper-binding capacity of the liver, the copper absorbed from food can no longer be taken up by the liver. This means that copper is stored in the brain, skeletal system, heart, cornea and kidneys — as is also the case when copper stored in the hepatocytes is released into the circulation on a large scale due to extensive liver cell necrosis. (332, 346)

CNS: Copper deposits affect the whole CNS. Degeneration and tissue loss as well as atrophy of the lenticular nucleus prevail. Occasionally, there are also small necrotic foci with a diffuse spot-like distribution. Microcavernous lesions occur due to the destruction of nerve cells. Myelinized fibres and oligodendrocytes are present, but there is also cellular hyperplasia and hypertrophy of astrocytes rich in protoplasm. The cerebral changes detectable in CT scanning do not correlate with the degree of severity of the functional disturbances (311, 328); however, there is a close correlation between the lesions detected by MRI and certain neurological findings. (313, 341, 359, 369) (s. p. 633)

Eyes: Copper is deposited in the form of a copper-sulphur complex in Descemet's membrane on the back of the cornea. Fine copper granules are observed, first as moderate colour changes at the upper limbus, then also at the lower limbus, with the ultimate development of a complete brown-green ring, 1–3 mm in width. (330, 331, 339) The **Kayser-Fleischer corneal ring** is nearly always found in adults with principally neurological and psychological problems, whereas it is generally not present in juveniles with a hepatic course. The best way to detect this ring is by slit-lamp examination. (s. fig. 4.17) The existence of such a ring is not in itself proof of Wilson's disease, as it is also found in CDNC-induced cirrhosis and primary sclerosing cholangitis; its absence does not, however, exclude Wilson's disease. • Occasionally (10–20%), a **sunflower cataract** is observed on the lens (E. SIEMERLING et al., 1922): a central gold-brown copper deposit in the frontal lens capsule with radial emanation into the posterior capsule areas. (321) Visual acuity is not compromised by these changes. Successful treatment leads to the regression of both ocular findings, making it possible to evaluate the course of disease (as well as to monitor inadequate treatment).

Kidneys: Dysfunction of the proximal tubule may occur as a late manifestation of Wilson's disease. Epithelial flattening, a loss of the brush-border membrane, mitochondrial anomalies and fatty cellular changes can be observed. These findings are, in turn, responsible for *proteinuria* with a predominance of *hyperaminoaciduria* (L. UZMAN et al., 1948). Enhanced *calciuria* and *phosphaturia* may cause osteomalacia as well as hypoparathyroidism. (322, 336) Glucosuria and uricosuria, if present, are without clinical relevance. Due to decreased bicarbonate resorption, *tubular acidosis* may occur, with a tendency towards osteomalacia as well as the development of nephrocalcinosis and renal stones (in some 15% of cases). (336, 348, 381) The intensity of the copper deposits in the kidneys correlates closely with the cellular changes and functional disorders. • The glomerular function is not compromised, with the result that substances normally excreted in the urine are not retained.

Skeleton: Renal phosphate diabetes associated with hypercalciuria may lead to osteomalacia or osteoporosis. Likewise, inflammatory or degenerative arthrosis is thought to be a late manifestation of Wilson's disease. (345) Often, these developments are combined with intra-articular calcium deposits and chondromalacia, in particular *patellar chondromalacia*. Bone fractures are frequently observed even with minor traumas. Calcification may occur in articular cartilage, capsule and tendinous insertions, and deposits of calcium pyrophosphate dihydrate can appear in the intervertebral disks.

Myocardium: Copper deposits in the myocardium causes interstitial fibrosis, the sclerosing of small vessels and focal inflammatory or degenerative lesions. This results in cardiac arrhythmia and cardiomyopathy.

Bone marrow: Leucopenia and thrombopenia may be a result of bone-marrow damage caused by copper deposits, although this can also be due to splenomegaly.

Skin and muscles: Acute *rhabdomyolysis* (355) and *dermatomyositis* are rare manifestations of Wilson's disease. • There may be evidence of *hyperpigmentation* and *acanthosis nigricans*. Bluish, lunular discolorations of the nails, so-called *azure lunulae,* are seldom. (315) (s. p. 88)

16.6 Clinical picture

The **symptoms** of Wilson's disease can hardly ever be recognized before the age of six. In most cases, the patients show symptoms between the 6th and 20th year of life — occasionally, however, as late as the 4th decade. About half the patients develop the disease before the age of 15. Sometimes, above-average growth in height is observed. Based on the prevailing symptoms, **three clinical forms** can be differentiated: *(1.) hepatic, (2.) neurological,* and *(3.) mixed courses.* The hepatic form is observed almost exclusively in children between the ages of 6 and 15, while the neurological form predominates in adults. • **Asymptomatic courses** are usually diagnosed only by chance. (319, 323, 332, 333, 357, 363, 370, 372)

> **Early diagnosis** is essential. This is true both for the recognition of *heterozygous carriers* and for the diagnosis of asymptomatic *homozygous carriers* — often, the two groups can only be differentiated by using complicated methods (e.g. specific DNA markers, gene linkage analysis, ^{64}Cu kinetics). (337, 342)

Once the diagnosis of Wilson's disease has been confirmed beyond doubt, all other **family members** have to be examined as well. During this process, occasional cases of a presymptomatic course of disease are detected. A reduction of ceruloplasmin in serum may even be present in carriers of heterozygous features. Genetic analysis can provide a diagnosis in some 95% of cases, even prenatally.

Liver diseases

Hepatic disorders are a prominent feature of Wilson's disease in childhood and adolescence. In the early stages, a **fatty liver** is often observed, the aetiology of which is at first unclear. • A slight increase in the transaminases may be the first biochemical sign, before any other symptoms appear. • In **acute hepatitis** of varying degrees of severity, Wilson's disease must always be ruled out. • In the natural course of disease, **chronic active hepatitis** may be found in the initial phase. In terms of clinical and laboratory examination, it can only be distinguished from other forms of chronic active hepatitis by way of aetiology-specific findings. (s. fig. 31.22) • **Fulminant hepatitis,** which is observed quite often, shows rapid progression with the development of pronounced jaundice; there is evidence of increased copper values in the serum and urine, while ceruloplasmin in the blood is decreased or normal. Ascites and growing liver insufficiency are evident. (328) The transaminases are only slightly elevated. A marked reduction in alkaline phosphatase is considered to be a characteristic feature. (367) At the same time, haemolysis is often present due to an abrupt discharge of cytosolic copper into the bloodstream. Fulminant hepatitis in Wilson's disease is usually fatal if there is no chance of liver transplantation. (312, 326, 327, 332, 344, 351, 361, 368, 371) • **Liver cirrhosis** develops slowly. (s. figs. 31.23–31.25) Non-specific general complaints and skin stigmata of liver disease (s. fig. 4.21), which are typical in chronic forms, as well as the symptoms and sequelae of portal hypertension are evident. In association with thrombopenia, cutaneous and mucosal bleeding may occur due to synthesis disorders of the coagulation factors. Occasionally, recurrent bouts of jaundice (generally due to haemolysis) are observed. An acute necrotizing episode may have a fatal outcome. • Hepatic injury is seen as a consequence of augmented oxidative stress. (349)

Neurological and psychiatric disorders

Neurological symptoms are not observed before an advanced stage of disease is reached, particularly in older juveniles or adults. In their case history, half of these patients have not shown any signs of haemolytic anaemia or hepatic symptoms which could have pointed to Wilson's disease. However, a very discrete symptomatology at the onset progresses continuously and ultimately characterizes the clinical picture of untreated Wilson's disease. (311, 364, 372) • *Psychiatric symptoms* (personality changes, behavioural disorders, neuroses, psychoses) are detected in 55–65% of cases. • A drop in *performance at school* may be one of the first signs of Wilson's disease. • The following symptoms are found in varying degrees of intensity and in different combinations (although some of the late features are no longer observed nowadays due to effective treatment techniques which are initiated at an early stage):

> - unsteady gait, balance disturbance, uncoordinated movements, grimacing
> - dysarthria, scanning speech, palilalia
> - dysphagia, salivation, raising and retracting of the upper lip
> - dysgraphia, micrographia
> - seizures
> - tremor, athetosis, resting and intention tremor, nystagmus, rigor, flexion contractures, spasticity
> - personality changes, behavioural disorders, neurotic or psychotic symptoms (including forgetfulness, irritability, emotional lability, inability to keep a distance)
> - hypomimia and amimia, mask-like face

Haemolysis

In about 15% of patients suffering from Wilson's disease, haemolysis with corresponding jaundice can be observed, sometimes as a relapse and occasionally as a haemolytic crisis. (s. tab. 12.3) The release of large amounts of copper from necrotized liver cells causes copper-induced damage to erythrocytes with subsequent haemolysis (due to enzyme deficiency). Haemolysis may even constitute the first manifestation of Wilson's disease (326, 327, 358) and precede the hepatic findings by several years. Usually, it is transitory and self-limiting. In severe cases, this non-spherocytic, Coombs-negative, intravascular haemolysis may be combined with haemoglobinuria. • Chronic haemolysis can lead to the formation of *pigment gallstones*.

16.7 Laboratory findings

When there are clinical signs suggesting the presence of Wilson's disease or corresponding differential diagnostic considerations, diagnosis (or diagnosis by exclusion) is established by laboratory parameters. AP is normal or slightly increased. The GPT/GOT quotient is generally > 4. (323, 332, 333, 346, 350, 377) (s. tab. 31.15)

Ceruloplasmin in the serum	↓	(< 20 mg/dl)
Copper content of the liver	↑	(> 250 µg/g)
Copper in the urine	↑	(> 70 µg/day)
Free copper in the serum	↑	(> 25 µg/dl)
Penicillamine test (600 mg)	+	(> 300 µg/6h)
Total copper in the serum	↓	(< 80 µg/dl)

Tab. 31.15: Decisive laboratory criteria for the diagnosis and follow-up of Wilson's disease

Ceruloplasmin: Usually, the serum value of ceruloplasmin is below 20 mg/dl in homozygous Wilson's disease; however, in about 15% of such symptomatic patients, the values are found in the lower normal range (20–30 mg/dl). In about 15% of heterozygous patients without manifestation of the disease, a slight decrease in the ceruloplasmin value is also observed. When the value is > 30 mg/dl, Wilson's disease can usually be ruled out. Nevertheless, in strongly compromised liver function, the ceruloplasmin value increases due to hyperoestrogenism, which develops subsequently and stimulates ceruloplasmin synthesis in the liver. A decrease to < 20 mg/dl is not confirmation of Wilson's disease. **Decreased values** are also found in nephrosis, Menkes' disease, aceruloplasminaemia (J.D. Gitlin, 1998), malabsorption syndrome, etc. **Increased values** are observed in cholestasis, during pregnancy, with oral contraceptives, in malignant and inflammatory processes, etc.

Cupruria: In pronounced liver cell decay, there is not only a rise in the copper value in serum, but more particularly in the amount of copper excretion in the urine. Cupruria of < 50 µg/day rules out the presence of Wilson's disease (differential diagnosis: e.g. kidney disease). • The **penicillamine test** has proved successful: after administration of 600 mg penicillamine, copper excretion increases to > 300 µg/6 hr (> 600 µg/24 hr). However, it should be noted that this test may show similar positive results in cholestatic liver diseases.

Copper content of the liver: The diagnosis of Wilson's disease is confirmed by determining the liver copper content (normal: 20–50 µg/g dry weight) with atomic absorption spectrometry. Firstly, the puncture instruments and glass vessels have to be free of copper (cleaned with a 0.1 EDTA solution). An inhomogenous distribution of copper in the liver, particularly in cirrhosis, has to be taken into account. • In addition, an increased hepatic copper content is also found in other liver diseases, e.g. bile-duct atresia, primary biliary or primary sclerosing cholangitis, bile-duct obstruction, chronic hepatitis, neoplasm, α_1-antitrypsin deficiency, Gilbert's disease, Dubin-Johnson syndrome.

16.8 Diagnostic measures

Suspicion: Detection of acute or chronic liver disease of unclear aetiology (above all in a fatty liver) and/or haemolysis, and/or neurological or psychological peculiarities in children above the age of 6, in juveniles and in adults up to the age of 40 suggest the presence of Wilson's disease *("give it thought!")*.

Hints: Detection of a Kayser-Fleischer corneal ring (in the early phase by slit-lamp examination) is considered to be the most important clinical finding of manifest Wilson's disease. (s. fig. 4.17)

Confirmation: The diagnosis is verified by laboratory parameters (determination of the serum values of copper and ceruloplasmin as well as of copper excretion in the urine, if necessary using the penicillamine test) and by demonstrating the copper content of the liver, with simultaneous differentiation of existing liver damage.

Organ involvement: The type and extent of organ involvement can be determined effectively by a broad spectrum of examinations. To a certain degree, these examinations are also important for monitoring progress and therapy. (s. tab. 31.16)

Sonography: At an advanced stage, ultrasound yields a metastasis-like picture: fatty degeneration together with areas of fibrosis (= echogenic) and normal parenchyma (= hypoechoic).

MRI: An MRI brain scan may demonstrate typical changes such as atrophy and densification in the basal ganglia and the lenticular nucleus (i.e. in the putamen and the globus pallidus). The cause of the particular sensitivity of these regions is unknown. (313)

1. **Liver**
   laboratory parameters,
   liver biopsy/laparoscopy,
   copper content of the liver
2. **CNS**
   EEG, ENG, EMG (CT), MRI
3. **Eyes**
   slit-lamp examination
4. **Kidneys**
   calciuria, phosphaturia, glucosuria,
   aminoaciduria, tubular acidosis
5. **Sonography**
   liver status, portal hypertension,
   kidney stones, nephrocalcinosis,
   gallstones
6. **Skeleton**
   osteomalacia, osteoporosis,
   chondrocalcinosis, arthropathy
7. **Blood**
   thrombocytes, leucocytes,
   coagulation factors,
   signs of haemolysis (s. tab. 12.3)
8. **Heart**
   ECG, echocardiography

Tab. 31.16: Diagnostic measures for detecting the type and extent of organ involvement in Wilson's disease

16.9 Prognosis

The prognosis depends essentially on **early diagnosis** and consistent treatment. (350, 363) If untreated, Wilson's disease is fatal. When treatment is initiated too late, irreversible, chronic damage is inevitable and the prognosis is poor. However, when **early treatment** is applied at an initial stage, the prognosis for Wilson's disease is relatively good; remissions over a period of seven years have even been reported. *(One of our own patients has now been in remission for more than 20 years.)* The prognosis is more favourable if copper excretion therapy is started in the preclinical phase. The life expectancy of the patients is not compromised if therapy is successful. After recovery, the patient's general condition and physical performance are usually unimpaired. (346)

16.10 Treatment

Early diagnosis and thus **early treatment** form the basis for (*1.*) establishing copper homoeostasis which is as stable as possible, (*2.*) avoiding chronic or irreversible organ damage, (*3.*) supporting the regression of still reversible lesions, and (*4.*) improving (perhaps even normalizing) functional disorders. Therapy must be continued lifelong, since copper reaccumulates, with the result that Wilson's disease becomes manifest, and there is a danger of acute liver failure. (312, 319, 324, 332, 364, 372)

16.10.1 Dietary measures

Nutrition should be *low in copper*. Patients must avoid foodstuffs and beverages containing copper, e. g. edible offal, nuts, cocoa products, mushrooms, potato crisps, rye flour, oat flakes, beans, dried figs, certain types of cheese, meat and fish, pineapple, mineral water (see relevant *lists* as to the composition of foodstuffs and copper content in food). Vegetarian food, from which copper cannot be easily mobilized, is therefore recommended. • Cooking utensils containing copper should not be used. • *Alcohol* is strictly forbidden.

16.10.2 Drug therapy

D-penicillamine: The first-choice medication is D-penicillamine (J. M. WALSHE, 1956). By forming copper chelate, it not only causes a reversal of copper deposition and cupruria (see penicillamine test), but also induces metallothionein synthesis, whereby the toxicity of the remaining copper is reduced, even though the copper content in the liver does not sink. Penicillamine reduces the activity of lysil oxidase, thus diminishing the deposition of collagen. As a result, however, the skin unfortunately becomes fragile and wounds heal more slowly. • The *initial dose* is adapted to the individual and ranges from 900–1,200 (−1,800) mg/day. The medication is given in three to four single doses per day, which have to be taken half an hour before meals. Therapeutic success is expected after six months at the earliest: there is continuous improvement with regard to abdominal complaints, neurological and psychological disorders, opthalmic findings and laboratory parameters. Occasionally, an initial worsening of the neurological symptoms is observed (most likely due to excessive copper mobilization), which, however, ultimately results in a constant improvement in the neurological status if treatment is carried on consistently. Whether or not the treatment has actually been successful can only be determined after about two years. • The removal of copper deposits is reflected in a normalization of copper excretion in the urine (after two days without medication) and serum parameters regarding copper metabolism. At this stage, a *maintenance dose* of 600–900 mg/day can be administered. Any interruption of treatment should not exceed a period of several weeks, since this would definitely result in a renewed overload of the organism with copper and possibly lead to acute and dangerous relapses. Treatment with penicillamine is continued even during pregnancy; breastfeeding is, however, not recommended. (312, 313)

In 20–25% of cases, **side effects** are observed, depending mainly on the dose (hypersensitivity reactions, aphthous lesions, arthralgia, nausea, fever). All in all, treatment of Wilson's disease with penicillamine is considered to be successful and safe. If penicillamine is not well tolerated or if serious side effects are observed (e. g. kidney or bone-marrow damage, polyneuropathy, pemphigus), treatment must be discontinued. • Penicillamine usually causes **pyridoxin deficiency**, so that substitution (25–40 mg/day) is recommended, particularly as chronic liver damage leads to vitamin B_6 deficiency. • If necessary, **electrolytes** and **trace elements** also have to be substituted.

Zinc: Treatment with zinc is seen as an alternative therapy for mobilizing copper deposits (T. U. HOOGENRAAD et al., 1978). (335) *Zinc inhibits intestinal copper resorption and stimulates the synthesis of metallothionein in the liver and intestinal mucosa.* The recommended dosage is 3 (−4) × 50 mg/day, one hour before meals. The duration of administration and the dose are adjusted in line with therapeutic success. Zinc can also be used in long-term treatment (i.e. maintenance of copper homoeostasis) following the initial release of copper deposits via penicillamine. Side effects have been reported in the form of gastrointestinal complaints. There is an increase in AP as well as amylase and lipase. (360, 378)

Potassium sulphide: A decrease in intestinal copper resorption can also be achieved by the administration of potassium sulphide (3 × 20 mg/day) (M. M. WINTROBE et al., 1954). However, this therapy is not readily accepted by patients because the substance has a bad taste and very unpleasant smell.

Triethylene tetramine: The copper-chelating agent triethylene tetramine (trientine) can be considered as an alternative therapy to penicillamine (J. M. WALSHE, 1982). (379) The initial dose is 3−4 × 600 mg/day; the recommended maintenance dose is 2 × 600 mg/day, administered about one hour before meals. The side effects are similar to those observed with penicillamine, but efficacy is lower. Iron-deficiency anaemia can occur. The substance is commercially available in the USA. (362) • *Further chelating agents being tested include 2,3,2-tetramine, APD and tetrathiomolybdate.*

16.10.3 Peritoneal dialysis

In acute copper toxicosis, peritoneal dialysis has been successfully implemented with simultaneous administration of penicillamine. In order to bridge the time until liver transplantation can be carried out, plasmapheresis and haemofiltrations are recommended.

16.10.4 Liver transplantation

In a fulminant course of Wilson's disease, MARS is a possible therapy. (366) In an advanced stage of cirrhosis with complications or where medication is not feasible, the only remaining alternative is liver transplantation. After successful transplantation, all clinical findings and laboratory parameters improve, and even neurological disorders become reversible. Transplantation is a causal therapy, which confirms that the primary metabolic defect of Wilson's disease is located in the liver. This means that no copper-releasing medication is required following transplantation. (317, 343, 354, 356, 365, 375)

16.11 Indian childhood cirrhosis

This condition, which is confined to India, leads to the development of childhood cirrhosis; it is fatal in almost all cases. Its aetiology is unknown. The condition affects children of both sexes between the ages of one and three years. Its familial occurrence points to genetic factors. There is increased copper ingestion through food and milk as well as from household utensils. Alkaloids may also be involved in aetiopathogenesis. • Initially, the symptoms include increased appetite, restlessness, sleep disturbances, bright and sticky stools as well as hepatomegaly. Kayser-Fleischer rings are not present. Serum ceruloplasmin is normal. The further course is characterized by jaundice, oedema and ascites, bouts of fever and liver atrophy. • The histological picture is similar to acute alcoholic hepatitis, but without fatty degeneration. Mallory's hyaline, which is surrounded by polymorphonuclear leucocytes, is detectable in 80−90% of hepatocytes. The liver shows the highest content of copper so far verified in humans; it is located in the cytoplasm. As a result of low-grade liver cell regeneration, only small nodules are formed in the extensive, dense connective tissue, so that micronodular cirrhosis results. • *Therapy* is based on a strict reduction in copper intake and the administration of D-penicillamine. (387)

Non-Indian childhood cirrhosis: This similar condition, found in other countries, is indistinguishable from Indian childhood cirrhosis. Therefore, it is also called *copper-related liver disease*. A genetic defect is probably involved. Any correlation with increased copper ingestion is unlikely. (386)

17 Haemochromatosis

▶ The first observation of haemochromatosis was made by Th. BONNET (1679). The first clinical case was described by A. TROUSSEAU (1865) with the *three main symptoms* of iron storage diseases: diabetes mellitus, bronze pigmentation of the skin and cirrhosis. In 1871 C. E. TROISIER termed this condition "la cirrhose pigmentaire dans le diabète sucré". In 1877 H. QUINCKE detected iron deposits in the liver parenchyma of these patients and called this clinical picture "siderosis". For the same condition, V. HANOT and A. M. CHAUFFARD (1892) coined the term "cirrhose hypertrophique pigmentaire dans le diabète sucré". In 1895 P. MARIE also described this illness as "diabète bronzé". The term "haemochromatosis" was suggested by F. D. v. RECKLINGHAUSEN in 1889. (453) Since 1935, haemochromatosis has been regarded as a genetically determined entity in itself and hypogonadism was added as a fourth cardinal symptom by J. H. SHELDON.

17.1 Definition

Haemochromatosis (HC) is a hereditary disease (autosomal recessive) affecting iron metabolism. It refers to pronounced iron deposition, mainly in the liver (> 50% of the total iron in the body), but also in other organs, e.g. pancreas, spleen, heart, endocrinium, bone marrow, lymph nodes, salivary glands, basal skin layers and gastrointestinal epithelia. • Besides these *hereditary* (HFE-related) or idiopathic (non-HFE-related) primary forms, there are numerous *acquired* secondary forms of HC. At first, the cells of the RES become laden with iron. Only when the capacity of the RES is exceeded is there iron deposition in the parenchymal cells; this leads to damage of the respective organs. (s. tab 31.17)

Haemosiderosis (HS) denotes iron storage in the organism, whereby iron deposition in the liver is < 0.5 g/100 g liver WW. Iron deposition occurs almost exclusively in the RES; parenchymal cells are rarely affected. Haemosiderosis exists in two forms: (*1.*) *absolute HS* resulting in generalized iron deposition in the body as a whole, or (*2.*) *relative HS* localized in a certain organ with the rest of the body showing normal iron distribution. Haemosiderosis does not cause haemochromatosis. (s. tab. 31.17)

17.2 Classification

Hereditary haemochromatosis (HC) can be differentiated in one HFE-related and three non-HFE-related types as well as in a few other forms. (s. tab. 31.17)

17.2.1 HFE-related haemochromatosis

Type 1 is the classic **HFE-related form** of HC. It has an autosomal recessive inheritance pattern. The gene mutation is localized on chromosome 6, directly next to the A-locus of the HLA system. (412, 413) It was originally termed HLA-H gene (M. Simon et al., 1976) and later called HFE gene (J. N. Feder et al., 1996). The exact interpretation of the letters HFE is unknown (human ferritin?). In about 90% of patients with haemochromatosis, a homozygote point mutation (Cys 282 Tyr) in the HFE gene is evident (= replacing cysteine with tyrosine causes the disulfide bridge to fall apart). A further point mutation (H 63 Asp) is found in 5−10% of HC patients. Its role in iron metabolism is still not clarified (= asparaginic acid is replaced by histidine). This mutation is often observed in HC together with a heterozygote status for Cys 282 Tyr mutation (= *compound heterozygosity*). For these two point mutations the terms C 282 Y and H 63 D have been used; the combined mutation of C 282 Y/H 63 D is often evident. • The phenotype of HC in northern Europe and the USA comprises the genotypes: (*1.*) C 282 Y/C 282 Y (85−95%), (*2.*) wildtype / wildtype (5−8%), (*3.*) C 282 Y/H 63 D (= *compound heterozygosity*) (<5%), (*4.*) C 282 Y/wildtype (<2%), (*5.*) H 63 D/wildtype (<2%), and (*6.*) H 63 D / H 63 D (<1%). In southern European populations, the frequency of C 282 Y homozygosity is lower (ca. 65%). • The localization of the HFE gene on chromosome 6 has

Hereditary (primary) haemochromatosis

HFE-related haemochromatosis
type 1   Hereditary haemochromatosis

Non-HFE-related haemochromatosis
type 2   Juvenile haemochromatosis
type 3   Transferrin-receptor-associated HC
type 4   Ferroportin-associated HC

Aceruloplasminaemia
Atransferrinaemia
Neonatal haemochromatosis

Acquired (secondary) haemochromatosis
(iron content of the liver > 0.5 g/100 g liver WW)

- extreme iron intake due to dietary habits
  e. g. Bantu disease or African iron overload (together with genetic basis), dietary iron overload
- extreme iron intake due to therapy
  e. g. frequent blood transfusions, chronic haemodialysis
- haemolytically induced
  e. g. thalassaemia
- metabolically induced
  e. g. tyrosinaemia, porphyria cutanea tarda, Zellweger's syndrome, glycogenoses, lipidoses, paraneoplastic ferritin production (such as in bronchiolar carcinoma)

Haemosiderosis
- liver siderosis
  (iron content of the liver < 0.5 g/100 g liver WW)
  e. g. chronic alcohol damage, portocaval anastomoses, hepatitis C, cirrhosis
- pulmonary haemosiderosis
- renal siderosis
  e. g. paroxysmal haemoglobinuria
- cerebral siderosis
  e. g. Alzheimer's disease, Pick's atrophy, Huntington's chorea

Tab. 31.17: Classification of haemochromatosis and haemosiderosis (WW = wet weight)

no close association to the receptor protein synthesis of ferritin or the iron-regulating factor. (391, 415, 439, 441, 443, 452, 468) (s. tab. 31.17)

17.2.2 Non-HFE-related haemochromatosis

Type 2 is **juvenile haemochromatosis**. This rare form of iron storage differs from type 1 through an earlier onset of clinical symptoms. It becomes manifest prior to the age of 30. Both sexes are affected equally. The gene defect is localized on chromosome 1 (= *hemojuvelin*) or 19 (= *hepcidin*). Compared to type 1, cardiomyopathy and hypogonadism are more frequent, the course of disease is more severe and cardiac-induced death is more common. HFE mutations are absent, and there is no association with the HLA system. This form of HC has an autosomal recessive inheritance. (s. tab. 31.17)

Type 3 is the **transferrin-receptor-associated** HE. The gene defect is localized on chromosome 7q22 and affects transferrin receptor 2. This form of HC probably has an autosomal recessive inheritance. The histomorphological and clinical findings are similar to those of type 1. (450) (s. tab 31.17)

Type 4 is the **ferroportin-associated** HC, an autosomal dominant variant. It has only been observed in Italy. The gene defect is located on chromosome 2q32 and affects iron export protein ferroportin 1. In contrast to types 1 and 3, there is early iron storage in the macrophages. A characteristic feature are the markedly increased values of ferritin together with a slight elevation of transferrin saturation. (s. tab. 31.17)

17.2.3 Aceruloplasminaemia

Aceruloplasminaemia is a very rare, autosomal recessive disease with diffuse iron overload. It is caused by a mutation of the ceruloplasmin gene. This leads to excessive iron storage, mainly in the brain, liver and pancreas. The principal symptoms are increased serum ferritin, decreased serum iron and transferrin saturation as well as extrapyramidal disturbances, retinal degeneration, cerebellar ataxia and diabetes mellitus. (469–471) (s. tab. 31.17)

17.2.4 Atransferrinaemia

Atransferrinaemia is an extremely rare inherited syndrome. The first case involving a seven-year-old girl was described in 1961 (472). Clinically, there is a serious hypochromic iron-deficiency anaemia with a reduction in iron-binding capacity together with marked iron storage in the tissue. (472, 473) (s. tab. 31.17)

17.2.5 Neonatal haemochromatosis

Neonatal haemochromatosis (NH) was first described by H. COTTIER in 1957. This fatal form of HC starts in utero and must be differentiated from the genetically induced types; it does not represent a variant of HC. Genetic markers are unknown, and the basic underlying defect is unclarified (inherited/acquired?). "Sporadic" cases have also been observed. Both sexes are affected with the same frequency. Even at birth, newborns have pronounced ferritin values, jaundice, hypalbuminaemia, hypoglycaemia, decreased transferrin, cholestasis, coagulopathy, oedemas and ascites as well as cirrhosis with iron storage. The babies affected die generally within the first few days or weeks. Pathogenetically, irregular transport of iron through the placenta or dysregulated iron metabolism in the foetal liver cells is assumed to be responsible. • The following *therapy* is recommended: acetylcysteine (100 mg/kg BW/day i.v. for 7 days), α-tocopherol (25 U/kg BW/day orally), desferrioxamine (30 mg/kg BW/day i.v. infusion over 8 hours until the serum ferritin is < 500 µg/l), selenium (3 µg/kg BW i.v. by continuous infusion) and prostaglandin E_1 (0.4 µg/kg BW i.v.). Liver transplantation, if successful, is curative. (388, 399, 423, 425, 432, 440, 460) (s. tab. 31.17)

17.3 Hereditary haemochromatosis

HFE-related haemochromatosis, which is synonymous with type 1, is the most frequent and most important form of HC.

17.3.1 Frequency

Hereditary haemochromatosis (HC) has an incidence of 0.25–0.5% in the Caucasian population. After Gilbert's disease, HC is the most common hereditary liver disease. Men are affected five to ten times more frequently than women. The gene mutation on chromosome 6 occurs with a frequency of 1:10 to 1:20 for the heterozygous type and of 1:200 up to 1:400 for the homozygous type, as far as this can be detected by current methods. The number of those affected with manifest HC is influenced by racial and exogenous factors (e.g. diet, alcohol, personal habits), which is an explanation for the variations in frequency between 1:500 to 1:4,000. Prevalence of the HC gene in the normal population is estimated at 6–7%. If both parents are heterozygous carriers, the probability of the children being homozygous is 1:4 and heterozygous 1:2. (391, 395, 398, 414, 437, 466, 468)

About 1:500 persons in Germany are carriers of homozygous HC. However, the number of clinically detected cases of HC only corresponds to a ratio of 1:5,000. A considerable number of homozygous carriers are diagnosed and treated far too late. • In 1% of patients with newly detected diabetes mellitus and in 3–15% of cirrhotic patients, the respective disease is aetiologically attributable to HC.

17.3.2 Pathogenesis

Iron storage is about 0.07 g per year in heterozygous carriers. In homozygous men, however, it is about ten times higher (0.6 g), whereas the rate in homozygous women is only 0.16 g due to loss of iron during menstruation, pregnancy and breastfeeding. Generally, men have stored a total of 20–30 g iron by the age of 50. As from 5–8 g, progredient organ damage begins. (420, 441, 447, 452, 468) (s. fig. 31.26)

A defect in the HFE gene leads to overenhanced (undesired) intestinal iron absorption. Thus the enteral absorption of iron is at a much higher level in HC (two-to fourfold) because of this dysregulation, although the iron content of the organism is increased. After being above average for several years, iron uptake returns to normal, even in HC patients. However, following venesection, the iron absorption in HC increases again. This disorder is primarily caused by the *HFE mutation* present in the crypts of the small intestine cells, where iron uptake usually occurs. • Iron absorption is regulated by the iron-responsive-elements-binding-protein. This *IREBP* shows a normal function in HC, since its gene is not localized on chromosome 6. In contrast, there is a disturbance of the association between C 282 Y mutation of HFE and the *β-microglobulin*, so that the normal function of HFE is reduced. In addition, the defect HFE gene does not interact with the transferrin receptor 1, with the result that iron is more easily absorbed in the cell. Both the transmembranous protein *Nramp 2* and the iron reductase (Dcyt = duodenal cytochrome B) are considered as apical iron transporters. • Intestinal uptake of iron is still influenced by the basolateral iron transporter *ferroportin 1*, whose gene defect causes type 4 HC. Iron is also transported by the multi-copper-iron-oxidase *hephaistin*, which creates the connection between iron and copper transport. • Transferrin receptor 2 is also involved in the regulation of intestinal iron transport; in the case of a gene defect, it is responsible for the development of type 3 HC. The modes of action behind iron absorption and iron transport based on the above-mentioned (and other?) proteins have only been partially clarified. (394, 397, 405, 438, 448)

Iron metabolism: Iron is the sixth most abundant element in the universe; it has two oxidation states: Fe(II) and Fe(III). Normal **diet** accounts for 10−30 mg iron/day, with about 1.5 mg/day of this amount being stored mainly in the bone marrow, skeletal musculature and liver (hepatocytes, Kupffer cells, endothelial cells); in HC, however, the amount is 3−5 mg/day. Thus HC produces an annual iron surplus of 500−1,000 mg. • **Resorption** of bivalent iron takes place in the mucosal cells of the duodenum and proximal jejunum. There, it is oxidized by ferroxidases into trivalent iron and bound (by means of apoferritin) reversibly to water-soluble **ferritin** (molecular weight 460,000, 50 Å in diameter, iron content about 20%). A single molecule of ferritin may contain up to 4,500 atoms of iron. The synthesis of ferritin, which enters the cell via ferritin receptors, is stimulated by iron; the site of synthesis is the RES. Ferritin is also formed on the polysomes of the hepatocytes and broken down in the lysosomes. The plasma ferritin value correlates with the total amount of iron stored in the body. Enteral iron resorption is controlled by the intracellular ferritin concentration: there is a negative correlation between these two quantities. In HC, ferritin is considerably decreased in or absent from the mucosal cells; there may be disturbed regulation of ferritin gene expression, i.e. ferritin-determined dysregulation is observed. • A second (but labile) intracellular storage form of iron is **haemosiderin,** a water-insoluble pigment of Fe(III) hydroxide (ca. 37%), protein, carbohydrate, lipids, copper and calcium. Haemosiderin is formed during the lysosomal breakdown of ferritin, a process by which released iron can be stored in the lysosomes. It is mainly stored in the peripheral area of the lobules and in the portal fields. In contrast to ferritin, haemosiderin shows a *positive Berlin-blue reaction*. (s. figs. 31.28, 31.29) • Intracellular iron is, to a certain extent, bound to **transferrin,** which is mainly produced in the hepatocytes. It is considered to be a carrier molecule for extracellular iron. Only one third of the total *iron-binding capacity* of transferrin (normal 250−370 µg/dl) is iron-saturated. The saturation capacity beyond this normal degree of transferrin saturation is called *free (latent) iron-binding capacity*. There is a negative correlation between the amount of iron in the organism and the transferrin synthesis rate. The absorption of transferrin into the target cells occurs by means of a specific receptor. (394, 405, 420, 433, 438, 450) (s. pp 54, 104)

An **additional pathogenetic factor** (apart from excessive iron supply or alcohol abuse) is *vitamin C*, which has different effects: on the one hand, it enhances intestinal iron resorption as well as iron excretion from the RES, but on the other hand, it is broken down due to an iron overload, which results in subsequent vitamin C deficiency. • *Alcoholic beverages* may support the development of haemochromatosis when the respective iron content is considerably increased (depending on the iron content of the soil or of the drinking water used in their production). Furthermore, alcohol-induced folate deficiency may cause ineffective erythropoiesis with enhanced endogenous iron storage. • A genetic association also exists between HC and the α_1-antitrypsin deficiency syndrome as well as *porphyria cutanea tarda*, which leads to a more rapid development of cirrhosis. • Any rise in iron storage is due to a **disturbed iron balance:** if the daily supply continues to be higher than the daily loss, the individual organs will absorb iron in line with their respective storage capacity.

17.3.3 Iron toxicity

It was O. WARBURG (1928) who first observed the toxic effects of "free" (ionized) iron on cell metabolism. Increased acid phosphatase, decreased glucose-6-phosphatase, disturbances in oxidative cell metabolism as well as augmented glycolytic breakdown processes in the liver and cardiac muscle cells have since been reported. • There are **three molecular mechanisms** which are important for the toxic effects of free iron on cell metabolism: (*1.*) increased formation of *reactive oxygen intermediates* (with release of lysosomal enzymes and indirect stimulation of fibrogenesis) (s. p. 71), (*2.*) direct *stimulation of collagen synthesis* (with enhanced fibrogenesis) (s. p. 410), and (*3.*) changes in or damage to *DNA* (with the possible induction of carcinogenesis). (s. fig. 31.26)

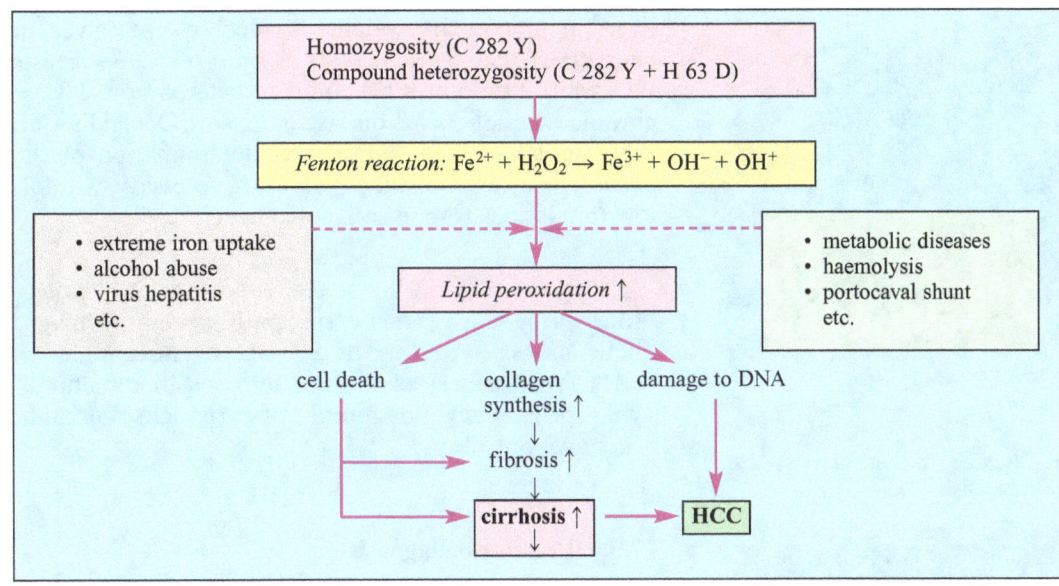

Fig. 31.26: Postulated pathogenetic and morphological cascade of damage in HC

17.3.4 Morphology

After being transported in increased quantities to the liver, iron is mostly stored as haemosiderin and ferritin in the hepatocytes of the lobular periphery. Initially, this *liver cell siderosis* does not impair the function of hepatocytes, as iron is absorbed by lysosomes. Iron storage commences in lobular zone 1 and progresses to zone 3. Gradually, the cells of the whole lobule become involved in iron deposition, mainly in the form of centroaxial pigment pathways, with enhanced iron deposition in the periportal area (haemosiderin granules). (409, 427)

When the storage capacity of the lysosomes is exhausted (usually with a liver iron content of >4,000 µg/g wet weight), there are unspecific inflammatory reactions in the portal field and lobular periphery, including single-cell necrosis as well as activation of fibroblasts and macrophages. Siderin, released from necrotized hepatocytes, is absorbed by Kupffer cells, which are usually increased in number and arranged in a nodular form. Coarse, grained siderosis of stellate cells likewise points to the extent of liver cell necrosis (= sideronecrosis). This phase may be called *acute siderophile hepatitis.* (408) Occasionally, there is formation of giant siderosomes and *glycogen vacuolations of the nuclei* in the hepatocytes of the peripheral lobules. (s. fig. 31.1) • Some excess iron is transported into the *bile ducts* and stored in their epithelial cells. The fainter and more finely granulated pigmentation (compared to hepatocytes) is important for the morphological diagnosis of HC.

The inflammatory mesenchymal reactions in the portal field and lobular periphery induce extremely low-cell perilobular and tylotic fibrosis. (427) Slowly, star-shaped **portal fibrosis,** so-called *holly-leaf fibrosis,* develops. This morphological picture, similar to that of chronic hepatitis, was termed *chronic siderophile hepatitis* by H. KALK (1962). • The hepatic lobules are gradually grouped into islet-like structures. Within the tylotic connective tissue, very fine epithelial tubuli, also known as pseudo bile ducts, are found; they are more strongly loaded with iron pigments than are the preformed bile ducts. These pseudo bile ducts are seen as minimal and ineffective attempts to regenerate the parenchyma, although the constant iron supply prevents epithelial substitution. This leads to the development of almost uniform, micronodular (later on mixed-nodular) and very coarse **pigment cirrhosis,** which is rich in fibres and poor in regeneration. (s. figs. 31.27 – 31.29)

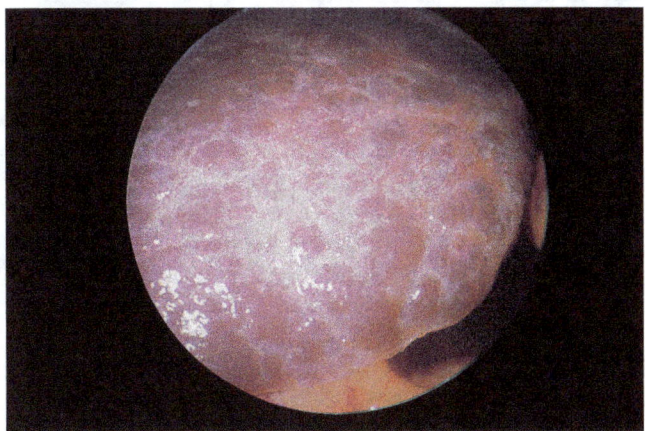

Fig. 31.27: Haemochromatotic cirrhosis: micronodular, slate-grey to brownish discolouration, rich in septate fibrosis, marked neovascularization

The morphological damage in other **iron-storing organs** (particularly the pancreas, heart and endocrinium) follows pathological mechanisms similar to those in the liver. These organs also show brown tissue changes with increasing fibrosis. HFE is expressed in all tissues involved in HC. • In HC, zinc is also stored in the liver at up to eight times the normal levels.

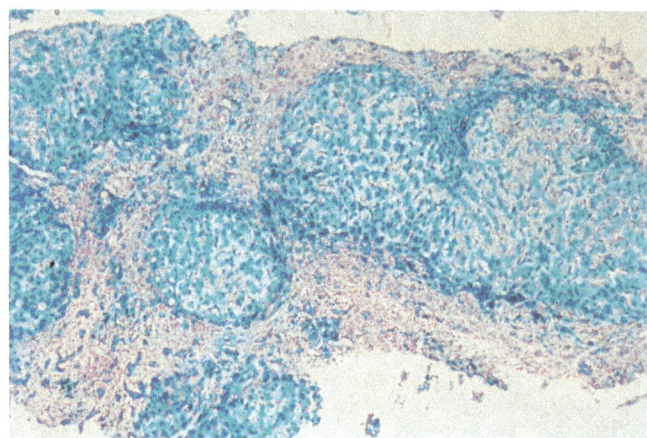

Fig. 31.28: Micronodular cirrhosis due to hereditary (HFE-related) haemochromatosis (Berlin blue)

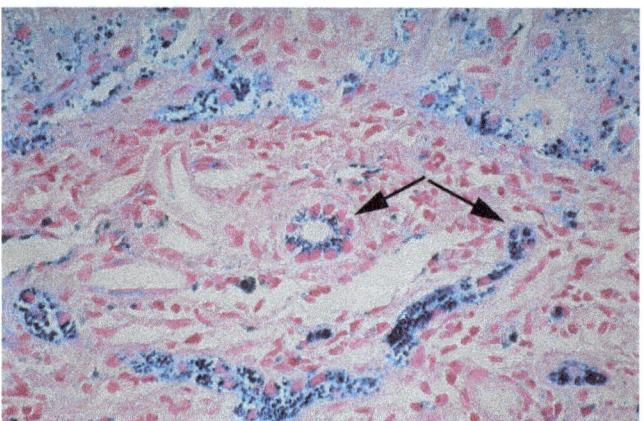

Fig. 31.29: Cirrhosis in hereditary haemochromatosis. Massive siderosis in hepatocytes and in epithelia of preformed bile ducts (arrows) (Berlin blue)

17.3.5 Early diagnosis

For successful treatment and thus also for prognosis, it is of the utmost importance to detect HC in its early phase. At this stage, however, neither subjective complaints nor clinical findings are apparent. The development of symptoms is slow and gradual — in men, not before the age of 30; in women, usually not before the menopause. • It is only by chance that an *increase in serum iron* (>160 µg/dl), *ferritin* (>200 µg/dl) or *transferrin saturation* (>45%) occasionally becomes evident. The combined determination of ferritin and transferrin saturation has a sensitivity of 90−95%, although specificity is lower. (s. tab. 31.18) These purely accidental findings, which initially appear as moderate deviations from normal values, are by no means conclusive, but they are nevertheless suggestive of HC. • However, *hepatic siderosis* can likewise be detected incidentally in liver biopsy, sometimes with an iron content of >1.7 mg/g dry weight, allowing the additional option of determining the hepatic iron index. (396, 398, 404, 441)

For the early diagnosis of HC, it has proved very useful to determine the **hepatic iron index:** iron content of the liver (in µmol/g dry weight) divided by age (given in years) (M. L. Bassett et al., 1984). A ratio of >2.0 suggests HC, while a ratio of <1.5 points to heterozygous HC or chronic alcoholic liver disease. (456, 461) Depending on the results obtained, subsequent determination of the *phenotype* or even of the *genotype*, if necessary, will follow (analogous to preventive diagnosis).

In the future, non-invasive **liver-iron quantification** (measuring the magnetic susceptibility as in "magnetic biopsy") by way of SQUID biosusceptimeter (BTi ferritometer) as a quick and sensitive method will open up new possibilities of early detection and therapy control.

17.3.6 Preventive diagnosis

The detection of HC requires targeted preventive diagnosis of family members (including siblings) and close relatives. Firstly, the **HFE genotype**, based on the determination of the *C282Y mutation*, shows a similarly high diagnostic sensitivity to that of a liver biopsy; HFE genotyping is therefore important for family screening. In heterozygosity, however, liver biopsy should be performed as a diagnostic marker instead of HFE genotyping. (391, 395−398, 404, 415, 420, 436, 441, 451, 452, 455, 457) • The **phenotype** varies considerably and is influenced by a number of factors (alcohol abuse, oestrogens, dietary iron intake, loss of iron, etc.). Elucidation of the phenotype focuses on the determination of *transferrin saturation* and *ferritin* concentration in the blood. With increased values, liver biopsy is indicated: an iron content of >1.7 mg/g dry weight points to HC, while a value of >4.5 mg/g or an iron index of >2.0 confirms the presence of HC and is also an indication for therapy.

HLA system: This system may have one of *three constellations*: (*1.*) when two alleles (A3 and B14 or B7) of the relative are identical to those of the patient, there is a high risk of HC (= annual check-ups are required); (*2.*) with only one HLA allele of the relative being identical to that of the diseased person, there is merely a minor risk (= check-ups every 4−5 years are sufficient); (*3.*) if neither allele of the relative is identical to those of the patient, there is no risk at all (= no further check-ups are required). (413, 428) • It should be noted, however, that the formerly recommended determination of the HLA types (A3, B7, B14) is no longer common.

17.3.7 Manifestation

Subjective complaints

When the organism is constantly overloaded with iron, subjective complaints gradually develop (in 5−40% of cases). These present a variety of uncharacteristic features, varying from individual to individual.

Fatigue	(40–60%)	Impaired potency	(10–20%)
Abdominal pain	(30–40%)	Nausea	(10–20%)
Stress dyspnoea	(20–30%)	Diarrhoea	(5–10%)
Weight loss	(15–25%)	Meteorism	(5–10%)
Heart problems	(15–25%)	Dysmenorrhoea	(5–10%)
Arthralgia	(15–25%)	Proneness to infection	(5–10%)
Thirst	(10–20%)		

Clinical findings

During the development of the disease, clinical findings appear which can be attributed to those organs primarily involved in iron storage and to their respective damaging mechanisms. (390, 395, 404, 415, 437, 441, 451, 468)

1. Liver involvement	(>90%)
2. Cutaneous pigmentation	(60–80%)
3. Diabetes mellitus	(50–70%)
4. Cardiomyopathy	(20–50%)
5. Arthropathy	(30–50%)
6. Endocrinopathy	(20–50%)

1. Liver involvement: The liver is enlarged and of firm consistency. Skin stigmata of liver disease occur with varying degrees of intensity. (s. p. 83) Portal hypertension with splenomegaly (30–50%), oesophageal varices and ascites develop. • Laboratory findings may include a slight increase in transaminases, P-III-P and IgG values as well as borderline pathological ICG and galactose tests. (s. p. 114) Occasionally, CA 19-9 levels are moderately increased. Vitamin E is reduced. A striking feature is the detection of normal parameters despite the presence of manifest cirrhosis. The existence of cirrhosis with a ferritin value of <1,000 µg/l is unlikely. • Determination of α_1-foetoprotein is recommended at long intervals.

2. Cutaneous pigmentation: "Bronze diabetes" (s. p. 635) is rare. The colour of the skin is usually grey-brown, particularly in areas exposed to light, but also in axillae and conjunctivae as well as in the genital area and oral cavity. The dirty grey discolouration is due to increased melanin and enhanced iron storage, particularly in the sweat glands. Pigmentation is most striking along the lines of the palms. (s. fig. 4.12!) (s. p. 88)

3. Diabetes mellitus: A glucose tolerance disorder is detectable at an early stage. Subsequently, 60–70% of the patients develop the distinct clinical picture of diabetes, including diabetic complications (retinopathy, polyneuropathy, nephropathy, arteriopathy). The β-cells show iron deposition and fibrosis, in contrast to the α-cells (so that glucagon secretion is still normal). It remains unclear whether an additional genetic defect is present in the β-cells. Usually, there is peripheral insulin resistance, which often becomes reversible as a result of successful treatment. With progressive destruction of the β-cells, insulin-dependent diabetes mellitus develops.

4. Cardiomyopathy: Iron deposition in the myocardium and/or the conduction system causes the walls of the heart, particularly of the ventricles, to thicken; apart from that, necrosis of the cardiac muscle cells with subsequent fibrosis can be observed. Dilatative cardiomyopathy is accompanied by tachyarrhythmias. Cases of sudden death have been described. Considerable improvement is generally achieved by the release of iron deposits. The aetiology of cardiomyopathy can be clarified by myocardial biopsy. (403, 446, 459, 465)

5. Arthropathy: Initially, the small joints (finger, toe and wrist) are affected. Subsequently, the large joints (knee, shoulder and hip) also become involved in the clinical picture of arthrosis. The patients complain at an early stage (in 30–50% of cases) of arthralgia located in the areas described above, but there seems to be no correlation with the degree of iron overload. X-ray scanning shows subchondral cysts and sclerotic changes, narrowing of the articular space, hypertrophic bone proliferations, chondrocalcinosis, and osteoporosis (particularly when hypogonadism is present). This kind of damage in the joints, cartilaginous parts and adjacent bones is caused by the formation of calcium phosphate crystals within the synovial cells, mainly due to iron-induced pyrophosphatase inhibition. Venesection treatment has little effect on arthropathy. (392, 448)

6. Endocrinopathy: Pronounced iron deposition can be found in the thyroid and parathyroid glands, the anterior lobe of the hypophysis and the adrenal cortex. Testicular atrophy is caused by insufficiency of the anterior lobe of the hypophysis, particularly since only a small (perivascular) amount of iron, or no iron at all, is deposited in the testes. Hypogonadism (loss of libido, menstrual disorders, impotency) may regress after the removal of iron deposits. In addition, signs of hypothyroidism, hypoparathyroidism and slight insufficiency of the adrenal cortex are found. Biochemical evidence showing decreased serum values of the relevant hormones (gonadotropins, testosterone, oestrogens, aldosterone, thyroid hormones) may provide an overview of the underlying endocrinopathy. Gynaecomastia has not been observed. (406, 430, 468)

Laboratory findings

There are many reasons why laboratory parameters of iron metabolism may deviate from normal values; they should always be checked to facilitate the differential diagnosis of HC or of acquired haemochromatosis and haemosiderosis. • In cases of HC, there are various deviations from normal values. (398, 404, 441, 451) (s. tab. 31.18)

The determination of **serum iron concentration** often shows normal values over a long period of manifest HC. In suspected HC, repeated examinations may be necessary due to daily fluctuations and circadian rhythms in the serum iron concentration as well as in factors influencing laboratory procedures. It is only in the later course of HC that serum iron is constantly and significantly increased. In 1953 H. KALK described **hypersiderinaemia** as the typical fifth cardinal symptom of HC. • When serum iron continues to fall, liver carcinoma can be suspected.

Determination of **transferrin saturation** (after 12 hours of fasting) supports a strong suspicion of manifest HC when the value is $>55\%$, while a saturation of $>75\%$ is almost diagnostic proof of homozygosity. This method is also seen as a reliable screening test. A value of $>55\%$ shows a specificity and sensitivity of 92% for HC. With a value of $>50\%$ in women and $>60\%$ in men, the ferritin level should be checked as well. An increased saturation value calls for liver biopsy, whereas a normal value requires a follow-up after one to two years.

> The **total iron-binding capacity** (TIBC) of transferrin can be calculated from the transferrin concentration in µg/dl or µmol/l: transferrin x 1.41 or transferrin x 25.2. This gives a normal value for men of 268–436 µg/dl or 48–78 µmol/l and for women of 257–402 µg/dl or 46–72 µmol/l. • The difference between TIBC and the amount of iron found before Fe^{3+} and magnesium carbonate are added is called **free iron-binding capacity**. This is the FIBC which is possible beyond the normal saturation capacity of about one third of the transferrin. • The **transferrin saturation** (in %) can be calculated as follows: serum iron (µg/dl) x 100 divided by transferrin (mg/dl) x 1.25. • *A free IBC of ≤ 50 µg/dl, i.e. transferrin saturation of >62%, suggests the presence of HC.*

The **ferritin value** corresponds well to the total value of body iron, whereby 1 µg/l ferritin is equivalent to about 7.5 mg body iron. The sensitivity of the ferritin value in HC is 85% and the specificity is 95%. A value of >700 µg/l points both to the presence of HC and to the development of liver fibrosis or cirrhosis. In contrast, a normal ferritin value and normal transferrin saturation rule out HC in about 95% of cases. (s. tab. 31.18)

Normal values		Haemochromatosis
1. **Serum iron**		
Men	59–158 µg/dl	
	10.6–28.3 mol/l	$>$ 180 µg/dl
Women	37–145 µg/dl	$>$ 32 µmol/l
	6.6–26.0 µmol/l	
2. **Ferritin**		
Men	35–217 µg/l	
Women	23–110 µg/l	$>$ 300 µg/l
3. **Transferrin**		
Men	210–340 mg/dl	
Women	200–310 mg/dl	$>$ 500 mg/dl
Saturation	16–45%	
Heterozygotes		$>$ 55%
Homozygotes		$>$ 70%
4. **Hepatic iron index**		
$\frac{\text{iron content of the liver (µmol/g)}}{\text{age (years)}}$		$>$ 2.0
5. **Deferoxamine test**		
500 mg i.m./iron excretion rate		$>$ 4 mg/6 hr

Tab. 31.18: Biochemical findings in hereditary haemochromatosis

Hypochromic anaemia with *poikilocytosis* may point to disturbed erythropoiesis as a result of iron overload. • Transferrin deficiency may, however, also be causally related to this disease.

While the **deferoxamine test** (s. p. 105) is often considered obsolete, it can nevertheless serve as another stone in the mosaic and prove helpful in the diagnostics or follow-up of HC, since it is an iron chelation test that is easy to apply, free of side effects and inexpensive. In healthy persons, this test reveals a urinary iron excretion of $<1-2$ mg; in haemosiderosis, the excreted amount is <4 mg, and in HC >4 mg. (450)

A **gastric mucosa biopsy** may facilitate differentiation between HC and secondary haemochromatosis, yet this examination is also regarded as obsolete today. (Iron in macrophages with HC = ∅, with secondary HC = ↑↑.)

Imaging techniques

CT determination of increased liver density due to iron overload in haemochromatosis yields values of 80–140 Hounsfield units (= white liver). The deposition of 1 g iron causes an increase in density of 1 HU. CT densitometry makes it possible to monitor the course of the blood-letting therapy. (447) (s. p. 181) • In **MRI**, a haemochromatotic liver appears dark grey to black (= *dark liver*) due to signal loss depending on the iron content. (s. fig. 8.8) With an iron concentration of 1 mg/g liver tissue, accuracy is 95–100%. (393, 402, 422, 424, 435) (s. p. 185) • Both examination techniques are of great importance in detecting liver cell carcinoma. • By using the newly developed **SQUID biosusceptimeter** (BTi ferritometer), even more reliable quantification of liver iron is expected.

Liver biopsy and laparoscopy

Laparoscopically, a dark brown liver surface with augmented fibrosis can be seen. (s. fig. 31.26) • Quantitative measuring of iron in the liver bioptate is the most reliable technique for diagnosing haemochromatosis. If possible, this kind of biopsy should be carried out under laparoscopic guidance, and *two biopsy punches* should be taken. The first sample is designed to serve as a histological specimen as well as to detect iron and iron localization, while the second sample is used for quantitative iron determination. • At the same time, the *hepatic iron index* is calculated arithmetically. This index also facilitates the differential diagnosis of chronic alcoholic disease, which is not always an easy task, particularly at the cirrhotic stage (index $<$ 1.4, in HC $>$ 2.0). (434, 464)

17.3.8 Prognosis

The following *three factors* are of decisive importance for course and prognosis:

1. early diagnosis
2. consistent long-term treatment
3. close (lifelong) cooperation between patient and physician

▶ Therapeutic results will be better if the morphological damage is less severe and the other organs have not been seriously affected. • It is necessary to regard HC treatment as a lifelong procedure requiring the joint therapeutic involvement of the patient and the general practitioner or specialist. (441)

Untreated HC has a slow course and follows certain patterns in its progression; spontaneous regressions are not to be expected. The 5-year survival rate after establishing the diagnosis is only 18%. The mean survival rate was about 1.5 years in 1935, about 4.4 years after the introduction of insulin treatment, and 8.2 years with consistent venesection therapy. (467)

However, with early diagnosis and consistent treatment, **HC** has a good prognosis. In a comparison of treated versus untreated patients with HC, 5-year survival rates of 89% (vs. 33%) or 92% and an overall 10-year survival rate of 76% were observed. When cirrhosis was already manifest, the survival rate was only 62% after 10 years, whereas it was 93% in non-cirrhotic patients. • We believe that normal life expectancy is indeed a realistic perspective. *One of our patients died after 19 years of ongoing treatment of causes apparently unrelated to HC.*

The greater the effect of iron depletion, the more likely it is that morphological liver changes or even fibrosis and hepatic transformation processes will be reversed. • Portal hypertension and oesophageal varices may also regress, and a decisive improvement in diabetic metabolism is often observed. • *One of our patients with diabetes mellitus showed a normal diurnal blood sugar profile after eight years of consistent treatment, while the glucose tolerance test (monitored over longer periods of time) produced a moderately pathological result.* • In contrast, arthropathy appears to be unresponsive to treatment and may cause considerable suffering.

The main **causes of death** in HC are related to the following developments which aggravate the clinical picture (particularly in those cases where alcohol consumption is continued):

1. complicative diabetes mellitus
2. cardiac insufficiency
3. primary liver cell carcinoma
4. hepatic coma, liver failure
5. bleeding oesophageal varices
6. intercurrent infections
7. acute abdomen

The correlation between **hepatocellular carcinoma** and haemochromatosis was described by M.J. Stewart in 1922. Primary liver cell carcinoma is seen as the most common cause of death in haemochromatosis. Its frequency ranges between 6–42% or 7.3–18.9% (mean value approx. 14%), i.e. the risk of developing liver cell carcinoma in HC is about 200 times higher than in the normal population. Nevertheless, carcinogenicity is not necessarily related to the presence of cirrhosis, nor to appropriate therapy or non-treatment (cf. potential cocarcinogens, alcohol or hepatitis viruses). HCC development is mainly multilocular. Manifestation of a sarcoma has only rarely been observed. The latency period is reported to be 20–30 years. Follow-up with sonography and AFP determination at six-month intervals is indicated. HCC can also develop some years after complete iron depletion. Long-term iron overload acts as a cocarcinogen, apparently by way of DNA impairment. (400, 401, 410, 416, 418, 421, 426, 431, 439, 462)

In HC, the frequency of **extrahepatic carcinoma** may also be increased: in one Italian study, the figure was 3.7%. This correlation, which has also been assumed by other authors, raises the question as to whether there are additional cocarcinogenic factors, such as alcohol or hepatitis viruses. (459) • It is a striking feature that **alcoholism** is much more frequently observed in patients with HC than in people suffering from liver cirrhosis or from hepatic carcinoma of different genesis. • It is also remarkable that prevalence of **HBsAg** and **anti-HCV** is two and three times higher respectively in HC patients than in the normal population. Presumably, the function of the immune system is blocked by iron. This would help to explain the high carcinoma rate in patients with HC, due to the procarcinogenicity of HBV and HCV on the one hand and of iron on the other hand. • In cases of iron overload, **yersiniosis** should also be considered as a typical concomitant infection, possibly with the development of liver abscesses: iron is of exceptional importance for the metabolism of yersinia and to a considerable extent conducive to their growth. (389, 467) (s. p. 486)

17.3.9 Treatment

The paramount aim of treatment is to reach a negative iron balance. This must be achieved before complications due to the chronic iron overload have their effect on the predisposed organs. • *The extreme uncontrolled increase in iron absorption is treatable by adjuvant measures, albeit with limited success.*

Venesection treatment

Venesection treatment (W.D. Davis et al., 1950) is the method of choice; it is the most effective therapy. Bloodletting of about 500 ml blood frees the body of some 250 mg iron. With an average accumulation of >25 g iron, *weekly venesection* should be considered over a period of at least two years. • In patients with haemochromatosis (without simultaneous anaemia), blood-letting of 500 ml is carried out weekly until the serum ferritin value has normalized. Experience shows that the de-ironing of the body using this technique takes about 18 months. Blood-letting is well-tolerated, and the patient's physical capacity is usually not affected. In general, the haemoglobin value does not fall below 12g/dl. • By the time the respective *blood values* (ferritin level and transferrin saturation) normalize, a large quantity of iron has been discharged. At this stage, blood-letting can be reduced to two or three times per three months, provided the ferritin value and transferrin saturation remain within the normal range. Subsequently, three to four venesections per year usually suffice to maintain the iron balance. *Proton pump inhibitors* suppress the absorption of dietary, non-haeme bound iron. This can reduce the frequency of phlebotomies. • *Plasmapheresis* is not required, since the plasmaproteins removed by blood-letting are easily replaced by the organism. However, in isolated cases, it may be necessary due to a cirrhosis-induced decrease in protein synthesis. The haemoglobin content should not (or only for a short period) fall below 11.5–12.0 g/dl, and the protein concentration should not fall below 6.0 g/dl. (404, 407, 415, 417, 431, 437, 441, 451) • *The number of venesections per year which are required to maintain the iron balance should be adhered to lifelong. This therapy must never be discontinued!*

Deferoxamine

This specific iron-chelating agent is obtained from actinomyces cultures. In a dose of 1.5 g, it is capable of mobilizing about 25 mg iron, i.e. the same amount as during a 500 ml venesection. • An *indication* may be given, even if only temporarily, when blood-letting cannot be carried out (e.g. anaemia, cardiac insufficiency). Deferoxamine binds iron in the tissue and in the serum; excretion occurs via the urine and faeces. However, it only has a biological half-life of about ten minutes, i.e. after this time merely half the pharmacon is still effective. Oral administration is ineffective. For this reason, subcutaneous injection is required as a slow infusion of 12 hours (using a portable infusion pump). With a daily dose of 25–50 mg/kg BW, removal of iron deposits will probably be successful. • Local irritations have been observed as *side effects*. Oculotoxicity (initial visual loss) may be evident, depending on the dose. Neurotoxic disturbances usually only occur when the dose is higher than 2–3 g/day (>90 mg/kg BW). This type of treatment is more complicated, less effective and much more expensive – it is intended as an alternative only when there is no possibility of venesection treatment. • In the foreseeable future, we can expect the development of other **iron-chelating agents** which will meet the ideal standards: oral administration, higher efficiency, lower costs and fewer side effects.

Adjuvant treatment measures

(1.) **Low-iron nutrition** is a basic requirement (there is practically no iron-free form of nutrition). However, intake of foodstuffs rich in iron is contraindicated when the iron balance has to be maintained. The iron balance is not greatly influenced by this measure, but it nevertheless has a certain effect: low-iron nutrition corresponds to two or three venesections per year! • *Every kind of adjuvant therapy should be used as a matter of principle – nothing can be said against such measures.*

(2.) This is also true of the daily consumption of **black tea** (1 cup with 5 g tea in the morning and at lunchtime). Tea is deemed to be an iron-chelating agent (iron tannate), which significantly reduces the resorption of iron, particularly in a low-iron diet – with or without ascorbic acid or milk added. (411, 429) • *We have always made sure that these adjuvant measures are strictly adhered to.*

(3.) **Deferoxamine** can also be used as an adjuvant agent in the initial treatment phase to reinforce venesection therapy. This is administered as an i.m. injection of 500 mg/week, usually by the family doctor, about two to three days before blood-letting is carried out.

(4.) **Abstention from alcohol** is absolutely essential and must be strictly adhered to. This is not only because of the minor amounts of iron usually found in alcoholic beverages, but also in order to avoid additional alcohol-induced lipid peroxidation and further stimulation of fibrosis already caused by iron.

(5.) The use of **antioxidants** is plausible from a pharmacological point of view, since lipid peroxidation due to iron intake may indeed lead to further tissue damage. (460) Silymarin (e.g. 2 x 140–170 mg), vitamin E (e.g. 100–200 mg) or β-carotene are good choices due to their lack of side effects and plausibility of efficacy.

(6.) HC patients who are **HBV-negative** should be actively immunized against hepatitis B. • As far as possible, patients should avoid any risk of HCV infection.

Normalization of the respective serum parameters, stabilization of the body's iron content at 3–5 g and improvement in the organ damage are to be expected in quite a short period of time when blood-letting therapy (if necessary, with deferoxamine as an option in long-term treatment) and adjuvant treatment measures (which may serve to support or speed up the successful outcome) are carried out consistently. The fact that better results can be achieved if the above-mentioned measures are applied has been shown by several impressive and carefully conducted studies. Therapeutic removal of iron overload is in any case not bound to a time factor! Generally, the faster and more constant the iron removal process is, the better. • Hypogonadism and arthropathies are less susceptible to treatment. Given the basic possibility of fibrosis regression, a certain optimism in this respect is definitely justified.

Simultaneous treatment

At the same time, consideration has to be given to the treatment of complaints or sequelae of organic manifestations, such as careful regulation of diabetes, management of cardiac insufficiency or dysrhythmia, hormone substitution, pain therapy in arthropathy, etc.

Liver transplantation

In principle, the indication for liver transplantation is limited to individual cases suitable for surgery (i.e. only in cases of early diagnosis and appropriate treatment). Unlike in Wilson's disease, the genetic defect is *not* removed by transplantation, and the transplanted liver may store iron again. • Consequently, a genuine indication is only given in acute liver failure and in an operable carcinoma restricted to the liver. The final stages of cirrhosis certainly continue to justify a transplantation, although the indication in this case is not based on HC, but on the fact that the diagnosis was established too late and/or that treatment was inadequate or not carried out at all. In young men with severe iron overload, a swift liver transplantation is always indicated. (419, 449)

A number of grave **mistakes** may occur in the treatment of HC. These include:

1. delay in reaching a precise diagnosis (including quantitative determination of iron in the liver bioptate)
2. blood-letting therapy carried out too hesitantly or inadequately
3. failure to carry out a family examination (preventive diagnosis)
4. merely monitoring family members who (still) show no signs of manifest disease instead of treating them properly

18 Haemosiderosis

Acquired ("secondary") haemochromatosis is caused by other diseases/conditions characterized by iron overload resulting from excessive iron storage in the organism (e.g. due to diet, medical treatment or haemolysis). The term acquired haemochromatosis should not be used unless the iron content of the liver is >0.5 g/100g wet weight. The causes are manifold. • In these patients, there is occasionally an HLA constellation which is identical to that of HC or a family history of iron storage. Therefore, it is postulated that these patients might be heterozygous HC carriers or that there might be another hitherto undetected triggering factor or a genetic defect in addition. (s. tab. 31.17)

18.1 Alcohol abuse

The most common cause (about 30% of cases) of hepatic siderosis is alcohol-induced liver disease. Its aetiology is unknown. With this form of acquired iron deposition, the more pronounced courses are characterized by stronger brownish cutaneous pigmentation, hypogonadism, glucose intolerance and hepatomegaly together with increased iron and ferritin values in the serum. This results in a similar symptomatology to that found in HC, only with a hepatic iron index clearly below 2.0. Blood-letting therapy is successful and reliable within a relatively short period of time. Iron deposition occurs mainly in the Kupffer cells, while the hepatocytes and the septa are largely free of iron.

18.2 Porphyria cutanea tarda

In porphyria cutanea tarda, iron deposition in the liver is generally low to moderate, predominantly in the hepatocytes of the acinar periphery. The cause is thought to be reduced activity of uroporphyrinogen decarboxylase resulting in decreased synthesis of porphyrin and haem. However, this variant of hepatic siderosis only becomes manifest as a result of various triggering factors. Treatment is also based on venesection.

18.3 Blood transfusion

Transfusional haemosiderosis (R.M. Kark, 1937) can occur following numerous blood transfusions. There are 200–250 mg iron in 500 ml (= 1 unit) blood. Thus numerous units (more than 50–60) must be transfused before siderin is clinically recognizable. It is initially deposited in the RES of the bone marrow, spleen and liver, ultimately in the hepatocytes as well.

18.4 Haemolytic anaemia

In all haemolytic anaemias, especially the genetically related forms, siderin is firstly deposited in Kupffer cells.

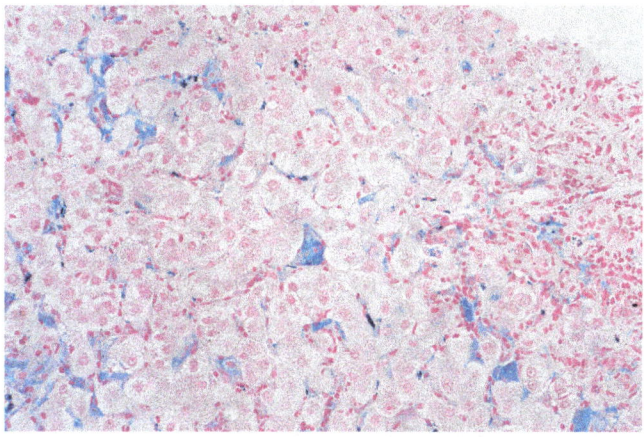

Fig. 31.30: Siderosis of Kupffer cells in haemolytic anaemia (Berlin blue)

The extent of siderosis depends on the duration and severity of the haemolysis. (s. fig. 31.30) In long-term haemolysis, iron is also stored increasingly in the hepatocytes. In such cases, the morphological and clinical picture of haemochromatosis can develop.

18.5 Chronic liver disease

Haemosiderosis can be found in several chronic liver diseases, such as chronic hepatitis (especially HVC leading to a reduced response rate to α-interferon), late-stage cirrhosis, spontaneous or surgical portal-systemic shunts, and non-alcoholic steatohepatitis.

18.6 African iron overload

In rural sub-Saharan Africa, there is a beer which is traditionally brewed in iron vats. The daily iron overload can be as much as 200 mg, with markedly increased iron absorption (T. H. BOTHWELL et al., 1965). • Such a condition is also observed in South Africa among the black population. Their diet consists of porridge fermented in iron pots with an acid pH value (V. R. GORDEUK et al., 1986). • In both cases, absorption of iron is facilitated by various factors, e.g. protein or vitamin C deficiency, alcohol abuse, acidic diet. It has been suggested that such iron overload is triggered by genetic factors.

References:

Fatty liver
1. Andersen, T., Gluud, C.: Liver morphology in morbid obesity: a literature study. Int. J. Obes. 1984; 8: 97–106
2. Angelico, F., del Ben, M., Conti, R., Francioso, S., Feole, K., Maccioni, D., Antonini, T.M., Alessandri, C.: Non-alcoholic fatty liver syndrome: a hepatic consequence of common metabolic diseases. J. Gastroenterol. Hepatol. 2003; 18: 588–594
3. Ballard, H., Bernstein, M., Farras, J.I.: Fatty liver presenting as obstructive jaundice. Amer. J. Med. 1961; 30: 196–201
4. Bedogni, G., Miglioli, L., Battistini, N., Masutti, F., Tiribelli, C., Bellentani, S.: Body mass index is a good predictor of an elevated alanine transaminase level in the general population: hints from the Dionysos study. Dig. Liver Dis. 2003; 35: 648–652
5. Braillon, A., Capron, J.P., Hervé, M.A., Degott, C., Quenum, C.: Liver in obesity. Gut 1985; 26: 133–139
6. Burt, A.D., Mutton, A., Day, C.P.: Diagnosis and interpretation of steatosis and steatohepatitis. Semin. Diagn. Pathol. 1998; 15: 246–258
7. Caturelli, E., Squillante, M.M., Andriulli, A., Cedrone, A., Cellerino, C., Pompili, M., Manoja, E.R., Rapaccini, G.L.: Hypoechoic lesions in the "bright liver": a reliable indicator of fatty change. A prospective study. J. Gastroenterol. Hepatol. 1992; 7: 469–472
8. Chong, V.F., Fan, Y.F.: Ultrasonographic hepatic pseudolesions: normal parenchyma mimicking mass lesions in fatty liver. Clin. Radiol. 1994; 49: 326–329
9. Christl, S.U., Müller, J.G.: Fatty liver in adult celiac disease. Dtsch. Med. Wschr. 1999; 124: 691–694
10. Clark, J.M., Brancati, F.L., Diehl, A.M.: Nonalcoholic fatty liver disease. An under-recognized cause of cryptogenic cirrhosis. J. Amer. Med. Ass. 2003; 289: 3000–3004
11. Dixon, J.B., Bhathal, P.S., Hughes, N.R., O'Brien, P.E.: Nonalcoholic fatty liver disease: Improvement in liver histological analysis with weight loss. Hepatology 2004; 39: 1647–1654
12. Giorgio, A., Francica, G., Aloisio, T., Tarantino, L., Pierri, P., Pellicano, M., Buscarini, L., Livraghi, T.: Multifocal fatty infiltration of the liver mimicking metastatic disease. Gastroenterol. Internat. 1991; 4: 169–172
13. Goland, S., Shimoni, S., Zornitzki, T., Knobler, H., Azoulai, O., Lutaty, G., Melzer, E., Orr, A., Caspi, A., Malnick, S.: Cardiac abnormalities as a new manifestation of nonalcoholic fatty liver disease. Echocardiographic and tissue Doppler imaging assessment. J. Clin. Gastroenterol. 2006; 40: 949–955
14. Hartroft, W.S., Sugioka, E., Porta, E.A.: Nutritional types of fatty livers in experimental animals and man. 5. Meeting-Internat. Assoc. Study of the Liver. Karlsbad 1968
15. Hautekeete, M.L., Degott, C., Benhamou, J.-P.: Microvesicular steatosis of the liver. Acta Clin. Belg. 1990; 45: 311–326
16. Jepsen, P., Vilstrup, H., Mellemkjall, L., Thulstrup, A.M., Olsen, J.H., Baron, J.A., Sorensen, H.T.: Prognosis of patients with a diagnosis of fatty liver. A registry-based cohort study. Hepato-Gastroenterol. 2003; 50: 2101–2104
17. Kemper, J., Jung, G., Poll, L.W., Jonkmanns, C., Luthen, R., Moedder, U.: CT and MRI findings of multifocal hepatic steatosis mimicking malignancy (case report). Abdom. Imag. 2002; 27: 708–710
18. Kral, J.G., Schaffner, F., Pierson, R.N.jr., Wang, J.: Body fat topography as an independent predictor of fatty liver. Metabolism 1993; 42: 548–551
19. Kuntz, E.: Fatty liver – a morphological and clinical review. Med. Welt 1999; 50: 406–413
20. Levenson, H., Greensite, F., Hoefs, J., Friloux, L., Applegate, G., Silva, E., Kanel, G., Buxton, R.: Fatty infiltration of the liver: quantification with phase-contrast MR imaging at 1.5 T vs biopsy. Amer. J. Roentgenol. 1991; 156: 307–312
21. Marchesini, G., Brizi, M., Morselli-Labate, A.M., Bianchi, G., Bugianesi, E., McCullogh, A.J., Forlani, G., Melchionda, N.: Association of nonalcoholic fatty liver disease with insulin resistance. Amer. J. Med. 1999; 107: 450–455
22. Mathiesen, U.L., Franzen, L.E., Aselius, H., Resjo, M., Jacobsson, L., Foberg, U., Fryden, A., Bodemar, G.: Increased liver echogenicity at ultrasound examination reflects degree of steatosis but not of fibrosis in asymptomatic patients with mild/moderate abnormalities of liver transaminases. Dig. Dis. Sci. 2002; 34: 516–522
23. Mofrad, P., Contos, M.J., Haque, M., Sargeant, C., Fisher, R.A., Luketic, V.A., Sterling, R.K., Shiffman, M.L., Stravitz, R.T., Sanyal, A.J.: Clinical and histologic spectrum of non-alcoholic fatty liver disease associated with normal ALT values. Hepatology 2003; 37: 1286–1292
24. Naschitz, J.E., Yeshurun, D., Zuckerman, E., Arad, E., Boss, J.H.: Massive hepatic steatosis complicating adult celiac disease: report of a case and review of the literature. Amer. J. Gastroenterol. 1987; 82: 1186–1189
25. Newman, J.S., Oates, E., Arora, S., Kaplan, M.: Focal spared area in fatty liver simulating a mass. Scintigraphic evaluation. Dig. Dis. Sci. 1991; 36: 1019–1022
26. Nomura, F., Ohnishi, K., Ochiai, T., Okuda, K.: Obesity-related nonalcoholic fatty liver: CT features and follow-up studies after low-calorie diet. Radiology 1987; 162: 845–847
27. Nussbaum, M.S., Li, S, Bower, R.H., McFadden, D.W., Dayal, R., Fischer, J.E.: Addition of lipid to total parenteral nutrition prevents hepatic steatosis in rats by lowering the portal venous insulin/glucagon ratio. J. Parent. Ent. Nutr. 1992; 16: 106–109
28. Quigley, E.M.M.M., Marsh, N., Shaffer, J.L., Markin, R.S.: Hepatobiliary complications of total parenteral nutrition. Gastroenterology 1993; 104: 286–301
29. Roediger, W.E.W.: New views on the pathogenesis of kwashiorkor: methionine and other amino acids. J. Pediatr. Gastroenterol. Nutr. 1995; 21: 130–136
30. Schulz, F., Hildebrand, E.: Exzessive generalisierte Fettembolie bei akut dystrophischer Fettleber. Med. Klin. 1977; 72: 59–63
31. Seifalian, A.M., Piasecki, C., Agarwal, A., Davidson, B.R.: The effect of graded steatosis on flow in the hepatic parenchymal microcirculation. Transplantation 1999; 68: 780–784
32. Silverman, J.F., Pories, W.J., Caro, J.F.: Liver pathology in diabetes mellitus and morbid obesity. Clinical, pathological, and biochemical considerations. Path. Ann. 1989; 24: 275–302
33. Tanaka, K., Kean, E.A., Johnson, B.: Jamaican vomiting sickness. Biochemical investigation of two cases. New Engl. J. Med. 1976; 295: 461–467
34. Teli, M.R., James, O.F.W., Burt, A.D., Bennett, M.K., Day, C.P.: The natural history of non-alcoholic fatty liver: a follow-up study. Hepatology 1995; 22: 1714–1719
35. Tendler, D., Lin, S., Yancy, W.S., Mavropoulos, J., Sylvestre, P., Rockey, D.C., Westman, E.C.: The effect of a low-carbohydrate, ketogenic diet on nonalcoholic fatty liver disease. A pilot study. Dig. Dis. Sci. 2007; 52: 589–593
36. Tsushima, Y., Endo, K.: Spleen enlargement in patients with nonalcoholic fatty liver – Correlation between degree of fatty infiltration in liver and size of spleen. Dig. Dis. Sci. 2000; 45: 196–200
37. Waterlow, J.C.: Kwashiorkor revisited: the pathogenesis of oedema in kwashiorkor and its significance. Trans. R. Soc. Trop. Med. Hyg. 1984; 78: 436–441
38. Younossi, Z.M., Gramlich, T., Matteoni, C.A., Boparai, N., McCullogh, A.J.: Non-alcoholic fatty liver disease in patients with type 2 diabetes. Clin. Gastroenterol. Hepatol. 2004; 2: 262–265
39. Zafrani, E.S.: Non-alcoholic fatty liver disease: an emerging pathological spectrum. Virch. Arch. 2003; 444: 3–12

Non-alcoholic steatohepatitis
40. Abdelmalek, M.F., Angulo, P., Jorgensen, R.A., Sylvestre, P.B., Lindor, K.D.: Betaine, a promising new agent for patients with nonalcoholic steato-hepatitis: results of a pilot study. Amer. J. Gastroenterol. 2001; 96: 2711–2717

41. **Angulo, P., Keach, J.C., Batts, K.P., Lindord, K.D.:** Independent predictors of liver fibrosis in patients with non-alcoholic steatohepatitis. Hepatology 1999; 30: 1356–1362
42. **Brunt, E.M., Janney, C.G., DiBisceglie, A.M., Neuschwander-Tetri, B.A., Bacon, B.R.:** Nonalcoholic steatohepatitis: A proposal for grading and staging the histological lesions. Amer. J. Gastroenterol. 1999; 94: 2467–2474
43. **Caldwell, S.H., Swerdlow, R.H., Khan, E.M., Iezzoni, J.C., Hespenheide, E.E., Parks, J.K., Parker, W.D.:** Mitochondrial abnormalities in non-alcoholic steatohepatitis. J. Hepatol. 1999; 31: 430–434
44. **Carson, K., Washington, M.K., Treem, W.R., Clavien, P.A., Hunt, C.M.:** Recurrence of non-alcoholic steatohepatitis in a liver transplant recipient. Liver Transpl. Surg. 1997; 3: 174–176
45. **Chen, S.W., Chen, Y.X., Shi, J., Lin, Y., Xie, W.F.:** The restorative effect of taurine on experimental nonalcoholic steatohepatitis. Dig. Dis. Sci. 2006; 51: 2225–2234
46. **Chitturi, S., Farrell, G., Frost, L., Kriketos, A., Lin, R., Liddle, C., Samarasinghe, D., George, J.:** Serum leptin in NASH correlates with hepatic steatosis but not fibrosis: a manifestation of lipotoxicity? Hepatology 2002; 36: 403–409
47. **Cotrim, H.P., Andrade, Z.A., Parana, R., Portugal, M., Lyra, L.G., Freitas, L.A.R.:** Nonalcoholic steatohepatitis: a toxic liver disease in industrial workers. Liver 1999; 19: 299–304
48. **Denk, H., Stumptner, C., Fuchsbichler, A., Zatloukal, K.:** Alcoholic and nonalcoholic steatohepatitis. Histopathologic and pathogenetic considerations. Pathologe 2001; 22: 388–398
49. **Eriksson, S., Eriksson, K.-F., Bondesson, L.:** Nonalcoholic steatohepatitis in obesity: a reversible condition. Acta Med. Scand. 1986; 220: 83–88
50. **George, D.K., Goldwurm, S., MacDonald, G.A., Cowley, L.L., Walker, N.I., Ward, P.J., Jazwinska, E.C., Powell, L.W.:** Increased hepatic iron concentration in non-alcoholic steatohepatitis is associated with increased fibrosis. Gastroenterology 1998; 114: 311–318
51. **Harrison, S.A., Torgerson, S., Hayashi, P., Ward, J., Schenker, S.:** Vitamin E and vitamin C treatment improves fibrosis in patients with non-alcoholic steatohepatitis. Amer. J. Gastroenterol. 2003; 98: 2485–2490
52. **Itoh, S., Yougel, T., Kawagoe, K.:** Comparison between non-alcoholic steatohepatitis and alcoholic hepatitis. Amer. J. Gastroenterol. 1987; 82: 650–654
53. **James, O., Day, C.:** Non-alcoholic steatohepatitis: another disease of affluence. Lancet 1999; 353: 1634–1636
54. **Koruk, M., Savas, C., Yilmaz, O., Taysi, S., Karokok, M., Gündogdu, C., Yilmaz, A.:** Serum lipids, lipoproteins and apolipoprotein levels in patients with nonalcoholic steatohepatitis. J. Clin. Gastroenterol. 2003; 37: 177–182
55. **Laurin, J., Lindor, K.D., Cripin, J.S., Gossard, A., Gores, G.J., Ludwig, J.:** Ursodeoxycholic acid or clofibrate in the treatment of non-alcoholic-induced steatohepatitis: a pilot study. Hepatology 1996; 23: 1464–1467
56. **Liangpunsakul, S., Chalasani, N.:** Is hypothyroidism a risk factor for non-alcoholic steatohepatitis? J. Clin. Gastroenterol. 2003; 37: 340–343
57. **Ludwig, J., Viggiano, T.R., McGill, D.B., Oh, B.J.:** Nonalcoholic steatohepatitis: Majo Clinic experiences with a hitherto unnamed disease. Majo Clin. Proc. 1980; 55: 434–438
58. **Molleston, J.P., White, F., Teckman, J., Fitzgerald, J.F.:** Obese children with steatohepatitis can develop cirrhosis in childhood. Amer. J. Gastroenterol. 2002; 97: 2460–2462
59. **Molloy, R.M., Komorowski, R., Varma, R.R.:** Recurrent non-alcoholic steatohepatitis and cirrhosis after liver transplantation. Liver Transpl. Surg. 1997; 3: 177–178
60. **Neuschwander-Tetri, B.A., Brunt, E.M., Wehmeier, K.R., Oliver, D., Bacon, B.R.:** Improved nonalcoholic steatohepatitis after 48 weeks of treatment with the PPAR-gamma ligand rosiglitazone. Hepatology 2003; 38: 1008–1017
61. **Ohbayashi, H.:** Twelve-month chronic administration of polyenephosphatidylcholine (EPL) for improving hepatic function of fatty liver patients. Progr. Med. 2004; 24: 1751–1756
62. **Perez-Carreras, M., del Hoyo, P., Martin, M.A., Rubio, J.C., Martin, A., Castellano, G., Colina, F., Arenas, J., Solis-Herruzo, J.A.:** Defective hepatic mitochondrial respiratory chain in patients with nonalcoholic steatohepatitis. Hepatology 2003; 38: 999–1007
63. **Powell, E.E., Cooksley, W.G., Hanson, R., Searle, J., Halliday, J.W., Powell, L.W.:** The natural history of non-alcoholic steatohepatitis: a follow-up study of forty-two patients for up to 21 years. Hepatology 1990; 11: 74–80
64. **Roberts, E.A.:** Nonalcoholic steatohepatitis in children. Curr. Gastroenterol. Rep. 2003; 5: 253–259
65. **Saibara, T.:** "Insuffient" leptin production for the fat mass: a risk factor for nonalcoholic steatohepatitis in obese patients? J. Gastroenterol. 2003; 38: 522–523
66. **Savas, M.C., Koruk, M., Pirim, I., Yilmaz, O., Karakok, M., Taysi, S., Yilmaz, A.:** Serum ubiquitin levels in patients with nonalcoholic steatohepatitis. Hepato-Gastroenterol. 2003; 50: 738–741
67. **Shimada, M., Hashimoto, E., Kaneda, H., Noguchi, S., Hayashi, N.:** Nonalcoholic steatohepatitis: risk factors for liver fibrosis. Hepatol. Res. 2002; 24: 429–438
68. **Sorbi, D., Boynton, J., Lindor, K.D.:** The ratio of aspartate aminotransferase to alanine aminotransferase: potential value in differentiating non-alcoholic steatohepatitis from alcoholic liver disease. Amer. J. Gastroenterol. 1999; 94: 1018–1021
69. **Struben, V.M.D., Espenheide, E.E., Caldwell, S.H.:** Nonalcoholic steatohepatitis and cryptogenic cirrhosis within kindreds. Amer. J. Med. 2000; 108: 9–13
70. **Sumida, Y., Nakashima, T., Yoh, T., Furutani, M., Hirohama, A., Kakisaka, Y., Nakajima, Y., Ishikawa, H., Mitsuyoshi, H., Okanoue, T., Kashima, K., Nakamura, H., Yodoi, J.:** Serum thioredoxin levels as a predictor of steatohepatitis in patients with nonalcoholic fatty liver disease. J. Hepatol. 2003; 38: 32–38
71. **Tajiri, K., Takenawa, H., Yamaoka, K., Yamane, M., Marumo, F., Sato, C.:** Nonalcoholic steatohepatitis masquerading as autoimmune hepatitis. J. Clin. Gastroenterol. 1997; 25: 538–540
72. **Thaler, H.:** Die Fettleber und ihre pathogenetische Beziehung zur Leberzirrhose. Virch. Arch. Path. Anat. 1962; 335: 180–210
73. **Yang, S.Q., Lin, H.Z., Lane, M.D., Clemens, M., Diehl, A.M.:** Obesity increases sensitivity to endotoxin liver injury: implications for the pathogenesis of steatohepatitis. Proc. Nat. Acad. Sci. 1997; 94: 2557–2562
74. **Zamin, I., Alves-de-Mattos, A., Zettler, C.G.:** Nonalcoholic steatohepatitis in nondiabetic obese patients. Can. J. Gastroenterol. 2002; 16: 303–307

Reye's syndrome

75. **Arrowsmith, J.B., Kennedy, D.L., Kuritsky, J.N., Faich, G.A.:** National patterns of aspirin use and Reye's syndrome reporting United States, 1980 to 1985. Pediatrics 1987; 79: 858–863
76. **Belay, E.D., Bresee, J.S., Holman, R.C., Khan, A.S., Shahriari, A., Schonberger, L.B.:** Reye's syndrome in the United States from 1981 through 1997. New Engl. J. Med. 1999; 340: 1377–1382
77. **Brain, W.R., Hunter, D., Turnbull, H.M.:** Acute meningo-encephalomyelitis of childhood: report of six cases. Lancet 1929/I: 221–227
78. **Casteels-van Daele, M., Eggermont, E.:** Reye's syndrome. Brit. Med. J. 1994; 308: 919–920
79. **Gauthier, M., Guay, J., Lacroix, J., Lortie, A.:** Reye's syndrome: a reappraisal of diagnosis in 49 presumptive cases. Amer. J. Dis. Child. 1989; 143: 1181–1185
80. **Glasgow, J.F.:** Reye's syndrome: The case for a causal link with aspirin. Drug Safety 2006; 29: 1111–1121
81. **Hall, S.M., Plaster, P.A., Glasgow, J.F., Hancock, P.:** Preadmission antipyretics in Reye's syndrome. Arch. Dis. Child. 1988; 63: 857–866
82. **Hardie, R.M., Newton, L.H., Bruce, J.C., Glasgow, J.F.T., Mowat, A.P., Stephenson, J.B.P., Hall, S.M.:** The changing clinical pattern of Reye's syndrome 1982–1990. Arch. Dis. Childh. 1996; 74: 400–405
83. **Heubi, J.E., Partin, J.C., Partin, J.S., Schubert, W.K:** Reye's syndrome: current concepts. Hepatology 1987; 7: 155–164
84. **Hilty, M.D., McClung, H.-J., Haynes, R.E., Romshe, C.A., Sherard, E.S.:** Reye's syndrome in siblings. J. Pediatr. 1979; 94: 576–579
85. **Meythaler, J.M., Varma, R.R.:** Reye's syndrome in adults. Diagnostic considerations. Arch. Intern. Med. 1987; 147: 61–64
86. **Pinsky, P.F., Hurwitz, E.S., Schonberger, L.B., Gunn, W.J.:** Reye's syndrome and aspirin. Evidence for a dose-response effect. J. Amer. Med. Ass. 1988; 260: 657–661
87. **Reye, R.D.K., Morgan, G., Baral, J.:** Encephalopathy and fatty degeneration of the viscera. A disease entity in childhood. Lancet 1963/II: 749–751
88. **Stillmann, A., Gitter, H., Shillington, D., Sobonya, R., Payne, C.M., Ettinger, D., Lee, M.S.:** Reye's syndrome in the adult: case report and review of the literature. Amer. J. Gastroenterol. 1983; 78: 365–368

Acute fatty liver of pregnancy

89. **Barton, J.R., Sibai, B.M., Mabie, W.C., Shanklin, D.R.:** Recurrent acute fatty liver of pregnancy. Amer. J. Obstet. Gynec. 1990; 163: 534–538
90. **Fesenmeier, M.F., Coppage, K.H., Lambers, D.S., Barton, J.R., Sibai, B.M.:** Acute fatty liver of pregnancy in 3 tertiary care centers. Amer. J. Obstetr. Gynecol. 2005; 192: 1416–1419
91. **Ko, H.H., Yoshida, E.:** Acute fatty liver of pregnancy. Can. J. Gastroenterol. 2006; 20: 25–30
92. **Kunelis, C.T., Peters, J.E., Edmondson, H.A.:** Fatty liver of pregnancy and its relation to tetracycline therapy. Amer. J. Med. 1985; 38: 359–377
93. **Mabie, W.C.:** Acute fatty liver of pregnancy. Gastroenterol. Clin. N. Amer. 1992; 21: 951–960
94. **McKee, C.M., Weir, P.E., Foster, J.H., Murnaghan, G.A., Callender, M.E.:** Acute fatty liver of pregnancy and diagnosis by computed tomography. Brit. Med. J. 1986; 292: 291–292
95. **Minuk, G.Y., Lui, R.C., Kelly, J.K.:** Rupture of the liver associated with acute fatty liver of pregnancy. Amer. J. Gastroenterol. 1987; 82: 457–460
96. **Moise, K.J., Shah, D.M.:** Acute fatty liver of pregnancy: etiology of fetal distress and fetal wastage. Obstetr. Gynec. 1987; 69: 482–485
97. **Ockner, S.A., Brunt, E.M., Cohn, S.M., Krul, E.S., Hanto, D.W., Peters, M.G.:** Fulminant hepatic failure caused by acute fatty liver of pregnancy treated by orthotopic liver transplantation. Hepatology 1990; 11: 59–64
98. **Reyes, H., Sandoval, L., Wainstein, A., Ribalta, J., Donoso, S., Smok, G., Rosenberg, H., Meneses, M.:** Acute fatty liver of pregnancy: a clinical study of 12 episodes in 11 patients. Gut 1994; 35: 101–106
99. **Riely, C.A., Latham, P.S., Romero, R., Duffy, T.P.:** Acute fatty liver of pregnancy. A reassessment based on observations in nine patients. Ann. Intern. Med. 1987; 106: 703–706

100. **Sheehan, H.L.:** The pathophysiology of acute yellow atrophy and delayed chloroform poisoning. J. Obstetr. Gynaec. Brit. Emp. 1940; 47: 49–62
101. **Sherlock, S.:** Acute fatty liver of pregnancy and the microvesicular fat diseases. Gut 1983; 24: 265–269
102. **Stander, H.J., Cadden, J.F.:** Acute yellow atrophy of liver in pregnancy. Amer. J. Obstetr. Gynec. 1934; 28: 61–69
103. **Tan, A.C.I.T.L., van Krieken, J.H.J.M., Peters, W.H.M., Steegers, E.A.P.:** Acute fatty liver in pregnancy (case report). Neth. J. Med. 2002; 60: 370–373
104. **Treem, W.R., Rinaldo, P., Hale, D.E., Stanley, C.A., Millington, D.S., Hyams, J.S., Jackson, S., Turnbull, D.M.:** Acute fatty liver of pregnancy and long-chain 3-hydroxyacyl coenzyme A dehydrogenase deficiency. Hepatology 1994; 19: 339–345
105. **Van Le, L., Podrasky, A.:** Computed tomographic and ultrasonographic findings in women with acute fatty liver of pregnancy. J. Reprod. Med. 1990; 35: 815–817
106. **Yang, W.W., Shen, Z.J., Peng, G.D., Chen, Y.G., Jiang, S.F., Kang, S.Y., Wu, J.C.:** Acute fatty liver of pregnancy: diagnosis and management of 8 cases. Chin. Med. J. 2000; 113: 540–543
107. **Zürcher, K.:** Unkomplizierte Zweitschwangerschaft nach akuter Schwangerschaftsfettleber. Schweiz. Med. Wschr. 1995; 125: 1003–1005

Mauriac syndrome
108. **Mandell, F., Berenberg, W.:** The Mauriac syndrome. Amer. J. Dis. Child. 1974; 127: 900–902

α_1-antitrypsin deficiency
109. **Bell, H., Schrumpf, E., Fagerhol, M.K.:** Heterozygous MZ alpha-1-antitrypsin deficiency in adults with chronic liver disease. Scand. J. Gastroenterol. 1990; 25: 778–792
110. **Carrell, R.W., Lomas, D.A.:** Mechanisms of disease-Alpha-1-antitrypsin deficiency. A model for conformational diseases (review). New Engl. J. Med. 2002; 346: 45–53
111. **Crystal, R.G.:** α_1-antitrypsin deficiency, emphysema and liver disease. Genetic basis and strategies for therapy. J. Clin. Invest. 1990; 85: 1343–1352
112. **Deutsch, J., Becker, H., Auböck, L.:** Histopathological features of liver disease in alpha-1 antitrypsin deficiency. Acta Paediatr. 1994; 393 (Suppl.): 8–12
113. **Eriksson, S., Elzouki, A.-N.:** α_1-Antitrypsin deficiency. Baill. J. Gastroenterol. 1998; 12: 257–273
114. **Filipponi, F., Soubrane, O., Labrousse, F., Devictor, D., Bernard, O., Valayer, J., Houssin, D.:** Liver transplantation for end-stage liver disease associated with α_1-antitrypsin deficiency in children: pretransplant natural history, timing and results of transplantation. J. Hepatol. 1994; 20: 72–78
115. **Fischer, H.-P., Ortiz-Pallardo, M.E., Ko, Y., Esch, C., Zhou, H.:** Chronic liver disease in heterozygous α_1-antitrypsin deficiency PiZ. J. Hepatol. 2000; 33: 883–892
116. **Francavilla, R., Castellaneta, S.P., Hadzic, N., Chambers, S.M., Portmann, B., Tung, J., Cheeseman, P., Heaton, N.D., Mieli-Vergani, G.:** Prognosis of alpha-1-antitrypsin deficiency-related liver disease in the era of pediatric liver transplantation. J. Hepatol. 2000; 32: 986–992
117. **Löhr, H.F., Schlaak, J.F., Dienes, H.P., Lorenz, J., Meyer zum Büschenfelde, K.-H., Gerken, G.:** Liver cirrhosis associated with heterozygous alpha-1-antitrypsin deficiency type PiMS and autoimmune features. Digestion 1995; 56: 41–45
118. **Lomas, D.A., Mahadeva, R.:** Alpha(1)-antitrypsin polymerization and the serpinopathies: pathobiology and prospects for therapy (review). J. Clin. Invest. 2002; 110: 1585–1590
119. **Mowat, A.P.:** Alpha-1-antitrypsin deficiency (PiZZ): features of liver involvement in childhood. Acta Paediatr. 1994; 393 (Suppl.): 13–17
120. **Pittschieler, K., Massi, G.:** Liver involvement in infants with PiSZ phenotype of α_1-antitrypsin deficiency. J. Pediatr. Gastro. Nutrit. 1992; 15: 315–318
121. **Prachalias, A.A., Kalife, M., Francavilla, R., Muiesan, P., Dhawan, A., Baker, A., Hadzic, D., Mieli-Vergani, G., Rela, M., Heaton, N.D.:** Liver transplantation for alpha-1-antitrypsin deficiency in children. Transplant. Internat. 2000; 13: 207–210
122. **Propst, T., Propst, A., Dietze, O., Judmaier, G., Braunsteiner, H., Vogel, W.:** Prevalence of hepatocellular carcinoma in alpha-1-antitrypsin deficiency. J. Hepatol. 1994; 21: 1006–1011
123. **Rudnick, D.A., Shikapwashya, O., Blomenkamp, K., Teckman, J.H.:** Indomethacin increases liver damage in a murine model of liver injury from alpha-1-antitrypsin deficiency. Hepatology 2006; 44: 976–982
124. **Sifers, R.N., Finegold, M.J., Woo, S.L.C.:** Molecular biology and genetic of α_1-antitrypsin deficiency. Semin. Liver Dis. 1992; 12: 301–310
125. **Steiner, S.J., Gupta, S.K., Croffie, J.M., Fitzgerald, J.F.:** Serum levels of alpha(1)-antitrypsin predict phenotypic expression of the alpha(1)-antitrypsin gene. Dig. Dis. Sci. 2003; 48: 1793–1796
126. **Sveger, T., Eriksson, S.:** The liver in adolescents with α_1-antitrypsin deficiency. Hepatology 1995; 22: 514–517
127. **Yoon, D., Kueppers, F., Genta, R.M., Klintmalm, G.B., Khaoustov, V.I., Yoffe, B.:** Role of alpha-1-antichymotrypsin deficiency in promoting cirrhosis in two siblings with heterozygous alpha-1-antitrypsin deficiency phenotype SZ (case report). Gut 2002; 50: 730–732
128. **Zhou, H., Ortiz-Pallardo, M.E., Ko, Y., Fischer, H.-P.:** Is heterozygous alpha-1-antitrypsin deficiency type PiZ a risk factor for primary liver carcinoma? Cancer 2000; 88: 2668–2676

Amyloidosis
129. **Arkenau, H.T., Widjaja, A.:** An unusual case of cholestasis and makrohematuria in a 52-year-old patient. Med. Klin. 2002; 97: 480–483
130. **Caballeria, J., Bruguera, M., Sole, M., Campistol, J.M., Rodes, J.:** Hepatic familial amyloidosis caused by a new mutation in the AL gene: clinical and pathological features. Amer. J. Gastroenterol. 2001; 96: 1872–1876
131. **Diel, R., Krüger, C.:** Primäre Amyloidose als seltene Ursache einer akuten Leberinsuffizienz. Dtsch. Med. Wschr. 1988; 113: 1433–1436
132. **Frank, H., Krammer, M., Fierlbeck, W., Rieß, R., Geiger, H.:** Unusual hepatorenal symptoms in amyloidosis. Med. Klin. 1999; 94: 274–278
133. **Gertz, M.A., Kyle, R.A.:** Hepatic amyloidosis: clinical appraisal in 77 patients. Hepatology 1997; 25: 118–121
134. **Harrison, R.F., Hawkins, P.N., Roche, W.R., MacMahon, R.F.T., Hubscher, S.G.:** "Fragile" liver and massive hepatic haemorrhage, due to hereditary amyloidosis. Gut 1996; 38: 151–152
135. **Hawkins, P.N., Pepys, M.B.:** Imaging amyloidosis with radiolabelled SAP. Eur. J. Nucl. Med. 1995; 22: 595–599
136. **Hoffmann, M.S., Stein, B.E., Davidian, M.M., Rosenthal, W.S.:** Hepatic amyloidosis presenting as severe intrahepatic cholestasis: a case report and review of the literature. Amer. J. Gastroenterol. 1988; 83: 783–785
137. **Holmgren, G., Ericzon, B.G., Groth, C.G., Stein, L., Suhr, O., Andersen, O., Wallin, B.G., Seymour, A., Richardson, S., Hawkins, P.N., Petys, M.B.:** Clinical improvement and amyloid regression after liver transplantation in hereditary transthyretin amyloidosis. Lancet 1993; 341: 1113–1116
138. **Iwai, M., Ishii, Y., Mori, T., Harada, Y., Kitagawa, Y., Kashiwadani, M., Ou, O., Okanoue, T., Kashima, K.:** Cholestatic jaundice in two patients with primary amyloidosis. Ultrastructural findings of the liver. J. Clin. Gastroenterol. 1999; 28: 162–166
139. **Jorquera Plaza, F., Fernandez Gundin, M.J., Espinel Diez, J., Munoz Nunez, F., Herrera Abian, A., Garcia Lagarto, E., Olcoz Goni, J.L.:** Ictericia colestasica como forma de presentacion de una amiloidosis sistemica. Rev. Esp. Enferm. Dig. 1997; 89: 859–861
140. **Kumar, K.S., Lefkowitch, J., Russo, M.W., Hesdorffer, C., Kinkhabwala, M., Kapur, S., Emond, J.C., Brown, R.S.:** Successful sequential liver and stem cell transplantation for hepatic failure due to primary AL amyloidosis. Gastroenterology 2002; 122: 2026–2031
141. **Llovat, L.B., Persey, M.R., Madhoo, S., Hawkins, P.N.:** The liver in systemic amyloidosis: insights from 123I serum amyloid P component scintigraphy in 484 patients. Gut 1998; 42: 727–734
142. **Mainenti, P.P., D'Agostino, L., Soscia, E., Romano, M., Salvatore, M.:** Hepatic and splenic amyloidosis: dual-phase spiral CT findings. Abdom. Imag. 2003; 28: 688–690
143. **Mohr, A., Miehlke, S., Klauck, S., Röcken, C., Malfertheiner, P.:** Hepatomegaly and cholestasis as primary clinical manifestations of an AL-kappa amyloidosis. Europ. J. Gastroenterol. Hepatol. 1999; 11: 921–925
144. **Monzawa, S., Tsukamoto, T., Omata, K., Hosoda, K., Araki, T., Sugimura, K.:** A case with primary amyloidosis of the liver and spleen: radiologic findings. Eur. J. Radiol. 2002; 41: 237–241
145. **Nowak, G., Westermark, P., Wernerson, A., Herlenius, G., Sletten, K., Ericzon, B.G.:** Liver transplantation as rescue treatment in a patient with primary AL kappa amyloidosis. Transpl. Internat. 2000; 13: 92–97
146. **Peters, R.A., Koukoulis, G., Glimson, A., Portamnn, B., Westaby, D., William, R.:** Primary amyloidosis and severe intrahepatic cholestatic jaundice. Gut 1994; 35: 1322–1325
147. **Sandberg-Gertzen, H., Ericzon, B.G., Blomberg, B.:** Primary amyloidosis with spontaneous splenic rupture, cholestasis, and liver failure treated with emergency liver transplantation. Amer. J. Gastroenterol. 1998; 93: 2254–2256
148. **Straub, R.F., Boyer, T.D.:** The liver-spleen scan in systemic amyloidosis: a clue to the diagnosis. J. Clin. Gastroenterol. 1993; 16: 340–343
149. **Ubina Aznar, E., Fernandez Moreno, N., Rivera Irigoin, R., Moreno Mejias, P., Fernandez Perez, F., Vera Rivero, F., Navarro Jarabo, J.M., Garcia Fernandez, G., de Sola Earle, C., Perez Aisa, A., Sanchez Santos, A.:** Massive hepatic amyloidosis with fatal hepatic failure (case report). Rev. Espan. Enferm. Dig. 2006; 98: 551–552

α_1-antichymotrypsin deficiency
150. **Callea, F., Brisigotti, M., Fabbretti, G., Bonino, F., Desmet, V.J.:** Hepatic endoplasmatic reticulum storage diseases. Liver 1992; 12: 357–362
151. **Eriksson, S., Lindmark, B., Lilja, H.:** Familial α_1-antichymotrypsin deficiency. Acta Med. Scand. 1986; 220: 447–453
152. **Lindmark, B., Eriksson, S.:** Partial deficiency of α_1-antichymotrypsin is associated with chronic cryptogenetic liver disease. Scand. J. Gastroenterol. 1991; 26: 508–512

Hereditary tyrosinaemia
153. **Dehner, L.P., Snover, D.C., Sharp, H.L., Ascher, N., Nakhleh, R., Day, D.L.:** Hereditary tyrosinemia type I (chronic form): Pathologic findings in the liver. Hum. Path. 1989; 20: 149–158
154. **Demers, S.I., Russo, P., Lettre, F., Tanguay, R.M.:** Frequent mutation reversion inversely correlates with clinical severity in a genetic liver disease, hereditary tyrosinemia. Hum. Pathol. 2003; 34: 1313–1320
155. **Freese, D.K., Tuchman, M., Schwarzenberg, S.J., Sharp, H.L., Rank, J.M., Bloomer, J.R., Ascher, N.L., Payne, W.D.:** Early liver transplan-

tation is indicated for tyrosinemia type I. J. Paediatr. Gastroenterol. Nutr. 1991; 13: 10−15
156. Grompe, M.: The pathophysiology and treatment of hereditary tyrosinemia type I. Semin. Liver Dis. 2001; 21: 563−571
157. Kvittingen, E.A.: Hereditary tyrosinemia type I − an overview. Scand. J. Clin. Lab. Invest. 1986; 46: 27−34
158. Lindstedt, S., Holme, E., Lock, E.A., Hjalmarson, O., Strandvik, B.: Treatment of hereditary tyrosinaemia type I by inhibition of 4-hydroxyphenylpyruvate dioxygenase. Lancet 1992; 340: 813−817
159. Macvicar, D., Dicks-Mireaux, C., Leonard, J.V., Wight, D.G.D: Hepatic imaging with computed tomography of chronic tyrosinaemia type 1. Brit. J. Radiol. 1990; 63: 605−608
160. Van Spronsen, F.J., Thomasse, Y., Smith, G.P.A., Leonard, J.V., Clayton, P.T., Fidler, V., Berger, R., Heymans, H.S.A.: Hereditary tyrosinemia type I: a new clinical classification with difference in prognosis on dietary treatment. Hepatology 1994; 20: 1187−1191

Disturbances of the urea cycle
161. Berry, G.T., Steiner, R.D.: Long-term management of patients with urea cycle disorders. J. Pediatr. 2001; 138: 56−60
162. Maestri, N.E., Brusilow, S.w., Clissold, D.B., Bassett, S.S.: Long-term treatment of girls with ornithine transcarbamylase deficiency. New Engl. J. Med. 1996; 335: 855−859
163. Mönch, E., Hoffmann, G.F., Przyrembel, H., Colombo, J.-P., Wermuth, B., Leonard, J.V.: Diagnosis and treatment of ornithine transcarbamylase (OTC)-deficiency. Mschr. Kinderheilkd. 1998; 146: 652−658
164. Takagi, H., Hagiwara, S., Hashizume, H., Kanda, D., Sato, K., Sohara, N., Kakizaki, S., Takahashi, H., Mori, M., Kaneko, H., Ohwada, S., Ushikai, M., Kobayashi, K., Saheki, T.: Adult onset type II citrullinemia as a cause of non-alcoholic steatohepatatis (case report). J. Hepatol. 2006; 44: 236−239
165. Tuchman, M., Matsuda, I., Munnich, A., Malcolm, S., Strautnieks, S., Briede, T.: Proportions of spontaneous mutations in males and females with ornithine transcarbamylase deficiency. Amer. J. Med. Genet. 1995; 55: 67−70

Glycogen storage diseases
166. Bodamer, O.A., Feillet, F., Lane, R.E., Lee, P.J., Dixon, M.A., Halliday, D., Leonard, J.V.: Utilization of cornstarch in glycogen storage disease type Ia. Eur. J. Gastroenterol. Hepatol. 2002; 14: 1251−1256
167. Burchell, A.: Glycogen storage diseases and the liver. Baill. Clin. Gastroenterol. 1998; 12: 337−353
168. Conti, J.A., Kemeny, N.: Type Ia glycogenosis associated with hepatocellular carcinoma. Cancer 1992; 69: 1320−1322
169. Demo, E., Frush, D., Gottfried, M., Koepke, J., Boney, A., Bali, D., Chen, Y.T. Kishnani, P.S.: Glycogen storage disease type III-hepatocellular carcinoma a long-term complication? J. Hepatol. 2007; 46: 492−498
170. De Moor, R.A., Schweizer, J.J., van Hoek, B., Wasser, M., Vink, R., Maaswinkel-Mooy, P.D.: Hepatocellular carcinoma in glycogen storage disease type IV. Arch. Dis. Childh. 2000; 82: 479−480
171. Fernandes, J.: Glycogen storage disease: recommendations for treatment. Europ. J. Pediat. 1988; 147: 226−228
172. Lee, P., Mather, S., Owens, J., Leonard, J., Dicksmireaux, C.: Hepatic ultrasound findings in the glycogen storage diseases. Brit. J. Radiol. 1994; 67: 1062−1066
173. Lei, K.-J., Pan, C.-J., Liu,J.-L., Shelly, L.L., Yang Chou, J.: Structure-function analysis of human glucose-6-phosphatase, the enzyme deficient in glycogen storage disease type Ia. J. Biol. Chem. 1995; 270: 11882−11886
174. Limmer, J., Fleig, W.E., Leupold, D., Bittner, R., Ditschuneit, H., Beger, H.G.: Hepatocellular carcinoma in type I glycogen storage disease. Hepatology 1988; 8: 531−537
175. Marfaing-Koka, A., Wolf, M., Boyer-Neumann, C., Meyer, D., Odièvre, T., Labrune, T.: Increased levels of hemostatic proteins are independent of inflammation in glycogen storage disease type Ia. J. Pediatr. Gastroenterol. Nutr. 2003; 37: 586−570
176. Martin, R., Schlotter, B., Müller-Höcker, J., Loeschke, K., Pongratz, D., Folwaczny, C.: 26-year old female patient with elevated liver enzymes. Z. Gastroenterol. 2002; 40: 885−890
177. Parker, P., Burr, I., Slonimi, A., Ghishan, F.K., Greene, H.: Regression of hepatic adenomas in type Ia glycogen storage disease with dietary therapy. Gastroenterology 1981; 81: 534−536
178. Rosh, J.R., Collins, J., Groisman, G.M., Schwersenz, A.H., Schwartz, M., Miller, C.M., LeLeiko, N.S.: Management of hepatic adenoma in glycogen storage disease Ia. J. Pediatr. Gastroenterol. Nutr. 1995; 20: 225−228
179. Selby, R., Starzl, T.E., Yunis, E., Todo, S., Tzakis, A.G., Brown, B.I., Kendall, R.S.: Liver transplantation for type I and type IV glycogen storage disease. Eur. J. Pediatr. 1993; 152 (Suppl. 1) 71−76
180. Siciliano, M., de Candia, E., Ballarin, S., Vecchio, F.M., Servidei, S., Annese, R., Landolfi, R., Rossi, L.: Hepatocellular carcinoma complicating liver cirrhosis in type IIIa glycogen storage disease. J. Clin. Gastroenterol. 2000; 31: 80−82
181. Talente, G.M., Coleman, R.A., Alter, C., Baker, L., Brown, B.I., Cannon, R.A., Chen, Y.-T., Crigler, J.F., Ferreira, P., Haworth, J.C., Herman, G.E., Issenman, R.M., Keating, J.P., Linde, R., Roe, T.F., Senior, B., Wolfsdorf, J.I.: Glycogen storage disease in adults. Ann. Intern. Med. 1994; 120: 218−226

Galactose intolerance
182. Berry, G.T., Nissim, I., Lin, Z., Mazur, A.T., Gibson, J.B., Segal, S.: Endogenous synthesis of galactose in normal men and patients with hereditary galactosaemia. Lancet 1995; 346: 1073−1074

183. Kumar, M., Yachha, S.K., Gupta, R.K.: Neonatal cholestasis syndrome due to galactosemia. Ind. J. Gastroenterol. 1996; 15: 26−27
184. Monk, A.M., Mitchell, A.J.H., Milligan, D.W.A., Holton, J.B.: The diagnosis of classical galactosaemia. Arch. Dis. Childh. 1977; 52: 943−946
185. Reichhard, J.K.V.: Mutations in galactosemia. Amer. J. Hum. Genet. 1995; 57: 978−979
186. Schweitzer, S., Shin, Y., Jakobs, C., Brodehl, J.: Long-term outcome in 134 patients with galactosaemia. Eur. J. Pediatr. 1993; 152: 36−43

Fructose intolerance
187. Ali, M., Rellos, P., Cox, T.M.: Hereditary fructose intolerance. J. Med. Genet. 1998; 35: 353−365
188. Mock, D.M., Perman, J.A., Thaler, M.M., Morris, R.C.: Chronic fructose intoxication after infancy in children with hereditary fructose intolerance. A cause of growth retardation. New Engl. J. Med. 1983; 309: 764−770
189. Odièvre, M., Gentil, C., Gautier, M., Alagille, D.: Hereditary fructose intolerance in childhood. Diagnosis, management and course in 55 patients. Amer. J. Dis. Childh. 1978; 132: 605−608
190. Stormon, M.O., Cutz, E., Furuya, K., Bedford, M., Yerkes, L., Tolan, D.R., Feigenbaum, A.: A six-month-old infant with liver steatosis. J. Pediatr. 2004; 144: 258−263
191. Tolan, D.R.: Molecular basis of hereditary fructose intolerance: mutations and polymorphisms in the human aldolase B gen. Hum. Mut. 1995; 6: 210−218

Wolman's disease
192. Fitoussi, G., Nègre-Salvayre, A., Pieraggi, M.-T., Salvayre, R.: New pathogenetic hypothesis for Wolman's disease: possible role of oxidized low-density lipoproteins in adrenal necrosis and calcification. Biochem. J. 1994; 301: 267−273
193. Lin, H.J., Jie, L.K., Ho, F.C.S.: Accumulation of glyceryl ether lipids in Wolman's disease. J. Lipid. Res. 1976; 17: 53−56
194. Wolf, H., Nolte, K., Nolte, R.: Wolman-Syndrom. Mschr. Kinderheilk. 1973; 121: 697−698

Cholesterol ester storage disease
195. Beaudet, A.L., Ferry, G.D., Nichols, B.F.jr., Rosenberg, H.S.: Cholesterol ester storage disease: clinical, biochemical, and pathological studies. J. Pediatr. 1977; 90: 910−914
196. Kale, A.S., Ferry, G.D., Hawkins, E.P.: End-stage renal disease in a patient with cholesteryl ester storage disease following successful liver transplantation and cyclosporine immunosuppression. J. Pediatr. Gastroenterol. Nutrit. 1995; 20: 95−97
197. Kelly, D.R., Hoeg, J.M., Demosky S.J.jr., Brewer, H.B.jr.: Characterization of plasma lipids and lipoproteins in cholesteryl ester storage disease. Biochem. Med. 1985; 33: 29−37
198. Kuntz, H.D., May, B., Schejbal, V., Assmann, G.: Cholesterinester-Speicherkrankheit der Leber. Leber Magen Darm 1981; 11: 258−263
199. Limbach, A., Stepperger, K., Naumann, A., Sandig, K., Lohse, P., Keller, E.: Cholesteryl ester storage disease as cause of hepatomegaly in childhood. Mschr. Kinderheilk. 2003; 151: 953−956

Cerebrotendinous xanthomatosis
200. Berginer, V.M., Salen, G., Shefer, S.: Long-term treatment of cerebrotendinous xanthomatosis with chenodeoxycholic acid. New Engl. J. Med. 1984; 311: 1649−1652
201. Berginer, V.M., Shany, S., Alkalay, D., Berginer, J., Dekel, S., Salen, G., Tint, G.S., Gazit, D.: Osteoporosis and increased bone fractures in cerebrotendinous xanthomatosis. Metabolism 1993; 42: 69−74
202. Cali, J.J., Hsieh, C.L.,Franke, U., Russel, D.W.: Mutations in the bile acid biosynthetic enzyme sterol 27-hydroxylase underlie cerebrotendinous xanthomatosis. J. Biol. Chem. 1991; 266: 7779−7783
203. Leitersdorf, E., Meiner, V.: Cerebrotendinous xanthomatosis. Curr. Opin. Lipidol. 1994; 5: 138−142
204. Nakamura, T., Matsuzawa, Y., Takemura, K., Kubo, M., Miki, H., Tarui, S.: Combined treatment with chenodeoxycholic acid and pravastatin improves plasma cholestanol levels associated with marked regression of tendon xanthomas in cerebrotendinous xanthomatosis. Metabolism 1991; 40: 741−746
205. Salen, G., Berginer, V.M., Shore, V., Horak, I., Horak, E., Tint, G.S., Shefer, S.: Increased concentrations of cholestanol and apolipoprotein B in the cerebrospinal fluid of patients with cerebrotendinous xanthomatosis. New Engl. J. Med. 1987; 316: 1233−1238

Abeta-hypobetalipoproteinaemia
206. Black, D.D., Hay, R.V., Rohwer-Nutter, P.L., Ellinas, H., Stephens, J.K., Sherman, H., Teng, B.-B., Whitington, P.F., Davidson, N.O.: Intestinal and hepatic apolipoprotein B gene expression in abetalipoproteinemia. Gastroenterology 1991; 101: 520−528
207. Castellano, G., Garfia, C., Gomez-Coronado, D., Arenas, J., Manzanares, J., Colina, F., Solis-Herruzo, J.A.: Diffuse fatty liver in familial heterozygous hypobetalipoproteinemia. J. Clin. Gastroenterol. 1997; 25: 379−382
208. Gregg, R.E., Wetterau, J.R.: The molecular basis of abetalipoproteinemia. Curr. Opin. Lipidol. 1994; 5: 81−86
209. Hagve, T.-A., Myrseth, L.-E., Schrumpf, E., Blomhoff, J.-P., Christophersen, B., Elgjo, K., Gjone, E., Prydz, H.: Liver steatosis in hypobetalipoproteinemia. A case report. J. Hepatol. 1991; 13: 104−111
210. Linton, M.F., Farese, R.V., Young, S.G.jr.: Familial hypobetalipoproteinemia. J. Lipid. Res. 1993; 34: 521−541

211. **Rader, D.J., Brewer, H.B.:** Abetalipoproteinemia: New insights into lipoprotein assembly and vitamin E metabolism from a rare genetic disease. J. Amer. Med. Ass. 1993; 270: 865–869
212. **Wetterau, J.R., Aggerbeck, L.P., Bouma, M.E., Eisenberg, C, Munck, A., Hermier, M., Gay, G., Rader, D.J., Gregg, R.E.:** Absence of microsomal triglyceride transfer protein in individuals with abetalipoproteinemia. Science 1992; 258: 999–1001

Hypoalphalipoproteinaemia
213. **Brooks-Wilson, A., Marcil, M., Clee, S.M. et al.:** Mutations in ABC1 in Tangier disease and familial high-density lipoprotein deficiency. Nature Genet. 1999; 22: 336–345
214. **Dechelotte, P., Kantelip, B., de Laguillamie, B.V.:** Tangier disease. A histological and ultrastructural study. Path. Res. Pract. 1985; 180: 424–430
215. **Velicia Llames, M.R., Gonzalez Hernandez, J.M., Sanz Santa Cruz, C., Fernandez Orcajo, P., Martinez Barrero, F.:** Elevacion de gammaglutamiltranspeptidasa en pacientes con hipoalfalipoproteinemia y dislipemias tipo IIa compensadas. Gastroenterol. Hepatol. 1995; 18: 319–322

Gaucher's disease
216. **Aderka, D., Garfinkel, D., Rothem, A., Pinkhas, J.:** Fatal bleeding from esophageal varices in a patient with Gaucher's disease. Amer. J. Gastroenterol. 1982; 77: 838–839
217. **Barton, N.W., Brady, R.O., Dambrosia, J.M., Di Bisceglie, A.M., Doppelt, S.H., Hill, S.C., Mankin, H.J., Murray, G.J., Parker, R.I., Argoff, C.E., Grewal, P.P., Yu, K.-T.:** Replacement therapy for inherited enzyme deficiency: macrophage targeted glucocerebrosidase for Gaucher's disease. New Engl. J. Med. 1991; 324: 1464.
218. **Beck, M., Valadares, E.R., Lotz, J.:** Gaucher's disease. Therapy by intravenous infusions of modified glucocerebrosidase. Clin. Invest. 1993; 71: 78.
219. **Beutler, E.:** Gaucher's disease: new molecular approaches to diagnosis and treatment. Science 1992; 256: 794–799
220. **Cox, T., Lachmann, R., Hollak, C., Aerts, J., van Weely, S., Hrebicek, M., Platt, F., Butters, T., Dwek, R., Moyses, C., Gow, I., Elstein, D., Zimran, A.:** Novel oral treatment of Gaucher's disease with N-butyl-deoxynojirimycin (OGT 918) to decrease substrate biosynthesis. Lancet 2000; 355: 1481–1485
221. **Fallet, S., Grace, M.E., Sibille, A., Mendelson, D.S., Shapiro, R.S., Hermann, G.; Grabowski, G.A.:** Enzyme augmentation in moderate to life-threatening Gaucher's disease. Pediat. Res. 1992; 31: 496–502
222. **Figueroa, M.L., Rosenbloom, B.E., Kay, A.C., Garver, P., Thurston, D.W., Koziol, J.A., Gelbart, T., Beutler, E.:** A less costly regimen of alglucerase to treat Gaucher's disease. New Engl. J. Med. 1992; 327: 1632–1636
223. **Harzer, K.:** Enzymic diagnosis in 27 cases with Gaucher's disease. Clin. Chim. Acta 1980; 106: 9–15
224. **James, S.P., Stromeyer, F.W., Chang, C., Barranger, J.A.:** Liver abnormalities in patients with Gaucher's disease. Gastroenterology 1981; 80: 126–133
225. **Kohn, D.B., Nolta, J.A., Weinthal, J., Bahner, I., Yu, X.J., Lilley, J., Crooks, G.M.:** Toward gene therapy for Gaucher's disease. Human Gene Ther. 1991; 2: 101–105
226. **Mistry, P.K.:** Genotype/phenotype correlations in Gaucher's disease. Lancet 1995; 346: 982–983
227. **Niederau, C., Holderer, A., Heintges, T., Strohmeyer, G.:** Glucocerebrosidase for treatment of Gaucher's disease: first German long-term results. J. Hepatol. 1994; 21: 610–617
228. **Peters, S.P., Lee, R.E., Glew, R.H.:** Gaucher's disease, a review. Medicine 1977; 56: 425–442
229. **Ringden, O., Groth, C.-G., Erikson, A., Bäckman, L., Granqvist, S., Mansson, J.-E., Svennerholm, L.:** Long-term follow-up of the first succesful bone marrow transplantation in Gaucher's disease. Transplantation 1988; 46: 66–70
230. **Stone, R., Benson, J., Tronic, B., Brennan, T.:** Hepatic calcifications in a patient with Gaucher's disease. Amer. J. Gastroenterol. 1982; 77: 95–98
231. **Tjhen, K.Y., Zillhardt, H.W.:** M. Gaucher Typ 1. Verlauf von 4 Geschwistererkrankungen vor und nach Splenektomie. Pädiat. Prax. 1977; 18: 247–260
232. **Zimran, A., Sorge, J., Gross, E., Kubitz, M., West, C., Beutler, E.:** Prediction of severity of Gaucher's disease by identification of mutations at DNA level. Lancet 1989/II: 349–352

Niemann-Pick disease
233. **Birch, N.C., Radio, S., Horslen, S.:** Metastatic hepatocellular carcinoma in a patient with Niemann-Pick disease, type C. J. Pediatr. Gastroenterol. Nutr. 2003; 37: 624–626
234. **Kulinski, A., Vance, J.E.:** Lipid homeostasis and lipoprotein secretion in Niemann-Pick C1-deficient hepatocytes. J. Biol. Chem. 2007; 282: 1627–1637
235. **Putterman, C., Zelingher, J., Shouval, D.:** Liver failure and the sea-blue histiocyte/adult Niemann-Pick disease. Case report and review of the literature. J. Clin. Gastroenterol. 1992; 15: 146–149
236. **Smanik, E.J., Tavill, A.S., Jacobs, G.H., Schafer, I.A., Farquhar, L., Weber, F.L., Mayes, J.T., Schulack, J.A., Petrelli, M., Zirzow, G.C., Oliver, J.W., Miller, S.P.F., Brady, R.O.:** Orthotopic liver transplantation in two adults with Niemann-Pick and Gaucher's disease: implications for the treatment of inherited metabolic disease. Hepatology 1993; 17: 42–49

237. **Tassoni, J.P., Fawaz, K.A., Johnston, D.E.:** Cirrhosis and portal hypertension in a patient with adult Niemann-Pick disease. Gastroenterology 1991; 100: 567–569
238. **Vellodi, A., Hobbs, J.R., O'Donnell, N.M., Coulter, B.S., Hugh-Jones, K.:** Treatment of Niemann-Pick disease type B by allogeneic bone marrow transplantation. Brit. Med. J. 1987; 295: 1375–1376
239. **Yerusalem, B., Sokol, R.J., Narkewicz, M.R., Smith, D., Ashmead, J.W., Wenger, D.A.:** Niemann-Pick disease type C in neonatal cholestasis at a North American center. J. Pediatr. Gastroenterol. Nutrit. 2002; 35: 44–50
240. **Zhou, H., Linke, R.P., Schaefer, H.E., Möbius, W., Pfeifer, U.:** Progressive liver failure in a patient with adult Niemann-Pick disease associated with generalized AL amyloidosis. Virchows Arch. 1995; 426: 635–639

Mucoviscidosis
241. **Akata, D., Akhan, O.:** Liver manifestations of cystic fibrosis (review). Eur. J. Radiol. 2007; 61: 11–17
242. **Brigman, C., Feranchak, A.:** Liver involvement in cystic fibrosis. Curr. Treat. Opin. Gastroenterol. 2006; 9: 484–496
243. **Colombo, C., Battezzati, P.M., Podda, M., Bettinardi, N., Giunta, A.:** Ursodeoxycholic acid for liver disease associated with cystic fibrosis: a double blind multicenter trial. Hepatology 1996; 23: 1484–1490
244. **Colombo, C., Battezzati, P.M., Crosignani, A., Morabito, A., Constantini, D., Padoan, R., Giunta, A.:** Liver disease in cystic fibrosis: a prospective study on incidence, risk factors, and outcome. Hepatology 2002; 36: 1374–1382
245. **Couetil, J.P., Houssin, D.P., Dousset, B.E., Chevalier, P.G., Guinvarch, A., Loumet, D., Achkar, A., Carpentier, A.F.:** Combined heart-lung-liver, double lung-liver, and isolated liver transplantation for cystic fibrosis in children. Transpl. Int. 1997; 19: 33–39
246. **Dray-Charrier, N., Paul, A., Veissiere, D., Mergey, M., Scoazec, J.-Y., Chapeau, J., Brahimi-Horn, C., Housset, C.:** Expression of cystic fibrosis transmembrane conductance regulator in human gallbladder epithelial cells. Lab. Invest. 1995; 73: 828–836
247. **Gelman, M.S., Kopito, R.R.:** Rescuing protein conformation: prospects for pharmacological therapy in cystic fibrosis (review). J. Clin. Invest. 2002; 110: 1591–1597
248. **Hultcrantz, R., Mengarelli, S., Strandvik, B.:** Morphological findings in the liver of children with cystic fibrosis: a light and electron microscopical study. Hepatology 1986; 6: 881–889
249. **Lindblad, A., Glaumann, H., Strandvik, B.:** Natural history of liver disease in cystic fibrosis. Hepatology 1999; 30: 1151–1158
250. **O'Connor, P.J., Southern, K.W., Bowler, I.M., Irving, H.C., Robinson, P.J., Littlewood, J.M.:** The role of hepatobiliary scintigraphy in cystic fibrosis. Hepatology 1996; 23: 281–287
251. **Strandvik, B., Hultcrantz, R.:** Liver function and morphology during long-term fatty acid supplementation in cystic fibrosis. Liver 1994; 14: 32–36
252. **Williams, S.G.J., Evanson, J.E., Hodgson, M.E., Boultbee, J.E., Westaby, D.:** An ultrasound scoring system for the diagnosis of liver disease in cystic fibrosis. J. Hepatol. 1995; 22: 513–521
253. **Yang, Y., Raper, S.E., Cohn, J.A., Engelhardt, J.F., Wilson, J.M.:** An approach for treating the hepatobiliary disease of cystic fibrosis by somatic gene transfer. Proc. Nat. Acad. Sci. USA 1993; 90: 4601–4605

Zellweger's syndrome
254. **Danks, D.M., Tippett, P., Adams, C., Campbell, P.:** Cerebro-hepato-renal syndrome of Zellweger. J. Pediatr. 1975; 86: 382–387
255. **Eyssen, H., Eggermont, E., van Eldere, J., Jaeken, J., Parmentier, G., Janssen, G.:** Bile acid abnormalities and the diagnosis of cerebro- hepato-renal syndrome (Zellweger's syndrome). Acta Paediatr. Scand. 1985; 74: 539–544
256. **Mathis, R.K., Watkins, J.B., van Szczepanik-van Leeuwen, P., Lott, I.T.:** Liver in the cerebro-hepato-renal syndrome: defective bile acid synthesis and abnormal mitochondria. Gastroenterology 1980; 79: 1311–1317
257. **Moser, A.E., Sing, I., Brown, F.R., Solish, G.I., Kelley, R.I., Benke, P.J., Moser, H.W.:** The cerebrohepatorenal (Zellweger) syndrome. Increased levels and impaired degradation of very-long-chain fatty acids and their use in prenatal diagnosis. New Engl. J. Med. 1984; 310: 1141–1146
258. **Santos, M.J., Moser, A.B., Drwinga, H., Moser, H.W., Lazarow, P.B.:** Analysis of peroxisomes in lymphoblasts: Zellweger's syndrome and a patient with a deletion in chromosome 7. Pediatr. Res. 1993; 33: 441–444

Porphyrias
259. **Andant, C., Puy, H., Bogard, C., Faivre, J., Soulé, J.C., Nordmann, Y., Deybach, J.C.:** Hepatocellular carcinoma in patients with acute hepatic porphyria: frequency of occurrence and related factors. J. Hepatol. 2000; 32: 933–939
260. **Andersson, C., Thunell, S., Floderus, Y., Forsell, C., Lundin, G., Anvret, M., Lannfelt, L., Wetterberg, L., Lithner, F.:** Diagnosis of acute intermittent porphyria in northern Sweden: an evaluation of mutation analysis and biochemical methods. J. Intern. Med. 1995; 237: 301–308
261. **Andersson, C., Innala, E., Backstrom, T.:** Acute intermittent porphyria in women: clinical expression, use and experience of exogenous hormones. A population-based study in northern Sweden. J. Intern. Med. 2003; 254: 176–183
262. **Bjersing, L., Andersson, C., Lithner, F.:** Hepatocellular carcinoma in patients from northern Sweden with acute intermittent porphyria:

morphology and mutations. Canc. Epidem. Biomark. Prev. 1996; 5: 393–397
263. **Bloomer, J.R., Rank, J.M., Payne, W.D., Snover, D.C., Sharp, H.L., Zwiener, R.J., Carithers, R.L.:** Follow-up after liver transplantation for protoporphyric liver disease. Liver Transplant. Surg. 1996; 4: 269–275
264. **Bloomer, J.R.:** Liver metabolism of porphyrins and haem. J. Gastroenterol. Hepatol. 1998; 13: 324–329
265. **Bonkovsky, H.L., Schned, A.R.:** Fatal liver failure in protoporphyria. Synergism between ethanol excess and the genetic defect. Gastroenterology 1986; 90: 191–201
266. **Bonkovsky, H.L., Barnard, G.F.:** Diagnosis of porphyric syndromes: a practical approach in the era of molecular biology. Semin. Liver Dis. 1998; 18: 57–65
267. **Brenner, D.A., Didier, J.M., Frazier, F., Christensen, S.R., Evans, G.A., Dailey, H.A.:** A molecular defect in human protoporphyria. Amer. J. Hum. Genet. 1992; 50: 1203–1210
268. **Bruguera, M.:** Liver involvement in porphyria. Semin. Dermatol. 1986; 5: 178–185
269. **Cox, T.M., Alexander, G.J.M., Sarkany, R.P.E.:** Protoporphyria. Semin. Liver Dis. 1998; 18: 85–93
270. **Da Silva, V., Simonin, S., Deybach, J.C., Puy, H., Nordmann, Y.:** Variegate porphyria: diagnostic value of fluometric scanning of plasma porphyrins. Clin. Chim. Acta 1995; 238: 163–168
271. **Doss, M.O., Frank, M.:** Hepatobiliary implications and complications in protoporphyria: a 20-year study. J. Clin. Biochem. 1989; 22: 223–239
272. **Doss, M.O., Kühnel, A., Groß, U., Sieg, I.:** Hepatic porphyrias and alcohol. Med. Klin. 1999; 94: 314–328
273. **Doss, M.O., Gross, U., Puy, H., Doss, M., Kuhnel, A., Jacob, K., Deybach, J.C., Nordmann, Y.:** Coexistence of hereditary coproporphyria and porphyria cutanea tarda: a new type of a dual porphyria. Med. Klin. 2002; 97: 1–5
274. **Egger, N.G., Goeger, D.E., Payne, D.A., Miskovsky, E.P., Weinman, S.A., Anderson, K.E.:** Porphyria cutanea tarda. Multiplicity of risk factors includes HFE mutations, hepatitis C, and inherited uroporphyrinogen decarboxylase deficiency. Dig. Dis. Sci. 2002; 47: 419–426
275. **Elder, G.H.:** Porphyria cutanea tarda. Semin. Liver Dis. 1998; 18: 67–76
276. **Fargion, S., Sergi, C., Bissoli, F., Fracanzani, A.L., Suigo, E., Carrazzone, A., Roberto, C., Cappellini, M.D., Fiorelli, G.:** Lack of association between porphyria cutanea tarda and α_1-antitrypsin deficiency. Europ. J. Gastroenterol. Hepatol. 1996; 8: 387–391
277. **Fargion, S., Fracanzani, A.L.:** Prevalence of hepatitis C virus infection in porphyria cutanea tarda. J. hepatol. 2003; 39: 635–638
278. **Ferri, C., Baicchi, U., La Civita, L., Greco, F., Zigneco, A.L., Manns, M.P.:** Hepatitis C virus-related autoimmunity in patients with porphyria cutanea tarda. Eur. J. Clin. Invest. 1993; 23: 851–855
279. **Gisbert, J.P., Garcia-Buey, L., Pajares, J.M., Moreno-Otero, R.:** Prevalence of hepatitis C virus infection in porphyria cutanea tarda: systematic review and meta-analysis. J. Hepatol. 2003; 39: 620–627
280. **Gorchein, A.:** Drug treatment in acute porphyria. Brit. J. Clin. Pharmacol. 1997; 44: 427–434
281. **Grandchamp, B., Puy, H., Lam oril, J., Deybach, J.C., Nordmann, Y.:** Review: Molecular pathogenesis of hepatic acute porphyrias. J. Gastroenterol. Hepatol. 1996; 11: 1046–1052
282. **Groß, U., Frank, M., Doss, M.O.:** Hepatic complications of erythropoietic protoporphyria. Photoderm. Photoimmun. Photomed. 1998; 14: 52–57
283. **Horie, Y., Norimoto, M., Tajima, F., Sasaki, H., Nanba, E., Kawasaki, H.:** Clinical usefulness of cimetidine treatment for acute relapse in intermittend porphyria. Clin. Chim. Acta 1995; 234: 171–175
284. **Ishibashi, A., Ogata, R., Sakisaka, S., Kumashiro, R., Koga, Y., Mitsuyama, K., Kuromatsu, R., Uchimura, Y., Ijuin, H., Tanaka, K., Iwao, T., Ishii, K., Sata, M., Inoue, O., Kin, Y., Oizumi, K., Nishida, H., Imaizumi, T., Tanikawa, K.:** Erythropoietic protoporphyria with fatal failure. J. Gastroenterol. 1999; 34: 405–409
285. **Kauppinen, R., Mustajoki, P.:** Acute porphyria and hepatocellular carcinoma. Brit. J. Cancer 1988; 57: 117–120
286. **Kauppinen, R., Mustajoki, P.:** Prognosis of acute porphyria: occurrence of acute attacks, precipitating factors, and associated diseases. Medicine 1992; 71: 1–13
287. **Kauppinen, R., Timonen, K., Mustajoki, P.:** Treatment of the porphyrias. Ann. Med. 1994; 26: 31–38
288. **Logan, G.M., Weimer, M.K., Ellefson, M., Pierach, C.A., Bloomer, J.R.:** Bile porphyrin analysis in the evaluation of variegate porphyria. New Engl. J. Med. 1991; 324: 1408–1411
289. **MacDonald, D.M., Germain, D., Perrot, H.:** The histopathology and ultrastructure of liver disease in erythropoetic protoporphyria. Brit. J. Dermatol. 1981; 104: 7–17
290. **Manzione, N.C., Wolkoff, A.W., Sassa, S.:** Development of porphyria cutanea tarda after treatment with cyclophosphamide. Gastroenterology 1988; 95: 1119–1122
291. **Moore, M.R.:** Biochemistry of porphyria. Int. J. Biochem. 1993; 25: 1353–1368
292. **Mustajoki, P., Nordmann, Y.:** Early administration of heme arginate for acute porphyric attacks. Arch. Intern. Med. 1993; 153: 2004–2008
293. **Navas, S., Bosch, O., Castillo, I., Marriott, E., Carreno, V.:** Porphyria cutanea tarda and hepatitis C and B viruses infection: a retrospective study. Hepatology 1995; 21: 279–284
294. **Poh-Fitzpatrick, M.B.:** Clinical features of the porphyrias. Clin. Dermatol. 1998; 16: 251–264

295. **Rank, J.M., Carithers, R., Bloomer, J.:** Evidence for neurological dysfunction in end-stage protoporphyric liver disease. Hepatology 1993; 18: 1404–1409
296. **Salata, H., Cortes, J.M., Enriquez de Salamanca, R., Oliva, H., Castro, A., Kusak, E., Carreno, V., Hernandez Guio, C.:** Porphyria cutanea tarda and hepatocellular carcinoma. Frequency of occurrence and related factors. J. Hepatol. 1985; 1: 477–487
297. **Samuel, D., Boboc, B., Bernuau, J., Bismuth, H., Benhamou, J.P.:** Liver transplantation for protoporphyria. Evidence for the predominent role of the erythropoetic tissue in protoporphyria overproduction. Gastroenterology 1988; 95: 816–819
298. **Sarkany, R.P.E., Alexander, G.J.M., Cox, T.M.:** Recessive inheritance of erythropoietic protoporphyria with liver failure. Lancet 1994; 343: 1394–1396
299. **Sassa, S., Kappas, A.:** Molecular aspects of the inherited porphyrias. J. Intern. Med. 2000; 247: 169–178
300. **Scarlett, Y.V., Brenner, D.A.:** Porphyrias. J. Clin. Gastroenterol. 1998; 27: 192–198
301. **Siersema, P.D., Rademakers, L.H.P.M., Cleton, M.I., ten Kate, F.J.W., de Bruijn, W.C., Marx, J.J.M., Wilson, H.J.P.:** The difference in liver pathology between sporadic and familial forms of porphyria cutanea tarda: the role of iron. J. Hepatol. 1995; 23: 259–267
302. **Stockinger, L.:** Elektronenmikroskopische Befunde bei Leberbiopsien bei Porphyria cutanea tarda. Wien. Zschr. Inn. Med. 1996; 47: 459–465
303. **Tefferi, A., Colgan, J.P., Solberg, L.A.:** Acute porphyrias: diagnosis and management. Mayo Clin. Proc. 1994; 69: 991–995
304. **Tenhunen, R., Mustajoki, P.:** Acute porphyria: treatment with heme. Semin. Liver Dis. 1998; 18: 53–55
305. **Toback, A.C., Sassa, S., Poh-Fitzpatrick, M.B., Schechter, J., Zaider, E., Harber, L.C., Kappas, A.:** Hepatoerythropoietic porphyria: clinical, biochemical, and enzymatic studies in a three-generation family lineage. New Engl. J. Med. 1987; 316: 645–650
306. **Todd, D.J.:** Molecular genetics of erythropoietic protoporphyria. Photoderm. Photoimmun. Photomed. 1998; 14: 70–73
307. **Verneuil de, H., Bourgeois, F., de Rooij, F., Siersema, P.D., Wilson, J.H., Grandchamp, B., Nordmann, Y.:** Characterization of a new mutation (R 292 G) and a deletion at the human uroporphyrinogen decarboxylase locus in two patients with hepatoerythropoietic porphyria. Hum. Genet. 1992; 89: 548–552
308. **Wagner, S., Doss, M.O., Wittekind, C., Bäcker, U., Meessen, D., Schmidt, F.W.:** Erythrohepatische Protoporphyrie mit rasch progredienter Leberzirrhose. Dtsch. Med. Wschr. 1989; 114: 1837–1841
309. **Wassif, W.S., Deacon, A.C., Floderus, Y., Thunell, S., Peters, T.J.:** Acute intermittent porphyria: diagnostic conundrums. Eur. J. Clin. Chem. Clin. Biochem. 1994; 32: 915–921
310. **Wells, M.M., Golitz, L.E., Bender, B.J.:** Erythropoietic protoporphyria with hepatic cirrhosis. Arch. Dermatol. 1980; 116: 429–432

Wilson's disease
311. **Akil, M., Brewer, G.J.:** Psychiatric and behavioral abnormalities in Wilson's disease. Adv. Neurol. 1995; 65: 171–178
312. **Ala, A., Walker, A.P., Ashkan, K., Dooley, J.S., Schilsky, M.L.:** Wilson's disease. Lancet 2007; 369: 397–408
313. **Akpinar, E., Akhan, O.:** Liver imaging findings of Wilson's disease (review). Eur. J. Radiol. 2007; 61: 25–32
314. **Badii, M., Wong, H., Steinbrecher, U.P., Freeman, H.J.:** Wilson's disease in an elderly patient. Can. J. Gastroenterol. 1995; 9: 78–80
315. **Bearn, A.G., McKusick, V.A.:** Azure lunulae. An unusual change in the fingernails in two patients with hepatolenticular degeneration (Wilson's disease). J. Amer. Med. Ass. 1958; 166: 904–906
316. **Bellary, S.V., van Thiel, D.H.:** Wilson's disease: a diagnosis made in two individuals greater than 40 years of age. J. Okla. State Med. Assoc. 1993; 86: 441–444
317. **Bellary, S.V., Hassanein, T., van Thiel, D.H.:** Liver transplantation for Wilson's disease. J. Hepatol. 1995; 23: 373–381
318. **Bowcock, A.M., Farrer, L.A., Herbert, J.M., Agger, M., Sternlieb, I., Scheinberg, I.H., Buys, C.H.C.M., Scheffer, H., Frydman, M., Chajek-Saul, T., Bonne-Tamir, B., Caralli-Sforza, L.L.:** Eight closely linked loci place the Wilson's disease locus within 13q14-q21. Amer. J. Human. Genet. 1988; 43: 664–674
319. **Brewer, G.J.:** Practical recommendations and new therapies for Wilson's disease. Drugs 1995; 50: 240–249
320. **Bull, P.C., Thomas, G.R., Rommens, J.M., Forbes, J.R., Wilson Cox, D.:** The Wilson's disease gene is a putative copper transporting P-type ATPase similar to the Menkes gene. Nat. Genet. 1993; 5: 327–337
321. **Cairns, J.E., Wiliams, H.P., Walshe, J.M.:** "Sunflower cataract" in Wilson's disease. Brit. Med. J. 1969/III: 95–96
322. **Carpenter, T.O., Carnes, D.L.jr., Anast, C.S.:** Hypoparathyroidism in Wilson's disease. New Engl. J. Med. 1983; 309: 873–877
323. **Cauza, E., Maier-Dobersberger, T., Polli, C., Kaserer, K., Kramer, L., Ferenci, P.:** Screening for Wilson's disease in patients with liver diseases by serum ceruloplasmin. J. Hepatol. 1997; 27: 358–362
324. **Dameron, C.T., Harrison, M.D.:** Mechanisms for protection against copper toxicity. Amer. J. Clin. Nutr. 1998; 67 (Suppl.): 1091–1097
325. **Davis, W., Chowrimootoo, G.F.E., Seymour, C.A.:** Defective biliary copper excretion in Wilson's disease: the role of caeruloplasmin. Eur. J. Clin. Invest. 1996; 26: 893–901
326. **De Andrade, D.R., Fujito Neto, F.G., Vieira, G.S., Tiberio, I.F., Warth, M.P., Carlich, I.:** Acute hemolytic crisis followed by fulminant hepatic

failure with fatal outcome, as a first clinical manifestation of Wilson's disease. Rev. Hosp. Clin. Fac. Med. Sao Paulo 1994; 49: 69–75
327. Degenhardt, S., Blomhard, G., Hefter, H., Kreuzpaintner, G., Lindemann, W., Lobeck, H., Schnaith, E., Stremmel, W., Grabensee, B.: Hämolytische Krise mit Leberversagen als Erstmanifestation eines Morbus Wilson. Dtsch. Med. Wschr. 1994; 119: 1421–1426
328. Duvoux, C.: Severe hepatitis during Wilson's disease. Gastroenterol. Clin. Biol. 2004; 28 (Suppl. 5): 202–205
329. Erhardt, A., Hoffmann, A., Hefter, H., Häussinger, D.: HFE gene mutations and iron metabolism in Wilson's disease. Liver 2002; 22: 474–478
330. Fleischer, B.: Zwei weitere Fälle von grünlicher Verfärbung der Kornea. Klin. Mbl. Augenheilk. 1903; 41: 489–491
331. Fleischer, B.: Die periphere braungrünliche Hornhautverfärbung als Symptom einer eigenartigen Allgemeinerkrankung. Münch. Med. Wschr. 1909; 56: 1120–1123
332. Gitlin, J.D.: Wilson disease (review). Gastroenterology 2003; 125: 1868–1877
333. Gow, P.J., Smallwood, R.A., Angus, P.W., Smith, A.L., Wall, A.J., Sewell, R.B.: Diagnosis of Wilson's disease: an experience over three decades. Gut 2000; 46: 415–419
334. Gu, M., Cooper, J.M., Butler, P., Walker, A.P., Mistry, P.K., Dooley, J.S., Schapira, A.H.V.: Oxidative-phosphorylation defects in liver of patients with Wilson's disease. Lancet 2000; 356: 469–474
335. Hoogenraad, T.U., van den Hamer, C.J.A., van Hattum, J.: Effective treatment of Wilson's disease with oral zinc sulphate: two case reports. Brit. Med. J. 1984; 289: 273–276
336. Hoppe, B., Neuhaus, T., Superti-Furga, A., Forster, I., Leumann, E.: Hypercalciuria and nephrocalcinosis, a feature of Wilson's disease. Nephron 1993; 65: 460–462
337. Houwen, R.H.J., Roberts, E.A., Thomas, G.R., Cox, D.W.: DNA markers for the diagnosis of Wilson's disease. J. Hepatol. 1993; 17: 269–276
338. Huster, D., Hoppert, M., Lutsenko, S., Zinke, J., Lehmann, C., Mössner, J., Berr, F., Caca, K.: Defective cellular localization of mutant ATP 7B in Wilson's disease patients and hepatoma cell lines. Gastroenterology 2003; 124: 335–345
339. Kayser, B.: Über einen Fall von angeborener grünlicher Verfärbung der Cornea. Klin. Mbl. Augenheilk. 1902; 40: 22–25
340. Lutsenko, S., Barnes, N.L., Bartee, M.Y., Dmitriew, O.Y.: Function and regulation of human copper-transporting ATPases. Physiol. Rev. 2007; 87: 1011–1046
341. Magalhaes, A.C., Caramelli, P., Menezes, J.R., Lo, L.S., Bacheschi, L.A., Barbosa, E.R., Rosemberg, L.A., Magalhaes, A.: Wilson's disease: MRI with clinical correlation. Neuroradiology 1994; 36: 97–100
342. Maier-Dobersberger, T., Mannhalter, C., Rack, S., Granditsch, G., Kaserer, K., Korninger, L., Steindl, P., Gangl, A., Ferenci, P.: Diagnosis of Wilson's disease in an asymptomatic sibling by DNA linkage analysis. Gastroenterology 1995; 109: 2015–2018
343. Mason, A.L., Marsh, W., Alpers, D.: Intractable neurological Wilson's disease treated with orthotopic liver transplantation. Dig. Dis. Sci. 1992; 38: 1746–1750
344. McCullough, A.J., Fleming, C.R., Thistle, J.L., Baldus, W.P., Ludwig, J., McCall, J.T., Dickson, E.R.: Diagnosis of Wilson's disease presenting as fulminant hepatic failure. Gastroenterology 1983; 84: 161–167
345. Menerey, K.A., Eider, W., Brewer, G.J., Braunstein, E.M., Schumacher, H.R., Fox, I.: The arthropathy of Wilson's disease: clinical and pathological features. J. Rheumatol. 1988; 15: 331–337
346. Merle, U., Schaefer, M., Ferencsi, P., Stremmel, W.: Clinical presentation, diagnosis and long-term outcome of Wilson's disease. A cohort study. Gut 2007; 56: 115–120
347. Myers, B.M., Prendergast, F.G., Holman, R., Kuntz, S.M., LaRusso, N.F.: Alterations in hepatocyte lysosomes in experimental hepatic copper overload in rats. Gastroenterology 1993; 105: 1814–1823
348. Nakada, S.Y., Brown, M.R., Rabinowitz, R.: Wilson's disease presenting as symptomatic urolithiasis: a case report and review of literature. J. Urol. 1994; 152: 978–979
349. Nagasaka, H., Inoue, I., Inui, A., Komatsu, H., Sogo, T., Murayama, K., Murakami, T., Yorifugi, T., Asayama, K., Katayama, S., Uemoto, S., Kobayashi, K., Takayanagi, M., Fujisawa, T., Tsukahara, H.: Relationship between oxidative stress and antioxidant systems in the liver of patients with Wilson's disease: Hepatic manifestation in Wilson's disease as a consequence of augmented oxidative stress. Pediatr. Res. 2006; 60: 472–477
350. Nazer, H., Ede, R.J., Mowat, A.P., Williams, R.: Wilson's disease: clinical presentation and use of prognostic index. Gut 1986; 27: 1377–1381
351. Okada, T., Morise, T., Takeda, Y., Mabuchi, H.: A new variant deletion of a copper-transporting P-type ATPase gene found in patients with Wilson's disease presenting with fulminant hepatic failure. J. Gastroenterol. 2000; 35: 278–283
352. Petrukhin, K., Fischer, S.G., Pirastu, M., Tanzi, R.E., Chernov, I., Devoto, M., Brzustowicz, L.M., Cayanis, E., Vitale, E., Russo, J.J., Matseoane, D., Boukhgalter, B., Wasco, W., Figus, A.L., Loudianos, J., Cao, A., Sternlieb, I., Evgrafov, O., Parano, E., Pavone, L., Warburton, D., Ott, J., Penchaszadeh, G.K., Scheinberg. I.H., Gilliam, T.C.: Mapping, cloning and genetic characterization of the region containing the Wilson's disease gene. Nat. Genet. 1993; 5: 338–343
353. Polio, J., Enriquez, R.E., Chow, A., Wood, W:M., Atterbury, C.E.: Hepatocellular carcinoma in Wilson's disease: Case report and review of the literature. J. Clin. Gastroenterol. 1989; 11: 220–224
354. Polson, R.J., Rolles, K., Calne, R.Y., Williams, R., Madsden, D.: Reversal of severe neurological manifestations of Wilson's disease following orthotopic liver transplantation. Quart. J. Med. 1987; 64: 685–691
355. Probst, A., Propst, T., Feichtinger, H., Judmaier, G., Willeit, J., Vogel, W.: Copper-induced acute rhabdomyolysis in Wilson's disease. Gastroenterology 1995; 108: 885–887
356. Rakela, J., Kurtz, S.B., McCarthy, J.T., Ludwig, J., Ascher, N.L., Bloomer, J.R., Claus, P.L.: Fulminant Wilson's disease treated with post-dilution hemofiltration and orthotopic liver transplantation. Gastroenterology, 1986; 90: 2004–2007
357. Roberts, E.A., Schilsky, M.L.: A practice guideline on Wilson disease. Hepatology 2003; 37: 1475–1492
358. Roche-Sicot, J., Benhamou, J.-P.: Acute intravascular hemolysis and acute liver failure associated as a first manifestation of Wilson's disease. Ann. Intern. Med. 1977; 86: 301–303
359. Roh, J.K., Lee, T.G., Wie, B.A., Lee, S.B., Park, S.H., Chang, K.H.: Initial and follow-up brain MRI findings and correlation with the clinical course in Wilson's disease. Neurology 1994; 44: 1064–1068
360. Rossaro, L., Sturniolo, G.C., Giacon, G., Montino, M.C., Lecis, P.E., Schade, R.R., Corazza, G.R., Trevisan, C.: Zinc therapy in Wilson's disease: observations in five patients. Amer. J. Gastroenterol. 1990; 85: 665–668
361. Sallie, R., Katsiyiannakis, L., Baldwin, D., Davies, S., O'Grady, J., Mowat, A., Mieli-Vergani, G., Williams, R.: Failure of simple biochemical index to reliably differentiate fulminant Wilson's disease from other causes of fulminant liver failure. Hepatology 1992; 16: 1206–1211
362. Scheinberg, I.H., Jaffe, M.E., Sternlieb, I.: The use of trientine in preventing the effects of interrupting penicillamine therapy in Wilson's disease. New Engl. J. Med. 1987; 317: 209–213
363. Schilsky, M.L.: Wilson disease: genetic basis of copper toxicity and natural history. Semin. Liver Dis. 1996; 16: 83–95
364. Schoen, R.E., Sternlieb, I.: Clinical aspects of Wilson's disease. Amer. J. Gastroenterol. 1990; 85: 1453–1457
365. Schumacher, G., Platz, K.P., Mueller, A.R., Neuhaus, R., Steinmüller, T., Bechstein, W.O., Becker, M., Luck, W., Schuelke, M., Neuhaus, P.: Liver transplantation: treatment of choice for hepatic and neurological manifestation of Wilson's disease. Clin. Transplant. 1997; 11: 217–224
366. Sen, S., Felldin, M., Steiner, C., Larsson, B., Gillett, G.T., Olausson, M., Williams, R., Jalan, R.: Albumin dialysis and molecular adsorbents recirculating system (MARS) for acute Wilson's disease (case report). Liver Transplant. 2002; 8: 962–967
367. Shaver, W.A., Bhatt, H., Combes, B.: Low serum alkaline phosphatase activity in Wilson's disease. Hepatology 1986; 6: 859–863
368. Stampfl, D.A., Munoz, S.J., Moritz, M.J., Rubin, R., Armenti, V.T., Jarrell, B.E., Maddrey, W.C.: Heterotopic liver transplantation for fulminant Wilson's disease. Gastroenterology 1990; 99: 1834–1836
369. Starosta-Rubinstein, S., Young, A.B., Kluin, K., Hill, G., Aisen, A.M., Gabrielsen, T., Brewer, G.J.: Clinical assessment of 31 patients with Wilson's disease. Correlations with structural changes on magnetic resonance imaging. Arch. Neurol. 1987; 44: 365–370
370. Sternlieb, I.: Wilson's disease and pregnancy. Hepatology 2000; 31: 531–532
371. Strand, S., Hofmann, W.J., Grambihler, A., Hug, H., Volkmann, M., Otto, G., Wesch, H., Mariani, S.M., Hack, V., Stremmel, W., Krammer, P.H., Galle, P.R.: Hepatic failure and liver cell damage in acute Wilson's disease involve CD 95 (APO-1/Fas)-mediated apoptosis. Nat. Med. 1998; 4: 588–593
372. Stremmel, W., Meyerrose, K.-W., Niederau, C., Hefter, H., Kreuzpainter, G., Strohmeyer, G.: Wilson's disease: clinical presentation, treatment, and survival. Ann. Intern. Med. 1991; 115: 720–726
373. Stromeyer, F.W., Ishak, K.G.: Histology of the liver in Wilson's disease. A study in 34 cases. Amer. J. Clin. Pathol. 1980; 73: 12–24
374. Tao, T.Y., Gitlin, J.D.: Hepatic copper metabolism: insights from genetic disease. Hepatology 2003; 37: 1241–1247
375. Terajima, H., Tanaka, K., Okajima, K., Inomata, Y., Yamaoka, Y.: Timing of transplantation and donor selection in living-related liver transplantation for fulminant Wilson's disease. Transplant. Proc. 1995; 27: 1177–1178
376. Thomas, G.R., Forbes, J.R., Roberts, E.A., Walshe, J.M., Cox, D.W.: The Wilson's disease gene: spectrum of mutations and their consequences. Nat. Genet. 1995; 9: 210–217
377. Turnland, J.R.: Human whole-body copper metabolism. Amer. J. Clin. Nutr. 1998; 67: 960–964
378. Veen, C., van den Hamer, C.J.A., de Leeuw, P.W.: Zinc sulphate therapy for Wilson's disease after acute deterioration during treatment with low-dose D-penicillamine. J. Intern. Med. 1991; 229: 549–552
379. Walshe, J.M.: Treatment of Wilson's disease with trientine (triethylene tetramine) dihydrochloride. Lancet 1982/I: 643–647
380. Walshe, J.M., Waldenstrom, E., Sams, V., Nordlinder, H., Westermark, K.: Abdominal malignancies in patients with Wilson's disease. Quart. J. Med. 2003; 96: 657–662
381. Wieber, D.O., Wilson, D.M., McLeod, R.A., Goldstein, N.P.: Renal stones in Wilson's disease. Am. J. Med. 1979; 67: 249–254
382. Wilkinson, M.L., Portmann, B., Williams, R.: Wilson's disease and hepatocellular carcinoma: Possible protective role of copper. Gut 1983; 24: 767–771
383. Wilson, S.A.K.: Progressive lenticular degeneration: A familiar nervous disease associated with cirrhosis of the liver. Brain 1912; 34: 295–509
384. Yamaguchi, Y., Heiny, M.E., Gitlin, J.D.: Isolation and characterization of a human liver cDNA as a candidate gene for Wilson's disease. Biochem. Biophys. Res. Commun. 1993; 197; 271–277

385. Yang, F., Naylor, S.L., Lum, J.B., Cutshaw, St., McCombs, J.L., Haberhaus, K.H., McGill, J.R., Adrian, G.S., Moore, J.L., Barnett, D.R., Bowman, B.H.: Characterisation, mapping and expression of the human caeruloplasmin gene. Proc. Natl. Acad. Sci. USA 1986; 83: 3257–3261

Indian childhood cirrhosis

386. Baker, A., Gormally, S., Saxena, R., Baldwin, D., Drumm, B., Bonham, J., Portmann, B., Mowat, A.P.: Copper-associated liver disease in childhood. J. Hepatol. 1995; 23: 538–543
387. Bavdekar, A.R., Bhave, S.A., Pradhan, A.M., Pandit, A.N., Tanner, M.S.: Long term survival in Indian childhood cirrhosis treated with D-penicillamine. Arch. Dis. Childh. 1996; 74: 32–35

Haemochromatosis

388. Adams, P.C., Searle, J.: Neonatal hemochromatosis: a case and review of the literature. Amer. J. Gastroenterol. 1988; 83: 422–425
389. Adams, P.C., Gregor, J.: Hemochromatosis and yersiniosis. Canad. J. Gastroenterol. 1990; 4: 160–162
390. Adams, P.C., Deugnier, Y., Moirand, R., Brissot, P.: The relationship between iron overload, clinical symptoms, and age in 410 patients with genetic hemochromatosis. Hepatology 1997; 25: 162–166
391. Adams, P.C., Kertesz, A.E., McLaren, C.E., Barr, R., Bamford, A., Chakrabarti, S.: Population screening for hemochromatosis: a comparison of unbound iron-binding capacity, transferrin saturation, and C282Y genotyping in 5,211 voluntary blood donors. Hepatology 2000; 31: 1160–1164
392. Aellen, P., Guerne, P.-A., Zenagui, D., Vischer, T.L.: L'arthropathie de l'hemochromatose: manifestation souvent inaugurale de la maladie. Schweiz. Med. Wschr. 1992; 122: 842–849
393. Alustiza, J.M., Artetxe, J., Castiella, A., Agirre, P., Emparanza, P., Otazua, P., Garcia-Bengoechea, M., Barrio, J., Mujica, F., Recondo, J.A.: MR quantification of hepatic iron concentration. Radiology 2004; 230: 479–484
394. Alustiza, J.M., Castiella, A., de Juan, M.D., Emparanza, J.I., Artetxe, J., Uranga, M.: Iron overload in the liver: diagnostic and quantification. Eur. J. Radiol. 2007; 61: 499–506
395. Baer, D.M., Simons, J.L., Staples, R.L., Rumore, G.J., Morton, C.J.: Hemochromatosis screening in asymptomatic ambulatory men 30 years of age and older. Amer. J. Med. 1995; 98: 464–468
396. Balan, V., Baldus, W., Fairbanks, V., Michels, V., Burritt, M., Klee, G.: Screening for hemochromatosis: a cost-effectiveness study based on 12,258 patients. Gastroenterology 1994; 107: 453–459
397. Beutler, E., Felitti, V., Gelbart, T., Ho, N.: The effect of HFE genotypes on measurements of iron overload in patients attending a health appraisal clinic. Ann. Intern. Med. 2000; 133: 329–337
398. Bhavnani, M., Lloyd, D., Bhattacharyya, A., Marples, J., Elton, P., Worwood, M.: Screening for genetic hemochromatosis in blood samples with raised alanine aminotransferase. Gut 2000; 46: 707–710
399. Blisard, K.S., Bartow, S.A.: Neonatal hemochromatosis. Hum. Path. 1986; 17: 376–383
400. Blumberg, R.S., Chopra, S., Ibrahim, R., Crawford, J., Farraye, F.A., Zeldis, J.B., Berman, M.D.: Primary hepatocellular carcinoma in idiopathic hemochromatosis after reversal of cirrhosis. Gastroenterology 1988; 95: 1399–1402
401. Boige, V., Castera, L., de Roux, N., Ganne-Carrie, N., Ducot, B., Pelletier, J., Beaugrand, M., Buffet, C.: Lack of association between HFE gene mutations and hepatocellular carcinoma in patients with cirrhosis. Gut 2003; 52: 1178–1181
402. Bonkovsky, H.L., Rubin, R.B., Cable, E.E., Davidoff, A., Pels Rijcken, T.H., Stark, D.D.: Hepatic iron concentration: noninvasive estimation by means of MR imaging techniques. Radiology 1999; 212: 227–234
403. Candell-Riera, J., Seres, L., Gonzales, J.B., Batille, J., Permanyer-Miralda, G., Garcia-del-Castillo, H., Soler-Soler, J.: Cardiac hemochromatosis: beneficial effects of iron removal therapy. Amer. J. Cardiol. 1983; 52: 824–829
404. Crawford, D.H.G., Leggett, B.A., Powell, L.W.: Haemochromatosis. Baill. Clin. Gastroenterol. 1998; 12: 209–225
405. Cremonesi, P., Acebron, A., Raja, K.B., Simpson, R.J.: Iron absorption: Biochemical and molecular insights into the importance of iron species for intestinal uptake. Pharm. Toxicol. 2002; 91: 97–102
406. Cundy, T., Butler, J., Bomford, A., Williams, R.: Reversibility of hypogonatotrophic hypogonadism associated with genetic haemochromatosis. Clin. Endocrin. 1993; 38: 617–620
407. Davis, W.D., Arrowsmith, W.R.: The effect of repeated bleeding in hemochromatosis. J. Lab. Clin. Med. 1950; 36: 814–815
408. De Bont, B., Walker, A.C., Carter, R.F., Oldfield, R.K., Davidson, G.P.: Idiopathic hemochromatosis presenting as acute hepatitis. J. Pediatr. 1987; 110: 431–434
409. Deugnier, Y.M., Loréal, O., Turlin, B., Guyader, D., Jouanolle, H., Moirand, R., Jacquelinet, C., Brissot, P.: Liver pathology in genetic hemochromatosis: a review of 135 homozygous cases and their bioclinical correlations. Gastroenterology 1992; 102: 2050–2059
410. Deugnier, Y.M., Guyader, D., Crantock, L., Lopez, J.-M., Turlin, B., Yaouanq, J., Jouanolle, H., Campion, J.-P., Launois, J., Halliday, J.W., Powell, L.W., Brissot, P.: Primary liver cancer in genetic hemochromatosis: a clinical pathological and pathogenetic study of 54 cases. Gastroenterology 1993; 104: 228–234
411. Disler, P.B., Lynch, S.R., Charlton, R.W., Torrance, J.D., Bothwell, T.H., Walker, R.B., Mayet, F.: The effect of tea on iron absorption. Gut 1975; 16: 193–200
412. Dugast, I.J., Papadopoulus, P., Zappone, E., Jones, C., Theriault, K., Handelman, G.J., Benarous, R., Drysdale, J.W.: Identification of two human ferritin H genes on the short arm of chromosome 6. Genomics 1990; 6: 204–211
413. Edwards, C.Q., Griffen, L.M., Dadone, M.M., Skolnick, M.H., Kushner, J.P.: Mapping the locus for hereditary hemochromatosis: localization between HLA-B and HLA-A. Amer. J. Genet. 1986; 38: 805–811
414. Edwards, C.Q., Griffen, L.M., Goldgar, D., Drummond, C., Skolnick, M., Kushner, J.P.: Prevalence of hemochromatosis among 11 065 presumably healthy blood donors. New Engl. J. Med. 1988; 318: 1355–1362
415. Eijkelkamp, E.J., Yapp, T.R., Powell, L.W.: HFE-associated hereditary hemochromatosis. Can. J. Gastroenterol. 2000; 14: 121–125
416. Elmberg, M., Hultcrantz, R., Ekborn, A., Brandt, L., Olsson, R., Lindgren, S., Lööf, L., Stal. P., Wallerstedt, S., Almer, S., Sandberg-Gertzen, H., Askling, J.: Cancer risk in patients with hereditary hemochromatosis and in their first-degree relatives. Gastroenterology 2003; 125: 1733–1741
417. Failla, M., Giannattasio, C., Piperno, A., Vergani, A., Grappiolo, A., Gentile, G., Meles, E., Mancia, G.: Radial artery wall alterations in genetic hemochromatosis before and after iron depletion therapy. Hepatology 2000; 32: 569–573
418. Fargion, S., Fracanzani, A.L., Piperno, A., Braga, M., D'Alba, R., Ronchi, G., Fiorelli, G.: Prognostic factors for hepatocellular carcinoma in genetic hemochromatosis. Hepatology 1994; 20: 1426–1431
419. Farrell, F.J., Nguyen, M., Woodley, S., Imperial, J.C., Garcia-Kennedy, R., Man, K., Esquivel, C.O., Keeffe, E.B.: Outcome of liver transplantation in patients with hemochromatosis. Hepatology 1994; 20: 404–410
420. Fletcher, L.M., Halliday, J.W.: Haemochromatosis: understanding the mechanism of disease and implications for diagnosis and patient management following the recent cloning of novel genes involved in iron metabolism. J. Intern. Med. 2002; 251: 181–192
421. Fracanzani, A.L., Conte, D., Fraquelli, M., Taioli, E., Mattioli, M., Losco, A., Fargion, S.: Increased cancer risk in a cohort of 230 patients with hereditary hemochromatosis in comparison to matched control patients with non-iron-related chronic liver disease. Hepatology 2001; 33: 647–651
422. Gandon, Y., Olivie, D., Guyader, D., Aube, C., Oberti, F., Sebille, V., Dlugnier, Y.: Non-invasive assessment of hepatic iron stores by MRI. Lancet 2004; 363: 357–362
423. Grabhorn, E., Richter, A., Burdelski, M., Rogiers, X., Ganschow, R.: Neonatal hemochromatosis: Long-term experience with favorable outcome. Pediatrics 2006; 118: 2060–2065
424. Guayder, D., Gandou, Y., Robert, J.Y., Heautot, J.F., Jouanolle, H., Jacquelinet, C., Messner, M., Deugnier, Y., Brissot, P.: Magnetic resonance imaging and assessment of liver iron content in genetic hemochromatosis. J. Hepatol. 1992; 15: 304–308
425. Hardy, L., Hansen, J.L., Kushner, J.P., Knisely, A.S.: Neonatal hemochromatosis. Genetic analysis of transferrin-receptor, H-apoferritin, and L-apoferritin loci and of the human leukocyte antigen class I region. Amer. J. Pathol. 1990; 137: 149–153
426. Hsing, A.W., McLaughlin, J.K., Olsen, J.H., Mellemkjar, L., Wacholder, S., Fraumemi, J.F.jr.: Cancer risk following primary hemochromatosis: a population-based cohort study in Denmark. Int. J. Cancer 1995; 60: 160–162
427. Hübscher, S.G.: Iron overload, inflammation and fibrosis in genetic haemochromatosis. (editorial) J. Hepatol. 2003; 38: 521–525
428. Jouanolle, A.M., Gandou, G., Jézéquel, P., Blayau, M., Campion, M.I., Yaouanq, J., Mosser, J., Fergelot, P., Chauvel, B., Bouric, P., Carn, G., Andrieux, N., Gicquel, I., Le Gall, J.-Y., David, V.: Haemochromatosis and HLA-H. Nat. Genet. 1996; 14: 251–252
429. Kaltwasser, J.P., Werner, E., Schalk, K., Hansen, C., Gottschalk, R., Seidl, C.: Clinical trial on the effect of regular tea drinking on iron accumulation in genetic haemochromatosis. Gut 1998; 43: 699–704
430. Kelly, T.M., Edwards C.Q., Meikle, A.W., Kushner, J.P.: Hypogonadism in hemochromatosis: reversal with iron depletion. Ann. Intern. Med. 1984; 101: 629–632
431. Kew, M.D.: Pathogenesis of hepatocellular carcinoma in hereditary hemochromatosis: occurence in noncirrhotic liver. Hepatology 1990; 11: 1086–1087
432. Knisely, A.S., Mieli-Vergani, G., Whitington, P.F.: Neonatal hemochromatosis. Gastroenterol. Clin. N. Amer. 2003; 32: 877–889
433. Lebron, J.A., Bennett, M.J., Vaughn, D.E., Chirino, A.J., Snow, P.M., Mintier, G.A., Feder, J.N., Bjorkman, P.J.: Crystal structure of the hemochromatosis protein HFE and characterization of its interaction with transferrin receptor. Cell 1998; 93: 111–123
434. Ludwig, J., Batts, K.P., Moyer, T.P., Baldus, W.P., Fairbanks, V.F.: Liver biopsy diagnosis of homozygous hemochromatosis: A diagnostic algorithm. Mayo Clin. Proc. 1993; 68: 263–267
435. Macfarlane, J.D., Vreugdenhil, G.R., Doornbos, J., van der Voet, G.B.: Idiopathic haemochromatosis: magnetic resonance signal intensity ratios permit non-invasive diagnosis of low levels of iron overload. Netherl. J. Med. 1995; 47: 49–53
436. McCune, C.A., Ravine, D., Worwood, M., Jackson, H.A., Erans, H.M., Hutton, D.: Screening for hereditary haemochromatosis within families and beyond. Lancet 2003; 362: 1897–1898
437. McDonnell, S.M., Preston, B.L., Jewell, S.A., Barton, J.C., Edwards, C.Q., Adams, P.C., Yip, R.: A survey of 2,851 patients with hemochromatosis: symptoms and response to treatment. Amer. J. Med. 1999; 106: 619–624

438. **Melefors, Ö., Hentze, M.W.:** Iron regulatory factor – the conductor of cellular iron regulation. Blood Rev. 1993; 7: 251–258
439. **Morcos, M., Dubois, S., Bralet, M.P., Belghiti, J., Terris, B.:** Primary liver carcinoma in genetic hemochromatosis reveals a broad histological spectrum. Amer. J. Clin. Path. 2001; 116: 738–743
440. **Muiesan, P., Rela, M., Kane, P., Dawan, A., Baker, A., Ball, C., Mowat, A.P., Williams, R., Heaton, N.D.:** Liver transplantation for neonatal haemochromatosis. Arch. Dis. Childh. 1995; 73: 178–180
441. **Nairz, M., Weis, G.:** Molecular and clinical aspects of iron homeostasis: from anemia to hemochromatosis. Wien. Klin. Wschr. 2006; 118: 442–462
442. **Niederau, C., Fischer, R., Pürschel, A., Stremmel, W., Häussinger, D., Strohmeyer, G.:** Long-term survival in patients with hereditary hemochromatosis. Gastroenterology 1996; 110: 1107–1119
443. **Nielsen, P., Carpinteiro, S., Fischer, R., Cabeda, J.M., Porto, G., Gabbe, E.E.:** Prevalence of the C282Y- and the H 63 D-mutations in the HFE-gene in patients with hereditary haemochromatosis and in control subjects from Northern Germany. Brit. J. Haematol. 1999; 103: 842–845
444. **Niemela, O., Parkkila, S., Britton, R.S., Brunt, E., Janney, C., Bacon, B.:** Hepatic lipid peroxidation in hereditary hemochromatosis and alcoholic liver injury. J. Lab. Clin. Med. 1999; 133: 451–460
445. **Olivieri, N.F., Berriman, A.M., Tyler, B.J., Davis, S.A., Francombe, W.H., Liu, P.P.:** Reduction in tissue iron stores with a new regime of continuous ambulatory intravenous deferoxamine. Amer. J. Hematol. 1992; 41: 61–63
446. **Olson, L.J., Edwards, W.D., Holmes, D.R.jr., Miller, F.A.jr., Nordstrom, L.A., Baldus, W.P.:** Endomyocardial biopsy in hemochromatosis: clinicopathologic correlates in six cases. J. Amer. Coll. Cardiol. 1989; 13: 116–120
447. **Olynyk, J., Hall, P., Sallie, R., Reed, W., Shilkin, K., Mackinnon, M.:** Computerized measurement of iron in liver biopsies: a comparison with biochemical iron measurement. Hepatology 1990; 12: 26–30
448. **Philpott, C.C.:** Molecular aspects of iron absorption: insights into the role of HFE in hemochromatosis. Hepatology 2002; 35: 993–1001
449. **Pillay, P., Tzoracoleftherakis, E., Tzakis, A.G., Kakizoe, S., van Thiel, D.H., Starzl, T.E.:** Orthotopic liver transplantation for hemochromatosis. Transplant. Proc. 1991; 23: 1888–1889
450. **Piperno, A., Arosio, C., Fossati, L., Vigano, M., Trombini, P., Vergani, A., Mancia, G.:** Two novel nonsense mutations of HFE gene in five unrelated Italian patients with hemochromatosis. Gastroenterology 2000; 119: 441–445
451. **Powell, L.W.:** Hereditary hemochromatosis and iron overload diseases. J. Gastroenterol. Hepatol. 2002; 17 (Suppl.): 191–195
452. **Ramrakhiani, S., Bacon, B.R.:** Hemochromatosis. Advances in molecular genetics and clinical diagnosis. J. Clin. Gastroenterol. 1998; 27: 41–46
453. **Recklinghausen, v.F.D.:** Über Hämochromatose. Berlin. Klin. Wschr. 1889; 26: 925
454. **Rivers, J., Garrahy, P., Robinson, W., Murphy, A.:** Reversible cardiac dysfunction in hemochromatosis. Amer. Heart J. 1987; 113: 216–217
455. **Rossi, E., Henderson, S., Chin, C.Y.B., Olynyk, J., Beilby, J.P., Reed, W.D., Jeffrey, G.P.:** Genotyping as a diagnostic aid in genetic haemochromatosis. J. Gastroenterol. Hepatol. 1999; 14: 427–430
456. **Sallie, R.W., Reed, W.D., Shilkin, K.B.:** Confirmation of the efficacy of hepatic tissue iron index in differentiating genetic hemochromatosis from alcoholic liver disease complicated by alcoholic hemosiderosis. Gut 1991; 32: 207–210
457. **Sanchez, M., Villa, M., Ingelmo, M., Sanz, C., Bruguera, M., Ascas, C., Oliva, R.:** Population screening for hemochromatosis: a study in 5370 Spanish blood donors. J. Hepatol. 2003; 38: 745–750
458. **Schumacher, H.R., Straka, P.C., Krikker, M.A., Dudley, A.T.:** The arthropathy of hemochromatosis: recent studies. Ann. N.Y. Acad. Sci. 1988; 526: 224–233
459. **Shaheen, N.J., Silverman, L.M., Keku, T., Lawrence, L.B., Rohlfs, E.M., Martin, C.F., Galanko, J., Sandler, R.S.:** Association between hemochromatosis (HFE) gene mutation carrier status and the risk of colon cancer. J. Nat. Canc. Inst. 2003; 95: 154–159
460. **Sigurdsson, I., Reyes, J., Kocoshis, S.A., Hansen, T.W.R., Rosh, J., Knisely, A.S.:** Neonatal hemochromatosis: outcomes of pharmacologic and surgical therapies. J. Pediatr. Gastroenterol. Nutrit. 1998; 26: 85–89
461. **Stremmel, W., Karner, M., Manzhalii, E., Gittes, W., Hermann, T., Merle, U.:** Liver and iron metabolism – A comprehensive hypothesis for the pathogenesis of genetic hemochromatosis (review). Zschr. Gastroenterol. 2007; 45: 71–75
462. **Terada, T., Nakamura, Y.:** Iron negative foci in siderotic macroregenerative nodules in human cirrhotic liver. A marker of incipient neoplastic lesion. Arch. Path. Lab. Med. 1989; 113: 916–920
463. **Vadillo, M., Corbella, X., Pac, V., Fernandez-Viladrich, P., Pujol, R.:** Multiple liver abscesses due to Yersimia enterocolitica discloses primary hemochromatosis: Three case report and review. Clin. Inf. Dis. 1994; 18: 938–941
464. **Villeneuve, J.-P., Bilodeau, M., Lepage, R., Cote, J., Lefebre, M.:** Variability in hepatic iron concentration measurements from needle-biopsy specimens. J. Hepatol. 1996; 25: 172–177
465. **Westra, W.H., Hruban, R.H., Baughman, K.L., Olson, J.L., Porterfield, J.K., Mitchell, M.C., Hutchins, G.M.:** Progressive hemochromatotic cardiomyopathy despite reversal of iron deposition after liver transplantation. Amer. J. Clin. Path. 1993; 99: 39–44
466. **Willis, G., Wimperis, J.Z., Lonsdale, R., Fellows, I.W., Watson, M.A., Skipper, L.M., Jennings, B.A.:** Incidence of liver disease in people with HFE mutations. Gut 2000; 46: 401–404
467. **Wojcik, J.P., Speechley, M.R., Kertesz, A.E., Chakrabarti, S., Adams, P.C.:** Natural history of C 282 Y homozygotes for hemochromatosis. Can. J. Gastroenterol. 2002; 16: 297–302
468. **Yen, A.W., Fancher, T.L., Bowlus, C.L.:** Revisiting hereditary hemochromatosis: Current concepts and progress. Amer. J. Med.. 2006; 119: 391–399

Acaeruloplasminaemia

469. **Loréal, D., Turein, B., Pigeon, C., Moisan, A., Ropert, M., Morice, P., Gandon, Y., Jouanolle, A.-M., Vérin, M., Hider, R.C., Yoshida, K., Brissot, P.:** Aceruloplasminemia: new clinical, pathophysiological and therapeutic insights. J. Hepatol. 2002; 36: 851–856
470. **Mariani, R., Arosio, C., Pelucchi, S., Grisoli, M., Piga, A., Trombini, P., Piperno, A.:** Iron chelation therapy in aceruloplasminemia: study of a patient with a novel missense mutation (case report). Gut 2004; 53: 756–758
471. **Yoshida, K., Furihata, K., Takeda, S., Nakamura, A., Yamamoto, K., Morita, H., Hiyamuta, S., Ikeda, S., Shimizu, N., Yanagisawa, N.:** A mutation in the ceruloplasmin gene is associated with systemic hemosiderosis in humans. Nature Genet. 1995; 9: 267–272

Atransferrinaemia

472. **Goya, N., Miyazaki, S., Kodate, S., Ushio, B.:** A family of congenital atransferrinemia. Blood 1972; 40: 239–245
473. **Heilmeyer, L., Keller, W., Vivell, O., Betke, K., Wöhler, F., Keiderling, W.:** Die kongenitale Atransferrinämie. Schweiz. Med. Wschr. 1961; 91: 1203

Clinical Aspects of Liver Diseases
32 Autoimmune hepatitis

		Page:
1	*Definition*	656
2	*Epidemiology*	656
3	***Aetiology***	656
3.1	Immunologic tolerance	656
3.2	Immunogenetic susceptibility	656
3.3	Trigger factors	656
4	***Pathogenesis***	656
4.1	HLA system	656
4.2	Cellular immune reaction	657
4.3	Autoantibodies	657
5	***Classification***	658
5.1	Type 1	658
5.2	Type 2	658
5.3	Type 3	659
5.4	Drug-induced AIH	659
5.5	Alcohol-related autoimmune reaction	659
5.6	Autoimmune polyendocrine syndrome	659
5.7	Association with HV infection	659
5.8	Cryptogenic chronic hepatitis	660
6	***Morphology***	660
7	***Clinical aspects***	661
7.1	Clinical symptoms	661
7.2	Laboratory diagnostics	661
7.3	Imaging techniques	661
7.4	Liver histology	662
8	***Course and prognosis***	662
8.1	Course of disease	662
8.2	Associated diseases	662
8.3	Hepatocellular carcinoma	662
8.4	Prognosis	662
9	***Therapy***	663
9.1	Detailed diagnostics	663
9.2	Immunosuppressive therapy	663
9.2.1	Glucocorticoids	663
9.2.2	Glucocorticoids and azathioprine	664
9.2.3	Ursodeoxycholic acid	664
9.2.4	Monitoring therapy	665
9.2.5	Non-responders to therapy	665
9.3	Liver transplantation	665
	• References (1–108)	665
	(Figures 32.1–32.6; tables 32.1–32.3)	

32 Autoimmune hepatitis

▶ A particular form of chronic liver disease prevalent among young women with an excessive increase in protein and γ-globulin was first described by S. AMBERG (1942) (2) and later by J. WALDENSTRÖM (1950), who used the name **"autoimmune hepatitis"**. (102). In 1951 H. G. KUNKEL et al. termed this condition **"hypergammaglobulinaemic chronic hepatitis"**. (47) This type of disease was confirmed by A. G. BEARN et al. (1956) (4) and, because of a positive LE-cell phenomenon in about 10% of cases (R. A. JOSKE et al., 1955) (43), was given the name **"lupoid hepatitis"** by I. R. MACKAY et al. (1956). (49) • During the following years, there were frequent reports of a particular form of active and necrotizing liver disease, which was assumed in many cases to be autoimmune due to the treatment success achieved with glucocorticoids and/or azathioprine. Laboratory parameters were characterized by increased transaminase values, GDH, γ-globulins and immunoglobulins as well as by distinct histological findings — *there was no possibility of obtaining immunologic evidence at that time.*

1 Definition

The cause of autoimmune hepatitis (AIH) is unknown. Autoimmune reactions lead to a chronic (rarely acute) inflammatory process (periportal piecemeal necrosis, infiltration of portal zones). AIH is frequently associated with autoimmune diseases of other organs. It occurs predominantly among women, particularly in younger years. Hypergammaglobulinaemia is invariably in evidence. Various autoantibodies to components of the liver parenchyma are found. The presence and specificity of these antibodies, together with the respective clinical symptoms, facilitate differentiation between the various subtypes of AIH. Diagnosis is substantiated by the response to immunosuppressive therapy. If left untreated, AIH progresses rapidly with transition to cirrhosis and/or liver failure. If treated adequately, the course taken by the disease is generally more favourable.

2 Epidemiology

AIH is present worldwide. Some 15–20% of all patients with chronic hepatitis can be classified as AIH. Prevalence and incidence differ in various geographic regions. In Europe and North America, *prevalence* ranges between 3–17/100,000 inhabitants, whereby the lowest rates are found in southern countries. The *incidence* in Europe and North America is estimated to be between 0.1–1.2/100,000 inhabitants per year. Women are four to five times and children seven to nine times more frequently affected. AIH can occur in all age groups. (7) In children, AIH mostly begins as an acute form; a fulminant course of disease has also been observed.

3 Aetiology

3.1 Immunologic tolerance

The aetiology of autoimmune hepatitis is (as yet) unresolved. • The immunologic tolerance of the body's own cell structures can be disturbed as a result of (*1.*) immunogenetic abnormalities in the **MHC system** (= major histocompatibility complex, i.e. the main complex in the HLA system, classes I and II), (*2.*) **clonal deletion** (= removal of so-called "mobile" genes from plasmids) as well as suppressor defects, and (*3.*) **molecular mimicry** (= partial correspondence of the molecular structure of a foreign antigen with a certain body-own protein structure). (s. p. 676)

3.2 Immunogenetic susceptibility

Genetic predisposition is paramount. • The existence of such a genetic factor can be deduced from occasional familial occurrence (25, 37), gender and age specificity as well as a close correlation with the HLA system. (65) Women are affected in 85–90% of cases, mainly between the ages of 40–55 years (women: men = 4:1).

3.3 Trigger factors

AIH must be triggered by an antigen. • Trigger factors include environmental noxae, medication, toxins, bacteria (e. g. salmonella antigen), hepatitis viruses HAV (74, 90, 96), HBV, HCV, Epstein-Barr (64, 97), lymphochoriomeningitis virus (39) and measles viruses (64, 97) as well as the Herpes simplex virus (type 1 of which is mainly responsible for AIH type 2). (78, 98) The development of AIH has also been precipitated by interferon therapy in chronic hepatitis B (13) and C (32, 67) even in children. (79) • The *viral trigger hypothesis* has recently aroused great interest, since various viruses (e. g. HAV, measles, Epstein-Barr) are known to persist "unnoticed" for years, e. g. in lymphocytes.

4 Pathogenesis

4.1 HLA system

Immunogenetic susceptibility is substantiated by the close association between autoimmune hepatitis and the HLA system. (24, 50, 65, 82) **Ethnic differences are evident:** an association with HLA-DR4 is frequent in Japan and in the Euro-Caucasian population. In patients with HLA-DR3 positivity, manifestation occurs in younger years, there is greater activity of disease and the outcome of therapy is less favourable (higher rate of non-responders and recurrences after ceasing immunosuppressive therapy, as well as more frequent indications for liver transplantation). In contrast, HLA-DR4 positivity correlates with manifestation at a more advanced age, a milder course of disease and a good response to immunosuppressives, albeit with the considerably more frequent occurrence of extrahepatic syndromes. The HLA markers DR3 and DR4 are hence characteristic of two different courses. • Further HLA types of importance include: HLA-A1, -B8, -DR4, -Bw54, -DR3, -DR13 (Brazil), -Dw3, -DR53, -C4AQO and -DQ4. • A close relationship was found between AIH and the CD 45 gene, which is considered quasi to be a *"modifier gene of human autoimmunity"*. (100)

4.2 Cellular immune reaction

Cellular alteration of the immune response is characterized by T lymphocytes infiltrating liver tissue. The target antigens of the T lymphocytes are deemed to be cytochrome P450 II D6, mitochondrial pyruvate dehydrogenase and asialoglycoprotein receptor proteins. (93) A loss of immune tolerance for autologous liver tissue can be attributed to the decrease in activity of T suppressor cells (with lymphocyte marker T8) and the preponderance of T helper cells (with lymphocyte marker T4) over the suppressor cells. Any existing suppressor defect in autoimmune hepatitis is eliminated by glucocorticoids – but not in cases of chronic viral hepatitis B. The suppressor T cell defect causes immunological hyperactivity against surface structures of the hepatocytes. T cells from the liver of autoimmune hepatitis patients are sensitized to asialoglycoprotein receptor proteins. (53, 54, 66, 88, 94, 104)

4.3 Autoantibodies

▶ There are various circulating autoantibodies to nuclear, cytoplasmatic and membranous antigens; they differ in their diagnostic and clinical significance. Autoantibodies are deemed to be secondary immunological phenomena of liver cell lesions and have no pathogenetic importance. Correlation of the antibody titres with AIH activity is unreliable. The antibodies may play a part in eliminating autoantigens. Their determination is essential for the diagnosis and classification of AIH as well as its overlap syndromes. (6, 17, 20, 66, 87, 89) (s. tabs. 5.19, 5.20; 32.1)

ANA: Antinuclear factors were first described by G.J. Friou et al. in 1957. These antibodies are mainly directed against nucleoprotein DNA histone and cycline A. They show a predominantly homogeneous or "speckled" pattern of fluorescence. ANA is not specific to the liver or to liver disease. (s. figs. 5.10, 5.11) (s. p. 124)

SMA: Smooth muscle antibodies were first described by G.D. Johnson et al. in 1965. They mostly possess anti-actin (generally F-actin) specificity, predominantly of the IgG type. Antibodies against troponin and α-actin may also be present. There is great heterogeneity, and a mixture of different antibodies can almost always be found. Evidence of anti-actin antibodies has a high diagnostic value, particularly with a titre of > 1:640 and in the presence of an IgG type. (s. fig. 5.12) (s. p. 125)

LKM: *Anti-LKM 1* were detected by M. Rizzetto et al. and W. B. Storch (87) in 1973. As liver/kidney microsomes, they are directed against an antigen of the ER (cytochrome P 450 II D 6) (anti-AER) as well as against proximal kidney tubuli. • There are also *anti-LKM 2* (antigen: P 450 II C 8 – II C 11 in tienilic acid-induced hepatitis) and *anti-LKM 3* (antigen: part of the UDP glucuronyltransferase in chronic hepatitis D as well as in hydralazine and carbamazepine-induced hepatitis against P 450 I A2). LKM antibodies are also directed against other microsomal antigens and consequently may be present in viral or toxic liver diseases. They constitute a heterogeneous group. (26, 38) (s. p. 125)

LP/SLA: Anti-LP antibodies were described by P.A. Berg et al. in 1981. They show a strong reaction against soluble antigens from the liver and pancreas. The specific antigen has not been identified. In autoimmune hepatitis, anti-LP antibodies are associated with ANA and/or SMA in >60% of cases; even when detected on their own, they are of diagnostic importance. (85) • Soluble liver-antigen antibodies (SLA) were first demonstrated by M.P. Manns et al. in 1987. (51) They seem to recognize cytokeratins as antigens and identify a target antigen of activated lymphocytes. SLA are probably identical to LP and possibly characterize the same patient group. Although they are of diagnostic relevance in AIH, they are not specific. LP/SLA are detectable in AIH in 25% of cases. (s. p. 126) • The postulated main antigen of cytosol antibodies has meanwhile been cloned. (101, 105) This group of cytosol antibodies was first described by W. Storch in 1975; they are probably identical to anti-LP and anti-SLA antibodies. (87)

▶ The autoantibodies ANA, SMA, LKM 1 and LP/SLA are of diagnostic relevance in autoimmune hepatitis. Moreover, they are usually detectable at a time when no clear diagnosis can be derived from clinical, laboratory or histological findings. This is important regarding early immunosuppressive therapy. Other autoantibodies are often associated with AIH, yet have no diagnostic relevance.

LC: These liver-specific antibodies (LC1 and LC2) react with a soluble cytosolic antigen in the liver cells (W. Storch, 1975, 1979). This was confirmed by E. Martini et al. in 1982. They are frequently associated with anti-LKM 1 antibodies (60–70%). The hepatocytes around the central vein of the liver lobule are left out of the otherwise homogeneous cytoplasmatic fluorescence. LC 1 antibodies are not present in chronic viral hepatitis C, and thus they are important in differentiating between (LC1-

positive) AIH and (LC1-negative) chronic HCV infection. LC1 is mainly seen in young patients presenting with AIH type 2. Only rarely are LC2 antibodies found in AIH; they react with periportal liver cells. (35, 45)

LMA: The liver membrane antibodies were first identified by W. STORCH in 1973 and confirmed by U. HOPF et al. in 1976. They are directed against various epitopes of the liver cell membrane, e.g. the ASGPR receptor. LMA are mostly associated with other (relevant) antibodies in AIH. (s. p. 125)

Asialoglycoprotein receptor: The antigen spectrum of anti-LSP antibodies is a heterogeneous group. The asialoglycoprotein receptor protein (anti-ASGPR) is a specific antigen of this LSP mixture (B.M. McFARLANE et al., 1986). In AIH, 80–85% of cases displayed antibodies against this purified protein. Yet, anti-ASGPR are also found in primary biliary cholangitis, primary sclerosing cholangitis and viral hepatitis. (93)

5 Classification

Autoimmune hepatitis may be classified into three (sometimes four) types according to the different antibody specificities in conjunction with the seromarkers of viral hepatitis. Further differentiation has also been made into subtypes (1a, 1b and 2a, 2b), although this remains controversial. In the future, it may well be possible to derive therapeutic indications or prognostic indices from these subtypes; at the moment, they offer no guidance in this respect. It is, however, remarkable that ANA, SMA and LKM 1 are not primarily detectable in 20% of patients with AIH, whereas other antibodies, such as LP/SLA and ASGPR antibodies, can often be identified. (52) • In this context, a more reliable definition of overlap syndromes might therefore be useful for therapy and prognosis. (s. tab. 32.1)

5.1 Type 1

This is the classical (formerly lupoid) form of autoimmune hepatitis. It shows a markedly genetic predisposition. Type 1 is the most frequently occurring form of AIH (70–80% of cases) and is mainly found in young women, especially between the ages of 20 and 40 years.

There is a marked increase in γ-globulins. ANA (40–70%), SMA (70–100%) (titre >1:80), LKM 1 and ASGPR (70–80%) are commonly present. AMA and pANCA are also occasionally detected. ANA often only appears during the course of disease. Antiactin antibodies (AAA) are a clear hint of AIH type 1. The condition is highly responsive to immunosuppressive therapy; that is why cirrhosis develops in "only" 40–45% of cases. HCV antibodies of groups 1a and 1b are found with the same frequency (14%). (16, 17, 36, 38, 61)

▶ **Subtype 1a:** This subtype is ANA-positive; it can be found with or without SMA. Its course is generally subclinical, so that the initial diagnosis can only be made later. Type 1a occurs more frequently in women than in men. Its frequency is distributed bimodally, with a peak between 10 and 30 years (= association with HLA-DR3) and again after 30 years of age or following the menopause (= association with HLA-DR4); occasionally, C4AQO is detectable. HLA-DR4 patients often have extrahepatic manifestations; they generally show higher IgH concentrations. Under therapy, the patients seldom suffer recurrence. The frequency of this subtype is 25–30% of cases.

▶ **Subtype 1b:** The SMA-positive subtype occurs particularly in children of all ages and of both sexes. In later life, men are more often affected. This classification is, however, still disputed.

5.2 Type 2

The main criterion of this type is the detection of LKM 1 (titre >1:80), which is exclusively found in AIH. ASGPR and LC 1 are sometimes also present. (26, 35, 45, 93, 108) In contrast, ANA and SMA antibodies are not detectable as a rule. Antithyroid and antiparietal cell antibodies can be frequently identified. Type 2 is 5–6 times less frequent (5–10%) than type 1. It occurs early in life (about 50% of cases involve children (34, 56) and adolescents) (69) and is often associated with extrahepatic manifestations. Type 2 usually commences like acute viral hepatitis, and genetically determined IgA deficiency is occasionally evident. Hypergammaglobulinaemia is not, however, as obvious as in type 1. Antibodies against thyroid and parietal cell antigens are frequently detectable. Type 2 is less responsive to immunosuppressive therapy than type 1. The prognosis is thus less favourable: cirrhosis develops frequently (approx. 80% of cases) and rapidly. Type 2 is associated in 10–15% of cases with autoimmune polyendocrine syndrome type 1. • Owing to a respective HCV positivity of 20–60% or 35%, differentiation into subtypes 2a

Subclassification	ANA	SMA	LKM1	SLA/LP	ASGPR	AMA	pANCA	AHA	HCV	anti-GOR
Autoimmune hepatitis										
1a	++	(+)	–	–	(+)+	–	(+)	–	(+)	(+)
1b	(+)	++	–	–	(+)+	–	(+)	–	(+)	(+)
2a	–	–	++	–	(+)+	–	–	–	–	–
2b	–	–	++	–	(+)+	–	–	–	+	+
3	(+)	(+)+	–	++	(+)+	(+)	–	–	–	–

Tab. 32.1: Differentiation of autoimmune hepatitis (s. tab. 5.20). • (AHA = anti-histone antibody; anti-GOR = anti-specific nuclear antigen in HCV) (see text for other abbreviations). –/(+) = no or occasional slight increase

and 2b was proposed. This may, however, not always be reliable.

Subtype 2a: The criteria of this subtype are positivity of LKM 1 and LC 1 with negativity of anti-HCV and HCV RNA. It becomes manifest early in life, and the course of disease is severe. Women are mainly affected. HLA-DR3, -B14 and -C4AQO are present.

Subtype 2b: The criteria of this subtype are positivity of LKM1 and anti-HCV as well as HCV RNA. It becomes manifest at a more advanced age. Men in particular are affected. In 70% of cases, it was possible to detect antibodies to certain nuclear HCV antigens, so-called **anti-GOR**. This is a fusion protein which is derived from a cDNA clone (GOR 47-1). (55) (s. pp 127, 452)

> ▶ The **explanation of the term GOR** is as follows: S. Mishiro et al. were trying at that time (before the discovery of HCV) to detect a new virus which could be the cause of NANB hepatitis by immunoscreening cDNA libraries which were derived from chimpanzees infected with NANB hepatitis. One of these chimpanzees had the name "Gabriel" ("G"). Two cDNA libraries were made from Gabriel's serum: one was primed with oligo-dT primer ("GO library") and the other with random primer ("GR library"). These two libraries were mixed to a combined one, "GO" + "GR" → GOR. Subsequently, an interesting clone was identified from the 47th plate of the GOR library: this was GOR 47-1. *(Personal information from S. Mishiro)*

5.3 Type 3

Type 3 is characterized by the positivity of LP/SLA. These antibodies are the only type found in 25% of patients with AIH. • Sometimes, SMA, ANA and ASGPR can also be detected, but at low titre levels. The frequency is 5–10%. Women are affected five times more often than men. There is a high concentration of γ-globulin. HCV antibodies were found in 11% of patients. (37) The clinical course is similar to type 1; as a rule, it progresses rapidly. The response to immunosuppressives is good. • Subtype 3, which was formerly classified as a separate entity, is now assigned to type 1. (s. tab. 32.1)

The clinical relevance of the subtypes is minimal. This is because (1.) the antibodies do not play any role in the pathogenesis of the subtypes, (2.) the antibodies do not offer any information regarding the aetiology of the respective subtype, (3.) the subtypes only account for a small proportion of the total number of AIH, and (4.) the subtypes do not play any role in the therapy of the disease. Up to now, it has only been possible to characterize type 1.

5.4 Drug-induced AIH

With a genetic or disease-related predisposition, the intake of medicaments and their subsequent catabolism in the biotransformatory system sometimes lead to the formation of reactive metabolites. (s. fig. 3.11) These can bind to components of the cytochrome system. After cytolysis, they may become the target antigens of antibodies. (s. fig. 29.1) This has already been ascertained, for example, for the following drugs:

Carbamazepine (LMK3)	Interferon
Clometazine	Isoniazide
Dantrolene	Ketoconazole
Diclofenac	Minocycline (33)
Halothane (LMK2)	Nitrofurantoin
Hydralazine (LMK3)	Ticrynafen (LMK2)

5.5 Alcohol-related autoimmune reaction

Approximately 80% of these patients display positive anti-histone 2 B antibodies. In alcoholic hepatitis, there is frequent evidence of LMA (60%) and LSP (30%) as well as ANA and/or SMA. In autoimmune hepatitis (15% of cases), high titres of IgA antibodies to histone 2 B can also be detected. • This autoimmune situation in alcoholic liver disease can indeed give rise to therapeutic problems *if, despite absolute abstinence, there is self-perpetuation of the morphological findings* (as we ourselves noticed in some cases).

5.6 Autoimmune polyendocrine syndrome

Approximately 20% of cases of the autosomal recessive APS type 1 are accompanied by autoimmune hepatitis. It is similar to AIH type 2. A loss of autoimmune regulator activity is considered to be the underlying cause. There are autoimmune reactions in the skin, ovaries, suprarenal glands, parathyroid glands, intestinal tract, etc.; generalized candidiasis is also evident. (s. tab. 32.2) Antibodies to LM (targeted against cytochrome P450 I A2) may be present. A combination of AIH and APS is more aggressive, with a tendency to an acute or subfulminant course, and shows a weak response to corticosteroid therapy.

Endocrine disorders
Diabetes insipidus (<1%)
Diabetes mellitus type 1 (1–2%)
Hypogonadism (40–45%)
Hypoparathyreoidism (85–90%)
Mucocutaneous candidiasis (70–75%)
Suprarenal insufficiency (55–65%)
Non-endocrine disorders
Chronic active hepatitis (20–30%)
Malabsorption syndrome (10–20%)

Tab. 32.2: Main endocrine and non-endocrine disorders in APS type 1

5.7 Association with HV infection

In **chronic hepatitis B**, 5–10% of cases display ANA and/or SMA. Due to the subtle differentiation achieved with HBV markers, it is possible to classify each individual case reliably. Prognosis and therapy are determined by chronic hepatitis B. Interferon therapy can trigger or exacerbate autoimmune hepatitis. (13, 67, 75, 79)

In **chronic hepatitis D,** 10—20% of cases displayed antibodies to LKM 3. The antigen is a part of UDP glucuronosyl transferase (T. PHILIPP et al. 1994).

In **chronic hepatitis C,** there is a strikingly frequent association with autoimmune hepatitis; this association, however, varies in different geographic regions. In ANA-positive AIH, HCV antibodies were detected in 40—50%, whereas in LKM-positive AIH, HCV markers were found in up to 88% of cases. Chronic hepatitis C showed ANA and/or SMA in 10—15% of patients, whereas 2—10% simultaneously displayed LKM 1 antibodies. This constellation, also classified as subtype 2b, has a relatively mild clinical course with relatively low LKM titres. Interferon therapy is indicated — yet caution is called for, since this can trigger acute inflammatory episodes of chronic hepatitis C as well as the development of AIH. (32, 67, 79) In the event of replicative HCV infection, immunosuppressive therapy is not indicated, since it is assumed that this is primarily chronic hepatitis C with concurrent autoimmunity. It is necessary to clarify the HCV infection by PCR and to differentiate the autoantibodies further. In assessing such an overlap retrospectively, consideration must be given to the fact that (*1.*) the determination of HCV antibodies has often been false owing to the still unreliable detection method, (*2.*) it has not yet been possible to verify HCV RNA by PCR, and (*3.*) hypergammaglobulinaemia produces higher false anti-HCV levels. (5, 31, 48, 55, 60, 61, 69, 92) (s. p. 449)

5.8 Cryptogenic chronic hepatitis

Occasionally, forms of autoantibody-negative chronic hepatitis are found with no detectable cause. They resemble autoimmune hepatitis in every respect and respond well to corticosteroid therapy. This special group (10—15%) possibly comprises cases of autoimmune hepatitis for which no immunoserologic markers are known as yet. In numerous cases of cryptogenic chronic hepatitis, AIH type 3 can be detected due to evidence of high-titric LP/LSA.

6 Morphology

Autoimmune hepatitis has no distinctive histology. The pattern resembles that of *chronic active hepatitis*: portal and periportal infiltration from some plasma cells as well as a high number of lymphocytes are evident. (s. figs. 32.1, 32.2) The lymphocytes are mainly of the T-cell type, whereby the ratio of subtypes CD4:CD8 is about 1:1. The lymphocytes reveal *emperipolesis* (= capable of infiltrating and surrounding other cells). (s. fig. 21.11) Hepatocytes often show hydrophic swelling

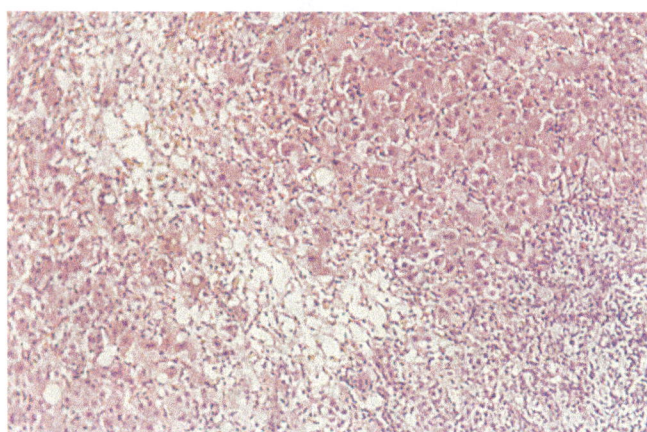

Fig. 32.1: Acute AIH type 1 (ANCA +) with pronounced centrilobular parenchymal loss. Rapid therapy success (clinically, biochemically) with immunosuppressives (HE)

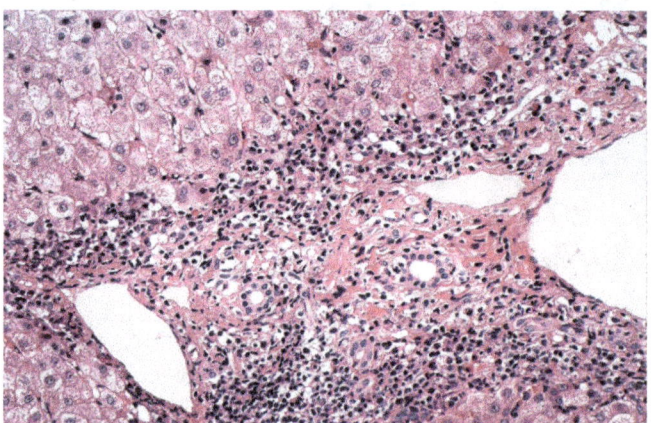

Fig. 32.2: Lymphoplasmocytic interface hepatitis in autoimmune hepatitis type 1 (HE)

and ballooning (s. fig. 21.4). Inflammatory activity varies, whereby some areas are near normal. In the lobule, there are infiltrates of lymphocytes with differing density together with activated Kupffer cells. As the degree of infiltration increases, with inflammatory activity varying from portal zone to portal zone, *piecemeal necroses* (= *interphase hepatitis*) and bridging necroses (between adjacent vascular structures) as well as *liver cell rosettes* (= hepatocytes surrounding a prominent canaliculus in a circular fashion) become more distinctive histologically. Whereas lytic necrosis leaves a "blank" in the trabecular texture, acidophilic necrosis shows residues containing *Councilman bodies*. (s. fig. 34.1) Early on in this process, it may be possible to detect pronounced *fibrosis*. (s. figs. 32.3 to 32.5) • Bile-duct lesions, granulomas and deposits of iron or copper are not present; their detection argues against AIH. (11, 23, 58, 84, 91) • *Non-alcoholic steatohepatitis* can resemble the picture of AIH.

▶ AIH is thus characterized by signs of *(1.) portal, (2.) periportal,* and *(3.) lobular hepatitis.* Due to the development of cirrhosis, both the entire liver structure (blood vessels, lymph vessels, bile ducts) and the parenchyma are transformed.

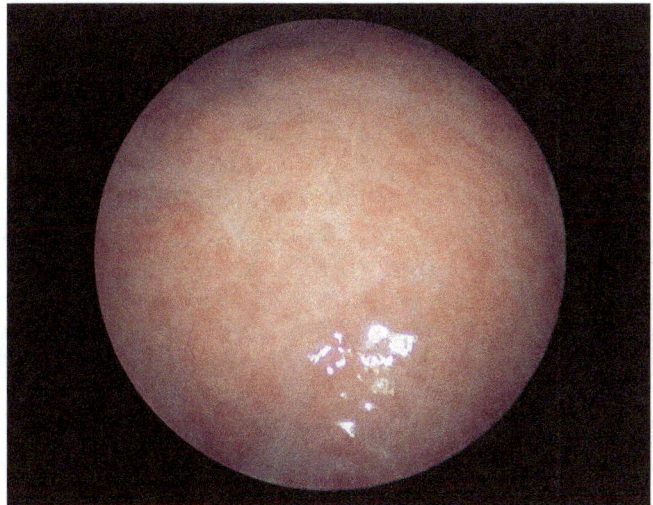

Fig. 32.3: AIH type 1 (so-called *lupoid hepatitis*). The left lobe of liver shows an irregularly rippled surface (scattered light reflex) with salmon-pink and yellow colouring; patchy red marking due to highly inflammatory parenchymal zones; fine vascular multiplication and whitish scarred areas with diffuse fibrosis

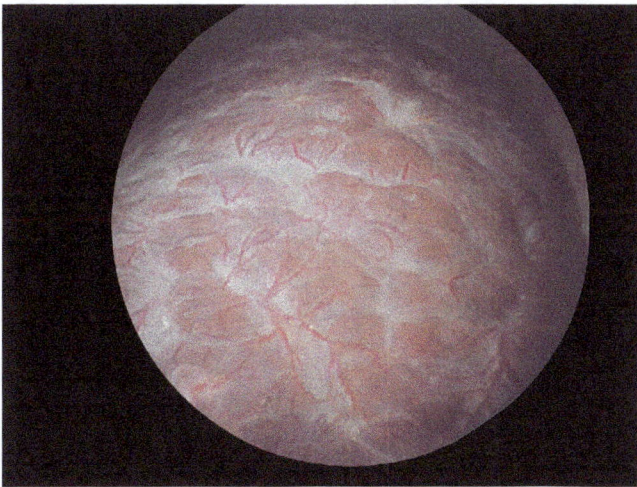

Fig. 32.5: Liver cirrhosis due to AIH: flat-nodular liver surface, highly cicatrized furrows, local neovascularization, signs of mild inflammation

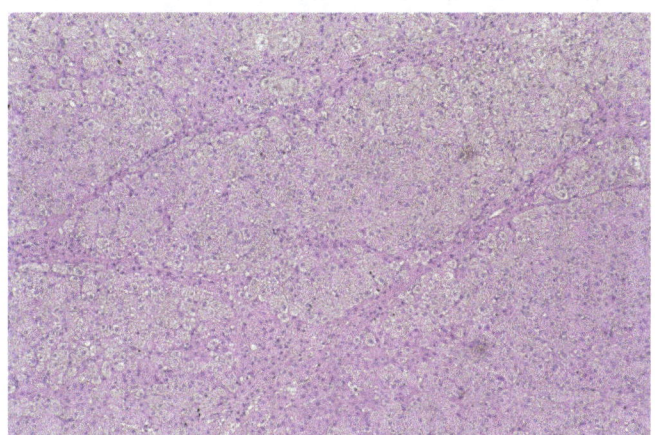

Fig. 32.4: Autoimmune hepatitis in remission under treatment: septal fibrosis and disarranged lobular structure (HE)

7 Clinical aspects

7.1 Clinical symptoms

Some 10−20% of patients with chronic active hepatitis can be categorized as autoimmune hepatitis cases. • Occasionally, the disease develops over a considerable period of time without being noticed subjectively. (36) This is why AIH is often not diagnosed before the stage of chronic hepatitis is reached. • Non-specific *complaints* have been reported, such as fatigue, languor, inappetence, decreased performance and sometimes arthralgia as well as myalgia, frequently accompanied by slight fever. • *Clinical findings* include hepato/splenomegaly, palmar erythema, facial teleangiectasia, hirsutism, amenorrhoea and spider naevi. In 25−40% of cases, AIH becomes manifest in the same way as acute viral hepatitis, but it presents more distinct subjective and clinical symptoms. At this point, scleral icterus or jaundice is usually present − as is generally the case in active phases of a disease. (31, 41, 66, 94, 99)

7.2 Laboratory diagnostics

Even at the subjective, asymptomatic stage, the *transaminases* are elevated to differing degrees. With the onset of symptomatic or acute hepatitis, high values can be detected for GPT, GOT and GDH (3 to 10 times, and more, above normal levels). The γ-GT value is only moderately or not at all increased; the same applies to bilirubin. Cholinesterase is often decreased. • Cholestasis-indicating enzymes (γ-GT, AP, LAP) are rarely elevated; clearly raised levels point to an overlap syndrome rather than to a (very infrequent) cholestatic form of autoimmune hepatitis. • A sharp rise in *γ-globulin* (1.5 to 2.0 times above normal) is a characteristic feature. This is almost solely due to an increase in the IgG fraction. IgA can be decreased. Hyperproteinaemia (>8g/dl) ensues. The blood sedimentation rate is greatly increased. • At this point, the serology of viral hepatitis (HBV, HCV, possibly HDV) has to be clarified. *Autoantibodies* (ANA, SMA, LKM, LP) and their titres are determined. When the presence of an overlap syndrome is suspected, the determination of specific autoantibodies is required (e.g. AMA with subtypes, LP, pANCA, anti-histone 2B, antinuclear antibodies). (s. tabs. 5.19, 5.20; 32.1) HLA typing (e.g. -A1, -B8, -DR3, -DR4) completes the diagnosis. • For the diagnosis of AIH, the **score system** of F. Alvarez et al. (1999) and E. M. Hennes et al. (2005) may be helpful.

7.3 Imaging techniques

Imaging techniques do not play any role in the diagnosis of AIH. A transition to cirrhosis can only be seen using sonography. With the help of elastography, it is possible to detect stiffening of the liver (fibrosis? cirrhosis?) (s. p. 135). A striking finding is the sonographic determination of enlarged abdominal (or periportal) inflammatory lymph nodes. (s. fig. 32.6)

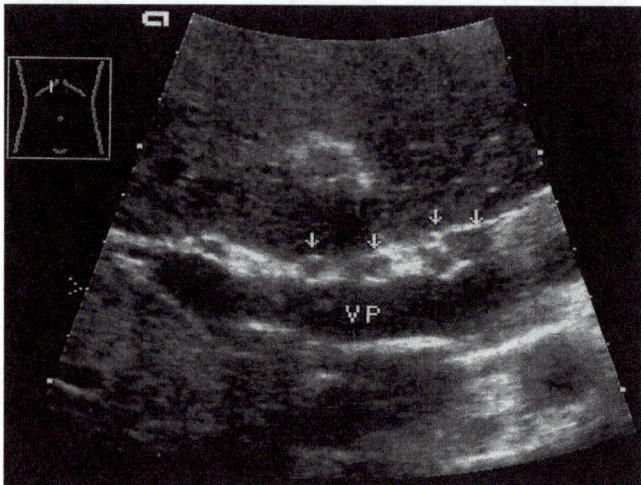

Fig. 32.6: Active autoimmune liver cirrhosis type 1 with enlarged periportal inflammatory lymph nodes (arrows) (VP = portal vein)

7.4 Liver histology

Histological examination of the liver and morphological clarification of the phase of disease (i.e. grading, staging) are imperative, although this does not facilitate the diagnosis of AIH. (11, 91) However, *liver biopsy* is recommended for the initial diagnosis; it should be carried out under *laparoscopy* to provide photodocumentation of the surface structure of the liver and to obtain several specimens (including some from the left lobe).

8 Course and prognosis

8.1 Course of disease

Autoimmune hepatitis displays a wide spectrum of clinical courses. Besides the subjective asymptomatic and insidious onset of the disease, acute manifestations similar to acute viral hepatitis may occur. Severe courses have also been described, including acute liver failure and extreme atrophy of the right lobe of liver. (36, 62) The course of disease is often characterized by acute intermittent phases. Other patients, however, experience uncharacteristic complaints over long periods of time together with aetiologically unexplained increases in the transaminases. • The effect of *pregnancy* on the course of AIH varies: deterioration, unchanged status and remission have been reported. Long-lasting spontaneous remissions were observed in up to 20% of cases (e. g. in placebo groups), but there were also cases of rapid transition into cirrhosis. In severe cases of AIH, the foetal mortality rate is increased and the number of abortions is higher. (9, 29, 41, 45, 94)

8.2 Associated diseases

A variety of immunopathies and diseases have been associated with AIH (20−30%). These association factors can render it more difficult to establish a diagnosis or differential diagnosis; as a result, therapy is more problematic, and the prognosis deteriorates. (s. tab. 32.3)

CREST	Myocarditis
Diabetes insipidus	Panniculitis
Diabetes mellitus (type I)	Pericarditis
Glomerulonephritis	Polyarthritis
Haemolytic anaemia	Polymyositis
Hypereosinophilic syndrome	Pulmonary fibrosis
Hyperthyroidosis	Sjögren's syndrome
Iridocyclitis	Thrombocytopenia
Lichen planus	Thyroidism
Lupus erythematodes	Ulcerative colitis
Mixed collagenoses	Vasculitis
Myasthenia gravis	Vitiligo

Tab. 32.3: Diseases or immunopathies which may be associated with autoimmune hepatitis (s. tabs. 22.2, 22.7, 22.8; 33.3, 33.6)

8.3 Hepatocellular carcinoma

Hepatocellular carcinoma is a rare occurrence (5−7%). (68, 80, 103, 107) It may not be due to AIH or related medication, but to concurrent HBV or HCV infection. An association of HCC with corticosteroid therapy is unusual (102); the same study group, however, reported an association of HCC with azathioprine therapy.

8.4 Prognosis

Prognosis depends on the time when the diagnosis is established and therapy can be initiated. *Risk factors* are considered to be manifestation in early years, severe hepatic inflammatory reactions with bridging necroses and the presence of HLA-DR3. Type 2 develops more rapidly into *cirrhosis* (up to 82% within 3 years). (38) If the condition is not treated, prognosis is poor; in such cases, cirrhosis inevitably develops. Approximately 50% of patients die after three to five years, and some 90% within ten years; mortality is highest during the first two years. It is obvious that prognosis is worst in those patients who have already reached the cirrhotic stage at the time of initial diagnosis. (46)

When immunosuppression is properly administered at an early stage, prognosis is good; such patients can anticipate normal life expectancy. It is even possible for liver *fibrosis* to recede. (19, 28) In general, a therapy-related *remission rate* of 80−90% can be achieved. • Relapse occurs in some two-thirds of successfully treated patients, yet this usually responds well to re-administration of the initial therapy at an adequately high dosage. So-called *non-responders* (approximately

15% of cases) should be critically reviewed in terms of detailed diagnosis, while additional exogenous or endogenous risk factors and patient compliance should be investigated anew. • The *survival rate* of treated patients (excluding cirrhosis and severe, well-advanced CAH at the time of initial diagnosis) is ca. 90% and 80% after 5 and 10 years respectively. In cirrhosis, despite properly administered therapy, the ten-year survival rate is reduced to <65% (relapse risk is 90%).

9 Therapy

Hardly any other autoimmunopathy responds so well to immunosuppressive treatment as does autoimmune hepatitis. Most patients can reckon with normal life expectancy. • However, this calls for the following *prerequisites*: (*1.*) early detailed diagnosis, (*2.*) appropriate, continuous therapy, and (*3.*) elimination and prevention of exogenous risk factors.

9.1 Detailed diagnosis

The diagnosis of autoimmune disease is in itself not difficult. • Nevertheless, the wide variety of autoimmunopathies and their multiple facets, their unpredictable preference for certain tissue, cellular or organ systems and the fact that they frequently overlap with a multitude of associated partners to differing degrees often give rise to problems which cannot be solved when setting up a detailed diagnosis. For this reason, depending on the respective level of knowledge, it is inevitable that "similar" immunopathies will be classified either as "identical" forms or possibly even as "entities" in their own right.

The occurrence of an autoimmunopathy is invariably based on a genetic predisposition with an inducibility that differs in intensity from case to case. • However, it is possible with great subtlety to detect the biochemical/biomolecular products of the cascade from the complement system, HLA system, antigen-antibody reactions, helper and suppressor cell functions, etc. (which in point of fact come *"at the end of the successful reaction"*). Furthermore, it is also possible to assess the respective interrelations of these products and to predict their immunopathogenetic significance. • Although the endocrine-autonomic-central nervous systems (in evidence *"at the beginning of humoral / cellular tolerance or defence"*) are generally accepted as a matter of course, they are still inadequately quantifiable.

The multiple reactions invoked *"on the biochemical pathway"* (*i.e. between the beginning and the end of an autoimmunopathy*) are definitely involved in the accumulation of other unknown intermediary products, which can in turn influence and manipulate a state of autoimmunopathy.

From their own experience, many clinicians are familiar with that often rapid and even insidious deterioration of an autoimmune disease as a result of extreme **overburdening of the endocrine or mental systems.** The cases of two patients, whose fate touched my staff and me deeply at the time, are briefly outlined below; as we experienced them, these were not merely post hoc, but propter hoc events, i.e. the one directly caused the other.

▶ *A female patient between 35 and 40 years of age with confirmed (in line with the methods of the time, including laparoscopy and biopsy) autoimmune hepatitis (ANA ++, SMA+, LMA+, LE factor+, IgG ++, γ-globulin++, GPT, GOT 80–100 U/l, GDH ca. 12 U/l, no cholestasis) had been undergoing treatment with prednisolone / azathioprine and had been in constant remission for over 3 years (maintenance dose of 4–6 mg prednisolone and 50 mg azathioprine for over 2 years). Physically and mentally stable, engaged in her profession, she had placed great confidence in us. Approximately 3 days after a sudden, severe emotional trauma with mental breakdown, the AIH deteriorated on a massive scale, and about 3 weeks later, the patient died in a coma hepaticum from acute liver failure.*

▶ *A female patient of approximately 45 years of age with autoimmune hepatitis and Sjögren's syndrome was in constant remission, having undergone treatment with prednisolone / azathioprine for more than 6 years. Physically and mentally stable, she was active at home, with her family and in her profession; compliance was excellent. The maintenance dose was 4–6 mg prednisolone and 50 mg azathioprine. A sudden, severe emotional trauma triggered an excessive and, despite all medication, progressive deterioration of her condition within a few days. A two-year period of suffering followed with progression of CAH, confirmed by laparoscopy and two biopsies, to florid complete cirrhosis, from which the patient died.*

The methods applied today allow precise differentiation of autoimmune hepatitis, thus providing the necessary **early diagnosis.** • Besides the "classical" or "pure" forms of autoimmune hepatitis and autoimmune cholangitis (s. p. 693), HBV-positive and HCV-positive individuals and possibly PCR-confirmed carriers should be strictly excluded from types 1–3 with their respective subgroups and classified in their own overlap groups. (s. tabs. 32.1, 33.1) (s. p. 694)

9.2 Immunosuppressive therapy

The primary target in treating autoimmune disease, especially autoimmune hepatitis, is to restore the immune balance. • When correctly administered, immunosuppression can effect the remission of autoimmune hepatitis and improve the survival rate — and even normalize individual life expectancy. But this requires an early detailed diagnosis and the widest possible differentiation of the immunological and serological profiles as well as histological investigation of the liver. (1, 14, 18, 53, 94, 99)

9.2.1 Glucocorticoids

Treatment of autoimmune hepatitis with glucocorticoids has been successfully carried out for about 45 years (A.R. PAGE et al., 1960). Fundamentally, prednisolone brings about remission of the condition in approx. 80%

of patients. A survival rate of 10 years has been observed in over 90% of precirrhotic patients under prednisolone therapy (G.L. DAVIES et al., 1989). A course of glucocorticoid monotherapy is indicated in (*1.*) young patients, (*2.*) minimal inflammatory activity in the initial phase, (*3.*) relevant bone-marrow depression, (*4.*) cholestasis under azathioprine therapy (very rare), and (*5.*) women contemplating pregnancy, but who have to avoid using azathioprine. (1, 15, 19, 70, 81, 86)

Dosage: Initial dose of approximately 1 mg/kg BW/day for about one week (until an obvious reduction in transaminase values has been achieved), ca. 40 mg/day for one week, ca. 30 mg/day for a further two weeks and then ca. 20 mg/day, depending on the decrease in activity and onset of remission. With continued acceptance of a lower dose, a further reduction should be made in steps of 2.5–5.0 mg at intervals of five to ten days until the desired maintenance dose of 4–8 mg is reached. A mean duration of treatment of two to three years is generally recommended. • Basically, we continued to administer the achieved maintenance dose ("only as much as required") as a *lifelong prednisolone therapy* unless, for any reason, it became necessary to stop treatment. In such cases, therapy should be phased out at a rate of 1 mg per week (!). On the principle of *"having respect for, but no fear of prednisolone"*, **osteoporosis prophylaxis** is of the utmost importance. Besides the administration of, for example, a combination of calcium and sodium fluorophosphates together with vitamin D, it is essential for the patients to exercise their muscles regularly every day. (s. p. 683) • *We also can confirm that the maintenance dose differs greatly for each individual patient – some patients remain in remission with 2–4 mg glucocorticoids.*

9.2.2 Glucocorticoids and azathioprine

Azathioprine should not be used initially as monotherapy. However, remission attained with prednisolone and azathioprine can be maintained by azathioprine on its own (100–200 mg/day). (5, 42, 86) • The combination of prednisolone with azathioprine (I.R. MACKAY, 1968) is just as effective as monotherapy with prednisolone. Moreover, with the above-mentioned initial dose of prednisolone (together with azathioprine), any subsequent dosage of prednisolone can be reduced more rapidly to a maintenance dose of 4–6 (–8) mg/day.

Dosage: An initial dose of azathioprine of 1–2 mg/kg BW/day (rounded off to the nearest 25 mg or 50 mg tablet) is recommended. A maintenance dose of 50–75 (–100) mg/day is sufficient. • We always administered the combination therapy from the outset and thereby did not observe any side effects from azathioprine – minor fluctuations in bone-marrow depression reverted to normal values spontaneously or after a short period of reduced dosage (25 mg). • With this maintenance dose, we retained a number of female patients in remission for over 16 years (!) – see the patient group treated with prednisolone and azathioprine for primary biliary cholangitis. (s. p. 683)

As a criterion of successful therapy, the following remission figures are given in the relevant literature: 50–60% after 6 months, 70–80% after 12 months and 80–90% after 24 months. The corresponding success figures in terms of liver histology are 10%, 30–40% and 50–60% respectively. At the end of successful therapy with a cessation of medication, ca. 50% of patients suffered a **relapse,** so that a new "initial dose" had to be applied – sometimes with less positive results. • Thus we consider a **lifelong maintenance dose** to be preferable. We have repeatedly noted that continued administration of the combination therapy eventually achieved a stabilized remission, even after a period of two to four years. *Particularly in immunopathies, patience is called for, while attention must focus on the current state of disease and on the patient "in his/her entirety".*

▶ Should *cirrhosis* be present at the time of initial diagnosis in the wake of confirmed "pure" autoimmune hepatitis (i.e. without HBV or HCV replication markers), it is advisable to implement combined immunosuppression – which is often successful in relatively low but sufficient dosage. Even if the morphological end-stage has already been reached, inflammatory activity can be repressed and clinical improvement achieved. • The question of whether (and when) a liver transplantation should be planned always has to be considered.

Budesonide: Initial results with the oral "topical" steroid budesonide have also proved remarkable in AIH. (21) In precirrhotic patients without collateral shunts, this substance achieves a first-pass effect in the liver of up to 90%, resulting in a satisfactory anti-inflammatory steroid impact with only minor side effects. • The dosage is 6–8 mg/day for 6–12 weeks.

9.2.3 Ursodeoxycholic acid

If cholestasis is not present, the additional application of ursodeoxycholic acid (UDCA) is worth considering because of its pharmacological properties and lack of side effects or interactions. • Initial results on the treatment of **chronic hepatitis** with UDCA were reported by F. ICHIDA (1961), T. NAKAHARA et al. (1975) and K. MIYAJI (1976). • In 1988 our study group also noted obvious and permanent effects of UDCA on the course of disease in terms of clinical and laboratory indices in severe **acute viral hepatitis B.** (s. p. 445) Such observations were confirmed by A. JORGE in 1993. • Owing to the multiple mechanisms of action of UDCA, in particular its immunomodulatory effect, adjuvant therapeutic efficacy can be anticipated in **autoimmune hepatitis,** as reported by P. JANOWITZ et al. in 1996. In autoimmune-associated chronic hepatitis C, UDCA proved to be a successful therapeutic agent (K. NAKAMURA et al., 1999).

9.2.4 Monitoring therapy

GPT is the main parameter for monitoring laboratory indices — initially at intervals of four to eight days and subsequently every two to four weeks (depending on the activity status). *GDH* is a good complementary value, possibly together with GOT (for the concurrent determination of the respective quotient). (s. tabs. 5.6, 5.7) • The *γ-globulin* value is a further important parameter. With these results, it is possible to assess the course of AIH reliably and thus monitor the success of therapy.

9.2.5 Non-responders to therapy

Patients in whom initial treatment was devoid of success (though a detailed diagnosis had been made) and increased dosage in a renewed course of therapy failed or in whom relapse therapy was not efficacious were administered **cyclosporin** A (3–6 mg/kg BW, twice daily) for about 10 weeks. However, there are divergent reports regarding the success rate of this treatment. (30, 40, 59, 69, 71, 83) • In individual cases, good results have been achieved with **cyclophosphamide** (100 mg and subsequently 50 mg/day). (44) • New, effective substances that have been successfully used in AIH type 1 include **tacrolimus** (2–3 mg, twice daily) for about 12 months. (95) and **mycophenolate mofetil** (250–1000 mg, twice daily) for several years. (8, 77) • In the case of treatment failure (prednisolone + azathioprine), the administration of **methotrexate** (7.5 mg/week) proved successful in type 1. (10) Good therapeutic efficacy was also achieved with **6-mercaptopurine** after failure with azathioprine. (73)

Boswellinic acids are seen as selective non-redox inhibitors of leukotriene biosynthesis. Leukotrienes are mediators of inflammation. Boswellic acids proved to be antiphlogistic, hepatoprotective and immunosuppressive in their impact (H. P. T. AMMON et al., 1991). • Although there has been no therapeutic application in hepatology up to now, it is likely that future discussion will focus on this pharmacologically interesting group of substances. (s. pp 685, 692)

A small percentage (5–15%) of patients can be defined at an early stage as **non-responders;** their condition and the laboratory parameters show no improvement within the first two to four weeks. Should histological investigation reveal bridging necroses that are already dilated as well as multilobular liver cell necroses, conservative therapy does not usually prove successful — such patients are candidates for liver transplantation.

This recently acquired knowledge gives new impetus to our **suggestion** of removing all patients with replicative HBV, HBV/HDV and HCV infections from their respective groups (1a, 1b, 2b, 3); they can then be redefined and treated as separate overlap groups.

• *These patients have "another immunology" — and indeed "other statistics".*

9.3 Liver transplantation

Liver transplantation is indicated in the terminal stage of cirrhosis, in acute liver failure and for non-responders to long-term therapy. The five-year survival rate is 80–90%. Determining the right time for transplantation is problematical, however. *All possibilities of medication should be exploited first.* It is remarkable that AIH reoccurs in the transplanted liver: in 7–10% of cases after 1 year and in 65–70% of cases after 5 years. In patients with HLA-DR3, there was no evidence of recurrence. Following transplantation, the autoantibodies may disappear from the serum. It is not possible to prevent recurrence after OLT despite correct therapy. The postoperative reappearance of antibodies does not necessary point to a recurrence. In approx. 50% of cases, there is recurrence without the formation of antibodies. (3, 12, 22, 27, 57, 63, 72, 76, 81, 106)

References:

1. **Alvarez, F.:** Treatment of autoimmune hepatitis: Current and future therapies. Curr. Treat. Opt. Gastroenterol. 2004; 7: 413–420
2. **Amberg, S.:** Hyperproteinemia associated with severe liver damage. Proc. Mayo Clin. 1942; 17: 360–362
3. **Ayata, G., Gordon, F.D., Lewis, W.D., Pomfret, E., Pomposelli, J.J., Jenkins, R.L., Khettry, U.:** Liver transplantation for autoimmune hepatitis: A long-term pathologic study. Hepatology, 2000; 32: 185–192
4. **Bearn, A.G., Kunkel, H.G., Slater, R.J.:** The problem of chronic liver disease in young women. Amer. J. Med. 1956; 21: 3–15
5. **Bellary, S., Schiano, T., Hartman, G., Black, M.:** Chronic hepatitis with combined features of autoimmune chronic hepatitis and chronic hepatitis C: favorable response to prednisone and azathioprine. Ann. Intern. Med. 1995; 123: 32–34
6. **Bianchi, F.B., Muratori, P., Muratori, L.:** New antibodies and autoantigens in autoimmune hepatitis. Clin. Liver Dis. 2002; 6: 497–509
7. **Boberg, K.M.:** Prevalence and epidemiology of autoimmune hepatitis. Clin. Liver Dis. 2002; 6: 347–359
8. **Brunt, E.M., di Bisceglie, A.M.:** Histological changes after the use of mycophenolate mofetil in autoimmune hepatitis. Hum. Path. 2004; 35: 509–512
9. **Buchel, E., van Steenbergen, W., Nevens, F., Fevery, J.:** Improvement of autoimmune hepatitis during pregnancy followed by flare-up after delivery. Amer. J. Gastroenterol. 2002; 97: 3160–3165
10. **Burak, K.W., Urbanski, S.J., Swain, M.G.:** Successful treatment of refractory type 1 autoimmune hepatitis with methotrexate. J. Hepatol. 1998; 29: 990–993
11. **Carpenter, H.A., Czaya, A.J.:** The role of histologic evaluation in the diagnosis and management of autoimmune hepatitis and its variants. Clin. Liver Dis. 2002; 6: 685–705
12. **Cattan, P., Berney, T., Conti, F., Calmus, Y., Homberg, J.C., Houssin, D., Soubrane, O.:** Outcome of orthotopic liver transplantation in autoimmune hepatitis according to subtypes. Transpl. Intl. 2002; 15: 34–38
13. **Cianciara, J., Laskus, T.:** Development of transient autoimmune hepatitis during interferon treatment of chronic hepatitis B. Dig. Dis. Sci. 1995; 40: 1842–1844
14. **Coverdale, S.A., Field, J., Farrell, G.C.:** How reversible is hepatic functional impairment in autoimmune hepatitis? J. Gastroenterol. Hepatol. 2003; 18: 371–375
15. **Czaja, A.J., Wang, K.K., Shiels, M.T., Katzmann, J.H.:** Oral pulse prednisone therapy after relapse of severe autoimmune chronic active hepatitis. J. Hepatol. 1993; 17: 180–186
16. **Czaja, A.J., Carpenter, H.A., Santrach, P.J., Moore, S.B.:** Significance of HLA DR4 in type 1 autoimmune hepatitis. Gastroenterology 1993; 105: 1502–1507
17. **Czaja, A.J., Cassani, F., Cataleta, M., Valentini, P., Bianchi, F.B.:** Frequency and significance of antibodies to actin in type 1 autoimmune hepatitis. Hepatology 1996; 24: 1068–1073
18. **Czaja, A.J.:** Treatment strategies in autoimmune hepatitis. Clin. Liver dis. 2002; 6: 799–824
19. **Czaja, A.J., Carpenter, H.A.:** Decreased fibrosis during corticosteroid therapy of autoimmune hepatitis. J. Hepatol. 2004; 40: 646–652
20. **Dalekos, G.N., Zachou, K., Liasko, C., Gatselis, N.:** Autoantibodies and defined target autoantigens in autoimmune hepatitis: an overview. Eur. J. Int. Med. 2002; 13: 293–303
21. **Danielsson, A., Prytz, H.:** Oral budesonide for treatment of autoimmune chronic active hepatitis. Aliment. Pharmacol. Ther. 1994; 8: 585–590

22. Devlin, J., Donaldson, P., Portmann, B., Heaton, N., Tan, K.-C., Williams, R.: Recurrence of autoimmune hepatitis following liver transplantation. Liver Transplant. Surg. 1995; 1: 162–165
23. Dienes, H.P., Autschbach, F., Gerber, M.A.: Ultrastructural lesions in autoimmune hepatitis and steps of the immune response in liver tissue. Semin. Liver Dis. 1991; 11: 197–204
24. Donaldson, P.T., Doherty, D.G., Hayllar, K.M., McFarlane, I.G., Johnson, P.J., Williams, R.: Susceptibility to autoimmune chronic active hepatitis: human leukocyte antigens DR4 and A1-B8-DR3 are independent risk factors. Hepatology 1991; 13: 701–706
25. Donaldson, P.T.: Genetics in autoimmune hepatitis. Semin. Liver Dis. 2002; 22: 353–364
26. Duchini, A., McHutchison, J.G., Pockros, P.J.: LKM-positive autoimmune hepatitis in the western United States: a case series. Amer. J. Gastroenterol. 2000; 95: 3238–3241
27. Duclos-Vallée, J.-C., Sebagh, M., Rifai, K., Johanet, C., Ballot, E., Guettier, C., Karam, V., Hurtova, M., Feray, C., Reynes, M., Bismuth, H., Samuel, D.: A 10 year follow-up study of patients transplanted for autoimmune hepatitis: histological recurrence precedes clinical and biochemical recurrence. Gut 2003; 52: 893–897
28. Dufour, J.-F., DeLellis, R., Kaplan, M.M.: Reversibility of hepatic fibrosis in autoimmune hepatitis. Ann. Intern. Med. 1997; 127: 981–985
29. Dufour, J.F., Zimmermann, M., Reichen, J.: Severe autoimmune hepatitis in patients with previous spontaneous recovery of a flare. J. Hepatol. 2002; 37: 748–752
30. Fernandes, N.F., Redeker, A.G., Vierling, J.M., Villamil, F.G., Fong, T.L.: Cyclosporine therapy in patients with steroid resistant autoimmune hepatitis. Amer. J. Gastroenterol. 1999; 94: 241–248
31. Fried, M.W., Draguesku, J.O., Shindo, M., Simpson, L.H., Banks, S.M., Hoofnagle, J.H., Di Bisceglie, A.M.: Clinical and serological differentiation of autoimmune and hepatitis C virus-related chronic hepatitis. Dig. Dis. Sci. 1993; 38: 631–636
32. Garcia-Buey, L., Garcia-Monzo·n, C., Rodriguez, S., Borque, M.J., Gar-cia-Sanchez, A., Iglesias, R., de Castro, M., Mateos, F.G., Vicario, J.L., Balas, A., Moreno-Otero, R.: Latent autoimmune hepatitis triggered during interferon therapy in patients with chronic hepatitis C. Gastroenterology 1995; 108: 1770–1777
33. Goldstein, N.S., Bayati, N., Silverman, A.L., Gordon, S.C.: Minocycline as a cause of drug-induced autoimmune hepatitis. – Report of four cases and comparison with autoimmune hepatitis. Amer. J. Clin. Path. 2000; 114: 591–598
34. Gregorio, G.V., Portmann, B., Reid, F., Donaldson, P.T., Doherty, D.G., McCartney, M., Mowat, A.P., Vergani, D., Mieli-Vergani, G.: Autoimmune hepatitis in childhood: a 20-year experience. Hepatology 1997; 25: 541–547
35. Han, S., Tredger, M., Gregorio, G.V., Mieli-Vergani, G., Vergani, D.: Anti-liver cytosolic antigen type 1 (LC1) antibodies in childhood autoimmune liver disease. Hepatology 1995; 21: 58–62
36. Herzog, D., Rasquin-Weber, A.-M., Debray, D., Alvarez, F.: Subfulminant hepatic failure in autoimmune hepatitis type 1: an unusual form of presentation. J. Hepatol. 1997; 27: 578–582
37. Hodges, S., Lobo-Yeo, A., Donaldson, P., Tanner, M.S., Vergani, D.: Autoimmune chronic active hepatitis in a family. Gut 1991; 32: 299–302
38. Homberg, J.-C., Abuaf, N., Bernard, O., Islam, S., Alvarez, F., Khalil, S.H., Poupon, R., Darnis, F., Lévy, V.-G., Grippon, P., Opolon, P., Bernuau, J., Benhamou, J.-P., Alagille, D.: Chronic active hepatitis associated with anti-liver/kidney microsome antibody type 1: a second type of "autoimmune hepatitis". Hepatology 1987; 7: 1333–1339
39. Hunziker, L., Recher, M., Andrew, J., Macpherson, A.J., Ciura, A., Freigang, S., Hengartner, H., Zinkernagel, R.M.: Hypergammaglobulinemia and autoantibody induction mechanisms in viral infection. Nat. Immunol. 2003; 4: 343–349
40. Jackson, L.D., Song, E.: Cyclosporine in the treatment of corticoid-resistant autoimmune chronic active hepatitis. Gut 1995; 36: 459–461
41. Johnson, P.J., McFarlane, I.G., Eddleston, A.L.W.F.: The natural course and heterogeneity of autoimmune-type chronic active hepatitis. Semin. Liver Dis. 1991; 11: 187–196
42. Johnson, P.J., McFarlane, I.G., Williams, R.: Azathioprine for long-term maintenance of remission in autoimmune hepatitis. New Engl. J. Med. 1995; 333: 958–963
43. Joske, R.A., King, W.E.: The L.E. cell phenomen in active viral hepatitis. Lancet 1955/II: 477–480
44. Kanzler, S., Gerken, G., Dienes, H.P., Meyer zum Büschenfelde, K.H., Lohse, A.W.: Cyclophosphamide as alternative immunosuppressive therapy for autoimmune hepatitis – report of three cases. Zschr. Gastroenterol. 1997; 35: 571–578
45. Klein, C., Philipp, T., Greiner, P., Strobelt, M., Müller, H., Trautwein, C., Brandis, M., Manns, M.: Asymptomatic autoimmune hepatitis associated with anti-LC-1 autoantibodies. J. Pediatr. Gastroenterol. Nutrit. 1996; 23: 461–465
46. Kogan, J., Safadi, R., Ashur, Y., Shouval, D., Ilan, Y.: Prognosis of symptomatic versus asymptomatic autoimmune hepatitis: a study of 68 patients. J. Clin. Gastroenterol. 2002; 35: 75–81
47. Kunkel, H.G., Ahrens, E.H., Eisenmenger, W.J., Bougiovanni, A.M., Slater, R.J.: Extreme hypergammaglobulinemia in young women with liver disease of unknown etiology. J. Clin. Invest. 1951; 30: 654–659
48. Lohse, A.W., Gerken, G., Mohr, H., Löhr, H.F., Treichel, U., Dienes, H.P., Meyer zum Büschenfelde, K.-H.: Relation between autoimmune liver diseases and viral hepatitis. Clinical and serological characteristics in 859 patients. Z. Gastroenterol. 1995; 33: 527–533
49. Mackay, I.R., Taft, L.I., Cowling, D.C.: Lupoid hepatitis. Lancet 1956/II: 1323–1326
50. Manabe, K., Donaldson, P.T., Underhill, J.A., Doherty, D.G., Mieli-Vergani, G., McFarlane, I.G., Eddleston, A.L., Williams, R.: Human leukocyte antigen A1-B8-DR3-DQ2-DPB1-0401 extended haplotype in autoimmune hepatitis. Hepatology 1993; 18: 1334–1337
51. Manns, M., Gerken, G., Kyriatsoulis, A., Staritz, M., Meyer zum Büschenfelde, K.-H.: Characterisation of a new subgroup of autoimmune chronic active hepatitis by autoantibodies against a soluble liver antigen. Lancet 1987/I: 292–294
52. McFarlane, I.G.: Definition and classification of autoimmune hepatitis. Semin. Liver Dis. 2002; 22: 317–324
53. Medina, J., Garcia-Buey, L., Moreno-Otera, R.: Immunopathogenetic and therapeutic aspects of autoimmune hepatitis (review). Amer. Pharm. Ther. 2003; 17: 1–16
54. Meyer zum Büschenfelde, K.H.: Autoimmune hepatitis: "Hepatitis sui generic". J. Hepatol. 2003; 38: 130–135
55. Michel, G., Ritter, A., Gerken, G., Meyer zum Büschenfelde, K.-H., Decker, R., Manns, M.P.: Anti-GOR and hepatitis C virus in autoimmune liver diseases. Lancet 1992; 339: 267–269
56. Mieli-Vergani, G., Vergani, D.: Autoimmune hepatitis in children. Clin. Liver Dis. 2002; 6: 247–259
57. Milkiewicz, P., Hubscher, S.G., Skiba, G., Hathaway, M., Elias, E.: Recurrence of autoimmune hepatitis after liver transplantation. Transplantation 1999; 68: 253–256
58. Misdraji, J., Thiim, M., Graeme-Cook, F.M.: Autoimmune hepatitis with centrilobular necrosis. Amer. J. Surg. Path. 2003; 28: 471–478
59. Mistilis, S.P., Vickers, C.R., Darroch, M.H., McCarthy, S.W.: Cyclosporine, a new treatment for autoimmune chronic active hepatitis. Med. J. Austr. 1985; 143: 463–465
60. Miyakawa, H., Kitazawa, E., Abe, K., Kawaguchi, N., Fuzikawa, H., Kikuchi, K., Kato, M., Komatsu, T., Hayashi, N., Kiyosawa, K.: Chronic hepatitis C associated with anti-liver/kidney microsome-1 antibody is not a subgroup of autoimmune hepatitis. J. Gastroenterol. 1997; 32: 769–776
61. Muratori, L., Lenzi, M., Cataleta, M., Giostra, F., Cassani, F., Ballardini, G., Zauli, D., Bianchi, F.B.: Interferon therapy in liver/kidney microsomal antibody type 1-positive patients with chronic hepatitis C. J. Hepatol. 1994; 21: 199–203
62. Nakadate, I., Nakamura, A., Endo, R., Iwai, M., Kaneta, H., Shimotono, H., Sasaki, S., Takikawa, Y., Yamazaki, K., Madarame, T., Kashiwabara, T., Suzuki, K., Sato, S.: Autoimmune hepatitis presenting with acute hepatic failure. Acta Hepatol. Japan. 1993; 34: 665–671
63. Neuberger, J., Portmann, B., Calne, R., Williams, R.: Recurrence of autoimmune chronic active hepatitis following orthotopic liver grafting. Transplantation 1984; 37: 363–365
64. Nobili, V., Comparcola, D., Sartorelli, M.R., Devito, R., Marcellini, M.: Autoimmune hepatitis type 1 after Epstein-Barr virus infection. Paediatr. Infect. J. 2003; 22: 387
65. Nouri-Aria, K.T., Donaldson, P.T., Hegarty, J.E., Eddleston, A.L.W.F., Williams, R.: HLA-A1-B8-DR3 and suppressor cell function in first degree relatives of patients with autoimmune chronic active hepatitis. J. Hepatol. 1985; 1: 235–241
66. Obermayer-Straub, P., Strassburg, C.P., Manns, M.P.: Autoimmune hepatitis. J. Hepatol. 2000; 32 (Suppl. 1) 181–197
67. Papo, T., Marcellin, P., Bernuau, J., Durand, F., Poynard, T., Benhamou, J.P.: Autoimmune chronic active hepatitis exacerbated by alpha-interferon. Ann. Intern. Med. 1992; 116: 51–53
68. Park, S.Z., Nagorney, D.M., Czaja, A.J.: Hepatocellular carcinoma in autoimmune hepatitis. Dig. Dis. Sci. 2000; 45: 1944–1948
69. Paroli, M., Franco, A., Santilio, I., Balsano, C., Levrero, M., Barnaba, V.: Cyclosporine A in the treatment of autoimmune chronic active hepatitis occurring with or without circulating antibodies against hepatitis C Virus. Int. J. Immunther. 1992; 8: 135–140
70. Perdigoto, R., Carpenter, H.A., Czaja, A.J.: Frequency and significance of chronic ulcerative colitis in severe corticosteroid-treated autoimmune hepatitis. J. Hepatol. 1992; 14: 325–331
71. Person, J.L., McHutchison, J.G., Fong, T., Redeker, A.G.: A case of cyclosporine-sensitive, steroid-resistant autoimmune chronic active hepatitis. J. Clin. Gastroent. 1993; 17: 317–320
72. Prados, E., Cuervas-Mons, U., de la Mata, M., Fraga, E., Rimola, A., Prieto, M., Clemente, G., Vicente, E., Casanova, J., Fabrega, J.E.: Outcome of autoimmune hepatitis after liver transplantation. Transplantation 1998; 66: 1645–1650
73. Pratt, D.S., Flavin, D.P., Kaplan, M.M.: The successful treatment of autoimmune hepatitis with 6-mercaptopurine after failure with azathioprine. Gastroenterology 1996; 110: 271–274
74. Rahaman, S.M., Chira, P., Koff, R.S.: Idiopathic autoimmune chronic hepatitis triggered by hepatitis A. Amer. J. Gastroent. 1994; 89: 106–108
75. Rehermann, B., Michitaka, K., Durazzo, M., Mergener, K., Velev, P., Manns, M.P.: Viruses and auto-immune hepatitis. Europ. J. Clin. Invest. 1994; 24: 11–19
76. Reich, D.J., Fiel, I., Guarrera, J.V., Emre, S., Schwartz, M.E., Miller, C.M., Sheiner, P.A.: Liver transplantation for autoimmune hepatitis. Hepatology 2000; 32: 693–700
77. Richardson, P.D., James, P.D., Ryder, S.D.: Mycophenolate mofetil for maintenance of remission in autoimmune hepatitis in patients resistant. J. Hepatol. 2000; 33: 371–375

78. **Robertson, D.A.F., Zhang, S.L., Guy, E.C., Wright, R.:** Persistent measles virus genome in autoimmune chronic active hepatitis. Lancet 1987/ I: 9–11
79. **Ruiz-Mureno, M., Rua, M.J., Carreno, V., Quironga, J.A., Manns, M., Meyer zum Büschenfelde, K.-H.:** Autoimmune chronic active hepatitis type 2 manifested during interferon therapy in children. J. Hepatol. 1991; 12: 265–266
80. **Ryder, S.D., Koskinas, J., Rizzi, P.M., McFarlane, I.G., Portmann, B.C., Naoumov, N.V., Williams, R.:** Hepatocellular carcinoma complicating autoimmune hepatitis: role of hepatitis C virus. Hepatology 1995; 22: 718–722
81. **Sanchez-Urdazpal, L., Czaja, A.J., von Hoek, B., Ruud, A.F., Krom and Russel, H., Wiesner, J.:** Prognostic features and role of liver transplantation in severe corticosteroid-treated autoimmune chronic active hepatitis. Hepatology 1991; 15: 215–221
82. **Seki, T., Kiyosawa, K., Inoko, H., Ota, M.:** Association of autoimmune hepatitis with HLA-Bw54 and DR4. Hepatology 1990; 12: 1300–1304
83. **Sherman, K.E., Narkewicz, M., Pinto, P.C.:** Cyclosporine in the management of corticosteroid-resistant type I autoimmune chronic active hepatitis. J. Hepatol. 1994; 21: 1040–1047
84. **Singh, R., Nair, S., Farr, G., Mason, A., Perrillo, R.P.:** Acute autoimmune hepatitis presenting with centrizonal liver disease: case report and review of the literature. Amer. J. Gastroenterol. 2002; 97: 2670–2673
85. **Stechemesser, E., Klein, R., Berg, P.A.:** Characterization and clinical relevance of liver-pancreas antibodies in autoimmune hepatitis. Hepatology 1993; 18: 1–9
86. **Stellon, A.J., Kreating, J.J., Johnson, P.J., McFarlane, I.G., Williams, R.:** Maintenance of remission in autoimmune chronic active hepatitis with azathioprine after corticosteroid withdrawal. Hepatology 1988; 8: 781–784
87. **Storch, W.B.:** New autoantibodies and their antigens in autoimmune diseases. Cell. Molec. Biol. 1997; 43: 337–344 • Autoantikörper und ihre diagnostische Bedeutung. Dtsch. Med. Wschr. 1998; 123: 1213–1216
88. **Storch, W.B.:** Autoimmune hepatitis – update 2004. Cell. Mol. Biol. 2004; 50: 569–580
89. **Strassburg, C.P., Manns, M.P.:** Autoantibodies and autoantigens in autoimmune hepatitis. Semin. Liver Dis. 2002; 22: 339–352
90. **Tagle Arrospide, M., Leon Barva, R.:** Viral hepatitis A as triggering agent of autoimmune hepatitis. Report of case and review of the literature. Rev. Gastroenterol. Peru 2003; 23: 134–137
91. **Terracciano, L.M., Patzina, R.A., Lehmann, F.S., Tornillo, L., Cathomas, G., Mhawech, P., Vecchione, R.; Bianchi, L:** A spectrum of histopathologic findings in autoimmune liver disease. Amer. J. Clin. Pathol. 2000; 114: 705–711
92. **Todros, L., Saracco, G., Durazzo, M., Abate, M.L., Touscoz, G., Scaglione, L., Verme, G., Rizetto, M.:** Efficacy and safety of interferon alfa therapy in chronic hepatitis C with autoantibodies to liver-kidney microsomes. Hepatology 1995; 22: 1374–1378
93. **Treichel, U., Gerken, G., Rossol, S., Rotthauwe, H.W., Meyer zum Büschenfelde, K.-H., Poralla, T.:** Autoantibodies against the human asialoglycoprotein receptor: effects of therapy in autoimmune and virus induced chronic active hepatitis. J. Hepatol. 1993; 19: 55–63
94. **Van den Berg, A.P.:** Autoimmune hepatitis: pathogenesis, diagnosis and treatment. Scand. J. Gastroenterol. 1998; 33 (Suppl. 225): 66–69
95. **Van Thiel, D.H., Wright, H., Carroll, P., Abu-Elmagd, K., Rodriguez, Rilo, H., McMichael, J., Irish, W., Starzl, T.E.:** Tacrolimus: a potential new treatment for autoimmune chronic active hepatitis: results of an open-label preliminary trial. Amer. J. Gastroenterol. 1995; 90: 771–776
96. **Vento, S., Garofano, T., di Perri, G., Dolci, L., Concia, E., Bassetti, D.:** Identification of hepatitis A virus as trigger for autoimmune chronic hepatitis type 1 in susceptible individuals. Lancet 1991; 337: 1183–1187
97. **Vento, S., Guella, L., Mirandola, F., Cainelli, F., di Perri, G., Solbiati, M., Ferraro, T., Concia, E.:** Epstein-Barr virus as a trigger for autoimmune hepatitis in susceptible individuals. Lancet 1995; 346: 608–609
98. **Vento, S., Cainelli, F., Ferraro, T., Concia, E.:** Autoimmune hepatitis type 1 after measles. Amer. J. Gastroenterol. 1996; 91: 2618–2620
99. **Vergani, D., Mieli-Vergani, G.:** Autoimmune hepatitis. Autoimmun. Rev. 2003; 2: 241–247
100. **Vogel, A., Strassburg, C.P., Manns, M.P.:** 77C/G mutation in the tyrosine phosphatase CD45 gene and autoimmune hepatitis: evidence for a genetic link. Genes Immun. 2003; 4: 79–81
101. **Wächter, B., Kyriatsouis, A., Lohse, A.W., Gerken, G., Meyer zum Büschenfelde, K.-H., Manns, M.P.:** Characterisation of liver cytokeratin as a major target of anti-SLA antibodies. J. Hepatol. 1990; 11: 232–239
102. **Waldenström, J.:** Leber, Blutproteine und Nahrungseiweiß. Dtsch. J. Verdau. Stoffwechselkr. 1950; 15: 113–119
103. **Wang, K.K., Czaja, A.J.:** Hepatocellular carcinoma in corticosteroidtreated severe autoimmune chronic active hepatitis. Hepatology 1988; 8: 1679–1683
104. **Wen, L., Peakman, M., Lobo-Yeo, A., McFarlane, B.M., Mowat, A.P., Mieli-Vergani, G., Vergani, D.:** T-cell-directed hepatocyte damage in autoimmune chronic active hepatitis. Lancet 1990; 336: 1527–1530
105. **Wies, I., Brunner, S., Henninger, J., Herkel, J., Kanzler, S., Meyer zum Büschenfelde, K.-H., Lohse, A.W.:** Identification of target antigen for SLA/LP autoantibodies in autoimmune hepatitis. Lancet 2000; 355: 1510–1515
106. **Wright, H.L., Bou-Abboud, C.F., Hassanein, T., Block, G.D., Demetris, A.J., Starzl, T.E., van Thiel, D.H.:** Disease recurrence and rejection following liver transplantation for autoimmune chronic active liver disease. Transplantation 1992; 53: 136–139
107. **Yamaoka, K., Koizumi, K., Asahina, Y., Tajiri, K., Sakai, Y., Tazawa, J.:** Hepatocellular carcinoma associated with autoimmune hepatitis – a case report and a review of the literature. Japan. J. Gastroenterol. 1994; 91: 1262–1267
108. **Zanger, U.M., Hauri, H.P., Loeper, J., Homberg, J.C., Meyer, U.A.:** Antibodies against human cytochrome P 450 db1 in autoimmune hepatitis type II. Proc. Nat. Acad. Sci. 1988; 27: 8256–8260

Clinical Aspects of Liver Diseases
33 Cholangitis and cholangiodysplasia

		Page:
1	*Definition*	670
2	*Systematics and aetiology*	670
3	***Cholangitis***	671
3.1	Infectious cholangitis	671
3.1.1	Bacterial cholangitis	671
3.1.2	Parasitic cholangitis	671
3.1.3	Viral cholangitis	671
3.1.4	Mycotic cholangitis	671
3.2	Obstructive cholangitis	671
3.3	Toxic cholangitis	672
3.4	Clinical aspects	672
3.5	Morphology	672
3.6	Diagnostics	673
3.7	Complications and prognosis	674
3.8	Therapy	674
4	***Primary biliary cholangitis***	675
4.1	Definition	675
4.2	Epidemiology	675
4.3	Aetiology	675
4.3.1	Genetic susceptibility	675
4.3.2	Hormone theory	676
4.3.3	Mycotoxin theory	676
4.3.4	Bacterial or viral theory	676
4.3.5	Elevation of leukotrienes	676
4.3.6	Increase in Mn-SOD	676
4.3.7	Immunologic factors	676
4.4	Pathogenesis	677
4.5	Morphology	678
4.6	Clinical courses	679
4.6.1	Asymptomatic stage	679
4.6.2	Oligosymptomatic stage	680
4.6.3	Symptomatic anicteric stage	680
4.6.4	Icteric stage	680
4.6.5	Final stage	680
4.7	Complications	680
4.8	PBC-associated immunologic diseases	681
4.9	Diagnostics	681
4.10	Prognosis	682
4.11	Therapy	683
4.11.1	Symptomatic therapy	683
4.11.2	Approaches to causal therapy	683
4.11.3	Therapy concepts	685
4.11.4	Liver transplantation	686

		Page:
5	***Primary sclerosing cholangitis***	686
5.1	Definition	686
5.2	Systematics	686
5.3	Epidemiology	686
5.4	Aetiopathogenesis	687
5.5	Morphology	688
5.6	Clinical aspects	689
5.7	Diagnostics	689
5.8	PSC-associated diseases	691
5.9	Complications	691
5.10	Course and prognosis	692
5.11	Therapy	692
5.11.1	Conservative therapy	692
5.11.2	Invasive therapy	693
5.11.3	Surgical measures	693
6	***Autoimmune cholangitis***	693
6.1	Clinical aspects	694
6.2	Hypothesis of pathogenesis	694
7	***Overlap syndrome***	695
7.1	Outlier syndrome	695
7.2	Conversion syndrome	695
7.3	Therapy	696
8	***Cholangiodysplasia***	696
8.1	Definition	696
8.2	Aetiopathogenesis	696
8.3	*Ductal plate malformation*	696
8.3.1	Caroli's disease	697
8.3.2	Congenital liver fibrosis	697
8.3.3	Childhood fibropolycystic disease	697
8.3.4	Adult polycystic disease	697
8.3.5	Solitary non-parasitic liver cyst	698
8.3.6	Microhamartoma	698
8.4	*Alagille's syndrome*	699
8.5	*North American Indian cirrhosis*	699
8.6	*Genetic-metabolic ductopenia*	699
8.6.1	α_1-antitrypsin deficiency	699
8.6.2	Mucoviscidosis	699
8.6.3	Zellweger's syndrome	699
8.7	*Acquired ductopenia*	699
8.8	*Idiopathic ductopenia*	700
	• References (1–534)	701
	(Figures 33.1–33.20; tables 33.1–33.7)	

33 Cholangitis

1 Definition

The term cholangitis subsumes localized or diffuse inflammatory changes of diverse aetiology, i.e. between the canal of Hering and the ampulla of Vater, affecting the intrahepatic and extrahepatic bile ducts. Cholangitis can be acute or chronic; it may originate as a primary disease in the bile ducts or develop as secondary concomitant cholangitis in the course of another underlying disease. Forms of cholangitis which exclusively affect the intrahepatic bile ducts lead to the clinical picture of liver disease in a great number of cases.

2 Systematics and aetiology

▶ *The bile is sterile under physiological conditions.* • Pathophysiological events can cause **asymptomatic bacteriocholia,** which is of no clinical importance. Microorganisms are verifiable in bile in 75–100% of patients with obstruction of the large bile ducts — whereas this applies only to 0–10% of patients with obstruction due to pancreatic carcinoma. Diagnostic or therapeutic endoscopic interventions in the bile ducts are often followed by **bacterial cholangitis**, attributable to the importation of microorganisms, particularly as a result of a (usually temporary) hindrance of bile flow. • *Cholangitis caused by infection is not a separate entity.*

Initially, **ascending cholangitis** has to be considered on account of its pathogenetic development. This condition originates in the gall bladder, duodenum or pancreas. Moreover, the bile ducts are liable to infection by bacteria or parasites as a consequence of cholestasis and/or achylia. • **Descending cholangitis** is considered to be less frequent, with the infection descending from a chronically infected gall bladder or from a primary infection of the liver, e.g. in salmonellosis. • An infection of the bile ducts may cause **pyogenic cholangitis,** which can take an acute, relapsing or chronic course, the latter mainly being caused by a hindrance of bile flow. • Depending on the time taken for an obstruction to develop, **obstructive cholangitis** manifests as either an acute or chronic disease. In the case of obstruction, the increase in intraductal pressure (>15–20 cm H_2O) causes a cholangiovenous or cholangiolymphatic *reflux* of bacteria or endotoxins into the blood circulation. As a result, signs of systemic and, in severe cases, septic disease appear. • **Toxic cholangitis** may be triggered by chemicals, medicaments or toxins. • Furthermore, there is also the clinical picture of **immunological cholangitis.**

This form includes (*1.*) *primary biliary cholangitis*, (*2.*) *primary sclerosing cholangitis*, (*3.*) *autoimmune cholangitis*, and (*4.*) *overlap syndromes*. (1, 27) (s. tab. 33.1)

1. Aetiology

• **Infections**
  – bacteria   – parasites
  – mycoses   – viruses
• **Obstruction**
  – benign stenoses
    (stenosis of the papilla of Vater, Mirizzi's syndrome, postoperative strictures, chronic pancreatitis, juxtapapillary diverticula, *etc.*)
  – malignant stenoses
    (histiocytosis X, Hodgkin's disease, CCC, *etc.*)
  – blood clots
  – mycoses
  – gallstones
  – oriental cholangiohepatitis
  – parasites
  – portal biliopathy
  – suture material, clips, sponges
  – highly viscous mucus
    (e.g. mucoviscidosis)
• **Immunological causes**
  – primary biliary cholangitis
  – primary sclerosing cholangitis
  – autoimmune cholangitis
  – graft-versus-host disease
  – rejection reaction
  – sarcoidosis
  – pharmacons
• **Toxic causes**
  – burn injury
  – cytostatics
  – pharmacons
• **Caroli's disease**

2. Clinical forms

• acute   • non-suppurative
• chronic   • suppurative
• relapsing
 	
    ▶ asymptomatic
    ▶ symptomatic

3. Pathogenesis

• **primary development**
  – genetic/congenital
  – immunological
  – toxic
• **secondary development**
  – ascending   – periductular lymphogenic
  – descending   – septicaemic via hepatic artery

Tab. 33.1: Classification, causes and pathogenesis of cholangitis

3 Cholangitis

3.1 Infectious cholangitis

3.1.1 Bacterial cholangitis

Based on the number of reported cases, bacterial cholangitis is by far the most frequent type. It can take an acute, relapsing or chronic course, and it may have a purulent (pyogenic, suppurative) or non-suppurative form. • There are **four routes** for bacteria, and hence infection, to spread: (*1.*) ascending, (*2.*) descending, (*3.*) periductular lymphogenetic, and (*4.*) in the case of sepsis, via the hepatic artery. The condition following Billroth's anastomosis II exposes patients to a particular risk, because the duodenal stump serves as a bacterial reservoir. Biliodigestive anastomoses are also regarded as risk factors. Older people are more frequently affected by cholangitis. In general, bacteriocholia only results in cholangitis in the case of disrupted bile flow. (s. tab. 33.1)

In bacterial cholangitis, bile culture is positive in 90–100% of cases, whereby several species of microorganisms are verifiable in 45–60%. Escherichia coli, Klebsiella pneumoniae, Aeromonas, Streptococcus faecalis and Pseudomonas are found most frequently. In up to 10% of cases, anaerobes may be the causative agents of cholangitis. Yersinia enterocolitica, Salmonella and tuberculosis bacilli are seen as rare causal pathogens. Under normal circumstances, bacteria from the intestinal tract can enter the portal blood. Migration of microorganisms into the bile is prevented by different defence mechanisms (e.g. intactness of tight junctions, normal phagocytic function of RES cells). Development of cholangitis is likewise impossible in the case of normal biliary flow and normal secretion of IgA into the bile. (8, 12, 14, 21, 25, 27, 35, 45, 52, 55) *(see chapter 24)*

3.1.2 Parasitic cholangitis

Ascaris lumbricoides, Clonorchis sinensis, Lamblia intestinalis, Fasciola hepatica, Opisthorchis felineus and viverrini, Lymnaea trunculata, Cryptosporidium, etc. have been identified as parasitic causes of cholangitis. The development of cholangitis is mainly due to a hindrance of bile drainage. Parasites induce inflammation and fibrosis of the bile ducts with partial or intermittent obstruction. During their migration into the biliary tree, parasites may physically introduce bacteria into the bile ducts, which often leads to secondary bacterial cholangitis. Cholangitis induced by Opisthorchis and Clonorchis predisposes to cholangiocarcinoma and liver cell carcinoma. Echinococcus cysts may break in the bile ducts. (8, 15) (s. tab. 33.1) *(see chapter 25)*

3.1.3 Viral cholangitis

Viral cholangitis is rare. It can be caused by primary hepatotropic viruses, such as HCV or HBV, and may also occur in systemic viral diseases. (5) Both immunocompetent and immunocompromised patients are affected. The effect on the bile ducts depends mainly on the status of the host immune system. Generally, bile ducts of 50–70 μm diameter are targeted. The cholangitic lesions can be divided in *four types*: (*1.*) granulomatous, (*2.*) lymphoid, (*3.*) fibrous, and (*4.*) pleomorphic (J. LUDWIG et al., 1984). In adults, cytomegaly is the sole cause of viral cholangitis, especially in HIV infections (= *HIV-associated cholangiopathy*) and in patients who have undergone liver transplantation. In the course of AIDS, biliary infections are frequently caused by opportunistic microorganisms, e.g. cryptosporidiosis, microsporidiosis (3, 11, 16, 30, 42, 54) and sclerosing cholangitis. (17, 48) • ERCP is important in the diagnosis of HIV-associated cholangiopathy. In acute viral hepatitis, HCV is more frequently associated with cholangitis (20–30%) than is HBV. There is mostly evidence of lymphocytic cholangitis, which is, as a rule, reversible and does not adversely influence the course of disease or response to therapy. The intraepithelial lymphocytes are of the T-cell type. • During the foetal period, viral cholangitis due to reoviruses (type 3) can cause bile-duct atresia, which may also be the result of rotaviruses (types A and C) and RS viruses. *(see chapter 23)*

3.1.4 Mycotic cholangitis

Various fungi have been found to cause (obstructive) cholangitis, e.g. Cryptococcus neoformans (4), Cryptosporidiosis (17, 54), Candida (10, 19), Microsporidium (42), Blastomyces. (46) (s. tab. 33.1) *(see chapter 26)*

3.2 Obstructive cholangitis

An obstruction in the bile ducts does not always result in cholangitis; however, a disorder of bile drainage is considered to be a prerequisite for the manifestation of cholangitis. In this case, the defence system is of particular importance with regard to bacterial infections. Further risk factors include advanced age and alcohol abuse. The causes of obstruction are manifold (e.g. due to hepatic artery ligation after abdominal trauma (37), with cholangiolithiasis being the most frequent. • An impaction of a gallstone in the cystic duct or neck of the gall bladder can narrow the choledochus, a condition known as *Mirizzi's syndrome* (P.L. MIRIZZI, 1948), with subsequent development of obstructive cholangitis or cholecystobiliary fistula. (s. fig. 33.1)

During cholecystectomy, choledocholithiasis was found in 12–24% of cases. A stone-free gall bladder does not exclude cholangiolithiasis. About 80% of the bile-duct stones are found in the choledochus, 15% in the common hepatic duct and 5% in the intrahepatic bile ducts. In obstructive cholangitis, the recognition and removal

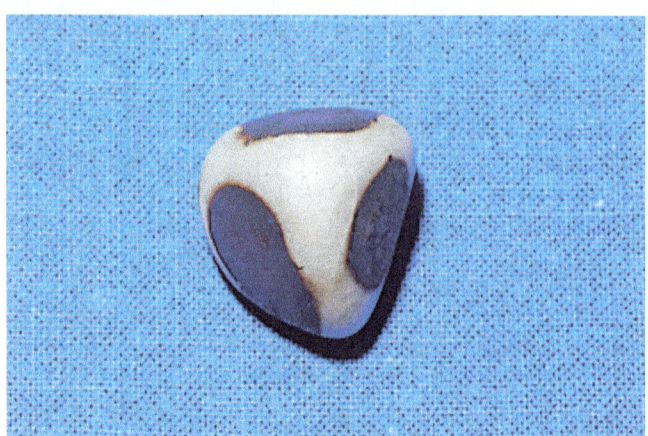

Fig. 33.1: Cholesterol-calcium-pigment stone: a rare specimen showing a striking coloured/chemical development (here: a socalled *tiger-eye stone*) *(at our disposal)*. Diagnosis: obstructive cholangitis due to *Mirizzi's syndrome*

of the obstruction constitutes causal therapy and is decisive for prognosis. (10, 15, 22, 28, 36, 41, 53, 59)

Oriental cholangiohepatitis: This particular type of cholangitis was first described by K. DIGBY in 1930. It develops from the formation of calcium bilirubinate stones, especially with intrahepatic localization (= *hepatolithiasis*). (s. fig. 33.7) It is mainly found in China, Japan, Malaysia and Taiwan. A nutritional cause together with a deficiency of glucaro-1,4-lactone is assumed, so that deglucuronidated bilirubin precipitates. Migration of parasites, especially Ascaris lumbricoides, into the bile ducts is probably an initiating event. (s. fig. 25.8!) Suppurative cholangitis develops. ERCP and MRCP are excellent diagnostic tools for depicting and examining the biliary tree. • *Treatment* consists of endoscopic stone removal, which often has to be repeated. The insertion of an expandable metallic stent has not proved effective in the long term. Surgical procedures include sphincteroplasty, biliointestinal bypass or hepatic resections. (7, 34, 50) • So-called *recurrent pyogenic cholangitis* is thought to be identical to oriental cholangiohepatitis. (13, 23, 29, 38, 51, 58, 59)

3.3 Toxic cholangitis

Toxic (especially sclerosing) cholangitis has been attributed to the effects of *aromatic amines*. Likewise, this condition can be caused by *lithocholic acid*. It may also be triggered by various *medicaments* acting as facultative toxins, e.g. allopurinol, antibiotics, carbamazepine, phenylbutazone, tolbutamide. (s. tab. 29.6) Toxic cholangitis sometimes occurs after intra-arterial administration of *cytostatics* (18, 20, 26, 40) and as a result of *burn injuries* (47) or *OLT.* (49) (s. tab. 33.4)

3.4 Clinical aspects

Acute cholangitis: The acute course is initially diagnosed clinically. It is characterized by **Charcot's triad:** (*1.*) sudden onset of pain (epigastric, right-sided), (*2.*) fever (also with shivers), and (*3.*) jaundice (J.M. CHARCOT, 1877: "intermittent gall fever"). This triad was expanded by B.M. REYNOLDS et al. (1959) to a **pentad,** which points to septic cholangitis: (*4.*) confusion, and (*5.*) coagulation disorder, occasionally with the development of disseminated intravascular coagulopathy (DIC). The course can be intermittent, or it may rapidly progress to sepsis with septic shock (in about 5%). However, a severe course of disease does not necessarily confirm the existence of suppurative cholangitis. In younger people, Charcot's triad is more clearly marked than in older patients, in whom jaundice is absent in 20−30% of cases. The liver is enlarged and tender upon pressure; splenomegaly is occasionally found. (27, 35, 55)

Suppurative cholangitis: Pyogenic (suppurative) cholangitis has the most severe course with a very poor prognosis. In general, there is complete bile obstruction with expanded pus-filled bile ducts (= bile-duct empyema). Clinically, *Reynold's pentad* is present in most cases. Hepatosplenomegaly, pronounced leucocytosis and hyperbilirubinaemia (in general >9 mg/dl) are found. Suspected severe or suppurative cholangitis requires instant diagnostic measures and, on confirmation of diagnosis, immediate therapeutic endoscopic (occasionally also surgical) intervention. (12, 14, 22) • *Severe or suppurative cholangitis is always an emergency!*

Chronic cholangitis: The symptomatology of chronic cholangitis is bland − particularly in older people. Younger people mostly suffer from a chronic relapsing course. Clinical symptoms include pain in the right upper abdomen, possibly also inappetence and nausea as well as verifiable hepatomegaly. Laboratory tests provide evidence of cholestasis with or without slight jaundice. It is postulated that damage to the bile duct leads to an increase in alkaline phosphatase. Symptom-free intervals and exacerbations with fever and jaundice can alternate. • Both acute and chronic cholangitis have a variable clinical picture with a wide spectrum of severity, including *cholangitis lenta*.

3.5 Morphology

Acute cholangitis: Thickened bile-duct walls with inflammatory infiltration as well as focal ulcerations are found histologically. The portal fields are expanded by oedema and reveal pericholangiolar and intracholangiolar infiltrations from leucocytes. Ductal tortuosity reflects increased pressure in the biliary ducts. Periductular abscesses can develop during the course of cholangitis. (s. fig. 33.2)

Chronic cholangitis: This disease shows dilated, proliferated, peripherally located ductules, which contain concentrated bile with degenerative epithelial changes. Large numbers of polymorphonuclear leucocytes are verifiable in the lumen and in the bile-duct wall; leucocytic infiltrations spread to the neighbouring parenchyma. Increasing (lamellar) periductular fibrosis and biliary strictures develop. (s. fig. 33.3) • *Laparoscopically*, progressive portal and portoportal fibrosis with cholestasis is characteristic of the macroscopic picture of chronic cholangitis. (s. fig. 33.4)

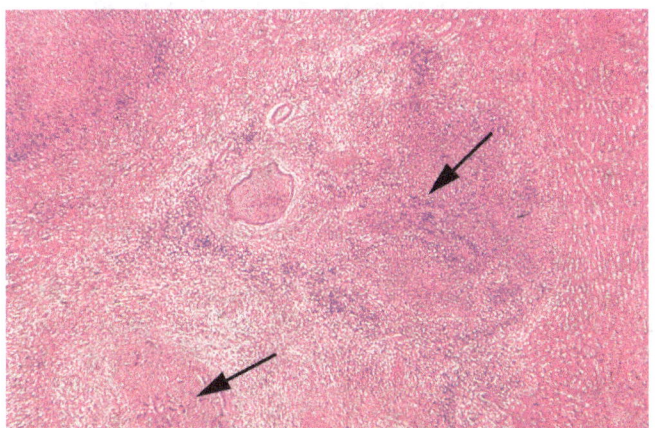

Fig. 33.2: Ascending, suppurative, destructive, relapsing cholangitis with abscess formation; the loose periportal fibre cuff (arrow) points to previous cholangitic episodes (HE)

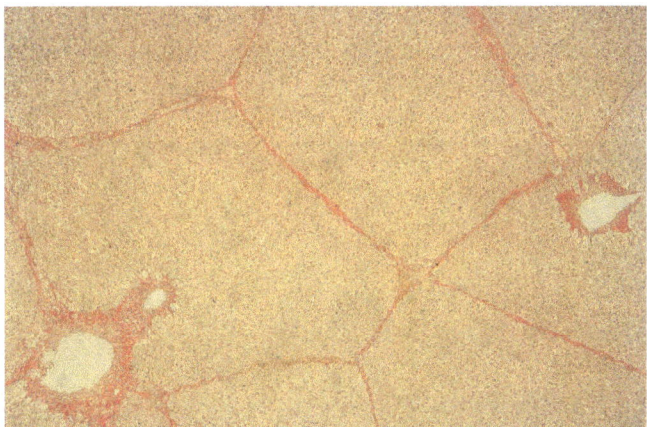

Fig. 33.3: Unusual form of slight fibrosis with septated pattern. Clinically: history of previous bile-duct inflammation (Sirius red)

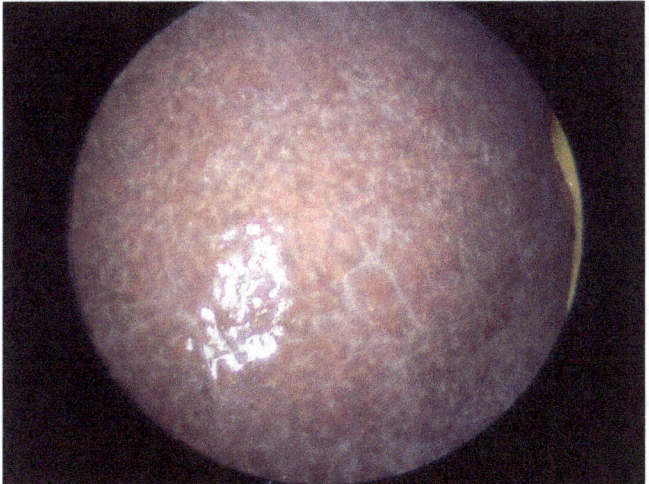

Fig. 33.4: Chronic cholangitis. Periportal fibrosis; dark red/brownish discolouration of the liver with greenish patches: finely nodular surface (= scattered light reflection)

If it is not possible to remove the obstruction and achieve defect healing (i.e. with fibrous residues) of the chronic (relapsing) cholangitis, the inflammatory destruction of periportal liver parenchyma will result in portoportal bridge formations and thus isolation of the hepatic lobules by means of connective tissue. • Monolobular, mostly micronodular *biliary cirrhosis* develops. (44, 57) (s. fig. 33.5)

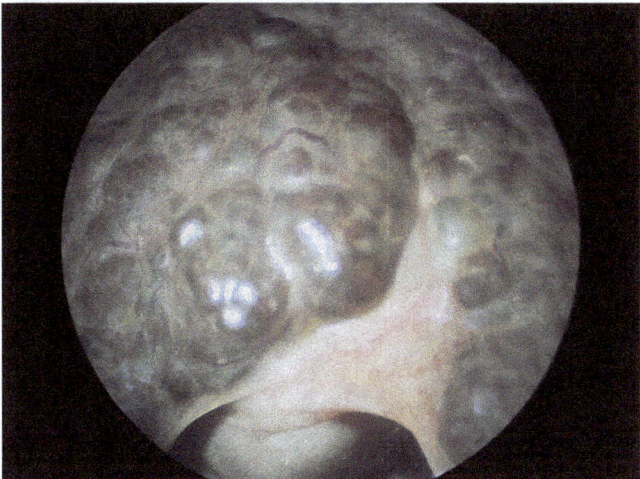

Fig. 33.5: Biliary cirrhosis following chronic relapsing and abscess-forming cholangitis; green and grey "dirty" colouration of the deformed micronodular surface. (Chronic cholecystitis with formation of a shrunken gall bladder)

3.6 Diagnostics

Diagnosis is initially based on detailed *anamnesis* focusing on the biliary system (preceding hepatobiliary diseases, endoscopic examinations, operative interventions). Previous examination results and surgical reports (if applicable) should be obtained. • With regard to *clinical findings*, the liver can be enlarged and/or tender on pressure, and jaundice may also be present. • *Laboratory investigations* reveal leucocytosis with inflammation criteria in the differential blood count, increased values for the erythrocyte sedimentation rate and CRP, elevated γ-GT, AP, LAP and bile acids, hyperbilirubinaemia, augmented $α_2$- and γ-globulins and IgM as well as increased GPT, GOT and GDH (pointing to involvement of the lobular periphery in the form of cholangiohepatitis). Occasionally, the amylase value and the tumour marker CEA 19-9 (due to cholestasis) are elevated. • *Bacteriaemia* is verifiable in 20—40% of patients during a fever episode, with the result that an antibiogram guarantees a more targeted therapy in these cases. • *Sonography* shows dilated bile ducts; normal bile ducts, however, do not exclude cholangitis! As a rule, the type and localization of an obstruction are verifiable and gas can occasionally be detected in the portal veins. Abscess foci are easily recognizable. (9, 19, 29, 33) • *Computer tomography* provides valuable evidence in difficult cases, for example in malignant obstruction. More recently, good results have been obtained by means of MRC. (27, 56)

Direct cholangiography by means of *ERCP* (s. p. 191) and *PTC* (s. p. 193) is a decisive examination with very high diagnostic reliability. These techniques should be carried out under antibiotic prophylaxis, the duration of which depends on the clinical picture. The important factor here is the well contrasted and complete visualization of the bile ducts. Using these two methods, it is possible to implement simultaneous therapeutic procedures, such as decompression of the bile ducts, flushing with antibiotics, papillotomy with stone extraction, nasobiliary or bilioduodenal drainage, stent implantation, etc. • If there is no suspicion of suppurative cholangitis (which calls for immediate invasive or surgical intervention!), antibiotic therapy is carried out for one or two days prior to ERCP and the result awaited, because ERCP can trigger complicative cholangitis in rare cases.

An inconspicuous cholangiogram now requires further diagnostic efforts to find the still unresolved cause of cholangitis, such as serological examination for viruses or bacteria, evidence of parasitic larvae or eggs in the bile or stool, autoantibodies (e.g. AMA, pANCA), toxins and colour-encoded Doppler sonography of the portal system.

▶ **Aerobilia** may have various causes, e.g. biliodigestive anastomosis or fistula, papillotomy, ERCP, cholangitis due to gas-forming bacteria. In aerobilia, there are sonographically echogenic, strand-like gas bubbles in the respective bile ducts. Linear reflexes together with reverberations are considered to be characteristic (= *ring-down artefact*). When the body is put into a different position, the microbubbles begin to move. (s. fig. 33.6)

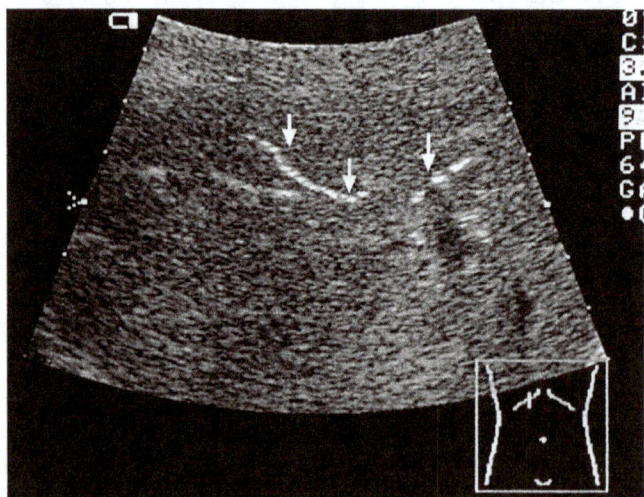

Fig. 33.6: Aerobilia: Sonography shows echogenic, strand-like gas bubbles in the respective bile ducts (↓)

This diagnostic programme, which has proved its worth in the case of cholangitis, can be incorporated into a **flow diagram** for the clarification of cholestasis or jaundice. (s. fig. 13.7) The individual characteristics of each case always have to be considered!

3.7 Complications and prognosis

The mild form of cholangitis frequently subsides spontaneously, mostly with antibiotic therapy, and can even be cured without morphological residues. • In rare cases, an extremely rapid development of secondary sclerosing cholangitis has been observed. (35) • Severe and progressive courses have a poor prognosis due to the development of **complications:** (*1.*) suppurative cholangitis, (*2.*) sepsis, possibly with septic shock, (*3.*) DIC, (*4.*) infected portal thrombosis, (*5.*) acute renal failure (= *biliorenal syndrome*), (*6.*) liver abscesses or metastatic abscess formation, and (*7.*) formation of intrahepatic gallstones (= *hepatolithiasis*) (s. fig. 33.7). • However, complications also have to be feared when using ERCP and PTC, since the inherent risks of these invasive techniques are greatly increased by bacterial infection of the bile duct (e.g. phlegmon, retroperitoneal or subphrenic abscess, pleural infection). There is a particular risk involved in the application of contrast medium under pressure (!) into the bile ducts, which may even result in death. • The **prognosis** is generally based on establishing whether (*1.*) the causal obstruction can be removed, (*2.*) decompression of the bile ducts can be achieved, (*3.*) effective drainage is guaranteed, and (*4.*) antibiotic therapy proves effective.

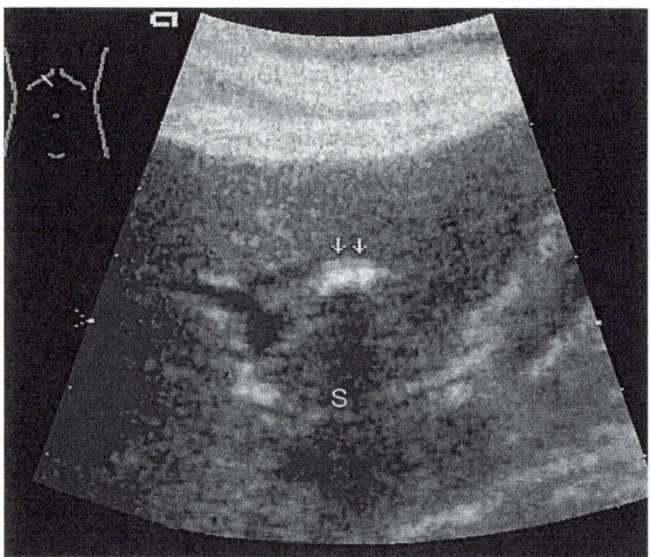

Fig. 33.7: Formation of intrahepatic gallstones (= hepatolithiasis) (arrows) in chronic bacterial cholangitis (S = acoustic shadow)

3.8 Therapy

1. **Standard therapy:** Intensive care treatment and monitoring is accepted as standard therapy; complications may appear unexpectedly and rapidly. In about 75% of patients with mild cholangitis, therapeutic success can be achieved by the substitution of fluid, electrolytes and zinc as well as vitamins, glucose (possibly also amino acids) and the (indispensable) administration of anti-

biotics. Analgesics and spasmolytics are generally necessary. • In addition, the administration of *fresh plasma* is recommended to stabilize haemostasis.

As long as there is no positive bacteriological result from the bile (or blood), **antibiotics** are administered on empirical and plausible principles. In this case, *mezlocillin* or *piperacillin* is initially recommended, 3 x 2 (−4 or −5) g/day, i.v. (55) These antibiotics are effective against virtually all bacteria in acute cholangitis, since they can reach high biliary concentrations. Once the course of disease has entered a more severe stage, an additional dose of *tobramycin*, for example, is indicated (e.g. 3 x 80 mg/day, i.v.). A septic clinical picture requires a course of *triple therapy* with ureidopenicillin + aminoglycoside + metronidazole (3 x 500 mg/day, i.v.).

2. **Invasive therapy:** If clinical improvement and defervescence do not occur within 12 (to 36) hours, **decompression** of the bile ducts becomes necessary. Decompression is carried out endoscopically by means of papillotomy. Providing there are no reasons against doing so, **bile drainage** should also be carried out at the same time via a nasobiliary tube or bilioduodenal endoprosthesis. Early decompression is recommended with a thrombocyte count of < 100,000/mm³ and an albumin value of < 3.0 g/dl. (24, 32, 50, 59) Under these circumstances, we regard the simultaneous administration of *fresh plasma* as a necessity. • If the bile ducts cannot be reached by retrograde endoscopy, **PTC** is available as an ideal alternative for decompression and drainage (and, occasionally, antibiotic instillation). Nevertheless, because of the bacterial (suppurative) situation, a higher complication rate has to be expected. (24, 39, 50) • **Surgical measures** carry a much higher risk than endoscopic papillotomy + drainage, which is why they are restricted to particular situations in special cases (e.g. Caroli's syndrome, liver abscess). (24, 31, 51)

4 Primary biliary cholangitis

▶ In 1826 P.F. RAYER reported on the peculiar appearance of xanthelasmas and xanthomas in middle-aged women. • In 1851 T. ADDISON et al. assumed a correlation between skin changes and liver disease. (61) In 1857 R. VIRCHOW pointed to a connection between these skin changes and cholestasis and cirrhosis. V. HANOT (1876) described the clinical picture of hypertrophic cirrhosis with chronic jaundice. (137) S.G. THANNHAUSER et al. (1938) postulated the combination of xanthomas and biliary cirrhosis as a separate entity. (271) In 1949 H.E. MACMAHON et al. used the term "xanthomatous biliary cirrhosis". (193) • A detailed description of this disease was presented by J.A. DAUPHINEE et al. (1949) (100) and E.H. AHRENS jr. et al. (1950), who coined the term **"primary biliary cirrhosis"**. (63) • In 1965 the group of H. POPPER introduced the expression **"chronic non-suppurative destructive cholangitis"**. (247)

4.1 Definition

Primary biliary cholangitis (PBC) is characterized by chronic, non-suppurative, destructive cholangitis (CNDC) of the small and medium-sized bile ducts (ductule, interlobular and septal). The cause is not yet known. • PBC proceeds slowly and does not cause any clinical symptoms for a long period of time. However, antimitochondrial antibodies (AMA) already appear at the preclinical stage, which allows a very early diagnosis to be made. During the further course of disease, the symptoms are those of chronic cholestasis. The final stage is characterized by the total destruction of the bile ducts. • In the case of a progressive (or unsuccessfully treated) course, primary biliary cholangitis gradually develops into *biliary cirrhosis* − as is also the case with primary and secondary sclerosing cholangitis.

4.2 Epidemiology

PBC is found in all races and social classes, although it is virtually unknown in Africa. Its *prevalence* ranges between 25−40/100,000 inhabitants (with regional differences). Its *incidence* is 2.7−3.5 cases per 100,000 inhabitants/year. The disease predominantly affects women (in about 90% of cases); the prevalence among women between the ages of 35 and 60 is >90/100,000. PBC is nearly always found in adults; it is extremely rare in children. (99) Close relatives have a prevalence of 4−6%. Patients with ulcerative colitis are affected thirty times more frequently than the general population. (152, 203)

4.3 Aetiology

The aetiology of PBC is still unknown. Possible causal factors include genetic susceptibility, infections, environmental influences and immunological reactions. (177) • *Probably, there is an individual concurrence of endogenous and exogenous factors.*

4.3.1 Genetic susceptibility

Isolated instances of **familial aggregation** of PBC involving siblings, twins, mother and daughter or father and daughter have been reported. The occurrence of AMA as well as an increase in IgM and γ-GT, or deficiency of IgA have occasionally been observed in relatives of PBC patients (genetics? close physical contact?), but it is not a hereditary disease. There is a genetic association with chromosome 6g 21.3. (62, 71, 86, 88, 90, 92, 93, 118, 128, 134, 149, 152, 275)

There is a certain **association with HLA,** such as HLA-DR8, -DR3, -DR4, -DPB1, -B8 or -DQB1, as well as with the formation of isohaemagglutinins −, however, not with the AB0 blood-group system or the Rhesus groups. The HLA-A class 2 antigen is significant in reducing susceptibility to and affording protection against PBC. HLA-DR8 is deemed a risk factor, particularly in the combination DR8/C4B2 and DR8/C4AQ0. (269, 278)

4.3.2 Hormone theory

The so-called **hormone theory** (J. AHLQVIST, 1980) is based on the impact of hyperoestrogenaemia on the biliary/canalicular system and bile acid metabolism. The question of sequential causality remains open. (quot. 79)

4.3.3 Mycotoxin theory

The so-called **mycotoxin theory** (E. KUNTZ, 1984) emerged from our examinations of stools for the presence of fungi in 54 female patients. (171, 172) • Normally, the lumen of the bile capillaries is surrounded by a network of actin-like filaments which radiate into the microvilli. The bile flow is essentially steered by this network. The mycotoxin cytochalasin B (possibly also other mycotoxins) causes loss of microvilli and dilatation of the canaliculi (M. J. PHILLIPS et al., 1975) — and, as a result, probably also retention of leukotrienes. (see 4.3.5) Mycotoxins can penetrate the intestinal mucosa and reach the liver cells through the portal vein. The frequent evidence of antiactin antibodies in PBC patients may be attributable to this. A (myco)toxic canalicular impairment as an "initiator" results sometimes in self-perpetuation in connection with (secondary) hyperoestrogenaemia due to a (tertiary) defect in the immunoregulatory mechanism. The formation of mitochondrial antibodies can be induced by a mycotoxic (?) (possibly bacterial?) antigen, which culminates in the formation of AMA with subsequent T-cell infiltration into the small bile ducts. Yet, the question remained unanswered for us as to whether this applies to (1.) markedly increased fungal colonization of the intestinal tract in individual cases, (2.) specific fungal species, (3.) increased perviousness of the (predamaged?) intestinal mucosa with regard to mycotoxins, or (4.) insufficient clearance function of the hepatic RES. • We were subsequently able to confirm this marked association on the basis of numerous mycological stool examinations — however, no further evidence could be obtained to substantiate our mycotoxic hypothesis at that time. • *It is of interest that AMA also react with PDH-E2 contained in mycoses.*

4.3.4 Bacterial or viral theory

The group of U. HOPF also examined the question of an **infectious toxic factor**, since there is a great similarity between bacterial and mitochondrial membranes. (79, 253, 266, 291) Evidence of so-called *R forms of E. coli* could be found in all PBC patients in the stool (with no relation to the severity of cholestasis), and A lipid could be detected frequently in hepatocytes and Kupffer cells. Mitochondrial antigens were present in the bacterial wall of Enterobacteriaceae. (143, 261) • Evidence of AMA in *tuberculosis patients* is of interest (R. KLEIN et al, 1993). *Urinary tract infections* with E. coli may also play a role in the development of anti-M_2 (A. K. BURROUGHS et al., 1984). • Anti-M_2 has also been observed after **bacterial** or **vival infections** with EBV, cytomegalovirus, Salmonella sp., toxoplasma, Chlamidia sp. (60), etc. Hepatitis viruses may also be "initiators". Propionibacterium acnes could be detected in granulomas. PBC is possibly caused by a coated retrovirus. This as yet unnamed virus has been detected in the epithelia of small bile ducts. It contains neither human nor viral DNA. Therefore, it is deemed to be an exogenous virus. (291) Thus antiviral treatment of patients with PBC may be considered a new therapy option.

4.3.5 Elevation of leukotrienes

Leukotrienes can form in hepatocytes, Kupffer cells and mastocytes. Their release, induced by endotoxins for example, correlates with the increase in AP, LAP and γ-GT. Leukotrienes have a marked inflammatory effect. Enhanced production together with reduced secretion of leukotrienes into the bile can result in severe lesions of the bile ducts. (202)

4.3.6 Increase in Mn-SOD

In PBC patients, manganese superoxide dismutase levels in the serum were found to be increased; it is secreted in greater quantities from damaged bile-duct epithelia. Free radicals were therefore assumed to play an aetiopathogenetic role regarding immunologically induced lipid peroxidations. (228)

4.3.7 Immunologic factors

1. Antimitochondrial antibodies (AMA): D. C. GAJDUSEK (1957) and J. R. MACKAY (1958) were able to determine different antibodies in the serum of patients suffering from PBC by means of a complement fixation test (CFT). • In 1965 J. G. WALKER et al. reported the occurrence of antimitochondrial antibodies in PBC patients. (281) These were directed against the antigens of the inner mitochondrial membrane. The antigen specific to PBC and sensitive to trypsin was termed *AMA-M_2*. The target antigen is an enzyme complex containing pyruvate dehydrogenase, keto acid dehydrogenase and branched chain keto dehydrogenase. In about 95% of cases, patients with PBC show a positive result. Four determinants (I–IV) are attributed to M_2: E_2, X, E_1, E_3. (75, 113, 140, 214, 263, 293) • The group of P. A. BERG identified an *anti-M_9* (1984) in PBC patients as well as a trypsin-resistant *anti-M_4* and a trypsin-sensitive *anti-M_8* (1985). Anti-M_9 was found almost exclusively in the early stage, often in family members who did not have an anti-M_2 — as well as in female laboratory assistants in frequent contact with AMA-positive serum. Anti-M_9 is verifiable in 10–15% of the population. (80, 284) (s. tab. 5.21) (s. fig. 5.14) It is still not clear whether AMA-

positivity is a sequela or a pathogenetic factor of PBC.
• Further *AMA subgroups* have been verified: anti-M_1 against syphilis (D.J. WRIGHT et al., 1970), anti-M_3 against pseudolupus (T.J. SAYERS et al., 1981), anti-M_5 against collagenosis, anti-M_6 against iproniacid (M.T. LABRO et al., 1982) and anti-M_7 against cardiomyopathies (R. KLEIN et al., 1984). • The typical antibodies for PBC (M_2, M_4, M_8, M_9) can be combined into **four constellation types** (A–D), which are probably of clinical importance. The sensitivity of detection ranges between 66–96%. • However, AMA are neither species-specific nor organ-specific. (132, 156, 166, 167, 198, 236, 262) (s. tab. 5.21)

2. Other antibodies: Antinuclear antibodies (ANA) in PBC are verifiable in 10–40% of cases. Antibodies to hepatocyte membranes (LMA) are present in about 40% of PBC patients. Furthermore, antibodies to microfilaments, intermediary filaments and microtubuli as well as to antiactin have been detected. In approx. 100% of PBC patients, antibodies against parietal cells can be identified (H.P. WIRTH et al., 1994). In 25% of cases, antibodies to thyreoglobulin have also been demonstrated. (98, 106, 146, 153, 262, 264) (s. tabs. 5.19–5.21)

3. Immunocomplexes: It has been suggested that complement activation with subsequent bile-duct lesions and an increased synthesis of immunoglobulins is evoked by immunocomplexes. They are even considered to be responsible for the formation of granulomas. However, they are certainly not the primary aetiological factors.

4. Immunoglobulin M: Virtually all PBC patients show increased serum IgM values. This IgM differs remarkably from the IgM of healthy persons. Elevated monomeric IgM was also detected in the skin, in hepatocytes and in the intestinal mucosa. Enhanced IgM serum values were likewise determined in relatives of PBC patients. (see 4.3.1) However, there was no correlation between IgM serum values and the tissue level values, cholestasis or morphological changes. Progressive PBC courses result in augmented IgG as well.

5. Cellular immunoreactions: Increased IgM values are a characteristic sign of enhanced B-lymphocyte activity, namely of an IgM-secreting subgroup, as well as a restriction in the normal transfer from type IgM to type IgG. Infiltrations are found in the hepatic tissue and consist mainly of T lymphocytes (activated, cytotoxic $CD8^+$ as well as $CD4^+$ helper cells). The portal field infiltrations predominantly show CD4 T lymphocytes, while the ductuli are surrounded by CD8 T lymphocytes. It is still not known which mechanisms are responsible for the bile-duct lesions brought about by the T lymphocytes, mainly of the CD8 type. The latter are assumed to react with M_2 antigens, which are expressed from the ductulus cells. • So-called MHC antigens are found on the surface of the bile-duct epithelia of PBC patients, i.e. they act as antigen-presenting (target) cells. This leads to the stimulation and proliferation of CD4 lymphocytes. These emit cytokines, which cause a proliferation of CD8 lymphocytes in the direct neighbourhood of the small bile ducts. However, the bile-duct epithelial cells are also target cells of the CD8 lymphocytes; the latter adhere to the bile-duct epithelia due to the expression of MHC antigens and adhesion molecules (ICAM), and enter the cells. Their cytotoxic impact destroys the small bile ducts and evokes an immunological inflammatory process with further secretion of cytokines, which are conducive to inflammation. However, with regard to cytokine production and response in PBC, the findings are still contradictory. Nor is it clear why these processes take place almost exclusively in the small bile ducts. (184, 214)

6. Selenium deficiency: The trace element selenium is also obligatory for the normal functioning of the immunological system. Selenium deficiency has been proposed as one of the aetiological factors in PBC – although this has not yet been verified.

4.4 Pathogenesis

In the pathogenesis of PBC, cellular immunoreactions, particularly the formation of autoantibodies, are probably of greater importance than humoral reactions. *Due to disturbed immunoregulation, the immune response is ineffective against both cell and humorally mediated cytotoxicity. On the one hand, therefore, causality is not eliminated and on the other hand, the initial damage still has an effect, so that the autoimmunological inflammatory reactions continue to target the organ in a self-perpetuating process.* • The frequent association with other autoimmunological diseases, infiltrations of activated CD4 and CD8 T lymphocytes in the portal fields and around the intralobular bile ducts as well as the expression of antigens of the MHC class II and ICAM class I on bile-duct cells point to the importance of autoimmunological reactions in the pathogenesis of PBC. • The involvement of M_2 antibodies in the pathogenesis of PBC has been discussed, but seems rather unlikely. A possible aspect would be the pathogenetic significance of AMA through antibody-transmitted cytotoxicity and the incorporation of complement factors. (102, 126, 149, 154)

Aetiopathogenetic hypothesis

The primary provocation of immunological phenomena by **toxins,** such as mycotoxins (E. KUNTZ, 1984) (171, 172), **bacteria** (U. HOPF et al., 1989) (143, 261) and **viral infection** (H.I. MASON et al., 1998) (197) – probably accompanied by hormone-induced bile-duct lesions (J. AHLQVIST, 1980) – can therefore be interpreted in terms of subsequent **self-perpetuation.** The expression of relevant mitochondrial epitopes in the small bile ducts caused by an external antigen through **molecular mimicry** (M.E. GERSHWIN, 1991, 1997) (121, 266) may support the chronic inflammatory process by way of autoaggression. Immunologically induced lipid peroxidations may be significant here. (228)

As early as 1979, it could be demonstrated by means of electron microscopy that mitochondria multiply in the epithelial cells of the canaliculi of PBC patients; this finally leads to obliteration of the affected canaliculi. The longitudinal consolidations of intercellular gaps point like fingers to the obliterated lumen (G. SCHWALBACH, 1979). • These results concurred with our concept at that time (172) which was based on the assumption that a *primary mycotoxic factor* (or *molecular mimicry*) constitutes an "initiator". (s. p. 676)

4.5 Morphology

▶ The morphological changes in *"primary biliary cirrhosis"* (PBC) (63) were deemed *"chronic non-suppurative destructive cholangitis"* (CNDC) by the study group of H. POPPER if the stage of cirrhosis was not yet reached. (247) The morphological classification of PBC, proposed by P.J. SCHEUER in 1967 (252), was modified in 1980. It differentiates **four stages,** which show fluid transition: ductal phase (I), ductular phase (II), fibrosing-cicatrizing (precirrhotic) stage (III), and cirrhotic stage (IV). Applying this classification, H. POPPER et al. (1970) described stage I as a cholangitic phase and stage II as a phase of ductular proliferation – they retained the original terms for stages III and IV. A modified classification was proposed by J. LUDWIG et al. in 1978. (191)

CNDC:	stage I	portal hepatitis
	stage II	periportal hepatitis
	stage III	septal fibrosis
PBC:	stage IV	cirrhosis

Electron microscopy: Focal destruction of the numerically diminished microvilli is evident. Spreading of the peribiliary canalicular ectoplasm is linked to an increase in filamentous structures. The mitochondria within the epithelial cells of the bile ducts multiply. Finally, the affected bile canaliculi are completely obliterated. • *Thus it would seem that the primary damage, which results in CNDC, actually originates from the canaliculi* (G. SCHWALBACH, 1979; K. TOBE, 1982). (212, 214, 292)

Stage I: *Laparoscopically*, the liver is of normal size and consistency. The surface colour is reddish-brown, possibly with yellowish spots; it may even have a "tiger skin-like" colouring. • *Histologically*, there is evidence of ductular lesions similar to cholangitis as well as portal and pericanalicular infiltrations (lymphocytes, histiocytes, plasma cells, eosinophilic leucocytes and, more rarely, polymorphonuclear granulocytes). The portal fields are affected regionally to different degrees and to a variably severe extent – sometimes, they are not affected at all. Mononuclear cells penetrate the walls of the small bile ducts. The histiocytes can form granulomas, mostly of the sarcoid type, which may also contain Langhans' giant cells. At first, the florid, interlobular and septa bile-duct lesions with follicular elements only develop focally. The liver parenchyma is hardly affected. The lesions are distributed irregularly in the liver. There is no evidence of cholestasis. (213–215, 251) (s. fig. 33.8)

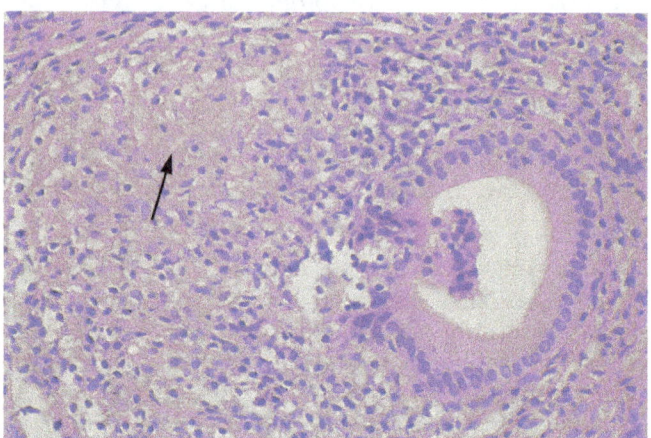

Fig. 33.8: PBC stage I: Epithelioid cell granuloma (↑) related to a septal bile duct; focal inflammatory destruction of the bile-duct epithelium; granuloma-like nodule of macrophages entering the lumen (HE)

Stage II: *Laparoscopically*, the liver now has a firmer consistency (ascertained by pressure of the probe). With the onset of cholestasis, the surface colour gradually becomes reddish-yellow to speckled green. There are clearly more subcapsular blood vessels. The surface is finely rippled or granulated. (119, 186, 206) (s. fig. 33.9)

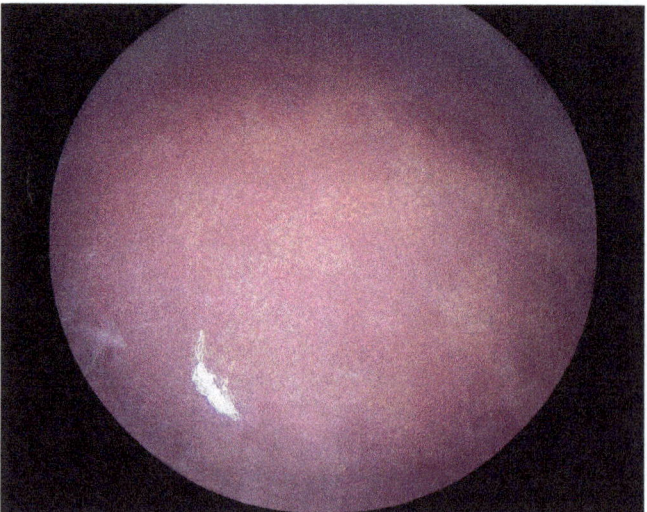

Fig. 33.9: Primary biliary cholangitis: Map-like marking of the liver surface (stage I); still largely smooth surface (see light reflex), dark red/livid blue colouring; tiger skin-like pattern in the irregular reddish areas

Histologically, there is a reduction in the periductular lesions, possibly with increasing proliferation of the cholangioles, and a drop in the number of portal bile ducts (= increasing appearance of arteries without concomitant bile ducts). There is often evidence of pigmentation and PAS-positive material in the bile-duct endothelia. A dense collagenous fibre network develops. The liver cells often contain Mallory-Denk bodies. Activated macrophages cause secondary cellular necroses. Proliferation of stellate cells and lymphocytic infiltrations develop in the sinusoids. The inflammatory infiltrations spread to the lobules and present as piecemeal necrosis (= interface hepatitis). (101, 111, 193, 234, 236, 256)

Stage III: *Laparoscopically,* the liver has a markedly firmer consistency; the granular, in parts finely tuberous surface has a reddish-brown colour with greyish-green speckling. There are noticeably more subcapsular blood and lymphatic vessels. The first evidence of commencing portal hypertension is found in the ligaments. The spleen is enlarged and of a dark red colour. • *Histologically,* periportal scarring and the formation of fibrosis predominate due to persistent stimulation of fibrogenesis. The bile ducts are greatly reduced in number, and countless small arteries are apparent. The inflammatory infiltrations and bile-duct proliferations gradually become less obvious. (s. fig. 33.10) • However, the different morphological stages can overlap in the same patient. Therefore it is very difficult (sometimes even impossible) to carry out grading or staging. Copper is increasingly deposited in the lysosomes (10−60 mg/100 g/dry weight) and subsequently in the liver, spleen and kidneys (but not in the brain). Severe lobular central cholestasis now becomes pronounced. Macrophages occasionally contain lipid and form pseudoxanthomatous cells. (s. fig. 33.10)

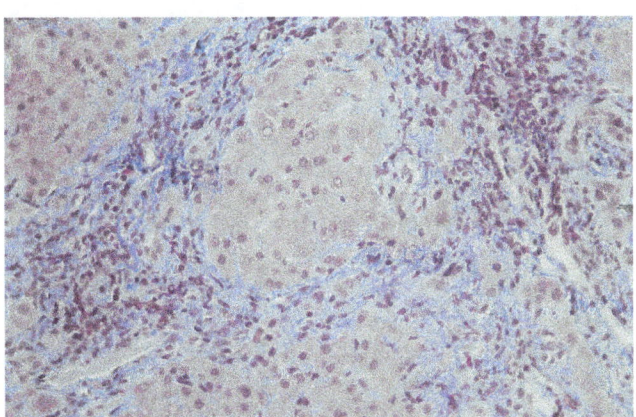

Fig. 33.10: Primary biliary cholangitis with cirrhotic transformation. Well-rounded parenchymal residues surrounded by collagenous fibre tissue; hardly recognizable bile ducts in the residual round cell-infiltrated portal fields (stages III−IV) (HE)

Stage IV: *Biliary cirrhosis,* also described as stage IV, is the possible morphological final stage of PBC (or CNDC), in which the remaining biliary ductules are now subject to destruction, and consequently disappear. Basically, CNDC is in itself "chronic cholangitis". • *Laparoscopically,* the liver surface shows irregular, finely rippled, micronodular (at selective sites also macronodular) cirrhosis. The vessels are more numerous and more clearly marked. The colour is brownish-grey to graphite-green, in some places more distinct. There are lymph cysts and signs of portal hypertension.

Histologically, one can find advanced scarred septation and regenerative growth in the form of a complete cirrhosis with almost no inflammatory activity. Cholestasis is severe. There is virtually no evidence of bile ducts; granulomas are rare. (64, 234, 246) (s. fig. 33.10)

▶ Strictly speaking, the historical term primary biliary "cirrhosis" (coined in 1950) (63) cannot be retained for primary biliary cholangitis with all its well-defined stages (CNDC I−III) − because there is no sign of cirrhosis during the precirrhotic stages I−III, and CNDC does not necessarily lead to cirrhosis. As early as 1965, E. RUBIN et al. objected to the definition of PBC as "cirrhosis" on the grounds that it was a "misnomer" (247). • All forms of "chronic cholangitis" (e.g. obstructive, primary biliary, primary or secondary sclerosing, and overlap syndromes) may develop into biliary cirrhosis − which can barely (or only unreliably) be differentiated histologically and in no way aetiologically. • *It is not justified to use a pathologically incorrect term simply because it once became established in a historical context.* Therefore it is finally time to eliminate the totally incorrect term "primary biliary cirrhosis" (PBC), which has been in use since 1950, for stages I−III of CNDC.

▶ *Cirrhosis is never "primary", but always has a relatively long developmental phase. Consequently, there is no "primary" and hence no "primary biliary" cirrhosis!*

▶ **Proposal:** Concerning the current term "primary biliary cirrhosis" (PBC), the word "cirrhosis" should be replaced by "cholangitis" (which has the same abbreviation!) together with the respective stage − I, II, III or IV.

4.6 Clinical courses

In general, the three morphological stages I−III (precirrhotic) are more or less equivalent to the clinical stages I−III, although fluid transitions understandably exist in each case. Stage IV (cirrhotic) would correspond to the clinical stages IV and V. • Assignment to a particular disease phase also yields prognostic information. From a clinical and morphological point of view, the division into a *precirrhotic* and a *cirrhotic* stage is significant (and generally adequate).

4.6.1 Asymptomatic stage (I)

In general, there is no evidence of PBC in this initial phase. About 60% of patients are asymptomatic at the time of diagnosis. Occasionally, some patients complain of *fatigue* (s. p. 243) and *weakness* But daytime fatigue is very similar to lethargy; it is often associated with depressive emotional response. Therapy with modafinil is recommended. (117, 123, 144, 240) • *Pruritus* can appear or spontaneously disappear in all stages of PBC. It mainly affects the extremities, the perigenital and perianal areas as well as the palms and soles. Pruritus becomes more intensive in warm conditions and at night. Therapy-resistent forms may cause the patient to become suicidal; in severe cases, liver transplantation may be necessary. (122) (s. pp. 243, 248) • Often, an (initially inexplicable) increase in γ-*GT* and *AP* is observed during investigations indicated for other reasons. The sulphated bile acids in the serum are elevated. • If the possibility of PBC is "taken into consideration" at this stage, evidence of *AMA* (>1:80), especially of the subtype M_2, can provide an early diagnosis. AMA are a very early marker of PBC – often a long time before other laboratory or clinical findings become evident. The PBC-specific AMA-M2 are directed against the mitochondrial pyruvate dehydrogenase complex E2 (PDC-E2). (80, 106, 113, 140, 153, 156, 166, 167, 204, 224, 246, 260, 262, 284, 293) • However, jaundice, gastrointestinal haemorrhages, bleeding oesophageal varices, osteoporosis and ascites have also been reported as *initial symptoms*. (41, 69, 73, 82, 94, 125, 242, 247)

4.6.2 Oligosymptomatic stage (II)

Clinically, pruritus becomes increasingly pronounced, above all at night, and is mainly localized in the extremities and perianal region. It is often the reason for a dermatological examination. Subjectively, arthralgia and steatorrhoea may also occur. Hepatomegaly is verifiable in about 50% of cases. The cholestasis-indicating enzymes are elevated; this correlates with the release of leukotrienes. Occasionally, (nearly) normal values of AP are found. The metabolism of bile acids is disturbed. The results of liver function tests are often pathological.

AMA are positive (ca. 95% of cases), so that the subtype M_2 can now be determined. (s. tab. 5.21) (s. fig. 5.14) There is no difference in the frequency of AMA between men and women. AMA are sometimes detectable in urine, bile and tears. About 10% of cases show no evidence of AMA. *ANA* appear in 25–50% of patients as a *multiple nuclear dot type* (MND-ANA) or a *nuclear ring standing form*. Their presence confirms an AMA-negative PBC. Furthermore, antibodies against Escherichia coli proteases are found in ca. 30% and a typical pANCA in ca 15% of patients. Antibodies against parietal cells *(anti-PCA)* are detectable in nearly all cases. Simultaneous negativity of AMA may suggest an overlap syndrome. (s. p. 694) As a rule, IgM is clearly increased. Elevated cholesterol and reduced HDL are often found together with an additional rise in LDL. Usually, lipoprotein X is present. (41, 65, 94, 204)

4.6.3 Symptomatic anicteric stage (III)

Pruritus and scratch wounds are a major impairment in daily life; the patients suffer enormously. With marked pruritus, a so-called *butterfly sign* is sometimes found on the patient's back, i.e. the area which cannot be reached by scratching (T. B. REYNOLDS, 1973). (s. pp 89, 243) • Gradually, hyperpigmentation of the skin occurs due to melanin. Hepatomegaly is verifiable in 70–80% of cases, splenomegaly in 20%. Portal hypertension develops, predominantly of the intrahepatic presinusoidal type. • Xanthelasmas and xanthomas form slowly, particularly on the lower and upper eyelids, on the tendons of the extensor muscles, on the elbows and heels as well as on the palms of the hands. They do not correlate with the serum values of cholesterol and triglycerides. Spontaneous regression is possible. (s. figs. 4.14–4.16) Biochemistry reveals increased values of AP, LAP, γ-GT and transaminases as well as enhanced values of cholesterol, LDL and IgM. In some patients, considerable eosinophilia occurs – in correlation with the activity of mast cells in the portal field. The galactose elimination capacity is reduced. Osteoporosis has reached an advanced stage. Fractures are found mainly on the vertebral column or ribs. Up to now, no factors predicting progression from the presymptomatic to the symptomatic stage are known. (94, 100, 204, 208, 224, 225, 246)

4.6.4 Icteric stage (IV)

Jaundice develops within six months in rapidly progressing forms or between two to three years after the onset of pruritus. In general, it suggests transition to the final stage. The bilirubin value mostly remains stable below 5.0 mg/dl for months or years, while clinical symptoms and hepatic erythema grow in intensity. Dark urine and acholic stool are observed. The AP, LAP and γ-GT levels are noticeably elevated; the transaminases stay within the range of 30–100 U/l. The parameters relating to the rate of synthesis (cholinesterase, Quick's value, albumin) decrease. The galactose elimination capacity is greatly reduced. (244) The γ-globulins and P-III-P are elevated. Serum copper is often increased, and copper secretion in urine is likewise higher.

4.6.5 Final stage (V)

Clinically, morphologically and biochemically, the overall picture of cirrhosis prevails (in 4 years: 30–50%); however, 20% of precirrhotic patients do not show any progression. PBC ends fatally either due to bleeding of oesophageal varices (50%) or liver insufficiency. This final stage is reached after a period of 8 to 15 years (depending on individual progression).

4.7 Complications

Owing to the greater sensitivity of PBC patients to pharmaceutical preparations, different pharmacons, e.g. phenothiazines, contraceptives, oestrogens and anabolic steroids, can reinforce cholestasis and the clinical symptoms, thus aggravating the course of disease. • *Gallstones* are frequently detectable (35−40%); as a rule, they are pigment gallstones. Administration of clofibrate is contraindicated; it gives rise to increased formation of gallstones due to enhanced cholesterol secretion into the bile. • *Xanthomas* can lead to mechanically induced neuropathy. (272) *Malabsorption* of fat-soluble vitamins due to steatorrhoea resulting from bile acid deficiency causes corresponding deficiency symptoms. (169) • *Osteopathies* are found in 20−60% (−100%) of cases; a decrease in bone density may be measurable at an early stage. Osteoporosis occurs twice as often as in the general population. The cause is multifactorial (e.g. deficiency of calcium, vitamin D and oestrogen, long duration of disease, genetic factors). Osteomalacia is less frequent. In both forms of osteopathy, excretion of hydroxyproline in urine is increased as a sign of the enhanced rate of bone absorption. (81, 107, 114, 129, 130, 136, 207, 216, 227, 232, 257) • About 20% of patients are suffering from asymptomatic urinary tract infection. Hepatocellular carcinoma develops in about 6% of PBC cases. PBC may be accompanied by severe complications, leading to a poorer prognosis. (s. tab. 33.2)

1. Cholelithiasis
2. Exocrine pancreatic insufficiency
3. Hemeralopia (vitamine A deficiency)
4. Carcinoma (116)
   − HCC (male > female) (151, 170, 220)
   − breast cancer (290)
5. Coagulopathy (vitamine K_1 deficiency)
6. Paramenia
7. Osteopathy
   with ostealgia, infraction of vertebral bodies, spontaneous fractures
   (predominantly in associated sprue: 5−10%)
   − osteoporosis
   − osteomalacia
8. Portal hypertension (69, 157)
   − oesophageal varices (125, 265, 293)
   − ascites
   − hepatic encephalopathy
9. Renal tubular acidosis
10. Xanthomatous neuropathy (272)

Tab. 33.2: Complications of PBC (with some references)

4.8 PBC-associated immunologic diseases

Apart from complicative developments, the course of PBC is also aggravated by associated diseases, which appear almost exclusively as immunologic disorders. About 25% (−40%) of all patients with PBC contract one or more such diseases. As a result, the quality of

1. Anaemia perniciosa
2. Ankylosing spondylitis (279)
3. CREST syndrome (195, 239)
   (= calcinosis cutis, Raynaud's phenomenon, oesophageal motility disorder, sclerodactyly, teleangiectasia)
4. Dermatitis herpetiformis (120)
5. Dermatomyositis
6. Glomerulonephritis (210, 243)
7. Grave's disease (219)
8. Haemolytic anaemia
9. IgA deficiency (149)
10. Immunocomplex capillaritis (243)
11. Intestinal manifestations
    − coeliac disease (74, 103, 120, 258)
    − ulcerative colitis (168)
    − jejunal villous atrophy
12. Lichen planus (125)
13. Lupus anticoagulant
14. Lupus erythematosus (135, 147)
15. Lymphadenopathy (105, 110, 192, 229)
16. Mixed collagenosis
17. Myelitis (66, 248)
18. Polymyalgia rheumatica
19. Polymyositis (85)
20. Pulmonary manifestations (91, 259, 282)
    − interstitial pulmonary fibrosis (285)
    − granulomatous lung infiltrates
    − pulmonary infiltrations
    − sarcoidosis (259)
21. Retroperitoneal fibrosis (268)
22. Rheumatoid arthritis (124, 196)
23. Sclerodermia (205, 233)
24. Sjögren's syndrome (66, 98, 106, 248, 274, 277)
25. Skin granulomas (150)
26. Teleangiectasia (138)
27. Thrombocytopenia
28. Thyreoiditis, hypothyroidism (98, 108)

Tab. 33.3: PBC-associated immunological diseases (with some references)

life is considerably impaired, further complications are induced or reinforced, and the prognosis worsens. (s. tabs. 33.3, 33.6)

4.9 Diagnosis

First of all, the diagnosis of PBC is based on the patient's **discomfort** in the form of fatigue, decline in functional capacity and pruritus, all of which, however, are uncharacteristic symptoms. PBC is verified if the following **laboratory parameters** can be demonstrated:

1. γ-GT ↑, AP ↑, LAP ↑
2. IgM ↑
3. Evidence of AMA
   − with subtypes (AMA profile)

The diagnosis of PBC should be supplemented by **laboratory values,** such as GPT, GOT, cholinesterase, cholesterol (especially HDL fraction), LP-X and/or α-lipoprotein, the galactose test, bilirubin as well as IgG and electrophoresis, possibly also P-III-P and the MEGX test. Because of their prognostic weighting, these values (including γ-GT and AP) are considered to be the main parameters for monitoring the course of disease and success of therapy. Furthermore, they co-determine the most suitable time for liver transplantation.

In the first instance, **morphological diagnostics** is based on *laparoscopy,* and, as a general principle, this method should be used for the initial diagnosis. All essential endoscopic findings are documented photographically. Naturally, laparoscopy does not produce a diagnosis of PBC, but it facilitates classification into the respective stages I–IV. (119, 186, 206) (s. p. 678) (s. fig. 33.9) • Targeted *liver biopsy* is then carried out by laparoscopy, whereby biopsy material is taken from both the right *and* left lobes of liver. The histological diagnosis of PBC is very unreliable because of the different patterns of morphological findings and the fact that criteria of the various stages can coexist. Nevertheless, targeted liver biopsy is imperative, even if the diagnosis is based upon reliable laboratory values: it facilitates an important additional assessment of inflammatory activity. (s. figs. 33.8, 33.10) • **Ultrasound** and **CT** do not yield any further diagnostic information. Lymphadenopathy is frequently present. (105, 110, 192, 229) Hepatobiliary sequential **scintigraphy** demonstrates a sevenfold to tenfold prolongation of the excretory phase in stages III and IV. (175, 223, 256) (s. fig. 13.7) • The **MRI** periportal halo sign is considered to be highly specific for PBC. (286) • Although **ERCP** plays an essential role in differential diagnosis, it cannot produce a diagnosis of PBC in itself. In the later course of disease, the bile ducts sometimes show certain irregularities and rarefaction (as ambiguous findings). (s. fig. 33.11)

4.10 Prognosis

Life expectancy ranges from 9–15 years following the diagnosis of PBC. The patient's life span is thus shorter than in the general population. The course of asymptomatic PBC is variable and difficult to predict. Some (25–35%) will never become symptomatic and others will run a progressive downhill course. The survival time of asymptomatic patients is generally longer than that of symptomatic patients; about 45% of cases were still asymptomatic at death. (242) Approximately 26% of PBC patients developed acute liver failure; in 39% of cases, liver transplantation could be kept until the censor date. (241) An individual prognostic assessment is desirable for the initiation of therapeutic measures. Indeed, several prognostic models have become established in recent years, e. g. Mayo model for survival (E.R. DICKSON et al., 1989). (87, 89, 126, 194, 224, 249, 256) • *Female patients* (only a very low number of males are affected) contract PBC in middle age (between 35 and 60 years). *Pregnancy* after the onset of PBC is very rare (so far <20 cases have been reported). (221) • An *early diagnosis* in the presymptomatic or, at the latest, in the oligosymptomatic stage offers the best prognosis. This is also true if the stage of disease is identified at a relatively early

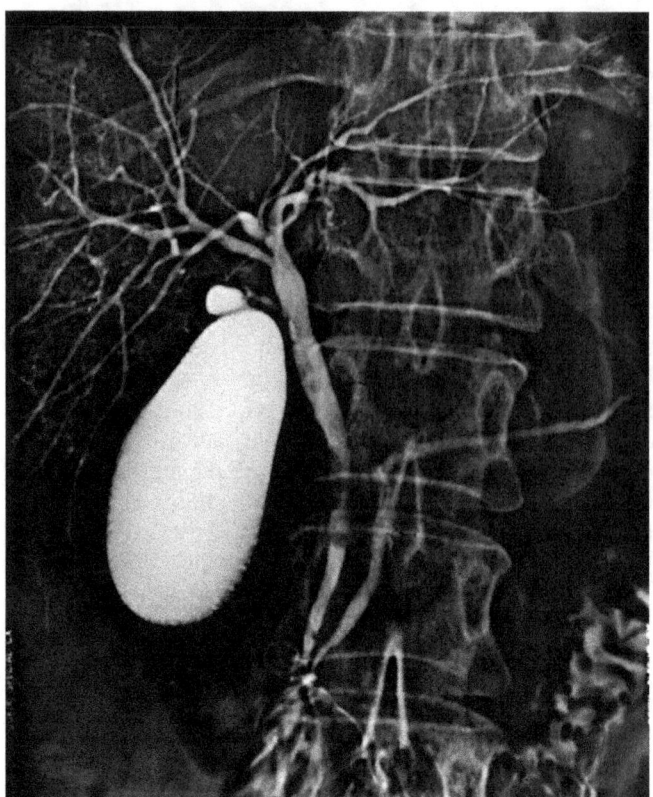

Fig. 33.11: ERCP shows smooth bile ducts of normal calibre; in later stages, there is rarefication of bile ducts, and certain irregularities appear

age (between 35 and 45 years). The *AMA profile* is apparently of some significance in early diagnosis (s. p. 126): in long-term follow-up over a period of up to 18 years, the poor prognosis of patients with profile C was only identifiable after 8–9 years, and with profile D after 6–7 years. In other studies, AMA profiles were not confirmed as a prognostic parameter. The profile of AMA subtypes does not change during the course of PBC. (s. tab. 5.21) • Those courses with less favourable prognoses showed a greater increase in *IgG values* as a sign of more distinct immunologic activity and correlated with increased TNF. • The presence of *SLA/LP antibodies* has a high specificity for the development of a secondary AIH overlap syndrome. (s. p. 694)

With regard to laboratory parameters, an increase in *bilirubin* to >5–6 mg/dl is seen as an essential prognostic factor. In such cases, the average life expectancy is now less than two years. A decline in the *synthesis rate* of the liver (cholinesterase, Quick's value, albumin) is usually also evident. Follow-up checks by means of the *galactose test* (244) are useful. Severe *cholestasis,* which can hardly or not at all be influenced, has to be rated just as poorly in terms of prognosis as a therapy-resistent and progressive pruritus. Increasing *portal hypertension* together with its complications, e. g. oesophageal varices, ascites and/or oedemas and hepatic encephalopathy, point to the final stage of PBC or to decompensated liver insufficiency. • Based on the pattern of these prognostic factors, important decisions can be taken with regard to drug therapy and possibly also the date of liver transplantation. • Histological findings are not suitable for the prognostic assessment of PBC.

4.11 Therapy

4.11.1 Symptomatic therapy

Pruritus: The relief or elimination of the unbearable itching is a top priority of any symptomatic therapy. (s. tab. 13.11) • Recommendations include: *cholestyramine* (4−24 g/day, gradually increasing dosage) or *cholestipol* (15−30 g/day), *phenobarbital* (5−10 mg/kg BW/day or 120 mg at night), *naloxone* (0.2 µg/kg BW/min i.v. infusion or 0.4−0.8 mg i.m.), *naltrexone* (50 mg/day), *rifampicin* (10 mg/kg BW/day) (121) *prednisolone* (10−20 mg/day), *metronidazole* (3 x 250 mg/day for 1 week), *antihistamines* and *propofol* in low doses, or *ultraviolet therapy* (9−12 min/day). The success rate of rifampicin was 80%, but 10−15% of patients suffered considerable side effects, including oedema of the lower leg (L. BACHS et al., 1992). *Ursodeoxycholic acid* (10−15 mg/kg BW/day) proved valuable; the success rate in stages I−II was 80−100% and in the precirrhotic stage III 40−60%. • In persistent PBC, there can be even more intensive pruritus despite treatment with UDCA. Itching which cannot be influenced or which becomes more intense generally points to an unfavourable prognosis. • In a case with refractory pruritus, a single **MARS** treatment effectively improved itching. Repetitive procedures are necessary to sustain this effect. (211)

Osteopathy: Prevention or improvement in osteopathy typical in PBC can be achieved by means of UDCA. In addition, sodium fluoride (50 mg/day), calcium (1,500 mg/day), alendronate (10 mg/day orally) (296), and vitamin D, e.g. 1.25 (OH)$_2$ D$_3$ (500−5000 units/day orally) should be administered. Calcitonin (50 units 3×/week i.m.) has also been used. (114) Substitution of oestrogens is advisable for postmenopausal women. (227) • Daily **muscular activity** is seen as the most important measure (e. g. regular physical exercise, stretching exercises, purposeful swimming). *Every patient should engage in physical exercise as a daily "must", because this is effective for the activation of the muscular system* (s. pp 551, 755):

> Twice a day, 10 to 15 slow knee-bends (= thigh muscles), plus 10 to 15 times standing on tiptoe (= calf muscles), plus 10 to 15 times upper arm flexing (= biceps), plus 10 to 15 times bending from the waist (= back muscles). This activates >60% of the total musculature on a daily basis without any special effort or expense, i.e. in the home environment, "in all weathers". Such regular exercise is essential for both prevention and treatment of osteopathy.

The administration of **medium-chain triglycerides** has a positive influence on the malabsorption of fat when accompanied by an adequate intake of proteins. Pancreas enzymes may be helpful. • **Simvastatin** or **bezafibrate** can be successful in the treatment of hypercholesterinaemia. (158, 159, 173, 245) • The deficiency of **fat-soluble vitamins** (A, D, E, K), accompanied by malabsorption of fatty acids, is treated by i.m. administration of these vitamins as combined medication (1−2 times a month). • **Zinc deficiency** requires substitution of this trace element. • The desired continuous detoxification of the intestine can be achieved using **lactulose.**

4.11.2 Approaches to causal therapy

Drug therapy is of little help except as a form of symptomatological or adjuvant treatment. Up to now, there is no causal or specific treatment for PBC. • Several substances, also in combination, have been used and partially tested in clinical studies over recent years. • *The therapeutic objectives in the choice of substances included prevention of an autoimmunologic inflammatory process, inhibition of fibrosis or improvement of chronic cholestasis with its unfavourable consequences.*

Azathioprine: As early as 1967, immunosuppression was attempted in PBC by means of azathioprine, but no positive influence on clinical course, laboratory parameters or morphological findings could be achieved. (112) • Subsequent studies have sometimes yielded encouragingly good results. Side effects are rare; despite occasional leucopenia, the risk of infection is not increased. (95)

Penicillamine: The high copper content of the liver led to the use of this substance in PBC. No positive effect on the disease could be ascertained. (83, 104, 217) In 46% of cases, severe side effects forced the discontinuation of therapy. (104) In individual cases, however, an improvement in the survival rate could be achieved with penicillamine during the late stages of PBC. (109)

Chlorambucil: A favourable influence on laboratory parameters and on inflammatory changes in histology was observed, but the morphological progression of PBC was not halted. Moreover, therapeutic use of chlorambucil is unacceptable owing to the danger of bone-marrow toxicity. (142)

Colchicine: This substance has been used in several studies over a period of up to 4 years (0.6−2.0 mg/day). There was an improvement both in laboratory values and in the survival rate (84% vs. 69% in the placebo group) (283) as well as in the mortality rate (21% vs. 47% in the placebo group). (160) Therapeutic efficacy was good. Side effects, mainly in the form of diarrhoea, were minimal (10−15%). (84, 161, 176, 297)

Prednisolone: There was no effect on laboratory values, progression or survival rate following an initial dosage of 30 mg/day and a maintenance dosage of 10 mg/day. Increased demineralization with the development of osteopathy only occurred during the first few months under high prednisolone doses. (201, 209) • In some patients, however, a favourable effect on laboratory values and histological inflammatory activity could be achieved using prednisolone. • This was confirmed by our own experience. (171) It is essential to keep the prednisolone dosage as low as possible – with consistent osteopathy prophylaxis (s. p. 683). • **We should have "respect" for, but no "fear" of prednisolone.**

Cyclosporine A: Cyclosporine was used for the first time by G. ROUTHIER et al. (1980) and by G.J.M. ALEXANDER et al. (1984) with encouraging results, yet with nephrotoxic side effects. In subsequent studies, the clinical picture and laboratory parameters as well as histological findings also showed significant improvement. However, an impairment of renal function and the occurrence of hypertension have to be anticipated. (182, 190, 287)

Methotrexate: The treatment of PBC with methotrexate was attempted for the first time by M.M. KAPLAN et al. (1988): the results were encouraging, but histology was unaffected. An initial dosage of 3 x 2.5 mg/week and a long-term dosage of 3 x 5 mg/week is recommended. Methotrexate should only be administered during the precirrhotic stages (I, II, II–III). (72) The hepatotoxicity of methotrexate, depression of bone marrow and possible development of interstitial pneumonia limit the use of this substance and may even force discontinuation of therapy. Administration of methotrexate led to better results regarding clinical symptoms, laboratory parameters and histology compared to a second group which received colchicine. (70, 101)

Ursodeoxycholic acid: F. ICHIDA et al. (1961) and T. NAKAHARA et al. (1975) were the first to report on the efficacy of UDCA in patients with *chronic hepatitis*. (s. p. 727) • In 1988 our group demonstrated obvious (and lasting) effects on the clinical and laboratory course with the use of UDCA in patients with a severe form of *acute viral hepatitis B*. (s. p. 445) • The first results of treatment of *primary biliary cholangitis* were submitted by the group of U. LEUSCHNER et al. (1985). During the following years (1986–1989), several clinical studies were published, all of them confirming the success of treatment in patients with PBC. The efficacy of hydrophilic UDCA is mainly based on the displacement of hydrophobic, potentially hepatotoxic bile acids. (174, 175, 294) So far, numerous clinically controlled studies regarding the use of UDCA in PBC have been carried out. The effects on clinical symptoms, laboratory parameters, AMA or IgM titres and histological findings ranged from good to very good, and a delayed formation of oesophageal varices was observed. Morphological lesions remained constant over a period of six years. (199) Progression was slowed down by UDCA, even though it was not possible to cure PBC. (178) However, contradictory results have also been submitted according to which PBC was only temporarily influenced by UDCA, and the development of cirrhosis could not be prevented. Nevertheless, UDCA proved to be significantly superior to all other substances and is now regarded as the drug of choice. The modes of action of UDCA are considered to be choleretic, hepatoprotective, immunomodulatory, membrane-stabilizing, anti-apoptic and membrane transporter-influencing. • A *dosage* of 12–16 mg/kg BW/day is recommended, divided into three single doses. Early commencement of therapy and lifelong application (without UDCA-free phases) are necessary! The survival rate has improved significantly (R.E. POUPON et al., 1997). Except for diarrhoea (about 2% of cases), no side effects are known. (67, 76–78, 96, 101, 115, 139, 145, 180, 188, 189, 200, 218, 226, 230, 231, 235, 237, 238, 254, 269, 270, 276, 294) (s. p. 886)

Tauro-ursodeoxycholic acid: This substance (TUDCA) has a hepatoprotective effect, even against toxic hydrophobic bile acids. In a dosage of 9 mg/kg BW/day, efficacy in PBC is similar to that of UDCA.

Mycophenolate mofetil: Esterification of the immuno-suppressive agent mycophenolic acid (MMA) leads to mycophenolate mofetil (MMF) as a prodrug with improved oral bioavailability. MMF (2 g/day) was first administered in PBC, combined with UDCA, by E.A. JONES et al. in 1999. In a later study, they were able to confirm their good results (based on selectively and reversibly inhibiting lymphocyte function) and the safety profile of MMF in long-term administration. (155)

Lamivudine + zidovudine: Because viruses are believed to play an important role in pathogenesis, lamivudine and zidovudine were added to the UDCA treatment which so far had been unsuccessful. After 12 months, most patients showed a normalization of the transaminases and alkaline phosphatase as well as a considerable improvement in histological findings. (197)

UDCA + colchicine: A combined application with colchicine was proposed in 1992 (600 mg UDCA + 1 mg colchicine/day) since the outcome of UDCA therapy had not been fully satisfactory. Good results were obtained with minor side effects. In a subsequent study, this combination therapy showed a slight advantage when the treatment was introduced in the early stages of PBC. (162, 235, 255, 280)

UDCA + methotrexate: It was frequently observed that not all patients with PBC responded to treatment with UDCA or that the disease even progressed. Therefore, a combination with methotrexate (1.5 mg/week) was introduced in 1993, which produced favourable results in some cases. (89) However, the side effects of methotrexate were considerable. This combination did not prove to be any more effective than UDCA alone, so that the application of methotrexate was considered to be inadvisable. (187)

UDCA + prednisone: In 1994 F.H.J. WOLFHAGEN et al. succeeded in favourably influencing the course of disease with a combination of UDCA and prednisone (10 mg/day) in those cases which had not previously been treatable in a satisfactory way. (288) • The combination of **UDCA + budesonide** has also proved successful. (68, 179) Budesonide shows a 15-times higher affinity to the glucocorticosteroid receptor as well as a distinct first-pass effect of >90%. The systemic side effects are low. • In cirrhosis, budesonide is contraindicated.

Azathioprine + prednisolone: As early as 1984, I reported on the good results obtained in 37 female patients (stages I–III) who had been treated with azathioprine (maintenance dose 1–2 x 50 mg/day) and prednisolone (initially 40 mg, maintenance dose 4–6 mg, intercurrently 8 mg) over a period of 2 to 13(!) years. Later on, a maintenance dose of 50 mg azathioprine every second day proved sufficient. (At that time, UDCA was not yet at our disposal.) The clinical and biochemical values during this long period can be described as good to very good; the histological changes likewise showed significant retrogression, and unspecific scarred residues were found. Consistent compliance with adjuvant measures (nutrition, fat-soluble vitamins, medium-chained triglycerides, muscular training) kept the side effects (osteopathy, diabetes, cataract, changes in the blood count) acceptably low. (171)

UDCA + prednisone + azathioprine: More recent results presented by F.H.J. WOLFHAGEN et al. on the first implementation of this triple therapy showed an impressive improvement in clinical, biochemical and histological findings. Dosage was as follows: UDCA (usual dose), prednisone (30 mg/day, gradually reduced to 10 mg/day) and azathioprine (50 mg/day). (289)

Prednimustine: The use of this substance (9 mg chlorambucil + 11 mg prednisolone) led to the normalization of bilirubin, IgM and alkaline phosphatase; however, these values increased again on discontinuation of prednimustine. (185)

Cyclosporine + prednisolone: Good treatment results were reported following the combined use of cylosporine (2.0–2.5 mg/kg BW/day) and prednisolone (4–8 mg/day).

UDCA + bezafibrate: This combination treatment also proved successful. The dose of UDCA was 600 mg/day and that of bezafibrate 400 mg/day over a period of 12 months. The administration of bezafibrate alone also produced good results. (159, 173) Recently, similar efficacy was reported in another study. (148)

UDCA + sulindac: The additional administration of sulindac, a non-steroidal antirheumatic agent (100–300 mg/day), showed an improvement in laboratory parameters – probably due to its choleretic effect. (181)

Alanine: In end-stage PBC, treatment with alanine (18 g/day) led to a remarkable improvement in jaundice, pruritus and laboratory values. (222)

Boswellinic acids: Leukotrienes appear to play a special role as inflammation mediators in the pathogenesis of PBC; they correlate closely with increasing cholestasis. Boswellinic acids are selective non-redox inhibitors of 5-lipoxygenase and therefore inhibit leukotriene biosynthesis. So far, they have not been used in PBC treatment. Based on existing pharmacological data, their application should now be considered.

4.11.3 Therapy concepts

The very extensive literature available on the treatment of PBC indeed provides valuable information for developing useful therapy concepts. *In this respect, the main aim is to apply a course of drug therapy which is as efficacious as possible with the fewest side effects.* • The following can be considered as evidence of **success:** (*1.*) improvement in life quality, (*2.*) tendency towards normalization of laboratory parameters (especially of bilirubin), (*3.*) regression of the inflammatory changes in histology or prevention of their progression, (*4.*) prolongation of life, and (*5.*) prolongation of the period of time prior to liver transplantation.

▶ In this respect, it must be remembered, that the **histological results** are extremely unreliable regarding both initial diagnosis and follow-up, because as a rule only one biopsy sample is taken percutaneously. The rate of error is so high in fact that the results are of little value, and thus initial diagnosis should also include targeted biopsy from both liver lobes by laparoscopy as well as photographic documentation of the liver surface.

At first, **symptomatic measures** (s. p. 680) are required in order to eliminate pruritus, prevent malnutrition, counteract osteopathy by means of regular physical exercise and eliminate the development of complications. This also includes careful observation with regard to any possible side effects of drugs or metabolic disorders. The intensity of these measures and the intervals between any necessary monitoring measures depend on the initial findings and the individual course of disease.

When applying the **substances** described above or their possible combinations, the efficacy spectrum of the remedy and the respective risk of side effects always have to be weighed against each other. In *long-term treatment*, a reduction in dosage may serve to lower the risk of side effects while maintaining a satisfactory level of success.

1. Irrespective of PBC stage and AMA profile, **UDCA** (12–16 mg/kg BW/day or 900 mg/day) is considered to be the drug of choice to be applied *as soon as possible and then continuously*! • Treatment with UDCA procedures led to a survival rate of 61%, which is similar to that of healthy persons. Therefore, special attention has

to be paid to non-responders (e.g. UDCA combined with methotrexate). (70)

2. At an advanced stage (II, III) with AMA profile B, the combination of **UDCA + prednisolone** (maintenance dose 4–8 mg/day in the morning) should be administered as first medication. • In the case of unsatisfactory therapeutic results or with AMA profiles C or D (= stages III or IV), we recommend the additional administration of **azathioprine** as a triple therapy. A dosage of 1 x 50 mg (up to 2 x 50 mg) per day is well-tolerated and, like prednisolone at this dosage, has relatively few side effects. A maintenance dose of 50 mg every second day may be sufficient. (171) • The *immunomodulatory action of UDCA* is thus combined with the *immunosuppressive effect of azathioprine*, while the *anti-inflammatory characteristics of the steroids* are also included, i.e. *the two-substance combination is extended to a triple combination if necessary, especially in profiles C or D.*

3. **Colchicine** (0.6–2.0 mg/day) has relatively minor side effects. As far as I know, the combination of **UDCA + prednisolone + colchicine** has never been applied in PBC stages II–IV or AMA profiles C and D, although this seems plausible from a pharmalogical point of view.

In the light of current knowledge and in view of the reinforced effect, there should be no objection to using a combination of **UDCA + methotrexate + colchicine**; nevertheless, the frequency of side effects due to methotrexate must be considered.

4.11.4 Liver transplantation

The symptomatic measures and a suitable combination of pharmacons are primarily aimed at preventing PBC progression and improving or even normalizing the findings. If this is not successful, the secondary aim is to achieve the longest possible period of time between initial diagnosis and *liver transplantation, which is the only chance in the late stages (IV, IV–V), and hence the therapy of choice.* The **optimal date** depends on general conditions, increase in the bilirubin value up to >6 mg/dl, but <9 mg/dl, extent of osteopathy, onset of water retention (oedema, ascites) and occurrence of drug-induced side effects, all of which rule out any further medication. If the bilirubin value exceeds 9 mg/dl, the patient should consult a transplantation centre.

The **success rate** of OLT is convincing in cases of PBC. However, consistent and regular osteopathy treatment during the postoperative phase, e.g. muscular training (s. p. 683) and drug therapy, is also of great importance. The 1-year survival rate was 93%, the 5-year survival rate was 76%, and the 8-year survival rate was 71%. About 80% of transplant patients become completely rehabilitated and are able to work again. Retransplantation is necessary in 10% of patients because of a "vanishing bile-duct syndrome". Most manifestations of PBC disappear, and even a reduction in bone changes may occur. In the first few months after LTX, osteoporosis becomes far more pronounced; the loss of bone density can be as much as 20%. There is a risk of spontaneous fractures. The rate of occurrence of PBC in the graft (granulomatous bile-duct damage, ductopenia, biliary-type fibrosis) increases with time: after 10 years, it is observed in 15–30% of patients. The risk factors are unknown. Cirrhosis has rarely been reported. Differentiation between PBC relapse and rejection of the transplant is difficult, because both present a similar morphological picture. However, patients with PBC show an increased frequency of chronic transplant rejection in comparison to other liver transplantation patients. After transplantation, AMA are still verifiable in the serum. (99, 107, 131, 133, 163–165, 183, 250, 273)

5 Primary sclerosing cholangitis

▶ The report by K. DELBET in 1924 is considered to be the first observation of a sclerosing cholangitis. (325) In 1958 J. SEYMOUR et al. distinguished between primary and secondary forms of the disease. (415)

5.1 Definition

Progressive, fibrous-stenosing and obliterating, mainly segmental inflammation of the intrahepatic (and extrahepatic) bile ducts is described as primary sclerosing cholangitis (PSC). The aetiology and pathogenesis of this chronic cholestatic disease are still unknown. In patients with a genetic predisposition, it is deemed to be an autoimmune disease. The course is slowly progressive, yet variable and unpredictable. PSC is a rare condition; it is closely associated with ulcerative colitis and less closely with Crohn's disease. In general, PSC develops into *biliary cirrhosis* with corresponding complications.

5.2 Systematics

Secondary sclerosing cholangitis (SSC) is distinguished from "classical" *primary sclerosing cholangitis* (PSC). SSC shows clinical, morphological and radiological findings identical to those of PSC. Manifest SSC is irreversible. While the origin of PSC has not yet been resolved, SSC can be attributed to various known causes. Until its aetiopathogenesis is clarified, PSC (like PBC) should continue to be defined as a particular form of "idiopathic" disease. (s. tab. 33.4)

5.3 Epidemiology

PSC, which was seldom described in the past, has been identified more frequently since the introduction of

1. **Primary sclerosing cholangitis (PSC)** • cause(s) unknown

2. **Secondary sclerosing cholangitis (SSC)**
• *mechanical causes*
  – choledochal tumour – postoperative factors
  – choledocholithiasis – stricture
  – papillitis stenosans
• *infectious causes*
  – AIDS – mycoses
  – bacteria – parasites
  – immunodeficiency – viruses (cytomegaly, REO)
• *toxic causes*
  – burn injuries – hydatidal obliteration
  – ethanol embolization – pharmacons (s. tab. 29.11)
• *vascular causes*
  – autoimmune vasculitis
  – collagenoses
  – cytostatics in hepatic artery
  – ischaemia (shock, surgery)
• *malignant causes*
  – amyloidosis – Hodgkin's lymphoma
  – CCC – mastocytosis
  – histiocytosis X
• *immunological causes*
  – autoimmune cholangiopathy
  – sarcoidosis
  – transplant rejection
    (allograft rejection, graft-versus-host reaction)
• *congenital causes*
  – Alagille syndrome
  – Caroli's disease
  – congenital liver fibrosis
  – cystic fibrosis
  – genetic metabolic ductopenia
  – microhamartoma
  – NAIC (s. fig. 33.18)

Tab. 33.4: Causes of sclerosing cholangitis

ERCP. • The prevalence of PSC is estimated at 2–8/100,000 inhabitants. About 70% of patients are males; they are affected twice as often as females. People aged between 25 and 45 years are most often affected. (318) PSC in childhood is a rarity. However, isolated cases have been diagnosed even at the neonatal stage. (327, 332, 334, 337, 366, 372, 407, 417, 434, 438) • There is a close association with simultaneous chronic inflammatory bowel disease (60–75%, up to 100%), whereby ca. 80% of cases involve ulcerative colitis, and only 10–15% Crohn's disease. PSC without concomitant CIBD affects mostly women. Smokers contract ulcerative colitis and PSC far less frequently than non-smokers (4% vs. 70%). (376) Perinuclear antineutrophilic cytoplasmic antibodies (pANCA) can also be detected in healthy members of the PSC patient's family.

5.4 Aetiopathogenesis

A **genetic disposition** is assumed for the occurrence of PSC. This idea is supported by the fact that the disease has indeed frequently been observed in certain races or families. (354, 361, 404)

HLA haplotypes: Frequent associations with special HLA haplotypes point to a specific immunological disposition in patients: HLA-B8 (60–80%), HLA-DR3 (25–70%) and HLA-DRw52a (DRB 1–1301) (100%) (the last-mentioned is said to be highly specific to PSC). HLA-DR2 is determined in up to 70% of HLA-B8-negative and HLA-DR3-negative patients. An association with HLA-DR4, HLA-DRb12, HLA-Drw17, HLA-Cw7, HLA-DQw2, HLA-A1 and HLA-DW has also been demonstrated. The discrepancy in findings may result from regional, individual, methodological and age differences within the patient cohorts. (315, 326, 384, 403) • A further specific feature is the aberrant expression of **blood group antigens** (A and B) on bile-duct epithelial cells and colon mucosa cells.

Cellular immunity: The decline in T lymphocytes resulting from a drop in the number of $CD8^+$ suppressor cells points to pre-existing cellular immunity (increase in the quotient $CD4^+ : CD8^+$), as does a rise in B lymphocytes (with an increase in T lymphocytes in the portal fields); an inhibition of leucocyte migration was likewise found. D.H. ADAMS et al. (1991) identified an elevated expression of the ICAM 1 on the bile-duct epithelia.

Humoral immunity: Indicators of the existence of humoral immunity are: hypergammaglobulinaemia with a predominance of IgM antibodies (321, 431); evidence of circulating immunocomplexes (>80% of cases), also in the bile; activation of the complement system. (414) • Antibodies were found with the following prevalence: SMA (<1:80) (60%), anticolon antibodies (60%) and ANA (<1:80) (35%). (440) The detection of these antibodies did not correlate with disease activity.

pANCA: The perinuclear antineutrophilic cytoplasmic antibodies, particularly types IgG_1 and IgG_3, are important. (362, 375, 413, 440) (s. p. 127) (s. tab. 5.20)

ARP: An anti-ribosomal P antibody was recently reported to be present in 80% of PSC patients.

It is still unclear whether these findings constitute disorders of pathogenetic relevance or immunological epiphenomena. Yet there is every reason to believe that PSC is an autoimmunological disease, which is triggered or initiated by different agents – e.g. toxins, infections (396, 401), viruses – in predisposed patients and in cases of reduced barrier function of the gut. • Due to increased permeability of the mucosa in CIBD, endotoxins reach the liver via the portal vein. However, it has not been confirmed that endotoxins are in any way pathogenetic. It is significant that the morphological changes appear predominantly segmental, even though immunological reactions are, in fact, systemically disturbed. • Ulcerative colitis and other inflammatory bowel diseases are of no primary pathogenetic importance. A connection with vascular components (e.g.

association of PSC with periarteriitis nodosa) is unlikely. A possible disorder of copper metabolism does not play any pathogenetic role.

5.5 Morphology

▶ However important the **liver biopsy** sample may be for the characterization of PSC (or PBC), the assessment of each individual finding can be problematic: liver changes often show a focal arrangement, while portal and lobular lesions can vary in degree; the signs of damage frequently overlap, depending on the stage of disease. No histological picture typical of PSC exists. In 25—50% of biopsies, no findings pointing to PSC are detected at all; in 40%, histology is generally decisive, but with almost the same frequency even stages III and IV were not recognized. • **Laparoscopically,** stages I and II display a liver surface which is still smooth. To an increasing degree (stages II, II—III), finely structured fibrosis and greyish-green maculation can be identified. Often, there are spider naevi on the liver surface. This finding is typical for PSC and only detectable in this condition. (s. fig. 33.13) The terminal stage is characterized by mixed-nodular *biliary cirrhosis* of a greyish-green to dirty grey colour. Liver biopsy, which is always regarded as a necessity, should be carried out as a targeted procedure during laparoscopy when establishing the initial diagnosis; in fact (as is the case with PBC), samples should be taken from *both* liver lobes in order to increase diagnostic reliability. The surface structure of the liver must be described in detail and documented by photography. (s. figs. 33.12, 33.13)

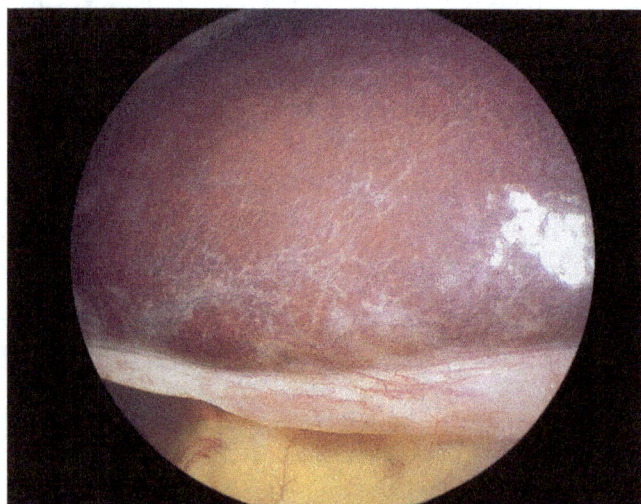

Fig. 33.12: Primary sclerosing cholangitis following cholecystectomy (due to involvement of the gall bladder); distinct periportal fibrosis with initial surface roughness

The **large bile ducts** are affected intrahepatically in 20%, intrahepatically and extrahepatically in 70—75%, and extrahepatically in 5% of cases. Differentiation between

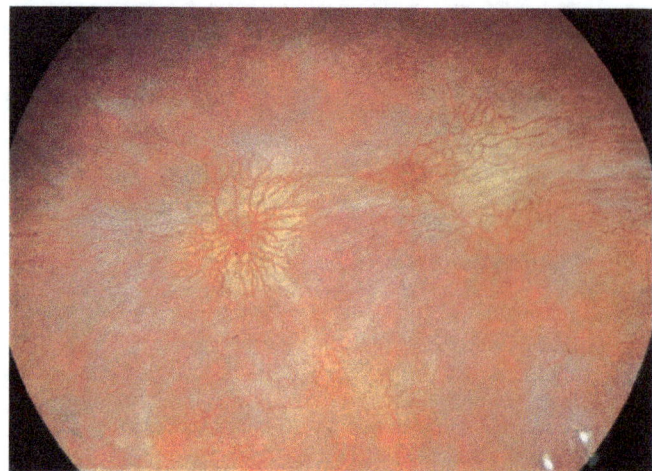

Fig. 33.13: PSC: two spider naevi are visible on the liver surface, which is typical for this condition. (s. fig. 31.19!) Additional pronounced vascularization and minor blood extravasates

"large-duct" and "small-duct" PSC by means of ERC or MRC may also be of importance.

Small-duct PSC (termed *pericholangitis* by A. WEE et al., 1985) is a variant of PSC involving only the small bile ducts. Therefore, it cannot be demonstrated by means of ERC, but with the help of liver biopsy. Marked cholestasis is evident. The course of disease is slower. Prognosis is better than in large-duct PSC. In rare cases, this condition can lead to cirrhosis. (303, 377, 378, 386)

Stage I: The **portal stage** is characterized by a widening of the portal field due to proliferations of the interlobular bile ducts, by formation of connective tissue and periductal oedema, and by portal infiltrations (= portitis + cholangitis). The bile-duct ephithelia show degenerative and atrophic changes, and even cell necrosis. Bile-duct ectasia is sometimes evident. (399, 433) (s. fig. 33.14)

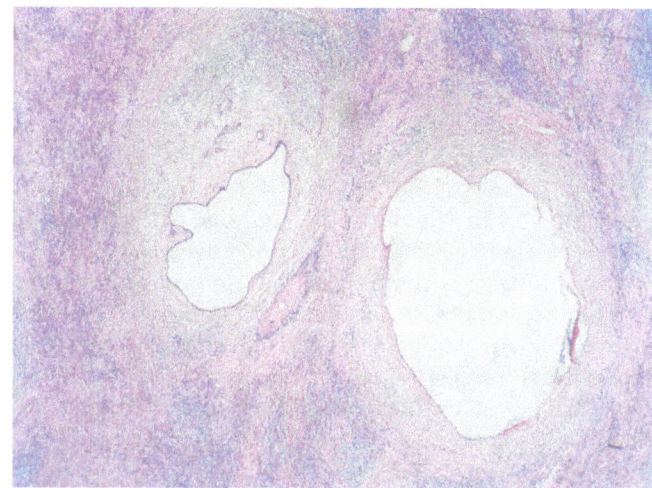

Fig. 33.14: PSC: periductal fibrosis and inflammatory infiltration; aneurysmal bile-duct ectasia (HE)

Stage II: The **periportal stage** presents an encroachment of the inflammatory changes on the parenchyma with piecemeal necrosis; connective tissue proliferations break into the lobule (= periportal hepatitis + fibrosis). Liver cell necroses are also found sporadically, whereby CD4 cells, CD56-NK cells and lymphocytes are markedly increased. In places, reduction in and fibrosis of the bile ducts are already evident. (335, 379) (s. fig. 33.15)

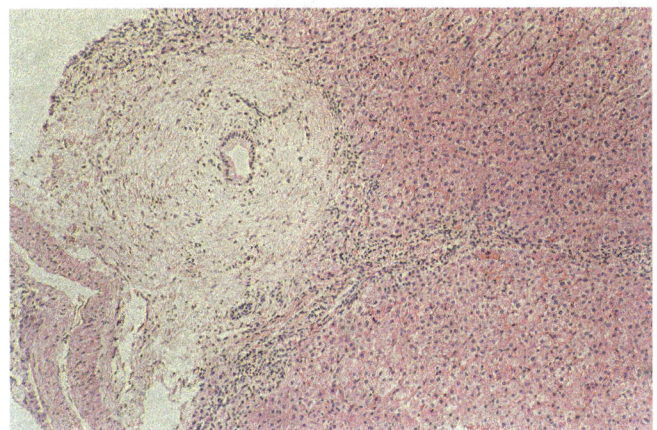

Fig. 33.15: PSC: marked concentric fibrosis around a septal bile duct together with slight periportal inflammation (HE)

Stage III: The **septal stage** displays periportal and bridging necrosis as well as an increasing loss of bile ducts with a simultaneous decline in portal inflammatory infiltrations. Dense concentric fibrosis develops around the bile ducts (so-called onion-skin appearance), and a portoportal band of connective tissue (bridging fibrosis) is subsequently formed. In some cases, segmental PSC is found. (349) • MRI and CT often show a focal atrophy of segments 2 and 3. (333, 360, 379)

▶ **Stage IV:** In this stage, **biliary cirrhosis** exhibits a loss of interlobular and septal bile ducts and the formation of regenerative nodes as well as distinct septation and connective tissue fields. As a result of cholestasis, the liver parenchyma contains high concentrations of copper. • The *extrahepatic bile ducts* appear as string-like thickened cords with a narrowing of the lumen. The *gall bladder* may be involved in a process of chronic fibrosing inflammation. (314, 352, 430) (s. fig. 33.12) • *Transitions* between the precirrhotic stages and biliary cirrhosis are found to be fluid in the *biopsy material*, and in part overlap; even normal intralobular bile ducts may alternate with inflammatory, periductal infiltrations or bile-duct scleroses. The *autoptic examination* sometimes conflicts with the result of liver biopsy. (333, 345, 359, 435)

5.6 Clinical aspects

In the early stages, PSC is clinically **asymptomatic** in 10—40% of cases. By chance, laboratory tests often reveal an inexplicable state of cholestasis. Cases with normal alkaline phosphatase have also been reported. (347, 360, 402)

The **symptomatic course** starts slowly, mostly with fatigue, loss of vitality, pruritus, occasional scleral icterus, upper abdominal pain on pressure, loss of weight, and fever. Hepatomegaly is verifiable in 50—75% of cases; splenomegaly is less frequent. The type and intensity of the discomfort as well as the clinical findings vary remarkably from patient to patient. Complications are principally due to damage of the bile ducts. In general, the symptoms have already existed for about two years prior to initial diagnosis. (347, 370, 435) • An increase in γ-GT and alkaline phosphatase is a first and important sign of the existence of hepatobiliary disease. But even in a symptomatic course, normal values of AP have been reported. This observation also confirms the importance of determining LAP in cases of an unresolved increase in γ-GT and normal AP values (AP non-response exists in 2—4% of patients with cholestasis!). IgM is rarely, but IgG4 often elevated (385). • In other patients, cholangitic episodes predominate in the clinical picture. In some cases, the diagnosis is only established in a more advanced course of disease or even during the stage of cirrhosis (with portal hypertension and oesophageal varices). (317, 330, 334, 347, 351, 370, 395, 412, 435, 436)

5.7 Diagnosis

The diagnosis of PSC is made on the basis of clinical, laboratory and morphological findings as well as by ERCP. The **main criteria** of PSC are: (*1.*) chronic cholestasis (γ-GT, AP, LAP), (*2.*) evidence of pANCA, and (*3.*) ERCP or MRC. (323, 334, 412) (s. tab. 33.5)

I. Suggestive factors	
1. Subjective discomfort	
2. Men, 20 to 45 years old	
3. Non-smoker (?)	
4. Association with chronic IBD	
5. Increased transaminases	
6. Hepato/splenomegaly	
II. Definite diagnosis	
1. *Chronic cholestasis*	3. *ERCP, MRC*
2. *pANCA +*	4. *Laparoscopy, liver biopsy*
III. Supplementary findings	
1. *Laboratory tests*	
– bilirubin ↑	– cholinesterase ↓
– IgM ↑, IgG4 ↑	– α-, γ-globulins ↑
– HLA haplotypes	– CRP +, ESR ↑
– ANA, SMA (+)	– haemoglobin ↓
– serum copper ↑	– eosinophilia
– cupruria	
2. *Sonography, CT*	

Tab. 33.5: Indicative, evidential and supplementary parameters for diagnosis of PSC

	ANA	SMA	LKM1	SLA/LP	ASGPR	AMA	pANCA	AHA	HCV	anti-GOR	specific nuclear antibody
Primary cholangitis											
• Primary biliary cholantitis (PBC)	(+)	–	–	–	(+)	++	(+)	–	–	–	
• Primary sclerosing cholangitis (PSC)	(+)	–	–	–	–	–	++	–	–	–	
Overlap syndrome											
AIH/PBC	+	(+)	–	(+)	(+)	+	–	–	–	–	
AIH/PSC	+	(+)	–	(+)	(+)	–	+	–	–	–	
AIH/HCV	(+)	(+)	+	(+)	+	–	–	–	–	(+)+	
AIH/alcohol	(+)	(+)	–	(+)	(+)	(+)	–	++	–	–	
AIH/collagenosis	++	++	–	(+)	(+)	–	–	–	–	–	++

Tab. 33.6: Differentiation of primary cholangitis and overlap syndromes by means of antibodies. (s. tab. 5.20) • (AHA = anti-histone antibody; anti-GOR = anti-specific nuclear antigen in HCV) (see text for other abbreviations). –/(+) = no or occasional slight increase

1. Association with CIBD: In 33–93% of cases (mean value 64%), PSC is associated with a chronic inflammatory bowel disease (CIBD). Ulcerative colitis predominates in 69–100% of cases (mean value 89%) compared to Crohn's disease in 0–31% (mean value 11%); however, a reversed rate of frequency regarding these two bowel diseases with 38% vs. 56% has also been reported. • The frequency of patients suffering from PSC in CIBD is about 3.7% (393), in ulcerative colitis 3.3%, and in Crohn's disease 2.5%. • PSC can occur before the determination of CIBD, after a long course of CIBD, and occasionally after colectomy. There is no correlation between the degree of severity of CIBD and the course of PSC. (331, 383, 386, 397, 404, 405, 424, 439) • Proctocolectomy does not influence the course of PSC. (319)

2. Cholestasis: The values of γ-GT, AP and LAP are elevated (with non-response of AP in 2–4% of cases). Hyperbilirubinaemia is verifiable in about half the patients at the time of initial diagnosis. Copper values in serum and urine are elevated. (298, 342) A slight rise in the transaminases is likewise observed. The first diagnostic step in determining cholestasis is sonography.

3. Sonography: Except in the late stage, there are generally no findings which point to PSC or explain the existing cholestasis. However, there is evidence of hepatomegaly and increased reflections from dilated intrahepatic bile ducts as well as a thickening of the bile duct walls; in addition, splenomegaly (380, 432) or intra-abdominal lymphadenopathy (300) are occasionally found. A nodular transformation of the liver can be detected. Tentative diagnosis by sonography now provides the indication for ERCP. • Compared to sonography, CT does not offer any fundamental advantages. (427)

4. ERC: This is the decisive examination for the final diagnosis of PSC (positive in >95% of cases). It is carried out under periendoscopic protection with antibiotics. Cholestasis can be accelerated by ERC. Typical findings include: *pearlstring-like changes* of the bile ducts with intermittent, diffusely distributed, multiple, irregular, circular strictures of different length (0.5–2.0 cm), with normal or only insignificantly widened bile-duct segments; *diverticular sacculation* of the bile ducts with or without preceding stenosis; segmental or diffuse rarefication of the bile ducts. Serious changes of the bile ducts are invariably found in more advanced stages of PSC. (s. fig. 33.16)

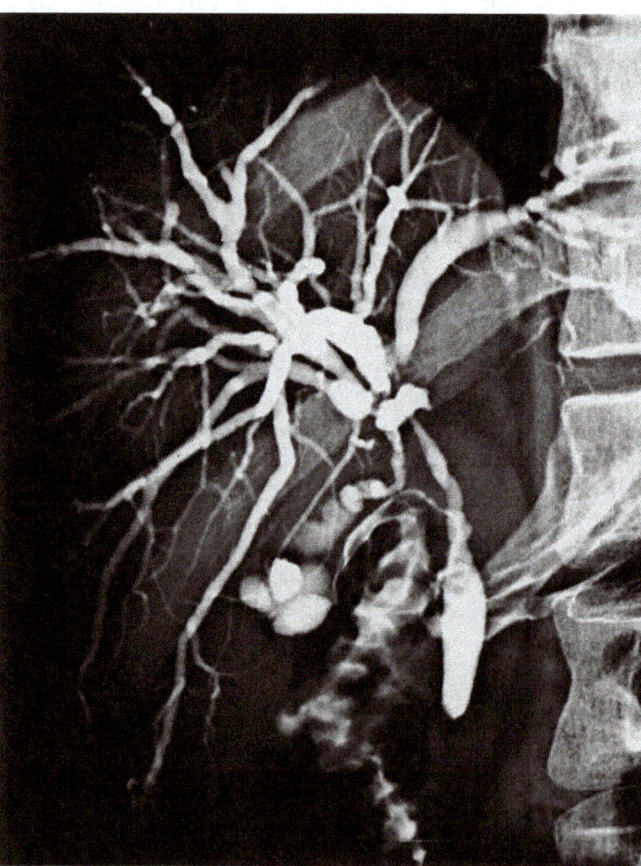

Fig. 33.16: ERC in primary sclerosing cholangitis: irregular wall contours, variable intrahepatic and extrahepatic duct stenoses with prestenotic dilatations (subsequently demonstrated bile-duct carcinoma on the basis of existing PSC)

About 80% of patients show both intrahepatic and extrahepatic changes; in 20% of cases, only the extrahepatic bile-duct system is affected. The severest changes are found in the area of the hepatic bifurcation (differential diagnosis: Klatkin's tumour). Distal bile-duct stenosis is frequent and almost characteristic. The gall bladder can also be involved. (391, 424) A *segmental PSC* is sometimes found, causing a difficult differential diagnosis, especially regarding CCC. (382)

5. pANCA: In 80–87% of cases, perinuclear antineutrophilic cytoplasmic antibodies are demonstrable with simultaneous PSC and CIBD. In PSC, detection of pANCA is possible in only 40% of patients, but in isolated CIBD in 85%. Thus pANCA correlates not with the activity of PSC, but with CIBD and portal inflammation. After colectomy or liver transplantation, antibodies are still evident in the serum. • pANCA are also found in AIH, PBC, LE, rheumatoid arthritis and autoimmune glomerulonephritis; cANCA is detectable in Wegener's disease. • Further antibodies may be present, e.g. ANA (10–70%), SMA (10–40%), anti-colon (10–60%), anticardiolipin, antithyroid antibodies. (302, 363, 375, 413, 440) (s. tab. 5.20) (s. fig. 5.15)

6. MRC: It is only at stages II–III, III and IV that MRC gives a reliable assessment of the intrahepatic and extrahepatic bile ducts — often even more reliable than ERC. MRC cannot replace ERC in primary diagnostics of PSC, but serves as an important supplementary examination. (305, 328, 335, 350, 388, 391, 406)

5.8 PSC-associated diseases

Like PBC, PSC is not limited to the hepatobiliary area. In about 25% of cases, it occurs as an independent disease; however, in more than 70% of patients, chronic IBD exists simultaneously. • Associations with **autoimmune diseases** have been observed far less frequently in PSC than in PBC. (s. tabs. 33.3, 33.7)

Coeliac disease	Myasthenia gravis
Collagenoses	Myelopathy
Diabetes mellitus (type 1)	Orbital pseudotumour
Folliculitis (356)	Pulmonary fibrosis (353)
Haemolytic anaemia (387)	Retroperitoneal fibrosis
Hodgkin's disease	Salivary pseudotumour
Hyperthyroidism (312)	Sarcoidosis
Lupus erythematosus (304)	Sjögren's syndrome
Lymphadenopathy (300)	Vasculitis
Mediastinal fibrosis	*etc.*

Tab. 33.7: Autoimmunological diseases associated with PSC (with some references)

5.9 Complications

The volume of the gall bladder is frequently increased. (314, 430) **Cholelithiasis** occurs in 20–25% of patients with PSC; in 30–35% of all cases, cholecystectomy was already carried out prior to initial diagnosis. (s. fig. 33.1) **Choledocholithiasis** (ca. 40%) is regarded as a complication of PSC or even as the cause of SSC. The following figure shows a rare finding in the form of a staghorn calculus taken from the bifurcation of the choledochus and the two branches of the common bile duct (still at our disposal). (s. fig. 33.17)

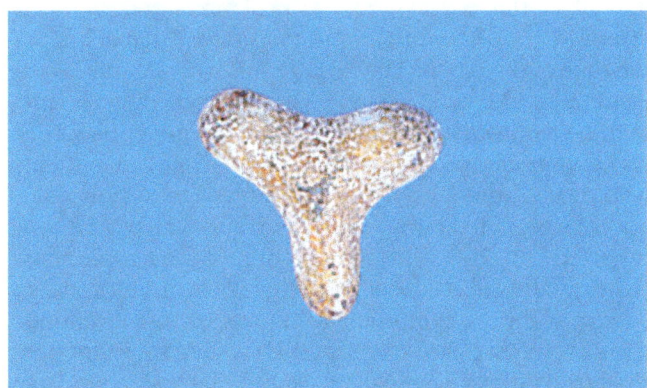

Fig. 33.17: Staghorn calculus in the common bile duct and the two branches of the common hepatic duct (so-called *Mercedes-star type*) in primary sclerosing cholangitis *(at our dsiposal)*

Chronic pancreatitis with typical changes in ERCP is verifiable in 10–12% of patients; exocrine pancreas insufficiency is rare.

PSC is seen as a pronounced form of precancerosis. The occurrence of **cholangiocarcinoma** must be anticipated in 6–23% of cases (1.5% per year, i.e. 161 times higher than in healthy persons). In autopsies and explanted livers, bile-duct carcinoma has been demonstrated in 30–50% of cases. Frequency increases with the duration of disease and the existence of CIBD. This complication is suspected in rapidly progressing cholestasis. Diagnosis is difficult; in > 80% of cases, CT yields evidence of cholangiocarcinoma, together with biliary brush cytology and findings of the late stage of PSC. If the formula *CA19-9 + (CEA x 40)* shows a value of >400 with a sensitivity of 86% (–100%), CCC is to be expected. (307, 313, 318, 320, 365, 369, 372, 381, 416, 420) PET is a new diagnostic procedure in this respect. In PSC patients with colitis ulcerosa, the frequency of colon carcinoma is 10 times and that of pancreas carcinoma 14 times higher than in healthy persons. Regular coloscopy and sonography is required. (419) Development of spindle cell carcinoma is extremely rare.

Osteopathy, which is expected in chronic cholestasis and often verifiable in PBC as well, is less frequently detected in PSC. (301, 346) **Xanthelasmas,** which are prevalent in PBC, are likewise less common in PSC (19% vs. 3%). • The frequency of **cholangitic episodes,** however, is about seven times higher in PSC than in PBC; there is a risk of liver abscess formation, strictures (310) and stenoses. A candida infection is sometimes found and may be the cause of suppurative cholangitis and biliary obstruction. (367) • In PSC, **hyperpigmentation** can be identified in only 25% of cases (compared to >50% in PBC). • Cirrhosis-related complications are more frequent in PSC (13%) than in PBC (8%).

5.10 Course and prognosis

The natural course of PSC showed a survival rate of 65−70% after 6 years, 75% after 9 years and 30−70% after 5 years, depending on the respective stage of PSC at the time of diagnosis. The average survival rate was calculated to be 12.9 or 17 and even 21 years, whereby patients with a symptomatic course at initial diagnosis had a far less favourable prognosis: 40−50% (−90%) of patients who died within a 6-year period underwent a symptomatic course. In contrast, a 5-year survival period was reported in 78−88% (and more) of asymptomatic patients. In 22−60% of cases with an asymptomatic course of PSC, a symptomatic clinical picture developed within 5 years. Based on current knowledge, it is not possible to predict which patients should be assigned to the risk group. (306, 317, 334, 347, 370, 372, 411, 428, 436)

These greatly differing figures in the literature reflect the fact that (*1.*) due to the inexact definition of PSC, the stage at initial diagnosis is based on different parameters and may vary greatly; (*2.*) the earlier the initial diagnosis is established and therapy is initiated, the more favourable the influence on survival time has proved to be (also true for PBC); (*3.*) monitoring and assessment of insidious PSC is inadequate despite such means as selected laboratory parameters, liver function tests, ERC and histology (the last-mentioned at long intervals). Elevated values of serum bilirubin and IgG4 (385) over a longer period as well as a decrease in albumin (428) relate to a poor prognosis. Evidence of DR4 points to rapid progression. (284) A fulminant course of PSC is rare. (308) • *Pregnancy* does not influence the course of PSC, nor does PSC impair the course of pregnancy or harm the embryo or foetus. • Any statement concerning prognosis depends on the following **criteria:** bilirubin value in the serum, concomitant chronic inflammatory bowel disease, histological stage of the biopsy specimen (if possible from both liver lobes), hepato/splenomegaly, duration of the symptomatic phase, and age.

There is no standardized evaluation of the valency of **cholestasis parameters:** the variations in weighting the prognosis parameters in the scores clearly show the difficulty of reliable assessment, especially as these parameters are not always obtained by uniform criteria (prospectively or retrospectively). However, the claim that cholestasis parameters do not permit any prognosis to be made must be seen as controversial. In our experience, cholestasis-indicating enzymes and the bilirubin value as well as GEC and the ICG tests (e.g. under UDCA or prednisolone therapy) facilitate an **evaluation of the course of disease** and provide valuable benchmarks for the planning or postponement of invasive and surgical measures. • Knowing the "natural" history of a disease and evaluating its course under therapeutic measures with regular laboratory tests are the two (essential and different) aspects of prognostic assessment.

5.11 Therapy

5.11.1 Conservative therapy

> Therapeutic measures are aimed at improving or normalizing the bile flow as well as reducing inflammatory tissue reactions in order to prevent the progression of biliary obstruction.

There is no specific or causal therapy of PSC. Reduction in or elimination of **pruritus** (339), elimination of **malabsorption** and, if necessary, replacement of fat-soluble vitamins (355), selenium (298) and zinc are the primary targets of therapy − as in PBC. (s. p. 683) • Relapsing cholangitis requires the administration of **broad-spectrum antibiotics;** however, antibiotic prophylaxis is not indicated. (316, 323, 324, 371, 412)

Therapeutic trials with **D-penicillamine** (e.g. 750 mg/day for three years) did not influence the course of disease. **Cyclosporine** and *azathioprine* were also ineffective.

Cyclosporine + prednisolone: A combination of cyclosporine and prednisolone, however, proved to be successful. (368)

Colchicine: The positive results achieved with colchicine could not be confirmed in a subsequent study. (394)

Methotrexate: The use of methotrexate (15 mg/week) led to an improvement in symptoms, cholestasis and histological findings. Application is worth considering in the early phase of PSC. (358, 364) However, occasional severe side effects have to be taken into account.

Prednisolone + colchicine: A combination of both substances (10 mg plus 1.2 mg per day) led to an improvement in biochemical findings, but no favourable long-term effect could be demonstrated. (373)

Ursodeoxycholic acid: In 1985 UDCA was used for the first time in PSC by the group of U. LEUSCHNER. (s. p. 684) Meanwhile, UDCA has proved to be the drug of choice. Clinical symptoms (322, 390), laboratory findings (cholestasis, bilirubin) (309, 337, 375, 390, 421), radiological changes and histology (309) could all be favourably influenced in numerous patients. An inhibition of the expression of HLA class II antigens on hepatocytes was also verified. However, lasting therapeutic success has not been achieved so far although the incidence of CCC was actually reduced after long-term treatment with UDCA. (409) Administration of UDCA (15−20 mg/kg BW/day) does not cause any side effects. Due to its beneficial effect, this substance should be used in the early phase of PSC (as in PBC), and thereafter continuously. (344, 392, 397, 422, 423, 429)

UDCA + prednisolone: UDCA (10–15 mg/kg BW/day) combined with prednisolone (initially about 40 mg/day, declining rapidly to a maintenance dose of 4–6 mg/day) is worth considering in view of the positive therapeutic effects recently reported.

UDCA + prednisolone + azathioprine: A triple therapy comprising azathioprine (1.0–1.5 mg/kg BW/day), prednisolone (1 mg/kg BW/day, decreasing to 5–10 mg/day) and UDCA (500–750 mg/day) has been reported for the first time. The (biochemical, histological, cholangiographic) results following an average observation period of 41 months were promising. (410)

UDCA + methotrexate: The combination of UDCA (13–15 mg/kg BW/day) and methotrexate (0.25 mg/kg BW/week) was ineffective, and side effects from methotrexate occurred frequently. (374)

UDCA + sulfasalazine: Using this combination as treatment, an improvement was achieved in three children with PSC. (366)

Budesonide, corticosteroids (312) or **pentoxifylline** appear to be of minimal, if any, benefit in PSC.

Boswellinic acids: The previous proposal regarding Boswellinic acids also applies to the treatment of PSC (s. p. 665, 685), particularly as this substance has already been used with some degree of success in patients with ulcerative colitis.

5.11.2 Invasive therapy

In isolated or short-length stenoses in the extrahepatic bile ducts, palliative but nevertheless effective treatment is possible by means of **balloon dilatation** and **stent insertion.** Generally, balloon dilatation is preferred. Due to the high risk of bacterial cholangitis, the stent should not be in position for longer than two weeks. Sphincterotomy may be necessary. This should precede surgical interventions. Repeated balloon dilatation and intermittent stenting may be indicated in order to bridge the period of time prior to liver transplantation (which is not negatively influenced as a result) and is generally applied in older patients. These measures should be supplemented by simultaneous administration of antibiotics and metronidazole as well as UDCA. (299, 306, 336, 343, 357, 398, 400, 408, 418, 422, 423)

5.11.3 Surgical measures

All reconstructive or resective interventions of the bile-duct system (and all abdominal operations) render subsequent orthotopic liver transplantation more difficult, or even impossible. (299, 348) • Intrahepatic **cholangiojejunostomy,** the influence of which on the survival rate could not be confirmed, should also be mentioned in this respect. (338) There is a significantly high perioperative risk with increased mortality regarding all of these surgical interventions, particularly in the late stages of PSC. For this reason, all possibilities of endoscopic therapy should be exhausted first.

Proctocolectomy may be indicated in the individual case of severe ulcerative colitis, but not in PSC. This operative intervention did not lead to an improvement in PSC in any of the patients. (319) Peristomal varicosis with a risk of haemorrhage sometimes occurs. The infection risk is significantly increased in subsequent liver transplantation.

Liver transplantation is the therapy of choice in the late stage of PSC. According to existing publications, the survival rate was 81% or 94% after one year, 71% or 92% after two years, 67–86% after five years and 70% after ten years. It is important to determine an optimal date for transplantation. End-to-end anastomosis of bile ducts is often impossible if PSC affects the extrahepatic bile ducts, which is why choledochojejunostomy must be carried out first in this special case. It has to be considered that PSC reoccurred in the transplanted liver in 5 out of 32 patients (340) and in 20–40% of cases. (311) At first, the pANCA values decrease after LTX, but they return to pre-transplantation levels after one year. The presence of colon carcinoma must be excluded prior to transplantation. After liver transplantation, colitis can exacerbate, and there may also be biliary complications. (311, 329, 340, 341, 389, 420, 425, 426, 437)

6 Autoimmune cholangitis

▶ The clinical picture of *autoimmune cholangitis (AIC)* was described by G. BRUNNER and O. KLINGE in 1987. (443) All patients were women. A genetic disposition was assumed, as all examined daughters and one granddaughter of the female patients had increased ANA and SMA titres as well (with AMA negativity). Treatment with azathioprine and prednisolone was successful.

Subsequently, this disease was also observed by others and described as *"autoimmune cholangiopathy"* (444, 457) or *"autoimmune cholangitis"*. AIC is not regarded as identical either to PBC and small-duct PSC or to AMA-negative PBC (448, 455) and idiopathic adulthood ductopenia. It may be a variant, i.e. transitional form between various autoimmune diseases, each of which manifests differently. It could also be an initial transitional stage in the early development of a classical syndrome. (445, 448) *AIC is generally considered to be an autoimmune enigma.* (451) Meanwhile, more cases of autoimmune cholangitis have been reported. (447, 452, 453, 458, 460)

The distinction between primary biliary cholangitis and primary or secondary sclerosing cholangitis by differential diagnosis may be made substantially more difficult at times owing to special courses of disease, autoimmune hepatitis or overlap syndromes.

6.1 Clinical aspects

In most aspects, immune cholangitis is similar to PBC: subjective *discomfort* corresponds to that of PBC, hepatomegaly is generally present, all the patients are female, the disease usually occurs after the age of 35 and there is a genetic disposition. Coexistent ulcerative colitis is rarely found. • *Laboratory findings* are similar to those of PBC. However, the levels of cholesterol and transaminases are increased to a lesser extent; the values of AP and γ-GT are generally higher, whereas the IgM values are lower. AMA are negative, while ANA and SMA are verifiable (17–71%). With the more sensitive AMA-immune blot test, 43% of AIC patients showed positive results. (451) Yet, ANA could also be determined in the above-mentioned daughters (and granddaughter) who had not been recognizably ill before (as is the case with AMA in numerous cases of PBC). There is an association with HLA-B8, -DR3 and -DR4. Thus the HLA risk factors are similar to those of AIH type I and PBC, but they differ from those of PSC. Differentiation between AIC and PBC by means of anticarbonic anhydrase II (449) could not be confirmed. (442) • In *histology*, and even in *immunohistochemistry*, immune cholangitis can hardly be differentiated from PBC. (450) However, it shows more substantial hepatocellular necrosis and distinct reactions of the stellate cells around the ductuli, which proliferate into the parenchyma. • Immune cholangitis differs markedly from the early forms of PSC. In particular, the fibre coats surrounding proliferated ductuli, which are typical of PSC and which develop early, and the PAS-positive colouring of the basal membrane are absent. *Biliary cirrhosis* must be anticipated as the final stage. (445, 459) (s. p. 679) • *Therapy* is with UDCA, first of all as monotherapy. With non-responders, the additional administration of azathioprine plus prednisolone is recommended. In coexistent chronic IBD, the administration of mesalazine (5' ASA) is indicated. Liver transplantation is required in the individual case. (446, 452, 454, 456)

6.2 Hypothesis of pathogenesis

The question arises as to whether *PBC* and *PSC* as well as *AIC* are "merely" **variations** (or subgroups) which can be subsumed under the generic clinical term **autoimmune cholangitis**. • The AIC has still not been defined (*1.*) as an entity in itself, (*2.*) as an overlap syndrome, or (*3.*) as an outlier syndrome.

In fact, very similar subjective discomfort or clinical findings as well as virtually identical laboratory parameters are found. Genetic disposition is generally verifiable. There is gender-related frequency: PBC and immune cholangitis are found almost exclusively in women, PSC (almost) exclusively in men. (441, 457, 461)

Immune reactions: A further difference exists in the variety of cellular and humoral immune reactions which can occur in the neuroendocrinologically influenced system. *Four serological types* are broadly distinguishable. (447)
• *Two additional serological types* may well appear as further variants of PSC. The association of PBC and PSC with numerous immunopathies should be noted. (s. tabs. 22.6, 22.7, 22.8; 33.3, 33.6, 33.7)

(1.) AMA + / ANA ∅	(3.) AMA ∅ / ANA +
(2.) AMA + / ANA +	(4.) AMA ∅ / ANA ∅
(5.) pANCA + / AMA ∅	
(6.) pANCA + / AMA +	

Morphology: While cellular and humoral immunity reactions exhibit a very broad spectrum of forms of manifestation, phenomena or epiphenomena and constellation types, this is not the case with liver morphology (which reacts in a relatively "monotonous" way). Given a *genetic* or *gender-related* disposition, the lesions, which seem to be primarily located either at the canaliculi or at the bile-duct epithelia, may be triggered by particular *causal factors*. The type, intensity and combination of the now developing cellular or humoral *immunity reactions* influence the histological changes at and around the bile ducts with their own particular characteristics – yet with a certain monotony peculiar to the biliary system. The result is "progressive cholangitis" with variations in the fine tissue structure in the respective morphological stages, but with the basic tendency of autoimmune cholangitis.

▶ **Liver biopsy:** The histological analysis of biopsy samples (which is sometimes overrated!) must be regarded critically in this context. It is often emphasized that (*1.*) PBC or PSC are focally and segmentally pronounced to different degrees, and (*2.*) different morphological stages are recognizable at the same time, in the same patient and in the same biopsy material. • In addition, (*1.*) percutaneous biopsy provides biopsy material only from the right liver lobe and only from a limited area (s. fig. 7.8), and (*2.*) follow-up biopsies can only reach this particular limited area of the liver, even if several biopsies are performed over a number of years. Not even initial diagnosis using laparoscopy and biopsy from both liver lobes can guarantee the definitive fine-tissue classification of autoimmune cholangitis. • *It should be noted that all percutaneous follow-up biopsies remain restricted to the small liver area.*

Therapy: The following therapeutic observations point to the independent status of AIC compared to PBC and PSC and are also suggestive of a close correlation with AIH: (*1.*) good response to corticosteroid therapy (443), (*2.*) tendency towards aggravation when the prednisolone dosage is too low, and (*3.*) successful administration of a prednisolone-azathioprine combination in the case of relapse after monotherapy. • Thus, depending on the respective finding, prednisolone therapy or additional administration of azathioprine is recommended right from the outset. • In cholestasis, which is generally present, *UDCA* is indicated in addition.

In view of the variety of possible immunological reactions directed towards the canaliculi or bile-duct epithelia and the difficulties involved in making a definitive histological diagnosis and classification, it would be feasible to include an overlap syndrome, outlier syndrome or conversion syndrome in the hypothesis of autoimmune cholangitis. • It is possible that AIC constitutes a conglomerate of different autoimmune liver diseases.

7 Overlap syndrome

Definition

There is currently no clear definition of the overlap syndrome (OLS). It is considered to be present if thorough assessment of biochemical, serologic, immunologic and histologic findings suggests the simultaneous occurrence of two chronic diseases in one liver. • This term was probably first used in connection with rheumatoid diseases as "mixed connective tissue disease" (MCTD) (H.-H. Peter, 1996). It was later introduced in hepatology by J. Woodward et al. in 2001. • The single findings may differ both qualitatively and quantitatively from patient to patient. Moreover, each of the two clinical pictures may predominate alternately. • One of the overlap diseases is always AIH.

AIH (type 1)	+ PBC: 7–9% (462, 465–467, 474–476, 481, 485, 489) 1st variant: AMA +/histology = AIH; therefore also termed "PBC, hepatic form" (481)
AIH (type 1)	+ PSC: 4–6% (469–473, 475, 477, 480, 482, 483, 491) Anti-ribosomal P (ARP) antibody is frequently found (ca. 80%). • Recently, further observations have been reported.
AIH (type 1)	+ AIC: 10–12%
AIH (type 2)	+ CAH-C: 10% (HCV +, ANA +, SMA +, LKM1 +)

Aetiology and pathogenesis are unknown. There is probably a genetic predisposition, whereupon OLS is caused by one or more triggers or pathogens. Subsequently, it becomes self-perpetuating. One of the two diseases of OLS is always type 1 or type 2 AIH. • *It is important for diagnosis that there is a constellation which consists of biochemical, serological, immunological and histological findings relating to both diseases.*

The prevalence of OLS in all hepatic immunopathies is 10–12%. (463, 488) • The following overlap syndromes have been confirmed:

AIH/PBC: This form usually develops in adults only, because children are not affected by PBC. Such an overlap syndrome can occur as two different variants:

Variant 1:
Histology generally like AIH
AMA M_2 +; IgM ↑↑, IgG ↑
ANA, SMA less frequent than in AIH
HLA factors as in AIH (B8, DR3, DR4)

Variant 2:
Histology generally like PBC
AMA ∅; IgM↑, IgG (↑)
IgM mostly lower than in PBC
ANA, SMA more frequent than in PBC
HLA factors as in AIH and PBC

Variant 1 can be seen as a variant of AIH or a variant of PBC. Variant 2 corresponds to AIC. There are various criteria pointing to the entity of AIC: IgM lower than in PBC, GOT is higher, HLA factors differ from those of PBC, lymphocytes in liver parenchyma express V β 5.1 Tc receptors.

AIH/PSC: This form is often found in children and has been adequately described. IgG are markedly higher. ANA, SMA and pANCA correspond to those of PSC. A typical feature is the evidence of the anti-ribosomal P antibody (80%). Rarely, there is an association with CIBD. Administration of prednisolone is contraindicated due to the danger of bacterial cholangitis.

AIH/HCV: The occurrence of HCV antibodies in LKM 1-positive AIH type 2 in up to 90% of cases may point to a viral genesis of AIH type 2. The antibody titres are, however, lower than in AIH, and the virus-associated LKM 1–3 may also have different features. Frequently, autoimmune syndromes appear at the same time. These diseases are not classified as OLS, but seen as autoimmune-associated chronic hepatitis C or a form of comorbidity.

7.1 Outlier syndrome

The following autoimmune diseases are summarized as an outlier syndrome (which has not yet been classified):

> PBC + CAH (468, 479, 484)
> PBC * PSC (464, 478)
> AIC + AMA-negative PBC
> AIC + CAH (487)
> AIH + M. Wilson
> PSC + CAH (486)
> PSC + autoimmune pancreatitis (490)

Cryptogenic chronic hepatitis is part of the outlier syndrome (about 13%); it is serologically unclassifiable. The condition of such patients is, however, similar to AIH. They often show positive evidence of SLP.

7.2 Conversion syndrome

There are reports that a defined and adequately treated autoimmune liver disease which has existed for a longer time (in general, for many years) can convert into a different type of autoimmune disorder. As a rule, this conversion only remains detectable for a few weeks or months, whereas the OLS continues to exist. Even after OLT, such a conversion from one disease to another is possible. The conversion syndrome comprises:

1. transition of PBC into AMA-negative PBC, then into ANA-positive AIH
2. transition of AIH into PSC

A progressive course of disease results in **biliary cirrhosis,** which does not, however, reveal whether the original diagnosis was PBC, PSC or AIH, or even an overlap syndrome.

▶ Regarding the therapeutic effects, it is per se unimportant whether the existing overlap is a coincidence, a subsequent sequela or a real overlap syndrome: *every PBC or PSC with the criteria of AIH requires immunosuppressive therapy.*

7.3 Therapy

In the presence of an overlap syndrome (or a conversion syndrome), the therapy concept depends on the respective predominant component, which as a rule is AIH. Consequently, prednisolone + UDCA or prednisolone + azathioprine + UDCA are applied. (463, 466)

Therapy becomes problematic when antibodies and markers of HCV infection are evident. It is imperative to complete the unambiguous identification of HCV antibodies by determination of HCV RNA. (The positivity of HCV antibodies may well be a methodologically related "false-positive" result.). If HCV RNA is detected, i.e. in florid HCV infection, interferon therapy (or a combination with ribavirin) should be considered. This antiviral therapy may be indicated despite positivity of LKM 1 following critical evaluation and close-meshed controls. There is a possibility of AIH activation under antiviral therapy. In this case, INF therapy has to be stopped as quickly as possible. It is not currently known whether this risk can be avoided by simultaneous administration of low-dose prednisolone. • The same problem arises in the (very rare) combination of AIH with coexistent florid HBV infection.

8 Cholangiodysplasia

▶ Remember that the intrahepatic bile-duct system is still immature at birth, and that the final development of the smallest ramifications takes place during the first few neonatal weeks. At this stage, the intrahepatic biliary system is therefore very susceptible to noxae, which can lead to paucity or even atresia of the bile ducts. (s. p. 16!)

8.1 Definition

Cholangiodysplasia can manifest as **atresia** of the intrahepatic or extrahepatic bile ducts ("vanishing bile-duct syndrome"), as **ductopenia** (or *paucity*) due to a marked decrease in the interlobular bile ducts (which may occur both in infancy and in early adulthood) and as **hypoplasia** or **ectasia** of the bile ducts. Destructive cholangitis (or cholangiolitis) may be an intermediate stage in the development of ductopenia. **Fibropolycystic diseases** must also be classified as cholangiodysplasia. • Generally, they do not appear as a single entity, but in various combinations; they also become manifest to a different extent.

8.2 Aetiopathogenesis

These forms of cholangiodysplasia can arise as a result of (*1.*) genetic defects of the ductal plate during embryonic development, (*2.*) congenital (prenatal or perinatal) disorders of the bile ducts, (*3.*) genetically determined metabolic diseases, and (*4.*) acquired destruction of the bile ducts in later life caused, for example, by viral, bacterial, immunological and toxic factors, or they can arise (*5.*) in an idiopathic form. • Causal factors may also combine and then act pathogenetically either at the same time or in sequence. (s. fig. 33.17)

8.3 Ductal plate malformation

Remodelling of the ductal plate can be arrested as a result of a genetic defect: in this case, a cuff-shaped cavity remains, which is coated with ductal cells. The portal vessel situated in this cavity is closed and obstructed by connective tissue. • The complete absence of bile ducts constitutes **biliary atresia.** It is rarely familial. This abnormality can commence at any time during ductal plate development, in most cases caused by extraneous noxae or infections. Thus atresia results from bile-duct destruction during intrauterine development or shortly after birth, but not from embryonic malformation of the biliary system. Biliary atresia may be located extrahepatically or intrahepatically. Generally, babies with complete atresia die during the first five years of life. (526)

A drastic reduction in numbers of interlobular bile ducts is termed **ductopenia** (= *paucity of bile ducts*). Ductopenia is considered to be present if the ratio of interlobular ducts to the number of portal tracts is < 0.5 (normal value: 0.9−1.8), i.e. in a sufficiently large biopsy specimen, no more than half of the portal fields should be without a bile duct. Ductopenia can appear as an isolated defect (= *non-syndromic*) or in combination with other extrahepatic (= *syndromic*) anomalies. Non-syndromic paucity constantly exhibits bile-duct dilatation with blunting of microvilli. Idiopathic neonatal hepatitis sometimes overlaps with non-syndromatic ductopenia. Children with ductopenia may survive into adulthood. (502, 526) (s. fig. 33.18)

8.3.1 Caroli's disease

A characteristic finding of this rare disease (J. CAROLI et al., 1958, 1964) (498) are the saccular multifocal dilatations of the large interlobular bile ducts. Cyst-like dilatations communicate with the remaining bile-duct system. There are no other morphological liver alterations. The bile ducts contain stagnated bile and sludge, so that cholangitis and intrahepatic calculi develop. This disease may spread diffusely in the liver, but mostly the left lobe or only a segment of the left lobe is affected. Fibroangiomatosis of the bile ducts with cholangiolithiasis and chronic cholangitis may develop as well as portal hypertension with oesophageal varices. • Caroli's disease has an autosomal recessive origin. An association with congenital liver fibrosis and medullary sponge kidney has been described. (494) About 75% of cases are men. • Diagnosis is confirmed by CT scanning (with the help of the characteristic *"central dot"* sign) (499) and by ERC, MRC or PTC. Hepatomegaly, abdominal pain and jaundice (e.g. during cholangitis-induced fever) may be present. (494, 496, 527, 531) Cholangiocarcinoma is found in about 7% of patients. • *Therapy:* Antibiotics are required in cholangitis. Intrahepatic stones are treated with UDCA (523), endoscopic and surgical procedures or extracorporeal shock wave lithotripsy. (512) Occasionally, liver resection (510, 517) or even liver transplantation is necessary. (496, 528) (s. pp 182, 785) (s. figs. 33.18; 36.15)

8.3.2 Congenital liver fibrosis

This is an autosomal recessive condition which can appear in a sporadic or familial form. Ductal plate malformation of interlobular bile ducts has been suggested as a pathogenetic mechanism of this disease (H. E. MACMAHON, 1929; R. G. F. PARKER, 1956). Histologically, congenital hepatic fibrosis is characterized by dense mature fibrous tissue of the considerably enlarged and restructured portal fields; subsequently, broad bands of connective tissue surround normal lobules and connect the portal fields with each other. These fibrous bands contain partly obliterated, partly dilated bile ducts, the latter often in the form of microcysts. (506) (s. fig. 33.19)

Generally, the portal vein branches are hypoplastic, and the arteries are more numerous. Both the architecture and function are normal, but the liver is enlarged, smooth and firm. Serum values of AP are sometimes increased. Sonographically, the dense fibrous bands are seen as bright areas of echogenicity. CT scanning may show cystic changes, often also in the kidneys. (534) Liver biopsy is essential for diagnosis, but laparoscopy together with biopsy gives additional important information. This disease can take a latent course or may cause presinusoidal portal hypertension with splenomegaly. There are associations with Caroli's disease (494), choledochal cysts, polycystic liver disease or microhamartoma. The slowly progressing destructive cholangitis leads to VBDS and "cholangiodysplastic pseudocirrhosis". Generally, the kidneys are involved as renal dysplasia or renal cysts. Due to their normal liver function, such patients are excellent candidates for portacaval shunts if subsequent oesophageal varix bleeding occurs. Hepatocellular and cholangiocellular carcinoma (492) as well as adenomatous hyperplasia (493) of the liver have been reported.

8.3.3 Childhood fibropolycystic disease

This polycystic degeneration is an inherited autosomal recessive disorder and its occurrence can be perinatal (at birth, renal cystic changes in 90%) neonatal (after ca. 1 month, renal cysts in 60%) and infantile (3−6 months of life, renal cysts in about 25% of cases). The incidence ranges between 1:6,000 and 1:40,000 births. Usually, there are only small liver cysts. Microscopically, enlarged portal fields due to connective tissue with ectatic bile ducts are found, which are erroneously regarded as cysts. These dilated ducts communicate with the remaining biliary system. The enlarged kidneys show cystically dilated collecting tubes. As a rule, children with a neonatal form die shortly after birth. The prognosis for the perinatal and infantile forms depends on the time of manifestation, i.e. it improves as age advances. A chronic course of disease develops into cholestasis, progressive fibrosis and portal hypertension.

8.3.4 Adult polycystic disease

This condition is an autosomal dominant disease. The liver cysts are mostly (50−60%) associated with (also dominantly inherited) polycystic kidneys. The prevalence of liver cysts increases with age (at < 20 years = less than 1%, at > 60 years = 75%). Isolated, dominantly inherited polycystic liver disease without renal involvement has been reported. Liver cysts are the result of a developmental disorder of the ductal plate at about the 23-mm stage of foetal life (i.e. fifth to eighth embryonic week). There is no biliary dysfunction. Liver cysts vary in size from a pinhead to ca. 10 cm in diameter, i.e. with a capacity of about 1 litre. They contain clear fluid secreted by the bile-duct epithelium lining the cysts or, occasionally, brown-coloured fluid due to haemolyzed and altered blood. The following complications are to

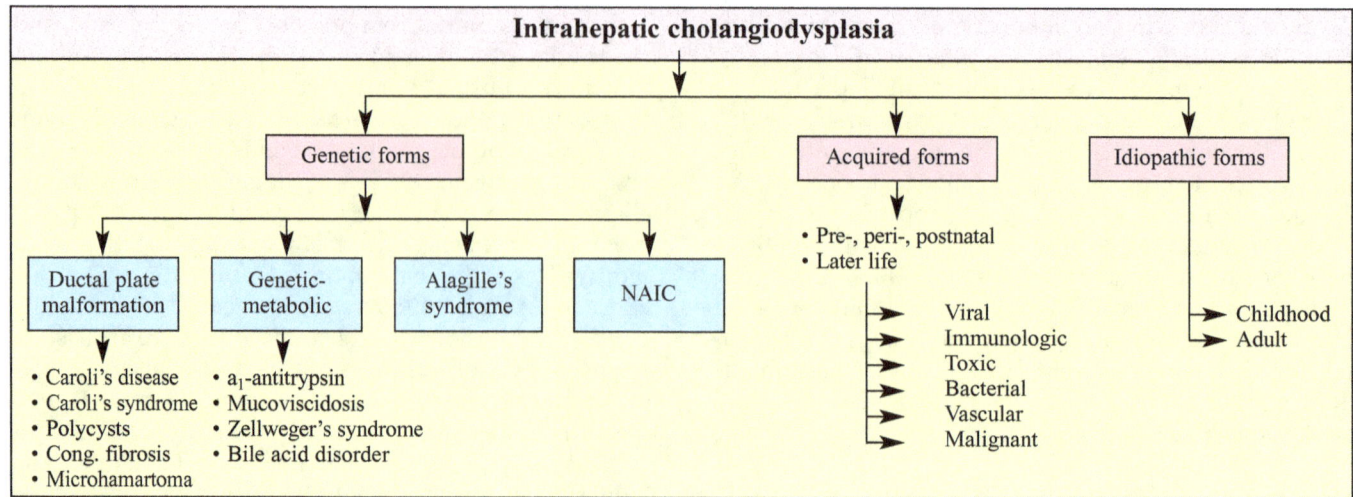

Fig. 33.18: Intrahepatic cholangiodysplasia – a proposed schematic classification. (NAIC = North American Indian cirrhosis)

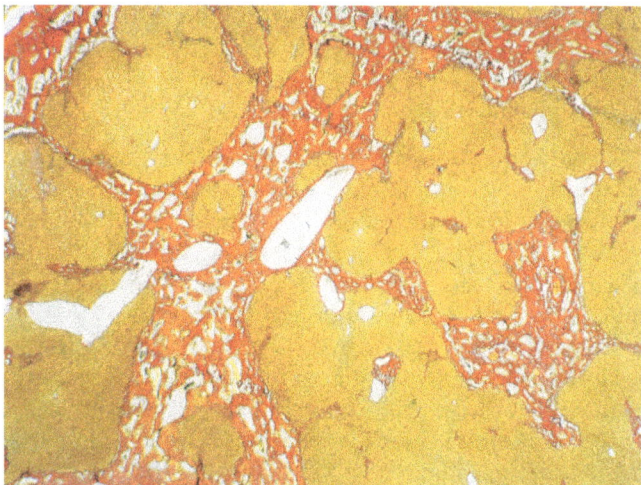

Fig. 33.19: Congenital liver fibrosis: onset of cirrhotic transformation, pathologically augmented bile-duct aggregates in portal and septal areas (Sirius red)

be feared: haemorrhage into a cyst, infection and rupture of cysts. • Liver function is normal; alkaline phosphatase and γ-GT may be elevated. Diagnosis is by sonography and CT scanning. The asymptomatic course is diagnosed by chance. Symptoms are usually caused by a considerable increase in the size of the cysts (dull abdominal pain, epigastric complaints, nausea and flatulence). Prognosis is determined by renal insufficiency due to renal cysts. • *Therapy:* Large cysts can be treated by instillation of minocycline, sclerotherapy with alcohol, operative or laparoscopic fenestration, liver resection and transplantation. (525) (s. p. 784)

8.3.5 Solitary non-parasitic liver cyst

This condition is probably a variant of polycystic liver disease. Aberrant bile ducts and blood vessels are noticeable in the fibrous cyst capsule. The cyst fluid is clear or brownish due to altered blood. Usually, the cyst develops in the inferior-anterior segment of the right lobe. The symptoms, which depend on the size of the cyst, include pressure effects on adjacent organs, cholestasis and obstructive jaundice.

8.3.6 Microhamartoma

A further disorder in ductal plate remodelling is seen in the *von Meyenburg complex* (H. von Meyenburg, 1918). These microhamartomas are the residues of malformed ductal plates (from which the peripheral branches of the intrahepatic bile ducts develop). They occur as groups of rounded biliary channels, which are lined with cuboid epithelium and embedded in fibrous tissue. The interlobular and terminal bile ducts are enlarged, often with inspissated bile. They communicate with the remaining, normal biliary system and are usually located directly in the portal tracts or nearby. The course of disease is asymptomatic; generally, the diagnosis is made by chance. Microhamartomas may be associated with polycystic disease or medullary sponge kidney. Portal hypertension is rare. (s. figs. 33.18, 33.20)

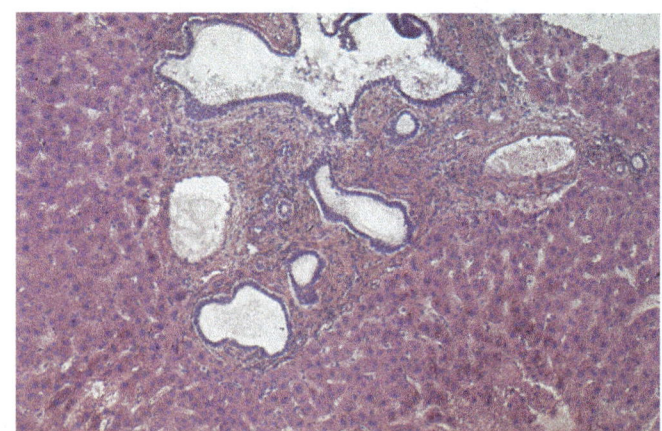

Fig. 33.20: von Meyenburg complex: biliary microhamartoma with ectatic bile ducts in an enlarged fibrous portal stroma (HE)

8.4 Alagille's syndrome

Arteriohepatic dysplasia (syndromic bile-duct hypoplasia) (G. Watson et al., 1973, D. Alagille et al., 1975, 1987) derives from dysfunction of the endoplasmic reticulum and the Golgi apparatus in the biligenetic area of the hepatocyte. This disorder is a dominant autosomal defect of the JAG-1 gen localized on chromosome 20 p 12. Components essential to the bile are retained at this site and result in secondary dysplasia or subsequent reduction in the interlobular bile flow system. The incidence is approx. 1 : 100,000 neonates. • The disease can be detected in all children during the first year of life. There is evidence of the following *symptoms*: chronic cholestasis with pronounced pruritus, xanthomas, intermittent jaundice, steatorrhoea, disturbance of mental development, deformities of the fingers, shortening of the ulna and radius, butterfly-shaped vertebrae, ataxia, chronic otitis and pigment changes in the retina. There are conspicuous facial anomalies, including deep-set eyes and a flat nose, prominent forehead and slender chin; various anomalies of the cardiovascular system (particularly hypoplasia of the peripheral pulmonary artery) and several renal anomalies also play an important role. Liver fibrosis with portal hypertension and hepatosplenomegaly can develop; in some 15% of cases, liver cirrhosis may occur. The 20-year survival rate is about 75%. Children without neonatal jaundice show a better prognosis with a longer survival rate; in these cases, liver transplantation is rarely indicated. • *Therapy* comprises UDCA, medium-chain fatty acids and fat-soluble vitamins. The possibility of liver transplantation always has to be considered. (497, 500, 508, 514, 520, 521, 524, 529) (s. fig. 33.18) (s. tab. 40.14)

8.5 North American Indian cirrhosis

North American Indian cirrhosis (NAIC) in children with a rapidly evolving form of familial cholestasis was first described by A. M. Weber et al. (1981) in aboriginal children from northwestern Quebec. Genetic investigations suggested autosomal recessive inheritance and showed that the NAIC gene is located on chromosome 16q22. There is a carrier frequency of 10% in this population. • Symptomatology consists of neonatal cholestasis with elevation of serum bile acids, alkaline phosphatase, LAP and γ-GT (ca. 70% of cases). Portal hypertension (ca. 90% of cases) develops rapidly due to early bile-duct proliferation, portal fibrosis and biliary cirrhosis. This results in variceal bleeding (ca. 50% of cases), which even occurs in children aged 10−12 months. Liver transplantation is therefore indicated. • On the basis of findings obtained from 30 patients, NAIC is regarded as a distinct entity and classified as "progressive familial cholangiopathy". (504)

8.6 Genetic-metabolic ductopenia

Some genetic defects can cause disturbed restructuring of the ductal plates in foetal development, so-called ductal plate malformations. (s. p. 16) • In contrast, in genetically determined metabolic disorders, secondary ductopenia (or *paucity of bile ducts*) may arise during the subsequent course of disease. (526)

8.6.1 α₁-antitrypsin deficiency

The deficiency may lead to a significant accumulation of non-secretable, abnormal α₁-antitrypsin. This causes cholestasis with inflammatory reactions in the region of the small bile ducts during the further course of disease. Destruction, obstruction and atrophy of the small bile ducts can therefore develop. (s. p. 607) (s. fig. 31.12)

8.6.2 Mucoviscidosis

Mucoviscidosis (or cystic fibrosis) is an autosomal recessive disease which is accompanied by the pathological production of viscous secretions in the excretory glands. Diagnosis is based on the sweat test (= pilocarpine iontophoresis; positive: chloride > 70 mmol/l, sodium > 60 mmol/l). There is a pronounced association with HLA types A2, B7, DR2 and DQw6. Serum cholic acid and the ratio of cholic acid/chenodeoxycholic acid correlate with histological liver damage and fibrosis. The further course of disease can lead to cholestasis and periportal inflammatory processes with fibrosis, which results in increasing destruction and obliteration of the bile ducts. Macrovesicular steatosis with hepatomegaly is often found. With advancing age, the frequency of hepatic damage (chronic cholestasis, fatty liver, fibrosis, cirrhosis) reaches 25−30% in adults. About 5% of patients develop biliary cirrhosis. Treatment with UDCA is recommended. Liver transplantation may be indicated. (s. p. 620)

8.6.3 Zellweger's syndrome

Peroxisomal disorders of bile acid synthesis, both in the side-chain decomposition process and at the steroid ring, can cause atrophy of the small bile ducts. This gives rise to Zellweger's syndrome with asyndromic bile-duct hypoplasia. (511) (s. pp 242, 620) (s. tabs. 13.3, 13.4)

▶ Bile-duct hypoplasia has also been observed in the **Aagenaes syndrome** of recurrent intrahepatic cholestasis (s. p. 241), in **Turkish non-syndromic paucity** of interlobular bile ducts (N. Kocak et al., 1997), etc.

8.7 Acquired ductopenia

Non-syndromic ductopenia is caused by the following events: (*1.*) degeneration and necrosis of bile-duct epithelia, (*2.*) hypoperfusion of the periductular capillary plexus, and (3.) inflammatory processes. However, there are close interactions between these three pathomorphological changes. • Degeneration and necrosis of bile-duct epithelia can be attributed to immunologic reactions or the influence of endogenous or exogenous toxins. This results in oxidative stress and hypercalcia with subsequent cell necrosis. • The hypoperfusion of the capillary plexus as a result of atrophy or arteritis also causes oxidative stress and hypercalcia. • Inflammatory processes (e.g. due to viruses, bacteria and toxins) damage the ductular cells and stimulate fibrogenesis ("vanishing bile ducts"). (495, 526, 530, 532)

Immunologic reactions: Primary biliary cholangitis, primary sclerosing cholangitis, overlap syndromes, allograft rejection, sarcoidosis, etc. are worth mentioning in this context.

Malignant diseases: Histiocytosis X and Hodgkin's disease (but not NHL) have been identified as causing ductopenia.

Vascular disorders: A decrease in the arterial blood supply, especially hypoperfusion of the periductular capillary plexus (501), can be caused by vasculitis, i.v. infusions of cytostatics (e.g. floxuridine) (18, 20, 26, 40) or alcohol into the hepatic artery, postoperative scarry strictures of the hepatic artery, allograft rejection, etc.

Foreign substances: Given an individual predisposition, chemicals or pharmacons (503) may trigger the syndrome of vanishing bile ducts. Numerous drugs can be included in this category. (s. tab. 29.3)

Virus infections: Viral cholangiopathy, sometimes with concomitant destruction of the intrahepatic bile ducts, has been reported to derive from several species of viruses, e.g. Epstein-Barr (522), HIV, cytomegaly, rotaviruses, respiratory syncitial virus (RS), hepatitis C, congenital rubella and reovirus 3. • **Bacteria** may, however, also be the cause of disease, as is the case with congenital syphilis.

8.8 Idiopathic ductopenia

Idiopathic adulthood ductopenia: The rare, non-syndromic form of ductopenia was described by J. Ludwig et al. in 1988. He subsequently diagnosed this condition in almost 60 patients. (513) Further cases have also been reported in the literature. (495, 505, 507, 515, 516, 518, 519, 532, 533) • This form of ductopenia does not reveal any congenital or acquired causes (see subchapters 7.4–7.7). All known causes of cholestasis must firstly be excluded and there should be no evidence of inflammatory bowel disease. The aetiology is (still) unclarified, i.e. *idiopathic*. • The onset of the disease is between the ages of 15 and 77, average 27 years, i.e. in adulthood. (511) Women are more often affected than men (1.8:1.0). •

The clinical symptoms vary; relatively long asymptomatic phases may precede diagnosis. Episodes of pruritus and jaundice are the first noticeable symptoms; occasionally, right upper quadrant pain develops. Signs of cholestasis are present: increase in the serum values of bile acids, alkaline phosphatase, γ-GT and LAP. There may be concomitant jaundice. The transaminases, which are suggestive of hepatocellular damage, vary from normal to a ten-fold increase.

Morphologically, diagnosis is based on a loss of interlobular or septal bile ducts in at least 50% of the portal fields. Nevertheless, 20 or more portal tracts should be evaluated, i.e. several needle biopsy samples must be obtained. The collection of biopsic material is best performed by laparoscopy, whereby specimens should be taken from both liver lobes. (s. fig. 7.8) The bile ducts can only be counted correctly if they are clearly distinguishable from the ductules (cholangioles). In most cases, the ductules have proliferated, i.e. bile-duct loss and ductular proliferation often coexist. At the same time, the biopsy samples should not display further findings, such as granulomas, PBC, PSC, histiocytosis, lymphoma, etc. • There may be a correlation between the cause of disease and the respective prognosis. Thus there have been reports of patients in adulthood presenting with a mild form of biliary idiopathic ductopenia. They showed no clinical findings and were largely asymptomatic. The values of γ-GT, AP and transaminases in these cases were normal or moderately increased. The prognosis was assessed as favourable. (515) However, the course of disease is usually progressive, culminating in biliary cirrhosis or acute liver failure. • *Treatment* with UDCA is recommended, although no favourable results have been reported. (507) Liver transplantation is the treatment of choice.

Idiopathic childhood ductopenia: The same criteria as established by J. Ludwig et al. for ductopenia in adulthood also apply to ductopenia in childhood. There is no clinical or biochemical difference between this form and the one found in infants. Chronic progressive cholestasis can occur in children as well, accompanied by pruritus, and sometimes by jaundice or xanthomas. Electron microscopic examination of livers taken from numerous premature infants (before 90 days of age) suggests that paucity in non-syndromic patients may result from primary ductal plate insult: there are undulations and breaks in the basal lamina and lymphocytic infiltration of the duct epithelium as well as canalicular dilatations with blunting of microvilli. (509) The cause of idiopathic childhood ductopenia is unknown. Apparently, one and the same event is involved, yet with different manifestation forms in childhood and in adulthood as well as with varying degrees of severity. (495)

References:

Cholangitis

1. **Abdalian, R., Heathcote, E.J.:** Sclerosing cholangitis: A focus on secondary causes. Hepatology 2006; 44: 1063–1074
2. **Arai, K., Kawai, K., Kohda, W., Tatsu, H., Matsui, O., Nakahama, T.:** Dynamic CT of acute cholangitis: early inhomogeneous enhancement of the liver. Amer. J. Roentgen. 2003; 181: 115–118
3. **Bouche, H., Housset, C., Dumont, J.-L., Carnot, F., Menu, Y., Aveline, B., Belghiti, J., Boboc, B., Erlinger, S., Berthelot, P., Pol, S.:** AIDS-related cholangitis: diagnostic features and course in 15 patients. J. Hepatol. 1993; 17: 34–39
4. **Bucuvalas, J.C., Bove, K.E., Kaufman, R.A., Gilchrist, M.J.R., Oldham, K.T., Balistreri, W.F.:** Cholangitis associated with Cryptococcus neoformans. Gastroenterology 1985; 88: 1055–1059
5. **Burgart, L.J.:** Cholangitis in viral disease. Mayo Clin. Proc. 1998; 73: 479–482
6. **Campbell, W.L., Ferris, J.V., Holbert, B.L., Thaete, F.L., Baron, R.L.:** Biliary tract carcinoma complicating sclerosing cholangitis: evaluation with CT, cholangiography, US, and MR imaging. Radiology 1998; 207: 41–50
7. **Carmona, R.H., Crass, R.A., Lim, R.C., Trunkey, D.D.:** Oriental cholangitis. Amer. J. Surg. 1984; 148: 117–124
8. **Carpenter, H.A.:** Bacterial and parasitic cholangitis. Mayo Clin. Proc. 1998; 73: 473–478
9. **Carroll, B.A., Oppenheimer, D.A.:** Sclerosing cholangitis: sonographic demonstration of bile duct wall thickening. Amer. J. Roentgenol. 1982; 139: 1016–1018
10. **Carstensen, H., Nilsson, K.O., Nettleblad, S.C., Cederlund, C.G., Hildell, J.:** Common bile duct obstruction due to an intraluminal mass of candidiasis in a previously healthy child. Pediatrics 1986; 77: 858–861
11. **Castiella, A., Iribarren, J.A., Lopez, P., Barrio, J., von Wichmann, M.A., Alzate, L.F., Arrizabalaga, J., Rodriguez, F., Arenas, J.I.:** AIDS-associated cholangiopathy in a series of ten patients. Rev. Esp. Enferm. Dig. 1998; 90: 425–430
12. **Chan, F.K.L., Ching, J.Y.L., Ling, T.K.W., Chung, S.C.S., Sung, J.J.Y.:** Aeromonas infection in acute suppurative cholangitis: review of 30 cases. J. Infect. 2000; 40: 69–73
13. **Chan, F.-L., Man, S.-W., Leong, L.L.Y., Fan, S.-T.:** Evaluation of recurrent pyogenic cholangitis with CT: analysis of 50 patients. Radiology 1989; 106: 165–169
14. **Csendes, A., Diaz, J.C., Burdiles, P., Maluenda, F., Morales, E.:** Risk factors and classification of acute suppurative cholangitis. Brit. J. Surg. 1992; 79: 655–658
15. **Danilewitz, M., Kotfila, R., Jensen, P.:** Endoscopic diagnosis and management of Fasciola hepatica causing biliary obstruction. Amer. J. Gastroenterol. 1996; 91: 2620–2621
16. **Da-Silva, F., Boudghene, F., Lecomte, I., Delage, Y., Grange, J.-D., Bigot, J.-M.:** Sonography in AIDS-related cholangitis: prevalence and cause of an echogenic nodule in the distal end of the common bile duct. Amer. J. Roentgenol. 1993; 160: 1205–1207
17. **Davis, J.J., Heyman, M.B., Ferrell, L., Kerner, R., Kerlan, R.jr., Thaler, M.M.:** Sclerosing cholangitis associated with chronic cryptosporidiosis in a child with a congenital immunodeficiency disorder. Amer. J. Gastroenterol. 1987; 82: 1196–1202
18. **Dikengil, A., Siskind, B.N., Morse, S.S., Swedlund, A., Bober-Sorcinelli, K.E., Burrell, M.I.:** Sclerosing cholangitis from intraarterial floxuridine. J. Clin. Gastroenterol. 1986; 8: 690–693
19. **Domagk, D., Fegeler, W., Conrad, B., Menzel, J., Domschke, W., Kucharzik, T.:** Biliary tract candidiasis: Diagnostic and therapeutic approaches in a case series. Amer. J. Gastroenterol. 2006; 101: 2530–2536
20. **Fukuzumi, S., Moriya, Y., Makuuchi, M., Terui, S.:** Serious chemical sclerosing cholangitis associated with hepatic arterial 5FU and MMC chemotherapy. Eur. J. Surg. Oncol. 1990; 16: 251–255
21. **Gigot, J.F., Leese, T., Dereme, T., Coutinho, J., Castaing, D., Bismuth, H.:** Acute cholangitis. Multivariate analysis of risk factors. Ann. Surg. 1989; 209: 435–438
22. **Gogel, H.K., Runyon, B.A., Volpicelli, N.A., Palmer, R.C.:** Acute suppurative obstructive cholangitis due to stones: treatment by urgent endoscopic sphincterotomy. Gastrointest. Endosc. 1987; 33: 210–213
23. **Harris, H.W., Kumwenda, Z.L., Sheen-Chen, S.-M., Shah, A., Schecter, W.P.:** Recurrent pyogenic cholangitis. Amer. J. Surg. 1998; 176: 34–37
24. **Himal, H.S., Lindsay, T.:** Ascending cholangitis: surgery versus endoscopic or percutaneous drainage. Surgery 1990; 108: 629–634
25. **Hoffmeister, B., Ockenga, J., Schachschal, G., Suttorp, N., Seybold, J.:** Rapid development of secondary sclerosing cholangitis due to vancomycin-resistant enterococci. J. Infect. 2007; 54: 65–66
26. **Hohn, D., Melnick, J., Stagg, R., Altman, D., Friedman, M., Ignoffo, R., Ferrell, L., Lewis, B.:** Biliary sclerosing in patients receiving hepatic arterial infusions of floxuridine. J. Clin. Oncol. 1985; 3: 98–102
27. **Jain, M.K., Jain, R.:** Acute bacterial cholangitis. Curr. Treat. Opt. Gastroenterol. 2006; 9: 113–121
28. **Kawada, N., Takemura, S., Minamiyama, Y., Inoue, M.:** Pathophysiology of acute obstructive cholangitis. Hepato-Bil.-Pancr.-Surg. 1996; 3: 4–8
29. **Khuroo, M.S., Dar, M.Y., Yattoo, G.N., Khan, B.A., Boda, M.I., Zargar, S.A., Javid, G., Allai, M.S.:** Serial cholangiographic appearances in recurrent pyogenic cholangitis. Gastrointest. Endosc. 1993; 39: 674–679
30. **Ko, W.F., Cello, J.P., Rogers, S.J., Lecours, A.:** Prognostic factors for the survival of patients with AIDS cholangiopathy. Amer. J. Gastroenterol. 2003; 98: 2176–2181
31. **Lai, E.C.S., Tam, P.-C., Paterson, I.A., Ng, M.M.T., Fan, S.-T., Choi, T.-K., Wong, J.:** Emergency surgery for severe acute cholangitis. The high-risk patients. Ann. Surg. 1990; 211: 55–59
32. **Lai, E.C.S., Mok, F.P.T., Tan, E.S.Y., Lo, C.-M., Fan, S.-T., You, K.-T., Wong, J.:** Endoscopic biliary drainage for severe acute cholangitis. New Engl. J. Med. 1992; 326: 1582–1586
33. **Lee, C.S., Kuo, Y.-C., Peng, S.-M., Lin, D.-Y., Sheen, I.-S., Lin, S.-M., Chuah, S.-K., Chien, R.-N.:** Sonographic detection of hepatic portal venous gas associated with suppurative cholangitis. J. Clin. Ultrasound 1993; 21: 331–334
34. **Lim, J.:** Oriental cholangiohepatitis: pathologic, clinical, and radiologic features. Amer. J. Roentgenol. 1991; 157: 1–8
35. **Lo, C.M., Lai, E.C.S.:** Causes and clinical manifestations of severe acute cholangitis. Hepato-Bil.-Pancr. Surg. 1996; 3: 9–11
36. **Lou, H.Y., Chang, C.C., Chen, S.H., Fang, C.L., Shih, Y.H., Liu, J.D., Pan, S.A.:** Acute cholangitis secondary to a common bile duct adenoma (case report). Hepato-Gastroenterol. 2003; 50: 949–951
37. **Martin de Carpi, J., Tarrado, X., Varea, V.:** Sclerosing cholangitis secondary to hepatic artery ligation after abdominal trauma (case report). Eur. J. Gastroenterol. Hepatol. 2005; 17: 987–990
38. **Mori, T., Sugiyama, M., Atomi, Y.:** Management of intrahepatic stones. Best Pract. Res. Clin. Gastroenterol. 2006; 20: 1117–1137
39. **Pessa, M.E., Hawkins, I.F., Vogel, S.B.:** The treatment of acute cholangitis. Percutaneous transhepatic biliary drainage before definitive therapy. Ann. Surg. 1987; 205: 389–392
40. **Pien, E.H., Zeman, R.K., Benjamin, S.B., Barth, K.H., Jaffe, M.H., Choyke, P.L., Clark, L.R., Paushter, D.M.:** Iatrogenic sclerosing cholangitis following hepatic arterial chemotherapy infusion. Radiology 1985; 156: 329–330
41. **Pokorny, C.S., McCaughan, G.W., Gallagher, N.D., Selby, W.S.:** Sclerosing cholangitis and biliary tract calculi–primary or secondary. Gut 1992; 33: 1376–1380
42. **Pol, S., Romana, C.A., Richard, S., Amouyal, P., Resportes-Livage, J.D., Carnot, F., Pays, J.-F., Berthelot, P.:** Microsporidia infection in patients with the human immunodeficiency virus an unexplained cholangitis. New Engl. J. Med. 1993; 328: 95–99
43. **Qureshi, W.A.:** Approach to the patient who has suspected acute bacterial cholangitis. Gastroenterol. Clin. North Amer. 2006; 35: 409–423
44. **Ramalho, L.N.Z., Ramalho, F.S., Zucoloto, S., Castro-e-Silva, O., Correa, F.M.A., Elias, J., Magalhaes, J.F.G.:** Effect of losartan, an angiotensin II antagonist, on secondary biliary cirrhosis. Hepato-Gastroenterol. 2002; 49: 1499–1502
45. **Rush, O., Sayed, H.I., Whitby, J.L., Wall, W.J.:** Cholangitis caused by Yersinia enterocolitica. Can. Med. Ass. J. 1980; 123: 1017–1018
46. **Ryan, M.E., Kirchner, J.P., Sell, T., Swanson, M.:** Cholangitis due to Blastomyces dermatitidis. Gastroenterology 1989; 96: 1346–1349
47. **Schmitt, M., Kölbel, C.B., Müller, M.K., Verbeke, C.S., Singer, M.V.:** Sclerosing cholangitis after burn injury. Z. Gastroenterol. 1997; 35: 929–934
48. **Schneiderman, D.J., Cello, J.P., Laing, F.C.:** Papillary stenosis and sclerosing cholangitis in the acquired immunodeficiency syndrome. Ann. Intern. Med. 1987; 106: 546–549
49. **Sebagh, M., Farges, O., Kalil, A., Samuel, D., Bismuth, H., Reynes, M.:** Sclerosing cholangitis following human orthotopic liver transplantation. Amer. J. Surg. Pathol. 1995; 19: 81–90
50. **Sonnenberg, van, E., Casola, G., Cubberly, D.A., Halasz, N.A., Cabrera, O.A., Wittich, G.R., Mattrey, R.F., Scheible, F.W.:** Oriental cholangiohepatitis: diagnostic imaging and interventional management. Amer. J. Roentgenol. 1986; 146: 327–331
51. **Stain, S.C., Incarbone, R., Guthrie, C.R., Ralls, P.W., Rivera-Lara, S., Parekh, D., Yellin, A.E.:** Surgical treatment of recurrent pyogenic cholangitis. Arch. Surg. 1995; 130: 527–533
52. **Sung, J.Y., Costerton, J.W., Shaffer, E.A.:** Defense system in the biliary tract against bacterial infection. Dig. Dis. Sci. 1992; 37: 689–696
53. **Takada, T., Yasuda, H., Hanyu, F.:** Pathophysiologic mechanisms in patients with cholangitis or obstructive jaundice: results of a cholangiographic study. Hepato-Bil.-Pancr. Surg. 1996; 3: 17–22
54. **Teixidor, H.S., Godwin, T.A., Ramirez, E.A.:** Cryptosporidiosis of the biliary tract in AIDS. Radiology 1991; 180: 51–56
55. **Thompson, J., Bennion, R.S., Pitt, H.A.:** An analysis of infectious failures in acute cholangitis. HPB Surgery 1994; 8: 139–145
56. **Vingan, H.:** Magnetic resonance cholangiopancreatography versus ERCP: the "superbowl" of pancreaticobiliary imaging. Amer. J. Gastroenterol. 1997; 92: 1396–1398
57. **Watson, C.J., Hoffbauer, F.W.:** The problem of prolonged hepatitis with particular reference to the cholangiolitic type and to the development of cholangiolitic cirrhosis of the liver. Ann. Intern. Med. 1946; 25: 195–227
58. **Wong, J., Choi, T.:** Recurrent pyogenic cholangitis. Dig. Surg. 1986; 3: 265–275
59. **Yoon, H.-K., Sung, K.-B., Song, H.-Y., Kang, S.-G., Kim, M.-H., Lee, S.-G., Lee, S.-K., Auh, Y.-H.:** Benign biliary strictures associated with recurrent pyogenic cholangitis: treatment with expandable metallic stents. Amer. J. Roentgenol. 1997; 169: 1523–1527

Primary biliary cholangitis

60. Abdulkarim, A.S., Petrovic, L.M., Kim, W.R., Angulo, P., Lloyd, R.V., Lindor, K.D.: Primary biliary cirrhosis: an infectious disease caused by Chlamydia pneumoniae? J. Hepatol. 2004; 40: 380–384
61. Addison, T., Gull, W.: On a certain affection of the skin, vitiligoidea plana and vitiligoidea tuberosa, with remarks. Guy's Hosp. Rep. 1851; 7: 265–276
62. Agarwal, K., Jones, D.E.J., Bassendine, M.F.: Genetic susceptibility primary biliary cirrhosis. Eur. J. Gastroenterol. Hepatol. 1999; 11: 603–606
63. Ahrens, E.H.jr., Payne, M.A., Kunkel, H.G., Eisenmenger, W.J., Blondheim, S.H.: Primary biliary cirrhosis. Medicine (Baltimore) 1950; 29: 299–364
64. Aishima, S., Kuroda, Y., Nishihara, Y., Taguchi, K., Yoshizumi, T., Taketomi, A., Maehara, Y., Tsuneyoshi, M.: Characteristic differences according to the cirrhotic pattern of advanced primary biliary cirrhosis: macronodular cirrhosis indicates slow progression. Hepatol. Res. 2006; 36: 188–194
65. Aly, A., Carlson, K., Johansson, C., Kirstein, P., Rössner, S., Wallentin,L.: Lipoprotein abnormalities in patients with early primary biliary cirrhosis. Eur. J. Clin. Invest. 1984; 14: 155–162
66. Anantharaju, A., Baluch, M., van Thiel, D.H.: Transverse myelitis occurring in association with primary biliary cirrhosis and Sjogren's syndrome (case report). Dig. Dis. Sci. 2003; 48: 830–833
67. Angulo, P., Batts, K.P., Therneau, T.M., Jorgensen, R.A., Dickson, E.R., Lindor, K.D.: Long-term ursodeoxycholic acid delays histological progression in primary biliary cirrhosis. Hepatology 1999; 29: 644–647
68. Angulo, P., Jorgensen, R.A., Keach, J.C., Dickson, E.R., Smith, C., Lindor, K.D.: Oral budesonide in the treatment of patients with primary biliary cirrhosis with a suboptimal response to ursodeoxycholic acid. Hepatology 2000; 31: 318–323
69. Arora, S., Kaplan, M.: Portal hypertension in early-stage primary biliary cirrhosis: a possible explanation. Amer. J. Gastroenterol. 1987; 82: 90–91
70. Babatin, M.A., Sanai, F.M., Swain, M.G.: Methotrexate therapy for the symptomatic treatment of primary biliary cirrhosis patients, who are biochemical incomplete responders to ursodeoxycholic acid therapy. Amer. Pharm. Ther. 2006; 24: 813–820
71. Bach, N., Schaffner, F.: Familial primary biliary cirrhosis. J. Hepatol. 1994; 20: 698–701
72. Bach, N., Bodian, C., Bodenheimer, H., Croen, E., Berk, P.D., Thung, S.N., Lindor, K.D., Themeau, T., Schaffner, F.: Methotrexate therapy for primary biliary cirrhosis. Amer. J. Gastroenterol. 2003; 98: 187–193
73. Balasubramaniam, K., Grambsch, P.M., Wiesner, R.H., Lindor, K.D., Dickson, E.R.: Diminished survival in asymptomatic primary biliary cirrhosis. A prospective study. Gastroenterology 1990; 98: 1567–1571
74. Bardella, M.T., Quatrieu, M., Zuin, M., Podda, M., Cesarini, L., Velio, P., Bianchi, P., Conte, D.: Screening patients with celiac disease for primary biliary cirrhosis and vice versa. Amer. J. Gastroenterol. 1997; 92: 1524–1526
75. Bassendine, M.F., Fussey, S.P.M., Mutimer, D.J., James, O.F.W., Yeaman, S.J.: Identification and characterization of four M2 mitochondrial autoantigens in primary biliary cirrhosis. Semin. Liver Dis. 1989; 9: 124–131
76. Bateson, M.C., Gedling, P.: Ursodeoxycholic acid therapy for primary biliary cirrhosis. A 10-year British single-centre population-based audit of efficacy and survival. Postgrad. Med. J. 1998; 74: 482–485
77. Batta, A.K., Salen, G., Mirchandani, R., Tint, G.S., Shefer, S., Batta, M., Abroon, J., O'Brien, C.B., Senior, J.R.: Effect of long-term treatment with ursodiol on clinical and biochemical features and biliary bile acid metabolism in patients with primary biliary cirrhosis. Amer. J. Gastroenterol. 1993; 88: 691–700
78. Battezzati, P.M., Podda, M., Bianchi, F.B., Naccarato, R., Orlandi, F., Surrenti, C., Pagliaro, L., Manenti, F.: Ursodeoxycholic acid for symptomatic primary biliary cirrhosis. Preliminary analysis of a doubleblind multicentre trial. J. Hepatol. 1993; 17: 332–338
79. Baur, G., Schwalbach, G., Tittor, W.: Neue Aspekte zur Pathogenese der primären biliären Zirrhose. Dtsch. Med. Wschr. 1982; 107: 378–382
80. Berg, P.A., Klein, R.: Antimitochondrial antibodies in primary biliary cirrhosis and other disorders: definition and clinical relevance. Dig. Dis. 1992; 10: 85–101 • Mitochondrial antigen/antibody systems in primary biliary cirrhosis: revisited. Liver 1995; 15: 281–292
81. Berkum, van, F.N.R., Beukers, R., Birkenhäger, J.C., Kooij, P.P.M., Schalm, S.W., Pols, H.A.P.: Bone mass in women with primary biliary cirrhosis: the relation with histological stage and use of glucocorticoids. Gastroenterology 1990; 99: 1134–1139
82. Beswick, D.R., Klatskin, G., Boyer, J.L.: Asymptomatic primary biliary cirrhosis. A progress report on long-term follow-up and natural history. Gastroenterology 1985; 89: 267–271
83. Bodenheimer, H.C., Schaffner, F., Sternlieb, I., Klion, F.M., Vernace, S., Pezzullo, J.: A prospective clinical trial of D-penicillamine in the treatment of primary biliary cirrhosis. Hepatology 1985; 5: 1139–1142
84. Bodenheimer, H.C., Schaffner, F., Pezzullo, J.: Evaluation of colchicine therapy in primary biliary cirrhosis. Gastroenterology 1988; 95: 124–129
85. Boki, K.A., Dourakis, S.P.: Polymyositis associated with primary biliary cirrhosis. Clin. Rheumatol. 1995; 14: 375–378
86. Bown, R., Clark, M.L., Doniach, D.: Primary biliary cirrhosis in brothers. Postgrad. Med. J. 1975; 51: 110–115
87. Boyer, T.D., Kokenes, D.D., Hertzler, G., Kutner, M.H., Henderson, J.M.: Effect of distal splenorenal shunt on survival of patients with primary biliary cirrhosis. Hepatology 1994; 20: 1482–1486
88. Brind, A.M., Bray, G.P., Portmann, B.C., Williams, R.: Prevalence and pattern of familial disease in primary biliary cirrhosis. Gut 1995; 36: 615–617
89. Buscher, H.-P., Zietzschmann, Y., Gerok, W.: Positive response to methotrexate and ursodeoxycholic acid in patients with primary biliary cirrhosis responding insufficiently to ursodeoxycholic acid alone. J. Hepatol. 1993; 18: 9–14
90. Chamuleau, R.A.F.M., van Berge Henegouwen, F.B., Bronkhorst, F.B., Brandt, K.H.: Primary biliary cirrhosis in sisters. Neth. J. Med. 1975; 18: 170–175
91. Chatte, G., Streichenberger, N., Boillot, O., Gille, D., Loire, R., Cordie, J.F.: Lymphocytic bronchitis/bronchiolitis in a patient with primary biliary cirrhosis. Eur. Respir. J. 1995; 8: 176–179
92. Chiaramonte, M., Floreani, A., Pasini, C.V., Ruffatti, A., Okolicsany, L., Naccarato, R.: Primary biliary cirrhosis in sisters: a case report. Ital. J. Gastroenterol. 1982; 14: 169–171
93. Chohan, M.R.: Primary biliary cirrhosis in twin sisters. Gut 1973; 14: 213–214
94. Christensen, E., Crowe, J., Doniach, D., Popper, H., Ranek, L., Rodes, J., Tygstrup, N., Williams, R.: Clinical pattern and course of disease in primary biliary cirrhosis based on an analysis of 236 patients. Gastroenterology 1980; 78: 236–246
95. Christensen, E., Neuberger, J., Crowe, J., Altman, D.G., Popper, H., Portmann, B., Doniach, D., Ranek, L., Tygstrup, N., Williams, R.: Beneficial effect of azathioprine and prediction of prognosis in primary biliary cirrhosis. Final results of an international trial. Gastroenterology 1985; 89: 1084–1091
96. Combes, B., Carithers, R.L., Maddrey, W.C., Lin, D., McDonald, M.F., Wheeler, D.E., Eigenbrodt, E.H., Munoz, S.J., Rubin, R., Garcia-Tsao, G., Bonner, F.G., West, A.B., Boyer, J.L., Luketic, V.A., Shiffman, M.L., Mills, S., Peters, M.G., White, H.M., Zetterman, R.K., Rossi, S.S., Hofmann, A.F., Markin, R.S.: A randomized double-blind, placebo-controlled trial of ursodeoxycholic acid in primary biliary cirrhosis. Hepatology 1995; 22: 759–766
97. Christensen, E., Gunson, B., Neuberger, J.: Optimal timing of liver transplantation for patients with primary biliary cirrhosis: use of prognostic modelling. J. Hepatol. 1999; 30: 285–292
98. Crowe, J.P., Christensen, E., Butler, J., Wheeler, P., Doniach, D., Keenan, J., Williams, R.: Primary biliary cirrhosis: the prevalence of hypothyroidism and its relationship to thyroid autoantibodies and sicca syndrome. Gastroenterology 1980, 78: 1437–1441
99. Dahlan, Y., Smith, L., Simmonds, D., Jewell, L.D., Wanless, I., Heathcote, E.J., Bain, V.G.: Pediatric-onset primary biliary cirrhosis (case report). Gastroenterology 2003; 125: 1476–1479
100. Dauphinee, J.A., Sinclair, J.C.: Primary biliary cirrhosis. Can. Med. Assoc. J. 1949; 61: 1–6
101. Degott, C., Zafrani, E.S., Callard, P., Balhau, R.E., Poupon, R.E., Poupon, R.: Histopathological study of primary biliary cirrhosis and the effect of ursodeoxycholic acid treatment on histology progression. Hepatology 1999; 29: 1007–1012
102. Di Leo, V., Venturi, C., Baragiotta, A., Martines, D., Floreani, A.: Gastroduodenal and intestinal permeability in primary biliary cirrhosis. Eur. J. Gastroenterol. Hepatol. 2003; 15: 967–973
103. Dickey, N., McMillan, St.A., Callender, M.E.: High prevalence of celiac sprue among patients with primary biliary cirrhosis. J. Clin. Gastroenterol. 1997; 25: 328–329
104. Dickson, E.R., Fleming, T.R., Wiesner, R.H., Baldus, W.P., Fleming, C.R., Ludwig, J., McCall, J.T.: Trial of penicillamine in advanced primary biliary cirrhosis. New Engl. J. Med. 1985; 312: 1011–1015
105. Dietrich, C.F., Leuschner, M.S., Zeuzem, S., Herrmann, G., Sarrazin, C., Caspary, W.F., Leuschner, U.F.H.: Peri-hepatic lymphadenopathy in primary biliary cirrhosis reflects progression of the disease. Eur. J. Gastroenterol. Hepatol. 1999; 11: 747–753
106. Dörner, T., Held, C., Trebeljahr, G., Lukowsky, A., Yamamoto, K., Hiepe, F.: Serologic characteristics in primary biliary cirrhosis associated with sicca syndrome. Scand. J. Gastroenterol. 1994; 29: 655–660
107. Eastell, R., Dickson, E.R., Hodgson, S.F., Wiesner, R.H., Porayko, M.K., Wahner, H.W., Cedel, S.L., Riggs, B.L., Krom, R.A.F.: Rates of vertebral bone loss before and after liver transplantation in women with primary biliary cirrhosis. Hepatology 1991; 14: 296–300
108. Elta, G.H., Seperky, R.A., Goldberg, M.J., Connors, C.M., Miller, K.B., Kaplan, M.M.: Increased incidence of hypothyroidism in primary biliary cirrhosis. Dig. Dis. Sci. 1983; 28: 971–975
109. Epstein, O., Jain, S., Lee, R.G., Cook, D.G., Boss, A.M., Jain, S., Scheuer, P.J., Sherlock, S.: D-penicillamine treatment improves survival in primary biliary cirrhosis. Lancet 1981/I: 1275–1277
110. Eustace, S., Buff, B., Kane, R., Jenkins, R., Longmaid, H.E.: The prevalence and clinical significance of lymphadenopathy in primary biliary cirrhosis. Clin. Radiol. 1995; 50: 396–399
111. Fickert, P., Trauner, M., Fuchsbichler, A., Stumptner, C., Zatloukal, K., Denk, H.: Mallory body formation in primary biliary cirrhosis is associated with increased amounts and abnormal phosphorylation and ubiquitination of cytokeratins. J. Hepatol. 2003; 38: 387–394
112. Fischer, J.A., Schmid, M.: Treatment of primary biliary cirrhosis with azathioprine. Lancet 1967/I: 421–424
113. Flannery, G.R., Burroughs, A.K., Butler, P., Chelliah, J., Hamilton-Miller, J., Brumfitt, W., Baum-Het, H.: Antimitochondrial antibodies in primary biliary cirrhosis recognize both specific peptides and shared

114. **Floreani, A., Chiaramonte, M., Giannini, S., Malvasi, L., Lodetti, M.G., Castrignano, R., Giacomini, A., D'Angelo, A., Naccarato, R.:** Longitudinal study on osteodystrophy in primary biliary cirrhosis (PBC) and a pilot study on calcitonin treatment. J. Hepatol. 1991; 12: 217–223
115. **Floreani, A., Zappala, F., Mazzetto, M., Naccarato, R., Plebani, M., Chiaramonte, M.:** Different response to ursodeoxycholic acid (UDCA) in primary biliary cirrhosis according to severity of disease. Dig. Dis. Sci. 1994; 39: 9–14
116. **Floreani, A., Baragiotta, A., Baldo, V., Menegon, T., Farinati, F., Naccarato, R.:** Hepatic and extrahepatic malignancies in primary biliary cirrhosis. Hepatology 1999; 29: 1425–1428
117. **Forton, D.M., Patel, N., Prince, M., Oatridge, A., Hamilton, G., Goldblatt, J., Allsop, J.M., Hajnal, J.V., Thomas, H.C., Bassendine, M., Jones, D.E.J., Taylor-Robinson, S.D.:** Fatigue and primary biliary cirrhosis: association of globus pallidus magnetization transfer ratio measurements with fatigue severity and blood manganese levels. Gut 2004; 53: 587–592
118. **Freeman, H.J., Bailey, R.J.:** Primary biliary cirrhosis in HLA-identical twin sisters. Can. J. Gastroenterol. 1994; 8: 88–91
119. **Friedrich, K., Henning, H.:** Stellenwert der Laparoskopie in der Diagnostik der chronischen nichteitrigen destruierenden Cholangitis. Z. Gastroenterol. 1986; 24: 364–374
120. **Gabrielsen, T.O., Hoel, P.S.:** Primary biliary cirrhosis associated with coeliac disease and dermatitis herpetiformis. Dermatologica 1985; 170: 31–34
121. **Gershwin, M.E., Mackay, I.R.:** Primary biliary cirrhosis: paradigm or paradox for autoimmunity. Gastroenterology 1991; 100: 822–833
122. **Ghent, C.N., Carruthers, S.G.:** Treatment of pruritus in primary biliary cirrhosis with rifampicin. Results of a double-blind crossover, randomized trial. Gastroenterology 1988; 94: 488–493
123. **Goldblatt, J., Taylor, P.J.S., Lipman, T., Prince, M.I., Baragiotta, A., Bassendine, M.F., James, O.F.W., Jones, D.E.J.:** The true impact of fatigue in primary biliary cirrhosis: a population study. Gastroenterology 2002; 122: 1235–1241
124. **Goldenstein, C., Rabson, A.R., Kaplan, M.M., Canoso, J.J.:** Arthralgias as a presenting manifestation of primary biliary cirrhosis. J. Rheumatol. 1989; 16: 681–684
125. **Gores, G.J., Wiesner, R.H., Dickson, E.R., Zinsmeister, A.R., Jorgensen, R.A., Langworthy, A.:** Prospective evaluation of esophageal varices in primary biliary cirrhosis: development, natural history and influence on survival. Gastroenterology 1989; 96: 1552–1559
126. **Goudie, B.M., Burt, A.D., Macfarlane, G.J., Boyle, P., Gillis, C.R., MacSween, R.N.M., Watkinson, G.:** Risk factors and prognosis in primary biliary cirrhosis. Amer. J. Gastroenterol. 1989; 84: 713–716
127. **Graham-Brown, R.A.C., Sarkany, I., Sherlock, S.:** Lichen planus and primary biliary cirrhosis. Brit. J. Dermatol. 1982; 106: 699–703
128. **Gregory, W.L., Bassendine, M.F.:** Genetic factors in primary biliary cirrhosis. J. Hepatol. 1994; 20: 689–692
129. **Guanabens, N., Pares, A., Del Rio, L., Roca, M., Gomez, R., Munoz, J., Rodes, J.:** Sodium fluoride prevents bone loss in primary biliary cirrhosis. J. Hepatol. 1992; 15: 345–349
130. **Guanabens, N., Pares, A., Ros, I., Alvarez, L., Pons, F., Caballeria, L., Monegal, A., Martinez-de-Osaba, M.J., Roca, M., Peris, P., Rodes, J.:** Alendronate is more effective than etidronate for increasing bone mass in osteopenic patients with primary cirrhosis. Amer. J. Gastroenterol. 2003; 98: 2268–2274
131. **Guy, J.E., Qian, P., Lowell, J.A., Peters, M.G.:** Recurrent primary biliary cirrhosis: Peritransplant factors and ursodeoxycholic acid treatment post-liver transplant. Liver Transplant. 2005; 11: 1252–1257
132. **Haagsma, E.B., Manns, M., Klein, R., Grond, J., Huizinga, J.R., Sloof, M., Meyer zum Büschenfelde, K.-H., Berg, P.A., Gips, C.H.:** Subtypes of antimitochondrial antibodies in primary biliary cirrhosis before and after orthotopic liver transplantation. Hepatology 1987; 7: 129–133
133. **Haagsma, E.B.:** Clinical relevance of recurrence of primary biliary cirrhosis after liver transplantation. Eur. J. Gastroenterol. Hepatol. 1999; 11: 639–642
134. **Hayase, Y., Iwasaki, S., Akisawa, N., Saibara, T., Kadokawa, Y., Omagari, K., Maeda, T., Onishi, S.:** Similar anti-mitochondrial antibody reactivity profiles in familial primary biliary cirrhosis. Hepatol. Res. 2005; 33: 33–38
135. **Hall, St., Axelsen, P.H., Larson, D.E., Bunch, T.W.:** Systemic lupus erythematosus developing in patients with primary biliary cirrhosis. Ann. Intern. Med. 1984; 100: 388–389
136. **Halmos, B., Szalay, F., Cserniczky, T., Nemesanszky, E., Lakatos, P., Barlage, S., Schmitz, G., Romics, L., Csaszar, A.:** Association of primary biliary cirrhosis with vitamin D receptor Bsml genotype polymorphism in a Hungarian population. Dig. Dis. Sci. 2000; 45: 1091–1095
137. **Hanot, V.:** Etude sur une forme de cirrhose hypertrophique du foie (cirrhose hypertrophique avec ictère chronique). J. B. Ballière, Paris, 1876
138. **Hays, S.B., Camisa, C.:** Rendu-Osler-Weber-like telangiectasia associated with primary biliary cirrhosis. Cutis 1985; 35: 152–153
139. **Heathcote, E.J., Cauch-Dudek, K., Walker, V., Bailey, R.J., Blendis, L.M., Ghent, C.N., Michieletti, P., Minuk, G.Y., Pappas, S.C., Scully, L.J., Steinbrecher, U.P., Sutherland, L.R., Williams, C.N., Witt-Sullivan, H., Worobetz, L., Milner, R.A., Wanless, I.R.:** The Canadian multicenter double-blind randomized controlled trial of ursodeoxycholic acid in primary biliary cirrhosis. Hepatology 1994; 19: 1149–1156
140. **Heseltine, L., Turner, I.B., Fussey, S.P.M., Kelly, P.J., James, O.F.W., Yeaman, S.J., Bassendine, M.F.:** Primary biliary cirrhosis. Quantitation of autoantibodies to purified mitochondrial enzymes and correlation with disease progression. Gastroenterology 1990; 99: 1786–1792
141. **Holtmeier, J., Leuschner, M., Schneider, A., Leuschner, U., Caspary, W.F., Braden, B.:** (13) C-methacetin and (13) C-galactose breath test can assess restricted liver function even in early stages of primary biliary cirrhosis. Scand. J. Gastroenterol. 2006; 41: 1336–1341
142. **Hoofnagle, J.H., Davis, G.L., Schafer, D.F., Peters, M., Avigan, M.I., Pappas, S.C., Hanson, R.G., Minuk, G.Y., Dusheiko, G.M., Campbell, G., MacSween, R.N.M, Jones, A.:** Randomized trial of chlorambucil for primary biliary cirrhosis. Gastroenterology 1986; 91: 1327–1334
143. **Hopf, U., Möller, B., Stemerowicz, R., Lobeck, H., Rodloff, A., Freudenberg, M., Galanos, C., Huhn, D.:** Relation between Escherichia coli R (rough) forms in gut, lipid A in liver, and primary biliary cirrhosis. Lancet 1989/II: 1419–1422
144. **Huet, P.M., Deslauriers, J., Tran, A., Faucher, C., Charbonneau, J.:** Impact of fatigue on the quality of life of patients with primary biliary cirrhosis. Amer. J. Gastroenterol. 2000; 95: 760–769
145. **Hwang, S.-J., Chan, C.-Y., Lee, S.-D., Wu, J.-C., Tsay, S.-H., Lo, K.-J.:** Ursodeoxycholic acid in the treatment of primary biliary cirrhosis: A short-term, randomized, double blind controlled, cross-over study with long-term follow up. J. Gastroenterol. Hepatol. 1993; 8: 217–223
146. **Invernizzi, P., Selmi, C., Ranftler, C., Podda, M., Wesierska-Gadek, J.:** Antinuclear antibodies in primary biliary cirrhosis. Semin. Liver Dis. 2005; 25: 298–310
147. **Islam, S., Riordan, J.W., McDonald, J.A.:** Case report: A rare association of primary biliary cirrhosis and systemic lupus erythematosus and review of the literature. J. Gastroenterol. Hepatol. 1999; 14: 431–435
148. **Itakura, J., Izumi, N., Nishimura, Y., Inoue, K., Ueda, K., Nakanishi, H., Tsuchiya, K., Hamano, K., Asahina, Y., Kurosaki, M., Uchihara, M., Miyake, S.:** Prospective randomized crossover trial of combination therapy with bezafibrate and UDCA for primary biliary cirrhosis. Hepatol. Res. 2004; 29: 216–222
149. **James, S.P., Jones, E.A., Schafer, D.F., Hoofnagle, J.H., Varma, R.R., Strober, W.:** Selective immunoglobulin A deficiency associated with primary biliary cirrhosis in a family with liver disease. Gastroenterology 1986; 90: 283–288
150. **Jardine, D.L., Chambers, S.T., Hart, D.J., Chapman, B.A.:** Primary biliary cirrhosis presenting with granulomatous skin lesions. Gut 1994; 35: 564–566
151. **Jones, D.E., Metcalf, J.V., Collier, J.D., Bassendine, M.F., James, O.F.W.:** Hepatocellular carcinoma in primary biliary cirrhosis and its impact on outcomes. Hepatology 1997; 26: 1138–1142
152. **Jones, D.E.J., Watt, F.E., Metcalf, J.V., Bassendine, M.F., James, O.F.W.:** Familial primary biliary cirrhosis reassessed: a geographically based population study. J. Hepatol. 1999; 30: 402–407
153. **Jones, D.E.:** Autoantigens in primary biliary cirrhosis. J. Clin. Pathol. 2000; 53: 813–821
154. **Jones, D.E.J.:** Pathogenesis of primary biliary cirrhosis. J. Hepatol. 2003; 39: 639–648
155. **Jones, E.A.:** Rationale for trials of long-term mycophenolate mofetil therapy for primary biliary cirrhosis. Hepatology 2002; 35: 258–262
156. **Joshi, S., Cauch-Dudek, K., Heathcote, E.J., Lindor, K., Jorgensen, R., Klein, R.:** Antimitochondrial antibody profiles: are they valid prognostic indicators in primary biliary cirrhosis? Amer. J. Gastroenterol. 2002; 97: 999–1002
157. **Kakizaki, S., Ishikawa, T., Koyama, Y., Yamada, H., Kobayashi, R., Sohara, N., Otsuka, T., Takagi, H., Mori, M.:** Primary biliary cirrhosis complicated with sigmoid colonic varices: the usefulness of computed tomographic angiography. Abdom. Imag. 2003; 28: 831–834
158. **Kamisako, T., Adachi, Y.:** Marked improvement in cholestasis and hypercholesterolemia with simvastatin in a patient with primary biliary cirrhosis. Amer. J. Gastroenterol. 1995; 90: 1187–1188
159. **Kanda, T., Yokosuka, O., Imazeki, F., Saisho, H.:** Bezafibrate treatment: a new medical approach for PBC patients? J. Gastroenterol. 2003; 38: 573–578
160. **Kaplan, M.M., Alling, D.W., Zimmerman, H.J., Wolfe, H.J., Sepersky, R.A., Hirsch, G.S., Elta, G.H., Glick, K.A., Eagen, K.A.:** A prospective trial of colchicine for primary biliary cirrhosis. New Engl. J. Med. 1986; 315: 1448–1454
161. **Kaplan, M.M., Schmid, C., Provenzale, D., Sharma, A., Dickstein, G., McKusick, A.:** A prospective trial of colchicine and methotrexate in the treatment of primary biliary cirrhosis. Gastroenterology 1999; 117: 1173–1180
162. **Kaplan, M.M., Cheng, S., Price, L.L., Bonis, P.A.L.:** A randomized controlled trial of colchicine plus ursodiol versus methotrexate plus ursodiol in primary biliary cirrhosis: ten-year results. Hepatology 2004; 39: 915–923
163. **Keiding, S., Ericzon, B.-G., Eriksson, S., Flatmark, A., Höckerstedt, K., Isoniemi, H., Karlberg, I., Keiding, N., Olsson, R., Samela, K., Schrumpf, E., Söderman, C.:** Survival after liver transplantation of patients with primary biliary cirrhosis in the Nordic countries. Comparison with expected survival in another series of transplantations and in an international trial of medical treatment. Scand. J. Gastroenterol. 1990; 25: 11–18
164. **Khettry, U., Anand, N., Faul, P.N., Lewis, W.D., Pomfret, E.A., Pomposelli, J., Jenkins, R.L., Gordon, F.D.:** Liver transplantation for primary biliary cirrhosis: a long-term pathologic study. Liver Transplant. 2003; 9: 87–96

165. Kim, W.R., Wiesner, R.H., Therneau, T.M., Poterucha, J.J., Porayko, M.K., Evans, R.W., Klintmalm, G.B., Crippin, J.S., Krom, R.A., Dickson, E.R.: Optimal timing of liver transplantation for primary biliary cirrhosis. Hepatology 1998; 28: 33–38
166. Klein, R., Huizenga, J.R., Gips, C.H., Berg, P.A.: Antimitochondrial antibody profiles in patients with primary biliary cirrhosis before orthotopic liver transplantation and titres of antimitochondrial antibody-subtypes after transplantation. J. Hepatol. 1994; 20: 181–189
167. Klein, R., Zilly, W., Glässner-Bittner, B., Breuer, N., Garbe, W., Fintelmann, V., Kalk, J.F., Müting, D., Fischer, R., Tittor, W., Pausch, J., Maier, K.P., Berg, P.A.: Antimitochondrial antibody profiles in primary biliary cirrhosis distinguish at early stages between a benign and a progressive course: a prospective study on 200 patients followed for 10 years. Liver 1997; 17: 119–128
168. Koulentaki, M., Koutroubakis, I.E., Petinaki, E., Tzardi, M., Oekonomaki, H., Mouzas, I., Kouroumalis, E.A.: Ulcerative colitis associated with primary biliary cirrhosis. Dig. Dis. Sci. 1999; 44: 1953–1956
169. Kowdly, K.V., Emond, M.J., Sadowski, J.A., Kaplan, M.M.: Plasma vitamin K level is decreased in primary biliary cirrhosis. Amer. J. Gastroenterol. 1997; 92: 2059–2061
170. Krasner, N., Johnson, P.J., Portman, B., Watkinson, G., MacSween, R.N.M., Williams, R.: Hepatocellular carcinoma in primary biliary cirrhosis: report of four cases. Gut 1979; 20: 255–258
171. Kuntz, E.: Klinik und Therapie der primär biliären destruierenden, nichteitrigen Cholangitis – neues Pathogenese- und Therapiekonzept. In: Die immunsuppressive Therapie der chronisch-aktiven Hepatitis. (Hrsg. W. Dölle; Springer) 1984: 101–118
172. Kuntz, E.: Mycotoxins – a primary immunological challenge involving molecular mimicry in primary biliary cholangitis (PBC)? Hepatol. Rap. Lit. Rev. (Falk-Foundation) 1998; 28 (3): IX–X
173. Kurihara, T., Furukawa, M., Tsuchiya, M., Akimoto, M., Ishiguro, H., Hashimoto, H., Niimi, A., Maeda, A., Shigemoto, M., Yamasha, K.: Effect of bezafibrate in the treatment of primary biliary cirrhosis. Curr. Therap. Res. 2000; 61: 74–82
174. Kurktschiev, D., Subat, S., Adler, D., Schenke, K.-U.: Immunomodulating effect of ursodeoxycholic acid therapy in patients with primary biliary cirrhosis. J. Hepatol. 1993; 18: 373–377
175. Lanzini, A., de Tavonatti, M.G., Panarotto, B., Scalia, S., Mora, A., Benini, F., Baisini, O., Lanzarotto, F.: Intestinal absorption of the bile acid analogue ^{75}Se-homocholic acid-taurine is increased in primary biliary cirrhosis, and reverts to normal during ursodeoxycholic acid administration. Gut 2003; 52: 1371–1375
176. Lee, Y.M., Kaplan, M.M.: Efficacy of colchicine in patients with primary biliary cirrhosis poorly responsive to ursodiol and methotrexate. Amer. J. Gastroenterol. 2003; 98: 205–208
177. Leung, P.S., Coppel, R.L., Gershwin, M.E.: Etiology of primary biliary cirrhosis: The search for the culprit. Semin. Liver Dis. 2005; 25: 327–336
178. Leuschner, U., Güldütuna, S., Imhof, M., Hübner, K., Benjaminov, A., Leuschner, M.: Effects of ursodeoxycholic acid after 4 to 12 years of therapy in early and late stages of primary biliary cirrhosis. J. Hepatol. 1994; 21: 624–633
179. Leuschner, M., Maier, K.P., Schlichting, J., Strahl, S., Herrmann, G., Dahm, H.H., Ackermann, H., Happ, J., Leuschner, U.: Oral budesonide and ursodeoxycholic acid for treatment of primary biliary cirrhosis: results of a prospective double-blind trial. Gastroenterology 1999; 117: 918–925
180. Leuschner, M., Dietrich, C.F., You, T., Seidl, C., Raedle, J., Herrmann, G., Ackermann, H., Leuschner, U.: Characterization of patients with primary biliary cirrhosis responding to long term ursodeoxycholic acid treatment. Gut 2000; 46: 121–126
181. Leuschner, M., Holtmeier, J., Ackermann, H., Leuschner, U.: The influence of sulindac on patients with primary biliary cirrhosis that responds incompletely to ursodeoxycholic acid: a pilot study. Eur. J. Gastroenterol. Hepatol. 2002; 14: 1369–1376
182. Lie, T.S., Preißinger, H.: Erfolgreiche Behandlung der primären biliären Zirrhose mit Ciclosporin. Dtsch. Med. Wschr. 1990; 115: 698–702
183. Liermann Garcia, R.F., Evangelista Garcia, C., McMaster, P., Neuberger, J.: Transplantation for primary biliary cirrhosis: retrospective analysis of 400 patients in a single center. Hepatology 2001; 33: 22–27
184. Lim, A.G., Jazrawi, R.P., Ahmed, H.A., Levy, J.H., Zuin, M., Douds, H.C., Maxwell, J.D., Northfield, T.C.: Soluble intercellular adhesion molecule-1 in primary biliary cirrhosis: relationship with disease stage, immune activity and cholestasis. Hepatology 1994; 20: 882–888
185. Lindgren, S., Danielsson, A., Olsson, R., Prytz, H., Eriksson, S.: Prednimustin treatment in primary biliary cirrhosis: a preliminary study. J. Intern. Med. 1992; 231: 139–141
186. Lindner, H., Dammermann, R., Klöppel, G.: The laparoscopic staging of primary biliary cirrhosis. Endoscopy 1977; 9: 68–73
187. Lindor, K.D., Dickson, E.R., Jorgensen, R.A., Andersen, M.L., Wiesner, R.A., Gores, G.J., Lange, S.M., Rossi, S.S., Hofmann, A.F., Baldus, W.P.: The combination of ursodeoxycholic acid and methotrexate for patients with primary biliary cirrhosis: the results of a pilot study. Hepatology 1995; 22: 1158–1162
188. Lindor, K.D., Jorgensen, R.A., Therneau, T.M., Malinchoc, M., Dickson, E.R.: Ursodeoxycholic acid delays the onset of esophageal varices in primary biliary cirrhosis. Mayo Clin. Proc. 1997; 72: 1137–1140
189. Lindor, K.D., Therneau, T.M., Jorgensen, R.A., Malinchoc, M., Dickson, E.R.: Effects of ursodeoxycholic acid on survival in patients with primary biliary cirrhosis. Gastroenterology 1996; 110: 1515–1518
190. Lombard, M., Portmann, B., Neuberger, J., Williams, R., Tygstrup, N., Ranek, L., Ring-Larsen, H., Rodes, J., Navasa, M., Trepo, C., Pape, G., Schou, G., Badsberg, J.H., Andersen, P.K.: Cyclosporine A treatment in primary biliary cirrhosis: results of a long-term placebo-controlled trial. Gastroenterology 1993; 104: 519–526
191. Ludwig, J., Dickson, E.R., McDonald, G.S.A.: Staging of chronic nonsuppurative destructive cholangitis (syndrome of primary biliary cirrhosis). Virchows Arch. (A) 1978; 379: 103–111
192. Lyttkens, K., Prytz, H., Forsberg, L., Hederström, E., Hägerstrand, I.: Ultrasound, hepatic lymph nodes and primary biliary cirrhosis. J. Hepatol. 1992; 15: 136–139
193. MacMahon, H.E., Thannhauser, S.J.: Xanthomatous biliary cirrhosis (a clinical syndrome). Ann. Intern. Med. 1949; 30: 121–179
194. Mahl, T.C., Shockcor, W., Boyer, J.L.: Primary biliary cirrhosis: survival of a large cohort of symptomatic and asymptomatic patients followed for 24 years. J. Hepatol. 1994; 20: 707–713
195. Martin Gabriel, J.C., Solis Herruzo, J.A.: Primary biliary cirrhosis and CREST syndrome (case report). Rev. Esp. Enferm. Dig. 2004; 96: 219–220
196. Marx, W.J., O'Connell, D.J.: Arthritis of primary biliary cirrhosis. Arch. Intern. Med. 1979; 139: 213–216
197. Mason, A.L., Farr, G.H., Xu, L., Hubscher, S.G., Neuberger, J.M.: Pilot study of single and combination antiretroviral therapy in patients with primaly biliary cirrhosis. Amer. J. Gastroenterol. 2004; 99: 2348–2355
198. Masuda, J.I., Omagari, K., Ohba, K., Hazama, H., Kadokawa, Y., Kinoshita, H., Hayashida, K., Ishibashi, H., Nakanuma, Y., Kohno, S.: Correlation between histopathological findings of the liver and IgA class antibodies to 2-oxo-acid dehydrogenase complex in primary biliary cirrhosis. Dig. Dis. Sci. 2003; 48: 932–938
199. Matsuzaki, Y., Doy, M., Tanaka, N., Shoda, J., Osuga, T., Nakano, M., Aikawa, T.: Biochemical and histological changes after more than four years of treatment of ursodeoxycholic acid in primary biliary cirrhosis. J. Clin. Gastroenterol. 1994; 18: 36–41
200. Mazzella, G., Parini, P., Bazzoli, F., Villanova, N., Festi, D., Aldini, R., Roda, A., Cipolla, A., Polimeni, C., Tonelli, A., Roda, E.: Ursodeoxycholic acid administration on bile acid metabolism in patients with early stages of primary biliary cirrhosis. Dig. Dis. Sci. 1993; 38: 896–902
201. Mazzella, G., Fusaroli, P., Pezzoli, A., Azzaroli, F., Mazzeo, C., Zambonin, L., Simoni, P., Festi, D., Roda, E.: Methylprednisolone administration in primary biliary cirrhosis increases cholic acid turnover, synthesis, and deoxycholate concentrations in bile. Dig. Dis. Sci. 1999; 44: 2478–2483
202. Menéndez, J.L., Giron, J.A., Manzano, L., Garrido, A., Abreu, L., Albillos, A., Dura·ntez, A., Alvarez-Mon, M.: Deficient interleukin-2 responsiveness of T-lymphocytes from patients with primary biliary cirrhosis. Hepatology 1992; 16: 931–936
203. Metcalf, J., James, O.: The geoepidemiology of primary biliary cirrhosis. Semin. Liver Dis. 1997; 17 13–1722
204. Metcalf, J.V., Mitchison, H.C., Palmer, J.M., Jones, D.E., Bassendine, M.F., James, O.F.W.: Natural history of early primary biliary cirrhosis. Lancet 1996; 348: 1399–1402
205. Miller, F., Lane, B., Soterakis, J., D'Angelo, W.A.: Primary biliary cirrhosis and scleroderma. Arch. Pathol. Lab. Med. 1979; 103: 505–509
206. Minami, Y., Seki, K., Nishikawa, M., Kawata, S., Mioshi, S., Imai, Y., Tarui, S., Kakiuchi, Y., Shinji, Y., Kiyonaga, G.: Laparoscopic findings of the liver in the diagnosis of primary biliary cirrhosis: "Reddish patch", a laparoscopic feature in the asymptomatic stage. Endoscopy 1982; 14: 203–208
207. Mitchison, H.C., Malcolm, A.J., Bassendine, M.F., James, O.F.W.: Metabolic bone disease in primary biliary cirrhosis at presentation. Gastroenterology 1988; 94: 463–470
208. Mitchison, H.C., Lucey, M.R., Kelly, P.J., Neuberger, J.M., Williams, R., James, O.F.W.: Symptom development and prognosis in primary biliary cirrhosis: a study in two centers. Gastroenterology 1990; 99: 778–784
209. Mitchison, H.C., Palmer, J.M., Bassendine, M.F., Watson, A.J., Record, C.O., James, O.F.W.: A controlled trial of prednisolone treatment in primary biliary cirrhosis. Three-year results. J. Hepatol. 1992; 15: 336–344
210. Morris, J.A., McIllmurray, M.B.: Primary biliary cirrhosis and focal glomerulonephritis. Brit. Med. J. 1981; 1: 1836–1837
211. Mullhaupt, B., Kullak-Ublick, G.A., Ambühl, P.M., Stocker, R., Renner, E.L.: Successful use of the molecular adsorbent recirculating system (MARS) in a patient with primary biliary cirrhosis (PBC) and treatment refractory pruritus (case report). Hepatol. Res. 2003; 25: 442–446
212. Nakanuma, Y., Ohta, G., Kono, N., Kobayashi, K., Kato, Y.: Electron microscopic observation of destruction of biliary epithelium in primary biliary cirrhosis. Liver 1983; 3: 238–248
213. Nakanuma, Y., Ohta, G.: Nodular hyperplasia of the liver in primary biliary cirrhosis of early histological stages. Amer. J. Gastroenterol. 1987; 82: 8–10
214. Nakanuma, T., Tsuneyama, K., Kono, N., Iloso, M., van de Water, J., Gershwin, M.E.: Biliary epithelial expression of pyruvate dehydrogenase complex in primary biliary cirrhosis: an immunohistochemical and immunoelectron study. Hum. Pathol. 1995; 26: 92–98
215. Nakamura, A., Yamazaki, K., Suzuki, K., Sato, S.: Increased portal tract infiltration of mast cells and eosinophils in primary biliary cirrhosis. Amer. J. Gastroenterol. 1997; 92: 2245–2249

216. Narayanan-Menon, K.V., Angulo, P., Boe, G.M., Lindor, K.D.: Safety and efficacy of estrogen therapy in preventing bone loss in primary biliary cirrhosis. Amer. J. Gastroenterol. 2003; 98: 889–892
217. Neuberger, J., Christensen, F., Portmann, B.: Double-blind controlled trial of D-penicillamine in patients with primary biliary cirrhosis. Gut 1985; 26: 114–119
218. Neuman, M.G., Cameron, R.G., Haber, J.A., Katz, G.G., Blendis, L.M.: An electron microscopic and morphometric study of ursodeoxycholic effect in primary biliary cirrhosis. Liver 2002; 22: 235–244
219. Nieri, S., Ricardo, G.G., Salvadori, G., Surrenti, C.: Primary biliary cirrhosis and Grave's Disease. J. Clin. Gastroenterol. 1985; 7: 434–437
220. Nijhawan, P.K., Therneau, T.M., Dickson, E.R., Boynton, J., Lindor, K.D.: Incidence of cancer in primary biliary cirrhosis: The Mayo experience. Hepatology 1999; 29: 1396–1398
221. Nir, A., Sorokin, Y., Abramovici, H., Theodor, E.: Pregnancy and primary biliary cirrhosis. Int. J. Gynaecol. Abstet. 1989; 28: 279–282
222. Nishiguchi, S., Habu, D., Kubo, S., Shiomi, S., Tatsumi, N., Tamori, A., Takeda, T., Ogami, M., Tanaka, T., Hirohashi, K., Kinoshita, H., Nakatani, T.: Effects of alanine in patients with advanced primary biliary cirrhosis: preliminary report. Hepatol. Res. 2003; 25: 8–13
223. Nishiguchi, S., Shiomi, S., Ishizu, H., Iwata, Y., Kawabe, J., Tamori, A., Habu, D., Takeda, T., Ochi, H.: Usefulness of scintigraphy with technetium-99m galactosyl human serum albumin in prediction of prognosis of primary biliary cirrhosis. Hepatol. Res. 2002; 22: 180–186
224. Nyberg, A., Lööf, L.: Primary biliary cirrhosis: clinical features and outcome, with special reference to asymptomatic disease. Scand. J. Gastroenterol. 1989; 24: 57–64
225. O'Connell, D.J., Marx, W.J.: Hand changes in primary biliary cirrhosis. Radiology 1978; 129: 31–35
226. Oka, H., Toda, G., Ikeda, Y., Hashimoto, N., Hasumura, Y., Kamimura, T., Ohta, Y., Tsuji, T., Hattori, N., Namihisa, T., Nishioka, M., Ito, K., Sasaki, H., Kakumu, S., Kuroki, T., Fujisawa, K., Nakanuma, Y.: A multi-center double-blind controlled trial of ursodeoxycholic acid for primary biliary cirrhosis. Gastroenterol. Jpn. 1990; 25: 774–780
227. Olsson, R., Mattsson, L.A., Obrant, K., Mellström, D.: Estrogen-progesteron therapy for low bone mineral density in primary biliary cirrhosis. Liver 1999; 19: 188–192
228. Ono, M., Sekiya, C., Ohhira, M., Namiki, M., Endo, Y., Suzuki, K., Matsuda, Y., Taniguchi, N.: Elevated level of serum Mn-superoxide dismutase in patients with primary biliary cirrhosis: possible involvement of free radicals in the pathogenesis in primary biliary cirrhosis. J. Lab. Clin. Med. 1991; 118: 476–483
229. Outwater, E., Kaplan, M.M., Bankoff, M.S.: Lymphadenopathy in primary biliary cirrhosis: CT observations. Radiology 1989; 171: 731–733
230. Pares, A., Caballeria, L., Rodes, J., Bruguera, M., Rodrigo, L., Garcia-Plaza, A., Berenguer, M., Rodriguez-Martinez, D., Mercader, J., Velicia, R.: Long-term effects of ursodeoxycholic acid in primary biliary cirrhosis: results of a double-blind controlled multicentric trial. J. Hepatol. 2000; 32: 561–566
231. Pares, A., Caballeria, L., Rodes, J.: Excellent long-term survival in patients with primary biliary cirrhosis and biochemical response to ursodeoxycholic acid. Gastroenterology 2006; 130: 715–720
232. Pereira, S.P., Bray, G.P., Pitt, P.I., Li, F.M., Moniz, C., Williams, R.: Non-invasive assessment of bone density in primary biliary cirrhosis. Eur. J. Gastroenterol. Hepatol. 1999; 11: 323–328
233. Pollak, C., Minar, E., Dragosics, B., Marosi, L.: Primäre biliäre Zirrhose und Sklerodermie: Langjähriger benigner Verlauf einer komplexen Autoimmunerkrankung. Leber Magen Darm 1985; 15: 85–89
234. Portmann, B., Popper, H., Neuberger, J., Williams, R.: Sequential and diagnostic features in primary biliary cirrhosis based on serial histologic study in 209 patients. Gastroenterology 1985; 88: 1777–1790
235. Poupon, R.E., Huet, P.M., Poupon, R., Bonnand, A.-M., Tran van Nhieu, J., Zafrani, E.S.: A randomized trial comparing colchicine and ursodeoxycholic acid combination to ursodeoxycholic acid in primary biliary cirrhosis. Hepatology 1996; 24: 1098–1103
236. Poupon, R., Chazouille'res, O., Balkau, B., Poupon, R.E.: Clinical and biochemical expression of the histopathological lesions of primary biliary cirrhosis. J. Hepatol. 1999; 30: 408–412
237. Poupon, R.E., Bonnand, A.M., Chretien, Y., Poupon, R.: Ten-year survival in ursodeoxycholic acid-treated patients with primary biliary cirrhosis. Hepatology 1999; 29: 1668–1671
238. Poupon, R.E., Lindor, K.D., Pares, A., Chazouillères, O., Poupon, R., Heathcote, E.J.: Combined analysis of the effect of treatment with ursodeoxycholic acid on histologic progression in primary biliary cirrhosis. J. Hepatol. 2003; 39: 12–16
239. Powell, F.C., Schroeter, A.L., Dickson, E.R.: Primary biliary cirrhosis and the CREST syndrome: A report of 22 cases. Quart. J. Med. 1987; 62: 75–82
240. Prince, M.I., James, O.F.W., Holland, N.P., Jones, D.E.J.: Validation of a fatigue impact score in primary biliary cirrhosis towards a standard for clinical and trial use. J. Hepatol. 2000; 32: 368–373
241. Prince, M., Chetwynd, A., Newman, W., Metcalf, J.V., James, O.F.W.: Survival and symptom progression in a geographically based cohort of patients with primary biliary cirrhosis: follow-up for up to 28 years. Gastroenterology 2002; 123: 1044–1051
242. Prince, M.I., Chetwynd, A., Craig, W.L., Metcalf, J.V., James, O.F.W.: Asymptomatic primary biliary cirrhosis: Clinical features, prognosis, and symptom progression in a large population based cohort. Gut 2004; 53: 865–870
243. Rai, G.S., Hamlyn, A.N., Dahl, M.G.C., Morley, A.R., Wilkinson, R.: Primary biliary cirrhosis, cutaneous capillaritis, and IgM-associated membranous glomerulonephritis. Brit. Med. J. 1977; I: 817
244. Reichen, J., Widmer, T., Cotting, J.: Accurate prediction of death by serial determination of galactose elimination capacity in primary biliary cirrhosis: a comparison with the Mayo Model. Hepatology 1991; 14: 504–510
245. Ritzel, U., Leonhardt, U., Nather, M., Schafer, G., Armstrong, V.W., Ramadori, G.: Simvastatin in primary biliary cirrhosis effects on serum lipids and distinct disease markers. J. Hepatol. 2002; 36: 454–458
246. Roll, J., Boyer, J.L., Barry, D., Klatskin, G.: The prognostic importance of clinical and histological features in asymptomatic and symptomatic primary biliary cirrhosis. New Engl. J. Med. 1983; 308: 1–7
247. Rubin, E., Schaffner, F., Popper, H.: Primary biliary cirrhosis: chronic non-suppurative destructive cholangitis. Amer. J. Pathol. 1965; 46: 387–407
248. Rutan, G., Martinez, A.J., Fieshko, J.T., van Thiel, D.H.: Primary biliary cirrhosis, Sjögren's syndrome, and transverse myelitis. Gastroenterology 1986; 90: 206–210
249. Rydning, A., Schrumpf, E., Abdelnoor, M., Elgjo, K., Jenssen, E.: Factors of prognostic importance in primary biliary cirrhosis. Scand. J. Gastroenterol. 1990; 12: 119–126 279
250. Sallie, R., O'Grady, J., Williams, R.: Transplantation in primary biliary cirrhosis. J. Gastroenterol. Hepatol. 1991; 6: 558–562
251. Saxena, R., Hytiroglou, P., Thung, S.N., Theise, N.D.: Destruction of canals of Hering in primary biliary cirrhosis. Hum. Pathol. 2002; 33: 983–988
252. Scheuer, P.J.: Primary biliary cirrhosis. Proc. R. Soc. Med. 1967; 60: 1257–1260
253. Selmi, C., Balkwill, D.L., Invernizzi, P., Ansari, A.A., Coppel, R.L., Podda, M., Leung, P.S., Kenny, T.P., van de Water, J.V., Nantz, M.H., Kurth, M.J., Gershwin, M.E.: Patients with primary biliary cirrhosis react against a ubiquitous xenobiotic-metabolizing bacterium. Hepatology 2003; 38: 1250–1257
254. Shi, J., Wu, C., Lin, Y.-X., Chen, L., Zhu, L., Xie, W.-F.: Long-term effects of mid-dose ursodeoxycholic acid in primary biliary cirrhosis: A meta-analysis of randomized controlled trials. Amer. J. Gastroenterol. 2006; 101: 1529–1538
255. Shibata, J., Fujiyama, S., Honda, Y., Sato, T.: Combination therapy with ursodeoxycholic acid and colchicine for primary biliary cirrhosis. J. Gastroenterol. Hepatol. 1992; 7: 277–282
256. Shiomi, S., Sasaki, N., Tamori, A., Habu, D., Takeda, T., Nishiguchi, S., Kuroki, T., Kawabe, J., Ochi, H.: Use of scintigraphy with (99m) technetium galactosyl human serum albumin for staging of primary biliary cirrhosis and assessment of prognosis. J. Gastroenterol. Hepatol. 1999; 14: 566–571
257. Solaymani-Dodaran, M., Card, T.R., Aithal, G.P., West, J.: Fracture risk in people with primary biliary cirrhosis: A population-based cohort study. Gastroenterology 2006; 131: 1752–1757
258. Sorensen, H.T., Thulstrup, A.M., Blomqvist, P., Norgaard, B., Fonager, K., Ekbom, A.: Risk of primary biliary liver cirrhosis in patients with celiac disease: Danish and Swedish cohort data. Gut 1999; 44: 736–738
259. Spiteri, M.A., Clarke, S.W.: The nature of latent pulmonary involvement in primary biliary cirrhosis. Sarcoidosis 1989; 6: 107–110
260. Springer, J., Cauch-Dudek, K., O'Rourke, K., Wanless, I.R., Heathcote, E.J.: Asymptomatic primary biliary cirrhosis: a study of its natural history and prognosis. Amer. J. Gastroenterol. 1999; 94: 47–53
261. Stemerowicz, R., Hopf, U., Möller, B., Wittenbrink, C., Rodloff, A., Reinhardt, R., Freudenberg, M., Galanos, C.: Are antimitochondrial antibodies in primary biliary cirrhosis induced by R (rough) mutants of enterobacteriaceae? Lancet 1988/II: 1166–1170
262. Strassburg, C.P., Jaeckel, E., Manns, M.P.: Antimitochondrial antibodies and other immunological tests in primary biliary cirrhosis. Eur. J. Gastroenterol. Hepatol. 1999; 11: 595–601
263. Sundin, U., Sundqvist, K.G.: Plasma membrane association of primary biliary cirrhosis mitochondrial marker antigen M2. Clin. Exp. Immunol. 1991; 83: 407–412
264. Szostecki, C., Will, H., Netter, H.J., Guldner, H.H.: Autoantibodies to the nuclear Sp 100 protein in primary biliary cirrhosis and associated disease: epitope specificity and immunoglobulin class distribution. Scand. J. Immunol. 1992; 36: 555–564
265. Takeshita, E., Kumagi, T., Matsui, H., Abe, M., Furukawa, S., Ikeda, Y., Matsuura, B., Michitaka, K., Horiike, N., Onji, M.: Esophagogastric varices as a prognostic factor for the determination of clinical stage in patients with primary biliary cirrhosis. J. Gastroenterol. 2003; 38: 1060–1065
266. Tanaka, A., Prindiville, T.P., Gish, R., Solnick, J.V., Coppel, R.L., Keeffe, E.B., Ansari, A., Gershwin, M.E.: Are infectious agents involved in primary biliary cirrhosis? A PCR approach. J. Hepatol. 1999; 31: 664–671
267. Tanaka, A., Quaranta, S., Mattalia, A., Coppel, R., Rosina, F., Manns, M., Gershwin, M.E.: The tumor necrosis factor-alpha promoter correlates with progression of primary biliary cirrhosis. J. Hepatol. 1999; 30: 826–829
268. Tang, K.H., Schofield, J.B., Powell-Jackson, P.R.: Primary biliary cirrhosis and idiopathic retroperitoneal fibrosis: a rare association. Eur. J. Gastroenterol. Hepatol. 2002; 14: 783–786
269. Terasaki, S., Nakanuma, Y., Ogino, H., Unoura, M., Kobayashi, K.: Hepatocellular and biliary expression of HLA-antigens in primary bili-

ary cirrhosis before and after ursodeoxycholic acid therapy. Amer. J. Gastroenterol. 1991; 86: 1194–1199
270. Ter Borg, P.C.J., Schalm, S.W., Hausen, B.E., van Buuren, H.R.: Prognosis of ursodeoxycholic acid-treated patients with primary biliary cirrhosis. Results of a 10-yr cohort study involving 297 patients. Amer. J. Gastroenterol. 2006; 101: 2044–2050
271. Thannhauser, S.J., Magendantz, H.: The different clinical groups of xanthomatous diseases; a clinical physiological study of 22 cases. Ann. Intern. Med. 1938; 11: 1662–1746
272. Thomas P.K., Walker, J.G.: Xanthomatous neuropathy in primary biliary cirrhosis. Brain 1965; 88: 1079–1088
273. Tinmouth, J., Tomlinson, G., Heathcote, E.J., Lilly, L.: Benefit of transplantation in primary biliary cirrhosis between 1985–1997. Transplantation 2002; 73: 224–227
274. Tsianos, E.V., Hoofnagle, J.H., Fox, P.C., Alspaugh, M., Jones, E.A., Schafer, D.F., Moutsopoulos, H.M.: Sjögren's syndrome in patients with primary biliary cirrhosis. Hepatology 1990; 11: 730–734
275. Tsuji, H., Murai, K., Akagi, K., Fujishima, M.: Familial primary biliary cirrhosis associated with impaired concanavalin A-induced lymphocyte transformation to relatives. Two family studies. Dig. Dis. Sci. 1992; 37: 353–360
276. Turner, I.B., Myszor, M., Mitchison, H.C., Bennet, M.K., Burt, A.D., James, O.F.W.: A two-year controlled trial examining effectiveness of ursodeoxycholic acid in primary biliary cirrhosis. J. Gastroenterol. Hepatol. 1994; 4: 162–168
277. Uddenfeldt, P., Danielsson, A., Forssell, A., Holm, M., Östberg, Y.: Features of Sjögren's syndrome in patients with primary biliary cirrhosis. J. Intern. Med. 1991; 230: 443–448
278. Underhill, J., Donaldson, P., Bray, G., Doherty, D., Portmann, B., Williams, R.: Susceptibility to primary biliary cirrhosis is associated with the HLA-DR8-DQB1*0402 haplotype. Hepatology 1992; 16: 1404–1408
279. Vargas, C.A., Medlina, R., Rübio, C.E., Torres, E.A.: Primary biliary cirrhosis associated with ankylosing spondylitis. J. Clin. Gastroenterol. 1994; 18: 263–264
280. Vuoristo, M., Färkkilä, M., Karronen, A.-L., Leino, R., Lehtola, J., Mäkinen, J., Mattila, J., Friman, C., Seppälä, K., Tuominen, J., Miettinen, T.A.: A placebo-controlled trial of primary biliary cirrhosis treatment with colchicine and ursodeoxycholic acid. Gastroenterology 1995; 108: 1470–1478
281. Walker, J.G., Doniach, D., Roitt, I.M., Sherlock, S.: Serological tests in the diagnosis of primary biliary cirrhosis. Lancet 1965/I: 827–831
282. Wallace, J.G.jr., Tong, M.J., Ueki, B.H., Quismorio, F.P.: Pulmonary involvement in primary biliary cirrhosis. J. Clin. Gastroenterol. 1987; 9: 431–435
283. Warnes, T.W., Smith, A., Lee, F.I., Haboubi, N.Y., Johnson, P.J., Hunt, L.: A controlled trial of colchicine in primary biliary cirrhosis. Trial design and preliminary report. J. Hepatol. 1987; 5: 1–7
284. Weber, P., Brenner, J., Stechemesser, E., Klein, R., Weckenmann, U., Kloppel, G., Kirchhof, M., Fintelmann, V., Berg, P.A.: Characterization and clinical relevance of a new complement-fixing antibody-anti-M8 in patients with primary biliary cirrhosis. Hepatology 1986; 6: 553–559
285. Weissman, E., Becker, N.: Interstitial lung disease in primary biliary cirrhosis. Amer. J. Med. Sci. 1983; 285: 21–27
286. Wenzel, J.S., Donohoe, A., Ford, K.L., Glastad, K., Watkins, D., Molmenti, E.: Primary biliary cirrhosis: MR imaging findings and description of MR imaging periportal halo sign. Amer. J. Roentgen. 2001; 176: 885–889
287. Wiesner, R.H., Ludwig, J., Lindor, K.D., Jorgensen, R.A., Baldus, W.P., Homburger, H.A., Dickson, E.R.: A controlled trial of cyclosporine in the treatment of primary biliary cirrhosis. New Engl. J. Med. 1990; 322: 1419–1424
288. Wolfhagen, F.H.J., van Buuren, H.R., Schalm, S.W.: Combined treatment with ursodeoxycholic acid and prednisone in primary biliary cirrhosis. Neth. J. Med. 1994; 44: 84–90
289. Wolfhagen, F.H.J., van Hoogstraten, H.J.F., van Buuren, H.R., van Berge-Henegouwen, G.P., Ten-Kate, F.J.W., Hop, W.C.J., van der Hoek, E.W., Kerbert, M.J., van Lijf, H.H., den Ouden, J.W., Smit, A.M., de Vries, R.A., van Zanten, R.A.A., Schalm, S.W.: Triple therapy with ursodeoxycholic acid, prednisone and azathioprine in primary biliary cirrhosis: a 1-year randomized, placebo-controlled study. J. Hepatol. 1998; 29: 736–742
290. Wolke, A.M., Schaffner, F., Kapelman, B., Sacks, H.S.: Malignancy in primary biliary cirrhosis. High incidence of breast cancer in affected women. Amer. J. Med. 1984; 76: 1075–1078
291. Xu, L.Z., Shen, Z.W., Guo, L.S., Fodera, B., Keogh, A., Joplin, R., Odonnell, B., Aitken, J., Carman, W., Neuberger, J., Mason, A.: Does a betaretrovirus infection trigger primary biliary cirrhosis? Proc. Nat. Acad. Sci. USA 2003; 100: 8454–8459
292. Yamada, G., Hyodo, I., Tobe, K., Mizuno, M., Nishihara, T., Kobayaski, T., Nagashimo, H.: Ultrastructural immunocytochemical analysis of lymphocytes infiltrating bile duct epithelia in primary biliary cirrhosis. Hepatology 1986; 6: 385–391
293. Yeaman, S.J., Fussey, S.P.M., Danner, D.J., James, O.F.W., Mutimer, D.J., Bassendine, M.F.: Primary biliary cirrhosis: identification of two major M2 mitochondrial autoantigens. Lancet 1988/I: 1067–1070
294. Yoshikawa, M., Tsujii, T., Matsumura, K., Yamao, J., Matsumura, Y., Kubo, R., Fukui, H., Ishizaka, S.: Immunomodulatory effects of ursodeoxycholic acid on immune responses. Hepatology 1992; 16: 358–364
295. Zeegen, R., Stansfeld, A.G., Dawson, A.M., Hunt, A.H.: Bleeding oesophageal varices as the presenting feature in primary biliary cirrhosis. Lancet 1969/II: 9–13
296. Zein, C.O., Jorgensen, R.A., Clarke, B., Wenger, D.E., Keach, J.C., Angulo, P., Lindor, K.D.: Alendronate improves bone mineral density in primary biliary cirrhosis: A randomized placebo-controlled trial. Hepatology 2005; 42: 762–771
297. Zifroni, A., Schaffner, F.: Long-term follow-up of patients with primary biliary cirrhosis on colchicine therapy. Hepatology 1991; 14: 990–993

Primary sclerosing cholangitis
298. Aaseth, J., Thomassen, Y., Aadland, E., Fausa, O., Schrumpf, E.: Hepatic retention of copper and selenium in primary sclerosing cholangitis. Scand. J. Gastroenterol. 1995; 30: 1200–1203
299. Ahrendt, St.A., Pitt, H.A., Kalloo, A.C., Venbrux, A.C., Klein, A.S., Herlong, H.F., Coleman, J., Lillemoe, K.D., Cameron, J.L.: Primary sclerosing cholangitis. Resect, dilate, or transplant? Ann. Surg. 1998; 227: 412–423
300. Alberti-Flor, J.J., Kalemeris, G., Dunn, G.D., Avant, G.R.: Primary sclerosing cholangitis associated with massive intraabdominal lymphadenopathy. Amer. J. Gastroenterol. 1986; 81: 55–60
301. Angulo, P., Therneau, T.M., Jorgensen, R.A., de Sotel, C.K., Egan, K.S., Dickson, E.R., Hay, J.E., Lindor, K.D.: Bone disease in patients with primary sclerosing cholangitis: prevalence, severity and prediction of progression. J. Hepatol. 1998; 29: 729–735
302. Angulo, P., Peter, J.B., Gershwin, M.E., DeSotel, C.K., Shoenfeld, Y., Ahmed, A.E.E., Lindor, K.D.: Serum autoantibodies in patients with primary sclerosing cholangitis. J. Hepatol. 2000; 32: 182–187
303. Angulo, P., Maor-Kendler, Y., Lindor, K.D.: Small-duct primary sclerosing cholangitis: a long-term follow-up study. Hepatology 2002; 35: 1494–1500
304. Audan, A., Bruley Des Varrannes, S., Georgelin, T., Sagan, C., Cloarec, D., Serraz, H., Le Bodic, L.: Cholangite sclerosante primitive et lupus erythemateux systemique. Gastroenterol. Clin. Biol. 1995; 19: 123–126
305. Bader, T.R., Beavers, K.L., Semelka, R.C.: MR imaging features of primary sclerosing cholangitis: patterns of cirrhosis in relationship to clinical severity of disease. Radiology 2003; 226: 675–685
306. Baluyut, A.R., Sherman, S., Lehman, G.A., Hoen, H., Chalasani, N.: Impact of endoscopic therapy on the survival of patients with primary sclerosing cholangitis. Gastrointest. Endosc. 2001; 53: 308–312
307. Bergquist, A., Ekbom, A., Olsson, R., Kornfeldt, D., Lööf, L., Danielsson, A., Hultcrantz, R., Lindgren, H., Prytz, H., Sandberg-Gertzen, H., Almer, S., Granath, F.Broomé, U.: Hepatic and extrahepatic malignancies in primary sclerosing cholangitis. J. Hepatol. 2002; 36: 321–327
308. Bergquist, A., Glaumann, H., Lindberg, B., Broome, U.: Primary sclerosing cholangitis can present with acute liver failure: Report of two cases. J. Hepatol. 2006; 44: 1005–1008
309. Beuers, U., Spengler, U., Kruis, W., Aydemir, Ü., Wiebecke, B., Heldwein, W., Weinzierl, M., Pape, G.R., Sauerbruch, T., Paumgartner, G.: Ursodeoxycholic acid for treatment of primary sclerosing cholangitis: A placebo-controlled trial. Hepatology 1992; 16: 707–714
310. Bjornsson, E., Lindqvist-Ottosson, J., Asztely, M., Olsson, R.: Dominant strictures in patients with primary sclerosing cholangitis. Amer. J. Gastroenterol. 2004; 99: 502–508
311. Bjoro, K., Brandsaeter, B., Foss, A., Schrumpf, E.: Liver transplantation in primary sclerosing cholangitis. Semin. Liver Dis. 2006; 26: 69–79
312. Boberg, K.M., Egeland, T., Schrumpf, E.: Long-term effect of corticosteroid treatment in primary sclerosing cholangitis. Scand. J. Gastroenterol. 2003; 38: 991–995
313. Boberg, K.M., Bergquist, A., Mitchell, S., Pares, A., Rosina, F., Broomé, U., Chapman, R., Fausa, O., Egeland, T., Rocca, G., Schrumpf, E.: Cholangiocarcinoma in primary sclerosing cholangitis: risk factors and clinical presentation. Scand. J. Gastroenterol. 2002; 37: 1205–1211
314. Brandt, D.J., MacCarty, R.L., Charboneau, J.W., LaRusso, N.F., Wiesner, R.H., Ludwig, J.: Gallbladder disease in patients with primary sclerosing cholangitis. Amer. J. Roentgenol. 1988; 150: 571–574
315. Broomé, U., Glaumann, H., Hultcrantz, R., Forsum, U.: Distribution of HLA-DR, HLA-DP, HLA-DQ antigens in liver tissue from patients with primary sclerosing cholangitis. Scand. J. Gastroent. 1990; 25: 54–58
316. Broomé, U.: Management of primary sclerosing cholangitis and its complications in adult patients. Acta Gastro-Enterol. Belg. 2002; 65: 37–44
317. Broomé, U., Glaumann, H., Lindström, E., Lööf, L., Almer, S., Prytz, H., Sandberg-Gertzen, H., Lindgren, S., Fork, F.T., Järnerot, G., Olsson, R.: Natural history and outcome in 32 Swedish patients with small duct primary sxlerosing cholangitis (PSC). J. Hepatol. 2002; 36: 586–589
318. Burak, K., Angulo, P., Pasha, T.M., Egan, K., Petz, J., Lindor, K.D.: Incidence and risk factors for cholangiocarcinoma in primary sclerosing cholangitis. Amer. J. Gastroenterol. 2004; 99: 523–526
319. Cangemi, J.R., Wiesner, R.H., Beaver, S.J., Ludwig, J., MacCarty, R.L., Dozois, R.R., Zinsmeister, A.R., LaRusso, N.F.: Effect of proctocolectomy for chronic ulcerative colitis on the natural history of primary sclerosing cholangitis. Gastroenterology 1989; 96: 790–794

320. **Chalasani, N., Baluyut, A., Ismail, A., Zaman, A., Sood, G., Ghalib, R., McCashland, T.M., Reddy, K.R., Zervos, X., Anbari, M.A., Hoen, H.:** Cholangiocarcinoma in patients with primary sclerosing cholangitis: a multicenter case-control study. Hepatology 2000; 31: 7–11
321. **Chapman, R.W.:** Role of immune factors in the pathogenesis of primary sclerosing cholangitis. Semin. Liver Dis. 1991; 11: 1–4
322. **Chazouillères, O., Poupon, R., Capron, J.-P., Metman, E.-H., Dhumeaux, D., Amouretti, M., Couzigou, P., Labayle, D., Trinchet, J.-C.:** Ursodeoxycholic acid for primary sclerosing cholangitis. J. Hepatol. 1990; 11: 120–123
323. **Colle, I., van Vlierberghe, H.:** Diagnosis and therapeutic problems of primary sclerosing cholangitis. Acta Gastro-Enterol. Belg. 2003; 66: 155–159
324. **Cullen, S.N., Rust, C., Fleming, K., Edwards, C., Bluers, U., Chapman, R.W.:** High dose ursodeoxycholic acid for the treatment of primary sclerosing cholangitis is safe and effective. J. Hepatol. 2008; 48: 792–800
325. **Delbet, K.:** Retrecissement du choledoque: Cholecystoduodenostomie. Bull. Mem. Soc. Nat. Chir. 1924; 50: 1144–1146
326. **Donaldson, P.T., Farrant, J.M., Wilkinson, M.L., Hayllar, K., Portmann, B.C., Williams, R.:** Dual association of HLA DR2 and DR3 with primary sclerosing cholangitis. Hepatology 1991; 13: 129–133
327. **El-Shabrawi, M., Wilkinson, M.L., Portmann, B., Mieli-Vergani, G., Chong, S.K.F., Williams, R., Mowat, A.P.:** Primary sclerosing cholangitis in childhood. Gastroenterology 1987; 92: 1226–1235
328. **Ernst, O., Asselah, T., Sergent, G., Calvo, M., Talbodec, N., Paris, J.C., L'Hermine·, C.:** MR cholangiography in primary sclerosing cholangitis. Amer. J. Roentgenol. 1998; 171: 1027–1030
329. **Farges, O., Malassagne, B., Sebagh, M., Bismuth, H.:** Primary sclerosing cholangitis: liver transplantation or biliary surgery. Surgery 1995; 117: 146–155
330. **Farrant, M., Williams, R.:** Natural history and prognosis in primary sclerosing cholangitis. Eur. J. Gastroenterol. Hepatol. 1992; 4: 272–275
331. **Fausa, O., Schrumpf, E., Elgjo, K.:** Relationship of inflammatory bowel disease and primary sclerosing cholangitis. Semin. Liver Dis. 1991; 11: 31–39 373
332. **Feldstein, A.E., Perrault, J., El-Youssif, M., Lindor, K.D., Freese, D.K., Angulo, P.:** Primary sclerosing cholangitis in children: a long-term follow-up study. Hepatology 2003; 38: 210–217
333. **Fleming, K.A.:** The hepatobiliary pathology of primary sclerosing cholangitis. Eur. J. Gastroenterol. Hepatol. 1992; 4: 266–271
334. **Floreani, A., Zancan, L., Melis, A., Baragiotta, A., Chiaramonte, M.:** Primary sclerosing cholangitis (PSC): clinical, laboratory and survival analysis in children and adults. Liver 1999; 19: 228–233
335. **Fulcher, A.S., Turner, M.A., Franklin, K.J., Shiffman, M.L., Sterling, R.K., Luketic, V.A.C., Sanyal, A.J.:** Primary sclerosing cholangitis: evaluation with MR cholangiography.– A case-control study. Radiology 2000; 215: 71–80
336. **Gaing, A.A., Geders, J.M., Cohen, S.A., Siegel, J.H.:** Endoscopic management of primary sclerosing cholangitis: review, and report of an open series. Amer. J. Gastroenterol. 1993; 88: 2000–2008
337. **Gilger, M.A., Gann, M.E., Opekum, A.R., Gleason, W.A.:** Efficacy of ursodeoxycholic acid in the treatment of primary sclerosing cholangitis in children. J. Pediatr. Gastroenterol. Nutr. 2000; 31: 136–141
338. **Goldenring, J.R., Cahow, C.E.:** Intrahepatic cholangiojejunostomy as a palliative procedure in primary sclerosing cholangitis. Arch. Surg. 1989; 124: 565–567
339. **Gomez, R.L., Griffin, M.D.J.W.jr., Squires, J.E.:** Prolonged relief of intractable pruritus in primary sclerosing cholangitis by plasmapheresis. J. Clin. Gastroenterol. 1986; 8: 301–303
340. **Graziadei, I.W., Wiesner, R.H., Marotta, P.J., Porayko, M.K., Hay, J.E., Charlton, M.R., Poterucha, J.J., Rosen, C.B., Gores, G.J., Lakusso, N.F., Krom, R.A.F.:** Long-term results of patients undergoing liver transplantation for primary sclerosing cholangitis. Hepatology 1999; 30: 1121–1127
341. **Graziadei, I.W.:** Recurrence of primary sclerosing cholangitis after liver transplantation. Liver Transplant. 2002; 8: 575–581
342. **Gross, J.B.jr., Ludwig, J., Wiesner, R.H., McCall, J.T., LaRusso, N.F.:** Abnormalities in tests of copper metabolism in primary sclerosing cholangitis. Gastroenterology 1985; 272–278
343. **Hadjis, N.S., Adam, A., Hatzis, G., Blenkharn, I., Thompson, I.W., Blumgart, L.H.:** Primary sclerosing cholangitis: Symptomatic and cholangiographic improvement after peripheral drainage. Amer. J. Gastroenterol. 1988; 83: 312–315
344. **Harnois, D.M., Angulo, P., Jorgensen, R.A., La Russo, N.F., Lindor, K.D.:** High-dose ursodeoxycholic acid as a therapy for patients with primary sclerosing cholangitis. Amer. J. Gastroenterol. 2001; 96: 1558–1566
345. **Harrison, R.F., Hübscher, S.G.:** The spectrum of bile duct lesions in end-stage primary sclerosing cholangitis. Histopathology 1991; 19: 321–327
346. **Hay, J.E., Lindor, K.D., Wiesner, R.H., Dickson, E.R., Krom, R.A.F., LaRusso, N.F.:** The metabolic bone disease of primary sclerosing cholangitis. Hepatology 1991; 14: 257–261
347. **Helzberg, J.H., Petersen, J.M., Boyer, J.L.:** Improved survival with primary sclerosing cholangitis: A review of clinicopathologic features and comparison of symptomatic and asymptomatic patients. Gastroenterology 1987; 92: 1869–1875
348. **Ismail, T., Angrisani, L., Powell, J.E., Hubscher, S., Buckels, J., Neuberger, J., Elias, E., McMaster, P.:** Primary sclerosing cholangitis: surgical options, prognostic variables and outcome. Brit. J. Surg. 1991; 78: 564–567
349. **Ito, H., Imada, T., Rino, Y., Kondo, J.:** A case of segmental primary sclerosing cholangitis. Hepato-Gastroenterol. 2000; 47: 128–131
350. **Ito, K., Mitchell, D.G., Outwater, E.K., Blasbalg, R.:** Primary sclerosing cholangitis: MR imaging features. Amer. J. Roentgenol. 1999; 172: 1527–1533
351. **Jeffrey, G.P., Reed, W.D., Laurence, B.H., Shilkin, K.B.:** Primary sclerosing cholangitis: clinical and immunopathological review of 21 cases. J. Gastroenterol. Hepatol. 1990; 5: 135–140
352. **Jeffrey, G.P., Reed, W.D., Carrello, S., Shilkin, K.B.:** Histological and immunohistochemical study of the gallbladder lesion in primary sclerosing cholangitis. Gut 1991; 32: 424–429
353. **Jonard, P., Geubel, A., Wallon, J., Rahier, J., Dive, C., Meunier, H.:** Primary sclerosing cholangitis and idiopathic pulmonary fibrosis: a case report. Acta Clin. Belg. 1989; 44: 24–30
354. **Jorge, A.D., Esley, C., Ahumada, J.:** Family incidence of primary sclerosing cholangitis associated with immunologic disease. Endoscopy 1987; 19: 114–117
355. **Jorgensen, R.A., Lindor, K.D., Sartin, J.S., LaRusso, N.F., Wiesner, R.H.:** Serum lipid and fat soluble vitamin levels in primary sclerosing cholangitis. J. Clin. Gastroenterol. 1995; 20: 215–219
356. **Kahana, M., Schewach-Millet, M., Trau, H., Gilon, E., Dolev, E.:** Perforating folliculitis in association with primary sclerosing cholangitis. Amer. J. Dermatopathol. 1985; 7: 271–276
357. **Kaya, M., Petersen, B.T., Angulo, P., Baron, T.H., Andrews, J.C., Gostout, C.J., Lindor, K.D.:** Balloon dilation compared to stenting of dominant strictures in primary sclerosing cholangitis. Amer. J. Gastroenterol. 2001; 96: 1059–1066
358. **Kaplan, M.M., Arora, S., Pincus, S.H.:** Primary sclerosing cholangitis and low-dose oral pulse methotrexate therapy. Ann. Intern. Med. 1987; 106: 231–235
359. **Katabi, N., Albores-Saavedra, J.:** The extrahepatic bile duct lesions in end-stage primary sclerosing cholangitis. Amer. J. Surg. Pathol. 2003; 27: 349–355
360. **Kawai, H., Aoyagi, Y., Nomoto, M., Takizawa, H., Suzuki, Y., Hama, A., Suda, T., Takahashi, T., Asakura, H.:** Asymptomatic primary sclerosing cholangitis with marked hepatic fibrosis. Dig. Dis. Sci. 2000; 45: 680–684
361. **Kelly, P., Patchett, S., McCloskey, D., Alstead, E., Farthing, M., Fairclough, P.:** Sclerosing cholangitis, race and sex. Gut 1997; 41: 688–689
362. **Kirby, D.F., Blei, A.T., Rosen, S.T., Vogelzang, R.L., Neiman, H.L.:** Primary sclerosing cholangitis in the presence of a lupus anticoagulant. Amer. J. Med. 1986; 81: 1077–1080
363. **Klein, R., Eisenburg, J., Weber, P., Seibold, F., Berg, P.A.:** Significance and specificity of antibodies to neutrophils detected by Western Blotting for the serological diagnosis of primary sclerosing cholangitis. Hepatology 1991; 14: 1147–1152
364. **Knox, T.A., Kaplan, M.M.:** A double-blind controlled trial of oral pulse methotrexate therapy in the treatment of primary sclerosing cholangitis. Gastroenterology 1994; 106: 494–499
365. **Kornfeld, D., Ekbom, A., Ihre, T.:** Survival and risk of cholangiocarcinoma in patients with primary sclerosing cholangitis. A population based study. Scand. J. Gastroenterol. 1997; 32: 1042–1045
366. **Kozaiwa, K., Tajiri, H., Sawada, A., Tada, K., Etani, Y., Miki, K., Okada, S.:** Case report: three paediatric cases of primary sclerosing cholangitis treated with ursodeoxycholic acid and sulphasalazine. J. Gastroenterol. Hepatol. 1998; 13: 825–829
367. **Kulaksiz, H., Rudolph, G., Kloeters-Plachky, P., Sauer, P., Geiss, H., Stiehl, A.:** Biliary candida infection in primary sclerosing cholangitis. J. Hepatol. 2006; 45: 711–716
368. **Kyokane, K., Ichihara, T., Horisawa, M., Suzuki, N., Ichihara, S., Suga, S., Nakao, A., Morise, K.:** Successful treatment of primary sclerosing cholangitis with cyclosporine and corticosteroid. Hepato-Gastroenterol. 1994; 41: 449–452
369. **Lazaridis, K.N., Gores, G.J.:** Primary sclerosing cholangitis and cholangiocarcinoma. Semin. Liver Dis. 2006; 26: 42–51
370. **Lebovics, E., Palmer, M., Woo, J., Schaffner, F.:** Outcome of primary sclerosing cholangitis. Analysis of long-term observation of 38 patients. Arch. Intern. Med. 1987; 147: 729–731
371. **Lee, Y.M., Kaplan, M.M.:** Management of primary sclerosing cholangitis. Amer. J. Gastroenterol. 2002; 97: 528–534
372. **Levy, C., Lindor, K.D.:** Primary sclerosing cholangitis: epidemiology, natural history, and prognosis. Semin. Liver Dis. 2006; 26: 22–30
373. **Lindor, K.D., Wiesner, R.H., Colwell, L.J., Steiner, B., Beaver, S., LaRusso, N.F.:** The combination of prednisone and colchicine in patients with primary sclerosing cholangitis. Amer. J. Gastroenterol. 1991; 85: 57–61
374. **Lindor, K.D., Jorgensen, R.A., Anderson, M.L., Gores, G.J., Hofmann, A.F., LaRusso, N.F.:** Ursodeoxycholic acid and methotrexate for primary sclerosing cholangitis: a pilot study. Amer. J. Gastroenterol. 1996; 91: 511–515
375. **Lo, S.K., Fleming, K., Chapman, R.W.G.:** A 2-year follow-up study of anti-neutrophil antibody in primary sclerosing cholangitis: relationship to clinical activity, liver biochemistry and ursodeoxycholic acid treatment. J. Hepatol. 1994; 21: 974–978
376. **Loftus, E.V.jr., Sandborn, W.J., Tremaine, W.J., Mahoney, D.W., Zinsmeister, A.R., Offord, K.P., Melton, L.J.:** Primary sclerosing cholangitis is associated with nonsmoking: a case-control study. Gastroenterology 1996; 110: 1496–1502
377. **Ludwig, J., MacCarty, R.L., LaRusso, N.F., Krom, R.A.F., Wiesner, R.H.:** Intrahepatic cholangiectases and large-duct obliteration in primary sclerosing cholangitis. Hepatology 1986; 6: 560–568

378. **Ludwig, J.:** Small-duct primary sclerosing cholangitis. Semin. Liver Dis. 1991; 11: 11–17
379. **Ludwig, J., Colina, F., Poterucha, J.J.:** Granulomas in primary sclerosing cholangitis. Liver 1995; 15: 307–312
380. **Majoie, C.B., Smits, N.J., Phoa, S.S., Reeders, J.W., Jansen, P.L.:** Primary sclerosing cholangitis: sonographic findings. Abdom. Imag. 1995; 20: 109–112
381. **Martins, E.B., Fleming, K.A., Garrido, M.C., Hine, K.R., Chapman, R.W.G.:** Superficial thrombophlebitis, dysplasia, and cholangiocarcinoma in primary sclerosing cholangitis. Gastroenterology 1994; 107: 537–542
382. **Matsumoto, T., Ajiki, T., Matsumoto, I., Tominaga, M., Hori, H., Mita, Y., Fujita, T., Fujino, Y., Suzuki, Y., Ku, Y., Kuroda, Y.:** Intrahepatic segmental primary sclerosing cholangitis: Report of a case. Surgery Today 2006; 36: 638–641
383. **McGarity, B., Bansi, D.S., Robertson, D.A.F., Millward-Sadler, G.H., Sherphed, H.A.:** Primary sclerosing cholangitis. an important and prevalent complication of Crohn's disease. Eur. J. Gastroenterol. Hepatol. 1991; 3: 361–364
384. **Mehal, W.Z., DennisLo, Y.-M., Wordsworth, B.P., Neuberger, J.M., Hubscher, S.C., Fleming, K.A., Chapman, R.W.:** HLA DR4 is a marker for rapid disease progression in primary biliary cholangitis. Gastroenterology 1994; 106: 160–168
385. **Mendes, F.D., Jorgensen, R., Keach, J., Katzmann, J.A., Smyrk, T., Donlinger, J., Chari, S., Lindor, K.D.:** Elevated serum IgG4 concentration in patients with primary sclerosing cholangitis. Amer. J. Gastroenterol. 2006; 101: 2070–2075
386. **Mistilis, G.P.:** Pericholangitis and ulcerative colitis. 1. Pathology, etiology and pathogenesis. Ann. Intern. Med. 1965; 63: 1–16
387. **Moeller, D.D.:** Sclerosing cholangitis associated with autoimmune hemolytic anemia and hyperthyroidism. Amer. J. Gastroenterol. 1985; 80: 122–125
388. **Moff, S.L., Kamel, I.R., Eustace, J., Lawler, L.P., Kantsevoy, S., Kalloo, A.N., Thuluvath, P.J.:** Diagnosis of primary sclerosing cholangitis: A blind comparative study using magnetic resonance cholangiography and endoscopic retrograde cholangiography. Gastroenterol. Endosc. 2006; 64: 219–223
389. **Narumi, S., Roberts, J.P., Emond, J.C., Lake, J., Ascher, N.L.:** Liver transplantation for sclerosing cholangitis. Hepatology 1995; 22: 451–457
390. **O'Brien, C.B., Senior, J.R., Arora-Mirchandani, R., Batta, A.K., Salen, G.:** Ursodeoxycholic acid for the treatment of primary sclerosing cholangitis: A 30-month pilot study. Hepatology 1991; 14: 838–847
391. **Oberholzer, K., Lohse, A.W., Mildenberger, P., Grebe, P., Schadeck, T., Bantelmann, M., Thelen, M.:** Diagnosis of primary sclerosing cholangitis: prospective comparison of MR cholangiography with endoscopic retrograde cholangiography. Fortschr. Roentgenstr. 1998; 169: 622–626
392. **Okolicsanyi, L., Groppo, M., Floreani, A., Morselli-Labate, A.M., Rusticali, A.G., Battocchia, A., Colombo, M., Galatola, G., Gasbarrini, G., Podda, M., Ricci, G., Rosina, F., Zuin, M.:** Treatment of primary sclerosing cholangitis with low-dose ursodeoxycholic acid: results of a retrospective Italian multicentre survey. Dig. Liver Dis. 2003; 35: 325–331
393. **Olsson, R., Danielsson, A., Järnerot, G., Lindström, E., Lööf, L., Rolny, P., Ryden, B.-O., Tysk, C., Wallerstedt, S.:** Prevalence of primary sclerosing cholangitis in patients with ulcerative colitis. Gastroenterology 1991; 100: 1319–1323
394. **Olsson, R., Broome·, U., Danielsson, A., Hagerstrand, I., Jarnerot, G.T., Lööf, L., Prytz, H., Ryden, B.O., Wallerstedt, S.:** Colchicine treatment of primary sclerosing cholangitis. Gastroenterology. 1995; 108: 1199–1203
395. **Olsson, R., Broome, U., Danielsson, A., Hägerstrand, I., Järnerot, G., Lööf, L., Prytz, H., Ryden, B.O.:** Spontaneous course of symptoms in primary sclerosing cholangitis: relationships with biochemical and histological features. Hepato-Gastroenterol. 1999; 46: 136–141
396. **O'Mahony, C.A., Vierling, J.M.:** Etiopathogenesis of primary sclerosing cholangitis. Semin. Liver Dis. 2006; 26: 3–21
397. **Pardi, D.S., Loftus, E.V., Kremers, W.K., Keach, J., Lindor, K.D.:** Ursodeoxycholic acid as a chemoprotective agent in patients with ulcerative colitis and primary sclerosing cholangitis. Gastroenterology 2003; 124: 889–893
398. **Petersen, K.M., Angulo, P., Baron, T.H.:** Balloon dilatation compared to stenting of dominant strictures in primary sclerosing cholangitis. Amer. J. Gastroenterol. 2001; 96: 1059–1066
399. **Ponsioen, C.Y., Kuiper, H., ten Kate, F.J., van Milligen-de-Witt, M., van Deventer, S.J., Tytgat, G.N.:** Immunohistochemical analysis of inflammation in primary sclerosing cholangitis. Eur. J. Gastroenterol. Hepatol. 1999; 11: 769–774
400. **Ponsioen, C.Y., Lam, K., Van Milligen de Wit, A.W.M., Huibregtse, K., Tytgat, G.N.J.:** Four years experience with short term stenting in primary sclerosing cholangitis. Amer. J. Gastroenterol. 1999; 94: 2403–2407
401. **Ponsioen, C.Y., Defoer, J., ten Kate, F.J.W., Weverling, G.J., Tytgat, G.N.J., Pannekoek, Y., Wertheim-Dillen, P.M.E.:** A survey of infectious agents as risk factors for primary sclerosing cholangitis: are Chlamydia species involved? Eur. J. Gastroenterol. Hepatol. 2002; 14: 641–648
402. **Porayko, M.K., Wiesner, R.H., LaRusso, N.F., Ludwig, J., MacCarty, R.L., Steiner, B.L., Twomey, C.K., Zinsmeister, A.R.:** Patients with asymptomatic primary sclerosing cholangitis frequently have progressive disease. Gastroenterology 1990; 98: 1594–1602
403. **Prochazka, E.J., Terasaki, P.I., Park, M.S., Goldstein, L.I., Busuttil, R.W.:** Association of primary sclerosing cholangitis with HLADRw52a. New Engl. J. Med. 1990; 322: 1842–1844
404. **Quigley, E.M.M., LaRusso, N.F., Ludwig, J., MacSween, R.N.M., Birnie, G.G., Watkinson, G.:** Familial occurence of primary sclerosing cholangitis and ulcerative colitis. Gastroenterology 1983; 85: 1160–1165
405. **Rasmussen, H.H., Fallingborg, J., Mortensen, P.B., Freund, L., Tage-Jensen, U., Kruse, V., Rasmussen, S.N.:** Primary sclerosing cholangitis in patients with ulcerative colitis. Scand. J. Gastroenterol. 1992; 27: 732–736
406. **Revelon, G., Rashid, A., Kawamoto, S., Bluemke, D.A.:** Primary sclerosing cholangitis: MR imaging findings with pathologic correlation. Amer. J. Roentgenol. 1999; 173: 1037–1042
407. **Roberts, E.A.:** Primary sclerosing cholangitis in children. J. Gastroenterol. Hepatol. 1999; 14: 588–593
408. **Rossi, P., Salvatori, F.M., Bezzi, M., Maccioni, F., Porcaro, M.L., Ricci, P.:** Percutaneous management of benign biliary strictures with balloon dilatation and selfexpanding metallic stents. Cardiovasc. Intervent. Radiol. 1990; 13: 231–239
409. **Rudolph, G., Kloeters,-Plachky, P., Rost, D., Stiehl, A:** The incidence of cholangiocarcinoma in primary sclerosing cholangitis after long-time treatment with ursodeoxycholic acid. Eur. J. Gastroenterol. Hepatol. 2007; 19: 487–491
410. **Schramm, C., Schirmacher, P., Helmreich-Becker, Gerken, G., Meyer zum Büschenfelde, K.H., Lohse, A.W.:** Combined therapy with azathioprine, prednisolone, and ursodial in patients with primary sclerosing cholangitis. – A case series. Ann. Intern. Med. 1999; 131: 943–946
411. **Schrumpf, E., Abdelnoor, M., Fausa, O., Elgjo, K., Jenssen, E., Kolmannskog, F.:** Risk factors in primary sclerosing cholangitis. J. Hepatol. 1994; 21: 1061–1066
412. **Schwegler, U., Kuntz, H.D., May, B.:** Primär-sklerosierende Cholangitis. Med. Welt 1986; 37: 1129–1132
413. **Seibold, F., Weber, P., Klein, R., Berg, P.A., Wiedmann, K.H.:** Clinical significance of antibodies against neutrophils in patients with inflammatory bowel disease and primary sclerosing cholangitis. Gut 1992; 33: 657–662
414. **Senaldi, G., Donaldson, P.T., Magrin, S., Farrant, J.M., Alexander, G.J., Vergani, D., Williams, R.:** Activation of the complement system in primary sclerosing cholangitis. Gastroenterology 1989; 97: 1430–1434
415. **Seymour, J., Schwartz, M.D., Dall, A.:** Primary sclerosing cholangitis. Review and report of six cases. Arch. Surg. 1958; 77: 439–451
416. **Shetty, K., Rybicki, L., Brzezinski, A., Carey, W.D., Lashner, B.A.:** The risk for cancer or dysplasia in ulcerative colitis patients with primary sclerosing cholangitis. Amer. J. Gastroenterol. 1999; 94: 1643–1649
417. **Sisto, A., Feldman, P., Garel, L., Seidman, E., Brochu, P., Morin, C.L., Weber, A.M., Roy, C.C.:** Primary sclerosing cholangitis in children: study of five cases and review of the literature. Pediatrics 1987; 80: 918–923
418. **Skolkin, M.D., Alspaugh, J.P., Casarella, W.J., Chuang, V.P., Galambos, J.T.:** Sclerosing cholangitis: palliation with percutaneous cholangioplasty. Radiology 1989; 170: 199–206
419. **Soetikno, R.M., Lin, O.S., Heidenreich, P.A., Young, H.S., Blackstone, M.O.:** Increased risk of colorectal neoplasia in patients with primary sclerosing cholangitis and ulcerative colitis. A meta-analysis. Gastrointest. Endosc. 2002; 56: 48–54
420. **Stieber, A.C., Marino, I.R., Iwatsuki, S., Starzl, T.E.:** Cholangiocarcinoma in sclerosing cholangitis. The role of liver transplantation. Int. Surg. 1989; 74: 1–3
421. **Stiehl, A., Walker, S., Stiehl, L., Rudolph, G., Hofmann, W.J., Theilmann, L.:** Effect of ursodeoxycholic acid on liver and bile duct disease in primary sclerosing cholangitis. A 3-year pilot study with a placebo controlled study period. J. Hepatol. 1994; 20: 57–64
422. **Stiehl, A., Rudolph, G., Sauer, P., Benz, C., Stremmel, W., Walker, S., Theilmann, L.:** Efficacy of ursodeoxycholic acid treatment and endoscopic dilation of major duct stenoses in primary sclerosing cholangitis. An 8-year prospective study. J. Hepatol. 1997; 26: 560–566
423. **Stiehl, A., Rudolph, G., Kloters-Plachky, P., Sauer, P., Walker, S.:** Development of dominant bile duct stenoses in patients with primary sclerosing cholangitis treated with ursodeoxycholic acid: outcome after endoscopic treatment. J. Hepatol. 2002; 36: 151–156
424. **Stockbrugger, R.W., Olsson, R., Jaup, B., Jensen, J.:** Forty-six patients with primary sclerosing cholangitis. Radiological bile duct changes in relationship to clinical course and concomitant inflammatory bowel disease. Hepatogastroenterol. 1988; 35: 289–294
425. **Strasser, S., Sheil, A.G.R., Gallagher, N.D., Waugh, R., McCaughan, G.W.:** Liver transplantation for primary sclerosing cholangitis versus primary biliary cirrhosis: a comparison of complications and outcome. J. Gastroenterol. Hepatol. 1993; 8: 238–243
426. **Tamura, S., Sugawara, Y., Kaneko, J., Matsui, Y., Togashi, J., Makuuchi, M.:** Recurrence of primary sclerosing cholangitis after living donor liver transplantation. Liver Internat. 2007; 27: 86–94
427. **Teefey, S.A., Baron, R.L., Rohrmann, C.A., Shuman, W.P., Freeny, P.C.:** Sclerosing cholangitis: CT findings. Radiology 1988; 169: 635–639
428. **Tischendorf, J.J.W., Hecker, H., Krüger, M., Manns, M.P., Meier, P.N.:** Characterization, outcome and prognosis in 273 patients with primary sclerosing cholangitis: A single-center study. Amer. J. Gastroenterol. 2007; 102: 107–114
429. **Tung, B.Y., Emond, M.J., Haggitt, R.C., Bronner, M.P., Kimmey, M.B., Kowdley, K.V., Brentnall, T.A.:** Ursodiol use is associated with lower prevalence of colonic neoplasia in patients with ulcerative colitis and primary sclerosing cholangitis. Ann. Intern. Med. 2001; 134: 89–95

430. Van den Meerberg, P.C., Portincasa, P., Wolfhagen, F.H.J., van Erpecum, K.J., van Berge-Henegouwen, G.P.: Increased gallbladder volume in primary sclerosing cholangitis. Gut 1996; 39: 594–599
431. Van Milligen de Witt, A.W.M., van Deventer, S.J., Tytgat, G.N.: Immunogenetic aspects of primary sclerosing cholangitis: implications for therapeutic strategies. Amer. J. Gastroenterol. 1995; 90: 893–900
432. Vrla, R.F., Gore, R.M., Schachter, H., Craig, R.M.: Ultrasound demonstration of bile duct thickening in primary sclerosing cholangitis. J. Clin. Gastroenterol. 1986; 8: 213–215
433. Watanabe, H., Ohira, H., Kuroda, M., Takagi, T., Ishikawa, H., Nishimaki, T., Kasukawa, R., Takahashi, K.: Primary sclerosing cholangitis with marked eosinophilic infiltration in the liver. J. Gastroenterol. 1995; 30: 524–528
434. Werlin, S.L., Glicklich, M., Jona, J., Starshak, R.J.: Sclerosing cholangitis in childhood. J. Pediatr. 1980; 96: 433–435
435. Wiesner, R.H., LaRusso, N.F., Ludwig, J., Dickson, E.R.: Comparison of the clinicopathologic features of primary sclerosing cholangitis and primary biliary cirrhosis. Gastroenterology 1985; 88: 108–114
436. Wiesner, R.H., Grambsch, P.M., Dickson, E.R., Ludwig, J., MacCarty, R.L., Hunter, E.B., Fleming, T.R., Fisher, L.D., Beaver, S.J., LaRusso, N.F.: Primary sclerosing cholangitis: natural history, prognostic factors and survival analysis. Hepatology 1989; 10: 430–436
437. Wiesner, R.H., Porayko, M.K., Dickson, E.R., Gores, G.J., LaRusso, N.F., Hay, J.E., Wahlstrom, H.E., Krom, R.A.F.: Selection and timing of liver transplantation in primary biliary cirrhosis and primary sclerosing cholangitis. Hepatology 1992; 16: 1290–1299
438. Wilschanski, M., Chait, P., Wade, J.A., Davis, L., Corey, M., Louis, P.St., Griffiths, A.M., Blendis, L.M., Moroz, St.P., Scully, L., Roberts, E.A.: Primary sclerosing cholangitis in 32 children: clinical, laboratory, and radiographic features, with survival analysis. J. Hepatol. 2004; 40: 857–859
439. Wurm, P., Dixon, A.D., Rathbone, B.J.: Ulcerative colitis, primary sclerosing cholangitis and coeliac disease: two cases and review of the literature. Eur. J. Gastroenterol. Hepatol. 2003; 15: 815–817
440. Zauli, D., Schrumpf, E., Crespi, C., Cassani, F., Fausa, O., Aadland, E.: An autoantibody profile in primary sclerosing cholangitis. J. Hepatol. 1987; 5: 14–18

Autoimmune cholangitis
441. Agarwal, K., Jones, D.E.J., Watt, F.E., Burt, A.D., Floreani, A., Bassendine, M.F.: Familial primary biliary cirrhosis and autoimmune cholangitis. Dig. Liver Dis. 2002; 34: 50–52
442. Akisawa, N., Nishimori, I., Miyaji, E., Iwasaki, S., Maeda, T., Shimizu, H., Sato, N.: The ability of anti-carbonic anhydrase II antibody to distinguish autoimmune cholangitis from primary biliary cirrhosis in Japanese patients. J. Gastroenterol. 1999; 34: 366–371
443. Brunner, G., Klinge, O.: Ein der chronisch-destruierenden nicht-eitrigen Cholangitis ähnliches Krankheitsbild mit antinukleären Antikörpern (Immuncholangitis). Dtsch. Med. Wschr. 1987; 112: 1454–1458
444. Colombato, L.A., Alvarez, F., Cote, J., Huet, P.M.: Autoimmune cholangiopathy: the result of consecutive primary biliary cirrhosis and autoimmune hepatitis? Gastroenterology 1994; 107: 1839–1843
445. Czaja, A.J., Carpenter, H.A., Santrach, P.J., Moore, S.B.: Autoimmune cholangitis within the spectrum of autoimmune liver disease. Hepatology 2000; 31: 1231–1238
446. Gisbert, J.P., Jones, E.A., Pajares, J.M., Moreno-Otero, R.: Is there an optimal therapeutic regimen for antimitochondrial antibody-negative primary biliary cirrhosis (autoimmune cholangitis)? (review) Alim. Pharm. Ther. 2003; 17: 17–27
447. Gogos, C.A., Nikolopoulou, V., Zolota, V., Siampi, V., Vagenakis, A.: Autoimmune cholangitis in a patient with celiac disease: a case report and review of the literature. J. Hepatol. 1999; 30: 321–324
448. Goodman, Z.D., McNally, P.R., Davis, D.R., Ishak, K.G.: Autoimmune cholangitis: a variant of primary biliary cirrhosis. Clinicopathologic and serologic correlations in 200 cases. Dig. Dis. Sci. 1995; 40: 1232–1242
449. Gordon, S.C., Quattrociocchi-Longe, T.M., Khan, B.A., Kodali, V.P., Chen, J., Silverman, A.L., Kiechle, F.L.: Antibodies to carbonic anhydrase in patients with immune cholangiopathies. Gastroenterology 1995; 108: 1802–1809
450. Kaserer, K., Exner, M., Mosberger, I., Penner, E., Wrba, F.: Characterization of the inflammatory infiltrate in autoimmune cholangitis. A morphological and immunhistochemical study. Virch. Arch. 1998; 432: 217–222
451. Kinoshita, H., Omagari, K., Whittingham, S., Kato, Y., Ishibashi, H., Sugi, K., Yano, M., Kohno, S., Nakanuma, Y., Penner, E., Wesierska-Gadek, J., Reynoso-Paz, S., Gershwin, M.E., Anderson, J., Jois, J.A., Mackay, I.R.: Autoimmune cholangitis and primary biliary cirrhosis – an autoimmune enigma. Liver 1999; 19: 122–128
452. Li, C.P., Tong, M.J., Hwang, S.J., Luo, J.C., Co, R.L., Tsay, S.H., Chang, F.Y., Lee, S.D.: Autoimmune cholangitis with features of autoimmune hepatitis: successful treatment with immunosuppressive agents and ursodeoxycholic acid. J. Gastroenterol. Hepatol. 2000; 15: 95–98
453. Marinho, R., Graca, H., Ramalho, F., Costa, A., Batista, A., Demoura, M.C.: Autoimmune cholangitis: case report. Hepato-Gastroenterol. 1999; 46: 1949–1952
454. Masumoto, T., Ninomiya, T., Michitaka, K., Horiike, N., Yamamoto, K., Akbar, S.M.F., Abe, M., Onji, M.: Three patients with autoimmune cholangiopathy treated with prednisolone. J. Gastroenterol. 1998; 33: 909–913
455. Michieletti, P., Wanless, I.R., Katz, A., Scheuer, P.J., Yeaman, S.J., Bassendine, M.F., Palmer, J.M., Heathcote, E.J.: Antimitochondrial antibody negative primary biliary cirrhosis: A distinct syndrome of autoimmune cholangitis. Gut 1994; 35: 260–265
456. Mohr, L., Heintges, T., Hensel, F., Niederau, C., Häussinger, D.: Treatment of autoimmune cholangitis. Dig. Dis. Sci. 1998; 53: 2160–2163
457. Noguchi, S., Hashimoto, E., Aoka, K., Taniai, M., Ishiguro, N., Hayashi, N.: Familial autoimmune cholangiopathy and primary biliary cirrhosis. (Japan.) Acta Hepatol. Jpn. 1996; 37: 336–342
458. Sanchez-Pobre, P., Castellano, G., Colina, F., Dominguez, P., Rodriguez, S., Canga, F., Solis Herruzo, J.A.: Antimitochondrial antibody-negative chronic nonsuppurative destructive cholangitis. Atypical primary biliary cirrhosis or autoimmune cholangitis. J. Clin. Gastroenterol. 1996; 23: 191–198
459. Sanchez-Pobre, P., Solis-Herruzo, J.A.: Autoimmune cholangitis nosological location. Rev. Esp. Enferm. Dig. 2003; 95: 791–794
460. Sedlack, R.E., Smyrk, T.C., Czaya, A.J., Talwalkar, J.A.: Celiac disease-associated autoimmune cholangitis (case report). Amer. J. Gastroenterol. 2002; 97: 3196–3198
461. Taylor, S.L., Dean, P.J., Riely, C.A.: Primary autoimmune cholangitis: An alternative to antimitochondrial antibody-negative primary biliary cirrhosis. Amer. J. Surg. Pathol. 1994; 18: 91–99

Overlap syndrome
462. Alric, L., Thebault, S., Selves, J., Peron, J.M., Mejdoubi, S., Fortenfant, F., Vinel, J.P.: Characterization of overlap syndrome between primary biliary cirrhosis and autoimmune hepatitis according to antimitochondrial antibodies status. Gastroenterol. Clin. Biol. 2007; 31: 11–16
463. Beuers, U., Rust, C.: Overlap syndromes. Semin Liver Dis. 2005; 25: 311–320
464. Burak, K.W., Urbanski, J.S., Swain, M.G.: A case of coexisting primary biliary cirrhosis and primary sclerosing cholangitis: A new overlap of autoimmune liver diseases. Dig. Dis. Sci. 2001; 46: 2043–2047
465. Chazouillères, O., Wendum, D., Serfaty, L., Montembault, S., Rosmorduc, O., Poupon, R.: Primary biliary cirrhosis – Autoimmune hepatitis overlap syndrome: clinical features and response to therapy. Hepatology 1998; 28: 296–301
466. Chazouillères, O., Wendum, D., Serfaty, L., Rosmorduc, O., Poupon, R.: Long term outcome and response to therapy of primary biliary cirrhosis – autoimmune hepatitis overlap syndrome. J. Hepatol. 2006; 44: 400–406
467. Duclos-Valleé, J.C., Hadengue, A., Ganne-Carrie, N., Robin, E., Degott, C., Erlinger, S.: Primary biliary cirrhosis - autoimmune hepatitis overlap syndrome. Corticoresistance and effective treatment by cyclosporine A. Dig. Dis. Sci. 1995; 40: 1069–1073
468. Floreani, A., Baragiotta, A., Leone, M.G., Baldo, V., Naccarato, R.: Primary biliary cirrhosis and hepatitis C Virus infection. Amer. J Gastroenterol. 2003; 98: 2757–2762
469. Gohlke, F., Lohse, A.W., Dienes, H.P., Lohr, H., Märker-Hermann, E., Gerken, G., Meyer zum Büschenfelde, K.-H.: Evidence for an overlap syndrome of autoimmune hepatitis and primary sclerosing cholangitis. J. Hepatol. 1996; 24: 699–705
470. Gopal, S., Nagral, A., Mehta, S.: Autoimmune sclerosing cholangitis: an overlap syndrome in a child. Indian J. Gastroenterol. 1999; 18: 31–32
471. Gregorio, G.V., Portmann, B., Karani, J., Harrison, P., Donaldson, P.T., Vergani, D., Mieli-Vergani, G.: Autoimmune hepatitis / sclerosing cholangitis overlap syndrome in childhood: a 16-year prospective study. Hepatology 2001; 33: 544–553
472. Griga, T., Tromm, A., Müller, K.M., May, B.: Overlap syndrome between autoimmune hepatitis and primary sclerosing cholangitis in two cases. Eur. J. Gastroenterol. Hepatol. 2000; 12: 559–564
473. Hatzis, G.S., Vassiliou, V.A., Delladetsima, J.K.: Overlap syndrome of primary sclerosing cholangitis and autoimmune hepatitis. Eur. J. Gastroenterol. Hepatol. 2001; 13: 203–206
474. Heurgue, A., Vitry, F., Diebold, M.D., Yaziji, N., Bernard-Chabert, B., Pennaforte, J.L., Picot, R., Louvet, H., Fremond, L., Geoffroy, P., Schmit, J.L., Cadiot, G., Thiefin, G.: Overlap syndrome of primary biliary cirrhosis and autoimmune hepatitis: A retrospective study of 115 cases of autoimmune liver disease. Gastroenterol. Clin. Biol. 2007; 31: 17–25
475. Joshi, S., Cauch-Dudek, K., Wanless, I.R., Lindor, K.D., Jorgensen, R., Batts, K., Heathcote, E.J.: Primary biliary cirrhosis with additional features of autoimmune hepatitis: response to therapy with ursodeoxycholic acid. Hepatology 2002; 35: 409–413
476. Kanda, T., Yokosuka, O., Hirasawa, Y., Imazeki, F., Nagao, K., Saisho, H.: Occurrence of autoimmune hepatitis during the course of primary biliary cirrhosis: Report of two cases. Dig. Dis. Sci. 2006; 51: 45–46
477. Kaya, M., Angulo, P., Lindor, K.D.: Overlap of autoimmune hepatitis and primary sclerosing cholangitis: an evaluation of a modified scoring system. J. Hepatol. 2000; 33: 537–542
478. Kingham, J.G.C., Abbasi, A.: Co-existence of primary biliary cirrhosis and primary sclerosing cholangitis: A rare overlap syndrome put in perspective. Eur. J. Gastroenterol. Hepatol. 2005; 17: 1077–1080
479. Klöppel, G., Seifert, G., Lindner, H., Dammermann, R., Sack, H.J., Berg, P.A.: Histopathological features in mixed types of chronic aggressive hepatitis and primary biliary cirrhosis. Virch. Arch. Pathol. Anat. Histol. 1977; 373: 143–160
480. Koskinas, J., Raptis, I., Manika, Z., Hadziyannis, S.: Overlapping syndrome of autoimmune hepatitis and primary sclerosing cholangitis

associated with pyoderma gangrenosum and ulcerative colitis. Eur. J. Gastroenterol. Hepatol. 1999; 11: 1421–1424
481. **Lohse, A.W., Meyer-zum-Büschenfelde, K.-H., Franz, B., Kanzler, S., Gerken, G., Dienes, H.P.:** Characterization of the overlap syndrome of primary biliary cirrhosis (PBC) and autoimmune hepatitis: evidence for it being a hepatitic form of PBC in genetically susceptible individuals. Hepatology 1999; 29: 1078–1084
482. **McNair, A.N.B., Moloney, M., Portmann, B.C., Williams, R., McFarlane, I.G.:** Autoimmune hepatitis overlapping with primary sclerosing cholangitis in five cases. Amer. J. Gastroenterol. 1998; 93: 777–784
483. **Minuk, G.Y., Sutherland, L.R., Pappas, S.C., Kelley, J.K., Martin, S.E.:** Autoimmunic chronic active hepatitis (lupoid hepatitis) and primary sclerosing cholangitis in two young adult females. Can. J. Gastroenterol. 1988; 2: 22–27
484. **Okuno, T., Seto, Y., Okanoue, T., Takino, T.:** Chronic active hepatitis with histological features of primary biliary cirrhosis. Dig. Dis. Sci. 1987; 32: 775–779
485. **Poupon, R., Chazouilleres, O., Corpechot, C., Chrétien, Y.:** Development of autoimmune hepatitis in patients with typical primary biliary cirrhosis. Hepatology 2006; 44: 85–90
486. **Rabinowitz, M., Demetris, A.J., Bou-Abboud, C.F., van Thiel, D.H.:** Simultaneous occurrence of primary sclerosing cholangitis and autoimmune chronic active hepatitis in a patient with ulcerative colitis. Dig. Dis. Sci. 1992; 37: 1606–1611
487. **Sanchez-Pobre, P., Gonzalez, C., Paz, E., Colina, F., Castellano, G., Munoz-Yague, T., Rodriguez, S., Yela, C., Alvarez, V., Solis-Herruzo, J.:** Chronic hepatitis C and autoimmune cholangitis: a case study and literature review. Dig. Dis. Sci. 2002; 47: 1224–1229
488. **Storch, W.B.:** So-called "overlap syndromes" in hepatology: combinations or associations of concurrent autoimmune liver and other diseases. Cell. Mol. Biol. 2003; 49: 645–648
489. **Suzuki, Y., Arase, Y., Ikeda, K., Saitoh, S., Tsubota, A., Suzuki, F., Kobayashi, M., Akuta, N., Somcya, T., Miyakawa, Y., Kumada, H.:** Clinical and pathological characteristics of the autoimmune hepatitis and primary biliary cirrhosis overlap syndrome. J. Gastroenterol. Hepatol. 2004; 19: 699–706
490. **Uehara, T., Hamano, H., Kawa, S., Sano, K., Honda, T., Ota, H.:** Distinct clinicopathological entity "autoimmune pancreatitis associated sclerosing cholaangitis" Pathol. Intern. 2005; 55: 405–411
491. **Van Buuren, H.R., van Hoogstraten, H.J.F., Terkivatan, T., Schalm, S.W., Vleggaar, F.P.:** High prevalence of autoimmune hepatitis among patients with primary sclerosing cholangitis. J. Hepatol. 2000; 33: 543–548

Cholangiodysplasia
492. **Bauman, M.E., Pound, D.C., Ulbright, T.M.:** Hepatocellular carcinoma arising in congenital hepatic fibrosis. Amer. J. Gastroenterol. 1994; 89: 450–451
493. **Bertheau, P., Degott, C., Belghiti, J., Vilgrain, V., Renard, P., Benhamou, J.P., Henin, D.:** Adenomatous hyperplasia of the liver in a patient with congenital hepatic fibrosis. J. Hepatol. 1994; 20: 213–217
494. **Braga, A.C., Calheno, A., Rocha, H., Lourenco-Gomes, J.:** Caroli's disease with congenital hepatic fibrosis and medullary sponge kidney. J. Pediatr. Gastroenterol. Nutr. 1994; 19: 464–467
495. **Bruguera, M., Llach, J., Rode·s, J.:** Nonsyndromic paucity of intrahepatic bile ducts in infancy and idiopathic ductopenia in adulthood: the same syndrome? Hepatology 1992; 15: 830–834
496. **Burt, M.J., Chambers, S.T., Chapman, B.A., Strack, M.F., Troughton, W.D.:** Two cases of Caroli's disease: diagnosis and management. J. Gastroenterol. Hepatol. 1994; 9: 194–197
497. **Cardona, J., Houssin, D., Gauthier, F., Devictor, D., Losay, J., Hadchouel, M., Bernard, O.:** Liver transplantation in children with Alagille syndrome – a study of twelve cases. Transplantation 1995; 60: 339–342
498. **Caroli, J., Soupault, R., Kossakowski, J., Plocker, L., Paradowska, L.:** La dilatation polycystique congenitale des voies biliaires intrahepatiques, essai de classification. Sem. Hop. Paris 1958; 34: 488–495
499. **Choi, B.I., Yeon, K.M., Kim, S.H., Han, M.C.:** Caroli disease: central dot sign in CT. Radiology 1990; 174: 161–163
500. **Crosnier, C., Lykavieris, P., Meunier-Rotival, M., Hadchouel, M.:** Alagille syndrome. The widening spectrum of arteriohepatic dysplasia. Clin. Liver Dis. 2000; 4: 765–778
501. **Deltenre, P., Valla, D.-C.:** Ischemic cholangiopathy (review). J. Hepatol. 2006; 44: 806–817
502. **Desmet, V.J.:** Congenital diseases of intrahepatic bile ducts: variations on the theme "ductal plate malformation". Hepatology 1992; 16: 1069–1083
503. **Desmet, V.J.:** Vanishing bile duct syndrome in drug-induced liver disease. J. Hepatol. 1997; 26 (Suppl.): 31–35
504. **Drouin, E., Russo, P., Tuchweber, B., Mitchell, G., Rasquin-Weber, A.:** North American Indian cirrhosis in children: a review of 30 cases. J. Pediatr. Gastroenterol. Nutr. 2000; 31: 395–404
505. **Faa, G., van Eyken, P.V., Demella, L., Vallebona, E., Costa, V., Desmet, V.J.:** Idiopathic adulthood ductopenia presenting with chronic recurrent cholestasis: a case report. J. Hepatol. 1991; 12: 14–20
506. **Giouleme, O., Nikolaidis, N., Tziomalos, K., Patsiaoura, K., Vassiliadis, T., Grammatikos, N., Papanikolaou, V., Eugenidis, N.:** Ductal plate malformation and congenital hepatic fibrosis. Clinical and histological findings in four patients (case report)
507. **Hartmann, H., Gröne, H.-J.:** Idiopathische Duktopenie des Erwachsenenalters: günstiger Effekt einer Ursodesoxycholsäure-Therapie. Z. Gastroenterol. 1993; 31 (Suppl. 2): 131–133
508. **Hoffenberg, E.J., Narkewicz, M.R., Sondheimer, J.M., Smith, D.J., Silverman, A., Sokol, R.J.:** Outcome of syndromic paucity of interlobular bile ducts (Alagille syndrome) with onset of cholestasis in infancy. J. Pediatr. 1995; 127: 220–224
509. **Kahn, E., Daum, F., Markowitz, J., Teichberg, S., Duffy, L., Harper, R., Aiges, H.:** Nonsyndromatic paucity of interlobular bile ducts: light and electron microscopic evaluation of sequential liver biopsies in early childhood. Hepatology 1986; 6: 890–901
510. **Knoop, M., Keck, H., Langrehr, J.M., Peter, F.J., Ferslev, B., Neuhaus, P.:** Therapie des unilobulären Caroli-Syndroms durch Leberresektion. Chirurg 1994; 65: 861–866
511. **Lazarow, P.B., Black, V., Shio, H., Fujiki, Y., Hajra, O.K., Dalta, N.S., Bangaru, B.S., Dancis, J.:** Zellweger syndrome: biochemical and morphological studies in two patients treated with clofibrate. Ped. Res. 1985; 19: 1356–1364
512. **Lointier, P.H., Kauffmann, P., Francannet, P., Pezet, D., Chippau, J.:** Management of intrahepatic calculi in Caroli's disease by extracorporeal shock wave lithotripsy. Brit. J. Surg. 1990; 77: 987–988
513. **Ludwig, J.:** Idiopathic adulthood ductopenia: an update. Mayo Clin. Proc. 1998; 73: 285–291
514. **Lykavieris, P., Hadchouel, M., Chardot, C., Bernard, O.:** Outcome of liver disease in children with Alagille syndrome: a study of 163 patients. Gut 2001; 49: 431–435
515. **Moreno, A., Carreno, V., Cano, A., Gonzalez, C.:** Idiopathic biliary ductopenia in adults without symptoms of liver disease. New Engl. J. Med. 1997; 336: 835–838
516. **Müller, C., Ulrich, W., Penner, E.:** Manifestation late in life of idiopathic adulthood ductopenia. Liver 1995; 15: 213–218
517. **Nagasue, N.:** Successful treatment of Caroli's disease by hepatic resection. Report of six patients. Ann. Surg. 1984; 200: 718–723
518. **Nakajima, K., Komatsu, M., Ono, T., Kuramitsu, T., Goto, M., Ito, R., Masamune, O.:** A case of idiopathic adulthood ductopenia. Endoscopy 1994; 26: 332–333
519. **Nakano, I., Fukuda, Y., Koyama, Y., Urano, F., Yamada, M., Katano, Y., Marui, A., Imada, K., Hayakawa, T., Ito, M., Yamashita, Y., Imoto, M., Nakanuma, Y.:** Idiopathic adulthood ductopenia. J. Gastroenterol. Hepatol. 1996; 11: 411–415
520. **Narula, P., Gifford, J., Steggall, M.A., Lloyd, C., van Mourik, I.D.M., McKiernan, P.J., Willshaw, H.E., Kelly, D.:** Visual loss and idiopathic intracranial hypertension in children with Alagille syndrome. J. Pediatr. gastroenterol. Nutr. 2006; 43: 348–352
521. **Oda, T., Elkahloun, A.G., Pike, B.L., Okajima, K., Krantz, I.D., Genin, A., Piccoli, D.A., Meltzer, P.S., Spinner, N.B., Collins, F.S., Chandrasekharappa, S.C.:** Mutations in the human Jagged 1 gene are responsible for Alagille syndrome. Nat. Genet. 1997; 16: 235–242
522. **Raftopoulos, S.C., Garas, G., Price, R., de Boer, W.B., Jeffrey, G.-P., Yusoff, I.F.:** Epstein-Barr virus associated cholangiopathy: A new disease entity? (case report). Gastrointest. Endosc. 2006; 63: 172–176
523. **Ros, E., Navarro, S., Bru, C., Gilabert, R., Bianchi, L., Bruguera, M.:** Ursodeoxycholic acid treatment of primary hepatolithiasis in Caroli's syndrome. Lancet 1993; 342: 404–406
524. **Schulte-Bockholt, A., Gebel, M., Wittekind, C., Burdelski, M., Schmidt, F.W.:** Das Alagille-Syndrom im Erwachsenalter. Dtsch. Med. Wschr. 1990; 115: 1276–1279
525. **Soravia, C., Mentha, G., Giostra, E., Morel, P., Rohner, A.:** Surgery for adult polycystic liver disease. Surgery 1995; 117: 272–275
526. **Strazzobosco, M., Fabris, L., Spirli, C.:** Pathophysiology of cholangiopathies. J. Clin. gastroenterol. 2005; 39: 90–102
527. **Taylor, A.C.F., Palmer, K.R.:** Caroli's disease. Eur. J. Gastroenterol. Hepatol. 1998; 10: 105–108
528. **Waechter, F.L., Sampaio, J.A., Pinto, R.D., Alvares-da-Silva, M.R., Cardoso, F.G., Francisconi, C., Pereira-Lima, L.:** The role of liver transplantation in patients with Caroli's disease. Hepato-Gastroenterol. 2001; 48: 672–674
529. **Witt, H., Neumann, L.M., Grollmuss, O., Luck, W., Becker, M.:** Prenatal diagnosis of Alagille syndrome (case report). J. Pediatr. Gastroenterol. Nutr. 2004; 38: 105–106
530. **Woolf, G.M., Vierling, J.M.:** Disappearing intrahepatic bile ducts: the syndromes and their mechanisms. Semin. Liver Dis. 1993; 13: 261–275
531. **Wu, K.L., Changchien, C.S., Kuo, C.M., Chuah, S.K., Chiu, Y.C., Kuo, C.H.:** Caroli's disease. A case report of two siblings. Eur. J. Gastroenterol. Hepatol. 2002; 14: 1397–1399
532. **Yehezkely-Schildkraut, V., Munichor, M., Mandel, H., Berkowitz, D., Hartmann, C., Eshach-Adiv, O., Shamir, R.:** Nonsynchronic paucity of interlobular bile ducts: Report of 10 patients. J. Pediatr. Gastroenterol. Nutr. 2003; 37: 546–549
533. **Zafrani, E.S., Metreau, J.-M., Douvin, C., Larrey, D., Massari, R., Reynes, M., Doffoel, M., Benhamou, J.-P., Dhumeaux, D.:** Idiopathic biliary ductopenia in adults: a report of five cases. Gastroenterology 1990; 99: 1823–1828
534. **Zeitoun, D., Brancatelli, G., Colombat, M., Federle, M.P., Valla, D., Wu, T., Degott, C., Vilgrain, V.:** Congenital hepatic fibrosis: CT findings in 18 adults. Radiology 2004; 231: 109–116

Clinical Aspects of Liver Diseases
34 Chronic hepatitis

		Page:
1	*Historical review*	712
2	*Definition*	712
3	**Histology**	712
3.1	Classification (1968)	712
3.2	Histological criteria	713
3.3	Problems of designation	713
3.4	Classification (1994)	714
4	*Aetiology and differential diagnosis*	716
5	**Diagnostics**	717
5.1	Clinical findings	717
5.2	Laboratory findings	717
5.3	Morphology	717
5.4	Imaging techniques	718
6	**Course and prognosis**	718
6.1	Course	718
6.2	Extrahepatic manifestations	719
6.3	Hepatocellular carcinoma	719
6.4	Prognosis	719
6.5	Chronic HBV infection	719
6.6	Chronic HCV infection	721
6.7	Chronic HBV/HDV infection	722
7	**Therapy**	722
7.1	*General treatment*	722
7.2	*Therapy of chronic hepatitis B*	723
7.2.1	Aims and forms of treatment	723
7.2.2	Interferon therapy	723
7.2.3	Lamivudine therapy	725
7.2.4	Treatment failure	725
7.2.5	Nucleoside analogues	725
7.2.6	Immunostimulants	726
7.2.7	Adjuvant substances	726
7.3	*Therapy of chronic hepatitis C*	727
7.3.1	Indication for therapy	727
7.3.2	Selection criteria for therapy	727
7.3.3	Combination therapy (IFN + ribavirin)	728
7.3.4	Therapy scheme	729
7.3.5	Treatment failure	730
7.4	*Therapy of chronic hepatitis D*	730
7.5	*Liver transplantation*	730
	• References (1–246)	731

(Figures 34.1–34.9; tables 34.1–34.14)

34 Chronic hepatitis

1 Historical review

▶ About 70 years ago (1932), the term **latent liver damage** was coined by H. KALK, who, without any knowledge of morphological findings, was the first clinician to attempt a classification of different chronic liver diseases into clinical groups. • This interpretation was the basis for G. v. BERGMANN's definition of **latent hepatopathy** (1936) (s.p. 78); the clinical observations made by him at that time indeed correspond closely to the picture of chronic hepatitis. • Based on clinical findings in eight patients, E. POLACK observed the transition of acute epidemic hepatitis into **chronic hepatitis** as early as 1937. • *Later, in 1942, K. ROHOLM et al. reported on the histological progression of acute hepatitis to chronic hepatitis in an extensive study involving twelve patients and even monitored the further course up to the development of cirrhosis.* • In 1942 A. KORNBERG used the nomenclature **chronic latent liver damage** following jaundice; F. GEBHARDT et al. (1944) reported on **posthepatitic residual damage** and M. D. ALTSCHULE et al. (1944) on **chronic latent hepatitis** following catarrhal jaundice. The occurrence of **late posthepatitic liver damage** was substantiated by W. VOLWILER et al. (1948). (quot. 17) • From 1947 onwards, H. KALK provided more basic knowledge about **chronic hepatitis**, which he considered to be a chronic interstitial inflammation (according to R. RÖSSLE). By means of laparoscopy, H. KALK distinguished between **four stages:** (*1.*) *large red liver*, (*2.*) *large white liver*, (*3.*) *large multicoloured liver*, and (*4.*) *large multicoloured tuberous liver*. (quot. 17)

2 Definition

Chronic hepatitis is *not an entity*, but a heterogeneous group of diseases of varying aetiology, pathogenesis, degree of activity and stage of progression. Thus, like acute hepatitis, this condition constitutes a *syndrome*. • The joint *histological picture* comprises predominant portal inflammation and subsequent periportitis (= interface hepatitis) with different degrees of focal, periportal, zonal or confluent liver cell necrosis, and progredient fibrosis. • *Duration* is long: chronic inflammatory liver diseases persist for more than 6 months. • *Prognosis* is doubtful. This condition may progress through a common final stage to cirrhosis, HCC or liver failure, but also to defective healing, whereby stationary liver fibrosis persists.

3 Histology

3.1 Classification (1968)

Based on the different histological criteria, chronic hepatitis was subdivided in 1968 into (*1.*) **chronic persistent hepatitis** (CPH) (a term coined by H. F. SMETANA as early as 1954) and (*2.*) **chronic active hepatitis** (CAH) (E. G. SAINT et al., 1953) with a *mild* (type A) and a *severe* (type B) course. (7) In this context, so-called **chronic necrotizing hepatitis** can be integrated. (23) (s. fig. 34.7) (s. tab. 34.1) • This classification was further refined by differentiation into **chronic lobular hepatitis** (CLH) (H. POPPER et al., 1971) and **chronic septal hepatitis** (CSH) (M. A. GERBER et al., 1974). (10) CLH and CSH are deemed to be variants of chronic persistent hepatitis. CPH exhibits septum formation with a clear inflammatory reaction, yet without piecemeal necrosis. The prognosis for CSH is poorer than that for CLH. • **Chronic minimal hepatitis** shows sparse hyaline necrosis and slight portal cellular infiltrations. Generally, these alterations remain unchanged for years. Morphologically, this term corresponds to so-called *non-specific reactive hepatitis* (V. DESMET, 1986). These reactions are of an inflammatory nature and attributable to primarily extrahepatic disease or to focal intrahepatic space-occupying lesions. (s. p. 398) • Sometimes, more severe inflammatory signs are found in CPH due to increased viral replication and immune reactions. This form was described as minimally active, chronic hepatitis (L. BIANCHI, 1986). (2) Thus, even CPH can develop into CAH.

Initially, this classification, which was based on well-defined **histological criteria**, proved useful – especially

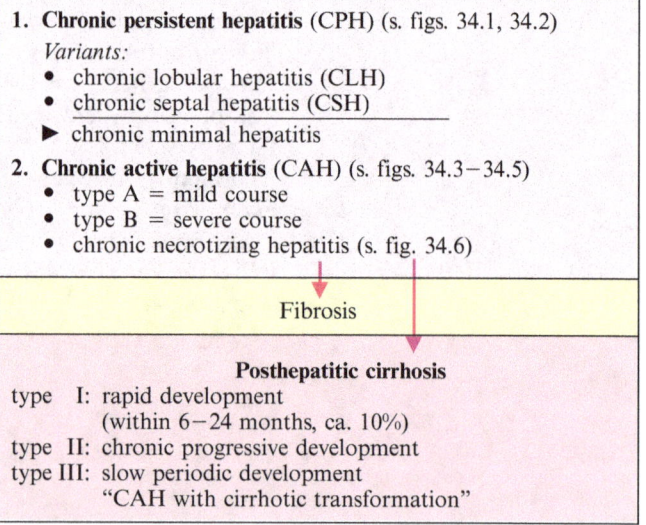

Tab. 34.1: Schematized morphological classification of chronic hepatitis and its potential to develop into fibrosis and cirrhosis

since reliable serological or immunological differentiation was not possible at that time. It should be mentioned that the differentiation of CLH was not generally accepted — although this condition is frequently seen in chronic hepatitis C. (17, 22, 24) (s. tab. 34.1)

3.2 Histological criteria

The histological criteria of chronic hepatitis are (*1.*) liver cell damage, (*2.*) inflammatory infiltration, and (*3.*) fibrosis formation. These chronic inflammatory reactions affect firstly the portal field, then the periportal region (i.e. zone 1) and finally the liver lobule. Such reactions constitute a dynamic process, whereby the intensity of the above-mentioned criteria and their topographical distribution pattern in the portal, periportal and azinar area vary considerably. (13, 15)

(*1.*) **Portal inflammation:** *Portal hepatitis* reveals varying inflammatory activity. It is common to all forms of chronic hepatitis and is composed mainly of a mixture of lymphocytes, plasma cells and macrophages. The portal inflammation may stop at the limiting plate, but can also penetrate it. In a long-term course, ductular proliferations sometimes appear at the edge of the portal field; they are accompanied by granulocytes. If the portal hepatitis shows no signs of periportal or lobular inflammation, the disease is deemed to be *inactive*. (1)

(*2.*) **Periportal inflammation:** *Periportal hepatitis* is characterized by penetration of the limiting plate. The border between the portal field and the lobule can appear irregular; sometimes it assumes the shape of a maple leaf. In this periportal zone (i.e. zone 1), piecemeal necroses may develop. They are, however, not true "necroses", but apoptoses. Today, periportal inflammation with piecemeal necrosis is termed *interface hepatitis*. This condition is not always accompanied by piecemeal necrosis; the inflammatory infiltrate can also enter the lobule without causing liver cell necroses. The composition of the inflammatory infiltrates is similar to that in the portal fields. Periportal inflammation contributes to the grading of chronic hepatitis. (1)

(*3.*) **Lobular inflammation:** Whereas lobular, diffusely distributed inflammation is more evident, in acute hepatitis portal and periportal inflammation predominates in chronic hepatitis and lobular hepatitis is less pronounced. Generally, it consists of separate small clusters of mononuclear cells. Scattered necrotic hepatocytes and *Councilman bodies* (s. p. 402) (s. fig. 34.1) are found; the hepatocellular nuclei are in disarray (= anisonucleosis); there is swelling of the hepatocytes, and mitoses are present. Marked lobular hepatitis in conjunction with considerable portal and periportal inflammation is typical of "flares" of chronic viral hepatitis or autoimmune hepatitis. In addition to single-cell necroses, there are confluent necroses, which affect entire lobules. Bridging necroses link portal tracts with other portal tracts or with terminal venules. (1)

▶ *Steatosis* is uncommon in chronic hepatitis; however, in chronic hepatitis C, steatosis is found in about 70% of cases (especially in genotype 3). Generally it is mild and non-zonal. • *Cholestasis* is rare in chronic hepatitis, but more frequent in autoimmune hepatitis.

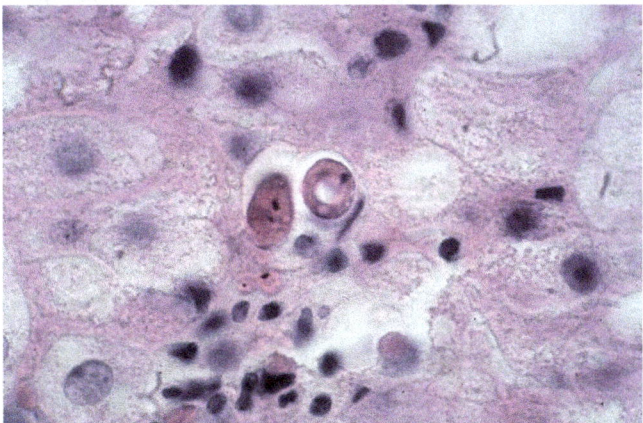

Fig. 34.1: Councilman bodies (= roundish, hyaline, eosinophilic bodies in the cytoplasm of degenerated hepatocytes) in chronic hepatitis C (HE)

3.3 Problems of designation

Various designations have been used in the literature for the multiform clinical picture of chronic hepatitis. This illustrates that in the absence of biochemical, serological and immunological test methods, chronic liver diseases with different aetiology or pathogenesis were defined almost exclusively on the basis of histological and, occasionally, laparoscopic findings as minimal chronic hepatitis, CPH, CAH, CLH or CSH. This inevitably led to widely **varying results** concerning the assessment and treatment of the different forms. • The five-year survival rate of CPH (97%), for instance, appeared to be nearly identical to that of CAH (87%) (55), i.e. these reference groups had been classified as CPH or CAH on the basis of "representative" biopsy specimens — yet according to current classification based on statistical evaluation, they showed a largely identical composition. • The chronic inflammatory reactions are by no means stationary, but constitute a fluent process with transitions and overlaps. • *Depending on the respective aetiopathogenesis, chronic hepatitis may vary greatly in its degree of severity with regard to segmental and focal lesions.* This significant finding, which was already made some 30 years ago(!), is most certainly worth recalling (s. p. 189 and there quot.: 155) • *The situation is further complicated by the fact that only a relatively small area of the right lobe of liver is accessible for histological examination by way of percutaneous biopsy.* Therefore, a specimen from this area is not necessarily representative for other parts of the liver! (s. fig. 7.8) (s. p. 697)

3.4 Classification (1994)

Increasing knowledge about HCV infection revealed that histological findings frequently suggest a seemingly favourable prognosis for CPH despite the high risk that chronic hepatitis and even cirrhosis may develop. (80) With the possibility of more exact serological and immunological differentiation, the previously used classification proved increasingly artificial and problematic. It was time to assess chronic hepatitis according to aetiopathogenetic criteria. • *The current classification of chronic hepatitis is based on:* (*1.*) aetiology of the disease, (*2.*) activity of the inflammatory process (= grading), and (*3.*) degree of fibrosis (= staging). (1, 8, 12) (s. tabs. 34.2, 34.3) (s. figs. 34.2 – 34.9)

(*1.*) **Aetiology** is based on laboratory parameters, serology, immunology or PCR. Immunohistochemical evidence of HBsAg and HBcAg may, in individual cases, confirm HBV infection as the cause of "cryptogenic" chronic hepatitis. By evaluating the number and the relative proportions of HBs-positive and HBc-positive cells, chronic hepatitis B can also be differentiated from HBs-carrier status or (acute or prolonged) HBV infection; the presence of antibodies against HAAg and HDAg also provides verification of a specific superinfection. • The term chronic hepatitis includes several different types: (*1.*) *chronic viral hepatitis*, (*2.*) *chronic toxic hepatitis*, (*3.*) *chronic autoimmune hepatitis*, (*4.*) *chronic metabolic hepatitis*, and (*5.*) *chronic cryptogenic hepatitis*. • Apart from that, there are numerous other pathological processes which can trigger chronic hepatitis. The coincidence of two (or three) causative factors may result in such a dis-

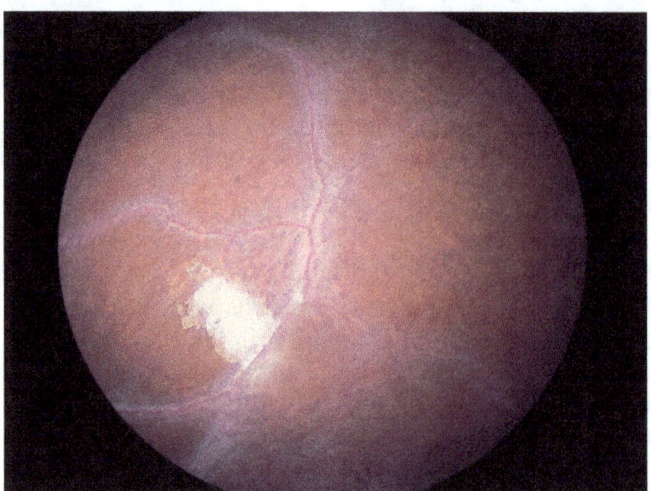

Fig. 34.2: Chronic persistent hepatitis: smooth liver surface with spotted, brick-red-coloured pattern. Clearly pronounced blood vessels with perivascular connective tissue, fine perilobular fibrosis

ease. Obviously, the severity and prognosis of chronic hepatitis primarily depend on the cause(s). (s. tab. 34.5)

(*2.*) **Grading** *describes the necroinflammatory activity*, which is based on (*1.*) hepatocellular damage, (*2.*) liver cell death, and (*3.*) inflammatory infiltration. Previously used terms such as CPH, CLH and CAH only represented grading, but not staging. The degree of activity ranges between minimal and severe. Various forms of *necrosis* are present: (*1.*) focal necrosis, (*2.*) confluent (bridging) necrosis, or (*3.*) periportal/periseptal piecemeal necrosis. (1) • The predominantly lymphocytic infiltrations of the portal fields can result in lesions of the bile ducts located in that area. The inflammatory changes

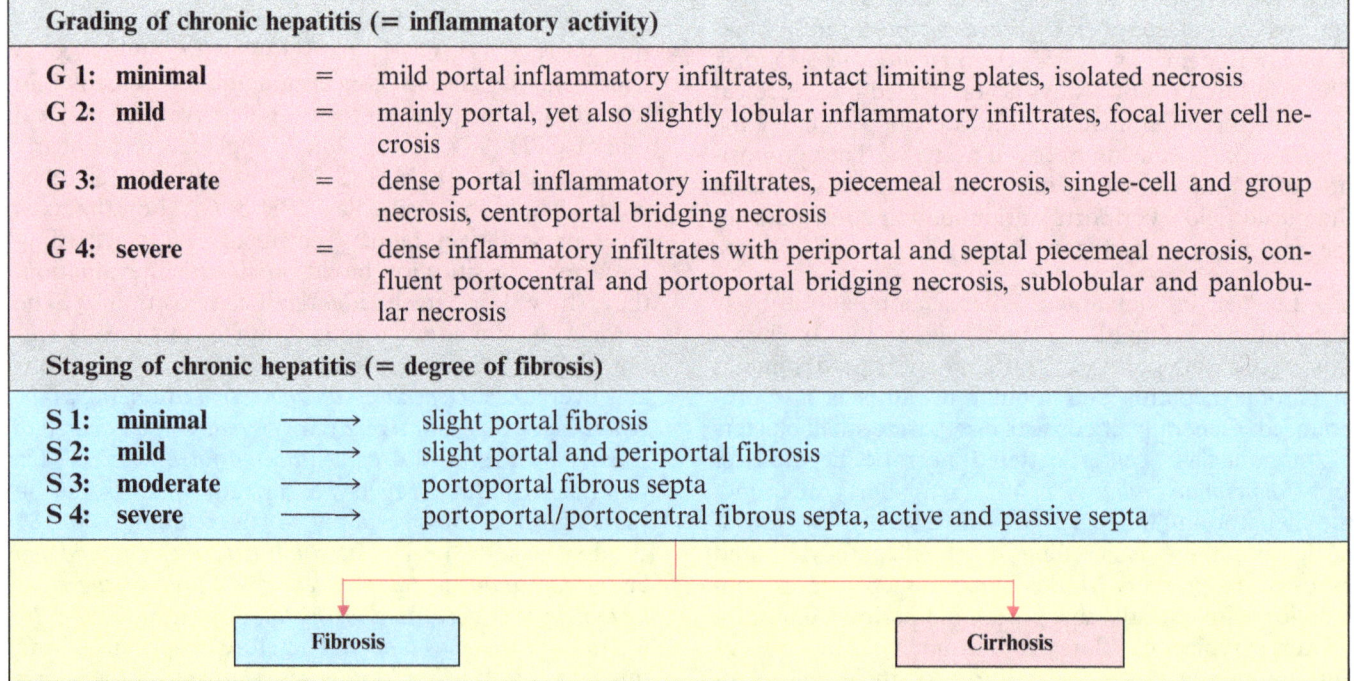

Tab. 34.2: Grades of activity and stages of fibrosis in chronic hepatitis (with abbreviations of classification: **G** 1–4, **S** 1–4)

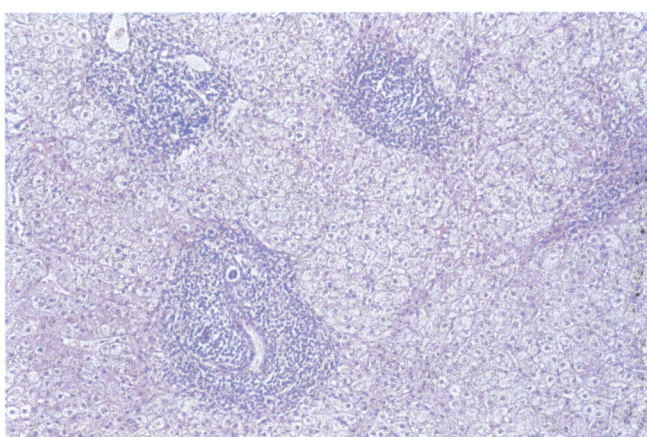

Fig. 34.3: Chronic portal hepatitis with dense lymphocytic infiltration of enlarged portal tracts (HE)

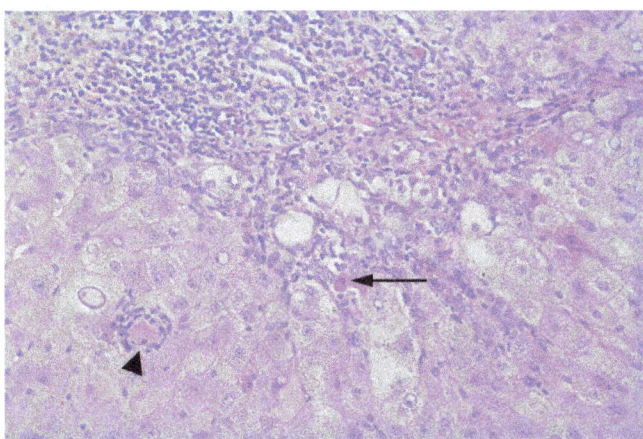

Fig. 34.5: Chronic active hepatitis with periportal piecemeal necrosis (→) and apoptosis (▶) in the lobular parenchyma (HE)

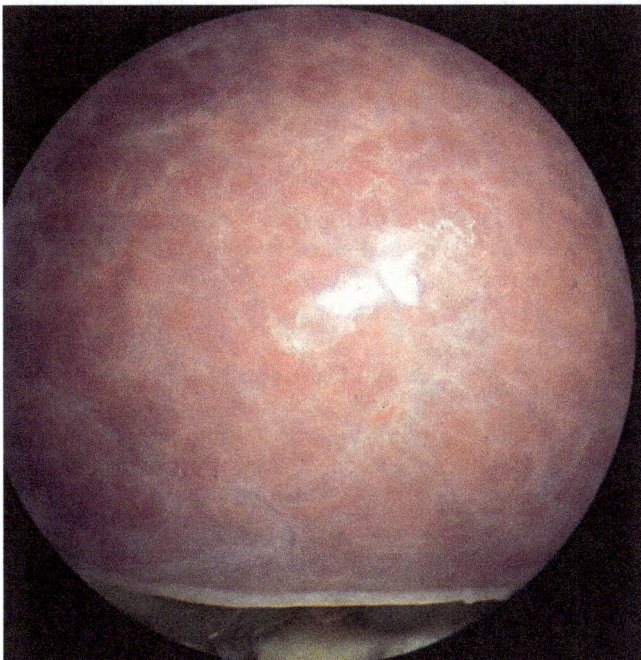

Fig. 34.4: Chronic active hepatitis: flat, undulatory liver surface ("scattered light reflection") with pronounced fibrosis, scarring and a marked rim of connective tissue in the left lobe of liver. Red spots due to highly inflammatory parenchymal areas. Isolated fine blood vessels and distinct lymphatic congestion

G 1: Minimal chronic hepatitis
- loose lymphocytic infiltrate, single-cell necroses
- slightly widened portal fields, intact limiting plate

G 2: Mild chronic hepatitis
- more dense lymphocytic infiltrates
- widening of portal fields
- lymphoid/pseudolymphoid follicles
- single-cell and (rare) group necroses
- damaged limiting plate (piecemeal necroses)

G 3: Moderate chronic hepatitis
- numerous piecemeal necroses, clearly widened portal fields
- dominant lymphocytes, liver cell rosettes
- pronounced necroses in the parenchyma
- dense inflammatory infiltrates in the lobule

G 4: Severe chronic hepatitis
- bridging necroses, greater number of piecemeal necroses
- street-like hepatocyte decay with lymphocytic infiltrates
- structural disorder of the liver

Tab. 34.3: Chronic hepatitis: grading of the inflammatory activity (G 1—4)

then spread to the limiting plate and subsequently to the lobule. Single-cell and group necrosis as well as confluent bridging necrosis occur. • If there are no or insufficient histological results, the values of the indicator enzymes (GPT, GOT, GDH) in combination with the DeRitis ratio and increases in γ-globulin and immunoglobulin levels (e.g. in autoimmune hepatitis) may serve as substitute parameters for assessing disease activity.

(*3.*) **Staging** reflects the degree of architectural alterations due to (*1.*) fibrosis and (*2.*) cirrhosis. Fibrosis may be portal, periportal, bridging portoportal or bridging portocentral. Glisson's capsule is also involved in fibrogenesis. The extent of fibrosis facilitates assessment of both the stage of chronic hepatitis and its progression to cirrhosis. Fibrosis is differentiated using the scale of "none" through to "severe". • *For reasons of simplification, the abbreviations G 1—4 and S 1—4 are suggested.* (s. tabs. 34.2—34.4) (s. figs. 34.2—34.9)

▶ **Fibrosis:** Due to the necroinflammatory process, fibrogenesis is activated (s. p. 410); it begins in the portal fields and leads to their fibrotic dilation. Fibrosis extends to the periportal zones and can ultimately link portal tracts to other portal tracts and to terminal hepatic venules. Reliable staging requires connective tissue stains, because with haemotoxylin and eosin stains, the true extent of the fibrosing process is often underestimated. Especially in chronic hepatitis C, fibrosis shows great variability. Subsequently, active and passive

> **S 1: Minimal fibrosis**
> – mild fibrous expansion of the portal fields
> – unchanged parenchyma
>
> **S 2: Mild fibrosis**
> – distinct fibrous widening of the portal fields
> – periportal fibrosis with fine strands in zone 1
>
> **S 3: Moderate fibrosis**
> – complete connective-tissue septa
> – portoportal and portocentral septa
>
> **S 4: Severe fibrosis**
> – pronounced formation of bridging fibrosis
> – transition into cirrhosis cannot be ruled out
> – nodular regeneration

Tab. 34.4: Chronic hepatitis: staging of the degree of fibrosis (S 1–4)

fibrous septa form (s. p. 414); regenerative nodules appear, pointing to the development of cirrhosis.

Due to the borderline morphology, it is impossible to draw a clear distinction between CPH and CAH, particularly with regard to chronic hepatitis C. Such cases should be classified as minimally active CAH (2), since they carry the risk of cirrhosis formation. The histological picture of CPH-C should therefore not be equated with continuous morphological inactivity and favourable prognosis; it is inadvisable to leave such a condition untreated, as is sometimes suggested. Chronic inflammation always has to be regarded as a fluent process, which may vary toporegionally. Histological findings are of great importance, but nevertheless only temporary (and possibly local) in nature. • The findings of *"chronic hepatitis"* (= chronic inflammatory process) and *"cirrhosis"* (= structural transformation of the hepatic lobular architecture) may overlap toporegionally. This problem of nomenclature is sometimes dealt with by using the term *"cirrhosis with CAH"*. (9)

Scoring systems: Semiquantitative systems have been proposed for classifying the results of grading and staging. (1, 3, 7, 16, 18–21, 24) They seem more practicable for scientific studies than for daily practice. (1) There is one particular system which can be recommended for histological scoring with regard to chronic hepatitis; it represents a modification of proposals. (s. tabs. 34.2, 34.3)

Histological activity index: The histological components of chronic hepatitis can be evaluated semiquantitatively and summarized in a histological activity index (HAI). This index combines the values for the inflammatory infiltrate, liver cell necrosis and fibrosis in an end score. (14) • The HAI modified in 1995 considers all aspects of criticism mentioned in this context and has proved very useful for comparative observations regarding the course of disease. (12)

At the end of the morphological development of chronic hepatitis, aetiologically defined **cirrhosis** occurs in a certain percentage of cases. In this connection, no "primary" cirrhosis exists (as with the exclusively historical term "primary" biliary cirrhosis). (s. p. 679) Even though cryptogenic cirrhosis may be in evidence, *the term "primary" is not acceptable because cirrhosis is not a "primary" occurrence!*

4 Aetiology and differential diagnosis

More than 600 million people are suffering from chronic hepatitis of different aetiology worldwide. Most of the diseases included in the syndrome of acute hepatitis (s. fig. 22.6) may also develop into chronic hepatitis. The latter is therefore considered to be a **syndrome**, i.e. *heterogeneous group* of chronic inflammatory liver diseases. • In most cases, chronic hepatitis is caused by the hepatitis viruses B, C, B/D, possibly also C/G and GB-C. • *However, a case of chronic hepatitis due to HAV infection was reported for the first time by K. INOUE et al. in 1996.* (25) • Isolated cases of chronic hepatitis caused by bacteria or secondary hepatotropic viruses are known, e.g. Q fever (P. ATIENZA et al., 1988), CMV (118), Epstein-Barr virus. • Chronic hepatic autoimmunopathies are more common than has hitherto been assumed (10–20%). Toxic liver damage may pose great problems in differential diagnosis. Fulminant liver failure can also develop into chronic hepatitis. Genetic and/or metabolic diseases are relatively rare, but should always be taken into account in the broad spectrum of chronic hepatitis. All of these possibilities which must be considered in the differential diagnosis require their own specific diagnostic parameters. (s. tab. 34.5)

Cryptogenic CAH: All chronic inflammatory liver diseases that have not yet been fully clarified as regards their aetiology are subsumed in the group of cryptogenic chronic hepatitis (15–20%). • As a result of improved biochemical, serological, immunological and histological/histochemical test procedures, this group is diminishing in terms of figures. *It can be expected that there will be further "revelations" concerning differential diagnostics in the near future and that the cryptogenic chronic hepatitis group will gradually disappear.*

Posthepatitic CAH: In terms of frequency, chronic hepatitis caused by hepatitis viruses (B, C, B/D) clearly predominates. (s. tab. 34.5) Because of their great epidemiological and prognostic relevance, treatment of these viral forms of chronic hepatitis has become a central issue, particularly since the use of newly-developed compounds has facilitated genuine therapeutic success for the first time. Until recently, no antiviral compounds were available – hence, a real breakthrough has now been achieved.

Non-viral CAH: It should be noted that the treatment of non-viral causes of chronic hepatitis is discussed in separate chapters covering the respective clinical pictures. (s. tab. 34.5)

---

1. **Primary hepatotropic viruses** *(see chapter 22)*
   - Hepatitis (A?) (s. p. 430!)   – Hepatitis C
   - Hepatitis B, B/D   – Hepatitis C/G
2. **Secondary hepatotropic viruses** *(see chapter 23)*
   - Cytomegalovirus   – Q fever
   - Epstein-Barr virus
3. **Bacterial infection** *(see chapter 24)*
4. **Parasitic infection** *(see chapter 25)*
5. **Toxic causes**
   - Alcohol *(see chapter 28)*
   - Drugs *(see chapter 29)*
   - Chemicals *(see chapter 30)*
6. **Genetic/metabolic aetiology** *(see chapter 31)*
   - Abetalipoproteinaemia
   - α_1-antitrypsin deficiency
   - Chronic hepatic porphyria
   - Glycogen storage disease
   - Galactosaemia
   - Haemochromatosis
   - Mucoviscidosis
   - Wilson's disease
7. **Autoimmunopathies**
   - Autoimmune hepatitis *(see chapter 32)*
   - Primary biliary cholangitis *(see chapter 33)*
   - Primary sclerosing cholangitis *(see chapter 33)*
   - Autoimmune cholangitis *(see chapter 33)*
   - Overlap syndrome *(see chapter 33)*
8. **Chronic cardiac liver congestion**
9. **Immunological rejection following transplantation**
10. **Malignant lymphoma mimicking CAH**
11. **Cryptogenic chronic hepatitis**

Tab. 34.5: Aetiology and differential diagnosis of chronic hepatitis (see respective chapter for more details)

5 Diagnosis

5.1 Clinical findings

Chronic hepatitis may take an **asymptomatic course** for several years, both subjectively and in terms of clinical findings. Frequently, it is only noticed by chance. In some cases, liver cirrhosis may be present at initial diagnosis. • **Symptomatic courses** are most commonly characterized by chronic fatigue (so-called *"pain of the liver"*), exhaustion and reduced performance; occasionally, patients suffer from malaise, loss of appetite, nausea, intolerance of certain foodstuffs and meteorism as well as myalgia and arthralgia. The complaints are often discrete and variable – but also non-specific, which easily leads to misinterpretation. (s. p. 81) • **Clinical findings**, such as hepatomegaly, skin stigmata of liver disease (s. p. 84) or urobilinogenuria, usually only become manifest after prolonged disease. In the majority of cases, acute episodes are accompanied by low-grade jaundice. (17, 41, 43)

5.2 Laboratory findings

Initially, laboratory findings are ambiguous. There is a moderate increase in GPT, GOT, GDH and γ-GT. In toxic and cholestatic forms, γ-GT and AP are correspondingly elevated. Cholinesterase is generally reduced. The rise in the transaminases is a sign of enzymatic activity, which usually correlates to a greater or lesser extent with histological activity. The elevation of γ-globulins and immunoglobulins is a sign of mesenchymal activity (s. p. 116); it is also an expression of the severity of fibrosis. The latter may be recognized by the rise in serum P III P and hyaluronic acid values. (103, 115) (s. p. 118) Zinc deficiency is frequently found, albeit less pronounced than in cirrhosis • However – as has been mentioned above – no exact diagnosis is possible yet. • Subsequent diagnostic procedures should include *specific parameters*. Viral serology is examined step by step and, in the case of suspicion, also the antibody profile (e.g. ANA, SMA, LKM, LP); in cholestatic forms, AMA and pANCA are likewise determined. (s. tabs. 5.20; 32.1) Metabolic liver diseases require individual laboratory tests, such as copper, ferritin, porphyrins or α_1-antitrypsin.

The *fourfold enzyme pattern*, which is compiled by adding alkaline phosphatase to the threefold pattern, has proved useful as a general screening test. Hereby, non-responders who do not show a γ-GT increase in cholestasis (2–3%) are also detected. Liver disease is confirmed or ruled out with a probability of 96–97%. (s. tab. 5.11) • Further diagnostic clues are rapidly and easily obtained by means of *enzyme ratios*. (s. tabs. 5.6, 5.7)

5.3 Morphology

It is beneficial to establish the morphological diagnosis during the first investigation by targeted **liver biopsy** (right and left lobes of liver) using **laparoscopy**. The structure of the liver surface should be recorded photographically. Examination of the biopsy specimens with UV light is essential. The sensitivity of percutaneous liver biopsy in chronic hepatitis is 75–80%, but 98% for laparoscopy plus biopsy (R. ORLANDO et al., 1990) and about 100% for biopsy specimens collected from both liver lobes. (5, 6, 9, 11, 63, 102) (s. fig. 7.10) (s. pp 151, 165, 720) • Any development of fibrosis must be detected. For this purpose, biochemical parameters (e.g. hyaluronic acid, P-III-P, platelet ratio index, GOT/platelet ratio index) and sonography (elastography, splenic arterial pulsatility index) are available. (98, 109)

▶ It should always be remembered that this method shows great variability (about 1 level in grading and staging) in some 30% of cases. (132) More precisely, the morphological result of the pathologist only applies to the examined biopsy specimen and cannot be seen as fully representative, e. g. in chronic hepatitis. This may lead to controversial results in different studies.

5.4 Imaging techniques

Imaging techniques (with the exception of ERC, e. g. in PSC) are generally of no diagnostic value in chronic hepatitis prior to the development of cirrhosis. • *Sonography* is regarded as a basic, routine examination and is always indicated in cholestatic diseases or suspected cirrhosis. (9) There is often evidence of abdominal lymphadenopathy (especially of the hepatoduodenal ligament), which points to a more severe histological picture. (23, 31) Examining the increase in liver stiffness by means of elastography makes it possible to minitor the development of fibrosis. • *CT* should be carried out in cases where α_1-foetoprotein, which is initially subject to regular monitoring at longer intervals, shows a continuous increase, thus arousing suspicion of the development of hepatocellular carcinoma. • Any further development of fibrosis or cirrhosis can be observed using xenon CT. In concordance with the histopathological stages, *^{1}H-MR spectroscopy* indicated the severity of fibrosis in chronic hepatitis. This imaging technique was suggested as a potential substitute for liver biopsy in staging chronic hepatitis. (4)

6 Course and prognosis

6.1 Course

The natural course and dynamics of chronic hepatitis are determined by the **underlying disease**. In line with the multiplicity of causes, the disease course is highly variable: on the one hand, there are courses which remain virtually static for years ("chronic persistent") – i. e. chronic hepatitis shows no changes in terms of clinical, biochemical and histological findings; on the other hand, there are chronic active courses, which progress rapidly ("chronic aggressive"), as well as "necrotic" hepatitis, which may result in cirrhosis within a few months (!). In contrast, remission periods of varying duration may also be observed. • The question of *"why"* the disease shows **chronification** in individual cases or *"why"* there is sometimes evidence of **exacerbation** remains unanswered. However, there are several possible causes which are cumulative or may even potentiate each other. Thus, course of disease and therapy success are strongly influenced by the individual genotype of HBV (39, 51, 58), lipid peroxidation (33) and microcirculatory disturbances. (36) (s. tab. 34.6)

Basis for initial prognosis
1. Early or late diagnosis
2. Underlying disease
3. Available therapy regimens
Risk factors
1. **Impaired immune system** • genetically determined • endogenously induced • exogenously induced
2. **Endogenous mechanisms of impairment** • hepatitis virus mutations • endocrine imbalance • toxins
3. **Exogenous factors** • alcohol • drug addiction • drugs • infections • chemicals • malnutrition
4. **Lipid peroxidation**
5. **Extrahepatic manifestations**

Tab. 34.6: Prognostic factors and possible causes of chronification, exacerbation or reactivation in hepatitis

The severity of *liver cell necrosis* is the focal point of the pathogenetic process; it determines both the dynamics and variability of the course of disease. Liver cell necrosis may result from (*1.*) direct damage by the causative factor, (*2.*) free radicals and lipid peroxidation (s. fig. 21.12) (s. pp 73, 408), and (*3.*) inadequate activation of CD4+ and CD8+ T lymphocytes in viral infection. • Lymphocytic infiltrates develop together with liver cell necrosis and the activation of phagocytosis. There is an increase in fibrosis with the associated deterioration in metabolic activity and thus further liver cell necrosis. (s. p. 407) Liver cells proliferate and regeneration nodes form, leading to more distortion and rarefaction of the vascular architecture. • Persistent liver cell necrosis continues to activate the cascade of proliferation processes and cause *fibrosis*: chronic inflammatory liver disease progresses to cirrhosis. Development of cirrhosis occurs with a probable frequency of 2–3% per year, i. e. a cumulative frequency of 15–20% in five years. In 2,215 patients with chronic viral hepatitis, the rate of development of cirrhosis was 7.6%, 21.7% and 32.2% in the 5th, 10th and 15th year respectively (K. IKEDA et al., 1998). Highly active CAH (type B) leads to the development of cirrhosis after seven years in 80–85% of cases, with a mortality rate of 40–45%. (32, 38, 44, 128) • Should the damaging process come to a halt with no further liver cell necrosis, *spontaneous remission* occurs in approx. 3% of cases per year, or partial recovery takes place with defective healing at the respective stage of (generally irreversible) liver fibrosis. (83, 88, 91, 101, 103, 114, 115, 164) Depending on the severity and localization of fibrosis and on the perfusion resistance, portal hypertension can develop. (17, 34, 44, 55, 133)

6.2 Extrahepatic manifestations

Extrahepatic disease manifestations associated with chronic hepatitis B and C are frequent; about 40 forms, mainly autoimmune disorders, have been reported up to now. (s. tabs. 22.2, 22.7, 22.8, 32.2, 33.3, 33.6,) A reliable association of these manifestations with HBV and HCV is not known, nor is a true frequency given. The most common association is found with HCV infection. Apparently, HCV has tropism for cells other than hepatocytes, particularly lymphocytes. Therefore it has been postulated that the HCV infection of lymphocytes may be the "cause" of a greater number of extrahepatic (especially autoimmune) diseases. A selection of extrahepatic manifestations shows the wide clinical spectrum of these disorders. (59, 81, 104, 111, 142) (s. tab. 34.7)

Mixed cryoglobulinaemia: The term cryoglobulinaemia was first used by A.B. LERNER et al. in 1947. Clinical manifestation consists of the *Meltzer triad*: *(1.)* weakness, *(2.)* arthralgias, and *(3.)* palpable purpura (M. MELTZER et al., 1966) as well as other clinical features, including glomerulonephritis, hepatomegaly, splenomegaly and lymphadenopathy. Morphologically, there is predominant leucocytoclastic vasculitis involving medium and small-sized arteries with deposition of immunocomplexes in the vessel walls and subsequent inflammatory reactions. An association with HBV infection was first described by Y. LEVO et al. in 1973 and with HCV infection by M. PASCUAL et al. in 1990. There are three forms of cryoglobulinaemia, whereby type II consists of monoclonal IgM and polyclonal IgG and type III of polyclonal IgM with RF activity. The *course* is mostly asymptomatic. The prognosis is unpredictable in the individual case. • *Therapy* of the HCV-associated form is with IFNα + ribavirin, more recently with anti-CD20 antibody rituximab (F. ZAJA et al., 1999). (124)

Antiphospholipid syndrome	Non-Hodgkin's lymphoma
Behcet's syndrome	Pancreatitis
Chronic fatigue syndrome	Pleural effusion (40)
CREST syndrome	Polyartheriitis nodosa
Cryoglobulinaemia (97, 134)	Polymyositis
Dermatomyositis (69)	Porphyria cutanea tarda
Diabetes mellitus	Pulmonary fibrosis
Fibromyalgia	Sarcoidosis
Glomerulonephritis	Schönlein-Henoch purpura
Guillain-Barré syndrome	Sialadenitis
Haemolytic anaemia	Sjögren's syndrome
Hypocholesterolaemia	Still's disease (35)
Lichen planus (69)	Thyreoiditis (61)
Lupus erythematodes	Urticaria
Multiple myeloma	Uveitis

Tab. 34.7: Selection of extrahepatic disease manifestations associated with HBV or HCV infection (with some references)

6.3 Hepatocellular carcinoma

It is likely that the development of hepatocellular carcinoma is predominantly due to chronic regeneration. Usually, cirrhosis precedes the development of HCC by several years. The risk of developing HCC in HBV or HCV infection with cirrhosis is about 3–5% of cases/year. However, individual cases of HCC without cirrhosis have also been reported. • Direct carcinogenic defects are assumed for hepatitis B (30) and hepatitis C (70) as well as for haemochromatosis and alcohol-related disease. In 2,215 patients with chronic viral hepatitis B or C, the rate of development to HCC was as follows: 2.1/4.8% in the 5th year, 4.9/13.6% in the 10th year and 18.8/26.0% in the 15th year (K. IKEDA et. al., 1998). • Vaccination against HBV infection prevents the development of HCC. (30) Successful treatment of chronic hepatitis C using IFN considerably lowers the risk of HCC. An increased frequency of HCC has been observed in all kinds of cirrhosis, regardless of aetiology. The period prior to the development of cirrhosis and the subsequent occurrence of HCC is decisively influenced by the underlying cause. • Regular, periodic monitoring of $α_1$-*foetoprotein* together with *sonography* is initially indicated. A continuous increase in $α_1$FP requires investigations by **CT** (and *laparoscopy*) for suspected HCC. (s. pp 442, 453, 799)

6.4 Prognosis

The prognosis for chronic hepatitis is unfavourable. Depending on its aetiology, the individual course varies and is therefore difficult to predict. Prognosis depends on: *(1.)* early diagnosis, *(2.)* the nature of the underlying disease, and *(3.)* the therapeutic possibilities available. The initial prognosis may be greatly worsened by immunological, endogenous and exogenous risk factors (s. tab. 34.5), e.g. childhood (29) and advanced age, high viral load and special viral characteristics. (34, 37, 39, 46, 51, 53, 133, 136)

It is noteworthy that HBV DNA may persist in the serum and liver despite the elimination of HBsAg. Contrary to early reports, carefully performed long-term studies have shown that the prognosis is essentially more favourable with exact diagnosis and appropriate long-term treatment. (47) • Coinfection with HGV and GBV-C or HCV is frequent, but it has no influence on the course and severity of chronic hepatitis C or on liver transplantation. (66)

6.5 Chronic HBV infection

Frequency: The frequency of chronic hepatitis following acute HBV infection is 5–10% of cases. The total number of patients with chronic infection B is estimated at 350–400 million worldwide, in Germany about 500,000. HBV infection in childhood leads to a higher rate of chronicity. The lethality rate can be as high as 1%. *(see chapter 22.4!)*

Causes: In addition to the basic risk factors (s. tab. 34.5), possible causes of chronicity in HBV infection also include weak or non-existent virus-specific T cell activation, reduced interferon production and the occurrence of an HBeAg-minus variant.

Morphology: There can be evidence of HBc-containing liver cell nuclei, (= *sanded nuclei*) and *ground glass hepatocytes*. The latter have homogeneous, glassy, slightly eosinophilic cytoplasm, which immunohistochemically displays a positive HBsAg reaction. This condition is probably a result of an abnormal composition of the HBsAg; in this special form, it cannot be discharged by hepatocytes. (54) (s. pp 120, 432) (s. fig. 22.8) HBsAg is stained with orcein in the hepatocytes only in HBV carriers and chronic hepatitis B (but not in the acute phase). (s. fig. 5.7) *Mallory-Denk bodies* are encountered more rarely than in chronic hepatitis C.

Serology: Based on quantitative determination of certain serological markers, **three stages** of chronic hepatitis B are distinguished: These are (*1.*) high-replication phase with excessive HBcAg expression in the liver, positivity of HBsAg, HBeAg and DNA, moderately increased transaminases (= immunotolerant), (*2.*) low-replication phase with increase in transaminases, decrease in DNA titre and positivity of anti-HBc (= immunoactive), and (*3.*) healing process. Minimal replication ($<10^5$ copies/ml in PCR) may persist with HBeAg negativity. This may cause a more severe course or even the much-feared "reinfection" of the liver transplant. (26, 49) • **Seroconversion** marks a transition from the high-replication phase to the low-replication phase: loss of HBeAg and presence of anti-HBe, with the transaminases simultaneously reduced or normalized. (28, 47) In the spontaneous course of chronic hepatitis B, seroconversion occurs every year in 1–3% (= HBsAg to anti-HBs) or 10–15% (= HBeAg to anti-HBe) of cases. Perinatally transmitted HBV may be spontaneously eliminated during a period of 30–40 years (K. ÖRDÖG et al., 2003). • Shortly before or during IFN-induced seroconversion, a transitory **inflammatory episode** with elevation of GPT, GOT and GDH in the serum (= *flare-up*) is frequently observed. With subsidence of this reaction and normalization of the transaminases, HBeAg is usually no longer detectable. Reactivation is rare, but can be triggered by various factors, such as cytostatics (56), etc. Carriers of chronic hepatitis B are quite frequent. (27, 53) Their urine may be infectious. (s. figs. 34.6, 34.7)

The **healing process**, which is the third phase (HBsAg, HBeAg and HBV RNA negativity as well as anti-HBs and anti-HBe positivity together with normalization of GPT), is rarely spontaneous. • After HBeAg elimination with permanent remission and anti-HBe positivity, **two serological courses** may also occur: (*1.*) persistence of

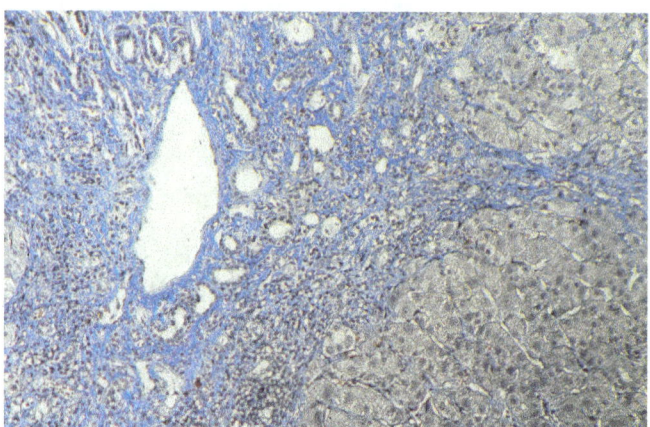

Fig. 34.6: Chronic, mildly active hepatitis B with pronounced periportal and septal fibrosis (as a sequela of previous inflammatory episodes) (Ladewig)

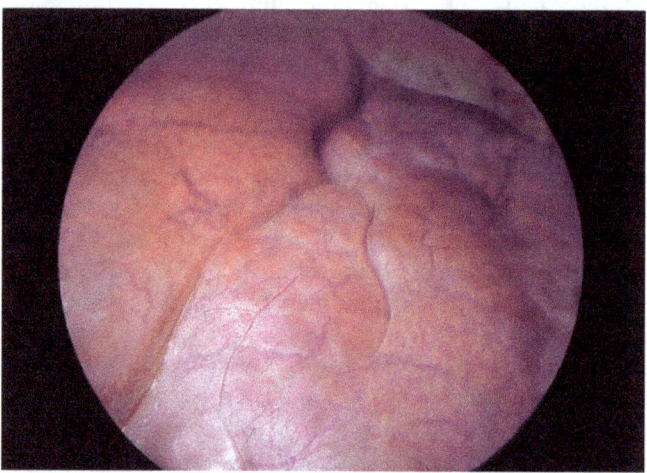

Fig. 34.7: Chronic necrotizing hepatitis B: marked postnecrotic cleft formation in the area of the left lobe of liver (10 months after severe, acute necrotic hepatitis). Brownish to brick-red colouring of the liver with a flat, undulatory surface, scarry indentations, proliferation of connective tissue and spots of capsular fibrosis. Fine hypervascular arteries, pronounced venous contours and isolated lymph vessel congestion

chronic hepatitis B despite the presence of anti-HBe and (*2.*) transient anti-HBe positivity with recurrence of HBeAg (30% of cases) as well as exacerbation and persistence of chronic hepatitis B.

In 10–30% of cases, **cirrhosis** appears with high morbidity and mortality, 3–6%/year. A clear reduction in the development of cirrhosis was achieved by administration of colchicine (5 mg/week) for a period of four years. The 10-year survival rate is 89% in CPH, 74% in CAH and as low as 47% in cirrhosis. • The frequency of **HCC** in patients with cirrhosis B is about 2%/year, i.e. the risk is approx. 200 times higher than in healthy subjects. (32, 46, 48, 52, 57) Development of HCC is closely associated with the seromarker status: the frequency of HCC was 87% in positivity of HBsAg and HBeAg, in HBsAg alone 12%, and in negativity of both markers only a rare event (1% of cases). (57)

6.6 Chronic HCV infection

The number of people suffering from chronic hepatitis C is estimated at approx. 200 million worldwide; in Germany the number is 600,000–800,000 (105, 136) If an HCV infection has not been registered, there is obligation of notification for chronic hepatitis. • Genotypes 1–3 have been observed worldwide, genotypes 4–5 predominantly in the Middle East or Africa, and genotype 6 in Asia. Different genotypes may be detected in a single patient at the same time or at different stages of the disease. The prognosis of an HCV infection differs in relation to the genotype *(see chapter 22.5!)*

Diagnosis: The level of *HCV-IgM antibody* titres correlates with the degree of severity of chronic hepatitis C. Evidence of anti-HCV is an important clue, but it can be interpreted as *(1.)* acute infection, *(2.)* chronic infection, *(3.)* carrier status, or *(4.)* non-infectious immune status. It should be noted that a negative test does not exclude viraemia. Infection can only be detected on the basis of HCV RNA using the PCR method; this is possible just a few days after infection. • A correlation (albeit only of minor significance) between the serum titre of HCV RNA and the level of the *transaminases* is controversial. Evidence of elevated transaminases requires differential diagnostic clarification, which may result in confirmation of HCV infection. The transaminases are a good marker for chronic hepatitis C (generally being threefold to fivefold the norm); the GPT/GOT ratio may point to the development of cirrhosis. Often (about 30%), however, stages of chronic hepatitis C with normal transaminases are found. (117) They correlate well with modest proliferation and apoptosis as well as with the development of low-degree fibrosis, particularly during simultaneous abstinence from alcohol.

In long-term follow-ups, the transaminases frequently display major fluctuations in activity (rise and fall before reaching their normal level). (43) Occasionally, there is a remarkable elevation of *γ-GT*, which is often even higher than GPT, initially raising suspicion of alcohol-induced liver damage. (131) In patients with increased γ-GT (particularly with a rise in AP), more severe damage of the bile ductules is evident. A decrease in hepatic function and a rise in gamma globulins and P III P can only be found during the development of cirrhosis. In most cases, the course of disease is anicteric. • Frequently, a rise in serum iron, ferritin and iron-binding capacity as well as increased iron resorption are observed. • *Autoantibodies* are often found: ANA and/or SMA (15–20%), LKM 1 (5–10%), AMA (1–2%); anti-GOR is detectable in 70–80% of patients. (67) (s. p. 659) Anti-GOR titres correlate with both therapeutic success and relapses. • Extrahepatic immunopathies are common and multifaceted. (59, 104, 111) (s. tab. 34.7) Cryoglobulinaemia was in evidence in 40–50% of cases. It did not influence IFN therapy. (97, 134)

Coinfections: HGV-C has no deleterious effect on the course or treatment of chronic hepatitis C (107) despite conflicting observations. The simultaneous detection of TT viruses in the serum or hepatocytes, particularly with type 1b and at an advanced stage of the disease, does not have an unfavourable effect (140). Coinfection with HBV leads to aggravation of the condition. Acute hepatic failure must also be anticipated, as is the case in HAV and HBV concomitance. (135) Active inoculation is therefore recommended for lack of immunity against HAV and HBV.

Perihepatic lymphadenopathy: This symptom was observed in chronic hepatitis in 1994 by K. LYTTKENS et al. using sonography. It is common in both chronic hepatitis C and (60–100% of cases) and chronic hepatitis B – even with normal liver values. (93) There is a correlation between lymph node volume and hepatic inflammatory activity or viraemia. A decrease in the total volume of lymph nodes is associated with a sustained virological response and an improvement in liver histology. (72, 108, 137, 141)

Morphology: After routine sonographic examination, morphology is clarified by **liver biopsy**. (62, 63, 65, 82, 85, 119, 130) Because the diagnosis is mostly established after a prolonged course of disease, liver biopsy should be carried out using **laparoscopy** to obtain more reliable morphological findings by taking specimens from both lobes of liver and inspecting the liver surface (with photodocumentation!). (s. figs. 7.16; 34.2, 34.4, 34.7) • In addition to the chronic inflammatory changes, which are often accompanied by *bile-duct lesions*, similar to PBC or AIC (76, 125!), and portal follicle-like lymphocyte aggregates, there is generally *steatosis* of the liver (40–50% of cases). Together with elevated γ-GT, this raises suspicion of alcohol-induced liver damage. (90, 99, 123) Fatty degeneration of the hepatocytes in different intensities (e.g. due to hypobetalipoproteinaemia) is attributable to chronic hepatitis C (directly or indirectly), various noxae, obesity, diabetes, etc. Genotype 3 is steatogenic. *Mallory bodies* (s. fig. 28.2!) are frequently detectable, whereas they are rare in chronic hepatitis B. Chronic lobular hepatitis accompanied by sinusoidal infiltration with lymphocytes in *single-file arrangement* is often present. • *Chronic HCV infection shows findings with great toporegional variation.* CPH and CAH (and also CLH) may therefore be present in the same liver, sometimes showing localized initial signs of transformation. Progressive fibrosis is decisive for both course and prognosis. (83, 88, 91, 101, 103, 114, 115) Lipid peroxidation products demonstrated in the liver correlate closely with fibrosis. (64, 71, 75, 95, 102, 103, 106, 127, 136) (s. tab. 34.4) (s. figs. 34.8, 34.9)

▶ *The morphological divergences in "chronic hepatitis" within the liver itself had already been noted by* L. WANNAGAT *in 1977 with the help of laparoscopy and segmental portography (s. p 189!) long before viral differentiation became possible.* • These divergences have now been taken into account in the new nomenclature.

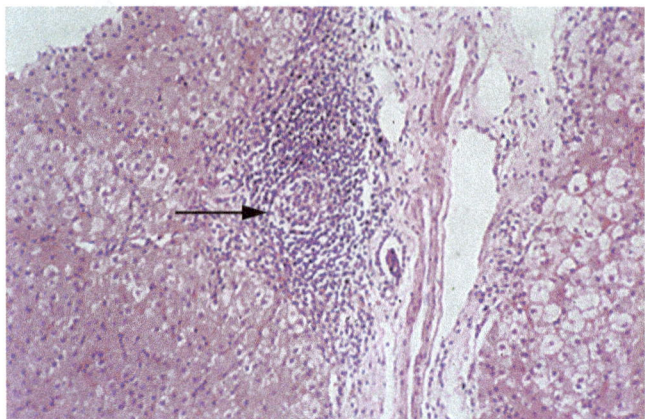

Fig. 34.8: Chronic, mildly active hepatitis C with portal lymph follicle (→) (HE)

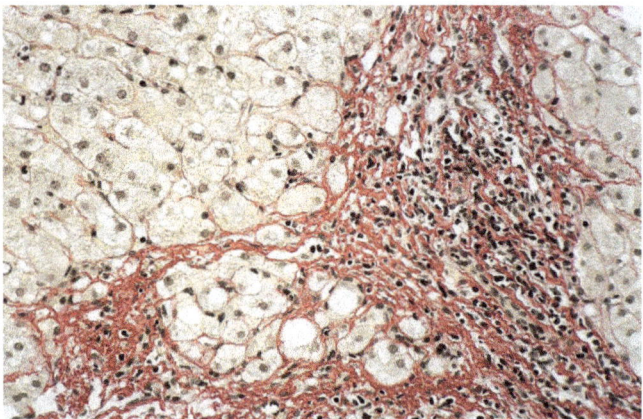

Fig. 34.9: Chronic hepatitis C with periportal and septal fibrosis (Sirius red)

Course and prognosis: The natural course of HCV infection varies from patient to patient; it is influenced by the specific *mode of infection* This remains unclarified (= sporadic) in 30−40% of cases. Possible routes of transmission for HCV infection include: i. v. drug abuse, mother-to-child infection, skin injuries, promiscuity, nosocomial infection, (122) (s. p. 450), contaminated blood products (129, 133), etc. Pregnancy and breast feeding are allowed (but not in the case of a high viral load). • Some 70−80% of acute HCV infections show an asymptomatic course, of which 50−85% develop into chronic hepatitis, i.e. HCV infection is the most frequent cause of chronic active hepatitis. • **Risk factors** are important for the course of disease. (128) Alcohol (112, 120, 121, 138, 213), iron (74, 126), obesity (88, 90, 110), insulin resistance (88, 91), smoking (87), lipid peroxidation (74) and copper overload (86) all play a decisive role. • The course itself is mostly insidious with uncharacteristic complaints such as fatigue (113, 116), decreased performance and loss of appetite. The quality of life is reduced. (78) If the regulations concerning hygiene are adhered to, there is principally no impairment in individual ability to go to work. *Neuropsychological impairment* is often observed. (77, 89, 96) In 10−30% of cases, chronic HCV infection is only recognized at the stage of cirrhosis. A total of 20−30% of patients with chronic hepatitis C develop cirrhosis within 20 years. HCC occurs in ca. 20% of cases, i.e. 2−6%/year. (70) Pretreatment fibrosis, elevated age and alcohol abuse are risk factors for development of HCC, even in SVR. About 10 (−50)% of cases develop non-Hodgkin lymphoma. (84) The development of associated lymphoproliferative diseases can be explained due to the binding of the HCV virus to the B-cell surface marker CD 81; this leads to a stimulation of B cells, resulting in lymphoproliferative disorders. (92) (s. tab. 34.7) • Some patients with anti-HCV and HCV RNA positivity did not present with pathological liver values or histological liver damage. Possibly, these cases involve a special type of HCV, or the HCV infection is not recognized by the patient's immune system. (60, 68, 73, 75, 94, 96, 106, 114, 139)

▶ **Differential diagnosis:** The following conditions should be excluded: (*1.*) alcohol-induced liver disease, (*2.*) primary biliary cholangitis (76), (*3.*) porphyria cutanea tarda (100), and (*4.*) autoimmune hepatitis (79) or autoimmune cholangitis (125) associated with anti-HCV.

6.7 Chronic HBV/HDV infection

Chronic hepatitis D generally takes a more severe course with striking histological findings. Prognosis is poor. Cirrhosis develops (particularly in superinfection with HBV replication) in 60−70% of cases − in about 15% already within one to two years. Serology shows anti-HDV, generally with HBsAg and HBeAg positivity. Serum HDV RNA is present, but often detectable only by PCR; the delta-antigen is also found in the liver tissue. CAH D cannot be reliably differentiated from CAH B by means of clinical and histological criteria. However, additional HDV infection with clear, lobular mesenchymal reactions must be considered in pronounced chronic hepatitis B. (143−146)

7 Therapy

7.1 General treatment

▶ **Physical exercise:** Excessive physical exercise should be avoided. During inflammatory episodes, which are mostly accompanied by subjective complaints, it is advisable to minimize physical effort and to lie down (= bed rest) as often as possible. Otherwise, patients may pursue their normal activities, i.e. light exercise, return to work (without overstrenuous tasks) or simple housework.

▶ **Diet:** No dietary measures are necessary in chronic hepatitis − there is no special diet for this condition. The physiological principles of nutrition should be used as a guideline. **Overweight** should be gradually reduced. • **Alcohol** is not permitted (aggravation of cell damage, increase in fibrogenesis, early development of cirrhosis,

HCC, etc.). **Hepatotoxic substances** and **smoking** should likewise be avoided.

> **Hygiene:** With potential infectiosity, all hygiene measures should be observed, if necessary in consultation with the Public Health Department. This applies to the work environment and to the question of active vaccination of family members or close contact persons against HBV (= **prophylactic vaccination ring**). (s. pp 430, 443) • In HAV or HBV negativity in chronic hepatitis C or in HAV negativity in chronic hepatitis B, the immunodeficiency should be compensated by corresponding active vaccination. • *It is essential to avoid additional viral infections.*

7.2 Therapy of chronic hepatitis B

Several compounds have been used in treating chronic viral hepatitis. Experimental and clinical studies have focused on **four groups of substances:** (*1.*) antiviral agents, (*2.*) immunostimulants, (*3.*) molecular biological agents, and (*4.*) adjuvant medicinal remedies. • *The rate of spontaneous seroconversion is 8–15%/year.*

7.2.1 Aims of treatment

An *indication for treatment* is given (*1.*) in chronic infection with considerable activity in order to avoid cirrhosis or HCC, (*2.*) in chronic infection with cirrhosis in order to avoid decompensation or HCC, and (*3.*) possibly for immunosuppressed patients or medical staff with chronic infection showing only slight activity. • The level of the transaminases and HBV-DNA values are important factors regarding the indication for therapy.

The *aims of treatment* are: (*1.*) normalization of the transaminases, (*2.*) negativity of HBeAg and reduction of HBV DNA to $<10^5$ copies/ml, and (*3.*) elimination of histological activity as well as avoidance of fibrosis. This leads to a better quality of life for the patient. The prognosis can be improved considerably if therapy-induced HBeAg negativity is reached. • Elimination of HBsAg by means of interferon is only achieved in 10–20% of cases.

▶ For the treatment of chronic hepatitis B, a fourfold **classification** has proved useful:

(1.) **Immunotolerant phase:** positivity of HBsAg and HBeAg, rise in HBV-DNA values ($>10^6$ copies/ml), normal to twofold elevated transaminases. • *No therapy* is necessary (but lamivudine or adefovir can be applied).

(2.) **Immunoactive phase:** Continued positivity of HBsAg and HBeAg, significantly elevated (>2-fold) transaminases, lower HBV-DNA values (but still $>10^5$ copies/ml). There is medium to strong necroinflammatory activity. • *Therapy* with interferon is indicated (possibly with lamivudine or adefovir).

(3.) **HBe-minus phase:** Predominance of minus mutants which can no longer synthesize HBeAg (= precore mutants). HBeAg is therefore negative, the transaminases are still more than twice the normal value, HBV-DNA levels are elevated ($>10^5$ copies/ml). • This HBeAg-negative form is found worldwide; it has a high replication rate and an increased histological index. Spontaneous remissions are less common than with the HBeAg-positive form. • *Therapy* is based on lamivudine or adefovir (possibly with interferon).

(4.) **Non-replicative phase:** HBeAg is negative, the transaminases are normal, HBV-DNA values are low ($<10^5$ copies/ml) or negative in a non-PCR procedure. • *No therapy* is required.

7.2.2 Interferon therapy

▶ Interferons (IFN) are glycoproteins with antiviral, antiproliferative and immunomodulatory properties. Besides the main types α, β and γ, other forms are available (lymphoblastoid IFNα, consensus IFNα, pegylated interferon alpha-2a). • Administration is subcutaneous. Bioavailability is about 90%. The serum peak is reached by using IFNα$_{2a}$ after 6–8 hours with a half-life of five hours or using IFNα$_{2b}$ after 3–12 hours with a half-life of three hours. Elimination is primarily via the kidneys. Interferons inhibit CYP1A2. There is no development of resistance. (154) *(see chapter 40.5.1.1!)*

Pegylated interferon: Significant improvement in the pharmacological properties of interferon was achieved by pegylation with polyethzylenglycol (PEG). (152, 176, 179, 186) (s. p. 729)

Some findings point to a good response regarding an *antiviral effect* of IFN (so-called "ideal patient") and other findings to a poor response. They are considered as selection criteria for IFN treatment. (s. tab. 34.8)

Good response ("ideal patient")
1. High GPT (>100 U/l)
2. Low HBV-DNA titre (<10^5 copies/ml)
3. Infection in adulthood
4. Short period since infection (<5 years)
5. Female
6. No coinfection, no noxae
7. Genotype A
Poor response
1. Low GPT (<100 U/l)
2. High HBV-DNA titre (>10^5 copies/ml)
3. Infection perinatally or in early childhood
4. Long period since infection (>5 years)
5. Increased hepatic iron content
6. Coinfection (e.g. HDV, HCV, HIV)
7. Coexistent noxae (e.g. alcohol, drugs)
8. Genotype C or D

Tab. 34.8: Selection criteria for IFN therapy in chronic hepatitis B with indicators of good or poor response

Therapy scheme: IFNα (or Peg IFNα$_{2a}$) is currently the antiviral agent of choice; it is applied as monotherapy. The following dosage is considered to be the most effective scheme of therapy: *IFNα at 5–6 million U/day* or *IFNα at 9–10 million U, 3 x/week*, preferably in the evening, usually self-administered (s.c.), in each case for four to six months. A seroconversion of HBeAg to anti-HBe is achieved in 35–40% of cases (vs. 8–13% spontaneous). In 80% of the responders, IFNα therapy leads to sustained viral response. A longer duration of therapy (> 6 months) is no more efficacious, whereas a shorter duration (< 4 months) produces a less successful result. Daily administration seems to be more favourable than an injection three times per week due to the half-life of IFNα. • Various *contraindications* should be heeded regarding the use of interferon. (s. tab. 34.9)

1. **Decompensated cirrhosis (Child C)**
2. **Depression, suicidal tendency, epilepsy** (200)
3. **Autoimmune diseases**
4. **Pregnancy, lactation period**
5. **Immunosuppression**
6. **Addiction problems**
7. **Serious extrahepatic disease**
– coronary insufficiency   – cardiac insufficiency (NYHA 3–4)
– dysthyreosis
– tachyarrhythmia   – HCC
– thrombopenia (<50,000 µl)   – leucopenia (<2,000 µl)
– renal insufficiency   – bacterial infection

Tab. 34.9: Contraindications to interferon therapy

Follow-up is firstly every two weeks, later at monthly intervals (physical status, haemogram, transaminases). After three and six months, HBeAg, anti-HBe and HBV DNA (quantitatively) as well as thyroid parameters (TSH, TAB) and calcium are determined.

Therapy success is seen in a reduction of the initial HBV-DNA titre by about 50% within three to five months. The transaminases show a sudden increase (= *flare-up*) after eight to ten weeks. (139) This results from the immunological destruction of HBV-replication hepatocytes, so that replication is terminated. Because flare-up is a favourable criterion, therapy continues unchanged.

If the course of disease remains successful, there will be a transition to the *low-replication phase* with a loss of HBeAg (i.e. HBeAg positivity = *incomplete response*) and HBV DNA as well as normalization of the transaminases after 10–14 months. It takes several years for the HBsAg to disappear completely: about 20% are HBsAg-negative after 12 months and about 65% after 6 years (i.e HBsAg positivity = *complete response*). At this point, HBV is considered to have been eliminated. Incomplete (*partial*) responders still have moderately increased transaminases, but show HBeAg and HBV-DNA negativity. However, anti-HBe may still be detectable in these patients after some years. Careful monitoring is required due to the danger of reactivation. • Generally, genotype A or B responds better to IFNα than type D or C, with earlier spontaneous seroconversion of HBeAg. (163, 174, 179, 193)

HBeAg-negative patients possess precore (minus) mutants. They show an initial response rate of up to 90%; there is no sign of flare-up. The aim of therapy is normalization of the transaminases and a loss of HBV DNA after more than 12 months. When IFNα therapy is stopped, reactivation usually occurs, even after several years. Only 15–25% of cases achieve sustained response. For this reason, IFN therapy lasting 12–24 months is recommended. • Patients with cirrhosis tolerate IFNα therapy in the same way as patients without cirrhosis and even show the same results.

Early side effects include fever and flu-like symptoms, which can be alleviated or eliminated by paracetamol; they are mostly temporary and of no clinical significance. • **Late side effects** depend on the individual case and dosage; they are influenced by coexistent diseases (e.g. diabetes) or psychic disposition. (192) There have been reports of numerous and different side effects. • *When such side effects occur, a dose reduction is necessary in 3–25% of cases (depending on the dose); IFN treatment has to be discontinued in 3–5%.* (s. tab. 34.10)

1. **Early side effects**
• Fever, flu-like symptoms
• Local inflammatory reaction
2. **Late side effects**
• *General*
– exhaustion, fatigue, sleep disturbances, loss of appetite, diarrhoea, loss of weight, hair loss, myalgia, arthralgia, tinnitus, anosmia, cough, headaches
• *Haematological*
– leucopenia, thrombopenia
• *Psychiatric* (200)
– irritability, affective lability, epileptic seizures, depression, suicidal tendency, loss of libido, changes in the EEG, schizoid psychoses, stroke syndrome
• *Infectious*
– infection (e.g. urinary tract, respiratory tract)
• *Endocrinological*
– impaired thyroid function, hypocalcaemia, insulin resistance
• *Cardiovascular*
– hypertension, hypotension, arrhythmia, cardiac insufficiency
• *Urogenital*
– proteinuria, impotence, nephritis
• *Immunological*
– IFN autoantibodies, autoimmunopathies, vasculitis, pleural effusion, pericarditis, sarcoidosis
• *Ophthalmological*
– retinal haemorrhagia, disturbed vision, conjunctivitis
• *Cutaneous*
– cutaneous necrosis, exanthema, pruritus, urticaria
• *Intestinal*
– eosinophilic enteritis, coeliac disease, pancreatitis

Tab. 34.10: Possible side effects of interferon therapy

Relapse: Reactivation is often associated with the presence of wildtype HBV (80−85%) or the occurrence of precore mutants (15−20%). This event (increase in the transaminases, evidence of replication markers such as HBeAg and HBV DNA, positive IgM anti-HBC, pronounced interface hepatitis) develops in 15−20% of cases one to three years after IFNα therapy has stopped. In such cases the question then arises of whether to apply lamivudine. This antiviral agent is administered in cases with an unfavourable constellation or contraindication regarding IFNα, or if the patient refuses IFN.

7.2.3 Lamivudine therapy

The daily dose of lamirudine amounts to 100 mg. Tolerance is good; no side effects have been observed up to now. HIV infection must be ruled out prior to therapy (danger of HIV resistance); a combination with ribavirin should be avoided (danger of lactate acidosis) or with trimethoprim (reduction in renal clearance of lamivudine); in HBeAg positivity, abrupt discontinuation is not allowed (danger of exacerbation or ALF). • The recommended duration of therapy is more than one year to long-term. If HBeAg seroconversion occurs at any time, therapy should be extended by about six months in order to improve the overall effect. The most reliable predictor of a good response is a transaminase value which is at least five times higher than normal. (149, 155, 157, 164, 167, 176, 178, 182, 183, 189, 194, 197)

HBeAg-positive patients: Some 90% of cases reach HBV-DNA elimination after about one year of treatment, but only 15−20% of cases achieve sustained HBV-DNA negativity. At the same time, a normalization of the transaminases (up to 70%) and inhibition of fibrosis may be observed. (164) Subsequent to seroconversion after 12 months of therapy, administration of lamivudine should be continued for a further 6 months due to the risk of relapse.

HBeAg-negative patients: These cases show no sign of seroconversion; therefore therapy should be continued for a further two years before being stopped. Generally, it seems reasonable to carry out long-term therapy until viral resistance develops in the form of mutants.

Viral mutants: As the duration of lamivudine therapy increases, the number of mutants rises, especially those resulting from YMDD-polymerase mutation. Viral mutants are found in about 20% of cases after 1 year, in 35−40% after 2 years and in 60−70% after 4 years. (153) Clinically, lamivudine resistance is recognizable due to an increase of the transaminases and a recurrence of viraemia. Risk factors include high GPT values, an elevated HBV-DNA level and a pathological body mass index. • In the case of resistance, the use of adefovir is recommended, since this nucleoside is also efficacious against HBV mutants.

7.2.4 Treatment failure

Treatment failure or reactivation leads to progressive fibrosis or development of cirrhosis/HCC; the patient's quality of life is also impaired. Responsibility towards the patient forces the physician to use any therapeutic approach available which is (*1.*) biomolecularly and pharmacologically plausible, (*2.*) free of or low in side effects and also suitable in a long-term regimen (the significance of a long-term follow-up should not be underrated), and (*3.*) justifiable in terms of cost.

Combination therapy: The combination of *IFNα + lamivudine* is superior to the corresponding monotherapy and yielded considerably better results in patients who were resistent to IFN. (158, 160, 180, 188, 189) Likewise *Peg-IFNα + lamivudine* was applied with success. (176) A combination of *lamivudine + ADV* led to a virological and biochemical improvement during treatment lasting up to 52 weeks (184, 185). In another study, however, therapy with *IFNα + lobucavir* (2 x 200 mg/day) had only little success. A combination of *lamivudine + famciclovir* sometimes produced a certain positive effect. (190) In the same way, *IFNα + famciclovir* improved initial values in some cases. (177) A combination of *famciclovir + thymosin* activates T-cell response in the immunotolerance phase. (166) The possibility that *IFNα + acyclovir* are synergistic in HBV infection has been suggested (S.W. SCHALM et al., 1985); acyclovir as monotherapy (45 mg/kg BW/day, i.v. infusion for 28 days) showed no benefit in chronic HBV carriers with stable disease. (147)

7.2.5 Nucleoside analogues

Because of their structural resemblance to natural nucleosides, these substances are integrated into the newly synthesized DNA strand by the enzymes of DNA synthesis (e. g. DNA polymerase, reverse transcriptase inhibition) in place of the natural nucleosides. The outcome is chain break. Virus mutation, however, may reduce the effectiveness of nucleoside analogue. • The clinical importance of these new antiviral substances, either as monotherapy or in combination, remain unclarified. A number of substances have been developed which have proved efficacious, but some of them have not yet been officially approved for the treatment of chronic hepatitis. (s. tab. 34.10)

Famciclovir is a quinine derivate and as such a prodrug, which is converted intracellularly to the efficacious substance penciclovir. It is administered orally; the daily dose amounts to 1,500 mg. Its effectiveness is low. (148, 166, 173)

Lamivudine is a nucleoside analogue, which acts as a reverse transcriptase inhibitor of HBV-DNA polymerase and causes a break in the molecular chain through its competitive integration in the DNA. Lamivudine is administered orally and well resorbed. The **half-life** is five to seven hours; it is eliminated unchanged via the kidneys. Therefore, the dose must be adjusted to the patient's creatinine clearance.

Adefovir is a nucleoside analogue, which causes a break in the molecular chain through its competitive integration in the newly synthesized HBV DNA. Adefovir dipivoxil (ADV) is a prodrug, which is converted into active ADV in the intestinal tract. Its half-life is 7–8 hours. Elimination is via the kidneys. Therefore, the dose must be adjusted in the case of renal insufficiency! It should be noted that the risk of damage to the kidneys is increased by simultaneous administration of aminoglycosides, vancomycin and antirheumatic agents.

Dosage is 10 mg/day orally; duration of treatment is 48 weeks. The effect of ADV is not impaired by a high viral load. In HBeAg-positive patients, it results in elimination of HBV DNA in 20–25%, seroconversion in 15–20% and normalization of the transaminases in 45–50% of cases. • In HBeAg-negative patients, ADV shows a loss of HBV DNA in approx. 50% and normalization of GPT in 70–75% of cases. In addition, a considerable improvement in histology was achieved. Viral resistance (due to mutants) was observed in <3% of cases after three years. ADV can also be applied in decompensated cirrhosis. Tolerance is good. As with lamivudine, abrupt discontinuation may lead to acute exacerbation (in about 25%). (156, 161, 162, 176, 195, 196)

Tenofovir is the active agent of the prodrug tenofovir disoproxil fumarate. Up to now, tenofovir (300 mg/day) has been used with HIV/HBV coinfected patients. In such cases, it proved effective regarding HBV DNA and the normalization of the transaminases.

Emtricitabine is a cytosine nucleoside with antiviral potency towards HBV and HIV. It is only slightly different from lamivudine. After 48 weeks of treatment (200 mg/day), it was possible to achieve HBV-DNA negativity in 60% and HBeAg negativity in 50% of cases. Tolerance is good (N. Leung et al., 2001). (170)

Entecavir is a guanosine nucleoside with strong antiviral activity. It is also effective in lamivudine-resistant patients. After 48 weeks of treatment comprising a daily dose of 0.5 or 1.0 mg, there was elimination of HBV DNA in 25–30% and normalization of the transaminases in 60–70% of lamivudine-resistant patients. Tolerance is good. Entecavir-induced mutants were not detected. (165, 186)

Telbuvidine: LdT proved to be effective and well tolerated in a dosage of 200–400 mg/day orally (C.L. Lai et al., 2001).

Clevudine is a pyrimidine-nucleoside analogue. It was effective in a dosage of 200 mg/day (P. Marcellin et al., 2003). (168)

An important risk factor concerning the development of resistant mutants is the incomplete suppression of HBC replication in the therapy. • In the case of primary treatment failure, HBV DNA does not fall below 103 copies/ml (= 200 IU/ml) after six months or does not fall constantly for a period of twelve months. Secondary treatment failure is given if initial therapy is successful, but HBV DNA subsequently increases at least tenfold (1 log power) in relation to the lowest level previously achieved despite continuous antiviral therapy. • It is necessary to recognize any resistance at the earliest possible stage, so that therapy can be adjusted – i.e. as soon as there is evidence of a virological (not biochemical!) relapse. (s. tab 34.11) • Antiviral therapy should be commenced as a permanent measure. Even in the case of HBeAg seroconversion, therapy should be combined for a further 6–12 months. The seroconversion of HBeAg is seen as a healing process for hepatitis B.

7.2.6 Immunostimulants

Immunostimulants activate the immune system – especially in cases of reduced immune defence. They can be (*1.*) endogenous substances, (*2.*) extracts of microorganisms, or (*3.*) substances of plant and chemical origin. • The use of **thymosin-α** has also proved promising (G.M. Mutchnick et al., 1991). It effects an improvement in the T-cell function. Promising biochemical, serological and histological results were obtained in chronic HBV infection. (150, 166) Good tolerance was recorded for this drug. • **Interleukins** are mediators of the induction and course of the T-cell-mediated cytotoxic immune reaction and of B-cell activation (antibody production). Interleukin 2 induces the proliferation and differentiation of T lymphocytes; the simultaneous induction of IFNγ triggers the activation of macrophages. A mixture of *interleukin 2, interleukin 6* and *anti-D3* may be considered as a further option in the future. • Good results have also been achieved with the **phyllanthus amarus extract**. Further studies are necessary to clarify the biological modes of action of this interesting plant. The same applies to the **bupleurum extract** as well as extracts from **glycyrrhiza** (used in chronic hepatitis C) (235), **schizandra, kurorinone** (151), etc. (s. pp 897, 898)

7.2.7 Adjuvant substances

Arguments: The following arguments justify the search for and use of adjuvant substances: (*1.*) the high number of patients with chronic viral hepatitis worldwide, (*2.*) the high morbidity and mortality associated with this disease, (*3.*) the high cost of treatment with interferon, ribavirin, lamivudine, etc., (*4.*) the occasionally severe side effects, and (*5.*) the still unsatisfactory therapeutic results and low success rate.

Criteria: The therapeutic agents should meet the following criteria: (*1.*) as far as possible, they should have no side effects or interactions, (*2.*) the adjuvant effects should be proven or at least deemed plausible by biochemical and/or pharmacological studies, and (*3.*)

the additional cost should be justifiable and within certain limits. • Because of their merely adjuvant modes of action, such substances must be used long-term (>2 years) to obtain positive effects in chronic hepatitis − as is also necessary with other chronic diseases. The main adjuvant substances include:

1. Colchicin
2. Essential phospholipids
3. Iron removal
4. N-acetylcystein
5. Silymarin
6. Tenoxicam
7. Ursodeoxycholic acid
8. Vitamin E

Iron removal: Increased iron and ferritin levels are found in approx. 30% of patients with chronic hepatitis B or C. Several studies have shown that the success rate of interferon therapy is reduced in the presence of elevated liver iron values. This is attributed to the fact that iron overload inhibits not only lymphocyte proliferation, but also the function of killer cells and B cells as well as the production of antibodies. Iron plays a role in the formation of free radicals and the occurrence of dangerous lipid peroxidations. Furthermore, iron, like oxygen radicals, promotes fibrogenesis. Iron removal leads to an improvement in laboratory parameters and better response to IFN-α therapy. (208, 231) On the other hand, the iron level is reduced as a result of successful IFN therapy. • In the case of a higher serum iron status before the initiation of interferon therapy, *venesections* at one-week intervals should be considered, if necessary until normal laboratory values (iron, ferritin, transferrin saturation) have been restored. During interferon therapy, a *low-iron diet* is advisable, as is the consumption of 2 x 1 cup of *black tea* (in the morning and at noon) to reduce iron absorption through chelate formation ("cheap, free of side effects and useful"). (s. p. 644) • *Silymarin* also leads to iron mobilization due to chelate formation.

Silymarin: The *hepatoprotective* and *hepatoregenerative* effects of silymarin have been demonstrated in numerous in-vitro and in-vivo studies. Its antioxidant properties have also been confirmed in recent years (C. DEHMLOW et al., 1996), especially in rats with iron overload (A. PIETRANGELO et al., 1995). The *antiperoxidative* efficacy of silymarin was found to be ten times greater than that of an equimolar concentration of α-tocopherol. This effect is attributed to biochemical interaction (chelate formation of silymarin with Fe^{2+}). Clinical studies also testified to the *antifibrogenetic* effect of silymarin in patients with chronic hepatitis (G. BUZZELLI et al., 1993). (see E. KUNTZ: footnote*, p. 895)

Ursodeoxycholic acid: As early as 1961, F. ICHIDA et al. reported on the successful treatment of chronic hepatitis with UDCA. Similar reports were published by T. NAKAHARA et al. in 1975 and two further Japanese groups in 1976. Furthermore, U. LEUSCHNER et al. (1985) noticed surprising improvements regarding biochemical parameters in chronic hepatitis. These effects were attributed to the immunomodulatory efficacy of UDCA. In principle, UDCA satisfies all the criteria for its combined use with interferon in chronic viral hepatitis. (s. p. 886)

Essential phospholipids: In a multicentre study, it could be demonstrated that essential phospholipids (EPL) not only significantly increased the proportion of IFN responders in patients with chronic hepatitis B and C, but also reduced the relapse rate. (181) (see E. KUNTZ: footnote*, p. 894)

7.3 Therapy of chronic hepatitis C

In **acute HCV infection**, which mostly develops asymptomatically, but sometimes with uncharacteristic complaints, HCV RNA is present within the first week after infection. Antibodies against HCV are detectable after six to eight weeks in >90% of cases. *(see chapter 22.5)*

Chronic hepatitis C manifests in 60−80% of infected patients and becomes active in 70−80% of cases. Of the latter, 20−30% gradually develop cirrhosis and 4−5% ultimately suffer from HCC. A higher risk of cirrhosis is given in patients with a high HCV-RNA concentration, with portal or bridging fibrosis accompanied by necroinflammatory activity and with permanently increased transaminases.

> Patients with chronic hepatitis C but without antibodies against HAV and/or HBV should be vaccinated immediately against the respective seronegative hepatitis form!

7.3.1 Indication for therapy

The indication for antiviral treatment of chronic hepatitis C is principally based on the following criteria: (*1.*) symptomatic course (subjective complaints, elevated transaminases, extrahepatic manifestations), (*2.*) inflammatory activity and progressive fibrosis or cirrhosis, and (*3.*) infection risk regarding contact persons.

Even in the case of *cirrhosis* (Child A, possibly also B), antiviral therapy should be used to achieve histological improvement of the findings and to reduce the frequency of HCC.

Half the patients with *normal transaminases* sometimes show both increased values and histological activity scores. Therefore, it is necessary to recheck the indications for these patients, especially because their sustained viral response (SVR) is comparable to that of patients with elevated transaminases.

7.3.2 Selection criteria for therapy

> Before commencing treatment of chronic hepatitis C, it is necessary to determine the genotype and HCV-RNA titre.

Reliable diagnosis: A definitive determination of the respective disease stage of HCV infection is often difficult regarding serological diagnostics; there are uncertain histological findings and only moderate correlation between histology and laboratory parameters. • The situation is further complicated by occasional difficulties in making a differential diagnosis based on the serological and autoimmune overlap findings. Erroneously indicated treatment with immunosuppressives or interferon may result in serious complications. • *The most important selection criterion is a reliable diagnosis!*

Liver biopsy: In this context, the actual nomenclature of chronic hepatitis promises better designation and classification. (s. tabs. 34.2, 34.3) Therefore, in patients with genotype 1 (and 4), liver biopsy is recommended before planning therapy, whereby in genotypes 2 and 3, liver biopsy is less important, because therapy is generally successful. • The value of the histological findings is based on (*1.*) determination of necroinflammatory activity and progressive fibrosis, (*2.*) assessment of prognosis and necessity of treatment, (*3.*) prediction for therapy success, (*4.*) comparison of initial findings with follow-ups, (*5.*) evaluation of therapy results, and (*6.*) exclusion of coexisting liver disease. • Disadvantages include (*1.*) sample error, (*2.*) extraction of biopsy specimen from a limited puncture area of the right lobe, and (*3.*) interobserver and intraobserver variability. (5, 6, 11, 62, 65, 119, 130) • A reliable morphological diagnosis and the all-important assessment of the liver surface regarding fibrosis progression or perhaps even the existence of cirrhosis are best achieved using *laparoscopy* (201) and one to two biopsies from both the right and left liver lobe. (s. pp 165, 716) • *Chronic hepatitis is not evenly spread in the liver in every case!* (s. pp 189, 697)

HCV genotype: The response rate to interferon therapy depends on the prevalent genotype. Genotypes 1 and 4 (but also 5, 6) show a poorer response to IFN than genotypes 2 and 3. The genotype reveals no relationship to the RNA titre or to histology. A change of type 1 to type 3 was also noted. (s. tab. 34.12)

Cofactors: *Coinfections* with HAV and HBV as well as with other viruses worsen the prognosis. By contrast, coinfections with HGV, GBV-C, SENV and TTV had no influence on the course of chronic hepatitis C. (107, 140) *Alcohol* impairs the cellular immune response unfavourably and leads to an aggravation of pathological liver morphology. (112, 120, 121, 138) • *Age* and *gender* play a special role. Generally, older patients are subject to a more severe course of disease. Women below the age of 40 benefitted significantly more from IFN therapy than women over 40 (75.0% vs. 15.6%). HCV clearance in women is better than in men (G. INOUE et al., 2000). There is also exacerbation of chronic hepatitis C due to pregnancy (H. FONTANE et al., 2000). • *HCV-RNA titres* of < 2 million copies/ml (or 0.8 million I U/ml) are considered more favourable, whereas an initial high viral load shows a worse response. • In comparison (low-titre) antibodies (e.g. ANA, AMA, LKM), are found more frequently in women than in men, but they had no influence on the response to IFNα therapy.

7.3.3 Combination therapy

The standard therapy for chronic hepatitis C is a combination of pegylated IFNα with ribavirin. (239) (s. tabs. 34.10, 34.11)

Nucleoside analogues	Dosage
Lamivudine	1 x 100 mg/day
Entecavir	1 x 0.5 mg/day
	1 x 1.0 mg/day with lamivudine resistance
Telbivudine	1 x 600 mg/day
Famciclovir	3 x 250 – 500 mg/day
Emtricitabine	1 x 200 mg/day
Nucleotide analogues	**Dosage**
Adefovir dipivoxil	1 x 10 mg/day
Tenofovir disoproxil	1 x 245 mg/day

Tab. 34.11: Nucleoside and nucleotide analogues as well as dosage for treatment of chronic hepatitis B (partly not approved as yet)

Treatment failure		Therapy options	
Lamivudine		Add on:	Adefovir Tenofovir
		Change to:	Tenofovir Entecavir Telbivudine
Adefovir	a) with lamivudine-naive patients	Add on:	Entecavir Telbivudine Lamivudine
	b) with non-lamivudine-naive patients	Change to: Add on:	Tenofovir Adefovir
Entecavir		Add on:	Adefovir Tenofovir
Telbivudine		Add on:	Adefovir Tenofovir
		Change to:	Entecavir
Tenofovir		Add on:	Entecavir Telbivudine Lamivudine

Tab. 34.12: Possible forms of therapy in the face of resistance development or insufficient treatment success with monotherapy (period of six months)

Interferon was used in the treatment of chronic hepatitis NANB as early as 1986 by J.A. HOOFNAGEL et al., i.e. three years before HCV was identified. The efficacy of IFNα for chronic hepatitis C could be proven in many studies. (203, 204, 207, 219, 230, 233, 238) • The **pegylation of IFNα** (= coupling to polyethylene glycol) leads to reduced enzymatic degradation, diminished antigenicity and delayed renal clearance; thus its half-life is prolonged.

As a result, a constant efficient level is achieved with only one or two injection(s) per week. This newly developed Peg IFNα led to a further improvement in the sustained viral response. (205, 221)

> ▶ **Peg IFNα$_{2a}$** (40 kDa) has a branched structure and is available in a ready-to-use solution. The dosage amounts to 180 µg, s.c., 1 x/week. Its efficient level lasts for 160 hours; half-life is approx. 80 hours. It can also be administered in cases of renal insufficiency due to its hepatic clearance.
>
> ▶ **Peg IFNα$_{2b}$** (12 kDa) has a linear structure. The solution comes in a two-chambered syringe and is prepared by mixing the contents of both compartments directly prior to injection. The dosage amounts to 1.0–1.5 µg/kg BW, s.c. 1 x/week. Half-life is approx. 40 hours. This substance should not be applied if creatinine clearance is <50 ml/min.

Ribavirin: This guanosine analogue was first used experimentally by O. REICHARD et al. (1991) and in chronic hepatitis C by J. ANDERSSON et al. (1991). Ribavirin is well resorbed. Half-life in patients with chronic hepatitis C is approx. 44 hours; once a steady state has been reached, the half-life is extended by up to 12 days. Elimination is mainly via the kidneys. Ribavirin is contraindicated in cases where creatinine clearance is <50 ml/min. As monotherapy, it effects a decrease in the transaminases and a slight improvement in histological activity during treatment. It inhibits the replication of RNA and DNA viruses. Dosage is 400–600 mg, 2 x/day; it depends on body weight, renal function and HCV genotype. Due to its potentially teratogenetic effect, pregnancy must be avoided before, during and for at least six months after therapy. This also applies to sexual partners of men treated with ribavirin. Ribavirin is also contraindicated during the lactation period. (241)

Using a combination of *IFNα + ribavirin*, it was possible to achieve a considerable improvement in comparison to former therapy results. (198, 201, 207, 211, 212, 226) • A combination of *Peg IFNα + ribavirin* led to a further enhancement of the sustained response including normalization of the transaminases and reduction of the inflammatory activity (70–75% after 1 year). Thus, the combination of Peg IFNα + ribavirin is considered to be standard therapy today.

▶ *Side effects* of ribavirin can appear in the form of nausea, pruritus, insomnia, irritability, haemolysis (216) and aggravation of IFNα-induced thrombopenia or leucopenia. In combination with other nucleoside analogues, there is a risk of lactate acidosis. • Side effects of Peg IFNα are similar to those of IFNα. (221, 223) The latter usually necessitates a reduction in dosage in about 20% and termination of therapy in 5–10% of cases. • Side effects of combined IFNα + ribavirin include pancreatitis (206), pulmonary toxicity (217), manifestation of sarcoidosis (210, 229), and mental disorders (224). *It should be noted that even in combination with ribavirin IFNα may show its own customary side effects.*

In an HBeAg-negative course, permanent therapy is needed. A withdrawal trial can be made after five years; a subsequent increase in HBV DNA is of no relevance. By contrast, an increase in HBV replication due to the development of resistance can lead to liver failure.

7.3.4 Therapy scheme

In summary, the "ideal patient" with good prognosis has to show various criteria. (s. tab. 34.12)

1. **Exact diagnosis**
2. **No contraindications**
3. **Good response** (ideal patient)
– genotype 2 or 3
– HCV RNA <2 million copies/ml
– slight fibrosis and inflammation
– normal hepatic iron level
– age <50 years (women <40 years)
– increase in GPT of >6 months
– exclusion of cirrhosis
– sporadic HCV infection
– no coinfection, no alcohol, no noxae
– no diabetes mellitus, no overweight
– short duration of infection (<10 years)

Tab. 34.13: Basic criteria for a prognostically good response

With the help of the current therapy scheme, SVR can be achieved in up to 55% of infected patients with genotype 1 or 4 and up to 80% of those with genotype 2 or 3. Even in patients with an initial high virus load, SVR is about 40% for genotype 1 and 4 and about 75% for genotype 2 and 3. If the virus load has not fallen by factor 100 (>2 log, i.e. <30,000 IU/ml), or has not gone below the absolute limit of verification after six months, therapy should be stopped. Early viral response (EVR) is a decisive factor regarding the success, failure or duration of therapy. If there is no EVR, it will probably not be possible to achieve SVR, even if therapy is continued for 12 months (or longer). • With genotype 2 and 3, therapy is stopped after 24 weeks, with genotype 1 (as well as 4, 5 and 6) after 48 weeks. Finally, the HCV-RNA titre should be measured anew. • The five-year survival rate of patients with SVR corresponds to that of the general population. After SVR has been achieved, subsequent reactivation is rare. (s. tab. 34.13)

Peg IFNα$_{2a}$	180 µg, s.c. 1 x/week	genotype 1, 4 = 48 weeks
Ribavirin	>75 kg = 2 x 600 mg/day	genotype 2, 3 = 24 weeks
	<75 kg = 2 x 500 mg/day	
Peg IFNα$_{2b}$	1.0–1.5 µg/kg BW, s.c., 1 x/week	genotype 1, 4 = 48 weeks
Ribavirin	>85 kg = 2 x 600 mg/day	genotype 2, 3 = 24 weeks
	65–85 kg = 2 x 500 mg/day	
	<65 kg = 2 x 400 mg/day	

Tab. 34.14: Scheme of combination therapy for chronic hepatitis C with Peg IFNα and ribavirin

Iron removal: In the case of increased iron storage in the liver or in hypersiderinaemia, iron removal has been reported to give better therapeutic results. (208, 231)

The **follow-ups** take place at first weekly, later at four-week intervals; they include leucocytes, thrombocytes, haemoglobin and the transaminases, in some cases calcium and TSH as well. At three-month intervals, HCV-RNA, TSH, TAB, creatinine and calcium should be determined.

The **aims of treatment** are firstly negativity of HCV RNA and secondly normalization of transaminases, reduction of inflammatory activity and fibrosis as well as prevention of cirrhosis.

7.3.5 Treatment failure

Relapse: In the case of relapse following successful treatment, it is advisable to wait for a certain time, since the relapse can be spontaneously limited in a number of patients. Some 80% of patients with genotype 2 or 3 and about 40% with genotype 1 or 4 show stable remission in the long term (up to 3 years). Follow-ups revealed that the risk of late relapse is relatively low after successful treatment. (199, 207)

Non-responders: As in the case of patients with relapse, it is advisable to weigh the slow progression of the disease against the side effects and costs of repeated combination therapy (particularly regarding higher dosage). The question also arises as to whether an improvement in the quality of life can be achieved. (198, 208, 226)

Repeat treatment: After repeat treatment had been decided on, increased dosage and prolonged duration of IFNα (226) or consensus IFN were used. • Other possible combinations were applied, such as *IFNα + thymosin* (225), *IFNα + cyclosporin* (215, 220), *IFNα + UDCA* (222) or *IFNα + amantadine* (237). In all these studies, positive results and an improvement in quality of life were described for some patients. • Even *iron removal* can be used as an additional measure. (208, 231) Good results have also been achieved with *immunostimulants, antioxidants* (218), and *adjuvant substances* (as in chronic hepatitis B) such as thymosin (150), kurorinone (151), bezafibrate (209), essential phospholipids (181) or glycyrrhizin (214, 225). Above all, adjuvant therapy using silymarin as a fibrosis inhibitor is worth mentioning.

Amantadine: The antiviral efficacy of amantadine was first reported by W. Davies et al. in 1964. The mode of action consists in preventing uncoating and viral maturation (inhibition of the release of the nucleic acids that have already penetrated the host cell). The active substance is almost completely absorbed following oral intake. It is eliminated unchanged via the kidneys. Half-life is about 16 hours. So far, it has been used to combat influenza virus type A. Tolerance is good. Amantadine on its own is only minimally effective against HCV; it is therefore not suitable for initial monotherapy.

Amantadine was administered for the first time in 31 patients with OLT due to chronic hepatitis C, who were suffering from severe reinfection of the transplant. Initial therapeutic success was already seen after three months: a significant fall in transaminases, bilirubin, AP and HCV-RNA titres, with improvement in liver histology (J.A. Goss et al., 1997). • In a further study, 22 patients with chronic hepatitis C who had failed to respond to IFN therapy were treated with amantadine (2 x 100 mg). After six months of treatment, GPT values showed a reduction in 64% and a normalization in 27% of cases; HCV RNA was no longer detectable. This situation was verifiable by PCR even six months after therapy in 18% of patients. (227) • *In combination with IFN, amantadine seems to be a well-tolerated and effective virustatic for HCV infection.* (228)

Triple combination: In non-responders, the triple therapy of *IFN + ribavirin + amantadine* may be effective. Sustained response can be achieved in 15–20% of cases. The additional costs for amantadine are relatively low; the number of side effects relating to IFNα + ribavirin has not proved higher than normal; the rate of SVR in initial therapy appears to be slightly better. Therefore, the question arises whether to use initial triple therapy in principle. (198, 202, 232, 234, 236, 240)

7.4 Therapy of chronic hepatitis D

Treatment consists of relatively high doses of interferon (generally 3 x 9–10 million U/week, s.c.) for a period exceeding 12 months. Even though normalization of GPT and HDV-RNA negativity as well as substantial histological improvement were achieved in 50% and 70% of cases and stabilized for over six years, HCV-RNA negativity was only maintained in 0% and 10% (−20%) of patients respectively. The relapse rate is higher than in chronic hepatitis B. (242–245) • An antiviral combination of IFN with lamivudine (246) or famciclovir (247) or aciclovir and ribavirin was not efficacious. • Liver transplantation should be planned in good time.

7.5 Liver transplantation

Reinfection occurs in about 50% of transplant recipients following chronic **HBV infection**; this seems to depend on presurgical replication activity. Some 83% of patients who were HBV RNA-positive prior to transplantation again showed viraemia and reinfection of the graft. In patients with preoperative HBeAg, HBsAg and HBV-DNA negativity, viraemia was found in only 53% of cases. The *survival rate* after three years is 45–50%. However, with presurgical IFN therapy for improving this problematical serological situation, the danger of IFN-induced liver cell necrosis developing in HBV-related cirrhosis proved to be high. Therapy with lamivudine (occasionally with HBIG) is advisable. (187) In the case of reinfection of the transplant, HBIG must be discontinued. (26, 49, 66, 80, 159) • In **chronic hepatitis D**, the situation is generally comparable to that of chronic HBV infection. • About 30% of liver transplantations are related to **HCV infection**. In these cases, *reinfection* of the graft is a frequent occurrence (6—28% after 5 years). However, this does not pose a serious clinical problem, since the histological finding in most cases was CPH. The difficulties regarding pretransplantation IFNα therapy with associated liver cell necrosis are of little relevance here. In individual cases, reinfection of the graft can progress to cirrhosis. Angiotensin-II receptor antagonist may help to reduce the development of graft fibrosis in recurrent hepatitis C. *Posttransplantation treatment with Peg IFNα* showed a complete response in 15—20% of cases; this correlated with a low HCV-RNA concentration prior to transplantation. (149)

Epilogue

Counselling of chronically ill patients is extremely important. The use of pharmacologically acceptable substances with a low frequency of side effects should always be preferred. *Medical efforts must focus on the individual criteria of the respective patient.* • In "treatment failure", we have always stressed that *this* treatment, at *this* dosage and for *this* period of time was not successful in *this* particular case (for whatever reason) and that further measures would now have to be initiated. • We can recall several patients with chronic hepatitis who felt that they had been left to their own devices and who were therefore trying out obscure, perhaps dangerous "therapeutic measures" and even consulting so-called "healers". • All these considerations on the part of both doctor and patient constitute an essential component of every individual treatment plan.

References:

Chronic hepatitis

1. **Batts, K.P., Ludwig, J.:** Chronic hepatitis — an update on terminology and reporting. Amer. J. Surg. Pathol. 1995; 19: 1409—1417
2. **Bianchi, L.:** Necroinflammatory liver diseases. Semin. Liver Dis. 1986; 6: 185—198
3. **Chevallier, M., Guerret, S., Chossegros, P., Gerard, F., Grimaud, J.-A.:** A histological semiquantitative scoring system for evaluation of hepatic fibrosis in needle liver biopsy specimens: comparison with morphometric studies. Hepatology 1994; 20: 349—355
4. **Cho, S.G., Kim, M.Y., Kim, H.J., Choi, W., Shin, S.H., Hong, K.C., Kim, Y.B., Lee, J.H., Suh, C.H.:** Chronic hepatitis: in vivo proton MR spectroscopic evaluation of the liver and correlation with histopathologic findings. Radiology 2001; 221: 740—746
5. **Colloredo, G., Guido, M., Sonzogni, A., Leandro, G.:** Impact of liver biopsy size on histological evaluation of chronic viral hepatitis: the smaller the sample, the milder the disease. J. Hepatol. 2003; 39: 239—244
6. **Crawford, A.R., Lin, X.Z., Crawford, J.M.:** The normal adult human liver biopsy: a quantitative reference standard. Hepatology 1998; 28: 323—331
7. **DeGroote, J., Desmet, V.J., Gedigk, P., Korb, G., Popper, H., Poulsen, H., Scheuer, P.J., Schmid, M., Thaler, H., Uehlinger, E., Wepler, W.:** A classification of chronic hepatitis. Lancet 1968/II: 626—628
8. **Desmet, F.J., Gerber, M., Hoofnagle, J.H., Manns, M., Scheuer, P.J.:** Classification of chronic hepatitis. Diagnosis, grading and staging. Hepatology 1994; 19: 1513—1520
9. **Gaiani, S., Gramantieri, L., Venturoli, N., Piscaglia, F., Siringo, S., D'Errico, A., Zironi, G., Grigioni, W., Bolondi, L.:** What is the criterion for differentiating chronic hepatitis from compensated cirrhosis? A prospective study comparing ultrasonography and percutaneous liver biopsy. J. Hepatol. 1997; 27: 979—985
10. **Gerber, M.A., Vernace, S.:** Chronic septal hepatitis. Virchows Archiv 1974; 363: 303—309
11. **Goldin, R.D., Goldin, J.G., Burt, A.D., Dhillon, P.A., Hubscher, S., Wyatt, J., Patel, N.:** Intra-observer and inter-observer variation in the histopathological assessment of chronic viral hepatitis. J. Hepatol. 1996; 25: 649—654
12. **Ishak, K., Baptista, A., Bianchi, L., Callea, F., De Groote, J., Gudat, F., Denk, H., Desmet, V., Korb, G., MacSween, R.N.M., Phillips, M.J., Portmann, B.G., Poulsen, H., Scheuer, P.J., Schmid, M., Thaler, H.:** Histological grading and staging of chronic hepatitis. J. Hepatol. 1995; 22: 696—699
13. **Ishak, K.G.:** Pathologic features of chronic hepatitis — A review and update. Amer. J. Clin. Path. 2000; 113: 40—55
14. **Knodell, R.G., Ishak, K.G., Black, W.C., Chen, T.S., Craig, R., Kaplowitz, N., Kiernan, T.W., Wollman, J.:** Formulation and application of a numerical scoring system for assessing histological activity in asymptomatic chronic active hepatitis. Hepatology 1981; 1: 431—435
15. **Korb, G.:** Chronic hepatitis B virus and hepatitis C virus infection. Histology, classification, examination. Pathologe 2001; 22: 124—131
16. **Krastev, Z.:** Liver damage score: a new index for evaluation of the severity of chronic liver diseases. Hepato-Gastroenterol. 1998; 45: 160—169
17. **Kuntz, E., Kühn, H.A.:** Systematik und Klinik der chronischen Hepatitis. Med. Klin. 1969; 64: 2227—2241
18. **Ludwig, J.:** The nomenclature of chronic active hepatitis: an orbituary. Gastroenterology 1993; 105: 274—278
19. **Rozario, R., Ramakrishna, B.:** Histopathological study of chronic hepatitis B and C: a comparison of two scoring systems. J. Hepatol. 2003; 38: 223—229
20. **Scheuer, P.J.:** Classification of chronic viral hepatitis: a need for reassessment. J. Hepatol. 1991; 13: 372—374
21. **Schmid, M., Flury, R., Bühler, H., Havelka, J., Grob, P.J., Heitz, Ph.U.:** Chronic viral hepatitis B and C: an argument against the conventional classification of chronic hepatitis. Virchows Archiv 1994; 425: 221—228
22. **Selmair, H., Vido, I., Wildhirt, E., Ortmans, H.:** Die chronisch-nekrotisierende Hepatitis. Dtsch. Med. Wschr. 1970; 95: 1397—1401
23. **Soresi, M., Bonfissuto, G., Magliarisi, C., Riili, A., Terranova, A., di Giovanni, G., Bascone, F., Carraccio, A., Tripi, S., Montalto, G.:** Ultrasound detection of abdominal lymph nodes in chronic liver diseases. A retrospective analysis. Clin. Radiol. 2003; 58: 372—377
24. **Thaler, H.:** Systematische, morphologische und klinische Probleme der chronischen Hepatitis. Internist 1973; 14: 604—614

Chronic hepatitis A

25. **Inoue, K., Yoshiba, M., Yotsuyanagi, H., Otsuka, T., Sekiyama, K., Fujita, R.:** Chronic hepatitis A with persistent viral replication. J. Med. Virol. 1996; 50: 322—324

Chronic hepatitis B

26. **Abdelmalek, M.F., Pasha, T.M., Zein, N.N., Persing, D.H., Wiesner, R.H., Douglas, D.D.:** Subclinical reactivation of hepatitis B virus in liver transplant recipients with past exposure. Liver transplant. 2003; 9: 1253—1257
27. **Bonino, F., Rosina, F., Rizzetto, M., Rizzi, R., Chiaberge, E., Tardanico, R., Callea, F., Verme, G.:** Chronic hepatitis in HBsAg carriers with serum HBV-DNA and anti-HBe. Gastroenterology 1986; 90: 1268—1273
28. **Bonino, F., Brunetto, M.R.:** Chronic hepatitis e antigen (HbeAg) negative, anti-Hbe positive hepatitis B: an overview. J. Hepatol. 2003; 39 (Suppl. 1): 160—163
29. **Bortolotti, F., Cadrobbi, P., Crivellaro, C., Guido, M., Rugge, M., Noventa, F., Calzia, R., Realdi, G.:** Long-term outcome of chronic type B hepatitis in patients who acquire hepatitis B virus infection in childhood. Gastroenterology 1990; 99: 805—810
30. **Chang, M.H.:** Decreasing incidence of hepatocellular carcinoma among children following universal hepatitis B immunization. Liver Internat. 2003; 23: 309—314
31. **Choi, M.S., Lee, J.H., Koh, K.C., Paik, S.W., Rhee, P.L., Kim, J.J., Rhee, J.C., Choi, K.W., Kim, S.H.:** Clinical significanca of enlarged perihepatic lymph nodes in chronic hepatitis B. J. Clin. Gastroenterol. 2001; 32: 329—332
32. **Chu, C.M.:** Natural history of chronic hepatitis B virus infection in adults with emphasis on the occurrence of cirrhosis and hepatocellular carcinoma. J. Gastroenterol. Hepatol. 2000; 15 (Suppl.) 25—30
33. **Demirdag, K., Yilmaz, S., Ozdarendeli, A., Ozden, M., Kalkan, A., Kilic, S.S.:** Levels of plasma malondialdehyde and erythrocyte antioxidant enzyme activities in patients with chronic hepatitis B. Hepato-Gastroenterol. 2003; 50: 766—770
34. **Fattovich, G., Brollo, L., Giustina, G., Noventa, F., Pontisso, P., Alberti, A., Realdi, G., Ruol, A.:** Natural history and prognostic factors for chronic hepatitis type B. Gut 1991; 32: 294—298
35. **Gambichler, T., Paech, V., Rotterdam, S., Stücker, M., Boms, S., Altmeyer, P.:** Hepatitis B-associated adult-onset Still's disease presenting with neutrophilic urticaria. Eur. J. Med. Res. 2003; 8: 527—530
36. **Hao, J.H., Shi, J., Ren, W.H., Han, G.Q., Zhu, J.R., Wang, S.Y., Xie, Y.B.:** Hepatic microcirculatory disturbances in patients with chronic hepatitis B. Chin. Med. J. 2002; 115: 65—68

37. Huo, T.L., Wu, J.C., Lee, P.C., Tsay, S.H., Chang, F.Y., Lee, S.D.: Diabetes mellitus as a risk factor of liver cirrhosis in patients with chronic hepatitis B virus infection. J. Clin. Gastroenterol. 2000; 30: 250–254
38. Huo, T.L., Wu, J.C., Hwang, S.J., Lai, C.R., Lee, P.C., Tsay, S.H., Chang, F.Y., Lee, S.D.: Factors predictive of liver cirrhosis in patients with chronic hepatitis B: a multivariate analysis in a longitudinal study. Europ. J. Gastroenterol. Hepatol. 2000; 12: 687–693
39. Kao, J.H., Chen, P.J., Lai, M.Y., Chen, D.S.: Genotypes and clinical phenotypes of hepatitis B virus in patients with chronic hepatitis B virus infection. J. Clin. Microbiol. 2002; 40: 1207–1209
40. Lee, H.-S., Yang, P.-M., Liu, B.-F., Lee, C.-L., Hsu, H.-C., Su, I.-J., Chen, D.-S.: Pleural effusion coinciding with acute exacerbations in a patient with chronic hepatitis B. Gastroenterology 1989; 96: 1604–1606
41. Maruyama, T., Schödel, F., Iino, S., Koike, K., Yasuda, K., Peterson, D., Milich, D.R.: Distinguishing between acute and symptomatic chronic hepatitis B virus infection. Gastroenterology 1994; 106: 1006–1015
42. McMahon, B.J.: The natural history of chronic hepatitis B virus infection. Semin. Liver Dis. 2004; 24 (Suppl.): 17–21
43. Merican, I., Guan, R., Amarapuka, D., Alexander, M.J., Chutaputti, A., Chien, R.N., Hasnian, S.S., Leung, N., Lesmana, L., Phiet, P.H., Noer, H.M.S., Sollano, J., Sun, H.S., Xu, D.Z.: Chronic hepatitis B virus infection in Asian countries. J. Gastroenterol. Hepatol. 2000; 15: 1356–1361
44. Moreno-Otero, R., Garcia-Monzon, C., Garcia-Sanchez, A., Garcia-Buey, L., Pajares, J.M., Di Bisceglie, A.M.: Development of cirrhosis after chronic type B hepatitis: a clinicopathologic and follow-up study of 46 HBe Ag-positive asymptomatic patients. Amer. J. Gastroenterol. 1991; 86; 560–564
45. Myers, R.P., Tainturier, M.H., Ratziu, V., Piton, A., Thibault, V., Imbert-Bismut, F., Messous, D., Charlotte, F., di Martino, V., Benhamou, Y., Poynard, T.: Prediction of liver histological lesions with biochemical markers in patients with chronic hepatitis B. J. Hepatol. 2003; 39: 222–230
46. Ohata, K., Hamasaki, K., Toriyama, K., Ishikawa, H., Nakao, K., Eguchi, K.: High viral load is a risk factor for hepatocellular carcinoma in patients with chronic hepatitis B virus infection. J. Gastroenterol. Hepatol. 2004; 19: 670–675
47. Peng, J., Luo, K.X., Zhu, Y.F., Guo, Y.B., Zhang, L., Hou, J.L.: Clinical and histological characteristics of chronic hepatitis B with negative hepatitis B e-antigen. Chin. Med. J. 2003; 116: 1312–1317
48. Pollicino, T., Squadrito, G., Cerenzia, G., Cacciola, I., Raffa, G., Craxi, A., Farinati, F., Missale, G., Smedile, A., Tiribelli, C., Villa, E., Raimondo, G.: Hepatitis B virus maintains its pro-oncogenic properties in the case of occult HBV infection. Gastroenterology 2004; 126: 102–110
49. Roche, B., Feray, C., Gigou, M., Roque-Alfonso, A.M., Arulnaden, J.L., Delvart, V., Dussaix, E., Guettier, C., Bismuth, H., Samuel, D.: HBV DNA persistence 10 years after liver transplantation despite successful anti-HBs passive immunoprophylaxis. Hepatology 2003; 38: 86–95
50. Schalm, S.W., Thomas, H.C., Hadziyannis, S.J.: Chronic hepatitis B. Prog. Liver Dis. 1990; 9: 443–462
51. Sumi, H., Yokosuka, O., Seki, N., Arai, M., Imazeki, F., Kurihara, T., Kanda, T., Fukai, K., Kato, M., Saisho, H.: Influence of hepatitis B virus genotypes on the progression of chronic type B liver disease. Hepatology 2003; 37: 19–26
52. Tang, B.Q., Kruger, W.D., Chen, G., Shen, F.M., Lin, W.Y., Mboup, S., London, W.T., Evans, A.A.: Hepatitis B viremia is associated with increased risk of hepatocellular carcinoma in chronic carriers. J. Med. Virol. 2004; 72: 35–40
53. Vegnente, A., Iorio, R., Guida, S., Cimmino, L.: Chronicity rate of hepatitis B virus infection in the families of 60 hepatitis B surface antigen-positive chronic carrier children: role of horizontal transmission. Europ. J. Pediatr. 1992; 151: 188–191
54. Wang, H.C., Wu, H.C., Chen, C.F., Fausto, N., Lei, H.Y., Su, I.J.: Different types of ground glass hepatocytes in chronic hepatitis B virus infection contain specific pre-S mutants that may induce endoplasmic reticulum stress. Amer. J. Path. 2003; 163: 2441–2449
55. Weissberg, J.I., Andres, L.L., Smith, C.I., Weick, S., Nichols, J.E., Garcia, G., Robinson, W.S., Merigan, T.C., Gregory, P.B.: Survival in chronic hepatitis B. An analysis of 379 patients. Ann. Intern. Med. 1984; 101: 613–616
56. Yeo, W., Chan, P.K.S., Hui, P., Ho, W.M., Lam, K.C., Kwan, W.H., Zhong, S., Johnson, P.J.: Hepatitis B virus reactivation in breast cancer patients receiving cytotoxic chemotherapy: a prospective study. J. Med. Virol. 2003; 70: 553–561
57. You, S.L., Yang, H.I., Chen, C.J.: Seropositivity of hepatitis B e antigen and hepatocellular carcinoma. Ann. Med. 2004; 36: 215–224
58. Yuen, M.F., Sablon, E., Wong, D.K.H., Yuan, H.J., Wong, B.C.Y., Chan, A.O.O., Lai, C.L.: Role of hepatitis B virus genotypes in chronic hepatitis B exacerbation. Clin. Infect. Dis. 2003; 37: 593–597

Chronic hepatitis C
59. Agnello, V., de Rosa, F.G.: Extrahepatic disease manifestations of HCV infection: some current issues (review). J. Hepatol. 2004; 40: 341–552
60. Alter, H.J., Seeff, L.B.: Recovery, persistence, and sequelae in hepatitis C virus infection: a perspective on long-term outcome. Semin. Liver Dis. 2000; 20: 17–35
61. Antonelli, A., Ferri, C., Pampana, A., Fallahi, P., Nesti, C., Pasquini, M., Marchi, S., Ferrannini, E.: Thyroid disorders in chronic hepatitis C. Amer. J. Med. 2004; 117: 10–13
62. Bain, V.G., Bonacini, M., Govindarajan, S., Ma, M., Sherman, M., Gibas, A., Cotler, S.J., Deschenes, M., Kaita, K., Ihangri, G.S.: A multicentre study of the usefulness of liver biopsy in hepatitis C. J. Viral Hepat. 2004; 11: 375–382
63. Bedossa, P., Bioulac-Sage, P., Callard, P., Chevallier, M., Degott, C., Deugnier, Y., Fabre, M., Reynés, M., Voigt, J.J., Zafrani, E.S.: Intraobserver and interobserver variations in liver biopsy interpretation in patients with chronic hepatitis C. Hepatology 1994; 20: 15–20
64. Bedossa, P., Poynard, T.: An algorithm for the grading of activity in chronic hepatitis C. Hepatology 1996; 24: 289–293
65. Bedossa, P., Dargere, D., Paradis, V.: Sampling variability of liver fibrosis in chronic hepatitis C. Hepatology 2003; 38: 1449–1457
66. Berenguer, M., Prieto, M., Rayon, J.M., Mora, J., Pastor, M., Ortiz, V., Carrasco, D., San-Juan, F., Burgueno, M.D.J., Mir, J., Berenguer, J.: Natural history of clinically compensated hepatitis C virus-related graft cirrhosis after liver transplantation. Hepatology 2000; 32: 852–858
67. Cassani, F., Cataleta, M., Valentini, P., Muratori, P., Giostra, F., Francesconi, R., Muratori, L., Lenzi, M., Bianchi, G., Zauli, D., Bianchi, F.B.: Serum autoantibodies in chronic hepatitis C: comparison with autoimmune hepatitis and impact on the disease profile. Hepatology 1997; 26: 561–566
68. Crespo, J., Rivero, M., Fabrega, E., Cayon, A., Amado, J.A., Garcia-Unzeta, M.T., Pons-Romero, F.: Plasma leptin and TNF-alpha levels in chronic hepatitis C patients and their relationship to hepatic fibrosis. Dig. Dis. Sci. 2002; 47: 1604–1610
69. Crowson, A.N., Nuovo, G., Ferri, C., Magro, C.M.: The dermatopathologic manifestations of hepatitis C infection: a clinical, histological, and molecular assessments of 35 cases. Hum. Pathol. 2003; 34: 573–579
70. Degos, F., Christidis, C., Ganne-Carrie, N., Farmachidi, J.P., Degott, C., Guettier, C., Trinchet, J.C., Beaugrand, M., Chevret, S.: Hepatitis C virus-related cirrhosis: time to occurrence of hepatocellular carcinoma and death. Gut 2000; 47: 131–136
71. Dhillon, A.P., Dusheiko, G.M.: Pathology of hepatitis C virus infection. Histology 1995; 26: 297–309
72. Dietrich, C.F., Stryjek-Kaminska, D., Teuber, G., Lee, J.H., Caspary, W.F., Zeuzem, S.: Perihepatic lymph nodes as a marker of antiviral response in patients with chronic hepatitis C infection. Amer. J. Roentgenol. 2000; 174: 699–704
73. DiMartino, V., Rufat, P., Boyer, N., Renard, P., Degos, F., Martinot-Peignoux, M., Matheron, S., LeMoing, V., Vachon, F., Degott, C., Valla, D., Marcellin, P.: The influence of human immunodeficiency virus coinfection on chronic hepatitis C in injection drug users: A long-term retrospective cohort study. Hepatology 2001; 34: 1193–1199
74. Erhardt, A., Hauck, K., Häussinger, D.: Iron as comorbid factor in chronic hepatitis. Med. Klin. 2003; 98: 685–691
75. Farinati, F., Cardin, R., de Maria, N., della Libera, G., Marafin, C., Lecis, E., Burra, P., Floreani, A., Cecchetto, A., Naccarato, R.: Iron storage, lipid peroxidation and glutathion turnover in chronic anti-HCV positive hepatitis. J. Hepatol. 1995; 22: 449–456
76. Floreani, A., Baragiotta, A., Leone, M.G., Baldo, V., Naccarato, R.: Primary biliary cirrhosis and hepatitis C virus infection. Amer. J. Gastroenterol. 2003; 98: 2757–2762
77. Forton, D.M., Taylor-Robinson, S.D., Thomas, H.C.: Central nervous system changes in hepatitis C virus infection. (review) Eur. J. Gastroenterol. Hepatol. 2006; 13: 441–448
78. Foster, G.R., Goldin, R.D., Thomas, H.C.: Chronic hepatitis C virus infection causes a significant reduction in quality of life in the absence of cirrhosis. Hepatology 1998; 27: 209–212
79. Fried, M.W., Draguesku, J.O., Shindo, M., Simpson, L.H., Banks, S.M., Hoofnagle, J.H., Di Bisceglie, A.M.: Clinical and serological differentiation of autoimmune and hepatitis C virus-related chronic hepatitis. Dig. Dis. Sci. 1993; 38: 631–636
80. Gane, E.J., Portmann, B.C., Naoumov, N.V., Smith, H.M., Underhill, J.A., Donaldson, P.T., Maertens, G., Williams, R.: Long-term outcome of hepatitis C infection after liver transplantation. New Engl. J. Med. 1996; 334: 815–820
81. Garcia-Carrasco, M., Escarcega, R.O.: Extrahepatic autoimmune manifestations of chronic hepatitis C virus infection. (editorial) Ann. Hepatol. 2006; 5: 161–163
82. Gebo, K.A., Herlong, H.F., Torbenson, M.S., Jenckes, M.W., Chander, G., Ghanem, K.G., El-Kamary, S.S., Sulkowski, M., Bass, E.B.: Role of liver biopsy in management of chronic hepatitis C: a systematic review. Hepatology 2002; 36 (Suppl.): 161–172
83. Ghany, M.G., Kleiner, D.E., Alter, H., Doo, E., Khokar, F., Promrat, K., Herion, D., Park, Y., Liang, T.J., Hoofnagle, J.H.: Progression of fibrosis in chronic hepatitis C. Gastroenterology 2003; 124: 97–114
84. Gisbert, J.P., Garcia-Buey, L., Pajares, J.M., Moreno-Otero, R.: Prevalence of hepatitis C virus infection in B-cell non-Hodgkin's lymphoma: systematik review and meta-analysis. Gastroenterology 2003; 125: 1723–1732
85. Gronbaek, K., Christensen, P.B., Hamilton-Dutoit, S., Federspiel, B.H., Hage, E., Jensen, O.J., Vyberg, M.: Interobserver variation in interpretation of serial liver biopsies from patients with chronic hepatitis C. J. Viral Hepat. 2002; 9: 443–449
86. Hatano, R., Ebara, M., Fukuda, H., Yoshikawa, M., Sugiura, N., Kondo, F., Yukawa, M., Saisho, H.: Accumulation of copper in the

liver and hepatic injury in chronic hepatitis C. J. Gastroenterol. 2000; 15: 786–791
87. Hezode, C., Lonjon, I., Roudot-Thoraval, F., Mavier, J.P., Pawlotsky, J.M., Zafrani, E.S., Dhumeaux, D.: Impact of smoking on histological liver lesions in chronic hepatitis C. Gut 2003; 52: 126–129
88. Hickman, I.J., Powell, E.E., Prins, J.B., Clouston, A.D., Ash, S., Purdie, D.M., Jonsson, J.R.: In overweight patients with chronic hepatitis C, circulating insulin is associated with hepatic fibrosis: implications for therapy. J. Hepatol. 2003; 39: 1042–1048
89. Hilsabeck, R.C., Perry, W., Hassanein, T.I.: Neuropsychological impairment in patients with chronic hepatitis C. Hepatology 2002; 35: 440–446
90. Hu, K.Q., Kyulo, N.L., Esrailian, E., Thompson, K., Chase, R., Hillebrand, D.J., Runyon, B.A.: Overweight and obesity, hepatic steatosis and progression of chronic hepatitis C: a retrospective study on a large cohort of patients in the United States. J. Hepatol. 2004; 40: 147–154
91. Hui, J.M., Sud, A., Farrell, G.C., Bandara, P., Byth, K., Kench, J.G., McCaughan, G.W., George, J.: Insulin resistance is associated with chronic hepatitis C and virus infection fibrosis progression. Gastroenterology 2003; 125: 1695–1704
92. Idilman, R., Colantoni, A., de Maria, N., Alkan, S., Nand, S., van Thiel, D.H.: Lymphoproliferative disorders in chronic hepatitis C. J. Viral Hepat. 2004; 11: 302–309
93. Ierna, D., D'Amico, R.A., Antoci, S., Campanile, E., Neri, S.: Perihepatic lymphadenopathy in chronic hepatitis C: a complementary diagnostic element? J. Gastroenterol. 2000; 15: 783–785
94. Jara, P., Resti, M., Hierro, L., Giacchino, R., Barbera, C., Zancan, L., Crivellaro, C., Sokal, E., Azzari, C., Guido, M., Bortolotti, F.: Chronic hepatitis C virus infection in childhood: clinical patterns and evolution in 224 white children. Clin. Infect. Dis. 2003; 36: 275–280
95. Jarmay, K., Karacsony, G., Ozsvar, Z., Lonovics, J., Schaff, Z.: Assessment of histological features in chronic hepatitis C. Hepato-Gastroenterol. 2002; 49: 239–243
96. Kramer, L., Bauer, E., Funk, G., Hofer, H., Jessner, W., Steindl-Munda, P., Wrba, F., Madl, C., Gangl, A., Ferenci, P.: Subclinical impairment of brain function in chronic hepatitis C infection. J. Hepatol. 2002; 37: 349–354
97. Leone, N., Pellicano, R., Maiocco, I.A., Modena, V., Marietti, G., Rizzetto, M., Ponzetto, A.: Mixed cryoglobulinaemia and chronic hepatitis C virus infection: the rheumatic manifestations. J. Med. Virol. 2002; 66: 200–203
98. Liu, C.H., Lin, J.W., Tsai, F.C., Yang, P.M., Lai, M.Y., Chen, J.H., Kao, J.H., Chen, D.S.: Noninvasive tests for the prediction of significant hepatic fibrosis in hepatitis C virus carriers with persistently normal alanine aminotransferases. Liver Intern. 2006; 26: 1087–1094
99. Lonardo, A., Loria, P., Adinolfi, L.E., Carulli, N., Ruggiero, G.: Hepatitis C and steatosis: a reappraisal. J. Vival Hepat. 2006; 13: 73–80
100. Martinelli, A.L.C., Villanova, M.G., Roselino, A.M.F., Figueiredo, J.F.C., Pasos, A.D.C., Covas, D.T., Zucoloto, S.: Abnormal uroporphyrin levels in chronic hepatitis C virus infection. J. Clin. Gastroenterol. 1999; 29: 327–331
101. McCaughan, G.W., George, J.: Fibrosis progression in chronic hepatitis C virus infection. Gut 2004; 53: 318–321
102. McCormick, S.E., Goodman, Z.D., Maydonovitch, C.L., Sjogren, M.H.: Evaluation of liver histology, ALT elevation, and HCV RNA titer in patients with chronic hepatitis C. Amer. J. Gastroenterol. 1996; 91: 1516–1522
103. McHutchison, J.G., Blatt, L.M., de Medina, M., Graig, J.R., Conrad, A., Schiff, E.R., Tong, M.J.: Measurement of serum hyaluronic acid in patients with chronic hepatitis C and its relationship to liver histology. J. Gastroenterol. Hepatol. 2000; 15: 945–951
104. Medina, J., Garcia-Buey, L., Moreno-Otero, R.: Review article: Hepatitis C virus-related extra-hepatic disease. Aetiopathogenesis and management. Alim. Pharm. Ther. 2004; 20: 129–141
105. Memon, M.I., Memon, M.A.: Hepatitis C: an epidemiological review. J. Viral Hepat. 2002; 9: 84–100
106. Merican, I., Sherlock, S., McIntyre, N., Dusheiko, G.M.: Clinical, biochemical and histologic features in 102 patients with chronic hepatitis C virus infection. Quart. J. Med. 1993; 86: 119–125
107. Moriyama, M., Matsumura, H., Shimizu, T., Shioda, A., Kaneko, M., Saito, H., Miyazawa, K., Tamaka, N., Sugitani, M., Komiyama, K., Arakawa, Y.: Hepatitis G virus coinfection influences the liver histology of patients with chronic hepatitis C. Liver 2000; 20: 397–404
108. Muller, P., Renou, C., Harafa, A., Jouve, E., Kaplanski, G., Ville, E., Bertrand, J.J., Masson, C., Benderitter, T., Halfon, P.: Lymph node enlargement within the hepatoduodenal ligament in patients with chronic hepatitis C reflects the immunological cellular response of the host. J. Hepatol. 2003; 39: 807–813
109. Nguyen-Khac, E., Capron, D.: Noninvasive diagnosis of liver fibrosis by ultrasonic transient elastography (Fibroscan) (review). Eur. J. Gastroenterol. Hepatol. 2006; 18: 1321–1325
110. Ortiz, V., Berenguer, M., Rayon, J.M., Carrasco, D., Berenguer, J.: Contribution of obesity to hepatitis C-related fibrosis progression. Amer. J. Gastroenterol. 2002; 97: 2408–2414
111. Pawlotsky, J.-M., Roudot-Thoraval, F., Simmonds, P., Mellor, J., Ben Yahia, M., André, C., Voisin, M.-C., Intrator, L., Zafrani, E.-S., Duval, J., Dhumeaux, D.: Extrahepatic immunologic manifestations in chronic hepatitis C and hepatitis C virus serotypes. Ann. Intern. Med. 1995; 122: 169–173
112. Pianko, S., Patella, S., Sievert, W.: Alcohol consumption induces hepatocyte apoptosis in patients with chronic hepatitis C infection. J. Gastroenterol. 2000; 15: 798–805

113. Piche, T., Gelsi, E., Schneider, S.M., Hebuterne, X., Giudicelli, J., Ferrua, B., Laffout, C., Benzaken, S., Hastier, P., Montoya, M.L., Longo, F., Rampal, P., Tran, A.: Fatigue is associated with circulating leptin levels in chronic hepatitis C. Gut 2002; 51: 434–439
114. Piche, T., Vandenbos, F., Abakar-Mahamat, A., Vanbiervliet, G., Barjoan, E.M., Calle, G., Giudicelli, J., Ferrua, B., Laffont, C., Benzaken, S., Tran, A.: The severity of liver fibrosis is associated with high leptin levels in chronic hepatitis C. J. Viral Hepat. 2004; 11: 91–96
115. Poynard, T., Bedossa, P., Opolon, P.: Natural history of liver fibrosis progression in patients with chronic hepatitis C. Lancet 1997; 349: 825–832
116. Poynard, T., Cacoub, P., Ratzin, V., Myers, R.P., Dezailles, M.H., Mercadier, A., Ghillani, P., Charlotte, F., Piette, J.C., Moussalli, J.: Fatigue in patients with chronic hepatitis C. J. Viral Hepat. 2002; 9: 295–303
117. Pradat, P., Alberti, A., Poynard, T., Esteban, J.-I., Weiland, O., Marcellin, P., Badalamenti, S., Trepo, C.: Predictive value of ALT levels for histologic findings in chronic hepatitis C: A European collaborative study. Hepatology 2002; 36: 973–977
118. Razonable, R.R., Burak, K.W., van Cruijsen, H., Brown, R.A., Charlton, M.R., Smith, T.F., Espy, M.J., Kremers, W., Wilson, J.A., Groettum, C., Wiesner, R., Paya, C.V.: The pathogenesis of hepatitis C virus is influenced by cytomegalovirus. Clin. Inf. Dis. 2002; 35: 974–981
119. Regev, A., Berho, M., Jeffers, L.J., Milikowski, C., Molina, E.G., Pyrsopoulos, N.T., Feng, Z.Z., Reddy, K.R., Schiff, E.R.: Sampling error and intraobserver variation in liver biopsy in patients with chronic HCV infection. Amer. J. Gastroenterol. 2002; 97: 2614–2618
120. Rigamonti, C., Mottaran, E., Reale, E., Rolla, R., Cipriani, V., Capelli, F., Boldorini, R., Vidali, M., Sartori, M., Albano, E.: Moderate alcohol consumption increases oxidative stress in patients with chronic hepatitis C. Hepatology 2003; 38: 42–49
121. Romero-Gomez, M., Grande, L., Nogales, M.C., Fernandez, M., Chavez, M., Castro, M.: Intrahepatic hepatitis C virus replication is increased in patients with regular alcohol consumption. Dig. Dis. Sci. 2001; 33: 698–702
122. Ross, R.S., Viazov, S., Gross, T., Hormann, F., Seipp, H.-M., Roggendorf, M.: Transmission of hepatitis C virus from a patient to an anaesthesiology assistant to five patients. New Engl. J. Med. 2000; 343: 1851–1854
123. Rubbia-Brandt, L., Quadri, R., Abid, K., Giostra, E., Malé, P.J., Mentha, G., Spahr, L., Zarski, J.P., Borisch, B., Hadengue, A., Negro, F.: Hepatocyte steatosis is a cytopathic effect of hepatitis C virus genotype J. Hepatol. 2000; 33: 106–115
124. Saadoun, D., Asselah, T., Resche-Rigon, M., Charlotte, F., Bedossa, P., Valla, D., Piette, J.C., Marcellin, P., Cacoub, P.: Cryoglobulinemia is associated with steatosis and fibrosis in chronic hepatitis C. Hepatology 2006; 43: 1337–1345
125. Sanchez-Pobre, P., Gonzalez, C., Paz, E., Colina, F., Castellano, G., Munoz-Yague, T., Rodriguez, S., Yela, C., Alvarez, V., Solis-Herruzo, J.: Chronic hepatitis C and autoimmune cholangitis: a case study and literature review. Dig. Dis. Sci. 2002; 47: 1224–1229
126. Sartori, M., Andorno, S., La Terra, G., Boldorini, R., Leone, F., Pi Hau, S., Zecchina, G., Aglietta, M., Saglio, G.: Evaluation of iron status in patients with chronic hepatitis C. Ital. J. Gastroenterol. Hepatol. 1998; 30: 396–401
127. Scheuer, P.J., Krawczynski, K., Dhillon, A.P.: Histopathology and detection of hepatitis C virus in liver. Semin. Immunpathol. 1997; 19: 27–45
128. Serfaty, L., Chazouillères, O., Poujol-Robert, A., Morand-Joubert, L., Dubois, C., Chrétien, Y., Poupon, R.E., Petit, J.-C., Poupon, R.: Risk factors for cirrhosis in patients with chronic hepatitis C virus infection: results of a case-control study. Hepatology 1997; 26: 776–779
129. Shakil, A.O., Conry-Cantilena, C., Alter, H.J., Hayashi, P., Kleiner, D.E., Tedeschi, V., Krawczynski, K., Conjeevaram, H.S., Sallie, R., DiBisceglie, A.M.: Volunteer blood donors with antibody to hepatitis C virus: clinical, biochemical, virologic, and histologic features. Ann. Intern. Med. 1995; 123: 330–337
130. Siddique, I., Abu-El-Naga, H., Madda, J.P., Memon, A., Hasan, F.: Sampling variability on percutaneous liver biopsy in patients with chronic hepatitis C virus infection. Scand. J. Gastroenterol. 2003; 38: 427–432
131. Silva, I.S.S., Ferraz, M.L.C.G., Perez, R.M., Lanzoni, V.P., Figueiredo, V.M., Silva, A.E.B.: Role of gamma-glutamyl transferase activity in patients with chronic hepatitis C virus infection. J. Gastroenterol. Hepatol. 2003; 19: 314–318
132. Skripenova, S., Trainer, T.D., Krawitt, E.L., Blaszyk, H.: Variability of grade and stage in simultaneous paired liver biopsies in patients with hepatitis C. J. Clin. Path. 2007; 60: 321–324
133. Tong, M.J., El-Farra, N.S., Reikes, A.R., Co, R.L.: Clinical outcomes after transfusion-associated hepatitis C. New Engl. J. Med. 1995; 332: 1463–1466
134. Trendelenburg, M., Schifferli, J.A.: Cryoglobulins in chronic hepatitis C virus infection. Clin. Exper. Immunol. 2003; 133: 153–155
135. Vento, S., Garofano, T., Renzini, C., Cainelli, F., Casali, F., Ghironzi, G., Ferraro, T., Concia, E.: Fulminant hepatitis associated with hepatitis A virus superinfection in patients with chronic hepatitis C. New Engl. J. Med. 1998; 338: 286–290
136. Verbaan, H., Widell, A., Lindgren, S., Lindmark, B., Nordenfelt, E., Eriksson, S.: Hepatitis C in chronic liver disease: an epidemiological study based on 566 consecutive patients undergoing liver biopsy during a 10-year period. J. Intern. Med. 1992; 232: 33–42

137. **Wedemeyer, H., Ockenga, J., Frank, H., Tillmann, H.L., Schuler, A., Caselitz, M., Gebel, M., Trautwein, C., Manns, M.P.:** Perihepatic lymphadenopathy: a marker of response to interferon alpha in chronic hepatitis C. Hepato-Gastroenterol. 1998; 45: 1062−1068
138. **Westin, J., Lagging, L.M., Spak, F., Aires, N., Svensson, E., Lindh, M., Dhillon, A.P., Norkrans, G., Wejstal, R.:** Moderate alcohol intake increases fibrosis progression in untreated patients with hepatitis C virus infection. J. Viral Hepat. 2002; 9: 235−241
139. **Zarski, J.P., McHutchinson, J., Bronowicki, J.P., Sturm, N., Garcia-Kennedy, R., Hoday, E., Truta, B., Wright, T., Gish, R.:** Rate of natural disease progression in patients with chronic hepatitis C. J. Hepatol. 2003; 38: 307−314
140. **Zein, N.N., Arslan, M., Li, H.J., Charlton, M.R., Gross, J.B., Poterucha, J.J., Therneau, T.M., Kolbert, C.P., Persing, D.H.:** Clinical significance of TT virus infection in patients with chronic hepatitis C. Amer. J. Gastroenterol. 1999; 94: 3020−3027
141. **Zhang, X.M., Mitchell, D.G., Shi, H.Y., Holland, G.A., Parker, L., Herrine, S.K., Pasqualin, D., Rubin, R.:** Chronic hepatitis C activity: correlation with lymphadenopathy on MR imaging. Amer. J. Roentgenol. 2002; 179: 417−422
142. **Zignego, A.L., Ferri, C., Pileri, S.A., Caini, P., Bianchi, F.B.:** Extrahepatic manifestations of hepatitis C virus infection: A general overview and guidelines for a clinical approach (review). Dig. Liver Dis. 2007; 39: 2−17

Chronic hepatitis D

143. **Ackerman, Z., Valinluck, B., McHutchison, J.G., Redeker, A.G., Govindarajan, S.:** Spontaneous exacerbation of disease activity in patients with chronic delta hepatitis infection: the role of hepatitis B, C or D? Hepatology 1992; 16: 625−629
144. **Elefsiniotis, I.S., Diamantis, I.D., Dourakis, S.P., Kafiri, G., Pantazis, K., Mavrogiannis, C.:** Anticardiolipin antibodies in chronic hepatitis B and chronic hepatitis D infection, and hepatitis B-related hepatocellular carcinoma. Relationship with portal vein thrombosis. Eur. J. Gastroenterol. Hepatol. 2003; 15: 721−726
145. **Gerken, G., Meyer zum Büschenfelde, K.-H.:** Chronic hepatitis delta virus (HDV) infection. Hepato-Gastroenterol. 1991; 38: 29−32
146. **Philipp, T., Durazzo, M., Trautwein, C., Alex, B., Straub, P., Lamb, J.G., Johnson, E.F., Tukey, R.H., Manns, M.P.:** Recognition of uridine diphosphate glucuronosyl transferases by LKM-3 antibodies in chronic hepatitis D. Lancet 1994; 344: 578−581

Therapy of chronic hepatitis B

147. **Alexander, G.J.M., Fagan, E.A., Hegarty, J.E., Yeo, J., Eddlestone, A.L.W.F., Williams, R.:** Controlled trial of acyclovir in chronic hepatitis B virus infection. J. Med. Virol. 1987; 21: 81−87
148. **Bartholomeusz, A., Groenen, L.C., Locarnini, S.A.:** Clinical experience with famciclovir against hepatitis B virus. Intervirology 1997; 40: 337−342
149. **Ben-Ari, Z., Mor, E., Tur-Kaspa, R.:** Experience with lamivudine therapy for hepatitis B virus infection before and after liver transplantation, and review of the literature. J. Intern. Med. 2003; 253: 544−552
150. **Chan, H.L.Y., Tang, J.L., Tam, W., Sung, J.J.Y.:** The efficacy of thymosin in the treatment of chronic hepatitis B virus infection: a meta-analysis. Alim. Pharm. Ther. 2001; 15: 1899−1905
151. **Chen, C., Guo, S.M., Liu, B.:** A randomized controlled trial of kurorinone versus interferon-α_{2a} treatment in chronic hepatitis B. J. Viral Hepat. 2000; 7: 225−229
152. **Cooksley, W.G.E., Piratvisuth, T., Lee, S.D., Mahachai, V., Chao, Y.C., Tanwandee, T., Chutaputti, A., Chang, W.Y., Zahm, F.E., Pluck, N.:** Peginterferon alpha-2a (40 k Da): An advance in the treatment of hepatitis B e antigen-positive chronic hepatitis B. J. Viral. Hepat. 2003; 10: 298−305
153. **Crowley, S., Tognanni, D., Desmond, P., Lees, M., Saat, G.:** Introduction of lamivudine for the treatment of chronic hepatitis B: expected clinical and economic outcomes based on 4-year clinical trial data. J. Gastroenterol. Hepatol. 2002; 17: 153−164
154. **Di Bisceglie, A.M., Fong, T.-L, Fried. M.W., Swain, M.G., Baker, B., Korenman, J., Bergasa, N.V., Waggoner, J.G., Park, Y., Hoofnagle, J.H.:** A randomized, controlled trial of recombinant α-Interferon therapy for chronic hepatitis B. Amer. J. Gastroenterol. 1993; 88: 1887−1892
155. **Dienstag, J.L., Goldin, R.D., Heathcote, E.J., Hann, H.W.L., Woessner, M., Stephenson, S.L., Gardner, S., Fraser-Gray, D., Schiff, E.R.:** Histological outcome during long-term lamivudine therapy. Gastroenterology 2003; 124: 105−117
156. **Fung, S.K., Chae, H.B.C., Fontana, R.J., Conjeecaram, H., Marrero, J., Oberhelman, K., Hussain, M., Lok, H.S.F.:** Virologic response and resistance to adefovir in patients with chronic hepatitis B. J. Hepatol. 2006; 44: 283−290
157. **Gaia, S., Marzano, A., Smedile, A., Barbon, V., Abate, M.L., Olivero, A., Lagget, M., Paganin, S., Fadda, M., Niro, G., Rizzetto, M.:** Four years of treatment with lamivudine: Clinical and virological evaluations in Hbe antigen-negative chronic hepatitis B. Alim. Pharm. Ther. 2004; 20: 281−287
158. **Genel, F., Unal, F., Ozgenc, F., Aksu, G., Aydogdu, S., Kutukculer, N., Yagci, R.V.:** Decreased ratio of CD4 / CD8 lymphocytes might be predictive for successful interferon alpha and lamivudine combined therapy in childhood chronic hepatitis B infection: A preliminary study. J. Gastroenterol. Hepatol. 2003; 18: 645−650

159. **Gish, R.G., McCashland, T.:** Hepatitis B in liver transplant recipients. Liver Transplant. 2006; 12 (Suppl. 2): 54−64
160. **Guptan, R.C., Thakur, V., Kazim, S.N., Sarin, S.K.:** Efficacy of granulocyte-macrophage colony-stimulating factor or lamivudine combination with recombinant interferon in non-responders to interferon in hepatitis B virus-related chronic liver disease patients. J. Gastroenterol. Hepatol. 2002; 17: 765−771
161. **Hadziyannis, S.J., Tassopoulos, N.C., Heathcote, E.J., Chang, T.T., Kitis, G., Rizzetto, M., Marcellin, P., Lim, S.G., Goodman, Z., Wulfsohn, M.S., Xiong, S., Fry, J., Brosgart, C.L.:** Adefovir dipivoxil for the treatment of hepatitis B e antigen-negative chronic hepatitis B. New Engl. J. Med. 2003; 348: 800−807
162. **Kimdo, Y., Kim, H.J., Lee, C.K., Suh, J.H., Kim, D.H., Cho, Y.S., Won, S.Y., Park, B.K., Park, I.S.:** Efficacy of adefovir dipivoxil in the treatment of lamivudine-resistant hepatitis B virus genotype C. Liver Intern. 2007; 27: 47−53
163. **Krogsgaard, K.:** The long-term effect of treatment with interferon-α_{2a} in chronic hepatitis B. J. Viral Hepatit. 1998; 5: 389−397
164. **Kweon, Y.O., Goodman, Z.D., Dienstag, J.L., Schiff, E.R., Brown, N.A., Burkhardt, E., Schoonhoven, R., Brenner, D.A., Fried, M.W.:** Decreasing fibrogenesis: an immunohistochemical study of paired liver biopsies following lamivudine therapy for chronic hepatitis B. J. Hepatol. 2001; 35: 749−755
165. **Lai, C.L., Rosmawati, M., Lao, J., van Vlierberghe, H., Anderson, F.H., Thomas, N., Dehertogh, D.:** Entecavir is superior to lamivudine in reducing hepatitis B virus DNA in patients with chronic hepatitis B infection. Gastroenterology 2002; 123: 1831−1838
166. **Lau, G.K.K., Nanji, A., Hou, J., Fong, D.Y.T., Au, W.S., Yuen, S.T., Lin, M., Kung, H.F., Lam, S.K.:** Thymosin-alpha 1 and famciclovir combination therapy activates T-cell response in patients with chronic hepatitis B virus infection in immune-tolerant phase. J. Viral Hepat. 2002; 9: 280−287
167. **Lau, G.K.K., Yiu, H.H.Y., Fong, D.Y.T., Cheng, H.C., Au, W.Y., Lai, L.S.F., Cheung, M., Zhang, H.Y., Lie, A., Ngan, R., Liang, R.:** Early is superior to deferred preemptive lamivudine therapy for hepatitis B patients undergoing chemotherapy. Gastroenterology 2003; 125: 1742−1749
168. **Lee, H.-S., Chung, Y.-H., Lee, K., Byun, K.S., Paik, S.W., Han, J.-Y., Yoo, K., Yoo, H.-W., Lee, J.H., Yoo, B.C.:** A 12-week clerudine therapy showed potent and durable antiviral activity in HBeAg-positive chronic hepatitis B. Hepatology 2006; 43: 982−988
169. **Liaw, Y.F.:** Hepatitis flares and hepatitis B e antigen seroconversion: implication in antihepatitis B virus therapy (review). J. Gastroenterol. Hepatol. 2003; 18: 246−252
170. **Lim, S.G., Ng, T.M., Kung, N., Krastev, Z., Volfova, M., Husa, P., Lee, S.S., Chan, S., Shiffman, M.L., Washington, M.K., Rigney, A., Anderson, J., Mondou, E., Snow, A., Sorbel, J., Guan, R., Rousseau, F.:** A double-blind placebo-controlled study of emtricitabine in chronic hepatitis B. Arch. Intern. Med. 2006; 166: 49−56
171. **Lok, A.S.F., McMahon, B.J.:** Chronic hepatitis B. Hepatoilogy 2007; 45: 507−539
172. **Main, J., Brown, J.L., Howels, C., Galassini, R., Crossey, M., Karayiannis, P., Georgiou, P., Atkinson, G., Thomas, H.C.:** A double-blind, placebo-controlled study to assess the effect of famciclovir on virus replication in patients with chronic hepatitis B virus infection. J. Viral Hepatit. 1996; 3: 211−215
173. **Malaguarnera, M., Restuccia, S., Receputo, G., Giugno, I., Pistone, G., Trovato, B.A.:** The efficacy of interferon alpha in chronic hepatitis B: a review and meta-analysis. Curr. Ther. Res. 1996; 57: 646−662
174. **Marcellin, P., Chang, T., Lim, S.G., Tong, M.J., Sievert, W., Shiffman, M.L., Jeffers, L., Goodman, Z., Wulfsohn, M.S., Xiong, S., Fry, J., Brosgart, C.L.:** Adefovir dipivoxil for the treatment of hepatitis B e antigen-positive chronic hepatitis B. New Engl. J. Med. 2003; 348: 808−816
175. **Marcellin, P., Lau, G.K.K., Bonino, F., Farci, P., Hadziyannis, S., Jin, R., Lu, Z.M., Piratvisuth, T., Germanidis, G., Yurdaydin, C., M., Gurel, S., Lai, M.Y., Button, P., Pluck, N.:** Peginterferon alfa-2a alone, lamivudine alone, and the two in combination in patients with HBeAg-negative chronic hepatitis B. New Engl. J. Med. 2004; 351: 1206−1217
176. **Marques, A.R., Lau, D.T.Y., McKenzie, R., Straus, S.E., Hoofnagle, J.H.:** Combination therapy with famciclovir and interferon-α for the treatment of chronic hepatitis B. J. Infect. Dis. 1998; 178: 1483−1487
177. **Mihm, U., Sarrazin, C., Herrmann, E., Teuber, G., von Wagner, M., Kronenberger, B., Zeuzem, S.:** Response predictors and results of a long-term treatment with lamivudine in patients with chronic hepatitis B. Z. Gastroenterol. 2003; 41: 249−254
178. **Munoz, R., Castellano, G., Fernandez, I., Alvarez, M.V., Manzano, M.L., Marcos, M.S., Cuenca, B., Solis-Herruzo, J.A.:** A pilot study of beta-interferon for treatment of patients with chronic hepatitis B who failed to respond to alpha-interferon. J. Hepatol. 2002; 37: 655−659
179. **Mutimer, D., Naoumov, N., Honkoop, P., Marinos, G., Ahmed, M., de Man, R., McPhillips, P., Johnson, M., Williams, R., Elias, E., Schalm, S.:** Combination alpha-interferon and lamivudine therapy for alpha-interferon resistant chronic hepatitis B infection: results of a pilot study. J. Hepatol. 1998; 28: 923−929
180. **Niederau, C., Strohmeyer, G., Heintges, T., Peter, K., Gopfert, F.:** Polyunsaturated phosphatidyl-choline and interferon alpha for treatment of chronic hepatitis B and C: a multicenter, randomized, double-blind, placebo-controlled trial. Hepato-Gastroenterol. 1998; 45: 797−804
181. **Oh, J.M., Kyun, J., Cho, S.W.:** Long-term lamivudine therapy for chronic hepatitis B in patients with and without cirrhosis. Pharmacotherapy 2002; 22: 1226−1234

182. Ohkoshi, S., Ogata, N., Ichida, T.: The long-term clinical outcome of 1-year treatment of chronic hepatitis B with lamivudine-5 years observation. Hepatol. Res. 2003; 27: 13–17
183. Perrillo, R., Hann, H.W., Mutimer, D., Willems, B., Leung, N., Lee, W.M., Moorat, A., Gardner, S., Woessner, M., Bourne, E., Brosgart, C.L., Schiff, E.: Adefovir dipivoxil added to ongoing lamivudine in chronic hepatitis B with YMDD mutant hepatitis B virus. Gastroenterology 2004; 126: 81–90
184. Peters, M.G., Hann, H.W., Martin, P., Heathcote, E.J., Buggisch, P., Rubin, R., Bourliere, M., Kowdley, K., Trepo, C., Gray, D.F., Sullivan, M., Kleber, K., Ebrahimi, R., Xiong, S., Brosgart, C.L.: Adefovir dipivoxil alone or in combination with lamivudine in patients with lamivudine-resistant chronic hepatitis B. Gastroenterology 2004; 126: 91–101
185. Robinson, D.M., Scott, L.J., Plosker, G.L.: Entecavir: A review of its use in chronic hepatitis B. Drugs 2006; 66: 1605–1622
186. Roche, B., Samuel, D., Gigou, M., Feray, C., Virot, V., Majno, P., Serraf, L., David, M.F., Dusseaix, E., Reynes, M., Bismuth, H.: Long-term ganciclovir therapy for hepatitis B virus infection after transplantation. J. Hepatol. 1999; 31: 584–592
187. Schalm, S.W., Heathcote, J., Cianciara, J., Farrell, G., Sherman, M., Willems, B., Dhillon, A., Moorat, A., Barber, J., Gray, D.F.: Lamivudine and alpha interferon combination treatment of patients with chronic hepatitis B infection: a randomized trial. Gut 2000; 46: 562–568
188. Schiff, E.R., Dienstag, J.L., Karayalcin, S., Grimm, I.S., Perrillo, R.P., Husa, P., de Man, R.A., Goodman, Z., Condreay, L.D., Crowther, L.M., Woessner, M.A., McPhillips, P.J., Brown, N.A.: Lamivudine and 24 weeks of lamivudine/interferon combination therapy for hepatitis B e antigen-positive chronic hepatitis B in interferon nonresponders. J. Hepatol. 2003; 38: 818–826
189. Shen, H., Alsatie, M., Eckert, G., Chalasani, N., Lumeng, L., Kwo, P.Y.: Combination therapy with lamivudine and famciclovir for chronic hepatitis B infection. Clin. Gastroenterol. Hepatol. 2004; 2: 330–336
190. Suzuki, Y., Arase, Y., Ikeda, K., Saitoh, S., Tsubota, T., Miyakawa, Y., Kumada, H.: Histological improvements after a three-year lamivudine therapy in patients with chronic hepatitis B in whom YMDD mutants did not or did develop. Intervirology 2003; 46: 164–170
191. Tamam, L., Yerdelen, D., Ozpoyraz, N.: Psychosis associated with interferon alfa therapy for chronic hepatitis B. Ann. Pharmacother. 2003; 37: 384–387
192. Vajro, P., Migliaro, F., Fontanella, A., Orso, G.: Interferon: a metaanalysis of published studies in chronic hepatitis B. Acta Gastroenterol. Belg. 1998; 61: 219–223
193. Villeneuve, J.-P., Condreay, L.D., Willems, B., Pomier-Layrargues, G., Fenyves, D., Bilodeau, M., Leduc, R., Peltekian, K., Wong, F., Margulies, M., Heathcote, E.J.: Lamivudine treatment for decompensated cirrhosis resulting from chronic hepatitis B. Hepatology 2000; 31: 207–210
194. Werle, B., Cinquin, K., Marcellin, P., Pol, S., Maynard, M., Trepo, C., Zoulim, F.: Evolution of hepatitis B viral load and viral genome sequence during adefovir dipivoxil therapy. J. Viral Hepat. 2003; 11: 74–83
195. Westland, C.E., Yang, H.L., Delaney, W.E., Gibbs, C.S., Miller, M.D., Wulfsohn, M., Fry, J., Brosgart, C.L., Xiong, S.: Week 48 resistance surveillance in two phase 3 clinical studies of adefovir dipivoxil for chronic hepatitis B. Hepatology 2003; 38: 96–103
196. Yokosuka, O.: Events occurring at the time of breakthrough hepatitis during lamivudine treatment for chronic hepatitis (editorial). J. Gastroenterol. 2004; 39: 813–814

Therapy of chronic hepatitis C
197. Adinolfi, L.E., Utili, R., Tonziello, A., Ruggiero, G.: Effects of alpha interferon induction plus ribavirin with or without amantadine in the treatment of interferon nonresponsive chronic hepatitis C: a randomized trial. Gut 2003; 52: 701–705
198. Arase, Y., Ikeda, K., Tsubota, A., Suzuki, Y., Saitoh, S., Kobayashi, M., Suzuki, F., Akuta, N., Someya, T., Hosaka, T., Kobayashi, M., Kumada, H.: Efficacy of interferon retreatment after relapse for chronic hepatitis C patients with biochemical response after first interferon therapy. J. Gastroenterol. 2004; 39: 455–460
199. Asnis, G.M., de la Garza, R.: Interferon-induced depression in chronic hepatitis C: A review of its prevalence, risk factors, biology, and treatment approaches. J. Clin. Gastroenterol. 2006; 40: 322–335
200. Bajaj, J.S., Molina, E., Regev, A., Schiff, E.R., Jeffers, L.J.: Pretreatment laparoscopic appearance of the liver can predict response to combination therapy with interferon alpha 2b and ribavirin in chronic hepatitis C. Gastrointest. Endosc. 2003; 58: 380–383
201. Berg, T., Kronenberger, B., Hinrichsen, H., Gerlach, T., Buggisch, P., Herrmann, E., Spengler, U., Goeser, T., Nasser, S., Wursthorn, K., Pape, G.R., Hopf, U., Zeuzem, S.: Triple therapy with amantadine in treatment-naive patients with chronic hepatitis C: a placebo-controlled trial. Hepatology 2003; 37: 1359–1367
202. Brok, J., Gluud, L.L., Gluud, C.: Effects of adding ribavirin to interferon to treat chronic hepatitis C infection: A systematic review and meta-analysis of randomized trials. Arch. Intern. Med. 2005; 165: 2206–2212
203. Calleja, J.L., Albillos, A., Moreno-Otero, R., Rossi, I., Cacho, G., Domper, F., Yebra, M., Escartin, P.: Sustained response to interferon-α or to interferon-α plus ribavirin in hepatitis C virus-associated symptomatic mixed cryoglobulinaemia. Aliment. Pharmacol. Ther. 1999; 13: 1179–1186
204. Camma, C., Di Bona, D., Schepis, F., Heathcote, E.J., Zeuzem, S., Pockross, P.J., Marcellin, P., Balart, L., Alberti, A., Craxi, A.: Effect of peginterferon α-2a on liver histology in chronic hepatitis C: a meta-analysis of individual patient data. Hepatology 2004; 39: 333–342
205. Chaudhari, S., Park, J., Anand, B.S., Pimstone, N.R., Dieterich, D.T., Batash, S., Bini, E.J.: Acute pancreatitis associated with interferon and ribavirin therapy in patients with chronic hepatitis C. Dig. Dis. Sci. 2004; 49: 1000–1006
206. Cheng, P.N., Chow, N.H., Hu, S.C., Young, K.C., Chen, C.Y., Jen, C.M., Chang, T.T.: Clinical comparison of high-dose interferon-alpha 2b with or without ribavirin for treatment of interferon-relapsed chronic hepatitis C. Dig. Dis. Sci. 2002; 34: 851–856
207. Di Bisceglie, A.M., Bonkovsky, H.L., Chopra, S., Flamm, S., Reddy, R.K., Grace, N., Killenberg, P., Hunt, C., Tamburro, C., Tavill, A.S., Ferguson, R., Krawitt, E., Banner, B., Bacon, B.R.: Iron reduction as an adjuvant to interferon therapy in patients with chronic hepatitis C who have previously not responded to interferon: a multicenter, prospective, randomized, controlled trial. Hepatology 2000; 32: 135–138
208. Fujita, N., Kaito, M., Kai, M., Sugimoto, R., Tanaka, H., Horiike, S., Konishi, M., Iwasa, M., Watanabe, S., Adadu, Y.: Effects of bezafibrate in patients with chronic hepatitis C infection: Combination with interferon and ribavarin. J. Vir. Hepat. 2006; 13: 441–448
209. Gitlin, N.: Manifestation of sarcoidosis during interferon and ribavirin therapy for chronic hepatitis C: a report of two cases. Eur. J. Gastroenterol. Hepatol. 2002; 14: 883–885
210. Hadziyannis, S.J., Settl, H., Morgan, T.R., Balan, V., Diago, M., Marcellin, P., Ramadori, G., Bodenheimer, H., Bernstein, D., Rizzetto, M., Zeuzem, S., Pockros, P.J., Lin, A., Ackrill, A.M.: Peginterferon-alpha 2a and ribavirin combination therapy in chronic hepatitis C. A randomized study of treatment duration and ribavirin dose. Ann. Intern. Med. 2004; 140: 346–356
211. Hasan, F., Asker, H., Al-Khaldi, J., Siddique, I., Al-Ajmi, M., Owaid, S., Varghese, R., Al-Nakib, B.: Peginterferon alfa-2b plus ribavirin for the treatment of chronic hepatitis C genotype 4. Amer. J. Gastroenterol. 2004; 99: 1733–1737
212. Hutchinson, S.J., Bird, S.M., Goldberg, D.J.: Influence of alcohol on the progression of hepatitis C virus infection: A meta-analysis. Clin. Gastroenterol. Hepatol. 2005; 3: 1150–1159
213. Ikeda, K., Arase, Y., Kobayashi, M., Saitoh, S., Someya, T., Sezaki, H., Akuta, N., Suzuki, Y., Suzuki, F., Kumada, H.: A long-term glycyrrhizin injection therapy reduces hepatocellular carcinogenesis rate in patients with interferon-resistant active chronic hepatitis C: A cohort study of 1249 patients. Dig. Dis. Sci 2006; 51: 603–609
214. Inoue, K., Sekiyama, K., Yamada, M., Watanabe, T., Yasuda, H., Yoshiba, M.: Combined interferon alpha 2b and cyclosporin A in the treatment of chronic hepatitis C: controlled trial. Gastroenterology. 2003; 38: 567–572
215. Itoh, Y., Okanoue, T.: Ribavirin-induced hemolytic anemia in chronic hepatitis C patients (editorial). J. Gastroenterol. 2004; 39: 704–705
216. Kumar, K.S., Russo, M.W., Borczuk, A.C., Brown, M., Esposito, S.P., Lobritto, S.J., Jacobson, I.M., Brown, R.S.: Significant pulmonary toxicity associated with interferon and ribavirin therapy for hepatitis C. Amer. J. Gastroenterol. 2002; 97: 2432–2440
217. Melhem, A., Stern, M., Shibolet, O., Israeli, E., Ackerman, Z., Pappo, O., Hemed, N., Rowe, M., Ohana, H., Zabrecky, G., Lohen, R., Ilan, Y.: Treatment of chronic hepatitis C virus infection via antioxidants – Results of a phase I clinical trial. J. Clin. Gastroenterol. 2005; 39: 737–742
218. Myers, R.P., Thibault, V., Poynard, T.: The impact of prior hepatitis B virus infection on liver histology and the response to interferon therapy in chronic hepatitis C. J. Viral Hepat. 2003; 10: 103–110
219. Nakagawa, M., Sakamoto, N., Enomoto, N., Tanabe, Y., Kanazawa, N., Koyama, T., Kurosaki, M., Maekawa, S., Yamashiro, T., Chen, C.H., Itsui, Y., Kakinuma, S., Watanabe, M.: Specific inhibition of hepatitis C virus replication by cyclosporin A. Biochem. Biophys. Res. Com. 2004; 313: 42–47
220. Pockros, P., Carithers, R., Desmond, P., Dhumeaux, D., Fried, M.W., Marcellin, P., Shiffman, M.L., Minuk, G., Reddy, K.R., Reindollar, R.W., Lin, A., Brunda, M.J.: Efficacy and safety of two-dose regimens of peginterferon alpha-2a compared with interferon controlled trial. Amer. J. Gastroenterol. 2004; 99: 1298–1305
221. Poupon, R.E., Bonnand, A.M., Queneau, P.E., Trépo, C., Zarski, J.P., Vetter, D., Raabe, J.J., Thieffin, G., Larrey, D., Grange, J.D., Capron, J.P., Serfaty, L., Chrétien, Y., St.-Girardin, M.F., Mathiex-Fortunet, H., Zafrani, E.S., Guéchot, J., Beuers, U., Paumgartner, G., Poupon, R.: Randomized trial of interferon-alpha plus ursodeoxycholic acid versus interferon plus placebo in patients with chronic hepatitis C resistant to interferon. Scand. J. Gastroenterol. 2000; 35: 642–649
222. Russo, M.W., Fried, M.W.: Side-effect of therapy for chronic hepatitis C. Gastroenterology 2003; 124: 1711–1719
223. Schaefer, M., Schmidt, F., Folwaczny, C., Lorenz, R., Martin, G., Schindlbeck, N., Heldwein, W., Soyka, M., Grunze, H., Koenig, A., Loeschke, K.: Adherence and mental side effects during hepatitis C treatment with interferon alfa and ribavirin in psychiatric risk groups. Hepatology 2003; 37: 443–451
224. Sherman, K.E., Sjogren, M., Creager, R.L., Damiano, M.A., Freeman, St., Lewey, S., Davis, D., Root, S., Weber, F.L., Ishak, K.G., Goodman, Z.D.: Combination therapy with thymosin α1 and interferon for the

treatment of chronic hepatitis C infection: a randomized, placebo-controlled double-blind trial. Hepatology 1998; 27: 1128–1135
225. **Shiffman, M.L., Hoffmann, C.M., Gabbay, J., Luketic, V.A., Sterling, R.K., Sanyal, A.J., Contos, M.J., Ryan, M.J., Yoshida, C., Rustgi, V.:** Treatment of chronic hepatitis C in patients who failed interferon monotherapy: effects of higher doses of interferon and ribavirin combination therapy. Amer. J. Gastroenterol. 2000; 95: 2928–2935
226. **Smith, J.P.:** Treatment of chronic hepatitis C with amantadine. Dig. Dis. Sci. 1997; 42: 1681–1687
227. **Smith, J.P., Riley, T.R., Bingaman, S., Mauger, D.T.:** Amantadine therapy for chronic hepatitis C: a dose escalation study. Amer. J. Gastroenterol. 2004; 99: 1099–1104
228. **Tahan, V., Ozseker, F., Guneylioglu, D., Baran, A., Ozaras, R., Mert, A., Ucisik, A.C., Cagatay, T., Yilmazbayhan, D., Senturk, H.:** Sarcoidosis after use of interferon for chronic hepatitis C-Report of a case and review of the literature. Dig. Dis. Sci. 2003; 48: 169–173
229. **Takimoto, M., Ohkoshi, S., Ichida, T., Takeda, Y., Nomoto, M., Asakura, A., Naito, A., Mori, S., Hata, K., Igarashi, K., Hara, H., Ohta, H., Soga, K., Watanabe, T., Kamimura, T.:** Interferon inhibits progression of liver fibrosis and reduces the risk of hepatocarcinogenesis in patients with chronic hepatitis C. A retrospective multicenter analysis of 652 patients. Dig. Dis. Sci. 2002; 47: 170–176
230. **Tanaka, N., Kiyosawa, K.:** Phlebotomy: a promising treatment for chronic hepatitis C (editorial). J. Gastroenterol. 2004; 39: 601–603
231. **Thuluvath, P.J., Pande, H., Maygers, J.:** Combination therapy with interferon-alpha (2b), ribavirin, and amantadine in chronic hepatitis C nonresponders to interferon and ribavirin. Dig. Dis. Sci. 2003; 48: 594–597
232. **Toccaceli, F., Laghi, V., Capurso, L., Koch, M., Sereno, S., Scuderi, M.:** Long-term liver histology improvement in patients with chronic hepatitis C and sustained response to interferon. J. Viral Hepat. 2003; 10: 126–133
233. **Ullerich, H., Avenhaus, W., Poremba, C., Domschke, W., Menzel, J.:** High-dose interferon alpha-2a with ribavirin and amantadine in naive chronic hepatitis C patients-results of a randomized, prospective, pilot study. Alim. Pharm. Ther. 2002; 16: 2107–2114
234. **Van Rossum, T.G.J., Vulto, A.G., de Man, R.A., Brouwer, J.T., Schalm, S.W.:** Review article: Glycyrrhizin as a potential treatment for chronic hepatitis C. Aliment. Pharm. Ther. 1998; 12: 199–205
235. **Younossi, Z.M., Mullen, K.D., Hodnick, S., Barnes, D.S., Carey, W.D., McCullough, A.C., Easley, K., Gramlich, T., Liebermann, B.Y.:** Triple combination of interferon alpha-2b, ribavirin, and amantadine for treatment of chronic hepatitis C. J. Clin. Gastroenterol. 2003; 36: 427–430
236. **Zeuzem, S., Teuber, G., Naumann, U., Berg, T., Raedle, J., Hartmann, S., Hopf, U.:** Randomized, double-blind, placebo-controlled trial of interferon alfa 2a with and without amantadine as initial treatment for chronic hepatitis C. Hepatology 2000; 32: 835–841
237. **Zeuzem, S., Heathcote, E.J., Shiffman, M.L., Wright, T.L., Bain, V.G., Sherman, M., Feinman, S.V., Fried, M.W., Rasenack, J., Sarrazin, C., Jensen, D.M., Lin, A., Hoffman, J.H., Sedarati, F.:** Twelve weeks of follow-up is sufficient for the determination of sustained virologic response in patients treated with interferon alpha for chronic hepatitis C. J. Hepatol. 2003; 39: 106–111
238. **Zeuzem, S., Hultcrantz, R., Bourliere, M., Goeser, T., Marcellin, P., Sanchez-Tapias, J., Sarrazin, C., Harvey, J., Brass, C., Albrecht, J.:** Peginterferon alfa-2b plus ribavirin for treatment of chronic hepatitis C in previously untreated patients infected with HCV genotypes 2 or 3. J. Hepatol. 2004; 40: 993–999
239. **Zilly, M., Lingenauber, C., Desch, S., Väth, T., Klinker, H., Langmann, P.:** Triple antiviral re-therapy for chronic hepatitis C with interferon-alpha, ribavirin and amantadine in nonresponders to interferon-alpha and ribavirin. Eur. J. Med. Res. 2002; 7: 149–154
240. **Zoulim, F., Zaem, J., Si Ahmed, S., Chossegros, P., Habersetzer, F., Chevallier, M., Bailly, F., Trépo, C.:** Ribavirin monotherapy in patients with chronic hepatitis C: a retrospective study of 95 patients. J. Viral Hepatit. 1998; 5: 193–198

Therapy of chronic hepatitis D
241. **Ehrhardt, A., Gerlich, W., Starke, C., Wend, U., Dunner, A., Sagir, A., Heintges, T., Häussinger, D.:** Treatment of chronic hepatitis delta with pegylated interferon-alpha 2b. Liver Intern. 2006; 26: 605–610
242. **Farci, P., Roskams, T., Chessa, L., Peddis, G., Mazzoleni, A.P., Scioscia, R., Serra, G., Lai, M.E., Loy, M., Caruso, L., Desmet, V., Purcell, R.H., Balestrieri, A.:** Long-term benefit of interferon-α therapy of chronic hepatitis D: regression of advanced hepatic fibrosis. Gastroenterology 2004; 126: 1740–1749
243. **Gaudin, J.L., Faure, P., Godinot, H., Gerard, F., Trepo, C.:** The French experience of treatment of chronic type D hepatitis with a 12-month course of interferon alpha-2b. Results of a randomized controlled trial. Liver 1995; 15: 45–52
244. **Kaymakoglu, S., Karaca, C., Demir, K., Poturoglu, S., Danalioglu, A., Badur, S., Bozaki, M., Besisik, F., Cakaloglu, Y., Okten, A.:** Alpha interferon and ribavirin combination therapy of chronic hepatitis D. Antimicrob. Ag. Chemother. 2005; 49: 1135–1138
245. **Wolters, L.M.M., van Nunen, A.B., Honkoop, P., Vossen, A.C.T.M., Niesters, H.G.M., Zondervan, P.E., de Man, R.A.:** Lamivudine-high dose interferon combination therapy for chronic hepatitis B patients co-infected with the hepatitis D virus. J. Viral Hepat. 2000; 7: 428–434
246. **Yurdaydin, C., Bozkaya, H., Gürel, S., Tillmann, H.L., Aslan, N., Okcu-Heper, A., Erden, E., Yalcin, K., Iliman, N., Uzunalimoglu, Ö., Manns, M.P., Bozdayi, A.M.:** Famciclovir treatment of chronic delta hepatitis. J. Hepatol. 2002; 37: 266–271

Clinical Aspects of Liver Diseases
35 Liver cirrhosis

		Page:
1	*Historical review*	738
2	*Definition*	738
3	*Aetiological classification*	738
4	*Morphological classification*	739
4.1	Liver size	739
4.2	Regeneration nodes	739
4.3	Morphological course	742
4.4	Completion	742
4.5	Pathogenetic development	742
4.6	Postdystrophic cirrhosis	742
4.7	Necrosis, fibrogenesis, regeneration	742
4.8	Morphological diagnostics	743
5	*Epidemiology*	743
6	*Aetiology*	743
7	*Clinical classification*	745
8	*Diagnostics*	746
8.1	Anamnesis	746
8.2	Complaints	746
8.3	Clinical findings	746
8.4	Laboratory findings	747
8.5	Imaging procedures	748
8.5.1	Sonography	748
8.5.2	Colour-encoded duplex sonography	749
8.5.3	Computer tomography	749
8.5.4	Magnetic resonance imaging	749
8.5.5	Radioisotope scanning	749
8.6	Liver biopsy and laparoscopy	749
8.7	Endoscopy	750
9	*Prognostic classification*	750
10	*Differential diagnosis*	751
11	*Consequences and complications*	751
11.1	Negative energy balance	751
11.2	Carbohydrate metabolism disorders	752
11.2.1	Hypoglycaemia	752
11.2.2	Hepatogenic diabetes mellitus	752
11.2.3	Glycogenolysis disorders	752
11.3	Protein metabolism disorders	752
11.3.1	Catabolism	753
11.3.2	Amino-acid imbalance	753
11.4	Lipid metabolism disorders	753
11.5	Hypovitaminoses	753
11.6	Endocrine disorders	754
11.7	Bacterial and viral infections	754
11.8	Hepatic osteopathy	754
11.8.1	Definition	754
11.8.2	Frequency	755
11.8.3	Pathogenesis	755
11.8.4	Clinical symptoms	755
11.8.5	Treatment	755
11.9	Hepatic encephalopathy	756
11.10	Ascites	756
11.11	Pleuropulmonary complications	757
11.11.1	Hepatopulmonary syndrome	758
11.11.2	Portopulmonary hypertension	758
11.11.3	Hydrothorax	759
11.12	Gastrointestinal bleeding	760
11.12.1	Portal hypertensive gastroenteropathy	760
11.12.2	Oesophagofundal varices	760
11.12.3	Ectopic varices	760
11.12.4	Anorectal varices	761
11.13	Febrile phases of disease	761
11.14	Cholelithiasis	761
11.15	Hepatocardiovascular syndrome	762
11.16	Hepatocellular carcinoma	762
12	*Prognosis*	763
13	*Therapy*	764
13.1	Causal treatment	764
13.2	Treatment of pathogenic reactions	764
13.3	Treatment of progression	764
13.4	Symptomatic treatment	764
13.4.1	Nutrition	765
13.4.2	Physical activity	765
13.4.3	Psychological guidance	766
13.4.4	Drug therapy	766
13.5	Monitoring	767
13.6	Liver transplantation	768
	• References (1–194)	768

(Figures 35.1–35.20; tables 35.1–35.10)

35 Liver cirrhosis

1 Historical review

▶ Aretaeus (2nd century AD) coined the term "skirros", because he thought that inflammation of the liver led to its **hardening (= skirros)**. • In 1543 A. Vesal described the granulation of the liver surface as being responsible for the compression of the small hepatic vessels. Even at that time, he associated these changes, which were thought to accompany a shrinking of the liver, with alcohol consumption. • When J. Posthius (1590) described ascites, he said that the changed liver was "all granulated inside". A drawing by J. Brown (1685) shows coarse nodular liver cirrhosis. G. B. Morgagni (1761) also wrote a treatise on cirrhosis, in which he described the small vessels as being compressed due to a shrinking and hardened liver. M. Baillie (1818) wrote an excellent description of the morphology of liver cirrhosis and, like A. Vesal, also postulated a causal connection with excessive alcohol consumption. • The first accurate report on atrophic, portal cirrhosis was given by R. T. H. Laennec (1819) as an incidental inclusion in his book «Traité d'auscultation». *Because of the* **yellow colour** *of the liver (=* **kirros**), *he coined the term* **cirrhosis.** • The first microscopic examinations were carried out by F. Kiernan (1833), R. Carswell (1838) and E. Hallmann (1839). F. Th. Frerichs differentiated between two stages of the cirrhotic course: stage of inflammation and stage of shrinking with formation of nodes. In 1911 F. B. Mallory defined cirrhosis as a "chronic, destructive, progressive process" with regeneration, accompanied by scarring and shrinking of the connective tissue. A. Ghon (1928) recognized the transformational processes in the liver as being an essential feature of cirrhosis. • In 1930 R. Rössle provided a morphological definition of cirrhosis by stating **three criteria:** (*1.*) destruction of liver parenchyma, (*2.*) connective tissue proliferation, and (*3.*) nodular compensatory hyperplasia together with regeneration of liver parenchyma. • In the following years, a **fourth criterion** was added: (*4.*) disturbance of the intrahepatic vascular system with consecutive formation of arteriovenous and portovenous anastomoses (H. Thaler, 1952, 1957, 1968; H. Popper et al., 1958; P. P. Anthony et al., 1977; A. M. Rappaport, 1980).

2 Definition

Cirrhosis is a gradually developing, chronic disease of the liver which always involves the organ as a whole. It is the irreversible consequence and final stage of various chronic liver diseases of different aetiology or the result of long-term exposure to various noxae. • The extent of the morphological changes depends on the cause and stage of cirrhosis. Accordingly, there is a wide spectrum of morphological findings and clinical symptoms. The variations of this disease range from symptom-free conditions, non-characteristic complaints and different laboratory findings through to life-threatening complications. Since, in most cases, no clear dividing line can be drawn between cirrhosis and the preceding liver disease, it is difficult to determine the exact point at which the cirrhotic stage begins; the transition is fluent.

Localized transformation processes such as those observed in **scarred liver** (s. p. 412) are not considered to be cirrhosis. The loss of parenchyma in scarred liver is generally the result of reduced blood supply in the respective area. Deep-set scars create the picture of a **funnel-shaped liver** (s. p. 413). Similarly, pronounced **liver fibrosis** (s. p. 412) does not fulfil the criteria of cirrhosis, since the lobular architecture as well as the intrahepatic and intra-acinar vascular supply are uncompromised. While fibrosis constitutes a precirrhotic stage, it does not necessarily progress to cirrhosis itself. Fibrosis can regress! • *Thus,* **liver cirrhosis** *is characterized by the following* **five criteria:**

1. Pronounced, insufficiently repaired necroses of the parenchyma (with or without inflammatory processes)
2. Diffuse connective tissue proliferation
3. Varying degrees of nodular parenchymal regeneration
4. *Loss and transformation of the lobular structure within the liver as a whole*
5. *Impaired intrahepatic and intra-acinar vascular supply*

Definitive classification of cirrhosis is difficult. It can be categorized according to its (*1.*) aetiology, (*2.*) morphology, (*3.*) pathogenetic development, (*4.*) clinical features, and (*5.*) prognostic criteria.

3 Aetiological classification

Classification of cirrhosis according to its **aetiology** would be desirable, as this approach may help determine prophylactic and therapeutic measures as well as prognosis. If all diagnostic options are employed and the patient cooperates optimally, an aetiological identification of cirrhosis is possible in almost all cases today. •

Due to improved detailed diagnostics, the group of so-called *cryptogenic cirrhoses* has been consistently reduced (< 10% of cases). (s. tab. 35.2)

However, classification of cirrhosis based on aetiology is limited for several reasons: (*1.*) the cause of cirrhosis cannot be determined in many cases, (*2.*) a certain cause gives rise to different morphological forms in individual patients, (*3.*) there may be several causes for the same form of cirrhosis, and (*4.*) various causes may frequently coincide in diverse combinations.

4 Morphological classification

Cirrhosis is an alteration which affects the whole liver. It is characterized by septa-forming fibrosis and the transformation of the lobular/acinar architecture into insular or nodular parenchyma.

So far, classification of cirrhosis by **morphology** has met with the most approval. (12) It is based on (*1.*) liver size, (*2.*) size of regeneration nodes, (*3.*) fine-tissue structure, (*4.*) progression, and (*5.*) completion of cirrhosis. (s. tab. 35.1) (12, 169) *(see chapter 21.5.2)*

I. Size of liver   1. Normotrophic cirrhosis   2. Hypertrophic cirrhosis   3. Atrophic cirrhosis (s. fig. 35.1)
II. Size of regeneration   1. Fine-nodular (granular) cirrhosis (s. figs. 28.13, 35.5)   2. Coarse-nodular (nodular) cirrhosis (s. fig. 35.2)   3. Coarse-bulbous (lobular) cirrhosis (s. fig. 35.4)   4. Mixed-nodular cirrhosis (s. fig. 35.8)   5. "Smooth" cirrhosis (s. fig. 14.3)
III. Structure of the fine tissue   1. Multilobular (multiacinar) cirrhosis   2. Monolobular (monoacinar) cirrhosis   3. Mixed forms
IV. Progression of cirrhosis   1. Active (= progressive) form   2. Inactive (= stationary) form
V. Completion of cirrhosis   1. Complete form   2. Incomplete form   3. Incomplete septal cirrhosis

Tab. 35.1: Criteria for the morphological classification of cirrhosis *(see chapter 21.5.2)*

4.1 Liver size

Liver size is determined by *sonography* (or *CT*). In cirrhosis, it varies from case to case and presents as *hepatomegaly, normal-sized liver* or *atrophy*. There may even be deviations due to a disproportion between the two lobes resulting in asymmetric enlargement or reduction in size. Usually, there is more functional parenchyma present in hypertrophic or normotrophic cirrhosis than in atrophic cirrhosis. *The majority of cirrhoses are assigned to the atrophic group. A progressive reduction in liver size tending towards atrophy is to be interpreted as a prognostically unfavourable sign,* particularly when the transaminase values decrease to a subnormal level. Determination of the liver size enables the course of disease to be evaluated in terms of the remaining parenchymal mass or its potential for regeneration.

Atrophic cirrhosis as described by R.T.H. LAENNEC (1819) was compared with **hypertrophic cirrhosis** as described by A. GUBLER (1853) and P. OLIVIER (1871); the latter condition was identified as *biliary cirrhosis* by V. HANOT (1875).

4.2 Regeneration nodes

Formation of nodes: While this conditions is a typical finding on the liver surface (s. figs. 28.13; 35.1, 35.2, 35.4, 35.8), in sectional preparations (s. fig. 35.6) and under the microscope (s. figs. 35.3, 35.7), it is not an obligate criterion. In many cases, it is hardly recognizable, e.g. in haemochromatotic, biliary and alcoholic cirrhosis. • **Smooth cirrhosis,** showing a smooth liver surface despite complete transformation, is likewise found; it is micronodular and poor in fibres. (s. fig. 14.3)

Proliferation is characterized by enlarged cells with great variability in the size of the nuclei (= anisonucleosis), occurrence of hepatocytes with two to three nuclei, and cell plates of varying thickness. The parenchyma which has remained undamaged is capable of regenerative proliferation. The vulnerability of the acinus structure is the prerequisite for the criterion *"transformation"*, and the tendency to proliferate is the criterion for *"nodes"*. • The **blood vessels** are also involved in this process: (*1.*) reduction in the distance between presinusoidal and postsinusoidal vessels, (*2.*) development of shunts, and (*3.*) formation of a perinodular plexus (E. GAUDIO et al., 1993). This plexus consisting of arterioles guarantees the arterial blood supply within the nodes. Due to the displacement effect of the nodes, arterial vessels also become compressed. This is particularly critical since the cirrhotic liver is almost exclusively supplied by arterial blood, so that some areas become increasingly hypoxic and are thus more prone to *coagulation necrosis*. This happens mainly under conditions of circulatory collapse caused, for instance, by haemorrhage or toxicosis. • In contrast, a favourable local arterial blood supply may lead to the formation of **gigantic regeneration nodes** similar to "proliferations". (s. fig. 35.1)

The following forms of cirrhosis are differentiated according to the **size of the regeneration nodes:** (*1.*) micronodular (granular), (*2.*) coarse-nodular (nodular),

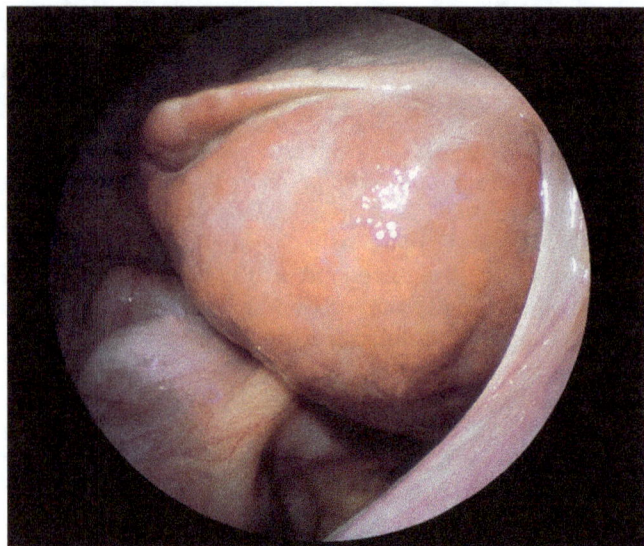

Fig. 35.1: Atrophic liver cirrhosis with pronounced, thick capsule callosity. Gigantic regeneration node "proliferating" from the underside of the right liver lobe, displacing the (duplicated!) gall bladder

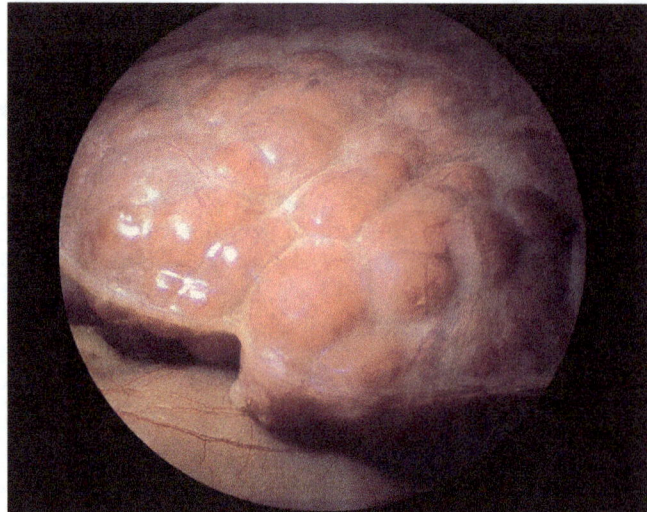

Fig. 35.2: Complete, coarse-nodular liver cirrhosis due to chronic viral hepatitis B

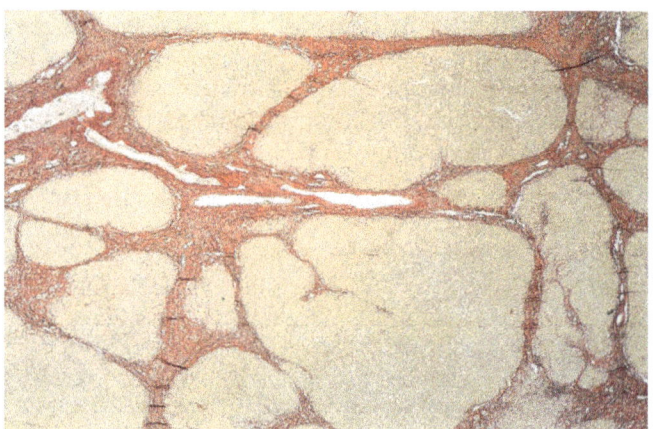

Fig. 35.3: Stationary macronodular liver cirrhosis in chronic non-active hepatitis C (Sirius red)

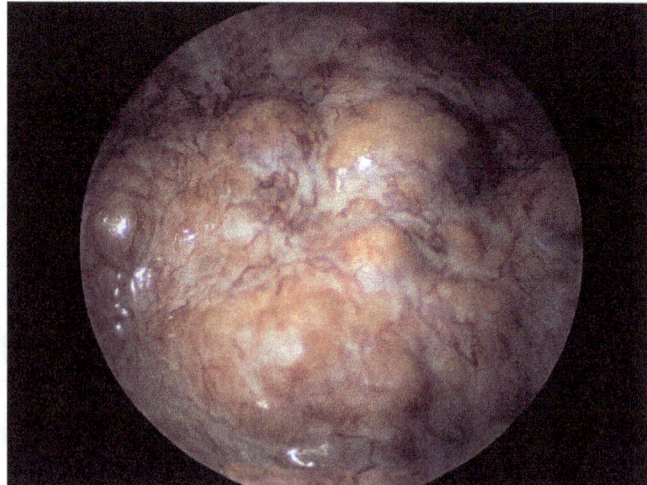

Fig. 35.4 Complete, coarse-bulbous cirrhosis after years of alcohol abuse and superimposed acute viral hepatitis B, showing a chronic course. Mild tendency towards cholestasis; pronounced subcapsular vascularization and vascular stasis. Occasional funnel-shaped parenchymal depressions

(*3.*) coarse-bulbous (lobular), and (*4.*) mixed-nodular. The classification into granular, nodular and lobular forms was proposed by A.H. BAGGENSTOSS et al. (1952). Despite complete transformation processes, cirrhosis with a smooth surface, completely or largely without intrahepatic nodes, is occasionally found. Various synonyms have been used for this kind of classification according to the type and size of the nodes. (quot. 89, 91)

Macronodular cirrhosis: In *multilobular cirrhosis*, the nodes develop from parts of several lobules or from larger parenchymal areas with intact lobular architecture. This group with nodes of >0.3 cm up to the size of a walnut is also called postnecrotic cirrhosis or Nagayo type A (M. NAGAYO, 1914). The liver is predominantly atrophic. The pseudolobules contain parts derived from several acini (= multiacinar or multilobular cirrhosis). Portal fields and central venules are present, however, in an abnormal topography. (s. figs. 35.2, 35.3)

A special form is **incomplete septal cirrhosis**; it is found especially as a result of chronic hepatitis B or in Wegener's granulomatosis. (190) The thin septa, which invade the parenchyma from the portal fields, contain no or only very few inflammatory infiltrates (= passive septa). (s. p. 414) • Lobular **coarse-bulbous cirrhosis** can likewise be assigned to this group, which, as posthepatitic cirrhosis, is also called Nagayo type B or may be referred to as *Marchand's hyperplasia* (F. MARCHAND, 1895) or *potato liver* (H. KALK, 1957) in the literature. Lobular nodes can reach such a size that they are mistaken for a normal hepatic lobe. (s. fig. 35.1) Macronodular forms may follow chronic viral hepatitis, chronic autoimmune hepatitis, metabolic diseases, toxic-necrotizing processes and alcohol abuse. (s. fig. 35.4)

Micronodular cirrhosis: Monolobular (monoacinar) cirrhosis consists of individual hepatic lobules separated by connective tissue, with the central vein maintained in the interior. In *pseudolobular cirrhosis*, no elements of the lobular architecture and no central vein can be detected; the nodules in this type of cirrhosis are small. The monolobular and pseudolobular forms are classified as micronodular cirrhosis, or Nagayo type C (with node size < 0.3 cm). A striking feature is the uniformity of the nodules. (s. figs. 35.5, 35.6)

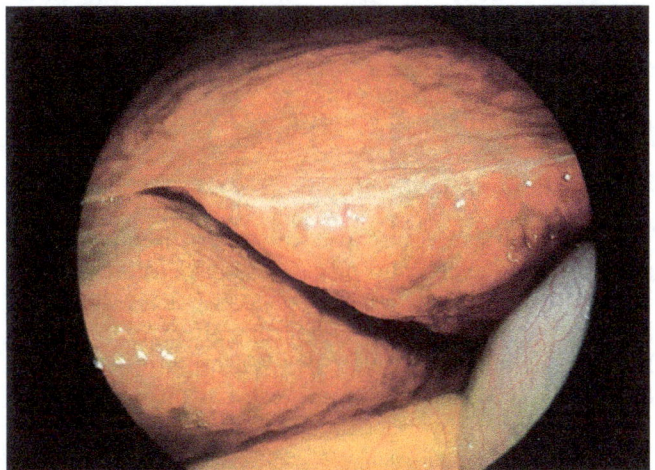

Fig. 35.5: Micronodular, alcohol-related liver cirrhosis with "simian cleft"; (s. figs. 2.3; 31.22) right lobe with rounded edge and thin fibrotic margin; numerous small scars (brandy drinker)

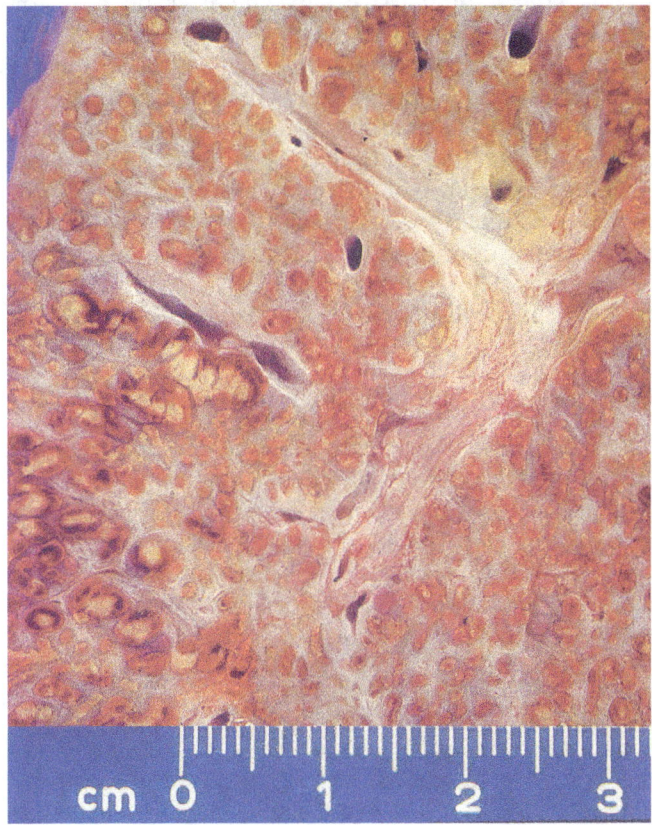

Fig. 35.6: Complete, micronodular to medium-nodular liver cirrhosis after chronic viral hepatitis B (section, native preparation)

The micronodular form can develop into a macronodular form, but not vice versa. Generally, micronodular cirrhosis contains more fibrosis than parenchyma; therefore it is firmer than macronodular cirrhosis. The development of micronodular cirrhosis, e.g. in alcohol abuse, may be caused by the fact that continuous alcohol intake blocks the protein synthesis, and thus the parenchyma has no time or chance for cellular proliferation. This form of cirrhosis mainly results from alcohol abuse, but may also be found in haemochromatosis, congestive liver, biliary cirrhosis, toxic liver damage due to pharmacons, metabolic diseases and chronic viral hepatitis. The liver is generally enlarged.

Mixed-nodular cirrhosis is considered to be a transitional form between micronodular and macronodular cirrhosis (V.J. DESMET et al., 1990). Due to variations in the regenerative capacity of the cirrhotic liver, 50% of micronodular forms with a diameter of 1.5 mm develop into macronodular forms after 2–4 years, whereas after 10 years, the rate is as high as 90%. • *Atrophic cirrhosis* is the most common form with regard to size (s. figs. 35.1, 35.14),

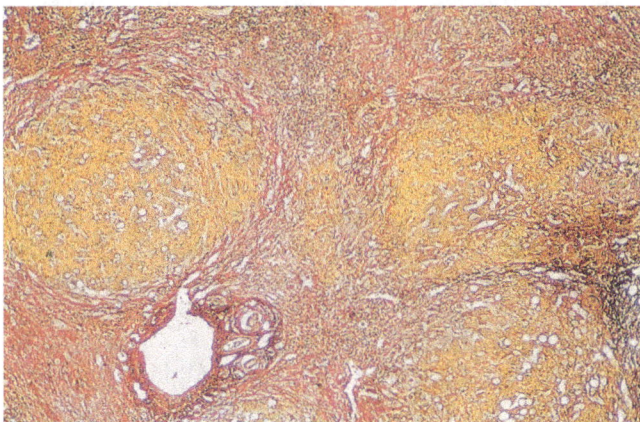

Fig. 35.7: Complete, micronodular, progressive liver cirrhosis with formation of pseudoacini (Sirius red)

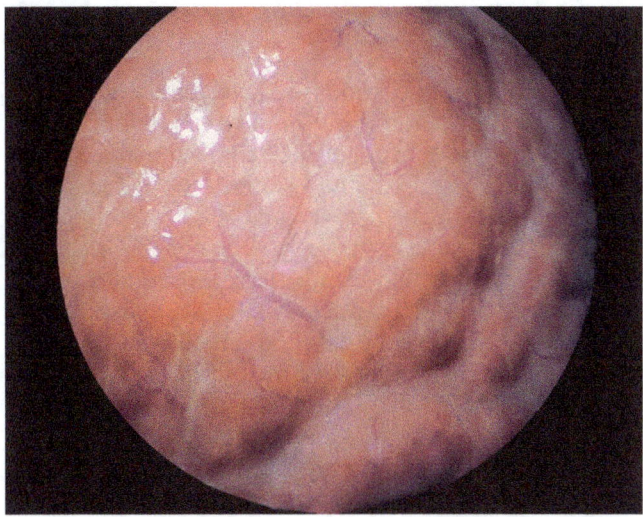

Fig. 35.8: Complete, mixed-nodular (toxin-induced) liver cirrhosis due to years of alcohol abuse and long-term oxyphenisatin abuse

whereas *mixed-nodular cirrhosis* is the most common form with regard to nodes. (s. tab. 35.1) (s. fig. 35.8)

4.3 Morphological course

Progression: The question as to the progression of cirrhosis is of crucial importance clinically and can only be answered by means of histology. There is evidence of dense, chronic inflammatory infiltration of the connective tissue; the boundary between connective tissue and parenchyma is blurred. Groups of damaged hepatocytes, liver cell necroses as well as nodules formed from the proliferation of Kupffer cells and round cells are found within the parenchyma. In places, piecemeal necroses infiltrate the parenchymal islands. Many cirrhoses only take a progressive course because of circulatory disturbances. *Clinical progression* frequently, but by no means always, corresponds to morphological progression. • **Stationary cirrhosis** is predominantly found in macronodular forms. It frequently exhibits round, clearly defined, nodular parenchymal areas within scar tissue. The boundary between the parenchyma and connective tissue is (relatively) clear-cut. (s. fig. 35.2) The scar tissue contains a small number of chronic inflammatory infiltrates of moderate and slightly varying density. The hepatocytes are conspicuously enlarged. Fully developed stationary cirrhosis may result, which is defined morphologically as defective healing. The morphological dynamics of progression or full-scale stationary cirrhosis has to be strictly differentiated from the respective clinical course. • **Remission** of the cirrhosis is possible, provided the cause of the disease is eliminated (e.g. abstention from alcohol, iron depletion in haemochromatotic cirrhosis, removal of biliary obstruction). However, nodular transformation processes cannot be reversed — restoration of normal lobular architecture is no longer possible.

4.4 Completion

Another important criterion is to determine whether the nodular transformation in the liver is complete or incomplete. This morphological characteristic can be found both in progressive and stationary cirrhoses. • In **complete cirrhosis,** the parenchyma is completely partitioned by connective tissue septa. The collapse of fibres (due to portocentral bridging necroses) results in the development of portocentral septa (= *passive septa*). Due to the spreading of the inflammation to the periportal parenchyma, septa develop and branch out from the portal fields (= *active septa*). Generally, they lead to capillarization of the sinusoidal walls as well. (s. fig. 35.9) **Incomplete cirrhosis** only displays the formation of short septa (= *subsepta*), with the result that there are occasional areas of incomplete (partial) subdivision of the parenchyma.

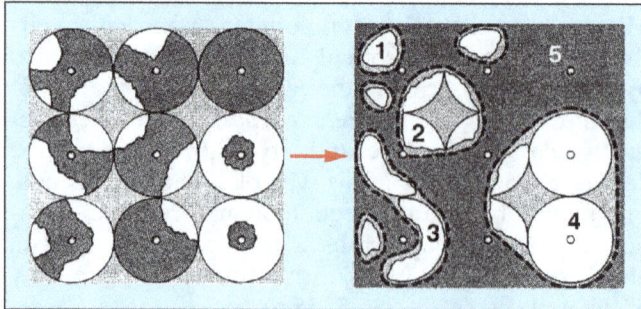

Fig. 35.9: Scheme of possibilities for hepatic transformation after parenchymal necroses: (1) formation of pseudolobuli, (2) nodes with enclosed portal field, (3) formation of parenchymal garlands, (4) development of a coarse node from several hepatic lobules which are, in part, completely intact, (5) scar formation after total lobular necrosis (H. THALER, 1975) (169)

4.5 Pathogenetic development

The development of cirrhosis can easily be understood by analysing the morphological findings. Differentiation is made between: (*1.*) *regular cirrhosis* (where the cause has a constant, long-term and strong effect, e.g. in alcohol abuse, haemochromatosis, Wilson's disease), (*2.*) *irregular cirrhosis* (where the cause has an intermittent effect interposed by inaction), (*3.*) *mixed forms,* (*4.*) *biliary forms,* and (*5.*) *vascular forms.*

4.6 Postdystrophic cirrhosis

In the course of massive subacute liver necrosis (or hepatic dystrophy), large parts of the hepatic parenchyma can be destroyed within a few months. Extensive regenerative nodes form from the remaining epithelium. Within these regenerations, the lobular architecture is either still maintained or has been partially restored. Areas of parenchymal loss are converted into fibre-dense scar tissue with embedded pseudoductuli and duct proliferations as well as irregularly located residual hepatocytes. This course is extremely rare. In the literature, it is also called *incomplete postnecrotic cirrhosis.*

4.7 Necrosis, fibrogenesis, regeneration

The mechanisms leading to *cell degeneration* and *cell death* have been described in detail. *(see chapter 21.3.4)* The processes of *regeneration (see chapter 21.3.5)* and *fibrogenesis (see chapter 21.3.6)* have also been discussed in depth. These three important events — cell death, regeneration and fibrogenesis — are involved in the development of cirrhosis.

Fibrogenesis commences with the activation of Ito cells by cytokines such as TGFβ1, PDGF, TNFα, IGF1. This induction of Ito cells leads to quantitatively increased (up to ten times the norm) and qualitatively altered synthesis of the extracellular matrix, which consists of collagens, glycoproteins, proteoglycans and glucosaminoglycans. • Degeneration of the matrix is reduced by a decrease in matrix metalloproteinases (MMP) with a simultaneous increase in the tissue inhibitors of metalloproteinases (TIMP). Both factors reduce further degradation of connective tissue. • The hepatocytes are now multilayered instead of normal single-layered cell plates and lose their microvilli. Fenestration of the sinusoids disappears, whereas the sinusoidal extracellular matrix increases, leading to **capillarization of the sinusoids.** (s. pp 410, 540) In this way, the distance between the hepatocytes and the blood becomes greater, and the clearance of macromolecular substances is reduced. Stronger flow resistance in the liver leads to portal hypertension. • Portoportal and portocentral bands of connective tissue form, in which portosystemic intrahepatic shunts develop.

Regeneration after liver resection follows a coordinated and limited course. This is not the case in cirrhosis: isolated and excessive regenerations of hepatocytes and bile ducts are formed, from which *adenomas* and *carcinomas* may develop.

4.8 Morphological diagnostics

In order to evaluate cirrhosis in terms of morphology, certain **requirements** have to be fulfilled. Occasional *diagnostic uncertainty* or *divergent classification* may arise from the fact that the biopsy material is insufficient and therefore not representative. This, in turn, is probably due to the fact that the techniques used in obtaining these inadequate samples were faulty or unsuitable. (s. pp 168, 169, 415, 750)

5 Epidemiology

Cirrhosis of the liver is a disease found all over the world, affecting all races, age groups and both sexes. • However, there are **geographical differences** regarding the most important causative factors: (*1.*) rate of alcohol consumption, and (*2.*) frequency of viral hepatitis. Few reliable figures concerning its incidence and prevalence are available, since cirrhosis is often symptom-free. Autopsy examinations suggest a **prevalence** of 4−10%. The **incidence** is about 240/million inhabitants/year. • The number of people suffering from cirrhosis in Germany is estimated at 600,000−700,000; some 25,000 patients die of cirrhosis every year, with **mortality** being twice as high in men as in women. Thus cirrhosis ranks ninth as a cause of death overall, and fifth for the age group 45−65 years. • Generally, the increasing mortality rate runs parallel to regional alcohol consumption. This correlation between alcohol consumption and cirrhosis-dependent mortality or morbidity applies equally to men and women. • The slight decrease in mortality in some countries observed during the past 10−15 years may be due to more effective prophylaxis and improved treatment options for complications. (65, 149)

6 Aetiology

The causes of "liver cirrhosis" are numerous; some of them are rare, appearing even in childhood (e.g. drinking water from copper pipes). Cirrhosis can be acquired or genetically based. Aetiological clarification, particularly with early diagnosis, should always be a priority, since it may aid treatment and thus prognosis. *Cirrhosis comes in many different forms!* • There is still no unequivocal answer to the question as to why these causal factors are responsible for the development of cirrhosis over such a widely varying period or why they may not cause cirrhosis at all in some individuals. There are even cases where cirrhosis develops despite effective elimination of the causes − probably as a result of self-perpetuation due to induced immunological mechanisms. • Although there are numerous causes with varying pathogenesis, it is possible to differentiate between three forms of cirrhosis from an aetiological viewpoint: (*1.*) parenchyma-related cirrhosis, including the so-called "common" cirrhosis (H.W. ALTMANN et al., 1986) and metabolic cirrhosis, (*2.*) bile duct-related cirrhosis (= biliary cirrhosis), and (*3.*) vessel-related cirrhosis (= vascular cirrhosis). (s. tab. 35.2)

Biliary cirrhosis: Biliary cirrhosis can be detected in 5−15% of cases. (s. pp 415, 673, 679, 696, 739, 743) (s. figs. 32.5; 35.10, 35.11)

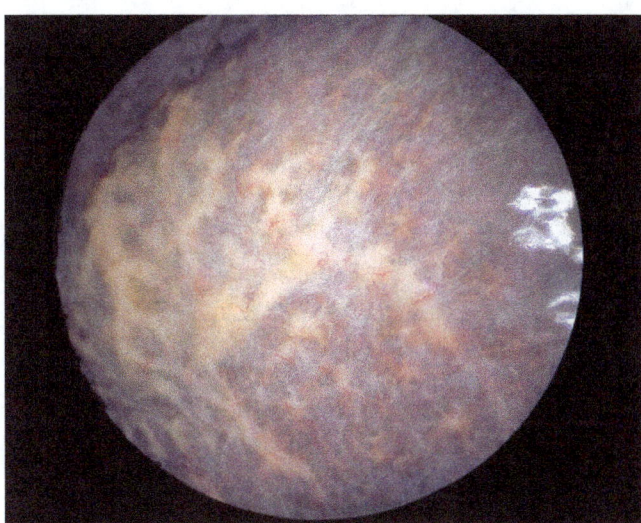

Fig. 35.10: Biliary liver cirrhosis after long-term chronic-recurrent cholangitis

Alcohol abuse: Alcohol abuse is the most common cause of cirrhosis. Nevertheless, no more than 40−60% of alcoholics contract the disease. Thus genetic factors must also be involved in the development of alcoholic cirrhosis. Alcohol itself can be a facilitative factor or cofactor. Moreover, "additives" contained in various alcoholic beverages in widely different quantities may be of greater importance than hitherto assumed. (99, 162, 175) (s. pp 542, 546) (s. figs. 28.13, 28.14; 35.3)

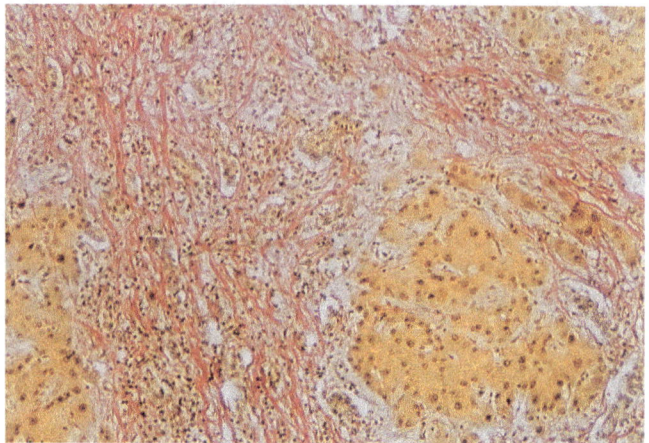

Fig. 35.11: Liver cirrhosis due to chronic-recurrent, ascending cholangitis (Sirius red)

Chronic autoimmune hepatitis: If untreated, AIH (especially type 2) develops almost inevitably into cirrhosis; the condition is further aggravated by the presence of multilobular necrosis and bridging necrosis. In bridging necrosis, development of cirrhosis is more rapid between the portal fields and the central vein than between the portal fields themselves. (s. p. 662) (s. fig. 32.4)

Chronic viral hepatitis: Within a period of five to six years, cirrhosis is caused by chronic viral hepatitis B in 15−30%, chronic viral hepatitis C in 20−50% and chronic viral hepatitis B/D in up to 60% of cases. The risk of cirrhosis is 4.2 times higher in HBsAg carriers and 2.3 times higher in carriers of anti-HCV than in people without these serum markers. (71, 81, 137)

Haemochromatotic cirrhosis: *Untreated* idiopathic haemochromatosis has an insidious course and, as a rule, leads to (micronodular) cirrhosis. Spontaneous remission has not been observed. The survival rate in haemochromatotic cirrhosis is 60−65% after ten years. (s. pp 639, 642) (s. figs. 31.24−31.26)

▶ We do not consider the terminological demarcation of "primary" cirrhosis or the differentiation into "primary" and "secondary" cirrhosis to be acceptable, because any kind of biliary cirrhosis constitutes the final stage of a preceding chronic biliary disease. (s. p. 679!)

Cryptogenic cirrhosis: Cirrhoses which cannot (yet) be clarified by means of current investigation techniques are subsumed under the term cryptogenic cirrhosis. (33) Earlier data regarding its frequency no longer apply. As a result of the methods of detailed diagnosis used nowadays, only a small number of cirrhoses remain truly "cryptogenic". (17) Modern hepatological detailed diagnostics yield an aetiological clarification rate of nearly 95% of all patients! (s. tab. 35.2) • In most of the remaining cases, **chemical substances** which are still unknown or which have not yet been identified as hepatotoxins are probably involved, so that the patient concerned

1. **Alcohol** (see chapter 28)
2. **Infections**
    Congenital syphilis (see chapter 24)
    Schistosomiasis (see chapter 25)
    Toxoplasmosis (see chapter 25)
    Viral hepatitis B, C, D (see chapter 22)
3. **Autoimmune diseases**
    Autoimmune hepatitis (see chapter 32)
    Autoimmune cholangitis (see chapter 33)
    Primary biliary cholangitis (see chapter 33)
    Primary sclerosing cholangitis (see chapter 33)
    Wegener's granulomatosis
4. **Pharmaceuticals** (see chapter 29)
    Amiodarone   Methotrexate
    Dantrolene   Methyldopa
    Halothane   Nitrofurantoin
    Isoniazid   Perhexiline
    MAO inhibitors   Propylthiouracil
5. **Chemical agents** (see chapter 30)
    Arsenic   Phosphorus
    Carbon tetrachloride   Phytotoxins
    Copper   Trichloroethylene
    Mycotoxins
6. **Cholestatic diseases** (see chapters 13, 33)
    Aagenaes syndrome   Byler's syndrome
    Arteriohepatic dysplasia Caroli's syndrome
    Bile-duct atresia   Choledochal cyst
    Bile-duct stenoses   Chronic cholangitis
7. **Venous congestion** (see chapters 14, 39)
    Budd-Chiari syndrome
    Constrictive pericarditis
    Right-sided heart failure
    Veno-occlusive disease
8. **Metabolic diseases** (see chapter 31)
    α_1-antitrypsin deficiency
    Abetalipoproteinaemia
    Acute intermittent porphyria
    Atransferrinaemia syndrome
    Cystinosis
    Erythrohepatic protoporphyria
    Fructose intolerance
    Galactosaemia
    Gaucher's disease
    Glycogenosis (types I, III, IV)
    Haemochromatosis
    Hurler's disease
    Hypermethioninaemia
    Mucoviscidosis
    Neonatal adrenoleucodystrophia
    Nieman-Pick disease
    Non-alcoholic steatohepatitis
    Porphyria cutanea tarda
    Seip-Lawrence syndrome
    Thalassaemia
    Tyrosinosis (type I)
    Wilson's disease
    Wolman's disease
    Zellweger syndrome
9. **Intestinal bypass**
10. **Rendu-Osler-Weber disease**
11. **Indian childhood cirrhosis**
12. **Cryptogenic cirrhosis** (< 10%)

Tab. 35.2: Possible causes of liver cirrhosis

remains unaware of them; furthermore, such substances might occur in combination with other noxae that cannot be identified. *(see chapter 30)* **Medication** may likewise cause chronic hepatitis and cirrhosis. This also applies to herbal remedies, e.g. wild germander. *(see chapter 29)* Knowledge in this field has been greatly improved by cooperation between clinicians, toxicologists and specialists in industrial and environmental medicine. **AIH** was the cause of cryptogenic cirrhosis in 20−25% of cases. • **Non-alcoholic steatohepatitis** is of particular aetiological importance in cryptogenic cirrhosis, especially in cases where obesity and diabetes coexist (30−35%). (17, 132, 136) *(see chapter 31.3.6)* • Owing to modern diagnostic options (and assuming the patient co-operates!), cryptogenic cirrhoses today constitute no more than 5−10% of cases.

7 Clinical classification

The following stages or courses of cirrhosis can be differentiated according to clinical criteria:

> 1. *Latent cirrhosis*
> 2. *Manifest cirrhosis*
>   - active form
>   - inactive form

Latent cirrhosis: There are no subjective complaints or clinical symptoms. This stage is identified by laboratory parameters, imaging procedures or histological examination of the liver. Frequency is between 10 and 20%.

Manifest cirrhosis: Manifest cirrhosis is characterized by subjective complaints and clinical findings. Hepatic haemodynamics are significantly altered, and other organs and organ systems as well as hormonal and humoral functions are affected. *Liver cirrhosis orchestrates a complex array of altered biochemical and physiological processes.* • Manifest cirrhosis can present in two forms:

> 1. *Stage of compensation*
> 2. *Stage of decompensation*
>   - portal decompensation
>   - metabolic decompensation

Apart from **histological activity** (= progressive) or **inactivity** (= stationary), **biochemical activity** must also be defined. The latter is determined by *(1.) enzymatic activity, (2.) mesenchymal activity,* and *(3.) immunological activity.* (s. p. 127) • Compensated cirrhosis may be either active or inactive. Even decompensated cirrhosis can sometimes be kept in an inactive (stationary) stage for a limited period of time. Jaundice (>3 mg/dl) is a typical sign of decompensation.

Portal hypertension derives from *microcirculatory disorders,* with increasing flow resistance in the sinusoids and postsinusoids. This condition is a consequence of the narrowing, rarefaction and compression of the sinusoids or central veins due to collagen deposition, fibrosis and nodulation as well as the presence of intrahepatic arterio-portovenous shunts. Elevated endothelin levels are involved in these processes. (15) Portal hypertension is also evoked or increased by (relatively common) **portal vein thrombosis.** (8, 22, 121, 183) Nitric oxide (5, 14, 21), endotoxins (36, 39), platelet-activating factor, prostacyclin, histamine, adenosine, serotonin, bile acids, secretin, glucagons, etc. are all considered to be mediators of **hyperdynamic splanchnic circulation.** (s. p. 762) The resulting portal hypertension with splenomegaly and collateral varicosis become detectable with progressive cirrhosis of the liver. An important factor is that in alcohol-induced liver diseases, portal hypertension may be present before cirrhosis develops. *(see chapter 14)*

Portal decompensation: Various forms manifest as *(1.)* hypersplenism, *(2.)* increasing collateral varicosis with a simultaneous rise in the splanchnic flow due to hyperdynamic circulation and vasodilatation in the area of the splanchnic vessels, *(3.)* hepatic encephalopathy, and *(4.)* oedema and ascites. *(see chapters 14, 15 and 16)*

Portal decompensation
• Hypersplenism • Collateral varicosis • Portal hypertensive gastropathy • Hepatic encephalopathy • Oedema and ascites

Tab. 35.3: Possible forms of portal decompensation in liver cirrhosis

By fulfilling a multitude of **metabolic functions,** the liver guarantees the survival of the organism. Some 70 metabolic partial functions grouped into 12 main metabolic areas need to be constantly maintained with the help of *some 500 biochemical processes* carried out separately within the hepatocytes. (s. p. 36)

Metabolic decompensation: Pronounced functional decrease or dysfunction in several metabolic areas result in *partial metabolic insufficiency.* With the failure of additional metabolic functions, there is a risk of *global metabolic insufficiency.* Development of metabolic insufficiency (also known as *cellular decompensation*) is due to a significant loss of hepatocytes (e.g. mass necroses) and/or a loss of function of the hepatocytes (e.g. insufficient numbers of hepatocytes and accumulation of waste products in cirrhotic transformation with the development of shunts).

Complications: Generally, complications can occur during the stages of compensation and decompensation. Some complications predominantly arise from a decompensated situation, whereas others do not necessarily occur at all in the natural course of cirrhosis. However, in view of the cirrhosis-induced lability of the metabolic functions, they may easily be provoked by the patient's inappropriate behaviour or by iatrogenic measures. Viruses, such as CMV or influenza A (55), can cause deterioration of the liver function or decompensation. (149) (s. tab. 35.4)

Metabolic decompensation
Disturbance of some or almost all *biochemical functions*, also with a *negative energy balance* (= **partial** or **global insufficiency**) *(see chapter 20)*: • Jaundice *(see chapter 12)* • Encephalopathy *(see chapter 15)* • Oedema, ascites *(see chapter 16)* • Disturbed coagulation *(see chapter 19)* • Impaired protein metabolism • Impaired carbohydrate metabolism • Disturbed biotransformation • Hormonal dysbalance • Altered pharmacokinetics • Bacterial and viral infections • States of deficiency (vitamins, trace elements, electrolytes, energy carrier substances)
1. HE and hepatic coma *(see chapter 15)* 2. Ascites *(see chapter 16)* 3. Spontaneous bacterial peritonitis *(see chapter 16)* 4. Hepatorenal syndrome *(see chapter 17)* 5. Hepatopulmonary syndrome *(see chapter 18)* 6. Coagulopathy (DIC) *(see chapter 19)* 7. Acute varix bleeding *(see chapter 19)* 8. Hepatocellular carcinoma *(see chapter 37)* 9. Hepatic osteopathy 10. Cholelithiasis 11. Impaired protein, carbohydrate, lipid, vitamin and hormonal metabolism 12. Portosystemic myelopathy and neuropathy

Tab. 35.4: Possible forms of metabolic decompensation in liver cirrhosis

8 Diagnosis

Liver cirrhosis is the final stage of a hepatic disease which has generally run a chronic course for several years. • Some 60—65% of cirrhoses are alcohol-induced (long-standing alcohol abuse does not go unnoticed!). Some 25—30% of cirrhoses are thought to be posthepatitic events. Although a very small number of anicteric HBV and particularly HCV infections remain unrecognized (the exact figure is impossible to estimate), most acute and icteric courses are diagnosed. • With today's diagnostic possibilities, **chronic liver disease** is mostly detected at an early stage, either due to general complaints by the patient or during medical examinations. Its course is then carefully monitored. • The point at which a chronic liver disease, particularly cirrhosis, is first detected depends on the patient's general attitude and the diagnostic interview, *which nowadays is far more effective than the standard was 20—30 years ago!*

Thus (subjectively and clinically symptom-free) **latent cirrhosis,** with a frequency of 10—20% of cases, need not remain undetected. Looking back on 40 years of experience, we can state that cirrhosis itself constituted the *first diagnosis* in no more than 10% of cases. The first diagnosis of cirrhosis at such a complicative stage as oesophageal varix bleeding or decompensation has fortunately become a rare event. • *The course of cirrhosis (progressing, stationary, or regressing) is monitored by clinical findings, liver function tests and sonography.*

8.1 Anamnesis

Targeted anamnesis can yield valuable diagnostic information as soon as liver disease is suspected. This may require insistent and intense questioning, involving additional consultations. Such an approach is especially helpful in determining risk factors concerning viral hepatitis infection and toxic effects. (s. p. 80) (s. fig. 4.21)

8.2 Complaints

Subjective complaints of cirrhosis are non-characteristic and ambiguous. Even determination of the severity of cirrhosis is only possible to a limited extent. *Fatigue* (= "pain of the liver") (60—80%), sleep disturbance (possibly due to an impaired melatonin rhythm) (44, 164), gastrointestinal complaints (50—60%) and mental disorders are sometimes mentioned. The most important subjective complaints are best noted on a **check list.** (s. p. 81) (s. fig. 4.21) • Frequently, however, the patient does not feel any noteworthy discomfort.

8.3 Clinical findings

As a rule, all cirrhosis-typical findings occur in the late course of the disease. Occasionally, patients report striking findings, such as changes in the consistency, colour or smell of *faeces*, cutaneous or mucous *bleeding* and unexplained *febrile episodes*. The senses of *taste and smell* are both impaired. (28) Eyelid retraction and eyelid lag are often increased. • The *liver* becomes harder; hepatomegaly is present in some 60% of patients, while in about 20% of cases, the liver is atrophic and therefore usually no longer palpable. Single nodes are sometimes detectable. • *Splenomegaly* is present in 50—75% of cases. Splenic infarction may also be detected (e.g. laparoscopically). (s. fig. 35.12) Generally, there is development of *hypersplenism* (= reticuloendothelial hyperplasia with increased fibrosis and hyperaemia). • *Muscle cramps* (F. Konikoff et al., 1985) may occur. Zinc deficiency or the administration of diuretics are not considered to be possible causes. These painful cramps happen mostly at night and mainly affect the gastrocnemius muscle and

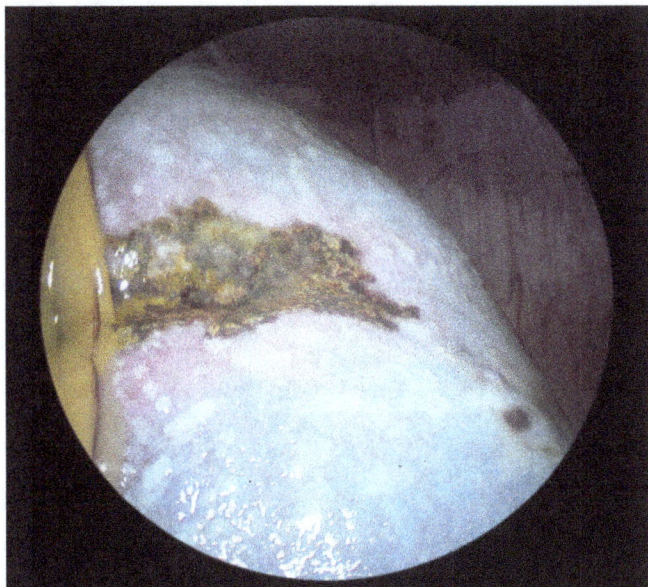

Fig. 35.12: Splenic infarction in splenomegaly due to complete liver cirrhosis. (Postpartum blood transfusion into the umbilical vein, with subsequent severe viral hepatitis B and rapid transition into early infantile cirrhosis.)

small muscles of the foot. Sometimes they are accompanied by increased activity of the renin system with a decrease in the effective blood volume. They usually respond to BCAA supplements in the late evening (143), quinine sulphate (oral application) or i.v. albumin infusion (1 x per week). (10) Hepatic *myelopathy* with spastic paraparesis is a rare event, especially in the advanced stage of cirrhosis. Pathogenesis is not yet clarified. Liver transplantation leads to complete recovery. • Symptoms of peripheral *neuropathy* have also been observed. (18, 85, 163) There is often *meteorism ("first the wind ...")*, and in many cases *ascites* develops *("... and then the rain")*. Tachycardia, hypotension and systolic murmur point to a *hyperdynamic circulation*. Pronounced spider naevi points to a significant disturbance of the systemic and pulmonary circulation. (21, 109) Occasional murmurs may be perceptible in the umbilical area (= Cruveilhier-Baumgarten syndrome). Men can display symptoms of feminization, while women display symptoms of hypogonadism. • Numerous **skin stigmata of liver disease**, which may be partially pathognomonic, are visible in varying intensities and combinations; they are best documented on a **check list**. (s. tab. 4.3) (s. figs. 4.6−4.11, 4.18−4.21) (s. pp 83−92)

8.4 Laboratory findings

Enzymatic activity: The enzymatic activity depends upon the extent of (*1.*) inflammatory or necrobiotic damage to the hepatocytes, and (*2.*) residual parenchymal mass. Accordingly, subnormal, normal or differently increased values of *GPT* and *GOT*, and in some cases also of *GDH*, are found. *Enzyme quotients* may be used for establishing the diagnosis. (s. tabs. 5.6, 5.7)

Cholestasis parameters are moderately elevated; in biliary diseases, however, the rise is significant. A progressive increase in γ-*GT* and *AP* suggests hepatocellular carcinoma and requires determination of α_1-*foetoprotein*. Disproportionally elevated γ-*GT* values generally indicate alcoholic or chemical-toxic aetiology or even HCV infection − but sometimes also regeneration of the hepatocytes. (89, 91, 160) With the progressive loss of liver parenchyma, the transaminase values fall to the normal range, and occasionally even to subnormal levels. This prognostically unfavourable sign correlates with a deterioration of the liver function test.

Mesenchymal activity: Mesenchymal activity is accompanied by an increase in γ-*globulins* and *immunoglobulins*. There is a broad-based, often dromedary-like humped γ-globulin peak (typically 22−35 rel.%). Albumins can be reliably determined by means of immunonephelometry. Generally, IgA is elevated in alcoholic cirrhosis, IgG in autoimmune cirrhosis and IgM in primary biliary cholangitis or CDNC-related cirrhosis. The rise in γ-globulins is due to reduced clearance of bacterial antigens in the RES, with increased antibody formation against intestinal bacteria, mainly E. coli. At the same time, elevated γ-globulins have a depressor effect on albumin synthesis and are indicators of the degree of portacaval anastomoses. The serum value of *copper* may be increased. In correlation with the dynamics of fibrogenesis, there is often a rise in *P-III-P* and hyaluronan. (88) • Increased γ-globulins and decreased cholinesterase may point to cirrhosis. (89, 91)

Liver function parameters: The most common endogenous liver function parameters, such as lowered *cholinesterase, albumin* (19) and *Quick's value*, are helpful for diagnosis. Since 1982, we have included the determination of *bile acids* as a relatively sensitive and specific follow-up procedure. Abnormal *coagulation factors* and *fibrinolysis values* are of particular diagnostic and prognostic importance. Factor 5 has a short half-life. (s. tab. 35.5) • These endogenous parameters can provide additional help in assessing the remaining liver function, especially when used in combination, and may thus facilitate prognostic evaluation. An increase in bilirubin and subsequent permanent *jaundice* are unfavourable prognostic signs. *Urobilinogenuria* is mostly present. • *Galactose elimination capacity* (141, 144) and the *indocyanine green test* are reliable exogenous liver function parameters. (69, 158) Good results have also been obtained using the *caffeine test, aminopyrine breath test* (47) and *MEGX test*. (118, 154) The formation of portosystemic collaterals can sometimes be assessed with the help of the *ammonium tolerance test*. (s. pp 113−116) • In more advanced cirrhosis, there is a decrease in BCAA (valine, leucine, isoleucine) and an increase in AAA (phenylalanine, tyrosine, methionine).

Additional parameters: Decreased serum values of *zinc* (103, 185) and *selenium* (30), *thrombopenia* or *thrombopa-*

Coagulation factors		Coagulation inhibitors		Fibrinolytic system	
Fibrinogen (I)	↓	Antithrombin III	↓	Plasminogen	↓
Factors II, IX, X	↓↓	Protein C	↓	$α_2$-antiplasmin	↓
Factor VII	↓↓	Protein C inhibitor		Prekallikrein	↓
Factors V, IX, XII, XIII	↓	Protein S	↓	HRGP	↓
Factor VIII	↑	Heparin cofactor	↓	t-PA	↑
TPT	↑			D dimer	↑
Quick's value	↓				
PTT	↑				

Tab. 35.5: Abnormal coagulation factors, coagulation inhibitors and fibrinolytic system values in hepatic cirrhosis (TPT = thromboplastin time; PTT = partial thromboplastin time; HRGP = histidine-rich glycoprotein; t-PA = tissue plasminogen activator)

thy (122) as well as increased values of *endotoxins* (36, 39) and *homocysteine* are also considered to be important laboratory parameters. Increased values of anticardiolipin antibodies are a hint of existing portal vein thrombosis. • Determination of $α_1$-*foetoprotein* (s. pp 112, 803) or *des-gamma-carboxy prothrombin* (s. p. 804) should be carried out to obtain a basic value, then checked at longer intervals; if values increase, they must be monitored at shorter intervals. This also applies if there is a progressive rise in AP and γ-GT.

8.5 Imaging procedures

Imaging techniques have greatly improved the diagnosis of cirrhotic diseases. They supply *detailed information* on (*1.*) structural changes in the liver, (*2.*) development of portal hypertension and formation of collaterals, (*3.*) occurrence of ascites at a very early stage, (*4.*) haemodynamics, and (*5.*) vascular changes. (s. tab. 35.6)

8.5.1 Sonography

Portal hypertension can be reliably detected and evaluated by way of sonographic criteria. (s. pp 139, 259) The sensitivity of sonography is limited by the extent of the cirrhosis-induced changes and reaches 85–90% in pronounced stages of cirrhosis. Specificity is high. The nodularity of the liver surface is, in general, easily visible, especially using a 7.5 MHz annular-array transducer. (114) Occasionally, however, the surface is so finely undulant that it appears smooth in sonography. The reflex echo is inhomogeneous, irregular and coarse; the vessels are rarefied, compressed and tortuous. A double-barrelled pattern (= prominent arteries) is sometimes evident. Splenomegaly and dilated portal vessels with

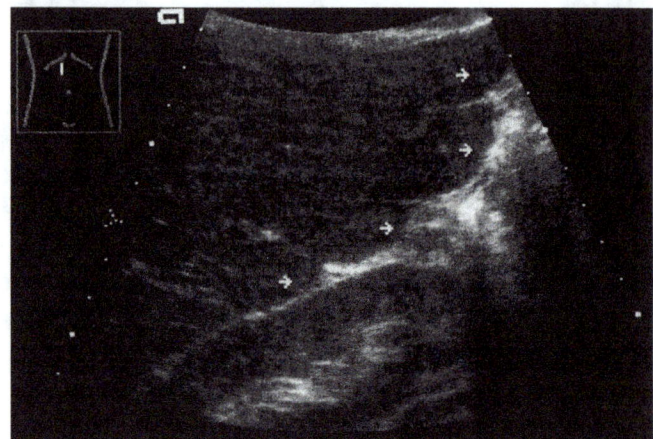

Fig. 35.13: Macronodular liver cirrhosis due to chronic hepatitis C with nodular surface (arrows) and inhomogeneous structure

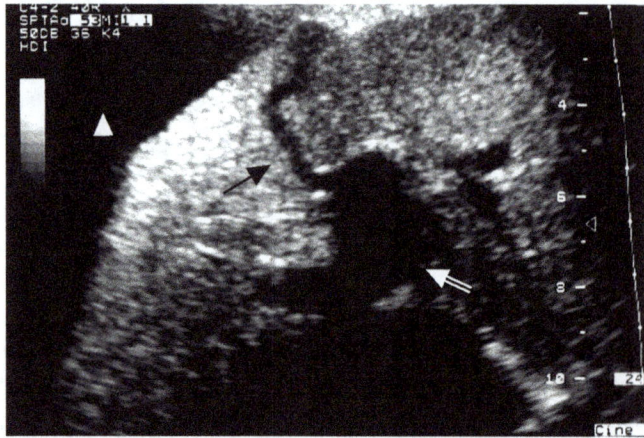

Fig. 35.14: Liver cirrhosis with ascites (▲). Re-opened umbilical vein (→), hepatic bifurcation and hilum of the liver with ramification of the portal vein (⇒)

	Diagnosis of cirrhosis	Diagnosis of portal hypertension			Diagnosis of HCC
		Portal vein	Splenomegaly	Collaterals	
1. Sonography	++	+	+++	++	+
2. Colour-encoded duplex sonography	++	++	+	++	+
3. CT	++	++	++	++	+++
4. MRI	++	+++	++	+++	++
5. Angiography	(+)	+++	+++	+++	+++

Tab. 35.6: Diagnostic reliability of imaging techniques in liver cirrhosis

collaterals can be observed. Any reduction in size of the quadrate lobe (segment IV) (<3 cm in diameter) is an important indicator. The caudate lobe (= segment I) is enlarged (especially in alcoholic cirrhosis) in relation to the right lobe. Regeneration nodes can appear as focal lesions; they may be misinterpreted as malignant foci. (s. figs. 6.6; 35.13, 35.14).

Sonography is also used as a routine technique for assessing the course of *cirrhosis*, but it does not provide information about the activity of disease or initial stage of a malignant process. The development of cirrhosis is best monitored by measuring liver stiffness with elastography. (60) (s. p. 135) (16, 42, 53, 83, 93, 94, 114, 159, 180) • EUS has proved successful in evaluating varices in the distal oesophagus and cardia area. (25) (s. pp 135, 360)

8.5.2 Colour-encoded duplex sonography

Colour-encoded duplex sonography facilitates characterization of the portal and hepatovenous haemodynamics and differentiation between the hepatofugal and hepatopetal direction of flow. (59) The flow wave flattens in hepatic veins. CEDS can show a shortened liver transit time (using sonographic contrast medium), collaterals, thrombosis or reopening of vessels, spontaneous portosystemic shunts (64, 139) and arterioportal fistulas (24) as well as determining the portacaval pressure gradient. (24, 64, 139, 160) (s. figs. 14.13; 35.15) (s. p. 134) • Colour-encoded duplex sonography is indispensable for establishing indications and excluding contraindications regarding TIPS; in addition, it can also be used for monitoring a TIPS placement.

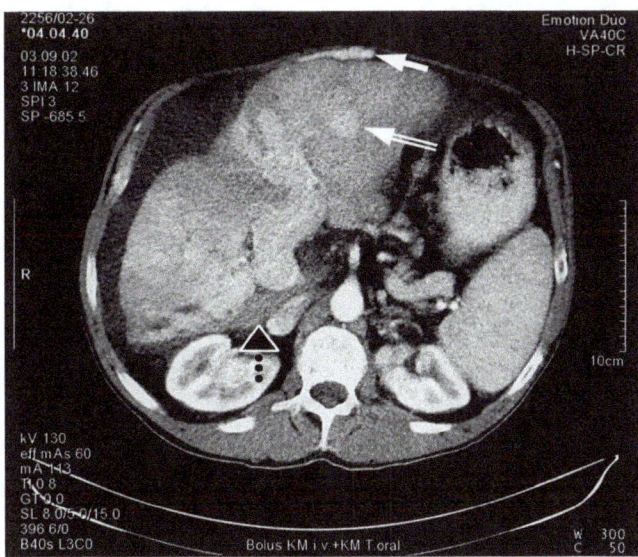

Fig. 35.16: Cirrhosis with regenerative node (⬅), recanalized umbilical vein (= caput Medusae) (⬅) and ascites (⬅⋯) in CT

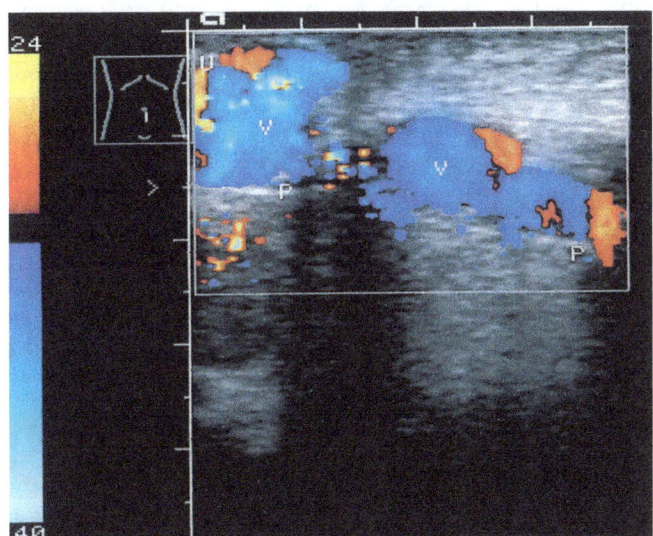

Fig. 35.15: Periumbilical venous convolutes (V) in abdominal wall (= caput Medusae) and subperitoneal area (P = peritoneum)

8.5.3 Computer tomography

CT scanning basically provides the same information as sonography, but the surface tubers or inhomogeneous internal structure are usually represented more clearly. Generally, regeneration nodes cannot be differentiated. The portal system and hepatic veins as well as collateral vessels are discernible. (86) Even small collections of ascitic fluid and some increases in density are recognizable. The caudate lobe is enlarged more in compensated than in decompensated cirrhosis. (83, 184) CT is useful in detecting small hepatocellular carcinomas. (26, 82, 101)

8.5.4 Magnetic resonance imaging

No further diagnostic information is gained by MRI, even though histological results can be improved to a certain extent by applying special techniques. By measuring the signal intensity of the liver, it is generally possible to quantify the extent of liver cirrhosis. Even the uptake of contrast medium as an expression of the still functioning proportion of the parenchyma may facilitate quantification. As a rule, liver perfusion is reduced in relation to the increase in arterial blood flow. The relative reduction in the volume of the right lobe of liver compared to the caudate lobe correlates closely with the extent of the cirrhosis. However, this has no relevance in the context of cirrhosis. (79, 82, 83, 101, 104, 163, 181)

8.5.5 Radioisotope scanning

This technique reveals decreased uptake of the radioisotope with an irregular pattern. Regeneration nodes cannot be visualized. There is enhanced storage in the spleen and bone marrow. (s. fig. 9.1)

8.6 Liver biopsy and laparoscopy

Laparoscopy: Direct visualization of the nodular liver by laparoscopy is the procedure of choice for primary morphological diagnosis. The diagnostic margin of error regarding percutaneous biopsy in cirrhosis is so high that there can be no indication for biopsy using a Menghini needle! *Only a compact biopsy sample turns histology into a diagnostic gold standard; furthermore, such a sample allows all other specific evaluation techniques to be carried out, if necessary.* • It is particularly important to obtain **photolaparoscopic documentation** of the liver surface, regeneration and scar areas, portal hypertension, spleen (or splenic infarction) (s. fig. 35.12) and other relevant, individual, abdominal findings. (90, 92, 123, 131) Although percutaneous biopsy using a Vim-Silverman needle usually produces a compact biopsy punch, it entails a higher and less controllable bleeding risk. Only an **adequate biopsy sample** yields the necessary results: (*1.*) confirmation of diagnosis, (*2.*) assessment of the degree of activity (= grading), (*3.*) evaluation of the extent of fibrosis (= staging), and (*4.*) specific histochemical examinations if a certain aetiology of cirrhosis is given.

Connective tissue collagen in biopsy specimens can be shown, for example, by the following staining:	
elastic fibres (e.g. sinusoids)	= elastin
reticulum fibres	= silver
portal and central zones	= van Gieson
basal membrane	= PAS

Both the risks and the possibility of obtaining uncertain results are far greater with percutaneous biopsy than with laparoscopically directed biopsy. The latter produces a detailed diagnosis in 97−100% of cases, a result also confirmed by our own observations. (50, 51, 91, 117, 123) • Insufficient training in laparoscopy or the non-availability of this examination technique do not constitute an indication for percutaneous biopsy in liver cirrhosis, at least for initial diagnosis. (s. figs. 7.8, 7.15; 16.5; 28.13; 35.2, 35.4, 35.5, 35.8)

8.7 Endoscopy

Gastroscopy (s. figs. 14.10, 14.14; 19.7, 19.9), rectocoloscopy (s. fig. 19.13) and, in certain cases, rectal endosonography are required for evaluating oesophageal varices, portal hypertensive gastroenteropathy (45, 68, 124, 127, 134, 179), gastric antral vascular ectasia (127), peptic ulcer (128, 161, 179), intestinal (23, 150) and anorectal (74) varices, etc.

9 Prognostic classification

The clinical picture of liver cirrhosis displays a great variety of forms. This makes it very difficult to judge the prognosis and to establish an appropriate treatment plan, particularly with regard to surgical intervention. It was indeed surgeons who proposed a classification suitable for improved evaluation of the risks involved in surgery (C.G. CHILD, J.G. TURCOTTE, 1964). By means of simple parameters, it is possible to assess the functional reserves of the liver with sufficient reliability. Some parameters show the severity of portal hypertension (e.g. ascites, encephalopathy), while others yield information about the metabolic functions of the liver (e.g. jaundice, albumin value, hyaluronan) (19, 88); these criteria were extended by the addition of Quick's value (R.N.H. PUGH et al., 1973). Clinicians hope to improve the value of this classification by multiplying the criteria of class A by 1, of class B by 2 and of class C by 3, so that an overall score ranging from 5 (= most favourable prognosis) to 15 (= worst prognosis) is achieved. A close correlation between the deterioration of the Child-Pugh grade and the increasing size of the oesophageal varices could be shown. (2, 39, 51, 81, 133, 137, 146, 149, 166, 192) (s. tab. 35.7)

Criteria: Criteria such as ascites, encephalopathy and nutritional status are obviously blurred and, to a certain extent, may be interpreted subjectively. For example, the degree of **ascites** (depending on the examination method chosen) and the determination of patient response to treatment (depending on the medication used) are criteria that are hard to standardize. By contrast, **encephalopathy** can be easily classified according to its stages. (s. tab. 15.5) • The occurrence of **hyponatraemia** is a severe complication with a worse prognosis, especially if it progresses into HRS. (11) • **Liver function tests**

Child-Turcotte stage and Pugh modification	A 1 point	B 2 points	C 3 points
1. Bilirubin (mg/dl, µmol/l) 2. Albumin (g/dl) 3. Ascites 4. Encephalopathy 5. Quick's value (%)*) (or INR)	<2.0 < 35 >3.5 none none >70 (<1.7)	2−3.0 35−51 2.8−3.5 easy to treat stages I, II 40−70 (1.8−2.3)	>3.0 > 51 <2.8 difficult to treat stages III, IV <40 (>2.3)
Points score (used by Pugh)	5−6	7−9	10−15
Survival rate: 1 and 2 year(s)	100%; 85%	80%; 60%	45%; 35%

Tab. 35.7: Classification of hepatic cirrhosis according to Child-Turcotte (1964) and Pugh (1973) (stage A = good compensation, stage B = significant functional loss, stage C = decompensation) *) Quick's value is additionally used by Pugh (INR = international normalized ratio)

may provide information about the severity of the functional disorder at an early stage of cirrhosis. We have always preferred to use the two liver function tests *GEC* and *ICG* as additional methods of evaluation, whereby ascites was determined sonographically and subjected to largely standardized treatment. Reproducible functional values make it much easier to distinguish between class A and B as well as between the scores 5–7 and 8–10. They are no substitute for classification (s. tab. 35.7), but may provide valuable information in individual cases. These two function tests are reliable in quantifying the **liver cell mass** (e. g. by means of GEC) as well as the effective **liver blood supply** (e. g. by means of ICG) as prognostically useful parameters.

10 Differential diagnosis

Differential diagnosis of liver cirrhosis is concerned with two questions: (*1.*) *confirmation of the diagnosis*, and (*2.*) *clarification of the aetiology*. (71, 91)

Diagnosis with an accuracy of almost 100% is guaranteed using **laparoscopy** and **biopsy,** whereby in the latter technique, samples are taken from both liver lobes, if necessary. It is important to obtain a compact biopsy sample – albeit in larger fragments. Crumbly material is of no use! If such tissue crumbs have been obtained by using a Menghini needle, the *Vim-Silverman needle* has to be used for a second biopsy (and should have been used in the first place in targeted biopsy in liver cirrhosis!). A reticulin preparation, which reveals the extent and distribution of connective tissue more clearly, is diagnostically valuable. • Differentiation has to be made between: (*1.*) **focal nodular hyperplasia,** which

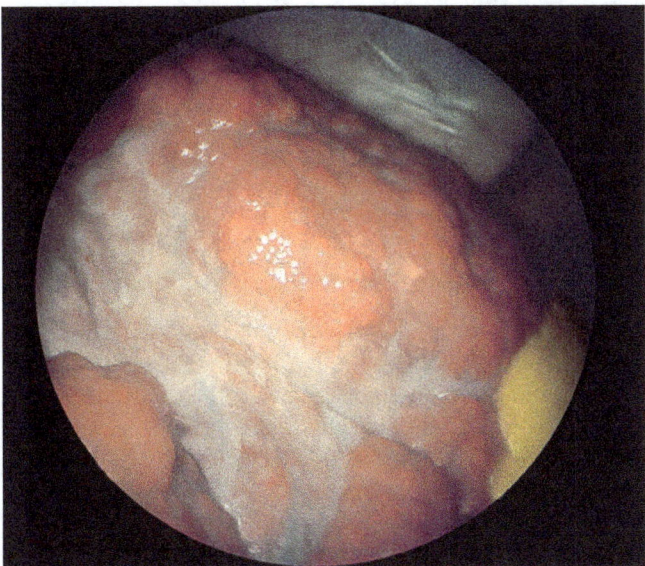

Fig. 35.17: Postnecrotic scarred liver after severe viral hepatitis B. Atrophy of the left liver lobe with regenerations, broad cicatricial areas and scarred furrows (s. figs. 21.13; 22.16; 35.1!)

does not show any lobular areas cut off by connective tissue, (*2.*) **liver fibrosis** (s. figs. 7.16; 21.14; 22.15; 28.6, 28.7), and (*3.*) **scar tissue** within cirrhosis, e. g. in a scarred liver. (s. p. 412) (s. fig. 35.17)

Clarification of the aetiology of cirrhosis is no problem as long as the potential causes are investigated carefully. In this context, an overview of the numerous causes of cirrhosis as a check list in chart form is very useful. (s. tab. 35.2) The necessary diagnostic parameters can then be applied efficiently. Specific histochemical investigations (e. g. in storage diseases) are carried out accordingly. It is important to categorize cirrhosis based on its aetiology, since some forms can then be treated more effectively. • Several sequelae or complications which impede a differential diagnosis are prevalent in certain types of cirrhosis; they are often the primary reason why the patient consults a physician. (s. tab. 35.2)

11 Consequences and complications

During the course of cirrhosis, it is almost impossible to differentiate between *metabolic consequences* and *complications* due to the fact that transitions are fluid both in terms of terminology and clinical features. Metabolic consequences may be complications in themselves, or play a special role in the occurrence of acute sequelae, or even turn a complicative event into a deleterious situation. The initial cause of such developments often remains unknown. Usually, a vicious circle of impaired mechanisms precedes relevant metabolic insufficiency or other complications. • The development of such events can be triggered by the course of disease itself or by the patient's behaviour, or even by therapeutic interventions.

The clinical picture of cirrhosis is overlapped by the symptomatology of the respective metabolic sequelae, or in some cases the complicative event predominates. Occasionally, a wide spectrum of symptoms and findings may be observed. This calls for detailed diagnostic clarification and varied medical treatment by an internal specialist as well as intensive care or sometimes invasive measures.

▶ In cirrhosis, both the overall hepatic *intermediary metabolism* (s. p. 36 and footnote *[)]*; s. tab. 3.1) and the *microcirculation* are severely impaired.

11.1 Negative energy balance

Cirrhotic patients often suffer from a negative energy balance even at an early stage, mainly due to protein deficiency, which is called *protein-energy malnutrition* (PEM). This pathological metabolic situation found in

70–80% of cases can be recognized by reduced oxygen consumption. The administration of β-blockers in patients with cirrhosis causes a favourable metabolic effect, whereby energy expenditure and catecholamine levels are decreased.

The energy required for hepatocellular metabolism is mainly provided by **oxidation** of short-chain fatty acids and amino acids via the citric acid cycle, usually in the mitochondria. Fructose and ethanol are also available for oxidation. In this process, O_2 **partial pressure** falls from 13% in the periportal area to 6% in the pericentral area, which means that the latter region is the most prone to hypoxic cellular damage.

The **energy supply** required by cirrhotic patients is achieved by mobilizing fats: the patient's fatty tissue is reduced and body weight decreases; the continuing energy requirement is met by the breakdown of muscle proteins with the result that amino acids are formed, which in turn are used for gluconeogenesis in the liver. Catabolism increases and leads to muscular atrophy, which is known as the *wasting syndrome*. (32, 35, 66, 87, 102, 110, 111, 120)

11.2 Carbohydrate metabolism disorders

The central role of the liver in carbohydrate metabolism is underlined by the term **glucostate** (K. JUNGERMANN, 1986). The ingestion of carbohydrates leads to the production and storage of glycogen; it is produced mainly in the pericentral area. A large amount of the glucose absorbed passes directly through the liver to the peripheral organs, where it is primarily utilized. The remaining C_3 bodies (alanine, lactate) are returned to the liver, where glycogen synthesis takes place predominantly in the periportal zone. Gluconeogenesis, i.e. hormone-regulated neoformation of glucose from lactate and glucoplastic amino acids, and glycolysis occur simultaneously and continuously in the same hepatocyte. Usually, about 80% of the glucose released comes from glucogenolysis and some 20% from gluconeogenesis. The energy yield from oxidative breakdown of fructose and glucose, for instance, is 34 and 38 ATP respectively; the energy from the β-oxidation of fatty acids, such as hexaonate or palmitate, is 44 and 129 ATP respectively. (s. p. 45) (s. figs. 3.6, 3.7) • In liver cirrhosis, **three forms** of *carbohydrate metabolic disorders* may be expected: (*1.*) hypoglycaemia, (*2.*) hepatogenic diabetes mellitus, and (*3.*) impaired glycogenolysis and gluconeogenesis (T. YOSHIDA et al., 1998).

11.2.1 Hypoglycaemia

Hypoglycaemia is a rare event. It is usually due to reduced gluconeogenesis, mainly following loss of parenchyma (>80%). Chronic alcohol abuse or acute alcohol intoxication can lead to hypoglycaemia. (s. p. 534)

11.2.2 Hepatogenic diabetes mellitus

Glucose intolerance is found in 50–80% and manifest diabetes in 10–15% of cirrhotic patients. Depending on the severity, glucose intolerance or manifest diabetes may also be observed in fatty liver in 40–70% and 10–40% of patients respectively; in haemochromatotic cirrhosis, the frequency of diabetes is 60–70%. The corresponding liver disease is generally the cause of the disturbed carbohydrate metabolism, which it precedes. • At the same time, increased insulin and glucagon values (two or three times above normal) can be detected; administration of insulin only causes a minor decrease in the glucose serum values. Thus there is no insulin deficiency, but *insulin resistance* (W. CREUTZFELDT et al., 1970); this may be caused by a TNF-induced disturbance in the tyrosine phosphorylation of the insulin receptor. Insulin resistance in cirrhosis is a multifactorial process. *Hyperinsulinaemia* is due to a reduced breakdown of insulin in the liver and may, among other things, be caused by increased insulin secretion stimulated by hyperglycaemia. In this process, however, hyperinsulinaemia is not sufficient to overcome peripheral insulin resistance; there is a reduction in insulin-dependent glucose absorption and its turnover in the skeletal musculature and fatty tissue. • *Treatment* of hepatogenic diabetes is by dietary measures or, depending on the case, by sulphonylurea (G. MARCHESINI et al., 1998) or (preferably) benzoic acid derivatives, e.g. repaglinide. Zinc leads to an improvement in glucose metabolism. Biguanides are contraindicated. (103, 132, 157, 167)

11.2.3 Glycogenolysis disorders

The glycogen content of the liver and glycogenolysis are reduced to 20–30% of the normal level. The clearly decreased glycogenolysis is compensated by increased gluconeogenesis (three or four times above normal). This requires amino acids from the breakdown of muscle protein. Absorption of glucose in the liver is reduced, particularly in portacaval anastomoses, while the release of glucose is unaffected.

11.3 Protein metabolism disorders

The protein and amino-acid metabolism of the liver is characterized by **three essential functions:** (*1.*) production and breakdown of proteins, (*2.*) production and breakdown of amino acids as well as regulation of their concentrations in the blood, and (*3.*) detoxification of ammonium via the synthesis of urea (= excretory form) and glutamine (= non-toxic transport or storage form) with simultaneous regulation of the acid-base balance. The breakdown of branched-chain amino acids occurs exclusively in the muscular system by way of deamination. (s. pp 42, 48)

11.3.1 Catabolism

In cirrhotic patients, a reduced synthesis rate of most proteins is found at an early stage, with albumin synthesis being the least compromised factor. Fat storage, muscle mass and protein turnover are reduced. This ultimately leads to *catabolism* (= stress metabolism) and increasing *muscular atrophy* (= wasting syndrome). The latter condition can also result from sympathicotonia with elevated catecholamine values; similarly, decreased values of IGF1 inhibit the formation of muscle tissue.

11.3.2 Amino-acid imbalance

The regulation of the amino-acid values in the blood plasma is increasingly disturbed, leading to significant changes in their distribution pattern. There is a decrease in **branched-chain amino acids,** probably due to greater absorption in the muscles and increased metabolic degradation (possibly as a consequence of hyperinsulinism). This can be prevented by the administration of β-blockers. • The rise in **aromatic amino acids** is thought to be caused by their reduced breakdown in the liver. They are the initial products for the formation of neurotransmitters and mediators; this explains the increase in serum values, e.g. of serotonin and noradrenaline, in liver cirrhosis. The plasma value of methionine is also elevated due to S-adenosylmethionine synthase deficiency, with simultaneously reduced methionine clearance. As a result, there is insufficient formation of glutathione; the phospholipid synthesis required for the biomembranes is reduced, and decreased polyamine synthesis compromises regeneration. (37) • A reduction in urea synthesis (by some 30%) results in hyperammonaemia and metabolic alkalosis. The turnover and concentration of alanine remain unchanged in cirrhosis; glutamine values are increased. Moreover, hyperinsulinism leads to a decrease in urea synthesis, as does zinc deficiency. (110, 111) (s. p 274)

11.4 Lipid metabolism disorders

The role of the liver in lipid metabolism is characterized by **five important functions:** (*1.*) β-oxidation and ketogenesis, (*2.*) lipogenesis, (*3.*) lipoprotein metabolism, (*4.*) cholesterol metabolism, and (*5.*) bile acid metabolism. • Short-chain fatty acids from the food are released in the intestine by lipolysis and transported to the liver. Beta-oxidation takes place in the mitochondria. In this process, acetyl coenzyme A is produced, which is oxidized to form CO_2 via the citric acid cycle or used to form **ketone bodies** in carbohydrate deficiency. After being resorbed in the enterocytes, long-chain fatty acids from the food are again incorporated into the triglycerides; they are passed on via the lymph to the periphery in the form of chylomicrons or transported to the liver as chylomicron remnants. They may also be β-oxidized in the mitochondria. • In **lipogenesis,** carbohydrates are converted via acetyl-coenzyme A, mainly on the cytoplasmic side of the endoplasmic reticulum. Lipogenesis is mainly controlled by the insulin-glucagon quotient. • **Lipoproteins** are required in order to transport water-insoluble lipids from the site of their synthesis to the site where they are used or broken down. (s. p. 46)

In **liver cirrhosis,** there are several changes: reduction in LCAT (with "cholesterol ester fall"), HDL, LDL and and VLDL, with a corresponding change in their distribution pattern; occurrence of hypertriglyceridaemia and atypical lipoproteins; reduction in phospholipid synthesis (31), possibly with greatly impaired structure and function of the biomembranes. Hepatic extraction of bile acids is reduced with the result that they reach the peripheral circulation – even in the early stages of cirrhosis! – and give rise to increased serum values. Bile acids have cholestatic and cytotoxic effects. When bile acid metabolism is markedly compromised, enteral absorption of fat-soluble vitamins is impeded, so that *A, D, E* and *K hypovitaminoses* may be observed.

11.5 Hypovitaminoses

The manifold relationships between the metabolic functions of the liver and the vitamins fulfil vital tasks in helping the organism to stay healthy. Nutrition low in vitamins or age-related reduction in intestinal vitamin resorption as well as chronic alcoholism may be responsible for the development of hypovitaminosis. Standard values of vitamins (including fat-soluble vitamins) in the serum do not exclude a deficit. Deficiency is often recognized for the first time owing to the manifestation of clinical symptoms, and now requires substitution. **Substitution therapy** may be recommended even if no vitamin deficiencies have become manifest at this stage. (s. p. 51) (s. tab. 28.2!)

Deficiency of **water-soluble vitamins** is far less precarious than a deficit of fat-soluble vitamins. While the first condition is generally rare, it can nevertheless often be observed in severe alcoholism. In liver cirrhosis, it was possible to detect a reduced amount of vitamins B_2, B_6, B_{12}, C and niacin or pantothenic acid in the liver as well as hypofunction of vitamins B_1, B_2, B_6, C and folic acid. Hypovitaminosis may develop due to the reduced formation of specific transport proteins or the decreased activation or secretion of vitamins despite the sufficient supply of water-soluble vitamins through food intake.

The **fat-soluble vitamins** D and K are activated in the liver, and vitamin A is stored there. Their cellular effect is seen in the cytosol (vitamins E, K) or in the nucleus (vitamins A, D). Transport to the target organs is facilitated by specific carrier proteins (vitamins A, D) or by VLDL (vitamins E, K).

Hypovitaminosis A: The vitamin A content of the liver and plasma as well as of the retinol-binding protein (RBP) is reduced in cirrhosis. The decreased plasma value of zinc, particularly in existing portacaval anastomoses, correlates with these findings. The **symptoms** observed in hypovitaminosis A and zinc deficiency are largely the same: night blindness, labyrinthine deafness and/or vertigo, disturbed sense of taste and smell (25), skin changes. Such deficiency symptoms in hypovitaminosis A should be treated primarily by substituting zinc. Possible **causes** of vitamin A deficiency are (*1.*) disturbed resorption, (*2.*) reduced formation of RBP in the endoplasmic reticulum, (*3.*) zinc deficiency, and (*4.*) increased breakdown of retinoids due to the enhanced activity of cytochrome P450.

Hypovitaminosis D: Some 20% of the daily vitamin D requirement are supplied by food intake, while about 80% are produced via endogenous synthesis through transformation of 7-dehydrocholesterol under the influence of ultraviolet light. Within the liver, D_3 (= cholecalciferol) is activated by 25-hydroxylation. It is excreted into the bile to become part of an enterohepatic circulation. In liver cirrhosis, and particularly in cholestasis, this circulation is impaired, so that vitamin D metabolites are activated in larger amounts and excreted in the faeces. The resulting clinical picture is usually a mixture of osteoporosis and osteomalacia.

Hypovitaminosis E: Vitamin E plays a key role in cell metabolism as an antioxidant for eliminating reactive oxygen intermediates. Subsequent to intestinal resorption, vitamin E is transported in chylomicrons into the liver, from where it reaches other organs together with VLDL. • Vitamin E deficiency is observed in chronic liver diseases caused by alcohol, Wilson's disease, haemochromatosis and abetalipoproteinaemia. In vitamin E deficiency, neurologic disturbances (areflexia, dysbasia, ocular palsy, reduced perception of vibration) occur; haemolysis can likewise be induced or become more pronounced due to epoxide formation of unsaturated fatty acids within the erythrocyte membranes.

Hypovitaminosis K: Vitamin K is necessary for the formation of coagulation factors II, VII, X and XI as well as of proteins C, S and M; in addition, it is indispensable for the production of osteocalcin, which stimulates osteoblast activity. It is transported from the liver to the bloodstream in the VLDL. • A deficiency is characterized by symptoms similar to those observed in haemorrhagic diathesis. It can be caused by intestinal resorption disturbance or loss of hepatocellular function (reduced carboxyl transfer to specific vitamin K-dependent proteins).

11.6 Endocrine disorders

Liver metabolism is controlled by hormones, and the plasma values of numerous hormones are controlled by the liver. The essential interactions of steroid, effector and thyroid hormones with the liver have already been discussed. *(see chapter 3.9)* (s. tabs. 3.9–3.12)

Patients with liver cirrhosis often suffer from endocrine disturbances, such as latent or even manifest diabetes mellitus; in most cases, the plasma levels of the growth hormone (STH) are increased; **low-T_3 syndrome** (with T_4 in the normal range) is generally accompanied by euthyroidism. Substitution therapy is not indicated in a euthyroid metabolic condition. • A disturbed sexual function is particularly significant. In the **hepatotesticular syndrome,** gynaecomastia (s. fig. 4.10) is found in about 50% and impotency or infertility in about 80% of cases. Such disturbances (especially testicular atrophy, which is often a direct consequence of alcohol abuse) are more frequent and more severe in cases of haemochromatotic and alcoholic cirrhosis. Feminization takes place. The analogous **hepato-ovarian syndrome** corresponds with an early onset of dysmenorrhoea or amenorrhoea and loss of libido. • The last two syndromes can be subsumed under the term **Silvestrini-Corda syndrome** (L. CORDA, 1925). Findings include a reduced breakdown of oestrogens and decreased testosterone synthesis or secretion.

11.7 Bacterial and viral infections

Bacterial infections are detected in 45–50% of patients with cirrhosis. Some 7% of fatalities in compensated cirrhosis and 20% of fatalities in decompensated cirrhosis are due to infections. The bacterial translocation to mesenteric lymph nodes is increased in relation to the Child stage. • The following *organic manifestations* predominate: (*1.*) spontaneous bacterial peritonitis in ascites, (*2.*) infections of the urogenital tract, and (*3.*) infections of the bronchopulmonary system. Tuberculosis (lungs, peritoneum, kidneys) and bacterial meningitis (108, 126) must also be taken into account in differential diagnosis. Diagnostic difficulties are often due to a lack of fever or leucocytosis. • This weakness of the endogenous immune system is likewise involved in **viral infections:** in 63% of patients with cirrhosis, for example, cytomegaly infection was observed prior to liver transplantation, while the infection rate was only 2.5% in the control group. (34, 57, 100, 116)

Causes: The following causes are seen as being responsible for an acquired immune deficiency syndrome in liver cirrhosis (B.A. RUNYON, 1995): (*1.*) hypofunction of the RES (a decrease in the filter or clearance function and phagocytosis capacity as well as reduced formation of immune modulators) (s. p. 69), (*2.*) reduction in hepatic synthesis of opsonins (s. p. 70), (*3.*) compromised function of leucocytes, (*4.*) impaired proliferation and activation of T lymphocytes, and (*5.*) increased mucosa permeability to bacteria. Both bacteria and bacterial lipopolysaccharides enter the organism in large numbers. They are responsible for increased serum levels of the cytokines (e.g. interleukins 1 and 6, TNF, γ-interferon), and there is increased production of these substances together with their reduced breakdown in the cirrhotic liver. Cytokines are formed in the monocytes of blood and in the mononuclear cells of various organs (above all in ascites).

11.8 Hepatic osteopathy

11.8.1 Definition

Osteoporosis is defined as an imbalance between the breakdown and neoformation of osseous substance, resulting in bone loss. Ostalgia is evident, and later, fractures of the vertebral bodies, femoral neck and antebrachial bones are observed.

In **osteomalacia,** the bone matrix is quantitatively and qualitatively normal, while the bones show a reduced content of minerals. There is ostalgia and muscle weakness as well as arcuation of the long tubular bones. X-ray imaging shows band-shaped zones of decalcification, usually in symmetrical arrangement, particularly at the ribs, femoral neck and pelvis (= *Looser-Milkman's syndrome*).

The term **hepatic osteopathy** (J. E. COMPSTON, 1986) describes skeletal changes in chronic liver diseases, including osteoporosis, which is by far the most prevalent form, and osteomalacia, which is detected very rarely, as well as their respective mixed forms.

11.8.2 Frequency

In cirrhosis, reduced bone density of the vertebral bodies could be observed in 16% and of the antebrachial bones in 23% of patients (compared to 7% and 5% respectively in the control group). Fractures of the vertebral bodies were detected in 16% and of the antebrachial bones in 21% of cases (compared to 8% and 8% respectively in the control group). Hepatic osteopathy usually occurs independently of the cause and type of the chronic liver disease. However, alcoholism, haemochromatosis and Wilson's disease result in osteoblastic hypofunction, so that osteopathy is more likely to appear in these patients, even prior to the development of cirrhosis. The occurrence of osteopathy is closely correlated with the severity of the liver disease and with hypogonadism. In liver cirrhosis, the prevalence of osteopenia is about 30%. (54, 77)

11.8.3 Pathogenesis

The pathogenesis of hepatic osteopathy is primarily characterized by disturbed bone formation due to (*1.*) reduced osteoblast surface (with the number of osteoblasts being in the normal range), and (*2.*) reduction in osteocalcin. The latter substance is a bone-matrix protein formed by the osteoblasts. Therefore, the serum value is seen as a marker of osteogenesis. There is no increase in osteoclasis. The causes and risk factors of disturbed bone metabolism are manifold and not totally understood as yet. (63)

▶ To date, we do not know what kind of changes in **vitamin D metabolism** or in the binding proteins may be (partially) responsible for these disturbances. Moreover, there are no reliable findings as to the role of **parathyroid hormone** and **calcitonin** in the development of hepatic osteopathy; this is also true for **gastrocalcin,** which (like calcitonin) makes the serum level of calcium decrease. Reduced enteral resorption of calcium is only observed in severe cholestasis, which causes no osteopathy however. While a deficiency of vitamin D can have pathogenetic effects, it does not in itself lead to osteopathy. An increased value of D_3 may be a predictor of a developing osteopathy. In addition, there is a correlation between the serum values of **gastrin** and osteopathy — but nothing else is known about this. • The intake of **antiepileptics** over a longer period of time triggers an induction of the cytochrome P 450 system, so that vitamin D is increasingly broken down, a loss which can, however, be substituted. • **Glucocorticoids** cause a reduction in enteral calcium resorption and the serum level of oestrogen; they are also responsible for calciuria and impeded osteoblast activity. These factors lead to a decrease in bone density and create what is called the *cortisone effect*. • By contrast, **cyclosporine** increases osteoblast activity.

11.8.4 Clinical symptoms

Hepatic osteopathy remains latent for a long time. *Backache* is considered to be the earliest hint of this type of complicative development in cirrhosis. The further course is characterized by trabecular osteopenia with loss of the cancellous bone structure. This causes *compression fractures* of the vertebral bodies with increasing kyphosis and a corresponding decrease in body height. Further sites susceptible to *fractures* are the femoral neck and the antebrachial bones. • Osteopathy does not yield any *biochemical findings*: the serum values of calcium, phosphate, parathyroid hormone, 25-hydroxycholecalciferol, osteocalcin and alkaline phosphatase are within the normal range. • Osteoporosis cannot be detected by *X-ray imaging* until the late stages. CT scanning allows density measurement of the skeleton. New radiological techniques (e. g. dual energy X-ray absorption) may provide an earlier diagnosis in the future.

Osteomalacia, a rare manifest form of hepatic osteopathy, causes pain mainly in the muscles, but less so in the bones. *Biochemically*, AP is markedly increased; there is a deficiency of calcium, phosphate and 25-hydroxycholecalciferol. *Radiologic diagnosis* shows signs of Looser-Milkman's syndrome: coarsening of cancellous bone structure, narrowing of the compacta in the tubular bones, reduced density of the skeletal system, and band-shaped zones of decalcification.

11.8.5 Treatment

The most important **prophylactic measures** for preventing the development of hepatic osteopathy are (*1.*) avoidance of harmful *noxae* (alcohol, nicotine), (*2.*) *avoidance of risk factors* (e. g. overweight; calcium, phosphate or vitamin D deficiency; use of glucocorticoids, cholestyramine and antacids containing aluminium), (*3.*) administration of vitamin K2 (menatetrenone) in women with risk factors, and (*4.*) routine **physical exercise**. (s. pp 551, 683, 765) Chronic liver patients should carry out the following exercises on a regular basis:

Two or three times per day: 10–15 slow knee-bending (= thigh muscles), 10–15 standing on tiptoe (= calf muscles), 10–15 upper arm flexing (= biceps), and 10–15 bending from the waist (= back muscles). This guarantees that about 60% of the musculature is trained under simple conditions at home.

The **drug therapy** used to date aims to achieve broad substitution. Therapy should be carried out for up to 24 months. • (*1.*) Daily *calcium requirement* is 1.2–1.6 g. Nutrition usually contains about 0.6 g, so that 3 x 200 mg to 3 x 300 mg per day should be substituted (e.g. with calcium carbonate). • (*2.*) In order to avoid *hypogonadism*, we recommend a daily administration of conjugated oestrogens (e.g. 2 mg, twice a week, applied dermally to avoid passage through the liver), possibly combined with gestagens. The daily requirement of oestrogen is about 0.6 mg. In men, the administration of testosterone may be indicated. • (*3.*) *Vitamin D* is only indicated when hypovitaminosis has been detected (e.g. as cholecalciferol, 1α- or 25-hydroxylated derivatives, or 1,25 dihydroxylated derivatives). These substances should only be applied as substitution therapy when there is a corresponding deficiency. • (*4.*) In individual cases, *calcitonin* (as nasal spray) and *biphosphonates* are further options. • In the osteomalacic form of osteopathy, treatment with calcium and vitamin D or its derivatives may be required. However, the serum value of calcium must not exceed 11.0–11.5 mg/dl.

11.9 Hepatic encephalopathy

Disturbances of personality, consciousness and intellectual functions are often observed in acute or chronic liver diseases. In 50–80% of cirrhosis patients, such neuropsychiatric signs of HE are found with varying intensity and duration (even with symptom-free intervals) as well as in different combinations. (s. tab. 10.1) While it is relatively easy to **diagnose** manifest HE *(stages I–IV)* (s. tab. 15.5), other potential causes of this clinical picture have to be excluded by differential diagnosis in each individual case (e.g. intracerebral bleeding, infections, metabolic imbalance, cerebral diseases). There is a close correlation between liver function and severity of HE — and thus also with quality of life. (13) Diagnosis of *latent HE (stages 0, 0–I)* can only be made with the help of psychometric test procedures (8) or special EEG techniques. Nuclear resonance imaging and SPECT (163) have been used in scientific studies. *(see chapter 10!)*

Numerous **biochemical factors** can be causal agents in HE. It may also be attributable to an increase in serum ammonia resulting from Helicobacter pylori. (s. tab. 15.2) Avoidance of causative factors is always the most important measure for the prevention of HE and their elimination is seen as a prerequisite for successful treatment. (s. p. 289)

The **pathogenesis** is multifactorial. In cirrhotic patients with latent HE, regional differences in cerebral ammonia uptake are present; this corresponds to histopathological changes in HE. Although increased ammonia values have a primary pathogenetic significance, other neurotoxins, neurotransmitter disturbances, amino-acid imbalances, high levels of benzodiazepines, zinc deficiency, increased manganese concentration, etc. also figure prominently. With the help of spin-lattice (T_1) relaxation time, significant correlation has been demonstrated between HE severity and the putative deposition of manganese in the globus pallidus, caudate nucleus and posterior limb of the internal capsule. (156) • Values of enterocyte phosphate-activated glutaminase are increased in cirrhosis and correlate closely with latent HE (stages 0, 0–I). H. pylori infection is not correlated with HE. (155) • *None of these substances or disturbances on its own has a comagenic effect. It is probable that the astrocytes are the pathogenetic end point upon which the cascade of causes has its impact.* (s. pp 273–278!)

The **clinical picture** comprises both *acute* and *chronic HE*. In addition, routine application of a simple test programme used for practical and clinical purposes (s. tab. 10.7) has repeatedly shown *"acute-on-chronic" stages* during long-term monitoring. Starting with the normal finding of "no HE", the stages are grouped, depending on their individual variability, as 0, 0–I (= latent HE) and I, I–II, II (= manifest HE). Furthermore, there is a link between extrapyramidal signs and the latent HE. Since HE can be detected quite reliably at an early stage during its latent period, therapeutic measures are also recommended in addition to the elimination of the causal factors. (s. pp 278–283)

Treatment is based on (*1.*) elimination of the causal factor(s) (s. tabs. 15.1, 15.2) and (*2.*) reduction or normalization of the ammonia level. The latter consists of: *intestinal detoxification* using lactulose (52, 98, 113), paramomycin, neomycin or metronidazole; *protein restriction* (0–30 g for the first to third day, gradually increased up to 1 g/kg BW/day) (despite some controversial results); sufficient *calorie* intake (glucose), *application of urea cycle intermediates* (138), administration of *zinc* (103, 185) and, if necessary, of *branched-chain amino acids* and *flumazenil*. Elimination of gastric infection due to *Helicobacter pylori* has proved effective for normalizing hyperammonaemia (caused by this condition). A decrease in ammonia is also achieved by *acetohydroxamic acid*, which is a powerful inhibitor of bacterial ureases of H. pylori. (155) Animal experiments have demonstrated that N-carbamoyl-L-glutamate plus L-arginine protects rats with cirrhosis from acute ammonia intoxication. Experience has shown that the very frequent occurrence of latent HE (stages 0, 0–I) can largely be avoided by careful prophylactic measures and that early treatment helps to prevent the latent phase from developing into a manifest one (stages I–IV), i.e. there is no necessity for inpatient treatment! *(see chapter 15.9!)*

11.10 Ascites

Impairment of **cerebral functions** and disturbances of the **water and electrolyte balance** are the two most important and most common manifestations of decompensated liver cirrhosis. • They may be reliably detected at an early stage by means of daily *body weight control* and simple *psychometric tests*. A **documentation sheet** filled in by the patient has proved to be worthwhile: latent oedemas, onset of ascites and latent encephalopathy can be detected in this way and thus treated at an early stage. **Long-term standing** leads to reduction of natriuresis with subsequent water retention and deterioration of renal blood flow (like a vicious circle). This is caused by activation of the RAAS and the sympathetic nervous system. Such a dangerous situation (which can arise for example after two hours of standing at a sports event with excessive emotional participation) is often underrated, as we ourselves observed in several patients! (s. p. 298) (s. fig. 16.3) *(see chapter 16!)*

About 50% of patients with cirrhosis develop ascites within ten years. In the case of a "simple" ascites (s. tab. 16.8), a therapy with diuretics is generally successful — in contrast to a "problematic" or refractory ascites.

Complications: The development of ascites causes many complications which greatly worsen the prognosis of cirrhosis. (s. tab. 16.9) • Every day, 40−80% of the ascitic fluid and 4% of the ascitic albumin are exchanged between the plasma and the ascites. In the absence of oedema, 400−500 ml (max. 750 ml) ascitic fluid can be removed from the abdominal cavity by diet and medication. (s. p. 312) • **Side effects** due to diuretic agents (hypovolaemia, hyponatraemia, hypokalaemia, disturbances of the acid-base balance) must be avoided. (s. p. 314) • The occurrence of **spontaneous bacterial peritonitis** is life-threatening. Prognosis could be markedly improved by early diagnosis, elimination of risk factors and efficient antibiotic treatment (e. g. amoxicillin-clavulanic acid) accompanied by simultaneous intestinal decontamination. (s. p. 310)

A step-by-step plan has proved effective for the **treatment** of ascites, with *therapeutic steps 1−4* being employed successively if the previous stage was unsuccessful. (s. tab. 35.8) However, progressing from step to step not only increases the effectiveness of the treatment, but also the frequency and severity of side effects. Nevertheless, a single paracentesis, during which an average of five litres of ascitic fluid were evacuated, resulted in normal cardiac, renal and hormonal parameters within two days. Paracentesis is considered to be a safe and efficient method. (129) *(see chapter 16.8)*

1. Basic therapy (s. tab. 16.11) (s. p. 311)
2. Diuretic therapy (s. tab. 16.12) (s. p. 312)
3. Osmotic diuresis (s. p. 314)
4. Paracentesis (s. p. 315)

Tab. 35.8: Therapeutic steps used in the treatment of ascites

Furosemide can cause hypovolaemia due to its rapid effect with subsequent unfavourable activation of the RAAS, especially after i.v. injection. Nevertheless, i.v. furosemide may be indicated in dilutional hyponatriaemia (s. p. 314). Generally, however, spironolactone on its own has proved more effective than in combination with (RAAS-activating?) furosemide. (147) We actually prefer a *combination* of spironolactone with xipamide, torasemide or clonidine. (s. p. 313)

Paracentesis should be combined with an i.v. solution of albumin (our own experience has shown that an i.v. solution of 20−40 ml plasma expander directly before i.v. albumin administration increases the oncotic pressure, so that albumin remains efficacious for a longer time in the blood circulation). • Apparently, 3 mg terlipressin is as effective as i.v. albumin in preventing a decrease in effective arterial blood volume. (s. p. 315)

Hydroxyethyl starch (HES) in repeated administration may be the cause of increased portal hypertension; liver insufficiency or sepsis can occur due to lysosomal storage of HES in Kupffer cells and hepatocytes.

Losartan is a highly selective angiotensin-2-receptor (type 1) antagonist; it decreases portal hypertension as well as improving glomerular filtration and natriuresis with good aquaretic response. (189) (s. p. 367)

When diuretics are administered at the same time, it is not absolutely necessary to adhere to strict **salt restriction**. We followed the recommended 6−8 g/day. Indeed, such a moderate restriction is usually observed more reliably by the patient. • Reducing **water intake** to 1.5−2.0 l/day is also sufficient. Only a hyponatraemic condition of <130 mmol/l requires a reduction in fluid intake to <1,000 ml/day. • Determination of **fractional sodium elimination** (FE_{Na}) may point to potential success even before treatment has begun: with a value of >0.5%, treatment steps 1 and 2 (see above) will achieve a probable success rate of about 95%. This favourable initial situation is supported by a still sufficient spontaneous **sodium excretion** of >40 mmol/day. Therapy resistance must be anticipated when fractional sodium elimination is <0.1% and sodium excretion is <10 mmol/day. • If treatment steps 1−4 are unsuccessful or renal function is clearly impaired initially and FE_{Na} is <0.1%, the insertion of a **peritovenous shunt** (PVS) should be considered. This procedure is designed to make use of the principle of ascites reinfusion for as long as possible. (s. tabs. 16.14−16.18) (s. p. 317) • **TIPS** may also prove to be an alternative to PVS, especially when using a polytetrafluoroethylene-covered stent to prevent occlusion. (107) (s. fig. 16.15) (s. pp 267, 320, 336, 368, 897)

Chronic hepatitis C is occasionally associated with cryoglobulinaemia and glomerulonephritis. • In all forms of cirrhosis, the intrarenal circulation is impaired and there is a redistribution of blood flow away from the cortex. A thickening of the mesangial stalk and capillary wall *(= cirrhotic glomerular sclerosis)* is often evident. These changes predispose to the hepatorenal syndrome. • It is essential to prevent the occurrence of the (particularly iatrogenic) **hepatorenal syndrome** with the following findings. (39, 96, 107) *(see chapter 17!)*:

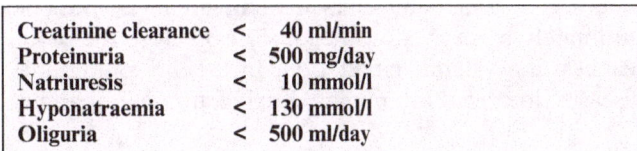

Creatinine clearance	<	40 ml/min
Proteinuria	<	500 mg/day
Natriuresis	<	10 mmol/l
Hyponatraemia	<	130 mmol/l
Oliguria	<	500 ml/day

11.11 Pleuropulmonary complications

In the course of primary **liver diseases** as well as during any requisite invasive measures, numerous pleuropulmonary disturbances or diseases may appear due to functional and/or mechanical conditions. They are closely associated with each other. Pleuropulmonary complications can have considerable adverse effects on the basic liver disease and thus worsen its prognosis. (3, 6, 72, 112, 151, 152) (s. tab. 35.9)

Pleuropulmonary complications	Liver disease
1. Hepatopulmonary syndrome (HPS)	Acute liver failure Chronic hepatitis Liver cirrhosis
2. Portopulmonary hypertension (PPH)	Alagille's syndrome Chronic hepatitis Focal nodular hyperplasia Hypoplastic portal vein Liver cirrhosis Schistosomiasis
3. Pleural effusions	Acute viral hepatitis After liver transplantation After varicosclerosation Chronic hepatitis Echinococcosis Liver abscess Liver cirrhosis
4. Pulmonary emphysema	α_1-antitrypsin deficiency
5. Chronic obstructive respiratory disease	α_1-antitrypsin deficiency Mucoviscidosis Sarcoidosis
6. Interstitial pneumonia	Autoimmune hepatitis Overlap syndrome PBC Sarcoidosis

Tab. 35.9: Common pleuropulmonary complications in the course of certain liver diseases

Primary **pulmonary diseases** (e.g. primary pulmonary hypertension, pulmonary fibrosis, chronic obstructive respiratory diseases) cause chronic **hepatic congestion** due to chronic pulmonary heart disease, possibly leading to insufficiency. • **Hypoxaemia** as a result of acute or chronic respiratory insufficiency can impair metabolic liver functions considerably. In 40–70% of patients with cirrhosis, hypoxaemia is found; in about 50% of cases with advanced cirrhosis, a reduced diffusion capacity for CO is detectable. • Furthermore, pulmonary tissue contains a high level of glutamine synthetase, so that **ammonia detoxification** is possible (ultimately by perivenous hepatocytes) before the blood reaches the systemic circulation. In existing pulmonary diseases, localized ammonia detoxification is impaired.

11.11.1 Hepatopulmonary syndrome

The hepatopulmonary syndrome (HPS) may occur in patients with chronic liver disease or in the course of acute liver failure. It is characterized by the following **criteria**: (*1.*) exclusion of an underlying pulmonary or cardiac disease, (*2.*) increase in the alveolocapillary oxygen difference with or without arterial hypoxaemia (<70 mm Hg O_2 partial pressure) and with a marked decrease in the O_2 value when the body position is changed from lying to standing, and (*3.*) evidence of intrapulmonary vascular dilatations and **arteriovenous shunts**, resulting in **ventilation-perfusion disturbance**. • The frequency of pulmonary gas exchange disturbance is 30–50% in cirrhosis patients. The most important clinical finding concerning HPS is **hypoxaemia**. Hypocapnia is also a frequent symptom and is generally associated with pulmonary vasodilation. (3) • Hypertrophic **osteoarthropathy** (hour-glass nails, drumstick fingers) (s. fig. 4.18) likewise belongs to this complex in terms of aetiopathogenesis. *(see chapter 18!)*

11.11.2 Portopulmonary hypertension

Definition

> Portopulmonary hypertension (PPH) is characterized by (*1.*) elevated pulmonary artery pressure (>25 mm Hg), (*2.*) increased pulmonary vascular resistance (>120 dyne/sec/cm^5), and (*3.*) normal pulmonary capillary wedge pressure (<15 mm Hg). • *The presence of portal hypertension is considered to be a prerequisite for the development of PPH.*

Frequency and causes

PPH was detected in 2.0% of patients with liver cirrhosis, compared to 0.1% in the control group, i.e. *the risk of PPH is 20 times higher in cirrhosis patients*. The prevalence of PPH in liver cirrhosis with portal hypertension was 0.73% in autopsy examinations, compared to 0.13% in all other autopsies. • PPH has not only been described in portal hypertension due to liver disease (cirrhosis, chronic hepatitis, fibrosis, etc.), but also (with or without portal hypertension) in *focal nodular hyperplasia, schistosomiasis, Alagille's syndrome* and *portal vein thrombosis*. Important extrahepatic causes of PPH include portal hypertension due to *hypoplasia of the portal vein* and *lupus erythematosus*. (112, 140) *(see chapter 18.7!)* (s. tab. 35.9) (s. fig. 35.18)

Morphology and pathogenesis

Morphology: In PPH, there is evidence of medial hypertrophy in the area of the pulmonary arteries and arterioles, intima fibrosis (= *plexogenic arteriopathy*) and fresh or recanalized thrombi. These changes are unevenly spread throughout the lung; they do not correlate with the severity of PPH. Plexiform damage of the small (50–300 µm) pulmonary arterial vessels is prevalent in patients who are also suffering from portal hypertension (J. R. RUTTNER et al., 1980).

▶ **Pathogenesis:** The mechanism responsible is based on the effect of vasoactive or toxic substances arriving directly at the pulmonary vascular system from the portal vein system by circumventing the liver (e.g. NO). Thus pulmonary hypertension is also detected surprisingly often in patients with shunt surgery. Endothelin-1 is considered to be a strong vasoconstrictor; this substance has been detected in high concentrations in the pulmonary vascular endothelia of PPH patients. In addition, microembolisms entering the pulmonary arterioles may also play a pathogenetic role; such emboli can reach the lungs via spontaneous or surgical portosystemic shunts (R. M. SENIOR et al., 1968). A similar mechanism may be responsible for this condition in drug addicts suffering from PPH who have developed pulmonary microembolisms due to water-insoluble drug components injected intravenously. (s. fig. 35.18) *(see chapter 18.7!)*

Complaints: In 80—85% of patients with PPH, there is stress dyspnoea and occasional syncopes, thoracic pain on palpation with a feeling of tightness, marked fatiguability, lack of concentration and vertigo.

Findings: In 80—85% of cases, a loud P_2 heart sound and systolic murmur can be heard on auscultation. Occasionally, there is haemoptysis or oedema; ascites is rare. • The *ECG* shows the signs of right ventricular overload (e. g. right bundle-branch block, P pulmonale). *Thoracic imaging* often displays prominent pulmonary arteries and cardiac hypertrophy. *Echocardiography* is of great diagnostic value. The diagnosis is confirmed by *right cardiac catheterization*.

Prognosis for PPH is poor: the mean survival time is about 15 months with a six-month mortality of 50%. The most common causes of death are right heart failure, dysrhythmia and infections.

Treatment still remains difficult, because few clinical studies are available. High doses of **calcium antagonists** are recommended, but their frequent side effects have to be taken into account, particularly with a cardiac output of <2 l/min. In severe cases, pulmonary pressure reduction by permanent infusion of **epoprostenol** over several weeks or long-term administration of **oxygen** may be helpful. Good experience has been made with the endothelin-receptor antagonist **bosentan** (2 × 125 mg/day). (40) (s. p. 344!) • On retrospective assessment of a large number of cirrhotic patients, some of whom we treated for more than ten years, it is our impression that long-term administration of **spironolactone + molsidomine + β-blocker** is of therapeutic value for portal hypertension and, at least as far as this problem is concerned, also for primary and progressive pulmonary hypertension. Such combination therapy is also pharmacologically plausible. (s. p. 767)

11.11.3 Hydrothorax

Hepatic hydrothorax (= absence of a non-hepatic cause) has been detected in 4—10% of patients suffering from **liver cirrhosis**. Two thirds of the pleural effusions were isolated and localized on the right side, whereas the remaining one third were found on the left side or on both sides with equal frequency. Ascites is present in almost all cases, but is not obligate. (35, 41, 58, 67) Hydrothorax is usually caused by small diaphragmatic defects through which ascitic fluid can penetrate into the pleural cavity (41); diaphragmatic lymphatic vessels may also play a causal role. An ascites-related pleural effusion can be confirmed by intraperitoneal injection of methylene blue or ^{99m}Tc-sulphur colloid due to the subsequent, rapid migration of the substrate into the hydrothorax. *Bacterial infection*, similar to spontaneous bacterial peritonitis, is possible. • Hydrothorax is sometimes observed in **acute viral hepatitis**. The frequency is 0.16%. We have encountered a total of six cases. (s. pp 304, 305) (s. tab. 35.9) (s. fig. 16.8)

Therapy includes paracentesis + thoracocentesis + i.v. albumin solution, pleural drainage or pleurodesis with talc. Recently, pleurodesis using argon beam coagulation + minocycline hydrochloride has been recommended. In the case of refractory hepatic hydrothorax, TIPS or liver transplantation may be indicated. (58)

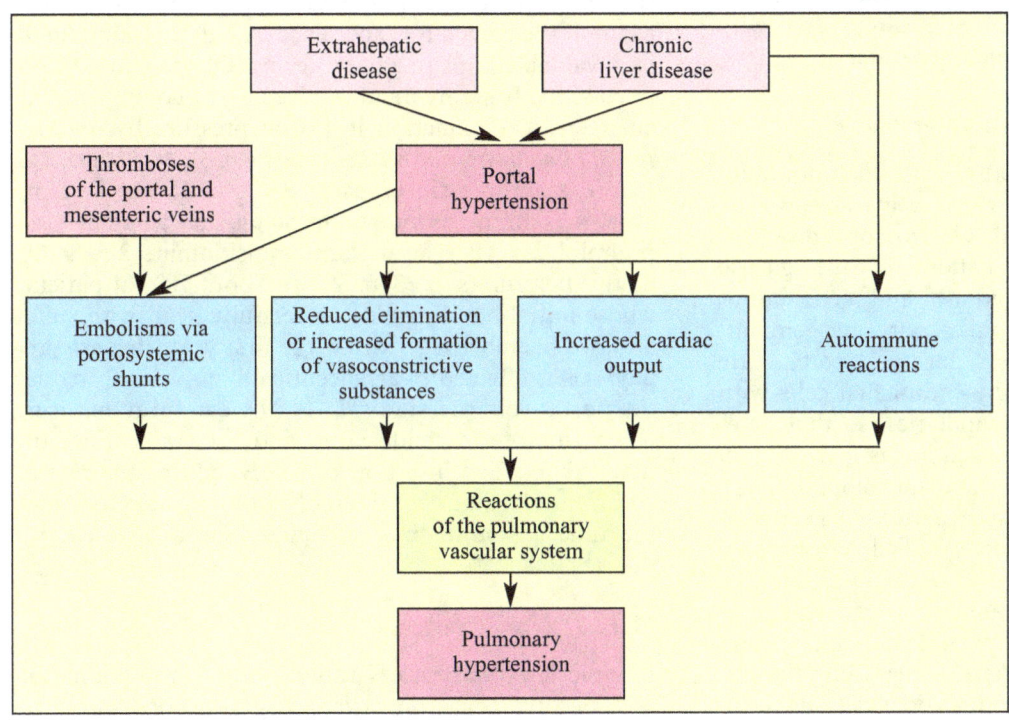

Fig. 35.18: Potential pathogenetic mechanisms associated with the coexistence of portal and pulmonary hypertension (based on B.J. ROBALINO et al., 1991 and M. WETTSTEIN et al., 1995)

> ▶ An evaluation of **25,682 clinical data sheets** from 1952−1963 (Dept. of Internal Medicine, University Hospital, Giessen) revealed the existence of pleural effusions (combination of "banal" effusion and hydrothorax) in 9.8% of cases (confirmed by X-ray imaging or autopsies). In **4.3%**, pleural effusion was found to be hepatogenous. • *Localization was bilateral in 69.0%, left-sided in 18.7%, and right-sided in 12.3% − a controversial result when compared with some statements made in the literature.* (s. p. 304 and footnote*))

11.12 Gastrointestinal bleeding

Acute upper or lower gastrointestinal bleeding is a common complication in liver cirrhosis and is often life-threatening. Several **bleeding sources** have to be taken into account, which may occur in combination in the individual case. *(see chapters 19.2−19.4!)*

1. Gastric antral vascular ectasia (GAVE)
2. Portal hypertensive gastroenteropathy
3. Oesophageal and/or fundus varices
4. Ectopic varices
5. Anorectal varices

Peptic ulcer is not cirrhosis-related. Duodenal ulcers are more common than gastric ulcers. Frequency of peptic ulceration in cirrhotic patients is 8−10%, but 60−70% of these cases are asymptomatic. Gastric ulcers heal more slowly and recur more frequently than in non-cirrhotic patients. This condition may be due to chronic alcohol abuse, portal hypertension or Helicobacter pylori infection (40−50%, with elevated gastrin in the serum). (128, 194) • **Mallory-Weiss syndrome** is often associated with cirrhosis, but there is in fact no causal relationship between the two. • **Gastroparesis** with delayed gastric emptying is sometimes observed. (179)

11.12.1 Portal hypertensive gastroenteropathy

Altered vascular microarchitecture with dilatation and/or narrowing of the capillaries and veins develops as a result of portal hypertension. Gastroscopy reveals a whitish-reticular, mosaic-like pattern of the gastric mucosa, containing limited reddish and oedematous areas. Frequently, there are pink spots and circumscribed red marks. In severe cases, dark pink patches are present. There are lesions of the endothelial cells with increased permeability of the capillaries, so that petechial or striated bleeding is observed in gastric (165) and/or intestinal mucosa (as well as in portal colopathy). (23, 150) These changes due to portal hypertensive gastropathy were previously (but incorrectly) called "erosive gastritis". They may cause gastric or intestinal paraesthesia or pain, but can also (less frequently) lead to occult bleeding or haematemesis. It is possible to achieve good results with the help of β-blockers. • Regarding the differential diagnosis, it is important to consider *angiodysplasia* (s. fig. 19.5) and *gastric antral vascular ectasia*. The latter resembles a watermelon with stripe-like haemorrhages. In the case of bleeding, endoscopic coagulation may be required. (45, 68, 124, 127, 134) (s. pp 357, 358) (s. tab. 19.4) (s. fig. 14.14)

11.12.2 Oesophagofundal varices

Acute bleeding must be anticipated in about 30% of patients with oesophagogastric varicosis and a pressure rise to >12 mm Hg. Physical overexertion can increase the portal vein pressure to dangerous levels. (20) Haemorrhaging mainly occurs in the lower third of the oesophagus and in the oesophagogastric transition zone, mostly due to venous anastomoses in the mucosa. Patients with small varices have a correspondingly lower bleeding risk. (s. figs. 14.8−14.10!) *(see chapter 19.3)* • There is a close association between **liver function** and relapse bleeding rate or mortality. Thus, all measures designed to improve **liver function** are beneficial, even though they are polypragmatic and perhaps of limited success. • **Primary prophylaxis** is indicated in patients with an increased bleeding risk (s. tab. 19.6); the portal vein pressure should be reduced by means of long-term pharmacological treatment. (73) In this context, the following drugs are recommended: propranolol (occasionally in combination with nitrate (62) or octreotide), nadolol (106), carvedilol (172), irbesartan (46), molsidomine and spironolactone. (s. p. 312) Primary prophylaxis using ligation (153) or sclerotherapy (119) ought to be started when small oesophageal varices are present. Primary shunt surgery is not indicated. • Mortality due to **initial bleeding** is 20−50%. The goal must be rapid and complete haemostasis. In principle, sclerotherapy and ligature are equally effective; the results depend upon the site of bleeding and the nature of the varices as well as upon the clinician's experience. A balloon tamponade is a valuable tool in guaranteeing the patient's transportability, bridging massive bleeding or coping with an emergency. A reduction in portal pressure by *previous (!) administration of medicaments* (20, 62, 76, 78, 109, 142, 153) (e. g. terlipressin bolus 1−2 mg and then 1−2 mg every 4−6 hr; octreotide bolus 50 µg, 25−50 µg/hr; propranolol 2 x 10−160 mg/day; molsidomine 2 x 8 mg/day) is helpful. (s. pp 366, 892) • About 70% of patients whose initial bleeding was successfully dealt with suffer another haemorrhage within the first year. **Relapse prophylaxis** is effected pharmaceutically in order to reduce the portal vein pressure (20, 109), by careful monitoring using (long-term) endoscopy and by eradicating any new varices. The insertion of **TIPS** reduces the rate of recurrent bleedings considerably and may help to bridge the time gap until **liver transplantation** can be carried out. (29, 148, 177)

11.12.3 Ectopic varices

Ectopic **intestinal varices** usually occur in combination with oesophagogastric varices. If gastroscopy shows no bleeding source, (rare) bleeding from ectopic intestinal varices should be suspected. Diagnosis is established by *scintigraphy* (accuracy is 90−95%). For more exact localization of bleeding detected by scintigraphy, *angiography* is subsequently used. In this context, CT angiography also provides much better diagnostic results. • This is also true of the (very rare) ectopic **peritoneal varices**, which can cause intra-abdominal haemorrhage. (s. pp 264, 265)

11.12.4 Anorectal varices

Anorectal varices originate from the **superior rectal vein**, which is connected to the portal vein system. This portacaval anastomosis drains the blood into the *iliac vein*. Occasionally, there is massive bleeding from rectal varices. Endoscopy is required for diagnosis and sclerotherapy. (74) (s. p. 264)

11.13 Febrile phases of disease

Patients suffering from cirrhosis often report fever episodes, similar to those observed in inpatients. Such episodes not only cause additional physical weakness and increase suffering, but also present a considerable **danger** for the patient. Among other things, fever causes (*1.*) catabolic metabolism, (*2.*) increased sympatheticotonia, (*3.*) disturbed water and salt balance (some 500 ml liquid and about 25 mmol salts are lost in 24 hours per degree of temperature rise!), and (*4.*) hypoxia of the hepatocytes. • This may lead to hepatic encephalopathy, portal ascites or hyperdynamic circulatory disturbance, with significant negative effects on renal function and hypoxia-induced metabolic liver insufficiency. The frequency of "cirrhosis-related fever" is 20%.

Cirrhosis patients often suffer from **bacterial infections**. (s. p. 754) The respiratory tract and urogenital system are mostly affected. Interleukin 6 may often increase in decompensated cirrhosis. Directed bacteriological diagnosis is required immediately; depending on the case, administration of antibiotics is recommended even before any evidence of bacteria has been obtained. (34)

Viral infection may likewise cause fever in cirrhosis. Even a mild viral infection can trigger viral hepatitis concomitant with underlying cirrhosis and produce a virotoxic effect with the risk of decompensation − in addition, the "fever" is in itself responsible for typical biochemical reactions in this condition.

Endotoxins are a further cause of fever episodes, particularly from gram-negative bacteria. The *spill-over effect* (*prehepatically* via portacaval anastomoses, the lymphatic system or mastocytes, and *intrahepatically* in RES insufficiency) leads to *endotoxinaemia*, which is responsible for numerous, even dangerous, biochemical reactions, e.g. hepatic encephalopathy and the activation of the coagulation cascade. • Long-term administration of *lactulose* can suppress a gram-negative intestinal flora and thus prevent the onset of endotoxaemia.

Protein degradation products may also trigger a febrile episode; aetiological differentiation of the fever caused by such metabolic products is usually impossible. There are no effective therapeutic measures. Differential diagnosis of "fever of unexplained origin" (R. G. PETERSDORF et al., 1961) can be very difficult in cirrhosis, a situation which presents an additional risk to the patient. • *In unexplained fever, laparoscopy is indicated.* (s. tab. 7.10)

> **Aetiocholanolone:** The degradation products of androgenous steroids are a further suspected cause of febrile episodes, since severe fever could be induced by i.m. injection of *aetiocholanolone* (3α-hydroxy-5β-H-androstane-17-on) (A. KAPPAS et al., 1957). In 1958 P. K. BONDY et al. for the first time detected an increase in aetiocholanolone in the plasma of patients with unexplained fever episodes, and thus they coined the term **aetiocholanolone fever**. Other steroids of the 5β-H configuration also revealed this pyrogenic feature. Aetiocholanolone may be the product of disturbed hepatocellular metabolism. Further observations and examinations have meanwhile been reported. (56, 130)

▶ *We detected markedly increased aetiocholanolone plasma values in numerous patients with liver cirrhosis and sudden febrile episodes* − but we could not show a direct correlation. • In 1966 F. SCHILLING reported that **aetiocholanolone fever** could be cured by *administration of indometacin. We were able to confirm this result (which had also been reported by* M. VLAHO et al. in 1976) *in those patients who had received indometacin as a suppository.* Indeed, we made use of this effect as differential therapy, but did not seek the underlying causes of a febrile episode unless the rectal administration of indometacin had been unsuccessful after one to three hours. Glucocorticoids, even when administered in a higher dosage, mostly proved ineffective, whereas a subsequent dose of indometacin caused the fever to subside within a very short time. While these may be *clinical observations*, they are remarkable enough to be reported. We suggest administering indometacin prior to any treatment with antibiotics. To our knowledge, renal insufficiency, as is known in cirrhosis (187), has not been observed following a single dose of indometacin.

11.14 Cholelithiasis

Cholelithiasis is found four to five times more often in patients with liver cirrhosis than in healthy persons. Follow-ups showed the development of cholelithiasis in 11.5% or 23.3% (−59%) of cases with women being mainly affected (♂ = 15−20%, ♀ 30−35%). In stages Child B and C, frequency is 35−45%. In more than 80% of cases, asymptomatic cholelithiasis is observed. (1, 7, 43, 48) Predominantly brownish-black bilirubin concrements (= calcium bilirubinate) are detectable. (s. figs. 35.19, 35.20) The duration and degree of severity of cirrhosis as well as prior alcohol abuse are important risk factors. Cholelithiasis has no influence on survival in cirrhosis. Surgical intervention poses a high risk and is therefore only indicated in life-threatening situations. • The cause is believed to be reduced contractility of the gall bladder in cirrhosis with disturbed emptying. (This can be checked with ^{99m}Tc-mebrofenin.) Hypersplenism, which is responsible for increased haemolysis and a reduction in UPD glucuronyltransferase activity in the liver, is assumed to be a further cause of this close association between cirrhosis and cholelithiasis. Hepatic secretion of unconjugated bilirubin is twice as high as normal and bile acid concentration is reduced, whereas the bile itself is oversaturated with cholesterol.*)

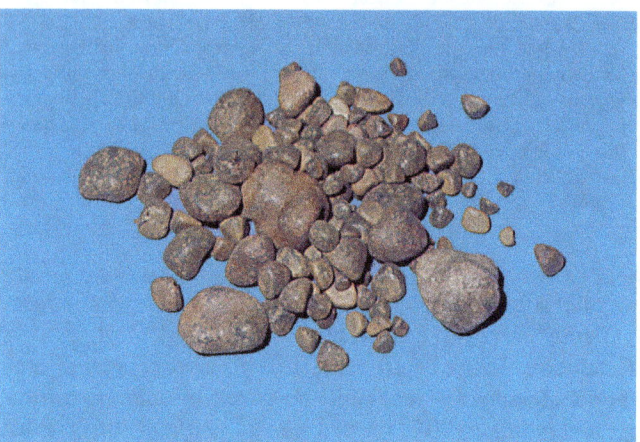

Fig. 35.19: Cholelithiasis in liver cirrhosis: pigment calculi

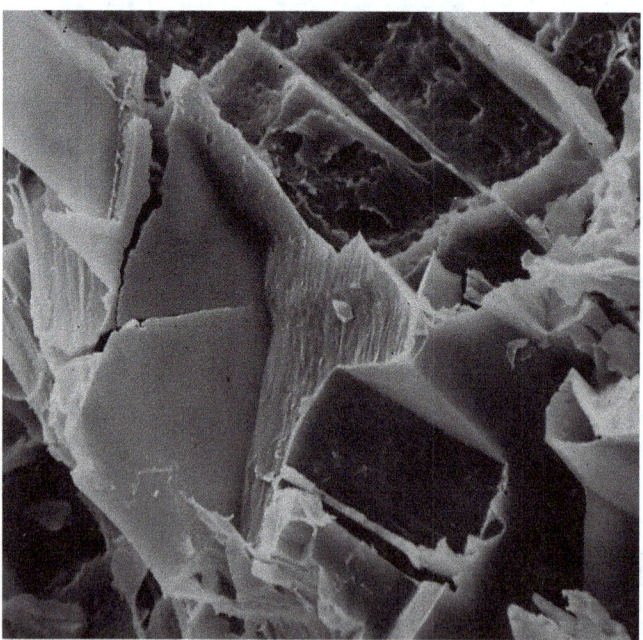

Fig. 35.20: Pigment calculus in liver cirrhosis, grid microscopy displaying characteristic plate-like bilirubin bodies

---

*) *Kuntz, E.:* Erkrankungen der Gallenblase und Gallenwege. (Diseases of the gall bladder and biliary tract) J.F. Lehmanns Verlag München, 1974. 344 pages, 126 figures.

11.15 Hepatocardiovascular syndrome

Apart from lung and kidney, heart and circulation are often involved, either primarily or secondarily, in liver diseases; this applies especially to cirrhosis.

Hyperdynamic circulation has a close correlation to portal hypertension, which results in (*1.*) reduction in vascular resistance and (*2.*) vasodilation of the splanchnic arteries and arterioles with increased blood volume in the vascular system. This leads to underfilling of the heart and reduction of the arteriovenous oxygen difference. The consequences are adaptive tachycardia, increased cardiac output and arterial hypotension. As a result of such a hyperdynamic circulation, there is a decrease in the *effective blood volume* (= central and peripheral blood volume in the cardiac ventricles, lungs and main arteries). The splanchnic hypervolaemia, in turn, increases the portal hypertension. The relative hypervolaemia in the arterial system and the hypotension cause a compensatory activation of the RAAS and the sympathetic nervous system. This is followed by an increase in the intrahepatic vascular resistance with continuous deterioration of the haemodynamics. This vicious circle finally leads to an enlargement of the collateral vessels with development of varices as well as to ascites and the hepatorenal syndrome.

Pathogenesis of vasodilation is multifactorial. The systemic or local vasodilators include: NO, glucagon, substance P, VIP, TNF, calcium-gene-related peptide, prostacyclin, etc. (14, 21, 36)

Clinical findings comprise: resting tachycardia and hypotension with large amplitude; dry and warm skin; flushed extremities, bounding pulses and capillary pulsations in the fingers; occasionally, an ejection systolic murmur is audible; QT time is often prolonged in correlation to the severity of cirrhosis. (171) • These cardiovascular findings are usually not a cause of heart insufficiency. After liver transplantation, there is complete regression. • Beta-blockers are recommended as therapy.

Cirrhotic cardiomyopathy: This term is defined as a left ventricular functional disorder due to stress (e. g. hyperdynamic circulation) or as pharmacological stimulation. But also the possibility of (toxically induced?) subclinical myocardial damage is discussed, especially because elevated troponin 1 serum values are detectable in every third patient. (4, 84, 135, 176) (Troponin is connected with propomyosin in the actin filaments at regular intervals and, as a "relaxing protein", has an important function in muscle metabolism, also in the heart).

Pericardial effusion: In ascites, there is often (50–60%) a generally small pericardial effusion, which can be recognized reliably with the help of echocardiography.

11.16 Hepatocellular carcinoma

HCC is the fourth most common tumour worldwide. In 68–89% of patients with HCC, cirrhosis was also detected, i.e. about six times more often than in non-cirrhotic patients. The incidence of HCC in cirrhosis is between 4% and 55% (2−5% per year), depending on (*1.*) aetiology of cirrhosis, (*2.*) type of cirrhosis, and (*3.*) observation period. Men are affected about eight times more often than women. (53, 95, 170) *(see chapter 37.3)*

Aetiology of cirrhosis: Cirrhosis due to hepatitis B, C and D as well as haemochromatosis, alcohol, NASH and α_1-antitrypsin deficiency increases the risk of developing HCC considerably; there is a less obvious association with primary and secondary cholangitis or with autoimmune hepatitis. (136, 168)

Type of cirrhosis: Macronodular cirrhosis (which is usually a posthepatitic form of cirrhosis) is the type most often associated with HCC (about 55% of cases). Compared to micronodular cirrhosis (usually alcohol-induced), development of HCC must be anticipated in 5−10% of patients. In this context, the actual presence of coarse-nodular cirrhosis seems to pose a greater risk of HCC than the aetiology of the underlying cirrhosis. • The adenomatous and hyperplastic transformations frequently found in cirrhosis tend to develop into HCC.

Observation period: The time lapse between the onset of cirrhosis and that of HCC is unpredictable. Small cancerous foci may be observed at a early stage of cirrhosis, which can only be demonstrated by SPECT in vivo. Clinically recognizable HCC is reported to take about four years on average to develop into HBV-induced cirrhosis (H. OBATA et al., 1980) and about eight years into alcoholic cirrhosis (C. M. LEEVY et al., 1964).

Diagnosis: Long-term monitoring of a cirrhotic patient is achieved by determination of α_1-**foetoprotein** (s. p. 112). As soon as the initial value has been established, follow-ups are carried out at long intervals (usually every six to twelve months if the values are normal) and at short intervals if the values are elevated. However, sensitivity is only about 60%, so that a normal value does not necessarily exclude HCC. Specificity is 75−90%. Despite unsatisfactory sensitivity, AFP determination is still useful for monitoring the development of "still normal" or "already moderately elevated" values. • The simultaneous determination of **des-gamma-carboxy prothrombin** (DCP) (sensitivity 50−60%, specificity 80−100%) can improve diagnostic value or assessment of the course. (s. p. 748) • **Sonography** serves as a tool in monitoring cirrhosis simultaneously, yet it should be noted that the sonographic differentiation of small-sized malignant foci is quite difficult in the cirrhotic liver. Sensitivity is 70−80% and specificity 90−95%. Follow-ups are recommended at six- to nine-month intervals. Regular monitoring at short intervals with the help of AFP determination and sonography is recommended in macronodular cirrhosis or in the presence of HCC risk factors. (94) • Suspected development of HCC is an indication for contrast-medium (= lipiodol) **computer tomography** (or spiral CT) in order to guarantee a relatively early diagnosis. (s. fig. 37.6) **MRI** (or spiral CT) has been used to distinguish between adenomatous hyperplastic nodes and HCC in cirrhosis. (82, 101, 186) • Cytologic confirmation of HCC can be substantiated by US/CT-guided **fine-needle biopsy**; this is especially true for intrahepatic foci. • In view of the bleeding risk, we would discourage clinicians from resorting to percutaneous biopsy and consider using **laparoscopy** instead. (s. figs. 37.1, 37.7, 37.8) The primary use of laparoscopy as a morphological tool (subsequent to imaging diagnostics) has the following *advantages*: (*1.*) inspection of the total liver surface facilitates a more reliable detection of foci, (*2.*) practically any superficial focus can be accessed by forceps biopsy, (*3.*) use of Robber's forceps is far less dangerous than any needle biopsy of the liver, (*4.*) explorative laparoscopy provides the required staging result, and (*5.*) any kind of "blind" percutaneous biopsy is more dangerous than forceps biopsy, which is carried out under visual control with the possibility of monitoring potential rebleeding and applying respective coagulative measures. *(see chapter 37.3)*

12 Prognosis

The prognosis for cirrhosis patients depends upon the respective complications. The underlying morphological processes, such as necrosis, fibrosis and regeneration, combine to widely differing degrees in the single cirrhotic patient. There are also individual divergencies in haemodynamic responses and the corresponding effects on the kidneys, lungs and liver, etc. Thus it is very difficult to give an accurate prognosis in each case. Furthermore, such a prognosis only covers a relatively short period of time (a few months up to a year). (2, 51, 81, 133, 137, 149, 166, 192, 193)

Various indices have been developed using weighted parameters to calculate the probability of fatality or survival in each case. **Classification** of cirrhosis according to the *criteria* devised by CHILD and TURCOTTE (1964) and the *modification* established by PUGH (1973) has been widely accepted. Our experience shows that the additional use of the *GEC test* and the *ICG test* makes the classification more reliable, particularly in stages A (= score 5−7) and B (= score 8−10). (s. tab. 35.7)

The prognosis of cirrhosis caused by toxins (alcohol or medicament abuse, chemical agents, iron storage, etc.) is much improved by *eliminating the causal noxa*. Recognition and treatment of *secondary immunoreactions*, which may occur concomitantly, are also important. Such reactions reduce the prognostically favourable effect of abstention (e. g. alcohol, pharmacons) if they are not adequately treated with corresponding drugs.

In compensated cirrhosis, the ten-year survival rate is 45−50%. Long-term compensation (for many years) can only be maintained in 40–45% of cases. Of the compensated patients, severe complications develop in 55–60% and decompensation occurs in 45–50% of cases. The mean survival rate for compensated cirrhosis is 8.9 years, for decompensated cirrhosis 1.6 years only. (133, 137, 166)

Complications such as variceal bleeding, hepatic encephalopathy, ascites, infections and reduced renal function also influence the **mortality rate** of liver cirrhosis (in Germany some 25,000/year). The main causes of death are hepatic coma or liver failure (25–40%), bleeding (20–30%), infections (about 10%) and HCC (about 5%). Spontaneous bacterial peritonitis is fatal in 50–70%, and with liver dysfunction in 90% of cases. Occurrence of the hepatorenal syndrome is almost invariably fatal.

> Prognosis of liver cirrhosis depends upon preventing complications as far as possible. • At the same time, all options should be used to stabilize compensation and improve liver function.

13 Therapy

In principle, **six treatment forms** can be implemented to combat the complex pathological events in liver cirrhosis, which may be extremely variable due to numerous complications. These are: (*1.*) causal treatment, (*2.*) treatment of pathogenetic primary reactions, (*3.*) treatment to prevent progression of cirrhosis, (*4.*) treatment of symptoms, (*5.*) treatment of complications, and (*6.*) liver transplantation.

13.1 Causal treatment

Once alcohol-induced cirrhosis has been detected, absolute **alcohol abstention** is essential. This abstention also includes the concealed amounts of alcohol in drinks and foodstuffs or in pharmaceuticals and tonics as well as the use of after-shave products, which may contain a high volume percentage of alcohol. Even fruit juices contain a certain amount of alcohol due to fermentation in the bottle. And so-called alcohol-free beer is in fact a beverage with a low alcohol content. Apart from that, intestinal fermentation caused by certain fungi may result in the production of considerable amounts of alcohol. All these factors can come together to produce "alarming" quantities of alcohol in the body and may even lead to a situation where a phase of abstinence is followed by renewed addiction. Women in general and patients with cirrhosis who have undergone gastric resection are mainly at risk with regard to this complex problem. All too often, these factors are underrated or go largely unnoticed as far as their cumulative effect is concerned. Beware of *cliché-ridden expressions* designed to trivialize the matter such as a "sip of wine", a "sip of beer" or a "nip of brandy" — this form of self-deception is simply not acceptable. (s. pp 64, 534–537)

Likewise, in cirrhosis due to medicaments or toxins, causal treatment entails elimination of the underlying **noxa(e)** (pharmaceuticals, chemicals, drugs) and a simultaneous "ban" on alcohol. Alcohol has an additive and sometimes intensifying effect as a noxa. • In a particular course and stage of cirrhosis due to viral hepatitis B or C, treatment with **interferon** may (still) be used as causal therapy. Hereby, the frequency of decompensation in HCV cirrhosis or of HCV-induced carcinoma could be lowered, although not significantly.

13.2 Treatment of pathogenic reactions

Treating pathogenic primary reactions does not cure the underlying cause of cirrhosis, but is an effective intervention in its pathogenesis. Continuous therapy may result in reduced inflammatory or immunological activity and decreased fibrogenesis despite the (regrettable) development of cirrhosis; thus it can create a tendency towards stabilization or inactivation of the overall process: e.g. *iron depletion* in haemochromatosis, *removal of copper* in Wilson's disease, *protection against ultraviolet light* in certain forms of porphyria cirrhosis, *immunosuppression* in autoimmune cirrhosis, and reduction in *portal hypertension* by medication.

13.3 Treatment of progression

The above-mentioned measures do not combat the cause(s) or eliminate the primary pathogenetic reactions (with a few exceptions). The general aim is to prevent progression of the disease, ideally until the cirrhosis comes to a halt. When such medication is administered effectively, complicative developments can also be prevented. Pathogenetic primary reactions often initiate a cascade of secondary mechanisms, in particular of a biochemical nature. This is true of the inhibition of concomitant cholestasis during the course of cirrhosis by *ursodeoxycholic acid* (97), the reduction in lipid peroxidation by *silymarin*, the inhibition of fibrogenesis by *colchicine* or *silymarin* (sometimes with improved quality of life), and the elimination of hyperammonaemia by *ornithine aspartate*. (138) (s. p. 287)

> Fundamentally, "treatment" of cirrhosis should begin during its chronic precursory stages, i.e. *chronic hepatitis* or *chronic cholangitis*. A chronic disease confirmed by detailed diagnostics usually still responds to effective treatment measures, which are, however, of no help once the cirrhotic stage has been reached.

13.4 Symptomatic treatment

From the subjective point of view concerning the pathological events, it is usually those symptoms which impair the state of health and lifestyle that are the most obvious. The patients "feel" tired, worn out, lack concentration, are unenthusiastic and unmotivated; they are inappetent and show muscular weakness; occasionally they suffer from pruritus; they "feel ill" or even "chronically poisoned" (as we were often told by such patients who used these words). Above all, the patient seeks advice and help, even polypragmatic help, in view of the often widely varying symptomatology.

▶ When liver cirrhosis has already been confirmed by detailed diagnosis and its (possible) secondary reactions or complicative developments have been determined (this is the *primary prerequisite* of "the physician"), it is possible to apply symptomatic treatment measures in a more effective and more targeted and thus more efficient way (which is what "the patient" *principally expects*). • In most cases, this forms a basis of mutual trust as it generally guarantees the patient's readiness to cooperate with regard to strict directions, certain treatment and follow-up measures as well as invasive therapy.

13.4.1 Nutrition

The question *"What can I eat?"* is nearly always of prime importance and it implicitly includes the basic idea of what the cirrhotic patient should avoid or what diet to give preference to. First of all, it should be clear that there is no such thing as a special **liver diet** designed to have instant curative effects on liver disease (despite the fact that many such diets have been extolled). • The diet of a cirrhotic patient is based on the principles of *nutritional physiology*, the *aetiology* of the cirrhosis, the patient's *body weight* and *age* as well as on any *complications*. (111) (s. pp 550, 878)

The calorie content of the diet should be adapted to the current body weight. As a rule, the percentage ratio between **calories** derived from carbohydrates, protein and lipids is considered well-balanced at 40:20:40 or 50:20:30, with a minimum of 2,000 calories per day. The recommended **protein** intake is about 0.8−1.2 (−1.5) g/kg BW; when there is a tendency towards encephalopathy, the protein content needs to be reduced accordingly, with an intake of mainly lactovegetative proteins. (s. p. 286) In catabolism or muscular atrophy, the protein intake must be increased to more than 100 g/day and/or **branched-chain amino acids** (37, 69, 80, 102, 105, 115, 143, 167, 188) or formula diets are recommended. The nitrogen balance must be in equilibrium. (87, 110) The daily intake of food should always be spread over **five meals** (i.e. three main meals and two snacks, as with diabetic patients): this makes digestion easier, and the catabolic phases become shorter. With regard to energy, a cirrhosis patient is basically in a condition of fasting. **Salt intake** should not exceed 7−8 g/day; as soon as signs of water retention in the tissue appear (s. fig. 16.2), salt consumption should be reduced further. (s. p. 311) • In addition, disease-induced **maldigestion/malabsorption** (e.g. deficiency of pancreatic enzymes or bile salts, portal hypertensive enteropathy) is responsible for a lack of essential nutritional components (often latent for a long time). In older people, reduced absorption of fat-soluble vitamins (173, 174) and arachidonic acid (125) (among other things) is also to be expected. However, one should not wait for a vitamin deficiency to arise; besides, biochemical evidence of reduced vitamin values is costly and unreliable. Daily intake of *multivitamin tablets* (as a dietary supplement) should thus be considered for obvious reasons. This is also true of a complementary supply of *electrolytes, zinc* (103, 185) and *selenium*. (30) • If steatorrhoea is observed, *MCT* (about 3 × 15 ml/day, equivalent to some 400 kcal) are given, possibly coupled with the administration of *"essential" phospholipids* to achieve the best results. (31)

> I have been told that **raw goat's milk** (2 × 0.25 l/day, stored in the refrigerator) is used "successfully" to treat liver cirrhosis in some regions. **Ubiquinone** (?) is thought to be the active substance − this agent is also said to have prevented the occurrence of cirrhosis in animal experiments.

Malnutrition, which is observed in 60−80% of cirrhotic patients, may be so severe that **parenteral nutrition** is called for. (32, 111) Glucose infusions as a main source of energy (6−10 g/kg BW/day), amino-acid solutions (1.0−1.5 g/kg BW/day) and lipid infusions (0.3 g/kg BW/day) can be used to guarantee a supply of about 2,270−3,000 kcal. • Parenteral nutrition should guarantee an adequate supply of *vitamins, electrolytes, zinc* and *choline* as well as *albumin*. (27) In encephalopathy, preference is usually given to *branched-chain amino acids* instead of total amino-acid solutions. Administration of *insulin* may be necessary in impaired glucose tolerance. • In pronounced catabolism, the nitrogen balance can be considerably improved by administering recombinant growth hormones. • *Laevulose, xylitol or sorbitol should not be administered as they are not sufficiently transformed into glucose in the cirrhotic liver, with the result that lactate acidosis and hypoglycaemia occur due to the increased formation of lactate. In addition, these substances lead to a further reduction in energy-rich phosphates, which are generally already decreased.*

13.4.2 Physical activity

Appropriate **physical activity** (with anabolic effects) is recommended for cirrhotic patients in order to prevent muscular atrophy and hepatic osteopathy. We had positive experience with a *muscle-training programme* carried out two (or even three) times a day. Almost 60% of the musculature is activated in this way − irrespective of age or weather conditions and without the need for particular clothing or equipment. (s. pp 551, 683, 755) • Swimming or water gymnastics are recommended activities, if possible. Physical overexertion must be avoided. (20, 61, 145) This also applies to the use of home-training equipment. An unfavourable rise in HVPG due to increased physical exercise can be prevented by propranolol. (20) • We recommend a **horizontal position** for about an hour after each of the three main meals. The positive effects of a recumbent position on numerous biochemical parameters, particularly in disturbed water and salt balance, remain undisputed – and are just as obvious as the negative effects of a long-term upright posture. (145) The latter may even trigger complications when there is simultaneous emotional (sympatheticotonic) excitement (e. g. when watching sports events!). • Vocational **rehabilitation** is the ultimate aim and the patient ought to be given tasks based on physical aptitude. If the physician agrees, patients should continue in their current profession. *The diagnosis "liver cirrhosis" does not automatically mean incapacity for work or vocational disability!* • Utmost care should be taken by the patient in keeping personal **records** (documentation sheet) in order to detect latent HE or latent water retention, which points to a commencement of decompensation. (s. fig. 15.3) (s. pp 283, 311)

13.4.3 Psychological guidance

▶ *Detailed and confirmed diagnosis* enables the physician to offer reliable guidance, which gives the patient the necessary confidence in the former's proficiency and experience. This is the first important *prerequisite* regarding active medical care. • The patients, who have various subjective complaints and are usually weakened by malnutrition, besides being severely restricted in their everyday lives, are mainly seeking *tangible help* to ease their own subjective suffering. The patient has more trust and readiness to cooperate if the physician shows understanding for these subjective complaints, takes them seriously and treats them (even if the treatment measures are gradual or polypragmatic). This is the second important *prerequisite* regarding active medical care. • Usually, it is the patient's desire to be informed in a comprehensible manner about the respective disease. The physician's patience and readiness with respect to *elucidation*, i.e. explaining the disease itself and the cirrhosis-related circumstances in an understandable manner, or even suggesting that a *second opinion* should be obtained from another hepatologist, reassure the patients that they are in the hands of a competent specialist. This is the third important *prerequisite* regarding active medical care.

Understandably, there are always questions concerning **prognosis**. *Cirrhoses come in many different shapes and sizes!* The individual *aetiology* of cirrhosis – more than thirty different causes are known (s. tab. 35.2) – initially determines the prognosis. This is all the more essential since certain forms respond well to treatment. In addition, prognosis is influenced by maintaining *compensation*, which, in turn, is supported by an *appropriate lifestyle*. The patient is fully aware of the fact that any kind of *active participation* is worthwhile, that even phases of decompensation can be overcome and that any early detection of such phases and complications offers the best chance of stabilization, provided that treatment commences as early as possible. The patient experiences how *aetiology* of the cirrhosis, personal *cooperation* and early detection of *complications* form an important **triad**, and that consequently the prognosis of liver cirrhosis need not be as poor as is generally assumed. • *We treated numerous cirrhotic patients over a long period, a large number of whom we accompanied for 10–15 years despite some interspersed "acute-on-chronic" events.*

Even an **infaust prognosis** should not be withheld from the patient, particularly in those cases where specific questions are asked about the true situation. In these conversations, the physician, who is naturally deeply involved, should explain the situation step by step, revealing one unfavourable fact after the other. In this way, all medical and nursing measures can be discussed frankly. The patients also need time to settle their personal and family affairs and to have a chance for contemplation as well as for finding spiritual support.

> A joint approach and communal experience concerning cirrhosis require the physician to show empathy and persuasion while discerning the degree to which the patient is able to grasp and understand the medical facts and findings intellectually and emotionally. Time and again, the three prerequisites described above have proved to be mainstays in the relationship between physician and patient.

13.4.4 Drug therapy

▶ A review of the past 60 years (since 1955), during which time we have experienced numerous developments in hepatology, shows that an unimaginable and fascinating spectrum of treatment options has been established. • This is true especially of the *treatment of pathogenetic primary reactions*, some examples of which have been outlined in the individual chapters describing the corresponding diseases. The same applies to the pharmacological treatment of *progressive tendencies* typical of cirrhosis, e. g. cholestasis, fibrosis, hyperammonaemia, electrolyte imbalance, lipid peroxidation.

> Dealing with complications is not what we consider to be the most important aspect of treating cirrhosis. A primary objective should be to carry out prophylactic measures for preventing such complications in the first place, insofar as this is possible.

As we have shown in the case of **encephalopathy** and **ascites** – *the two earliest and thus most common decompensation syndromes* – successful **prophylaxis** for about one year is less of a financial burden than (just) one week of inpatient treatment after manifestation. Even more important is the absolute danger to the patient inherent in a progressive course. • *Prevention of complications is always better and cheaper — for all parties involved!*

The use of the following substances has proved suitable in terms of pharmacological plausibility and clinical results, provided there are no particular circumstances, forms of treatment, intolerance or individual imponderables to contraindicate their application.

Step 1: (*1.*) *lactulose* (2–3 stools/day) and (*2.*) *spironolactone* (50 mg per day or every second day). This therapy is practically free of side effects — even during long-term administration. (s. pp 287, 312, 887)

Step 2: Additional administration of (*3.*) *ornithine aspartate* (1–3 x 6 g/day). This may be indicated by the detection of latent HE (stages 0, 0–I). Usually, the administration of (*4.*) *zinc* (15–30 mg/day) is also indicated in this context. (s. pp 287, 885, 890)

Step 3: Reduction in portal pressure (46, 78, 109) and prevention of variceal bleeding are important measures as part of a primary prophylaxis. In our experience, the development of pulmonary hypertension can be delayed (or even prevented). This might be achieved, for example, by administering (*5.*) *molsidomine* and (*6.*) *beta blockers* (in combination with spironolactone as in Step 1). The frequent occurrence of portal colopathy (30–40%), even with colitis-like abnormalities, can be reduced by propanolol. (23, 150) • A combination of isosorbide-5-mononitrate with nadolol has been successful in cases where treatment with beta blockers alone did not prove effective. (s. pp, 267, 366)

Fat-soluble vitamins: Oral intake of vitamins A, D and E is usually sufficient — as is the dosage contained in multivitamin preparations when taken daily. Biochemical evidence of deficiency or the occurrence of diseases due to deficiency usually require vitamins *A, D, E* and *K* to be supplied parenterally as a compound preparation.

Silymarin: At present, there is no unequivocal confirmation of the positive effects of silymarin as a cytoprotective agent against various noxae; in particular, the scavenger effects attributed to this substance and its alleged regenerative properties have not been confirmed in cirrhosis. (s. p. 895)

Phosphatidylcholine: As is the case with silymarin, there is a vast amount of information in the literature about this substance. Animal experiments have shown that the development of septal fibroses and the occurrence of cirrhosis could be prevented despite chronic alcohol consumption. The studies available to date on cirrhotic patients provide insufficient information. (s. p. 894)

Colchicine: Inhibition of progressive fibrosis in cirrhotic patients with a markedly improved survival time was reported (dosage: 1 mg/day, 5 days/week). However, this was not confirmed in a later study. We have no information about potential side effects, particularly during long-term treatment (which is usually desirable in cirrhosis therapy). (s. p. 897) • The use of **proline-4-hydroxylase** results in the significant inhibition of collagen synthesis in animal experiments. No clinical data are available to date.

Coagulation parameters: Detection of pathological laboratory values is not an indication for substitution. Such measures are unnecessary before clinical manifestations are observed. Propranolol ameliorates thrombopenia. (142) (s. pp 352, 353)

Liver cirrhosis is the final stage of disease of the largest metabolic organ, with diverse functionally, biochemically and morphologically related complications. Decompensation mechanisms should therefore be avoided with the help of targeted treatment. The aim is to maintain the stage of compensation for as long as possible and to recognize complications at their onset. • *The costly and complex treatment strategies for dealing with cirrhotic complications, often involving intensive care, are described in the respective chapters.*

13.5 Monitoring

Regular monitoring is essential and should always be carried out in a targeted and economical way. The basic parameters used in the follow-up should be limited to obtaining really informative results!

▶ In the course of some 40 years, we have accompanied cirrhotic patients for considerable periods of their lives, many for more than 10 years, some even for more than 15 years. This often resulted in experiences that modified and ultimately standardized our follow-up programme. • Basic control parameters, i.e. parameters important in all forms of cirrhosis, are supplemented by more informative investigations (such as iron, copper or phosphatase values) in cases with a particular aetiology.

Such a **standard programme**, *which nevertheless leaves room for individual concepts, has proved successful over many years.* (s. tab. 35.10)

1. Interim anamnesis: Important events during a certain period of time have to be noted in a concise manner — otherwise the abbreviation n.a.d. (= no abnormality detected) is sufficient.

2. Therapeutic status: The name and dosage of the pharmacons used in the meantime; the name and date of any medicine discontinued or newly prescribed; side effects and intolerances observed, if any. All relevant details concerning the remedies are recorded, which facilitates interim repeat prescriptions.

1. Interim anamnesis:	....	
2. Therapeutic status:	....	
3. Clinical findings:	....	
4. Documentation sheet:	....	

5. Laboratory parameters		
GPT	γ-GT	every (2–)4 weeks
Na	P	every (2–)4 weeks
ChE	Quick	every (4–)8 weeks
Electrophoresis		every (3–)6 months

6. Particular values:	....
	....
	....

Doctor's orders:	....
	....
	....

Tab. 35.10: Standardized (uniform and easy-to-document) evaluation programme for the long-term follow-up of compensated cirrhotics. (Time intervals in accordance with the current situation, particular values in accordance with the given cirrhosis aetiology)

3. Clinical findings: Relevant changes in findings are recorded tersely; unchanged status is noted with the abbreviation n.c. (= no changes).

4. Documentation sheet: Presentation of the documentation sheet by the patient containing details of body weight and handwriting specimens during the respective follow-up phase. This form (which can easily be drawn up by the patient) may contain, on the front and back, daily entries for two follow-up months. This patient-own documentation is the *cheapest and most reliable follow-up method* with regard to early detection of the two most sensitive signs of decompensation: latent HE and latent ascites. (s. fig. 15.3) (s. pp 283, 311)

5. Laboratory parameters: These are of *secondary importance* in the long-term follow-up of compensated liver cirrhosis. *GPT* is sufficient for evaluating enzymatic activity, while *γ-GT* is suitable for initial detection of concomitant cholestasis or toxic components (in some cases, there are also hints of malignancy or even regeneration). Depending on the individual situation, these two values have to be checked at intervals of (2–)4 weeks. In order to monitor liver function, *cholinesterase* and *Quick's value* are determined at intervals of (4–)8 weeks, while *electrophoresis* (for evaluating mesenchymal activity and albumin synthesis) is conducted every (3–)6 months. • Control of *sodium* (Na) and *potassium* (P) is carried out according to the individual situation. However, these two electrolytes are nearly always within the normal range if the findings in the above mentioned documentation sheet referring to latent HE or latent oedema are also normal – a fact which can be explained in terms of pathophysiology. • With specific forms of cirrhosis, one or two *additional parameters* of particular significance are applied.

The aim is to maintain the **stage of compensation** in an undisturbed state for as long as possible, to use all possible measures to prevent negative effects, and to detect and treat the onset of any decompensation mechanisms as early as possible. This is essential and decisive both for prognosis and for structuring a worthwhile daily life. • The requirements of *quality management* are met by adhering to a standardized **follow-up programme**, which can be documented. • This well-established overall concept has also been successful in reducing the expense involved. The **costs** of caring for one cirrhotic patient have been calculated at more than 13,000 US dollars per year (T. Szucs et al., 1997).

13.6 Liver transplantation

All patients with end-stage cirrhosis should be considered for liver transplantation in good time. Selection initially requires a thorough and critical evaluation of the indication with regard to the patient's general physical and mental condition. The **risk factors**, which have to be assessed in advance, include: (*1.*) cardiac, pulmonary and renal function, (*2.*) coagulation system, (*3.*) albumin value, (*4.*) obesity, (*5.*) prior complex hepatobiliary surgery, (*6.*) portal vein thrombosis, (*7.*) autoimmune disease, (*8.*) viral infection, (*9.*) coexisting diseases, (*10.*) problems relating to addiction, (*11.*) unfavourable familial and social environment, and (*12.*) individual unwillingness to cooperate. • These twelve evaluation criteria provide an initial overview of the extent of the risk factors which can be identified in advance and which are of significance for the patient's registration at a transplantation centre. • For many patients in a life-threatening situation, liver transplantation remains the only chance of survival.

References:

1. **Acalovschi, M., Badea, R., Pascu, M.:** Incidence of gallstones in liver cirrhosis. Amer. J. Gastroenterol. 1991; 86: 1179–1181
2. **Adler, M., Verset, D., Bouhdid, H., Bourgeois, N., Gulbis, B., Moine, O. le Stadt, J., van de Gelin, M., Thiry, P.:** Prognostic evaluation of patients with parenchymal cirrhosis. J. Hepatol. 1997; 26: 642–649
3. **Agusti, A.G.N., Roca, J., Bosch, J., Rodriguez-Roisin:** The lung in patients with cirrhosis. J. Hepatol. 1990; 10: 251–257
4. **Al Hamoudi, W., Lee, S.S.:** Cirrhotic cardiomyopathy. (review). Ann. Hepatol. 2006, 5: 132–139
5. **Al Sarela, Mihaimeed, F.M.A., Batten, J.J., Davidson, B.R., Mathie, R.T.:** Hepatic and splanchnic nitric oxide activity in patients with cirrhosis. Gut 1999, 44: 749–753
6. **Aller, R., Moya, J.L., Moreira, V., Boixeda, D., Picher, J., Garcia-Rull, S., de Luis, D.A.:** Etiology and frequency of gas exchange abnormalities in cirrhosis. Rev. Esp. Enf. Digest. 1999; 91: 564–568
7. **Alvaro, D., Angelico, M., Gandin, C., Corradini, S.G., Capocaccia, L.:** Physico-chemical factors predisposing to pigment gallstone formation in liver cirrhosis. J. Hepatol. 1990; 10: 228–234
8. **Amitrano, L., Guardascione, M.A., Brancaccio, V., Margaglione, M., Manguso, F., Iannaccone, L., Grandone, E., Balzano, A.:** Risk factors

and clinical presentation of portal vein thrombosis in patients with liver cirrhosis. J. Hepatol. 2004; 40: 736–741
9. **Amodio, P., del Piccolo, F., Marchetti, P., Angeli, P., Iemmolo, R., Caregaro, L., Merkel, O., Gerunda, G., Gatta, A.:** Clinical features and survival of cirrhotic patients with subclinical cognitive alterations detected by the number connection test and computerized psychometric tests. Hepatology 1999; 29: 1662–1667
10. **Angeli, P., Albino, G., Carraro, P., dalla Pria, M., Merkel, C., Caregaro, L., de Bei, E., Bortoluzzi, A., Plebani, M., Gatta, A.:** Cirrhosis and muscle cramps: evidence of a causal relationship. Hepatology 1996; 23: 264–273
11. **Angeli, P., Wong, F., Watson, H., Gines, P.:** Hyponatremia in cirrhosis: Results of a patient population survey. Hepatology 2000; 44: 1535–1542
12. **Anthony, P.P., Ishak, K.G., Nayak, N.C., Poulsen, H.E., Scheuer, P.J., Sobin, L.H.:** The morphology of cirrhosis: definition, nomenclature and classification. Bull. WHO 1977; 55: 521–524
13. **Arguedas, M.R., DeLawrence, T.G., McGuire, B.M.:** Influence of hepatic encephalopathy on health-related quality of life in patients with cirrhosis. Dig. Dis. Sci. 2003; 48: 1622–1626
14. **Arkenau, H.-T., Stichtenoth, D.O., Fröhlich, J.C., Manns, M.P., Böker, K.-H.W.:** Elevated nitric oxide levels in patients with chronic liver disease and cirrhosis correlate with disease stage and parameters of hyperdynamic circulation. Z. Gastroenterol. 2002; 40: 907–912
15. **Asbert, M., Gines, A., Gines, P., Jimenez, W., Claria, J., Salo, J., Arroyo, V., Rivera, F., Rodes, J.:** Circulating levels of endothelin in cirrhosis. Gastroenterology 1993; 104: 1485–1491
16. **Aubé, C., Oberti, F., Korali, N., Namour, M.A., Loisel, D., Tanguy, J.Y., Valsesia, E., Pilette, C., Rousselet, M.C., Bedossa, P., Rifflet, H., Maiga, M.Y., Penneau-Fontbonne, D., Caron, C., Cales, P.:** Ultrasonographic diagnosis of hepatic fibrosis or cirrhosis. J. Hepatol. 1999; 30: 472–478
17. **Ayata, G., Gordon, F.D., Lewis, D., Pomfret, E., Pomposelli, J.J., Jenkins, R.L., Khettry, U.:** Cryptogenic cirrhosis: Clinicopathologic findings at and after liver transplantation. Human Path. 2002; 33: 1098–1104
18. **Bajaj, B.K., Agarwal, M.P., Ram, B.K.:** Autonomic neuropathy in patients with hepatic cirrhosis. Postgrad. Med. J. 2003; 79: 408–411
19. **Ballmer, P.E., Walshe, D., McNurlan, M.A., Watson, H., Brunt, P.W., Garlick, P.J.:** Albumin synthesis rate in cirrhosis: correlation with Child-Turcotte classification. Hepatology 1993; 18: 292–297
20. **Bandi, J.-C., Garcia-Pagan, J.C., Escorsell, A., Francois, E., Moithinho, E., Rodes, J., Bosch, J.:** Effects of propranolol on the hepatic hemodynamic response to physical exercise in patients with cirrhosis. Hepatology 1998; 28: 677–682
21. **Battista, S., Bar, F., Mengozzi, G., Zanon, E., Grosso, M., Molino, G.:** Hyperdynamic circulation in patients with cirrhosis: direct measurement of nitric oxide levels in hepatic and portal veins. J. Hepatol 1997; 26: 75–80
22. **Belli, L., Sansalone, C.V., Aseni, P., Romani, F., Rondinara, G.:** Portal thrombosis in cirrhosis. Ann. Surg. 1986; 203: 286–291
23. **Bini, E.J., Lascarides, C.E., Micale, P.L., Weinshel, E.H.:** Mucosal abnormalities of the colon in patients with portal hypertension: an endoscopic study. Gastrointest. Endosc. 2000; 52: 511–516
24. **Bolognesi, M., Sacerdoti, D., Bombonato, G., Chiesura-Corona, M., Merkel, C., Gatta, A.:** Arterioportal fistulas in patients with liver cirrhosis: usefulness of color Doppler US for screening. Radiology 2000; 216: 738–743
25. **Boustière, C., Dumas, O., Jouffre, C., Letard, J.C., Patouillard, B., Etaix, J.P., Barthélémy, C., Audigier, J.C.:** Endoscopic ultrasonography classification of gastric varices in patients with cirrhosis. Comparison with endoscopic findings. J. Hepatol. 1993; 19: 268–272
26. **Brancatelli, G., Federle, M.P., Ambrosini, R., Lagala, R., Carriero, A., Midivi, M., Vilgrain, V.:** Cirrhosis CT and MR imaging evaluation. Eur. J. Radiol. 2007; 61: 57–69
27. **Brinch, K., Moller, S., Bendtsen, F., Becker, U., Henriksen, J.H.:** Plasma volume expansion by albumin in cirrhosis. Relation to blood volume distribution, arterial compliance and severity of disease. J. Hepatol. 2003; 39: 24–31
28. **Burch, R.E., Sackin, D.A., Ursick, J.A., Jetton, M.M., Sullivan, J.F.:** Decreased taste and smell acuity in cirrhosis. Arch. Intern. Med. 1978; 138: 743–746
29. **Bureau, C., Garcia-Pagan, J.C., Otal, P., Pomier-Layrargues, G., Chabbert, V., Cortez, C., Perreault, P., Peron, J.M., Abraldes, J.G., Bouchard, L., Bilbao, J.I., Bosch, J., Rousseau, H., Vinel, J.P.:** Improved clinical outcome using polytetrafluoroethylene-coated stents for TIPS: Results of a randomized study. Gastroenterology 2004; 126: 469–475
30. **Burk, R.F., Early, D.S., Hill, K.E., Palmer, I.S., Boeglin, M.E.:** Plasma selenium in patients with cirrhosis. Hepatology 1998; 27: 794–798
31. **Cabrè, E., Abad-Lacruz, A., Nunez, M.C., Gonzalez-Huix, F., Fernandez-Banares, F., Gil, A., Esteve-Comas, M., Moreno, J., Planas, R., Guilera, M., Gassull, M.A.:** The relationship of plasma polyunsaturated fatty acid deficiency with survival in advanced liver cirrhosis: multivariate analysis. Amer. J. Gastroenterol. 1993; 88: 718–722
32. **Cabrè, E., Gonzalez-Huix, F., Abad-Lacruz, A., Esteve, M., Acero, D., Fernandez-Banares, F., Xiol, X., Gassull, M.A.:** Effect of total enteral nutrition on the short-term outcome of severely malnourished cirrhotics. A randomized controlled trial. Gastroenterology 1990; 98: 715–720
33. **Caldwell, S.H., Oelsner, D.H., Iezzoni, J.C., Hespenheide, E.E., Battle, E.H., Driscoll, C.J.:** Cryptogenic cirrhosis: clinical characterization and risk factors for underlying disease. Hepatology 1999; 29: 664–669
34. **Caly, W.R., Strauss, E.:** A prospective study of bacterial infections in patients with cirrhosis. J. Hepatol. 1993; 18: 353–358
35. **Campillo, B., Bories, P., Devanlay, M., Sommer, F., Wirzuin, E., Fouet, P.:** The thermogenic and metabolic effect of food in liver cirrhosis: Consequences on the storage of nutrients and the hormonal counterregulatory response. Metabolism 1992; 41: 472–482
36. **Campillo, B., Bories, P.N., Benvenuti, C., Dupeyron, C.:** Serum and urinary nitrate levels in liver cirrhosis: endotoxemia, renal function and hyperdynamic circulation. J. Hepatol 1996; 25: 707–714
37. **Campollo, O., Sprengers, D., McIntyre, N.:** The BCAA/AAA ratio of plasma amino acids in three different groups of cirrhotics. Rev. Invest. Clin. 1992; 44: 513–518
38. **Cardenas, A., Kelleher, T., Chopra, S.:** Review article: hepatic hydrothorax. Aliment. Pharmacol. Ther. 2004; 20: 271–279
39. **Chan, C.C., Hwang, S.J., Lee, F.Y., Wang, S.S., Chang, F.Y., Li, C.P., Chu, C.J.:** Prognostic value of plasma endotoxin levels in patients with cirrhosis. Scand. J. Gastroenterol. 1997; 32: 942–946
40. **Channick, R.N., Simonneau, G., Sitbon, O., Robbins, I.M., Frost, A., Tapson, V.F., Badesch, D.B., Roux, S., Rainisio, M., Bodin, F., Rubin, L.J.:** Effects of the dual endothelin-receptor antagonist bosentan in patients with pulmonary hypertension: a randomized placebo-controlled study. Lancet 2001; 358: 1119–1123
41. **Chen, A., Ho. Y., Tu. Y., Tang, H., Cheng, T.:** Diaphragmatic defect as a cause of massive hydrothorax in cirrhosis of the liver. J. Clin. Gastroenterol. 1988; 10: 663–666
42. **Colli, A., Fraquelli, M., Andreoletti, M., Marino, B., Zuccoli, E., Conte, D.:** Severe liver fibrosis or cirrhosis: Accuracy of US for detection. – Analysis of 300 cases. Radiology 2003; 227: 89–94
43. **Conte, D., Fraquell, M., Fornari, F., Lodi, L., Bodini, P., Buscarini, L.:** Close relation between cirrhosis and gallstones. Arch. Intern. Med. 1999; 159: 49–52
44. **Cordoba, J., Cabrera, J., Lataif, L., Penev, P., Zel, P., Blei, H.T.:** High prevalence of sleep disturbance in cirrhosis. Hepatology 1998; 27: 339–345
45. **D'Amico, G., Montalbano, L., Traina, M., Pisa, R., Menozzi, M., Spano, C., Pagliaro, L.:** Natural history of congestive gastropathy in cirrhosis. Gastroenterology 1990; 99: 1558–1564
46. **Debernardi-Venon, W., Barletti, C., Alessandria, C., Marzano, A., Baronio, M., Todros, L., Saracco, G., Repici, A., Rizzetto, M.:** Efficacy of irbesartan, a receptor selective antagonist of angiotensin II, in reducing portal hypertension. Dig. Dis. Sci. 2002; 47: 401–404
47. **Degre, D., Bourgeois, N., Boon, N., LeMoine, O., Louis, H., Donckier, V., El Nakadi, I., Closset, J., Lingier, P., Vereerstraeten, P., Gelin, M., Adler, M.:** Aminopyrine breath test compared to the MELD and Child-Pugh scores for predicting mortality among cirrhotic patients awaiting liver transplantation. Transplant. Internat. 2004; 17: 31–38
48. **Del Olmo, J.A., Garcia, F., Serra, M.A., Maldonado, L., Rodrigo, J.M.:** Prevalence and incidence of gallstones in liver cirrhosis. Scand. J. Gastroenterol. 1997; 32: 1061–1065
49. **Del Olmo, J.A., Serra, M.A., Rodriguez, F., Escudero, S., Gilabert, S., Rodrigo, J.M.:** Incidence and risk factors for hepatocellular carcinoma in 967 patients with cirrhosis. J. Canc. Res. Clin. Oncol. 1998; 124: 560–564
50. **Denzer, U., Arnoldy, A., Kanzler, S., Galle, P.R., Dienes, H.P., Lohse, A.W.:** Prospective randomized comparison of minilaparoscopy and percutaneous liver biopsy: Diagnosis of cirrhosis and complications. J. Clin. Gastroenterol. 2007; 41: 103–110
51. **Desmet, V.J., Sciot, R., van Eyken, P.:** Differential diagnosis and prognosis of cirrhosis: role of liver biopsy. Acta Gastroenterol. Belg. 1990; 53: 198–208
52. **Dhiman, R.K., Sawhney, I.M.S., Chawla, Y.K., Das, G., Ram, S., Dilawari, J.B.:** Efficacy of lactulose in cirrhotic patients with subclinical hepatic encephalopathy. Dig. Dis. Sci. 2000; 45: 1549–1552
53. **Di Lelio, A., Cestari, C., Lomazzi, A., Beretta, L.:** Cirrhosis: diagnosis with sonographic study of the liver surface. Radiology 1989; 172: 389–392
54. **Diamond, T.H., Stiel, D., Lunzer, M., McDowall, D., Eckstein, R.P., Posen, S.:** Hepatic osteodystrophy. Static and dynamic bone histomorphometry and serum bone Gla-Protein in 80 patients with chronic liver disease. Gastroenterology 1989; 96: 213–221
55. **Duchini, A., Viernes, M.E., Nyberg, L.M., Hendry, R.M., Pockros, P.J.:** Hepatic decompensation in patients with cirrhosis during infection with influenza A. Arch. Intern. Med. 2000; 160: 113–115
56. **Essers, U., Bleifeld, W., Kaiser, E.:** Rezidivierendes Fieber und Erhöhung des ungebundenen Ätiocholanolons im Blut. Dtsch. Med. Wschr. 1971; 96: 107–117
57. **Fernandez, J., Navasa, M., Gomez, J., Colmenero, J., Vila, J., Arroyo, V., Rodes, J.:** Bacterial infections in cirrhosis. Epidemiological changes with invasive procedures and norfloxacin prophylaxis. Hepatology 2002; 35: 140–148
58. **Ferrante, D., Arguedas, M.R., Cerfolio, R.J., Collins, B.G., van Leeuwen, D.J.:** Video-assisted thoracoscopy surgery with talc pleurodesis in the management of symptomatic hepatic hydrothorax. Amer. J. Gastroenterol. 2002; 97: 3172–3175
59. **Gaiani, St., Bolondi, L., li Bassi, S., Zironi, G., Siringo, S., Barbara, L.:** Prevalence of spontaneous hepatofugal portal flow in liver cirrhosis. Clinical and endoscopic correlation in 228 patients. Gastroenterology 1991; 100: 160–167
60. **Gaune-Carrie, N., Ziol, M., de Ledinghen, V., Douvin, C., Marcellin, P., Castera, L., Drumeaux, D., Truchet, J.C., Beaugrand, M.:** Accuracy

of liver stiffness measurement for the diagnosis of cirrhosis in patients with chronic liver diseases. Hepatology 2006; 44: 1511–1517
61. Garcia-Pagán, J., Santos, C., Barberá, J.A., Luca, A., Roca, J., Rodriguez-Roisin, R., Bosch, J., Rodés, J.: Physical exercise increases portal pressure in patients with cirrhosis and portal hypertension. Gastroenterology 1996; 111: 1300–1306
62. Garcia-Pagan, J.C., Morillas, R., Banares, R., Albillos, A., Villanueva, C., Vila, C., Genesca, J., Jimenez, M., Rodriguez, M., Calleja, J.L., Balanzo, J., Garcia-Duran, F., Planas, R., Bosch, J.: Propranolol plus placebo versus propranolol plus isosorbide-5-mononitrate in the prevention of a first variceal bleed: A double-blind RCT. Hepatology 2003; 37: 1260–1266
63. Giouleme, O.I., Vyzantiadis, T.A., Nikolaidis, N.L., Vasiliadis, T.G., Papageorgiou, A.A., Eugenidis, N.P., Harsoulis, F.I.: Pathogenesis of osteoporosis in liver cirrhosis. Hepato-Gastroenterology 2006; 53: 936–943
64. Golli, M., Kriaa, S., Said, M., Belguith, M., Zbidi, M., Saad, J., Nouri, A., Ganouni, A.: Intrahepatic spontaneous portosystemic venous shunt: value of color and power Doppler sonography. J. Clin. Ultrasound 2000; 28: 47–50
65. Graudal, N., Leth, P., Marbjerg, L., Galloe, A.M.: Characteristics of cirrhosis undiagnosed during life: a comparative analysis of 73 undiagnosed cases and 149 diagnosed cases of cirrhosis, detected in 4929 consecutive autopsies. J. Intern. Med. 1991; 230: 165–171
66. Greco, A.V., Mingrone, G., Benedetti, G., Capristo, E., Tataranni, P.A., Gasbarrini, G.: Daily energy and substrate metabolism in patients with cirrhosis. Hepatology 1998; 27: 346–350
67. Gur, C., Ilan, Y., Shibolet, O.: Hepatic hydrothorax. Pathophysiology, diagnosis and treatment. Review of the literature. Liver Internat. 2004; 24: 281–284
68. Guslandi, M., Foppa, L., Soirghi, M., Pellegrini, A., Fanti, L., Tittobello, A.: Breakdown of mucosal defences in congestive gastropathy in cirrhotics. Liver 1992; 12: 303–305
69. Habu, D., Nishiguchi, S., Nakatani, S., Kawamura, E., Lee, C., Enomoto, M., Tamori, A., Takeda, T., Tanaka, T., Shiomi, S.: Effect of oral supplementation with branched-chain amino acid granules on serum albumin level in the early stage of cirrhosis: a randomized pilot trial. Hepatol. Res. 2003; 25: 312–318
70. Haitjema, T., de Maat, C.E.M.: Pleural effusion without ascites in a patient with cirrhosis. Neth. J. Med. 1994; 44: 207–209
71. Herold, C., Heinz, R., Radespiel-Tröger, M., Schneider, H.T., Schuppan, D., Hahn, E.G.: Quantitative testing of liver function in patients with cirrhosis due to chronic hepatitis C to assess disease severity. Liver 2001; 21: 26–30
72. Herve, P., Le Pavec, J., Sztrymf, B., Decante, B., Savale, L., Sitbon, O.: Pulmonary vascular abnormalities in cirrhosis. Best Pract. Res. Clin. Gastroenterol. 2007; 21: 141–159
73. Hicken, B.L., Sharara, A.I., Abrams, G.A., Eloubeidi, M., Fallon, M.B., Arguedas, M.R.: Hepatic venous pressure gradient measurements to assess response to primary prophylaxis in patients with cirrhosis: A decision analytical study. Alim. Pharm. Ther. 2003; 17: 145–153
74. Hosking, S.W., Smart, H.L., Johnson, A.G., Triger, D.R.: Anorectal varices, hemorrhoids, and portal hypertension. Lancet 1989/I: 349–352
75. Hourani, J.M., Bellamy, P.E., Tashkin, D.P., Batra, M.S., Simmons, M.S.: Pulmonary dysfunction in advanced liver disease. Frequent occurrence of an abnormal diffusing capacity. Amer. J. Med. 1991; 90: 693–700
76. Huang, L.Y., Cui, J., Wu, C.R., Liu, Y.X.: Embolization combined with endoscopic variceal ligation for the treatment of oesophagogastric variceal bleeding in patients with cirrhosis. Clin. Med. J. 2007; 107: 36–40
77. Idilman, R., de Maria, N., Uzunalimoglu, O., van Thiel, D.H.: Hepatic osteodystrophy: a review. Hepatogastroenterology 1997; 44: 574–581
78. Ikegami, M., Toyonaga, A., Tanikawa, K.: Reduction of portal pressure by chronic administration of isosorbide dinitrate in patients with cirrhosis: effects on systemic and splanchnic hemodynamics and liver function. Amer. J. Gastroenterol. 1992; 87: 1160–1164
79. Ito, K., Mitchell, D.G.: Hepatic morphologic changes in cirrhosis: MR imaging findings. Abdom. Imag. 2000; 25: 456–461
80. Iwasa, M., Matsumura, K., Watanabe, Y., Yamamoto, M., Kaito, M., Ikoma, J., Gabazza, E.C., Takeda, K., Adachi, Y.: Improvement of regional cerebral blood flow after treatment with branched-chain amino acid solutions in patients with cirrhosis. Eur. J. Gastroenterol. Hepatol. 2003; 15: 733–737
81. Jongh, de, F.E., Janssen, H.L.A., de Man, R.A., Hop, W.C.J., Schalm, S.W., van Blankenstein, M.: Survival and prognostic indicators in hepatitis B surface antigen-positive cirrhosis of the liver. Gastroenterology 1992; 103: 1630–1635
82. Kanematsu, M., Hoshi, H., Murakami, T., Inaba, Y., Kim, T., Yamada, T., Kato, M., Yokoyama, R., Nakamura, H.: Detection of hepatocellular carcinoma in patients with cirrhosis: MR imaging versus angiographically assisted helical CT. Amer. J. Roentg. 1997; 169: 1507–1515
83. Kanematsu, M., Hoshi, H., Yamada, T., Kim, T., Kato, M., Yokoyama, R., Nakamura, H.: Small hepatic nodules in cirrhosis: ultrasonographic, CT, and MR imaging findings. Abdom. Imag. 1999; 24: 47–55
84. Kaya, D., Kockar, M.C., Bavbek, N., Dagli, M., Kovar, A.: Cardiac dysfunction in cirrhosis. Hepatol. Res. 2003; 26: 181–185
85. Kharbanda, P.S., Prabhakas, S., Chawla, Y.K., Das, C.P., Syal, P.: Peripheral neuropathy in liver cirrhosis. J. Gastroenterol. Hepat. 2003; 18: 922–926
86. Kim, Y.J., Raman, S.S., Yu, N.C., To'o, K.J., Jutabha, R., Lu, D.S.: Esophageal varices in cirrhotic patients: Evaluation with liver CT. Amer. J. Roentgenol. 2007; 188: 139–144
87. Kondrup, J., Nielsen, K., Juul, A.: Effect of long-term refeeding on protein metabolism in patients with cirrhosis of the liver. Brit. J. Nutr. 1997; 77: 197–212
88. Körner, T., Kropf, J., Kosche, B., Kristahl, H., Jaspersen, D., Gessner, A.M.: Improvement of prognostic power of the Child-Pugh classification of liver cirrhosis by hyaluronan. J. Hepatol. 2003; 39: 947–953
89. Kuntz, E.: Systematik und Ätiologie der Leberzirrhose. Münch. Med. Wschr. 1984; 126: 983–987
90. Kuntz, E.: 30 Jahre Erfahrung bei 6000 Laparoskopien (1955–1986). Fortschr. Med. 1987; 105: 521–524
91. Kuntz, E.: Klinische Aspekte, Prognose und Therapie der Leberzirrhose. Lebensversicherungsmed. 1990; 42: 52–55
92. Kuntz, E.: Der aktuelle Stellenwert der Laparoskopie in der Hepatologie. Med. Welt 1999; 50: 42–47
93. Lafortune, M., Matricardi, L., Denys, A., Favret, M., Déry, R., Ponnier-Layrargues, G.: Segment 4 (the quadrate lobe): a barometer of cirrhotic liver disease at US. Radiology 1998; 206: 157–160
94. Larcos, G., Sorokopud, H., Berry, G., Farell, G.C.: Sonographic screening for hepatocellular carcinoma in patients with chronic hepatitis or cirrhosis: an evaluation. Amer. J. Roentg. 1998; 171: 433–435
95. Le Bail, B., Bernard, P.-H., Carles, J., Balabaud, C., Bioulac-Sage, P.: Prevalence of liver cell dysplasia and association with HCC in a series of 100 cirrhotic liver explants. J. Hepatol. 1997; 27: 835–842
96. Lenz, K., Hörtnagel, H., Druml, W., Reither, H., Schmid, R., Schneeweiss, B., Laggner, A., Grimm. G., Gerbes, A.L.: Ornipressin in the treatment of functional renal failure in decompensated liver cirrhosis. Effects on renal hemodynamics and atrial atriuretic factor. Gastroenterology 1991; 101: 1060–1067
97. Lirussi, F., Nassuato, G., Orlando, R., Iemmolo, R.M., Beccarello, A., Bortolato, L., Rusticali, A.G., Okolicsanyi, L.: Treatment of active cirrhosis with ursodeoxycholic acid and a free radical scavenger: a two year prospective study. Med. Sci. Res. 1995; 23: 31–33
98. Liu, Q., Duan, Z.P., Ha, D.K., Bengmark, S., Kurtovic, J., Riordan, S.M.: Synbiotic modulation of gut flora: Effect on minimal hepatic encephalopathy in patients with cirrhosis. Hepatology 2004; 39: 1441–1449
99. Ludwig, J., Hashimoto, E., Porayko, M.K., Moyer, T.P., Baldus, W.P.: Hemosiderosis in cirrhosis: a study of 447 native livers. Gastroenterology 1997; 112: 882–888
100. Malnick, S.D.H., Attali, M., Israeli, E., Gratz, R., Geltner, D.: Spontaneous bacterial arthritis in a cirrhotic patient. J. Clin. Gastroenterol. 1998; 27: 364–366
101. Marcato, N., Abergel, A., Alexandre, M., Boire, J.Y., Darcha, C., Duchene, B., Chipponi, J., Boyer, L., Viallet, J.F., Bommelaer, G.: Hepatocellular carcinoma in patients with cirrhosis: performance and semiology of magnetic resonance imaging and lipiodol computerized tomography. Gastroenterol. Clin. Biol. 1999; 23: 114–121
102. Marchesini, G., Bianchi, G., Merli, M., Amodio, P., Panella, C., Loguericio, C., Rossi Fanelli, F., Abbiati, R.: Nutritional supplementation with branched-chain amino acids in advanced cirrhosis: A double-blind randomized trial. Gastroenterology 2003; 124: 1792–1801
103. Marchesini, G., Bugianesi, E., Ronchi, M., Flamia, R., Thomaseth, K., Pacini, G.: Zinc supplementation improves glucose disposal in patients with cirrhosis. Metabolism 1998; 47: 792–798
104. Marti-Bonmati, L., Talens, A., del Olmo, J., del Val. A., Serra, M., Rodrigo, J.M., Fernandez, A., Torres, V., Rayon, M.: Chronic hepatitis and cirrhosis. Evaluation by means of MR imaging with histological correlation. Radiology 1993; 188: 37–43
105. Matsuoka, C., Tanaka, N., Arakawa, Y.: Beneficial effects of branched-chain amino acids on altered protein and amino acid metabolism in liver cirrhosis: Evaluation in a model of liver cirrhosis induced in rats with carbon tetrachloride. Hepatol. Res. 2003; 27: 117–123
106. Merkel, C., Marin, R., Angeli, P., Zanella, P., Felder, M., Bernardinello, E., Cavalarin, G., Bolognesi, M., Donada, C., Bellini, B., Torboli, P., Gatta, A.: A placebo-controlled clinical trial of nadolol in the prophylaxis of growth of small esophageal varices in cirrhosis. Gastroenterology 2004; 127: 476–484
107. Michl, P., Gülberg, V., Bilzer, M., Waggershauser, T., Reiber, M., Gerbes, A.L.: Transjugular intrahepatic portosystemic shunt for cirrhosis and ascites: effects in patients with organic or functional renal failure. Scand. J. Gastroenterol. 2000; 35: 654–658
108. Molle, I., Thulstrup, A.M., Svendsen, N., Schonheyder, H.C., Sorensen, H.T.: Risk and case fatality rate of meningitis in patients with liver cirrhosis. Scand. J. Infect. Dis. 2000; 32: 407–410
109. Morillas, R.M., Planas, R., Cabré, E., Galan, A., Quer, J.C., Feu, F., Garcia Pagan, J.C., Bosch, J., Gassull, M.A.: Propranolol plus isosorbid-5-mononitrate for portal hypertension in cirrhosis: long term hemodynamic and renal effects. Hepatology 1994; 20: 1502–1508
110. Morrison, W.L., Bouchier, I.A.D., Gibson, J.N.A., Rennie, M.J.: Skeletal muscle and whole-body protein turnover in cirrhosis. Clin. Sci. 1990; 78: 613–619
111. Müller, M.J.: Malnutrition in cirrhosis. J. Hepatol. 1995; 23 (Suppl. 1): 31–35
112. Murata, K., Shimizu, A., Takase, K., Nakano, T., Tameda, Y.: Asymptomatic primary pulmonary hypertension associated with liver cirrhosis. J. Gastroenterol. 1997; 32: 102–104
113. Murawaki, Y., Kobayashi, M., Koda, M., Kawasakia, H.: Effects of lactulose on intestinal bacterial flora and fecal organic acids in patients with liver cirrhosis. Hepatol. Res. 2000; 17: 56–64

114. Nagata, N., Miyachi, H., Nakano, A., Nanri, K., Kobayashi, H., Matsuzaki, S.: Sonographic evaluation of the anterior liver surface in chronic liver diseases using a 7.5-MHz annular-array transducer: correlation with laparoscopic and histopathologic findings. J. Clin. Ultrasound 2003; 31: 393–400

115. Nakamura, I., Ochiai, K., Imawari, M.: Phagocytic function of neutrophils of patients with decompensated cirrhosis is restored by oral supplementation of branched-chain amino acids. Hepatol. Res. 2004; 29: 207–211

116. Navasa, M., Fernandez, J., Rodes, J.: Bacterial infections in liver cirrhosis. Ital. J. Gastroenterol. 1999; 31: 616–625

117. Nord, H.J.: Biopsy diagnosis of cirrhosis: blind percutaneous versus guided direct vision techniques – a review. Gastrointest. Endosc. 1982; 28: 102–104

118. Oellerich, M., Burdelski, M., Lautz, H.U., Schulz, M., Schmidt, F.W., Herrmann, H.: Lidocaine metabolite formation as a measure of liver function in patients with cirrhosis. Ther. Drug Monit. 1990; 12: 219–226

119. Ogusu, T., Iwakiri, R., Sakata, H., Matsunaga, K., Shimoda, R., Oda, K., Watanabe, K., Ootani, H., Kikkawa, A., Ootani, A., Tsunada, S., Fujimoto, K.: Endoscopic injection sclerotherapy for esophageal varices in cirrhotic patients without hepatocellular carcinoma: A comparison of long-term survival between prophylactic therapy and emergency therapy. J. Gastroenterol. 2003; 38: 361–364

120. Okamoto, M., Sakaida, I., Tsuchiya, M., Suzuki, C., Okita, K.: Effect of a late evening snack on the blood glucose level and energy metabolism in patients with liver cirrhosis. Hepatol. Res. 2003; 27: 45–50

121. Okuda, K., Ohnishi, K., Kimura, K., Matsutani, S., Sumida, M., Goto, N., Musha, H., Takashi, M., Suzuki, N., Shinagawa, T., Suzukui, N., Ohtsuki, T., Arakawa, M., Nakashima, T.: Incidence of portal vein thrombosis in liver cirrhosis. An angiographic study in 708 patients. Gastroenterology 1985; 89: 279–286

122. Ordinas, A., Escolar, G., Cirera, I., Viñas, M., Cobo, F., Bosch, J., Terés, J., Rodés, J.: Existence of a platelet-adhesion defect in patients with cirrhosis independent of hematocrit: studies under flow conditions. Hepatology 1996; 24: 1137–1142

123. Orlando, R., Lirussi, F., Okolicsanyi, L.: Laparoscopy and liver biopsy: further evidence that the two procedures improve the diagnosis of liver cirrhosis. J. Clin. Gastroenterol. 1990; 12: 47–52

124. Panés, J., Bordas, J.M., Pique, J.M., Bosch, J., Garcin-Pagan, J.C., Feu, F., Casaderall, M., Teres, J., Rodes, J.: Increased gastric mucosal perfusion in cirrhotic patients with portal hypertensive gastropathy. Gastroenterology 1992; 103: 1875–1882

125. Pantaleo, P., Marra, F., Vizzutti, F., Spardoni, S., Ciabattoni, G., Galli, C., la Villa, G., Gentilini, P., Laffi, G.: Effects of dietary supplementation with arachidonic acid on platelet and renal function in patients with cirrhosis. Clin. Sci. 2004; 106: 27–34

126. Pauwels, A., Pines, E., Abboura, M., Chiche, I., Levy, V.-G.: Bacterial meningitis in cirrhosis – review of 16 cases. J. Hepatol. 1997; 27: 830–834

127. Payen, J.-L., Cales, P., Voigt, J.-J., Barbe, S., Pilette, C., Dubuisson, L., Desmorat, H., Vinel, J.-P., Kervran, A., Chayvialle, J.-A., Pascal, J.-P.: Severe portal hypertensive gastropathy and antral vascular ectasia are distinct entities in patients with cirrhosis. Gastroenterology 1995; 108: 138–144

128. Pellicano, R., Leone, N., Berrutti, M., Cutufia, M.A., Fiorentino, M., Rizzetto, M., Ponzetto, A.: Helicobacter pylori seroprevalence in hepatitis C virus positive patients with cirrhosis. J. Hepatol. 2000; 33: 648–650

129. Peltekian, K.M., Wong, F., Liu, P.P., Logan, A.G., Sherman, M., Blendis, L.M.: Cardiovascular, renal and neurohumoral response to single large-volume paracentesis in patients with cirrhosis and diuretic-resistant ascites. Amer. J. Gastroenterol. 1997; 92: 394–399

130. Plewe, G., Beyer, J.: Ätiocholanolon und Fieber. Dtsch. Med. Wschr. 1984; 109: 589–591

131. Poniachik, J., Bernstein, D.E., Reddy, K.R., Jeffers, L.J., Coelho-Little, M.-E., Civaertos, F., Schiff, E.R.: The role of laparoscopy in the diagnosis of cirrhosis. Gastrointest. Endosc. 1996; 43: 568–571

132. Poonawala, A., Nair, S.P., Thuluvath, P.J.: Prevalence of obesity and diabetes in patients with cryptogenic cirrhosis: A case-control study. Hepatology 2000; 32: 689–692

133. Powell, W.J., Klatskin, G.: Duration of survival in patients with Laennec's cirrhosis. Amer. J. Med. 1968; 44: 406–420

134. Primignani, M., Carpinelli, L., Preatoni, P., Battaglia, G., Carta, A., Prada, A., Cestari, R., Angeli, P., Gatta, A., Rossi, A., Spinzi, G., de Franchis, R.: Natural history of portal hypertensive gastropathy in patients with liver cirrhosis. Gastroenterology 2000; 119: 181–187

135. Rasaratnam, B., Kaye, D., Jennings, G., Dudley, F., Chin-Dusting, J.: The effect of selective intestinal decontamination on the hyperdynamic circulatory state in cirrhosis. Ann. Intern. Med. 2003; 139: 186–193

136. Ratziu, V., Bonyhay, L., di Martino, V., Charlotte, F., Cavallaro, L., Sayegh-Tainturier, M.H., Giral, P., Grimaldi, A., Opolon, P., Poynard, T.: Survival, liver failure, and hepatocellular carcinoma in obesity-related cryptogenic cirrhosis. Hepatology 2002; 35: 1485–1493

137. Realdi, G., Fattovich, G., Hadziyannis, S., Schalm, S.W., Almasio, P., Sanchez-Tapias, J., Christensen, E., Giustina, G., Noventa, F.: Survival and prognostic factors in 366 patients with compensated cirrhosis type B.: a multicenter study. J. Hepatol. 1994; 21: 656–666

138. Rees, C.J., Oppong, K., Al-Mardini, H., Hudson, M., Record, C.O.: Effect of L-ornithine-L-aspartate on patients with and without TIPS undergoing glutamine challenge: a double blind, placebo controlled trial. Gut 2000; 47: 571–574

139. Riehl, J., Bongartz, D., Nguyen, H., Sieberth, H.G.: Spontaneous portosystemic shunts in liver cirrhosis: demonstration by color coded Duplex ultrasonography. Ultraschall Med. 1997; 18: 272–276

140. Robalino, B.J., Moodie, D.S.: Association between primary pulmonary hypertension and portal hypertension: analysis of its pathophysiology and clinical, laboratory and hemodynamic manifestations. J. Amer. Coll. Cardiol. 1991; 17: 492–498

141. Saadeh, S., Behrens, P.W., Parsi, M.A., Carey, W.D., Connor, J.T., Grealis, M., Barnes, D.S.: The utility of the (13) C-galactose breath test as a measure of liver function. Alim. Pharm. Ther. 2003; 18: 995–1002

142. Sakai, K., Iwao, T., Oho, K., Toyonaga, A., Sata, M.: Propranolol ameliorates thrombocytopenia in patients with cirrhosis. J. Gastroenterol. 2002; 37: 112–118

143. Sako, K., Imamura, Y., Nishimata, H., Tahara, K., Kubozono, O., Tsubouchi, H.: Branched-chain amino acids supplements in the late evening decrease the frequency of muscle cramps with advanced hepatic cirrhosis. Hepatol. Res. 2003; 26: 327–329

144. Salerno, F., Borroni, G., Moser, P., Sangiovanni, A., Almasio, P., Budillon, G., Capuano, G., Muraca, M., Marchesini, G., Bernardi, M., Marenco, G., Molino, G., Rossaro, L., Solinas, A., Ascione, A.: Prognostic value of the galactose test in predicting survival of patients with cirrhosis evaluated for liver transplantation. J. Hepatol. 1996; 25: 474–480

145. Salo, J., Gines, A., Anibarro, L., Jimenez, W., Bataller, R., Claria, J., Gines, P., Rivera, F., Arroyo, V., Rodes, J.: Effect of upright posture and physical exercise on endogenous neurohormonal systems in cirrhotic patients with sodium retention and normal supine plasma renin, aldosterone, and norepinephrine levels. Hepatology 1995; 22: 479–487

146. Sangiovanni, A., Prati, G.M., Fasani, P., Ronchi, G., Romeo, R., Manini, M., del Ninno, E., Morabito, A., Colombo, M.: The natural history of compensated cirrhosis due to hepatitis C virus: A 17-year cohort study of 214 patients. Hepatology 2006; 43: 1303–1310

147. Santos, J., Planas, R., Pardo, A., Durandez, R., Cabre, E., Morillas, R.M., Granada, M.L., Jimenez, J.A., Quintero, E., Gassull, M.A.: Spironolacton alone or in combination with furosemide in the treatment of moderate ascites in non azotemic cirrhosis. A randomized comparative stucy of efficacy and safety. J. Hepatol. 2003; 39: 187–192

148. Sanyal, A.J., Freedman, A.M., Luketic, V.A., Purdum, P.P., Shiffman, M.L., Demeo, J., Cole, P.E., Tisnado, J.: The natural history of portal hypertension after transjugular intrahepatic portosystemic shunts. Gastroenterology 1997; 112: 889–898

149. Saunders, J.B., Walters, J.R., Davies, A.P., Paton, A.: A 20 year prospective study of cirrhosis. Brit. Med. J. 1981; 282: 263–266

150. Scandalis, N., Archimandritis, A., Kastanas, K., Spiliadis. C., Delis, B., Manika, Z.: Colonic findings in cirrhotics with portal hypertension. J. Clin. Gastroenterol. 1994; 18: 325–329

151. Schenk, P., Madl, C., Rezaie-Majd, S., Lehr, S., Müller, C.: Methylene blue improves the hepatopulmonary syndrome. Ann. Intern. Med. 2000; 133: 701–706

152. Schenk, P., Schöniger-Hekele, M., Fuhrmann, V., Madl, C., Silberhumer, G., Müller, C.: Prognostic significance of the hepatopulmonary syndrome in patients with cirrhosis. Gastroenterology 2003; 125: 1042–1052

153. Schepke, M., Kleber, G., Nürnberg, D., Willert, J., Koch, L., Veltzke-Schlieker, W., Hellerbrand, C., Kluth, J., Schanz, S., Kahl, S., Fleig, W.E., Sauerbruch, T.: Ligation versus propranolol for the primary prophylaxis of variceal bleeding in cirrhosis. Hepatology 2004; 40: 65–72

154. Schinella, M., Guglielmi, A., Veraldi, G.F., Boni, M., Frameglia, M., Caputo, M.: Evaluation of the liver function of cirrhotic patients based on the formation of monoethylglycine xylidide (MEGX) from lidocaine. Europ. J. Clin. Chem. Clin. Biochem. 1993; 31: 553–557

155. Scotinoitis, I.A., Lucey, M.R., Metz, D.C.: Helicobacter pylori infection is not associated with subclinical hepatic encephalopathy in stable cirrhotic patients. Dig. Dis. Sci. 2001; 46: 2744–2751

156. Shah, N.J., Neeb, H., Zaitsev, M., Steinhoff, S., Kircheis, G., Amunts, K., Häussinger, D., Zilles, K.: Quantitative T1 mapping of hepatic encephalopathy using magnetic resonance imaging. Hepatology 2003; 38: 1219–1226

157. Shmueli, E., Miell, J.P., Stewart, M., Alberti, K.G.M.M., Record, C.O.: High insulin-like growth factor binding protein 1 levels in cirrhosis: link with insulin resistance. Hepatology 1996; 24: 127–133

158. Shresta, R., McKinley, C., Showalter, R., Wilner, K., Marsano, L., Vivian, B.R., Everson, G.T.: Quantitative liver function tests define the functional severity of liver disease in early stage cirrhosis. Liver Transplant. Surg. 1997; 3: 166–173

159. Simonovsky, V.: The diagnosis of cirrhosis by high resolution ultrasound of the liver surface. Brit. J. Radiol. 1999; 72: 29–34

160. Siringo, S., Bolondi, L., Gaiani, St., Sofia, S., di Febo, G., Zironi, G., Rigamonti, A., Migliolo, M., Cavalli, G., Barbara, L.: The relationship of endoscopy, portal Doppler ultrasound flowmetry, and clinical and biochemical tests in cirrhosis. J. Hepatol. 1994; 20: 11–18

161. Siringo, S., Vaira, D., Menegatti, M., Piscaglia, F., Sofia, S., Gaetani, M., Miglioli, M., Corinaldesi, R., Bolondi, L.: High prevalence of Helicobacter pylori liver cirrhosis. Relationship with clinical and endoscopic features and the risk of peptic ulcer. Dig. Dis. Sci. 1997; 42: 2024–2030

162. Sorensen, T.I.A., Orholm, M., Bentsen, K.D., Hoybye, G., Eghoje, K., Christoffersen, P.: Prospective evaluation of alcohol abuse and alcoholic liver injury in men as predictors of development of cirrhosis. Lancet 1984/II: 241–244

163. **Spahr, L., Vingerhoets, F., Lazeyras, F., Delavelle, J., du Pasquier, R., Giostra, E., Mentha, G., Terrier, F., Hadengue, A.:** Magnetic resonance imaging and proton spectroscopic alterations correlates with parkinsonian signs in patients with cirrhosis. Gastroenterology 2000; 119: 774–781
164. **Steindl, P.E., Finn, B., Bendok, B., Rothke, S., Zee, P.C., Blei, A.T.:** Disruption of the diurnal rhythm of plasma melantonin in liver cirrhosis. Wien. Klin. Wschr. 1997; 109: 741–746
165. **Such, J., Guardiola, J.V., de Juan, J., Casellas, J.A., Pascual, S., Aparicio, J.R., Sola-Vera, J., Perez-Mateo, M.:** Ultrastructural characteristics of distal duodenum mucosa in patients with cirrhosis. Eur. J. Gastroenterol. Hepatol. 2002; 14: 371–376
166. **Sugimura, T., Tsuji, Y., Sakamoto, M., Kotoh, K.:** Long term prognosis and prognostic factors of liver cirrhosis in the 1980s. J. Gastroenterol. Hepatol. 1994; 9: 154–161
167. **Tabaru, A., Shirohara, H., Moriyama, A., Otsuki, M.:** Effects of branched-chain-enriched amino acid solution on insulin and glucagon secretion and blood glucose level in liver cirrhosis. Scand. J. Gastroenterol. 1998; 33: 853–859
168. **Tarao, K., Rino, Y., Ohkawa, S., Tamai, S., Miyakawa, K., Takakura, H., Endo, O., Yoshitsugu, M., Watanabe, N., Matsuzaki, S.:** Close association between high serum alanine aminotransferase levels and multicentric hepatocarcinogenesis in patients with hepatitis C virus-associated cirrhosis. Cancer 2002; 94: 1787–1795
169. **Thaler, H.:** Hepatitis und Zirrhose. Dtsch. Med. Wschr. 1975; 100: 1018–1025
170. **Thorgeirsson, S.S., Grisham, J.W.:** Molecular pathogenesis of human hepatocellular carcinoma. Nature Genet. 2002; 31: 339–343
171. **Trevisani, F., Merli, M., Savelli, F., Valeriano, V., Zambruni, A., Riggio, O., Caraceni, P., Domenicali, M., Bernardi, M.:** QT interval in patients with non-cirrhotic portal hypertension and in cirrhotic patients treated with transjugular intrahepatic portosystemic shunt. J. Hepatol. 2003; 38: 461–467
172. **Tripathi, D., Therapondos, G., Lui, H.F., Stanley, A.J., Hayes, P.C.:** Haemodynamic effects of acute and chronic administration of low-dose carvedilol, a vasodilating beta-blocker, in patients with cirrhosis and portal hypertension. Alim. Pharm. Ther. 2002; 16: 373–380
173. **Ukleja, A., Scolapio, J.S., McConnell, J.P., Dickson, R.C., Nguyen, J.H., O'Brien, P.C.:** Serum and hepatic vitamin E assessment in cirrhotics before transplantation. J. Parent. Ent. Nutr. 2003; 27: 71–73
174. **Ukleja, A., Scolapio, J.S., McConnell, J.P., Spivey, J.R., Dickson, R.C., Nguyen, J.H., O'Brien, P.C.:** Nutritional assessment of serum and hepatic A levels in patients with cirrhosis. J. Parent. Ent. Nutr. 2002; 26: 184–188
175. **Urbain, D., Muls, V., Makhoul, E., Jeghers, O., Thys, O., Ham. H.R.:** Prognostic significance of hepatic venous pressure gradient in medically treated alcoholic cirrhosis: comparison to aminopyrine breath test. Amer. J. Gastroenterol. 1993; 88: 856–859
176. **Valeriano, V., Funaro, S., Lionetti, R., Riggio, O., Pulcinelli, G., Fiore, P., Masini, R., deCastro, S., Merli, M.:** Modification of cardiac function in cirrhotic patients with and without ascites. Amer. J. Gastroenterol. 2000; 95: 3200–3205
177. **Van Buuren, H.R., ter Borg, P.C.J.:** Transjugular intrahepatic portosystemic shunt (TIPS); Indications and long-term patency. Scand. J. Gastroenterol. 2003; 38 (Suppl. 239): 100–104
178. **Venturini, I., Cioni, G., Turrini, F., Gandolfo, M., Modonesi, G., Cosenza, R., Miglioli, L., Cristani, A., D'Alimonte, P., de Santis, M., Zeneroli, M.L.:** Mesenteric vein thrombosis: a rare cause of abdominal pain in cirrhotic patients. Two case reports. Hepato-Gastroenterol. 1998; 45: 44–47
179. **Verne, G.N., Soldevia-Pico, C., Robinson, M.E., Spicer, K.M., Reuben, A.:** Autonomic dysfunction and gastroparesis in cirrhosis. J. Clin. Gastroenterol. 2004; 38: 72–76
180. **Vilgrain, V., Lebrec, D., Menu, Y., Scherrer, A., Nahum, H.:** Comparison between ultrasonographic signs and the degree of portal hypertension in patients with cirrhosis. Gastrointest. Radiol. 1990; 15: 218–222
181. **Vitellas, K.M., Tzalonikou, M.T., Bennett, W.F., Vaswani, K.K., Bova, J.G.:** Cirrhosis: Spectrum of findings on unenhanced and dynamic gadolinium-enhanced MR imaging. Abdom. Imag. 2001; 26: 601–615
182. **Wagner, S., Doss, M.-O., Wittekind, C., Bäcker, U., Meessen, D., Schmidt, F.W.:** Erythrohepatische Protoporphyrie mit rasch progredienter Leberzirrhose. Dtsch. Med. Wschr. 1989; 114: 1837–1841
183. **Wanless, I.R., Wong, F., Blendis, L.M., Greig, P., Heathcote, E.J., Levy, G.:** Hepatic and portal vein thrombosis in cirrhosis: possible role in development of parenchymal extinction and portal hypertension. Hepatology 1995; 21: 1238–1247
184. **Watanabe, S., Kimura, Y., Nishioka, M., Ohkawa, M., Kozeki, M., Yano, M., Hashimoto, N.:** Assessment of hepatic functional reserve in cirrhotic patients by computer tomography of the caudate lobe. Dig. Dis. Sci. 1999; 44: 2554–2563
185. **Weismann, K., Christensen, E., Dreyer, V.:** Zinc supplementation in alcoholic cirrhosis. A double-blind clinical trial. Acta Med. Scand. 1979; 205: 361–366
186. **Winston, C.B., Schwartz, L.H., Fong, Y.M., Blumgart, L.H., Panicek, D.M.:** Hepatocellular carcinoma: MR imaging findings in cirrhotic livers and noncirrhotic livers. Radiology 1999; 210: 75–79
187. **Wong, F., Massie, D., Hsu, P., Dudley, F.:** Indometacin-induced renal failure in patients with well-compensated cirrhosis. Gastroenterology 1993; 104: 869–876
188. **Yamauchi, M., Takeda, K., Sakamoto, K., Ohata, M., Toda, G.:** Effect of oral branched chain amino acid supplementation in the late evening on the nutritional state of patients with liver cirrhosis. Hepatol. Res. 2001; 21: 199–204
189. **Yang, Y.A., Lin, H.C., Lee, W.C., Hou, M.C., Lee, F.Y., Chang, F.Y., Lee, S.D.:** One-week losartan administration increases sodium excretion in cirrhotic patients with and without ascites. J. Gastroenterol. 2002; 37: 194–199
190. **Zen, Y., Sunagozaka, H., Tsuneyama, K., Matsutomi, K., Terasaki, S., Kaneko, S., Kobayashi, K., Nakanuma, Y.:** In complete septal cirrhosis associated with Wegener's granulomatosis (case report). Liver 2002; 22: 388–393
191. **Zhang, S.C., Wang, W., Ren, W.Y., Dai, Q.A., He, B.M., Zhou, K.:** Effects of lactulose on intestinal endotoxin and bacterial translocation in cirrhotic rats. Clin. Med. J. 2003; 116: 767–771
192. **Zoli, M., Cordiani, M.R., Marchesini, G., Iervese, T., Morselli Labate, A.M., Bonazzi, C., Bianchi, G., Pisi, E.:** Prognostic indicators in compensated cirrhosis. Amer. J. Gastroenterol. 1991; 86: 1508–1513
193. **Zoli, M., Merkel, C., Magalotti, D., Gueli, C., Grimaldi, M., Gatta, A., Bernardi, M.:** Natural history of cirrhotic patients with small esophageal varices: a prospective study. Amer. J. Gastroenterol. 2000; 95: 503–508
194. **Zullo, A., Rinaldi, V., Meddi, P., Folino, S., Lauria, V., Diana, F., Winn, S., Attili, A.F.:** Helicobacter pylori infection in dyspeptic cirrhotic patients. Hepatogastroenterol. 1999; 46: 395–400

Clinical Aspects of Liver Diseases
36 Benign hepatic lesions and tumours

		Page:
1	*Definition*	774
2	***Classification***	774
2.1	Sonomorphological classification	774
2.2	Histological classification	774
3	***Diagnostics***	775
3.1	Anamnesis	775
3.2	Complaints	775
3.3	Findings	775
3.4	Imaging procedures	775
3.5	Biopsy and laparoscopy	776
4	***Differential diagnosis***	776
4.1	Adenoma	776
4.2	Focal nodular hyperplasia	777
4.3	Nodular regenerative hyperplasia	779
4.4	Haemangioma	779
4.5	Infantile haemangioendothelioma	781
4.6	Fat-containing tumours	782
4.6.1	Focal fatty changes	782
4.6.2	Lipoma	782
4.6.3	Myelolipoma	782
4.6.4	Angiolipoma	782
4.6.5	Angiomyolipoma	782
4.7	Chondroma	782
4.8	Leiomyoma	783
4.9	Schwannoma	783
4.10	Glomangioma	783
4.11	Mesenchymal hamartoma	783
4.12	Mesothelioma	783
4.13	Fibrous tumour	783
4.14	Cysts	783
4.14.1	Polycystic liver disease	784
4.14.2	Parasitic cysts	784
4.15	Cholangiocellular tumours	785
4.15.1	Caroli's disease/syndrome	785
4.15.2	Hepatobiliary cystadenoma	785
4.15.3	Bile-duct adenomas	785
4.15.4	Bile-duct papillomatosis	786
4.15.5	Biliary hamartoma	787
4.16	Abscesses	787
4.17	Lymphangioma	787
4.18	Peliosis hepatis	787
4.19	Granulomas	787
4.19.1	Sarcoidosis	788
4.20	Inflammatory pseudotumour	789
4.21	Erdheim-Chester disease	789
4.22	Calcareous foci	789
5	***Surgical treatment***	790
	• References (1−210)	791
	(Figures 36.1−36.24; tables 36.1−36.5)	

36 Benign hepatic lesions and tumours

1 Definition

The term **lesion** denotes a circumscribed impairment of function or tissue structure, while the word **tumour** describes a circumscribed swelling or the growth of body tissue. • **Benign hepatic focal lesions** are circumscribed alterations. They differ markedly from the surrounding hepatic tissue, which shows a normal or diffusely changed structure. Differences in tissue type or chemical composition are revealed by imaging procedures. Benign hepatic coin lesions can appear either in solitary or multiple form. They may be only 1–2 mm in size or cover large hepatic areas, and even a complete lobe.

2 Classification

Benign hepatic focal lesions are usually detected as an incidental finding in sonography. As a rule, there are no subjective or characteristic complaints, no identified neoplastic disease and no objective clinical findings.

2.1 Sonomorphological classification

Sonomorphological differentiation may be helpful in classifying incidentally detected liver foci: (*1.*) anechoic, (*2.*) hypoechoic, and (*3.*) echogenic lesions. (s. tab. 36.1)

Anechoic lesions	Hypoechoic lesions
Caroli's syndrome	Adenoma
Cysts	Echinococcus alveolaris
Echinococcus alveolaris	FNH
Fresh haematoma	Focal non-fatty changes
Liquefied abscess	Fresh abscess
Osler's disease	Hamartoma
Echogenic lesions	Lymphoma
Fibroma	NRH
Focal fatty changes	Old haematoma
Granuloma	Peliosis hepatis
Haemangioma	Regenerative nodes
Hamartoma	
Lipoma	
Regenerative nodes	

Tab. 36.1: Sonomorphological classification of benign hepatic focal lesions according to their (predominant) echogenicity

As a typical anechoic focus, a cyst displays a delicate margin, dorsal sound reduction and a completely anechoic lumen. • Focal hepatic lesions or coin lesions are variable in size, number, internal echo (homogeneous or structured), demarcation from the surrounding hepatic tissue and secondary findings (displacement effects, compression). • *It is important to rule out malignant hepatic tumours.*

2.2 Histological classification

Differential diagnosis of circular hepatic foci helps to decide whether therapeutic measures are necessary, not required, or not feasible. • The histological *classification* of benign coin-like hepatic lesions differentiates between (*1.*) hepatocellular tumours, (*2.*) cholangiocellular tumours, (*3.*) mesenchymal tumours, and (*4.*) tumour-like lesions. There may also be evidence of (*5.*) calcareous foci. (2, 3, 6, 11, 14) (s. tab. 36.2)

1. **Hepatocellular tumours**
   Adenoma
   Focal nodular hyperplasia
   Nodular regenerative hyperplasia
   Regenerative nodes
2. **Cholangiocellular tumours**
   Bile-duct papillomatosis
   Biliary hamartoma
   Caroli's disease/syndrome
   Intrahepatic bile-duct adenoma
   Intrahepatic bile-duct cystadenoma
3. **Mesenchymal tumours**
   Angiolipoma
   Angiomyolipoma
   Benign haemangioendothelioma
   Cavernous haemangioma
   Chondroma
   Fibrous tumour
   Focal fatty changes
   Glomangioma
   Leiomyoma
   Lipoma
   Lymphangioma
   Mesenchymal hamartoma
   Mesothelioma
   Myelolipoma
   Myolipoma
   Myxoma
   Schwannoma
4. **Tumour-like lesions**
   Abscess
   Cyst
   Granuloma
   Haematoma
   Inflammatory pseudotumour
   Peliosis hepatis
5. **Calcareous foci**

Tab. 36.2: Histological classification of benign hepatic coin lesions

3 Diagnostics

3.1 Anamnesis

In most cases, benign liver tumours are detected by chance during sonography. Any *information* elicited during anamnesis about the long-term use of contraceptives, androgens or medication as well as any possible intake of chemicals, potential infections with parasites or zoonoses, abdominal trauma or febrile diseases and previous episodes of jaundice may be important.

3.2 Complaints

There are usually no subjective complaints – except when there are large space-occupying lesions which cause anorexia, weight loss, upper abdominal pain upon pressure, haemorrhaging in the tumour or tumour rupture. Febrile conditions and pain may point to infection, liver abscess or echinococcosis.

3.3 Findings

Anamnesis and **complaints** are of little diagnostic value. Clinical examination frequently reveals non-characteristic findings, such as hepatomegaly, abdominal pain on pressure, diaphragmatic elevation, right-sided pleural effusion or hepatic vascular murmur (e. g. in large haemangiomas). **Laboratory parameters** are mostly normal. Sometimes the transaminases and γ-GT are elevated; AP and respective values relating to cholestasis can be higher. In an inflammatory process, CRP and BSR are often elevated, while ChE and iron may be lower.

3.4 Imaging procedures

The following imaging procedures can be used for the detection and differential diagnosis of benign hepatic lesions or tumours: (*1.*) sonography, (*2.*) computer tomography, (*3.*) scintigraphy, and (*4.*) magnetic resonance imaging. These methods show clear differences in their ability to detect tumours of minimum size, in their sensitivity and specificity, and in the costs involved. • Echogenic and anechoic foci can obviously be detected by sonography at a much smaller diameter than hypoechoic foci. In scintigraphy, hepatic tumours in the portal area and in the centre of the liver must have a larger diameter in order to be visualized. By combining scintigraphy and CT, it is generally possible to differentiate FNH from adenoma. In CT and MRI, detection of a tumour depends on its structure. • Sensitivity, i.e. the rate of correct positive results, should be as high as possible, but there are clear differences here. The specificity of these diagnostic procedures is high at 90 to 95%.

Sonography is the method of choice on the basis of the following *criteria*: (*1.*) it has a high diagnostic yield (including extrahepatic areas), (*2.*) it is cost-effective, (*3.*) it can be used in various locations, (*4.*) it is not time-consuming, and (*5.*) it does not burden the patient. The use of new techniques (contrast-enhanced power Doppler sonography, phase-invasion harmonic imaging) can help to make the assessment more reliable in individual cases. US is clearly inferior to CT when it comes to diagnosing metastases. (5) • *It should be noted that the respective diagnostic reliability is highly dependent upon the investigator's experience.* (s. tab. 36.3)

Computer tomography has a greater sensitivity than sonography; however, there are higher costs involved, it takes more time, requires more space and entails exposure to radiation. More sophisticated methods such as helical CT or CT arterioportography allow a more differentiated application in certain constellations (e. g. malignant lymphoma, metastases of parvicellular bronchial carcinoma, or breast cancer). Permanent-location CT with administration of bolus contrast medium is suitable for the differentiation of haemangioma. Sonography and CT are considered to be useful complementary techniques in diagnosing hepatic focal lesions, since in this way foci can be detected which are missed by the respective other method. (1) (s. tab. 36.3)

Criterion	US	CT	MRI	SC	FNB	Lap
Detectable size of focus (cm)	>0.5	>0.8	>1.0	>2.0	>1.5	>0.1
Sensitivity (%)	50–70	60–90	70–95	40–60	75–90	ca. 100
Specificity (%)	90	>95	>95	>95	ca. 100	ca. 100
Additional information	+	+	+	∅	∅	++
Costs	(+)	++	+++	++	(+)	+

Tab. 36.3: Respective values of the different diagnostic methods regarding the detection of hepatic focal lesions (US = ultrasound, CT = computer tomography, MRI = magnetic resonance imaging, SC = scintigraphy, FNB = fine-needle biopsy, Lap = laparoscopic findings at the liver surface)

Magnetic resonance imaging may provide e. g. extra differentiation of unclarified findings (particularly in diagnosis of haemangioma). Hypovascular lesions are detected more easily with SPIO-enhanced MRI, whereas detection and characterization of hypervascular lesions are best with gadolinium-enhanced MRI. (1, 7, 13) (s. tab. 36.3)

Scintigraphy can be indicated for differentiating an adenoma from FNH (combination of colloid scintigram and hepatobiliary sequential scintigraphy) and for diagnosing haemangioma. (12)

Angiography: Visualization of hepatic veins or arteries is rarely required. Angiography is indicated for diagnosing metastases of active endocrine tumours. This technique may also be necessary in the planning phase of liver surgery. A further possible indication is its use in carrying out therapeutic measures.

3.5 Biopsy and laparoscopy

Reliable differentiation between benign and malignant hepatic tumour is not possible using imaging procedures; thus, an indication is given for US-guided or CT-controlled **fine-needle biopsy**. (s. tab. 36.3) (s. pp 133, 156) However, FNB is diagnostically inferior to thick-needle biopsy (>1.2 mm) − although the bleeding risk is clearly much lower. The indication for **biopsy** should be viewed critically, particularly when considering the use of a thick needle. (4) • *In all cases where the findings cannot be substantiated by imaging procedures and where treatment implications can be expected as a result of diagnostic clarification, laparoscopy is indicated. The combination of laparoscopy and biopsy yields the highest diagnostic sensitivity and specificity. The diagnostic reliability is almost 100% in focal lesions on the liver surface.* (9, 10) Tissue samples for histological examination can be gained from selected tumour areas by careful, directed **forceps biopsy** (also by FNB). Laparoscopy makes possible the photographic documentation of the findings as well as of any additional important pathological changes in the abdominal cavity − this may prove very helpful. (s. tab. 36.3.) *(see chapter 7!)*

4 Differential diagnosis

4.1 Adenoma

Epidemiology and aetiology: Adenomas have an incidence of 4−10/100,000 inhabitants/year. They are almost exclusively found in women during their reproductive years. Children are rarely affected. (29) In men, the risk is higher when they take anabolic agents. In about 90% of cases, there is a correlation with the intake of oral contraceptives over many years; this was pointed out for the first time by J.K. BAUM et al. in 1973. (19, 22, 26, 33, 34) There is also an association with the polycystic ovary syndrome. (35) An adenoma can develop in glycogenosis types I and III (with multilocular nodulation) (30) as well as in type IV. (15) The administration of various other drugs (e.g. carbamazepine) has also been associated with adenomas.

Morphology: Adenomas are mostly solitary (75%) and located mainly in the right liver lobe (65−70%). The rare occurrence of multiple adenomas (>3 lesions) is termed *adenomatosis* of the liver. (20) A familial form has been observed, showing the association with germline hepatocyte nuclear factor alpha. (17) Usually, adenomas develop close to the surface beneath the liver capsule. They vary greatly in size, but have an average diameter of 10 cm (2 cm to >30 cm); even pediculate nodes have been observed. Adenomas are hypervascularized and have a firm, rubber-like consistency. Due to their bright red to light brown colour, they stand out from the rest of the hepatic tissue. (s. fig. 29.11!)

Histology: The parenchyma is formed from pluricellular trabeculae and two (or three) layers of hepatocytes, the width of which varies from location to location. The hepatocytes are rich in glycogen, often pleomorphic and enlarged, and usually show fine-droplet fatty deposits. No evidence of acinar architecture or Kupffer cells is found; very few preexisting and incorporated portal fields, central veins or bile ducts are detectable. There are numerous arteries and ectatic sinusoids (without Kupffer cells). This is the site of haemorrhages into necroses which are mostly found in larger nodes. These haemorrhages may also penetrate the adjacent liver parenchyma and rupture into the abdominal cavity. There are no fibroses or inflammatory reactions. Reticular fibres are delicate or have disappeared completely. Adenomas often possess a capsule made of fibre tissue or compressed liver parenchyma, so that adenoma nodes are easy to enucleate from their hepatic bed. (20, 23, 25)

▶ According to recent studies, adenomas can be classified into four forms: (1.) **archtypical adenoma** (monoclonal, no atypias, no inflammation, no ductular structures), (2.) **variant 1** (mutation of HNFα gene, steatosis ++, no atypias, no inflammation), (3.) **variant 2** (mutation of β-catenin gene, minor atypias, slight metaplasias), and (4.) **variant 3** (monoclonal, previously "telangiectatic type of FNH", ductular structures, inflammatory infiltrates, sinus ectasias). (18)

Diagnosis: Small adenomas do not cause any discomfort. Large adenomas may become palpable or cause pain upon pressure and have displacement effects. **Laboratory parameters** are generally normal, although AP is sometimes increased; the serum value of AFP remains unchanged. The administration of oestrogen results in a subnormal γ-GT value. • **Sonography, CT** and **MRI** do not show any abnormalities, since the tissue is hepatogenic and thus somewhat hypoechoic or hypodense on a non-enhanced CT scan, but hyperdense in the arterial phase. In some cases, a space-occupying lesion is detectable. There may be evidence of circular vascularization, from which irregular vessels penetrate the adenoma. (16, 28, 32) (s. pp 142, 181) Hypervascularized adenomas can be seen in colour Doppler sonography (as well as in coeliacography or MR angiography). Differential diagnosis of haemangioma, HCC or metastases may be rendered more difficult by haemorrhages. • **Scintigraphy** using ^{99m}Tc sulphur colloid shows no activity enhancement. Functional scintigraphy reveals a normal flow and reduced or no enhancement in the parenchymal and excretory phases. • **Laparoscopy** facilitates a *"split-second visual diagnosis"*, with histological confirmation by forceps biopsy, if required. (s. tab. 36.3) (s. fig. 29.11!)

Complications: Intense pain may occur due to haemorrhage in the adenoma or haemorrhagic penetration of the neighbouring liver parenchyma. A rupture causes haemoperitoneum with symptoms typical of acute abdomen and circulatory shock. (s. fig. 36.1) • An association between

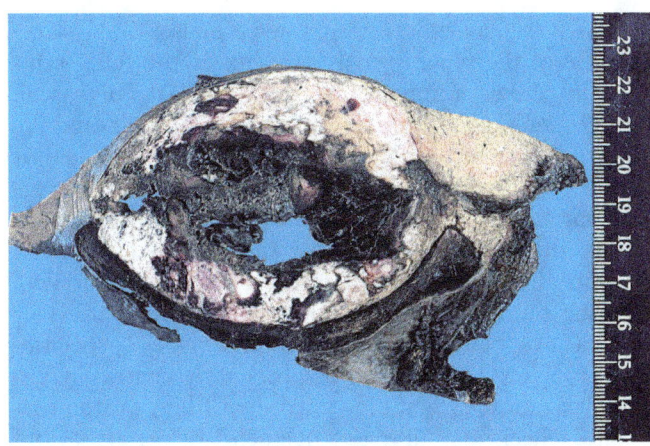

Fig. 36.1: Spontaneously ruptured hepatocellular adenoma in non-cirrhotic liver tissue (30-year-old woman, 15 year's use of oral contraceptives)

menstruation and adenoma rupture has been reported. The risk of bleeding is 30–40%. Malignant degeneration is a potential danger (approx. 10%). (24, 26, 31, 33) • *We can add one observation of our own regarding malignant degeneration.* (s. p. 563) (s. fig. 29.14!)

Prognosis: All in all, prognosis is relatively good. While some adenomas became smaller or even went into remission as soon as oral contraceptives were discontinued (19), there were other cases in which the tumour maintained its size or indeed continued to grow. Even after regression of the adenoma, there is always a danger of hepatocellular carcinoma developing. Systemic AA amyloidosis or paraneoplastic symptoms are rare complications. (22) Monitoring is effected by US or CT, as appropriate. Determination of hormone receptors could provide an additional prognostic criterion in the future. Alkaline phosphatase, γ-GT and ChE, for example, may serve as laboratory parameters.

Treatment: Imaging procedures cannot exclude the presence of malignant adenoma degeneration. This uncertainty, together with a high risk of haemorrhage and rupture, which increases with further growth of the tumour, provides the basic indication for enucleation or resection of the adenoma, particularly in the event of an unexpected trauma of the liver. Embolization prior to resection leads to a reduction in size of larger adenomas, thus giving better results. Surgery is indicated from the outset: (*1.*) when an already large adenoma (>5 cm) is present at initial diagnosis, (*2.*) in pediculate tumours, (*3.*) in cases of proven haemorrhage or subcapsular haematoma, (*4.*) when there is an increased risk of abdominal trauma in everyday life, and (*5.*) prior to a planned pregnancy. • *As a rule, every resectable adenoma should be removed surgically.* (20, 23, 29, 31, 38, 40)

4.2 Focal nodular hyperplasia

Epidemiology and aetiology: Focal nodular hyperplasia (FNH) was first described by M. Simmonds in 1884. It is about twice as common as adenoma and is the second most frequent type of benign liver tumour. Its incidence is 20 (−30)/100,000 inhabitants/year; in autopsy statistics, frequency is 0.3−8.0%. FNH has also been observed in children (53), as has the simultaneous occurrence of FNH and adenoma. Cigarette smoking is deemed to be a risk factor. FNH affects mainly women (80%); in some 60−70% of women, there is a connection with the long-term intake of oral contraceptives (48) and the Klinefelter syndrome. (56) When the contraceptives are discontinued, FNH (like adenoma) often goes into remission. A hyperplastic reaction to a pre-existing arterial malformation is thought to be one of the pathogenetic possibilities. This view is substantiated by evidence of other concomitant vascular abnormalities (e.g. haemangioma in 20−25% of cases, aneurysm, teleangiectasia) and malformations (e.g. brain tumour) or indeed the occurrence of FNH among family members. FNH is caused by increased arteriohepatic perfusion and additional local portovenous thrombosis, resulting in nodular hyperplasia of the hyperperfused parenchyma. (8, 49) In a recent study, increased values of the genes angiopoietin 1 and 2 have been reported. (51)

Morphology: FNH is usually solitary; multiple nodes of varying sizes (up to 20 cm) are only detected in about 20% of cases. (41, 55) FNH is present mainly in the right liver lobe (50−60%), in individual cases also as a pediculate tumour. There is generally no capsule. FNH has a firm consistency. In two thirds of cases, strikingly large arteries can be seen supplying the tumour. Tumours located close to the surface are reddish-brown to yellowish-brown in colour. (s. fig. 29.12!) • A **progressive type** of FNH is a rare variant; however, this type may recur following partial liver resection. (56) The **teleangiectatic type** of FNH displays a molecular pattern closer to that of adenomas than to FNA; therefore these atypical lesions should be referred to as "teleangiectatic hepatocellular adenomas". (s. p. 776) (s. fig. 36.2)

▶ **Histology:** Hepatocytes are rich in glycogen. There is no lobular structure, since portal fields and central veins

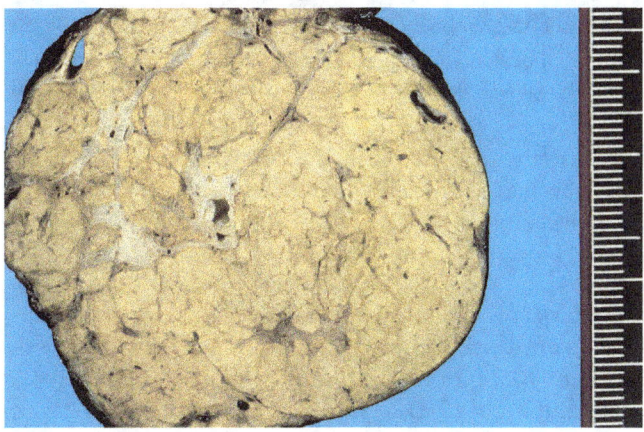

Fig. 36.2: Focal nodular hyperplasia: sharply delineated, ochre-coloured, non-encapsulated, nodulated lesion with star-shaped radiating septa

are absent. But there are Kupffer cells and sinusoids with varying dilatations. Many bile-duct proliferations are found, e.g. within the connective tissue septa. These findings may lead to *misdiagnosing* "cholangiocarcinoma in cirrhosis", since numerous, sometimes chaotic, blood vessels are present. Connective tissue bands originating from a *central scar* and directed towards the periphery contain biliary tract elements, arteries and veins, infiltrates and occasional epithelioid cell granulomas. Thick-walled blood vessels show mucoid media degenerations. These *hypervascular septa* cut off parenchymal areas of varying sizes and form pseudoacini. The result is a wheelspoke-like structure and the clinical picture of *pseudocirrhosis*. (36, 41, 42, 43, 49) (s. fig. 29.13!)

Diagnosis: When FNH reaches a certain size (7–10 cm or more), upper abdominal pain upon pressure, displacement effects and hepatomegaly occur, i.e. FNH remains asymptomatic for a long period of time. Laboratory parameters are normal. Cholestasis is a rare finding. • **Sonography** shows a hypoechoic image corresponding to that of the liver. (s. figs. 6.14; 36.3)

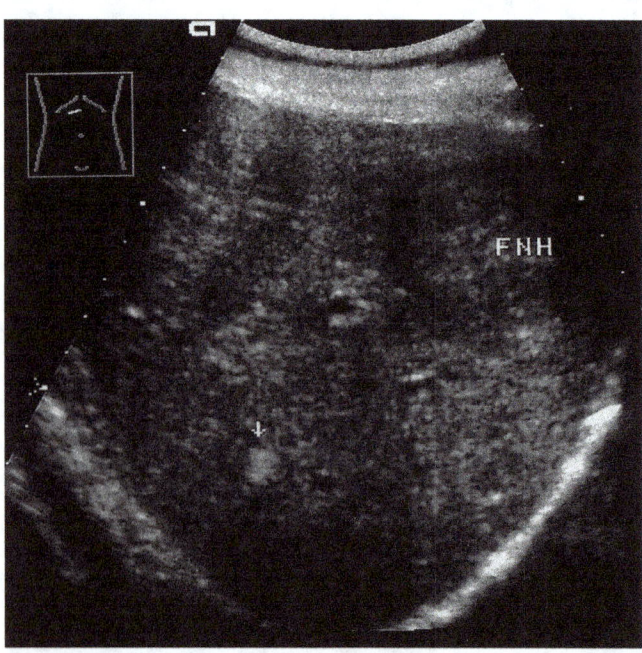

Fig. 36.3: Focal nodular hyperplasia (FNH). (There is also evidence of a small hyperechoic focal lesion, probably haemangioma)

It is often possible to identify a fibrous *"vascular star"* with vessels in a radial or circular arrangement similar to a *"wheelspoke pattern"*. This is clearly visualized by colour Doppler sonography. (s. fig. 36.4) (44, 45, 47, 57) **CT** usually shows a hypodense tumour with smooth boundaries and short, inhomogeneous, massive enhancement during the arterial phase (12–25 sec), with contrast adaptation to the neighbouring parenchyma occurring after 45–120 sec. There may also be signs of the central scar. Spiral CT increases diagnostic accuracy. (36, 37, 39, 58, 59) (s. fig. 36.5) • Following administration of Gd-DTPA, **MRI** yields similar results to CT. The fibrous vascular star appears hyperdense (T_2). (44) • Because of the phagocytosis capacity of the RES, **scintigraphy** shows storage of colloids (in 70% of cases), whereby enhanced storage is seen as pathognomonic. Some 30% remain "cold" due to increasing weakness of the RES. Functional scintigraphy helps to detect hypervascularization as well as (mild to normal) enhancement during the parenchymal phase and retarded excretion (= trapping) as a result of rarefied bile ducts, showing that the remaining liver tissue has long been freed of ^{99m}Tc IDA (= afterstorage). Sensitivity is 87%, specificity is 100%. • **Angiography** displays early central hypervascularization with rapid centrifugal filling of the tortuous, wheelspoke-like arrangement of arteries and delayed venous visualization. • Clear differentiation, e.g.

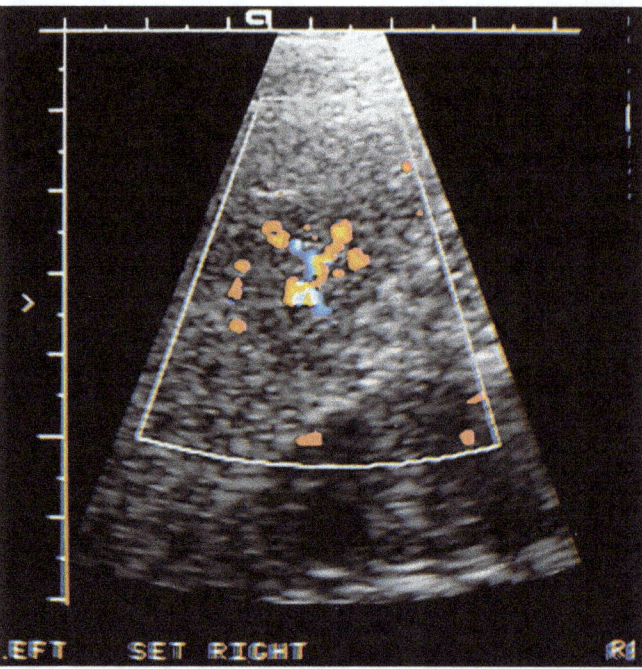

Fig. 36.4: Colour-encoded Doppler sonography of FNH with wheelspoke pattern (s. fig. 6.14!)

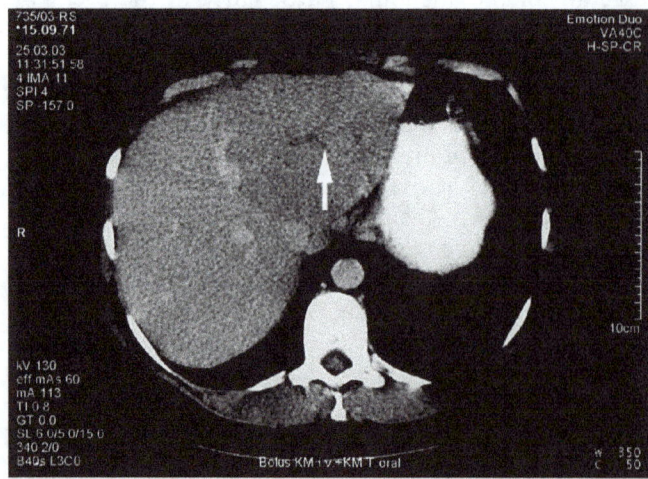

Fig. 36.5: CT in the portal venous phase: FNH with star-shaped scar

from HCC, is often impossible with imaging procedures. An unclear diagnosis calls for **laparoscopy** (9, 10), (s. figs. 29.12, 29.13), possibly with refined forceps biopsy or fine-needle biopsy. (54) • Thick-needle biopsy is contraindicated due to the risk of bleeding (and because FNH does not require histological examination).

Complications: In 10% of cases, there is a potential risk of vein obstruction (52) or bleeding. Portal hypertension can develop, in some cases with pulmonary hypertension. Spontaneous regression has been reported. (50) • Malignant degeneration is extremely rare.

Treatment: Monitoring by imaging procedures suffices in the first instance. A marked increase in size and particularly haemorrhage or rupture are indications for embolization or surgery. (38, 40, 46)

4.3 Nodular regenerative hyperplasia

▶ The first description was given in 1953 by S. Ranström, who called this condition "miliary hepatocellular adenomatosis". The term "nodular regenerative hyperplasia" was introduced by P. E. Steiner in 1959.

In nodular regenerative hyperplasia (NRH), the liver is interspersed with numerous diffuse nodes, which are 1–3 mm in size (occasionally up to 3 cm) and yellow to yellowish brown in colour with blurred boundaries; they consist of hyperplastic hepatocytes. No fibroses or perinodal connective tissue septa are evident. The multilayered, disordered trabeculae do not have a lobular structure. (69, 72) CD 8^+ cytotoxic T cells infiltrate the acinus. The nodes lack central veins and bile duct proliferations. The internodular parenchyma becomes atrophied due to pressure. It is possible with reticulin staining to show nodes containing irregular trabeculae, whereas the altered vessels are best seen using elastica staining. The liver surface is smooth. In the course of disease, presinusoidal, and later sinusoidal, portal hypertension with hepatosplenomegaly and oesophageal varices are usually observed. (67, 68, 70) (s. fig. 36.6)

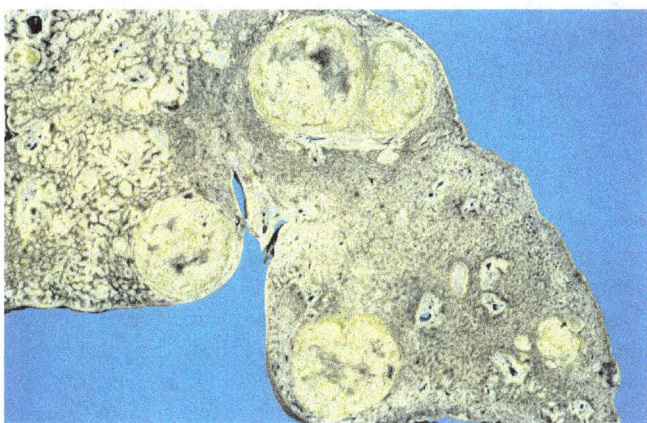

Fig. 36.6: Macroregenerative nodes in liver cirrhosis with Budd-Chiari syndrome

Men and women are affected with the same frequency at almost any age. Familial forms have been described. (65) There is an association with polyarthritis, coeliac disease (60), PSC, PBC (63), sarcoidosis, Budd-Chiari syndrome (s. fig. 36.6), and collagenoses or myeloproliferative diseases. A connection with thorotrast (61), immunosuppressives, cytostatics and contraceptives or androgens as well as with antirheumatics, arsenic, vinyl chloride and the so-called "toxic oil syndrome" is also postulated. • As a pathogenetic factor, disturbance of the microcirculation is discussed: reduced blood perfusion can lead to atrophy of the ischaemic acini with subsequent stimulation of hyperperfused areas, resulting in nodular hyperplasia. (8, 43) • Occasionally, transaminases, AP and γ-GT are increased. Using sonography, it is possible to find an inhomogeneous reflex pattern in the case of larger nodules. CT may show hypodense lesions with peripheral-central enhancement of the contrast medium. Imaging techniques can misjudge the NRH as a micronodular cirrhosis. (64, 71) Diagnosis is confirmed by laparoscopy (62, 66) with forceps biopsy or two to three large biopsy specimens. (9, 10) • As a rule, NHR progresses slowly and has at least one stationary stage. However, ALF has been reported in four patients. • *Therapy* consists of treating portal hypertension (TIPS or surgical shunt); liver transplantation may be indicated. (67)

▶ **Partial nodular transformation:** This form is characterized by morphological changes similar to those observed in NRH, but with only partial liver involvement. (70) Formation of nodes is limited to the area where the larger vessels begin, i.e. perihilar region. The pale nodes can reach a size of up to 4 cm. Haemorrhage and necrosis may occur in larger nodes.

4.4 Haemangioma

Epidemiology and aetiology: F. Th. Frerichs (s. fig. 1) described a haemangioma for the first time in 1861. • With a frequency of 2–8% and an incidence of 800/100,000 inhabitants/year, it is the most common benign tumour of the liver and is about 40 (−100) times more frequent than adenoma. It occurs in all ages, but is observed slightly more often in women than in men. There is no association with the intake of oestrogen or progesterone, although a higher frequency has been recorded in multiparous women. Puberty, pregnancy and oestrogens may cause an increase in tumour size. The aetiology is unknown. Haemangiomas have also been detected in children (85); this finding suggests that these tumours are true neoformations. There is no known malignant degenerative tendency. Haemangiomas may become thrombosed, fibrosed or calcified.

Histology: Due to vascular malformation, thin-walled spaces, which are filled with blood and lined with endothelium, develop; they are separated by septa. The blood is thrombosed or the thrombus becomes organized. The surrounding liver parenchyma is unchanged. (s. fig. 36.7)

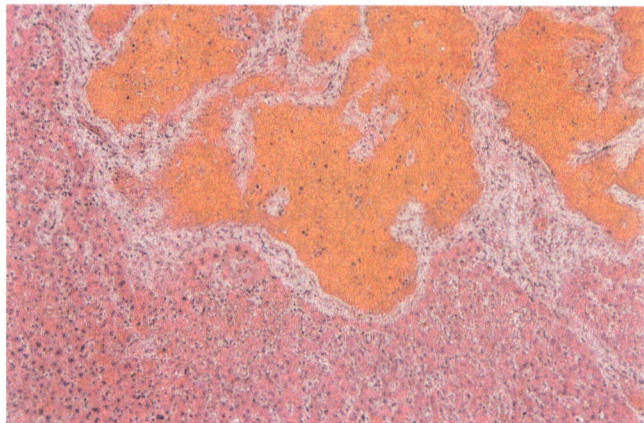

Fig. 36.7: Cavernous haemangioma: thin-walled spaces lined with endothelium, partially septated, filled with blood. The surrounding parenchyma appears to be unchanged (HE)

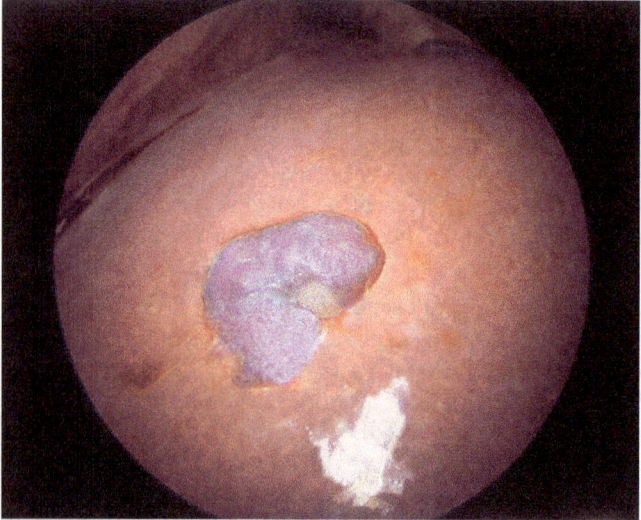

Fig. 36.8: Grape-shaped, multi-chambered, livid bluish haemangioma (right liver lobe)

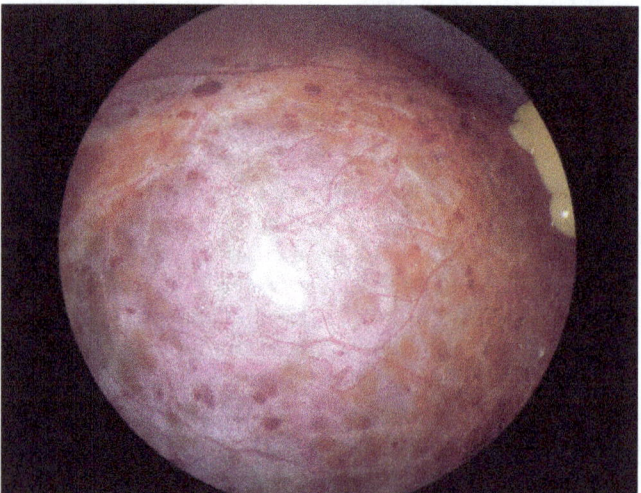

Fig. 36.9: Giant (larger than a fist) cavernous haemangioma with a smooth surface in the left liver lobe. Numerous blood vessels and peliosis-like livid blue foci of up to 0.5 cm in size in the capsule area

Morphology: Haemangiomas appear in solitary or (in some 20—30% of cases) multiple form. (87) They are usually located beneath the liver capsule and are clearly differentiated from the parenchyma by a pseudocapsule. Their usual size is 1—4 cm and they are found in both liver lobes, apparently with a higher frequency in the left lobe. It is worth mentioning that the haemangiomas situated in the right lobe are predominantly found in the usual percutaneous biopsy area (which needs to be taken into account in prepuncture sonography). Haemangiomas continue to grow due to enlargement of the respective cavernous spaces. *Laparoscopically,* haemangiomas appear as bluish red or crimson red structures, sometimes tuberous, usually protruding slightly beyond the liver capsule; a multi-chambered structure is visible in most cases. (s. fig. 36.8, 36.9) • More rarely (about 7%), voluminous tumours, which may spread over the whole liver lobe, develop (= *giant haemangioma*, with a size of > 10 cm). (76, 77, 81, 86, 88, 89, 94) Up to now, only about 20 cases involving *giant pedunculated forms* have been observed.

Diagnosis: Haemangiomas are usually asymptomatic and, as a rule, discovered incidentally. Having reached a particular size, however, they may cause upper abdominal pain, nausea and inappetence. Acute pain results from bleeding in the tumour, thrombosis or rupture. Palpation may suggest hepatomegaly or an unusual kind of resistance. • Laboratory values are within the normal range. Thrombopenia and/or a reduction in fibrinogen may be present in thrombosis. (79, 84, 90, 97)

Sonography shows a hyperechoic structure (60—70%) with smooth boundaries, but no hypoechoic margin or sound shadow (= *white tumour*). There may be an efferent and an afferent vessel. As the size of the haemangioma increases, thrombosis develops, while connective tissue organisation and regressive liquefaction become evident. Inhomogeneous and irregular internal structures result from this, making diagnostic classification difficult. Sensitivity is about 80%. (78, 79, 83, 96, 98) (s. fig. 6.15) • **Computer tomography** shows a hypodense tumour. After intravenous bolus contrast-medium injection, enhancement increases in a peripheral-central direction followed by a focal globular contrast and subsequently a rapid reduction of the contrast-rich zone *("iris diaphragm phenomenon")*; this occurs in ca. 60% of cases. The haemangioma becomes isodense with the liver parenchyma. The isodense phase may last up to 90 minutes. The sensitivity of this examination is about 90%. (93) (s. figs. 8.5, 8.9) • **MRI** displays a low-signal T_1 time and pronounced hyperintensity in the T_2-weighted picture with well-defined margins, which means that even haemangiomas smaller than 1.0 cm can be detected. The *"cotton wool sign"* is followed by the *"light bulb sign"*. The heterogeneous structure points to thrombosis, fibrosis, etc. Both the specificity and sensitivity of MRI are 85—95%. (75, 98) (s. figs. 8.7; 36.10 a—c) • In the blood pool scintigram (Tc^{99m}-

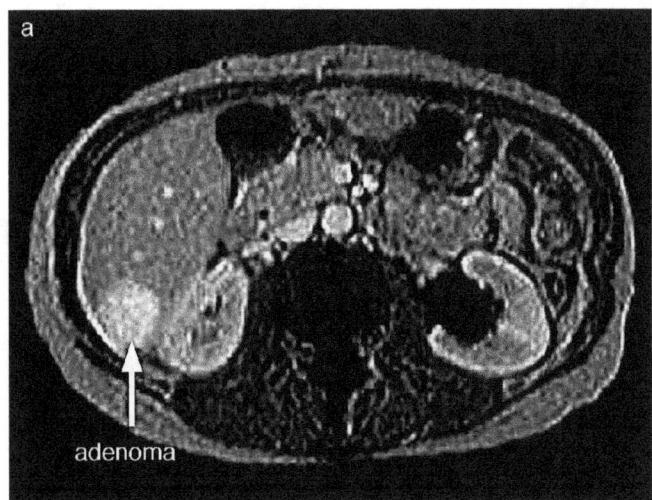

Fig. 36.10: a) Adenoma (↑), (not visible) haemangioma (the same female patient as in b and c)

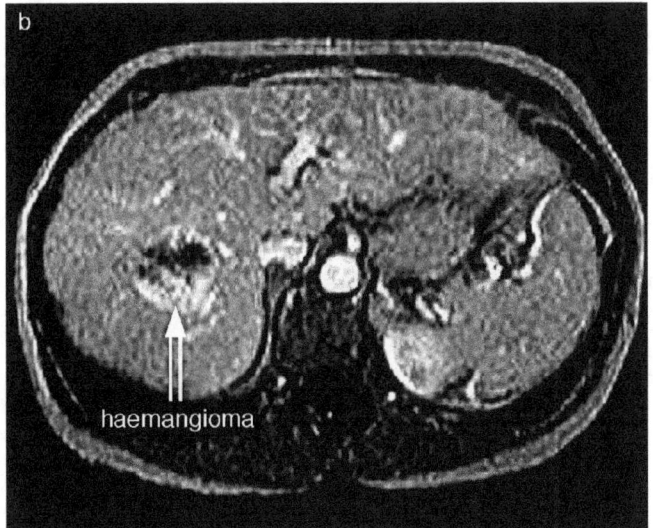

b) Haemangioma (↑) in MRI: T_1-weighted axial (portovenous) ("cotton wool sign") (the same female patient as in a and c)

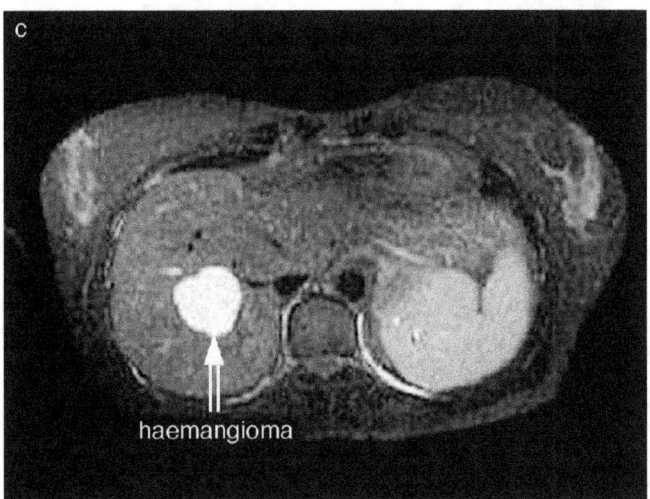

c) Haemangioma (↑): T_2-weighted ("light bulb sign"), with fat suppression (the same female patient as in a and b)

marked autologous erythrocytes), **scintigraphy** shows the pathognomonically useful filling-in phenomenon. Activity enhancement increases from the periphery towards the centre and is detectable for several hours. By contrast, the haemangioma remains negative both in static and liver-function scintigraphy; this is because the haemangioma has neither hepatocytes nor RES cells. (73, 75, 83, 89) • **Fine-needle biopsy** (82) is occasionally favoured. *We consider percutaneous biopsy, particularly thick-needle biopsy, to be contraindicated because of the risk of bleeding (it is indeed of little help from a diagnostic viewpoint, since better diagnostic tools are available); we also feel that there is no justification in using exploratory laparotomy for diagnostic purposes.* • In order to obtain a definitive diagnosis, **exploratory laparoscopy** is the method of choice, since haemangiomas are usually situated in the subcapsular area, which means that a *"split-second visual diagnosis"* is possible ("one-second biopsy" is not indicated!). (9, 10) (s. figs. 36.5, 36.6)

Complications: Blunt abdominal trauma increases the risk of rupture, which can also occur spontaneously. The mortality rate is 60–80%. (74) Large shunt volumes may give rise to the development of cardiac insufficiency, particularly during childhood. The development of portal hypertension has also been observed. (97) Anaemia, thrombopenia and hypofibrinogenaemia may occur due to the haemangioma-thrombocytopathy syndrome (= *Kasabach-Merritt syndrome*). (86)

Treatment: A ruptured haemangioma requires immediate surgical intervention; it is often necessary to ligate the hepatic artery. Enucleation is sometimes possible. (80, 90) Resection or arterial embolization are recommended for very large and symptomatic haemangiomas. Inoperable tumours should be reduced in size by external irradiation or interferon-α therapy. Liver transplantation is a rare indication. (91, 92, 95) • All in all, prognosis is good. (97)

4.5 Infantile haemangioendothelioma

This benign infantile tumour is of embryonic origin and usually diagnosed within the first months of life, whereby girls are twice as often affected as boys. In most cases, capillary haemangiomas of the skin and mucosa as well as of other organs are also in evidence. Cardiac and vascular malformations are often found.

Morphology: Haemangioendotheliomas appear in solitary or (seldom) multiple form and may reach a size of some 15 cm. The unencapsulated tumour foci have blurred boundaries. They are sponge-like and reddish brown in colour, but may become firm and grey in bigger tumours. Vascular segments of differing width are connected with each other and embedded in loose, cell-rich mesenchyma. • Two **histological types** can be differentiated: *type I* is characterized by a layer of cuboid endothelial cells, while *type II* shows papillary proliferations and several layers of pleomorphic cells (which are similar to those found in angiosarcoma). Malignant degeneration of the haemangioendothelioma is possible.

Diagnosis: Hepatomegaly and an occasional systolic vascular murmur above the tumour are clinically detectable. Patients suffer from anorexia, vomiting, weight loss and lethargy. Laboratory investigation often reveals thrombopenia, haemolytic jaundice and anaemia. Disseminated intravascular coagulopathy (= *Kasabach-Merrit syndrome*) can occur. Signs of cardiac insufficiency are present at an early stage due to arteriovenous shunts with cardiac volume overload. Acute pain is a sign of haemorrhage in the tumour or of a ruptured tumour. Diagnosis is established by imaging techniques; angiography has been widely replaced by colour Doppler sonography or angio-MR. Occasionally, laparoscopy has also been used. (99–105)

Treatment: If it is possible, elective resection is indicated. (103) However, due to cardiac or (increasing) hepatic insufficiency, invasive techniques cannot usually be attempted. External irradiation may be used in an effort to minimize the tumour. Ligature or embolization of the afferent hepatic artery is sometimes indicated. Steroid therapy has proved unsuccessful. The use of interferon-α is a new therapeutic approach: tumour regression is accelerated and cardiac insufficiency is compensated. (106) Liver transplantations have also been carried out successfully. This infantile, benign tumour may regress with increasing age.

4.6 Fat-containing tumours

4.6.1 Focal fatty changes

Circumscribed fatty foci ("yellow spots") were seen relatively often during laparoscopy in the past. (13) We ourselves also observed them on many occasions. (s. fig. 31.6) • Sonography and CT have shown these rare benign foci to be more frequent than previously supposed. They may occur in focal or segmental form. (s. figs. 8.3, 8.4)

4.6.2 Lipoma

Hepatic lipoma is very rare. Research of the literature shows that S. Young was the first to publish a documented observation of this tumour in 1951. Although lipomas grow slowly, they may reach a considerable size. They consist of fatty tissue (adipocytes) with a lobular structure; according to (rare) observations made to date, there is no capsule. The lipoma is hyperechoic, which usually makes it easily identifiable by sonography and CT. There is no evidence of vascularization and no tendency towards malignant degeneration. Larger lipomas should be removed surgically, particularly when they have become symptomatic. (107, 108)

4.6.3 Myelolipoma

This rare type of mesenchymal tumour, which contains adipocytes and blood-forming tissue, can grow to an enormous size (e.g. 26 x 16 x 12 cm). When reaching a certain diameter in a specific location, it usually becomes symptomatic. It has a yellowish colour and contains fatty tissue as well as myeloid elements. Due to its echogenicity, the presence of this benign focus can be demonstrated by sonography and CT. Angiography shows a tumour that is usually avascular. Large or symptomatic tumours require surgical treatment. • Definitive diagnosis of these forms of fat-containing tumours is provided by biopsy, with thick-needle biopsy being the most reliable technique. (109, 110)

4.6.4 Angiolipoma

This benign mesenchymal tumour consists of fatty cells and numerous blood vessels, which have a tendency to thrombose. In general, angiolipomas occur singly in both liver lobes.

4.6.5 Angiomyolipoma

The first observation of an angiomyolipoma was reported by K.G. Ishak in 1976. Up to now, about 100 cases have been published. Owing to its fat content, this benign tumour has a yellowish-red colour. The largest tumour reported to date was 36 cm in diameter. Women are mainly affected. (120, 122) The right liver lobe is the preferred location. Fatty cells, blood vessels and smooth muscle cells can be demonstrated histologically. (126) The vessels may be thick-walled and are usually arranged in an island-like configuration. The tumour appears as a hyperechoic focus in sonography and as a hypodense focus in CT and MRI. (111, 121, 124, 127, 129) Hypervascularity is observed in arteriography. Multiple angiomyolipomas have been reported (125), occasionally also in kidneys and lungs. (116) The occurrence of spontaneous rupture (118) or disseminated intravascular coagulopathy was reported as a rare complication. Due to their vascular richness, diagnostic evidence of angiolipomas and angiomyolipomas should be obtained by fine-needle biopsy (114, 121), possibly together with immunohistochemistry. Malignant degeneration has not been observed. (112, 113, 115–117, 119, 123, 128)

4.7 Chondroma

To date, there has only been one single observation of a chondroma in the liver. (130) This tumour was excessively large (19 x 15 x 9.5 cm); it was hypervascularized, had a multilobular structure and did not possess a capsule. Focal calcifications were detectable. Chondrocyte-like cells and a chondroid matrix were found. Such a tumour can be visualized by imaging procedures. Laparoscopically, a hard, nodular surface is detectable. Diagnosis can only be confirmed histologically.

4.8 Leiomyoma

Up to now, only very few cases have been described. These tumours also become symptomatic once they have acquired a certain size and may grow to excessive proportions in the liver (e.g. 19.5 x 12 x 12 cm). (131)

4.9 Schwannoma

Schwannoma (neurinoma) is a benign tumour originating from Schwann cells. It is very rare. (132) Recently, a schwannoma of the bile duct causing obstructive jaundice was reported. (133)

4.10 Glomangioma

Glomus organs are small a.v. anastomoses for thermoregulation of the extremities. Glomangiomas are therefore most frequently located in the toes and fingers. However, they are also found in the respiratory, gastrointestinal and genital organs. A glomangioma was recently reported for the first time as a benign solitary tumour in the liver. This smooth, well-defined subcapsular lesion could be clarified histologically with the help of imaging-guided biopsy and later on confirmed by evaluation of the surgically excised tumour. (134) Malignant transformation of glomangioma is possible.

4.11 Mesenchymal hamartoma

▶ R. Maresch described hamartoma as a cystic tumour structure in 1903; it was termed mesenchymal hamartoma by H. A. Edmondson in 1956.

This benign tumour is caused by faulty tissue composition of certain organs, including the liver. The tumour is mostly found in the right liver lobe; it grows rapidly and progressively. This type of cystic tumour is mainly observed within the first year of life. Boys are more often affected than girls. In adults, mesenchymal hamartoma is very rare. Pre-existing composition disorders of the liver tissue can be stimulated into growth by steroids. Hamartomas remain asymptomatic until attainment of a certain size results in compressional or displacement phenomena. In their interior, they contain cysts filled with a yellowish, gelatinous substance. The stroma presumably derives from the connective tissue of the portal fields, from which the hamartoma may also originate. Malignant degeneration has been reported. Due to its tendency to grow, early surgical removal of the tumour is indicated. (135–137)

4.12 Mesothelioma

Mesotheliomas of the liver are extremely rare. They consist of parallel bundles of collagenous and reticular fibres as well as fibroplastic and epithelial cells. (138) The reported observation of a hepatic mesothelioma weighing some 2,800 g remains a rarity. (139)

4.13 Fibrous tumour

A solitary fibrous tumour was first described in pleural tissue by P. Klemperer et al. in 1931. Meanwhile, this rare entity has been reported in various organs, with the liver being affected in 26 cases. The tumour shows cellular areas (consisting of bundles of spindle cells arrayed haphazardly or in a storiform pattern) and relatively acellular areas (containing abundant collagen bundles). There is evidence of cellular atypia, mitotic activity and ectatic vessels. This tumour possesses malignant potential with the ability to metastazise. (140)

4.14 Cysts

Liver cysts can occur in solitary or in multiple form. They may be congenital or acquired. The reported frequency varies between 1% and 20%. The cysts are lined with a layer of cuboid cells and mostly filled with fluid. They are usually detected by chance. When cysts compress bile ducts or vessels, they become symptomatic. (142) • In *sonography*, the cyst appears as an anechoic (black) space with well-defined margins and distal sound amplification. (s. fig. 6.10) Haemorrhage into the cyst cavity and debris can mimic a cystadenoma or even cystadenocarcinoma. The presence of septa suggests a neoplastic cyst. (142) • In *computer tomography*, their content can generally be determined at +0 to +15 Houndsfield units. The i.v. administration of a contrast medium shows no evidence of enhancement. (s. figs. 8.6; 36.11) • Cysts are easily detected by *magnetic resonance imaging* (T_1 image = dark; T_2 image = light with high signal intensity). *Laparoscopy* provides a very impressive view of cysts. (s. figs. 36.12, 36.13)

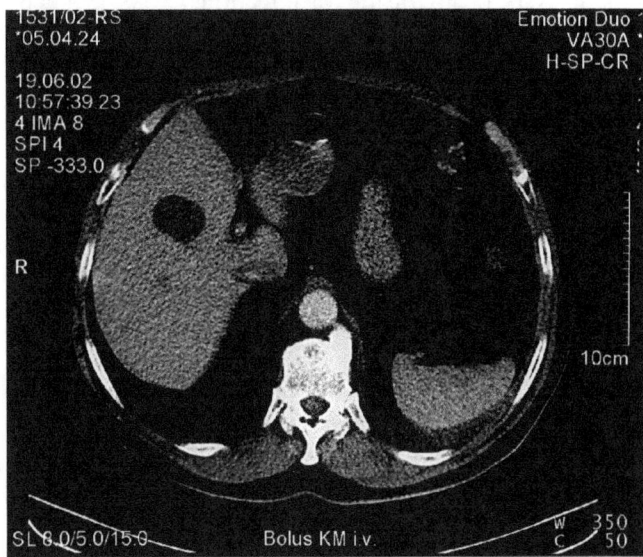

Fig. 36.11: CT with contrast medium: solitary liver cyst. (s. fig. 8.6)

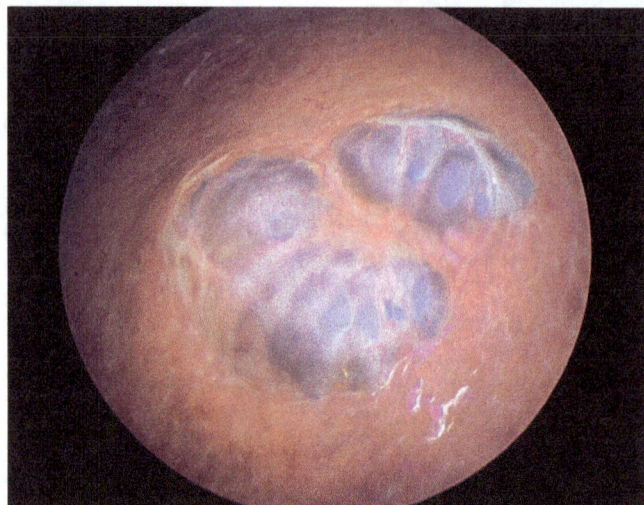

Fig. 36.12: Multiple cysts with several chambers in the area of the right liver lobe

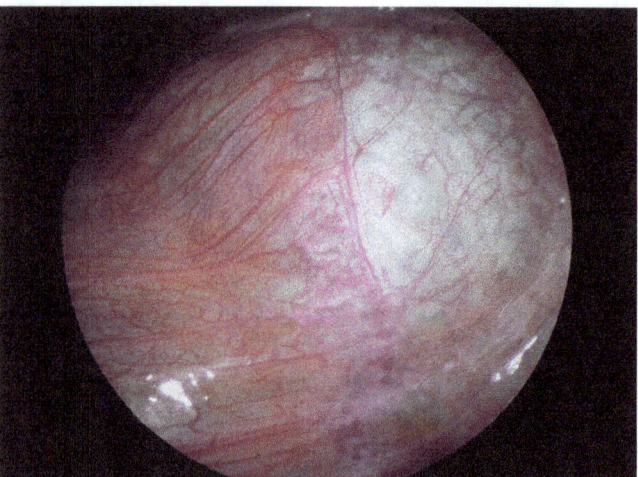

Fig. 36.13: Giant (fist-sized) solitary cyst in the right liver lobe

Four **types of cysts** can be differentiated: (*1.*) dysontogenetic cysts, (*2.*) parasitic (or infectious) cysts, (*3.*) neoplastic cysts, and (*4.*) post-traumatic cysts. The cause of cystic neoplasms is unknown. Traumatic cysts (C. WHIPPLE, 1898) occur from an injured intrahepatic bile duct after blunt abdominal trauma. (142)

Treatment: *Asymptomatic cysts* do not require treatment; large cysts which might rupture are an exception. • *Symptomatic cysts* (usually > 5 cm) are generally sclerosed. Reliable sclerotherapeutic agents include aethoxysclerol (1%), alcohol (95%) (153), minocycline hydrochloride (141, 156), tetracycline hydrochloride (1 g), and sodium chloride solution (10%). The sclerosing procedure is successful and low in side effects. Percutaneous aspiration of the cysts has a high relapse rate. Sclerotherapy does not prevent relapse, since a sclerotherapeutic agent destroys the cells, but not the cyst walls. Parasitic cysts require specific therapeutic measures. • Under laparoscopy, cysts which prove to be problematic may be treated reliably by fenestration (T.Y. LIN et al., 1968).

Surgical procedures (e.g. cyst excision, resection, cystjejunostomy, cystenterostomy) are rarely indicated and involve a much higher risk. (142, 148, 155)

4.14.1 Polycystic liver disease

The incidence is 1:500 to 1:5,000 births/100,000/per year. The gene responsible is located on chromosome 16; often another gene located on chromosome 4 is also involved. This autosomal dominant polycystic disease of the liver and kidneys can occur in (*1.*) children and (*2.*) adults (♂: ♀ = 1:5). The intrahepatic bile ducts are widely dilated and lined with bile-duct epithelium. Each liver segment may be interspersed by cysts of varying sizes which are connected with the biliary duct system. The cysts are surrounded by a fibrous capsule. Both the number and size of the cysts increase in later life. Usually, polycystic degeneration of the kidneys also occurs. (142) (s. fig. 8.6) Pancreatic cysts or colonic diverticulosis are less frequent. Occasionally, the cysts cover the liver in a balloon-like manner. (s. fig. 36.14) Rupture of large cysts may give rise to the clinical picture of acute abdomen. Compression leads to portal hypertension, jaundice (145), cholestasis and leg oedema. • Renal insufficiency is also a dangerous complication.

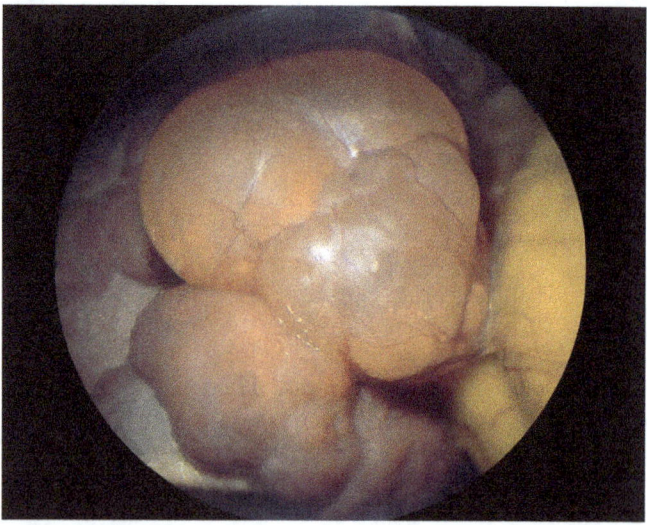

Fig. 36.14: Polycystic liver with spheroid, balloon-like cysts in the right liver lobe

Treatment may be by laparoscopic or surgical fenestration (143, 144–147, 149–152), injection of alcohol (40%) (153) or minocycline hydrochloride (141, 156), as well as surgical management. (148) Liver transplantation is a rare indication. (154)

4.14.2 Parasitic cysts

The cysts of Echinococcus granulosus (cysticus) (s. figs. 25.16, 25.17, 25.19) and Echinococcus multilocularis (alveolaris) (s. fig. 25.21) are of particular clinical importance. *(see chapter 25.2.3)*

4.15 Cholangiocellular tumours

4.15.1 Caroli's disease/syndrome

▶ This congenital clinical picture was first described in the form of intrahepatic stones by H. R. VACHELL et al. in 1906. • Later on, in 1958, J. CAROLI et al. were able to establish an association between characteristic congenital bile-duct alterations, cholangitis, cholangiolithiasis and renal cyst formation. In 1964 J. CAROLI et al. differentiated a particular form with simultaneous congenital liver fibrosis (which had already been described by D. V. S. KERR et al. in 1961). Both forms are autosomal recessive.

Caroli's disease is characterized by congenital, segmental dilatation of the intrahepatic bile ducts, causing bile sludge formation and the development of gallstones. Clinical findings include hepatomegaly, cholestasis and subicterus as well as cholangitis with upper abdominal pain and biochemical signs of inflammation. (158, 160) (s. tab. 38.2) Diagnosis is by CT (157, 159) (s. pp 182, 696), Doppler sonography (159) and ERC. (s. fig. 36.15)

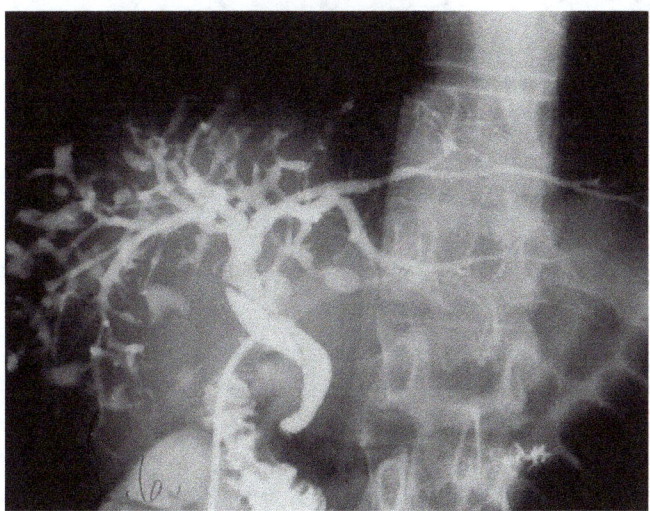

Fig. 36.15: ERC findings in Caroli's disease: mainly segmental, sack-like dilatations of the intrahepatic bile ducts with some small-diameter connections to the efferent bile ducts

Caroli's syndrome is additionally characterized by congenital liver fibrosis. (s. p. 697) There may be fibroangiomatosis of the bile ducts and microcysts in the kidneys. The condition can lead to portal (presinusoidal) hypertension. • Choledochal cysts, polycystic degeneration of the liver and kidneys, Laurence-Moon-Biedl syndrome and ectasia of the renal tubules may all appear. • Apart from cholangitis and hepatolithiasis, potential complications include liver abscess, pancreatitis, amyloidosis, malignant tumours and liver failure. • *Treatment* consists of biliary drainage, antibiotics, surgical procedures and liver transplantation. Ursodeoxycholic acid may be used as an adjuvant.

4.15.2 Hepatobiliary cystadenoma

This rare benign tumour probably develops from congenital bile-duct malformations. It is found mostly in women (>90%), mainly after the age of 45–50 years. The tumour grows very slowly, yet can reach a considerable size (5–25 cm). Cystadenomas occur as solitary, but multilobular cystic tumours. The cysts are frequently separated by septa. The *mucous type* consists of a mucous/gelatinous, bile-coloured fluid, often containing old blood. Occasionally, a *serous type* of cystadenoma without mesenchymal stroma is found. There is evidence of ovary-like stroma together with unilaminar bile epithelium, which is folded in a polyploid or papillary manner in places. (161) (s. fig. 36.16) The collagenic capsule is rich in vessels. Surrounding the tumour, numerous abnormal bile ducts and arterial vascular clusters are evident. • Cholestasis or even obstructive jaundice develops. (162) Diagnosis of this cystic lesion (mainly in the right lobe) is by imaging techniques. Differential diagnosis may be extremely difficult (and is often only possible by means of surgery). • Due to the tendency of cystadenoma towards malignant degeneration, resection should be carried out as soon as possible. (163–167)

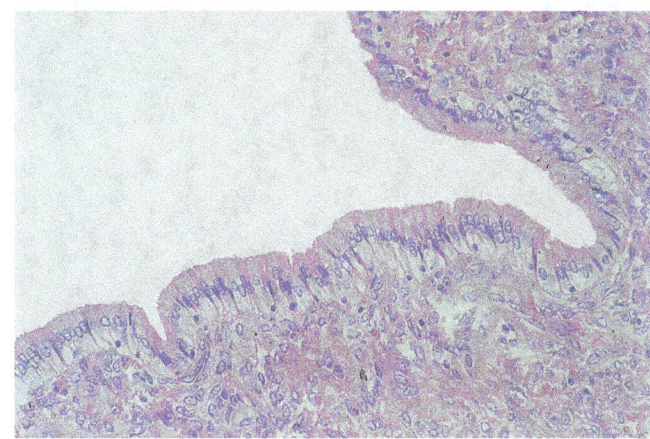

Fig. 36.16: Hepatobiliary cystadenoma with ovary-like stroma (HE)

4.15.3 Bile-duct adenomas

Bile-duct adenomas are rare. Usually, they are solitary and <2 cm in size. This type of adenoma is more often detected in men than in women (3:1), and it occurs in patients mainly over the age of 50. It is nearly always localized beneath the liver capsule. Sonography shows roundish, hypoechoic foci of different sizes with relatively unclear contours (s. fig. 36.17). They are visible in MRT as hypotense (T_1-weighted) lesions (s. fig. 36.18). Imaging procedures do not reveal any characteristic features. With the help of laparoscopical examination, roundish, greyish-white, well-defined foci are visible. The lesions cause slight bulging on the liver surface. The surrounding tissue is unchanged and without vascularization. The biopsy material taken from the foci turned out to be crumbly (!). (s. fig. 36.19) This adenoma has the form of a firm, whitish or whitish-grey node and consists of bile-duct proliferations. It contains biliary acini and tubules which are lined with a layer of cuboid epithelium within loose fibrous, partially hyaline stroma.

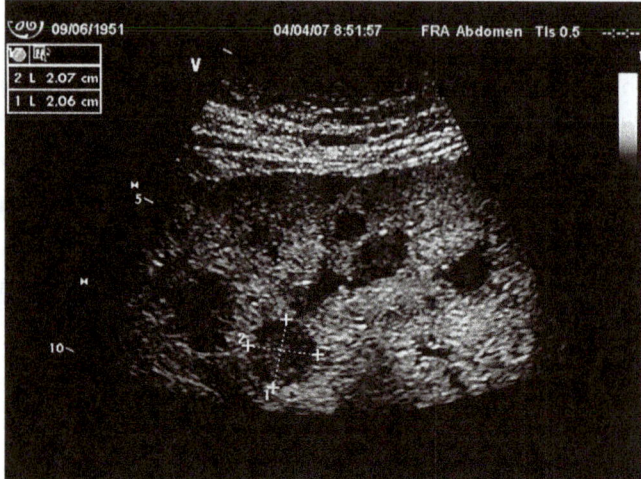

Fig. 36.17: Several roundish, hypoechoic foci of different sizes with relatively blurred contours. Unclear aetiology. (50-year-old man; the same patient as in figures 36.18–36.21)

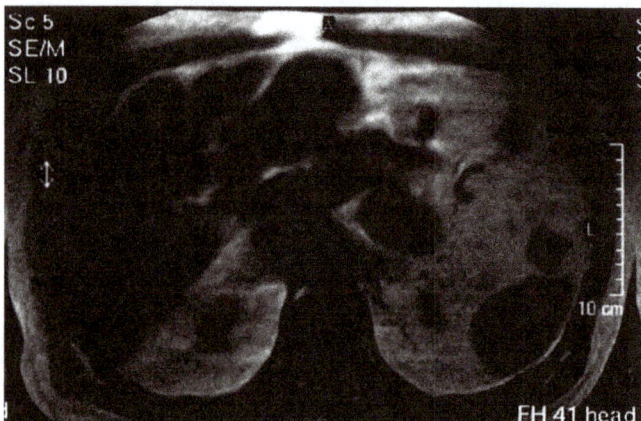

Fig. 36.18: Axial T_1-weighted MRT showing at least three hypointense roundish foci with slightly hazy edges in the right liver lobe. One focal lesions is subcapsular, causing minimal bulging on the surface. There are no signs of any radiological features which might facilitate a diagnosis

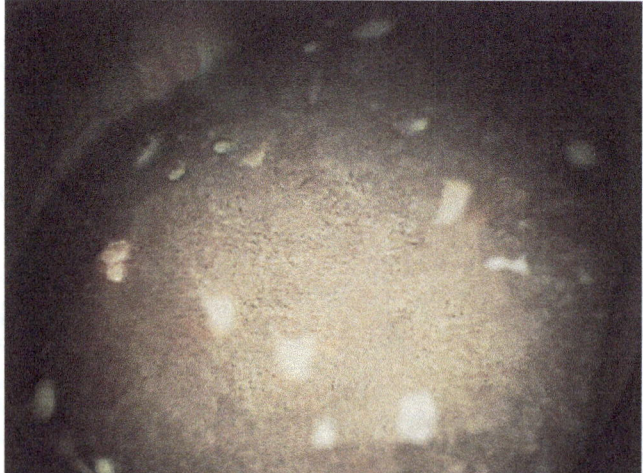

Fig. 36.19: Diffusely disseminated greyish-white foci of different sizes in both liver lobes with relatively sharp contours. The liver surface shows slight bulging (about 1–2 mm), but no central dipping; no vascularisation is visible. The perifocal tissue is unchanged

There is evidence of mononuclear inflammatory cells and, occasionally, lymph follicles. (s. figs. 36.20, 36.21) • It is discussed that such biliary adenomas are peribiliary gland hamartomas. (169) There are no clinical or biochemical abnormalities, nor is there any tendency towards malignant degeneration. (168, 170)

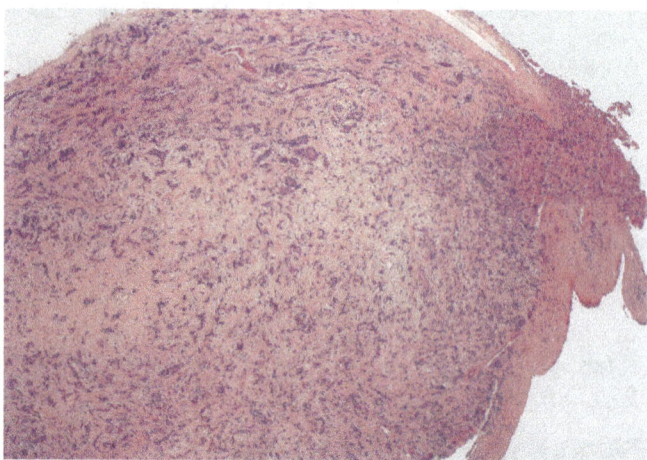

Fig. 36.20: Bile-duct adenoma in subcapsular liver tissue (HE)

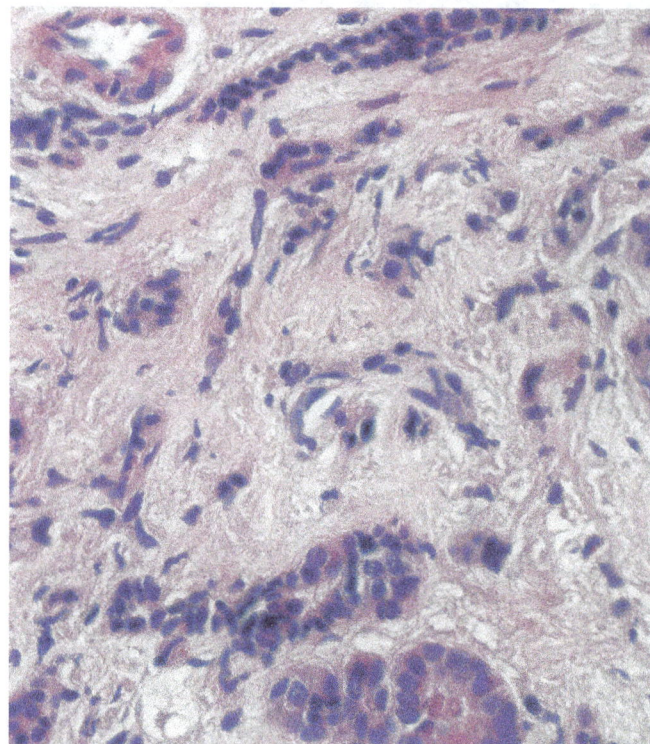

Fig. 36.21: Bile-duct adenoma composed of small tubules, which are lined by a single layer of slightly irregular epithelial cells. The ducts are embedded in a dense collagenous stroma (HE)

4.15.4 Bile-duct papillomatosis

Bile-duct papillomatosis is a very rare finding (up to now about 50 cases have been reported) which occurs mainly in elderly women. There are papillomatous proliferations in both intrahepatic and extrahepatic bile ducts. Clinically, it is characterized by recurrent episodes of jaundice and cholestasis as well as ascending cholangitis and haemobilia. The bile ducts can be dilated; their wall surface is irregular. The course is progredient; the prognosis is poor. (173) Recently, encouraging results have been reported following intraluminal iridium[192] therapy (172) and liver transplantation (171). Malignant degeneration into cholangiocarcinoma is possible.

4.15.5 Biliary hamartoma

Benign biliary microhamartomas (= *Meyenburg's complex*) were described by H. von MEYENBURG in 1918. (s. p. 698 and fig. 33.20) They consist of small cysts developing from dilatations of the small (interlobular) bile ducts and are surrounded by fibrous stroma. The cysts are remnants of ductal plate malformations. Sometimes typical ductal plates are also detected. The hamartomas can reach a diameter of up to 0.5 (−1.0) cm. Macroscopically, they appear as firm, greyish-white nodules which are clearly delineated from the liver parenchyma. Subcapsular nodules may also be detected by laparoscopy. (176) They are sometimes misinterpreted as small metastases. Here, MRI is of great diagnostic value. (175)
• Microhamartomas are often associated with malformations of the small branches of the portal veins. They may represent a transition to the autosomal dominant form of polycystic degeneration. These tumours have a tendency to develop into cholangiocarcinoma. (174−177)

4.16 Abscesses

Depending on their cause, liver abscesses are classified as (*1.*) pyogenic or (*2.*) parasitic. This factor largely determines differential diagnosis, diagnosis and therapy. Fresh abscesses usually have blurred margins; following consolidation, they have a round to elliptical form. Evidence of gas bubbles is seen as pathognomonic. The abscesses are generally hypoechoic and hypodense. *(see chapter 27!)*

4.17 Hepatic lymphangioma

This rare, congenital benign tumour consists of multiple, small (1−4 mm in diameter) dilations of intrahepatic lymph vessels, which communicate with each other. They contain chylous fluid. Mostly, there are lymphangiomas in other organs as well. (178)

4.18 Peliosis hepatis

Peliosis hepatis may be caused by various kinds of medication (181) or chemical agents and is associated with numerous diseases (of a viral, bacterial, parasitic or metabolic nature). Its aetiopathogenesis is unknown. It has also been detected in small children. (180, 182) *Histologically*, there are spaces lined with endothelium corresponding to dilated sinusoids and Disse's spaces. They are filled with blood (= "globoid bleeding"). Their size varies from

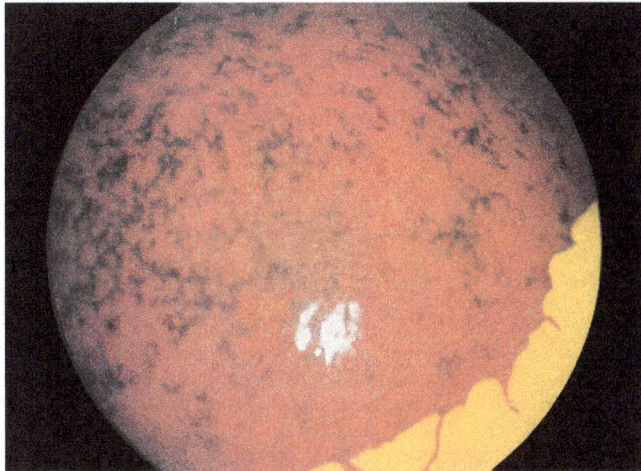

Fig. 36.22: Hepatic peliosis composed of a network of dark-blue to livid-reddish vessels below a yellowish-red surface of a fatty liver

0.5−2.0 mm and can even reach > 1 cm. The hepatocytes and venules are unchanged. (s. p. 404!) (s. figs. 21.8; 36.22)

Clinical findings include fever, abdominal pain and hepatomegaly. *Laboratory values* reveal occasional subicterus and elevated transaminases. (180) *Imaging procedures* often yield no findings or merely uncharacteristic changes. (179) Definitive results are obtained by *laparoscopy* (183): characteristic foci of a livid-reddish to dark-blue colour are found, mostly rounded and subcapsular, often with net-like confluence (s. fig. 36.23). The findings are so typical and distinctive that histological examination is no longer necessary; however, biopsy may be justified under visual control. The most important *complications* are haemorrhages and, especially following trauma, rupture of the liver capsule with bleeding into the abdominal cavity. (180, 181)

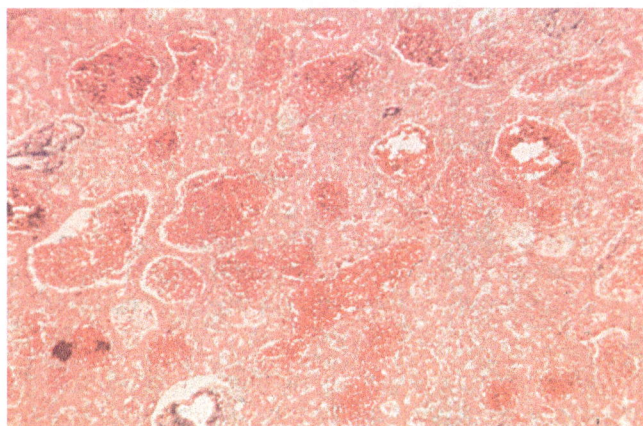

Fig. 36.23: Peliosis hepatis: non-endothelialized cavernous blood-filled cavities surrounded by hepatocellular trabeculae (HE)

4.19 Granulomas

It is generally not possible to detect granulomas using imaging procedures. When the foci are densely grouped, it is possible to see an inhomogeneous reflex pattern during sonography and a variable pattern in the CT scan. The causes are manifold and vary greatly. (s. tab. 21.1) • Diagnosis is facilitated by laparoscopy and forceps biopsy, provided the foci are located on the surface (which is mostly the case). If the surface is free of foci, multiple biopsies from both liver lobes done under laparoscopy yield reliable results. (s. p. 405) (s. figs. 21.9, 21.10; 24.14; 29.6; 38.5)

4.19.1 Sarcoidosis

▶ A cutaneous form of sarcoidosis ("Mortimer's disease"), first described by A. HUTCHINSON in 1877, was observed in further courses of disease by E. BESNIER ("lupus pernio") and C.P. MOELLER-BOECK ("sarcoidosis", "miliary lupoid") in 1899. In 1917 these single findings were synthesized by J. SCHAUMANN. Various terms, such as Besnier-Boeck-Schaumann disease, benign lymphogranulomatosis or Boeck's disease, have been used in the past to describe this condition. However, the term sarcoidosis has gained more and more acceptance.

Definition

Sarcoidosis is a primary multisystemic, granulomatous disease of (still) unknown aetiology with enhanced immunity at the site of manifestation. The lungs and the intrathoracic lymph nodes are nearly always affected. In many cases, the extrathoracic organs are involved as well. Sarcoidosis is characterized by the presence of epithelioid cell granulomas, which do not show caseous changes.

▶ Since 1964, our study group, consisting of L. MANDI et al. (Debrecen/Hungary) and E. KUNTZ, has been intensively involved in investigating the striking regional differences in sarcoidosis. We postulated an **immune reaction** — with a *genetic disposition* — against a **mycobacterial substrate**. • Among other things, we found **Ziehl-Neelsen positivity** of pollen obtained from numerous trees and plants. A high correspondence of sarcoidosis frequency with certain ZN-positive pollen locations became obvious as we catalogued our findings. This might also explain familial aggregation as a result of similar exogenous exposure. • **Injection** of ZN-positive pollen, embedded in paraffin, into the testicles of guinea pigs resulted in the *dissemination* of histological findings fully corresponding to sarcoidosis. By contrast, ZN-negative pollen did not elicit this reaction in animal experiments.

Frequency: Men and women are affected with the same frequency. Manifestation mainly occurs between the ages of 20 to 40, predominantly in winter. The incidence is highest in Scandinavian countries, the USA and Japan (always with considerable regional variations) at 5–40/100,000 inhabitants/year.

Localization: Based on X-ray findings, *intrathoracic sarcoidosis* can be divided into four stages: 0, I–III. • The *extrathoracic manifestation* of sarcoidosis affects the lymphatic system, bone marrow, bones, skin, eyes, lacrimal and salivary glands, urogenital system, musculature, nervous system and endocrine glands. Extrathoracic manifestations without thoracic findings are rare. At least two organs must exhibit granulomas to substantiate the diagnosis of sarcoidosis.

Aetiopathogenesis: Development of sarcoidosis has been observed during treatment with *interferon*-α. (187) • Mycobacteria were also seen as a possible cause of sarcoidosis, which was recently reinforced when *mycobacterial DNA* and *RNA* were found in sarcoidosis tissue (H. H. POPPER et al., 1994) and the presence of *acid-fast L forms* was detected in patients' blood (P. L. ALMENOFF et al., 1996).

Liver: The liver is involved in sarcoidosis in 60–80% of cases. Initially, loosely concentrated *epithelioid cells* are found which combine to form small *epithelioid granulomas* mainly in the portal and periportal area. These small granulomas may join together and form conglomerates up to the size of lentils. Within the epithelioid cell granulomas, there is evidence of one or more *Langhans' giant cells*, which are rich in the angiotensin-converting enzyme. Epithelioid cells and giant cells release α_1-antitrypsin and lysozymes as well as other substances; epithelioid cells also release interleukin-I. Within the giant cells (displaying a rosette-like arrangement of nuclei), *asteroid bodies* (5–20 µm) resembling a sea anemone are often found. Moreover, there is evidence of *Schaumann bodies* (25–200 µm) (more frequently in lymph nodes than in the liver) and small *vesicles*. • Inflammatory *cellulation* is low: it consists of eosinophils, T lymphocytes ($CD4^+$) and plasma cells. Granulomas may increase in size, but may also heal by way of fibrosis. (190) • Chronic cholestasis (ductopenia, cholate stasis, copper storage) as well as the histological picture of PBC (or less frequently of PSC) can be found in 50–60% of cases. (quot: 188) • *This would suggest a connection with the mycotoxin theory of PBC (E. KUNTZ, 1984), whereby molecular mimicry (M. E. GERSHWIN, 1991) is of potentially pathogenetic significance in sarcoidosis as well.* (s. p. 676) • Pronounced fibrosis leads to *portal hypertension*. Formation of *NRH* was evident in 9% and *cirrhosis* in 6% of cases.

Clinical findings: Usually, there are no subjective complaints. As the lungs become increasingly affected, fatigue and (exercise-related) dyspnoea may occur. Extrathoracic manifestations can cause corresponding symptoms. Hepato(spleno)megaly is observed in 5–10% of cases. In an acute stage, polyarthralgia, erythema nodosum and fever are generally found. Kveim's test is positive, while the BCG test is clearly reduced or negative. (184–186, 189–191)

Biochemistry: In most cases, eosinophilia and monocytosis are present in leukopenia and lymphopenia. BSR and CRP are normal or only slightly elevated. The γ-globulins may be increased. Cholestasis is often found, whereas jaundice is rare. Hypercalcaemia is a striking feature; occasionally there is evidence of augmented ACE and lysozymes in the serum.

Histology: The best method of obtaining the prominent, whitish granulomas on the liver surface, the size of a pin-head up to a lentil (= *fly agaric liver*), is by *laparoscopy* and *forceps biopsy*; otherwise, *thick-needle biopsies* can be performed on suspicious areas of the right and left liver lobe. The diagnostic accuracy of this procedure is more than 98%, while that of percutaneous liver biopsy is 30−70%. (s. figs. 21.9, 21.10) (s. pp 405, 486, 561) • *Bronchoscopy* used for taking mucosa samples also facilitates histological diagnosis.

Imaging procedures: Enlargement of abdominal lymph nodes can occasionally be detected by sonography, CT or MRI. (185, 189) The liver may exhibit an inhomogeneous reflex pattern due to fibrosis.

Treatment: Intrathoracic sarcoidosis has a high rate of spontaneous remission with possible fibrosis residues. • Extrathoracic manifestations may cause considerable symptoms and secondary disorders, depending on the organs affected. This is also true of the liver. Treatment consists of monitored waiting and administration of glucocorticoids (usually as long-term therapy). Liver transplantation is necessary in some cases.

4.20 Inflammatory pseudotumour

The synonyms used for inflammatory pseudotumour include myofibroblastic inflammatory tumour, histiocytoma, pseudolymphoma, fibroxanthoma and plasma cell granuloma. This condition was first described by G. T. PACK et al. in 1953. It is a rare type of tumour (about 100 reports so far) which can occur at any age (but mainly between 30 and 40), with men being affected three times more often than women. The tumour mostly affects the liver (90%), but also numerous other organs (lung, stomach, parotis, pleura, ovaries, thyroid gland, lacrimal glands, etc.). A tumour size of up to 25 cm has been reported. Its pathogenesis is not clear. (192) Bacterial and viral infections (e. g. EBV) are possible trigger factors. An association with systemic inflammatory diseases, e. g. Crohn's disease (194), has been reported.

Histology: There are obvious fusiform cells, foamy histiocytes, plasma cells and lymphocytes, but no irregular mitosis. Extensive connective tissue may form incomplete capsular boundaries. The pseudotumour is vascularized despite the presence of numerous obliterated vessels. (196) The bile ducts exhibit inflammatory alterations. Fatty degeneration and occasional central necrosis as well as bleeding are evident. This gives rise to simulated HCC. Malignant degeneration is rare. (195) • The main symptoms include fever, epigastric pain, weight loss, elevated transaminases, inflammatory laboratory parameters, cholestasis and increased gamma globulins. (193, 196−198) Sonographically, a hypoechoic space-occupying lesion can be seen. In CT, the tumour is hypodense with a blurred margin; following CM application, it shows mild, heterogeneous and delayed enhancement. MRI displays low signal intensity in T_1 images and significant signal enhancement in T_2 images. A thick hyperintensive periphery may be present.

Treatment: Spontaneous regression is rare. The administration of prednisolone and antibiotics has been used with controversial results. In general, there is an indication for surgical resection, which is deemed a successful method of treatment.

4.21 Erdheim-Chester disease

This condition is a rare form of non-Langerhans histiocytosis. The foamy histiocytes are lipid-laden and affect the lower extremities, lungs and kidneys, causing progressive disseminated, granulomatous lesions. In a first report of biliary manifestation of ECD, these granulomatous lesions were embedded in extended periductular fibrosis. A remarkable cholestasis was found with moderate increase of the transaminases. (199)

4.22 Calcareous foci

Calcareous foci in the liver are detected incidentally in X-ray or sonographic examination of the abdomen. It may be quite difficult to identify their aetiology, since calcification can be observed in numerous diseases. Diagnostic clarification often has no prognostic or therapeutic implications. However, in many cases, the irrelevance of such a diagnosis can only be determined retrospectively after numerous examinations (imaging procedures, laparoscopy with targeted biopsy) have been

Calcification of benign lesions
Aneurysm of the hepatic artery
Arteriovenous fistula
Calcification of the hepatic artery
Cavernous haemangioma
Echinococcus cysts
Granulomas: histoplasmosis, brucellosis, tuberculosis
Gumma (hepar lobatum)
Haemangiomatosis
Haematoma
Haemochromatosis
Intrahepatic bile-duct calculus
Intrahepatic dislocated staghorn calculus
Liver abscess
Microlithiasis in cystic fibrosis
Portal vein thrombosis
Posttraumatic cysts
Calcification of malignant tumours

• Primary liver tumours
• Metastases
  − vipoma
  − ovarian cystadenocarcinoma
  − gastric or colon carcinoma

Porcelain liver

Tab. 36.4: Calcification of benign and malignant liver foci

carried out. (202, 204) Different calcified foci, such as calcified vipoma (201), calcified metastasis (s. figs. 37.24, 37.25), microlithiasis in cystic fibrosis (203) or calcification of the hepatic artery (205), are rare observations. Calcification of an echinococcus cyst is the most common type of calcareous focus. (s. fig. 25.18) (s. tab. 36.4)

A so-called **porcelain liver** should be clarified by differential diagnosis. (200) This condition is characterized by focal calcareous deposits in the liver capsule, which can be detected by X-ray examination as well as by sonography and CT. It may be caused by phleboliths, pseudolipoma, histoplasmosis, calcified larvae, small capsule haematomas, small abscesses, etc.

▶ A case involving an **unusual calcification of tremendous size** in the right liver lobe was the subject of much speculation. It was not until laparotomy was carried out that this case was resolved (s. fig. 36.24):

What was discovered was a **monstrous gall-bladder staghorn calculus** *which had migrated to and become embedded in the liver parenchyma. In order to be removed, it had to be cut into four parts (which are well-preserved and still at our disposal). With a length of 12 cm, a diameter of 4–5 cm and a dry weight (!) of some 120 g, it may well be the largest gallstone ever reported.* • *Our investigations of the literature revealed a previous maximum weight of 110 g (published in 1917).* (s. p. 761, footnote*): E. KUNTZ)

5 Surgical treatment

Most benign tumours are asymptomatic and do not require surgical intervention. A smaller group of benign liver foci are treated conservatively or require interventional treatment. • Other tumours are difficult to differentiate as either benign or malignant, or they tend towards malignant degeneration and should be removed surgically. Surgery is indicated in unresolved findings, or when the tumour increases in size with secondary compressional effects, or if there are complications. Postoperative morbidity is low with negligible mortality; life expectancy and quality of life are not compromised.

It is important that the *preoperative examination* is carried out meticulously and that the tumour can be adequately assessed by imaging techniques regarding its intrahepatic location, size, extent and segmental affiliation. When

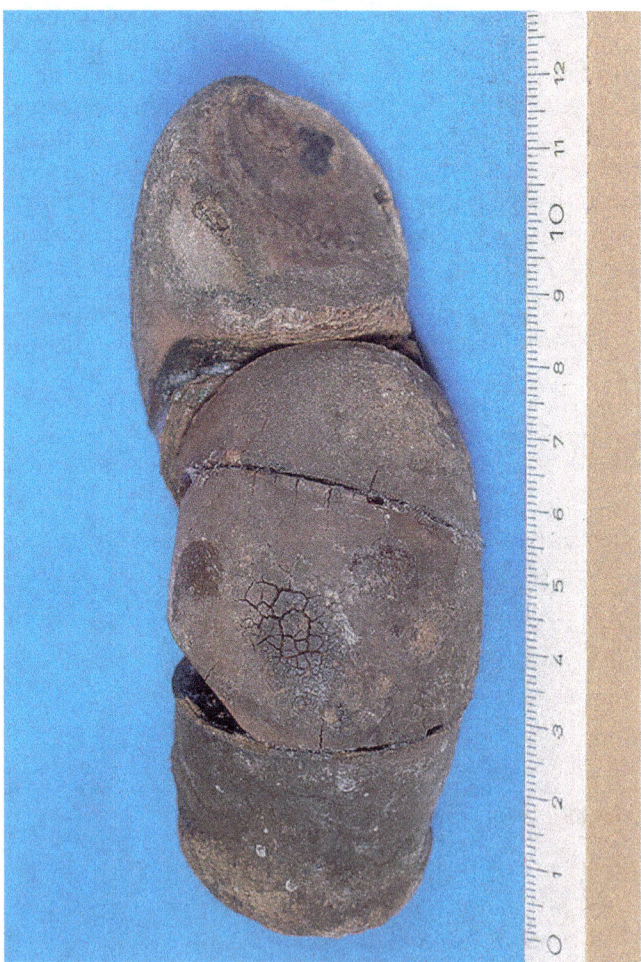

Fig. 36.24: Giant gall-bladder staghorn calculus, dislocated into the right liver lobe and embedded in the parenchyma. *(at our disposal)* — **Probably the largest gallstone reported to date: 12 x 5 cm, 120 g dry weight!**

1. **Ligature or embolization of the hepatic artery**
   – in acute bleeding
   – in angiomatosis with large, functionally effective arteriovenous shunts
2. **Atypical liver resection, enucleation, local tumour excision**
   (without liver hilus preparation)
   – method of choice and relative indication in clearly benign hepatic tumours showing symptoms and a clear increase in size of tumour (haemangioma, FNH, lipoma, *etc.*)
3. **Anatomical, segment-oriented liver resection**
   (including liver hilus preparation in most cases)
   – necessary in unresolved or ambiguous hepatic tumours (e.g. suspected adenoma) as absolute indication due to risk of malignancy and in complications (e.g. haemorrhage, rupture). The aim is radical removal of the tumour with a sufficient safety margin (as in malignant tumours)
4. **Partial/total vascular ligation**
   – useful additional technique for better intraoperative control of haemorrhage and haemostasis, particularly suitable for well-vascularized tumours or those close to the inferior vena cava
5. **Various modifications of in/ante/ex situ resection**
   – relatively rare techniques which may, however, be useful (with additional protection of the liver and possible autotransplantation) for improving technical resectability when the size or location of the tumour presents problems (e.g. confluence of the hepatic veins)
6. **Hepatectomy and allogenic liver transplantation**
   – exceptional techniques applied in multiple tumours, diffuse changes (e.g. haemangiomatosis) or concomitant liver diseases often of a metabolic nature (e.g. glycogenosis). Radical oncological treatment for eliminating the risk of malignant tumour development

Tab. 36.5: Surgical treatment options for benign hepatic tumours (according to B. RINGE et al., 1997) (209)

participation of vascular or biliary structures or involvement of extrahepatic organs is suspected, additional investigations are called for. • The *hepatological status* is determined as follows: enzymatic and mesenchymal activities, cholestasis and jaundice, functional test values (e. g. cholinesterase, albumin, coagulation status, indocyaninegreen test, galactose elimination capacity). • The surgical strategy is chosen in accordance with the tumour type and any additional individual factors. Atypical resection, enucleation or excisional separation of the local tumour are considered to be less invasive and therefore less inconvenient for the patient. (205–210) (s. tab. 36.5)

References:

Diagnosis

1. **Barakos, J.A., Goldberg, H.I., Brown, J.J., Gilbert, T.J.:** Comparison of computed tomography and magnetic resonance imaging in the evaluation of focal hepatic lesions. Gastrointest. Radiol. 1990; 15: 93–101
2. **Biecker, E., Fischer, H.P., Strunk, H., Sauerbruch, T.:** Benign hepatic tumours. Z. Gastroenterol. 2003; 41: 191–200
3. **Ferrell, L.D., Crawford, J.M., Dhillon, A.P., Scheuer, P.J., Nakanuma, Y.:** Proposal for standardized criteria for the diagnosis of benign, borderline, and malignant hepatocellular lesions arising in chronic advanced liver disease. Amer. J. Surg. Path. 1993; 17: 1113–1123
4. **Francque, S.M., de Pauw, F.F., van den Steen, G.H., van Marck, E.A., Pelckmans, P.A., Michielsen, P.P.:** Biopsy of focal liver lesions: Guidelines, comparison of techniques and cost-analysis. Acta Gastro-Enterol. Belg. 2003; 66: 160–165
5. **Hohmann, J., Albrecht, T., Hoffmann, C.W., Wolf, K.J.:** Ultrasonographic detection of focal liver lesions: increased sensitivity and specificity with microbubble contrast agents. Eur. J. Radiol. 2003; 46: 147–159
6. **Ishak, K.G., Rabin, L.:** Benign tumors of the liver. Med. Clin. N. Amer. 1975; 59: 995–1013
7. **Kim, M.J., Kim, J.H., Chung, J.J., Park, M.S., Lim, J.S., Oh, Y.T.:** Focal hepatic lesions: Detection and characterization with combination gadolinium- and superparamagnetic iron oxide-enhanced MR imaging. Radiology 2003; 228: 719–726
8. **Kondo, F., Koshima, Y., Ebara, M.:** Nodular lesions associated with abnormal liver circulation. Intervirology 2004; 47: 277–287
9. **Kuntz, E.:** 30 Jahre Erfahrung bei 6000 Laparoskopien (1955–1986). Fortschr. Med. 1987; 105: 521–524
10. **Kuntz, E.:** Der aktuelle Stellenwert der Laparoskopie in der Hepatologie. Med. Welt 1999; 50: 42–47
11. **Nichols, F.C., van Heerden, J.A., Weiland, L.H.:** Benign liver tumors. Surg. Clin. N. Amer. 1989; 69: 297–314
12. **Rubin, R.A., Lichtenstein, G.R.:** Hepatic scintigraphy in the evaluation of solitary solid liver masses. J. Nucl. Med. 1993; 34: 697–705
13. **Tom, W.W., Yeh, B.M., Cheng, J.C., Qayyum, A., Joe, B., Coakley, F.V.:** Hepatic pseudotumor due to nodular fatty sparing: the diagnostic role of opposed-phase MRI. Amer. J. Roentgenol. 2004; 183: 721–724
14. **Wanless, I.R.:** Terminology of nodular hepatocellular lesions. International working party. Hepatology 1995; 22: 983–993

Adenoma

15. **Alshak, N.S., Cocjin, J., Podesta, L., van de Velde, R., Makowka, L., Rosenthal, P., Geller, S.A.:** Hepatocellular adenoma in glycogen storage disease type IV. Arch. Pathol. Lab. Med. 1994; 118: 88–91
16. **Arrive, L., Flejou, J.F., Vilgrain, V., Belghiti, J., Najmark, D., Zins, M., Menu, Y., Tubiana, J.-M., Nahum, H.:** Hepatic adenoma: MR findings in 51 pathologically proved lesions. Radiology 1994; 193: 507–512
17. **Bacq, Y., Jacquemin, E., Balabaud, C., Jeannot, E., Scotto, B., Branchereau, S., Laurent, C., Bourlier, P., Pariente, D., de Muret, A., Fabre, M., Bioulac-Sage, P., Zucman-Rossi, J.:** Familial liver adenomatosis associated with hepatocyte nuclear factor 1 alpha inactivation (case report). Gastroenterology 2003; 125: 1470–1475
18. **Boulac-Sage, P., Balabaud, C., Bedossa, P., Scoazec, J.Y., Chiche, L., Dhillon, A.P., Ferrell, L., Paradis, V., Roskams, T., Vilgrain, V., Wanless, I.R., Zucman-Rossi, J.:** Pathological diagnosis of liver cell adenoma and focal nodular hyperplasia: Bordeaux Update. J. Hepatol. 2007; 46: 521–527
19. **Bühler, H., Pirovino, M., Akovbiantz, A., Altorfer, J., Weitzel, M., Maranta, E., Schmid, M.:** Regression of liver cell adenoma. A follow-up study of three consecutive patients after discontinuation of oral contraceptive use. Gastroenterology 1982; 82: 775–782
20. **Chiche, L., Dao, T., Salamé, E., Galais, M.P., Bouvard, N., Schmutz, G., Rousselot, P., Bioulac-Sage, P., Ségol, P., Gignoux, M.:** Liver adenomatosis: Reappraisal, diagnosis, and surgical management. – Eight new cases and review of the literature. Ann. Surg. 2000; 231: 74–81
21. **Colovic, R., Grubor, N., Micev, M., Radak, V.:** Hepatocellular adenoma with malignant alteration (case report). Hepatogastroenterology 2007; 54: 386–388
22. **Cosme, A., Horcajada, J.P., Vidaur, F., Ojeda, E., Torrado, J., Arenas, J.I.:** Systemic amyloidosis induced by oral contraceptive-associated hepatocellular adenoma: a 13 year follow-up. Liver 1995; 15: 164–167
23. **Eckhauser, F.E., Knol, J.A., Raper, S.E., Thompson, N.W.:** Enucleation combined with hepatic vascular exclusion is a safe and effective alternative to hepatic resection for liver cell adenoma. Amer. Surg. 1994; 60: 466–472
24. **Foster, J.H., Berman, M.M.:** The malignant transformation of liver cell adenomas. Arch. Surg. 1994; 129: 712–717
25. **Gouysse, G., Frachon, S., Hervieu, V., Fiorentino, M., dπErrico, J., Dumortier, J., Boillot, O., Partensky, C., Grigioni, W.F., Scoazec, J.F.:** Endothelial cell differentiation in hepatocellular adenomas: implication for histopathological diagnosis. J. Hepatol. 2004; 41: 259–266
26. **Gyorffy, E.J., Bredtfeldt, J.E., Black, W.C.:** Transformation of hepatic cell adenoma to hepatocellular carcinoma due to oral contraceptive use. Ann. Intern. Med. 1989; 110: 489–490
27. **Hashimoto, L., Dabbs, A., Sewell, P., Doherty, M.:** Resection and radio frequency ablation of multiple liver adenomas secondary to anti-conceptive pills (case report). Hepato-Gastroenterol. 2004; 51: 837–838
28. **Ichikawa, T., Federle, M.P., Grazioli, L., Nalesnik, M.:** Hepatocellular adenoma: multiphasic CT and histopathologic findings in 25 patients. Radiology 2000; 214: 861–868
29. **Janes, C.H., McGill, D.B., Ludwig, J., Krom, R.A.F.:** Liver cell adenoma at the age of 3 years and transplantation 19 years later after development of carcinoma: A case report. J. Hepatol. 1993; 17: 583–585
30. **Labrune, P., Trioche, P., Duvaltier, I., Chevalier, P., Odièvre, M.:** Hepatocellular adenomas in glycogen storage disease type I and III: a series of 43 patients and review of the literature. J. Pediatr. Gastroenterol. Nutr. 1997; 24: 276–279
31. **Leese, T., Farges, O., Bismuth, H.:** Liver cell adenomas. A 12-year surgical experience from a specialist hepato-biliary unit. Ann. Surg. 1988; 208: 558–564
32. **Lewin, M., Handra-Luca, Arrive, L., Wendum, P., Paradis, V., Bridel, E., Flejou, J.F., Belghiti, J., Tubiana, J.M. Vilgrain, V.:** Liver adenomatosis: Classification of MR imaging features and comparison with pathologic findings. Radiology 2006; 241: 433–440
33. **Perret, A.G., Mosnier, J.-F., Porcheron, J., Cuilleron, M., Berthoux, P., Boucheron, S., Audigier, J.-C.:** Role of oral contraceptives in the growth of a multilobular adenoma associated with a hepatocellular carcinoma in a young woman. J. Hepatol. 1996; 25: 976–979
34. **Tao, L.C.:** Oral contraceptive-associated liver cell adenoma and hepatocellular carcinoma: cytomorphology and mechanism of malignant transformation. Cancer 1991; 68: 341–347
35. **Toso, C., Rubbia-Brandt, L., Negro, F., Morel, P., Mentha, G.:** Hepatocellular adenoma and polycystic ovary syndrome (case report). Liver Internat. 2003; 23: 35–37

Focal nodular hyperplasia

36. **Attal, P., Vilgrain, V., Brancatelli, G., Paradis, V., Terris, B., Belghiti, J., Taouli, B., Menu, Y.:** Telangiectatic focal nodular hyperplasia: US, CT, and MR imaging findings with histopathologic correlation in 13 cases. Radiology 2003; 228: 465–472
37. **Carlson, S.K., Johnson, C.D., Bender, C.E., Welch, M.J.:** CT of focal nodular hyperplasia of the liver. Amer. J. Roentg. 2000; 174: 705–712
38. **Cherqui, D., Rahmouni, A., Charlotte, F., Boulahdour, H., Métreau, J.M., Meignan, M., Fagniez, P.L., Zafrani, E.S., Mathieu, D., Dhumeaux, D.:** Management of focal nodular hyperplasia and hepatocellular adenoma in young woman: a series of 41 patients with clinical, radiological, and pathological correlations. Hepatology 1995; 22: 1674–1681
39. **Choi, C.S., Freeny, P.C.:** Triphasic helical CT of hepatic focal nodular hyperplasia: incidence of atypical findings. Amer. J. Roentg. 1998; 170: 391–395
40. **Closset, J., Veys, I., Peny, M.O., Braude, P., van Gansbeke, D., Lambilliotte, J.P., Gelin, M.:** Retrospective analysis of 29 patients surgically treated for hepatocellular adenoma or focal nodular hyperplasia. Hepato-Gastroenterol. 2000; 47: 1382–1384
41. **Colle, I., Op-de-Beeck, B., Hoorens, A., Hautekeete, M.:** Multiple focal nodular hyperplasia. J. Gastroenterol. 1998; 33: 904–908
42. **Fabre, A., Audet, P., Vilgrain, V., Nguyen, B.N., Valla, D., Belghiti, J., Degott, C.:** Histologic scoring of liver biopsy in focal nodular hyperplasia with atypical presentation. Hepatology 2002; 35: 414–420
43. **Fukukura, Y., Nakashima, O., Kusaba, A., Kage, M., Kojiro, M.:** Angioarchitecture and blood circulation in focal nodular hyperplasia of the liver. J. Hepatol. 1998; 29: 470–475
44. **Ko, S.F., Ng, S.H., Lee, T.Y., Wan, Y.L., Lin, J.W., Chen, C.L.:** Hepatic focal nodular hyperplasia: The "star sign" on gadolinium-enhanced magnetic resonance angiography. Hepatogastroenterol. 2002; 49: 1377–1381
45. **Kudo, M., Tomita, S., Tochio, H., Kashida, H., Hirasa, M., Todo, A.:** Hepatic focal nodular hyperplasia: specific findings at dynamic contrast-enhanced US with carbon dioxide microbubbles. Radiology 1991; 179: 377–382
46. **Landen, S., Siriser, F., Bardaxoglou, E., Maddern, G.J., Chareton, B., Campion, J.P., Launois, B.:** Focal nodular hyperplasia of the liver: a retrospective review of 20 patients managed surgically. Acta Chir. Belg. 1993; 93: 94–97
47. **Learch, T.J., Ralls, P.W., Johnson, M.B., Jeffrey, R.B., Nino Murcia, M., Lee, K.P., Radin, D.R.:** Hepatic focal nodular hyperplasia: findings with color Doppler sonography. J. Ultrasound Med. 1993; 12: 541–544
48. **Mathieu, D., Kobeiter, H., Maison, P., Rahmouni, A., Cherqui, D., Zafrani, E.S., Dhumeaux, D.:** Oral contraceptive use and focal nodular hyperplasia of the liver. Gastroenterology 2000; 118: 560–564

49. Ngujen, B.N., Flejou, J.F., Ferris, B., Belghiti, J., Degott, C.: Focal nodular hyperplasia of the liver – a comprehensive pathologic study of 305 lesions and recognition of new histologic forms. Amer. J. Surg. Pathol. 1999; 23: 1441–1454
50. Ohmoto, K., Honda, T., Hirokawa, M., Mitsui, Y., Iguchi, Y., Kuboki, M., Yamamoto, S.: Spontaneous regression of focal nodular hyperplasia of the liver (case report). J. Gastroenterol. 2002; 37: 849–853
51. Paradis, V., Bieche, I., Dargere, D., Laurendeau, I., Nectoux, J., Degott, C., Belghiti, J., Vidaud, M., Bedossa, P.: A quantitative gene expression study suggests a role for angiopoietins in focal nodular hyperplasia. Gastroenterology 2003; 124: 651–659
52. Rangheard, A.S., Vilgrain, V., Audet, P., O'Toole, D., Vullierme, M.P., Valla, D., Belghiti, J., Menu, Y.: Focal nodular hyperplasia inducing hepatic vein obstruction. Amer. J. Roentgenol. 2002; 179: 759–762
53. Reymond, D., Plaschkes, J., Luthy, A.R., Leubundgut, K., Hirt, A., Wagner, H.P.: Focal nodular hyperplasia of the liver in children: review of follow-up and outcome. J. Pediadr. Surg. 1995; 30: 1590–1593
54. Ruschenburg, I., Droese, M.: Fine needle aspiration cytology of focal nodular hyperplasia of the liver. Acta Cytol 1989; 33: 587–860
55. Sadowski, D.C., Lee, S.S., Wanless, I.R., Kelly, J.K., Heathcote, E.J.: Progressive type of focal nodular hyperplasia characterized by multiple tumors and recurrence. Hepatology 1995; 21: 970–975
56. Santarelli, L., Gabrielli, M., Orefice, R., Nista, E.C., Serricchio, M., Nestola, M., Rapaccini, G., de Ninno, M., Pola, P., Gasbarrini, G., Gasbarrini, A.: Association between Klinefelter syndrome and focal nodular hyperplasia. J. Clin. Gastroenterol. 2003; 37: 189–191
57. Tohara, K., Sakaguchi, S., Hatono, N., Mitsuyasu, Y., Miyajima, Y., Tanaka, M., Yao, T.: Usefulness of power Doppler imaging in the diagnosis of small focal nodular hyperplasia of the liver. Hepatol. Res. 1999; 14: 26–34
58. Yen, Y.H., Wang, J.H., Lu, S.N., Chen, T.Y., Changchien, C.S., Chen, C.H., Hung, C.H, Lee, C.M.: Contrast-enhanced ultrasonographic spoke-wheel sign in hepatic focal nodular hyperplasia. Eur. J. Radiol, 2006; 60: 439–444
59. Yoshida, T., Ono, N., Nishimura, H., Hayabuti, N., Tanikawa, K.: Diagnostic imaging of patients with focal nodular hyperplasia of the liver. Hepatol. Res. 1997; 9: 209–217

Nodular regenerative hyperplasia
60. Austin, A., Campbell, E., Lane, P., Elias, E.: Nodular regenerative hyperplasia of the liver and celiac disease: potential role of IgA anticardiolipin antibody. Gut 2004; 53: 1032–1034
61. Beer, T.W., Carr, N.J., Buxton, P.J.: Thorotrast associated nodular regenerative hyperplasia of the liver. J. Clin. Pathol. 1998; 51: 941–942
62. Cano-Ruiz, A., Martin-Scapa, M.A., Larraona, J.L., Gonzalez-Martin, J.A., Moreno-Caparros, A., Garcia-Plaza, A.: Laparoscopic findings in seven patients with nodular regenerative hyperplasia of the liver. Amer. J. Gastroenterol. 1985; 80: 796–800
63. Colina, F., Pinedo, F., Solis, J.A., Moreno, D., Nevado, M.: Nodular regenerative hyperplasia of the liver in early histological stages of primary biliary cirrhosis. Gastroenterology 1992; 102: 1319–1324
64. Dachman, A.H., Ros, P.R., Goodman, Z.D., Olmsted, W.W., Ishak, K.G.: Nodular regenerative hyperplasia of the liver: clinical and radiologic observations. Amer. J. Roentgenol. 1987; 148: 717–722
65. Dumortier, J., Boillot, O., Chevallier, M., Berger, F., Potier, P., Valette, P.J., Paliard, P., Scoazec, J.Y.: Familial occurrence of nodular regenerative hyperplasia of the liver: a report on three families. Gut 1999; 45: 289–294
66. Fujii, H., Sakaguchi, H., Enomoto, M., Yamamori, K., Inagawa, M., Watanabe, T., Kawada, N., Seki, S., Arakawa, T.: Laparoscopic observation of 2 cases of nodular regenerative hyperplasia of the liver (case report). Gastrointest. Endosc. 2007; 65: 171–173
67. Loinaz, C., Colina, F., Musella, M., Lopez-Rios, F., Gomez, R., Jimenez, C., Gonzales Pinto, I., Garcia, I., Moreno Gonzales, E.: Orthotopic liver transplantation in 4 patients with portal hypertension and noncirrhotic nodular liver. Hepatogastroenterol. 1998; 45: 1787–1794
68. Naber, A.H., van Haelst, U., Yap, S.H.: Nodular regenerative hyperplasia of the liver: an important cause of portal hypertension in noncirrhotic patients. J. Hepatol. 1991; 12: 94–99
69. Nakamura, Y.: Nodular regenerative hyperplasia of the liver: retrospective survey in autopsy series. J. Clin. Gastroenterol. 1990; 12: 460–465
70. Sherlock, S., Feldman, C.A., Moran, B., Scheuer, P.J.: Partial nodular transformation of the liver with portal hypertension. Amer. J. Med. 1966; 40: 195–203
71. Trauner, M., Stepan, K.M., Resch, M., Ebner, F., Pristautz, H., Klimpfinger, M.: Diagnostic problems in nodular regenerative hyperplasia (nodular transformation) of the liver. Review of the literature and report of two cases. Z. Gastroenterol. 1992; 30: 187–194
72. Wanless, I.R.: Micronodular transformation (nodular regenerative hyperplasia) of the liver: a report of 64 cases among 2500 autopsies and a new classification of benign hepatocellular nodules. Hepatology 1990; 11: 787–797

Haemangioma
73. Achong, D.M., Oates, E.: Hepatic hemangioma in cirrhotics with portal hypertension: evaluation with Tc-99m red blood cell SPECT. Radiology. 1994; 191: 115–117
74. Aiura, K., Ohshima, K., Matsumoto, K., Ishii, S., Arisawa, Y., Nakagawa, M.: Spontaneous rupture of liver hemangioma: risk factors for rupture. Hepatobil. Pancr. Surg. 1996; 3: 308–312
75. Birnbaum, B.A., Weinreb, J.C., Megibow, A.J., Sanger, J.J., Lubat, E., Kanamüller, E., Noz, M.E., Bosniak, M.A.: Definitive diagnosis of hepatic hemangiomas: MR imaging versus Tc-99 m-labeled red blood cell SPECT. Radiology 1990; 176: 95–101
76. Coumbaras, M., Wendum, D., Monnier-Cholley, L., Dahan, H., Tubiana, J.M., Arrive, L.: CT and MR imaging features of pathologically proven atypical giant hemangiomas of the liver. Amer. J. Roentgenol. 2002; 179: 1457–1463
77. Demircan, O., Demiryurek, H., Yagmur, O.: Surgical approach to oymptomatic giant cavernous hemangioma of the liver. Hepato. Gastroenterol. 2005; 52: 183–186
78. Dietrich, C.F., Mertens, J.C., Braden, B., Schuessler, G., Ott, M., Ignee, A.: Contrast-enhanced ultrasound of histologically proven liver hemangiomas. Hepatology 2007; 45: 1139-1145
79. Gandolfi, L., Leo, P., Solmi, L., Vitelli, E., Verros, G., Colecchia, A.: Natural history of hepatic haemangiomas: clinical and ultrasound study. Gut 1991; 32: 677–680
80. Gedaly, R., Pomposelli, J.J., Pomfret, E.A., Lewis, W.D., Jenkins, R.L.: Cavernous hemangioma of the liver – Anatomic resection vs. enucleation. Arch. Surg. 1999; 134: 407–411
81. Hanazaki, K., Kajikawa, S., Matsushita, A., Monma, T., Koide, N., Nimura, Y., Yazawa, K., Watanabe, H., Nishio, A., Adachi, W., Amano, J.: Hepatic resection of giant cavernous hemangioma of the liver. J. Clin. Gastroenterol. 1999; 29: 257–260
82. Heilo, A., Stenwig, A.E.: Liver hemangioma: US-guided 18-gauge core-needle biopsy. Radiology 1997; 204: 719–722
83. Jacobson, A.F., Teefey, S.A.: Cavernous hemangiomas of the liver. Association of sonographic appearance and results of Tc-99m labeled red blood cell SPECT. Clin. Nucl. Med. 1994; 19: 96–99
84. Joon, S.S., Charny, C.K., Fong, Y., Jarnagin, W.R., Schwartz, L.H., Blumgart, L.H., de Matteo, R.P.: Diagnosis, management, and outcomes of 115 patients with hepatic hemangioma. J. Amer. Coll. Surg. 2003; 197: 392–402
85. Kassarjian, A., Zurakowski, D., Dubois, J., Paltiel, H.J., Fishman, S.J., Burrows, P.E.: Infantile hepatic hemangiomas: Clinical and imaging findings and their correlation with therapy. Amer. J. Roentgenol. 2004; 182: 785–795
86. Klompmaker, I.J., Slooff, M.J.H., van der Meer, J., de Jong, G.M.T., de Bruijn, K.M., Bams, J.L.: Orthotopic liver transplantation in a patient with a giant cavernous hemangioma of the liver and Kasabach-Merritt syndrome. Transplantation 1989; 48: 149–151
87. Langner, C., Thonhofer, R., Hegenbarth, K., Trauner, M.: Diffuse hemangiomatosis of the liver and spleen in an adult. Pathologe 2001; 22: 424–428
88. Lerner, S.M., Hiatt, J.R., Salamandra, J., Chen, P.W., Farmer, D.G., Ghobrial, R.M., Buouttil, R.W.: Giant cavernous liver hemangiomas. Effect of operative approach on outcome. Arch. Surg. 2004; 139: 818–821
89. Middleton, M.L.: Scintigraphic evaluation of hepatic mass lesions: emphasis on hemangioma detection. Semin. Nucl. Med. 1996; 26: 4–15
90. Nghiem, H.V., Bogost, G.A., Ryan, J.A., Lund, P., Freeny, P.C., Rice, K.M.: Cavernous hemangiomas of the liver: enlargement over time. Amer. J. Roentgenol. 1997; 169: 137–140
91. Özden, I., Emre, A., Alper, A., Tunaci, M., Acarli, K., Bilge, O., Tekant, Y., Ariogul, O.: Long-term results of surgery for liver hemangiomas. Arch. Surg. 2000; 135: 978–981
92. Pietrabissa, A., Giulianotti, P., Campatelli, A., Di Candio, G., Farina, F., Signori, S., Mosca, F.: Management of follow-up of 78 giant haemangiomas of the liver. Brit. J. Surg. 1996; 83: 915–918
93. Quinn, S.F., Benjamin, G.G.: Hepatic cavernous hemangiomas: simple diagnostic sign with dynamic bolus CT. Radiology 1992; 182: 545–548
94. Takahashi, T., Katoh, H., Dohke, M., Okushiba, S.: A giant hepatic hemangioma with secondary portal hypertension. A case report of successful surgical treatment. Hepato-Gastroenterol. 1997; 44: 1212–1214
95. Tsai, H.P., Jeng, L.B., Lee, W.C., Chen, M.F.: Clinical experience of hepatic hemangioma undergoing hepatic resection. Dig. Dis. Sci. 2003; 48: 916–920
96. Yeh, W.C., Yang, P.M., Huang, G.T., Sheu, J.C., Chen, D.S.: Long-term follow-up of hepatic hemangiomas by ultrasonography: With emphasis on the growth rate of the tumor. Hepato-Gastroenterol. 2007; 54: 475–479
97. Yoon, S.S., Charny, C.K., Fong, Y., Jarnagin, W.R., Schwartz, L.H., Blumgart, L.H., de Matteo, R.P.: Diagnosis, management, and outcomes of 115 patients with hepatic hemangioma. J. Amer. Surg. 2003; 197: 392–402
98. Yu, J.S., Kim, M.J., Kim, K.W., Chan, J.C., Jo, B.J., Kim, T.H., Lee, J.T., Yoo, H.S.: Hepatic cavernous hemangioma: Sonographic patterns and speed of contrast enhancement on multiphase dynamic MR imaging. Amer. J. Roentgenol. 1998; 171: 1021–1025

Infantile haemangioendothelioma
99. Becker, J.M., Heitler, M.S.: Hepatic hemangioendothelioma in infancy. Surg. Gynec. Obstetr. 1989; 168: 189–200
100. Dachman, A.H., Lichtenstein, J.E., Friedman, A.C., Hartman, D.S.: Infantile hemangioendothelioma of the liver: a radiologic-pathologic-clinical correlation. Amer. J. Roentgenol. 1983; 140: 1091–1096
101. Daller, J.A., Bueno, J., Gutierrez, J., Dvorchik, I., Towbin, R.B., Dickman, P.S., Mazariegos, G., Reyes, J.: Hepatic hemangioendothelioma: clinical experience and management strategy. J. Pediatr. Surg. 1999; 34: 98–105
102. Diment, J., Yurim, O., Pappo, O.: Infantile hemangioendothelioma of the liver in an adult. Arch. Pathol. Lab. Med. 2001; 125: 931–932
103. Kaniklides, C., Dimopoulos, P.A., Bajic, D.: Infantile hemangioendothelioma. A case report. Acta Radiol. 2000; 41: 161–164

104. **Kardoff, R., Fuchs, J., Peuster, M., Rodeck, B.:** Infantile hemangioendothelioma of the liver: Sonographic diagnosis and follow-up. Ultrasch. Med. 2001; 22: 258–264
105. **Selby, D.M., Stocker, J.T., Waclawiw, M.A., Hitchcock, C.L.:** Infantile hemangioendothelioma of the liver. Hepatology 1994; 20: 39–45
106. **Woltering, M.C., Robben, S., Egeler, R.M.:** Hepatic hemangioendothelioma of infancy: treatment with interferon α. J. Pediatr. Gastroenterol. Nutrit. 1997; 24: 348–351

Lipoma
107. **Marti-Bonmati, L., Menor, F., Vizcaino, I., Vilar, J.:** Lipoma of the liver: US, CT, and MRI appearance. Gastrointest. Radiol. 1989; 14: 155–157
108. **Sonsuz, A., Ozdemir, S., Akdogan, M., Sentürk, H., Özbay, G., Akin, P., Gürakar, M.:** Lipoma of the liver. Z. Gastroenterol. 1994; 32: 348–350

Myelolipoma
109. **Moreno Gonzales, E., Seoane Gonzalez, J.B., Bercedo Martinez, J., Santoyo Santoyo, J., Gomez Sanz, R., Vargas Castrijon, J., Ballestin Carcavilla, C., Garcia Maurino, M.L., Colina Ruiz-Delgado, F.:** Hepatic Myelolipoma; new case and review of the literature. Hepato-Gastroenterol. 1991; 38: 60–63
110. **Rubin, E., Russinovich, N.A.E., Luna, R.F., Tishler, J.M.A., Wilkerson, J.A.:** Myelolipoma of the liver. Cancer 1984; 54: 2043–2046

Angiomyolipoma
111. **Ahmadi, T., Itai, Y., Takahashi, M., Onaya, H., Kobayashi, T., Tanaka, Y.O., Matsuzaki, Y., Tanaka, N., Okada, Y.:** Angiomyolipoma of the liver: significance of CT and MR dynamic study. Abdom. Imag. 1998; 23: 520–526
112. **Block, S., Theilmann, L.:** Angiomyolipoma of the liver. Dtsch. Med. Wschr. 2000; 125: 743–745
113. **Carloni, A., Tranchart, H., Beauthier, V., Mas, A.E., Daguer, I., Dumas de la Roque, A., Landau, A., Franco, D.:** Angiomyolipome hepatique symptomatique. Gastroenterol. Clin. Biol. 2007; 31: 555–556
114. **Cha, I., Cartwright, D., Guis, M., Miller, T.R., Ferrell, L.D.:** Angiomyolipoma of the liver in fine-needle aspiration biopsies. Cancer 1999; 87: 25–30
115. **Croquet, V., Pilette, C., Aubé, C., Bouju, B., Oberti, F., Cervi, C., Arnaud, J.P., Rousselet, M.C., Boyer, J., Cales, P.:** Late recurrence of a hepatic angiomyolipoma. Eur. J. Gastroenterol. Hepatol. 2000; 12: 579–582
116. **Garcia, T.R., de Juan, M.J.M.:** Angiomyolipoma of the liver and lung: a case explained by the presence of perivascular epithelioid cells. Pathol. Res. Pract. 2002; 198: 363–367
117. **Goodman, Z.D., Ishak, K.G.:** Angiomyolipomas of the liver. Amer. Surg. Pathol. 1994; 8: 745–750
118. **Guidi, G., Catalano, O., Rotondo, A.:** Spontaneous rupture of a hepatic angiomyolipoma: CT findings and literature review. Eur. Radiol. 1997; 7: 335–337
119. **Hoffmann, A.L., Emre, S., Verham, R.P., Petrovic, L.M., Eguchi, S., Silverman, J.L., Geller, S.A., Schwartz, M.E., Miller, C.M., Makowka, L.:** Hepatic angiomyolipoma: two case reports of caudate-based lesions and review of the literature. Liver Transplant. Surg. 1997; 3: 46–53
120. **Ju, Y., Zhu, X.Z., Xu, J.F., Zhou, J., Tan, Y.S., Wang, J., Fan, J., Zhou, Y.N.:** Hepatic angiomyolipoma: a clinicopathologic study of 10 cases. Chin. Med. J. 2001; 114: 280–285
121. **Messiaen, T., Lefebvre, C., van Beers, B., Sempoux, C., Cosyns, J.P., Geubel, A.:** Hepatic angiomyo(myelo)lipoma: difficulties in radiological diagnosis and interest of fine needle aspiration biopsy. Liver 1996; 16: 338–341
122. **Ng, K.K.C., Poon, R.T.P., Lam, K.Y., Trendell-Smith, N.J., Fan, S.T.:** Hepatic angiomyolipoma. Surgery 2003; 133: 594–595
123. **Nonomura, A., Mizukami, Y., Kadoya, M., Matsui, O., Shimizu, K., Izumi, R.:** Angiomyolipoma of the liver: Its clinical and pathological diversity. J. Hep. Bil. Pancr. Surg. 1996; 3: 122–132
124. **Takayama, Y., Moriura, S., Nagata, J., Hirano, A., Ishiguro, S., Tabata, T., Matsumoto, T., Sato, T.:** Hepatic angiomyolipoma: radiologic and histopathologic correlation (case report). Abdom. Imag. 2002; 27: 180–183
125. **Tang, L.H., Hui, P., Garcia-Tsao, G., Salem, R.R., Jain, D.:** Multiple angiomyolipomata of the liver: a case report. Modern Pathol. 2002; 15: 167–171
126. **Wang, S.N., Tsai, K.B., Lee, K.T.:** Hepatic angiomyolipoma with trace amounts of fat. A case report and literature review. J. Clin. Path. 2006; 59: 1190–1199
127. **Yan, F.H., Zeng, M.S., Zhou, K.R., Shi, W.B., Zheng, W.W., Da, R.R., Fan, J., Ji, Y.:** Hepatic angiomyolipoma: various appearances of two-phase contrast scanning of spiral CT. Eur. J. Radiol. 2002; 41: 12–18
128. **Yang, C.Y., Ho, M.C., Jeng, Y.M., Hu, R.H., Wu, Y.M., Lee, P.H.:** Management of hepatic angiomyolipoma. J. Gastrointest. Surg. 2007; 11: 452–457
129. **Yoshimura, H., Murakami, T., Kim, T., Nakamura, H., Hirabuki, N., Sakon, M., Wakasa, K., Inoue, Y.:** Angiomyolipoma of the liver with least amount of fat component: imaging feature of CT, MR, and angiography (case report). Abdom. Imag. 2002; 27: 184–187

Chondroma
130. **Fried, R.H., Wardzala, A., Willson, R.A., Sinanan, M.N., Marchioro, T.L., Haggitt, R.:** Benign cartilaginous tumor (chondroma) of the liver. Gastroenterology 1992; 103: 678–680

Leiomyoma
131. **Herzberg, A.J., MacDonald, J.A., Tucker, J.A., Humphrey, P.A., Myers, W.C.:** Primary leiomyoma of the liver. Amer. J. Gastroenterol. 1990; 85: 1642–1645

Schwannoma
132. **Hytiroglou, P., Linton, P., Klion, F., Schwartz, M., Miller, C., Thung, S.N.:** Benign schwannoma of the liver. Arch. Pathol. Lab. Med. 1993; 117: 216–218
133. **Jakobs, R., Albert, J., Schilling, D., Nuesse, T., Riemann, J.F.:** Schwannoma of the common bile duct: a rare cause of obstructive jaundice (case report). Endoscopy 2003; 35: 695–697

Glomangioma
134. **Gassel, H.J., Klein, I., Timmermann, W., Kenn, W., Gassel, A.M., Thiede, A.:** Presentation of an unusual benign liver tumor: primary hepatic glomangioma (case report). Scand. J. Gastroenterol. 2002; 37: 1237–1240

Hamartoma
135. **Cook, J.R., Pfeifer, J.D., Dehner, L.P.:** Mesenchymal hamartoma of the liver in the adult: Anociation with distinct clinical features and histological changes. Hum. Pathol. 2002; 33: 893–898
136. **DeMaioribus, C.A., Lally, K.P., Sim, K., Isaacs, H., Mahour, G.H.:** Mesenchymal hamartoma of the liver. A 35-year review. Arch. Surg. 1990; 125: 598–600
137. **Lack, E.E.:** Mesenchymal hamartoma of the liver. A clinical and pathological study of nine cases. Amer. J. Pediatr. Hematol./Oncol. 1986; 8: 91–98

Mesothelioma
138. **Flemming, P., Becker, T., Klempnauer, J., Hogemann, D., Kreft, A., Kreipe, H.H.:** Benign cystic mesothelioma of the liver. Amer. J. Surg. Pathol. 2002; 26: 1523–1527
139. **Kim, H., Damjanov, I.:** Localized fibrous mesothelioma of the liver. Report of a giant tumor studied by light and electron microscopy. Cancer 1983; 52: 1662–1665

Fibrous tumour
140. **Neeff, H., Obermaier, R., Technaulhling, K., Werner, M., Kurtz, C., Imdahl, A., Hopf, U.T.:** Solitary fibrous tumour of the liver: case report and review of the literature. Langenbecks Arch. Surg. 2004; 389: 293–298

Cysts
141. **Cellier, C., Cuenod, C.A., Deslandes, P., Auroux, J., Landi, B., Siauve, N., Barbier, J.-P, Frija, G.:** Symptomatic hepatic cysts: treatment with single-shot injection of minocycline hydrochloride. Radiology 1998; 206: 205–209
142. **Cowles, R.A., Mulholland, M.W.:** Solitary hepatic cysts. Amer. Coll. Surg. 2000; 191: 311–321
143. **De Simone, M., Cioffi, U.:** Laparoscopic Lin operation for the treatment of polycystic liver disease. Hepato-Gastroenterol. 1998; 45: 1846–1848
144. **Diez, J., Decoud, J., Gutierrez, L., Suhl, A., Merello, J.:** Laparoscopic treatment of symptomatic cysts of the liver. Brit. J. Surg. 1998; 85: 25–27
145. **Dmitrewski, J., Olliff, S., Buckels, J.A.C.:** Obstructive jaundice associated with polycystic liver disease. HPB Surg. 1996; 10: 117–120
146. **Garcea, G., Pattenden, C.J., Stephenson, J., Dannison, A.R., Berry, D.P.:** Nine-year single-center experience with non-parasitic liver cysts: Diagnosis and management, Dig. Dis. Sci. 2007; 52: 185–191
147. **Gigot, J.-F., Jadoul, P., Que, F., van Beers, B.E., Etienne, J., Horsmans, Y., Collard, A., Geubel, A., Pringot, J., Kestens, P.-J.:** Adult polycystic liver disease. Is fenestration the most adequate operation for long-term management? Ann. Surg. 1997; 225: 286–294
148. **Henne-Bruns, D., Klomp, H.-J., Kremer,B.:** Non-parasitic liver cysts and polycystic liver disease: results of surgical treatment. Hepatogastroenterology 1993; 40: 1–5
149. **Kathouda, N., Hurwitz, M., Gugenheim, J., Mavor, E., Mason, R.J., Waldrep, D.J., Rivera, R.T., Chandra, M., Campos, G.M.R., Offerman, S., Trussler, A., Fabiani, P., Mouiel, J.:** Laparoscopic management of benign solid and cystic lesions of the liver. Ann. Surg. 1999; 229: 460–466
150. **Klingler, P.J., Gadenstätter, M., Schmid, T., Bodner, E., Schwelberger, H.G.:** Treatment of hepatic cysts in the era of laparoscopy surgery. Brit. J. Surg. 1997; 84: 438–444
151. **Konstadoulakis, M.M., Gomatos, I.P., Albanopoulos, K., Alexakis, N., Leandros, E.:** Laparoscopic fenestration for the treatment of patients with severe adult polycystic liver disease. Amer. J. Surg. 2005; 189: 71–75
152. **Kwon, A.H., Matsui, Y., Inui, H., Imamura, A., Kamiyama, Y.:** Laparoscopic treatment using an argon beam coagulator for nonparasitic liver cysts. Amer. J. Surg. 2003; 185: 273–277
153. **Okano, A., Hajiro, K., Takakuwa, H., Nishio, A.:** Alcohol sclerotherapy of hepatic cysts: its effect in relation to ethanol concentration. Hepatol. Res. 2000; 17: 179–184
154. **Swenson, K., Seu, P., Kinkhabwala, M., Maggard, M., Martin, P., Goss, J., Bussutil, R.:** Liver transplantation for adult polycystic liver disease. Hepatology 1998; 28: 412–415
155. **Tocchi, A., Mazzoni, G., Costa, G., Cassini, D., Bettelli, E., Agostini, N., Miccini, M.:** Symptomatic nonparasitic hepatic cysts. Options for and results of surgical management. Arch. Surg. 2002; 137: 154–158
156. **Yoshida, H., Onda, M., Tajiri, T., Arima, Y., Mamada, Y., Taniai, N., Akimaru, K.:** Long-term results of multiple minocycline hydrochloride injections for the treatment of symptomatic solitary hepatic cyst. J. Gastroenterol. Hepatol. 2003; 18: 595–598

Caroli's disease
157. **Choi, B.I., Yeon, K.M., Kim, S.H., Han, M.C.:** Caroli disease: central dot sign in CT. Radiology 1990; 174: 161–163
158. **Dagli, Ü., Atalay, F., Sasmaz, N., Bostanoglu, S., Temucin, G., Sahin, B.:** Caroli's disease: 1977–1995 experiences. Eur. J. Gastroenterol. Hepatol. 1998; 10: 109–112
159. **Inui, A., Fujisawa, T., Suemitsu, T., Fujikawa, S., Ariizumi, M., Kagimoto, S., Kinoshita, K.:** A case of Caroli's disease with special reference to hepatic CT and US findings. J. Pediatr. Gastroenterol. Nutr. 1992; 14: 462–406
160. **Taylor, A.C.F., Palmer, K.R.:** Caroli's disease. Eur. J. Gastroenterol. Hepatol. 1998; 10: 105–108

Cystadenoma
161. **Akwari, O.E., Tucker, A., Seigler, H.F., Itani, K.M.F.:** Hepatobiliary cystadenoma with mesenchymal stroma. Ann. Surg. 1990; 211: 18–27
162. **Beretta, E., de Franchis, R., Staudacher, C., Faravelli, A., Primignani, M., Vecchi, M., Conti, E., di Carlo, V.:** Biliary cystadenoma: an uncommon cause of recurrent cholestatic jaundice. Amer. J. Gastroenterol. 1986; 81: 138–140
163. **Devaney, K., Goodman, Z.D., Ishak, K.G.:** Hepatobiliary cystadenoma and cystadenocarcinoma. A light microsopig and immunohistochemical study of 70 patients. Amer. J. Surg. Pathol. 1994; 18: 1078–1091
164. **Lewis, W.D., Jenkins, R.L., Rossi, R.L., Munson, L., Re Mine, S.G., Cady, B., Braasch, J.W., McDermott, W.V.:** Surgical treatment of biliary cystadenoma. A report of 15 cases. Arch. Surg. 1988; 123: 563–568
165. **Subramony, C., Herrera, G.A., Turbat-Herrera, E.A.:** Hepatobiliary cystadenoma. A study of five cases with reference to histogenesis. Arch. Pathol. Lab. Med. 1993; 117: 1036–1042
166. **Thomas, K.T., Welch, D., Trueblood, A., Sulur, P., Wise, P., Gorden, D.L., Chari, R.S., Wright, J.K., Washington, K., Pinson, C.W.:** Effective treatment of biliary cystadenoma. Ann. Surg. 2005; 241: 769–775
167. **Tressallet, C., Jordi-Galais, P., Nguyen-Thanh, Q., Aubriot-Lorton, M.H., Costedoat-Chalumeau, N., Chigot, J.P., Menegaux, F.:** Cystadenoma of the liver with high levels of ACE and CA 19-9 in the cyst (case report). Gastroenterol. Clin. Biol. 2003; 27: 413–415

Bile duct adenoma
168. **Allaire, G.S., Rabin, L., Ishak, K.G., Sesterhenn, I.A.:** Bile duct adenoma. A study of 152 cases. Amer. J. Surg. Path. 1988; 12: 708–715
169. **Bhathal, P.S., Hughes, N.R., Goodman, Z.D.:** The so-called bile duct adenoma is a peribiliary gland hamartoma. Amer. J. Surg. Pathol. 1996; 20: 858–864
170. **Tajima, T., Honda, H., Kuroiwa, T., Yoshimitsu, K., Irie, H., Aibe, H., Taguchi, K., Shimada, M., Masuda, K.:** Radiologic features of intrahepatic bile duct adenoma: a look at the surface of the liver. J. Comput. Assist. Tomogr. 1999; 23: 690–695

Papillomatosis
171. **Beavers, K.L., Fried, M.W., Johnson, M.W., Zacks, S.L., Gerber, D.A., Weeks, S.M., Fair, J.H., Odell, P., Shresta, R.:** Orthotopic liver transplantation for biliary papillomatosis. Liver Transplant. 2001; 7: 264–265
172. **Gunven, P., Gorsetman, J., Ohlsen, H., Ruden, B.-I., Lundell, G., Skoog, L.:** Six-year recurrence free survival after intraluminal iridium 192 therapy for human bilobar biliary papillomatosis. Cancer 2000; 89: 69–73
173. **Lee, S.S., Kim, M.H., Lee, S.K., Jang, S.J., Song, M.H., Kim H.J., Seo, D.W., Song, D.E., Yu, E., Lee, S.G., Min, Y.I.:** Clinicopathologic review of 58 patients with biliary papillomatosis. Cancer 2004; 100: 783–793

Biliary hamartoma
174. **Burns, C.D., Kuhns, J.G., Wieman, T.J.:** Cholangiocarcinoma in association with multiple biliary microhamartomas. Arch. Pathol. Lab. Med. 1990; 114: 1287–1289
175. **Maher, M.M., Dervan, P., Keogh, B., Murray, J.G.:** Bile duct hamartomas (von Meyenburg complexes): value of MR imaging in diagnosis. Abdom. Imag. 1999; 24: 171–173
176. **Ohta, W., Ushio, H.:** Histological reconstruction of a von Meyenburg's complex as the liver surface. Endoscopy 1984; 16: 71–76
177. **Orii, T., Ohkohchi, N., Sasaki, K., Satomi, S., Watanabe, M., Moriya, T.:** Cholangiocarcinoma arising from preexisting biliary hamartoma of liver. – Report of a case. Hepato-Gastroenterol. 2003; 50: 333–336

Lymphangioma
178. **Van Steenbergen, W., Joosten, E., Marchal, G., Baert, A., Vanstapel, M.J., Desmet, V., Wijnants, P., de Groote, J.:** Hepatic lymphangiomatosis. Report of a case and review of the literature. Gastroenterology 1985; 88: 1968–1972

Peliosis hepatis
179. **Ferrozzi, F., Tognini, G., Zuccoli, G., Cademartiri, F., Pavone, P.:** Peliosis hepatis with pseudotumoral and hemorrhagic evolution: CT and MR findings. Abdom. Imag. 2001; 26: 197–199
180. **Jacquemin, E., Pariente, D., Fabre, M., Huault, G., Valayer, J., Bernard, O.:** Peliosis hepatis with initial presentation as acute hepatic failure and intraperitoneal hemorrhage in children. J. Hepatol. 1999; 30: 1146–1150
181. **Loomus, G.N., Aneja, P., Bota, R.A.:** A case of peliosis hepatis in association with tamoxifen therapy. Amer. J. Clin. Pathol. 1983; 80: 881–882
182. **Samyn, M., Hadzic, N., Davenport, M., Verma, A., Karani, J., Portmann, B., Mieli-Vergani, G.:** Peliosis hepatis in childhood: case report and review of the literature. J. Pediatr. Gastroenterol. Nutr. 2004; 39: 431–434
183. **Solis-Herruzo, J.A., Colina, F., Munoz-Yagüe, M.T., Castellano, G., Morillas, J.D.:** Reddish-purple areas on the liver surface: the laparoscopic picture of peliosis hepatis. Endoscopy 1983; 15: 96–100

Sarcoidosis
184. **Afifi, R., Benelbarhdadi, I., Ibrahimi, A., Fall, A.B., Benazzouz, M., Essaid, A., Sebti, M.F.:** Les granulomatoses hépatiques. Ann. Gastroéntérol. Hépatol. 1997; 33: 218–222
185. **Ayyala, U.S., Padilla, M.L.:** Diagnosis and treatment of hepatic sarcoidosis. Curr. Treat. Opin. Gastroenterol. 2006; 9: 475–483
186. **Blich, M., Edoute, Y.:** Clinical manifestations of sarcoid liver disease. J. Gastroenterol. Hepatol. 2004; 19: 732–737
187. **Hoffmann, R.M., Jung, M.-C., Motz, R., Gößl, C., Emslander, H.-P., Zachoval, R., Pape, G.R.:** Sarcoidosis associated with interferon-α therapy for chronic hepatitis C. J. Hepatol. 1998; 28: 1058–1063
188. **Ishak, K.G.:** Sarcoidosis of the liver and bile ducts. Mayo Clin. Proc. 1998; 73: 467–472
189. **Jung, G., Brill, N., Poll, L.W., Koch, J.A., Wettstein, M.:** MRI of hepatic sarcoidosis: large confluent lesions mimicking malignancy. Amer. J. Roentgenol. 2004; 183: 171–173
190. **Karagiannidis, A., Karavalaki, M., Koulaouzidis, A.:** Hepatic sarcoidosis (review). Ann. Hepatol. 2006; 5: 251–256
191. **Mueller, S., Boehme, M.W., Hofmann, W.J., Stremmel, W.:** Extrapulmonary sarcoidosis primarily diagnosed in the liver. Scand. J. Gastroenterol. 2000; 35: 1003–1008

Inflammatory pseudotumour
192. **Hoosein, M.M., Tapuria, N., Standish, R.A., Koti, R.S., Webster, G.J.M., Millar, A.D., Davidson, B.R.:** Inflammatory pseudotumour of the liver: The residuum of a biliary cystadenoma? (case report) Eur. J. Gastroenterol. Hepatol. 2007; 19: 333–336
193. **Noi, I., Loberant, N., Cohen, I.:** Inflammatory pseudotumor of the liver. Clin. Imag. 1994; 18: 283–285
194. **Papachristou, G.I., Wu, T., Marsh, W., Plevy, S.E.:** Inflammatory pseudotumor of the liver associated with Crohn's disease (case report). J. Clin. Gastroenterol. 2004; 38: 818–822
195. **Pecorella, I., Ciardi, A., Memeo, L., Trombetta, G., de Quarto, A., de Simone, P., di Tondo, U.:** Inflammatory pseudotumor of the liver – evidence for malignant transformation. Pathol. Res. Pract. 1999; 195: 115–120
196. **Seki, S., Kitada, T., Sakaguchi, H., Iwai, S., Hirohashi, K., Higaki, I., Nakamura, K., Wakasa, K., Kinoshita, H.:** A clinicopathological study of inflammatory pseudotumors of the liver with special reference to vessels. Hepato-Gastroenterol. 2004; 51: 1140–1143
197. **Shek, W.H., Ng, O.L., Chan, K.W.:** Inflammatory pseudotumor of the liver. Report of four cases and review of the literature. Amer. J. Surg. Pathol. 1993; 17: 231–238
198. **Zamir, D., Jarchowski, J., Singer, C., Abumoch, S., Groisman, G., Ammar, M., Weiner, P.:** Inflammatory pseudotumor of the liver – a rare entity and a diagnostic challenge. Amer. J. Gastroenterol. 1998; 93: 1538–1540

Erdheim-Chester disease
199. **Gundling, F., Nerlich, A., Heitland, W.U., Schepp, W.:** Biliary manifestation of Erdheim-Chester disease mimicking Klatskin's carcinoma (case report). Amer. J. Gastroenterol. 2007; 102: 452–454

Calcareous foci
200. **Delamarre, J., Capron, J.-P., Sevestre, H., Davion, T., Deschepper, B., Jouet-Gondry, C.:** "Porcelain-liver" appearance due to Glisson's capsule phleboliths. Gastrointest. Radiol. 1989; 14: 339–340
201. **Faßbender, C.M., Büchsel, R., Seelis, R., Hofstädter, F., Matern, S.:** Leberverkalkungen bei metastasierendem Vipom. Dtsch. Med. Wschr. 1989; 114: 1445–1449
202. **Kim, M.H., Sekijima, J., Lee, S.P.:** Primary intrahepatic stones. Amer. J. Gastroenterol. 1995; 90: 540–548
203. **Magruder, M.J., Munden, M.M.:** Intrahepatic microlithiasis: another gastrointestinal complication of cystic fibrosis. J. Ultrasound Med. 1997; 16: 763–765
204. **Pitt, H.A., Venbrux, A.C., Coleman, J., Prescott, C.A., Johnson, M.S., Osterman, F.A., Cameron, J.L.:** Intrahepatic stones. The transhepatic team approach. Ann. Surg. 1994; 219: 527–537
205. **White, L.M., Wilson, S.R.:** Hepatic arterial calcification: a potential pitfall in the sonographic diagnosis of intrahepatic biliary calculi. J. Ultrasound Med. 1994; 13: 141–144

Treatment
206. **Belghiti, J., Paterson, D., Panis, Y., Vilgrain, V., Fléjou, J.F., Benhamou, J.P., Fékété, F.:** Resection of presumed benign liver tumours. Brit. J. Surg. 1993; 80: 380–383
207. **Gibbs, J.F., Litwin, A.M., Kahlenberg, M.S.:** Contemporary management of benign liver tumors. Surg. Clin. North Amer. 2004; 84: 463–480
208. **Mangiante, G., Nicoli, N., Marchiori, L., Procacci, C., Giorgetti, Colombari, R., Aurola, P.P., Serio, G.:** La strategia terapeutica dei tumori epatici benigni: esperienza di 20 anni. Chir. Ital. 1994; 46: 50–60
209. **Ringe, B., Canelo, R., Lorf, T., Klinge, B., Schulze, F.-P., Fischer, U., Herrmann, A., Ramadori, G.:** Chirurgische Therapie von benignen Lebertumoren. Internist 1997; 38: 944–953
210. **Weimann, A., Ringe, B., Klempnauer, J., Lamesch, P., Gratz, K.F., Prokop, M., Maschek, H., Tusch, G., Pichlmayr, R.:** Benign liver tumors: differential diagnosis and indications for surgery. World. J. Surg. 1997; 21: 983–990

Clinical Aspects of Liver Diseases
37 Malignant liver tumours

		Page:
1	*Historical review*	796
2	*Classification*	796
2.1	Systematization	796
2.2	TNM staging system	797
3	*Hepatocellular carcinoma*	798
3.1	Definition	798
3.2	Epidemiology and frequency	798
3.3	Risk factors and causes	798
3.4	Pathogenesis	800
3.5	Morphology	801
3.5.1	Macroscopic forms	801
3.5.2	Microscopic forms	801
3.5.3	Cytological differentiation	802
3.5.4	Metastatic spread	802
3.6	Symptomatology	802
3.6.1	Subjective complaints	802
3.6.2	Clinical findings	803
3.7	Diagnostics	803
3.7.1	Laboratory findings	803
3.7.2	Imaging procedures	804
3.7.3	Morphological diagnosis	805
3.8	Prognosis	806
3.9	Therapy	807
3.9.1	Surgical therapy	807
3.9.2	Interventional therapy	809
3.9.3	Medicinal therapy	811
3.9.4	Adjuvant measures	811
3.10	*Fibrolamellar carcinoma*	813
4	*Cholangiocellular carcinoma*	814
4.1	Definition	814
4.2	Morphology	814
4.3	Epidemiology	815
4.4	Pathogenic risk factors	815
4.5	Clinical features and diagnostics	815
4.6	Therapy	816
4.6.1	Invasive and surgical techniques	816

		Page:
4.6.2	Chemotherapy and radiotherapy	816
4.6.3	Adjuvant measures	817
5	*Cystadenocarcinoma*	817
6	*Hepatablastoma*	817
7	*Mesenchymal liver tumours*	817
7.1	Embryonal sarcoma	817
7.2	Epithelioid haemangioendothelioma	818
7.3	Angiosarcoma	818
7.4	Leiomyosarcoma	818
7.5	Rhabdomyosarcoma	819
7.6	Fibrosarcoma	819
7.7	Fibrous histiocytoma	819
7.8	Malignant schwannoma	819
7.9	Hepatic liposarcoma	819
7.10	Hepatic osteosarcoma	819
8	*Neuroendocrine tumours*	820
8.1	Hepatic gastrinoma	820
8.2	Primary hepatic carcinoid	820
9	*Malignant lymphoma*	820
10	*Liver metastases*	821
10.1	Definition	821
10.2	Morphology	821
10.3	Symptomatology	822
10.4	Diagnostics	823
10.5	Metastases in children	825
10.6	Therapy	825
10.6.1	Resection therapy	825
10.6.2	Cryotherapy	826
10.6.3	Liver transplantation	826
10.6.4	Local treatment	826
10.6.5	Local chemotherapy	827
10.6.6	Systemic therapy	827
10.6.7	Systemic chemotherapy	827
10.6.8	Adjuvant measures	828
	• References (1—379)	828

(Figures 37.1—37.36; tables 37.1—37.12)

37 Malignant liver tumours

1 Historical review

▶ C. A. Rokitansky (1849) was probably the first author to refer to primary liver carcinoma as an independent disease. Until then, the problem had been to accept the existence of both primary and secondary (metastatic) liver tumours and to differentiate between them histologically. • In 1854 E. Noeggerath described a congenital hepatic carcinoma as being a mechanical obstetric obstacle. In 1859 T. Billroth reported the presence of hepatic metastases from a cylindroma. A. Kelsch and B. L. Kliener presented the first case reports of a primary liver tumour in 1876. A short time later, in 1881, C. Sabourin made significant histological progress by differentiating between hepatocellular and cholangiocellular carcinomas. He reported on four more patients suffering from primary hepatic carcinoma and coined the term "hepatoma". In 1883 J. A. P. Price described the development of carcinoma from cirrhosis, which led to the introduction of the term *"cirrhosis hepatis carcinomatosa"*. In 1888 V. C. Hanot et al. attempted to differentiate liver tumours according to macroscopic and microscopic criteria.

H. Eggel (1901) confirmed the association between cirrhosis and liver carcinoma, actually finding cirrhosis in 85% of all liver carcinomas. He distinguished carcinomas according to nodular, massive or diffuse growth, evaluating all cases that had been published since 1865. (5) Primary cystadenocarcinoma of the liver was initial differentiated in 1909 (P. Bascho). To our knowledge, the first right-sided lobectomy for hepatic carcinoma was carried out in 1911 (W. Wendel). • In 1932 T. Yoshida succeeded in creating a hepatocellular carcinoma in animal experiments by using o-amidoazotoluol: this marks the beginning of the search for chemotoxicological causes. M. M. Steiner (1938) wrote a detailed report on primary liver carcinoma in children. (243) L. Lisa et al. (1942) observed that metastases were rarely found in a cirrhotic liver. In 1952 C. Berman presented an overview of about 2,000 cases of primary liver cell carcinoma reported up to that time. • In 1950 G. M. Findlay postulated an association with chronic viral hepatitis, which he had detected in his epidemiologic examination of soldiers stationed in regions south of the Sahara desert, a finding that was also reported by M. Payet et al. in 1956. This supposition was confirmed when the hepatitis B virus was discovered (J. B. Smith et al., 1965; S. Sherlock et al., 1970). (4, 13, 149)

2 Classification

Morphologically speaking, the liver is (1.) origin of benign or malignant tumours, (2.) important target organ for metastatic spread, and (3.) susceptible to reactive nodulation due to its ability to regenerate.

Final differentiation between these three types of tissue formation is only possible with histomorphological techniques, and not with imaging procedures. The latter, however, are able to determine small foci (< 1.0 cm), which is required for US- and CT-guided biopsy.

Macroregenerative nodules are generally reactive benign tumours without any malignant tendency. They are found in various conditions, e.g. Budd-Chiari syndrome (s. fig. 36.6), congenital hepatic fibrosis, focal nodular hyperplasia, and appear in different forms: (1.) monoacinar nodules, (2.) multiacinar nodules, (3.) lobar or segmental hyperplasia, (4.) focal nodular hyperplasia, and (5.) monoacinar or multiacinar cirrhotic nodes. • The common pathogenetic principle is a pathological perfusion of the liver parenchyma.

2.1 Systematization

Malignant liver tumours may be grouped as follows: (*1.*) primary forms, i.e. originating in the liver (s. figs. 29.14; 30.2; 37.1, 37.9, 37.10), (*2.*) secondary forms, i.e. arising from metastases (s. figs. 37.2, 37.18, 37.19, 37.24, 37.33–37.35), and (*3.*) extrahepatic tumours infiltrating the liver from the outside (e.g. gall-bladder carcinoma). (s. fig. 37.3)

Primary liver tumours originate in principle from all histogenetic cell elements found in the liver: hepatocytes, bile-duct epithelia, periductal biliary glands, neuroendocrine cells and mesodermal structures (such as endothelial cells, Ito cells, Kupffer cells) as well as fibroblasts, nerve cells and muscle cells. However, they may also occur as mixed forms. In rare cases, ectopic tissue in the liver may be the starting point for malignant tumours. (s. tab. 37.1)

Primary liver tumours can be categorized according to macroscopic criteria. The solitary coarse-granulomatous type is predominantly found in the right lobe, while the

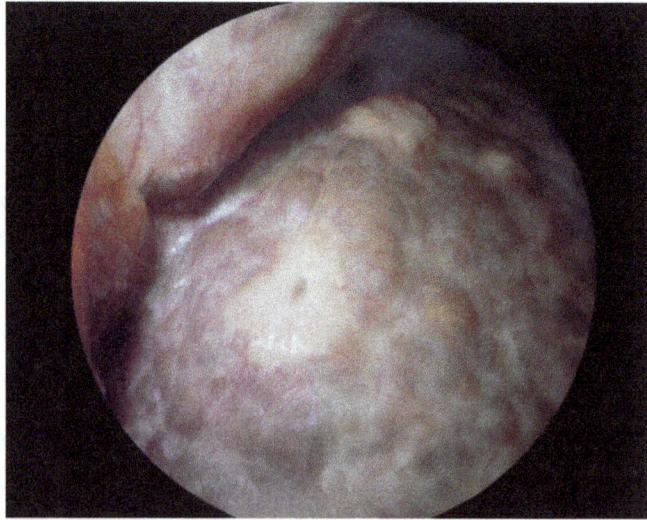

Fig. 37.1: Grey-coloured, medium-coarse tubercular cirrhosis in haemochromatosis with hepatocellular carcinoma: in the foreground, white, flat tumour granuloma of the right hepatic lobe with vascularization at the tumour margin and small "cancer umbilicus"; in the background, two additional tumour granulomas. Carcinomas infiltrating the peritoneal serosa in the right upper abdomen

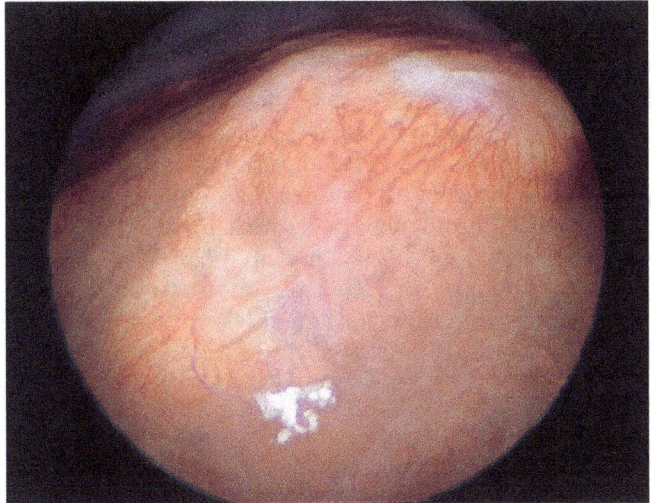

Fig. 37.2: Liver metastases in the right hepatic lobe in breast cancer with pronounced chaotic vascularization. Dissipated light reflex due to tumourous tubercles on the surface

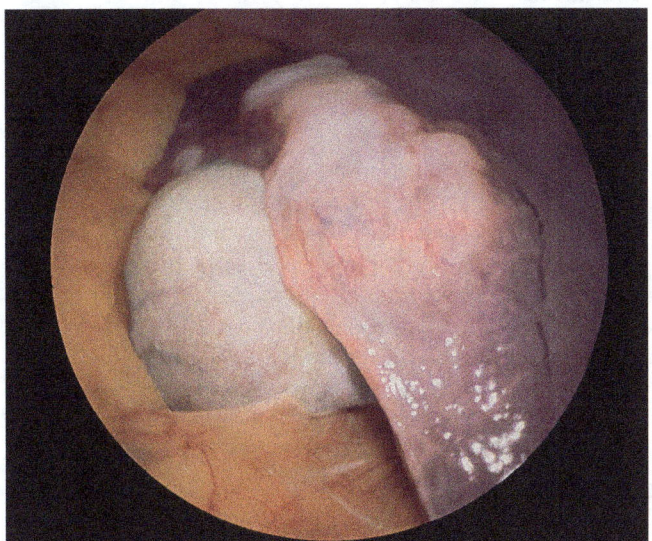

Fig. 37.3: Gall-bladder carcinoma subsequent to cholelithiasis with chronic cholecystitis and shrunken gall bladder. Bulbous carcinoma infiltrating the right lobe of liver

nodular multi-granulomatous type is most common in cirrhosis. The diffuse infiltrative type is relatively rare (5−10% of cases). A combined type is observed on occasions. The right lobe is affected seven times more frequently than the left lobe. Some 3−5% of malignant liver tumours are of primary origin.

Secondary liver tumours: In contrast, 95−97% of all malignant liver tumours are assumed to be secondary liver tumours, so-called *liver metastases*. (s. tab. 37.1)

2.2 TNM staging system

In medical letters/reports, an identified tumour is (correctly) classified according to the TNM staging system. In this process, unclear or incorrect interpretations are sometimes given due to inconsistent use of the terminology or lack of sufficient experience with this kind of classification. Thus it is appropriate to explain this system with interpretations. The anatomical spread of malignant liver tumours is also described according to the TNM staging system. It is important to assess the histologically verifiable invasion of vessels in the preparation and, at the same time, to clarify the question of whether the resected tissue still contains tumourous foci. (s. tab. 37.2)

The TNM staging system comprises the following stages with a respective survival time of three years after resection of HCC:

stage I	= T_1 No Mo (83%)
stage II	= T_2 No Mo (70−75%)
stage III A	= T_3 No Mo (45−50%)
stage III B	= T_1 N_1 Mo (20−40%)
stage IV A	T_4 N, Mo (10−25%)
stage IV B	T, N, M_1

Primary malignant liver tumours
Epithelial tumours
1. Hepatocellular carcinoma
Special type: fibrolamellar carcinoma
2. Cholangiocellular carcinoma
3. Combined HCC/CCC
4. Biliary cystadenocarcinoma
5. Hepatoblastoma
Mesenchymal tumours
1. Embryonal sarcoma
2. Malignant epithelioid haemangioendothelioma
3. Angiosarcoma
4. Leiomyosarcoma
5. Rhabdomyosarcoma
6. Fibrosarcoma
7. Malignant fibrous histiocytoma
8. Malignant schwannoma
9. Hepatic liposarcoma
10. Hepatic osteosarcoma
Malignant lymphoma
− hepatic B-cell lymphoma
− hepatosplenic T-cell lymphoma
Neuroendocrine tumours
1. Hepatic gastrinoma
2. Hepatic carcinoid tumour
Mixed tumours
1. Mixed liver tumour
2. Carcinosarcoma
Secondary liver tumours
1. Metastases
2. External infiltration per continuitatem
3. Malignant lymphoma and leukaemia

Tab. 37.1: Systematization of primary and secondary malignant liver tumours

T1	Single nodule without vascular invasion
T2	Single nodule with vascular invasion or multiple nodules, none more than 5 cm in diameter
T3	Multiple tumours more than 5 cm or tumour involving a major branch of the portal or hepatic vein
T4	Tumour with direct invasion of an adjacent organ other than the gall bladder or perforation of visceral peritoneum
N0	No regional lymph node metastases
N1	Regional lymph nodes metastases
M0	No distant metastases
M1	Distant metastases
Stage I	T1 N0 M0
Stage II	T2 N0 M0
Stage IIIa	T3 N0 M0
Stage IIIb	T4 N0 M0
Stage IIIc	Any T N1 M0
Stage IV	Any T or N M1

Tab. 37.2: TNM staging of liver tumours (Tumour/Nodules/Metastases). • In postoperative morphologic TNM staging, T, N and M are preceded by the letter "p"

3 Hepatocellular carcinoma

3.1 Definition

Hepatocellular carcinoma (HCC) originates in the hepatocytes; HCC thus resembles liver parenchyma in morphology. It may present as highly differentiated, moderately differentiated or undifferentiated (anaplastic). The most common (and basic) structure is the trabecular aggregation of tumour cells around a capillary vascular bed. Clinically, HCC is seen as an extremely malignant, rapidly progressing tumour. Therapeutic measures remain limited, with surgery being the only potentially curative treatment.

3.2 Epidemiology and frequency

Epidemiology: HCC is one of the most common malignant primary liver tumours worldwide. It ranks fifth in frequency in men and eighth in women (♂ = 6%, ♀ = 3%). Between 500,000 and one million new cases are reported each year. The annual mortality rate is virtually the same as its annual incidence. Its *geographical distribution* varies greatly and correlates almost 100 per cent with the regional incidence rates of HBV and HCV infection. There are areas showing low incidence with <5/100,000 inhabitants/year (e.g. Scandinavia, Australia, USA., Central Europe), moderate incidence with 5−20/100,000 inhabitants/year (e.g. East/South-East Europe, Mediterranean region) and high incidence with 20−150/100,000 inhabitants/year (e.g. Asia, Africa).

Frequency: During the course of the 20th century, the statistical frequency of HCC rose constantly − owing to an increase in autopsies and improvements in diagnostic procedures. • In 1910, for example, autopsy records showed HCC in only 0.04% of cases; in 1930 the figure was 0.13%, in 1960 0.23%, and in 1970 0.6−0.8%. In 1986 the frequency of HCC was given at about 1% of cases based on autopsy findings. The ratio of HCC to liver metastases is about 1:50.

Age: HCC affects persons of all age groups. In Asian and African countries, the morbidity peak is reached in adolescence or between the ages of 20 and 40 years, corresponding to predominantly perinatal or postnatal infection with hepatitis viruses. (176) In countries with a low incidence, the morbidity peak is between the ages of 50−60 years. • HCC has also been observed in babies and infants.

The HCC **gender ratio** between men and women is about 3:1, but up to 8:1 in countries with a high incidence. In a cirrhosis-free liver, however, men and women are equally affected by HCC, i.e. the gender ratio of cirrhosis seems to determine the ratio of HCC. Androgens are thought to be of aetiopathogenetic significance, since carcinoma cells have been shown to carry androgen receptors which display qualities favouring growth, and a carcino-protective effect was observed in animal experiments when androgen was withdrawn. Sex hormones appear to be cocarcinogens. (25, 41, 45, 80)

3.3 Risk factors and causes

▶ **Animal experiments:** A considerable number of chemical agents have proved to be directly carcinogenic in animal experiments. This is most likely to apply to humans as well (but as yet no supporting evidence has been presented). Both a linear dosage-effect relationship and a respective time-exposure relationship can be observed: the higher the dosage and the longer the exposure, the greater is the likelihood of carcinoma formation. Carcinomatous degeneration occurs predominantly in epithelial or mesenchymal tissues. (s. tab. 37.3)

Risk factors: The figures and observations relating to the epidemiology and frequency of HCC are the result of individual or combined risk factors. The extent of risk correlates with (*1.*) aetiology, (*2.*) duration, and (*3.*) inflammatory activity of the liver disease. In 10−15% of patients, no risk factor could actually be determined in the development of HCC. (s. tab. 37.4)

Genetic mechanisms: A *genetic disposition* is suspected in HCC, as in other malignant tumours. Some 22% of patients suffering from HCC had other organ tumours as well. (133) • Several *hereditary metabolic diseases*, with or without cirrhosis, may increase the risk of HCC considerably. These include tyrosinaemia (type I), glycogenosis (type I), alpha$_1$-antitrypsin deficiency, galactos-

Azo-compounds
1. 2,2-azonaphthalin
2. 2,2-diamino-1,1-naphthyl
3. m-methyl-p-dimethylaminoazobenzene
4. o-aminoazotoluene
5. p-aminoazobenzene
6. p-dimethylaminoazobenzene (butter yellow)
7. p-monomethylaminobenzene

Hydrocarbon compounds
1. 2-aminofluorene
2. 4-aminostilben
3. 2-anthramine
4. 1,2-benzanthracene
5. 1,2,5,6-dibenzanthracene
6. 3,4,5,6-dibenzkarbazole
7. Acetylaminofluorene
8. Carbon tetrachloride
9. Ethylurethane
10. Methylcholanthrene
11. Thioacetamide

Tab. 37.3: Chemical substances displaying carcinogenicity, as has been demonstrated in experiments or is very probable

1. **Hepatitis viruses**
   HBV, HCV
2. **Liver diseases**
   Chronic hepatitis
   Cirrhosis
   NASH
3. **Mycotoxins or phytotoxins**
   Aflatoxin (46, 109, 173)   Microcystin
   Cycasin   Ochratoxin
   Luteoskyrin   Safrol
   Maltrozym
4. **Nutrition, social drugs**
   Alcohol (157)   Ethionine surplus
   Betel quid chewing (166)   Tobacco smoke
   B_6 and choline deficiency
5. **Metabolic diseases**
   $alpha_1$-antitrypsin deficiency (47)
   Colon polyposis
   Galactosaemia
   Glycogenosis (type I) (38, 102)
   Haemochromatosis (28)
   Neurofibromatosis
   Porphyria (51)
   Tyrosinaemia (type I) (170)
6. **Chemical agents**
   Alkylating substances   Nitrose compounds
   Aromatic amines   Vinyl chloride (146)
   Azo-compounds   *etc.*
7. **Inorganic substances**
   Arsenic, asbestos,
   Cadmium, chromium,
   Lead, manganese, nickel
8. **Medication**
   Androgens, anabolics   Methotrexate
   Contraceptives (50, 167)   Methyldopa
   Cyproterone acetate
9. **Ionizing radiation**
   Thorium (52, 70)
   X-rays

Tab. 37.4: Risk factors (carcinogens and cocarcinogens) regarding hepatocellular carcinoma, which have already been proved (including some references) (s. tabs. 29.10; 37.3)

aemia, porphyria cutanea tarda, acute intermittent porphyria and idiopathic haemochromatosis. Patients with diabetes mellitus and obesity (30, 62) also have a higher risk of developing hepatocellular carcinoma. • HCC has only rarely been associated with Wilson's disease; copper seems to have a carcino-protective effect. (171) (s. tab. 37.4)

Chemicals: A number of chemicals can cause malignant hepatic tumours, including HCC, both in animal experiments and in the everyday life of humans. These include vinyl chloride, aromatic amines, nitrogen compounds, polycyclic aromatic hydrocarbons and alkylating substances. Similarly, mycotoxins and phytotoxins (aflatoxin, cycasin, ochratoxin, safrol, etc.), betel quid chewing as well as inorganic substances (arsenic, asbestos, cadmium, chromium, etc.) can have a carcinogenic effect. In addition, substances emitting ionizing radiation must be mentioned in this context. (s. tab. 37.4)

Medication: The aetiological relationship between the intake of certain types of medication and the development of HCC is well known. These include methotrexate, methyldopa, androgens/anabolic steroids, oestrogen derivatives/oral contraceptives and cyproterone acetate. (s. tabs. 29.9; 37.4)

Alcohol and tobacco: Alcohol is seen as a *cocarcinogen*, i.e. it requires additional noxae (e.g. tobacco smoke, aflatoxin) to be able to induce HCC as a carcinogen. The combined effects of alcohol and aflatoxin result in a 35-fold increase in carcinogenicity. Aflatoxin may cause a specific type of mutation within the tumour suppressor gene p53 and thus trigger initiation (i.e. the first step in the development of a tumour). The risk of HCC developing with underlying alcoholic cirrhosis is about 15% or 22.6% (i.e. there is approximately a fourfold increase in the HCC risk); abstention from alcohol does not lower the risk of HCC significantly. (157) • Interestingly, regular coffee intake is probably a protective factor in HCC.

Hepatitis viruses: In chronic infections, **HBV DNA** may become integrated into the genetic material of the hepatocytes; this has a strong, time-dependent carcinogenic effect. Alcohol speeds up the incorporation of viral DNA into the host genome. HBV carriers (those suffering from liver disease as well as healthy persons) have an HCC risk which is 200 times higher than that of other people. Integration of viral DNA into the tumour cells is well documented. Integrated HBV DNA shows a number of modifications. Genetic damaging of hepatocytes by the integrated viral DNA (also in serologically HBV-negative patients, who may be molecular-biologically positive) is considered to be the initiation of carcinogenesis. In this process, the HBV subtypes apparently behave like the HBV type itself. HBxAg is undoubtedly of pathogenic significance; possibly it also damages p53. HBV protein (and the core protein of HCV) are able to activate NF-kappa B, which is considered to be important in HCC pathogenesis. *Vaccination against HBV infection is thought to be an effective prophylactic measure against the development of HCC.* • Superinfection with **HDV** has a potentiating effect, resulting in the earlier occurrence of both cirrhosis and HCC — but not in a higher incidence of HCC. Animal experiments show that HBV can induce HCC without further cofactors. This evidence of the strong carcinogenicity of HBV also explains why, for example, HBsAg-positive men have a risk of developing HCC which is 98 times higher than that of an HBsAg-negative control group of the same age. A higher familial frequency has also been observed. (64, 109, 149, 165) • **HCV** is equally carcinogenic; in certain regions, its carcinogenicity is actually 2.7 times higher than that of HBV, whereby different molecular mechanisms are responsible for the development of HCC. HCV is not integrated into the hepatocellular genome. Prevalence of HCV antibodies in HCC patients has been shown to be considerable (albeit varying between individual countries), e.g. 27% vs 4%, 55% vs 10%, 30% vs 1%, and 71% vs 5%. This corresponds to a 27-fold increase in the risk of HCC. Genotype 1 b is associated with a higher risk of HCC as well as a decrease in IGF. Simultaneous infection with GBV-C does not increase the HCC risk. The likelihood of HCC occurring subsequent to an HCV infection is 21.5% after 5 years, 53.2% after 10 years, and 75.2% after 15 years. HCV cirrhosis is associated with HCC at a malignant transformation rate of 2–8% per year. (64, 125, 155, 162, 165)

Liver diseases: An association with AIH and with secondary biliary or CDNC-induced biliary cirrhosis has been reported (91, 115, 153), albeit as a rare event.

Cirrhosis: In 70–80% of cases, HCC develops in underlying (mainly multicentred, coarse-granulomatous) liver cirrhosis, i.e. some 20% of cirrhotic patients suffer from HCC. • *Cirrhosis of any aetiology must thus be considered a precarcinogenic factor.* • In Europe and the USA, cirrhosis is mostly alcohol-induced. In HCC patients in Africa or Asia, cirrhosis is less common: generally perinatal, postnatal or juvenile HBV infections, most likely involving large numbers of viruses, result in the formation of HCC before cirrhosis can develop. Chronic viral hepatitis, just like cirrhosis, causes an increase in hepatocellular proliferation. Unless the genetic damage induced by viral DNA can be repaired by enzymes produced in the hepatocytes, it is passed on via mitoses to the daughter cells. An increased DNA synthesis rate within the cirrhosis is accompanied by an elevated risk of malignant transformation. Cirrhosis increases the susceptibility of the liver tissue to other carcinogens. A rise in the mitosis rate thus also results in an increase in genetic alterations. This causes oncogens to be activated, while tumour suppressor genes or mutation repair genes become inactivated. (20, 41)

3.4 Pathogenesis

Development of HCC begins in the small diploid hepatocytes, which have a higher growth rate. Pathogenesis is a multifactorial event. The sequential course has three main phases: (*1.*) **initiation**: various noxae cause a genetic defect, which can be repaired by endogenous mechanisms and is thus reversible; (*2.*) **promotion**: if the genetic damage is beyond repair, the initiated hepatocytes are stimulated and mitosis begins, with the result that the genetic damage is transferred to the daughter cells; (*3.*) **progression**: clonal expansion of the altered ("malignatized") cells occurs.

Tumour-suppressor gene: The tumour-suppressor gene p53 is located on chromosome 17. Noxae may cause mutations of this gene, which results in the loss of its suppressor effect. (6) • *An autosomal dominant mutation of p53 is also encountered in humans, so that a tumour can develop during adolescence*, the so-called **Li-Fraumeni syndrome**.

Carcinogens are cancer-causing substances which are able to initiate genetic damage of the hepatocytes (or of bile-duct epithelia or sinusoidal endothelial cells) without the assistance of additional noxae. **Cocarcinogens** require other cocarcinogens or carcinogens in order to cause malignant transformation. • The **interaction** between hepatitis viruses, alcohol, chemical agents, hormones, etc. is a crucial factor in the development of manifest HCC. In this context, constituents of tobacco smoke, nutritional factors (e.g. choline deficiency, vitamin B_6 deficiency, aethionine surplus) or occasionally enhanced fatty acid synthesis (128) may act as cocarcinogenic factors.

Growth factors (HGF, IGF, etc.) are also of crucial importance in pathogenesis, as is a compromised immune defence system. Increased expression of angiopoietin 1 and 2 plays an important role in the vascular development of HCC. (163)

3.5 Morphology

▶ *Aetiopathogenesis is multifactorial as an interaction of genetic, exogenous and/or endogenous factors. In a molecular-biological context, HCC is regarded as an extremely heterogeneous tumour.*

3.5.1 Macroscopic forms

The macroscopic or histologic differences in the morphology of individual hepatocellular carcinoma types are of little epidemiological or clinical significance. • Macroscopically, HCC has a whitish-yellow colour, is often permeated by bile and shows a soft consistency. There are often haemorrhages in the nodes as well as central necrosis. HCC is mainly supplied with arterial blood. Its doubling time is 30 to 400 days, with an average of 120 days. Occasionally, infiltration into the portal vein system or the hepatic veins occurs (s. fig. 6.16), with intrahepatic metastases and thromboses in the branches of the portal or hepatic veins. (137) HCC may also become manifest simultaneously with cholangiocarcinoma. • **Three forms** (nearly identical with the three forms described by H. EGGEL in 1901) (5) can be differentiated: (*1.*) expansive type, (*2.*) infiltrative type, and (*3.*) combination type. • A rare form is the **pedunculated HCC** (only about 100 cases have been reported). It occurs mostly on the underside of the right lobe and protrudes beyond the upper edge of the liver. This form (occasionally >1 kg in weight) can be more easily resected, leading to a better prognosis. (123, 177) (s. tab. 37.5)

Macroscopic forms	Microscopic forms
1. *Expansive type* (ca. 18%) • solitary coarse-nodular • multiple coarse-nodular 2. *Infiltrative type* (ca. 33%) • diffuse infiltrative (ca. 5%) 3. *Combination type* (ca. 42%)	1. Trabecular type 2. Pseudoglandular type 3. Scirrhous type 4. Solid type 5. Fibrolamellar type 6. Spindle-cell type
Degree of tumour differentiation	
1. High differentiation 2. Moderate differentiation 3. Low differentiation 4. No differentiation (anaplastic type)	
Cytologic differentiation	
1. Polygonal 2. Pleomorphic	3. Clear-cellular 4. Small-cellular

Tab. 37.5: Macroscopic forms, microscopic typing and degree of tumour differentiation in hepatocellular carcinoma

3.5.2 Microscopic tissue types

Dysplasia: Dysplasia is defined as variably large, different-shaped hepatocytes, mostly in localized groups, with enlarged, pleomorphic and hyperchromatic nuclei as well as enlarged nucleoli. These dysplastic hepatocytes are often polyploid. Dysplasia can occur as a *macrocellular* (with eosinophilic cytoplasm) or *microcellular* (with basophilic cytoplasm and increased proliferation) variant. The latter is a precancerous stage. • **Dysplastic foci** with a diameter of 1(−2) mm consist of enriched, mainly small-cellular dysplastic hepatocytes. • **Dysplastic nodes** with a diameter of 0.3−1.0 cm have an atypical architecture and cellular atypias; trabecular or pseudoglandular structures are evident. Atypical hepatocytes are often clear-cellular, basophilic or steatotic. Fluent transition into HCC is seen occasionally. (84, 93)

Growth forms: Histologically, there are six growth forms of HCC. (s. tab. 37.5) The most common form is the **trabecular type**, usually comprising highly differentiated carcinomas with polygonal tumour cells similar to hepatocytes; they grow in multilayered trabeculae and enclose blood spaces lined with endothelium (usually without Kupffer cells). • The **pseudoglandular type** is often found in combination with the trabecular form. It is characterized by the formation of gland-like structures containing detritus and bilic or liquid material. • The **scirrhous type** shows excessive deposits of sclerosed connective tissue, which is relatively low in cells. There are no necroses or haemorrhages. The moderately differentiated tumour cells lie between the septa, which resemble connective tissue. This type is mostly found after chemotherapy or radiation therapy. (92) • The **solid type** is an undifferentiated HCC, with the tumour cells displaying considerable cellular polymorphism; the trabecular tissue pattern has disappeared. The tumour is compact due to compression of the sinusoids. • Differentiation is, however, only possible in rare cases, since there is often great heterogenicity within the tumour, i.e. different tissue types may be found in the same HCC. (s. figs. 37.4, 37.5) • **Fibrolamellar HCC** is rare; it consists of solid cell trabeculae with connective-tissue septation and a capsule. (s. p. 813) (s. figs. 37.12, 37.13) • **Spindle cell-like differentiated HCC** is likewise a rare histological form with a fascicular-sarcomatous growth pattern. (110) Prognosis is significantly poorer than with other forms of HCC (S. KAKIZOE et al., 1987).

Tumour differentiation: Histological tumour differentiation ranges from the highly differentiated grade 1 to the undifferentiated grade 4. (s. tab. 37.5) It does not provide sufficiently reliable information for giving a prognosis of HCC. This also applies to the above-mentioned histological growth forms — with the exception of the fibrolamellar type, which has a more favourable prognosis in the majority of cases.

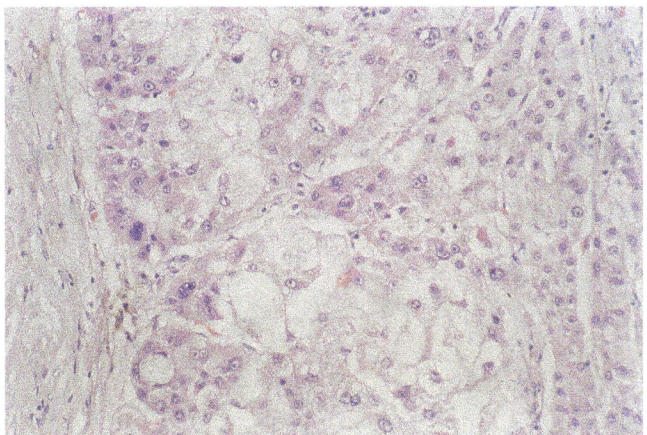

Fig. 37.4: Highly differentiated, macrotrabecular hepatocellular carcinoma with hydropic swelling of the tumour cells (condition after alcohol injection) (HE)

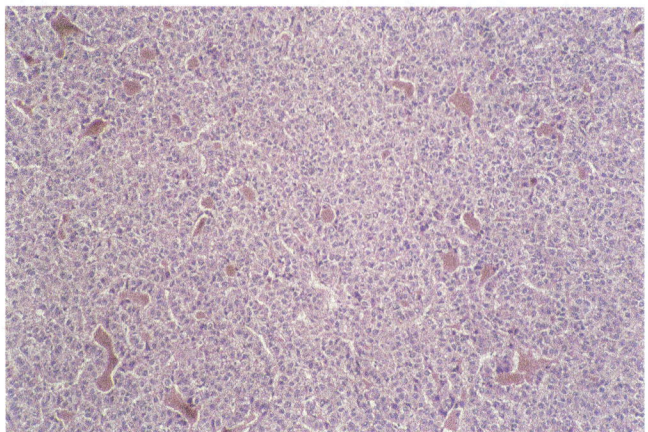

Fig. 37.5: Partly solid, partly pseudoacinar hepatocellular carcinoma with bile pigment in canalicular structures (HE)

3.5.3 Cytological differentiation

Polygonal cells are predominantly found in HCC. They have dense nuclei and lumpy, eosinophilic cytoplasm, which subsequently becomes basophilic. Bile canaliculi are often observed. Sometimes there are haemorrhagic necroses. (s. fig. 37.6) • **Pleomorphous** cells are present in immature tumours. They are generally smaller than the hepatocytes and may vary in their overall cell size as well as in the size of the nucleus; occasionally, they grow to form multinuclear cells or multinuclear giant cells containing bizarre nuclei. • Typical **hyaline inclusion bodies** with autofluorescence are sometimes detected, pointing to disturbed protein secretion; they can be differentiated immunohistochemically, e.g. in the form of ferritin, α_1-foetoprotein or α_1-antitrypsin. The detection of **Mallory-Denk bodies** in tumour cells is likewise typical for HCC. (158) They are caused by disturbed metabolism of the intermediate filaments. **Ground glass cells** are also found (due to HBsAg expression or enhancement of fibrin). **Nuclear inclusion bodies** are caused by invaginated cytoplasmic substances. Bile may still be produced, particularly within a highly differentiated HCC; this is expressed in the formation of **bile thrombi**, as is shown by morphology.

The glycogen content in the tumour cells varies. When a large amount of glycogen (and water or lipids) is stored, HCC takes on a **clear-cellular** "hypernephroid" form. • **Small-cellular** carcinomas are also occasionally in evidence. (s. tab. 37.5)

A **grading of HCC** with regard to these different forms is usually without clinical importance: (*1.*) the forms do not necessarily correlate with the clinical course and (*2.*) different forms can appear in one and the same patient.

3.5.4 Metastatic spread

HCC metastasizes intrahepatically, haematogenically (50–60%) and lymphogenically (30%) into the regional lymph nodes, mainly (and also initially) below the diaphragm. • Haematogenous metastases affect the lungs (40–50%) and skeletal system; metastases are only rarely found in the kidneys or brain. • However, infiltrating growth affects neighbouring organs (e.g. gall bladder, diaphragm, kidneys, hepatic vessels, bile ducts). (75, 178)

3.6 Symptomatology

3.6.1 Subjective complaints

HCC develops without subjective complaints. Even further tumour growth often remains undetected; alternatively, the complaints are explained as general symptoms relating to cirrhosis or to an existing chronic liver disease. HCC is hence usually detected late. *Complaints* are very varied:

• pain in the upper abdomen	• weight loss
• bloating, flatulence	• fatigue, weakness
• inappetence, nausea	• stool irregularities

The patient is suspected to be suffering from HCC when the subjective complaints continue to worsen and when an increase in complaints, which may occur quite abruptly in some cases, cannot be explained by the progression of cirrhosis. Most patients are affected by pain radiating into the right side of the back or into the right shoulder and neck area. This is due to an irritation of the phrenic nerve caused by expansion of the tumour towards or even into the liver capsule. Anorexia is more pronounced. Occasionally, the course of HCC is acute, resembling liver failure or liver abscess.

3.6.2 Clinical findings

The clinical situation deteriorates rapidly: febrile temperatures and leucocytosis as well as subicterus are observed; there are also signs of encephalopathy. An arterial murmur can often be heard on auscultation,

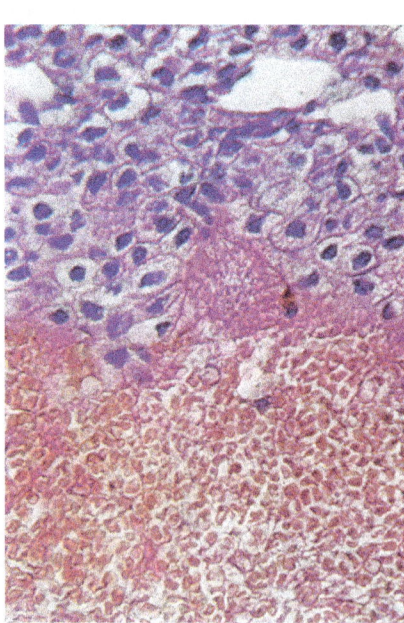

Fig. 37.6: Haemorrhage and polygonal tumour cells with hyperchromatic nuclei in HCC (HE)

since the tumour is mainly supplied with blood from the hepatic artery. A sudden "blossoming" of vascular spider naevi is frequently seen with underlying cirrhosis. *Virchow-Troisier's lymphadenopathy* may be present. (81) Fever and leucocytosis frequently occur in tumour necrosis. Clinical findings include:

- fever
- subicterus
- meteorism/ascites
- latent encephalopathy
- arterial murmur
- tenderness upon pressure
- palpable tumour
- perihepatic friction

Paraneoplastic findings: Occasionally, there are paraneoplastic symptoms or syndromes which vary greatly from individual to individual, such as erythrocytosis (due to enhanced expression of erythropoietin), polycythaemia, hyperparathyroidism with hypercalcaemia, hyperthyroidism, painful gynaecomastia (14), osteoarthropathy, pseudoporphyria, hypercholesterolaemia, hypertension (16), polyneuropathy, polymyositis (61), water diarrhoea syndrome, dermatomyositis, and an increase in the vitamin B_{12}-binding protein. Large and glycogen-rich tumours cause hypoglycaemia (possibly due to enhanced expression of IGF2).

3.7 Diagnosis

The efficacy of therapeutic measures, particularly the prospect of curative treatment and thus prognosis, depend upon the *early diagnosis* of HCC.

3.7.1 Laboratory findings

While **non-specific signs of inflammation** may also be present in liver cirrhosis, they are much more obvious in HCC. For example, positive CRP values as well as an increase in the BSR, α-globulins, $α_1$-antitrypsin and fibrinogen can be found. A constellation of decreased serum iron and elevated serum copper (139) points to a consuming inflammatory process or malignant tumour. (s. tab. 5.10) Usually, the haemogram shows leucocytosis and anaemia. Nitric oxide values in the plasma are elevated in correlation with tumour size. (s. tabs. 37.6, 37.11, 37.12)

Conspicuous **enzyme activities** include a disproportionate increase in γ-GT, AP (especially the Regan isoenzyme, which is identical to the placenta isoenzyme) and LDH. This constellation is thought to be an important indicator of HCC, particularly when HBDH is also elevated. Intrahepatic cholestasis is invariably present in HCC. More and more foetal γ-GT is produced in carcinomatous hepatocytes and is detectable at the biliary pole of the cells. The transaminases rise only slowly; the enzyme quotients may provide revealing information. (s. tab. 5.6) • Hepatic **synthesis capacity** (albumin, cholinesterase, Quick's value) decreases progressively. ChE is also greatly reduced in cases of malignant ascites. The

1. **Non-specific parameters**
   - CRP +, BSR ↑, $α_2$-globulins ↑, γ-globulins ↑, fibrinogen ↑, cholinesterase ↓, D-dimer ↑
2. **Iron/copper constellation**
   - iron ↓, copper ↑, ferritin ↑
3. **Cholestasis**
   - γ-GT ↑, AP ↑
4. **Enzyme constellation**
   - GPT ↑, GOT ↑, LDH ↑, GDH ↑
5. • GOT/GPT = >2
   • γ-GT/GOT = >12
   • (GPT + GOT)/GDH = <15
5. **Serology**
   - $α_1$-foetoprotein ↑ (+ ferritin ↑) = ↑↑
   - des-γ-carboxy prothrombin ↑
   - aldolase A ↑
   - α-L-fucosidase ↑

Tab. 37.6: Laboratory findings arousing suspicion in HCC, with increasing diagnostic reliability given by continuous deviation from normal values

indocyanine green test is considered to be conclusive for evaluating the residual liver parenchyma prior to hepatectomy. A combination of the *ICG test* and *galactose elimination capacity* (s. p. 114) is an even more reliable tool, according to our experience.

$α_1$-**foetoprotein** has gained great importance as a laboratory value pointing to HCC. (s. p. 112) First discovered in hepatomas by G. ABELEV et al. in animal experiments in 1963, this type of oncofoetal protein was also detected in human HCC by Y.S. TATARINOV in 1964. AFP is a glycoprotein formed initially within the yolk sac and later in the liver and gastrointestinal tract of the foetus. Serum values of about 70,000 µg/l are found in neonates, decreasing to the normal value of < 10 µg/l within 9−12 months. Higher values can be detected in liver cell regeneration (acute and chronic hepatitis, cirrhosis) and particularly in HCC (>20 µg/l). Thus, a continuous increase in AFP values arouses suspicion; a value of >100 µg/l is highly suspicious for HCC. There is only a moderate correlation between AFP and the respective tumour size and doubling time. A false-negative AFP value is detected in about 20% of patients suffering from HCC. The response to chemotherapy usually corresponds to decreasing AFP values. • Specificity is between 76−91%, sensitivity 39−64% (approx. 85% when ferritin is increased at the same time). Serum values of >2,000 µg/l may ultimately be reached. Liver metastases usually show values of <150 µg/l, with no tendency to rise. AFP values in the normal range exclude HCC in 90−95% of cases. No AFP is produced in very mature or very immature tumour cells. AFP production in elder patients is lower; it is mostly higher in virus-related cirrhosis than in alcoholic cirrhosis. (39, 72, 150, 152)

Diagnostic importance is also attributed to **des-γ-carboxy prothrombin** (60—80% positivity in HCC) (H.A. LIEBMAN et al., 1984). (87, 119, 131, 152) It is synthesized in the normal hepatocytes and therefore also in HCC. The diagnostic accuracy in small hepatocellular carcinomas (<3 cm) could be greatly improved by determining this precursor prothrombin (PIVKA II) in combination with AFP. • A decrease in the **factor-II index**, i.e. (factor VII + factor X) − (factor II) = >15, has proved to be a specific and independent marker of HCC. • In addition, isoferritins, Regan-AP, telomerase activity (97), leptin receptor (168) and L-fucosidase as well as CEA variants may be helpful in the demarcation of HCC. • *Laboratory diagnosis of HCC is indeed much more reliable if various important parameters are added.* (s. tab. 37.6)

3.7.2 Imaging procedures

Sonography: *Sonography is the method of choice in monitoring the course of risk patients, particularly in combination with AFP determination at four- to six-month intervals.* In this way, a longer survival time could be achieved. Under optimal examination conditions with an experienced investigator, foci are detectable at a size of 1 cm. However, demarcation of HCC in a cirrhotic liver is very difficult, if not impossible, due to its inhomogeneous reflex pattern. Small foci (<2 cm) are usually hypoechoic; when they grow, their echogenicity increases (due to deposition of fat, connective tissue formation or necrosis) and a hypoechoic margin with a rather blurred *halo* (= tumour cells plus compressed liver parenchyma) is often in evidence. A *bull's eye* is also detectable (= hypoechoic centre surrounded by a hyperechoic edge). At a size of >4 cm, the reflex pattern becomes inhomogeneous. However, HCC has no typical image. In 50 to 70% of cases, diagnosis is successful at a size of 2 cm and more. Detection of HCC also depends on its degree of differentiation: well-differentiated liver carcinomas are barely distinguishable from normal liver tissue. A hypoechoic halo points to a fibrous capsule and − in combination with a mosaic structure within the focus − arouses suspicion of a carcinoma. (2, 26, 35, 39, 43, 84) • The use of **colour-encoded Doppler sonography** shows hypervascularization even in the early tumour stage and thus provides diagnostic differentiation from regeneration nodes and adenomatous hyperplasia. Visualization of tumour vessels is improved by intravenous injection of a contrast medium. When HCC infiltrates the portal vein, arterial vessels can be identified in the tumour thrombus in 60−70% of cases. (8, 11, 53, 58, 67, 122) • The use of **intraoperative US** as well as **laparoscopic US** (21, 65) results in a 20% higher detection rate of HCC than in preoperative diagnostics. When all space-occupying lesions of the liver are included, the diagnostic results are up to 40% better than those gained by conventional sonography. The haemodynamic pattern *"nodule-in-nodule"* (= a vascular spot in a hypovascular nodule) is a sign of a suspicious node − this could, in turn, be an early stage of HCC. (88, 181) • Characterization of liver tumours with contrast-enhanced sonography and digital grey-scale analysis offers the possibility of an investigator-independent differential diagnosis. (11)

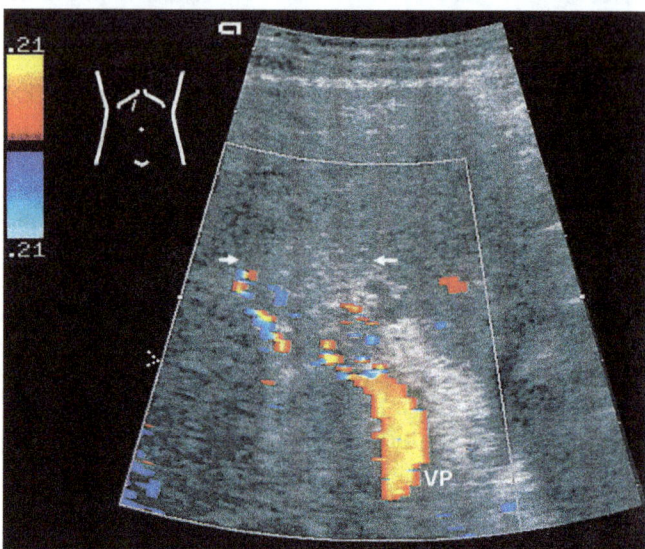

Fig. 37.7: Thrombosis inside the blood vessels of a diffuse hepatocellular carcinoma resulting from alcoholic cirrhosis (arrows). Spot-like neovascularization in the thrombosed blood vessels. (VP = portal vein)

Computer tomography: The detection of small carcinomas, especially of tumours in cirrhosis, is unreliable using conventional CT scanning. However, when the tumour has reached a certain size, capsule formation, fatty transformation of the tumour mass, vascular infiltration and development of arterioportal shunts are evident. Abdominal lymph node metastases can be found. Sensitivity is about 60%. (s. fig. 37.8) • The introduction of **lipiodol CT** has resulted in a considerable improvement in HCC diagnosis: the oily contrast

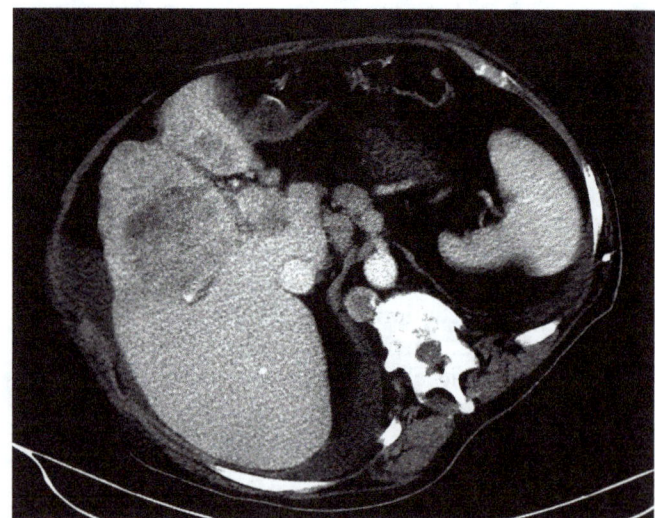

Fig. 37.8: HCC: nodular liver surface in cirrhosis. Tumour formation in the right lobe of liver, in parts at the margin; central hypodensity with peripheral hypervascularization (CT after CM)

medium injected into the hepatic artery under angiographic monitoring is stored within the tumour tissue, so that any tumour above a size of 3 mm can be identified in conventional CT scanning in full contrast for a period of one to two weeks. Sensitivity is about 70%, specificity about 80%. (24, 112) • **Spiral CT** has proved to be most effective (sensitivity 90%). This technique offers a biphasic examination supported by contrast medium, with the first (hepatic-arterial) phase showing mainly hypervascularized HCC and the second (portal-venous) phase showing mainly hypovascularized HCC. (10, 37) • **CTAP** (CT following arterioportography) is considered to be a very sensitive method for the detection of HCC in a non-cirrhotic liver (CTAP is not suitable in cases of portal hypertension and portosystemic shunts). The sensitivity of CTAP is 85–90%. • Although **CT arteriography** is an invasive procedure, it shows the highest sensitivity in extensive cirrhosis, because HCC is predominantly supplied with arterial blood.

Angiography: HCC appears as a hypervascularized tumour in angiography via the hepatic artery. The vessels show irregular internal diameters; due to arteriovenous anastomoses, the hepatic veins are rapidly filled, giving retrograde visualization of the portal vein. Poorly vascularized or non-vascularized areas present in the tumour develop due to necrosis or bleeding. Evidence of a hypervascularized *"bush pattern"* in a cirrhotic liver is considered to be an obvious sign of HCC. In terms of sensitivity, angiography is, however, inferior to other imaging techniques. There is no alternative to angiography when assessing surgical strategies or chemoperfusion and chemoembolization; angiography is often combined with simultaneous regional tumour treatment.

Magnetic resonance imaging: Malignant tumours generally show longer relaxation times compared to healthy liver tissue. This results in hypointensity in T_1-weighting and hyperintensity in T_2-weighting – in contrast to healthy liver parenchyma. T_2-signal intensity is more sensitive in the diagnosis of advanced HCC and in the assessment of a tumour capsule; this is prognostically significant. Early stages of highly differentiated HCC are better defined in T_1-weighting. Diagnosis is further improved with contrast medium. (29, 112, 169, 172)

Scintigraphy: The approaches used to date in scintiscanning have proved to be inadequate for diagnosing HCC and are also inferior to other imaging techniques. • New methods (Tc-GSA) as well as immunoscintigraphy, ^{18}F-FDG PET or SPECT (3, 83, 100, 154, 159) have not yet been evaluated with regard to their diagnostic sensitivity or specificity in detecting HCC or in preoperative staging. Their main value consists in better detection of extrahepatic tumours; they may also have a direct impact on operative management. (1)

Plain X-ray: The rare event of HCC calcification is characterized by the so-called *sunburst sign*.

3.7.3 Morphological diagnosis

Percutaneous fine-needle biopsy: This technique is associated with the risk of tumour cell spreading. The frequency of subcutaneous implantation metastases is reported to be 2%; they mostly appear within three months. When this procedure is indicated, the bleeding risk from the usually hypervascularized tumour must also be taken into account. The cytologic-diagnostic sensitivity is 80–85% of cases; specificity is 97–100%. (32–34, 126)

Percutaneous thick-needle biopsy: We consider this technique to be *contraindicated*, mainly because of the bleeding risk involved: (*1.*) HCC is usually a densely vascularized tumour, (*2.*) the tumour tissue does not possess the requisite spontaneous contractility for mechanical closure of the biopsy canal, (*3.*) local coagulation is usually disturbed in the tumour tissue. Punctures into the necrotic centre of a tumour may cause uncontrollable haemorrhagic oozing. The risk of implantation metastases is the same as in FNB. (34) • This raises the question of whether histological or cytological confirmation of the diagnosis is really necessary. In this context, cytological assessment of the malignancy is equal or even superior to histology. However, cytological delimitation of highly differentiated HCC from adenomatous hyperplasia may be very difficult in certain cases. Diagnosing the tumour type is much more accurate by histological examination than by cytology.

Surgery is indicated if a resectable space-occupying lesion in liver cirrhosis with sufficient evidence of HCC has been determined by imaging techniques and the AFP value is >400 µg/l. Operability in terms of internal medicine as well as hepatology has to be established. • Provided laboratory, sonographic and radiological findings are largely unambiguous, surgery is indicated even without an increase in AFP values; preoperative percutaneous biopsy should *not* be carried out in such cases.

Morphological clarification of the findings is necessary if differential diagnosis of a hepatic space-occupying lesion is unclear. • Cytological or histological confirmation of tumour malignancy is likewise required prior to palliative therapy, even in patients with no chance of curative treatment.

Laparoscopy: This technique should always be used to achieve the required morphological clarification. (s. figs. 37.1–37.3, 37.9, 37.10, 37.18, 37.19) (9, 85, 155) • It initially serves as **explorative laparoscopy** in the careful inspection of the abdominal cavity using various body positions in order to gain as reliable a picture as possible of malignant metastases, particularly in the region of diaphragm, peritoneum and ligaments. (s. figs. 37.33, 37.34) Inspecting large areas of the visible surface of the liver as well as certain parts of the underside when lifted by a probe allows excellent differentiation of all the respective findings – especially in cirrhosis. *Explorative*

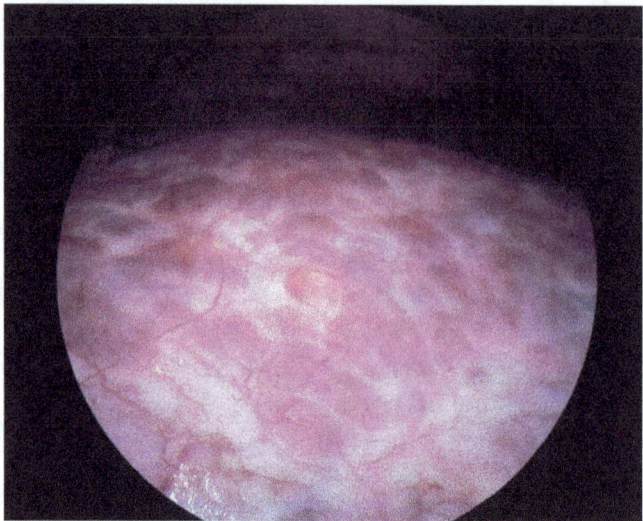

Fig. 37.9: Small to medium-nodular, alcoholic cirrhosis with undifferentiated, multilobular hepatocellular carcinoma and subcapsular vascularization

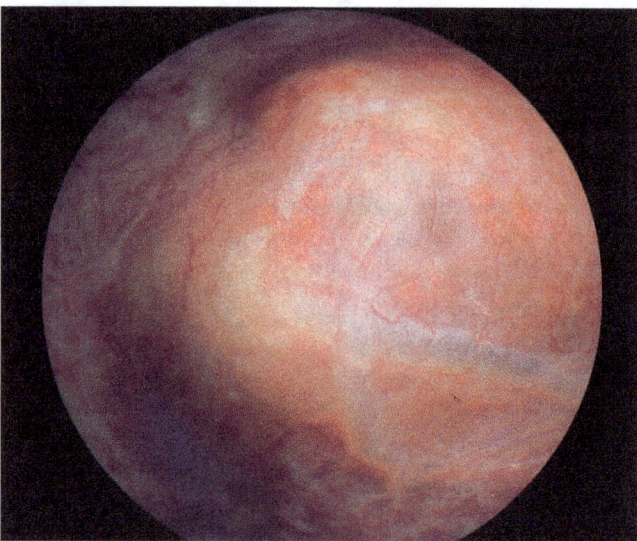

Fig. 37.10: Large-bulbous hepatocellular carcinoma due to alcohol abuse and active chronic hepatitis B with cirrhotic transformation in some places

laparoscopy also facilitates **staging**, which cannot be achieved as effectively by imaging diagnostics.

All findings are documented by **photolaparoscopy**. (s. p. 164) Sufficiently large and compact tissue particles can be obtained from foci lying close to the surface by using **biopsy forceps**. Highly vascularized areas are thus avoided. The site of extraction can be coagulated immediately, so that prolonged biopsy bleeding or late bleeding is excluded. • Foci that lie at a deeper level or those which cannot be reached with forceps should be evaluated by **fine-needle biopsy**. Assisted by sonography, this can be carried out at the same time as or after deflating the pneumoperitoneum, while the position of the trocar (or alternatively the Veres needle) is maintained. If necessary, a clear view into the abdominal cavity can be regained by quick insufflation using the trocar.

> **Explorative laparotomy**, as is often recommended in older literature, is *contraindicated* in our opinion. • *All* comparisons with respect to the degree of risk, stress or inconvenience to the patient, expenditure of time, material, staff and the costs involved, and particularly the diagnostic benefits, speak *against* laparotomy and *in favour of* **explorative laparoscopy**.

3.8 Prognosis

The prognosis of HCC is determined by the tumour mass and its speed of growth at the time of diagnosis. Signs of a *poor prognosis* are included in the (p)TNM classification. (s. tab. 37.2)

> 1. Considerable size of tumour (> 5 cm)
> 2. Infiltrative or multilocular growth
> 3. Metastatic spread

The **natural course** of disease shows an average survival rate of five months (2–8 months). Longer courses of HCC have only been observed occasionally; some 3% of patients survive for five years. • The number of tumour nodes and the existing cirrhosis correlate with the likelihood of recurrence. In contrast, the histological degree of tumour differentiation as well as potential capsule or bile formation by the tumour are unlikely or still disputed risk factors for a relapse. This is also true of the biological features of the tumour, such as ploidy, mitosis rate and proliferation marker index. (54, 107)

By including clinical and laboratory parameters (ascites, jaundice, hyperalbuminaemia), K. OKUDA et al. (1985) introduced a **classification** into stages in order to improve prognostic accuracy regarding survival time. (s. tab. 37.7) The survival rate in the untreated course was calculated to be 11 months in stage I, 3 months in stage II, and 1 month in stage III. The corresponding 1-year survival rates are 39%, 12%, and 3%. A survival rate of 29 months can be expected for tumours with <25% invasion of the liver in stage I; the corresponding figure for 25–50% liver invasion is 8 months. With smaller tumours (< 3 cm), the survival rates are slightly better: 1 year = 91%, 2 years = 55%, 3 years = 13%. In older patients and in those with moderately increased γ-GT values, tumour growth is retarded. Evidence of antibodies against the tumour suppressor gene p53 point to an unfavourable prognosis.

Another alternative HCC staging system is the so-called **CLIP score** (36). This also combines morphological criteria of the HCC with liver functions (Child-Pugh) and, additionally, with portal vein thrombosis and AFP. (s. tab. 37.8) • **BCLC classification** can be recommended for staging-adapted management of HCC. (106, 107)

Complications: Acute liver failure, arterioportal fistula formation, oesophageal varices (15) and pulmonary

	0 points	1 point
A: Liver invasion	≤ 50%	> 50%
B: Ascites	no	yes
C: Bilirubin	≤ 3 mg/dl	> 3 g/dl
D: Albumin	> 3 mg/dl	< 3 g/dl
A+B+C+D =	0 points:	stage I = 8.3
A+B+C+D =	1–2 points:	stage II = 2.0
A+B+C+D =	3–4 points:	stage III = 0.7

Tab. 37.7: Classification of the stages of hepatocellular carcinoma and survival time in months (untreated) (K. Okuda et al., 1985)

Criteria	Points 0	1	2
1. Child-Pugh	A	B	C
2. HCC morphology	solitary < 50% of liver	multifocular < 50% of liver	multifocular > 50% of liver
3. α_1-fetoprotein	< 400 µg/l	> 400 µg/l	
4. portal vein thrombosis	no	yes	
Survival rate			
points	mean rate	1 year (%)	2 year (%)
0	36	84	65
1	22	66	45
2	9	45	17
3	7	36	12
4–6	3	9	0

Tab. 37.8: CLIP staging system of HCC and the respective survival rate (36)

hypertension have been reported as complications. • In most cases, the **cause of death** is anorexia with *tumour cachexia*, accompanied by signs of circulatory and renal failure. Occasionally, there is intraperitoneal haemorrhage, portal vein thrombosis (137, 144) and *tumour rupture* with formation of haemorrhagic ascites. (120)

Spontaneous regression: As far as I know, it was E.B. Gottfried et al. (1982) who first reported spontaneous regression of HCC. In the meantime, further (> 25) unusual observations of this kind have been published. However, recurrence after such regression has also been reported. (49, 59, 66, 73, 103, 111, 118, 161, 164)

3.9 Therapy

Surgical, local-interventional, regional and systemic procedures and palliative measures are available for the treatment of HCC. • Longer survival periods can be achieved by surgery, which is seen as the only form of potentially curative treatment for small tumours (< 3 cm, or even < 5 cm). • At present, merely 5% of patients suffering from HCC have any chance of being cured. Some 25–30% of *inoperable* patients were rendered *operable* by means of preoperative selective irradiation with yttrium[90] microparticles (intra-arterially) or by several cycles of cisplatin + IFNα_{2b} + doxorubicin + 5-fluorouracil. The results could be further improved by postoperative treatment with lipiodol-J[131]. • In this context, the overall chance of recovery is reported to be 15%.

▶ An **interdisciplinary consensus conference** to decide upon the best therapy possible must be held before any treatment of a carcinoma begins. A gastroenterologist, a surgeon, an oncologist and a radiologist should participate, irrespective of the department in which the patient is being cared for. The treatment plan must then be explained to the patient and (with the patient's consent) also to the closest relatives. • So-called *"virtual liver surgery"* will play an important role in this connection in the foreseeable future.

3.9.1 Surgical therapy

Resection

About 30% of tumours are still resectable by the time HCC is diagnosed. • The following conditions are given as **contraindications** for resection: (*1.*) multicentric tumours, (*2.*) metastases, (*3.*) invasion of the tumour into the portal or hepatic vein, (*4.*) liver malfunction (jaundice, hypoalbuminaemia, considerable reduction in Quick's value and cholinesterase), and (*5.*) decompensated portal hypertension (ascites, encephalopathy). • **Surgical techniques** include (*1.*) right-sided or left-sided hemihepatectomy, (*2.*) right-sided or left-sided lobectomy, (*3.*) segment IVb resection, and (*4.*) atypical resections and wedge excisions. (s. pp 825, 900) Resection of the small left lobe of liver is tolerated best. When the larger right lobe is resected, there is a risk of liver insufficiency due to inadequate residual functional capacity. Preoperative administration of [131]J-lipiodol (60 mCi/injection) showed promising results. (142) • The following procedure was recommended for the safe removal of liver parenchyma: first, embolization of the portal vein branch associated with the tumour is carried out; this results in atrophy of the embolized lobe and hypertrophy of those segments to be maintained, with a correspondingly better functional capacity. • If non-resectability is revealed during the operation, a catheter should immediately be implanted in the hepatic artery for regional chemotherapy. • For non-cirrhotic patients, **mortality** is 1–3%, for those with cirrhosis 7–25%. The **survival rate** is 25–60% after five years, depending on tumour size; this rate sinks to 25–35% when the capsule or the portal vein are infiltrated. Decisive factors are the radicalness of the intervention and the functional capacity of the residual liver parenchyma. Intraoperative blood loss should be kept as low as possible in order to limit morbidity. Patients in **Child-Pugh** stage A showed a five-year survival rate of 27–53% (cf. disease-free survival rate of 20—33%), and in stage B of about 30%; stage C is usually non-resectable or has no surgical benefits. Preoperative staging using laparoscopy is absolutely necessary. It is decisive for choosing the correct management (the original procedure had to be changed in 20—30% of patients due to the laparoscopic findings). (7, 9, 17, 60, 77, 85, 94, 96, 116, 124, 140, 182) (s. p. 825)

The **radicalness of the intervention** is assessed by the pathologist based on the findings of the resected preparation and the surgical report. First, the pTNM stage is determined. (s. tab. 37.2) Then, the **R classification** is made to establish whether the resection was curative. *R0 resection* means that the tumour was fully removed, no tumourous residues were left behind, and the resection margin is tumour-free. *R1 resection* implies that there are still tumour cells at the resection margin. *R2 resection* signifies that macroscopically visible tumour tissue is left. When the tumour markers normalize within the first four postoperative months after R0 resection, this is defined as *R0a resection*, and without normalization as *R0b resection*. (7) • In cirrhosis patients with small HCC, **liver function** is the most important factor for long-term survival. In this context, the indocyanine green test, MEGX test and the Okuda stage system have proved useful. Under favourable conditions, *relapse resections* are also possible. (69) • Resection therapy can be used as "bridging" prior to a liver transplantation.

Recidivation is generally due to undetected small intrahepatic foci. Especially in cirrhosis, the recurrence rate is very high as a result of this factor. A further cause of recidivation after primary R0 resection is attributed to the multicentricity of the HCC, i.e. synchronic or metachronic development of additional tumours which are independent of the primary tumour. Therefore, the **secondary prophylaxis** takes on a special meaning (systemic or intra-arterial chemotherapy, interferon, retinoids, autologous lymphocyte transfusion, etc.). An increase in ornithine decarboxylase and spermidine is apparently a high risk factor for recurrence. • Even after recidivation, repeated resection or interventional procedures (e.g. RFTA) are sometimes successful.

Cryosurgery: Cryotherapy of tumours was introduced by I. S. Cooper in 1963. • Intraoperative insertion of a probe into the liver tumour is carried out directly. Necrosis is induced in the tumour tissue by the application of fluid nitrogen and the subsequent rethawing of the iced area (ca. $-50\,°C$). This procedure is usually repeated. It is indicated in cases of non-resectable liver tumours and for the freezing of margins following resection. (22, 174) (s. p. 826)

Liver transplantation

With insufficient functional reserve capacity of the liver and/or non-curative resectability of the tumour, liver transplantation is generally indicated. However, such a procedure does not yield better long-term results than resection, particularly since the frequency of **relapse** (some 65% of cases) in the transplanted liver is higher due to the fact that *immunosuppression* is constantly required. A further problem is that the tumour-doubling time (102—195 days) is shortened to about 26 days. Relapses originate from preoperatively undetected metastases, which show strikingly rapid growth.

In order to limit these relapses, **neoadjuvant chemotherapy** has been recommended, e.g. intra-arterial or systemic administration of cisplatin and doxorubicin, possibly in combination with interferon. The survival rates after 1, 2 and 3 years were reported as 70%, 60%, and 59% respectively. Another form of neoadjuvant therapy was based on 5-FU (continuous infusion for 6 months), with intermittent administration of adriamycin and cisplatin prior to transplantation. This procedure had a survival rate after 1, 2 and 4 years of 73% vs 55%, 61% vs 40%, and 61% vs 22% respectively. The relapse rate was only 18%. *Indications for liver transplantation should always be considered with great caution.*

Careful preoperative examination regarding **HBV** or **HCV infection** (PCR, if necessary) is recommended, since there is a very high risk of the transplanted liver being infected by viruses from extrahepatic tissues under immunosuppression. • **Survival rates** in HCC cases without and with cirrhosis are almost equal at up to 85% after 1 year, 30% after 3 years, 20—45% after 5 years, and about 20% after 10 years. A long-term survival rate is only to be expected in patients with small solitary tumour nodes (< 5 cm) or not more than 3 nodes of < 3 cm in diameter and without signs of vascular invasion (so-called Milano or Mazzaferro criteria). (113) A hyperextended indication is only given in rare cases. These rates largely correspond to the results obtained in non-malignant liver diseases. Transplantation is regarded as being better than resection in cirrhosis patients with early detected HCC, since the precancerous potential of cirrhosis is totally eliminated at an early stage. In every case, preoperative and/or postoperative chemotherapy should be considered. The previous **operative mortality rate** of 15—20% has now been further reduced. (23, 53, 85, 116, 121, 151, 156)

3.9.2 Interventional therapy

After discussing the clinical and imaging findings as well as the result of exploratory laparoscopy, it is important to decide on the most promising management in the interdisciplinary conference. • Once resection techniques and liver transplantation have been ruled out, the next alternative are interventional procedures. (s. tab. 37.9)

Percutaneous injection therapy

Percutaneous injection therapy has meanwhile proved effective in a number of cases. Two principal methods are important in this respect.

1. **Percutaneous injection therapy**
   - ethanol
   - acetic acid
2. **Transcatheter arterial therapy**
   - transarterial chemotherapy
   - transarterial embolization
   - transarterial chemoembolization
   - transarterial radiation
     - ^{131}J-lipiodol
     - ^{90}yttrium
3. **Percutaneous thermoablation therapy**
   - laser-induced thermotherapy
   - microwave coagulation
   - radiofrequency ablation

Tab. 37.9: Local-interventional procedures in HCC management

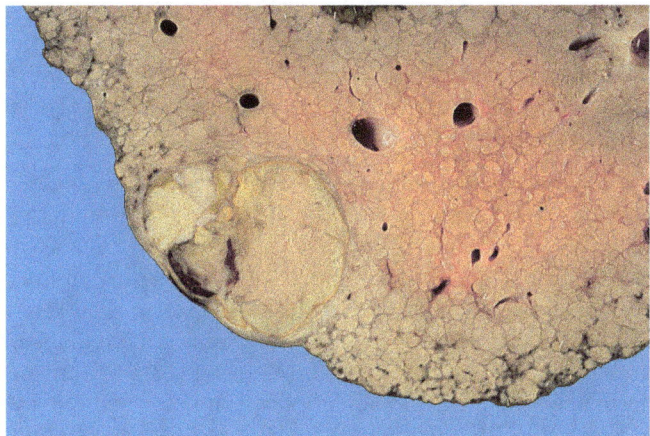

Fig. 37.11: Subcapsular HCC in liver cirrhosis: mostly necrotic following ethanol injection

▶ **Percutaneous ethanol injection** (PEI): This procedure was described by N. SUGIURA et al. in 1983. In solitary HCC with a size of <3 (−5) cm in diameter, alcohol (96 vol.%) is injected into the tumour using sonographic, laparoscopic (76) or CT monitoring. This technique (5−10 ml, about 3 times a week, regularly over a period of 3−4 months) is a relatively inexpensive procedure which is technically simple and well tolerated (albeit usually very painful!). Due to the fact that HCC has a soft consistency compared to the firmer liver tissue, it is possible to a large extent to infiltrate the tumour selectively and limit necrosis as desired. (s. fig. 37.11)

Imaging findings after PEI are: in US, alcohol distribution appears like an echogenic cloud and the tumour becomes relatively hyperechoic; in Doppler sonography, the colour signals disappear; in CT, gas formation is sometimes visible. More than 70% of the tumour mass may be necrotized. Under favourable conditions, a complete response can be achieved in 80% of cases. • Adverse events include acute cholecystitis, cholangitis, haemorrhages, liver abscess, pleural effusion, portal vein thrombosis, etc. • The PEI technique has no significant effect on tumours with a size of > 5 cm and multilocular tumours. Some cases of stitch-track metastases have been reported. The relapse rate is approx. 60%. The survival rate is 68−80% after 3 years and about 50% after 5 years. Long-term success depends upon the number and size of the tumours as well as on the respective liver function. PEI is contraindicated in Child-Pugh stage C. (18, 68, 76, 82, 86, 104, 114, 117, 132, 138, 175)

▶ **Percutaneous acetic acid injection** (PAI): Injection of acetic acid (40−50%, 2−5 ml, two to four sessions) into the tumour also resulted in necrotic destruction of the tumour tissue (M. IMAMURA et al., 1995). PAI is considered to be just as effective as PEI; the success was most evident when the intratumoural retention of acetic acid persisted for about three days after completion of the treatment. (63, 101, 130)

Transcatheter arterial therapy

As an alternative to percutaneous injection therapy, there is a possibility to develop new local-interventional treatment strategies by selectively exploring the tumour-feeding branch of the proper hepatic artery.

Transarterial chemotherapy (TAC): The systemic administration of cytostatics, both as monochemotherapy or polychemotherapy, led to unsatisfactory results with considerable side effects. By transporting cytostatics transarterially to the tumour itself, it was possible to build up a high concentration of these substances in the arteries supplying the HCC. Because there were far fewer side effects, the dosage of cytostatics could be optimized. A further advantage of this method is that the extratumoural parenchyma has a portal venous blood supply; thus the arterially transported cytostatics do not cause any significant peritumoural liver damage. This transarterial chemoperfusion could be improved even more by positioning the selective-arterial catheter exactly and by implanting a port system. (s. p. 827)

Lipiodol (= iodized ester of poppyseed oil) used as a contrast medium for lymphography accumulates selectively in the tumour over a longer period. As a result, local-interventional (oily) *lipiodol chemotherapy* (TOCE) was developed. Lipiodol acts as a carrier for the admixed cytostatic agents, so that the latter retain their effect in the tumour long-term in a high (systematically unacceptable) dose. Hereby, cisplatin or epidoxorubicin (99) is emulgated in lipiodol. It was possible to achieve 1-year survival rates of 36−55%. Other cytostatics did not prove to be any more effective.

Transarterial embolization (TAE): By occluding the smaller tumour-feeding arteries, it is possible to achieve a hypoxia-induced necrosis of the HCC. This is more successful if the tumour is encapsulated. Such embolization is effected using collagen particles, polyvinyl alcohol, gelfoam or galactose spheres. However, the HCC cannot be eliminated completely, because the malignant cells in its periphery, which are supplied by the portal venous system, remain intact, so that recidivation often occurs (30-50%) at the same place. (108) With (repeat) embolization, 1-year and 2-year survival rates of 65% and 38% respectively were achieved. (s. p. 827)

Transarterial chemoembolization (TACE): The direct application of a cytostatic agent (using the DSA technique via the femoral artery) into the tumour-feeding artery, followed by temporary occlusion of the vessel, leads to (*1.*) high intratumoural concentration of the cytostatic agent, (*2.*) longer action time of this substance, and (*3.*) therapeutically important ischaemia of the HCC. As a rule, lipiodol is applied together with cisplatin (or mitomycin-C, epiduricin, doxorubicin); this is followed by embolization (see above). Evaluation of therapy success is best carried out using MRI, but coded phase-inversion harmonic sonography is likewise highly sensitive and accurate. TACE is also possible under outpatient conditions. *Repeated embolization* is recommended at intervals of about four weeks; this creates extensive tumour necroses. Remission was achieved in 30-60% of patients.

The following *side effects* have been observed: fever, nausea, vomiting, upper abdominal pain (= *post-embolization syndrome*), lipiodol embolisms, pancreatitis, gall-bladder infarction, tumour rupture and liver failure. (74) Chemoembolization is thus a very aggressive form of treatment and should only be considered in patients with a well-functioning liver. The administration of BCAA after TACE has proved beneficial (increase in serum albumin, reduction in mortality, improvement in quality of life). (142) • The 1-year and 2-year survival rates were given as 82% and 63% respectively.

A further improvement in the survival rate was observed following the oral administration of pravastatin (20-40 mg/day). (78) For HCC which is primarily supplied by venous blood, chemotherapy is contraindicated, as is also the case with portal vein thrombosis and renal insufficiency. • It is open to question whether it is possible (and whether it makes sense) to improve the results of a subsequent resection by primary reduction in the tumour mass through chemoembolization or even by treating resectable HCC with chemoembolization from the onset. (31, 48, 74, 130, 143, 180) (s. p. 827)

Combination therapy: The use of local-interventional procedures is restricted to a maximum tumour size of 5 cm in diameter. Therefore, a combination of two local techniques may be promising. • The joint application of PEI and TAE has proved efficacious. (175) Similarly, there have been reports about the successful use of TACE following laser thermal ablation. (134) Further encouraging options include a combination of TACE and RFTA, TACE with microwave coagulation (147) or TACE with cryotherapy. Using TACE, the size of the HCC can be reduced in some cases, making it possible to carry out subsequent ablation with better results.

Transarterial radiation (TAR): Intra-arterial radiation of ^{131}*iodine lipiodol* into the tumour tissue has shown good results with a six-month survival rate of 48-52%. This procedure has hardly any influence on hepatic arterial perfusion. For this reason, the technique can also be used in portal vein thrombosis. (27, 95, 142) • Transarterial injection of ^{90}*yttrium* particles did not lead to tumour regression in the first study carried out in 1992. (148) A new administration form consisting of 30 μm-sized particles of resin loaded with ^{90}yttrium was recently developed. The radiation dose amounts to approx. 2 gigabecquerel. The rays penetrate the tissue to a depth of about 2.4 mm. The results obtained so far have proved excellent (A. KENNEDY et al., 2004).

Percutaneous thermoablation therapy

Targeted, temperature-related tumour necrotization can be achieved either through extreme refrigeration (= *cryotherapy*) or overheating (= *thermotherapy*). In the latter case, microwaves, laser-induced radiation or high-frequency current are generally used. The energy is applied with the help of a specially developed probe.

Laser-induced thermotherapy (LITT): In 1983, S.G. BOWN applied this technique for the first time as minimally invasive percutaneous ablation therapy. By means of quartz fibres, Nd : YAG laser light (1,064 nm) is conducted directly into the tumour via a probe. The laser light is converted into heat, thus causing a coagulation necrosis of the tumour. Necroses of up to 4-5 cm in diameter may result. Probe application is carried out by MR-guiding; this technique is also used for monitoring success. The procedure is considered to be both safe and efficacious. (42, 127) (s. p. 826)

Microwave coagulation therapy (MCT): Necrotization of liver tumours by means of microwave coagulation (2,450 ± 50 MHz) is another thermoablation technique (T. SEKI et al., 1994). The tumour is punctured using a 14 G needle, through which a special probe is inserted. Good results were obtained by using this US-guided procedure. The four-year survival rate of patients with superficial HCC was 64.2%; the local recurrence rate was 27.1%. In 12.8% of cases, no evidence of surviving tumour tissue was observed following treatment. (44, 71, 129) When MCT was compared with RFTA, the results, side effects and complications proved to be more or less equal. MCT is also recommended in metastases. (371)

Radiofrequency thermal ablation (RFTA): S. ROSSI et al. (1990, 1993) were the first to introduce this procedure. Under analgosedation and local anaesthesia, an expandable, cooled-tip needle electrode is inserted percutaneously into the tumour with the help of US, CT or MR guidance. There are various types of probes with some differences. Due to high-frequency alternating current (480-500 kHz), the tumour tissue is gradually heated (up to max. 105 °C). A necrosis volume of 4-5 cm in diameter can be achieved. An indication is given for one to three foci, each with a maximum size of 5 cm in diameter. This also applies to compromised liver function. One or more sessions are necessary for this treatment. Morbidity is <10%, lethality 1–2%. The 3-year survival rates were 80–85% in Child A and 30–35% in Child B. After ablation of the tumour, success is monitored using CT plus CM: in the case of complete ablation, there is no enhancement of CM. Local recidivation is observed in 10–15% of cases. Therefore, a regular monitoring (laboratory parameter together with US or MRI) is required. In the case of recidivation, subsequent therapy with the help of TACE is promising. The following adverse events have been observed: liver insufficiency, colon perforation, portal vein thrombosis, liver abscess, pleural effusion, pneumothorax, haematoma, haemoperitoneum, needle-tract seeding, etc. RFTA can also be carried out laparoscopically (145) or operatively. • Overall, the results of RFTA are better than those of PEI (2-year survival rate: 64% vs. 43%); this is especially true of the disease-free survival rate. It would appear that RFTA is just as effective as resection therapy. (22, 56, 57, 79, 105) (s. p. 826)

3.9.3 Medicinal therapy

Systemic chemotherapy: This kind of treatment yielded a response rate of 5–15% only, irrespective of whether monotherapy or polytherapy was used. (98) A major cause of the low efficacy is the considerable quantity of mixed-functional oxidases in the tumour cells together with an overexpression of the multidrug resistance gene localized on chromosome 7. This MDR can be compensated to a large extent by chemosensitizers (e. g. calcium antagonists). However, there was no clinical success and the side effects were stronger. • In a recent study, the combination of gemcitabine plus oxaliplatin seemed promising. (160) The application of 5′fluorouracil + cisplatin + IFN also proved well-tolerated and favourable. (89) With such chemotherapy, there are generally considerable side effects, particularly in the case of an underlying cirrhosis. • Overall, HCC shows hardly any response to systemic chemotherapy, so that this treatment does not really represent a therapeutic option.

Hormone receptor antagonist: The hepatocytes possess oestrogen receptors and react to oestrogen with proliferation. Therefore, it seemed advisable to apply anti-oestrogens as part of the therapy. However, the efficacy of these substances, e. g. tamoxifen at 10–20 mg twice daily, could not be confirmed. *Toremifen* appeared to be more successful. • *Cyproterone acetate* proved inefficacious as an anti-androgenic agent. *Flutamide* likewise showed no effect.

Immunotherapy: *Interferon-alpha* has an antiproliferative effect on tumour cells. Previous studies, however, have shown no success in HCC, not even when IFN was combined with cytostatics. • In order to improve the severely weakened immune system of tumour patients, *immunostimulants* (e. g. autologous lymphocyte infusion, thymostimulin) were used. (135) The incorporation of liposomes loaded with monoclonal antibodies into tumour cells is a further therapeutic option. • In *gene therapy*, the application of so-called suicide genes by means of retroviruses (possibly even adenoviruses) has aroused particular interest. So far, however, the experimental gene transfer has not been sufficient to eliminate the respective tumour mass.

Somatostatin: Somatotropin release inhibiting factor (SRIF) displays antimitotic effects regarding various non-endocrine tumours. In animal experiments, *octreotide* retards tumour growth. The subcutaneous administration of octreotide (250 µg, 2x/day) led to a considerable improvement in survival time and quality of life. (90) This result could not, however, be confirmed. (19) There are still no clinical results available regarding the use of *lanreotide*, which has a longer action time.

3-bromopyruvate, a potent inhibitor of ATP, has proved efficacious as an intra-arterial injection. (55) Likewise, i.m. administration of **arginine deiminase** (160 IU/m^2) was effective and well-tolerated. (40) • In recent studies, two further groups of substances have proved efficacious with good tolerance: *bevacizumab* for angiogenesis inhibition, and *sorafenib* as the dual inhibitor of Raf kinase and VEGF. They may well represent a new approach in the systemic chemotherapy of HCC.

3.9.4 Adjuvant measures

There are several adjuvant measures which are deemed unconventional, i.e. the purported therapeutic efficacy has not yet been confirmed in controlled clinical studies. In the field of oncology, many treatment approaches (cancer-related diets, medication, physical or instrumental therapy forms, psychological methods, etc.) have been propagated. • These should not be seen as alternative techniques, since they cannot replace the frequently tested and well-established methods used in surgery, radiology and chemotherapy. Thus they are known as "supplementary", "additive", "adjuvant", and "complementary" measures or "best supportive care". • It is understandable that many tumour patients or their relatives demand these treatment options besides the traditional mainstream medical care when the diagnosis of "cancer" has been made. Up to 70% of all tumour patients try out such unconventional methods in the course of their disease. • Numerous cancer-related diets have been extolled – none of which came up to previous expectations. Everybody is, however, at liberty to add various supplements (beetroot, probiotics, vitamins C and E, etc.) to their daily diet in line with the physiological principles of nutrition. • Moreover, special psychological treatment methods have been used, such as autosuggestion, crisis therapy, meditation and visualization. Psychotherapeutic and spiritual assistance can, without doubt, have positive effects on tumour symptomatology. A combination of *dietary recommendations*

+ *physiotherapy* + *psychotherapy* should indeed be included in the overall concept of cancer therapy.

▶ Both physician and patient are confronted with a wide range of *unconventional therapeutic measures*. It is logical that patients and their relatives resort, in their desperation, to any methods which may offer a therapeutic chance: "We have nothing to lose, but maybe we can defeat the cancer in the end; time and again, one hears of such healing or remission." And which doctor would want to destroy hope even in the face of oncological reality? • The alternatives indeed cover a broad spectrum. (s. tab. 37.10)

Immunobiological tumour therapy	
• Selenium	• Zinc
• Organ lysates	• Mistletoe extracts
• Rhodococcus rodochrous	• Tumour vaccines
• Fungi belonging to	• G-SH + anthocyane
– tricholomataceae	+ L-cysteine
– polyporaceae	• VEGF blockage
Holistic tumour therapy	
• Hyperthermia	• Ozone therapy
• Oxygen multi-step therapy	• Enzymes
Naturopathy	
• Muscular training	• Nutritional therapy
• Physiotherapy	• Relaxation therapy
Psycho-oncological care	
Spiritual care	

Tab. 37.10: Some adjuvant or unconventional therapeutic methods used in malignant diseases

▶ Experiencing and coping with the diagnosis of carcinoma (and also "accepting" it) puts any patient under severe stress. As a consequence, the **immune system,** which is of essential significance in fighting the malignant disease, is usually weakened. • Subsequent *surgery* burdens the immune system even more. Unfortunately, *chemotherapy*, in addition to its cytostatic effectiveness, also results in massive long-term suppression of the immune system. This is equally true of *radiology*. • The **survival time** varies considerably both in the natural course of disease and/or subsequent to invasive therapeutic measures mainly as a result of differences in individual defence systems. • In comparative studies, the patients treated symptomatically (*how?* and *with what?*) often fare better in terms of survival time and the remaining quality of life — without painful therapeutic interventions, which often involve numerous side effects. The greatly varying efficiency of individual immune systems makes it difficult to compare the clinical and thus also statistical data obtained from group studies, and this might also account for the divergent results. • The tested, carefully considered and (largely) well-established techniques of (*1.*) *surgery*, (*2.*) *radiology*, and (*3.*) *chemotherapy* continue to serve as unchallenged pillars in the treatment of malignant tumours. In future, (*4.*) *immunotherapy* will also play a more important (perhaps decisive) role — even though the patient's "immune status" cannot (unfortunately) be measured adequately.

Nevertheless, all possibilities of activating the **immune system** should be made use of. These adjuvant measures can (and should) precede or simultaneously supplement any invasive treatment procedures.

Selenium: As a main constituent of glutathion peroxydase and thioredoxin reductase, selenium is a valuable antioxidant. The daily requirement of 75 µg is often not reached, especially by tumour patients, and substitution is necessary. In addition, malignant diseases generally show a reduction in the serum value of selenium. Moreover, it intensifies the cytotoxicity of T lymphocytes and natural killer cells, leading to a corresponding effect on tumour cells. This effect is enhanced through the stimulation of IFN-γ. The application of cytostatics thus becomes more favourable. A daily dose of 200 µg (−1,000 µg) selenium is recommended. (s. pp 55, 310, 388)

Zinc is of greatest importance for the normal functioning of the immune system. (s. pp 55, 635) In abdominal surgery, we usually detected pronounced *zincuria* (s. tab. 3.15), which, in our experience, could not be prevented by intravenous (even high-dosage) administration of zinc. Zinc deficiency, however, has negative effects on the immune system. • We found that postoperative zincuria could mostly be prevented in abdominal surgery by the peri- and postoperative administration of the aldosterone antagonist **potassium canrenoate**. *At the same time, major postoperative intestinal atonicity (probably due to potassium deficiency in the cells) was no longer observed in this condition!* • This was the rationale for administering zinc and potassium canrenoate intravenously in all cases involving abdominal surgery one day prior to and three or four days after the operation. *We wish to share these positive clinical experiences, which are free from side effects.*

At this point, it is worth mentioning several efforts aimed at preventing **metastasis formation** subsequent to surgical manipulation of the organ containing the primary tumour. • In 1984 **D-galactose-specific lectin** was discovered on hepatocytes. Lectins seem to play a major part in the "docking" of tumour cells on other organ cells. Apparently, the organ specificity of malignant cells is determined by the lectin pattern on the surface of their target cells, with which the corresponding sugars on the tumour cells link up. Animal experiments based on the **lectin-receptor theory** (G. UHLENBRUCK et al., 1986) showed that the formation of liver metastases was almost completely prevented by administering D-galactose prior to tumour inoculation. In two pioneering clinical studies (compared to a control group), formation of liver metastases subsequent to colorectal tumour surgery was suppressed in 50% of patients within three years. A 5% D-galactose solution (1.6 g/kg BW) was infused 1 hour prior to surgery, and this was repeated until the third postoperative day. (365) • This use of galactose (or other carbohydrates?), which is free from side effects, should indeed be investigated. Such procedures can probably also be recommended in the puncture of tumours as a means of preventing tumour cell spread.

3.10 Fibrolamellar carcinoma

In 1956 this rare tumour was described by H. A. EDMONDSON in a 14-year-old girl as a "fibrosing variant of HCC in adolescents" (238); subsequent to tumour resection, the patient was without relapse for two years. J.R. CRAIG et al. (1980) outlined the specific clinical and histological criteria of fibrolamellar hepatocellular carcinoma (FHCC). Some 2–3% of HCC cases are assigned to FHCC; frequency is 20–60 cases/year in Germany. • FHCC shows the following features: (1.) it develops in a non-cirrhotic liver (cirrhosis frequency about 4%); (2.) it is found in younger people (between the ages of 5 and 35); (3.) men and women are affected with the same frequency; (4.) it is not associated with HBV or HCV infection (HBsAg is positive in 6–8% of cases); (5.) AFP values are not at all or only rarely increased (7–11%); (6.) FHCC is most often localized in the left liver lobe, generally as a grey, firm tumour. • With increasing growth, abdominal pain and weight loss occur. As the tumour grows in size, the transaminases, AP, γ-GT and copper values increase. (188, 194, 195) • With regard to **imaging procedures,** sonography yields a hyperechoic pattern, while CT and MRI show FHCC as a large, solitary and solid tumour. (184, 186, 187) The tumour resembles FNH by virtue of a generally recognizable central scar and multiple fibrous septa. FHCC was therefore suspected to be a malignant variant of FNH. In MRI, both the scar and the septa show hypodense signal intensity in T_1 and T_2 images. In contrast to FNH, haemorrhages, necroses or central fibrous scars and calcifications are occasionally observed in this hypervascularized tumour. Metastatic spread occurs late and initially into the abdominal lymph nodes.

The **diagnosis** is based on histology (because of hypervascularization using FNB or targeted biopsy under laparoscopy): large eosinophilic tumour cells with large nuclei and dense nucleoli are found. The polygonal tumour cells contain a copper protein as well as inclusion bodies (consisting of α_1AT, α_1FP, fibrinogen, ferritin, etc.). Granular eosinophilia is caused by a surplus of mitochondria. Lamellar connective tissue lies between the trabecular formations. (183, 185, 191, 193–195) (s. figs. 37.12, 37.13)

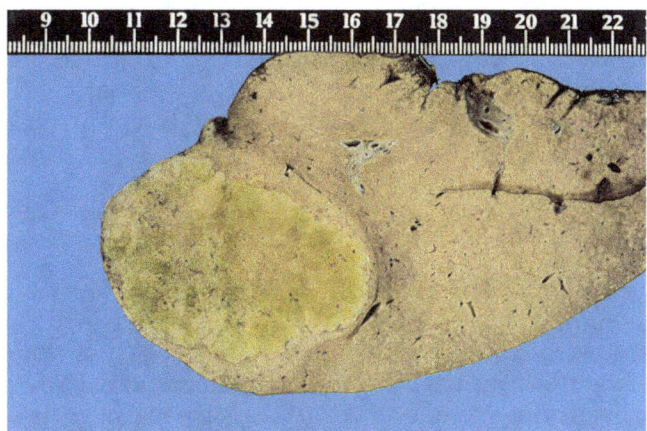

Fig. 37.12: Fibrolamellar hepatocellular carcinoma as is usually seen in a non-cirrhotic liver

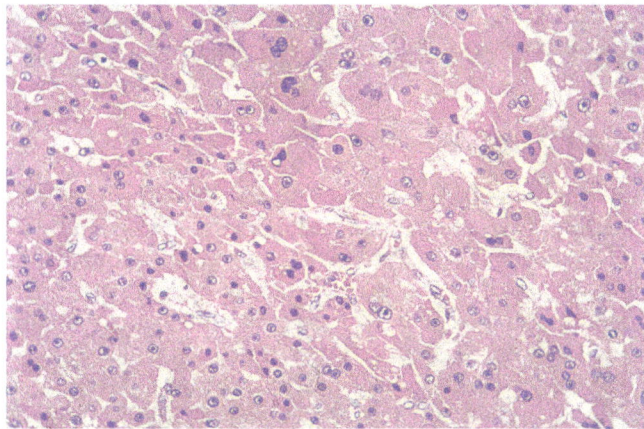

Fig. 37.13: Fibrolamellar hepatocellular carcinoma: large, polygonal cells with granular-eosinophilic cytoplasm (based on a surplus of mitochondria) (HE)

A high vitamin B_{12} value in the serum is typical, because the tumour cells trigger enhanced synthesis of transcobalamin I. Neurotensin and ceruloplasmin are also seen as tumour markers. • The **prognosis** of FHCC is generally more favourable than that of HCC and cholangiocarcinoma. Some 50–80% of patients are resectable. The survival rate after 5 years was 40–60% (the overall survival rate equals 3–16 years following surgery, but is no more than two years without surgery). After liver transplantation, the prognosis of FHCC is better than in HCC and CCC. (189, 190, 192, 195)

4 Cholangiocellular carcinoma

Intrahepatic localizations must be distinguished from extrahepatic CCC. They are subdivided into **three areas** of the large bile duct: (1.) the upper third from the liver hilum to the opening of the cystic duct (frequency about 49%); (2.) the medial third of the common bile duct (frequency about 25%); (3.) the lower third reaching to the opening into the duodenum (frequency about 19%). Diffuse involvement of the whole extrahepatic area was found in 7% of cases. • Tumours situated in the upper third are designated proximal, central or hilar CCC and are also known as **Klatskin tumours**. (206) • Distal localizations of the extrahepatic CCC must be clearly differentiated from carcinomas of Vater's ampulla and pancreas head.

4.1 Definition

Cholangiocellular carcinoma (CCC) is a malignant tumour originating from the cholangiocytes of the intrahepatic small bile ducts *(peripheral CCC)* or the larger bile ducts *(hilar CCC)*. Intrahepatic CCC is found with a frequency of 10%; this type is far more rare than hepatocellular carcinoma. More than 90% are adenocarcinomas. CCC occurs mainly between the ages of 60–70, with men and women being equally affected. Prognosis is poor; the survival time is one to two years.

4.2 Morphology

In more than 90% of cases, a (rather slow-growing) adenocarcinoma can be detected. Evidence of glandular and trabecular structures with substantial connective tissue-like stroma is typical. A reliable histologic diagnosis is only possible if carcinomatous changes in the bile ducts can be demonstrated, a process which is very rarely observed in a liver biopsy specimen. Usually, a highly differentiated tumour is present; lesser degrees of differentiation are only seldom found. Distinguishing between CCC and metastases or adenocarcinomas (e.g. of the gastrointestinal tract or pancreas) can prove extremely difficult. Evidence of keratin 7, 19 or 903 in the tumour cells is characteristic of CCC. Expression of lamina-γ-2 is believed to play an important role in growth-related morphology. (196, 197) (s. fig. 37.14)

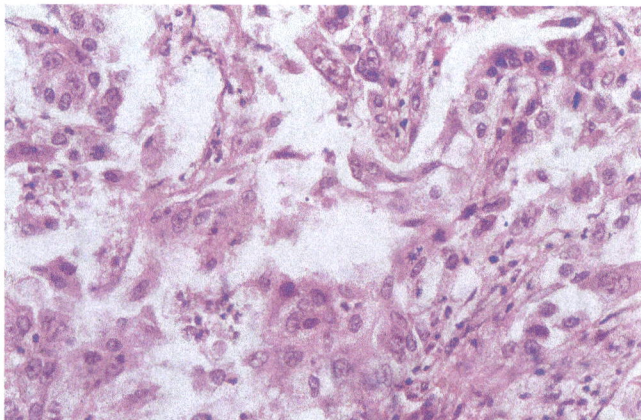

Fig. 37.14: Cholangiocellular carcinoma with tubular glands (HE)

Morphological classification: Precise characterization of CCC in terms of growth pattern and staging is very important for optimal treatment planning and for determining a prognosis. (205, 208, 209, 211)

(1.) Mass-forming type: This form appears firm and coarse due to profusely developed stroma. The tumour is only slightly vascularized. It generally has a greyish-white, sometimes dark green colour and can reach a size of up to 15 cm in diameter; the margins are well circumscribed, but irregular. Central necrosis may be present. Satellite or daughter nodules are frequent and vary in size. Usually, this tumour type does not produce bile. Evidence of keratin 903 is considered to be typical. (196) In comparison to the other types of CCC, metastases are more frequently found in hilar and parapancreatic lymph nodes as well as in the peritoneum; the tumour itself often has a haematogenous spread. Vascular invasion is rare. (207, 215)

(2.) Periductal-infiltrating type: This form grows along the bile ducts; it is therefore elongated, spiculated or branch-like. The bile ducts proximal to this CCC may be dilated if the lumen is narrowed or even obstructed. The tumour remains unidentifiable for a long time.

(3.) Intraductal-growing type: This form is mostly a papillary adenocarcinoma. It comprises innumerable frond-like infoldings of proliferated columnar epithelial cells and a slender fibrovascular core. The tumour is generally small, but often spreads superficially along the mucosal surface, forming a kind of "papillomatosis". Mostly, it produces a profuse amount of mucous, resulting in focal or segmental biliary obstruction with respective dilatations. Such a papillary adenocarcinoma has low-grade malignancy. • Some papillary tumours produce a large amount of mucin. This *mucinous tumour* is seen as a variant of the intraductal-growing type. (198)

Cholangiohepatocellular carcinoma arising from both cell types is a mixed form. (216) It sometimes appears as a subtype with two separate tumour forms or as a subtype with mixed HCC and CCC components. This type of carcinoma can develop in different parts of the liver; its subtypes may also be seen in close proximity to one another or even appear within the same tumour. It is rarely found in liver cirrhosis. Typically, there is extensive mucin production and evidence of glandular biliary epithelia. With the help of specific keratin patterns, these tumours can be identified immunohistochemically. Prognosis is poorer than in the case of the respective singular form.

Mucoepidermoid carcinoma was first described by L.E. PIANZOLA et al. in 1971. (225) It is a rare entity; this subtype constitutes only 2–3% of all CCC. Up to now, 41 cases have been reported. The tumour contains components of both adenocarcinoma and squamous cell carcinoma. It is discussed that this condition derives from a squamous metaplasia of the terminal ramifications of the bile canaliculi or from adenocarcinoma cells. A combination of HCC and mucoepidermoid carcinoma has been observed. (222) This tumour contains components of both cell types. A male predominance was found. The clinical findings and laboratory data are similar to CCC. Pathogenesis is unknown; various congenital cysts of the biliary tract (221) and non-parasitic cysts (224, 226) as well as hepatic cholelithiasis (usually associated with infection) have been proposed as aetiological factors. (220) • Although its resectability was shown to be better than that of CCC, the prognosis is poor. (200, 223, 227) (s. tab. 37.1)

4.3 Epidemiology

CCC is rare, comprising about 7% of malignant liver tumours. The tumour is most commonly found between the ages of 60—70. Men and women are affected with the same frequency. Incidence is largely dependent upon regional risk factors; on average, it ranges from 1-8/100,000 inhabitants.

4.4 Pathogenic risk factors

The pathogenesis of CCC is associated with numerous risk factors. (*1.*) *Intrahepatic cholelithiasis* results in CCC in 5—10% of cases; chronic cholangitis is usually present. (219) (*2.*) *Parasitic infestation* of the bile ducts, e.g. Clonorchis sinensis, Opisthorchis felineus and Opisthorchis viverrini (204), may be associated with CCC in up to 60% of cases when it has been present for several years. (*3.*) *Congenital anomalies* of the bile ducts (biliary atresia, cysts, dilatations, Caroli's syndrome, Alagille's syndrome) (201) pose a much higher carcinoma risk. (*4.*) *Primary sclerosing cholangitis* increases the morbidity risk to 15—30%. (212, 213) Subsequent diagnosis of CCC was confirmed in 40% of a group of patients who had died from PSC and in 35% of liver transplant patients. The prevalence of CCC in patients suffering from chronic inflammatory intestinal diseases also rose by 0.2—1.4% with pathogenic association between PSC and ulcerative colitis, whereby CCC occurred earlier in these cases (i.e. from the age of 40). A higher frequency of mutations of the oncogenes (e.g. K-ras, c-myc, p16) and tumour suppressor gene p53 (213), with a strong expression of p53 in tumour tissue, was confirmed in patients with PSC-associated CCC. (*5.*) *Thorium dioxide,* which is stored lifelong in the RES, led to the development of CCC in many cases, with an average latency period of 35 years. (*6.*) *Chemical agents* such as dioxin, nitrosamine and aflatoxin are seen as risk factors for the development of CCC. (*7.*) *Medication* (isoniazid, anabolic steroids, methyldopa, contraceptives) has often also been associated with an increase in CCC.

4.5 Clinical features and diagnosis

Symptoms: The clinical symptomatology principally depends on the localization of the tumour. Extrahepatic CCC manifests in most cases as obstructive jaundice. In intrahepatic localization of CCC, the developing clinical picture reveals abdominal pain, nausea, inappetence, loss of weight and weakness; cholangitis is often observed. (199)

Biochemistry: Non-specific signs of inflammation, cholestasis parameters and increasing jaundice are found. The tumour markers AFP and CEA are normal, while the tumour markers CA 19—9 and CA 50 are usually elevated. There may also be mutations of the cyclin-dependent kinase inhibitor p16/MTS1. (s. tab. 37.11)

Laboratory findings
1. *Non-specific signs of inflammation*
   - BSG ↑, CRP +, serum iron ↓, copper ↑, haptoglobin ↑, fibrinogen ↓, D-dimer ↑, α_2-globulins ↑, ChE ↓, anaemia
2. *Cholestasis*
   - AP ↑, LAP ↑, γ-GT ↑
3. *Jaundice*
   - Serum bilirubin ↑
4. *Tumour markers*
   - α_1FP normal, CEA normal, CA 19—9 ↑, CA 50 ↑

Imaging diagnostics
1. Sonography
   ↓
2. CT and CT angiography - - - → MR
   ↓
3. ERCP (or PTC)

Morphological diagnostics
1. Laparoscopy and biopsy
2. Percutaneous biopsy
3. Percutaneous fine-needle biopsy
4. ERC with brush biopsy

Tab. 37.11: Diagnostic parameters and examination techniques in cholangiocellular carcinoma

Sonography: In this biochemical constellation, sonography (also colour-encoded duplex sonography with visualization of the intrahepatic bile ducts) is the examination technique of choice, particularly when obstructive jaundice is suspected. There is evidence of prestenotically dilated bile ducts and, in some cases, accompanying strand-like, hyperechoic, infiltrating structures, which may be surrounded by a hypoechoic margin. The tumour itself can be identified in most cases, especially when it is localized in the liver hilum.

CT: This technique is useful for assessing intrahepatic carcinoma and detecting peripheral CCC. Occasionally, proximally dilated bile ducts can also be visualized. The gall bladder and the common bile duct are inconspicuous. Differential diagnosis of metastases or HCC can be extremely difficult. (217, 218) • **MR** cholangiography has become an important procedure due to more sophisticated technology. (s. fig. 37.15)

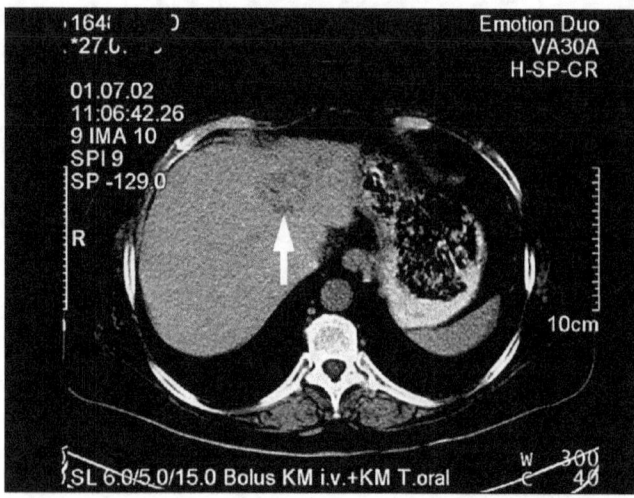

Fig. 37.15: Cholangiocellular carcinoma (↑) in CT with contrast medium

Cholangiography: If *ERCP* proves unsuccessful or if it is not possible to assess the bile ducts or the extent of tumour expansion, *PTC* is indicated. Nevertheless, ERC remains the method of choice, especially when combined with brush biopsy.

Scintigraphy: Hepatobiliary sequential scintigraphy imaging using ^{99m}T-etifenin can often provide additional information about tumour localization. Fluoro-2-deoxy-D glucose PET may be helpful in the diagnosis of perihilar CCC or metastatic spread.

Angiography: CT arteriography, CT arterioportography or MR angiography may help to detect vascular invasion and irregularities. Cholangiocellular carcinomas are poorly vascularized.

Laparoscopy: Laparoscopy should be used to confirm the diagnosis morphologically. This technique provides photodocumentary findings and also affords the possibility of targeted thick-needle, fine-needle or forceps biopsy. Tumour biopsy is only deemed necessary prior to palliative therapy. Moreover, *explorative laparoscopy* offers a much better overview of the whole abdominal area than does explorative laparotomy — and the risk involved is considerably lower. Carrying out laparotomy staging prior to liver transplantation is, in our opinion, also far less efficient and thus not indicated; instead, laparoscopy should be the technique of choice. (s. pp 158, 163, 169, 806)

4.6 Therapy

Resection or liver transplantation are considered to be the only curative forms of treatment for cholangiocellular carcinoma. • External or intracavitary radiation therapy is the method of choice when it comes to palliative measures. • The spectrum of adjuvant or alternative therapy procedures used in HCC is broad, as it is for all oncological conditions.

4.6.1 Invasive and surgical techniques

Classification of intrahepatic CCC is also made according to the TNM staging system. Due to the low frequency rate of CCC, experience of treating this tumour surgically by **resection** is limited. Patients with resectable tumours were reported to have a survival time of 12—24 months — which is not essentially longer than the normal course of disease. Survival times of more than 5 years have been reported in about 10% of cases. In 80—85% of patients, however, the tumour was not resectable at the time of diagnosis. (199, 203, 205, 210, 214)

Results to date concerning **liver transplantation** have been disappointing, so that this treatment is not considered to be indicated for CCC. Recurrence of CCC in a transplanted liver is most likely caused by immunosuppression. Attempts are hence being made to prevent such recurrence by combining liver transplantation with subsequent irradiation of the portal liver hilum and simultaneous administration of 5-FU.

Drainage therapy results in subjective improvement and decreases the risk of cholangitis. Techniques used include *biliodigestive anastomosis, percutaneous transhepatic drainage* or an *endoprosthesis* to bridge bile-duct stenosis.

4.6.2 Chemotherapy and radiotherapy

To date, **chemotherapy** for CCC has remained unsuccessful, no matter what kind of substance is used in monotherapy or polytherapy (e.g. 5-FU plus leucoverin). Local chemotherapy using arterial infusion of cytostatics may be indicated in individual cases. • **Radiotherapy** has no influence on survival time, but usually reduces pain.

4.6.3 Adjuvant measures

Even in cases of CCC which appear to be hopeless in terms of oncology, both the patient and the attending physician still have a broad spectrum of **adjuvant** and/or **unconventional therapeutic approaches** at their disposal. It is essential to provide sympathetic counselling and guidance for the desperate patient, who is prepared to seize any chance of preventing unnecessary suffering and harm. (s. p. 811) (s. tab. 37.10)

5 Cystadenocarcinoma

Primary biliary cystadenocarcinoma (CC) was first described by P. Bascho in 1909. It is a rare tumour (about 120 cases have been reported) which occurs in malformations of the bile ducts. CC mainly affects women and is predominantly found in the right liver lobe. Cystadenomas or choledochal cysts are seen as a probable precursor. (229, 232, 233, 235) Diagnosis is reached using imaging techniques (228, 231) and histology (229, 235).

Sometimes, CC develops without ovarian-like stroma. (230) The marker CA 19-9 may be increased. The tumour is usually made up of plurilocular cysts with papillary folds lined with carcinomatous biliary epithelium and contains bile-stained mucinous material. It is surrounded by a fibrous capsule consisting of dense hyaline stroma. (229) CC with a "pseudosarcomatous growth pattern" has been described (P.D. UNGER et al., 1987). After resection, the survival rate can be as high as five years. (234) (s. tab. 37.1)

6 Hepatoblastoma

The most common liver tumour in children is malignant foetal hepatoblastoma. (238) (s. tab. 37.1) It constitutes 30−45% of all primary liver tumours and 50−60% of all malignant tumours occurring in childhood. (239, 240, 241, 243) Hepatoblastoma is often associated with a congenital anomaly, especially with familial adenomatous polyposis coli. (236) The tumour is partially lobulated by fibrous septae and well-vascularized. Arising in the endodermal liver epithelium, it usually becomes manifest prior to the third year of life, but rarely in older children or adults. (242, 245) Boys are affected twice as often as girls. • *Histologically*, there are *three types*: (*1.*) epithelial type with embryonal hepatocytes or foetal hepatocytes, (*2.*) mixed-cellular type containing epithelial and mesenchymal components, and (*3.*) anaplastic type with small, undifferentiated cells. • *Embryonic hepatocytes* are small, partially spindle cell-like, cuboidal or polygonal, and display uniform hyperchromic cell nuclei. The sparse cytoplasm is easy to stain. The cells have band-like or rosette-like structures. *Foetal hepatocytes* are larger and possess a marked cytoplasm; they contain abundant glycogen and form canaliculi as well as cellular trabeculae between the sinusoids. Epithelial cell nests of bright and dark cell elements alternate. Haematopoietic foci are detectable in the area of the foetal hepatocytes. (s. fig. 37.16)

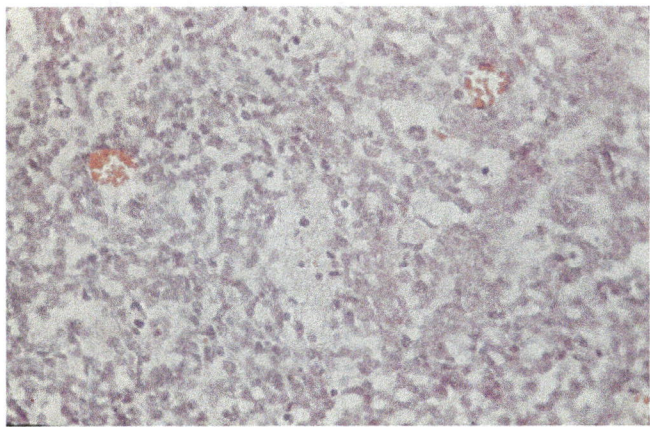

Fig. 37.16: Hepatoblastoma (three-year-old boy) with mainly foetal differentiation (HE)

Macroscopically, there is usually a solitary medullar tumour, 5−15(−25) cm in size, which mostly develops in the right liver lobe. A tumour capsule is found in 50% of cases. It may contain necroses, haemorrhages and calcifications. This tumour grows relatively rapidly. Metastatic spread affects the infradiaphragmal lymph nodes, lungs and brain. Immunohistochemistry shows an expression of cytokeratin 7, 8, 18 and 19, or AFP as well as vimentin. • Hepatomegaly, fever, anaemia, growth retardation, sexual precocity (due to ectopic gonadotropin), abdominal pain and high or non-decreasing values of α_1-foetoprotein (which normally decreases in the first years of life in healthy infants) are suggestive of the kind of tumour. Imaging techniques and biopsy facilitate the diagnosis. (237) Cystathionine is increased in the urine in most cases. Early detection allows curative resection in about 20% of children. Preoperative chemotherapy may help to reduce the tumour size, thus leading to better surgical results. (238, 239, 244) Liver transplantation is sometimes indicated. (240)

7 Mesenchymal liver tumours

7.1 Embryonal sarcoma

Undifferentiated embryonal sarcoma (UES) was first described by J.T. STOCKER et al. in 1978. (251) (s. tab. 37.1) This mesenchymal tumour is the third most frequent tumour in childhood and adolescence; occurrence in adults is a rare event. (248) There are no gender-related differences. It is predominantly localized in the right hepatic lobe. The tumour presents as a well-circumscribed node with a size up to 20 cm in diameter comprising cystic zones (of necrotic tissue and blood). An association with a mesenchymal hamartoma is discussed (249), especially since alterations in chromosome 19q have been detected in both conditions. • The polynuclear tumour cells are star-shaped or fusiform with numerous mitoses. In addition, there are large cells with PAS-positive, diastase-resistant globular inclusions. The tumour cells show no differentiation; they are surrounded by pronounced myxoid stroma. (12, 250, 252) • In a CT scan, the tumour appears hypodense with a peripheral capsule. (247) This malignancy is not (or only slightly) vascularized. It grows rapidly and can infiltrate the neighbouring organs or metastasize in the lung or abdomen. US shows a solid space-occupying lesion with an inhomogeneous reflex pattern and circumscribed cystic areas. • If feasible, resection is indicated, possibly in combination with chemotherapy. (246) A ligature of the hepatic artery may also be applied. Recidivation after resection therapy is frequent. The three-year survival rate is about 30%. (252, 253)

7.2 Epithelioid haemangioendothelioma

Epithelioid haemangioendothelioma is a malignant mesenchymal tumour, which was first described in the liver by S.W. WEISS et al. in 1982. (s. tab. 37.1) It is probably a variant of haemangiosarcoma, but with a much better prognosis (approx. 50% of patients survive for more than 5 years). This multifocal, vascularized tumour with low-grade malignancy can affect the liver primarily or appear in the liver as a metastasis. Women are more affected than men. Usually, the liver is interspersed with multiple, firm and greyish-white lesions up to 3-11cm in diameter. (12) There are no differences in frequency with respect to age. The tumour cells grow along the vessels, whereby the portal fields and the acinar structure are unchanged. These cells are irregular-shaped, dendritic or spindle-like; they may display intracytoplasmatic vacuoles and *Weibel-Palade bodies* (E.R. WEIBEL et al., 1964) as markers of arterial endothelia. The stroma contains collagenous fibres, mucopolysaccharides and, later on, calcifications as well. (255) Often, a Budd-Chiari syndrome is mimicked. (268) Immunohistochemical demonstration of factor VIII antigen is helpful in differential diagnosis. An association with vinyl chloride and contraceptives as well as with NRH has been postulated. (263) • Some laboratory parameters (AP, GPT, GOT, bilirubin) are increased. • Imaging procedures show a space-occupying lesion without characteristic findings. (261, 266, 267) Diagnosis can only be reached by means of histology (254, 256–258, 260, 262, 265), best guaranteed with (forceps) biopsy under laparoscopy. (257) • The tumour grows slowly, but may metastasize. (254, 258, 259) Resection mostly cannot be carried out. Liver transplantation is the therapy of choice, occasionally combined with IFN. The five-year survival rate is >75%. (259, 260, 264)

7.3 Angiosarcoma

Angiosarcoma is the most frequent mesenchymal tumour; it has a soft consistency. (12) *Macroscopically*, conglomerate sponge-like nodes are found, which are partially greyish-white and interspersed with haemorrhages or central necroses. They are highly vascularized and show blurred margins. Smaller satellite nodes may also form. • *Histologically*, this tumour consists of polymorphous, fusiform sinusoidal endothelial cells, which line blood spaces and grow in a confluent infiltrative manner. The rate of mitoses is high. There are peliosis-like dilated cavities. Polynuclear giant cells may be present. Infiltration of tumour cells in portal or central veins and extramedullary foci of haemopoiesis are usually demonstrable. Liver cell plates, provided they remain in position, are characteristically enwrapped by tumour cells. Immunohistochemically, factor VIII-associated antigen can be detected. (s. figs. 30.1; 37.17)

Angiosarcoma is closely associated with the effects of thorium dioxide (273) (s. p. 586!), chronic arsenic poisoning (278) (s. p. 586!) and exposure to vinyl chloride (276) (s. p. 584) or radium as well as with neurofibromatosis

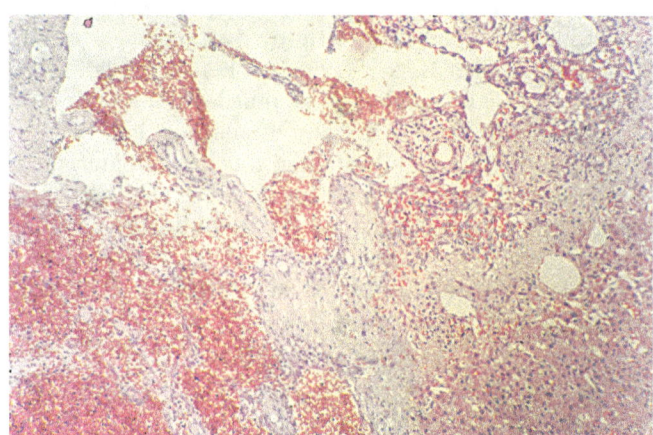

Fig. 37.17: Hepatic haemangiosarcoma (s. fig. 30.1) (HE)

or haemochromatosis. Transition of infantile haemangioendothelioma and cavernous haemangioma into angiosarcoma has been reported. It has also been observed following the intake of phenylhydrazine and anabolic (271) or contraceptive steroids. Older people are mainly affected, men more than women (3–4:1). In childhood, girls are the main sufferers. (269) • The tumour progresses quickly, grows multicentrically (in the shape of a cavernoma or node) and is localized in both hepatic lobes. The survival time is less than one year. Metastatic spread occurs in the lungs and hilar lymph nodes as well as, occasionally, in the spleen and bones. (277) Diagnostic biopsy (even as FNB) is contraindicated in this highly vascularized tumour. (272) Diagnosis is made by CT angiography, FDG PET or MR angiography. (274) Vascular murmur "over" the liver may be audible. A sudden complication is a rupture with haemoperitoneum; DIC sometimes develops. The course is irrepressibly progressive; the prognosis is poor.

7.4 Leiomyosarcoma

Leiomyosarcoma originates from smooth-muscular elements of the liver, which are located in the walls of vessels and around bile ducts. (12) Men and women are affected with the same frequency, predominantly in middle age. It is a very rare mesenchymal tumour (only about 50 cases have been reported so far). This tumour grows slowly, the colour is greyish-white and the consistency is firm; it can reach up to 35 cm (!) in diameter. Occasionally, there are multiple nodes. (281) It not only occurs in the liver (mainly in the right liver lobe), but is also found in the round ligament, the hepatic or portal veins (280) and inferior vena cava (283) (possibly together with the Budd-Chiari syndrome). The tumour cells appear homogeneous and spindle-like with eosinophilic cytoplasm. Clinical findings or imaging results are non-specific; splenomegaly and ascites may occur. (279, 281, 282, 284) Therapy consists of tumour resection.

7.5 Rhabdomyosarcoma

Rhabdomyosarcoma is a mesenchymal tumour of grey colour with partially cystic growth. (12) It mainly occurs during childhood. (285) The tumour cells appear small, round or spindle-like, hyperchromatic, sometimes with eosinophilic cytoplasm. (287) They show various stages of differentiation of embryonal skeletal muscle cells. This tumour originates from peribiliary located muscular structures. (285) • An association with the long-term use of oral contraceptives has been reported. (286)

7.6 Fibrosarcoma

Fibrosarcoma is a mesenchymal tumour originating from fibroblasts; it can therefore occur ubiquitously in the whole body. (12) It was first described by R.H. Jaffe in 1924. About 35 cases have been reported so far. This type of tumour has a firm consistency and contains cystic structures with focal necroses and haemorrhages. It possesses a fibrous pseudocapsule and consists of fascicularly arranged, spindle-like or fusiform tumour cells embedded in parallel collagen fibres. The non-epithelial stroma marker vimentin is overexpressed. These cells may exhibit marked polymorphism. Fibrosarcoma mainly occurs in men of advanced age. Therapy consists of tumour resection and adjuvant chemotherapy. (288, 289)

7.7 Fibrous histiocytoma

Malignant fibrous histiocytoma (MFH) is a rare mesenchymal tumour of histiocytic origin. This tumour was first described by L. Ozello et al. (1963) and J.E. O'Brien et al. (1964). It has not yet been clarified which cell type this tumour derives from and whether it is a single entity. The tumour tends to develop in the tissue of the extremities and in the retroperitoneum. MFH rarely occurs in the liver (so far, reports of 22 cases have been published). (12) The tumour cells contain a vacuolated cytoplasm with oval-polymorphic nuclei; giant cells may be present. (291, 292) MFH shows a firm consistency and greyish-yellow colour. There are no typical findings. (290, 293, 294) It appears mainly in patients of advanced age. Diagnosis is confirmed immunohistochemically. The prognosis for this extremely aggressive tumour is poor. Resection at an early stage with subsequent chemotherapy is the only possible therapeutic option.

7.8 Malignant schwannoma

Malignant schwannoma is a very rare mesenchymal tumour derived from the Schwann cells or nerve-sheath cells. It is also termed neurilemmoma or neurinoma. Only about ten cases involving the liver have been reported. This tumour is mostly associated with neurofibromatosis. Men are more frequently affected than women. Schwannoma usually occurs in the ages between 20−50 years. It shows a firm consistency and has a greyish-white colour. Generally, there are multiple lesions. In the tumour itself, necroses and haemorrhages are found. Schwannoma consists of strands of spindle cells which interweave to form a herringbone pattern. The stroma contains strong bundles of collagen fibres. There are cell polymorphisms and mitoses as well as areas of densely grouped cells. Expression of S-100 antigen from the tumour cells is increased. A high level of alkaline phosphatase is a characteristic finding in spite of normal transaminases. Prognosis is relatively poor. (295, 296)

7.9 Hepatic liposarcoma

The first liposarcoma observed in the liver was reported by J.I. Kim et al. in 1987. (297) Up to now, about 10 cases have been published. Bright yellow tissue containing mature fat cells admixed with scattered immature lipoblasts were found in various stages of development. Moreover, hyperchromatic nuclei in pleomorphic tumour cells, eosinophilic cytoplasm and fusiform cells were evident. (298) On US, liposarcoma is generally inhomogeneous with hypoechoic or hyperechoic features. Also on CT, this myxoid tumour is inhomogeneous and has Hounsfield units ranging from near-water density to that of muscle and may exhibit contrast enhancement. In addition, cystic areas and septated areas may be seen in MRI.

7.10 Hepatic osteosarcoma

Primary hepatic osteosarcoma is a very rare mesenchymal tumour, which was first described by J.H. Maynard et al. in 1969. It is of greyish-white to pale yellow colour and shows a gritty consistency. It grows rapidly with an aggressive behaviour. The survival time is short. • Histologically, there are different components, such as osteoblastic, chondroblastic and fibroblastic cells. Numerous osteoblastic-like giant cells are present. Expression of vimentin is positive, whereas actin, desmin and cytokeratin are not detectable. The tumour cells produce lace-like osteoid. (299, 300)

8 Neuroendocrine tumours

These tumours generally grow slowly. They develop from the neuroendocrine system, which is considered to be part of the APUD system (= **a**mine **p**recursor **u**ptake and **d**ecarboxylation) (A.G.E. Pearse et al., 1978). However, due to the secretion of biologically active hormones, they give rise to manifold clinical symptoms. Such tumours very seldom develop primarily in the liver. They meanwhile present a real diagnostic challenge even for today's sophisticated imaging procedures. (305) (s. fig. 37.28)

8.1 Hepatic gastrinoma

This primary hepatic gastrinoma is a rare event, although the liver is a very common site for gastrinoma metastases. Hepatic gastrinoma is a subtype of the neuroendocrine tumour. It tends to occur in slightly younger patients or those with a Zollinger-Ellison syndrome. Males are more frequently affected than females. Gastrin levels in the serum are high. Imaging procedures for diagnosis include somatostatin-receptor scintigraphy with ^{111}In DTPA octreotide. Because of the slow growth and the feasibility of resection, the prognosis is relatively good. (301–304)

8.2 Primary hepatic carcinoid

The term "carcinoid" was coined by S. OBERNDORFER in 1907 as a result of observations involving tumours in the small intestine. H. HARTMANN first reported a primary hepatic carcinoid in 1920. To date, only few cases have been described in the literature. Its histology is similar to that of adenocarcinoma, but it is aggressive. • Hepatic carcinoids are mostly metastases arising from primary carcinoids in the area of the appendix, stomach or colon. Such carcinoids may infiltrate the liver diffusely or form nodes and cysts. Both primary and metastatic forms have a brownish colour and grow slowly. Endocrine tumour cells show ribbon-like or rosette-like patterns; they may develop along the intrahepatic bile ducts and lead to the formation of hepatic carcinoid tumour. The inclination to infiltrative growth and metastatic spread apparently depends on the localization and size of the tumour. (306, 309) Expression of neuroendocrine marker proteins (chromogranin A, synaptophysin, neuro-specific enolase, etc.), but also of CEA, is found. (308) A specific marker is the enhanced excretion of 5-hydroxyindolacetic acid in the urine (> 30 ng/24 hr).

Biochemical parameters are only slightly altered. Imaging techniques show space-occupying lesions. In sonography, this tumour is echogenic with many cystic areas. Lesions are markedly hypervascular on colour Doppler US and angiography. (307) The diagnosis, however, is only secured histologically or by scintigraphy with I^{131}-meta-iodobenzylguanidine or octreotide. The *carcinoid syndrome* is triggered by the release of serotonin from the tumour cells into the blood circulation. A larger amount of serotonin in the blood causes a "flush" (= pronounced redness of the face and upper body due to vascular dilatation, which may last several hours) as well as sweats, hypotension and bronchiospasms. • Octreotide or ketanserin are useful medicinal agents. Surgery (resection or possibly transplantation) is indicated. Chemoembolization also shows good results.

9 Malignant lymphoma

Primary malignant lymphoma of the liver is rare (A.A. ATA et al., 1965); so far, about 100 cases have been described. It occurs both in children and adults; however, men older than 50 years are mainly affected. There is a close association to immunosuppressed patients, especially in HIV infection. (312) Single observations regarding a pathogenetic relationship with EBV infection, hepatitis B and C, PBC (319), coeliac disease and lupus erythematosus have not been confirmed Lymphadenopathy is absent. • *Histology* shows lymphomatoid infiltrations in the portal fields; they can penetrate the neighbouring parenchyma. These lymphomas derive from the lymphocytes and Kupffer cells of the portal fields. About two-thirds of the hepatic lymphomas are B cell type and one-third are T cell type, the latter usually consisting of anaplastic large cells (H. STEIN et al., 1985). Malignant lymphomas generally develop as solitary nodes, less frequently in the form of multiple nodes, and, occasionally, as diffuse infiltrations throughout the entire liver. (316) Special forms include low-grade malignant B cell lymphoma of the *MALT type* and *γδ-T cell lymphoma*. (314, 318) The latter affects mainly younger adults, and its course is more aggressive. In this subtype, the spleen and bone marrow are also involved. • Clinical and imaging findings are not characteristic (313); in most cases, fever, loss of weight and night sweats are found. The transaminases may be increased. Diagnosis is confirmed by histology and with the help of immunohistochemical examinations of epithelial and lymphatic antigens. Reactive lymphatic hyperplasia must be ruled out as a differential diagnosis. • The mean survival time is one to two years. Therapy consists of resection and chemotherapy. (310, 311, 315, 317, 320)

10 Liver metastases

10.1 Definition

Metastasis ("tumour spread") is a secondary focus of disease caused by haematogenic, lymphogenic or ductal transport of living or dead matter from the primary focus of disease. • In the narrow sense of the term, **metastasis** is the secondary or "daughter" focus ("filia") of a malignant primary tumour. It may manifest as *local metastasis* (with a local relationship to the primary tumour as a neighbouring metastasis due to continuous tumour growth, e.g. in gall-bladder carcinoma), *regional metastasis* (within the regional lymphatic system) or *distant metastasis*. Metastases occur spontaneously or due to mechanical transportation. • **Liver metastasis** develops via the portal vein (particularly in carcinomas of the gastrointestinal tract), via the hepatic artery (e.g. from the lung, breast, oesophagus, pancreas, and in melanomas) or via retrograde lymphatic permeation and extension along the vascular lumen. This occurs in 30–35% of all malignancies and in 45–50% of abdominal tumours. In 95–97% of cases, liver metastases cause malignant hepatic lesions.

10.2 Morphology

Liver metastases may occur as well-demarcated solitary or multiple nodes and can ultimately infiltrate almost the whole liver tissue. This metastasis itself results in extreme *hepatomegaly* (> 5,000 g). In most cases, there are clearly limited nodes of a greyish-white colour and firm consistency. The consistency depends on the ratio of cancer cells to fibrous stroma. Metastases tend to bulge from the liver surface; localization is very rarely confined to the interior of the liver. A solitary node is found in some 10% of patients at the time of diagnosis; in 15—20% of cases, only one lobe is affected. • There is often a central depression due to tumour necrosis caused by insufficient blood supply within the tumour (= *cancer umbilicus*). (s. figs. 37.18, 37.19) Sometimes, the metastases are enclosed in a fibrous pseudocapsule. (362) The immediate surroundings of the metastases are occasionally characterized by a dark, bluish-red discolouration due to venous hyperaemia (= **Zahn's infarct**).

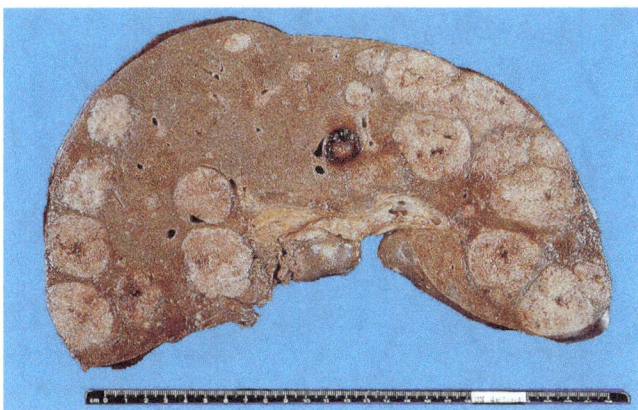

Fig. 37.20: Liver metastases of G3 prostatic carcinoma

In rare cases (particularly in small-cellular bronchial carcinoma), diffuse metastasis develops (s. figs. 37.19, 37.21), which resembles liver cirrhosis and may cause acute liver failure. (324, 342) • *Histology* is often similar to that of a primary tumour. (s. figs. 37.22, 37.23) However, there may also be considerable deviation, which makes classification of the primary tumour difficult and uncertain, or indeed impossible. (326) • In *liver cirrhosis*, metastases are less frequent, whether due to the altered vascular structure of the cirrhotic liver, an enhanced content of metalloproteinases, decreased expression of adhesion molecules or the fact that the patients do not survive long enough for the formation of metastases to become evident — the short survival time is a result of the combination of cirrhosis and carcinoma. (363) Fatty liver or angiostatin suppresses angiogenesis in metastases. (348) By contrast, alcohol consumption enhances liver metastasis in colon carcinoma. (357) • *Spontaneous regression* has also been reported. (334, 346)

Adjacent tissue often shows local, *non-specific reactive hepatitis* (activation of Kupffer cells, small round-cellular infiltration of the sinusoids and portal fields, single-cell necroses, nodular infiltrations). (s. fig. 21.1)

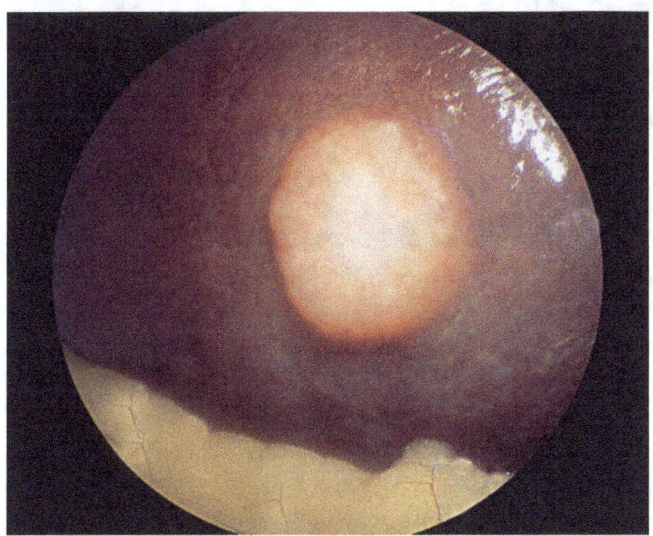

Fig. 37.18: Large metastasis in the right hepatic lobe with distinct "cancer umbilicus" subsequent to breast cancer (serosa, peritoneum and ligaments without pathological findings)

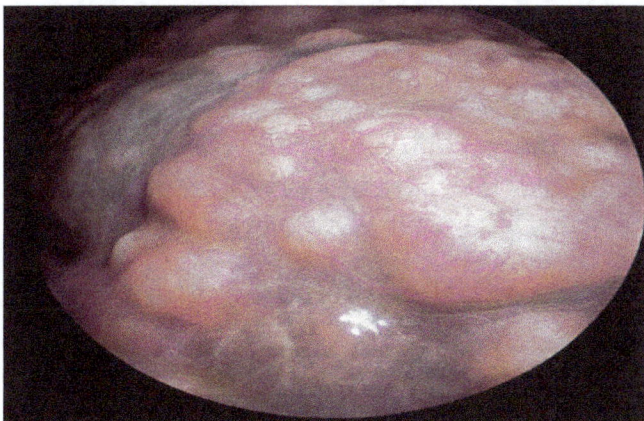

Fig. 37.19: Pronounced liver invasion by metastases of varying sizes partly with "cancer umbilicus" and neovascularization. Clinical diagnosis: bronchial carcinoma

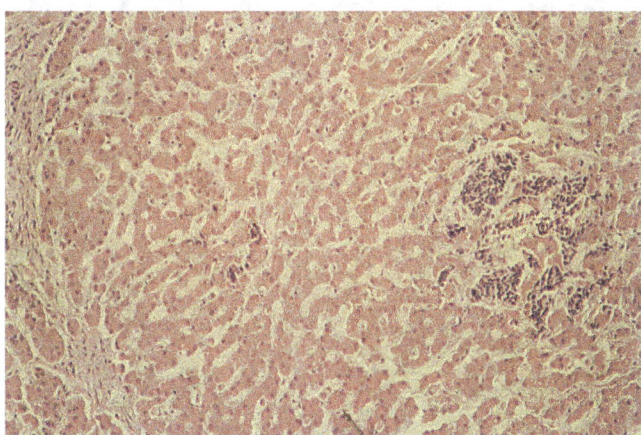

Fig. 37.21: Sinusoidal infiltrates of a small-cell carcinoma of the lung (HE)

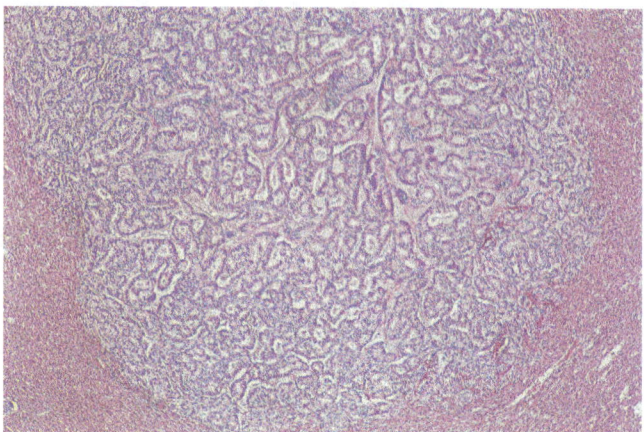

Fig. 37.22: Metastasis of a highly differentiated colonic adenocarcinoma (HE)

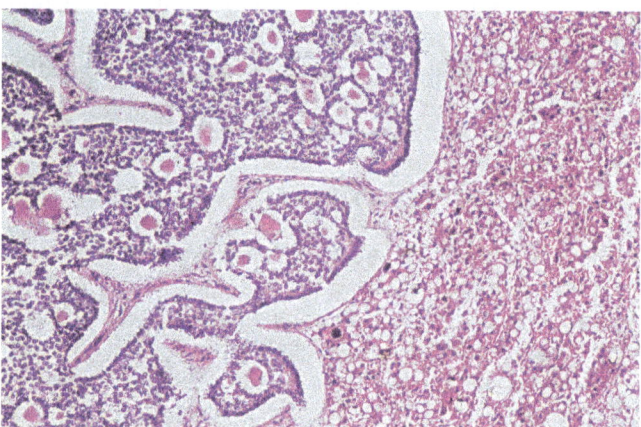

Fig. 37.23: Metastasis of a malignant granulosa cell tumour of the ovary (HE)

10.3 Symptomatology

The occurrence and growth of liver metastases are accompanied by increasing lassitude and malaise, a pervasive feeling of weakness, febrile attacks, upper abdominal pain, inappetence, night sweats and weight loss. Pronounced hepatomegaly is often found, together with a hardening of the liver and occasional palpability of the tumour nodes. The spleen may also be enlarged. Jaundice usually develops as the tumour continues to grow. Pleural effusion, oedema (reflecting obstruction of the inferior vena cava), ascites (reflecting peritoneal metastases) (s. figs. 37.24, 37.25), haemoperitoneum (368) and thrombosis of the portal vein may occur. Sometimes, there is a swelling of the lymph nodes, especially in the right supraclavicular region. • Tumour cells have a limited lifespan in the blood circulation (< 24 hr) if the defence system of the body is intact. Even if a peritoneovenous shunt is carried out in malignant ascites, metastatic spread is rare.

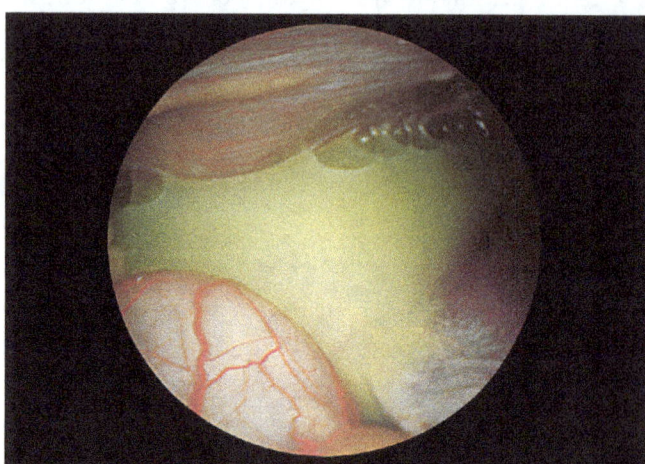

Fig. 37.25: Chylous ascites, greenish-coloured due to bile, in colon carcinoma, with metastases in the liver and peritoneal cavity

10.4 Diagnosis

Biochemistry: Non-specific signs of inflammation become more pathological. A rise in γ-GT, initially as an isolated value, is characteristic; this is then accompanied by higher cholestasis-related parameters. (328) In addition, there is an increase in LDH, GPT, GOT and the DeRitis quotient. Gamma GT is also seen as a control parameter in chemotherapy. In colorectal liver metastases, the serum value of endothelin-1 is often elevated. (370) • While **tumour markers** can be helpful in establishing the diagnosis and for classifying metastases, they are of even greater importance in monitoring the course of disease. (s. tab. 37.12)

Sonography: Metastases can be detected from a size of > 0.5 cm. Diffuse infiltration is not visible. Due to their high water content, metastases appear as hypoechoic lesions. (s. p. 144) (s. figs. 6.20; 37.26−37.28) With continued growth, central echo amplifications occur due to regressive tissue changes. In metastasis, a halo has a specificity of 86% and a sensitivity of 88% − a finding which, however, also applies to benign tumours. A bulging liver surface or displacement of the vessels and bile ducts may also point indirectly to metastases. Normal sonographic findings do not exclude metastasis of the

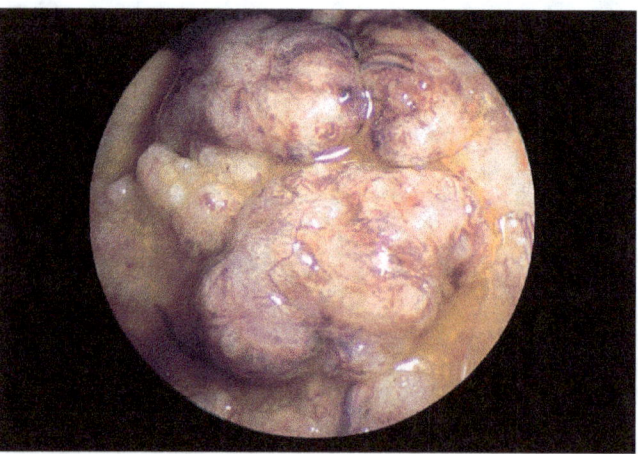

Fig. 37.24: Pronounced peritoneal metastasis (with simultaneous liver metastases) in ovarian carcinoma

Non-specific signs of inflammation
BSR ↑, CRP +, iron ↓, copper ↑, α-globulins ↑, fibrinogen ↑, haptoglobin ↓, γ-GT ↑, anaemia, D-dimer ↑
Cholestasis parameters
AP ↑, LAP ↑, γ-GT ↑
Enzymes
LDH ↑, GPT ↑, GOT ↑, ChE ↓
GOT/GPT   = >2
γ-GT/GOT   = >12
(GPT + GOT)/GDH = <15
Tumour markers
Bronchial system   CEA, calcitonin, CYFR 21−4
Colon   CEA, CA 19−9, CA 50, CA 72−4
Stomach   CA 72−4, CA 19−9, CEA
Breast   CA 15−3, CEA
Pancreas   CA 19−9, CEA
Ovary   CA 125, CA 72−4
Prostate   PSA
Melanoma   S−100
APUDomas   NSE
Thyroid gland   Calcitonin

Tab. 37.12: Laboratory findings and tumour markers arousing suspicion in liver metastasis

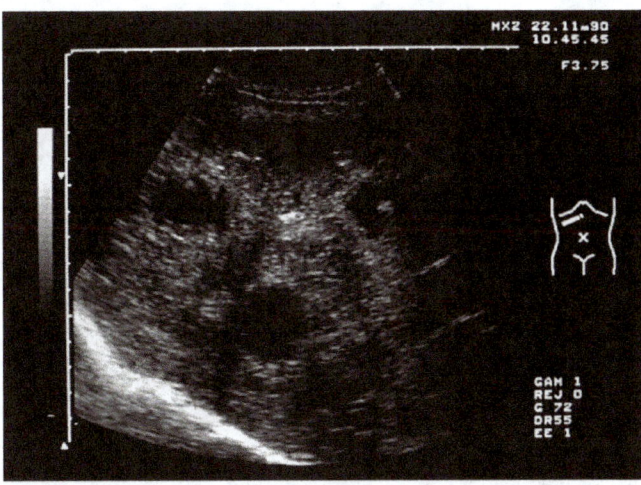

Fig. 37.27: Numerous centrally liquefied liver metastases (differential diagnosis: liver abscesses)

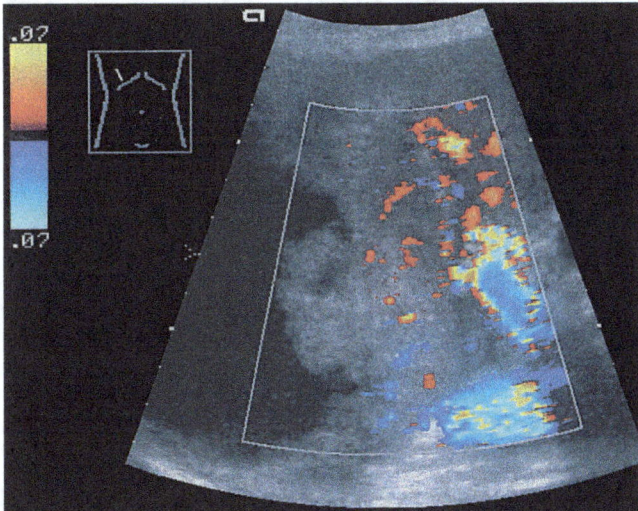

Fig. 37.28: Metastases of a neuroendocrine tumour (carcinoid): typically complex space-occupying structure with echo-free and echo-rich parts. Colour-coded duplex sonography shows intensive tumour vascularisation

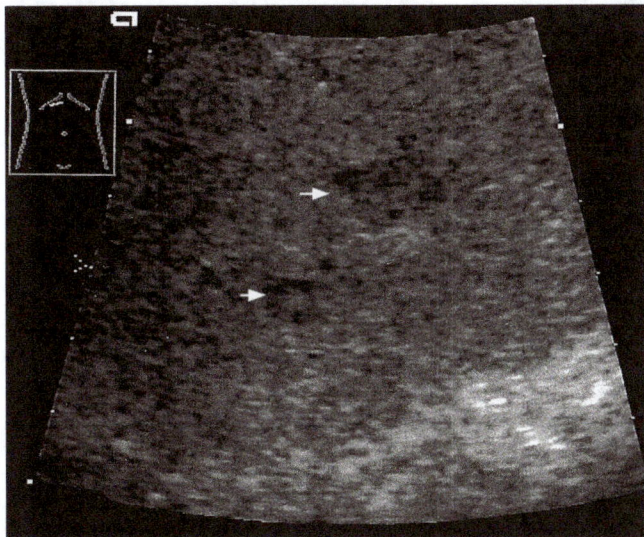

Fig. 37.26: Early metastases (0.7−1.0 cm (↑)) detected during aftercare following sigmoid carcinoma surgery

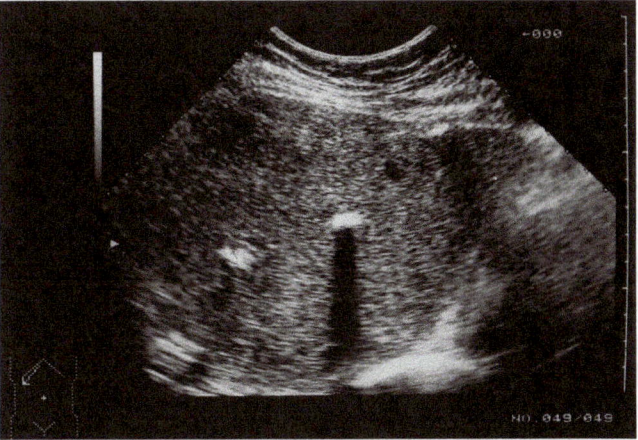

Fig. 37.29: Calcified liver metastasis and other small hypoechoic tumours; condition after resection of a colon carcinoma

liver. Ascites or haemoperitoneum (368) can occasionally be found. • With a sensitivity of 96%, *endosonography* is the gold standard. (343, 352, 360, 364) • Detection of *calcified liver metastases* by sonography or CT is rare (340); we were able to observe this event subsequent to surgical removal of a colon carcinoma and a breast carcinoma. (s. figs. 37.29, 37.30)

CT: Most metastases are hypodense prior and subsequent to the application of contrast medium. Sensitivity

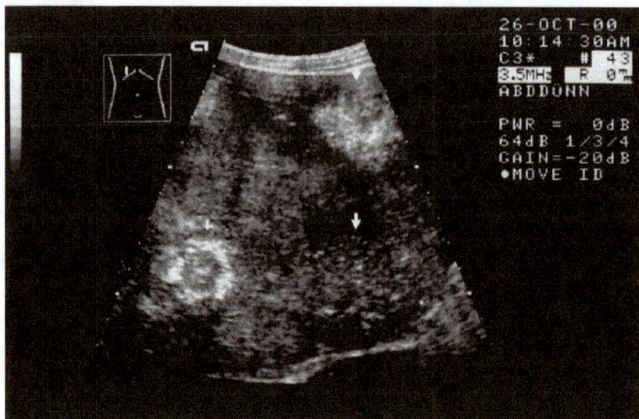

Fig. 37.30: Calcified metastasis after treatment of breast cancer: hyperechoic pattern and numerous white nodules representing microcalcifications (↑)

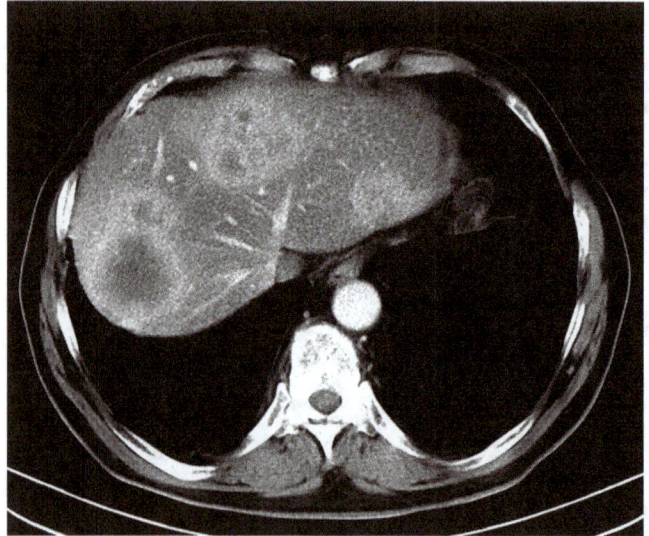

Fig. 37.31: Liver metastases in colon carcinoma with fatty liver: foci in both liver lobes, hyperdense margin formation with central hypodensity

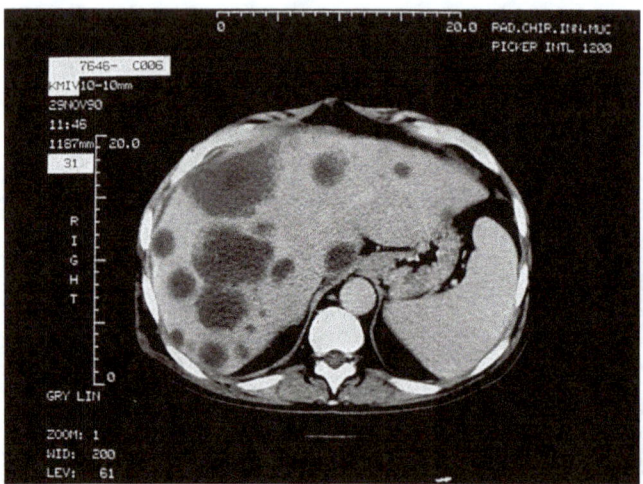

Fig. 37.32: Numerous cystoid liver metastases due to a central necrotizing process (differential diagnosis: liver abscesses)

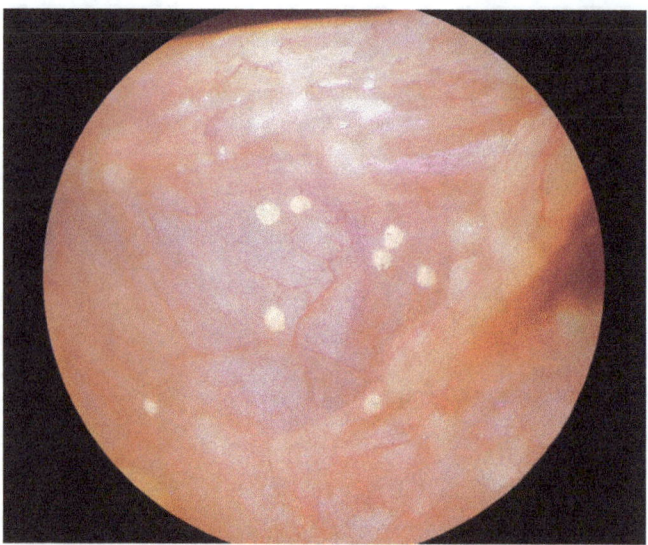

Fig. 37.33: Laparoscopic staging: peritoneal metastases in gastric carcinoma

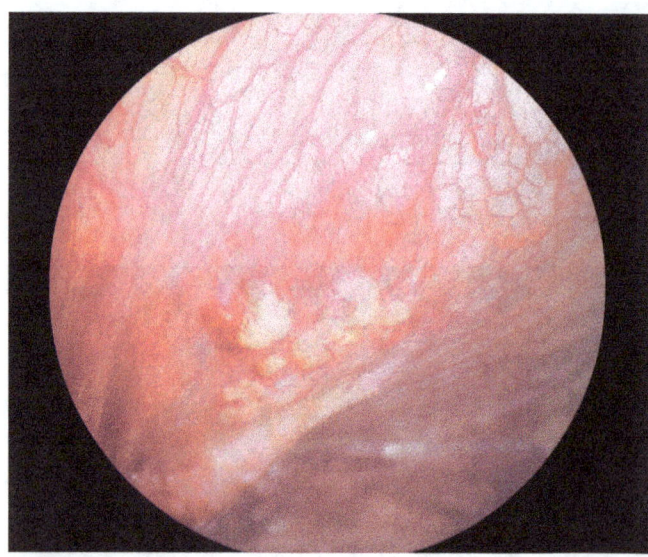

Fig. 37.34: Laparoscopic staging: metastases at the falciform ligament in oesophageal carcinoma

is 92% in foci of > 15 mm, but only 55% in smaller ones. When there is concomitant fatty degeneration, CT is inferior to sonography for the detection of metastases. The best results were achieved by using spiral CT and *CTAP* with a sensitivity of 92–93%; all metastases larger than 6 mm could be identified. (335, 350, 360, 372) (s. p. 183) (s. figs. 37.31, 37.32)

MRI: Metastases usually show low signal intensity in T_1-weighted images and high signal intensity in T_2-weighted images. Necrotic metastases may show a signal intensity in T_2-weighted images similar to that of haemangioma. In contrast-amplified T_1-weighted images, perifocal oedemas can be distinguished from the tumour. Haemorrhages are signal-intense in T_1-weighted images. Sensitivity is 85–95% and can be further improved when superparamagnetic iron oxides are used. (335, 350, 373) (s. p. 186) (s. fig. 8.8)

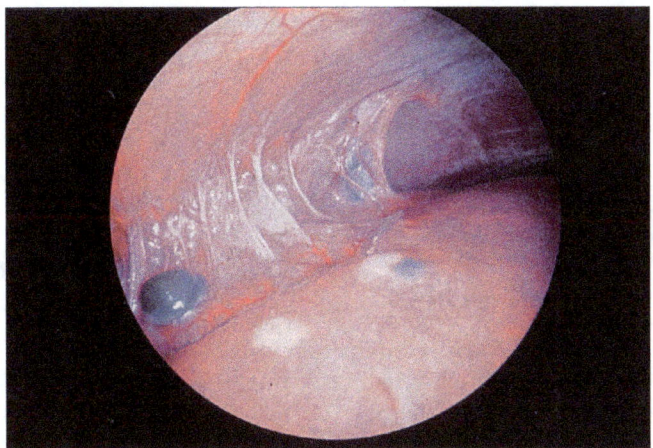

Fig. 37.35: Laparoscopic staging: Melanotic and non-melanotic metastases of melanoma (right liver lobe with transition to right abdominal peritoneum; liver capsule/peritoneal adhesions)

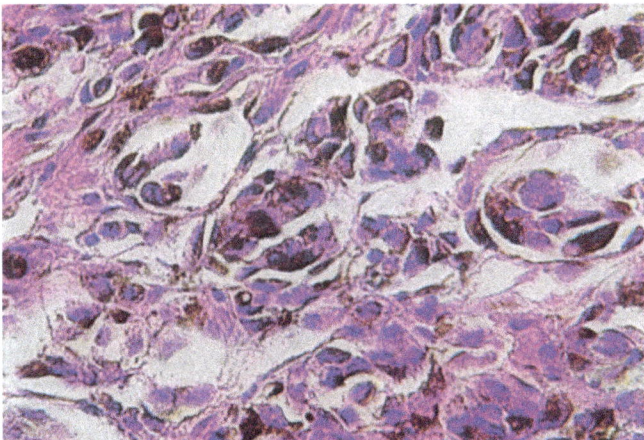

Fig. 37.36: Liver metastasis of a malignant melanoma: dark-brown coarse-grained pigment in melanoma cells (HE)

Laparoscopy: If it has not been possible to make a clear diagnosis, explorative laparoscopy now becomes the method of choice. (s. figs. 37.18, 37.19, 37.35) This technique allows excellent *inspection* of the whole abdominal cavity, also for the purpose of **staging,** as well as facilitating targeted, low-risk biopsies, preferably using forceps. With the help of this method, we very often found small metastatic foci, for example on the peritoneum (s. fig. 37.33) or the falciform ligament (s. fig. 37.34), which could not be detected prior to surgery by any other technique (not even by explorative laparotomy).

All findings are documented using **photolaparoscopy** and, together with histology, they can facilitate a more reliable assessment both for the pathologist and for *interdisciplinary discussion* of any therapy concept which may be necessary — this applies to other diseases as well. (347, 359, 367) (s. p. 164) • **Fine-needle biopsy** allows cytological diagnosis in a high percentage of cases.

10.5 Metastases in children

In children, metastases are also found far more frequently than primary liver tumours. Generally, we may expect metastases from the same tumour types in children as are observed in adults. However, two types of tumour are particularly important in this respect.

(1.) **Wilms' tumour:** This extremely malignant embryonic adenosarcoma of the kidney causes liver metastases in 20–25% of cases.

(2.) **Neuroblastoma:** Liver metastases develop with extreme rapidity within the first six to nine months of life. The general condition is not compromised until later. This metastatic spread is a result of a sympathogonioma which has its origin in the adrenal medulla or autonomic ganglia. Such a clinical picture is also termed *Pepper's syndrome* (W. PEPPER, 1901).

10.6 Therapy

The manifestation of liver metastases and their prognosis are largely determined by the localization and degree of malignancy of the primary tumour. The survival time subsequent to the detection of metastases is about one year. Patients with liver metastases from colon carcinoma have the most favourable prognosis.

> As a general principle, treatment of liver metastases should be preceded by an **interdisciplinary consensus conference** — this also applies to primary liver tumour. (s. p. 807)

10.6.1 Resection therapy

The choice of resection procedure is based on the size, location and number of the metastases. (321, 330, 332, 361) (s. pp 807, 825, 900)

Metastasectomy: Using this method, small and superficial metastases can be removed without having to pay attention to vessels; a safety margin of 1 cm around the metastases should be adhered to. (374)

Segmental resection: In some cases only a monosegment is resected, in other cases bisegmental or polysegmental resections are carried out to remove adjacent segments. Under certain conditions, multi-segmental resection is used for removing several segments from different areas of the liver at the same time. Perisegmental resection is necessary when a metastasis is located on the boundary between two separate segments. • In all these resection procedures, it is also necessary to adhere to a safety margin of 1cm (although the technique of parenchymal dissection used today makes it possible to resect with a smaller safety margin). (322, 329, 330, 336, 337, 344, 355, 378)

Parenchymal dissection: Instead of the parenchymal-fracture technique used in the past, ultrasound dissection or aqua-jet dissection is now applied.

Parenchymal sealing is usually carried out by means of fibrin spray if the wound surface is "dry" or by means of argon beamer if the wound surface is still bleeding.

To date, resection of liver metastases of colorectal or neuroendocrine tumours is the only treatment option which may result in definitive removal of the cancerous disease. Resection is indicated in those cases in which the primary tumour can be removed completely and when no further metastases are detectable. Repeated resection is also possible. Extrahepatic metastases or involvement of neighbouring organs are generally no longer regarded as contraindications. (322, 323, 329, 330)

Morbidity should not exceed 30%. Lethality is between 0—3%. The 5-year survival rate following **R0 resection** in metastatic colorectal carcinoma is 20—40%, in neuroendocrine tumours 90—100%, in malignant melanoma 15—25%, and in breast cancer 10—30%. Prognosis is poor in metastasizing renal cell carcinoma and in gastric or pancreatic carcinoma. Both **R1** and **R2 resection** worsen the prognosis to the same extent.

The following factors are decisive for the success rate: (*1.*) age of the patient, (*2.*) distribution pattern and number of metastases, (*3.*) size of the largest metastasis, (*4.*) stage of primary tumour, (*5.*) extrahepatic metastases, (*6.*) lymph node involvement, (*7.*) respective value of the tumour marker, and (*8.*) intraoperative blood loss. (336)

For the follow-up after resection, sonography and determination of CEA and CA 19-9 (or other relevant markers) are necessary. In about 60% of cases, resected liver metastases recur; in about 30% of these patients, repeat resection is possible. (379)

> In patients undergoing surgical resection of colorectal liver metastases, haematogenous tumour cell dissemination could be detected in preoperative blood samples in 30%, in intraoperative blood samples in 46% and in postoperative blood samples in 22% as well as in bone marrow samples in 16% of cases. • Thus, there are once again good reasons for using *neoadjuvant systemic chemotherapy* together with perioperative administration of *i.v. galactose infusions*. (351)

10.6.2 Cryotherapy

This technique, first described by J. ARNOTT in 1945, was applied by I.S. COOPER in 1963 for liver metastases. The treatment uses a probe, introduced (possibly by laparoscopy) into the tumour, which is subsequently frozen with liquid nitrogen at a temperature of $-196\,°C$. The result is necrotic degeneration of the tumerous tissue. Usually, two freezing procedures lasting 15 minutes each are carried out. The risk of damaging the large vessels is relatively low. The advantage of cryotherapy is that the tumour cells are kept in place mechanically with the help of the extracellular ice matrix, thus inhibiting dissemination of the tumour cells. The method is painless. However, there are some disadvantages, including the high costs and the more pronounced parenchymal trauma. (339, 349, 358, 366, 369) (s. p. 808)

10.6.3 Liver transplantation

In the case of diffuse metastasizing in the liver due to a neuroendocrine tumour, transplantation may be indicated.

10.6.4 Local treatment

There are no clear recommendations concerning indications for percutaneous interventional procedures. It is uncertain whether the metastases have been completely removed when guiding is based on imaging techniques. Moreover, the extent of the placed necrosis can only be assessed in a limited way; however, evaluation is more exact if the resected tissue is analyzed histologically.

RFTA: The monopolar system which has been used up to now will probably be replaced in the near future by a bipolar system. Coagulation necrosis of up to 5 cm can be achieved. However, RFTA sometimes has a negative impact in areas near the large vessels, since the cooling effect may cause the tumour cells close to the vessel walls to survive, with a risk of recidivation. In special cases, RFTA can also be applied as an open (operative) technique. A combination of ablation therapy and resection is possible. RFTA has several advantages: it is relatively low in cost, there is less parenchymal loss, the procedure is safe and can be repeated. (353) (s. p. 811)

LITT: Even in the case of liver metastases, the laser applicator is positioned using a percutaneously or laparoscopically inserted puncture needle. The procedure lasts 15—20 minutes. Repeat treatment is possible. (331, 356, 376) (s. p. 810)

PEI: Percutaneous ethanol injection therapy with alcohol or acetic acid is not recommendable in liver metastases. (338)

10.6.5 Local chemotherapy

TAC: Application of cytostatics is generally carried out using a port-catheter system via the gastroduodenal artery and the proper hepatic artery (R.D. SULLIVAN et al., 1964). Foci in excess of 2 mm are supplied by this artery in 80—100% of cases. Moreover, the blood flow can be slowed down by administering starch microspheres or similar substances, so that a higher concentration of cytostatics is achieved in the tumours. In order to avoid toxic damage, the right gastric artery must be ligated and a cholecystectomy carried out; cholangitis may develop as a side effect. (327) In about 30% of patients, positioning of the catheter is not possible or must be modified due to vascular anomalies. Therefore, it is necessary to perform a coeliacography preoperatively to check the anatomy of the vessels. TAC has been applied for the treatment of colorectal liver metastases using 5-FU/folinic acid, 5-FU/mitomycin or fluordesoxyuridin as a continuous i.v. infusion based on (still) varying schemes. This therapy option is not regarded as effective for liver metastases. (325, 341, 344, 345, 354, 375) (s. p. 810)

TAE, TACE: Both transarterial embolization and chemoembolization with the help of a port-catheter system via the proper hepatic artery (analogous to TAC) might be a therapeutic option regarding non-resectable liver metastases. An indication is also given if there is a high surgical risk involved. Embolization can be repeated several times. In metastatic neuroendocrine tumours, preoperative treatment with somatostatin analogues is recommended. The response rate in colorectal liver metastases is usually low. In combination with lipiodol, however, a response rate of 45% can be achieved in solitary metastasis. It should be noted that lipiodol enrichment only occurs at the margins of metastases. More positive results have been obtained with a combination of collagen + cisplatin + doxorubicin + mitomycin, particularly when administered at intervals of six to eight weeks. (s. p. 810)

10.6.6 Systemic therapy

In special kinds of tumours, the application of a certain substance can be helpful as adjuvant therapy.

Anti-hormone therapy: Gastroenteropancreatic tumours show a good response to the systemic administration of anti-hormonal substances, especially those which are directed against the biological activity and peptide secretion of these tumours. • As a result, **octreotide** therapy can be applied as s.c. injection for a longer time. Follow-up is possible by determining serotonin and chromogranin A in the serum as well as 5-hydroxyindole acetic acid in the urine. • In metastasized insulinoma, **diazoxide**, a benzothiazide analogue, can block the release of insulin and increase glycogenolysis. However, this substance has considerable side effects.

Interferon therapy: The application of IFN is based on inhibiting protein synthesis and thus cell proliferation. Its indication is recommended in metastatic neuroendocrine tumours.

10.6.7 Systemic chemotherapy

Systemic chemotherapy is usually not indicated in non-colorectal liver metastases due to lack of response. The systemic administration of cytostatics (also in combination) possesses the status of palliative therapy. • However, in metastatic neuroendocrine tumours, a combination of octreotide + IFN had a positive effect on the survival time. Systemic chemotherapy produced remission rates of up to 60%. (333) • In metastatic breast cancer, systemic chemotherapy is indicated, usually in combination with hormonal and immune therapy. (329, 356)

• In metastatic gastric carcinoma, palliative chemotherapy can achieve a remission rate of up to 40%, with a slight extension of survival time.

> As a rule, the suitability of a combination of cytostatics following operative or local interventional therapy should be discussed at an interdisciplinary conference.

5-FU monotherapy: In metastatic colorectal carcinoma, 5-FU/folinic acid has constituted the basis of systemic chemotherapy for more than 40 years: survival time is prolonged, tumour-related symptoms are diminished and quality of life improves. Folinic acid is seen as the main modulator of 5-FU efficacy. Various schemes are used in different dosages and forms: (*1.*) *O'Connel scheme*, (*2.*) *Ardalan scheme*, (*3.*) *Machover's scheme*, and (*4.*) *Rougier's scheme*. • In the meantime, the *De Gramont scheme* has been introduced in France (200 mg/m^2 folinic acid, 400 mg/m^2 5-FU [bolus] and 600 mg/m^2 [22 hr i.v. infusion] on day 1 and 2, repeated on day 15), and the *AIO scheme* has been introduced in Germany (500 mg/m^2 folinic acid, 2.6 g/m^2 5-FU [24 hr i.v. infusion] 6 x/week, 1-week interruption of therapy).

Fluoropyrimidine-based prodrugs: A new development are the oral prodrugs *ftorafur* and *capecitabin*. Both substances have already proved effective. Capecitabin should not be combined with folinic acid.

Irinotecan-based combination: Irinotecan is a camptothecin-derivative, which as a prodrug is converted into a cytotoxic agent by means of carboxylesterase. It is considered to be one of the most active cytostatics in advanced colon carcinoma. The combination with 5-FU as an i.v. continuous infusion is recommended as a preferential form of treatment.

Oxaliplatin-based combination: Oxaliplatin has likewise been used successfully in combination with 5-FU. The most important limiting side effects of a long-term therapy are cumulative neuropathic symptoms.

▶ In metastatic colorectal carcinoma, it is possible to achieve complete surgical removal (R0) of the metastases in initially incurable resected patients due to the relatively successful systemic chemotherapy schemes used today. In about 20% of the patients with oligotropic metastatic spread, this **therapy triad** consisting of resection + chemotherapy +' resection can lead to a 5-year survival rate of 25% (cf. primary curative resection).

10.6.8 Adjuvant measures

The information presented in section 3.9.4 (s. p. 811) similarly provides a basis for adjuvant or unconventional treatment and for general care of tumour patients with metastases. (s. tab. 37.10) • In addition, the perioperative use of **galactose** may be worth considering in surgical (or invasive) treatment of metastases, especially since it is without side effects and does not involve undue costs. • Furthermore, we would like to point out that the administration of **zinc** and **selenium** as well as **potassium canrenoate** is useful when planning a resection of metastases. (s. p. 813)

References:

Diagnostic

1. **Bohm, B., Voth, M., Georghegan, J., Heltfritzsch, H., Petrovich, A., Scheele, J., Gottschild, D.:** Impact of positron emission tomography on strategy in liver resection for primary and secondary liver tumors. J. Canc. Res. Clin. Oncol. 2004; 130: 266–272
2. **Cosgrove, D., Blomley, M.:** Liver tumors: Evaluation with contrast-enhanced ultrasound. Abdom. Imag. 2004; 29: 446–454
3. **Delbeke, D., Martin, W.H., Sandler, M.P., Chapman, W.C., Wright, J.K., Pinson, C.W.:** Evaluation of benign vs malignant hepatic lesions with positron emission tomography. Arch. Surg. 1998; 133: 510–516
4. **Edmondson, H.A., Steiner, P.E.:** Primary carcinoma of the liver. A study of 100 cases among 48900 autopsies. Cancer 1954; 7: 462–503
5. **Eggel, H.:** Über das primäre Carcinom der Leber. Beitr. Pathol. Anat. Allg. Pathol. 1901; 30: 506–604
6. **Harris, C.C., Hollstein, M.:** Clinical implications of the p53 tumor suppressor gene. New Engl. J. Med. 1993; 321: 1318–1327
7. **Hermanek, P., Wittekind, C.:** Residual tumour (R) classification and prognosis. Semin. Surg. Oncol. 1994; 10: 12–20
8. **Konno, K., Ishida, H., Hamashima, Y., Komatsuda, T., Sato, M., Furuya, T., Asanuma, Y., Masamune, O.:** Color Doppler findings of tumor seeding after US-guided liver tumor biopsy. Abdom. Imag. 1999; 24: 401–403
9. **Kuntz, E.:** 30 years' experience with 6000 laparoscopies (1955–1986). Fortschr. Med. 1987; 105: 521–524 • Current status of laparoscopy in hepatology. Med. Welt 1999; 50: 42–47
10. **Kuszyk, B.S., Bluemke, D.A., Urban, B.A., Choti, M.A., Hruban, R.H., Sitzmann, J.V., Fishman, E.K.:** Portal-phase contrast-enhanced helical CT for the detection of malignant hepatic tumors. Amer. J. Roentgenol. 1996; 166: 91–95
11. **Lemke, A.J., Chopra, S.S., Hengst, S.A., Brinkmann, M.J., Steinmüller, T., Felix, R.:** Characterization of hepatic tumors with contrast-enhanced ultrasound and digital grey-scale analysis. Fortschr. Röntgenstr. 2004; 176: 1607–1616
12. **Mani, H., van Thiel, D.H.:** Mesenchymal tumors of the liver. Clin. Liver Dis. 2001; 5: 219–257
13. **Steiner, P.E.:** Cancer of the liver and cirrhosis in trans-Saharan Africa and the United States of America. Cancer 1960; 13: 1085–1166
14. **Summerskill, W.H.J., Adson, M.A.:** Gynecomastia as a sign of hepatoma. Amer. J. Dig. Dis. 1962; 74: 250–254

Hepatocellular carcinoma

15. **Akanuma, M., Yoshida, H., Okamoto, M., Ogura, K., Maeda, S., Hata, Y., Sato, S., Shiina, S., Kawabe, T., Shiratori, Y., Omata, M.:** Risk factors for esophageal variceal bleeding in patients with hepatocellular carcinoma. Hepato-Gastroenterol. 2002; 49: 1039–1044
16. **Arai, H., Saitoh, S., Matsumoto, T., Makita, F., Mitsugi, S., Yuasa, K., Takagi, H., Mori, M.:** Hypertension as a paraneoplastic syndrome in hepatocellular carcinoma. J. Gastroenterol. 1999; 34: 530–534
17. **Arii, S., Tanaka, J., Yamazoe, Y., Minematsu, S., Morino, T., Fujita, K., Maetani, S., Tobe, T.:** Predictive factors for intrahepatic recurrence of hepatocellular carcinoma after partial hepatectomy. Cancer 1992; 69: 913–919
18. **Bartolozzi, C., Lencioni, R., Ricci, P., Paolicchi, A., Rossi, P., Passariello, R.:** Hepatocellular carcinoma treatment with percutaneous ethanol injection: evaluation with contrast-enhanced color Doppler US. Radiology 1998; 209: 387–393
19. **Becker, G., Allgaier, H.P., Olschewski, M., Zähringer, A., Blum, H.E.:** Long-acting octreoide versus placebo for treatment of advanced HCC: A randomized controlled double-blind study. Hepatology 2007; 45: 9–15
20. **Benvegnu, L., Noventa, F., Bernardinello, E., Pontisso, P., Gatta, A., Alberti, A.:** Evidence for an association between the aetiology of cirrhosis and pattern of hepatocellular carcinoma development. Gut 2001; 48: 110–115
21. **Berber, E., Garland, A.M., Engle, K.L., Rogers, S.J., Siperstein, A.E.:** Laparoscopic ultrasonography and biopsy of hepatic tumors in 310 patients. Amer. J. Surg. 2004; 187: 213–218
22. **Bilchik, A.J., Wood, T.F., Allegra, D., Tsioulias, G.J., Chung, M., Rose, D.M., Ramming, K.P., Morton, D.L.:** Cryosurgical ablation and radiofrequency ablation for unresectable hepatic malignant neoplasms – a proposed algorithm. Arch. Surg. 2000; 135: 657–664
23. **Bismuth, H., Majno, P.E., Adam, R.:** Liver transplantation for hepatocellular carcinoma. Semin. Liver Dis. 1999; 19: 311–322
24. **Bizollon, T., Rode, A., Bancel, B., Gueripel, V., Ducerf, C., Baulieux, J., Trepo, C.:** Diagnostic value and tolerance of lipiodol-computed tomography for the detection of small hepatocellular carcinoma: correlation with pathologic examination of explanted livers. J. Hepatol. 1998; 28: 491–496
25. **Bosch, F.X., Ribes, J., Diaz, M., Cleries, R.:** Primary liver cancer: worldwide incidence and trends. Gastroenterology 2004; 127 (Suppl. 1): 5–16
26. **Botelli, R., Tibballs, J., Hochhauser, D., Watkinson, A., Dick, R., Burroughs, A.K.:** Ultrasound screening for hepatocellular carcinoma (HCC) in cirrhosis: the evidence for an established clinical practice. Clin. Radiol. 1998; 53: 713–716
27. **Boucher, E., Corbinais, S., Rolland, Y., Bourguet, P., Guyader, D., Boudjema, K., Meunier, B., Raoul, J.L.:** Adjuvant intra-arterial injection of iodine-131-labelled lipiodol after resection of hepatocellular carcinoma. Hepatology 2003; 38: 1237–1241
28. **Britto, M.R.C., Thomas, L.A., Balaratnam, N., Griffiths, A.P., Duane, P.D.:** Hepatocellular carcinoma arising in non-cirrhotic liver in genetic haemochromatosis. Scand. J. Gastroenterol. 2000; 35: 889–893
29. **Burkill, G.J.C., Mannion, E.M., Healy, J.C.:** Lymph node enhancement at MRI with MnDPDP in primary hepatic carcinoma. Clin. Radiol. 2001; 56: 67–71
30. **Caldwell, S.H., Crespo, D.M., Kang, H.S., Al-Osaimi, A.M.S.:** Obesity and hepatocellular carcinoma. Gastroenterology 2004; 127 (Suppl. 1): 97–103
31. **Camma, C., Schepis, F., Orlando, A., Albanese, M., Shalied, L., Trevisani, F., Andreone, P., Craxi, A., Cottone, M.:** Transarterial chemoembolization for unresectable hepatocellular carcinoma: Meta-analysis of randomized controlled trials. Radiology 2002; 224: 47–54
32. **Caturelli, E., Bisceglia, M., Fusilli, S., Squillante, M.M., Castelvetere, M., Siena, D.A.:** Cytological vs. microhistological diagnosis of hepatocellular carcinoma. Comparative accuracies in the same fine-needle biopsy specimen. Dig. Dis. Sci. 1996; 41: 2326–2331
33. **Caturelli, E., Solmi, L., Anti, M., Fusilli, S., Roselli, P., Andriulli, A., Fornari, F., del Vecchio Blanco, C., de Sio, I.:** Ultrasound guided fine needle biopsy of early hepatocellular carcinoma complicating liver cirrhosis: A multicentre study. Gut 2004; 53: 1356–1362
34. **Chapoutot, C., Perney, P., Fabre, D., Taourel, P., Bruel, J.M., Larrey, D., Domergue, I., Ciurana, A.J., Blanc, F.:** Needle-tract seeding after percutaneous ultrasound guided needle biopsy of hepatocellular carcinoma. A study of 150 patients. Gastroenterol. Clin. Biol. 1999; 23: 552–556
35. **Choi, B.I., Lee, J.Y., Han, J.K., Lee, J.M., Kim, S.H.:** Contrast-enhanced sonography for hepatocellular carcinoma. Intervirology 2004; 47: 162–168
36. **CLIP: The Cancer of the Liver Italian Program investigators.** Prospective validation of the CLIP score: a new prognosis system for patients with cirrhosis and hepatocellular carcinoma. Hepatology 2000; 31: 840–845
37. **Colagrande, S., la Villa, G., Bartolucci, M., Lanini, F., Barletta, G., Villari, N.:** Spiral computed tomography versus ultrasound in the follow-up of cirrhotic patients previously treated for hepatocellular carcinoma: A prospective study. J. Hepatol. 2003; 39: 93–98
38. **Conti, J.A., Kemeny, N.:** Type Ia glycogenosis associated with hepatocellular carcinoma. Cancer 1992; 69: 1320–1322
39. **Cottone, M., Turri, M., Parisi, P., Orlando, A., Fiorentino, G., Virdone, R., Fusco, G., Grasso, R., Simonetti, R.G., Pagliaro, L.:** Screening for hepatocellular carcinoma in patients with child's A cirrhosis: an 8-year prospective study by ultrasound and alpha fetoprotein. J. Hepatol. 1994; 21: 1029–1034
40. **Curley, S.A., Bomalaski, J.S., Ensor, C.M., Holtsberg, F.W., Clark, M.A.:** Regression of hepatocellular cancer in a patient treated with arginine deiminase (case report). Hepato-Gastroenterol. 2003; 50: 1214–1216
41. **Del Olmo, J.A., Serra, M.A., Rodriguez, F., Escudero, K., Gilabert, S., Rodrigo, J.M.:** Incidence and risk factors for hepatocellular carcinoma in 96 patients with cirrhosis. J. Canc. Res. Clin. Oncol. 1998; 124: 560–564
42. **Dick, E.A., Joarder, R., de Jode, M., Taylor-Robinson, S.D., Thomas, H.C., Foster, G.R., Gedroyc, W.M.W.:** MR-guided laser thermal ablation of primary and secondary liver tumours. Clin. Radiol. 2003; 58: 112–120
43. **Ding, H., Kudo, M., Onda, H., Suetomi, Y., Minami, Y., Maekawa, K.:** Contrast-enhanced subtraction harmonic sonography for evaluating treatment response in patients with hepatocellular carcinoma. Amer. J. Roentgenol. 2001; 176: 661–666
44. **Dong, B.W., Liang, P., Yu, X.L., Su, L., Yu, D.J., Cheng, Z.G., Zhang, J.:** Percutaneous sonographically guided microwave coagulation therapy for hepatocellular carcinoma: results in 234 patients. Amer. J. Roentgenol. 2003; 180: 1547–1555
45. **El-Serag, H.B.:** Hepatocellular carcinoma. An epidemiologic view. J. Clin. Gastroenterol. 2002; 35 (Suppl. 2): 72–78
46. **Enwonwu, C.O.:** The role of dietary aflatoxin in the genesis of hepatocellular cancer in developing countries. Lancet 1984/II: 956–958
47. **Eriksson, S.J., Carlson, J., Velez, R.:** Risk of cirrhosis and primary liver cancer in alpha$_1$-antitrypsin deficiency. New Engl. J. Med. 1986; 314: 736–779
48. **Farinati, F., de Maria, N., Marafin, C., Herszenyi, L., del Prato, St., Rinaldi, M., Perini, L., Cardin, R., Naccarato, R.:** Unresectable hepatocellular carcinoma in cirrhosis. Survival, prognostic factors, and unexpected side effects after transcatheter arterial chemoembolization. Dig. Dis. Sci. 1996; 41: 2332–2339
49. **Feo, C.F., Marrosu, A., Scanu, A.M., Ginesu, G.C., Fancellu, A., Migaleddu, V., Porcu, A.:** Spontaneous regression of hepatocellular carcinoma: report of a case. Eur. J. Gastroenterol. Hepatol. 2004; 16: 933–936

50. Fiel, M.I., Min, A., Gerber, M.A., Faire, B., Schwartz, M., Thung, S.N.: Hepatocellular carcinoma in long-term oral contraceptive use. Liver 1996; 16: 372–376
51. Francanzani, A.L., Taioli, E., Sampietro, M., Fatta, E., Bertelli, C., Fiorelli, G., Fargion, S.: Liver cancer risk is increased in patients with porphyria cutanea tarda in comparison to matched control patients with chronic liver disease. J. Hepatol. 2001; 35: 498–503
52. Frank, I.L., Tharakan, J., Vasudev, K.S., Isaacs, P.E.T.: Malignant hepatic tumours associated with previous exposure to thorotrast: four cases. Eur. J. Gastroenterol. Hepatol. 1996; 8: 1121–1124
53. Gambarin-Gelwan, M., Wolf, D.C., Shapiro, R., Schwartz, M.E., Min, A.D.: Sensitivity of commonly available screening tests in detecting hepatocellular carcinoma in cirrhotic patients undergoing liver transplantation. Amer. J. Gastroenterol. 2000; 95: 1535–1538
54. Gelatti, U., Donato, F., Tagger, A., Fantoni, C., Portolani, N., Ribero, M.L., Martelli, C., Trevisi, P., Covolo, L., Simonati, C., Nardi, G.: Etiology of hepatocellular carcinoma influences clinical and pathologic features but not patient survival. Amer. J. Gastroenterol. 2003; 98: 907–914
55. Geschwind, J.F., Ko, Y.H., Torbenson, M.S., Magee, C., Pedersen, P.L.: Novel therapy for liver cancer: direct intraarterial injection of a potent inhibitor of ATP production. Cancer 2002; 62: 3909–3913
56. Giorgio, A., Tarantino, L., de Stefano, G., Scala, V., Liorre, G., Scarano, F., Perrotta, A., Farella, N., Aloisio, V., Mariniello, N., Coppola, C., Francica, G., Ferraioli, G.: Percutaneous sonographically guided saline-enhanced radiofrequency ablation of hepatocellular carcinoma. Amer. J. Roentgenol. 2003; 181: 479–484
57. Grasso, A., Watkinson, A.F., Tibballs, J.M., Burroughs, A.K.: Radiofrequency ablation in the treatment of hepatocellular carcinoma – a clinical viewpoint. J. Hepatol. 2000; 33: 667–672
58. Gritzmann, N.: Small hepatocellular carcinomas in patients with liver cirrhosis: potential and limitations of contrast-enhanced power Doppler sonography. Eur. J. Gastroenterol. Hepatol. 2003; 15: 881–883
59. Halteren, van, H.K., Salemans, J.M.J.I., Peters, H., Vreugdenhil, G., Driesser, W.M.M.: Spontaneous regression of hepatocellular carcinoma. J. Hepatol. 1997; 27: 211–215
60. Hanazaki, K., Kajikawa, S., Shimozawa, N., Mihara, M., Shimada, K., Hiraguri, M., Koide, N., Adachi, W., Amano, J.: Survival and recurrence after hepatic resection of 386 consecutive patients with hepatocellular carcinoma. Amer. J. Surg. 2000; 191: 381–388
61. Hasegawa, K., Uesugi, H., Kubota, K., Ugawa, Y., Murayama, S., Kobayashi, T., Hippo, Y., Gunji, T., Ohnishi, S., Mori, M., Makuuchi, M.: Polymyositis as a paraneoplastic manifestation of hepatocellular carcinoma. Hepato-Gastroenterol. 2000; 47: 1425–1427
62. Hassan, M.M., Hwang, L.Y., Hatten, C.J., Swaim, M., Li, D., Abbruzzese, J.L., Beastley, P., Patt, Y.Z.: Risk factors for hepatocellular carcinoma: Synergism of alcohol with viral hepatitis and diabetes mellitus. Hepatology 2002; 36: 1206–1213
63. Huo, T.I., Huang, Y.H., Wu, J.C., Lee, P.C., Chang, F.Y., Lee, S.D.: Persistent retention of acetic acid is associated with complete tumour necrosis in patients with hepatocellular carcinoma undergoing percutaneous acetic acid injection. Scand. J. Gastroenterol. 2004; 39: 168–173
64. Idilman, R., de Maria, N., Colantoni, A., van Thiel, D.H.: Pathogenesis of hepatitis B and C-induced hepatocellular carcinoma. J. Viral Hepatitis 1998; 5: 285–299
65. Ido, K., Nakazawa, Y., Isoda, N., Kawamoto, C., Nagamine, N., Ono, K., Hozumi, M., Sato, Y., Kimura, K., Sugano, K.: The role of laparoscopic US and laparoscopic US-guided aspiration biopsy in the diagnosis of multicentric hepatocellular carcinoma. Gastrointest. Endosc. 1999; 50: 523–526
66. Iiai, T., Sato, Y., Nabatame, N., Yamamoto, S., Makino, S., Hatakeyama, K.: Spontaneous complete regression of hepatocellular carcinoma with portal vein tumor thrombus (case report). Hepato-Gastroenterol. 2003; 50: 1628–1630
67. Imamura, M., Shiratori, Y., Shiina, S., Sato, S., Obi, S., Okudaira, T., Teratani, T., Kato, N., Akahane, M., Ohtomo, K., Minami, M., Omata, M.: Power Doppler sonography for hepatocellular carcinoma: factors affecting the power Doppler signals of the tumors. Liver 1998; 18: 427–433
68. Ishii, H., Okada, S., Okusaka, T., Yoshimori, M., Nakasuka, H., Shimada, K., Yamasaki, S., Nakanishi, Y., Sakamoto, M.: Needle tract implantation of hepatocellular carcinoma after percutaneous ethanol injection. Cancer 1998; 82: 1638–1642
69. Itamoto, T., Nakahara, H., Amano, H., Kohashi, T., Ohdan, H., Tashiro, H., Asahara, T.: Repeat hepatectomy for recurrent hepatocellular carcinoma. Surgery 2007; 141: 589–597
70. Ito, Y., Kojiro, M., Nakashima, T., Mori, T.: Pathomorphologic characteristics of 102 cases of thorotrast-related hepatocellular carcinoma, cholangiocarcinoma, and hepatic angiosarcoma. Cancer 1988; 62: 1153–1162
71. Izumi, N., Asahina, Y., Noguchi, O., Uchihara, M., Kanazawa, N., Itakura, J., Himeno, Y., Miyake, S., Sakai, T., Enomoto, N.: Risk factors for distant recurrence of hepatocellular carcinoma in the liver after complete coagulation by microwave or radiofrequency ablation. Cancer 2001; 91: 949–956
72. Kaibori, M., Matsui, Y., Yanagida, H., Yokoigawa, N., Kwon, A.H., Kamiyama, Y.: Positive status of alpha-fetoprotein and des-gamma-carboxy prothrombin: important prognostic factor for recurrent hepatocellular carcinoma. World J. Surg. 2004; 28: 702–707
73. Kato, H., Nakamura, M., Muramatsu, M., Orito, E., Ueda, R., Mizokami, M.: Spontaneous regression of hepatocellular carcinoma: Two case reports and a literature review. Hepatol. Res. 2004; 29: 180–190
74. Katsushima, S., Inokuma, T., Oi, H., Okamura, J., Higashi, T., Takeuchi, R., Hidaka, A., Shigeno, C., Iida, Y., Konishi, J.: Acute hepatic failure following transcatheter arterial embolization for the treatment of hepatocellular carcinoma. Digestion 1997; 58: 189–195
75. Katyal, S., Oliver, J.H., Peterson, M.S., Ferris, J.V., Carr, B.S., Baron, R.L.: Extrahepatic metastases of hepatocellular carcinoma. Radiology 2000; 216: 698–703
76. Kawamoto, C., Ido, K., Isoda, N., Nagamine, N., Hozumi, M., Ono, K., Nakazawa, Y., Sato, Y., Kimura, K.: Prognosis of small hepatocellular carcinoma after laparoscopic ethanol injection. Gastrointest. Endosc. 1999; 50: 214–220
77. Kawasaki, S., Makuuchi, M., Miyagawa, S., Kakazu, T., Hayashi, K., Kasai, H., Miwa, S., Hui, A., Nishimaki, K.: Results of hepatic resection of hepatocellular carcinoma. World J. Surgery 1995; 19: 31–34
78. Kawata, S., Yamasaki, E., Nagase, T., Inui, Y., Ito, N., Matsuda, Y., Inada, M., Tamura, S., Noda, S., Imai, Y., Matsuzawa, Y.: Effect of pravastatin on survival in patients with advanced hepatocellular carcinoma. A randomized controlled trial. Brit. J. Canc. 2001; 84: 886–891
79. Kettenbach, J., Kostler, W., Rucklinger, E., Gustorff, B., Wolf, F., Peer, K., Weigner, M., Lammer, J., Muller, W., Goldberg, S.N.: Percutaneous saline-enhanced radiofrequency ablation of unresectable hepatic tumours: Initial experience in 26 patients. Amer. J. Roentgenol. 2003; 180: 1537–1545
80. Kew, M.C.: Epidemiology of hepatocellular carcinoma. Toxicology 2002; 181: 35–38
81. Kew, M.C.: Virchow-Troisier's lymph node in hepatocellular carcinoma. J. Clin. Gastroenterol. 1991; 13: 217–219
82. Khan, K.N., Yatsuhashi, H., Yamasaki, K., Yamasaki, M., Inoue, O., Koga, M., Yano, M.: Prospective analysis of risk factors for early intrahepatic recurrence of hepatocellular carcinoma following ethanol injection. J. Hepatol. 2000; 32: 269–278
83. Khan, M.A., Combs, C.S., Brunt, E.M., Lowe, V.J., Wolverson, M.K., Solomon, H., Collins, B.T., DiBisceglie, A.M.: Positron emission tomography scanning in the evaluation of hepatocellular carcinoma. J. Hepatol. 2000; 32: 792–797
84. Kim, C.K., Lim, J.H., Lee, W.J.: Detection of hepatocellular carcinomas and dysplastic nodules in cirrhotic liver: accuracy of ultrasonography in transplant patients. J. Ultrasound Med. 2001; 20: 99–104
85. Kim, R.D., Nazarey, P., Katz, E., Chari, R.S.: Laparoscopic staging and tumor ablation for hepatocellular carcinoma in Child C cirrhotics evaluated for orthotopic liver transplantation. Surg. Endosc. 2004; 18: 39–44
86. Koda, M., Murawaki, Y., Mitsuda, A., Ohyama, K., Horie, Y., Suou, T., Kawasaki, H., Ikawa, S.: Predictive factors for intrahepatic recurrence after percutaneous ethanol injection therapy for small hepatocellular carcinoma. Cancer 2000; 88: 529–537
87. Koike, Y., Shiratori, Y., Sato, S., Obi, S., Teratani, T., Imamura, M., Yoshida, H., Shiina, S., Omata, M.: Des-gamma-carboxy prothrombin as a useful predisposing factor for the development of portal vein invasion in patients with hepatocellular carcinoma – A prospective analysis of 227 patients. Cancer 2001; 91: 561–569
88. Kojiro, M.: "Nodule-in-nodule" appearance in hepatocellular carcinoma: Its significance as a morphologic marker of dedifferentiation. Intervirology 2004; 47: 179–183
89. Komorizomo, Y., Kohara, K., Oketani, M., Maeda, M., Shibathou, S., Shigenobu, S., Hiramine, Y., Yamasaki, N., Arima, T., Katzuaki, I., Arima, T.: Systemic combined chemotherapy with low dose of 5-fluorouracil, cisplatin, and interferon-alpha for advanced hepatocellular carcinoma. – A pilot study. Dig. Dis. Sci. 2003; 48: 877–881
90. Kouroumalis, E., Skordilis, P., Thermos, K., Vasilaki, A., Moschandrea, J., Manousos, O.N.: Treatment of hepatocellular carcinoma with octreotide: a randomized controlled study. Gut 1998; 42: 442–447
91. Krasner, N., Johnson, P.J., Portmann, B., Watkinson, G., MacSween, R.N.M., Williams, R.: Hepatocellular carcinoma in primary biliary cirrhosis: report of four cases. Gut 1979; 2: 255–258
92. Kurogi, M., Nakashima, O., Miyaaki, H., Fujimoto, M., Kojiro, M.: Clinicopathological study of scirrhous hepatocellular carcinoma. J. Gastroenterol. Hepatol. 2006; 21: 1470–1477
93. Kwon, Y., Lee, S.K., Kim, J.S., Ro, J.Y., Yu, E.S.: Synchronous hepatocellular carcinoma and cholangiocarcinoma arising in two different dysplastic nodules. Modern Pathol. 2002; 15: 1096–1101
94. Lai, E.C.-S., Ng, I.O.-L., Ng, M.M.-T., Lok, A.S.-F., Tam, P.-C., Fan, S.-T., Choi, T.-K., Wong, J.: Long-term results of resection for large hepatocellular carcinoma: a multivariate analysis of clinicopathological features. Hepatology 1990; 11: 815–818
95. Lau, W.Y., Leung, T.W.T., Ho, S.K.W., Chan, M., Lau, J., Chan, A.T.C., Yeo, W., Mok, T.S.K., Yu, S.C.H.: Adjuvant intra-arterial iodine-131-labelled lipiodol for resectable hepatocellular carcinoma: a prospective randomized trial. Lancet 1999; 353: 797–801
96. Lau, W.Y., Leung, T.W.T., Lai, B.S., Liew, C.T., Ho, S.K.W., Yu, S.C.H., Tang, A.M.Y.: Preoperative systemic chemoimmunotherapy and sequential resection for unresectable hepatocellular carcinoma. Ann. Surg. 2001; 233: 236–241
97. Lee, C.M., Hsu, C.Y., Eng, H.L., Huang, W.S., Lu, S.N., Changchien, C.S., Chen, C.L., Cho, C.L.: Telomerase activity and telomerase catalytic subunit in hepatocellular carcinoma. Hepato-Gastroenterol. 2004; 51: 796–800
98. Leung, T.W.T., Patt, Y.Z., Lau, W.Y., Ho, S.K.W., Yu, S.C.H., Chan, A.T.C., Mok, T.S.K., Yeo, W., Liew, C.T., Leung, N.W.Y., Tang, A.M.Y., Johnson, P.J.: Complete pathological remission is possible

with systemic combination chemotherapy for inoperable hepatocellular carcinoma. Clin. Canc. Res. 1999; 5: 1676–1681
99. **Leung, W.T., Shiu, W.C., Leung, N., Chan, M., Tsao, M., Li, A.K., Metreweli, C.:** Treatment of inoperative hepatocellular carcinoma by intra-arterial lipiodol and 4-epidoxorubicin. Canc. Chemother. Pharmacol. 1992; 29: 401–404
100. **Li, S., Beheshti, M., Peck-Radosavljevic, M., Oezer, S., Grumbeck, E., Schmid, M., Hamilton, G., Kapiotis, S., Dudczak, R., Kletter, K.:** Comparison of 11C-acetate positron emission tomography and 67Gallium citrate scintigraphy in patients with hepatocellular carcinoma. Liver Internat. 2006; 26: 920–927
101. **Liang, H.L., Yang, C.F., Pan, H.B., Lai, K.H., Cheng, J.S., Lo, G.H., Chen, C.K.H., Lai, P.H.:** Small hepatocellular carcinoma: safety and efficacy of single high-dose percutaneous acetic acid injection for treatment. Radiology 2000; 214: 769–774
102. **Limmer, J., Fleig, W.E., Leupold, D., Bittner, R., Ditschuneit, H., Beger, H.G.:** Hepatocellular carcinoma in type I glycogen storage disease. Hepatology 1998; 8: 531–537
103. **Lin, T.J., Liao, L.Y., Lin, C.L., Shih, L.S., Chang, T.A., Tu, H.Y., Chen, R.C., Wang, C.S.:** Spontaneous regression of hepatocellular carcinoma: A case report and literature review. Hepato-Gastroenterol. 2004; 51: 579–582
104. **Livraghi, T., Giorgio, A., Marin, G., Salmi, A., de Sio, I., Bolondi, L., Pompili, M., Brunello, F., Lazzaroni, S., Torzilli, G., Zucchi, A.:** Hepatocellular carcinoma and cirrhosis in 746 patients: long-term results of percutaneous ethanol injection. Radiology 1995; 197: 101–108
105. **Livraghi, T., Goldberg, S.N., Lazzaroni, F., Meloni, F., Solbiati, L., Gazelle, G.S.:** Small hepatocellular carcinoma: Treatment with radiofrequency ablation versus ethanol injection. Radiology 1999; 210: 655–661
106. **Llovet, J.M., Bru, C., Bruix, J.:** Prognosis of hepatocellular carcinoma: The BCLC staging classification. Semin. Liver Dis. 1999; 19: 329–338
107. **Llovet, J.M., Fuster, J., Bruix, J.:** Prognosis of hepatocellular carcinoma (review). Hepato-Gastroenterol. 2002; 49: 7–11
108. **Llovet, J.M., Bruix, J.:** Unresectable hepatocellular carcinoma: meta-analysis of arterial embolization. Radiology 2004; 230: 300–301
109. **Lutwick, L.I.:** Relation between aflatoxin, hepatitis-B virus, and hepatocellular carcinoma. Lancet 1979/I: 755–757
110. **Maeda, T., Adachi, E., Kajiyama, K., Sugimachi, K., Tsuneyoshi, M.:** Spindle cell hepatocellular carcinoma. A clinicopathological analysis of 15 cases. Cancer 1996; 77: 51–57
111. **Magalotti, D., Gueli, C., Zoli, M.:** Transient spontaneous regression of hepatocellular carcinoma. Hepato-Gastroenterology 1998; 45: 2369–2371
112. **Marcato, N., Abergel, A., Alexandre, M., Boire, J.Y., Darcha, C., Duchene, B., Chipponi, J., Boyer, L., Viallet, J.F., Bommelaer, G.:** Hepatocellular carcinoma in patients with cirrhosis: performance and semiology of magnetic resonance imaging and lipiodol computerized tomography. Gastroenterol. Clin. Biol. 1999; 23: 114–121
113. **Mazzaferro, V., Regalia, E., Doci, R., Morabito, A., Gennari, L., Andreola, S., Pulvirenti, A., Bozzetti, F., Montalto, F., Ammatuna, M.:** Liver transplantation for the treatment of small hepatocellular carcinomas in patients with cirrhosis. New Engl. J. Med. 1996; 334: 693–699
114. **Mazzanti, R., Arena, U., Pantaleo, P., Antonuzzo, L., Cipriani, G., Neri, B., Giordano, C., Lanini, F., Marchetti, S., Gentilini, P.:** Survival and prognostic factors in patients with hepatocellular carcinoma treated by percutaneous ethanol injection: A 10-year experience. Can. J. Gastroenterol. 2004; 18: 611–618
115. **Melia, W.M., Johnson, P.J., Neuberger, J.:** Hepatocellular carcinoma in primary biliary cirrhosis: detection by α-fetoprotein estimation. Gastroenterology 1984; 87: 660–663
116. **Michel, J., Suc, B., Montpeyroux, Hachemanne, S., Blanc, P., Domergue, J., Mouiel, J., Gouillat, C., Ducerf, C., Saric, J., Le Treut, Y.P., Fourtanier, G., Escat, J.:** Liver resection or transplantation for hepatocellular carcinoma? Retrospective analysis of 215 patients with cirrhosis. J. Hepatol. 1997; 26: 1274–1280
117. **Miki, K., Makuuchi, M., Takayama, T., Matsukura, A., Minagawa, M., Kubota, K., Hirata, M.:** Peritoneal seeding of hepatocellular carcinoma after ethanol injection therapy. Hepato-Gastroenterol. 2000; 47: 1428–1430
118. **Misawa, K., Hata, Y., Manabe, K., Matsuoka, S., Saito, M., Takada, J., Sano, F.:** Spontaneous regression of hepatocellular carcinoma. J. Gastroenterol. 1999; 34: 410–414
119. **Mita, Y., Aoyagi, Y., Yanagi, M., Suda, T., Suzuki, Y., Asakura, H.:** The usefulness of determining des-γ-carboxy prothrombin by sensitive enzyme immunoassay in the early diagnosis of patients with hepatocellular carcinoma. Cancer 1998; 82: 1643–1648
120. **Miyamoto, M., Sudo, T., Kuyama, T.:** Spontaneous rupture of hepatocellular carcinoma: a review of 172 Japanese cases. Amer. J. Gastroenterol. 1991; 86: 67–71
121. **Mor, E., Tur Kaspa, R., Sheiner, P., Schwartz, M.:** Treatment of hepatocellular carcinoma associated with cirrhosis in the era of liver transplantation. Ann. Intern. Med. 1998; 129: 643–653
122. **Morimoto, Y., Kubo, K., Shuto, T., Tanaka, H., Hirohashi, K., Yamamoto, T., Yamada, R., Kinoshita, H.:** Power Doppler ultrasonographic diagnosis of small hepatocellular carcinoma. Dig. Surg. 2002; 19: 379–387
123. **Moritz, M.W., Shoji, M., Sicard, G.A., Shioda, R., DeSchyver, K.:** Surgical therapy in two patients with pedunculated hepatocellular carcinoma. Arch. Surg. 1988; 123: 772–774
124. **Nagasue, N., Ono, T., Yamanoi, A., Kohno, H., El-Assal, O.N., Taniura, H., Uchida, M.:** Prognostic factors and survival after hepatic resection for hepatocellular carcinoma without cirrhosis. Brit. J. Surg. 2001; 88: 515–522
125. **Naoumov, N.V., Chokshi, S., Metivier, E., Maertens, G., Johnson, P.J., Williams, R.:** Hepatitis C virus infection in the development of hepatocellular carcinoma in cirrhosis. J. Hepatol. 1997; 27: 331–336
126. **Navarro, F., Taourel, P., Michel, J., Perney, P., Fabre, J.-M., Blanc, F., Domerque, J.:** Diaphragmatic and subcutaneous seeding of hepatocellular carcinoma following fine-needle aspiration biopsy. Liver 1998; 18: 251–254
127. **Nikfarjam, M., Christophi, C.:** Interstitial laser thermotherapy for liver tumours (review). Brit. J. Surg. 2003; 90: 1033–1047
128. **Ockner, R.K., Kaikaus, R.M., Bass, N.M.:** Fatty-acid metabolism and the pathogenesis of hepatocellular carcinoma: review and hypothesis. Hepatology 1993; 18: 669–676
129. **Ohmoto, K., Miyake, I., Tsuduki, M., Shibata, N., Takesue, M., Kunieda, T., Ohno, S., Kuboki, M., Yamamoto, S.:** Percutaneous microwave coagulation therapy for unresectable hepatocellular carcinoma. Hepato-Gastroenterol. 1999; 46: 2894–2900
130. **Ohnishi, K., Yoshioka, H., Kosaka, K., Toshima, K., Nishiyama, J., Kameda, C., Ito, S., Fujiwara, K.:** Treatment of hypervascular small hepatocellular carcinoma with ultrasound-guided percutaneous acetic acid injection: comparison with segmental transcatheter arterial embolization. Amer. J. Gastroenterol. 1996; 91: 2574–2579
131. **Okuda, H., Nakanishi, T., Takatsu, K., Saito, A., Hayashi, N., Takasaki, K., Takenami, K., Yamamoto, M., Nakano, M.:** Serum levels of des-gamma-carboxy prothrombin measured using the revised enzyme immunoassay kit with increased sensitivity in relation to clinicopathologic features of solitary hepatocellular carcinoma. Cancer 2000; 88: 544–549
132. **Orlando, A., Cottone, M., Virdone, R., Parisi, P., Sciarrino, E., Maringhini, A., Caltagirone, M., Simonetti, R.G., Pagliaro, L.:** Treatment of small hepatocellular carcinoma associated with cirrhosis by percutaneous ethanol injection. A trial with a comparison group. Scand. J. Gastroenterol. 1997; 32: 598–603
133. **Ozturk, M.:** Genetic aspects of hepatocellular carcinogenesis. Semin. Liver Dis. 1999; 19: 235–242
134. **Pacella, C.M., Bizzarri, G., Cecconi, P., Caspani, B., Magnolfi, F., Bianchini, A., Anelli, V., Pacella, S., Rossi, Z.:** Hepatocellular carcinoma: long-term results of combined treatment with laser thermal ablation and transcatheter arterial chemoembolization. Radiology 2001; 219: 669–678
135. **Palmieri, G.B.E., Morabito, A., Rea, A., Gravina, A., Bianco, A.R.:** Thymostimulin treatment of hepatocellular carcinoma in liver cirrhosis. Int. J. Canc. 1996; 8: 827–832
136. **Pang, R., Poon, R.T.:** Angiogenesis and antiangiogenic therapy in hepatocellular carcinoma. Cancer Lett. 2006; 242: 151–167
137. **Pirisi, M., Avellini, C., Fabris, C., Scott, C., Bardus, P., Soardo, G., Beltrami, C.A., Bartoli, E.:** Portal vein thrombosis in hepatocellular carcinoma: age and sex distribution in an autopsy study. Cancer Res. Clin. Oncol. 1998; 124: 397–400
138. **Pompili, M., Rapaccini, G.L., de Luca, F., Caturelli, E., Astone, A., Siena, D.A., Villani, M.R., Grattagliano, A., Cedrone, A., Gasbarrini, G.:** Risk factors for intrahepatic recurrence of hepatocellular carcinoma in cirrhotic patients treated by percutaneous ethanol injection. Cancer 1997; 79: 1501–1508
139. **Poo, J.L., Rosas-Romero, R., Montemayor, A.C., Isoard, F., Uribe, M.:** Diagnostic value of the copper/zinc ratio hepatocellular carcinoma: a case control study. J. Gastroenterol. 2003; 38: 45–51
140. **Poon, R.T.P., Fan, S.T., Wong, J.:** Selection criteria for hepatic resection in patients with large hepatocellular carcinoma larger than 10 cm in diameter. J. Amer. Coll. Surg. 2002; 194: 592–602
141. **Poon, R.T.P., Yu, W.C., Fan, S.T., Wong, J.:** Long-term oral branched chain amino acids in patients undergoing chemoembolization for hepatocellular carcinoma: A randomized trial. Aliment. Pharm. Ther. 2004; 19: 779–788
142. **Raoul, J.L., Messner, M., Boucher, E., Bretagne, J.F., Campion, J.P., Boudjema, K.:** Preoperative treatment of hepatocellular carcinoma with intra-arterial injection of (131)J-labelled lipiodol. Brit. J. Surg. 2003; 90: 1379–1383
143. **Rose, D.M., Chapman, W.C., Brockenbrough, A.T., Wright, J.K., Rose, A.T., Meranze, S., Mazer, M., Blair, T., Blanke, C.D., Debelak, J.P., Wright Pinson, C.:** Transcatheter arterial chemoembolization as primary treatment for hepatocellular carcinoma. Amer. J. Surg. 1999; 177: 405–410
144. **Samonakis, D.N., Koutroubakis, I.E., Sfiridaki, A., Malliaraki, N., Antoniou, P., Romanos, J., Kouroumalis, E.A.:** Hypercoagulable states in patients with hepatocellular carcinoma. Dig. Dis. Sci. 2004; 49: 854–858
145. **Santambrogio, R., Podda, M., Zuin, M., Bertolini, E., Bruno, S., Cornalba, G.P., Costa, M., Montorsi, M.:** Safety and efficacy of laparoscopic radiofrequency of hepatocellular carcinoma in patients with liver cirrhosis. Surg. Endosc. 2003; 17: 1826–1832
146. **Saurin, J.C., Tanière, P., Mion, F., Jacob, P., Partensky, C., Paliard, P., Berger, F.:** Primary hepatocellular carcinoma in workers exposed to vinyl chloride. A report of two cases. Cancer 1997; 79: 1671–1677
147. **Seki, T., Tamai, T., Nakagawa, T., Imamura, M., Nishimura, A., Yamashiki, N., Ikeda, K., Inoue, K.:** Combination therapy with transcatheter arterial chemoembolization and percutaneous microwave

coagulation therapy for hepatocellular carcinoma. Cancer 2000; 89: 1245–1251
148. **Shepherd, F.A., Rotstein, L.E., Houle, S., Yip, T.C.K., Paul, K., Suiderman, K.W.**: A phase 1 dose escalation trial of yttrium^{90} microspheres in the treatment of primary hepatocellular carcinoma. Cancer 1992; 70: 2250–2254
149. **Sherlock, S., Fox, R.A., Niazi, S.P., Scheuer, P.J.**: Chronic liver disease and primary liver-cell cancer with hepatitis-associated (Australia) antigen in serum. Lancet 1970/I: 1243–1247
150. **Sherman, M., Takayama, Y.**: Screening and treatment for hepatocellular carcinoma. Gastroenterol. Clin. N. Amer. 2004; 33: 671–691
151. **Shetty, K., Timmins, K., Brensinger, C., Furth, E.E., Rattan, S., Sun, W.J., Rosen, M., Soulen, M., Shaked, A., Reddy, K.R., Olthoff, K.M.**: Liver transplantation for hepatocellular carcinoma validation of present selection criteria in predicting outcome. Liver Transplant. 2004; 10: 911–918
152. **Shimada, M., Takenaka, K., Fujiwara, Y., Gion, T., Kajiyama, K., Maeda, T., Shirabe, K., Sugimachi, K.**: Des-γ-carboxy prothrombin and α-fetoprotein positive status as a new prognostic indicator after hepatic resection for hepatocellular carcinoma. Cancer 1996; 78: 2094–2100
153. **Shimizu, A., Koyama, M., Okuda, Y., Takase, K., Nakano, T., Tameda, Y.**: Hepatocellular carcinoma in primary biliary cirrhosis: A case report and review of the Japanese literature. Hepato-Gastroenterology 1998; 45: 2352–2355
154. **Shiomi, S., Nishiguchi, S., Ishizu, H., Iwata, Y., Sasaki, N., Tamori, A., Habu, D., Takeda, T., Kubo, S., Ochi, H.**: Usefulness of positron emission tomography with fluorine-18-fluorodeoxyglucose for predicting outcome in patients with hepatocellular carcinoma. Amer. J. Gastroenterol. 2001; 96: 1877–1880
155. **Shiraki, K., Shimizu, A., Takase, K., Suzuki, A., Tameda, Y., Nakano, T.**: Prospective study of laparoscopic findings with regard to the development of hepatocellular carcinoma in patients with hepatitis C virus-associated cirrhosis. Gastrointest. Endosc. 2001; 53: 449–455
156. **Srinivasan, P., McCall, J., Pritchard, J., Dhawan, A., Baker, A., Vergani, G.M., Muriesan, P., Rela, M., Heaton, N.D.**: Orthotopic liver transplantation for unresectable hepatoblastoma. Transplantation 2002; 74: 652–655
157. **Stickel, F., Schuppan, D., Hahn, E.G., Seitz, H.K.**: Cocarcinogenic effects of alcohol in hepatocarcinogenesis. Gut 2002; 51: 132–139
158. **Stumptner, C., Heid, H., Fuchsbichler, A., Hauser, H., Mischinger, H.J., Zatloukal, K., Denk, H.**: Analysis of intracytoplasmatic hyaline bodies in a hepatocellular carcinoma. Demonstration of p62 as major constituent. Amer. J. Path. 1999; 154: 1701–1710
159. **Sugiyama, M., Sakahara, H., Torizuka, T., Kanno, T., Nakamura, F., Futatsubashi, M., Nakamura, S.**: (18)F-FDG PET in the detection of extrahepatic metastases from hepatocellular carcinoma. J. Gastroenterol. 2004; 39: 961–968
160. **Taieb, J., Bonyhay, L., Golli, L., Ducreux, M., Boleslawski, E., Tigaud, J.M., de Baere, T., Mansourbakht, T., Delgado, M.A., Hannoun, L., Poynard, T., Boige, V.**: Gemcitabine plus Oxaliplatin for patients with advanced hepatocellular carcinoma using two different schedules. Cancer 2003; 98: 2664–2670
161. **Takeda, Y., Togashi, H., Shinzawa, H., Miyano, S., Ishii, R., Karasawa, T., Takeda, I., Saito, Y., Saito, K., Haga, H., Matsuo, T., Aoki, M., Mitsuhashi, H., Watanabe, H., Takahashi, T.**: Spontaneous regression of hepatocellular carcinoma and review of literature. J. Gastroenterol. Hepatol. 2000; 15: 1079–1086
162. **Tanaka, Y., Mizokami, M., Kato, T., Matsumoto, Y., Ishihama, T., Sugauchi, F., Suzuki, S., Miyata, N.**: GB virus C/hepatitis C virus infection among patients with hepatocellular carcinoma. Hepatol. Res. 1997; 8: 44–51
163. **Torimura, T., Ueno, T., Kin, M., Harada, R., Taniguchi, E., Nakamura, T., Sakata, R., Hashimoto, O., Sakamoto, M., Kumashiro, R., Sata, M., Nakashima, O., Yano, H., Kojiro, M.**: Overexpression of angiopoietin-1 and angiopoietin-2 in hepatocellular carcinoma. J. Hepatol. 2004; 40: 799–807
164. **Trenn, G., Utz, D., Reis, H.E.**: Spontaneous remission of a hepatocellular carcinoma. Onkologie 1998; 21: 156–159
165. **Tsai, J.-F., Chang, W.-Y., Jeng, J.-E., Ho, M.-S., Lin, Z.-Y., Tsai, J.-H.**: Hepatitis B and C virus infection as risk factors for liver cirrhosis and cirrhotic hepatocellular carcinoma: a case-control study. Liver 1994; 14: 98–102
166. **Tsai, J.F., Chuang, L.Y., Jeng, J.E., Ho, M.S., Hsieh, M.Y., Lin, Z.Y., Wang, L.Y.**: Betel quid chewing as a risk factor for hepatocellular carcinoma: a case control study. Brit. J. Canc. 2001; 84: 709–713
167. **Vana, J., Murphy, G.P., Aronoff, B.L., Baker, H.W.**: Primary liver tumors and oral contraceptives. Results of a survey. J. Amer. Med. Ass. 1977; 238: 2154–2158
168. **Wang, S.N., Chuang, S.C., Yeh, Y.T., Yang, S.F., Chai, C.Y., Chen, W.T., Kuo, K.K., Chen, J.S., Lee, K.T.**: Potential prognostic value of leptin receptor in hepatocellular carcinoma. J. Clin. Path. 2006; 59: 1267–1271
169. **Ward, J., Guthrie, J.A., Scott, D.J., Atchley, J., Wilson, D., Davies, M.H., Wyatt, J.I., Robinson, P.J.**: Hepatocellular carcinoma in the cirrhotic liver: Double-contrast MR imaging for diagnosis. Radiology 2000; 216: 154–162
170. **Weinberg, A.G., Mize, C.E., Worthan, H.G.**: The occurrence of hepatoma in the chronic form of hereditary tyrosinemia. J. Pediatr. 1976; 88: 434–438
171. **Wilkinson, M.L., Portmann, B., Williams, R.**: Wilson's disease and hepatocellular carcinoma: possible protective role of copper. Gut 1983; 24: 767–771
172. **Winston, C.B., Schwartz, L.H., Fong, Y.M., Blumgart, L.H., Panicek, D.M.**: Hepatocellular carcinoma: MR imaging findings in cirrhotic livers and noncirrhotic livers. Radiology 1999; 210: 75–79
173. **Wogan, G.N.**: Aflatoxins as risk factors for hepatocellular carcinoma in humans. Canc. Res. 1992; 52: 2114–2118
174. **Wong, W.S., Patel, S.C., Cruz, F.S., Gala, K.V., Turner, A.F.**: Cryosurgery as a treatment for advanced stage hepatocellular carcinoma. Cancer 1998; 82: 1268–1278
175. **Yamamoto, K., Masuzawa, M., Karo, M., Kurosawa, K., Kaneko, A., Ishida, H., Imamura, E., Park, N.J., Shirai, Y., Fujimoto, K., Michida, T., Hayashi, N., Ikeda, M.**: Evaluation of combined therapy with chemoembolization and ethanol injection for advanced hepatocellular carcinoma. Semin. Oncol. 1997; 24 (Suppl. 6): 50–55
176. **Yamazaki, Y., Kakizaki, S., Sohara, N., Sato, K., Takagi, H., Arai, H., Abe, T., Katakai, K., Kojima, A., Matsuzaki, Y., Mori, M.**: Hepatocellular carcinoma in young adults: The clinical characteristics, prognosis, and findings of a patient survival analysis. Dig. Dis. Sci. 2007; 52: 1103–1107
177. **Yeh, C.N., Lee, W.C., Jeng, L.B., Chen, M.F.**: Pedunculated hepatocellular carcinoma: Clinicopathologic study of 18 surgically resected cases. World J. Surg. 2002; 28: 1133–1138
178. **Yuki, K., Hirohashi, S., Sakamoto, M., Kanai, T., Shimosato, Y.**: Growth and spread of hepatocellular carcinoma. A review of 240 consecutive autopsy cases. Cancer 1990; 66: 2174–2179
179. **Yuki, N., Hijikata, Y., Kato, M., Kawahara, K., Wakasa, K.**: Squamous cell carcinoma as a rare entity of primary liver tumor with grave prognosis (case report). Hepatol. Res. 2006; 36: 322–327
180. **Zangos, S., Gille, T., Eichler, K., Engelmann, K., Woitaschek, D., Balzer, J.O., Mack, M.G., Thalhammer, A., Vogl, T.J.**: Transarterial chemoembolization in hepatocellular carcinoma: technique, indications, results. Radiologe 2001; 41: 906–914
181. **Zheng, R.Q., Zhou, P., Kudo, M.**: Hepatocellular carcinoma with nodule-in-nodule appearance: Demonstration by contrast-enhanced coded phase inversion harmonic imaging. Intervirology 2004; 47: 184–190
182. **Zhou, X.D., Tang, Z.Y., Yang, B.H., Lin, Z.Y., Ma, Z.C., Ye, S.L., Wu, Z.Q., Fan, J., Qin, L.X., Zheng, B.H.**: Experience of 1000 patients who underwent hepatectomy for small hepatocellular carcinoma. Cancer 2001; 91: 1479–1486

Fibrolamellar carcinoma
183. **Berman, M.A., Burnham, J.A., Sheahan, D.G.**: Fibrolamellar carcinoma of the liver. An immunohistochemical study of nineteen cases and a review of the literature. Hum. Pathol. 1988; 19: 784–794
184. **Brandt, D.J., Johnson, C.D., Stephens, D.H., Weiland, L.H.**: Imaging of fibrolamellar hepatocellular carcinoma. Amer. J. Radiol. 1988; 151: 295–299
185. **Chang, Y.C., Dai, Y.C., Chow, N.H.**: Fibrolamellar hepatocellular carcinoma with a recurrence of classic hepatocellular carcinoma: a case report and review of oriental cases. Hepato-Gastroenterol. 2003; 50: 1637–1640
186. **Hui, M.-S., Choi, W.-M., Perng, H.-L., Chen, L.-K., Yang, K.-C., Chen, T.-F.**: Fibrolamellar hepatocellular carcinoma – an atypical MR manifestation. Hepato-Gastroenterol. 1998; 45: 514–517
187. **Ichikawa, T., Federle, M.P., Grazioli, L., Marsh, W.**: Fibrolamellar hepatocellular carcinoma: pre- and posttherapy evaluation with CT and MR imaging. Radiology 2000; 217: 145–151
188. **Katzenstein, H.M., Krailo, M.D., Malogolowkin, M.H., Ortega, J.A., Qu, W.C., Douglass, E.C., Feusner, J.H., Reynolds, M., Quinn, J.J., Newman, K., Finegold, M.J., Haas, J.E., Sensel, M.G., Castleberry, R.P., Bowman, L.C.**: Fibrolamellar hepatocellular carcinoma in children and adolescents. Cancer 2003; 97: 2006–2012
189. **Martinez Isla, A., Ferrara, A., Badia, J.M., Holloway, I., Tanaka, H., Riaz, A., Habib, N.A.**: Fibrolamellar hepatocellular carcinoma: results of partial liver resection. Rev. Esp. Enf. Digest. 1997; 89: 703–705
190. **Pinna, A.D., Iwatsuki, S., Lee, R.G., Todo, S., Madariaga, J.R., Marsh, J.W., Casavilla, A., Dvorchik, I., Fung, J.J., Starzl, T.E.**: Treatment of fibrolamellar hepatoma with subtotal hepatectomy or transplantation. Hepatology 1997; 26: 877–883
191. **Soreide, O., Czerniak, Al, Bradpiece, H., Bloom, S., Blumgart, L.**: Characteristics of fibrolamellar hepatocellular carcinoma. A study of nine cases and a review of the literature. Amer. J. Surg. 1986; 151: 518–523
192. **Starzl, T.E., Iwatsuki, S., Shaw jr., B.W., Nalesnik, M.A., Farhi, D.C., van Thiel, D.H.**: Treatment of fibrolamellar hepatoma with partial or total hepatectomy and transplantation of the liver. Surg. Gyn. Obstetr. 1986; 162: 145–148
193. **Vecchio, F.M.**: Fibrolamellar carcinoma of the liver: a distinct entity within the hepatocellular tumors. A review. Appl. Pathol. 1988; 6: 139–148
194. **Yamaguchi, R., Tajika, T., Kanda, H., Nakanishi, K., Kawanishi, J.**: Fibrolamellar carcinoma of the liver. Hepato-Gastroenterology 1999; 46: 1706–1709
195. **Yoshimi, F., Asato, Y., Amemiya, R., Itabashi, M., Nakamura, K.**: Fibrolamellar hepatocellular carcinoma in a Japanese man: Report of a case. Surg. Today 2002; 32: 174–179

Cholangiocellular carcinoma

196. Aishima, S., Asayama, Y., Taguchi, K., Sugimachi, K., Shirabe, K., Shimada, M., Sugimachi, K., Tsuneyoshi, M.: The utility of keratin 903 as a new prognostic marker in mass-forming-type intrahepatic cholangiocarcinoma. Mod. Pathol. 2002; 15: 1181–1190
197. Aishima, S., Matsuura, S., Terashi, T., Taguchi, K., Shimada, M., Maehara, Y., Tsuneyoshi, M.: Aberrant expression of laminin gamma 2 chain and its prognostic significance in intrahepatic cholangiocarcinoma according to growth morphology. Mod. Pathol. 2003; 17: 938–945
198. Chen, M.-F., Jan, Y.-Y., Chen, T.-C.: Clinical studies of mucin-producing cholangiocellular carcinoma. Ann. Surg. 1998; 227: 63–69
199. Chu, K.-M., Lai, E.C.S., Al-Hadeedi, S., Arciall, jr., C.E., Lo, C.-M., Liu, C.-L., Fan, S.-T., Wong, J.: Intrahepatic cholangiocarcinoma. World J. Surg. 1997; 21: 301–306
200. DeOliveira, M.L., Cunningham, S.C., Cameron, J.L., Kamangar, F., Winter, J.M., Lillemoe, K.D., Choti, M.A., Yeo, C.J., Schulick, R.D.: Cholangiocarcinoma: Thirty-one-year experience with 564 patients at a single institution. Ann. Surg. 2007; 245: 755–762
201. Goto, N., Yasuda, I., Uematsu, T., Kanemura, N., Takai, S., Ando, K., Kato, T., Osada, S., Takao, H., Saji, S., Shimokawa, K., Moriwaki, H.: Intrahepatic cholangiocarcinoma arising 10 years after the excision of congenital extrahepatic biliary dilation. J. Gastroenterol. 2001; 36: 856–862
202. Haas, S., Gütgemann, I., Wolff, M., Fischer, H.P.: Intrahepatic clear cell cholangiocarcinoma. Immunohistochemical aspects in a very rare type of cholangiocarcinoma. Amer. J. Surg. Path. 2007; 31: 902–906
203. Harrison, L.E., Fong, Y., Klimstra, D.S., Zee, S.Y., Blumgart, L.H.: Surgical treatment of 32 patients with peripheral intrahepatic cholangiocarcinoma. Brit. J. Surg. 1998; 85: 1068–1070
204. Haswell-Elkins, M.R., Satarug, S., Elkins, D.B.: Opisthorchis viverrini infection in northeast Thailand and its relationship to cholangiocarcinoma. J. Gastroenterol. 1992; 7: 538–548
205. Hirohashi, K., Uenishi, T., Kubo, S., Yamamoto, T., Tanaka, H., Shuto, T., Kinoshita, H.: Macroscopic types of intrahepatic cholangiocarcinoma: Clinicopathologic features and surgical outcome. Hepato-Gastroenterol. 2002; 49: 326–329
206. Klatskin, G.: Adenocarcinoma of the hepatic duct and its bifurcation within the porta hepatis. An unusual tumor with distinctive clinical and pathological features. Amer. J. Med. 1965; 38: 241–256
207. Kubo, S., Uenishi, T., Yamamoto, S., Hai, S., Yamamoto, K., Ogawa, M., Takemura, S., Shuto, T., Tanaka, H., Yamazaki, O., Hirohashi, K., Kinoshita, H.: Clinicopathologic characteristics of small intrahepatic cholangiocarcinomas of mass-forming type. Hepatol. Res. 2004; 29: 223–227
208. Lim, J.H.: Cholangiocarcinoma: morphologic classification according to growth pattern and imaging findings. Amer. J. Roentgenol. 2003; 181: 819–827
209. Okami, J., Dono, K., Sakon, M., Tsujie, M., Hayashi, N., Fujiwara, Y., Nagano, H., Umeshita, K., Nakamori, S., Monden, M.: Patterns of regional lymph node involvement in intrahepatic cholangiocarcinoma of the left lobe. J. Gastrointestin. Surg. 2003; 7: 850–856
210. Otto, G.: Diagnostic and surgical approaches in hilar cholangiocarcinoma (review). Internat. J. Colorect. Dis. 2007; 22: 101–108
211. Polizos, A., Kelekis, N., Sinani, C., Patsiaoura, G., Papadamou, G., Dalekos, G.N.: Advanced intrahepatic cholangiocarcinoma in hepatitis C virus-related decompensated cirrhosis: Case report and review of the literature. Eur. J. Gastroenterol. Hepatol. 2003; 15: 331–334
212. Ramage, J.K., Donaghy, A., Farrant, J.M., Iorns, R., Williams, R.: Serum tumor markers for the diagnosis of cholangiocarcinoma in primary sclerosing cholangitis. Gastroenterology 1995; 108: 865–869
213. Rizzi, P.M., Ryder, S.D., Portmann, B., Ramage, J.K., Naoumov, N.V., Williams, R.: p53 protein overexpression in cholangiocarcinoma arising in primary sclerosing cholangitis. Gut. 1996; 38: 265–268
214. Roayaie, S., Guarrera, J.V., Ye, M.Q., Thung, S.N., Emre, S., Fishbein, T.M., Guy, S.R., Sheiner, P.A., Miller, C.M., Schwartz, M.E.: Aggressive surgical treatment of intrahepatic cholangiocarcinoma: Predictors of outcomes. J. Amer. Coll. Surg. 1998; 187: 365–372
215. Sasaki, A., Kawano, K., Aramaki, M., Ohno, T., Tahara, K., Kitano, S.: Correlation between tumor size and mode of spread in mass-forming intrahepatic cholangiocarcinoma. Hepato-Gastroenterol. 2004; 51: 224–228
216. Shiraishi, M., Takushi, Y., Simoji, H., Oshiro, T., Shinzato, S., Tanigawa, N., Kusano, T., Muto, Y.: Combined hepatocellular and cholangiocellular carcinoma in a non-cirrhotic liver. J. Gastroenterol. 1998; 33: 593–596
217. Soyer, P., Bluemke, D.A., Hruban, R.H., Sitzmann, J.V., Fishman, E.K.: Intrahepatic cholangiocarcinoma: findings on spiral CT during arterial portography. Eur. J. Radiol. 1994; 19: 37–42
218. Valls, C., Guma, A., Puig, I., Sanchez, A., Andia, E., Serrano, T., Figueras, J.: Intrahepatic peripheral cholangiocarcinoma: CT evaluation. Abdom. Imag. 2000; 25: 490–496
219. Yoshimoto, H., Ikeda, S., Tanaka, M., Matsumoto, S.: Intrahepatic cholangiocarcinoma associated with hepatolithiasis. Gastroint. Endosc. 1985; 31: 260–263

Mucoepidermoid carcinoma

220. Choi, D., Kim, H., Lee, K.S., Lee, K.G., Park, C.K.: Mucoepidermoid carcinoma of the liver diagnosed as a liver abscess: report of a case. Surg. Today 2004; 34: 968–972
221. De Lajarte-Thirouard, A.S., Rioux-Leclercq, N., Boudjema, K., Gandon, Y., Ramee, M.P., Turlin, B.: Squamous cell carcinoma arising in a hepatic forgut cyst (case report). Pathol. Res. Pract. 2002; 198: 697–700
222. Kang, H.Y., Park, Y.N., Kim, S.E., Sohn, K.R., Yoo, N.C., Park, J.Y., Kim, K.S., Park, C.: Double primary mucoepidermoid carcinoma and hepatocellular carcinoma of the liver. A case report. Hepato-Gastroenterol. 2003; 50: 238–241
223. Maeda, T., Takenaka, K., Taguchi, K., Kajiyama, K., Shirabe, K., Shimada, M., Tsuneyoshi, M., Sugimachi, K.: Adenosquamous carcinoma of the liver. Clinicopathologic characteristics and cytokeratin profile. Cancer 1997; 80: 364–371
224. Monteagudo, M., Vidal, G., Moreno, M., Bella, R., Diaz, M.J., Colomer, O., Santesmasses, A.: Squamous cell carcinoma and infection in a solitary hepatic cyst. Eur. J. Gastroenterol. Hepatol. 1998; 10: 1051–1053
225. Pianzola, L.E., Drut, R.: Mucoepidermoid carcinoma of the liver. Amer. J. Clin. Pathol. 1971; 56: 758–761
226. Yagi, H., Ueda, M., Kawachi, S., Tanabe, M., Aiura, K., Wakabayashi, G., Shimazu, M., Sakamoto, M., Kitajima, M.: Squamous cell carcinoma of the liver originating from non-parasitic cysts after a 15 year follow-up (case report). Eur. J. Gastroenterol. Hepatol. 2004; 16: 1051–1056
227. Yeh, C.-N., Jan, Y.-Y., Chen, M.-F.: Adenosquamous carcinoma of the liver: Clinicopathologic study of 10 surgically treated cases. World J. Surg. 2003; 27: 168–172

Biliary cystadenocarcinoma

228. Choi, B.I., Lim, J.H., Han, M.C., Lee, D.H., Kim, S.H., Kim, Y.I., Kim, C.-W.: Biliary cystadenoma and cystadenocarcinoma: CT and sonographic findings. Radiology 1989; 171: 57–61
229. Devaney, K., Goodman, Z.D., Ishak, K.G.: Hepatobiliary cystadenoma and cystadenocarcinoma. A light and microscopic and immunohistochemical study of 70 patients. Amer. J. Surg. Pathol. 1994; 18: 1078–1091
230. Horsmans, Y., Laka, A., van Beers, B.E., Descamps, C., Gigot, J.F., Geupel, A.P.: Hepatobiliary cystadenocarcinoma without ovarian stroma and normal CA 19-9 levels. Dig. Dis. Sci. 1997; 42: 1406–1408
231. Kinoshita, H., Tanimura, H., Onishi, H., Kasano, Y., Uchiyama, K., Yamaue, H.: Clinical features and imaging diagnosis of biliary cystadenocarcinoma of the liver. Hepato-Gastroenterol. 2001; 48: 250–252
232. Kubota, E., Katsumi, K., Iida, M., Kishimoto, A., Ban, Y., Nakata, K., Takahashi, N., Kobayashi, K., Andoh, K., Takanashi, A., Joh, T.: Biliary cystadenocarcinoma followed up as benign cystadenoma for 10 years (case report). J. Gastroenterol. 2003; 38: 278–282
233. Sato, M., Watanabe, Y., Tokui, K., Kohtani, T., Nakata, Y., Chen, Y., Kawachi, K.: Hepatobiliary cystadenocarcinoma connected to the hepatic duct: a case report and review of the literature. Hepato-Gastroenterol. 2003; 50: 1621–1624
234. Shrikhande, S., Kleeff, J., Adyanthaya, K., Zimmermann, A., Shrikhande, V.: Management of hepatobiliary cystadenocarcinoma. Dig. Surg. 2003; 20: 60–63
235. Wee, A., Nilsson, B., Kang, J.Y., Tan, L.K., Rauff, A.: Biliary cystadenocarcinoma arising in a cystadenoma. Report of a case diagnosed by fine needle aspiration cytology. Acta Cytol. 1993; 37: 966–970

Hepatoblastoma

236. Bernstein, I.T., Bulow, S., Mauritzen, K.: Hepatoblastoma in two cousins in a family with adenomatous polyposis. Report of two cases. Dis. Colon Rectum 1992; 35: 373–374
237. Boechat, M.I., Kangarloo, H., Ortega, J., Hall, T., Feig, St., Stanley, P., Gilsanz, V.: Primary liver tumors in children: comparison of CT and MR imaging. Radiology 1988; 169: 727–732
238. Edmondson, H.A.: Differential diagnosis of tumors and tumor-like lesions of liver in infancy and childhood. Amer. J. Dis. Child. 1956; 91: 168–189
239. Fish, J.C., McCary, R.G.: Primary cancer of the liver in childhood. Arch. Surg. 1966; 93: 355–359
240. Koneru, B., Flye, M.W., Busuttil, R.W., Shaw, B.W., Lorber, M.I., Emond, J.C., Kalayoglu, M., Freese, D.K., Starzl, T.E.: Liver transplantation for hepatoblastoma. The American experience. Ann. Surg. 1991; 213: 118–121
241. Manivel, C., Wick, M.R., Abenoza, P., Dehner, L.P.: Teratoid hepatoblastoma. The nosologic dilemma of solid embryonic neoplasms of childhood. Cancer 1986; 57: 2168–2174
242. Remes-Troche, J.M., Montano-Loza, A., Meza-Dunco, J., Garcia-Leiva, J., Torre-Delgadillo, A.: Hepatoblastoma in adult age. A case report and literature review. Ann. Hepatol. 2006; 5: 179–181
243. Steiner, M.M.: Primary carcinoma of the liver in childhood. Report of two cases, with a critical review of the literatur. Amer. J. Dis. Child. 1938; 55: 807–824
244. Weinberg, A.G., Feingold, M.J.: Primary hepatic tumors of childhood. Hum. Pathol. 1983; 14: 512–537
245. Yamazaki, M., Ryu, M., Okazumi, S., Kondo, F., Cho, A., Okada, T., Takayama, W., Kawashima, T., Furuki, A., Hirata, T.: Hepatoblastoma in an adult – a case report and clinical review of literature. Hepatol. Res. 2004; 30: 82–188

Embryonal sarcoma

246. Baron, P.W., Majlessipour, F., Bedros, A.A., Zuppan, C.W., Ben-Youssef, R., Yanni, G., Ojogho, O.N., Concepcion, W.: Undifferentiated embryonal sarcoma of the liver successfully treated with chemotherapy and liver resection. J. Gastrointest Surg. 2007; 11: 73–75
247. Buetow, P.C., Buck, J.L., Pantongrag-Brown, L., Marshall, W.H., Ros, P.R., Levine, M.S., Goodman, Z.D.: Undifferentiated (embryonal) sar-

coma of the liver. Pathologic basis of imaging findings in 28 cases. Radiology 1997; 203: 779–783
248. Houry, S., Gharbi, L., Huguier, M., Callard, P., André, T.: Undifferentiated embryonal sarcoma in the liver of adults. Presse Med. 1998; 27: 518–520
249. Lauwers, G.Y., Grant, L.D., Donnelly, W.H., Meloni, A.M., Foss, R.M., Sanberg, A.A., Langham, M.R.: Hepatic undifferentiated (embryonal) sarcoma arising in a mesenchymal hamartoma. Amer. J. Surg. Pathol. 1997; 21: 1248–1254
250. Leuschner, I., Schmidt, D., Harms, D.: Undifferentiated sarcoma of the liver in childhood: morphology, flow cytometry and literature review. Hum. Pathol. 1990; 21: 68–76
251. Stocker, J.T., Ishak, K.G.: Undifferentiated (embryonal) sarcoma of the liver. Report of 31 cases. Cancer 1978; 42: 336–348
252. Walker, N.I., Horn, M.J., Strong, R.W., Lynch, S.V., Cohen, J., Ong, T.H., Harris, O.D.: Undifferentiated (embryonal) sarcoma of the liver. Pathologic findings and long-term survival after complete surgical resection. Cancer 1992; 69: 52–59
253. Webber, E.M., Morrison, K.B., Pritchard, S.L., Sorensen, P.H.B.: Undifferentiated embryonal sarcoma of the liver: results of clinical management in one center. J. Pediatr. Surg. 1999; 34: 1641–1644

Epithelioid haemangioendothelioma
254. Demetris, A.J., Minervini, M., Raikow, R.B., Lee, R.G.: Hepatic epithelioid hemangioendothelioma. Amer. J. Surg. Pathol. 1997; 21: 263–270
255. Den Bakker, M.A., den Bakker, A.J., Beenen, R., Mulder, A.H., Eulderink, F.: Subtotal liver calcification due to epithelioid hemangioendothelioma. Path. Res. Pract. 1998; 194: 189–195
256. Dietze, O., Davies, S.E., Williams, R., Portmann, B.: Malignant epithelioid hemangioendothelioma of the liver: A clinicopathological and histochemical study of 12 cases. Histopathology 1989; 15: 225–237
257. Furuta, K., Sodeyama, T., Usuda, S., Yoshizawa, K., Kiyosawa, K., Furuta, S., Imai, Y., Itoh, N., Fukuzawa, M., Hotchi, M.: Epithelioid hemangioendothelioma of the liver diagnosed by liver biopsy under laparoscopy. Amer. J. Gastroenterol. 1992; 87: 797–800
258. Ishak, K.G., Sesterhenn, I.A., Goodman, M.Z.D., Rabin, L., Stromeyer, F.W.: Epithelioid hemangioendothelioma of the liver: a clinicopathologic and follow-up study of 32 cases. Hum. Pathol. 1984; 15: 839–852
259. Kayler, L.K., Merion, R.M., Arenas, J.D., Magee, J.C., Campbell, D.A., Rudich, S.M., Punch, J.D.: Epithelioid hemangioendothelioma of the liver disseminated to the peritoneum treated with liver transplantation and interferon alpha-2b. Transplantation 2002; 74: 128–130
260. Kelleher, M.B., Iwatsuki, S., Sheahan, D.G.: Epithelioid hemangioendothelioma of liver: clinicopathological correlation of 10 cases treated by orthotopic liver transplantation. Amer. J. Surg. Pathol. 1989; 13: 999–1008
261. Lyburn, I.D., Torreggiani, W.C., Harris, A.C., Zwirewich, C.V., Buckley, A.R., Davis, J.E., Chung, S.W., Scudamore, C.H., Ho, S.G.F.: Hepatic epithelioid hemangioendothelioma: sonographic, CT, and MRT imaging appearances. Amer. J. Roentgenol. 2003; 180: 1359–1364
262. Makhlouf, H.R., Ishak, K.G., Goodman, Z.D.: Epitheloid hemangioendothelioma of the liver. A clinicopathologic study of 137 cases. Cancer 1999; 85: 562–582
263. Malamut, G., Perlemuter, G., Buffet, C., Bedossa, P., Joly, J.P., Colombat, M., Kuoch, V., Pelletier, G.: Epithelioid hemangioendothelioma in a patient with nodular regenerative hyperplasia. Gastroenterol. Clin. Biol. 2001; 25: 1105–1107
264. Marino, I.R., Todo, S., Tzakis, A.G., Klintmalm, G., Kelleher, M., Iwatsuki, S., Starzl, T.E., Esquivel, C.O.: Treatment of hepatic epithelioid hemangioendothelioma with liver transplantation. Cancer 1988; 62: 2079–2084
265. Mehrabi, A., Kashfi, A., Fonouni, H., Schemmer, P., Schmied, B.M., Hallscheidt, P., Schirmacher, P., Weitz, J., Friess, H., Büchler, M.W., Schmidt, J.: Primary malignant hepatic epithelioid haemangioendothelioma: A comprehensive review of the literature with emphasis on the surgical therapy. Cancer 2006; 107: 2109–2121
266. Mermuys, K., Vanhoenacker, P.K., Roskams, T., Dhaenens, P., Van Hoe, L.: Epithelioid hemangioendothelioma of the liver: Radiologic-pathologic correlation. Abdom. Imag. 2004; 29: 221–223
267. Miller, W.J., Dodd, G.D., Federle, M.P., Baron, R.L.: Epitheloid hemangioendothelioma of the liver: imaging findings with pathologic correlation. Amer. J. Roentg. 1992; 159: 53–57
268. Walsh, M.M., Hytiroglou, P., Thung, S.N., Fiel, I., Siegel, D., Emre, S., Ishak, K.G.: Epithelioid hemangioendothelioma of the liver mimicking Budd-Chiari syndrome. Arch. Pathol. Lab. Med. 1998; 122: 846–848

Angiosarcoma
269. Awan, S., Davenport, M., Portmann, B., Howard, E.R.: Angiosarcoma of the liver in children. J. Pediatr. Surg. 1996; 31: 1729–1732
270. Bolt, H.M.: Vinylchlorid – a classical industrial toxicant of new interest. Crit. Rev. Toxicol. 2005; 35: 307–323
271. Falk, H., Thomas, L.B., Popper, H., Ishak, K.G.: Hepatic angiosarcoma associated with androgenic-anabolic steroids. Lancet 1979/II: 1120–1123
272. Hertzanu, Y., Peiser, J., Zirkin, H.: Massive bleeding after fine needle aspiration of liver angiosarcoma. Gastrointest. Radiol. 1990; 15: 42–46
273. Kojiro, M., Nakashima, T., Ito, Y., Ikezaki, H., Moni, T., Kido, C.: Thorium dioxide-related angiosarcoma of the liver: Pathomorphologic study of 29 autopsy cases. Arch. Path. Lab. Med. 1985; 109: 853–857
274. Koyama, T., Fletcher, J.G., Johnson, C.D., Kuo, M.S., Notohara, K., Burgart, L.J.: Primary hepatic angiosarcoma: Findings at CT and MR imaging. Radiology 2002; 222: 667–673
275. Maeda, T., Tateishi, U., Hasegawa, T., Ojima, H., Arai, Y., Sugimura, K.: Primary hepatic angiosarcoma on coregistered FDG PET and CT images (case report). Amer. J. Roentgenol. 2007; 188: 1615–1617
276. Mark, L., Delorme, F., Creech, J.L., Odgen, L.L., Fadell, E.H., Songster, C.L., Clanton, J., Johnson, M.N., Christopherson, W.M.: Clinical and morphological features of hepatic angiosarcoma in vinyl chloride workers. Cancer 1976; 37: 149–163
277. Molina, E., Hernandez, A.: Clinical manifestations of primary hepatic angiosarcoma. Dig. Dis. Sci. 2003; 48: 677–682
278. Salgado, M., Sans, M., Forns, X., Bruguera, M., Castells, A., Navasa, M., Rodes, J.: Hepatic angiosarcoma: A report of a case associated treatment with arsenic salts and a review of the literature. Gastroenterol. Hepatol. 1995; 18: 132–135

Leiomyosarcoma
279. Baur, M., Pötzi, R., Lochs, H., Neuhold, N., Walgram, M., Gangl, A.: Primary leiomyosarcoma of the liver – a case report. Z. Gastroenterol. 1993; 31: 20–23
280. Celdran, A., Frieyro, O., del Rio, A., Franco, A., Bosch, O., Sarasa, J.L.: Leiomyosarcoma of the portal venous system: A case report and review of literature. Surgery 2004; 135: 455–456
281. Cioffi, U., Quattrone, P., de Simone, M., Bonavia, L., Segalin, A., Masini, T., Montorsi, M.: Primary multiple epithelioid leiomyosarcoma of the liver. Hepato-Gastroenterol. 1996; 43: 1603–1605
282. Civardi, G., Cavanna, L., Iovine, E., Buscarini, E., Vallisa, D., Buscarini, L.: Diagnostic imaging of primary hepatic leiomyosarcoma: A case report. Ital. J. Gastroenterol. 1996; 28: 98–101
283. Griffin, A.S., Sterchi, J.M.: Primary leiomyosarcoma of the inferior vena cava: a case report and review of the literature. J. Surg. Oncol. 1987; 34: 53–60
284. Maki, H.S., Hubert, B.C., Sajjad, S.M., Kirchner, J.P., Kuehner, M.E.: Primary hepatic leiomyosarcoma. Arch. Surg. 1987; 122: 1193–1196

Rhabdomyosarcoma
285. Burrig, K.F., Knauer, S.: Rhabdomyosarcoma of the liver in adulthood. Case report and review of the literature. Pathologe 1994; 15: 54–57
286. Cote, R.J., Urmacher, C.: Rhabdomyosarcoma of the liver associated with long-term oral contraceptive use. Amer. J. Surg. Pathol. 1990; 14: 784–790
287. Huang, F.C., Eng, H.L., Chen, C.L., Ko, S.F.: Primary pleomorphic rhabdomyosarcoma of the liver: A case report. Hepato-Gastroenterol. 2003; 50: 73–76

Fibrosarcoma
288. Ito, Y., Uesaka, Y., Takeshita, S., Fujino, H., Uta, Y., Yasuda, H., Oshima, M., Kawabe, T., Tagawa, K., Unuma, T., Nakahama, M., Takanashi, R.: A case report of primary fibrosarcoma of the liver. Gastroenterol. Jpn. 1990; 25: 753–757
289. Nakahama, M., Takanashi, R., Yamazaki, I., Machinami, R.: Primary fibrosarcoma of the liver. Acta Pathol. Japon. 1989; 39: 814–820

Fibrous histiocytoma
290. Ferrozzi, F., Bova, D.: Hepatic malignant fibrous histiocytoma: CT findings. Clin. Radiol. 1998; 53: 699–701
291. Fujita, S., Lauwers, G.Y.: Primary hepatic malignant fibrous histiocytoma: report of a case and review of the literature. Pathol. Inst. 1998; 48: 225–229
292. Katsuda, S., Kawahara, E., Matsui, Y., Ohyama, S., Nakanishi, I.: Malignant fibrous histiocytoma of the liver: a case report and review of the literature. Amer. J. Gastroenterol. 1988; 83: 1278–1282
293. Schweyer, S., Meyer-Venter, R., Lorf, T., Sattler, B., Fayyazi, A.: Malignes fibröses Histiozytom der Leber. Z. Gastroenterol. 2000; 38: 243–248
294. Yu, J.S., Kim, K.W., Kim, C.S., Yoon, K.H., Jeong, H.J., Lee, D.G.: Primary malignant fibrous histiocytoma of the liver. Imaging features of five surgically confirmed cases. Abdom. Imag. 1999; 24: 386–391

Schwannoma
295. Morikawa, Y., Ishihara, Y., Matsuura, N., Miyamoto, H., Kakudo, K.: Malignant schwannoma of the liver. Dig. Dis. Sci. 1995; 40: 1279–1282
296. Young, S.J.: Primary malignant neurilemma (schwannoma) of the liver in a case of neurofibromatosis. J. Pathol. 1975; 117: 151–153

Liposarcoma
297. Kim, Y.I., Yu, E.S., Lee, K.W., Park, E.U., Song, H.G.: Dedifferentiated liposarcoma of the liver. Cancer 1987; 60: 2785–2790
298. Wright, N.B., Skinner, R., Lee, R.E., Craft, A.W.: Myxoid liposarcoma of the porta hepatis in childhood. Pediatr. Radiol. 1993; 23: 620–621

Osteosarcoma
299. Govender, D., Rughubar, K.N.: Primary hepatic osteosarcoma: case report and literature review. Pathology 1998; 30: 323–325
300. Hochstetter, A.R., Hattenschwiler, J., Vogt, M.: Primary osteosarcoma of the liver. Cancer 1987; 60: 2312–2317

Hepatic Gastrinoma
301. Diaz, R., Aparicio, J., Pous, S., Dolz, J.F., Calderero, V.: Primary hepatic gastrinoma. Dig. Dis. Sci. 2003; 48: 1665–1667
302. Moriura, S., Ikeda, S., Hirai, M., Naiki, K., Fugioka, T., Yokochi, K., Gotou, S.: Hepatic gastrinoma. Cancer 1993; 72: 1547–1550

303. Smyrniotis, V., Kehagias, D., Kostopanagiotou, G., Tripolitsioti, P., Paphitis, A.: Primary hepatic gastrinoma. Amer. J. Gastroenterol. 1999; 94: 3380–3382
304. Tiommy, E., Brill, S., Baratz, M., Messer, G., Greif, F., Moshkowitz, M., Gilat, T.: Primary liver gastrinoma. J. Clin. Gastroenterol. 1997; 24: 188–191
305. Van der Hoef, M., Crook, D.W., Marincek, B., Weishaupt, D.: Primary neuroendocrine tumours of the liver: MRI features in two cases. Abdom. Imag. 2004; 29: 77–81

Carcinoid tumour

306. Asakawa, T., Tomioka, T., Abe, K., Yamaguchi, T., Tsunoda, T., Kanematsu, T.: Primary hepatic carcinoid tumor. J. Gastroenterol. 1999; 34: 123–127
307. Hirata, M., Ishida, H., Konno, K., Naganuma, H., Nakajima, K., Igarashi, K., Onji, M., Iuchi, H., Nishiura, S., Maeda, T.: Primary carcinoid tumor of the liver: Report of two cases with an emphasis on US findings. Abdom. Imag. 2002; 27: 325–328
308. Kim, S.R., Imoto, S., Maekawa, Y., Matsuoka, T., Hayashi, Y., Ando, K., Mita, K., Shintani, S., Kim, H.B., Ku, K., Koterazawa, T., Fukuda, K., Yano, Y., Nakaji, M., Ikawa, H., Ninomiya, T., Kudo, M., Kim, K.I., Hirai, M.: CEA producing primary hepatic carcinoid. Hepatol. Res. 2002; 22: 313–321
309. Mizuno, Y., Ohkohchi, N., Fujimori, K., Doi, H., Orii, T., Asakura, T., Kimura, N., Pilichowska, M., Inomata, M., Satomi, S.: Primary hepatic carcinoid tumor: a case report. Hepato-Gatroenterol. 2000; 47: 528–530

Malignant lymphoma

310. Anthony, P.P., Sarsfield, P., Clarke, T.: Primary lymphoma of the liver: clinical and pathological features of 10 patients. J. Clin. Pathol. 1990; 43: 1007–1013
311. Avlonitis, V.S., Linos, D.: Primary hepatic lymphoma: a review. Eur. J. Surg. 1999; 165: 725–729
312. Baschinsky, D.Y., Weidner, N., Baker, P.B., Frankel, W.L.: Primary hepatic anaplastic large-cell lymphoma of T-cell phenotype in acquired immunodeficiency syndrome: a report of an autopsy case and review of the literature. Amer. J. Gastroenterol. 2001; 96: 227–232
313. Castroagudin, J.F., Molina, E., Abdulkader, I., Forteza, J., Delgado, M.B., Dominguez-Munoz, J.E.: Sonographic features of liver involvement by lymphoma. J. Ultrasound. Med. 2007; 26: 791–796
314. Dargent, J.L., de Wolf-Petersen, C.: Liver involvement by malignant lymphoma. Identification of a distinctive pattern of infiltration related to T-cell / histiocyte-rich B-cell lymphoma. Ann. Diagn. Path. 1998; 2: 363–369
315. DeMent, S.H., Mann, R.B., Staal, S.P., Kuhadja, F.P., Boitnott, J.K.: Primary lymphoma of the liver: Report of six cases and review of the literature. Amer. J. Clin. Pathol. 1987; 88: 255–263
316. Loddenkemper, C., Longerich, T., Hummel, M., Ernestus, K., Anagnostopoulos, I., Dienes, H.P., Schirmacher, P., Stein, H.: Frequency and diagnostic patterns of lymphomas in liver biopsies with respect to the WHO classification. Virchows Arch. 2007; 450: 493–502
317. Matsumoto, S., Mori, H., Takaki, H., Ishitobi, F., Shuto, R., Yokoyama, S.: Malignant lymphoma with tumor thrombus in the portal venous system. Abdom. Imag. 2004; 29: 460–462
318. Salhany, K.E., Feldman, M., Kahn, M.J., Peritt, D., Schretzmair, R.D., Wilson, D.M., DiPaola, R.S., Glick, A.D., Kant, J.A., Nowell, P.C., Kamoun, M.: Hepatosplenic γδ T-cell lymphoma: ultrastructural immunophenotypic, and functional evidence for cytotoxic T-lymphocyte differentiation. Hum. Pathol. 1997; 28: 674–685
319. Sato, S., Masuda, T., Oikawa, H., Satoh, T., Suzuki, Y., Takikawa, Y., Yamazaki, K., Suzuki, K., Sato, S.: Primary hepatic lymphoma associated with primary biliary cirrhosis. Amer. J. Gastroenterol. 1999; 94: 1669–1673
320. Zafrani, E.S., Gaulard, P.: Primary lymphoma of the liver. Liver 1993; 13: 57–61

Liver metastases

321. Adam, R., Bismuth, H., Castaing, D., Waechter, F., Navarro, F., Abascal, A., Majno, P., Engerran, L.: Repeat hepatectomy for colorectal liver metastases. Ann. Surg. 1997; 225: 51–62
322. Ambiru, S., Miyazaki, M., Isoni, T., Ito, H., Nakagawa, K., Shimizu, H., Kusashio, K., Furuya, S., Nakajima, N.: Hepatic resection for colorectal metastases – Analysis of prognostic factors. Dis. Colon Rect. 1999; 42: 632–639
323. Antoniou, A., Lovegrove, R.P., Tilney, H.S., Heriot, A.G., John, T.G., Rees, M., Tekkis, P.P., Welsh, F.K.S.: Metaanalysis of clinical outcome after first and second liver resection for colorectal metastases. (review). Surgery 2007; 141: 9–18
324. Athanasakis, E., Mouloudi, E., Prinianakis, G., Kostaki, M., Tzardi, M., Georgopoulos, D.: Metastatic liver disease and fulminant hepatic failure: Presentation of a case and review of the literature. Eur. J. Gastroenterol. Hepatol. 2003; 15: 1235–1240
325. Bartlett, D.L., Libutti, S.K., Figg, W.D., Fraker, D.L., Alexander, H.R.: Isolated hepatic perfusion for unresectable hepatic metastases from colorectal cancer. Surgery 2001; 129: 176–187
326. Bläker, H., Hofmann, W.J., Theuer, D., Otto, H.F.: Pathohistologic findings in liver metastases. Radiology 2001; 41: 1–7
327. Botet, J.F., Watson, R.C., Kemeny, N., Daly, J.M., Yeh, S.: Cholangitis complicating intraarterial chemotherapy in liver metastases. Radiology 1985; 156: 335–337
328. Bramkamp, M., Dedes, K.J., Strobel, K., Pahnke, J., Breitenstein, S., Clavien, P.A.: Cholestasis from malignant melanoma. J. Clin. Oncol. 2007; 25: 725–726
329. Carlini, M., Leonardo, M.T., Carboni, F., Petric, M., Vitucci, C., Santoro, R., Lepiane, P., Ettorre, G.M., Santoro, E.: Liver metastases from breast cancer. Results of surgical resection. Hepato-Gastroenterol. 2002; 49: 1597–1601
330. Cavallari, A., Vivarelli, M., Bellusci, R., Montalti, R., De Ruvo, N., Cuccetti, A., De Vivo, A., De Raffele, E., Salone, M.C., La Barba, G.: Liver metastases from colorectal cancer: Present surgical approach. Hepato-Gastroenterol. 2003; 50: 2067–2071
331. Christophi, C., Nikfarjam, M., Malcontenti-Wilson, C., Muralidharan, V.: Long-term survival of patients with unresectable colorectal liver metastases treated by percutaneous interstitial laser thermotherapy. World J. Surg. 2004; 28: 987–994
332. Drixler, T.A., Rinkes, I.H.M., Ritchie, E.D., van Vroonhoven, T.J.M.V., Gebbink, M.F.B.G., Voest, E.E.: Continuous administration of angiostatin inhibits accelerated growth of colorectal liver metastases after partial hepatectomy. Canc. Res. 2000; 60: 1761–1765
333. Dromain C., de Baere, T., Lumbroso, J., Caillet, H., Laplanche, A.S., Boige, V., Ducreux, M., Duvillard, P., Elias, D., Schlumberger, M., Sigal, R., Baudin, E.: Detection of liver metastases from endocrine tumors: a prospective comparison of somatostatin receptor scintigraph, computed tomography, and magnetic resonance imaging. J. Clin Oncol. 005; 23: 70–78
334. Francis, A., Temple, J.G., Hallissey, M.T.: Spontaneous resolution of histologically proven liver metastases from colorectal cancer. Brit. J. Surg. 1997; 84: 818
335. Fretz, C.J., Stark, D.D., Metz, C.E., Elizondo, G., Weissleder, R., Shen, J.-H., Wittenberg, J., Simeone, J., Ferrucci, J.T.: Detection of hepatic metastases: comparison of contrast-enhanced CT, unenhanced MR imaging and iron oxide enhanced MR imaging. Amer. J. Roentgenol. 1990; 155: 763–770
336. Fujii, K., Fujioka, S., Kato, K., Machiki, Y., Kutsuna, Y., Ishikawa, A., Takamizawa, J., Mizutani, K., Ko, K., Youshida, K.: Factors influencing survival in 33 patients undergoing resection of hepatic metastases from colorectal cancer. Hepato-Gastroenterol. 2000; 47: 607–611
337. Fusai, G., Davidson, B.R.: Strategies to increase the resectability of liver metastases from colorectal cancer. Dig. Surg. 2003; 20: 481–496
338. Giovannini, M., Seitz, F.J.: Ultrasound-guided percutaneous alcohol injection of small liver metastases. Results in 40 patients. Cancer 1994; 73: 294–297
339. Haage, P., Tacke, J.: MR-guided percutaneous cryotherapy of liver metastases. Radiologe 2001; 41: 77–83
340. Hale, H.L., Husband, J.E., Gossios, K., Norman, A.R., Cunningham, D.: CT of calcified liver metastases in colorectal carcinoma. Clin. Radiol. 1998; 53: 735–741
341. Hanazaki, K., Kawamura, N., Wakabayashi, M., Sodeyama, H., Yokoyama, S., Sode, Y., Miyazaki, T.: Long-term survivor with liver metastases from rectal cancer treated by hepatectomy after hepatic arterial infusion chemotherapy. Hepato-Gastroenterol. 1998; 45: 816–820
342. Harrison, H.B., Middleton, H.M. III, Crosby, J.H., Dasher, M.N. jr.: Fulminant hepatic failure: an unusual presentation of metastatic liver disease. Gastroenterology 1981; 80: 820–825
343. Hartley, J.E., Kumar, H., Drew, P.J., Heer, K., Avery, G.R., Duthie, G.S., Monson, J.R.T.: Laparoscopic ultrasound for the detection of hepatic metastases during laparoscopic colorectal cancer surgery. Dis. Colon Rect. 2000; 43: 320–325
344. Heslin, M.J., Medina-Franco, H., Parker, M., Vickers, S.M., Aldrete, J., Urist, M.M.: Colorectal hepatic metastases – Resection, local ablation, and hepatic artery infusion pump are associated with prolonged survival. Arch. Surg. 2001; 136: 318–323
345. Howell, J.D., Warren, H.W., Anderson, J.H., Kerr, D.J., McArdle, C.S.: Intra-arterial 5-fluorouracil and intravenous folinic acid in the treatment of liver metastases from colorectal cancer. Eur. J. Surg. 1999; 165: 652–658
346. Ikuta, S., Miki, C., Ookura, E., Tonouchi, H., Kusunoki, M.: Spontaneous regression of a metastatic liver tumor: Report of a case. Surg. Today 2002; 32: 844–848
347. Jarnagin, W.R., Conlon, K., Bodniewicz, J., Dougherty, E., DeMatteo, R.P., Blumgart, L.H., Fong, Y.: A clinical scoring system predicts the yield of diagnostic laparoscopy in patients with potentially resectable hepatic colorectal metastases. Cancer 2001; 91: 1121–1128
348. Karube, H., Masuda, H., Hayashi, S., Ishii, Y., Nemoto, N.: Fatty liver suppressed the angiogenesis in liver metastatic lesions. Hepato-Gastroenterol. 2000; 47: 1541–1545
349. Kerkar, S., Carlin, A.M., Sohn, R.L., Steffes, C., Tyburski, J., Littrup, P., Weaver, D.: Long-term follow up and prognostic factors for cryotherapy of malignant tumours. Surgery 2004; 136: 770–779
350. Kinkel, K., Lu, Y., Both, M., Warren, R.S., Thoeni, R.F.: Detection of hepatic metastases from cancer of the gastrointestinal tract by using noninvasive imaging methods (US, CT, MR imaging, PET): a metaanalysis. Radiology 2002; 224: 748–756
351. Koch, M., Kienle, P., Hinz, U., Antolovic, D., Schmidt, J., Hefarth, C., von Knebel doeberitz, M., Weitz, J.: Detection of hematogenous tumor cell dissemination predicts tumor relapse in patients undergoing surgical resetion of colorectal liver metastases. Ann. Surg. 2005; 241: 199–205
352. Larsen, L.P., Rosenkilde, M., Christensen, H., Bang, N., Bolvig, L., Christiansen, T., Laurberg, S.: The value of contrast enhanced ultraso-

nography in detection of liver metastases from colorectal cancer. A prospective double-blind study. Eur. J. Radiol. 2007; 62: 302–307
353. **Livraghi, T., Goldberg, S.N., Monti, F., Bizzini, A., Lazzaroni, S., Meloni, F., Pellicano, S., Solbiati, L., Gazelle, G.S.:** Saline-enhanced radiofrequency tissue ablation in the treatment of liver metastases. Radiology 1997; 202: 205–210
354. **Lorenz, M., Hochmuth, K., Müller, H.H.:** Hepatic arterial infusion of chemotherapy for metastatic colorectal cancer. New Engl. J. Med. 2000; 342: 1525–1526
355. **Lygidakis, N.J., Spentzouris, N., Dedemadi, G.:** Resectional liver surgery in metastatic liver disease. Hepato-Gastroenterology 1998; 45: 1034–1038
356. **Mack, M.G., Straub, R., Eichler, K., Söllner, O., Lehnert, T., Vogl, T.J.:** Breast cancer metastases in liver: Laser-induced interstitial thermotherapy. Local tumor control rate and surival data. Radiology 2004; 233: 400–409
357. **Maeda, M., Nagawa, H., Maeda, T., Koike, H., Kasai, H.:** Alcohol consumption enhances liver metastasis in colorectal carcinoma patients. Cancer 1998; 83: 1483–1488
358. **Mala, T., Edwin, B., Mathisen, O., Tillung, T., Fosse, E., Bergan, A., Soreide, O., Gladhaug, I.:** Cryoablation of colorectal liver metastases: minimally invasive tumour control. Scand. J. Gastroenterol. 2004; 39: 571–578
359. **Middleton, W.D., Hiskes, S.K., Teefey, S.A., Boucher, L.D.:** Small (1.5 cm or less) liver metastases: US-guided biopsy. Radiology 1997; 205: 729–732
360. **Milsom, J.W., Jerby, B.L., Kessler, H., Hale, J.C., Herts, B.R., O'Malley, C.M.:** Prospective blinded comparison of laparoscopic ultrasonography vs. contrast-enhanced computerized tomography for liver assessment in patients undergoing colorectal carcinoma surgery. Dis. Colon Rect. 2000; 43: 44–49
361. **Nave, H., Mössinger, E., Feist, H., Lang, H., Raab, H.R.:** Surgery as primary treatment in patients with liver metastases from carcinoid tumours: a retrospective, unicentric study over 13 years. Surgery 2001; 129: 170–175
362. **Okano, K., Yamamoto, J., Kosuge, T., Yamamoto, S., Sakamoto, M., Nakanishi, Y., Hirohashi, S.:** Fibrous pseudocapsule of metastatic liver tumors from colorectal carcinoma – clinicopathological study of 152 first resection cases. Cancer 2000; 89: 267–275
363. **Pereira-Lima, J.E., Lichtenfels, E., Barboso, F.S., Zettler, C.G., Uldrich-Kulczynski, J.M.:** Prevalence study of metastases in cirrhotic livers. Hepato-Gastroenterol. 2003; 50: 1490–1495
364. **Prasad, P., Schmulewitz, N., Patel, A., Varadarajulu, S., Wildi, S.M., Roberts, S., Tutuian, R., King, P., Hawes, R.H., Hoffman, B.J., Wallace, M.B.:** Detection of occult liver metastases during EUS for staging of malignancies. Gastrointest. Endosc. 2004; 59: 49–53
365. **Pulverer, G., Ko, H.L., Beuth, J., Uhlenbruck, G., Oette, K., Isenberg, J., Pichlmaier, H.:** Blockage of the liver lectines due to i.v. galactose infusions: therapeutic concept regarding metastazation prophylaxis (in German). Onkologie 1995; 18 (Suppl. 1): 51–54
366. **Rivoire, M., de Cian, F., Meeus, P., Negrier, S., Sebban, H., Kaemmerlen, P.:** Combination of neoadjuvant chemotherapy with cryotherapy and surgical resection for the treatment of unresectable liver metastases from colorectal carcinoma. Long-term results. Cancer 2002; 95: 2283–2292
367. **Rodgers, M.S., Collinson, R., Desai, S., Stubbs, R.S., McCall, J.L.:** Risk of dissemination with biopsy of colorectal liver metastases. Dis. Colon Rect. 2003; 6: 454–459
368. **Schoedel, K.E., Dekker, A.:** Hemoperitoneum in the setting of metastatic cancer of the liver. A report of two cases with review of the literature. Dig. Dis. Sci. 1992; 37: 153–154
369. **Seifert, J.K., Achenbach, T., Heintz, A., Böttger, T.C., Junginger, T.:** Cryotherapy for liver metastases. Internat. J. Colorectal Dis. 2000; 15: 161–166
370. **Shankar, A., Loizidou, M., Aliev, G., Fredericks, S., Holt, D., Boulos, P.B., Burnstock, G., Taylor, I.:** Raised endothelin 1 levels in patients with colorectal liver metastases. Brit. J. Surg. 1998; 85: 502–506
371. **Shibata, T., Murakami, T., Ogata, N.:** Percutaneous microwave coagulation therapy for patients with primary and metastatic hepatic tumors during interruption of hepatic blood flow. Cancer 2000; 88: 302–311
372. **Sica, G.T., Ji, H., Ros, P.R.:** CT and MR imaging of hepatic metastases. Amer. J. Roentgenol. 2000; 174: 691–698
373. **Soyer, P., Riopel, M., Bluemke, D.A., Scherrer, A.:** Hepatic metastases from leiomyosarcoma: MR features with histopathologic correlation. Abdom. Imaging 1997; 22: 67–71
374. **Su, W.T., Rutigliano, D.N., Gholizadeh, M., Jarnagin, W.R., Blumgart, L.H., La Quaglia, M.P.:** Hepatic metastasectomy in children. Cancer 2007; 109: 2089–2092
375. **Van Riel, J.M.G.H., van Groeningen, C.J., Giaccone, G., Pinedo, H.M.:** Hepatic arterial chemotherapy for colorectal cancer metastatic to the liver. Oncology 2000; 59: 89–97
376. **Vogl, T.J., Straub, R., Eichler, K., Söllner, O., Mack, M.G.:** Colorectal carcinoma metastases in liver: Laser-induced interstitial thermotherapy. Local tumor control rate and survival data. Radiology 2004; 230: 450–458
377. **Wein, A., Riedel, C., Bruckl, W., Merkel, S., Ott, R., Hanke, B., Baum, U., Fuchs, F., Gunther, K., Reck, T., Papadopoulos, T., Hahn, E.G., Hohenberger, W.:** Neadjuvant treatment with weekly high-dose 5-fluorouracil as 24-hour infusion, folinic acid and oxaliplatin in patients with primary resectable liver metastases of colorectal cancer. Oncology 2003; 64: 131–138
378. **Witte, R.S., Cnaan, A., Mansour, E.G., Barylak, E., Harris, J.E., Schutt, A.J.:** Comparison of 5-fluorouracil alone, 5-fluorouracil with levamisole, and 5-fluorouracil with hepatic irradiation in the treatment of patients with residual, nonmeasurable, intra-abdominal metastasis after undergoing resection for colorectal carcinoma. Cancer 2001; 91: 1020–1028
379. **Yamamoto, J., Kosuge, T., Shimada, K., Yamasaki, S., Moriya, Y., Sugihara, K.:** Repeat liver resection for recurrent colorectal liver metastases. Amer. J. Surg. 1999; 178: 275–281

Clinical Aspects of Liver Diseases
38 Systemic diseases and the liver

		Page:
1	***Systemic haematological diseases***	838
1.1	Extramedullary haemopoiesis	838
1.2	Acute leukaemia	838
1.3	Myeloproliferative syndrome	839
1.3.1	Osteomyelofibrosis	839
1.3.2	Chronic myeloid leukaemia	839
1.3.3	Polycythaemia vera	839
1.3.4	Essential thrombocytosis	840
1.4	Haemolytic syndrome	840
1.4.1	Sickle-cell anaemia	840
1.4.2	Thalassaemia	840
1.4.3	Paroxysmal haemoglobinuria	840
2	***Systemic lymphatic diseases***	840
2.1	Hodgkin lymphoma	840
2.2	Non-Hodgkin lymphoma	842
2.2.1	Low-grade malignant NHL	843
2.2.2	High-grade malignant NHL	845
3	***Systemic rheumatic diseases***	845
3.1	Rheumatoid arthritis	845
3.2	Still's disease	846
3.3	Adult Still's disease	846
3.4	Sjögren's syndrome	846
3.5	Felty's syndrome	846
3.6	Polymyalgia rheumatica	846
3.7	Polymyositis	846
3.8	Periarteritis nodosa	847
3.9	Lupus erythematosus	847
3.10	Wegener's granulomatosis	847
3.11	Eosinophilic granulomatous vasculitis	847
4	***Mastocytosis***	848
5	***Histiocytosis X***	848
	• References (1–123)	848
	(Figures 38.1–38.18; tables 38.1–38.4)	

38 Systemic diseases and the liver

Systemic diseases originating in the *haemopoietic* or *lymphatic* systems and those belonging to the category of *rheumatic diseases* can affect the liver either directly or indirectly. (s. tab. 38.1)

Haematopoietic system
1. *Direct effects on the liver*
   = pathological extramedullary haemopoiesis in the liver
   = disturbed liver haemodynamics following haemolysis
2. *Indirect effects on the liver*
   = reduced defence against infections facilitates bacterial, viral or mycotic liver damage
   = toxic liver damage caused by drugs (e.g. cytostatics, immunosuppressants)
   = graft-versus-host reaction in bone-marrow transplants

Lymphatic system
1. *Direct effects on the liver*
   = pathological formation and deposition of lymphocytes or lymphoblasts with formation of infiltrates or focal lesions
   = cholestasis following mechanically mediated biliary dyskinesia
2. *Indirect effects on the liver*
   = reduced defence against infections facilitates bacterial, viral or mycotic liver damage
   = toxic liver damage caused by drugs (e.g. cytostatics, immunosuppressants)

Rheumatic diseases
1. *Direct effects on the liver*
   = rheumatism-related inflammatory or immunologically induced intrahepatic vasculitis with sequelae
   = non-specific reactive hepatitis
2. *Indirect effects on the liver*
   = toxic liver damage caused by drugs (e.g. antirheumatic agents, immunosuppressants)

Tab. 38.1: Relationship of the liver to the haematopoietic and lymphatic systems and to the category of rheumatic diseases

1 Systemic haematological diseases

1.1 Extramedullary haemopoiesis

Intrahepatic haemopoiesis is a **physiological process** in foetuses and neonates. From 6th to 24th week of pregnancy, haemopoiesis takes place in the liver (and spleen) in a diffuse manner within the sinusoids. Thereafter, focal haemopoiesis may still continue in the liver up to about the second week of life.

Myeloid metaplasia beyond this physiological endpoint of intrahepatic haemopoiesis is regarded as a **pathological event.** Haemopoietic foci are seen in the sinusoids, in Disse's spaces and sometimes to a minor degree in the portal fields; they consist of erythropoietic and myeloproliferative precursors as well as polynuclear giant cells of the megakaryocyte type. This variety of cells provides important evidence in histological differential diagnosis for excluding leukaemic infiltrates and mononuclear hepatitis. Myeloid metaplasia accompanies displacement of the bone marrow, e.g. in osteomyelofibrosis, bone-marrow carcinomatosis and myeloproliferative diseases. Occasionally, megakaryocytes are also present in the liver. Naphtol-AS-D chloracetate esterase-positive cells of granulopoiesis are a striking feature in this context. Hepatomegaly is generally found. Ascites can develop due to portal hypertension. (s. fig. 38.1)

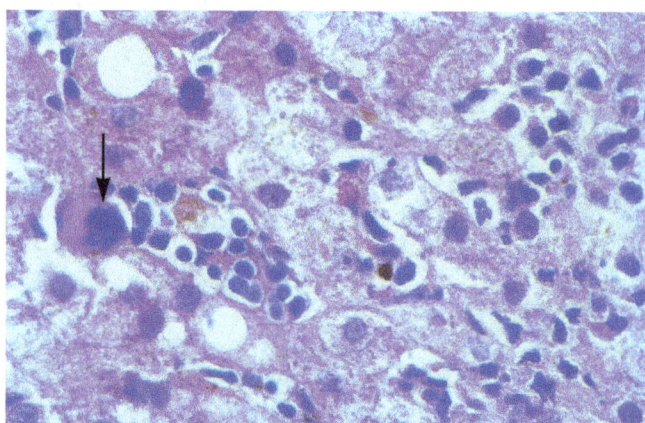

Fig. 38.1: Extramedullary haemopoiesis in the liver with erythropoiesis precursors and intrasinusoidal megakaryocyte (↑) due to the so-called marrow-replacement syndrome or chronic myeloproliferative disease (HE)

1.2 Acute leukaemia

In acute myeloid leukaemia or lymphatic leukaemia as well as in acute leukaemic episodes in non-Hodgkin lymphoma, involvement of the liver may only be detectable clinically by the presence of hepatomegaly and subicterus. • **Laboratory parameters** usually show slightly elevated transaminase as well as bilirubin values, and distinct cholestasis is occasionally observed. (7) Acute hepatic failure can occur during the course of acute leukaemia. (1, 8, 27, 65) • **Histologically,** there are massive, yet uniform blast-cell infiltrates; these are found mainly within the portal fields in acute lymphatic leukaemia (about 95%) and within the sinusoids in acute myeloid leukaemia (about 75%). • Involvement of the liver is of no consequence with regard to the underlying disease and its therapy. Secondary infections require systemic treatment with antibiotics and/or antimycotics.

1.3 Myeloproliferative syndrome

The term myeloproliferative syndrome encompasses the following forms: (*1.*) chronic myeloid leukaemia, (*2.*) idiopathic osteomyelofibrosis and sclerosis, (*3.*) polycythaemia vera, and (*4.*) essential thrombocytosis. Intermediate forms of these manifestations are possible. The pathogenesis is based on the transformation of a stem cell and its clonal proliferation. • Chronic lymphatic leukaemia is classified as malignant non-Hodgkin lymphoma. Overlaps between the different forms of disease are frequent. There is a tendency for fibrosis to develop in all types of the myeloproliferative syndrome with subsequent sclerosis of bone marrow in later stages. Certain forms may progress to acute leukaemia, which is termed *blast crisis*.

1.3.1 Osteomyelofibrosis

Osteomyelofibrosis is a chronic, progressive, fibrous obliteration of the bone marrow. Greyish-white discolouration appears with an increase in collagenous fibrils and later also in reticular fibrils. Clinically, there is hepatomegaly (and generally also splenomegaly) correlating with the stage of disease. Arthralgia occurs occasionally. • *Laboratory parameters* may show a slight elevation of γ-GT, AP, transaminases and bilirubin. Leucocyte alkaline phosphatase is enhanced. • *Histologically*, extramedullary haemopoiesis, comprising erythrocyte and granulocyte precursors as well as dysplastic megakaryocytes, is found in the liver in >90% of cases. (14, 17) (s. fig. 38.1) Infiltrates appear in the sinusoids, which are partly dilated and display fibrosis and deposits of haemosiderin. This results in portal hypertension (6, 13); ascites (10) and oesophageal varices are rare (about 7% of cases). Further potential complications include cholelithiasis (its relationship has not been clarified so far), Budd-Chiari syndrome and portal vein thrombosis. (2) • Diagnosis is established by liver histology. Imaging procedures are of no significance here.

1.3.2 Chronic myeloid leukaemia

In CML, granulopoiesis is markedly accelerated, with increased formation of immature precursors. This occurs mainly in the bone marrow. Accordingly, there is only a rare and slight involvement of the *liver* in CML, with the exception of a terminal myeloblast crisis. (s. fig. 38.2) Hepatomegaly is pronounced in some cases. Massive splenomegaly is generally evident; it often presents as a sugar-icing spleen *(= perisplenitis cartilaginea)*. (s. fig. 38.3) • Infiltrations of immature granulocytes and erythrocytes as well as of megakaryocytes are identifiable above all in the (generally dilated) sinusoids. Biochemically, there is an elevation of alkaline phosphatase and LDH. Complications include portal hypertension following obstruction of the sinusoids and as a result of increased hepatic blood flow. (19) Acute liver failure has been observed. (16) In the final stage, metastasis-like structures can appear in the liver (= *chloroma*). Imaging procedures reveal no abnormalities in the area of the liver parenchyma. (5, 12) • *Therapy* with imatinib was recently reported as being successful.

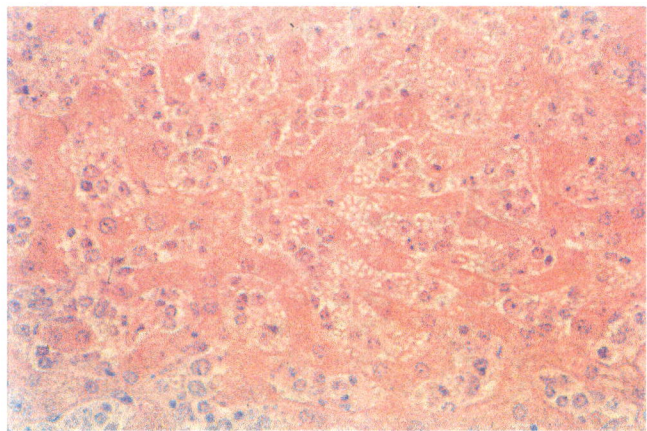

Fig. 38.2: Terminal blast crisis of chronic myeloid leukaemia: numerous myeloid blasts in the sinusoids (HE)

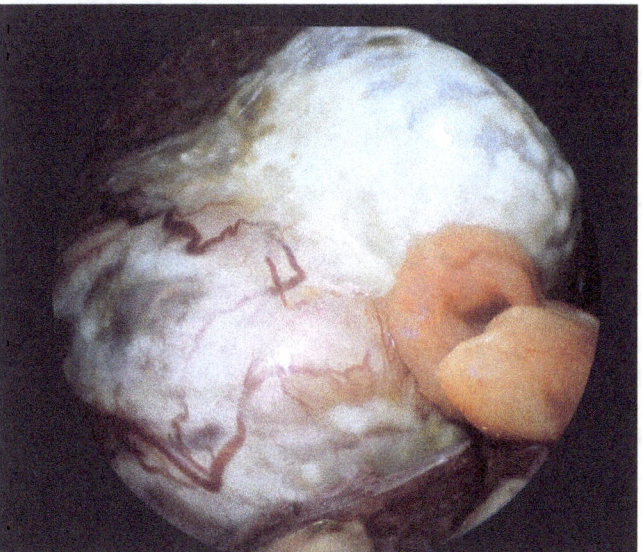

Fig. 38.3: Splenomegaly with perisplenitis cartilaginea (sugar-icing spleen) in chronic myeloid leukaemia

1.3.3 Polycythaemia vera

Liver involvement in Osler-Vaquez disease is rare or not detectable at all. There is, however, evidence of *hepatosplenomegaly* due to extramedullary haemopoiesis. Of importance here is the association with the *Budd-Chiari syndrome* and *veno-occlusive disease*. Polycythaemia vera should be considered in cases of aetiologically unclarified *portal vein thrombosis*. (s. fig. 39.11)

1.3.4 Essential thrombocytosis

With the exception of occasional hepatosplenomegaly, liver involvement is rare. There is again an association with the *Budd-Chiari syndrome* and *veno-occlusive disease*.

1.4 Haemolytic syndrome

▶ Numerous congenital or acquired diseases lead to *haemolysis*. (s. p. 226) (s. tab. 12.3) They are subsumed under the term haemolytic syndrome. Sickle-cell anaemia, thalassaemia and paroxysmal nocturnal haemoglobinuria are worthy of mention in this context.

1.4.1 Sickle-cell anaemia

This form of genetic *haemoglobinopathy* is characterized by chronic haemolysis and haemolytic crises. • **Acute haemolysis** is associated with acute right upper quadrant pain, leucocytosis, jaundice and elevated transaminases, AP and LDH. This hepatic crisis can mimic acute cholecystitis. It lasts two to three weeks. The condition is caused by a slowing down of the sinusoidal blood flow, which contains sickle cells, and, in addition, by a multiplication of the Kupffer cells. The liver is enlarged, rich in blood and violet-red. The sinusoids are dilated and contain agglutinates of sickle cells. The Kupffer cells contain ceroid, siderin and phagocytosed erythrocytes. Single-cell necroses of hepatocytes with Councilman bodies are detectable. Acute liver failure, usually with cholestasis and deep jaundice, is a rare event. (s. fig. 38.4)

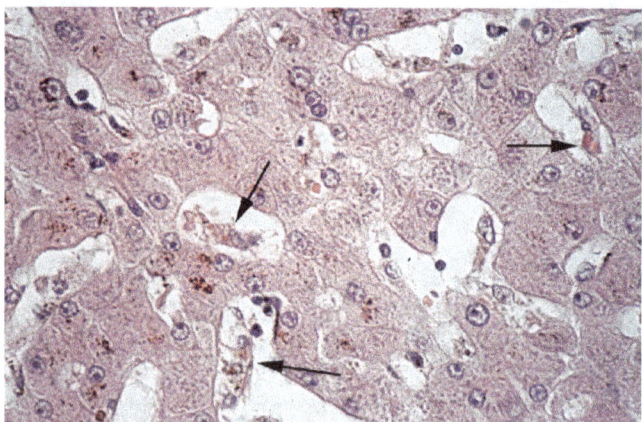

Fig. 38.4: Erythrophagocytosis in Kupffer cells (arrows) in haemolytic anaemia (HE)

Chronic haemolysis can lead to mostly asymptomatic gallstones (approx. 25% in children, 50–70% in adults). Furthermore, portal hypertension and portal fibrosis may develop. There is a slight elevation of the transaminases in a steady state of the disease. Higher values of AP may be due to associated veno-occlusive crises involving the bones. (3, 4, 9, 11, 15, 20) • *Therapy:* Exchange transfusion is indicated. Surgery must be avoided in cases where acute cholecystitis is only mimicked. Successful liver transplantation has been reported.

1.4.2 Thalassaemia

As a result of the crises entailing destruction of the red blood cells and the frequently required blood transfusions, liver siderosis develops. This may lead to fibrosis in some cases. Episodic cholestasis can be observed. In progressive siderosis, treatment with deferoxamine is indicated. *Pigment gallstones* (s. figs. 35.16, 35.17) can appear in the course of chronic haemolysis. (4)

1.4.3 Paroxysmal haemoglobinuria

Paroxysmal nocturnal haemoglobinuria may also give rise to chronic haemolysis. This membrane defect of the erythrocytes is due to mutation of the PIG-A gene on chromosome X resulting in deficient biosynthesis of the glycosylphosphatidlinositol anchor. The erythrocytes are sensitive to lysis when the pH of the blood becomes more acidic during sleep. This clinical picture can lead to hepatomegaly, a rise in the transaminases, iron deficiency, siderosis and centrizonal necrosis. *Thrombosis* of the portal and splenic veins as well as the *Budd-Chiari syndrome* are possible complications. Sclerosing cholangitis is likely to develop due to ischaemia. (18)

2 Systemic lymphatic diseases

Hodgkin's disease and non-Hodgkin's lymphomas belong to this group. Liver involvement due to these diseases consists of lymphocytic infiltrates or their precursors as well as the formation of lymphatic tissue nodes. The liver itself has no organ-specific lymphatic tissue.

2.1 Hodgkin lymphoma

▶ TH. HODGKIN first described this condition in 1832; in 1865 S. WILKS coined the term Hodgkin lymphoma. R. PALTAUF reported on lymphosarcomatosis in 1897. • The aetiology of this malignant systemic disease is unknown. Hodgkin's lymphoma invariably begins in the lymphatic tissue (= *lymphogranulomatosis*), mainly in the neck and mediastinum. The lymph node swelling is not painful.

Typical **Hodgkin cells** derive from undifferentiated reticular cells. They have a slightly basophilic cytoplasm and one or two glowing red or violet nucleoli in a very light, almost unstained nucleus. These cells are the mononuclear precursors of the polynuclear **Paltauf-Sternberg giant cells** (R. PALTAUF, 1897; C. V. STERNBERG, 1936). Such reticular giant cells are seen as a reliable symptom of Hodgkin lymphoma in the liver (stage IV) when they are found in the typical cellular environment of a Hodgkin's granuloma. • **Five forms** of Hodgkin lymphoma are distinguishable histologically:

1. nodular sclerosis	40–80%
2. mixed cellular form	20–40%
3. lymphocytotic type	2–10%
4. lymphocytopenic type	2–5%
5. unclassifiable form	1–5%

The **liver** is the most frequently affected non-lymphatic organ in Hodgkin lymphoma (30–50% of cases). Liver involvement is highest in the lymphocytopenic type (which also has a particularly unfavourable prognosis) and in nodular sclerosis. It is lowest in the lymphocytotic type. There is evidence of large, irregularly delineated tumour nodes and multiple, diffusely distributed nodules or even subcapsular miliary nodules. These macroscopic forms also occur in combination; their histological properties are largely identical. Acute liver failure can develop. (36, 39) *Hepatomegaly* is frequently observed. *Splenomegaly* is generally associated with liver involvement. Non-involvement of the spleen is rare (35); a normal-sized spleen mostly rules out liver involvement. • *Hodgkin infiltrates* originate in the portal fields; they are arranged irregularly. Numerous reticulin fibres and dilatations of the sinusoids are frequently found in zones 2 and 3. The infiltrates consist of focally arranged histiocytes, epithelioid cells, eosinophils and small lymphocytes as well as *Hodgkin cells* and *Sternberg cells*. Central venous obstruction and endophlebitis can appear as a consequence of Hodgkin lymphoma in the liver. (21, 28, 40, 51, 57) (s. figs. 38.5–38.9)

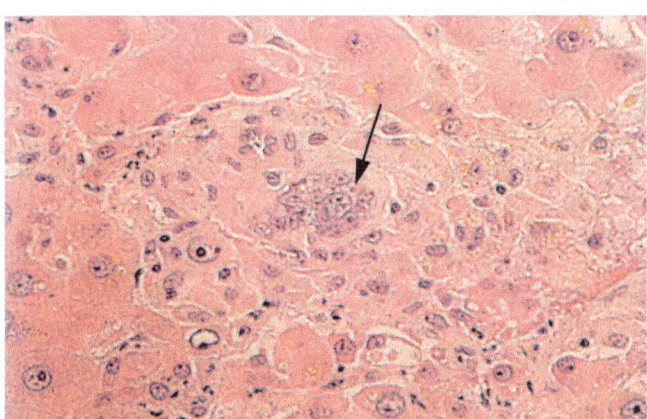

Fig. 38.5: Hodgkin lymphoma: portal granuloma with Paltauf-Sternberg giant cell (↑) (HE)

Clinically, there is *loss of weight* (>10% within 6 months), *fever* (= Pel-Ebstein type, i.e. periodic fever at short intervals), *night sweats*, weakness, pain in the lymph nodes (following intake of alcohol) and pruritus (particularly in the later stages). The so-called *B-symptomatology* (= (1.) weight loss, (2.) fever, (3.) night sweats) is mostly given when the liver is involved. (34)

Laboratory investigation reveals highly pathological "inflammatory criteria", which probably point to a con-

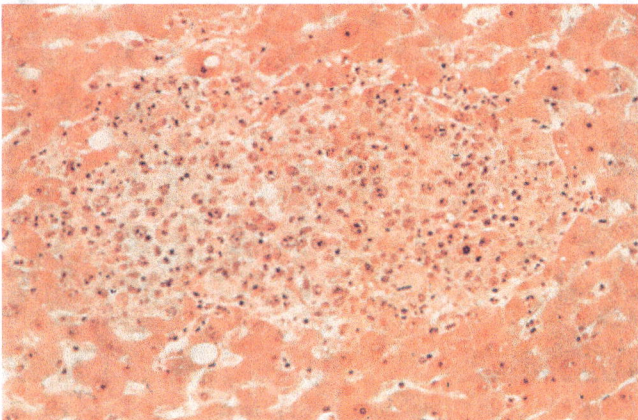

Fig. 38.6: Hodgkin lymphoma: relatively well-defined, large intralobular granuloma with numerous Hodgkin cells (HE)

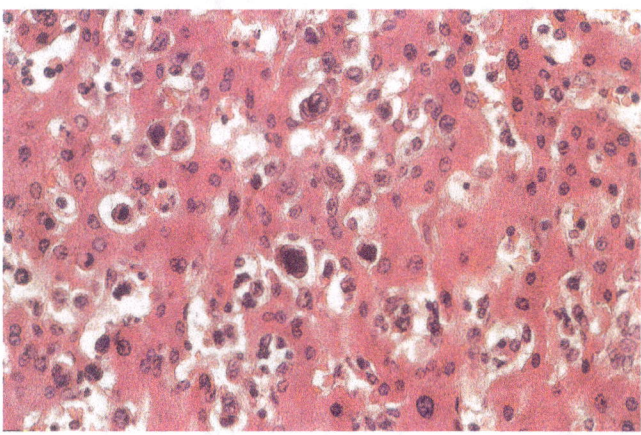

Fig. 38.7: Late stage of lymphocyte depleted Hodgkin lymphoma (HE)

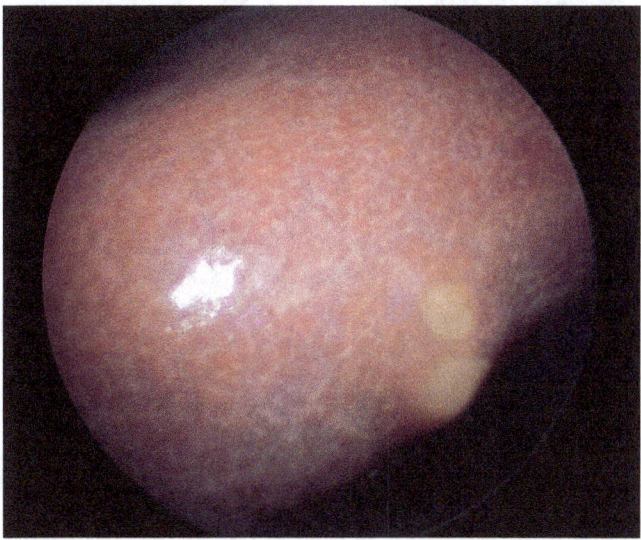

Fig. 38.8: Hodgkin lymphoma: node at the margin of the left liver lobe; clear, diffuse (reticular) fibrosis of the liver

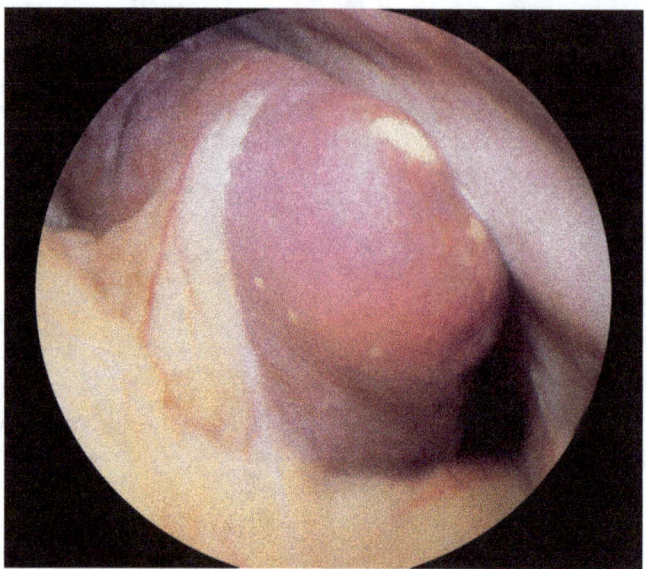

Fig. 38.9: Hodgkin lymphoma: several foci up to the size of a lentil and a 1.5 cm tumour node in the greatly enlarged spleen

suming or malignant process. Alkaline phosphatase and bilirubin rise in the further course of disease (about 80% of cases). Lymphopenia and eosinophilia are often in evidence. (37, 39, 42) (s. tab. 38.2)

Non-specific "inflammatory criteria" (or indicators of a consuming process)	
ESR ↑	α-globulins ↑
CRP +	haptoglobin ↓
fibrinogen ↑	copper ↑
iron ↓	cholinesterase ↓
haemoglobin ↓	D-dimer ↑

Tab. 38.2: Non-specific "inflammatory criteria" (or indicators of a consuming process) (s. tabs. 37.6, 37.11, 37.12)

Imaging procedures display focal lesions, which appear hypoechoic and generally without a halo in sonography; in the further course of disease, the centre can yield a more hyperechoic structure. MR-SPECT has proved especially reliable in this connection. (26, 58, 62) • The diagnosis is established morphologically. This can be achieved most reliably by **laparoscopy** and targeted biopsy. (23, 51) Percutaneous biopsy has low specificity; it must be carried out, if at all, under US or CT guidance (several samples should be obtained from both liver lobes). Liver involvement always corresponds to *Hodgkin stage IV* (= non-localized, diffuse or disseminated disease of one or more extralymphatic organs or tissues with or without involvement of the lymphatic system). (44) • **Therapy** consists of polychemotherapy and/or intercurrent small-field irradiation, if applicable. The recurrence rate can be significantly reduced by mild chemotherapy prior to irradiation. In the case of recidivation, however, high-dose chemotherapy clearly shows greater efficacy. (53)

2.2 Non-Hodgkin lymphoma

The term non-Hodgkin lymphoma (NHL) subsumes a large number of different malignant diseases of the lymphatic system. Taken together, they have more or less the same frequency as Hodgkin's lymphoma itself. The annual incidence of the disease in Germany is about 15 per one million inhabitants.

▶ According to their clinical progression, they are classified into lymphomas of low and high malignancy. **Classification** was formerly based on the Kiel Classification (K. LENNERT, 1978), the USA Classification (H. RAPPAPORT et al., 1978) or the New Working Formulation (1980). This whole system has now been replaced by the WHO classification (2001). Staging corresponds to that of Hodgkin's lymphoma, i.e. liver involvement represents the prognostically critical stage IV. (s. tab. 38.3)

1. Diffuse large B-cell lymphoma (DLBCL)
2. T-cell rich B-cell lymphoma (TCRBCL)
3. B-cell chronic lymphocytic leukaemia (B-CLL)
4. Classical Hodgkin lymphoma (cHL)
5. Follicular lymphoma (FL)
6. Marginal zone lymphoma (MZL)
7. Leukemic plasmacytoma (PL)
8. Burkitt lymphoma (BL)
9. Mantic cell lymphoma (MCL)
10. B-lymphoblastic leukaemia (B-ALL)
11. Hairy cell leukaemia (HCL)
12. Peripheral T-cell lymphoma, unspecified (pTCL)
13. Anaplastic large cell lymphoma (ALCL)
14. Hepatosplenic T-cell lymphoma (HSTCL)

Tab. 38.3: Entities of lymphomas based on the WHO classification

NHL occurs in **three macroscopic forms**
1. **disseminated micronodular infiltrates** (s. fig. 38.10)
2. **multiple macronodular nodes** (s. fig. 38.11)
3. **solitary tumour masses** (s. fig. 38.12)

Liver: There is (primary or secondary) involvement of the liver in about 50% of NHL patients (initially in approx. 20%, postmortem in >60%). The liver is seldom affected without simultaneous involvement of the spleen. However, liver involvement in NHL is less important than in Hodgkin's lymphoma. Lymphocytic lymphomas mostly result in miliary foci, whereas histiocytic lymphomas mainly develop into tumour nodes. Macronodular, greyish-white (or yellowish-white) nodes and solitary, greyish-white tumour masses are rare. Micronodular, disseminated infiltrates are produced by involvement of the portal fields, especially in low-grade malignant forms of NHL. They appear as barely recognizable, fine-grained, white foci on the cut surface of the liver. • *Diagnosis* is confirmed morphologically using laparoscopy and targeted biopsy or forceps biopsy (23, 51), or by percutaneous biopsy under US or CT guidance. Immunohistochemical methods allow further differentiation and a more reliable diagnosis. (21, 22, 38, 52) (s. figs. 38.10, 38.11, 38.12)

Systemic diseases and the liver

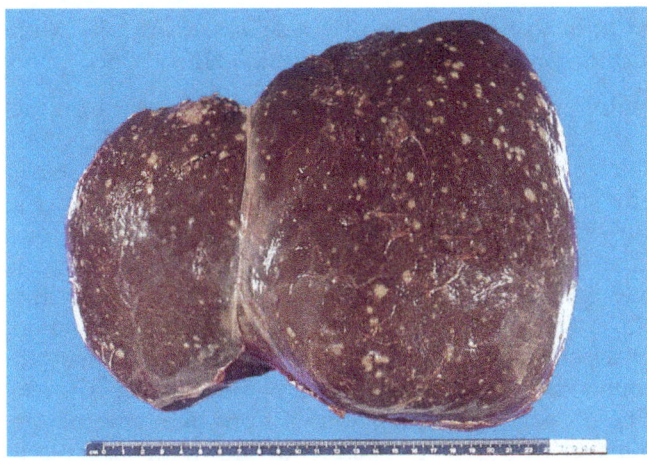

Fig. 38.10: Micronodular infiltration of the liver by disseminated non-Hodgkin lymphoma

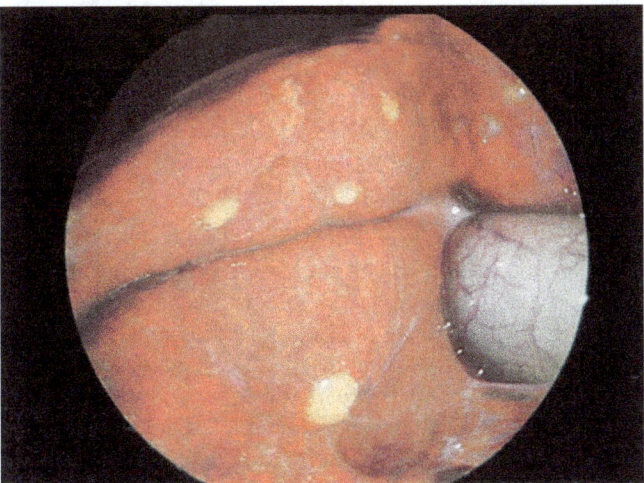

Fig. 38.11: Nodular involvement of the liver by a highly malignant B-cell non-Hodgkin lymphoma. Laparoscopy shows macronodular nodes of yellowish-white colour and different sizes; whitish fibrin deposits; furrowing of the liver

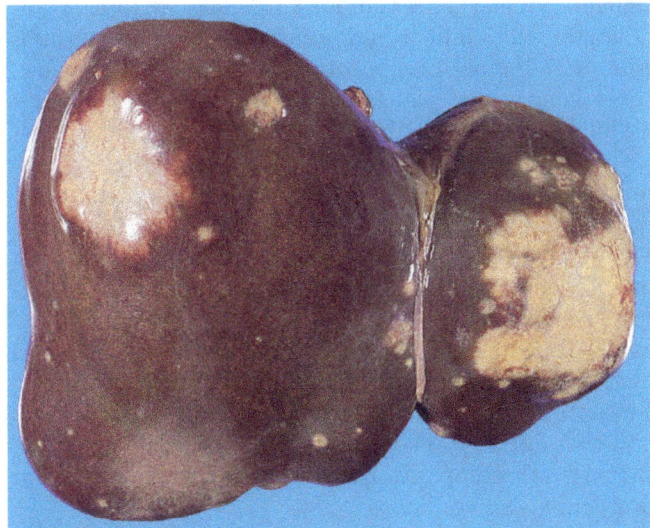

Fig. 38.12: Large tumour masses formed by a highly malignant B-cell non-Hodgkin lymphoma

Clinically, general symptoms of illness, such as fatigue, weakness, lack of appetite, loss of weight and fever are in evidence. A tentative diagnosis is based on hepato-(spleno)megaly and peripheral lymphadenopathy. • **Laboratory investigations** reveal "inflammatory criteria" in relation to the severity and form of NHL, as in Hodgkin lymphoma. (s. tab. 38.2) LDH and alkaline phosphatase are generally elevated; a slight rise in transaminase values is sometimes evident. There is a strikingly frequent association with HCV infection (29, 30, 33, 45, 55, 60), AIDS, and possibly also azathioprine. • **Imaging procedures** can provide diagnostic evidence by displaying local lesions, usually as a singular space-occupying process of varying echogenicity and density. (43, 54, 58, 62) • The majority of cases are not diagnosed until they have reached an advanced stage. The symptomatology, course and prognosis depend on the type of NHL. Fulminant liver failure is relatively frequent – sometimes as the initial manifestation. (25, 31, 32, 41, 46, 50, 63) • New methods of **treatment** – in addition to or instead of interferon – are continuously being sought in the therapy of NHL. This includes transplantation of blood stem cells following whole-body irradiation combined with chemotherapy, chemoembolization or possibly tumour resection. Moreover, *rituximab* is available as an antibody against lymphoma cells.

2.2.1 Low-grade malignant NHL

The incidence of low-grade malignant lymphoma shows an increasing tendency. There are signs of a causal relationship with environmental factors (e.g. pesticides). Low-grade malignant NHL leads more often to liver involvement than do the other forms.

Chronic lymphatic leukaemia: CLL occurs as B-cell and T-cell types. B-CLL is the most common form (approx. 95%); it is based on the malignant transformation of B-lymphocytes and occurs mainly in older people. The surface of B-cells is coated with immunoglobulins of the heavy chain type. T-CLL results from malignant transformation of T-lymphocytes; it is comparatively rare (5%). All in all, CLL is the most common form of both leukaemia (approx. 30%) and NHL. The liver is involved in >40% of cases. (s. figs. 38.13)

Histologically, there are dense, uniform portal field infiltrates of small lymphoid tumour cells, whereas lymphoblasts are generally not detectable. The portal fields are extended, but the limiting plates usually remain intact and are only penetrated by the lymphocytic tumour cells in the later course of disease. (s. figs. 38.14, 38.15) Bridge-like infiltrates can then develop between the portal fields. Small infiltrates also occur in the liver lobule. The sinusoids show a cumulation of round cells. Jaundice and cholestasis develop following obstruction of the portal bile ducts. These findings can also be caused by compression of enlarged lymph nodes. (59) • *Complications* include portal hypertension (following fibrosis) (47), nodular regenerative hyperplasia and cholelithiasis (due to chronic haemolysis). Micronodular cirrhosis may also develop. • *Therapy* is carried out in accordance with haemato-oncological guidelines, especially with *alemtuzumal* (= antibody campath-1 H).

Hairy cell leukaemia: This designation is based on the microvillar "hairy" surface of the tumour cells. It is considered to be a special form of B-CLL. The disease begins insidiously, mainly at an advanced age, and has a chronic progressive course. (24) Men are affected four times more often than women. Massive splenomegaly and panmyelophthisis are already detectable at an early stage. • In the **liver,** there is characteristic infiltration of the sinusoids with intralobular angiomatous changes, simulating the clinical picture of peliosis hepatis. (66) The associated angiomatous lesions are covered by hairy cells. (49, 64) A special feature of the hairy cell infiltrates is the presence of tartrate-resistant acid phosphatase, which is a reaction product of the tumour cells. Hepatomegaly is often present (in 40% of cases), whereas lymphadenopathy is very rare. In severe forms of infiltration, the picture of a nutmeg liver can develop. Colliquation of liver parenchyma with formation of lacunas can be detected as focal lesions by means of sonography and CT. Ascites can occur. • *Therapy* (with a generally favourable prognosis) consists of interferon-α or deoxycoformycin. Hairy cell leukaemia is resistant to radiation treatment and chemotherapy.

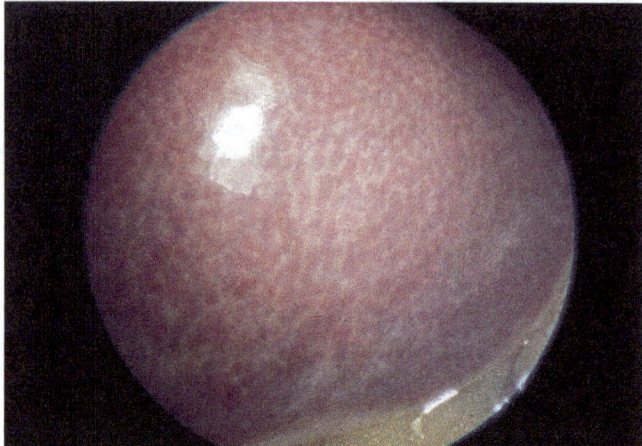

Fig. 38.13: Chronic lymphatic leukaemia: smooth liver surface, greyish-red colour with slight cholestasis; reticular fibrosis. (Three different patients in 38.13–38.15)

Mycosis fungoides: This malignant T-cell lymphoma begins in the skin, but may also affect internal organs. The liver is rarely involved; this is more frequently the case with a leukaemic variant, the so-called **Sezary syndrome.** In the final stage of mycosis, however, portal field infiltrations are frequently detectable. They consist of atypical polymorphic lymphoid *Lutzner cells* (M.A. LUTZNER et al., 1971) and of larger cells containing hyperchromic and highly polymorphic nuclei (= *mycosis cells*). The disease is apparently caused by retroviruses. The prognosis is unfavourable; radiation therapy and cytostatic agents are ineffective.

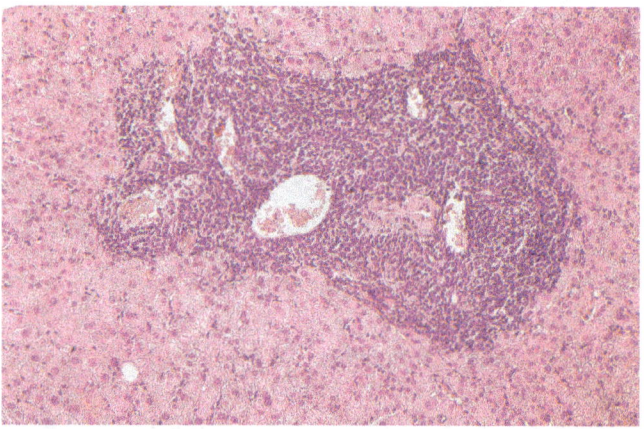

Fig. 38.14: Chronic lymphatic leukaemia: dense portal lymphoid cell infiltration (HE)

Immunocytoma: This tumour originates in three types of immunoglobulin-secreting cells: (*1.*) lymphoplasmocytic, (*2.*) lymphoplasmocytoid, and (*3.*) polymorphic. In isolated cases, patients with Waldenström's macroglobulinaemia can also be assigned to this category. • *Clinical* symptoms include lymphadenopathy, splenomegaly, infiltration of the skin, fever, night sweats and pruritus. Immunoglobulins M and G are elevated. • The *liver* is involved in >90% of cases. The portal fields are only focally affected. The infiltrates are loosely and diffusely arranged. They frequently contain (50–80% of cases) PAS-positive, globular, nuclear and cytoplasmic inclusions, which represent retained immunoglobulins. The infiltrates also comprise a scattering of mast cells and eosinophils. The limiting plates remain intact. Increased flooding of the sinusoids is regarded as a sign of a leukaemic course.

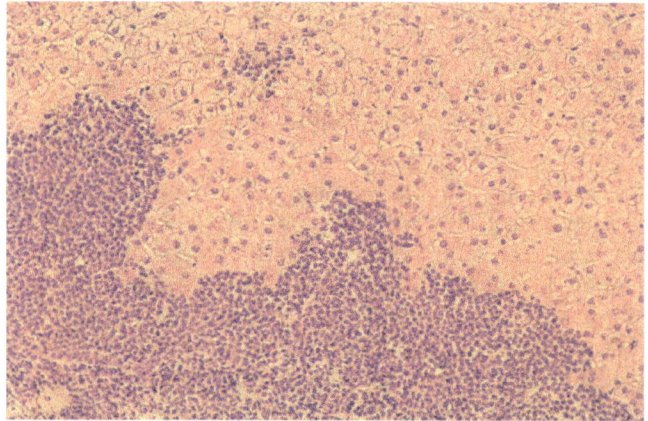

Fig. 38.15: Chronic lymphatic leukaemia: dense portal lymphocytic infiltration extending into the liver parenchyma (HE)

Plasmocytoma: Extramedullary plasmocytic lymphoma likewise has its origin in immunoglobulin-secreting B-lymphocytes. It is also termed *multiple myeloma*. The condition occurs most frequently in the 7th decade of life and ends fatally after 1−2 (−3) years. • In the *liver*, there are sometimes sinusoidal and portal infiltrations of B-lymphocytes and plasmocytic tumour cells; nodular formation can also occur. Generally, however, liver involvement is found in 40% of cases. (48, 61) (s. fig. 38.16) • Recently, patients with non-response or relapse after high-dose chemotherapy were treated successfully with *thalidomide* (starting with 200 mg daily, the dose was increased by 200 mg every two weeks until it reached 800 mg per day). (56) • **Plasma cell leukaemia** is a rare complicative variant which tends to have its own individual course.

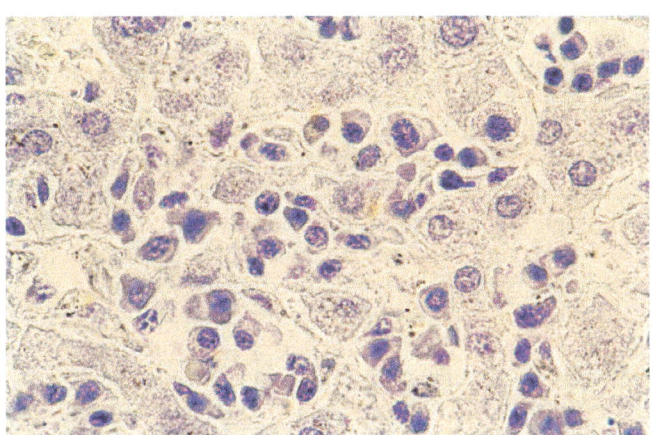

Fig. 38.16: Intrasinusoidal accumulation of atypical plasma cells in plasmocytoma (HE)

Centrocytic lymphomas: These have their origin in lymphatic germ centre cells. *Liver involvement* occurs in about 50% of patients. The portal infiltrates consist of small cells with bright, irregularly shaped, indented nuclei. The portal fields are globularly distended as a result of the infiltration; the limiting plates remain intact, however, and the portal bile ducts are also undamaged.

Centroblastic-centrocytic lymphomas: This tumour type also develops from lymphatic germ centre cells. *Liver involvement* occurs in about 30% of cases. The portal fields are rounded due to infiltration; the limiting plates are penetrated in places. Follicular structures can occasionally be recognized.

2.2.2 High-grade malignant NHL

High-grade malignant lymphomas in the *liver* bring about destruction of the periportal limiting plates and fragmentation or neogenesis of the portal reticular fibres. All of these extremely malignant forms of NHL were classified as reticulosarcomas in the past, but only immunoplastic lymphoma can strictly be assigned to this category. High-grade malignant NHL is usually characterized by irregular portal infiltrates, which penetrate the limiting plates and show (rapid) destructive growth. (29, 38) Fulminant liver failure has also been observed. There is usually far less liver involvement in high-grade malignant NHL than in low-grade forms. • Good results (complete remission in up to 75% of cases) could be achieved by shortened CHOP 14 therapy (cyclophosphamide + hydroxydaunorubicin + vincristine + prednisolone) in six cycles every two weeks.

3 Systemic rheumatic diseases

Rheumatic diseases can also cause direct or indirect liver damage (s. tab. 38.4). A common denominator is the occurrence of HLA type B8. There is often a close association between rheumatic diseases or collagenoses and chronic viral hepatitis (B, C), autoimmune hepatitis, primary biliary cholangitis as well as cirrhosis.

1. Rheumatoid arthritis	7. Polymyositis
2. Still's disease	8. Periarteritis nodosa
3. Adult Still's disease	9. Lupus erythematosus
4. Sjögren's syndrome	10. Wegener's granulomatosis
5. Felty's sydrome	11. Churg-Strauss vasculitis
6. Polymyalgia rheumatica	

Tab. 38.4: Rheumatic diseases causing direct or indirect liver damage

3.1 Rheumatoid arthritis

The cause of this systemic disease, which has a chronic course, is unknown. Generally, several small and large peripheral joints are affected, usually symmetrically. Women suffer far more frequently than men. **Clinically,** there is arthralgia of varying intensity and symptoms of chronic proliferative inflammation of the synovial fluid in the diseased joints. Systemic manifestations can be recognized on the basis of haematological, neurological, pulmonary, renal, cardiovascular and hepatic symptoms. **Laboratory parameters** show marked "inflammatory criteria" (s. tab. 38.2) as well as a rise in γ-globulins and immunoglobulins M and G. The *rheumatoid factor* is often detectable. (s. p. 124) Alkaline phosphatase may be elevated. (100)

Liver involvement occurs in 10−20% of cases. There is hepatomegaly and a slight elevation of the transaminases. Histologically, inflammatory infiltrates and fatty changes in the liver cells may be present together with *non-specific reactive hepatitis*. (s. figs. 21.1; 38.17) Slight fibrosis or rheumatic nodules also occur in some cases after a lengthy period of disease. (67, 76, 79, 85, 91, 94, 101, 107)

3.2 Still's disease

Juvenile rheumatoid arthritis is termed Still's disease (G.F. STILL, 1897). The disease begins in the finger joints and attacks the large joints and the cervical vertebral

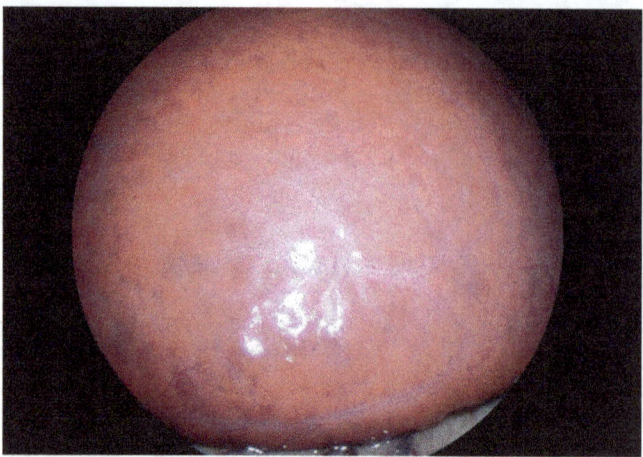

Fig. 38.17: Acute exacerbation of chronic rheumatoid arthritis. Laparoscopy shows light red liver with slightly uneven surface (see scattered light reflex); fine reticular and perivascular fibrosis; isolated red (= inflammatory) foci. Histology shows slight steatosis and non-specific reactive hepatitis

column in progressive steps. Lymphadenopathy is also present. • The *liver* and spleen may be considerably enlarged. Despite this, there are few histological findings, such as periportal lymphocytic infiltrates and Kupffer cell proliferations. (103)

3.3 Adult Still's disease

Adult Still's disease presents with seronegative polyarthritis, febrile attacks, lymphadenopathy, skin symptoms, hepatosplenomegaly, jaundice and involvement of the pleura and pericardium. • The *liver* is enlarged in about 30% of patients; the transaminases may be slightly elevated. Periportal lymphocytic infiltrates and Kupffer cell proliferation can be demonstrated histologically. (68, 69)

3.4 Sjögren's syndrome

Sjögren's syndrome (H.S.C. Sjögren, 1933) is characterized by reduced secretion from the salivary and lacrimal glands with parotid enlargement (and occasional formation of calculi) together with chronic polyarthritis. Women in the menopause are mainly affected. Hyperfibrinogenaemia is common. The cause of the syndrome is unknown. • The *liver* is involved in 5−20% of patients with "sicca" syndrome. (88) Hepatomegaly and elevated alkaline phosphatase (25−40%) are detectable. Liver involvement can be ascertained on the basis of the findings of non-specific reactive hepatitis. (96, 99, 106, 107) An association with the Budd-Chiari syndrome has also been reported. (89)

3.5 Felty's syndrome

Felty's syndrome (A.R. Felty, 1924) is a special form of seropositive polyarthritis. It leads to considerable changes in the articular structures. Characteristic findings include splenomegaly, leucopenia, lymphadenopathy and skin pigmentation. Men are mainly affected. • The *liver* is involved in about 70% of patients. The transaminases and γ-GT values are moderately elevated, and there is an occasional rise in alkaline phosphatase. Lymphocytic infiltrates of the sinusoids, proliferation of Kupffer cells and periportal fibrosis are detectable histologically. Nodular regenerative hyperplasia can develop, which may subsequently cause portal hypertension and macronodular cirrhosis. (71, 95, 104)

3.6 Polymyalgia rheumatica

Clinically, this pathological picture is characterized by severe pain in the area of the shoulder/upper arm, pelvic girdle and femoral musculature. Symptoms include fatigue, weakness, fever and loss of appetite. Women are affected far more frequently than men − generally after the age of 50. • *Laboratory parameters* show highly pathological "inflammatory criteria" (s. tab. 38.2) and greatly elevated AP, but no antibodies or rheumatoid serological findings. • *Temporal arteritis,* which is a special form of polymyalgia rheumatica, is frequently found. • If larger arteries emanating from the aortic arch are likewise affected, this condition is known as **giant-cell arteritis.** (78, 81, 86, 87, 92) The thickened intima and the media contain histiocytic, lymphocytic and epithelioid cell infiltrates with polynuclear giant cells and plasma cells. Thrombosis often occurs in the affected arteries − also in the liver.

Liver involvement is common. Granulomatous arteritis of the hepatic artery and its intrahepatic branches gives rise to the clinical picture of granulomatous hepatitis. There are lymphocytic infiltrates in the portal fields together with liver cell necroses, so that chronic persistent hepatitis is in evidence. Fatty changes in the liver cells together with hypertrophy of the perisinusoidal lipocytes can also be observed. • *Therapy* is with glucocorticosteroids. (83, 86)

3.7 Polymyositis

Polymyositis can occur as a primary disease or a paraneoplastic syndrome. *Clinically,* there is weakness and pain in the shoulder and hip musculature, with muscular atrophy. *Laboratory parameters* show greatly elevated "inflammatory criteria" (s. tab. 38.2) and a rise in myosin AB. • *Liver involvement* is characterized by hepatomegaly, inflammatory infiltration of the portal fields, fatty changes in the liver cells and single-cell necrosis as well as necrotic foci.

3.8 Periarteritis nodosa

Necrotizing inflammation of small and medium-sized arteries as well as of the perivascular tissue (= periarteritis) with inclusion of adjacent veins leads to nodular-aneurysmal changes in the diseased arteries. The arterial capillaries remain unaffected. The vessel walls are permeated by polymorphonuclear leucocytes and monocytes; the inflammatory infiltration does not always involve the entire circumference of the vessel. Vascular branches are particularly affected. The aneurysmal distensions of the vessels show a tendency to rupture. • *Clinically*, there is evidence of fatigue, weakness, fever, lack of appetite, myalgia and arthralgia, together with abdominal pain. *Laboratory parameters* show highly pathological "inflammatory criteria" (s. tab. 38.2), e.g. greatly elevated ESR and alkaline phosphatase.

If the *liver* is involved, the respective enzymes (GPT, GOT, γ-GT, GDH) are increased. There is frequently an association with HBV or HCV infection (50—75% of cases). Together with the skin and the kidneys, the liver is one of the most affected organs. There are cell necroses. Vascular involvement can lead to infarction, intrahepatic bleeding (98), acute cholecystitis (leading to perforation) (72) and thrombosis. Nodular regenerative hyperplasia can develop. • Aneurysms in the area of the medium arteries are detectable by arteriography. Percutaneous liver biopsy is not recommended because of the bleeding risk and the low success rate. • *Therapy* is with glucocorticosteroids in combination with azathioprine or cyclophosphamide. (70, 75)

3.9 Lupus erythematosus

Lupus erythematosus (LE) is a systemic autoimmune disease, occurring mainly in young women. Its aetiology is unknown. The *clinical* symptoms are chronic recurrent arthralgia with febrile attacks, lack of appetite, fatigue, decreased performance, skin changes on areas of the body exposed to light, lymphadenopathy and renal findings following localized vasculitis. Its *biochemistry* is characterized by highly pathological "inflammatory criteria" (s. tab. 38.2) as well as by the detection of antinuclear antibodies, DNA-AB and the LE factor. Anaemia, leucopenia and thrombopenia are also frequently in evidence. In rare cases, jaundice due to haemolysis occurs. LE cells may be present in the blood or bone marrow (M. M. Hargraves et al., 1948).

The *liver* is involved in 40—60% of cases, but with greatly varying intensity. Hepatomegaly is frequently present. Even acute liver failure has been observed. Discrete laboratory or histological findings relating to the liver can precede the diagnosis of LE by several years in some cases. The clinical picture of acute hepatitis with cholestasis has also been observed. Histologically, there is a broad spectrum of changes comprising fatty degeneration in the liver cells, chronic persistent hepatitis, giant cell hepatitis (73, 77), hepatic infarction (82), cholestasis, veno-occlusive disease (93), nodular regenerative hyperplasia, and cirrhosis with portal and pulmonary hypertension. (108) Lupus anticoagulans (antiphospholipid antibody) can lead to hepatic vein thrombosis. The activity of LE correlates well with the activity of the liver changes. It is a striking feature that patients with liver involvement complain less frequently of arthralgia, but more frequently have gastric, thyroid and haematological complications. It should be noted that there is hepatic idiosyncrasy towards nonsteroidal antirheumatics. (90, 97, 102, 105)

3.10 Wegener's granulomatosis

Wegener's granulomatosis (F. Wegener, 1936, 1939) is a necrotizing form of granulomatous vasculitis originating in the upper respiratory tract and lungs (rhinitis and sinusitis with sanguineous secretion, repeated nosebleeds, ulcers, encrustations and pulmonary infiltrations). Glomerulonephritis subsequently develops. Finally, generalized vasculitis can be detected. (80)

The *liver* shows vasculitis with necrotizing epithelioid cell granulomas. Non-specific reactive hepatitis is also present. *Therapy* is with cyclophosphamide (1—2 mg/kg BW/day). • We have given an extensive description of this clinical picture based on 132 cases in the literature as well as on our own experience. (84)

3.11 Eosinophilic granulomatous vasculitis

Churg-Strauss vasculitis (J. Churg et al., 1951) is characterized by angitis with extravascular granulomas, eosinophilia and bronchial asthma. Allergic factors are held to be responsible for this disease. Reports on about 200 cases have been published so far; men are affected twice as often as women. • Histologically, there is necrotizing inflammation of the small arteries and accompanying veins with paravascularly arranged granulomas deriving from macrophages and giant cells as well as leucocytes and lymphocytes; the centre of a granuloma is strikingly rich in eosinophils. • Such changes also occur in the *liver*. Concurrent involvement of the liver and the omentum can result in a palpable tumour. *Therapy* is with glucocorticosteroids. (74)

4 Mastocytosis

Mast cell hyperplasia can affect several organ systems. Regarding the liver, 50% of cases present as hepatomegaly. Mast cell infiltrates are found in the portal fields. They can lead to occlusion of the small vessels with subsequent fibrosis or cirrhosis. (112) Moreover, there is evidence of marked lymphadenopathy and skin lesions. Polygonal cells with eosinophilic granules are present in the portal fields. On staining with Giemsa and toluidine blue, the typical metachromatic cytoplasmic granules are sometimes identified. NRH, VOD and marked fibrosis have been reported and may be the cause of portal hypertension and ascites. (114, 116) Cirrhosis occurs in 5% of cases. (112)

5 Histiocytosis X

In 1938 A.H.T. ROBB-SMITH mentioned this condition for the first time. One year later, he and R.B. SCOTT together described a disease characterized by "fever, wasting, generalized lymphadenopathy and hepatosplenomegaly, which in the final stages was associated with jaundice, purpura, anaemia and leucopenia". This disease almost always resulted in death after an average duration of 15 weeks. The authors termed the condition "histiocytic medullary reticulosis". (117) • The term "histiocytosis X" was introduced by L. LICHTENSTEIN in 1953 (115), summarizing (1.) Letterer-Siwe disease (reticulosis in infancy), (2.) Hand-Schüller-Christian disease (lipogranulomatosis), and (3.) eosinophilic granuloma of bone. Overlapping syndromes and mixed forms of these three diseases exist. The first two disease forms are mainly disseminated, while eosinophilic granulomas mostly appear as solitary bone lesions (with a better prognosis). • The term "malignant histiocytosis" was introduced by H. RAPPAPORT in 1966. These disseminated forms were distinguished as being benign or malignant and acute or chronic by W.A. NEWTON et al. in 1973.

Histiocytosis X is considered to be a form of reticulosis because of the proliferation and aggregation of Langerhans' cells in the RES. These cells contain so-called *Birbeck granules* and the neural-specific protein S-100. The involvement of the liver and spleen (which is not evident in every case) becomes visible as hepatosplenomegaly. In most cases, there are diffuse, sinusoidal infiltrations consisting of large, mostly multinucleated, atypical histiocytes (usually with hyperchromatic nuclei) and widespread phagocytosis of erythrocytes. (s. fig. 38.4) The Kupffer cells show hyperplasia. Periportal infiltration and cell necrosis are sometimes found. (s. fig. 38.18)

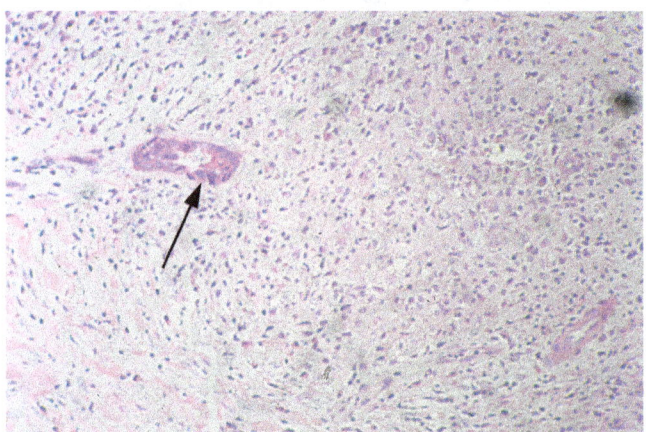

Fig. 38.18: Histiocytosis X: distinct portal inflammation and periductal infiltration by Langerhans cells simulating cholangitis (↑) (HE)

Gross tumour-nodule formation in the liver and spleen is rare. (122) Mild portal fibrosis may be present. (111, 113, 118, 121) In some two-thirds of cases, periportal cholestasis with portal-duct proliferation can be demonstrated. The clinical picture of primary sclerosing cholangitis may appear. (119) Occasionally, pronounced fibrosis with portal hypertension and oesophageal varices develops. (110) Transition into cirrhosis is possible. A suitable form of chemotherapy resulted in a 30–40% decrease in lethality. In portal hypertension, shunt surgery has been applied. Liver transplantation was successfully carried out without evidence of recurrent disease during a seven-year follow-up. (123)

References:

Haematopoietic system
1. **Anderson, S.H.C., Richardson, P., Wendon, J., Pagliuca, A., Portmann, B.:** Acute liver failure as the initial manifestation of acute leukemia. Liver 2001; 21: 287–292
2. **Anger, B.R., Seifried, E., Scheppach, J., Heimpel, H.:** Budd-Chiari syndrome and thrombosis of other abdominal vessels in chronic myeloproliferative diseases. Klin. Wschr. 1989; 67: 818–825
3. **Banerjee, S., Owen, C., Chopra, S.:** Sickle cell hepatopathy. Hepatology 2001; 33: 1021–1028
4. **Brittenham, G.M., Cohen, A.R., McLaren, C.E., Martin, M.B., Griffith, P.M., Nienhuis, A.W., Young, N.S., Allen, C.J., Farrell, D.E., Harris, J.W.:** Hepatic iron stores and plasma ferritin concentration in patients with sickle-cell anemia and thalassemia major. Amer. J. Hematol. 1993; 42: 81–85
5. **Cervantes, F., Rozman, C.:** A multivariate analysis of prognostic factors in chronic myeloid leukemia. Blood 1982; 60: 1298–1304
6. **Dubois, A., Dauzat, M., Pignodel, C.:** Portal hypertension in lymphoproliferative and myeloproliferative disorders: hemodynamics and histological correlation. Hepatology 1993; 17: 246–250
7. **Goor, Y., Goor, O., Michalewitcz, R., Cabili, S.:** Acute myeloid leukemia presenting as obstructive jaundice. J. Clin. Gastroenterol. 2002; 34: 485–486
8. **Hess, C.E., Joyce, R.A.:** Acute myeloblastic leukemia presenting as progressive hepatic failure. South Med. J. 1981; 74: 1028–1029
9. **Johnson, C.S., Omata, M., Tong, M.J., Simmons, J.F., Weiner, J., Tatter, D.:** Liver involvement in sickle-cell disease. Medicine 1985; 64: 349–356
10. **Knobel, B., Melamud, E., Virag, I., Meytes, D.:** Ectopic medullary hematopoiesis as a cause of ascites in agnogenic myeloid metaplasia. Case report and review of the literature. Acta Haematol. 1993; 89: 104–107
11. **Kotila, T., Adedapo, K., Adedapo, A., Oluwasola, O., Fakunle, E., Brown, B.:** Liver dsyfunction in steady state sickle cell disease. Ann. Hepatol. 2005; 4: 261–263
12. **Ligumski, M., Polliack, A., Benbassat, J.:** Nature and incidence of liver involvement in agnogenic myeloid metaplasia. Scand. J. Haematol. 1978; 21: 81–93
13. **Muller, E.U., De Wolf, J.T.M., Haagsma, E.B.:** Portal hypertension as presenting feature of a myeloproliferative disorder. Diagnosis and therapeutic dilemmas. Scand. J. Gastroenterol. 1993; 28 (Suppl.) 74–79
14. **Navarro, M., Crespo, C., Perez, L., Martinez, C., Galant, J., Gonzalez, I.:** Massive intrahepatic extramedullary hematopoiesis in myelofibrosis. Abdom. Imag. 2000; 25: 184–186
15. **Olivieri, N.F.:** Progression of iron overload in sickle cell disease. Semin. Haematol. 2001; 38 (Suppl. 1): 57–62
16. **Ondreyco, S.M., Kjeldsberg, C.R., Fineman, R.M., Vaninetti, S., Kushner, J.P.:** Monoplastic transformation in chronic myelogenous leukemia: presentation with massive hepatic involvement. Cancer 1981; 48: 957–963
17. **Pereira, A., Bruguera, M., Cervantes, F., Rozman, C.:** Liver involvement at diagnosis of primary myelofibrosis: A clinicopathological study of twenty-two cases. Eur. J. Haematol. 1988; 40: 355–361
18. **Rosse, W.F.:** Paroxysmal nocturnal haemoglobinuria as a molecular disease. Medicine 1997; 76: 63–93
19. **Roux, D., Merlio, J.P., Quinton, A., Lamouliatte, H., Balabaud, C., Bioulac-Sage, P.:** Agnogenic myeloid metaplasia, portal hypertension, and sinusoidal abnormalities. Gastroenterology 1987; 92: 1067–1072
20. **Shao, S.H., Orringer, E.P.:** Sickle cell intrahepatic cholestasis: Approach to a difficult problem. Amer. J. Gastroenterol. 1995; 90: 2048–2050

Lymphatic system
21. **Aderka, D., Kraus, M., Avidor, I., Sidi, Y., Weinberger, A., Pinkhas, J.:** Hodgkin's and non-Hodgkin's lymphomas masquerading as "idiopathic" liver granulomas. Amer. J. Gastroenterol.1984; 79: 642–644

22. Bachmeyer, C., Harry, G., Cazier, A., Bonnard, P., Cadranel, J.F.: Portal hypertension due to intrahepatic obstruction as non-Hodgkin's lymphoma. Eur. J. Gastroenterol. Hepatol. 2001; 13: 1491–1493
23. Bagley, C.M., Thomas, L.B., Johnson, R.E., Chretien, P.B., DeVita, V.T.: Diagnosis of liver involvement by lymphoma: results in 96 consecutive peritoneoscopies. Cancer 1973; 31: 840–847
24. Bouroncle, B.A.: Unusual presentations and complications of hairy cell leukemia. Leukemia 1987; 1: 288–293
25. Braude, S., Gimson, A.E.S., Portmann, B., Williams, R.: Fulminant hepatic failure in non-Hodgkin's lymphoma. Postgrad. Med. J. 1982; 58: 301–304
26. Castellino, R.A.: Imaging techniques for staging abdominal Hodgkin's disease. Cancer Treat. Rep. 1982; 66: 697–700
27. Conway, E.E., Santorineou, M., Mitsudo, S.: Fulminant hepatic failure in a child with acute lymphoblastic leukemia. J. Pediatr. Gastroenterol. Nutr. 1992; 15: 194–197
28. Dich, N.H., Goodman, Z.D., Klein, M.A.: Hepatic involvement in Hodgkin's disease. Clues to histologic diagnosis. Cancer 1989; 64: 2121–2126
29. Ellenrieder, V., Beckh, K., Müller, D., Klatt, S., Adler, G.: Intrahepatic high-grade malignant non-Hodgkin lymphoma in a patient with chronic hepatitis C infection. Z. Gastroenterol. 1996; 34: 283–285
30. Ferri, C., LaCivita, L., Caracciolo, F.: Non-Hodgkin's lymphoma: possible role of hepatitis C. J. Amer. Med. Ass. 1994; 272: 355–356
31. Gargot, D., Maitre, F., Causse, X., Goralski, M., Festin, D., Legoux, J.L.: Primary liver non-Hodgkin's lymphoma presenting as fulminant hepatitis. Eur. J. Gastroenterol. Hepat. 1994; 6: 843–846
32. Ghosh, P., Fox, I.J., Rader, A.M., Sorrell, M.F.: Fulminant hepatic failure as the initial manifestation of non-Hodgkin's lymphoma. Amer. J. Gastroenterol. 1995; 90: 2207–2209
33. Gisbert, J.P., Garcia-Buey, L., Pajares, J.M., Moreno-Otero, R.: Prevalence of hepatitis C virus infection in B-cell non-Hodgkin's lymphoma: systematic review and meta-analysis. Gastroenterology 2003; 125: 1723–1732
34. Gobbi, P.G., Parrinello, G.A., Di Prisco, U., Federico, M., Bonacorsi, G., Dini, D., Marabelli, S., Rizzo, S.C., Ascari, E.: New clinical criteria for the assessment of liver involvement in Hodgkin's disease. Eur. J. Cancer Clin. Oncol. 1982; 18: 1443–1449
35. Gordon, C.D., Sidawy, M.K., Talarico, L., Kondi, E.: Hodgkin's disease in the liver without splenic involvement. Arch. Intern. Med. 1984; 144: 2277–2278
36. Gunasekaran, T.S., Hassall, E., Dimmick, J.E., Chan, K.W.: Hodgkin's disease presenting with fulminant liver disease. J. Pediatr. Gastroenterol. Nutr. 1992; 15: 189–193
37. Hubscher, S.G., Lumley, M.A., Elias, E.: Vanishing bile-duct syndrome: a possible mechanism for intrahepatic cholestasis in Hodgkin's lymphoma. Hepatology 1993; 17: 70–77
38. Jaffe, E.S.: Malignant lymphomas: pathology of hepatic involvement. Semin. Liver Dis. 1987; 7: 257–268
39. Lefkowitch, J.H., Falkow, S., Whitlock, R.T.: Hepatic Hodgkin's disease simulating cholestatic hepatitis with liver failure. Arch. Pathol. Lab. Med. 1985; 109: 424–426
40. Leslie, K.O., Colby, T.V.: Hepatic parenchymal lymphoid aggregates in Hodgkin's disease. Hum. Pathol. 1984; 15: 808–809
41. Lettieri, C.J., Berg, B.W.: Clinical features of non-Hodgkin's lymphoma presenting with acute liver failure: a report of five cases and review of published experience. Amer. J. Gastroenterol. 2003; 98: 1641–1646
42. Lieberman, D.A.: Intrahepatic cholestasis due to Hodgkin's disease. An elusive diagnosis. J. Clin. Gastroenterol. 1986; 8: 304–307
43. Maher, M.M., McDermott, S.R., Fenlon, H.M., Conroy, D., O'Keane, J.C., Carney, D.N., Stack, J.P.: Imaging of primary non-Hodgkin's lymphoma of the liver. Clin. Radiol. 2001; 56: 295–301
44. Mauch, P., Larson, D., Osteen, R., Silver, B., Yeap, B., Canellos, G., Weinstein, H., Rosenthal, D., Pinkus, G., Jochelson, M., Coleman, C.N., Hellmann, S.: Prognostic factors for positive surgical staging in patients with Hodgkin's disease. J. Clin. Oncol. 1990; 8: 257–265
45. Mazzaro, C., Zagonel, V., Monfardini, S., Tulissi, P., Pussini, F., Fanni, M., Sorio, R., Bortolus, R., Crovatto, M., Santini, G., Tiribelli, C., Sasso, F., Masutti, R., Pozzato, G.: Hepatitis C virus and non-Hodgkin's lymphomas. Brit. J. Haematol. 1996; 94: 544–550
46. Morali, G.A., Rozenmann, E., Ashkenazi, J., Munter, G., Braverman, D.Z.: Acute liver failure as the sole manifestation of relapsing non-Hodgkin's lymphoma. Eur. J. Gastroenterol. Hepatol. 2001; 13: 1241–1243
47. Pauwels, M., Pauwels, S., Capron, J.P., Sevestre, H., Desablens, B.: Intra-hepatic portal hypertension during chronic lymphatic leukemia. Gastroenterol. Clin. Biol. 2000; 24: 221–224
48. Perez-Soler, R., Esteban, R., Allende, E., Tornos Salomon, C., Julia, A., Guardia, J.: Liver involvement in multiple myeloma. Amer. J. Hematol. 1985; 20: 25–29
49. Roquet, M.-L., Zafrani, E.-S., Farcet, J.-P., Reyes, E., Pinaudeau, Y.: Histopathological lesions of the liver in hairy cell leukemia: a report of 14 cases. Hepatology 1986; 5: 496–500
50. Salo, J., Nomdedeu, B., Bruguera, M., Ordi, J., Gines, P., Castells, A., Villela, J., Rodes, J.: Acute liver failure due to non-Hodgkin's lymphoma. Amer. J. Gastroenterol. 1993; 88: 774–776
51. Sans, M., Andreu, V., Bordas, J.M., Llach, J., Lopez-Guillermo, A., Cervantes, F., Bruguera, M., Mondelo, F., Montserrat, E., Teres, J., Rodes, J.: Usefulness of laparoscopy with liver biopsy in the assessment of liver involvement at diagnosis of Hodgkin's and non-Hodgkin's lymphomas. Gastrointest. Endosc. 1998; 47: 391–395
52. Scheimberg, I.B., Pollock, D.J., Collins, P.W., Doran, H.M., Newland, A.C., van der Walt, J.D.: Pathology of the liver in leukaemia and lymphoma. A study of 110 autopsies. Histopathology 1995; 26: 311–321
53. Schmitz, N., Pfistner, B., Sextro, M., Sieber, M., Carella, A.M., Haenel, M., Boissevain, F., Zschaber, R., Müller, P., Kirchner, H., Lohrl, A., Decker, S., Koch, B., Hasenclever, D., Goldstone, A.H., Diehl, V.: Aggressive conventional chemotherapy compared with high-dose chemotherapy with autologous haemopoietic stem-cell transplantation for relapsed chemosensitive Hodgkin's disease: a randomized trial. Lancet 2002; 359: 2065–2071
54. Scoazec, J.-Y., Degott, C., Brousse, N., Barge, J., Molas, G., Potet, F., Benhamou, J.-P.: Non-Hodgkin's lymphoma presenting as a primary tumor of the liver: presentation, diagnosis and outcome in eight patients. Hepatology 1991; 13: 870–875
55. Silvestri, F., Pipan, C., Barillari, G., Zaja, F., Fanin, R., Infanti, L., Russo, D., Falasca, E., Botta, G.A., Baccarani, M.: Prevalence of hepatitis C virus infection in patients with lymphoproliferative disorders. Blood 1996; 87: 4296–4301
56. Singhal, S., Mehta, J., Desikan, R., Ayers, D., Roberson, P., Eddlemon, P., Munshi, N., Anaissie, E., Wilson, C., Dhodapkar, M., Zeldis, J., Barlogie, B.: Antitumor activity of thalidomide in refractory multiple myeloma. New Engl. J. Med. 1999; 341: 1565–1571
57. Skovsgaard, T., Brinckmeyer, L.M., Vesterarger, L., Thiede, T., Nissen, N.I.: The liver in Hodgkin's disease – II. Histopathologic findings. Eur. J. Cancer Clin. Oncol. 1982; 18: 429–435
58. Soyer, P., van Beers, B., Teillet-Thiebaud, F., Grandin, C., Kazerouni, F., Barge, J., Pringot, J., Levesque, M.: Hodgkin's and non-Hodgkin's hepatic lymphoma: sonographic findings. Abdom. Imag. 1993; 18: 339–343
59. Sweet, D.L., Golomb, H.M., Ultmann, J.E.: The clinical features of chronic lymphocytic leukaemia. Clin. Haematol. 1987; 6: 185–202
60. Thalen, D.J., Raemaekers, J., Galama, J., Cooreman, M.P.: Abscence of hepatitis C virus infection in non-Hodgkin's lymphoma. Brit. J. Haematol. 1997; 96: 872–973
61. Thomas, F.B., Clausen, K.P., Greenberger, N.J.: Liver disease in multiple myeloma. Arch. Intern. Med. 1973; 132: 195–202
62. Wernecke, K., Peters, P.E., Krüger, K.-G.: Ultrasonographic patterns of focal hepatic and splenic lesions in Hodgkin's and non-Hodgkin's lymphoma. Brit. J. Radiol. 1987; 60: 655–660
63. Woolf, G.M., Petrovic, L.M., Rojter, S.E., Villamil, F.G., Makowka, L., Podesta, L.G., Sher, L.S., Memsic, L., Vierling, J.M.: Acute liver failure due to lymphoma. A diagnostic concern when considering liver transplantation. Dig. Dis. Sci. 1994; 39: 1351–1358
64. Yam, L.T., Janckila, A.J., Chan, C.H., Li, C.-Y.: Hepatic involvement in hairy cell leukemia. Cancer 1983; 51: 1497–1504
65. Zafrani, E.S., Leclercq, B., Vernant, J.P., Pinaudeau, Y., Chomette, G., Dhumeaux, D.: Massive blastic infiltration of the liver: a cause of fulminant hepatic failure. Hepatology 1983; 3: 428–432
66. Zafrani, E.S., Degos, F., Guigui, B., Durand-Schneider, A.-M., Martin, N., Flandrin, G., Benhamou, J.-P., Feldmann, G.: The hepatic sinusoid in hairy cell leukemia: an ultrastructural study of 12 cases. Hum. Pathol. 1987; 18: 801–807

Rheumatic diseases

67. Agarwal, R.K., O'Neil, K.M., Bedi, D.: Focal radiolucent hepatic lesions in a patient with juvenile rheumatoid arthritis. J. Rheumatol. 1994; 21: 580–581
68. Andres, E., Kurtz, J.E., Perrin, A.E., Pflumio, F., Ruellan, A., Goichot, B., Dufour, P., Blickle, J.F., Grogard, J.M., Schlienger, J.L.: Retrospective monocentric study of 17 patients with adult Still's disease, with special focus on liver abnormalities. Hepato-Gastroenterol. 2003; 50: 192–195
69. Atsukawa, K., Tsukada, N., Yonei, Y., Inagaki, Y., Miyamoto, K., Suzuki, O., Kiryu, Y., Sato, S., Kano, S.: Two cases of adult-onset Still's disease accompanied with centrilobular liver damage. Acta Hepatol. Japon. 1995; 36: 53–57
70. Barquist, E.S., Goldstein, N., Ziner, M.J.: Polyarteritis nodosa presenting as a biliary stricture Surgery 1991; 109: 16–19
71. Blendis, L.M., Lovell, D., Barnes, C.G., Ritland, S., Cattan, D.: Oesophageal variceal bleeding in Felty's syndrome associated with nodular regenerative hyperplasia. Ann. Rheum. Dis. 1978; 37: 183–186
72. Blidi, M., Quang Tri, N., Cassan, P., Guillevin, L.: Les cholécystites aiguës de la périartérite noueuse. Huit observations. Ann. Med. Interne 1996; 147: 304–312
73. Cairns, A., McMahon, R.F.T.: Giant-cell hepatitis associated with systemic lupus erythematosus. J. Clin. Pathol. 1996; 49: 183–184
74. Chumbley, L.C., Harrison, E.G., DeRemee, R.A.: Allergic granulomatosis and angiitis (Churg-Strauss syndrome). Report and analysis of 30 cases. Mayo Clin. Proc. 1977; 52: 477–484
75. Cowan, R.E., Mallinson, C.N., Thomas, G.E., Thomson, A.D.: Polyarteritis nodosa of the liver: a report of two cases. Postgrad. Med. J. 1977; 53: 89–93
76. Dietrichson, O., From, A., Christoffersen, P., Juhl, E.: Morphological changes in liver biopsies from patients with rheumatoid arthritis. Scand. J. Rheum. 1976; 5: 65–69
77. Dohmen, K., Ohtsuka, S., Nakamura, H., Arase, K., Yokogawa, Y., Asayama, R., Kuroiwa, S., Ishibashi, H.: Post-infantile giant-cell hepatitis in an elderly female patient with systemic lupus erythematosus. J. Gastroenterol. 1994; 29: 362–368
78. Duerksen, D.R., Jewell, L.D., Bain, V.G.: Hepatic giant-cell arteritis and polymyalgia rheumatica. Can. J. Gastroenterol. 1994; 8: 36–38

79. **Ellmann, M.H., Weis, M.J., Spelberg, M.A.:** Liver disease in rheumatoid arthritis. Amer. J. Gastroenterol. 1974; 62: 46–53
80. **Fauci, A.S., Haynes, B.F., Katz, P., Wolff, S.M.:** Wegener's granulomatosis: prospective clinical and therapeutic experience with 85 patients for 21 years. Ann. Intern. Med. 1983; 98: 76–85
81. **Ilan, Y., Ben-Chetrit, E.:** Liver involvement in giant-cell arteritis. Clin. Rheumat. 1993; 12: 219–222
82. **Khoury, G., Tobi, M., Oren, M., Traub, Y.M.:** Massive hepatic infarction in systemic lupuserythematosus. Dig. Dis. Sci. 1990; 35: 1557–1560
83. **Kosolcharoen, P., Magnin, G.E.:** Liver dysfunction and polymyalgia rheumatica. A case report. J. Rheumat. 1976; 3: 50–53
84. **Kuntz, E., Benecke, G., Knoth, W.:** Die Wegenersche Granulomatose (in German). Med. Welt 1967; 18: 295–304
85. **Kuntz, H.D., Oellig, W.P., Thiel, H., May, B.:** Leberveränderungen bei akutem rheumatischem Fieber. Med. Klin. 1981; 76: 504–507
86. **Kyle, V., Wraight, E.P., Hazleman, B.L.:** Liver scan abnormalities in polymyalgia rheumatica/giant-cell arteriitis. Clin. Rheumatol. 1991; 10: 294–297
87. **Leong, A.S., Alp, M.H.:** Hepatocellular disease in the giant cell arteriitis/polymyalgia rheumatica syndrome. Ann. Rheum. Dis. 1981; 40: 92–95
88. **Lindgren, S., Manthorpe, R., Eriksson, S.:** Autoimmune liver disease in patients with primary Sjögren's syndrome. J. Hepatol. 1994; 20: 354–358
89. **Matsuura, H., Matsumoto, T., Hashimoto, T.:** Budd-Chiari syndrome in a patient with Sjögren's syndrome. Amer. J. Gastroenterol. 1983; 78: 822–825
90. **Miller, M.H., Urowitz, M.B., Gladman, D.D., Blendis, L.M.:** The liver in systemic lupus erythematosus. Quart. J. Med. 1984; 53: 401–409
91. **Mills, P.R., Sturrock, R.D.:** Clinical associations between arthritis and liver disease. Ann. Rheum. 1982; 41: 295–307
92. **Ogilvie, A.L., James, P.D., Toghill, P.J.:** Hepatic artery involvement in polymyalgia arteritica. J. Clin. Pathol. 1981; 314: 769–772
93. **Pappas, S.C., Malone, D.G., Rabin, L., Hoofnagle, J.H., Jones, E.A.:** Hepatic veno-occlusive disease in a patient with systemic lupus erythematosus. Arthr. Rheum. 1984; 27: 104–108
94. **Rau, R.:** Leberbefunde bei juveniler chronischer Polyarthritis. Schweiz. Med. Wschr. 1977; 107: 1235–1237
95. **Rau, R.:** Leberbefunde beim Felty-Syndrom. Eine Übersicht. Z. Rheumatol. 1978; 37: 267–273
96. **Rau, R.:** Leberbefunde beim Sjögren-Syndrom. Schweiz. Rundschau Med. 1977; 66: 1437–1477
97. **Runyon, B.A., LaBreque, D.R., Anuras, S.:** The spectrum of liver disease in systemic lupus erythematosus: report of 33 histologically-proved cases and review of the literature. Amer. J. Med 1980; 69: 187–194
98. **Schröder, W., Brandstetter, K., Vogelsang, H., Nathrath, W., Siewert, J.R.:** Massive intrahepatic hemorrhage as first manifestation of polyarteritis nodosa. Hepato-Gastroenterol. 1997; 44: 148–152
99. **Skopouli, F.N., Barbatis, C., Moutsopoulos, H.M.:** Liver involvement in primary Sjögren's syndrome. Brit. J. Rheum. 1994; 33: 745–748
100. **Spooner, F.J., Smith, D.H., Bedford, D., Beck, P.R.:** Serum gamma-glutamyltransferase and alkaline phosphatase in rheumatoid arthritis. J. Clin. Pathol. 1982; 35: 638–641
101. **Sullivan, S., Hamilton, E.B.D., Williams, R.:** Rheumatoid arthritis and liver involvement. J. Roy. Coll. Phycns. 1978; 12: 416–422
102. **Sutton, E., Malatjalian, P., Hayne, O.A., Hanly, I.G.:** Liver lymphoma in systemic lupus erythematosus. J. Rheumatol. 1989; 16: 1584–1588
103. **Tesser, J.R.P., Pisko, E.J., Hartz, J.W., Weinblatt, M.E.:** Chronic liver disease and Still's disease. Arthr. Rheum. 1982; 25: 579–582
104. **Thorne, C., Urowitz, M.B., Wanless, I., Roberts, E., Blendis, L.M.:** Liver disease in Felty's syndrome. Amer. J. Med. 1982; 73: 35–40
105. **Van Hoek, B.:** The spectrum of liver disease in systemic lupus erythematosus. Nederl. J. Med. 1996; 48: 244–253
106. **Viogel, C., Wittenborg, A., Reichart, R.:** The involvement of the liver in Sjögren's syndrome. J. Oral Surg. 1980; 50: 26–29
107. **Webb, J., Whaley, K., MacSween, R.N.M., Nuki, G., Dick, W.C., Buchanan, W.W.:** Liver disease in rheumatoid arthritis and Sjögren's syndrome. Ann. Rheum. Dis. 1975; 34: 70–81
108. **Woolf, D., Voigt, M.D., Jaskiewicz, K., Kalla, A.A.:** Pulmonary hypertension associated with non-cirrhotic portal hypertension in systemic lupus erythematosus. Postgrad. Med. J. 1994; 70: 41–43

Mastocytosis and histiocytosis
109. **Granot, E., Cohen, P., Asli, Y., Bar-Ziv, J.:** Histiocytosis X presenting as prolonged cholestatic jaundice in childhood. Eur. J. Gastroenterol. Hepatol. 1994; 6: 275–279
110. **Grosfeld, J.L., Fitzgerald, J.F., Wagner, V.M., Newton, W.A., Baehner, R.L.:** Portal hypertension in infants and children with histiocytosis X. Amer. J. Surg. 1976; 131: 108–113
111. **Guthery, S.L., Heubi, J.E.:** Liver involvement in childhood histiocytotic syndromes. Curr. Opin. Gastroenterol. 2001; 17: 474–478
112. **Horny, H.-P., Kaiserling, E., Campbell, M., Parwaresch, M.R., Lennert, K.:** Liver findings in generalized mastocytosis. A clinicopathologic study. Cancer 1989; 63: 532–538
113. **Kaplan, K.J., Goodman, Z.D., Ishak, K.G.:** Liver involvement in Langerhans' cell histiocytosis: a study of nine cases. Mod. Pathol. 1999; 12: 370–378
114. **Kyriakou, D., Kouroumalis, E., Konsolas, J., Oekonomaki, H., Tzardi, M., Kanavaros, P., Manoussos, O., Eliopoulos, G.D.:** Systemic mastocytosis: a rare cause of non cirrhotic portal hypertension simulating autoimmune cholangitis – report of four cases. Amer. J. Gastroenterol. 1998; 93: 106–108
115. **Lichtenstein, L.:** Histiocytosis X: integration of eosinophilic granuloma of bone: "Letterer-Siwe" disease and "Schüller-Christian" disease as related manifestations of a single nosologic entity. Arch. Path. 1953; 56: 84–102
116. **Mican, J.M., DiBisceglie, A.M., Fong, T.-L., Travis, W.D., Kleiner, D.E., Baker, B., Metcalfe, D.D.:** Hepatic involvement in mastocytosis: clinicopathologic correlations in 41 cases. Hepatology 1995; 22: 1163–1170
117. **Scott, R.B., Robb-Smith, A.H.T.:** Histiocytic medullary reticulosis. Lancet 1939/II: 194–198
118. **Serck-Hanssen, A., Purchit, G.P.:** Histiocytic medullary reticulosis. Report of 14 cases from Uganda. Brit. J. Canc. 1968; 22: 506–516
119. **Thompson, H.H., Pitt, H.A., Lewin, K.J., Longmire, W.P.:** Sclerosing cholangitis and histiocytosis X. Gut 1984; 25: 526–530
120. **Vogel, J.M., Vogel, P.:** Idiopathic histiocytosis: a discussion of eosinophilic granuloma, the Hand-Schüller-Christian syndrome and the Letterer-Siwe syndrome. Semin. Hematol. 1972; 9: 349–369
121. **Warnke, R.A., Kim, H., Dorfman, R.F.:** Malignant histiocytosis (histiocytic medullary reticulosis). I. Clinicopathological study of 29 cases. Cancer 1975; 35: 215–230
122. **Yagita, K., Iwai, M., Yagita-Toguri, M., Kimura, H. Taniwaki, M., Misawa, S., Okanoue, T., Kashima, K., Tsuchihashi, Y.:** Langerhans cell histiocytosis of an adult with tumors in liver and spleen. Hepato-Gastroenterol. 2001; 48: 581–584
123. **Zandi, P., Panis, Y., Debray, D., Bernard, O., Houssin, D.:** Paediatric liver transplantation for Langerhans' cell histiocytosis. Hepatology 1995; 21: 129–133

Clinical Aspects of Liver Diseases

39 Cardiovascular diseases and the liver

		Page:
1	*Cardiocirculatory disorders of the liver*	852
1.1	Acute heart insufficiency	853
1.1.1	Shock liver	853
1.1.2	Acute liver congestion	853
1.2	Chronic heart insufficiency	854
2	*Disorders of the hepatic veins*	856
2.1	*Budd-Chiari syndrome*	856
2.1.1	Historical review	856
2.1.2	Definition	856
2.1.3	Aetiology	856
2.1.4	Morphology	857
2.1.5	Clinical features	857
2.1.6	Diagnostics	858
2.1.7	Treatment	858
2.2	*Veno-occlusive disease*	859
2.2.1	Definition	859
2.2.2	Aetiology	859
2.2.3	Morphology	859
2.2.4	Clinical features	859
2.2.5	Treatment	860
2.3	*Inferior vena cava syndrome*	860
3	*Disorders of the portal vein*	860
3.1	Anomalies of the portal vein	860
3.1.1	Cavernous transformation	861
3.1.2	Cruveilhier-Baumgarten disease	861
3.1.3	Arterioportal venous fistula	861
3.2	Pylephlebitis	862
3.3	Portal vein thrombosis	862
3.4	Portal vein aneurysm	863
3.5	Zahn's pseudoinfarct	863
3.6	Hepatic portal venvous gas	864
4	*Disorders of the hepatic arteries*	864
4.1	Aneurysm	864
4.1.1	Definition	864
4.1.2	Aetiology	864
4.1.3	Clinical features	864
4.1.4	Diagnostics	865
4.1.5	Treatment	865
4.2	Arterial occlusion	865
4.2.1	Aetiology	865
4.2.2	Clinical features	865
4.3	Nodular periarteritis	865
4.4	Arteriosclerosis	866
5	*Hereditary haemorrhagic telangiectasia*	866
	● References (1−180)	866
	(Figures 39.1−39.13; tables 39.1−39.6)	

39 Cardiovascular diseases and the liver

Due to its twofold vascular supply (portal vein, hepatic artery), the liver is closely integrated into the systemic circulation. The total blood flow through the liver is 1,500 ± 300 ml/min. Oxygen consumption amounts to 6 ml/min/100g LWW. (s. pp 21, 252) The portal vein supplies about two-thirds of the hepatic flow volume and is thus responsible for 50% of the oxygen requirement of the liver. The ratio between portal and arterial perfusion is about 2:1; this may, however, be reversed by compensatory autoregulation in cirrhosis patients. Blood from the portal and arterial systems reaches the sinusoids, where both mixing and pressure compensation occur. The hepatic blood flow is mainly regulated by inflow from the hepatic artery, which can be doubled when more oxygen is required. With continued demand for oxygen, the high capacity of the liver cell to extract oxygen (up to 95%) compensates for a limited blood flow. The hepatic flow volume is about 20—25% of the cardiac output (CO). • In addition, the pressure in the lesser circulation is transferred directly to the pressure in the hepatic vein, so that the latter is almost equal to the pressure in the right atrium. The oxygen saturation of the arterioportal mixed blood in the sinusoids decreases continually with the flow of blood from the periportal zone to the central vein. The venous blood is then carried from the central veins and the venous branches into the inferior vena cava, usually through three (valveless) hepatic veins. • This anatomical proximity explains disturbances of the liver function as well as morphological damage resulting from shock situations, acute flow block in the hepatic veins and global heart failure. • **Cardiovascular diseases** may thus affect the heart or each of the three vascular systems:

1. Diseases of the hepatic vein
2. Diseases of the portal vein
3. Diseases of the hepatic artery

4. Hereditary haemorrhagic telangiectasia
5. Impaired cardiac function

1 Cardiocirculatory disorders of the liver

Historical review

▶ The functional relationship between the heart and the liver has been known since ancient times. In animal experiments conducted in 1914, C. BOLTON examined the effects of a ligation of the inferior vena cava on liver histology for the first time. • N. JOLLIFFE (1929) detected clinically measurable changes of the hepatic function in congestive heart failure. (11) • Systematic investigations by S. SHERLOCK (1951) showed the consequences of passive liver congestion on hepatic morphology: complete cirrhosis was observed in 25.5% and an increase in reticular fibres in 27.5% of cases; the liver was without pathological findings in 47% of cases. • Autopsies carried out by P. KOTIN (1951) showed "cardiac cirrhosis" in 10% of patients suffering from right heart insufficiency. (14) • Subsequently, the effects of cardiocirculatory disturbances on various partial functions and on the morphology of the liver, including the effects of drug metabolism, were presented in numerous publications.

Pathophysiology

▶ The close functional relationship between the heart and the liver is based upon **two physiologic facts:**

(1.) The *hepatic flow volume* is 20—25% of the CO and is thus directly dependent on the cardiac ejection volume.

(2.) The *pressure* in the lesser circulation is transferred directly to the valveless hepatic veins and may thus also reach the central veins.

▶ Even though the pathophysiology of hepatic changes during circulatory shock and in chronic liver congestion is very complex, **two single mechanisms** may be held jointly responsible for the impairment of metabolic and excretory liver functions:

(1.) Reduction in blood flow through the liver with hypoxia.

(2.) Increase in hepatic vein pressure with centrilobular hyperaemia.

▶ Circulatory disturbances within the hepatic lobules are of central pathophysiological importance; **three forms** can be differentiated:

(1.) *Disturbed outflow:* the microscopic correlate is centrilobular hyperaemia; macroscopically, the liver is enlarged and has a dark red colour.

(2.) *Disturbed inflow:* hypoperfusion due to arterial, portovenous or combined oligaemia results in centrilobular necrosis or even anaemic liver infarction.

(3.) *Disturbed flow:* primarily, this occurs intralobularly due to various disorders (e.g. DIC, intrasinusoidal fibrin precipitation, centrilobular increase in fibres).

The liver may be involved in numerous ways due to acute, short-term disturbances of the cardiocirculatory function or due to chronic, long-term heart failure:

Acute heart insufficiency	Chronic heart insufficiency
1. Shock liver	1. Chronic liver congestion
2. Acute liver congestion	2. Congestive fibrosis
	3. Cardiac cirrhosis

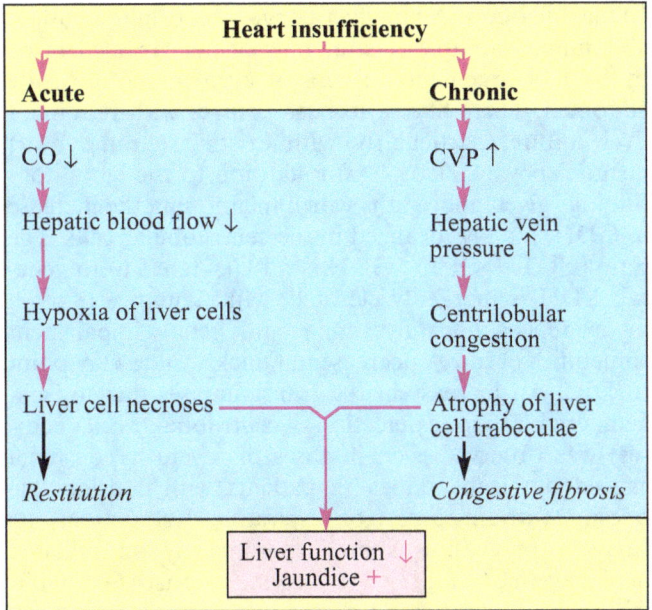

Tab. 39.1: Pathophysiology of cardiocirculatory changes in the liver

1.1 Acute heart insufficiency

Shock liver and acute liver congestion often display very similar histological changes, while the pathophysiologic features, such as laboratory findings, functional tests and drug metabolism, vary considerably. • Cardiogenic shock resulting from myocardial infarction is considered to be both a typical and frequent cause of shock liver, while acute liver congestion (acute right heart insufficiency) is in most cases the consequence of pulmonary embolism. • During shock, the liver is involved in two ways: (*1.*) it is an important regulatory organ (= *liver in shock*), and (*2.*) its function and morphology are compromised by shock mechanisms (= *shock liver*).

1.1.1 Shock liver

This condition is characterized by a reduced hepatic blood flow (CO ↓) and hepatocellular hypoxia, resulting in a loss of glycogen, the formation of hypoxic vacuoles in the hepatocytes and membrane blebbing; there are also coagulation necroses in acinar zone 3. Strikingly, the function of the liver is only mildly compromised and recovers quickly once the circulation is stabilized. Since the lattice fibre framework is generally intact, the centrolobular necroses do not leave behind any scars. During this phase, we only detected slightly delayed indocyanine green (ICG) elimination, while galactose elimination capacity and theophylline clearance were slightly inhibited. (19) This means that essential partial functions of the liver are relatively independent of the blood flow and that short-term hypoxia can be compensated by increased extraction of oxygen. By contrast, we also found greatly increased GOT and GPT values similar to those present in "hepatitis", with low-grade cholestasis and jaundice. The terms ischaemic hepatitis, hypoxic hepatitis or acute hepatic infarction are alternative definitions. (4, 6, 7, 12, 26, 30) In shock liver, there is therefore a marked discrepancy between a relatively slight reduction in excretory and metabolic functions and considerable liver cell damage detectable by enzyme analysis. • The hepatic blood flow is decreased due to shock-induced hyperperfusion of the heart and brain with simultaneous vasoconstriction in the splanchnic nerve area (= *centralization of circulation*). However, liver cell damage often develops or intensifies as a result of subsequent reperfusion, whereby the substances that are introduced in increased amounts at this point (endotoxins, cytokines, biogenic amines, degradation products, etc.) are probably the main cause of such liver cell damage. (27) A diffuse hepatic microcalcification as a sequela to shock liver can sometimes be found. (28) The damage occurring in shock liver and acute liver congestion may thus be due to ischaemia and/or ischaemic-toxic factors. (2, 3, 5, 29) (s. fig. 39.1)

1.1.2 Acute liver congestion

In our investigations, patients suffering from acute right heart insufficiency showed considerable delays in ICG half-times. In an earlier study, we were able to demonstrate a close correlation with right-sided atrial pressure. Theophylline clearance was likewise delayed. Standard enzymes revealed only slightly increased or even normal values; hyperbilirubinuria, which is seen as the most sensitive laboratory value in liver congestion, was generally present. Thus there is also a discrepancy between "liver function" and "cell damage" in this context — albeit exactly the reverse of that found in shock liver. (17, 19) Patients with acute liver congestion have greatly impaired metabolic and excretory functions, even after clinical recompensation. Perisinusoidal oedema due to elevated hepatic vein pressure is of utmost pathogenetic significance in acute liver congestion, because it lengthens the transit route. In acute congestion, the liver is capable of taking up blood equivalent to 70% of its own weight (1.0–1.5 l), so that both circulatory overload and tachycardia are reduced.

Morphology: Within the first day following the onset of acute liver congestion, massive sinusoidal hyperaemia and perivenous cell necroses occur due to the fact that centrilobular oxygen saturation is lower than that of the lobular periphery. The reticular fibre framework usually remains intact. Venous stasis may also occur, especially in acute congestion, including dilatation of the central veins and sinusoids with blood pooling, resulting in hepatomegaly. Macroscopically, the liver appears heavy and dark red. Microthrombi may be present due to disseminated intravascular coagulation. They can form the basis of later diffuse calcification. This might be related to the disturbance of intracellular calcium homoeostasis

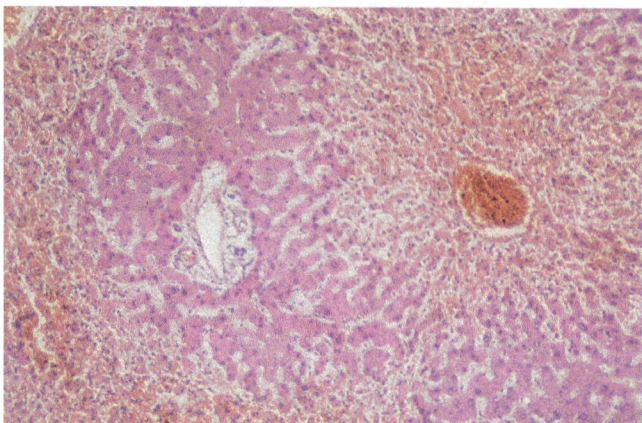

Fig. 39.1: Centroacinar shock necrosis and acute haemostasis in the liver (HE)

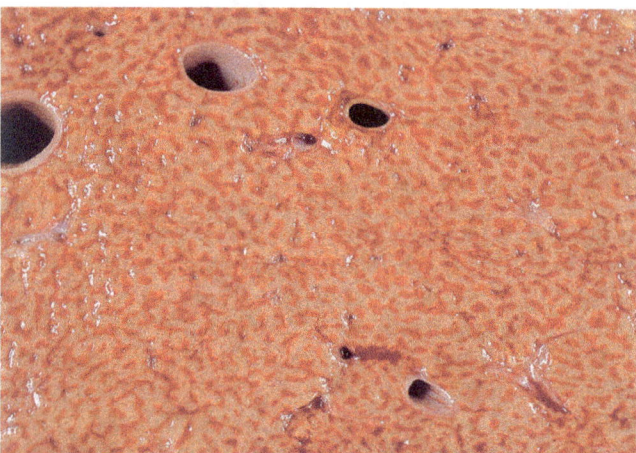

Fig. 39.2: Acute blood stasis with centrilobular congestion and centricentral congestion paths

Clinical features: Acute liver congestion results in upper abdominal pain due to stretching of the capsule caused by liver enlargement; this might even mimic an acute abdomen. There have also been courses with fulminant liver failure, particularly with existing chronic heart insufficiency. (9, 21, 25, 27) In addition to the laboratory findings given above, it is worth mentioning the increase in GDH, mainly localized in the centrilobular cells. The ratio (GOT + GPT) : GDH is < 10. (s. tab. 5.6) In general, LDH is markedly elevated. Mild jaundice is often in evidence; hyperglycaemia and renal impairment sometimes occur. A decrease in Quick's value may point to DIC. An increase in the transaminases due to ischaemia (with bioptic detection of centrilobular cell necroses) was observed even in cases of severe hypoxaemia caused by sleep apnoea in patients with considerable obesity (without cardiac or respiratory dysfunction!). (6) Imaging procedures show hepatomegaly and dilated hepatic veins. (s. fig. 39.3) • *Treatment* consists of stabilizing the circulation and eliminating the causes.

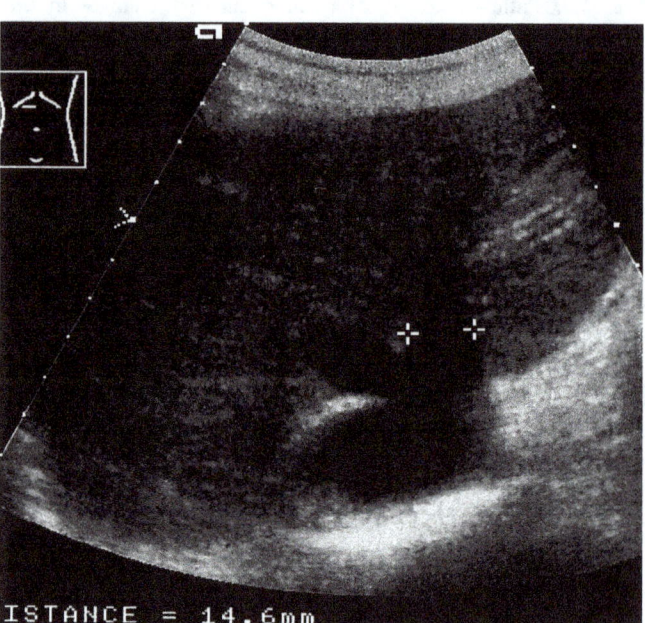

Fig. 39.3: Massive cardiac congestion of the hepatic veins with distinct dilatation up to 14.6 mm (++) (normally up to 10 mm)

due to ischaemia. (28) After recompensation, numerous granulocytes and pigment-loaded macrophages appear, followed by proliferating epithelial cells. The necrotized cells and erythrocytes are phagocytized by the Kupffer cells. Morphological repair starts after about five days and is completed within three to four weeks. (1, 17, 20) (s. tab. 39.1) (s. figs. 39.1, 39.2)

Drug metabolism: According to present knowledge, there is a delay in the elimination of certain drugs in patients with acute heart insufficiency. Thus, a *dose reduction* may have to be considered in some cases. In particular, these drugs include quinidine, cumarin/warfarin, digoxin, hydrochlorothiazide, lidocaine, mexiletine, procainamide and theophylline. (17, 19) • Our studies demonstrated a 30% reduction in the elimination rate of flow-limited (= ICG) and capacity-limited (= galactose, theophylline) substances. • We found a normal glucuronidization capacity for **4-methylumbelliferone**, but a significant delay in the biliary excretion of *4-MU-monoglucuronide*. (16) These findings are considered to be the cause of conjugated hyperbilirubinaemia, which is common in patients suffering from a congested liver.

1.2 Chronic heart insufficiency

The hepatic blood flow is decreased in chronic heart insufficiency, and there is disturbed venous outflow, i.e. cardiac output is diminished. There is also a pressure increase in the splanchnic nerve area with subsequent blood pooling as a result of the rise in CVP. The markedly reduced hepatic blood flow at first evokes an increase in oxygen extraction, but after its elimination, hypoxia with centrilobular cell necroses follows. The elevated CVP extends as far as the central veins, so that dilatation and hyperaemia of the sinusoids occur. Pericentral atrophy in the liver cell trabeculae develops at a later stage. (s. tab. 39.1) (s. fig. 39.4)

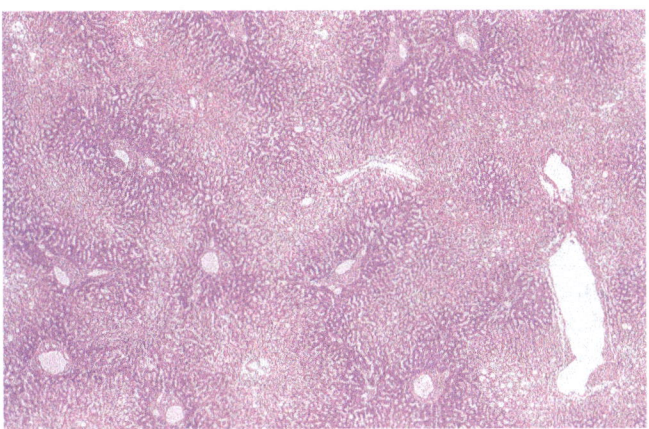

Fig. 39.4: Chronic passive congestion with centroacinar parenchymal atrophy and fibrosis (HE)

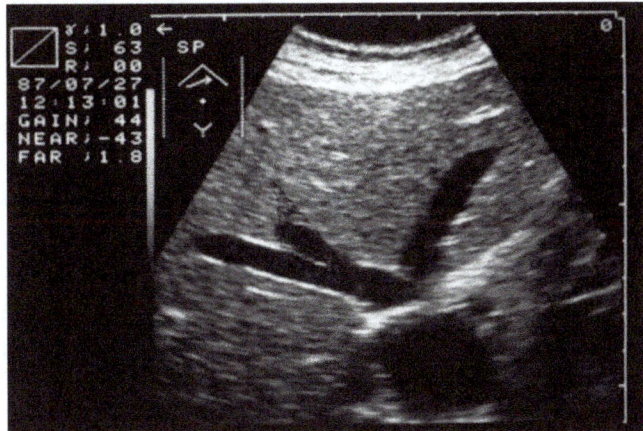

Fig. 39.5: Sonographic image of chronic liver congestion with dilated hepatic veins and inferior vena cava

Chronic congestion leads to an enlarged and plump liver with a dark red (purplish) colour. The central veins are dilated. In continued congestion, stasis paths develop between the central veins, resulting in the formation of confluent stasis areas. Various degrees of fatty changes in the liver cells as well as pigment deposits (lipofuscin, ceroid) appear. In the course of time, fibrosis of sinusoidal reticular fibres takes place; fibroses can also be observed along the stasis paths. In about 15% of cases, periodic acid-Schiff positive and diastase-resistant hyaline globules can be found. They are typically located directly around the zones of centrilobular congestion in hepatocytes. These globules range in size from 3 to 20 μm; they occur either as one or two large globules or as clusters of smaller inclusion bodies. (13) The extent of the **congestive fibrosis** depends largely upon the degree of cardiac congestion. (s. fig. 39.4) In 147 patients with chronic pulmonary heart disease, it was possible to demonstrate congestive fibrosis by autopsy in 14−42% of cases (depending on the degree of severity and duration of disease). (8) • Chronically indurated **nutmeg liver** (F. KIERNAN, 1833) develops gradually; the cut surface of such a diseased liver shows sunken, dark red centrilobular zones and slightly raised bulging, yellowish to pale brown (depending on the degree of fatty changes) peripheral areas of the lobules. • **Cardiac cirrhosis** was mentioned in older studies in up to 10% of cases. (14) Our own studies did not yield a single case of cardiac cirrhosis. (8) This clinical picture must be considered rare and is most likely in cases of constrictive pericarditis or in long-standing tricuspid valve insufficiency. It is assumed that the development of cardiac cirrhosis originates in sinusoidal thrombosing processes which extend to the vascular bed of the hepatic veins. (24, 31) Distinct regenerative nodes are not found in cardiac cirrhosis; this condition generally does not lead to extrahepatic cirrhosis-related complications.

Clinical features: With regard to the main findings of chronic heart insufficiency, the liver is symptom-free, apart from tenderness upon pressure in the right upper abdomen corresponding to *hepatomegaly*. On palpation, the liver is hard and has a smooth surface. *Splenomegaly* is detected in about 20% of patients.

In this condition, **hepato-jugular reflux** is *positive* if the venous channels between the hepatic and jugular veins are patent (i.e. long-standing pressure below the right costal arch accelerates the filling of the jugular veins, since the insufficient right ventricle is incapable of transporting the rising amount of blood supplied by the liver). • When the result is *negative*, the free passage between the hepatic veins and the jugular vein is interrupted. This sign is useful for diagnosing tricuspid regurgitation.

According to our own investigations, **P-III-P concentration** is the most important laboratory parameter (18): it is significantly higher in patients suffering from chronic liver congestion (due to the activity of fibrogenesis). There was also a correlation with the pressure in the right atrium. Moreover, the P-III-P value allowed a follow-up of chronic liver congestion or chronic congestive fibrosis. No correlation with hepatic biochemical standard values was found − these were normal or just marginally elevated. (15, 17, 18) Only the serum bilirubin was slightly increased in most cases. ICG elimination and the galactose elimination capacity were significantly reduced. Severe jaundice may occur in heart failure (23), in some cases with massive liver cell necroses.

Hepato(spleno)megaly is detected by **sonography.** The liver margin is rounded, the reflex pattern is dense and inhomogeneous. The hepatic veins are enlarged (at the confluence >10 mm) and show a systolic − diastolic pendular blood flow with predominant hepatopetal flow. (s. figs. 39.5, 39.6) The inferior vena cava presents a rigid wall without respiratory-dependent lumen fluctuations. Smaller amounts of ascites are frequently detectable. *Echocardiography* and *colour-encoded Doppler sonography* are the most important diagnostic and monitoring methods. (10) *CT* may yield additional findings of chronic liver congestion. (22)

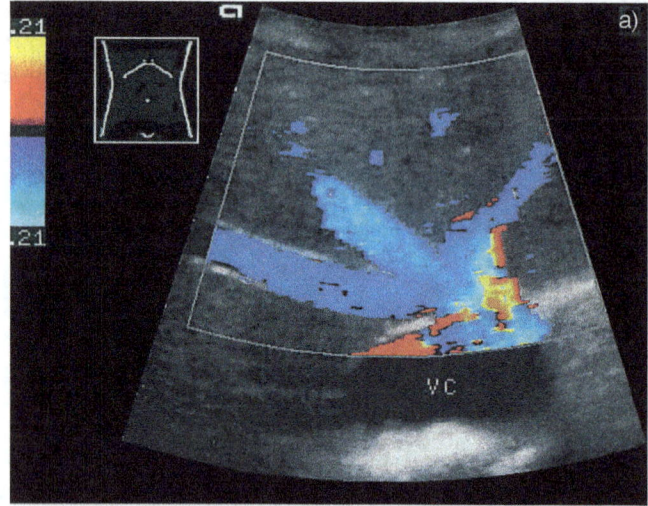

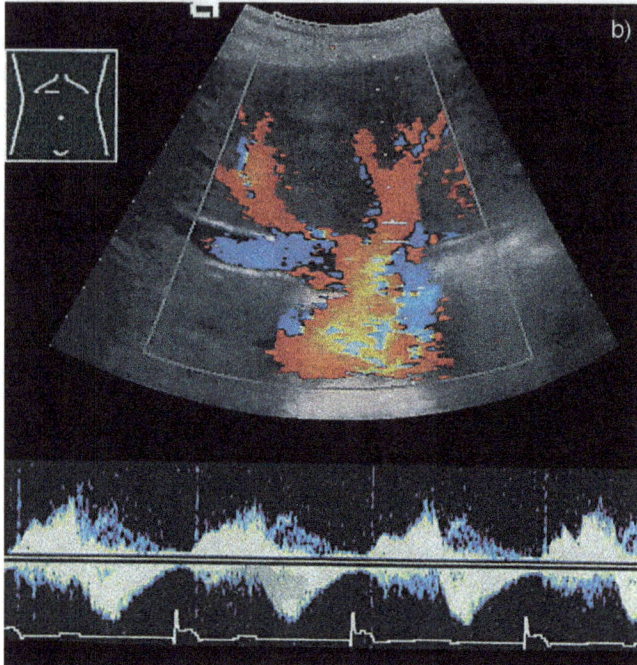

Fig. 39.6: *"Hepatic vein star"* • a) Normal finding: blue-coded right, medial and left hepatic veins indicate the hepatofugal flow. (VC = vena cava) • b) Right heart insufficiency: systolic-diastolic pendular blood flow with predominant hepatopetal flow

2 Disorders of the hepatic veins

The hepatic venous blood flow begins in the **central vein** of the lobules (= terminal hepatic vein), drains into the *sublobular veins* (= intercalated veins), from there into the *collecting veins* and then into the *truncal veins*. Perivenous connective tissue increases with the diameter of the vein. Venous blood reaches the *inferior vena cava* via three (valveless) **hepatic veins**; the confluence is below or within the diaphragm. From the **caudate lobe,** one to two small veins open directly into the inferior vena cava, as do a few small veins from the posterior segment of the right lobe of liver. (s. p. 21) • There are generally no **anastomoses** between the hepatic veins and the portal vein, except in liver cirrhosis. Similarly, no anastomoses are present between the hepatic veins and arteries either in a healthy liver or in a cirrhotic liver. • Normal **hepatic vein pressure** is about 6 mm Hg. **Oxygen saturation** of the hepatic veins amounts to approx. 67%.

With regard to the main diseases of the hepatic venous system, there are **three types** worthy of mention:

1. Budd-Chiari syndrome
2. Veno-occlusive disease
3. Endophlebitis obliterans hepatica

2.1 Budd-Chiari syndrome

2.1.1 Historical review

▶ REYNAUD (1829) was the first to report thrombosis in the vena cava with involvement of hepatic veins and the development of collateral circulation. In 1842 E. LAMBRON described inflammation of the hepatic veins concomitant with a liver abscess. • In 1845 the English internist G. BUDD reported three further cases: in two of them, hepatic vein thrombosis was likewise caused by liver abscesses, whereas no cause was evident in the third case although membranes were detected in the hepatic veins. • In 1899 the German pathologist H. CHIARI, who was working in Prague at that time, gave an account of two of his own patients and assessed the 8 cases which were known to him from the literature. However, more than 25 cases of veno-occlusive disease had already been reported prior to Chiari's publication. • The above-mentioned clinical picture with unclarified aetiology was defined by H. CHIARI (1899) as primary phlebitis of the large hepatic veins with secondary thrombosis, which he regarded as a separate entity. This gave rise to the term *endophlebitis obliterans hepatica*, also called Chiari's disease.

2.1.2 Definition

The Budd-Chiari syndrome (BCS) is defined as partial or complete obstruction of the hepatic veins due to thrombosis. This may affect the whole hepatic venous system from the central vein to the large hepatic veins, even as far as the opening of the inferior vena cava into the right atrium. However, the obstruction can simply occur in individual branches of the hepatic veins and thus affect only certain areas of the liver. The syndrome may have an acute onset or begin insidiously and take a chronic course. The clinical picture is usually characterized by the *Chiari triad*: (*1.*) hepatomegaly, (*2.*) abdominal pain, and (*3.*) ascites.

2.1.3 Aetiology

Aetiologically, BCS is characterized by an extremely heterogeneous clinical picture, even though it is initially possible to categorize the majority of causes into four groups: (*1.*) hypercoagulopathies, (*2.*) infections, (*3.*) malignant diseases, and (*4.*) endotheliotoxic substances. In 80–90% of patients, BCS can be attributed to a specific cause. The disease has often been detected during pregnancy as well. The observation that women contract the disease twice as often as men following the introduction of oral contraceptives supports the aetiological theory that it is linked to an increase in the oestrogen/progesterone level. The discovery of new genetic defects causing hypercoagulability can also explain some cases of BCS. (60) • A membranous obstruction, especially close to the opening of the middle and left hepatic veins into the inferior vena cava, is considered to be an aetiological peculiarity. Such a "web" varies from a thin membrane to a thick fibrous band. This unusual phenomenon is often encountered in India, Japan and South Africa (congenital?, phytotoxins?). A chronic course develops. (s. tabs. 14.5; 39.2) (s. pp 257, 562)

2.1.4 Morphology

Laparoscopy: The liver is enlarged and displays a dark reddish cyanotic surface with a rounded margin. Congested veins and collaterals in the abdominal region suggest portal hypertension. Transformational processes may occur in a chronic course (in 30—40% of cases) or when the liver is only partially affected, so that even the picture of a cirrhosis has been observed. Ascites, occasionally also in its sanguinolent form, is detected in most patients.

Liver biopsy: Histology reveals pronounced centrilobular congestion as well as sinus ectasia, necroses and thrombi in the central veins, which are either fresh or already organized. Parenchymal atrophies and nodal transformational processes can be observed after a longer period of time. (s. figs. 29.9; 39.7)

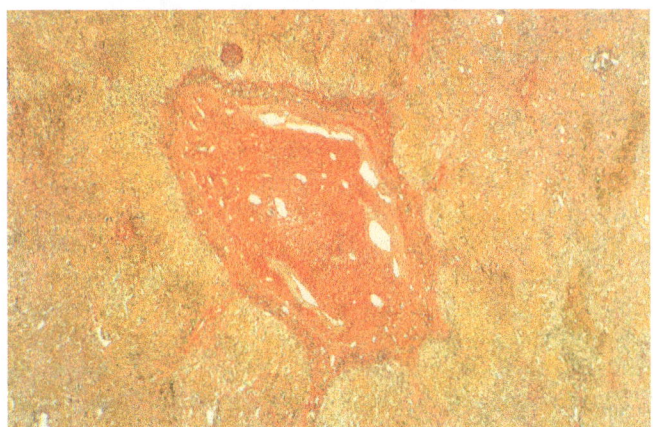

Fig. 39.7: Budd-Chiari syndrome due to essential thrombocythaemia. Long-standing thrombotic occlusion of a liver vein (Sirius red) (s. fig. 29.9!)

2.1.5 Clinical features

BCS is a rare disease and responsible for about 5% of all cases of portal hypertension. The highest incidence is observed in the third and fourth decades. Frequency varies considerably in different countries and regions depending on its aetiology. • The clinical picture is determined by the course of disease and therefore there

1. **Hypercoagulopathies**
   Antiphospholipid syndrome (63)
   Antithrombin III deficiency
   Essential thrombocytosis
   Factor V mutation (42)
   Hyperhomocysteinaemia
   Lupus anticoagulant
   Myeloproliferative disease (32)
   Paroxysmal nocturnal haemoglobinuria
   Polycythaemia vera
   Protein C deficiency (71)
   Protein S deficiency
   Sickle-cell anaemia
2. **Infections**
   Amoebic liver abscess
   Aspergillosis
   Crohn's disease
   Echinococcosis
   Hepatic abscess
   Pyogenic abscess (49)
   Schistosomiasis
   Syphilis
   Tuberculosis
3. **Malignant diseases**
   Adrenal carcinoma
   Bronchogenic carcinoma
   Fibrolamellar carcinoma
   Hepatocellular carcinoma
   Leiomyosarcoma
   Leukaemia
   Renal cell carcinoma
   Rhabdomyosarcoma
4. **Endotheliotoxic substances**
   Cytostatics (66)
   Azathioprine
   Phytotoxins
5. **Hormonal factors**
   Oral contraceptives (60)
   Pregnancy (50)
6. **Immunological factors**
   Behçet's disease (36)
   Hypereosinophilia
   Sarcoidosis (67)
   Sjögren's syndrome (57)
7. **Other aetiological observations**
   Abdominal trauma (56)
   Laparoscopic cholecystectomy
   Membranous obstruction
   Polycystic liver disease (37)
   Retroperitoneal neurilemmoma (68)
   Tumour in the right atrium (45)
8. **Cryptogenic**

Tab. 39.2: Possible causes of the Budd-Chiari syndrome (including some references) (s. figs. 29.9; 39.7)

is great variability in findings. In **chronic BCS,** abdominal pain is mild, and hepatomegaly develops only gradually. Splenomegaly, diarrhoea and ascites, including oedema in the legs, are occasionally in evidence. Oesophageal varices may develop as a result of postsinusoidal portal hypertension. Non-characteristic symptoms (fatigue, inappetence, weakness, meteorism) are present in most cases. All laboratory parameters may remain in the normal range for a long time. • A far smaller percentage of patients suffer from **acute BCS** with severe pain in the upper abdomen, nausea, vomiting and malaise. Jaundice is often present. Hepatomegaly develops rapidly. Acute BCS can present clinically as acute liver failure. (64) The *caudate lobe* is enlarged as it has efferent hepatic veins of its own, which circumvent the main branches of the hepatic vein and lead directly to the inferior vena cava. (35) As a rule, in an enlarged caudate lobe, which may also compress the inferior vena cava, it is technically impossible to apply a portacaval shunt. In cases of severe parenchymal deterioration, there is a risk of hepatic encephalopathy and hepatorenal syndrome. The prognosis of acute BCS is very poor; the dramatic course of the disease rapidly leads to liver failure. (40, 43, 54, 55, 58, 64, 72, 76, 77)

2.1.6 Diagnostics

Laboratory parameters are irrelevant for diagnosis! Transaminases, LDH, GDG and alkaline phosphatase are in general moderately increased, and hyperbilirubinaemia can be detected in 20—25% of cases. The albumin level is usually reduced; hypoproteinaemia may be caused by protein-losing enteropathy. Evidence of disturbances in *blood coagulation*, with regard to both hypercoagulopathic status and haemorrhagic diathesis, is of significance. *P-III-P* serum values rise in chronic courses with increasing fibrosis. Liver function tests, however, generally show normal results.

Sonography shows hepatomegaly and inhomogeneous, hypoechoic zones. The hepatic veins are invisible or present as narrow structures. The caudate lobe is enlarged and often causes an hourglass-like constriction of the inferior vena cava. Ascites is confirmed. Colour-encoded duplex (or Doppler) sonography provides extra information, e.g. high flow velocities in areas of stenosis in the IVC or hepatic veins. Diagnosis proves to be correct in 85—90% of cases; the results are further improved by CT angiography or MR angiography. (38, 41, 58, 72, 77)

Computer tomography, especially when coupled with a contrast medium and in the form of CTAP, is an excellent tool for analyzing the venous blood flow and detecting any disturbances in inflow or outflow. Thrombosed hepatic veins are not visible, whereas intrahepatic collateral vessels are detectable. The parenchyma is characterized by an inhomogeneous, patch-like enhancement. (39, 44) (s. fig. 39.8) • **MRI** provides reliable evaluation by means of multiphase, contrast-enhanced, three-dimensional MR angiography. (76, 77)

Angiography, coupled with cavography and venography of the liver, is the most reliable examination method: venous obstructions can easily be localized, and the residual venous blood circulation always displays a spider web-like picture. • In some 20% of cases, the portal vein is also thrombosed, indicating arteriography in the form of indirect splenoportography. In addition, angiography also offers the therapeutic possibilities of interventional radiology. (47, 50)

Histology: In cases where histological evidence is required, samples should be taken from both liver lobes, since the expressivity of the histological picture can vary greatly in different sections of the liver in BCS. The best technique in this connection is **laparoscopy** (possibly combined with *targeted biopsy*). Although the risk of haemorrhage is generally high in biopsy, intense bleeding or delayed coagulation can be effectively reduced and more easily controlled under laparoscopy. As a rule, however, the laparoscopic image of BCS is impressive enough per se — especially if supported by imaging procedures — so that biopsy and the accompanying risks can indeed be avoided altogether.

2.1.7 Treatment

There are very few reports of **spontaneous remission** even in partial BCS. • The *therapeutic principle* in all cases is to remove liver congestion, limit and lyse any thromboses as well as eliminate ascites. (43, 55, 72) • Medication includes immediate **lysis treatment** followed by heparinization. Despite initial success, frequent complications have been reported (e.g. pulmonary embolism, re-occlusion, intraperitoneal bleeding). (69) • **Percutaneous balloon angioplasty** was first used by S. EGUCHI et al. in 1974 in membranous obstruction of the inferior vena cava and was subsequently applied in BCS. (s. fig. 39.8)

In some cases, a *stent implantation* proved to be successful. (53, 73—75) The significance of *percutaneous transluminal angioplasty* is not only based on its long-term therapeutic effect, but also on its combination with operative shunts or other surgical techniques. (47) This method was improved by laser assistance (S. FURUI et al., 1988) • To date, a total of 23 different **surgical techniques** have been reported (33, 51, 54, 58, 62, 72, 76), consisting mainly of shunt placements, preferably the mesocaval shunt, bypass operations, resections, thrombectomies and liver transplantation. Even though it is technically difficult, dorsocranial liver resection with direct hepatoatrial anastomosis successfully corrects the venous perfusions of the liver physiologically. Meanwhile, urgent covered (polytetrafluoroethylene) TIPS and portal vein thrombectomy have proved effective. (46, 48, 59, 61, 65) It is relatively quick and easy to apply, has proved to be a low-risk procedure and can be carried out before resorting to other invasive or surgical techniques. Thus it is possible to bridge the time required for planning any surgical intervention or **liver transplantation.** The latter is urgently indicated in an acute course. Continuous long-term anticoagulation is necessary even after transplantation, as is invariably the case with all of the above-mentioned treatment measures. (48, 52, 70)

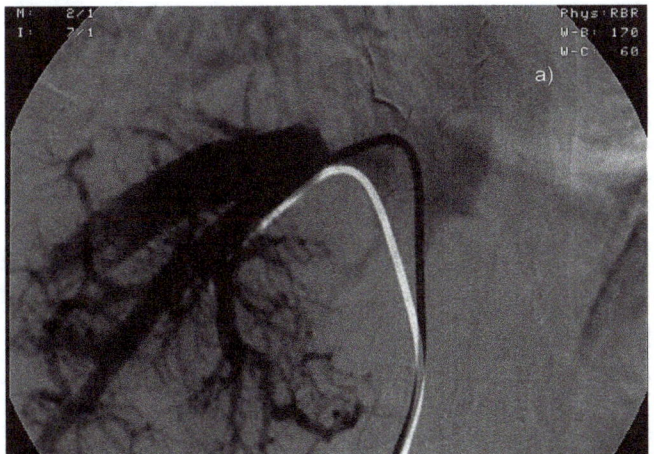

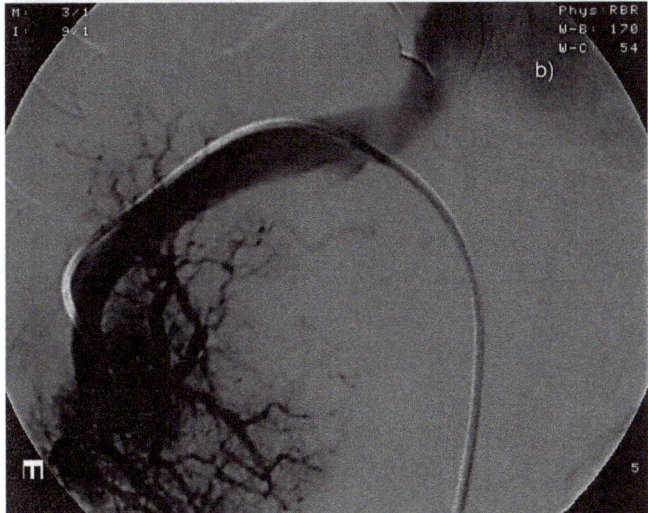

Fig. 39.8: Budd-Chiari syndrome • a) Pronounced collateral circulation resulting from thrombotic occlusion of the right hepatic vein. • b) Re-opening of the vessel and rapid reduction of the collateral vessels following successful balloon dilatation

Constrictive pericarditis
The clinical picture and hepatic changes are like those of the Budd-Chiari syndrome. Considerable thickening of the liver capsule resembles *sugar icing*. The liver is enlarged and firm. Tense ascites is present. Histologically, the changes are similar to those of cardiac cirrhosis.

2.2 Veno-occlusive disease

2.2.1 Definition

Veno-occlusive disease (VOD) is characterized by thrombosis of the central and small (sublobular) hepatic veins. It is also known as the *radicular form* of the Budd-Chiari syndrome or as the *Stuart-Bras syndrome*. (s. tab. 14.5) (79, 96–98)

2.2.2 Aetiology

Toxic substances or physical impact cause direct damage to the centrilobular veins and the small branches of the hepatic veins, resulting in thrombosis. • The first reports were published simultaneously in South Africa (G. SELZER et al.) and Jamaica (K.R. HILL) in 1951. This disease is due to chronic intoxication with pyrrolizidine alkaloids, which are found in plants like Senecio, Crotalaria, Heliotropium and Cynoglossum. Intake occurs by drinking medicinal tea or through consuming contaminated pulses and cereals. In 1974 and 1978, epidemic-like outbreaks of VOD were observed in Afghanistan and India after local inhabitants had eaten cereals contaminated with pyrrolizidine alkaloids. The real toxicity of these alkaloids is based upon their transformation into alkylating pyrrole derivatives, which are toxic to endothelial cells and hepatocytes. • Other causes of VOD include cytostatics, immunosuppressives, radiotherapy (> 30 Gy), immunological reactions and alcoholic hepatitis. (s. tab. 39.3) (s. pp 562, 587)

1. Alcoholic hepatitis
2. Bone-marrow transplantation (84, 88, 89, 91)
3. Cytostatics (80, 82, 83, 90, 92)
4. Immunosuppressives
5. Lupus erythematosus (94)
6. Oral contraceptives (78)
7. Pyrrolizidine alkaloids (93, 95)
8. Radiotherapy
9. Stem-cell transplantation (87)

Tab. 39.3: Possible causes of veno-occlusive disease (VOD) (including some references) (s. fig. 29.10)

2.2.3 Morphology

Histology provides useful diagnostic evidence. Sinusoidal endothelial damage can be found, including extravascular accumulation of erythrocytes in Disse's spaces as well as subendothelial oedema and cellulation. After two to three days, delicate fibres appear within the central and sublobular veins, occasionally also in the medium-sized hepatic veins, ultimately resulting in occlusion of the lumen. Fibrotic thickening of the vessel walls occurs. Stenosis and thrombosis of the small hepatic veins cause extensive sinusoidal congestion. The liver cells become necrotic or atrophic. • Micronodular cirrhosis develops in a chronic course. (s. fig. 29.10)

2.2.4 Clinical features

The clinical symptomatology is similar to that of chronic Budd-Chiari syndrome. About 10% of cases display an asymptomatic clinical picture over an extended period of time. • Spontaneous reversibility of VOD has been observed following administration of pyrrolizidine. (95) However, the disease may also progress rapidly to liver failure. A chronic course generally leads to liver cirrhosis with postsinusoidal portal hypertension. • *Laboratory values* reveal a slight increase in the transaminases and occasionally in alkaline phosphatase as well as thrombocytopenia with a rapid decrease in haemoglobin. A rise in P-III-P is also significant in VOD, both for early diagnosis and monitoring purposes. (84) • The *wedged hepatic vein pressure* is increased. Due to its localization in the small hepatic veins, VOD cannot be diagnosed by means of *imaging techniques.* However, these techniques, particularly CEDS and CTAP, provide reliable evidence of gradually developing portal hypertension as well as the reduction or reversal of the portal blood flow during normal flow in the hepatic veins and the inferior vena cava. (85, 86, 98) • *Histology* makes it possible to achieve a reliable diagnosis. (s. fig. 29.10)

2.2.5 Treatment

Once the cause of VOD has been found, it must be eliminated (if possible). Treatment is symptom-oriented and directed towards the sequelae of portal hypertension. In order to reduce portal hypertension, medication (spironolactone, molsidomin, beta blockers, etc.) and TIPS are recommended. (81) Ultimately, indications for liver transplantation have to be considered. (91)

2.3 Inferior vena cava syndrome

An obstruction of the IVC above the influx of the hepatic veins can be caused by a congenital anomaly or the presence of "webs". The latter may also be acquired in the case of membranous obstruction. Sometimes, a hepatopulmonary syndrome develops; in this case, balloon cavoplasty is a possible indication for treatment. • Such an obstruction passes over into HCC in 30−40% of cases. This is probably caused by the ongoing liver cell necrosis and regeneration processes. An important diagnostic hint is the formation of whorls in the obstructed area of the IVC, as shown by colour-encoded Doppler sonography. This finding points to an infiltrating, usually malignant process in the caudate lobe. (s. fig. 39.9)

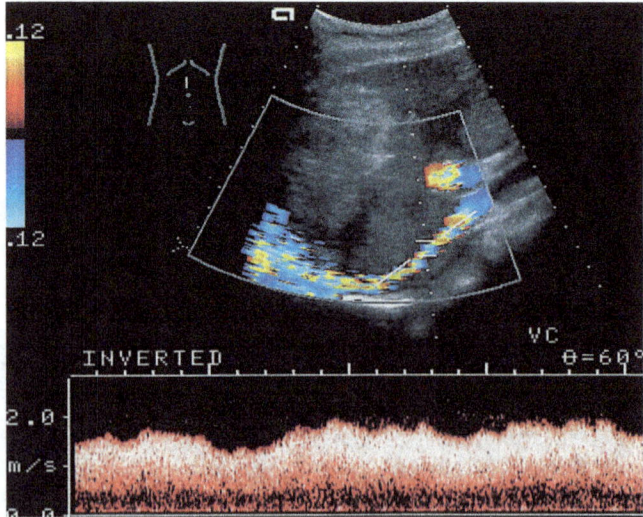

Fig. 39.9: Inferior vena cava syndrome with infiltration and stenosis: blue-red-yellow colour changes as a sign of whorl formation due to an infiltrating malignant process in the caudate lobe

3 Disorders of the portal vein

▶ The **portal vein** is formed by the retropancreatic union of the right and left gastric veins, the pyloric vein, the superior and inferior mesenteric veins and the splenic vein. Its trunk runs inside the **hepatoduodenal ligament** to the liver. Within the porta hepatis, the portal vein divides into a **right branch** (which also receives the cystic vein) and a **left branch** (into which the paraumbilical veins contained in the round ligament and the ventroflexus ramus from the left sagittal fossa open). • The rami of the portal vein branch out and reach the portal fields where they become **interlobular veins,** which generally fork into **two interlobular venules** (= leading veins). The latter transport the blood into distributory veins which continue in Y-form into the **afferent venules** (final ramifications) and transport portal blood into the **sinusoids.** • The portal vein is 5−8 cm in *length* and has a *diameter* of 1.2 ± 0.2 cm. The normal *portal pressure* is 3−6 (−8) mmHg. (s. fig. 2.6) The portal blood flow amounts to 1150−1300 ml/min. (s. pp 21, 252)

> Portal vein diseases may be *congenital* or *acquired,* or arise as a sequela of portal hypertension: (*1.*) portal vein anomalies, (*2.*) pylephlebitis, (*3.*) portal vein thrombosis, and (*4.*) portal venous gas.

3.1 Anomalies of the portal vein

Congenital anomalies of the portal vein are very rare. This also applies to accessory portal veins with their individually varying patterns.

Accessory portal veins are small veins at the surface of the hepatic serosa and in the surrounding peritoneal folds which normally originate in the diaphragm and the stomach. They can either open into the portal vein or enter the liver parenchyma independently. • **Anomalous accessory portal veins** may sometimes originate in the area of the portal veins around the gall bladder, the porta hepatis, the omentum, the interior surface of the abdominal wall or the hepatorenal ligament, etc.

Anomalies include missing portal vein and intrahepatic branches with simultaneous hyperplasia of the hepatic artery. • *Abernethy malformation:* The congenital aplasia of the portal vein was first described more than 200 years ago (J. ABERNETHY, 1793). In this condition, the portal vein connects with the inferior vena cava, generally at the same point as the renal veins. (99) • The portal vein and its branches may also be located in front of the duodenum and the pancreatic head. Sometimes, a multitude of small vessels are found instead of a single portal vein. Another anomaly is a faulty opening of the portal vein into the renal vein, with the enlarged hepatic artery taking over the entire blood supply to the liver. • Moreover, there may be anomalous anastomoses between the portal vein and the branches of the greater circulation. (100) • Besides aplasia or obliteration of the portal vein, congenital arterioportal fistulas (s. tab. 14.2) (s. p. 253) or portal vein stenoses also cause portal hypertension with subsequent *phlebosclerosis*.

In addition to the congenital anomalies, various other clinical features are considered to be responsible for disorders affecting the portal vein system. (s. tab. 39.4)

1. Anomalous accessory portal veins
2. Aplasia
3. Arterioportal fistula
4. Cavernous transformation
5. Cruveilhier-Baumgarten syndrome
6. Faulty openings of the portal vein
7. Displacement
8. Obliteration
9. Portal vein stenosis

Tab. 39.4: Clinical features responsible for disorders of the portal vein system

3.1.1 Cavernous transformation

This condition is primary angiomatosis of the portal vein: a spongy convolution of venous vessels branching in a tendril-like manner has formed instead of a trunk – predominantly in the area of the hepatoduodenal ligament. (101, 102) • Prehepatic portal hypertension develops as a result of the disturbed outflow from the splanchnic nerve area. However, both liver function and histology are normal. Occasionally, considerable mechanical jaundice has been observed. Clinical symptoms include abdominal pain, splenomegaly, haematemesis and oesophageal varices. (103) The internal pressure in the spleen is increased, while the wedged hepatic vein pressure remains in the normal range. Successful diagnosis is based upon imaging techniques and colour-encoded duplex Doppler sonography. (105) There is often an atrophy of the left lateral segment and right liver lobe as well as a hypertrophy of the caudate lobe and segment IV can be found. (104) (s. tab. 14.2) (s. p. 253)

3.1.2 Cruveilhier-Baumgarten disease

In the absence of physiological postnatal closure of the umbilical vein, an anastomosis will form between the portal vein and the abdominal wall. Hypoplasia of the portal system and liver can also be observed. Prehepatic portal hypertension develops with visible and palpable venectasia in the abdominal skin (= *Medusa's head*) (M.A. SEVERINO, 1632). (s. p. 91) (s. fig. 14.13) A venous murmur (= *venous hum*) is often heard periumbilically, generally in the centre of the Medusa's head. Splenomegaly causes splenogenous maturation arrest. Diagnosis is confirmed by imaging techniques. (s. p. 254!)

Cruveilhier-Baumgarten syndrome: This is a secondary syndrome observed in liver cirrhosis with pronounced portal hypertension. Recanalization of the umbilical vein and of the paraumbilical veins develops. (s. fig. 39.10) • Clinical symptoms include splenomegaly, Medusa's head, periumbilical vascular murmur and ascites.

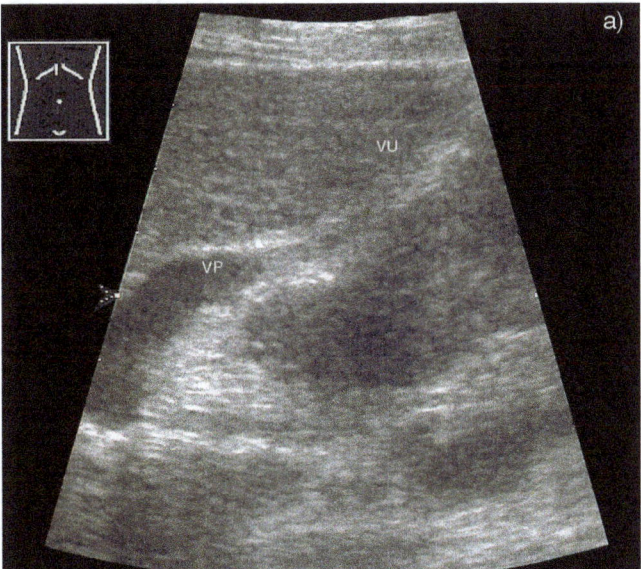

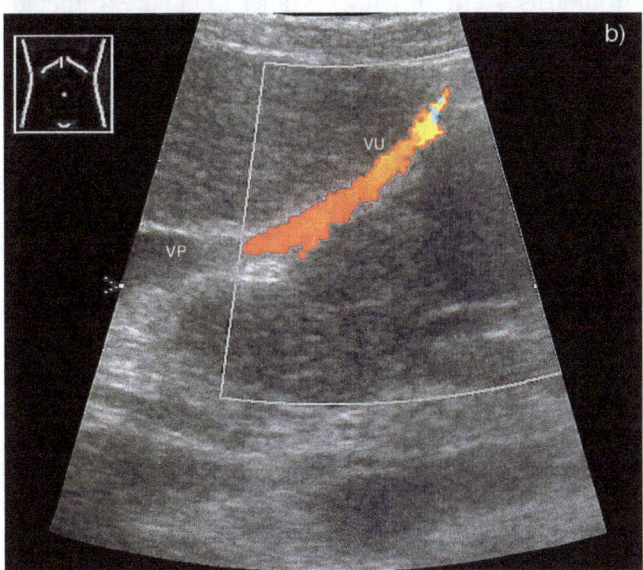

Fig. 39.10: a) Re-opened umbilical vein (VU) due to pronounced portal hypertension in haemochromatotic cirrhosis. (VP = umbilical branch of the left portal vein) • b) Hepatofugal blood flow in the umbilical vein (VU) depicted by colour-encoded duplex sonography

Acquired causes may also be responsible for some of the congenital anomalies described above. Mention should be made of (*1.*) arterioportal fistulas, (*2.*) cavernous transformation of the portal vein (in portal vein thrombosis), (*3.*) fibrous obliteration of the portal vein, and (*4.*) cicatricial portal vein stenosis. These may also cause prehepatic hypertension. (s. tab. 14.2) (s. p. 254!)

3.1.3 Arterioportal venous fistula

Arterioportal venous fistulas (R. SACHS, 1892) between the arterial and portal system may occur following puncture, trauma, HCC, HHT, invasive surgery and tumour growth. Congenital arterioportal fistula is rare. About 12 cases have been reported. (106) Clinical symptoms include prehepatic portal hypertension (111, 113), vascular murmur in the right hypochondrium, abdominal pain (113) and signs of hyperdynamic circulation. Sonography shows dilation of both the hepatic artery and the intrahepatic portal vein branches, often with hepatofugal flow. (110) Calcification of a liver biopsy-related fistula may occur. (109) Diagnosis is made by duplex Doppler sonography and confirmed by angiography, with the possibility of simultaneous embolization of the fistula. Diffuse forms are usually congenital, whereas solitary fistulas are typically acquired. The latter are more frequent. (108, 112) If treatment fails, selective resection of the fistula is indicated. (107) There is normally no change in portal hypertension after the development of *hepatoportal sclerosis*. (s. p. 254)

3.2 Pylephlebitis

Purulent inflammation of the branches of the portal vein is usually accompanied by subsequent portal vein thrombosis. Aetiologically, intrahepatic and extrahepatic purulent pylephlebitis share certain similarities. • Portal vein infections have their *origin* in inflammatory processes of neighbouring structures such as appendicitis, cholecystitis, liver abscesses (as was already postulated by H. CHIARI in the first cases published) (s. p. 856), suppurative hydatid cysts, colitis, diverticulitis, infected haemorrhoids, covered perforations (gall bladder, gastric ulcer) and malignant tumours (gall bladder, pancreas). • *Clinical symptoms* include fever, chills, abdominal pain, meteorism, enlarged and tender liver as well as splenomegaly. In most cases, inflammation parameters are clearly pathological. (s. tab. 37.6) Bacteriological haemocultures only yield positive results when the defence mechanisms of the liver RES have been overwhelmed. The clinical picture of septic portal vein thrombosis can often be observed. • *Treatment* with local fibrinolysis and TIPS has proved successful.

3.3 Portal vein thrombosis

Thromboses in the vessels of the portal system are the most common cause of prehepatic portal hypertension. • Even in the **postpartal** phase, portal vein thrombosis may occur due to the obliteration of the umbilical vein spreading to the portal vein or due to an infection of the umbilical vein with subsequent pylephlebitis. • In the **adult**, this clinical picture is often observed in liver diseases that cause the portal blood flow to slow down (or even reverse). All diseases accompanied by hypercoagulopathies also have a strong tendency to cause portal vein thrombosis. (117, 118, 120, 122, 124, 129, 132, 133, 136) Patients with HCC due to cirrhosis frequently develop thrombosis. Septic processes (e.g. appendicitis, diverticulitis, colitis) are a further cause, particularly in immunocompromised patients. In addition, inflammatory tissue, tumours, lymphomas or fibrosis may narrow the lumen of the portal vein and trigger thrombosis. Thrombosis of the portal vein can also result from progressive thrombosis of the splenic vein. (s. tab. 14.2) Portal vein thrombosis is hence caused by many factors. (119, 133, 136–138) (s. tab. 39.5)

1. **Hypercoagulopathy**	
Antiphospholipid sydrome	Oral contraceptives
Antithrombin III deficiency	Protein C deficiency
Factor V mutation	Protein S deficiency
Factor VIII elevation	Pregnancy
Hyperhomocysteinaemia	Thromboembolism
Myeloproliferative diseases	
2. **Inflammatory processes**	
Appendicitis	Crohn's disease
Behçet's disease	Diverticulitis
Cholangitis	Pancreatitis
Cholecystitis	PSC
Collagenoses	Ulcerative colitis
3. **Infections**	
Actinomycosis	Schistosomiasis
Candida albicans	Tuberculosis
Echinococcus	
4. **Invasive treatment**	
Abdominal surgery	Liver transplantation
Alcohol injection	Portography
Chemoembolization	Sclerotherapy
Dialysis	Splenectomy
Islet-cell injection	TIPS
Liver resection	
5. **Progressive splenic vein thrombosis**	
Pancreatitis	Splenectomy
Pancreatic carcinoma	
6. **Malignant processes**	
Cholangiocarcinoma	Hepatocellular carcinoma
Cystic carcinoma	Pancreatic tumour
7. **Intoxications**	
Arsenic	Radiation
Cytostatics	
8. **Delayed portal blood flow**	
Congenital fibrosis	
Liver cirrhosis	
Lymphoma	
Nodular regenerative hyperplasia	
Retroperitoneal fibrosis	
Stenoses/strictures	
9. **Haematologic diseases**	
Paroxysmal nocturnal haemoglobinuria	
Sickle cell anaemia	
10. **Cardiovascular diseases**	
Constrictive pericarditis	
Obstruction of inferior vena cava	
Pylephlebitis	
Tricuspid insufficiency	
Tumour of the right atrium	
Umbilical vein infection	
Veno-occlusive disease	
11. **Trauma**	
12. **Cryptogenic**	

Tab. 39.5: Possible causes of portal vein thrombosis

The severity of the clinical picture depends upon how rapidly and to what extent the portal vein obstruction develops. • Haemorrhagic infarction of the intestine, due to sudden thrombotic occlusion, causes severe abdominal pain, haematemesis and melaena, circulatory shock and, ultimately, the death of the patient. • In gradual obstruction, splenomegaly and hypersplenism develop, accompanied by collateral vessels in the form of a sponge-like venous network (= *cavernous transformation*), which makes partial compensation possible. Gallbladder varices, even with rupture and bleeding, have also been observed. (115, 121) Pronounced gastric varices can sometimes be found. (s. fig. 39.11). The size of the liver is normal, as are the wedged hepatic vein pressure (with increased intrasplenic pressure) and histology.

of disease), TIPS (possibly with local thrombolysis) or a shunt operation. Prognosis is poor.

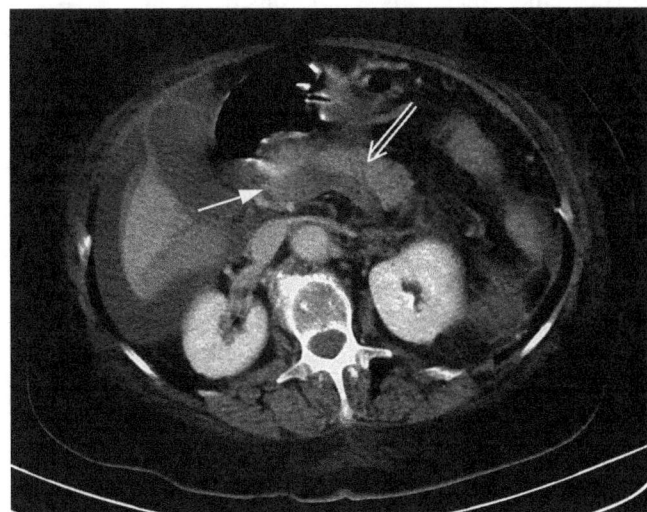

Fig. 39.12: Thrombosis of the portal vein (⇐) and splenic vein (→): contrast medium-free, hypodense structure; evidence of ascites

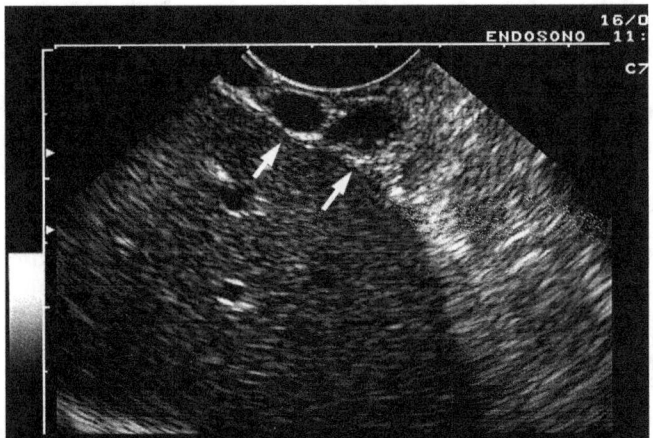

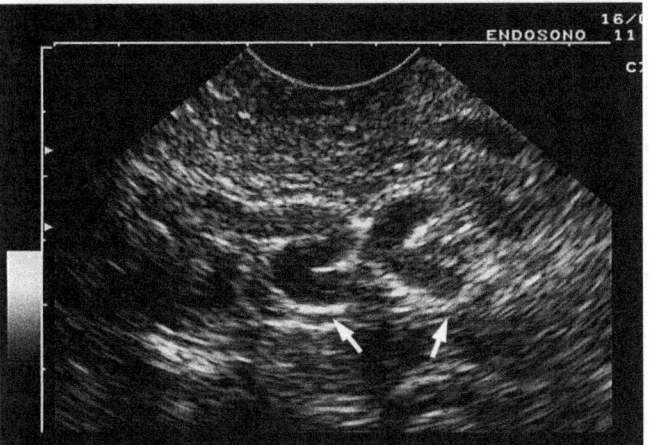

Fig. 39.11: Pronounced gastric varices (arrows) in portal vein thrombosis (= prehepatic block) caused by polycythaemia vera

Impairment of liver function only occurs at a later stage (131), and *hepatoportal sclerosis* develops. • Diagnosis is made by colour Doppler sonography (sensitivity >90%) (126), CT (s. fig. 39.12) and angiography (e.g. CTAP). Angiographic findings are also useful for deciding on the respective *therapy*: thrombolysis with subsequent anticoagulant treatment (if possible!) (116, 125, 128), percutaneous transhepatic angioplasty and thrombectomy (both procedures can only be applied in the early stages

3.4 Portal vein aneurysm

Aneurysms of the portal vein are very rare. However, since the introduction of imaging procedures, this generally asymptomatic finding has been detected more frequently, in most cases by chance. In **intrahepatic localization** (first reported by H.S. VINE et al., 1979), the aneurysms are mainly situated in the right lobe and reach a size of up to 4 cm in diameter. The cause is not clear. Congenital malformation with subsequent portal hypertension has been postulated, as has acquired vessel wall weakness (e.g. in pancreatitis). The diagnosis is made by sonography and MRI. (139, 140) Caroli's syndrome has to be ruled out by differential diagnosis. Spontaneous rupture of such an aneurysm has been reported. (142) Treatment is not primarily required, but regular monitoring is necessary. In portal hypertension, however, the application of a shunt (surgically, transjugal-portacavally) may be indicated. (141)

3.5 Zahn's pseudoinfarct

This well-demarcated hyperaemic area in the liver was first described by F.W. ZAHN in 1897. He called the phenomenon "atrophic red liver infarction", but without necrosis. Such a form of infarct is an oddity. (123, 130) Sudden intrahepatic occlusion of the portal vein branches with simultaneous reduction of the arterial blood flow results in a narrowing and atrophy of the liver cell trabeculae and consecutive dilation of the associated sinusoids. A wedge-shaped, dark bluish-red area of the liver appears, which is most clearly visible when the liver is simultaneously congested. The thin end of the wedge points to the occluded branch of the portal vein. Despite the term "infarct", no necrosis can be observed! • Zahn's infarct may also be found in the area surrounding liver metastases due to compression of the portal vein branches by tumourous tissue.

3.6 Hepatic portal venous gas

This rare condition, which has a high mortality rate (up to 80%), was first described by J.N. WOLF et al. in 1955. (146) • In cases of diverticulitis, bowel-wall fistulas, necrotizing enterocolitis, intraperitoneal abscesses, etc., gas-forming pathogens may pass into the portal vein system. These gas bubbles are visible using US and CT. (s. fig. 39.13) At the same time, thrombosing processes may develop in the portal veins. • Therapy depends on the underlying disease and is based on antibiotics. In isolated cases, it is also necessary to administer anticoagulants and apply interventional methods. (143–145)

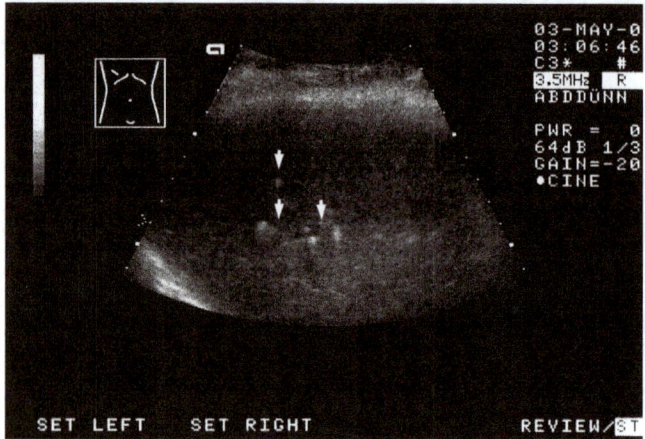

Fig. 39.13: Pylephlebitis with gas bubbles (arrows) in the portal vein system in intestinal gangrene

4 Disorders of the hepatic arteries

▶ The **common hepatic artery,** a branch of the coeliac artery, runs in a retroperitoneal direction above the pancreas into the hepatoduodenal ligament. It continues as the **proper hepatic artery,** which branches into the **right hepatic artery** (with the cystic artery) and the **left hepatic artery** to supply the two liver lobes. Ramification of the hepatic artery varies greatly. • The branches of the hepatic artery accompany the bile ducts and the portal vein as far as the portal fields. Radicular branches subsequently fork off forming the **peribiliary plexus** within the connective tissue of the portal paths. The peripheral, medial and central areas of the hepatic lobules are supplied by **intralobular arterioles.** • A small percentage of the arterial blood supply is also guaranteed by influx from the superior mesenteric, inferior pancreatic-duodenal and supraduodenal arteries. • Only 40–50% of the oxygen requirement and 35% of the blood volume of the liver (350–500 ml/min.) are supplied by the hepatic artery. Hence, the clinical picture of diseased liver arteries is usually relatively mild, apart from bleeding caused by ruptures. (s. p. 20) • The most important clinical disorders of the hepatic artery are:

1. Aneurysm	3. Nodular periarteritis
2. Occlusion	4. Arteriosclerosis

4.1 Aneurysm

4.1.1 Definition

While aneurysms of the hepatic arteries are in themselves rare, they nevertheless constitute 20% of all aneurysms of the splanchnic arteries. They are located extrahepatically in 80% and intrahepatically in 20% of cases. At 60%, the common hepatic artery is most frequently involved, followed by the right hepatic artery, which is affected in 30% of cases. A rupture (up to 80% of cases) constitutes a great risk to the afflicted, but often symptom-free patients. After confirmation of the diagnosis, treatment should begin immediately.

4.1.2 Aetiology

Congenital anomalies and aneurysms in the hepatic arteries are very rare. (148) **Acquired** aneurysms are the result of vessel wall damage, injuries or inflammatory processes. (150, 152, 156) • **Pseudoaneurysms** may occur after acute pancreatitis and the formation of pseudocysts. (155) (s. tab. 39.6)

1. **Congenital aneurysms**	5. **Infections**
2. **Vascular wall degeneration**	Endocarditis
Arteriosclerosis	Mycosis
Fibromuscular dysplasia	Pancreatitis
Media degeneration	Syphilis
	Tuberculosis
3. **Abdominal traumas**	
4. **Iatrogenic causes**	6. **Vasculitis**
Bile-duct surgery	Periarteritis nodosa
Intra-arterial chemotherapy	Vasculitis
Liver biopsy	
Transhepatic interventions	7. **Multiple pregnancies**

Tab. 39.6: Possible causes of hepatic artery aneurysm

4.1.3 Clinical features

Symptomatology depends on the extent and localization of the aneurysm, which can vary greatly in size, ranging from the diameter of a millet seed to that of a walnut (there have been cases with aneurysms as big as a grapefruit). Small aneurysms do not cause any symptoms and are only discovered incidentally during imaging procedures or surgery. Patients mostly complain of uncharacteristic abdominal pain, which may precede a rupture by several months. Large aneurysms are characterized by a continuous murmur. (151)

After **perforation** (60–80% of patients), an aneurysm becomes manifest in the form of abdominal pain, which can be very severe. (148) When an intrahepatic haematoma reaches the bile ducts, haemobilia may result (about 40% of cases) (152), just as compression of the excretory bile ducts may lead to the development of jaundice (in some 50% of cases). (154, 158) Heavy bleeding into the free abdominal cavity constitutes an acute abdomen with signs of circulatory shock. Bleeding into the intestinal tract or into the portal vein is less frequent. Lethality due to rupture is 30—50%; the prognosis for massive bleeding with haemoperitoneum is even poorer.

4.1.4 Diagnosis

Laboratory findings are normal. However, alkaline phosphatase (and LAP) and possibly also bilirubin may be increased in biliary stasis.

With unclarified abdominal pain, **sonography** is usually the diagnostic procedure of choice. An aneurysm appears as a round or oval focus either intrahepatically or extrahepatically between the portal hilum and the pancreas. The hypoechoic, cystic focus may contain hyperechoic, thrombotic material. Occasionally, there is a connection to an afferent vessel. (147) A suspected aneurysm can be confirmed by **colour Doppler sonography,** with the possibility of distinguishing blood flow and arterial blood. An echo-free aneurysm provides a typical arterial sphygmogram.

CT scanning reveals a hypodense to hyperdense focal space-occupying lesion, with the hyperdense parts corresponding to the thrombotic structures within the aneurysm. Diagnostic accuracy is considerably improved by using contrast-medium CT.

Angiographic scanning of the hepatic artery confirms the diagnosis as well as giving an indication of the most appropriate therapeutic measures. • Due to the development of modern MRI techniques, invasive angiography is no longer necessary in most cases.

4.1.5 Treatment

Once detected, an aneurysm of the hepatic artery requires immediate treatment. Up to a certain size, intrahepatic aneurysms are treated by angiographic embolization. Coagulation by means of direct thrombin injection has also been described. (149) Larger aneurysms are treated by vascular surgery (ligation, vascular reconstruction, resection). (151, 153, 157)

4.2 Arterial occlusion

Occlusion of the hepatic artery is responsible for a 50% reduction in oxygen supply. Even if an unimpaired oxygen supply via the portal vein is guaranteed, arterial occlusion usually causes ischaemic infarction. The clinical and morphological pictures are characterized (1.) by the speed with which an occlusion develops, and (2.) by the presence of variants that can be used as a bypass or of collaterals that have already been established in gradual vascular occlusion. This results in a broad clinical spectrum, which may range from a symptom-free condition to liver hypoxia, including infarction up to hepatic coma.

4.2.1 Aetiology

Causes of occlusion are as follows: (1.) primary vascular diseases (nodular periarteritis, giant-cell arteritis, etc.), (2.) iatrogenic measures (intra-arterial catheterization, i.v. cytostatic infusions, surgical interventions, etc.), (3.) traumas (dissections), (4.) embolisms (bacterial endocarditis, severe arteriosclerosis, mitral valve defect), and (5.) fibromuscular hyperplasia.

4.2.2 Clinical features

In acute occlusion with infarction, there is dull upper abdominal pain, often coupled with shock symptoms; the liver is tender upon pressure. Fever, jaundice and leucocytosis rapidly develop; Quick's value decreases, and haemorrhages develop. Transaminase and alkaline phosphatase levels rise. Liver failure is imminent. Apart from possibly detecting hypoechoic foci, sonography provides no diagnostic information. Contrast-medium CT reveals hypodense regions with mostly blurred boundaries. In MRI, the infarct is low T_1-weighted, with a high signal intensity in the T_2 image. The diagnosis is confirmed by arteriography, which should be carried out without delay if there is suspicion of acute occlusion. • *Treatment* is symptomatic and aimed at stabilizing the liver function in order to allow time for the formation of collaterals (within a few days). A lethal course must be anticipated if the openings of the gastric and gastroduodenal arteries are involved in the occlusion. The prognosis for distal occlusions in the area of the right or left hepatic artery is more favourable.

Ischaemic infarction: Ischaemic infarction with haemorrhagic marginal zones not only occurs after occlusion (159—161), but also *without* vascular obstruction, e. g. in shock, diabetic ketoacidosis, pre-eclampsia or lupus erythematosus. Small infarctions have also been described as complications following liver biopsy. • Morphologically, fresh anaemic infarctions appear as coagulation necroses. Large infarctions may cause "bile lakes" with evidence of air. From the second day, a wall of leucocytes forms at the infarction margins, and pigment-loaded macrophages can be observed. The reticular fibre structures collapse, and the granulation tissue is vascularized. Ultimately, indrawn scars develop.

4.3 Nodular periarteritis

This *primary vascular disease* is a febrile systemic autoimmune reaction, presumably caused by excessive immune activities. In this process, immune complexes are deposited in the walls of vascular arterioles as well as in the larger arteries, giving rise to a progressive inflammatory reaction with round-cell infiltrates, pearl string-like thickening and proliferations of the intima. The narrowing of the lumen results in ischaemic necroses, which are also present in the liver in up to 65% of patients. Non-specific reactive inflammation in the portal fields may also be observed. As a rule, the gall bladder is involved just as frequently. Nodular periarteritis often leads to the development of aneurysms. • *Clinically*, there are highly pathological inflammation parameters. (s. tab. 39.2) Marked increases in BSR and alkaline phosphatase are characteristic. Various pains generally develop in the abdomen, joints and renal areas; weight loss adds to a distinct feeling of being ill. If the liver is affected, transaminase values may be slightly increased. • *Treatment* consists of prednisolone and azathioprine, unless active viral hepatitis is present.

4.4 Arteriosclerosis

Arteriosclerosis affects the extrahepatic liver arteries with the same frequency as the mesenteric arteries, but less frequently than the splenic artery. • The intrahepatic branches of the hepatic artery are usually only involved in cases of pronounced arterial hypertension. In these patients, thickening of the media can be found in the small arteries of the portal fields.

5 Hereditary haemorrhagic telangiectasia

This *dysvascular state*, also known as *Osler's disease* or *Rendu-Osler-Weber disease*, was first observed by the Canadian internist W. OSLER in 1901. (173) It is a rare autosomal dominant hereditary disease (1 : 100,000) with high penetrance (almost 100%). The homozygous presence of the affected allele is a lethal factor. All types of vessels are affected by these vascular malformations. Thus, for example, arteriovenous fistulas, aneurysms and telangiectasias of the arterial and venous terminal vessels as well as phlebectasias are found. The liver is involved in 40–70% of cases. Star-shaped vascular ectasias appear on the liver surface. Polymorphism of these angiodysplasias is caused by genetically determined damage to fibroelastic fibres within the vascular walls and the perivascular tissue. There is no evidence of any mesenchymal reaction or inflammatory activity. (162, 163, 166, 168, 175, 176, 179) • Osler's disease usually progresses through three phases: the asymptomatic *latent period* extends from childhood into puberty: the subsequent *haemorrhagic phase* is generally characterized by recurrent nasal bleeding; *manifest angiomatosis* has its onset in the third or fourth decade. Various clinical features can be observed, including posthaemorrhagic anaemia, hyperdynamic circulatory problems due to arteriovenous fistulas with cardiac insufficiency, signs of portal hypertension with hepatomegaly (157), phases of hepatic encephalopathy and, in some cases, gastrointestinal bleeding. Dense vascular networks with vascular anomalies are found especially in the region of the mesenteric arteries. Diagnosis is based on colour-encoded Doppler sonography (163, 164, 165, 169, 172, 177), CTAP, MRF and arteriography. (167, 179) The common artery is dilated (180); a giant aneurysm can develop. (171) The CO level is high, so that right-sided cardiac catheterization is indicated in these patients. Following a protracted course, which requires frequent blood transfusions, secondary biliary cirrhosis may appear. (170) • Embolization or surgical interventions (ligation of afferent vessels, partial liver resection) and even liver transplantation (166, 174, 178) are indicated, provided such procedures are technically possible.

References:

Cardiocirculatory disorders

1. **Arcidi, J.M., Moore, G.W., Hutchins, G.M.:** Hepatic morphology in cardiac dysfunction. A clinicopathologic study of 1000 subjects at autopsy. Amer. J. Pathol. 1981; 104: 159–166
2. **Bulkley, G.B., Oshima, A., Bailey, R.W.:** Pathophysiology of hepatic ischemia in cardiogenic shock. Amer. J. Surg. 1986; 151: 87–96
3. **De La Monte, S.M., Arcidi, J.M., Moore, G.W., Hutchins, G.M.:** Midzonal necrosis as a pattern of hepatocellular injury after shock. Gastroenterology 1984; 86: 627–631
4. **Gibson, P.R., Dudley, F.J.:** Ischemic hepatitis: clinical features, diagnosis and prognosis. Aust. NZ. J. Med. 1984; 14: 822–825
5. **Helling, T.S.:** The liver and hemorrhagic shock. J. Amer. Coll. Surg. 2005; 201: 774–783
6. **Henrion, J., Colin, L., Schapira, M., Heller, F.R.:** Hypoxic hepatitis caused by severe hypoxemia from obstructive sleep apnea. J. Clin. Gastroenterol. 1997; 24: 245–249
7. **Hickman, P.E., Potter, J.M.:** Mortality associated with ischaemic hepatitis. Aust. NZ. J. Med. 1990; 20: 32–34
8. **Hinrichs, S., Hüppe, D., Reitemeyer, E., Jäger, D., Kuntz, H.-D., May, B.:** Leberveränderungen bei akutem und chronischem myokardialen Pumpversagen: Klinische und histologische Befunde. Intensivmed. 1990; 27: 186–192
9. **Hoffman, B.J., Pate, M.B., Marsh, W.H., Lee, W.M.:** Cardiomyopathy unrecognized as a cause of hepatic failure. J. Clin. Gastroenterol. 1990; 12: 306–309
10. **Hosoki, T., Arisawa, J., Marukawa, T., Tokunaga, K., Kuroda, C., Kozuka, T., Nakano, S.:** Portal blood flow in congestive heart failure: pulsed duplex sonographic findings. Radiology 1990; 174: 733–736
11. **Jolliffe, N.:** Liver function in congestive heart failure. J. Clin. Invest. 1929; 8: 419–433
12. **Kamiyami, T., Miyakawa, H., Tajiri, K., Marumo, F., Sato, C.:** Ischemic hepatitis in cirrhosis. Clinical features and prognostic implication. J. Clin. Gastroenterol. 1996; 22: 126–130
13. **Klatt, E.C., Koss, M.N., Young, T.S., Macauley, L., Martin, S.E.:** Hepatic hyaline globules associated with passive congestion. Arch. Pathol. Lab. Med. 1988; 112: 510–513
14. **Kotin, P., Hall, E.M.:** "Cardiac" or congestive cirrhosis of the liver. Amer. J. Pathol. 1951; 27: 561–568
15. **Kubo, S.H., Walter, B.A., John, D.H.A., Clark, M., Cody, R.J.:** Liver function abnormalities in chronic heart failure. Influence of systemic hemodynamics. Arch. Int. Med. 1987; 147: 1227–1230
16. **Kuntz, H.D.:** Glukuronidierungskapazität der Leber. Beurteilung mit dem Modellsubstrat 4-Methylumbelliferon. Fortschr. Med. 1987; 105: 149–152
17. **Kuntz, H.D., Matthes, U., Reitemeyer, E., Tönissen, R., May, B.:** Leber und Herz. Pathophysiologie, Morphologie und Klinik zirkulatorisch bedingter Lebererkrankungen. Med. Welt 1987; 38: 1410–1415
18. **Kuntz, H.D., Braun, B.E., Hüppe, D.:** Chronische Stauungsleber bei obstruktiven Atemwegserkrankungen: Beurteilung der Fibrogenese mit Prokollagen-III-Peptid. Atemw.- Lungenkrkh. 1989; 15: 436–439
19. **Kuntz, H.-D., May, B., Hüppe, D.:** Zirkulationsstörungen der Leber. Pathophysiologie und Klinik von Schockleber und Stauungsleber. Verdauungskrankh. 1993; 11: 13–17
20. **Lefkowitch, J.H., Mendez, G.:** Morphologic features of hepatic injury in cardiac disease and shock. J. Hepatol. 1986; 2: 313–327
21. **Moriel, M., Morali, G., Rosenmann, E., Shaheen, J., Tzivoni, D.:** Cardioversion-induced fulminant hepatitis. Eur. J. Gastroenterol. Hepatol. 2001; 13: 1481–1483
22. **Moulton, J.S., Miller, B.L., Dodd, G.D., Vu, D.N.:** Passive hepatic congestion in heart failure: CT abnormalities. Amer. J. Roentgenol. 1988; 151: 939–942

23. Moussavian, S.N., Dincsoy, H.P., Goodman, S., Helm, R.A., Bozian, R.C.: Severe hyperbilirubinemia and coma in chronic congestive heart failure. Dig. Dis. Sci. 1982; 27: 175–180
24. Myers, R.P., Cerini, R., Sayegh, R., Moreau, R., Degott, C., Lebres, D., Lee, S.S.: Cardiac hepatopathy: Clinical hemodynamic, and histologic characteristics and correlations. Hepatology 2003; 37: 393–400
25. Nouel, O., Henrion, J., Bernuau, J., Degot, C., Rueff, B., Benhamou, J.P.: Fulminant hepatic failure due to transient circulatory failure in patients with chronic heart disease. Dig. Dis. Sci. 1980; 25: 49–52
26. Seeto, R.K., Fenn, B., Rockey, D.C.: Ischemic hepatitis: Clinical presentation and pathogenesis. Amer. J. Med. 2000; 109: 109–113
27. Shibayama, Y.: The role of hepatic venous congestion and endotoxinemia in the production of fulminant hepatic failure secondary to congestive heart failure. J. Pathol. 1987; 151: 133–138
28. Shibuya, A., Unuma, T., Sugimoto, T., Yamakado, M., Tagawa, H., Tagawa, K., Tanaka, S., Takanashi, R.: Diffuse hepatic calcification as a sequela to shock liver. Gastroenterology 1985; 89: 196–201
29. Strassburg, C.P.: Shock liver. Best Pract. Res. Clin. Gastroenterol. 2003; 17: 369–381
30. Valla, D.C.: Hypoxic hepatitis-passive liver congestion in heart disease (in French). Gastroenterol. Clin. Biol. 2003; 27 (Suppl.): 33–40
31. Wanless, I.R., Liu, J.J., Butany, J.: Role of thrombosis in the pathogenesis of congestive hepatic fibrosis (cardiac cirrhosis). Hepatology 1995; 21: 1232–1237

Budd-Chiari syndrome
32. Anger, B.R., Seifried, E., Scheppach, J., Heimpel, H.: Budd-Chiari syndrome and thrombosis of other abdominal vessels in the chronic myeloproliferative diseases. Klin. Wschr. 1989; 67: 818–825
33. Balducci, G., Lucandri, G., Mercantini, P., di Giacomo, G., Amodio, P.M., D'Amico, G., Salvatori, F.M., Ziparo, V.: Caval stenting and side-to-side portocaval shunt in the treatment of Budd-Chiari syndrome. Eur. J. Surg. 2002; 168: 651–653
34. Balta, Z., Nattermann, J., Flacke, S., Sauerbruch, T.: Budd-Chiari syndrome in a patient with paroxysmal nocturnal haemoglobinuria. (case report) (in German). Dtsch. Med. Wsch. 2005; 130: 2257–2260
35. Bargallo, X., Gilabert, R., Nicolau, C., Garcia-Pagan, J.C., Bosch, J., Bru, C.: Sonography of the caudate vein: value in diagnosing Budd-Chiari syndrome. Amer. J. Roentgenol. 2003; 181: 1641–1645
36. Bayraktar, Y., Balkanci, F., Bayraktar, M., Calguneri, M.: Budd-Chiari syndrome: a common complication of Behcet's disease. Amer. J. Gastroenterol. 1997; 92: 858–862
37. Bhupalan, A., Talbot, K., Forbes, A., Owen, M., Samson, D., Murray-Lyon, I.M.: Budd-Chiari syndrome in association with polycystic disease of the liver and kidneys. J. Royal Soc. Med. 1992; 85: 296–297
38. Bolondi, L., Gaiani, S., Li Bassi, S., Zironi, G., Bonino, F., Brunetto, M., Barbara, L.: Diagnosis of Budd-Chiari syndrome by pulsed Doppler ultrasound. Gastroenterology 1991; 100: 1324–1331
39. Brancatelli, G., Vilgrain, V., Federle, M.P., Hakime, A., Iannaccone, R., Valla, D.: Budd-Chiari syndrome: Spectrum of imaging findings. Amer. J. Roentgenol. 2007; 188: 168–176
40. Cazals-Halem, D., Vilgrain, V., Genin, P., Denninger, M.L., Durand, F.O., Belghiti, J., Valla, D., Degott, C.: Arterial and portal circulation and parenchymal changes in Budd-Chiari syndrome: A study in 17 explanted livers. Hepatology 2003; 37: 510–519
41. Chaubal, N., Dighe, M., Hanchate, V., Thakkar, H., Desmukh, H., Rathod, K.: Sonography in Budd-Chiari syndrome. J. Ultrasound Med. 2006; 25: 373–379
42. Deltenre, P., Denninger, M.H., Hillaire, S., Guilin, M.C., Casadevall, N., Brière, J., Erlinger, S., Valla, D.C.: Factor V Leiden related Budd-Chiari syndrome. Gut 2001; 48: 264–268
43. Dilawari, J.B., Bambery, P., Chawla, Y., Kaur, U., Bhusnurmath, S.R., Malhotra, H.S., Sood, G.K., Mitra, S.K., Khanna, S.K., Walia, B.S.: Hepatic outflow obstruction (Budd-Chiari syndrome). Experience with 177 patients and a review of the literature. Medicine 1994; 73: 21–36
44. Erden, A.: Budd-Chiari syndrome. A review of imaging findings. Eur. J. Radiol. 2007; 61: 44–56
45. Feingold, M.L., Litwak, R.L., Geller, S.S., Baron, M.M.: Budd-Chiari-syndrome caused by a right atrial tumor. Arch. Intern. Med. 1971; 127: 292–295
46. Gandini, R., Konda, D., Simonetti, G.: Transjugular intrahepatic portosystemic shunt patency and clinical outcome in patients with Budd-Chiari syndrome: Covered versus uncovered stents. Radiology 2006; 241: 298–305
47. Griffith, J.F., Mahmoud, A.E.A., Cooper, S., Elias, E., West, R.J., Olliff, S.P.: Radiological intervention in Budd-Chiari syndrome: techniques and outcome in 18 patients. Clin. Radiol. 1996; 51: 775–784
48. Hemming, A.W., Langer, B., Greig, P., Taylor, B.R., Adams, R., Heathcote, E.J.: Treatment of Budd-Chiari syndrome with portosystemic shunt or liver transplantation. Amer. J. Surg. 1996; 171: 176–181
49. Karadag, O., Akinci, D., Aksoy, D.Y., Bayraktar, Y.: Acute Budd-Chiari syndrome resulting from a pyogenic liver abscess (case report). Hepato-Gastroenterol. 2005; 52: 1554–1556
50. Khuroo, M.S., Datta, D.V.: Budd-Chiari syndrome following pregnancy. Report of 16 cases, with roentgenologic, hemodynamic and histologic studies of the hepatic outflow tract. Amer. J. Med. 1980; 68: 113–121
51. Klein, A.S., Molmenti, E.P.: Surgical treatment of Budd-Chiari syndrome (review). Liver Transplant. 2003; 9: 891–896
52. Knoop, M., Lemmens, H.-P., Bechstein, W.O., Blumhardt, G., Schattenfroh, N., Keck, H., Neuhaus, P.: Treatment of the Budd-Chiari syndrome with orthotopic liver transplantation and long-term anticoagulation. Clin. Transplant. 1994; 8: 67–72
53. Lopez, R.R., Benner, K.G., Hall, L., Rösch, J., Pinson, C.W.: Expandable venous stents for treatment of the Budd-Chiari syndrome. Gastroenterology 1991; 100: 1435–1441
54. Mahmoud, A.E.A., Mendoza, A., Meshikhes, A.N., Olliff, S., West, R., Neuberger, J., Buckels, J., Wilde, J., Elias, E.: Clinical spectrum, investigations and treatment of Budd-Chiari syndrome. Quart. J. Med. 1996; 89: 37–43
55. Mahmoud, A.E.A., Helmy, A.S., Billingham, L., Elias, E.: Poor prognosis and limited therapeutic options in patients with Budd-Chiari syndrome and portal venous system thrombosis. Eur. J. Gastroenterol. Hepatol. 1997; 9: 485–489
56. Markert, D.J., Shanmuganathan, K., Mirvis, S.E., Nakajima, Y., Hayakawa, M.: Budd-Chiari syndrome resulting from intrahepatic IVC compression secondary to blunt hepatic trauma. Clin. Radiol. 1997; 52: 384–387
57. Matsuura, H., Matsumoto, T., Hashimoto, T.: Budd-Chiari syndrome in a patient with Sjögren's syndrome. Amer. J. Gastroenterol. 1983; 78: 822–825
58. Menon, K.V.N., Shah, V., Kamath, P.S.: The Budd-Chiari syndrome. New Engl. J. Med. 2004; 350: 578–585
59. Michl, P., Bilzer, M., Waggershauser, T., Gülberg, V., Rau, H.G., Reiser, M., Gerbers, A.L.: Successful treatment of chronic Budd-Chiari syndrome with a transjugular intrahepatic portosystemic shunt. J. Hepatol. 2000; 32: 516–520
60. Minnema, M.C., Janssen, H.L.A., Niermeijer, P., de Man, R.A.: Budd-Chiari syndrome: combination of genetic defects and the use of oral contraceptives leading to hypercoagulability. J. Hepatol. 2000; 33: 509–512
61. Murad, S.D., Valla, D.C., de Groen, P.C., Zeitoun, G., Hopmans, J.A.M., Haagsma, E.B., van Hock, B., Hansen, B.E., Rosendaal, F.R., Janssen, H.L.A.: Determinants of survival and the effect of portosystemic shunting in patients with Budd-Chiari syndrome. Hepatology 2004; 39: 500–508
62. Orloff, M.J., Daily, P.O., Orloff, S.L., Girard, B., Orloff, M.S.: A 27-year experience with surgical treatment of Budd-Chiari syndrome. Ann. Surg. 2000; 232: 340–350
63. Pelletier, S., Landi, B., Piette, J.-C., Ekert, P., Coutellier, A., Desmoulins, C., Fadlallah, J.-P., Herson, S., Valla, D.: Antiphospholipid syndrome as the second cause of non-tumorous Budd-Chiari syndrome. J. Hepatol. 1994; 21: 76–80
64. Powell-Jackson, P.R., Ede, R.J., Williams, R.: Budd-Chiari syndrome presenting as fulminant hepatic failure. Gut 1986; 27: 1101–1105
65. Rössle, M., Olschewski, M., Siegerstetter, V., Berger, E., Kurz, K., Grandt, D.: The Budd-Chiari syndrome: outcome after treatment with the transjugular intrahepatic portosystemic shunt. Surgery 2004; 135: 394–403
66. Runne, U., Doepfmer, K., Antz, H., Groth, W., Féaux de Lacroix, W.: Budd-Chiari-Syndrom unter Dacarbazin. Dtsch. Med. Wschr. 1980; 105: 230–233
67. Russi, E.W., Bansky, G., Pfaltz, M., Spinas, G., Hammer, B., Senning, A.: Budd-Chiari syndrome in sarcoidosis. Amer. J. Gastroenterol. 1986; 81: 71–75
68. Schoen, U.: Budd-Chiari-Syndrom bei retroperitonealem Neurinom. Dtsch. Med. Wschr. 1972; 97: 335–338
69. Sharma, S., Texeira, A., Texeira, P., Elias, E., Wilde, J., Olliff, S.P.: Pharmacological thrombolysis in Budd-Chiari syndrome: A single centre experience and review of the literature (case report). J. Hepatol. 2004; 40: 172–180
70. Srinivasan, P., Rela, M., Prachalias, A., Muiesan, P., Portmann, B., Mufti, G.J., Pagliuca, A., O'Grady, J., Heaton, N.: Liver transplantation for Budd-Chiari syndrome. Transplantation 2002; 73: 973–977
71. Sugano, S., Suzuki, T., Makino, H., Yanagimoto, S., Nishio, M., Onmura, H., Iinuma, M., Matuda, T., Shinozawa, Y.: Budd-Chiari syndrome attributed to protein C deficiency. Amer. J. Gastroenterol. 1996; 91: 777–779
72. Wang, Z., Zhu, Y., Wang, S., Pu, L., Du, Y., Zhang, H., Yuan, C., Chen, Z., Wei, M., Pu, L.Q., Du, W., Liu, M., Liu, X., Johnson, G.: Recognition and management of Budd-Chiari syndrome: report of one hundred cases. J. Vasc. Surg. 1989; 10: 149–156
73. Weernink, E.E.M., Huisman, A.B., van Baarlen, J., ten Napel, C.H.H.: Treatment of the Budd-Chiari syndrome by insertion of a wall-stent in the hepatic vein after percutaneous transluminal angioplasty: the necessity of follow-up. Eur. J. Gastroenterol. Hepatol. 1996; 8: 85–88
74. Witte, A.M.C., Schultze Kool, L.J., Venendaal, R., Lamers, C.B.H.W., van Hoek, B.: Hepatic vein stenting for Budd-Chiari syndrome. Amer. J. Gastroenterol. 1997; 92: 498–501
75. Xu, K., He, F.-X., Zhang, H.-G., Zhang, X.-T., Han, M.-J., Wang, C.-R., Kaneko, M., Takahashi, M., Okawada, T.: Budd-Chiari syndrome caused by obstruction of the hepatic inferior vena cava: immediate and 2-year treatment results of transluminal angioplasty and metallic stent placement. Cardiovasc. Intervent. Radiol. 1996; 19: 32–36
76. Zhang, X.M., Li, Q.L.: Etiology, treatment, and classification of Budd-Chiari syndrome. Chin. Med. J. 2007; 120: 159–161
77. Zimmerman, M.A., Cameron, A.M., Ghobrial, R.M.: Budd-Chiari syndrome. Clin. Liver Dis. 2006; 10: 259–273

Veno-occlusive disease
78. Alpert, L.I.: Veno-occlusive disease of the liver associated with oral contraceptives: case report and review of the literature. Hum. Path. 1976; 7: 709–718

79. Bras, G., Jelliffe, D.B., Stuart, K.L.: Veno-occlusive disease of the liver with non-portal type of cirrhosis occurring in Jamaica. Arch. Pathol. 1954; 57: 285–300
80. Essell, J.H., Thompson, J.M., Harman, G.S., Halvorson, R.D., Snyder, M.J., Johnson, R.A., Rubinsak, J.R.: Marked increase in veno-occlusive disease of the liver associated with methotrexat use for Graft-Versus-Host disease prophylaxis in patients receiving busulfan/cyclophosphamide. Blood 1992; 79: 2784–2788
81. Fried, M.W., Connaghan, D.G., Sharma, S., Martin, L.G., Devine, St., Holland, K., Zuckerman, A., Kaufman, S., Wingard, J., Boyer, T.D.: Transjugular intrahepatic portosystemic shunt for the management of severe venoocclusive disease following bone marrow transplantation. Hepatology 1996; 24: 588–591
82. Gill, R.A., Onstad, G.R., Cardamone, J.M., Maneval, D.C., Sumner, H.W.: Hepatic veno-occlusive disease caused by 6-thioguanine. Ann. Intern. Med. 1982; 96: 58–60
83. Griner, P.F., Elbadawi, A., Packman, C.H.: Veno-occlusive disease of the liver after chemotherapy of acute leukemia: a report of two cases. Ann. Intern. Med. 1976; 85: 578–582
84. Heikinheimo, M., Halila, R., Fasth, A.: Serum procollagen typ III is an early and sensitive marker for veno-occlusive disease of the liver in children undergoing bone marrow transplantation. Blood 1994; 83: 3036–3040
85. Hommeyer, S.C., Teefey, S.A., Jacobson, A.F., Higano, C.S., Bianco, J.A., Colacurcio, C.J., McDonald, G.B.: Venocclusive disease of the liver: prospective study of US evaluation. Radiology 1992; 184: 683–686
86. Jansen, T.L.T.A., de Vries, R.A., Kesselring, F.O.H.W., Meijer, J.W.R.: Magnetic resonance imaging in the staging of hepatic veno-occlusive disease. Eur. J. Gastroenterol. Hepatol. 1994; 6: 453–456
87. Kumar, S., Deleve, L.D., Kamath, P.S., Tefferi, A.: Hepatic veno-occlusive disease (sinusoidal obstruction syndrome) after hematopoetic stem cell transplantation (review). Mayo Clin. Proc. 2003; 78: 589–598
88. Lassau, N., Leclère, J., Auperin, A., Bourhis, J.H., Hartmann, O., Valteau-Couanet, D., Benhamou, E., Bosq, J., Ibrahim, A., Girinski, T., Pico, J.L., Roche, A.: Hepatic veno-occlusive disease after myeloablativ treatment and bone marrow transplantation: value of Gray-scale and Doppler US in 100 patients. Radiology 1997; 204: 545–552
89. McDonald, G.B., Hinds, M.S., Fisher, L.D., Schoch, H.G., Wolford, J.L., Banaji, M., Hardin, B.J., Shulman, H.M., Clift, R.A.: Veno-occlusive disease of the liver and multiorgan failure after bone marrow transplantation: a cohort study of 355 patients. Ann. Intern. Med. 1993; 118: 255–267
90. Modzelewski, J.R., Daeschner, C., Joshi, V.V., Mullick, F.G., Ishak, K.G.: Veno-occlusive disease of the liver induced by low-dose cyclophosphamide. Modern Pathol. 1994; 7: 967–972
91. Norris, S., Crosbie, O., McEntee, G., Traynor, O., Molan, N., McCann, S., Hegarty, J.: Orthotopic liver transplantation for veno-occlusive disease complicating autologous bone marrow transplantation. Transplantation 1997; 63: 1521–1524
92. Ortega, J.A., Donaldson, S.S., Ivy, S.P., Pappo, A., Maurer, H.M.: Venoocclusive disease of the liver after chemotherapy with vincristine, actinomycin D, and cyclophosphamide for the treatment of rhabdomyosarcoma: a report of the intergroup rhabdomyosarcoma study group. Cancer 1997; 79: 2435–2439
93. Ortiz Cansado, A., Crespo Valades, E., Morales Blanco, P., Saenz de Santamaria, J., Gonzalez Campillejo, J.M., Ruiz Tellez, T.: Enfermedad venooclusiva hepatica por ingestion de infusiones de senecio vulgaris. Gastroenterol. Hepatol. 1995; 18: 413–416
94. Pappas, S.C., Malone, D.G., Rabin, L., Hoofnagel, Y.H., Jones, E.A.: Hepatic veno-occlusive disease in a patient with systemic lupus erythematosus. Arthr. Rheumat. 1984; 27: 104–108
95. Sperl, W., Stuppner, H., Gassner, I., Judmaier, W., Dietze, O., Vogel, W.: Reversible hepatic veno-occlusive disease in an infant after consumption of pyrrolizidine-containing herbal tea. Eur. J. Pediatr. 1995; 154: 112–116
96. Stein, H., Isaacson, C.: Veno-occlusive disease of the liver. Brit. Med. J. 1962/I: 372–374
97. Stuart, K.L., Bras, G.: Veno-occlusive disease of the liver. Quart. J. Med. 1957; 26: 291–315
98. Wadleigh, M., Ho, V., Momtaz, P., Richardson, P.: Hepatic veno-occlusive disease: Pathogenesis, diagnosis and treatment. Curr. Opin. Hepatol. 2003; 10: 451–462

Portal vein anomalies
99. Oei, M., Wessling, J.: Abernethy malformation – congenital aplasia of the portal vein in a 29-year-old patient (case report) (in German). RöFo 2007; 179: 167–169
100. Remer, E.M., Motta-Ramirez, G.A., Henderson, J.M.: Imaging findings in incidental intraheptaic portal venous shunts. Amer. J. Roentgenol. 2007; 188: 162–167

Cavernous transformation
101. Bayraktar, Y., Balkanci, F., Kayhan, B., Özenc, A., Arslan, S., Telatar, H.: Bile duct varices or "pseudo-cholangiocarcinoma sign" in portal hypertension due to cavernous transformation of the portal vein. Amer. J. Gastroenterol. 1992; 87: 1801–1806
102. Caturelli, E., Pompili, M., Squillante, M.M., Sperandeo, G., Carughi, St., Sperandeo, M., Perri, F., Andriuli, A., Cellerino, C., Rapaccini, G.L.: Cruveilhier-Baumgarten syndrome: an efficient spontaneous portosystemic collateral preventing oesophageal varices bleeding. J. Gastroenterol. Hepatol. 1994; 9: 236–241
103. Chang, C.Y., Yang, P.M., Hung, S.P., Tsay, W., Lin, L.C., Lin, J.T., Wang, H.P.: Cavernous transformation of the portal vein: Etiology determines the outcome. Hepato-Gastroenterol. 2006; 53: 892–897
104. Vilgrain, V., Condat, B., Bureau, C., Hakime, A., Plessier, A., Cazals-Hatem, D., Valla, D.C.: Atrophy-hypertrophy complex in patients with cavernous transformation of the portal vein: CT evaluation. Radiology 2006; 241: 149–155
105. Weltin, G., Taylor, K.J.W., Carter, A.R., Taylor, C.R.: Duplex Doppler: identification of cavernous transformation of the portal vein. Amer. J. Roentgenol. 1985; 144: 999–1001

Arteriovenous fistula
106. Agarwala, S., Dutta, H., Bhatnagar, V., Gulathi, M., Paul, S., Mitra, D.: Congenital hepatoportal arteriovenous fistula: report of a case. Surg. Today 2000; 30: 268–271
107. Eickhoff, U., Kemen, M., Kollig, E., Zumtobel, V., Senkal, M.: The posttraumatic arterioportal intrahepatic fistula. Zbl. Chir. 2000; 125: 983–986
108. Guzman, E.A., McCabill, L.E., Rogers, F.B.: Arterioportal fistulas: Introduction of novel classification with therapeutic implications. J. Gastroenterol. Surg. 2006; 10: 543–550
109. Hurwitz, L.M., Thompson, W.M.: Calcified hepatic arteriovenous fistula found after biopsy of the liver: unusual cause of calcification in the right upper quadrant. Amer. J. Roentgenol. 2002; 179: 1293–1295
110. Mallant, M.P.J.H., van den Berg, F.G., Verbeke, J.I.M.L., Bökenkamp, A.: Pulsatile hepatofugal flow in the portal vein: Hallmark of a congenital hepatoportal arteriovenous fistula. (case report) J. Pediatr. Gastroenterol. Nutrit. 2007; 44: 143–145
111. Michalowicz, B., Pawlak, J., Malkowski, P., Zieniewicz, K., Nyckowsk, P., Leowska, E., Rowinski, O., Pracho, R., Krawczyk, M.: Intraabdominal arteriovenous fistulae and their relation to portal hypertension. Hepato-Gastroenterol. 2003; 50: 1996–1999
112. Norton, S.P., Jacobson, K., Moroz, S.P., Culham, G., Ng, V., Turner, J., John, P.: The congenital intrahepatic arterioportal fistula syndrome: Elucidation and proposed classification. J. Pediatr. Gastroenterol. Nutrit. 2006; 43: 248–255
113. Pohle, T., Fischbach, R., Domschke, W.: Arterioportal fistula: A rare cause of portal hypertension and abdominal pain. Scand. J. Gastroenterol. 2003; 36: 1227–1229
114. Takayasu, K., Muramatsu, Y., Mizuguchi, Y., Moriyama, N., Okusaka, T.: Multiple non-tumorous arterioportal shunts due to chronic liver disease mimicking hepatocellular carcinoma: Outcomes and the associated elevation of alpha-fetoprotein. J. Gastroenterol. Hepatol. 2006; 21: 288–294

Portal vein thrombosis
115. Chawla, Y., Dilawari, J.B., Katariya, S.: Gallbladder varices in portal vein thrombosis. Amer. J. Roentgenol. 1994; 162: 643–645
116. Condat, B., Pessione, F., Hillaire, S., Denninger, M.H., Guillin, M.C., Poliquin, M., Hadengue, A., Erlinger, S., Valla, D.: Current outcome of portal vein thrombosis in adults: risk and benefit of anticoagulant therapy. Gastroenterology 2001; 120: 490–497
117. Condat, B., Valla, D.: Nonmalignant portal vein thrombosis in adults (review). Nat. Clin. Pract. Gastroenterol. Hepatol. 2006; 3: 505–515
118. Egesel, T., Büyükasik, Y., Dündar, S.V., Gürgey, A., Kirazli, S., Bayraktar, Y.: The role of natural anticoagulant deficiencies and factor V Leiden in the development of idiopathic portal vein thrombosis. J. Clin. Gastroenterol. 2000; 30: 66–71
119. Fidler, H., Booth, A., Hodgson, H.J.F., Calam, J., Luzatto, L., Hughes, J.M.B.: Portal vein thrombosis in myeloproliferative disease. Brit. Med. J. 1990; 300:590–592
120. Harmanci, O., Ersoy, O., Gurgey, A., Buyukasik, Y., Gedikoglu, G., Balkanci, F., Sivri, B., Bayraktar, Y.: The etiologic distribution of thrombophilic factors in chronic portal vein thrombosis. J. Clin. Gastroenterol. 2007; 41: 521–527
121. Hellerich, U., Pollak, S.: Spontaneous gallbladder rupture caused by variceal hemorrhage: an unusual complication of portal vein thrombosis. Beitr. Gerichtl. Med. 1991; 49: 319–323
122. Hirohata, Y., Murata, A., Abe, S., Otsuki, M.: Portal vein thrombosis associated with antiphospholipid syndrome. J. Gastroenterol. 2001; 36: 574–578
123. Horrocks, P., Tapp, E.: Zahn's "infarcts" of the liver. J. Clin. Path. 1966; 19: 475–478
124. Julapalli, V.R., Bray, P.F., Duchini, A.: Elevated factor VIII and portal thrombosis (case report). Dig. Dis. Sci. 2003; 48: 2369–2371
125. Lagasse, J.-P., Bahallah, M.L., Salem, N., Debillon, G., Labarrière, D., Serve, M.-P., Advenier, V., Causse, X., Legoux, J.-L.: Acute thrombosis of the portal venous system. Systematic treatment with heparin and a recombinant tissue plasminogen activator or heparin alone in 10 patients. Gastroenterol. Clin. Biol. 1997; 21: 919–923
126. Lai, L., Brugge, W.R.: Endoscopic ultrasound is a sensitive and specific test to diagnose portal venous system thrombosis (PVST). Amer. J. Gastroenterol. 2004; 99: 40–44
127. Leong, R.W.L., House, A.K., Jeffrey, G.P.: Chylous ascites caused by portal vein thrombosis treated with octreotide (case report). J. Gastroenterol. Hepatol. 2003; 18: 1211–1213
128. Malkowski, P., Pawlak, J., Michalowicz, B., Szczerban, J., Wroblewski, T., Leowska, E., Krawczyk, M.: Thrombolytic treatment of portal thrombosis. Hepato-Gastroenterol. 2003; 50: 2098–2100
129. Mangia, A., Villani, M.R., Cappucci, G., Santoro, R., Ricciardi, R., Facciorusso, D., Leandro, G., Caruso, N., Andriuli, A.: Causes of portal

venous thrombosis in cirrhotic patients: the role of genetic and acquired factors. Eur. J. Gastroenterol. Hepatol. 2005; 17: 745–751
130. Matsumoto, T., Kuwabara, N., Abe, H., Fukuda, Y., Suyama, M., Fujii, D., Kojima, K., Futagawa, S.: Zahn infarct of the liver resulting from occlusive phlebitis in portal vein radicles. Amer. J. Gastroenterol. 1992; 87: 356–368
131. Rangari, M., Gupta, R., Jain, M., Malhotra, V., Sarin, S.K.: Hepatic dysfunction in patients with extrahepatic portal venous obstruction. Liver Internat. 2003; 23: 434–439
132. Shibahara, K., Tatsuta, K. Orita, H., Yonemura, T., Kohno, H.: Superior mesenteric and portal vein thrombosis caused by congenital antithrombin III deficiency. Report of a case. Surg. Today 2007; 37: 308–310
133. Sobhonslidsuk, A., Reddy, K.R.: Portal vein thrombosis: a concise review. Amer. J. Gastroenterol. 2002; 97: 535–541
134. Tan, K.J., Chow, P.K.H., Tan, Y.M., Thng, C.H.: Portal vein thrombosis secondary to hyperhomocysteinemia. A case report. Dig. Dis. Sci. 2006; 51: 1218–1220
135. Valla, D., Casadevall, N., Huisse, M.G., Tulliez, M., Grange, J.D., Muller, O., Binda, T., Varet, B., Rueff, B., Benhamou, J.P.: Etiology of portal vein thrombosis in adults. A prospective evaluation of primary myeloproliferative disorders. Gastroenterology 1988; 94: 1063–1069
136. Valla, D.C., Condat, B.: Portal vein thrombosis in adults: pathophysiology, pathogenesis and management. J. Hepatol. 2000; 32: 865–871
137. Van't Riet, M., Burger, J.W.A., van Muiswinkel, J.M., Kazemier, G., Schipperus, M.R., Bonjer, H.J.: Diagnosis and treatment of portal thrombosis following splenectomy. Brit. J. Surg. 2000; 87: 1229–1233
138. Yerdel, M.A., Gunson, B., Mirza, D., Karayalcin, E., Olliff, S., Buckels, J., Mayer, D., McMaster, P., Pirenne, J.: Portal vein thrombosis in adults undergoing liver transplantation. Risk factors, screening, management, and outcome. Transplantation 2000; 69: 1873–1881

Portal vein aneurysm
139. Ascenti, G., Zimbaro, G., Mazziotti, S., Visalli, C., Lamberto, S., Scribano, E., Gaeta, M.: Intrahepatic portal vein aneurysm: three-dimensional power Doppler demonstration in four cases. Abdom. Imag. 2001; 26: 520–523
140. Erdem, C.Z., Erdem, L.O., Comert, M., Ustundag, Y., Gundogu, S.: Multiple intra-hepatic portal vein aneurysms – findings on magnetic resonance angiography. Clin. Radiol. 2003; 58: 899–901
141. Lee, H.C., Yang, Y.C., Shih, S.L., Chiang, H.J.: Aneurysmal dilatation of the portal vein. J. Pediatr. Gastroenterol. Nutr. 1989; 8: 387–389
142. Okur, N., Inal, M., Akgul, E., Demircan, O.: Spontaneous rupture and thrombosis of an intrahepatic portal vein aneurysm. Abdom. Imag. 2003; 28: 675–677

Hepatic portal venous gas
143. Chiu, H.H., Chen, C.M., Lu, Y.Y., Lin, J.C.T., Mo. L.R.: Hepatic portal venous gas. Amer. J. Surg. 2005; 189: 501–503
144. Huurman, V.A.L., Visser, L.G., Steens, S.A., Terpstra, O.T., Schaapherder, A.F.M.: Persistent portal venous gas. J. Gastroenterol. Surg. 2006; 10: 783–785
145. Negro, U., Verdecchia, M., Paci, E., Antico, E., Valeri, G., Risaliti, A., Vecchi, A., Svegliati-Baroni, G., Giovagnoni, A.: Hepatic portal venous gas in a patient with enterovascular fistula (case report). Abdom. Imag. 2006; 31: 706–709
146. Wolf, J.N., Evans, W.A.: Gas in the portal veins of the liver in infants: A roentgenographic demonstration with post-mortem anatomical correlation. Amer. J. Roentgenol. 1955; 74: 486–489

Hepatic artery aneurysm
147. Athey, P.A., Sax, S.L., Lamki, N., Cadavid, G.: Sonography in the diagnosis of hepatic artery aneurysms. Amer. J. Roentgenol. 1986; 147: 725–727
148. Cooper, S.G., Richman, A.H.: Spontaneous rupture of a congenital hepatic artery aneurysm. J. Clin. Gastroenterol. 1988; 10: 104–107
149. Cope, C., Zeit, R.: Coagulation of aneurysms by direct percutaneous thrombin injection. Amer. J. Roentgenol. 1986; 147: 383–387
150. Countryman, D., Norwood, S., Register, D., Torma, M., Andrassy, R.: Hepatic artery aneurysm: report of an unusual case and review of the literature. Amer. Surg. 1983; 49: 51–54
151. Dougherty, M.J., Gloviczki, P., Cherry, K.J., Bower, T.C., Hallett, J.W., Pairolero, P.C.: Hepatic artery aneurysm: evaluation and current management. Int. Angiol. 1993; 12: 178–184
152. Ferrari, A.P., Ferreira, J.P.A., de Paulo, G.A., della Libera, E.: Hemobilia caused by a mycotic aneurysm of the hepatic artery treated by enbucrilate injection during ERCP (case report). Gastrointest. Endosc. 2003; 57: 260–263
153. Jung, N.C., Kim, S.K., Chung, E.C., Park, H., Cho, Y.K.: Endovascular treatment for rupture of intrahepatic artery aneurysm in a patient with Behcet's syndrome. (case report). Amer. J. Roentgenol. 2007; 188: 400–402
154. Mazziotti, S., Blandino, A., Gaeta, M., Lamberto, S., Vinci, V., Ascenti, G.: Hepatic artery aneurysm, an unusual cause of obstructive jaundice: MR cholangiography findings. Abdom. Imag. 2003; 28: 835–837
155. Pinsky, M.A., May, E.S., Taxier, M.S., Blackford, J.: Late manifestation of hepatic artery pseudoaneurysm: case presentation and review. Amer. J. Gastroenterol. 1987; 82: 467–469
156. Sukerkar, A.N., Dulay, C.C., Anandappa, E., Asokan, S.: Mycotic aneurysm of the hepatic artery. Radiology 1977; 124: 444
157. Van den Steen, G., Michielsen, P., van Outryve, M., Corthouts, B., de Backer, A., D'Archambeau, O., van den Brande, F., Ysebaert, D.: Asymptomatic aneurysm of the hepatic artery. Management options (case report). Acta Gastro-Enterol. Belg. 2003; 66: 298–302
158. Zachary, K., Geier, S., Pellecchia, C., Irwin, G.: Jaundice secondary to hepatic artery aneurysm: radiological appearance and clinical features. Amer. J. Gastroenterol. 1986; 81: 295–298

Arterial occlusion
159. Khoury, G., Tobi, M., Oren, M., Traub, Y.M.: Massive hepatic infarction in systemic lupus erythematosus. Dig. Dis. Sci. 1990; 35: 1557–1560
160. Kitagawa, T., Iriyama, K.: Hepatic infarction as a complication of gastric cancer surgery: report of four cases. Jpn. J. Surg. Today 1998; 28: 542–546
161. Smith, G.S., Birnbaum, B.A., Jacobs, J.E.: Hepatic infarction secondary to arterial insufficiency in native livers: CT findings in 10 patients. Radiology 1998; 208: 223–229

Hereditary haemorrhagic telangiectasia
162. Bernard, G., Mion, F., Henry, L., Plauchu, H., Paliard, P.: Hepatic involvement in hereditary hemorrhagic telangiectasia: clinical, radiological, and hemodynamic studies of 11 cases. Gastroenterology 1993; 105: 482–487
163. Buscarini, E., Danesino, C., Olivieri, C., Lupinacci, G., Zambelli, A.: Liver involvement in hereditary haemorrhagic telangiectasia or Rendu-Osler-Weber disease. Dig. Liver Dis. 2007; 37: 835–845
164. Caselitz, M., Bahr, M.J., Bleck, J.S., Chavan, A., Manns, M., Wagner, S., Gebel, M.: Sonographic criteria for the diagnosis of hepatic involvement in hereditary hemorrhagic telangiectasia (HHT). Hepatology 2003; 37: 1139–1146
165. Garcia-Tsao, G.: Liver involvement in hereditary hemorrhagic telangiectasia (HHT) (review). J. Hepatol. 2007; 46: 499–507
166. Hillert, C., Broering, D.C., Gundlach, M., Knoefel, W.T., Izbicki, J.R., Rogiers, X.: Hepatic involvement in hereditary haemorrhagic telangiectasia: An unusual indication for liver transplantation. Liver Transplant. 2001; 7: 266–268
167. Ianora, A.A.S., Memeo, M., Sabba, C., Cirulli, A., Rotondo, A., Angelelli, G.: Hereditary hemorrhagic telangiectasia: multi-detector row helical CT assessment of hepatic involvement. Radiology 2004; 230: 250–259
168. Larson, A.M.: Liver disease in hereditary hemorrhagic telangiectasia (review). J. Clin. Gastroenterol. 2003; 36: 149–158
169. Matsuo, M., Kanematsu, M., Kato, H., Kondo, H., Sugisaki, K., Hoshi, H.: Osler-Weber-Rendu disease: Visualizing portovenous shunting with three-dimensional sonography. Amer. J. Roentgenol. 2001; 176: 919–920
170. Mendoza, A., Oliff, S., Elias, E.: Hereditary haemorrhagic telangiectasia and secondary biliary cirrhosis. Eur. J. Gastroenterol. Hepatol. 1995; 7: 999–1002
171. Milot, L., Dumortier, J., Boillot, O., Pilleul, F.: Giant aneurysm of the main hepatic artery secondary to hereditary hemorrhagic telangiectasia: 3 D contrast-enhanced MR angiography features. (case report). Gastroenterol. Clin. Biol. 2007; 31: 297–299
172. Ocran, K., Rickes, S., Heukamp, I., Wermke, W.: Sonography findings in hepatic involvement of hereditary haemorrhagic telangiectasia. Ultrasound. Med. 2004; 25: 191–194
173. Osler, W.: On a familiary form of recurring epistaxis associated with multiple teleangiectasias of the skin and mucous membranes. Bull. John's Hopk. Hosp. 1901; 12: 333–337
174. Pfitzmann, R., Heise, M., Langrehr, J.M., Jonas, S., Steinmüller, T., Podrabsky, P., Ewert, R., Settmacher, U., Neuhaus, R., Neuhaus, P.: Liver transplantation for treatment of intrahepatic Osler's disease: first experiences. Transplantation 2001; 72: 237–241
175. Saluja, S., White, R.I.: Hereditary hemorrhagic telangiectasia of the liver: hyperperfusion with relative ischemia. Poverty amidst plenty. Radiology 2004; 230: 25–27
176. Saurin, J.C., Dumortier, J., Menard, Y., Henry, L., Boillot, O., Plauchu, H., Paliard, P.: Hepatic vascular malformations in Rendu-Osler disease. Gastroenterol. Clin. Biol. 2000; 24: 89–93
177. Secil, M., Göktay, A.Y., Dicle, O., Pirnar, T.: Splenic vascular malformations and portal hypertension in hereditary hemorrhagic telangiectasia: sonographic findings. J. Clin. Ultrasound 2001; 29: 56–59
178. Thevenot, T., Vnlemmens, C., Di Martino, V., Becker, M.C., Denue, P.O., Kantelip, B., Bresson-Hadni, S., Heyd, B., Mantion, G., Miguet, J.P.: Liver transplantation for cardiac failure in patients with hereditary hemorrhagic telangiectasia (case report). Liver Transplantation 2005; 11: 834–838
179. Weik, C., Greiner, L.: The liver in hereditary hemorrhagic telangiectasia (Weber-Rendu-Osler disease). Scand. J. Gastroenterol. 1999; 34: 1241–1246
180. Wu, J.S., Saluja, S., Garcia-Tsao, G., Chong, A., Henderson, K.J., White, R.I.: Liver involvement in hereditary hemorrhagic telangiectasia: CT and clinical findings do not correlate in symptomatic patients. Amer. J. Roentgenol. 2006; 187: 399–405

Clinical Aspects of Liver Diseases
40 Treatment of liver diseases

		Page:			Page:
1	***From mythology to provable treatment***	872	5.6	*Branched-chain amino acids*	888
1.1	In global medicine	872	5.7	*Amino acids of the urea cycle*	890
1.2	In hepatology	872	5.8	*D-penicillamine*	892
2	***Clinical studies***	873	5.9	*Somatostatin*	892
2.1	Types of clinical studies	873	5.10	*Terlipressin*	892
2.2	Problems of clinical studies	873	5.11	*S-adenosyl-L-methionine*	893
2.3	Placebo	874	5.12	*Haemarginate*	893
2.4	Difficulty of evaluation	874	5.13	*Phytotherapeutics*	894
2.5	Provability of treatment	874	5.13.1	Essential phospholipids	894
3	***Principles of liver therapy***	875	5.13.2	Silymarin	896
3.1	Basic considerations	875	5.13.3	Glycyrrhiza glabra	897
3.1.1	Liver therapy	875	5.13.4	Colchicine	897
3.1.2	Liver therapeutic agents	875	5.13.5	Betaine	897
3.1.3	Protective therapy of the liver	875	5.13.6	Cynara scolymus	898
3.2	Preconditions	875	5.13.7	Bupleurum falcatum	898
3.3	Forms of "liver therapy"	876	5.13.8	Phyllanthus amarus	898
3.4	Aims of treatment	876	5.13.9	Schizandra chinensis	898
3.5	Categories of "liver therapeutics"	876	5.13.10	Catechin	898
3.6	Active substances	876	6	***Surgical therapy of liver diseases***	898
3.7	Dose adjustment of medicaments	877	6.1	*TIPS*	899
3.8	Significance of quality of life	878	6.2	*Shunt operation*	899
3.9	Assessment of survival rate	878	6.3	*Block surgery*	900
4	***Nutritional therapy of liver diseases***	878	6.4	*Liver resection*	900
4.1	Artificial feeding	879	6.4.1	Basic principles	900
4.1.1	Enteral feeding	879	6.4.2	Classification and indications	901
4.1.2	Parenteral feeding	879	6.4.3	Regeneration	902
4.2	Diet in malnutrition	880	6.5	*Liver injuries*	902
4.3	Special diets	880	7	***Liver transplantation***	903
5	***Drug therapy of liver diseases***	881	7.1	Indications	903
5.1	*Virustatics*	881	7.2	Contraindications	905
5.1.1	Interferon	882	7.3	Preoperative diagnostics	905
5.1.2	Nucleoside analogues	883	7.4	Preparation of patients	906
5.2	*Immunosuppressants*	884	7.5	Surgical aspects	906
5.2.1	Glucocorticoids	884	7.6	Postoperative features	908
5.2.2	Azathioprine	884	7.7	Aftercare and rehabilitation	910
5.2.3	Cyclosporine A	885	8	***Sociomedical aspects***	911
5.2.4	Tacrolimus	885	8.1	Health awareness	911
5.2.5	Cyclophosphamide	885	8.2	Preventive medicine	912
5.2.6	Methotrexate	885	8.3	Rehabilitation	912
5.3	*Immunostimulants*	885	8.4	Capacity for work	912
5.3.1	Selenium	885	8.5	Self-help groups	914
5.3.2	Zinc	886		• References (1–445)	914
5.3.3	Thymosin	886		(Figures 40.1–40.11; tables 40.1–40.19)	
5.4	*Ursodeoxycholic acid*	886			
5.5	*Lactulose*	887			

40 Treatment of liver diseases

1 From mythology to provable treatment

1.1 In global medicine

▶ Recommendations and discussions on the treatment of diseases and injuries are as old as medicine itself. According to our knowledge of earlier times, medicine has its origins in **mythological therapy.** This also applies to the treatment of liver diseases. • Understandably, *"surgical medicine"*, especially traumatology, enjoyed the highest scientific status in antiquity, since the actual "cause" and medical "effect" were most obvious in this field. • Mythological ideas and rituals were therefore of minor significance to the barber surgeon: in general, practical experience, manual skill and (mostly self-developed) appropriate instruments produced the desired result. By contrast, *"conservative medicine"* was characterized by mythology, steeped in ritual as well as (mantic) divination and, for many epochs, mostly left in the hands of the "priest doctor". In spite of sometimes astonishingly good diagnostic capabilities and prognostic accuracy, medicine on the whole – especially treatment of the individual patient – was subject to the prevailing mythology of the respective epoch. (s. tab. 40.1)

With the gradual rejection of "mythos" and a stronger tendency to "logos", therapeutic measures of a mythological and ritual nature were increasingly abandoned. At the same time, however, the absurd ideas of **speculative therapy** reached an unimaginable level of odiousness. Obscure mixtures, fantastic preparations as well as nauseating and even cruel treatment methods were more and more propagated and applied. An insight into these abnormalities of speculative medicine is given by K. F. PAULLINI (1699) in his book: „Neu-vermehrte, heilsame Dreck-Apotheke" ("Revised and Enlarged Curative Dirty Pharmacy").

With the coming of the Age of Enlightenment in the middle of the 18th century, accompanied by a rapid increase in medical knowledge, the calls for confirmed results became more and more urgent. This led to the advent of **empirical therapy**, which required subtle observation, critical analysis, careful examination and, above all, a written record of case histories. In this connection, surgical empiricism was more strongly based on morphological facts and objective methodological experience than the therapeutic empiricism of conservative medicine.

▶ Preventive therapeutic empiricism was applied for the first time around 1600, when it was discovered by "therapy comparison" that those seamen of the East India Company who drank lemon juice as a supplementary beverage did not contract scurvy. *This was the basis of (probably) the first* **"statistical" therapeutic study,** *which J. LIND carried out in 1747 in order to confirm the theory of a lemon-juice therapy in several groups of people by administering various substances, including a "placebo".* This theory was also confirmed by J. COOK in 1776, using a similar study design. • Further therapeutic milestones of medical history include the comparative studies with *digitalis* (W. WITHERING, 1785), *smallpox vaccine* (E. JENNER, 1798) and *mercury treatment* of syphilis (J. PEARSON, 1800). • Such comparative studies, which were based on individual observations, aimed at proving the effectiveness of treatments; this development ended the epoch of empirical therapy. (2) (tab. 40.1)

1.2 In hepatology

▶ During a period of about 3,000 years, hepatology also experienced these **historical medical epochs** of therapy, (*1.*) mythological, (*2.*) speculative, (*3.*) empirical, and (*4.*) provable. (s. tab. 40.1) • In addition to cataplasms – consisting of various herbs, oils or products derived from animals, mostly prepared and used according to mythologically related ideas – cupping, scarification, enemas, blood-letting and sternutators, the following materials were also used: dried wolf liver with honey, donkey liver with parsley, raw ox liver dipped in honey, ox blood, etc. Some highly complex and fantastic mythological diets were applied as well. Therapeutic measures were often based on certain mythological numbers or ritual-dependent points in time and performed before statues of gods or in connection with animal sacrifice. *(see chapter 1.)* • From the mediaeval "dirty pharmacy" came numerous, disgusting therapeutic recommendations for patients with liver disease, e. g. consumption of the excrement of certain animals, ear wax, dirt scraped off sheep udders, earthworms, polypods dissolved in wine, or a certain number of live sheep's lice. (s. p. 446) • Empirical treatment increasingly made use of substrates of plant origin or extracts of Hyoscamus, Cheliodonium, dandelion or milk thistle, etc. To my knowledge, *comparative therapeutic investigations* such as those mentioned above were not performed in hepatology. Until modern times, treatment of liver diseases remained almost exclusively empirical – and thus scientifically unproven.

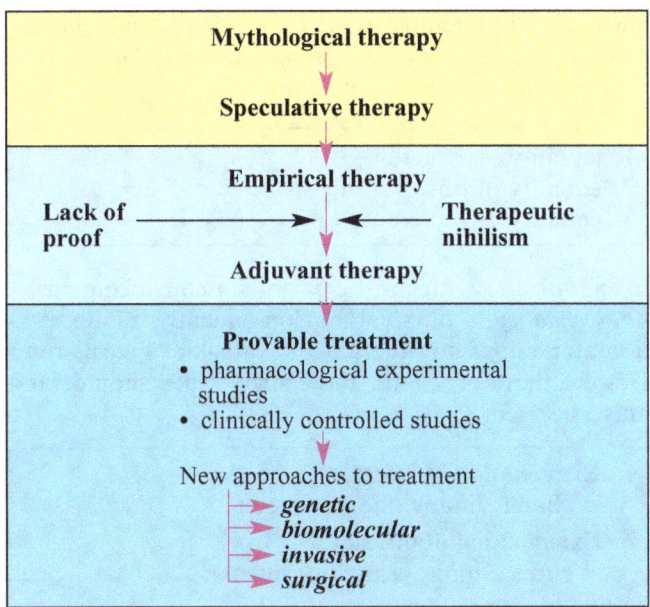

Tab. 40.1: Epochs of medicine: (*1.*) mythological, (*2.*) speculative, and (*3.*) empirical therapy, through to (*4.*) provable treatment

The occasionally pronounced **"polypragmatism"** was confronted by the opposite extreme of **"therapeutic nihilism"** in the sense of treatment based on expectation. This inevitably led to frustration on the part of the physician and to resignation on the part of the patient suffering from a liver disease. • Thus, the realization of provable treatment also became an urgent challenge in hepatology.

2 Clinical studies

▶ The first ethical principles of biomedical research had already been developed in Germany prior to World War I: relevant instructions were issued by the Prussian Education Office in 1900. • At the proposal of the German National Health Board, guidelines for modern curative treatment and for the performance of scientific studies in humans were issued in 1931 by the Ministry of Internal Affairs in Germany.

This measure was indeed the beginning of *scientifically based therapy*. • In 1932 P. MARTINI published his methodology of therapeutic research (8), and in 1937 A. B. HILL established the principles of medical statistics. (6)

2.1 Types of clinical studies

Significant contributions have since been made concerning the importance, performance and evaluation of **clinical studies.** (5, 7) In recent years, statistical and legal issues in particular have been discussed. (3, 10, 11, 12) • Controlled clinical studies are rightly called for and they are indispensable for avoiding therapeutic misjudgement deriving from "trial and error" and for creating an objective basis for official decisions. They may be carried out, as far as possible comparatively, as a retrospective or prospective investigation. • A **retrospective study** is a backward-looking review of facts and effects, i.e. against a time axis, to identify preceding causes. The data can be collected according to a fixed plan (**= prolective**) or generated before the study begins (**= retrolective**). Furthermore, a distinction is made between following the individual course from the time the causative factor appears through to the onset of effect (**= cohort**) and following the individual course from the onset of effect back to the earliest possible point in time when the causative factor appeared (**= trohoc**) (A. R. FEINSTEIN, 1977). Thus, a retrospective study is deemed scientifically correct if its execution is justified and the methodology is clearly defined. • A **prospective study** starts from causative factors, observing the effect over the course of time. (7, 10, 12)

Special cases are the *open (non-blind) study* on the one hand and the *crossover study* on the other hand. • This means that the controlled clinical study is "fundamentally" (i.e. with some exceptions) the sole and most essential tool for obtaining proof of the efficacy of a given substance. If the conditions for a controlled clinical study cannot be met, then it must be dispensed with.

The **typology** of clinical studies differentiates four types according to their aims: (*1.*) pharmacological studies, (*2.*) therapeutic explorative studies, (*3.*) therapeutic confirmative studies, and (*4.*) drug-monitoring studies. The purpose of the last-mentioned group is to define the cost/benefit ratio more precisely, identify rare side effects and provide better dosage recommendations.

2.2 Problems of clinical studies

There is a vast array of literature dealing with still controversial aspects of controlled clinical studies. • *We should be aware that on the one hand, medicine is not an exact science and on the other hand, humans do not represent a quantifiable model with data on call as needed.* Problems in clinical studies often arise in **different fields:**

1. ethical	4. psychological
2. methodological	5. heuristic
3. legal	6. economic

Proof in the strict sense cannot be delivered by a controlled clinical study, which has been called the "sacred cow". (5) However, the probability of statistical error in terms of the chosen target criteria can be fixed in advance. In clinical studies, different interpretations of results are still possible, since *"intuitive medical observation and judgement remain indispensable in the individual case"* (E. BUCHBORN, 1982). • The **triad** of *empiricism, intuition* and *logic* is necessary in both diagnosis and treatment (R. GROSS, 1988).

2.3 Placebo

A placebo (Latin, "I shall please") or ADT (= **a**ny what you **d**esire **t**hing) is a "dummy" without any active substance, identical in appearance to the respective active drug and not designed to be effective. This term has been known since the 14th century. (4) • In medicine, a placebo assumes **two roles**: (*1*.) as a therapeutic agent in the practical treatment of patients, intended to have an "effect" on a disease or a symptom, or exerting such effects without the physician's knowledge, and (*2*.) as a control substance in clinical studies with drugs. • In individual cases, even **objective** changes in physiological functions and **specific** effects may be demonstrable. The form of administration and the dosage of a placebo, the physician's personality (and that of the patient) and the intensity of the disease situation may lead to a weakening or potentiation of the placebo effect. The important (individual and social) ethical issues associated with placebo administration concern both the patient and the physician, who have to be informed in general about such procedures. These issues have been clarified by law after being discussed in detail and assessed on the basis of experimental findings.

> ▶ The placebo effect in controlled clinical studies should never be regarded as "zero", even though this is, of course, desired (or even imputed) from the statistical viewpoint.

Within the scope of clinical studies, valuable economic information on medical procedures can (and should) be obtained. Today, **economic assessment** assumes a special role in clinical studies, and because of its complex stratification and the general need for rationalization, e.g. in terms of the cost/benefit analysis, it is likely to become more and more important. The quality-adjusted life year (G. W. TORRANCE, 1987) should be included in the assessment. (s. p. 878)

2.4 Difficulty of evaluation

Proving the efficacy of a (surgical or medicinal) therapeutic measure — *and this also applies in hepatology* — is very difficult, as it mainly depends on **two factors**:

> 1. non-comparability of individual humans
> 2. non-comparability of individual diseases

Statistical methods cannot render either **non-comparability** of individual humans or that of diseases comparable — at best, they may compensate it by means of large patient numbers or are able to assess sameness under certain circumstances. (1, 5) • Statistical **comparability** of different patient groups can only be achieved if **three requirements** are met:

> 1. equality of structure
> 2. equality of observation
> 3. equality of representation

Even with great diagnostic effort, no convincing *structural equality* is obtainable. Consequently, randomization alone does not guarantee a valuable clinical study. Despite these problems, **three study types** should (and must) be used:

> 1. **Examination of effect**
>   = change in any one parameter
> 2. **Examination of efficacy**
>   = cure or improvement of disease
> 3. **Examination of superiority**
>   = improvement of parameters, or cure, or improvement of disease by conventional therapy vs. new therapy

2.5 Provability of treatment

In clinical studies involving drugs — *this also applies to hepatology* — the terms "effect" and "efficacy" have not always been appropriately distinguished, but were often (erroneously) considered identical. • The **effect** of a specific drug (or "liver therapeutic") showing changes in any measured parameters or reactions is easier to prove than its efficacy in the sense of cure or improvement of disease. Therapeutic **efficacy** (or efficacy of "liver therapy") is defined by the difference between the uninfluenced disease course (i.e. possible or usual course) and the disease course changed by therapeutic measures (i.e. actual course). *There is, however, no chance of ever observing and assessing the "possible" and the "actual" disease course simultaneously.*

(*1*.) The **marketability** of a pharmaceutical preparation is controlled by an act of administration. In this context, **three criteria** must be satisfied for the licensing of medicaments, including "liver therapeutics":

> 1. *quality*   2. *safety*
>   3. **efficacy**

(*2*.) The term **"quality"** is defined by various criteria: purity, identity, content, galenic properties and temperature stability of a substance. • The term **"safety"** is defined in relation to acute and chronic toxicity, foetal toxicity and fertility, mutagenic and carcinogenic potential.

(*3*.) As regards the term **"efficacy"**, no legal definition exists. As a rule, efficacy is defined by the sum of desired effects with regard to a certain therapeutic aim. Thus, in terms of the licensing regulations, the efficacy of a drug, including "liver therapeutics", may be defined as *"the abstract quality of medicine to achieve therapeutic success with proper use, accidental and placebo success having been excluded"* (K. J. HENNING, 1978). The US Food, Drug and Cosmetic Act defines the term "efficacy" in a similar manner. • Mere proof of quality and safety is sufficient for medicine that does not have be licensed, but only registered; no proof of efficacy is required. This applies to homoeopathic remedies, for example.

(*4.*) The efficacy of medicinal remedies, including "liver therapeutics", may be regarded as a **continuum**, i.e. from *"very weak"* to *"highly potent"*. Thus, efficacy is also proven when the substance is shown to be only slightly effective or is only effective in some patients (individual cases). Principally (= exceptions are possible), proof of efficacy is to be provided by controlled clinical studies. No proof of superiority of the drug under investigation over the standard preparation is required by law. Nor does the licensing procedure check whether there is a potential need for the drug in question.

> *Thus the aim of clinical studies is to provide proof of safety and appropriate efficacy. • However, it is essential to ensure the quality of the randomized, controlled trials in every respect!* (9)

3 Principles of liver therapy

3.1 Basic considerations

> First of all, two terms need rectifying, since the superficial yet incorrect use of the designations *"liver therapy"* and *"protective therapy of the liver"* have rendered it fundamentally more difficult to make accurate statements. These terms are relics from the epochs of speculative or empirical therapy and constitute the origin of the catchword "therapeutic nihilism". (s. tab. 40.1)

3.1.1 Liver therapy

There has never been and there still is not any "liver therapy" in the true sense — and no such therapy will exist in future either. The liver as the largest biochemical performance centre of the body is constantly active in some 11 major metabolic areas with 60–70 integrated partial functions. In order to accomplish the many tasks, about 300 billion liver cells undertake approx. 500 biomolecular reactions daily — indeed an unbelievable feat. Consequently, it is not possible for drugs to have an effect on the liver as a whole. *However,* **therapies for liver diseases** *or therapies for hepatological symptoms are available.* With this linguistic correctness, our therapeutic efforts in hepatology become *realistic* and *objectifiable*. There are far more than 100 liver diseases plus variants and diverse complications. A large number of them can be treated successfully with pharmacological regimens — sometimes with strikingly good results — as well as, of course, by invasive and surgical therapy.

3.1.2 Liver therapeutic agents

In the strict linguistic and hepatological sense, there is no such thing as liver therapeutic agents. However, this *unfortunate term* is frequently — and indeed deliberately — used rhetorically in publications or for administrative reasons. Here, the expression **"hepatic agents"** (analogous to cardiac, otologic and diuretic agents, etc.) would be more correct and not so promising in the popular sense as the designation "liver therapeutic agents". • *In any case, one ought to be aware of the possible psychological effect of such a term, especially with regard to a "placebo".* (s. p. 874)

3.1.3 Protective therapy of the liver

Similarly, there is no generally protective therapy of the liver. Liver "protection" as such may include active vaccination against viral hepatitis A or B, for example, and, in a wider sense, also passive immunization after exposure or general avoidance of typical liver noxae. This can "protect" the liver from diseases. (16)

In **in-vitro** and **in-vivo experiments,** certain substances can be studied for their protective effect on the hepatocytes or endothelial cells (including biomembranes and organelles) under the influence of various noxae or toxins. *Many substances have been shown to display distinct protective properties experimentally under various investigative conditions.* Such studies are not, however, admissible in humans. • These experimental protective properties may also be of therapeutic value in individual cases (e.g. application of *silibinin* in Amanita poisoning).

A "liver-protective preparation" must therefore be capable of protecting the hepatocytes (as well as the sinus endothelium) from a particular liver toxin, or from two to three clearly defined (or, in the optimal case, all obligate) liver toxins, *by administration before or, at the latest, when the damage occurs*. The use of a substance in existing cellular damage would be classified as "therapy" and no longer "protection". The term protective liver therapy clearly implies prophylaxis — which, apart from the above exceptions (e.g. vaccination), is usually not feasible under the provisions of the respective health insurance system. (16)

3.2 Preconditions

The question of provability of a certain therapy is also dependent on various **factors** in hepatology: (*1*.) knowledge of the spontaneous course of a liver disease (not known in individual cases, but only globally assessable), (*2.*) endogenous factors (gender, age, genetics), and (*3.*) exogenous influence (e.g. lifestyle, noxae, patient compliance). These imponderables can scarcely (if at all) be integratively assessed or excluded even using subtle statistical methods. Randomization and double-blind clinical trials can do no more than balance out these differences. In order to obtain usable data, certain **statistical conditions** should be fulfilled as far as possible:

- homogeneous findings
  in
- homogeneous patients
  with
- homogeneous disease

These requirements are difficult to meet even in controlled clinical studies in hepatology. Moreover, the use of medication in liver disease is based on further essential **clinical conditions:**

1. Detailed hepatic diagnosis with exact classification of the liver disease
2. Identification and elimination of the causative noxa(e)
3. Elimination of concomitant negative factors or additional noxae

Therapeutic uncertainties or differing conclusions regarding drug effects or efficacy may thus be attributed to varying degrees of methodological **inaccuracy**:

- different disease courses
  with
- different pathogenesis
  in
- different patients
  and an
- insufficient detailed diagnosis
  were submitted
  to
- joint statistical evaluation

3.3 Forms of "liver therapy"

Causal treatment of liver diseases, which is rarely (if ever) feasible, should achieve the complete elimination of the actual cause(s) (e.g. elimination of the causative noxa, antiviral treatment, gene therapy in hereditary liver diseases). • **Treatment of pathogenetic primary reactions** (e.g. with interferon, immunosuppressants or penicillamine) is aimed at interrupting the "postcausal" pathogenesis. • **Treatment of disease progression** intervenes in the pathological process in a lasting and efficient manner and thus prevents or slows down the generally dangerous consequences (e.g. inhibition of cholestasis, fibrogenesis and portal hypertension). •

Almost all substances used in hepatology are classed as **symptomatic treatment.** These substances help (*1.*) to combat malaise and disturbances secondary to the liver disease (e.g. antipruritics), and (*2.*) to influence the structures and functions of the hepatocytes and endothelial cells as well as the bile capillaries (e.g. antioxidants, essential phospholipids, UDCA, silymarin). (16)

3.4 Aims of treatment

Drug therapy of a particular liver disease or complicative development must have basic **treatment aims.** The primary therapeutic aim is to eliminate the existing causative factors and pathogenetic mechanisms. The final goal is always the *rehabilitation* of the liver patient. (s. tab. 40.2) (s. p. 912)

1. Eliminating or definitively overcoming the cause of disease (as far as possible) as well as promoting and speeding up its cure
2. Inhibition of inflammatory reactions
3. Curbing of mesenchymal reactions
4. Modulation of immunological reactions
5. Support/normalization of liver cell functions
6. Stimulation of hepatic regeneration

Rehabilitation

Tab. 40.2: Treatment aims in liver diseases

3.5 Categories of "liver therapeutics"

A number of substances and preparations are available for the treatment of liver diseases. They can be categorized in various ways. (s. tab. 40.3)

1. **Prophylactics:** e.g. immunoglobulins or vaccines against hepatotropic virus infections
2. **Antidotes:** e.g. silibinin against Amanita poisoning or N-acetylcysteine in paracetamol intoxication, haemarginate in acute porphyria
3. **Primary liver therapeutics:** e.g. penicillamine, glucocorticoids, azathioprine, interferon-α, aimed at primary intervention in the aetiology or pathomechanism of liver disease.
4. **Secondary liver therapeutics:** e.g. fat-soluble vitamins in impending deficiency states, drugs to reduce portal hypertension, substances to relieve hyperammoniaemia, aimed at secondary prevention of the various sequelae of liver disease.

Tab. 40.3: Categories of liver therapeutic agents

3.6 Active substances

For several years, (negative) claims appeared in the press stating that the pharmaceutical market was oversaturated with more than 600 liver preparations. Although the originator of this claim was not identified, this utopian number made the rounds. • In fact, there are merely **25 substances** or **groups of substances** (of chemical or plant origin) listed in the pharmacopoeia. Here, the various preparations containing the same substance are numbered separately, which gives a total of **90—100 listed preparations**. • It is irresponsible that some "liver therapeutics" still have an **alcohol content** of 25—66 vol.% (particularly homoeopathic and phytotherapeutic remedies). (s. p. 64) Although the often quantitatively low intake of alcohol in a preparation may be "harmless" (even "3 times daily"), it will usually cause a relapse in an abstinent alcoholic. *In principle, there is no justifiable argument for keeping the alcohol content in a hepatological preparation!*

Some drugs with **special indications** are used in liver diseases or in certain complications. They are not found in the special category of liver therapeutics (pharmacopoeia), but are listed according to their main indication. Treatment with some of these active substances may be accompanied by side effects. (s. tab. 40.4)

Chemical substances (or groups)
1. AA of the urea cycle
2. Beta blockers
3. Bile acids
4. BCAA
5. Deferoxamine
6. D-penicillamine
7. Diuretics
8. Glucocorticoids
9. Haemarginate
10. Immunosuppressants
11. Immunostimulants
12. Lactulose
13. Nucleoside analogues
14. S-adenosyl-L-methionine
15. Somatostatin
16. Spironolactone
17. Virustatics
18. Vitamins (A—K)
19. Zinc
Phytotherapeutic agents (or groups)
1. Colchicine
2. Essential phospholipids
3. Glycyrrhizin
4. Silymarin
5. Various herbal preparations

Tab. 40.4: Active chemical substances (or groups) and phytotherapeutic agents used in some liver diseases or their complications

Active substances with proven efficacy in hepatology *are only administered as "treatment" and not as "liver protec-tion" (apart from the prophylactics mentioned above).* These active substances are used in patients when, according to the diagnosed disease and the clinical and pharmacological results, they are actually indicated. • *Thus, it is the existing liver disease and/or complication and not the medication budget or the patient's wishes which decides the therapeutic indication.* • Anything else would go against the principles of a physician or be uneconomical, and legally problematic in individual cases.

The second dimension of controlled studies, **"time"**, is frequently given insufficient consideration in evaluating therapeutic results. In fact, it is only possible to assess whether the substances used in chronic liver disease have the required efficacy after an adequate treatment period. In the drug therapy of patients with chronic liver disease as carried out by the clinician and general practitioner, evaluation periods invariably extend over several years. In such cases, positive or negative results can be obtained "empirically", but because they are not "statistically" confirmed, they are not "provable". In this context as well,

- *empiricism*
- *intuition*
- *logic*

may diverge (s. p. 873), so that statistics, which as such are indispensable, may indeed prove to be an obstacle.

Perhaps the expectations or requirements of "liver therapy" are too high. With regard to other organs and their respective diseases, established medication often does not really achieve a "cure", but merely "functional improvements" (e. g. recompensation, inhibition of progression, stabilization in everyday life, improvement in quality of life, rehabilitation). In principle, these fully acceptable therapy aims apply to the treatment of liver diseases as well.

3.7 Dose adjustment of medicaments

Liver and medicaments are interrelated in **three ways**:

1. Medication *inducing* liver diseases
2. Medication *for* liver diseases
3. Medication *changed by* liver diseases

Apart from the kidneys, the liver is the most important excretory organ for drugs. In contrast to other mechanisms of drug elimination, which are relatively well understood, **liver metabolism** of drugs has proved extremely complicated. (s. pp 56—60) *Biotransformation* is influenced by variable and non-variable factors under physiological and pathological conditions. (s. tab. 3.18) • **Changes in pharmaceutical preparations** are alterations in the respective properties which occur due to the disturbed metabolization function of the liver cells and/or hepatic blood flow secondary to liver disease. Additionally, drug metabolism may be drastically modified by coexisting hypoalbuminaemia or cholestasis. Liver diseases do not only affect the elimination parameters (e. g. half-life, clearance), but also absorption (e. g. bioavailability) and distribution of the drug in the body. A further factor are the interactions of certain drugs with receptors at the site of action (e. g. increased sensitivity of the brain to diazepam in cirrhosis patients). Biotoxometabolites and lipid peroxidation, which are not normally typical of a certain medicament, must also be anticipated. • In principle, a **dose reduction** should be considered in severe and chronic liver disease, especially when the medicament is used regularly. On the other hand, a **dose increase** may be required in i.v. administration owing to reduced hepatic blood flow and using medication with a high elimination rate. • Disturbed drug metabolism may be further aggravated by alcohol consumption with its multiple biochemical effects. (s. p. 65) (s. tabs. 28.2, 28.3)

Despite great efforts, it has not been possible so far to make single **dose calculations** (*1.*) for a *certain* medicament, (*2.*) in a *certain* liver disease, and (*3.*) in a *certain* patient. Some drugs have been classified into three groups on the basis of their hepatic extraction rate and route as well as their form of administration: drugs with a high, with a moderate and with a low risk of overdosage — however, such information is given with reservations. The difficulties regarding the correct dose adjustment of a medicinal remedy in therapeutic use require careful **monitoring** of the individual patient, sometimes also determination of the blood values, or consultation with a pharmacologist. (16)

▶ **Clinical studies:** In view of the above-mentioned difficulties, it may be problematic to administer the *same* dose to *all* volunteers and to obtain pharmacologically *equivalent* results in clinical studies. • This might also explain the occasionally great variation in study results (despite a carefully chosen trial design) and any potential "inefficacy" or undesired effect of the drug. (s. pp 60, 873, 878)

3.8 Significance of quality of life

Of the two dimensions of life, quantity and quality, clinical studies have inevitably paid far more attention to the former (i.e. length of life). The **quantity of life** (judged by survival probability, mortality rate or survival curves) seems to be the most important parameter for assessing treatment efficacy. A review of 99 publications which appeared in leading surgical journals from 1981–1986 revealed that in 97% of the papers, no mention was made of quality of life after surgical procedures — in 341 publications on cardiac surgery, this was mentioned in only 8% of cases (J. O'YOUNG et al., 1985, 1987). Obviously, the prolongation of life was paramount in fixing therapeutic aims. (1, 13, 14, 18, 19)

Defining and measuring the **quality of life** has become important in recent years. This also applies to the conservative or invasive treatment of liver disease, and, in future, more attention will have to be paid to criteria for assessing the changed quality of life under certain therapies as well as the choice of certain treatment strategies (M. LUDWIG, 1988). • The *definition* of good life quality implies that (*1.*) a person experiences the least possible impairment and handicap under a given therapy (= *clinical norm*), (*2.*) this person functions in accordance with existing social roles and derives satisfaction from this (= *social norm*), and (*3.*) the hopes and expectations of this person are fulfilled (= *individual norm*) (M. BULLINGER, 1988). • In one comprehensive survey of the literature, not one single study focusing on the quality of life in liver disease is cited. • Remarkably, a later study mentioned a significant reduction in the quality of life in *patients with chronic hepatitis C*. (14) In a further study, interferon treatment was not only shown to improve the disease, but also to enable the patients to resume their normal daily routine.

3.9 Assessment of survival rate

In the treatment of liver diseases which have a fulminant course or which are chronically progressive (and the respective complications), the question of survival arises. In this context, the classification according to *Child-Turcotte* (1964) and *Pugh* (1973) has proved its worth worldwide. (s. fig. 35.7) • We have used this classification on a regular basis.

In 2000 a score was published giving a prediction of the survival chances in patients with TIPS. (16) Subsequently, this score was validated in several cohorts of patients suffering from different forms of liver disease with varying degrees of severity. The studies included inpatients and outpatients in many different geographical regions. The new model was initially termed "Mayo end-stage liver disease" (MELD). This name was later changed into "Model for end-stage liver disease" *(MELD)*, although the acronym MELD remained unaltered. (18) MELD is based on values relating to creatinine, bilirubin and INR (international normalized ratio). These values are included in the original mathematical formula for MELD:

$$9.57 \times \log_e (\text{creatinine}) + 3.78 \times \log_e (\text{bilirubin}) + 11.2 \times \log_e (\text{INR}) + 6.43 = \ldots\ldots$$

4 Nutritional therapy of liver diseases

The Hippocratic idea that *"dyscrasia"* was the cause of nearly all diseases meant that **dietetics** (= diaita) was necessary for the *"restoration to normal of the life order"*.

(s. p. 6) Even in antiquity, special forms of nutrition were of great importance in the treatment of liver diseases. In addition to those dietary prescriptions which were within the reach of everyone (e.g. donkey liver with parsley and honey) (s. pp 7, 872), there were also extremely complicated diets for the treatment of jaundice which only "kings" could afford (CELSUS called jaundice the *morbus regius*). (s. p. 7) • During all historical epochs of medicine, dietetic measures have played an essential role in the treatment of liver diseases — even in the so-called "dirty pharmacy" of mediaeval times. (s. p. 872) Because dietetics assumed such an important role in hepatology, nutrition, i.e. enteral intake of special beverages and food, was mainly based on mythological and, at a later date, also on speculative ideas.

From the beginning of the 20th century, a **mild liver diet** was propagated, which in some cases was pursued with scientific meticulousness. The purists issued strict nutritional rules for patients concerning liver diets. In those days, we young clinicians often had great difficulty in implementing such guidelines in practical terms. • This one extreme was set against the other extreme of therapeutic nihilism, i.e. a **free choice of food** by the patient ("eat what you like"). (s. tab. 40.1)

▶ *Neither extreme is acceptable — in fact, certain liver diseases or complicative developments require special forms of nutrition.*

4.1 Artificial feeding

Artificial feeding is indicated when the liver patient (*1.*) is no longer *able* to, (*2.*) does not *want* to, or (*3.*) is not *allowed* to eat anything because of certain complications. It may also be necessary to prevent malnutrition as well as to eliminate manifest dietary deficits rapidly and successfully. • Artificial feeding can be performed **enterally** by nasogastric tubes, percutaneous-endoscopic gastrotomy (PEG) or jejunostomy (PEJ), and **parenterally** by central-venous catheter systems. This measure is carried out **short term** during inpatient treatment or **long term** on an outpatient basis at home.

4.1.1 Enteral feeding

Should artificial feeding be necessary, the enteral route of application should be given preference. This is feasible in 90% of hepatological problem cases. Nutrition consists of high or low molecular weight formula diets. Feeding may be continuous or in four to five phases. Nasogastric tubes (i.e. 7–8 Ch) are harmless even when oesophageal varices exist. The correct position has to be checked and documented, preferably using radiology! • Artificial enteral feeding must correspond with the principles of energy and metabolism as well as containing vitamins, electrolytes and trace elements in optimum amounts. It must be appropriate with regard to the underlying liver disease. • Enteral feeding has significant trophic effects on the intestinal mucosa in terms of stimulating local IgA production, improving its integrity as a barrier against bacterial translation, regulating the physiologically adapted intake of nutritional components (which are subsequently made available to the liver in a physiological first pass effect) as well as steering secretion and hormone production. Serious metabolic disturbances must be avoided; other complications occur only rarely. (22, 29, 31)

4.1.2 Parenteral feeding

Indications for artificial feeding via a central-venous catheter must be considered carefully. As a rule, it is possible only for a brief time, since the application period is limited by several **complications:** (*1.*) venous thrombosis, (*2.*) local infection, and (*3.*) systemic infection (in the usually immunocompromised liver patient). With prolonged parenteral alimentation, (*4.*) complications in the form of various liver damage must be anticipated. (28, 42) • The reported frequency of **liver damage** is 15–100%. This generally depends on the duration of parenteral feeding, but occasionally the composition of the infusion solution proves to be inappropriate. Laboratory parameters show increases in GPT, GOT and γ-GT as well as in alkaline phosphatase and bilirubin. As a rule, these changes are reversible; however, excessive elevations, especially catheter-associated infections, may necessitate the discontinuation of parenteral feeding. Deaths have occurred in up to 3% of cases. (20, 21, 23, 27) • Various forms of *morphological liver damage* may develop, possibly in combination:

1. Cholangitis	6. Fibrosis
2. Cholelithiasis	7. Hepato/splenomegaly
3. Cholestasis	8. Jaundice
4. Chronic hepatitis	9. Liver cirrhosis
5. Fatty liver disease	10. Steatohepatitis

The **pathogenetic mechanisms** of liver disease caused by artificial feeding are not fully understood. Various **theories** have been postulated: (*1.*) deficiency of essential fatty acids or essential phospholipids, (*2.*) exceeding the maximum glucose oxidation rate, (*3.*) lack of important substances (e.g. choline, taurine, glutamine, inositol, carnitine), (*4.*) in individual cases, the presence of toxic metabolic components (e.g. methionine, plant sterols) or newly formed biotoxometabolites. • It must be borne in mind that cirrhosis patients usually show *endogenous hyperinsulinaemia*. A high intake of glucose should thus be avoided, as should the additional administration of insulin. • *The so-called **sugar substitutes** (e.g. sorbitol, mannitol, xylit, maltit) are not to be recommended.* (26) (s. p. 387)

The calculated glucose requirement of the brain is 1.5 mg/kg BW per minute (i.e. 140–160 g carbohydrates, 560–700 kcal). Blood glucose and lactate levels must be monitored. Fats are the most important energy carriers; 20–50% of the total calorie requirement should be provided in the form of lipids, preferably as MCT/LCT emulsion (1 g fat/kg BW). The latter are also readily metabolized by cirrhosis patients. (25–27) In acute liver failure, disturbances in amino-acid metabolism often occur. Amino-acid infusions should be avoided in this phase – coma-adapted or liver-adapted amino-acid infusions may be indicated (0.4 g AA/kg BW/day with a possible dose increase up to 1.0 (–1.5) g/kg BW/day). Vitamins, electrolytes and trace elements must be sufficiently substituted. The adjuvant use of essential phospholipids and ornithine aspartate is pharmacologically plausible. The regimen of parenteral nutrition must be monitored daily. (23, 26)

The daily requirement of energy, substrate and electrolytes is based on fixed values. (s. tab. 40.5)

Water	25–45 ml/kg BW
Energie	25–30 kca/kg BW
• Carbohydrate	50–55%
• Lipids	30–35%
• Protein	15–20%
• Standard	0.8–1.5 kca/kg BW
Elextrolytes	
– Natrium	550 mg
– Chloride	830 mg
– Potassium	2,000 mg
– Calcium	1,000 mg
– Phosphorus	700 mg
– Magnesium	400 mg

Tab. 40.5: Daily requirement of water, energy and electrolytes under normal conditions

4.2 Diet in malnutrition

Chronic liver diseases, especially cirrhosis and alcohol-induced conditions, are accompanied by (protein-caloric) malnutrition in 65–90% of cases. The prognosis of the liver disease largely depends on the nutritional state – there is also a direct relationship between the degree of malnutrition and the progression of the disease and/or complications as well as the probability of survival after liver transplantation. (22, 23, 25, 26, 31–34, 36, 39) • *A BMI of less than 20.5 denotes malnutrition.*

Causes of malnutrition include: (*1.*) reduced quantity and quality of nutrition, (*2.*) maldigestion and malabsorption, (*3.*) accelerated protein breakdown and protein loss as well as *reduced protein synthesis,* (*4.*) increased energy requirement, especially in the case of complications, and (*5.*) metabolic disturbances (e.g.

insulin resistance, sympathicotonia, loss of metabolic efficiency). (s. p. 765)

The **resting energy expenditure** (REE) (in kcal) in chronic liver disease can be calculated according to the *Harris-Benedict equation* (1918), considering the patient's body weight, kg (W), height, cm (H) and age, years (A). • Multiplying the REE (kcal) by **activity factor** 1.2–1.4 gives the energy requirement under normal daily conditions (in e.g. trauma, sport up to factor 6.0 or even more).

Men	= $66.47 + (13.7 \times W) + (5.0 \times H) - (6.8 \times A)$
Women	= $655.1 + (9.6 \times W) + (1.8 \times H) - (4.7 \times A)$

The **proportions** of carbohydrates (4.0–5.0), fats (1.0–2.0) and proteins (0.8–1.5) (each in g/kg BW/day) in patients with chronic liver disease correspond to those of an ordinary diet; the basic calorie requirement is 25–30 kcal/kg BW/day. • From the metabolic viewpoint, and in the case of diabetes, daily **food intake** should be divided into three main meals and two snacks. As a prophylactic measure, it is advisable to restrict the use of common salt to 7–8 g (because of the very high NaCl content in the usual diet). Moreover, a preponderance of lactovegetarian proteins over proteins derived from meat and fish (with their higher production of ammonia) is recommended. A sufficient intake of vitamins, electrolytes, trace elements and roughage should be guaranteed. (29, 35, 37, 40, 41) (s. p. 765)

Principles of lifestyle
1. Alcohol abstinence
2. Avoidance of noxae and toxins
3. Reaching and maintaining a normal BMT
4. Paying attention to the sensitive water-electrolyte balance (s. figs. 16.1, 16.3) (s. pp 294, 311, 765)
5. Avoidance of malnutrition and undernourishment (s. pp 604, 751)

List of instructions: These "principles of lifestyle" should be closely observed by the patient; they apply to every liver disease. We have always included these principles on a *list of instructions* given to our patients together with the *documentation sheet.* (s. fig. 15.3)

4.3 Special diets

Special dietary measures are of major, often even of decisive importance for several types of liver disease or associated complications. • Here, too, the false, universal claim that "there is no liver diet" is invalid. In the same way that treatment of a liver condition is indeed possible, there are also dietary measures for certain forms or complications of liver disease. • After an exact diagnosis has been made, there is often a necessity for dietary therapy based on the respective situation.

At this point, we would like to emphasize once again that a strict lactovegetarian protein supply must be adhered to not only in latent encephalopathy, but also in (acute or chronic) liver diseases in which insufficient detoxification of ammonia is anticipated. When assessing the so-called protein tolerance threshold (s. p. 286), the *documentation sheet* (s. fig. 15.3) as well as a *psychomotoric test programme* (s. p. 211) can be of great help.

Metabolic diseases: A *fatty liver* does not require a low-fat diet, but standard nutrition based on general reference values for usual daily routine. With a normal body weight and an increased energy requirement (work, sports), the calorie intake has to be adjusted accordingly. • In *overweight patients,* a slow, continuous, yet systematic weight reduction should be striven for. Coexistent *hyperlipoproteinaemia* may require supportive treatment. *Diabetes mellitus* must be properly controlled. This also applies to concomitant *gout*.

Cirrhosis: In compensated liver cirrhosis without obvious malnutrition or undernourishment, no special diet is necessary, and normal balanced nutrition is adequate. In liver cirrhosis, a lactovegetarian protein supply always has to be given preference; ammonia-forming animal proteins should only be present in the food in low quantities and consumed every few days. *Malnutrition* has to be eliminated by corresponding dietetic measures. In severe cases of disease, artificial feeding (enteral, or for a short time parenteral) may be recommended. (24, 30, 33, 37–39) (s. pp 765, 879)

Haemochromatosis: Iron is ubiquitous in food. A *low-iron* diet must be observed (using available food tables). Although a lactovegetarian diet is desirable, attention should be paid to the high iron content of pulses, green vegetables and dried fruit. • *Black tea* (2–3 cups per day) should be drunk regularly. (s. p. 644)

Wilson's disease: With a normal diet, the daily copper supply amounts to 3–6 mg. In Wilson's disease, however, the copper content should be reduced to <1 mg/day (using the available food tables). As in haemochromatosis, a lactovegetarian diet is important, but attention should be paid to the high copper content of coarse-grained wholemeal products, nuts, cheese (Emmental, Edam) and cocoa. The intestinal absorption of copper can be reduced further by potassium sulphide (3 × 20 mg). (s. p. 635)

Encephalopathy: The diagnosis of HE, even in the stage of latency (s. p. 280) (s. fig. 15.3), requires an adjustment of protein intake. This applies to both the daily amount (= cutting down) and the type of protein (= only lactovegetarian proteins). No reduction in fats is necessary. (34) Carbohydrates should be restricted to 2.5–3.5 g/kg BW. The return to standard nutrition should correspond to the gradually improving quantitative and later also qualitative protein tolerance threshold, varying from case to case. Should no nitrogen balance and no improvement in the HE symptoms be achieved with lactovegetarian protein intake, supplementation with *branched-chain amino acids* is indicated. The latter also stimulate muscular protein synthesis and promote the formation of glutamine in the brain. However, they are not equivalent to substitution by balanced amino-acid solutions. Commercially available protein preparations should be low in common salt. (s. pp 285, 754)

Ascites: The occurrence of a disturbed water-electrolyte balance in the late stage of latent oedema (s. fig. 15.3) requires immediate restriction of the salt intake (<3–6 g/day) – depending on the level of natriuresis: the intake of fluid is limited to 1.0 (−1.5) l/day, especially in hyponatriaemia. An intermittent *fruit and rice diet* (generally for 1–2 days) is recommended because it is extremely low in sodium, but rich in potassium. Marked *NaCl restriction* simultaneously leads to a reduction in protein intake. The use of commercially available low-salt protein preparations is therefore advisable (e.g. 60 g protein/100 g + 5 mval sodium/100 g, or 48 g protein/100 g + 13 g, or 15 g sodium/100 g). NaCl restriction is contraindicated in natriuresis of <25 mmol/day. (s. p. 314)

Storage diseases: Some genetic metabolic diseases require special dietary measures: e.g. (*1.*) *disorders of the urea cycle* are treated with a diet similar to that used in encephalopathy (s. p. 611), (*2.*) *Gierke's disease* needs a high-carbohydrate diet (s. p. 612), (*3.*) *Cori's disease* is treated with formula diets and a starch diet (s. p. 613), (*4.*) *galactosaemia* wants a galactose- and lactose-free diet (s. p. 614), and (*5.*) in *fructose intolerance*, a fructose- and saccharose-free diet must be given. (s. p. 615)

5 Drug therapy of liver diseases

Many different **active substances** have been discussed in connection with the treatment of the various liver diseases or their complications in the respective chapters. The effectiveness of these substances has either been *statistically confirmed* in controlled trials, or they have been *tested empirically*, or they seem to be *pharmacologically plausible* for a specific application. • Some of these therapeutic substances and their uses are presented in the following.

5.1 Virustatics

Viruses have no metabolism of their own; and they just contain DNA or RNA and envelope proteins. They are only able to replicate in living host cells, whereby they need to make use of the enzymes, synthesis mechanisms, amino acids and nucleic acids of the host cell. Replication can be inhibited by virustatics. Generally, however, viruses cannot be completely inactivated; as a rule, this is only possible by means of the body's own defences. •

The viruses attach themselves to the cell membranes via specific receptors (= **adsorption**). Viruses enter the cells by means of **endocytosis**. The virus coat opens, with the result that viral nucleic acid and enzymes are liberated (= **uncoating**). This is followed by **transcription** of viral nucleic acid to mRNA, the formation of enzymes (= early-phase proteins) and structural proteins (= late-phase proteins) as well as nucleic acids for virus multiplication (= **replication**). After maturation, the viruses are released from the host cells by exosomes.

Virustatics are substances which inhibit viral replication without inactivating the viruses themselves (i.e. they are not virucidal). Chemically speaking, they are either derivates of nucleic acids or glycoproteins (e.g. interferon). Virustatics have no effect until the virus has been taken up in the host cell. They can therefore have the following *points of attack*: (*1.*) prevention of viral attachment to the host cells, (*2.*) inhibition of penetration, (*3.*) inhibition of uncoating, (*4.*) inhibition of nucleic acid synthesis, (*5.*) inhibition of protein synthesis, and (*6.*) prevention of virus liberation. • *Any therapeutic impact on viruses is also an attack on the metabolism of the host cell.* (s. tab. 40.6)

Due to their various modes of action and viral targets, some first and second generation virustatics have also been employed for treating hepatitis viruses. Thus, various virustatics are indicated in infections with **secondary hepatotropic viruses** (s. pp 118, 474):

Aciclovir	HSV, VZV (EBV)
Amantadine	Influenza A, B
Didanosine	HIV
Famciclovir	HSV
Foscarnet	HSV, CMV, HIV
Ganciclovir	CMV, HSV, VZV (EBV)
Vidarabine	HSV, VZV (EBV)
Zidovudine	HIV

Virustatics are indicated in *acute* viral hepatitis C, with interferon being the therapy of first choice in this connection. They are used as early as possible. Their application is also recommended in *chronic* hepatitis B, C and B/D. • In infections with hepatotropic viruses, the following virustatics have already been introduced or are under discussion:

1. Aciclovir	6. Famciclovir	11. Lobucavir
2. Adefovir	7. Foscarnet	12. Ribavirin
3. Amantadine	8. Ganciclovir	13. Tenofir
4. Emtricitabine	9. Interferon α, β	14. Vidarabine etc.
5. Entecavir	10. Lamivudine	

5.1.1 Interferon

Interferons (IFN) were discovered in England by A. Isaacs et al. in 1957. (46) They are low molecular weight glycoproteins acting as cytokines (so-called intercellular mediators) with clear species-specific effects.

		DNA-dependent polymerase	Reverse transcriptase	Chain break
Amantadin	Uncoating			
Aciclovir	Replication	+		+
Adefovir	"	+		+
Famciclovir	"			+
Foscarnet	"	+		
Ganciclovir	"	+		+
Interferon	"	+		
Lamivudine	"	+	+	
Lobucavir	"	+		+
Vidarabine	"	+		
Didanosine	Transcription of RNA to DNA		+	+
Foscarnet			+	
Zalcitabine			+	+
Zidovudine			+	+
Interferon	Maturation			
Ribavirin	Replication	Inosinmonophosphat-Dehydrogenase		

Tab. 40.6: Some modes of action and points of attack of virustatics

Interferon type I includes the subtypes IFN-α and IFN-β. They are formed by nearly all cells, whereby *IFN-α* is mainly produced by monocytes and B-lymphocytes, and *IFN-β* mainly by fibroblasts. Both subtypes bind to the same receptor at the target cells and are taken up in the hepatocytes by endocytosis. Prior to degradation, IFN activates many genes, thus causing a broad spectrum of proteins to be synthesized. This explains its multiple biological effects. The antiviral effect of IFN-α is evident in all the important steps of virus replication. However, the various cell types form different IFN-α subtypes; so far, more than 30 subtypes are known. IFN-α and IFN-β have a half-life of three to four hours.

Interferon type II includes IFN-γ, which is probably only produced by T lymphocytes and natural killer cells. IFN-γ is of no importance for the therapy of viral hepatitis. (44) (s. p. 723!) • Recently, *IFN-ω* was isolated, but its biological role is not yet understood.

Recombinant IFN is produced from a clone of E. coli, which carries a plasmid that possesses a gene for IFN$_{-α2b}$. The molecular weight amounts to 19,200 daltons. It has a high level of purity (>99%). If antibodies against recombinant IFN occur, natural IFN may prove useful. Recombinant interferons differ in only one single amino-acid position:

	Position 23	Position 34
IFN-α$_{2a}$	lysine	histidine
IFN-α$_{2b}$	arginine	histidine
IFN-α$_{2c}$	histidine	arginine

Lymphoblastoid IFN-α is a mixture of natural IFN-α subtypes with different structures of the carbohydrate chains. • A **consensus IFN-α** has also been developed; this is a genetically modified IFN-α, which has the properties of various IFN-α subtypes. Thus its biological activity is increased (by ca. 30% in chronic hepatitis C, probably due to better receptor affinity).

Pegylated IFN optimizes the biological effects of IFN. The term "pegylation" denotes covalent linkage of polyethylglycol (PEG) to IFN. Thus IFN is protected from proteolysis, and its half-life is extended approx. tenfold (to about 40 hours). This "depot interferon" therefore has improved efficacy due to prolonged persistence in the body. (43, 45, 51) (s. pp 723, 728)

	Peginterferon alpha-2a (40 kDa)	Peginterferon alpha-2b (12 kDa)
Volume of distribution (units)	8–12 l	0.99 l
Clearance (units)	94 ml/h	22.0 ml/h
Absorption half-life	50 h	4.6 h
Elimination half-life	80 h	~40 h
Peak-to-trough ratio	1.5	>10
Time to maximum concentration (T_{max})	72–96 h	15–44 h

1. **Antiviral effects**
   - Reduction in cellular uptake of viruses
   - Inhibition of intracellular processing of viruses
   - Reduction in viral mRNA synthesis
   - Reduction in protein synthesis
   - Induction of ribonuclease
2. **Immunostimulation**
   - Induction of substances inhibiting cell division and reducing oncogene expression
     - cytokines
     - complement factors (B, C_2)
     - nuclear proteins
   - Increase in the activity of
     - macrophages and natural killer cells
     - cytotoxic T lymphocytes
   - Hypothalamus-mediated fever
3. **Increased expression of membrane proteins**
   - HLA classes I, II − antigens
   - β_2-microglobulin
   - Fc-receptor
4. **Antineoplastic effect**
   - Inhibition of cell division
   - Decrease in oncogene expression
   - Direct cytotoxicity
5. **Inhibition of fibrosis**

Tab. 40.7: Biological modes of action of interferons

▶ The interferons display multiple **biological modes of action.** Each of these effects (or their sum) contributes to therapeutic efficacy. It is still unclear which actions or mechanisms assume a central role in the treatment of chronic viral hepatitis. (47–45) (s. tab. 40.7)

5.1.2 Nucleoside analogues

Nucleosides (e. g. adenosine, cytidine, guanosine, pyrimidine, thymidine, uridine) consist of a nitrogenous purine or pyrimidine base linked to a 5-carbon sugar (ribose or deoxyribose). **Nucleotides** (adenine, cytosine, guanine, thymine, uracil), the phosphate esters of nucleotides, form the basis of RNA and DNA. As infectious viral nucleic acids, they are capable of penetrating the cells and using available enzyme systems for replication.

As modified nucleoside components, the **nucleoside analogues** inhibit the replication of viral nucleic acids. Therefore, they belong to the group of virustatics. They are phosphorylated by means of cellular or viral kinases, thus becoming biologically active. As regards their clinical application as virustatics, it must be ensured that endogenous DNA synthesis is not inhibited along with viral nucleic acid synthesis. Otherwise, severe mitochondrial lesions with lactic acidoses and irreversible liver damage may occur, possibly with a fatal outcome, as was the case with fialuridine used in chronic hepatitis B (R. MCKENZIE et al., 1995).

Many of these nucleoside analogues have already been used clinically as **virustatics** against secondary hepatotropic viruses, influenza A or HIV infection. (s. p. 882). The development of nucleoside analogues is of great importance for the treatment of chronic hepatitis B and C or D. Their virustatic efficacy can be studied in chronic hepatitis B using standardized in-vitro systems and animal experiments. (56) In hepatitis C, no such models exist, so that efficacy studies are only possible in infected patients. Several new developments have already been incorporated into clinical studies in hepatology. They are generally used in combination with interferon; in some cases, two nucleoside analogues may be used together. (51, 56, 58, 61)

(*1.*) **Famciclovir:** After absorption, this guanine derivative is converted to its active form *penciclovir*. The biologically active metabolite penciclovir triphosphate, which effects the inhibition of viral DNA polymerase, is only formed in the infected liver cell. The dosage is 3 × 500 mg/day. • After discontinuation of this substance, the previous findings usually reappear, i.e. it is only effective as an ongoing treatment. It is used therapeutically in combination with IFN. (53) (s. p. 725)

(*2.*) **Lamivudine:** This is a cytosine(cytidine)-nucleoside analogue. Its effect is based on the inhibition of reverse transcriptase in HIV and of DNA polymerase in HBV. The daily oral dosage is 1 (−3) × 100 mg/day. After discontinuation of lamivudine, the previous findings recur; here, too, efficacy only exists with continued therapy. A combination with famciclovir seems promising.

Its clinical application is mainly in combination with IFN. Long-term monotherapy over several years may be necessary. (54, 60) (s. p. 725)

(*3.*) **Lobucavir:** This guanosine derivative has proved very effective against HBV. The dosage is $1-4 \times 200$ mg/day. After discontinuation of the one-month therapy, values returned to their initial levels. A combination with IFN is also recommended for this substance, and indeed has a very good action profile.

(*4.*) **Aciclovir:** After oral application, only about 20% of the applied dose of this guanosine derivative is absorbed. Aciclovir is mainly eliminated via the kidneys (ca. 85% of the dose within 48 hours). Its half-life, which is approximately three hours, depends on renal function. The substance is employed especially in HSV and VZV infections. This agent inhibits DNA polymerase (i.e. replication) and effects a chain break. As a monotherapy in HBV infection, aciclovir only shows moderate efficacy. Side effects are rare.

(*5.*) **Ganciclovir:** This is a guanosine derivative with a good action profile in HBV, EBV, CMV and VZV infection. Ganciclovir triphosphate inhibits virus replication. Half-life is about four hours. Elimination is via the kidneys. Only a fraction of this substance is absorbed after oral administration; application (e. g. in CMV infection) is intravenous (10 mg/kg BW/day). It has severe toxic side effects. Ganciclovir was given successfully as early as 1989 in chronic hepatitis B. Subsequently, good results were achieved in combination with IFN.

(*6.*) **Ribavirin:** This guanosine analogue was first used experimentally by O. REICHARD et al. (1991) and in chronic hepatitis C by J. ANDERSSON et al. (1991). It is rapidly absorbed and distributed in the body, but excreted slowly (half-life is 79 hours). Bioavailability is 45−65%. As a monotherapy, it only leads to a decrease in the transaminases and a slight improvement in histological activity. Ribavirin may not exhibit a direct antiviral effect, but can trigger a favourable response to interferon. When combined with IFN, ribavirin proved far more efficacious in chronic hepatitis C (immunomodulation?) without any increase in the typical side effects of IFN. (55, 57, 59) (s. p. 729)

(*7.*) **Amantadine:** The antiviral efficacy of amantadine (1-adamantanamine) was reported for the first time by W. L. DAVIES et al. in 1964. The mode of action consists in preventing uncoating and viral maturation (i. e. inhibiting the release of the nucleic acids that have already penetrated the host cell). The active substance is almost completely absorbed following oral administration. It is eliminated unchanged via the kidney. The half-life is about 15 hours. So far, it has only been indicated to combat influenza virus type A. (s. p. 730)

5.2 Immunosuppressants

Immunosuppressants are substances that suppress the immune response. Inhibition or neutralization of the major part of the body's defence system is essential in (*1.*) organ transplantation, and (*2.*) autoimmune diseases. The following are considered to be some of the most important immunosuppressants:

1. Antilymphocytic globulin	6. Glucocorticoids
2. Anti-CD 3 antibodies	7. Methotrexate
3. Azathioprine	8. Sirolimus
4. Cyclophosphamide	9. Tacrolimus
5. Cyclosporine A	

5.2.1 Glucocorticoids

The immunosuppressive effect of glucocorticoids is based on the reduced formation of interleukins 2 and 6 with inhibition of T lymphocyte proliferation and on a decrease in IL-2 release. The glucocorticoids are therefore effective at a very early phase of the immune response. • At the same time, phospholipase A_2, and thus prostaglandin synthesis, is inhibited, and leucocyte migration is reduced (= anti-inflammatory effect). The clinical use of glucocorticoids is indicated in (*1.*) autoimmune hepatitis, (*2.*) immunocholangitis, (*3.*) PBC with a progressive course, (*4.*) florid alcohol-induced hepatitis or progressive alcoholic liver disease with evidence of antihistone B2, and (*5.*) drug-induced idiosyncrasy of the immunological type. In the diseases mentioned under points (*4.*) and (*5.*), the use of glucocorticoids should be reviewed critically.

5.2.2 Azathioprine

The effect of azathioprine is based on inhibition of T lymphocyte proliferation and differentiation of activated B and T cells. This results in a change in interleukin expression. Azathioprine suppressed CD 28-dependent Rac-1 activation, resulting in suppression of bcl-x expression and a consecutive induction of T cell apoptosis. These results have important implications for the development of novel substances showing higher affinity to Rac-1 with more specific therapy in autoimmune diseases and organ transplantation. Azathioprine is converted in the hepatocytes to 6-mercaptopurine, the actual active agent. Half-life is five hours. It can take several weeks until a steady state is reached in the blood, which explains the delayed effect of azathioprine (3−6 months). It is assumed that (due to genetic determination?) the imidazole residue of azathioprine is capable of binding sulphhydryl groups, resulting in an additional antimetabolic effect. (62) Pharmacological differences are further suggested by a report stating that treatment failure with azathioprine in autoimmune hepatitis was successfully overcome by subsequent treatment with 6-mercaptopurine. (68) A short time after the introduction of azathioprine, results of comparative studies with azathioprine and 6-mercaptopurine in CAH (probably autoimmune hepatitis) were reported. (66) • Azathioprine is used clinically in autoimmune hepatitis, immunocholangitis and progressive PBC. Combined use with prednisolone yields even better results. (68) These two substances administered at a low maintenance dosage can ensure remission for many years. Maintenance of remission achieved with azathioprine following discontinuation of prednisolone has likewise been reported. Hepatological side effects include bone-marrow depression, allergic reactions, greater susceptibility to infection, cholestasis, destructive cholangitis, VOD and nodular regenerative hyperplasia. (s. pp 664, 683)

5.2.3 Cyclosporine A

This active substance suppresses the release of interleukin 1 from monocytes and the synthesis of interleukins 2, 3 and 4 as well as of TNF-α from T helper cells; T cell proliferation, macrophage stimulation and B cell activation are inhibited. Even at an early stage of the immune reaction, this leads to the suppression of both humoral and cellular immune responses. The body's bacterial defence is still not significantly influenced, as the phagocytic activity of the RES is barely inhibited by cyclosporine. Bioavailability is about 35% following oral application; it is almost completely metabolized in the body and eliminated predominantly via the bile. Clinically, its main indication is the prevention of transplant rejection. (63, 67, 69) Occasionally, it has also been used in liver diseases, particularly in autoimmune hepatitis and PBC. (70) As in the case of azathioprine, cholestasis also constitutes a major hepatological side effect when using cyclosporine. Canalicular damage demonstrated in animal experiments could be prevented by S-adenosyl-L-methionine. Cyclosporine may cause elevated as well as reduced blood values in combination with many other medicaments. (72) (s. pp 665, 684)

5.2.4 Tacrolimus

Tacrolimus was introduced for clinical use in 1989 as a new, well-tolerated immunosuppressive substance that can be administered orally or intravenously. Its immunosuppressive effect is based on the inhibition of the lymphokinin synthesis of interleukins 2 and 3, interferon-γ and TNF-α as well as a reduction in interleukin-2 receptor expression. Tacrolimus leads to inhibition of T cell activation, the formation of cytotoxic T lymphocytes, the induction of specific T helper cells and T helper cell-dependent B cell proliferation. Its bioavailability is about 20%. A number of studies have meanwhile been published reporting the superiority of tacrolimus over cyclosporine. (64, 67) Experimentally, tacrolimus has been found to effect a decrease in free radicals, cytokines, tumour necrosis factor and neutrophilic infiltration in liver tissue. A possible increase in blood values (hitherto) occurring with about 20 drugs and a fall in blood values with numerous other drugs must be considered. Tacrolimus may cause manifestation of diabetes, or even trigger it. Initially only intended as an immunosuppressant against graft rejection (65), tacrolimus has meanwhile also been used successfully in PSC and autoimmune hepatitis. (71) (s. p. 684)

5.2.5 Cyclophosphamide

Cyclophosphamide is a prodrug which is converted into active metabolites in the liver. Urotoxic side effects must be anticipated; they can be suppressed by the additional administration of sodium-2 mercaptoethanesulphonate.
• This alkylating substance has a strong immunosuppressive effect; therefore, it is occasionally used to prevent graft rejection or (at a low dosage) in autoimmune hepatitis. (s. p. 684)

5.2.6 Methotrexate

This folic acid antagonist belongs to the group of antimetabolites which suppress endogenous substances (metabolites) and trigger the formation of functionally incompetent macromolecules. Because of their largely non-specific effect, all rapidly dividing cells are adversely affected and toxically damaged. At a low dosage, methotrexate has been used in autoimmune diseases. (s. pp 665, 684, 692)

5.3 Immunostimulants

Immunostimulants are defined as substances which stimulate immunological responses and improve a weakened immune system. They include interferon, thymus factor, interleukins, extracts of microorganisms, chemically defined substances (e.g. levamisole, selenium, zinc) and plant-derived substances (extracts from Phyllanthus, Bupleurum, Glycyrrhiza, Schizandra, etc.). (s. pp 726, 898)

5.3.1 Selenium

Discovered by J.J. BERZELIUS as early as 1817, selenium was only recognized as being an essential trace element for humans in 1957. So far, glutathione peroxidase (G.C. MILLS, 1957) and 5-deiodase (D. BEHNE et al., 1990) have been defined as selenium-containing enzymes. The daily requirement ranges from 20 to 100 µg, which is met mainly by animal protein; in the case of a lactovegetarian diet and a simultaneously increased need (e.g. due to liver cirrhosis or malabsorption), cellular selenium deficiency may occur. (77) Of the thirteen selenium proteins known so far, only two glutathione peroxidases have been closely defined: one membrane-bound and one cytosol-bound enzyme. They are components of an antioxidative system in that they catalyze the reduction in hydrogen peroxide, organic hydroperoxides and fatty acid hydroperoxides. Further biochemical effects include stimulation of the immune system (increased activity of the natural killer cells, stimulation of IFN-γ synthesis, enhanced capability to phagocytize) (76), hepatoprotection, detoxication of heavy metals, regulation of lipid peroxidation (scavenger of free radicals), inhibition of carcinogenesis and tumour growth, etc. (76, 77, 79) (s. pp 55, 812) • *Sodium selenite* seems to be most appropriate for infections. (s. p. 310)

5.3.2 Zinc

Zinc is an essential trace element, 98% of which is deposited in the intracellular space. The various organs differ significantly in their zinc concentration. The total body content amounts to 1.5−4.0 g. The daily zinc requirement ranges between 10 and 15 mg. A high content of certain amino acids (alanine, cysteine, glycine, histidine) greatly facilitates the intestinal absorption of zinc, whereas phytate-containing pulses and cereals as well as chronic alcohol abuse impair its absorption to a considerable extent. Zinc is readily excreted and hardly accumulates in the body. All in all, there are many factors leading to relative or absolute zinc deficiency. (s. p. 55) (s. tab. 3.15) • Zinc is an essential component of about 200 enzymes. It plays a major role in the metabolism of carbohydrates, proteins, lipids, vitamin A and alcohol as well as influencing DNA and RNA synthesis and stimulating the immune system. It activates ornithine carbamoyltransferase, alkaline phosphatase, δ-ALA synthetase and carboanhydrase, and especially superoxide dismutase. Zinc metabolism primarily occurs in the liver. It is largely governed by hormones (e.g. glucagon, insulin, glucocorticoids, ACTH, STH, sex hormones) and regulated by interleukins 1 and 4 as well as TNF. Its close relationship with the immune system thus becomes evident. Among other things, zinc influences thymulin, DNA and RNA polymerase (= gene expression in cell differentiation and proliferation) and the mediator functions in the immune response. (79) Understandably, zinc deficiency in liver cirrhosis or alcoholic liver diseases may well contribute to the patient's susceptibility to infections or febrile conditions (e. g. spontaneous bacterial peritonitis) and possibly even the induction of carcinogenesis. • The multiple biochemical roles of over 200 zinc-containing enzymes explain the wide spectrum of manifestations associated with zinc deficiency in hepatology. This is of great importance for the pathogenesis of hepatic encephalopathy and the therapeutic use of zinc. (73, 74, 80, 82) (s. pp 105, 277, 286, 812)

5.3.3 Thymosin

Of the group of thymosins, a mixture of various thymus hormones (or factors), fraction 5 has been well defined. It is already used, for example, for the synthetic manufacture of **thymosin-α**. Further thymus factors include *thymulin* and *thymostimulin* (G. M. MUTCHNICK et al., 1991). • Thymus factors effect the maturation of thymus T cells, which migrate to the lymphatic system as immune cells. The clinical use of thymosin-α is indicated in impaired immune defence with a decreased count or reduced function of T lymphocytes. (78) Clear effects on HBV DNA and on the transaminases were demonstrated in chronic hepatitis B. (75) • In combination with IFN, good results were also obtained in chronic hepatitis C. (83) In a recent study, the use of thymosin as monotherapy in chronic hepatitis C did not prove to have any beneficial effect. Generally, good tolerance was recorded for this drug. (81) (s. p. 726)

5.4 Ursodeoxycholic acid

The secondary bile acid *7-keto-lithocholic acid* is transported from the intestinal tract via the portal vein to the liver, where it is converted to **ursodeoxycholic acid** (UDCA) by bacterial enzyme action. (s. pp 40, 684) (s. fig. 3.3!) • The *molecular formula* of UDCA is identical to that of CDCA (= $C_{24}H_{40}O_4$); however, it has the hydroxyl group at the C_7 atom in the β-position and not in the α-position like chenodeoxycholic acid. The tertiary bile acid UDCA thus constitutes the 7β-epimer of the secondary bile acid CDCA. This changes the steric arrangement: the molecule possesses a *higher polarity* and is thus less able to form micelles. UDCA is hydrophilic and only slightly lipophilic, and therefore practically non-toxic to the organism. With its *molecular weight* of 392.6, it constitutes 0.5−1.0 (−5.0)% of human bile. Following oral administration, UDCA is passively absorbed in the jejunum and in the proximal portion of the ileum and, through active transport, in the distal ileum; in addition, approx. 20% of the UDCA can be absorbed in the colon. In portal blood, UDCA is transported bound to protein and conjugated in the liver with taurine (to a small extent also with glycine). These conjugates reach the bile. The *half-life* is 3.5−5.8 days. Like its breakdown product isoursodeoxycholic acid, UDCA is excreted predominantly in faeces and to a lesser degree in urine. (90, 92, 93, 100, 111, 117)

Functioning as detergents, **hydrophobic (lipophilic) bile acids** (cholic acid, chenodeoxycholic acid, deoxycholic acid, lithocholic acid) exert toxic effects on the biomembranes of liver cells and mitochondria. At the same time, these bile acids display an immunosuppressive effect and influence the humoral and cell-mediated defence (e. g. inhibition of monocytes). As in the case of PBC, hydrophobic bile acids also induce an excessive expression of MHC-I and MHC-II molecules from hepatocytes and biliary cells.

Modes of action: The mechanisms of UDCA and its effects in cholestatic liver diseases are not yet fully understood − even though a number of different effects have been demonstrated. (87, 101) These include (*1.*) hepatoprotective (99, 109, 110), (*2.*) cytoprotective (96, 114), and (*3.*) biliary-metabolic effects (88, 102, 120, 121), as well as (*4.*) an influence on the immune system. (119) In ligature of the bile duct in rats, UDCA was found to reduce the occurrence of histological changes and biliary cirrhosis as well as of portal hypertension. (s. tab. 40.8)

1. Inhibition of the enteral absorption of hydrophobic bile acids
2. Induction of bicarbonate hypercholeresis
   – increase in bile flow (hypercholeresis)
   – increase in the cholehepatic circulation of UDC (= cholehepatic shunt) (s. p. 40)
3. Incorporation into the lipid membranes of liver cells and mitochondria, preventing loss of phospholipids and cholesterol
   – stabilization of membranes
   – improvement of bile acid transport
   – amelioration of immunological membrane functions
4. Influence on calcium-mediated intracellular signal transfer
5. Interaction with the glucocorticoid receptor
6. Influence on protein kinase C
7. Reduction in MHC-I and MHC-II molecule overproduction (= decrease in T lymphocyte toxicity)
8. Inhibition of interleukins 1, 2, 4 and 6, TNF-α and immunoglobulin formation
9. Synergistic effect with IFN-α

Tab. 40.8: Biochemical and pharmacological modes of action of ursodeoxycholic acid

Cholestatic liver diseases
1. Alcoholic liver disease with cholestasis
2. Chemically induced cholestasis
3. Cholestasis with complete enteral feeding (84)
4. Drug-induced cholestasis
5. Secondary sclerosing cholangitis

Genetically determined cholestasis
1. Alagille's syndrome
2. Byler's syndrome
3. Cholestasis of pregnancy (95)
4. Disturbances of the steroid ring
   – 7α-hydroxylase deficiency
   – 4δ-3-oxosteroid-5β-reductase deficiency
   – 3β-hydroxysteroid-5δ-dehydrogenase
5. Mucoviscidosis (91)
6. Recurrent benign cholestasis

Organ transplantation
1. After liver transplantation (85, 89)
2. Refractory graft vs. host reaction (116)

Prevention of carcinoma
1. Colorectal carcinoma (107, 118)
2. Cholangiocarcinoma (112)

Tab. 40.9: Demonstrated, empirically confirmed or pharmacologically justified indications for the therapeutic use of ursodeoxycholic acid (with some references)

Contraindications: The following contraindications should be observed: acute cholecystitis, acute cholangitis, obstruction of the cystic duct and common bile duct as well as frequent biliary colic.

Indications: The indications for the clinical use of UDCA are either already well-documented, empirically proven or pharmacologically justified. (98, 103, 105, 108, 113–115, 117) • Practically *no side effects* are to be expected. From the therapeutic viewpoint, it is possible to achieve an improvement in the clinical symptoms (fatigue, pruritus, gastrointestinal symptoms, steatorrhoea), especially in cholestasis with decreased values of AP, LAP, γ-GT and bilirubin. (104–106) • There is a similar improvement in further laboratory parameters (transaminases, GDH, IgM, cholesterol, etc.) together with an amelioration of histological alterations. (86) Special attention should be paid when administering UDCA in cirrhosis with ascites. (s. pp 664, 684, 692) (s. tabs. 13.10; 40.9)

Viral hepatitis
Acute viral hepatitis (94)
Chronic hepatitis (86, 106, 115)

Autoimmune diseases
1. Autoimmune cholangitis
2. Autoimmune hepatitis
3. Overlap syndrome (s. p. 709)
4. Primary biliary cholangitis (89, 103, 113) (s. p. 705)
5. Primary sclerosing cholangitis (97, 118) (s. p. 707)

5.5 Lactulose

Chemistry: Lactulose does not occur in nature, nor is it present in breast milk or fresh cow's milk. Small amounts of lactulose are, however, found in heated dairy products, especially in condensed milk (an average of 660 mg, up to a maximum of 940 mg, per 100 ml). • The initial substance for the synthetic manufacture of lactulose is **lactose**. This disaccharide consists of D-glucose and D-galactose. • **Lactulose** was originally manufactured as a keto-analogue of lactose (E. Montgomery et al., 1929). As a disaccharide, it is composed of D-galactose and D-fructose. The **molecular formula** is $C_{12}H_{22}H_{11}$, with a **molecular weight** of 342.3. Lactulose has a high **degree of sweetness** (0.48–0.62, compared with 1.0 for sucrose). The **pH value** ranges between 3.4 and 4.0. (122)

Pharmacokinetics: Lactulose can be neither absorbed nor broken down by enzymatic or bacterial action in the small intestine; after one to two hours, it reaches the colon unchanged. There is no influence on the lactase activity in the intestinal mucosa. Following oral intake of lactulose, 0.5–1.0% is taken up by the intestinal mucosa through **passive diffusion** and completely excreted unaltered in the urine. However, its absorption is increased by intestinal disease or damage to the intestinal mucosa due to cytotoxic chemotherapy. With simultaneous oral ingestion of hyperosmotic solutions, elevated lactulose levels are likewise detectable in the urine. The amount of lactulose thus excreted provides clues to the degree of damage caused to the intestinal mucosa. After oral administration of 20–25 ml lactulose, there is only a slight rise in the **blood sugar level** of 1–12 mg%; therefore, no clinically relevant aggravation of diabetes need be feared with lactulose therapy, nor are any systemic effects evident. • Lactulose is not demonstrable in the stool; this suggests that a complete **breakdown** takes place in the colon owing to saccharolytic bacteria. The following bacteria have proved effective for lactulose catabolism: Lactobazillus species, Bifidobacterium, Clostridium perfringens and the Bacteroides species. Up to 80 ml lactulose can be broken down per day by bacterial enzyme action under physiological conditions. Long-term treatment with lactulose stimulates the formation of bacterial β-galactosidase, whereby higher bacterial metabolization rates of lactulose are achieved. (122) The main metabolites include **lactic acid**, resulting from anaerobic fermentation, and **pyruvic acid**, resulting from aerobic metabolism. This leads to a **fall in the pH value** in the colon (dose-dependent) to 5–6. The pH value is not in the desired therapeutic acid range until an **increase in osmotic pressure** with an evacuation frequency of two to three times/day has been achieved at the respective lactulose dosage. • Degradation of lactulose in the colon with enhanced formation of organic acids results in an **inhibition of growth** of gram-negative proteolytic microorganisms responsible for the formation of endotoxins. There is also promoted growth of saccharolytic bacteria, creating bifidus flora typical of breast-fed babies. (126)

"Wrong idea, good results (the lactulose story)" (U. P. HAEMMERLI et al., 1969); "Lactulose works, but why?" (K. A. HUBEL, 1973); "In several aspects lactulose is an unusual drug"; "Lactulose is a fascinating hybrid of a nutrient and a drug" (J. BIRCHER et al., 1988); "Lactulose is a many splendored thing ... with many other beneficial actions in its bag of tricks" (H. O. CONN, 1992). (s. fig. 40.1)

Pharmacology: Unchanged lactulose is pharmacologically inert. Its multiple effects are only evident after breakdown by bacterial enzymes in the colon. (122) • The ability to **break down** lactulose varies greatly from one bacterial species to another, and even from strain to strain, depending on their enzyme endowment. Therefore, the quantity and the predominant type of organic acids formed on breakdown depend on the lactulose dose and the enzyme endowment of the saccharolytic bacteria. The total acid content of the colon is also influenced by individual factors, such as the absorption rate into the colon mucosa or the buffering caused by secreted bicarbonates, and possibly also by retroactive effects of the lactulose metabolites on the intestinal bacteria with potential changes in their metabolism. • The organic acids and the bacterial formation of gas as well as the increase in osmotic pressure account for the **laxative effect** (F. MAYERHOFER et al., 1959). This action occurs within 8 hours of lactulose administration. With a rise in the bacterial count of more than 50%, there is also (1–2 days after lactulose application) a rise in the stool mass and thus an additional acceleration of defaecation. • The **formation of ammonia** in the intestine is due to

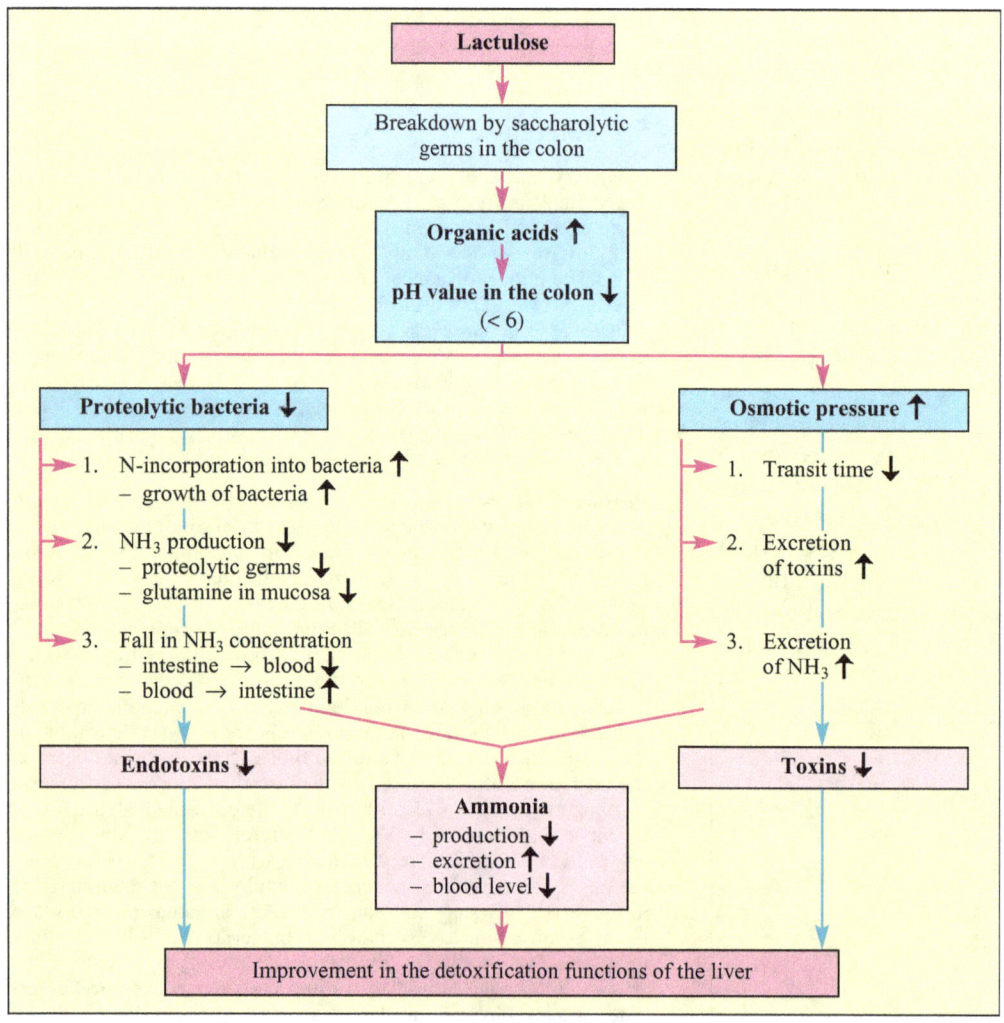

Fig. 40.1: Reduction in the blood ammonia levels with a corresponding improvement in the detoxification functions of the liver as a result of multifactorial influence exerted by lactulose on ammonia metabolism

the breakdown of proteins or amino acids, nucleic acids and biogenic amines. The intestinal formation of ammonia is inhibited by intraluminal acidosis and promoted by alkalosis. Independently of the intestinal flora, ammonia is also formed in the intestinal mucosa through glutamine uptake and the release of ammonia, alanine and glutaminic acid. This metabolic NH_3 production with hyperammonaemia was also demonstrable in microbe-free and hepatectomized experimental animals. With an intestinal pH value of <6, non-ionized ammonia (NH_3) diffuses from the blood to the intestine, while the diffusion of non-ionized ammonia from the intestine into the bloodstream is simultaneously decreased. This results in an elevated excretion of ammonium cations (NH_4^+) in faeces and a **reduction in hyperammonaemia**. The rapid onset of effect on hyperammonaemia following lactulose enemas can also be explained by the influence on non-ionic diffusion. A further mechanism underlying the lactulose-induced decrease in hyperammonaemia may be based on the fact that lactulose constitutes a valuable carbon and energy source for intestinal bacteria. Bacterial growth is thereby promoted and a substantial quantity of nitrogen is included in the protein synthesis of bacteria, which leads to a measurable consumption of ammonia. A fall in the colonic ammonia level may also be the result of a marked reduction in proteolytic intestinal bacteria by lactulose. (123, 125, 129)

The therapeutic efficacy of lactulose in the treatment of **hepatic encephalopathy** was demonstrated by J. BIRCHER et al. in 1966. Numerous publications dealing with this indication have appeared. (s. p. 287) Such favourable experience has been further supported by recent studies. (123, 124, 127, 128) • The efficacy of lactulose in **endotoxinaemia** shown by D. SCEVOLA et al. (1979) was later confirmed in various publications, and recently demonstrated anew. Different explanations for this anti-endotoxin effect of lactulose have been put forward: (*1.*) increased removal of endotoxins due to higher evacuation frequency, (*2.*) blocking of endotoxin receptors by lactulose, and (*3.*) influence on the number and metabolic performance of gram-negative intestinal bacteria. (s. fig. 40.1)

▶ A therapeutic drop in the pH value to <6 is generally achieved when *evacuation occurs two or three times per day*. In order to guarantee this condition, respective quantities of lactulose should be administered in two to three daily doses. • In principle, evacuation frequency should be *"no less than two and no more than four times per day"*. With this regimen, no major side effects need to be feared.

A **reduction in the cholesterol level** due to lactulose was observed by N. EBNER in 1973 and confirmed by D. CONTE et al. in 1977. Lactulose can also be used in hepatogenic disturbances of lipid metabolism. • **Translocation** of gram-negative bacteria to the mesenterial lymph nodes was significantly suppressed in experimental obstructive jaundice under lactulose treatment compared to the reference group without lactulose. Furthermore, galactosaemia-induced liver damage and bacterial conveyance could be prevented by lactulose therapy. (129)

Indications: The multiple modes of action of lactulose, which are based on an interplay of several effects, require a sufficiently acidic pH value in the colon.

Lactulose is administered as long-term therapy. The indications are derived from its modes of action. (s. tab. 40.10)

1. Reducing or normalizing hyperammonaemia in hepatic encephalopathy
2. Eliminating endotoxinaemia
3. Prophylactic use in cirrhosis (and other chronic liver diseases)
4. Decreasing susceptibility to infections in cirrhosis by inhibiting the translocation of intestinal bacteria
5. Reducing the cholesterol level and influencing lipid metabolic disturbances in primary biliary cholangitis (and other liver diseases accompanied by hyperlipidaemia)
6. Improving the absorption of calcium in malabsorption

Tab. 40.10: Indications for the therapeutic use of lactulose

5.6 Branched-chain amino acids

The cirrhosis patient is in a **vicious circle** regarding protein metabolism: *cirrhosis → hepatic encephalopathy → protein restriction → malnutrition → catabolism →*. Thus, prolonged protein restriction and catabolism may considerably worsen the prognosis of cirrhosis. • *In this hazardous situation, the dietary and therapeutic use of branched-chain amino acids (BCAA), i. e. valine, leucine and isoleucine, is a logical therapeutic intervention.*

The **urea cycle** is the most important process in biological ammonia detoxification. (s. pp 61, 274) (s. figs. 3.12, 3.13) • It is directly linked with **amino-acid metabolism** and thus also with NH_2 donors and precursors through specific amino acids and transamination processes. Here, the major transamination processes are those involving glutamate and oxalacetate as well as α-ketoglutarate and aspartate.

The **ammonia hypothesis** postulates that a high ammonia concentration in the tissue inevitably leads to a clear increase in glutamine. This results in a marked intracellular **decrease in glutamate** (and α-ketoglutarate). This glutamate pool can be refilled by a more intensive **degradation of BCAA** as NH_2 donors. At the same time, transamination effects the **formation of branched-chain**

keto-analogues of the respective amino acids. • Succinyl CoA is also facultatively involved, providing **α-ketoglutarate** via the citric acid cycle; this is the starting substrate of glutamate prior to transamination. These reactions occur mainly in the muscles. (135, 142) (s. fig. 40.2)

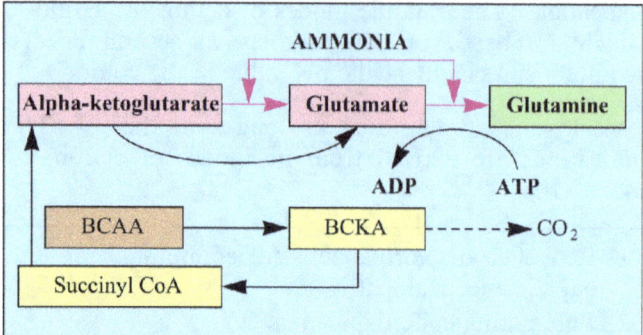

Fig. 40.2: Indirect influence of ammonia on the metabolism of branched-chain amino acids (so-called *ammonia hypothesis*) (BCAA = branched-chain amino acids, BCKA = branched-chain keto acids)

Branched-chain amino acids apparently stimulate the urea cycle. Carbamoylphosphate synthetase, which channels ammonia into the urea cycle, is induced by ornithine and N-acetylglutamate as a cofactor of urea synthesis. Here, BCAA follow **two modes of action:** (*1.*) they stimulate the synthesis of N-acetylglutamate via synthetase formed from glutamate and acetyl CoA, and (*2.*) they inhibit ornithine-keto acid transferase, which is the enzyme responsible for ornithine degradation, leading to an increase in ornithine concentration. • **Ammonia detoxication is thus stimulated by two regulatory mechanisms.** (s. fig. 40.2)

As a rule, cirrhosis patients show reduced plasma BCAA levels and unchanged BCAA concentrations in the brain, whereas methionine and aromatic amino acids (AAA) (phenylalanine, tyrosine, tryptophan) are elevated in the plasma and brain. (s. p. 288) • The **fall in BCAA levels** is attributable to its increased degradation, which, in turn, is caused or aggravated by hyperinsulinaemia. Methionine and AAA compete with BCAA for the same transport system at the **blood-brain barrier.** Lowered BCAA levels in the blood therefore favour the passage of elevated methionine and AAA concentrations. The influx of these amino acids is increased by concomitant hyperammonaemia. Ammonia crosses the blood-brain barrier freely. In the astrocytes of the brain, BCAA effect an increase in glutamate by transamination with α-ketoglutarate. Glutamine formation rises, permitting the removal of ammonia from the brain. Glial swelling could be reduced in animal experiments. • **Anabolic protein metabolism** in the muscles is responsible for (*1.*) reduction in muscle protein breakdown products which contribute to the formation of ammonia, and (*2.*) higher amounts of ammonia being taken up by the musculature and converted via glutamate to glutamine, which is harmless. • Hyperammonaemia in liver cirrhosis cannot be influenced by **keto-analogue amino acids,** which are N-free precursors of protein synthesis. However, the keto-analogue of leucine can inhibit the breakdown of muscle protein, which means that favourable effects might still be achieved by using BCKA in decompensated cirrhosis – without any discernible impact on the ammonia level itself. (130, 131, 134, 135, 147)

The use of branched-chain amino acids is based on different **modes of action**. (s. tab. 40.11)

1. Compensation of the amino-acid imbalance
2. Restoration of the competitive transport mechanisms at the blood-brain barrier
3. Stimulation of glutamine synthesis in the brain, muscle and liver (= transitory ammonia detoxication)
4. Inhibition of ornithine breakdown in the liver with a favourable effect on urea synthesis (= definitive ammonia detoxication)
5. Anabolic and anticatabolic effects, especially in muscles
6. Stimulation of the HGF, favouring liver regeneration

Tab. 40.11: Modes of action of branched-chain amino acids

The **indication** for administering BCAA in patients with hepatic encephalopathy to compensate amino-acid imbalance was proposed by J. E. Fischer et al. in 1974, and implemented parenterally. However, oral application of BCAA for an adequate treatment period also has *beneficial effects* on cirrhosis and HE: (*1.*) improvement in protein tolerance and the nutritional condition (140), (*2.*) improvement in cerebral functions (132, 136, 138), probably due to an amelioration of liver function, (*3.*) stimulation of ammonia detoxification with a positive nitrogen balance (132, 136), (*4.*) reduction in or normalization of AAA levels, and (*5.*) promotion of glutamine synthesis with a favourable effect on the cells of the immune system and on renal function. • Using BCAA, it was possible to prolong survival time and delay liver failure in rats with CCl_4-induced cirrhosis. (139, 144) • However, there are diverging results, which need further clarification. Nocturnal administration of BCAA is primarily used for protein synthesis (and therefore advisable), whereas intake during the day is preferentially used for physical exercise. In principle, the use of BCAA is seen as a necessary form of supplementary treatment for catabolic metabolism in cirrhosis (142, 143, 145, 146, 148–151), in (also latent) HE and after curative resection of hepatocellular carcinoma. (137, 141) (s. p. 288)

5.7 Amino acids of the urea cycle

As early as 1932, H. A. Krebs and K. Henseleit discovered in their investigation of the amino acids that *ornithine*, even in small amounts, was capable of increasing urea synthesis from (toxic) ammonia. Otherwise, only *argi-*

nine had a slight effect in this respect. (157) The following table shows which of the **amino acids involved in the urea cycle** are available for therapeutic purposes:

Arginine Ornithine aspartate (OA) = *available*	Arginine aspartate Arginine malate Aspartic acid Citrulline Ornithine Ornithine α-ketoglutarate = *not available at present*
Arginine + citrulline + ornithine = *available*	

▶ The ammonia-reducing effect of the amino acids involved in the urea cycle has been strikingly well demonstrated in a variety of **experimental studies** by several research groups. In most of these studies, ornithine aspartate was used, although arginine, ornithine and ornithine α-ketoglutarate have also been investigated. (153, 156, 160, quot. 158) • The greatest effect on ammonia reduction was achieved with **ornithine aspartate,** the combination of these two amino acids being more effective than the administration of either substance alone. The above results were confirmed in experimental studies by K. ZICHA et al. (1968) and G. HERMANN (1972). In healthy dogs, the increased ammonia levels due to ammonia overload were lowered to normal by ornithine aspartate; in dogs with Eck's fistula, the occurrence of toxic ammonia levels could be prevented (C.E. GROSSI et al., 1967). • Further experimental studies revealed that the liver content of ornithine, citrulline, arginine, glutamate and urea rose following exposure to ammonium chloride in rats. The urea synthesis rate exceeded the norm by 50%, while glutamate concentration doubled as a result of α-ketoglutaric acid, which increased to the highest possible limit. With simultaneous administration of *arginine* or *ornithine*, hepatic ornithine concentration increased considerably, and urea synthesis rose by 80–85%. • In healthy volunteers, administration of *ornithine α-ketoglutarate* led to elevated renal excretion of urea and ornithine α-ketoglutarate, i.e. a clear stimulation of urea synthesis was attained.

Since the **clinical studies** of L. ZIEVE et al. in 1960, the use of these amino acids or their salts has been indicated in hyperammonaemia. (165) Thus, following protein overload in alcoholic cirrhosis patients, a reduction in ammonia levels was achieved by administering 60 g ornithine α-ketoglutarate. (154, 159) • *Since the first clinical use of* **ornithine aspartate** *more than 30 years ago (1968), a series of studies has been published.* (155, 161–164) This ammonia-reducing substance is the stable salt of L-ornithine and L-aspartic acid with the *empirical formula* $C_9H_{19}N_3O_6$ and a *molecular weight* of 265.3. *Bioavailability* is $82.2 \pm 28.0\%$. The substance is rapidly absorbed, with subsequent splitting into its two component amino acids. Its *half-life* is 40 minutes.

The **biomolecular modes of action** of ornithine have been the subject of several experimental investigations.

Ornithine activates the enzymes carbamylphosphate synthetase and ornithine carbamyltransferase, which are necessary for the liver-specific process of **urea synthesis** (153, 158); this occurs mostly in the *periportal hepatocytes* (= definitive ammonia detoxification). Glutamine synthesis (binding of ammonia to glutamate) takes place mainly in the *perivenous hepatocytes* (= transitory ammonia detoxification). Large amounts of glutamate are needed for this. Aspartate, ornithine (via α-ketoglutarate), glutamate and other dicarboxylates are taken up almost exclusively by the perivenous hepatocytes responsible for glutamine synthesis. In addition, aspartate and dicarboxylates are seen as activators of glutamine synthesis, a process which is disturbed in cirrhosis patients. (s. pp 62, 274) (s. figs. 3.12, 3.13)

Aspartic acid is not only involved in the urea cycle, but following oxidative deamination to α-ketoglutarate, it is also a component of the citric acid cycle. More energy is thus made available in the form of ATP for the energy-consuming urea cycle. More the energy cycle is additionally stimulated by transamination of aspartic acid to oxalacetate. The increased channelling of aspartic acid into the urea cycle facilitates the release of fumaric acid, which is also a substrate of the citric acid cycle, and thus further enhances the formation of ATP. Moreover, aspartic acid binds the ammonia which is present in the musculature; as a result, asparagine is formed, and free toxic ammonia is bound. • Aspartic acid is a glucoplastic amino acid and an important initial substrate for pyrimidine synthesis in liver cell regeneration. Following condensation with carbamylphosphate and the formation of the intermediate product L-dihydroorotic acid, orotic acid, the central product in the biosynthesis of pyrimidine nucleotides, is formed by oxidation. (s. tab. 40.12)

There are several biochemical and clinical **modes of action** associated with ornithine aspartate. (s. tab. 40.12)

---

1. Increase in urea synthesis by ornithine
   – substrate of the urea cycle
   – activator of carbamylphosphate synthetase
   – activator of ornithine carbamyltransferase
   – activator of glutamine synthesis
2. Increase in glutamine synthesis by aspartate
   – substrate of glutamine synthesis
   – activator of glutamine synthetase
3. Increase in the energy balance by aspartate
   – substrate of the citric acid cycle
   – formation of oxalacetate
   – channelling of fumaric acid into the citric acid cycle
4. Increase in NH_3 detoxification in the musculature
5. As a component of pyrimidine nucleotide synthesis leading to liver cell regeneration

Tab. 40.12: Modes of action of ornithine aspartate

The various modes of action provide the basis for the following **therapeutic indications** of ornithine aspartate:

1. Hepatic encephalopathy
   – with improvement in the mental condition and psychometric test results
2. Relief of NH_3 intoxication symptoms
   – e.g. fatigue, weakness

5.8 D-penicillamine

D-penicillamine is a **non-physiological amino acid.** It is a dimethyl derivative of cysteine, which is a structural component of many proteins. Metabolically, penicillamine is relatively stable. In addition to the amino group ($-NH_2$) and the carboxyl group ($-COOH$), it contains a sulphhydryl group ($-SH$) as a further reactive centre. The underlying biochemical **modes of action** are:

1. Chelate formation with heavy metals
2. Exchange reactions with disulphides
   – with low molecular weight substances
   – with proteins
3. Binding with aldehyde to form
   – pyridoxal phosphate
   – aldehyde groups in collagen and other proteins

Penicillamine may effect **chelate formation** with the heavy metals copper, lead, zinc, gold and mercury. This complex formation is accompanied by simultaneous reduction processes, e.g. copper is reduced to copper-1-ion. From the biochemical viewpoint, an influence on **collagen synthesis** is also conceivable, as the amino-oxydase involved in the formation of collagen contains copper, so that this enzyme is inactivated through the binding of copper to penicillamine. To my knowledge, this process has not yet been confirmed in vivo. • The **mesenchyma suppression effect** of penicillamine with a decrease in the formation of connective tissue is based on the inhibition of the cross-linkage between fibre protein precursors and hydroxyproline synthesis. However, it appears that the process of hepatic fibrosis is not influenced. • Of relevance is the reaction with macro-globulins, which is accompanied by the breaking of the disulphide (S-S) bridges through exchange reactions; this leads to depolymerization. An example of the binding of penicillamine to an aldehyde group is its binding to pyridoxal phosphate – a coenzyme which is formed in the body from vitamin B_6. Equally important is the reaction of penicillamine with the aldehyde groups of tropocollagen, which causes the formation of thiazolidine, thus preventing synthesis of insoluble collagen. (168) • Intestinal **absorption** is rapid and relatively high. The *half-life* is three to four hours. The greater part of the orally applied substance is eliminated within 24 hours. In particular, diseases with high hepatic copper concentrations are an indication for penicillamine. • *Side effects* occur frequently; the use of vitamin B_6 may be necessary.

The principal **indications** for penicillamine are:

1. Wilson's disease (s. p. 634)
2. Indian childhood cirrhosis (166) (s. p. 635)
3. Primary biliary cholangitis (167) (s. p. 683)
4. Heavy metal poisoning

5.9 Somatostatin

▶ Somatostatin was first isolated from the *hypothalamus* of sheep for use as a growth hormone-inhibiting factor in 1973 (P. BRAZEAU et al.). In the same year, its synthetic production was also reported (H. D. CROY et al., 1973). The *molecular weight* is 1,638. The *empirical formula* of this substance, which is composed of 14 amino acids, is $C_{76}H_{106}N_{18}O_{19}S_2$. To my knowledge, somatostatin was used *clinically* for the first time in 1974 in a patient with acromegaly (S. S. C. YEN et al.). • Since 1979, somatostatin has been recommended for **oesophageal variceal bleeding** (L. THULIN et al.). Its plasma half-life is one to two minutes; the substance is broken down by endopeptidases and aminopeptidases, with a renal excretion rate of about 80%. • The following **organ-specific effects** are worth mentioning: (*1.*) inhibition of endocrine and exocrine functions (in the area of the pancreas, stomach and small intestine – especially inhibition of insulin and glucagon release), and (*2.*) inhibition of the blood supply to the gastric mucosa and splanchnic vessels.

In **oesophageal variceal bleeding,** somatostatin is recommended immediately after emergency admission to hospital at the following dosage: an i.v. bolus injection of 250 (−500) µg and subsequently 250 µg per hour (possibly with two-minute bolus injections). In this way, sclerotherapy or ligation is technically facilitated and the effectiveness of the therapy improved; fewer blood products are needed. No major side effects have occurred at this dosage. (170, 171) The bolus injection rapidly effects a reduction in portal venous and intravaricose pressure as well as a decrease in the blood flow in the azygous vein. (169) It is worth noting that intestinal blood is eliminated more slowly and virtually unchanged, since somatostatin inhibits the release of digestive enzymes and prolongs the intestinal transit time. Continued passage of tarry stool may at first be erroneously interpreted as an effect of somatostatin – unless systemic problems or a fall in Hb actually suggest further bleeding. (s. p. 366)

5.10 Terlipressin

▶ Terlipressin, chemical name N-α-triglycyl-8-lysine-vasopressin, consists of 12 amino acids. The *molecular weight* is 1,377.5, and the *empirical formula* is $C_{52}H_{74}N_{16}O_{15}S_2 \cdot C_2H_4O_2 \cdot 5H_2O$. Through hydrolytic removal of the glycyl residues, the vasoconstrictor hormone *lysine-vasopressin* is slowly released as an active substance. Peak concentrations are obtained after 120 minutes. The breakdown of lysine-vasopressin into inactive metabolites, effected by hepatic and renal endopeptidases and exopeptidases, is almost total, so that only about 1% is excreted in the urine. • The *plasma half-life* is 12 minutes, the elimination time is 40−180 minutes. The effect persists for four to five hours. The *vasoconstriction* is particularly intensive in the splanchnic system; as a result, arterial blood flow is reduced, and portal hypertension is lowered (by up to 35% with 1 mg terlipressin). (172, 174) The smooth muscles of the oesophageal sphincter are contracted with consecutive compression of the existing varices. At the same time, increased peristalsis occurs, leading to a more rapid evacuation of intestinal blood and of ammonia formed by intestinal bacteria. • The *renal blood flow* is elevated in hypovolaemia. The elevated WHVP and HVPG become reduced and hepatic arterial blood flow increases.

The following dosage is recommended for acute **oesophageal variceal bleeding:** 1–2 mg terlipressin as an i.v. bolus (if possible in the ambulance or upon emergency admission) followed by 1 mg as an i.v. bolus every four to six hours for a total period of two to three days. Terlipressin reduces the elevated blood levels of renin and aldosterone and increases the GFR. The combined use of vasoconstrictor therapy with local mechanical haemostasis gives the best results — and a higher chance of survival. The side effects are slight. (175, 176) (s. p. 366) • Application is recommended in the case of the *hepatorenal syndrome.* (173)

5.11 S-adenosyl-L-methionine

S-adenosyl-L-methionine (SAMe) is present in nearly all **body cells.** About 30% of hepatic SAMe is localized in the mitochondria. It is formed from methionine and ATP by SAMe synthetase (G. L. Cantoni, 1952). Transport from the cytosol to the mitochondria takes place via a specific phospholipid carrier system in the biomembranes. (178, 184) • Metabolically, S-adenosyl-L-methionine is an important initial substrate for numerous **synthesis pathways** (178):

1. **Transmethylation:** The transfer of methyl groups is of great relevance for phospholipid synthesis in the biomembranes and for the synthesis of hormones, nucleinic acids, proteins, porphyrins, etc.
2. **Transsulphuration:** The involvement of SAMe leads to the formation of glutathione, cysteine, etc. These substances play an important metabolic role in detoxification processes and in the elimination of reactive oxygen intermediates.
3. **Aminopropylation:** The transfer of decarboxylated SAMe is crucial to the synthesis of polyamines (spermine, spermidine, putrescine). Together with ornithine decarboxylase, SAMe determines the synthesis rate of polyamines, which are essential for cell regeneration. At 30–60 minutes, the half-life of SAMe decarboxylase is very short and thus readily adaptable to various metabolic situations.

In **experiments,** SAMe was found to prevent lipid peroxidation and to normalize the reduced glycogen content of hepatocytes in liver damage. In further studies, its cytoprotective effect was also confirmed. (177, 180, 182, 183, 185, 189–192) This protective effect likewise applied to preneoplastic cell damage. The results concerning the prevention of cholestasis were impressive. • In cirrhosis or severe liver disease, there is a reduction in SAMe synthetase, glutathione, cysteine and phospholipid methyltransferase (together with a simultaneous deficiency in phosphatidylcholine formation, accompanied by disturbed membrane fluidity and decreased activity of Na^+/K^+-ATPase and Ca^{2+}-ATPase).

The pharmacological effects and therapeutic uses of SAMe in hepatology are discussed in a detailed review. (181) The impressive outcome of various experiments led to numerous **clinical studies,** which, however, had some negative results. (179, 181, 186–188) On the whole, there was a significant decrease in bilirubin, bile acids, alkaline phosphatase and transaminases. Pruritus, a frequent symptom in cholestasis, also showed regression.

S-adenosyl-L-methionine is an interesting substance which deserves further clinical investigation. The recommended *dosage* is 800 mg/day with intravenous administration or 1,200 mg/day orally. No major *side effects* have been noted. The studies available so far suggest the following *indications*:

1. Alcoholic liver disease, especially in cholestasis (s. p. 552)
2. Drug-induced cholestasis (s. p. 569)
3. Chemically induced cholestasis (s. p. 589)
4. Recurrent intrahepatic cholestasis (s. p. 241)
5. Recurrent intrahepatic cholestasis of pregnancy (s. p. 241)
6. Gilbert-Meulengracht syndrome (s. p. 229)
7. Compensated liver cirrhosis (s. p. 765)

5.12 Haemarginate

The requirements for successfully treating clinically manifest acute porphyria are: (*1.*) elimination of the causative factor(s), (*2.*) use of supportive therapeutic measures (fluid and electrolyte balance, analgesics, anticonvulsants, antihypertensive agents, antiemetics, antiarrhythmics), (*3.*) i.v. glucose infusion (approx. 400 g/day), and (*4.*) haemarginate. (s. p. 625)

Haemarginate is produced from erythrocyte concentrate. It compensates the loss of the intracellular haem balance, which regulates haem synthesis. In this way, the overproduction of porphyrin precursors is reduced. Haemarginate is relatively stable; following i.v. administration, it is bound to haemopexin and albumin, and thus made available to the liver cells. (195) • *Dosage* is 3 mg/kg BW/day, administered per daily i.v. infusion (for about 15 minutes) exclusively in 0.9% NaCl solution (100 ml). Haemarginate is stabilized by arginine and contains 96 vol.% ethanol (1,000 mg/ampoule) as well as propyleneglycol (4,000 mg/ampoule). It is degraded into bilirubin and excreted via the bile. The application period depends on the degree of severity of acute porphyria; as a rule, it extends over three to five days. With successful use of haemarginate, the excessive elimination of PBG and ALA is restored to normal, as is the excretion of uroporphyrinogen and coproporphyrin. These values should be monitored in the urine under haemarginate therapy. (193, 194) • *Side effects* may appear in the form of phlebitis. This is, however, rare when haemarginate is administered intravenously into large veins. Minor, clinically insignificant effects on blood coagulation have only seldom been observed.

Important: Haemarginate treatment should be initiated as early as possible before any neuronal damage, which may be irreversible, occurs.

5.13 Phytotherapeutics

> Plant extracts have been used in the treatment of liver diseases for over 2,000 years. • So far, more than 170 plant-derived substances from some 55 plant families have been well documented regarding their **hepatoprotective efficacy.** (197) Recently, the Rosmarinus species (196) and Salvia miltiorrhiza (199) were added to this list as antifibrinogenetic agents. • In controlled **clinical studies,** many of these active substances proved effective in various liver diseases. Some of them are already listed in the pharmacopoeia. • *Two points* should be made here: (*1.*) in the plant kingdom, there are no doubt other substances with specific agents which would act on liver structures or against liver diseases, but have not yet been recognized as such; (*2.*) more sophisticated biochemical/biomolecular procedures now allow more exact characterization and a more precise description of known and previously unknown active substances, so that their targeted therapeutic use may be made possible. (198)

Phytotherapeutics are defined by law as substances derived from plants, plant parts or plant components in a processed or unprocessed form and used medicinally. As substances, phytogenic preparations are treated in the same way as synthetic chemical compounds or substances of other origin. Phytopharmaceuticals must likewise comply with the usual safety standards, such as quality, harmlessness and efficacy. (s. p. 567)

Phytotherapeutic agents are used as *primary preparations* (e. g. tinctures) or as a concentration of various *active substance fractions* and as *pure substances*. Monoextracts are complicated mixtures of chemical substances. They contain primary active agents, secondary active agents and inert accompanying substances. The **main active agents** wholly or predominantly determine the therapeutic properties of phytopharmaceuticals. **Secondary active agents** present in addition to the main active agent(s) may attenuate, potentiate or modify the effects of the main active agent. The overall therapeutic effect generally results from the synergy of several constituents. **Accompanying substances** include cellulose, lignin and starch as well as various forms of sugar, protein and fat. • The active constituents of plants essentially depend on climate, location and other exogenous factors. Therefore, isolating the main active agent is a prerequisite for clarifying its composition, synthesis and pharmacosynthetic modification. Should an active substance be unknown or not well-documented, a quantatively predominant substance (or several substances) amenable to analysis is then defined as the **key substance.** This is to ensure that a certain phytopharmaceutical preparation is offered at a standardized quality. According to the legal requirements, the key substances may also be defined as so-called *"other scientifically proven material"*.

▶ Pharmaceuticals of plant origin also form part of rational drug therapy in science-oriented medicine. They are used in the treatment of certain defined diseases and complaints. The more carefully the various pharmacological characteristics of phytogenic remedies are elucidated, the more reliably their clinical effects can be evaluated (e. g. digitalis, rauwolfia, hyoscyamine, senna). • *This is also true of the phytotherapeutic preparations used in hepatology.*

5.13.1 Essential phospholipids

> ▶ Essential phospholipids (EPL) are isolated from the **soya bean.** This plant was mentioned in the books of Pen Ts'ao Kong Mu (during the reign of Emperor Sheng Nung, 2838 BC). It was one of the five "holy cereals" considered essential for human life. • Today, about 800 soya bean species are known. Depending on the species, location and extraction method, the seeds contain 35–40% proteins, 20–30% carbohydrates, 5–10% accompanying substances (amines, vitamins, triterpene saponins, glycopeptides, lectin, flavonoids, xanthines, etc.) and 12–18% crude fats. The crude oil contains 90–95% fatty acid glycerides, predominantly unsaturated fatty acids (oleic acid, linoleic acid). Refining crude oil yields 30–45% phosphatides (soya lecithin). The phosphatides contain 15–20% phosphatidylcholine ("lecithin"), which represents an important constituent of cell membranes and is also involved in lipid metabolism in the liver (H. EIKERMANN, 1939). *(Detailed account: 200)*

Essential phospholipids are a highly purified phosphatidylcholine fraction from soybean containing essential (unsaturated) fatty acids, especially linoleic acid (about 70%), in the C_1 and C_2 positions. The main active ingredient in EPL is 1,2 dilinoleoylphosphatidylcholine (DLPC) (40–52% of the phosphatidylcholine molecules). Standardization is performed with reference to 3-sn-phosphatidylcholine (73–79% or 92–96%). In the literature, the designation PPC (polyenylphosphatidylcholine) is also used; this is intended to emphasize the special fatty acid composition. DLPC has a high bioavailability and an affinity for cell membranes. The phosphatidylcholines constitute a typical lipid bilayer and are thus the main structural component of cellular and subcellular membranes. • Moreover, the proportion of phosphatidylcholines with highly unsaturated (essential) fatty acids is a decisive factor in determining membrane fluidity/flexibility and thus also the biological membrane functions (see figure 40.3 regarding the multiple functions of essential phospholipids). Endogenous phospholipids are substituted by EPL, which may be administered by the oral route or, in a highly purified form, by the intravenous route. (222, 223, 241) (s. fig. 2.19)

EPL administration has protective, curative and/or regenerative effects on the biomembranes of hepatocytes and sinus endothelia following damage to the cell membrane through toxic, inflammatory, allergic, metabolic or immunological reactions. The cytoprotective effect of EPL has been demonstrated in 19 in-vitro and 121 in-vivo experiments including 33 different models and 8

Intoxications due to chemical substances			Intoxication due to drugs		
CCl_4	acute/subacute	17	1. Paracetamol	acute	1
	chronic	10	2. Tetracycline	subacute	2
CCl_4 + ethanol	chronic	1	3. Rifampicin	subacute	1
Ethanol	acute/subacute	20	4. Cholic acid	chronic	1
Ethanol + triton, INH/rifampicin	chronic	18	5. Indomethacin	acute	2
			6. Choline deficiency	subacute	1
Cyanate, Carbonyl-Fe	acute/chronic	4	7. Anaesthetics	subacute	3
Galactosamine	acute/subacute	10	8. INH	subacute	1
Allyl alcohol	acute	5	9. Platidium +/− CCl_4	acute	1
Allyl alcohol	acute	5	10. Reye syndrome	acute	1
Allyl alcohol	acute	5	11. Cyclosporine A (205)	subacute	1
Ethionine	subacute	1			
Organic solvents	chronic	2	Cholestasis intoxication		4
Carbon disulphide	chronic	1	Antigen-antibody reaction		1
Thioacetamide	chronic	1	Intoxication due to radiation		8
Sodium glutamate	chronic	1	Lipid peroxidation due to $FeSO_4$		2
Hexachlorcyclohexane	chronic	1	Endogenous oxidative stress		2
Ammonium fluoride	chronic	1	Ischemia/reperfusion (211)		1

Tab. 40.13: Cytoprotective effects of EPL in in-vivo investigations (121 experiments, 33 different models, 8 different animal species) (status 1988: E. Kuntz; status 2008: K.-J. Gundermann)

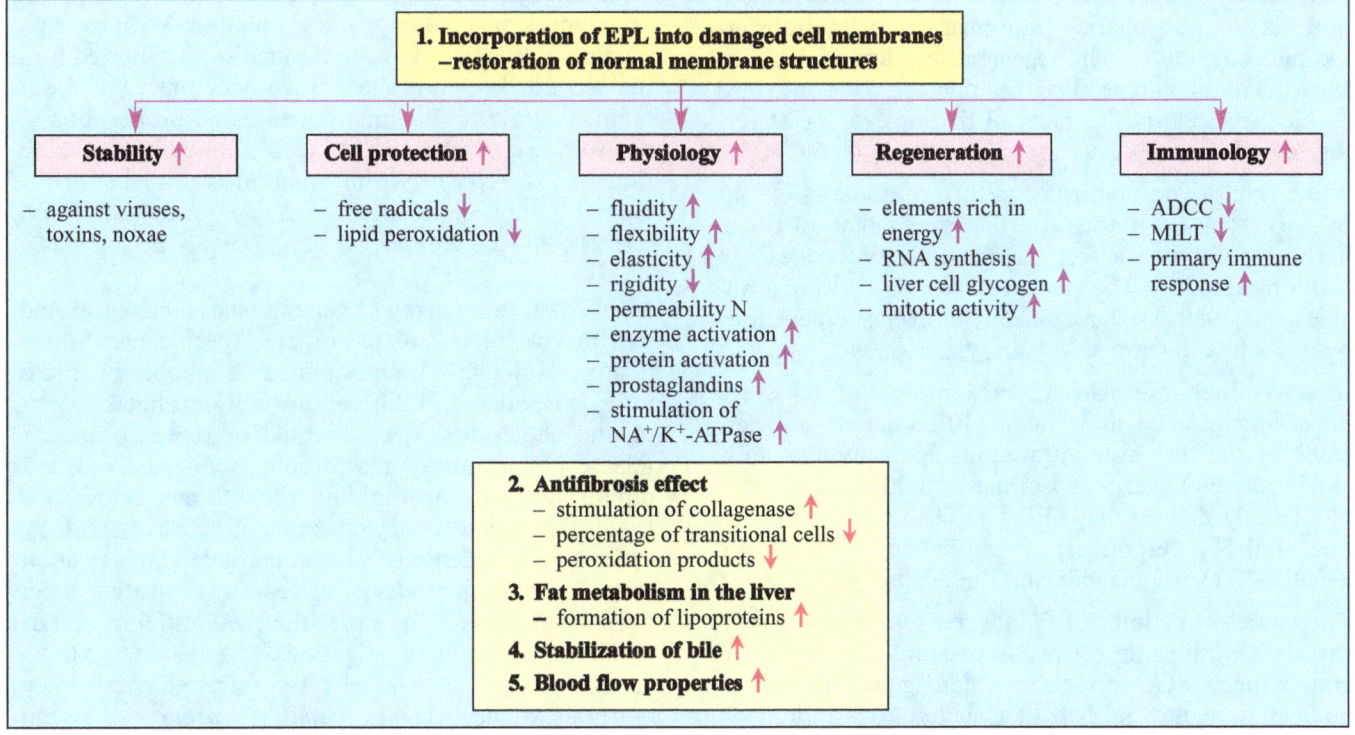

Fig. 40.3: Putative and demonstrated hepatic modes of action of EPL in vitro and in vivo. (ADCC = antibody-dependent cell-mediated cytotoxicity, MILT = mitogen-induced lymphocytotoxicity, N = normal)

different animal species. They were conducted using EPL together with various chemicals (201, 233, 244), alcohol (204, 208, 225, 227, 228, 230, 236–238), narcotic drugs, cytostatics, ionizing rays, etc. (s. tab. 40.13) These experiments clearly demonstrated the notable **hepatoprotective** and **curative effects** of EPL in vivo. Remarkably good results were also obtained with EPL as an antifibrogenic agent. (209, 224–226, 229, 232) The earlier EPL was given, the more pronounced the effects were. Inhibition of lipid peroxidation in the liver membranes was likewise verified. In animal experiments, it could be demonstrated that PPC increases SAMe and GSH levels in alcohol-induced hepatic oxidative stress. (203) Similarly, it was possible to diminish the antiapoptotic action against ethanol-induced hepatocyte apoptosis. (234) In a further study, the alcohol-induced increase in peroxinitrite hepatotoxicity and the concomitant production of oxide and superoxide could be prevented by PPC. (204) Furthermore, it has been shown that PPC activates enzymes such as hepatic triglyceride lipase, which is responsible for triglyceride degradation in the liver. (210) Dilinoleoylphosphatidylcholine, which is the main active ingredient in PPC, diminishes the activity of acylcoenzyme A: cholesterol acyltransferase, an enzyme that leads to the storage of cholesterol in the liver. (235) • Based on these pharmacological and clinical data, PPC would appear to be the drug of choice for significantly reducing or abolishing fatty liver of different origin, e.g. due to alcohol or obesity, even if the causing noxa cannot be eliminated, as is the case with diabetes-associated steatosis. (214, 216, 220) Interestingly, it could be observed that administration of betaine attenuates alcoholic steatosis by restoring the phosphatidylcholine generation via the phosphatidylethanolamine methyltransferase pathway. (219) • The **regenerative effect** of EPL on experimentally induced liver cell damage was confirmed by biochemical and histological findings. (215) (for further details, see 200, 209, 223) (s. tab. 40.13) (s. fig. 40.3)

These results were confirmed in further studies. (206, 240, 242, 243, 245, 246) It was also discovered that EPL can have an inhibitory effect on alcoholic fibrogenesis in baboons. (226, 230) The **clinical studies** which were available up to 1988 (200) have meanwhile been supplemented by other investigations. (207, 213, 218, 231, 239)

In **severe liver insufficiency,** we were able to achieve a life-saving reversal in 7 out of 10 seemingly hopeless cases by the first ever intravenous application of PPC (3,000 mg/day). (221) • A European multicentre double-blind study showed that EPL significantly increased the rate of IFN-α responders among patients with **chronic hepatitis C** as well as reducing the relapse rate. (239)

The modes of action of EPL suggest the following **indications:** curative, protective/curative and curative/regenerative therapy (*1.*) in toxic liver damage and fatty liver, and (*2.*) in acute viral hepatitis, acute intoxication, liver insufficiency, as well as (*3.*) as a supportive flanking therapy in chronic viral hepatitis and cirrhosis.

5.13.2 Silymarin

The name "sillybon" was given by ancient Greek writers — and later by THEOPHRASTUS (372–287 BC) — to a thistle species, without its being defined more closely. In "De Materia Medica" by DIOSCORIDES (about 50 AD), the plant later called milk thistle is described as a medical remedy for the bites of poisonous snakes. In his book "Historia Naturalis", PLINIUS THE ELDER (23–79 AD) was the first to mention the choleretic effect of milk thistle. The extract was recommended as a liver remedy by H. BRUNFELS (1434) and P. A. MATHIOLUS (1590), and also in the herbals of H. BOCK (1560) and A. LONICERUS (1564). • As a result of the investigations of F. MAYER et al. (1949) and O. EICHLER et al. (1949), the year 1949 can be regarded as the "hour of birth" of silymarin concerning liver treatment. *(Detailed account: 247)*

Silymarin is a mixture of three chemically related *flavanolignoids*; it is extracted from the seeds of the milk thistle (Silybum marianum Gaertn. or Carduus marianus [L]). These flavanolignoids include: (*1.*) *silibinin*, (*2.*) *silidianin*, and (*3.*) *silicristin*. **Silibinin** is the main active constituent. Its molecular weight is 482.5, the empirical formula is $C_{25}H_{22}O_{10}$. • The *major pharmacokinetic characteristics* are rapid absorption and a calculated absorbed fraction of 23–47%. Peak plasma concentrations are achieved after one to two hours. In plasma, 90–95% of silymarin is bound to protein. Half-life is 6.3 hours. Due to its relatively high molecular weight, >90% is excreted via the bile. About 10% of the given dose enters the enterohepatic circulation. With repeated administration, steady state elimination is achieved from the second day; thus there is no accumulation of silibinin. • *Silicristin* has pharmacokinetic properties similar to those of silibinin, yet with a lower biliary excretion rate (4–10%). No information is available on the second minor component *silidianin* (and *isosilibinin*). (248, 250, 261–263, 267, 280, 282, 285) *(Detailed account: 247)*

In addition to an array of general **pharmacological findings** in vivo or in isolated organs, specific hepatology-related results have been obtained. A number of studies provided evidence of different membrane effects; experimental cholestasis was prevented or reduced, and the release of histamine or serotonin from mast cells was diminished. Silymarin inhibits the different cytochrome P-450 enzymes to a varying extent. (248, 250, 262, 263, 270, 280, 282, 285) Evidence of **membranotropia** and **hepatoprotection** is of major relevance: respective positive effects have been shown in more than 30 different model studies in over 120 investigations. (252–256, 258–260, 266, 269, 274–276, 278, 279, 281, 286, 288) • The efficacy of silymarin as an **antioxidant** (= *radical scavenger*) was confirmed in recent studies. (249, 257, 271, 273, 275, 277, 287) Furthermore, an **antifibrosis effect** (251, 264, 268, 272) and the inhibition of β-glucuronidase (256) have been demonstrated. The modes of action of silymarin are based on several cellular targets. (s. tab. 40.14)

The **clinical studies** (approximately 120) available up to 1988 (247) have meanwhile been supplemented by further investigations. (256, 262, 266, 283, 284) Silymarin did not prove beneficial to patients with PBC.

▶ The **combination** of *essential phospholipids* and *silymarin* is of special clinical interest because of the cellular targets and modes of action of these two drugs. (289, 291, 292, 294, 295) (s. fig. 40.3) (s. tab. 40.14) In patients with chronic hepatitis, this combination was applied with success. (290) Thus, the available results of clinical studies suggest a number of **indications.**

Silibinin (intravenous)
▶ Amanita poisoning

Silymarin (oral)
- Toxic liver damage
  - alcohol toxicity
  - drug toxicity
  - chemical toxicity
- Supportive therapy
  - chronic hepatitis
  - liver cirrhosis

1. **Protection of biological membranes from noxae**
   - Inhibition of toxin uptake
   - Stabilization of biological membranes
     - influence on phospholipid turnover
     - biochemical interactions with membranes
     - decrease in enzyme induction
     - inhibition of phosphodiesterase
2. **Support of cellular detoxication mechanisms**
   - Stimulation of superoxide dismutase
   - Maintenance of the glutathione pool (GSH) of hepatocytes
3. **Antioxidative effect**
   - Interactions with free radicals
   - Reduction in lipid peroxidation
     - inhibition of lipoxygenase
     - decrease in malondialdehyde
     - diminution of glutathione consumption
4. **Inhibition of fibrogenesis**
5. **Increase in protein biosynthesis**
6. **Inhibition of cholesterol synthesis**
   - fall in microsomal hydroxylmethylglutaryl-CoA reductase

Tab. 40.14: Cellular tackling points and modes of action of silymarin

---

5.13.3 Glycyrrhiza glabra

Glycirrhizin was first used in hepatology in 1977 by H. Suzuki et al., who achieved good results in patients with chronic hepatitis. The main constituents isolated from the roots of Glycyrrhiza glabra are triterpene saponins, including glycyrrhizin (5–20%), and triterpene sapogenins. Glycyrrhizin is a conjugate of 1 molecule of glycyrrhetinic acid with 2 molecules of glucuronic acid. It is metabolized by β-glucuronidase, predominantly in the intestine (by bacteria) and to a lesser extent in the liver (by lysosomes). Half-life is three to five hours, in chronic liver disease four to ten hours. The following modes of action are postulated: (*1.*) it acts as a radical scavenger, (*2.*) it decreases cell-membrane permeability, and (*3.*) it prevents membrane penetration by viral particles. (297) The antiviral cytoprotective and immunomodulatory effects are based on these modes of action. Although its previously known pharmacological effects were not considered to be of any consequence for hepatology, glyzyrrhizin has meanwhile surprisingly proved its worth as a hepatoprotective compound. The agent induces interferon formation and, in this way, also has an antiviral effect. Good therapeutic results were recorded in several clinical studies on chronic hepatitis B, NANB and C and for prophylactic use in transfusion hepatitis (with administration both before and after blood transfusions) as well as in subacute viral liver failure (200–600 mg/day). Glycyrrhizin inhibited HAV replication and improved the immunological identification of HBsAg; HBeAg-positive patients showed more rapid seroconversion. A mixture of glycyrrhizin (40 mg) + cysteine (20 mg) + glycine (400 mg) has also been used as therapy. • With long-term administration, **pseudoaldosteronism** may appear, which can be eliminated by spironolactone (e. g. 50 mg/day). (296, 298, 299)

5.13.4 Colchicine

▶ Colchicine is an alkaloid obtained from the *autumn crocus* (Colchicum autumnale). It is a nitrogen-containing, tricyclic compound with a tropolone structure. The results of the pharmacokinetic studies available so far are summarized in a review. (310) Colchicine inhibits the function of the microtubuli (301) and acts as a toxin on cells, mitoses and capillaries. (300, 304, 308, 311) Albumin synthesis is apparently only slightly affected. In existing iron overload, further iron uptake is greatly increased by colchicine. Trimethylcolchicinic acid proved less toxic. The antifibrotic effect of colchicine is probably based on a reduction in collagen secretion and an increase in collagenase activity with elevated collagen breakdown. (307) In existing liver disease, the pharmacokinetics of colchicine is influenced. (309, 310) A potential antilipid peroxidative effect was observed in experimentally induced acetaminophen liver damage. (304)

The results obtained from the *clinical use* of colchicine are controversial. Good results in preventing cirrhosis in chronic hepatitis B and, when combined with UDCA, in primary biliary cholangitis are counterbalanced by unfavourable results in chronic hepatitis (303, 312), primary biliary cirrhosis (302), primary sclerosing cholangitis (306) and alcoholic hepatitis. • A beneficial effect of colchicine on hepatic fibrogenesis should be the subject of further debate. (305) (s. pp 683, 692, 766)

5.13.5 Betaine

Betaine is a quarternary ammonium compound. This substance is widely found in nature; it was first isolated from *sugar beet* (Beta vulgaris). • Like choline and methionine, betaine belongs to the group of *lipotropic substances.* Choline plays a major role in the mobilization of neutral fats in the liver, using them to form transportable phospholipids with neutral fats. In order to give up its methyl group, choline requires betaine. Thus it assumes an important function in the transmethylation cycle of lipid metabolism. It could be demonstrated that betaine attenuates alcoholic steatosis by restoring the phosphatidylcholine generation (219), particularly since it is also essential for the resynthesis of methionine. Within the therapeutic dosage range, betaine is in no way toxic.

5.13.6 Cynara scolymus

Cynarine is the main active agent of artichoke extract. It is a cinnamic acid derivative; the substitution pattern of its aromatic rings is similar to that of dopamine. Caffeic acid is also regarded as a major active substance. It has not yet been clarified to which constituents the known *modes of action* are attributable: (*1.*) increase in choleresis, (*2.*) inhibition of cholesterol biosynthesis, (*3.*) hepatoprotection due to antioxidative effects, and (*4.*) activation of the urea cycle.

5.13.7 Bupleurum falcatum

An extract of *Bupleurum falcatum* with the active agent saiko has for a long time been used in hepatobiliary diseases in Eastern Asia. The substance is commercially available in China under the name Sho-Saiko-To. The active components are attributed to the saiko-saponins (M. Yamamoto et al., 1981, 1985). Inhibition of fibrogenesis was demonstrated in animal experiments. (313–315) A good effect was achieved in chronic hepatitis in several clinical studies. Significantly more rapid HBeAg elimination was attained in children with chronic hepatitis B. (316) (s. pp 567, 726)

5.13.8 Phyllanthus amarus

Extracts from Phyllanthus amarus and Phyllanthus niruri have been used in India for more than 20 years in acute viral hepatitis, apparently with success. Compared with essential phospholipids, Ph. niruri was equally effective in improving laboratory values, while Ph. amarus proved to be even more efficacious. Phyllanthus extracts inhibit HBV reduplication (319, 320) and DNA polymerase in HBV and WHV infection (321), whereas this effect was not verified in DHV hepatitis. (318) HBsAg carriers also exhibited a loss of HBsAg in 50% of cases and a significant rise in anti-HBs titres. (317) These good results contrast with a number of unfavourable experiences, which may be attributable to the fact that the Phyllanthus species contain varying amounts of active substances in different countries. This was also believed to explain the better efficacy of Phyllanthus urinaria compared to Ph. amarus and Ph. niruri.

5.13.9 Schizandra chinensis

The hepatoprotective efficacy of Schizandra chinensis is based on its lignoids Gomisines A, C, N, Wuweizisu C and Schisanthesin D. (323) A rapid decrease in the transaminases was verified in chronic viral hepatitis. (329) Hepatoprotective and anticarcinogenic effects were demonstrated in experimental studies. (322, 324–328)

5.13.10 Catechin

The active substance (+)-catechin is the main component of the plant *Uncaria gambir*. In the systematic chemical nomenclature, this natural substance is called (+)-cyanidanol-3. Pure (+)-catechin is considered completely non-toxic. Catechin is readily absorbed and rapidly degraded in the liver. So far, 11 metabolites have been identified. Because of its low molecular weight, catechin is mainly eliminated via the kidney. • The following *modes of action* have been demonstrated: (*1.*) increase in ATP concentration in the liver, and (*2.*) inhibition of lipid peroxidation. This is the basis of the marked hepatoprotective effect. It was used clinically as an adjuvant in acute viral hepatitis, chronic hepatitis and toxic (also alcohol toxic) liver damage. The results reported seemed promising. • Although catechin was regarded as totally non-toxic on the basis of experimental studies, major (unexplained) **side effects** including haemolytic anaemia, idiosyncratic reactions and even deaths occurred (K. A. Neftel et al., 1980; N. Brattig et al., 1981). The preparation, which had already been introduced in many countries, was thereupon **withdrawn from the market.**

6 Surgical therapy of liver diseases

▶ Even in antiquity, liver injuries were considered to be fatal due to the uncontrollable bleeding. Proof of an enemy's death was not furnished until his liver could be presented. (s. p. 5) As far as we know, Celsus (30 BC–50 AD) gave the first, remarkable description of *liver surgery*, which, due to the high volume of blood, was carried out using a cautery knife. • Surgical treatment techniques for liver diseases were not included in textbooks on hepatology until 1965. The two-volume book by F. Th. Frerichs (1861) (s. fig. 1.19), the textbook by H. Eppinger (1937) (s. fig. 5.1) and the two-volume textbook by I. Magyar (1961) *contained no descriptions of liver surgery* — apart from the treatment of echinococcus cysts — although extensive liver or portal vein system surgery had been carried out since the second half of the 19th century.

▶ Since the first surgical treatment of refractory ascites by **hepatopexy** (C. T. Billroth, 1894) and, in the same year, of bleeding oesophageal varices using **resection of the short gastric veins** (G. Banti, 1894), vast numbers of surgical techniques have been developed in order to manage both of these emergency situations.

*The attempt to compile a **systematic list** of all procedures is bound to be incomplete despite thorough investigations. However, it is worth the effort to include the ingenious —*

and seemingly logical – surgical methods of our worthy predecessors, so that their approaches to the operative management of ascites or bleeding oesophageal varices are not forgotten. (s. tabs. 16.19 and 19.7!)

An important prerequisite for liver surgery was knowledge of the **vascular system,** which was first described by F. GLISSON in 1654 (s. fig. 1.16) and again by R. REX in 1888, and which is known in detail today. • For the **segmental classification** of the liver, the system according to C. COUINAUD (1954) and A. PRIESCHING (1986), using the branches of the portal vein as orientation, gained prevalence. The caudate lobe is designated as segment I. Segment IV is situated on the right side of the falciform ligament (it is exclusively oriented to venous drainage via the intermediate hepatic vein). This sets limits for surgical techniques, and the haematogenous route of liver metastases is also taken into account. • Hjortsjö's concept (C. H. HJORTSJÖ, 1948) referring to the division of the anterior segment into two vertical subsegments could be confirmed by recent investigations. (356) (s. figs. 2.5, 40.4) (s. p. 19)

During the past 30 years, surgical treatment of liver diseases or injuries has made enormous **progress** due to the introduction of more sophisticated techniques, newly developed instruments and anaesthetic procedures as well as better management of intraoperative haemodynamics. These options regarding superior liver surgery have only been made possible by modern imaging procedures, endoscopic techniques and angiography. As with the use of laparoscopy, such examination methods guarantee far more exact presurgical staging than was conceivable in the past. • It should be noted that an appropriate **shunt operation** creates a more stable situation than TIPS, especially in the long term. Indeed, shunt surgery, rehabilitated by C. E. ZÖCKLER et al. (1985), is experiencing a revival in many places.

6.1 TIPS

The most common **indication** for the placement of TIPS is as a prophylaxis for or therapy of oesophagovariceal bleeding, ascites, Budd-Chiari syndrome, HRS, hepatic hydrothorax and complications associated with portal vein thrombosis. (331, 333, 336, 337) • **Contraindications** include a bilirubin value of >3 mg/dl, HE (in secondary symptomatic HE, TIPS placement is possible), cardiac insufficiency (due to the shunt-related blood overload) and a MELD score of >24. The frequency of **complications** is 2–5%, the mortality rate is <1%. A common occurrence is HE; about 90% appear in the first seven days after the placement of a shunt. They generally respond well to conservative treatment. In 10% of cases, a chronic progressive course of HE develops. If uncovered stents are used, stenosis occurs in 5% of patients within one year. Stenosis can mostly be avoided by using covered (albeit expensive) shunts – the rate of stenosis is merely 10% after one year. (332) Follow-up is performed by means of sonography. (s. figs. 16.15, 16.16) (s. pp 267, 320, 336, 343, 368)

Ascites in portal hypertension: Even though conservative therapy proves efficacious in 85–90% of ascites cases, 5–15% are unresponsive to such treatment. • These patients can be treated successfully using invasive or surgical measures, since the prognosis for ascites which is really refractory is poor. However, in each case, surgical options have to be carefully considered, taking into account all individual facts and deciding about indications with respect to (*1.*) peritoneovenous shunt, (*2.*) TIPS, or (*3.*) liver transplantation. • The first two methods contribute to recompensation and help to bridge the time gap until liver transplantation can be carried out, whereby the liver function should be maintained as effectively as possible. • After **peritoneovenous shunt** (s. p. 317) (s. figs. 16.12–16.14) (s. tabs. 16.14–16.18) or **TIPS** (320, 331, 335) (s. fig. 16.15, 16.16), a subsequent transplantation no longer poses a problem.

Bleeding in portal hypertension: The causal spectrum of upper or lower gastrointestinal bleeding is extremely broad. (s. tab. 19.4) (s. pp 354, 372) The most common sources of bleeding in portal hypertension are varices of the oesophagus and stomach (s. pp 262, 358), portal hypertensive gastropathy or intestinal vasculopathy (s. p. 265), and intestinal varices. (s. p. 264) It is particularly the unexpected and massive variceal bleeding which is life-threatening and requires intensive care, i.e. a combination of medication and mechanical measures. Of greatest importance are drugs to reduce portal vein pressure, sclerotherapy or variceal ligation, and (if necessary) balloon tamponade. (s. p. 365) • Whether or not surgical techniques are indicated is determined after definitive haemostasis and should be based on a critical evaluation of individual risk factors and the respective liver status. However, surgical treatment is needed for variceal bleeding which lasts longer than two days (requiring a daily supply of more than four units of blood) and which could not be stopped despite all conservative measures; this also applies to early relapse bleeding. • From a haemodynamic point of view, TIPS, which is a non-surgical connection between the hepatic and portal vein, represents a *portacaval side-to-side shunt*. This results in a sustained decrease in portal vein pressure. Relapse bleeding is reduced to 10–20%. Such an approach does not complicate subsequent liver transplantation. TIPS is thought to be the ideal technique for bridging the time gap before liver transplantation can be carried out. (331, 333)

6.2 Shunt operation

The importance of surgical treatment for oesophageal or gastric variceal bleeding is still controversial. Nevertheless, according to the findings to date, shunt surgery with a relapse bleeding risk of 5 (−10)% is deemed to be the best **prophylaxis against bleeding,** so that >50% of Child A and B patients reach their fifth postoperative year. In the only comparative prospective study carried out so far, the small-calibre, portacaval H-graft prosthetic shunt proved superior to TIPS in all relevant aspects. • Good **selection criteria** are: (*1.*) Child A and B patients, (*2.*) liver volume between 1,000−2,500 ml (as a close correlation to the O_2 consumption of the liver), (*3.*) portal vein perfusion of 10−30% of the total hepatic blood flow (for a distal splenorenal shunt of >30%) in sequential scintigraphy or duplex Doppler sonography, (*4.*) selective panangiography to check if the arteries and veins have a sufficient length and lumen, and (*5.*) use of a shunt technique which does not harm liver function and at the same time facilitates subsequent liver transplantation. • The most efficient techniques are the **distal splenorenal shunt** (particularly in high portal vein residual perfusion), using the same procedure as with splenopancreatic disconnection and gastric transection (343), and the small-calibre **mesocaval interpositional prosthetic shunt** (especially in cases of decreased portal vein blood flow). Chylous ascites was observed as a rare complication of a distal splenorenal shunt. If, for surgical reasons, these methods cannot be applied, the portacaval side-to-side shunt using a small-calibre stent is now recommended when there is no possibility of liver transplantation. (340) The partial portacaval shunt is preferred to the direct shunt. (339) The **survival rate** after 5 and 10 years is reported to be 75−80% and 65−70% respectively. • The outcome of shunt surgery is determined by the **preoperative liver function** and the arterial compensation capacity (which still cannot be measured exactly). The preoperative portal vein pressure is obviously not a risk factor during surgery or postoperatively. (338, 341, 342, 344) • Treatment of multiple arterioportal fistulas by shunt surgery should be mentioned as a **rarity** here. (s. p. 370!) (s. tab. 19.7)

6.3 Block surgery

Block surgery prevents the portal blood from flowing to the oesophagus and thus intervenes directly at the site of bleeding. However, it does not reduce portal hypertension and portal vein residual perfusion is not decreased. • The numerous methods or modifications may be put into **three groups**: (*1.*) simple block operations, in which the oesophagus is divided close to the cardia and re-anastomosed, (*2.*) extended block operations, which comprise additional skeletization of the stomach in order to avoid fundus variceal bleeding, and (*3.*) the Sugiura method, which also includes splenectomy in addition to gastric devascularization and oesophageal section. (338) • Block operations are only indicated when TIPS or shunt surgery could not be carried out or were unsuccessful. Devascularization procedures are worth considering as emergency interventions. (s. p. 370)

6.4 Liver resection

▶ The first liver resection in the form of a lobectomy was carried out on a dog by G. ZAMBECCARI as early as 1680. The first resection in humans (removal of an adenoma) was also performed in Italy, but the outcome was fatal (A. LIUS, 1886). The first successful resection of a large, benign, pedicled lobular constriction was carried out by C. v. LANGENBUCH (Germany) in 1888, while successful resections were performed in the USA by W. W. KEEN as from 1892.

6.4.1 Basic principles
Definition

A liver resection is defined as the surgical removal of tissue components of the liver in order to eliminate a localized disease process. • The left hepatic lobe (segments I−IV) contains 40% and the right lobe (segments V−VIII) contains 60% of the total liver mass. (s. fig. 40.4) Removal of >80% of a healthy liver is (in principle) fatal. • Hyperplasia of the remaining liver can be expected, while regeneration of the resected portion of the liver is also possible.

Functional reserve: The method of choice and the extent of the resection depend upon the residual function of the remaining liver tissue. As a rule, it is relatively easy to determine the loss of tissue caused by surgical intervention, but this is not equivalent to the functional loss: on the one hand, the tumourous or diseased tissue which has been removed had no function and therefore cannot be evaluated as a functional loss; on the other hand, the neighbouring tissue, which was displaced by the growth process, might indeed experience functional recovery after tumour resection. It should be noted that healthy liver tissue usually has to be removed due to the necessity of allowing a safety margin. This is especially true when keeping to the respective segmental boundaries. Evaluation of the remaining functional reserve is extremely difficult in a diffusely diseased liver. This is above all true in cirrhosis; here, it is first of all necessary to determine the *Child Pugh stage.* (s. tab. 35.6) Several *laboratory parameters* (e.g. ChE, GEC, ICG, aminopyrin ^{14}C test) (363, 364) as well as CT volumetry or ^{99m}Tc GSA (363) − and, in the future, *virtual liver surgery* (360) − are suitable for assessing preoperative liver function and its postoperative functional reserve (even though functional values cannot be directly related to the functional hepatocyte mass). (345, 357, 358, 365)

Parenchyma setting: When incisions are made in the parenchyma, all structures within the tissue (arteries, portal veins, hepatic veins, bile ducts) must remain intact. Apart from the well-established method called "finger fracture" (W. ANSCHÜTZ, 1903), ultrasonic cutters, water beam dissectors or laser scalpels are used nowadays in order to distinguish between hepatic parenchyma and vascular structures. • **Haemostasis** can be

extended left hemihepatectomy, segment V or VIII is also resected. (s. fig. 40.4)

Right hemihepatectomy: This procedure was successfully carried out for the first time by W. WENDEL (Germany) in 1911 in order to remove a large adenoma. • The technique involves the resection of segments V, VI, VII and VIII, i.e. right liver lobe is removed. • *Extended right hemihepatectomy* also includes segment IV (left middle segment). (s. fig. 40.4)

Lobectomy: In left lobectomy, segments II and III are removed, while in right lobectomy, segments IV–VIII are resected (whereby the right and left halves of the liver are incorrectly called "lobes"). (s. fig. 40.4)

Segmentectomy: This surgical technique involves the removal of a single liver segment or a combination of segments. Both marginal and central segments may be involved. Another surgical option includes going beyond the boundaries of the segments, such as removal of segment V and the lower half of segment IV. • Resection of segment VIII is the most difficult procedure; usually, segment VII is removed at the same time, since the venous blood flow is interrupted in any case. • Segmentectomy IV divides the liver into two parts as far as the vena cava. The cava/gall-bladder line serves as orientation. • **Left lateral segment resection** involves segments II and III (also known as left lobectomy, see above). • **Segment I** cannot be assigned to either of the two halves of the liver. Its boundaries are difficult to determine; in general, the anterior boundary is defined by the hilar ramification of the portal vein structures, while the posterior boundary line is deemed to be the vena cava. Segment I varies in size, and sometimes it is nothing more than a thin layer of tissue. (368) • As a rule, it is possible to define the segmental boundaries by targeted puncture of the portal vein branches to show colour contrast in the respective segment and also by intrasurgical sonography. (350) (s. fig. 40.4)

Dorsocranial resection, a special technique with simultaneous hepato-atrial anastomosis, may be indicated in the Budd-Chiari syndrome (G. BANSKY et al., 1986; S. MEYER et al., 1988). (s. p. 856)

A wide spectrum of *focal lesions* of varying sizes provides the **indication** for liver resection (347, 349, 352, 354, 355, 357, 361):

1. Benign liver tumour (s. fig. 40.5)
2. Congenital malformations
3. Focal bile-duct processes
4. Liver metastasis (s. fig. 40.6)
5. Malignant liver tumour (s. fig. 40.7)
6. Parasitic foci
7. Traumatic liver injury

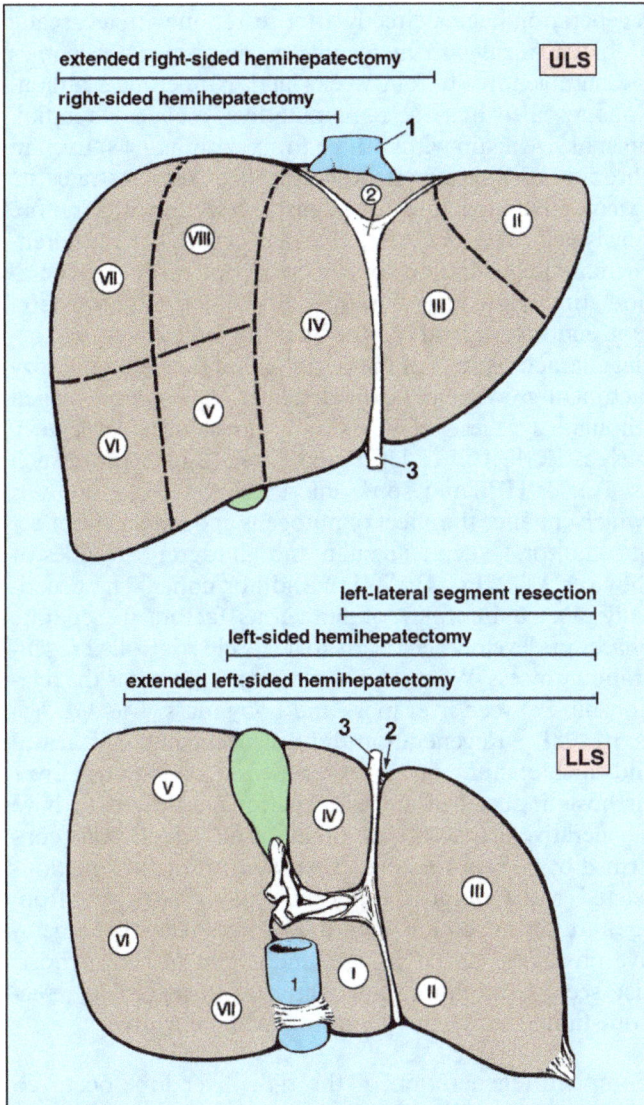

Fig. 40.4: Representation of the liver segments (according to C. COUINAUD, 1954) (ULS = upper liver surface, LLS = lower liver surface). (351) Left liver lobe: I–IV (segment I corresponds to the caudate lobe and can only be delimited at the LLS; segment IV is actually located to the right of the falciform ligament). Segment IV is subdivided into an apical part (IVa) and a caudal part (quadrate lobe) (IVb). Right hepatic lobe: segments V–VIII. (1 = inferior vena cava; 2, 3 = falciform ligament) (s. figs. 2.1, 2.5)

achieved by surgical techniques and electrocoagulation, infrared coagulation, argon beamer or fibrin glue. • The insertion of **drainage tubes** allows the removal of postoperative lymph, gall, residual haematomas and (possibly) oozing blood. Even if these surgical methods are carefully managed, it is not possible to avoid such fluid discharge completely. • The post-resection **methylene blue test** helps to reduce the postoperative biliary leakage rate. (359) (s. pp 807, 825!)

6.4.2 Classification and indications

Left hemihepatectomy: This procedure includes segments II, III and IV, i.e. left liver lobe is removed. • In

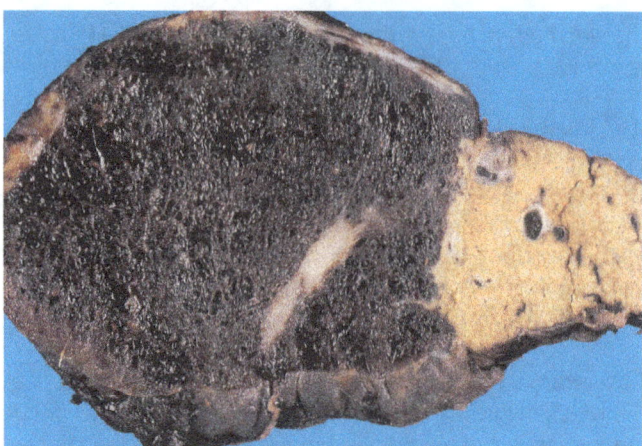

Fig. 40.5: Cavernous haemangioma in a liver resection specimen

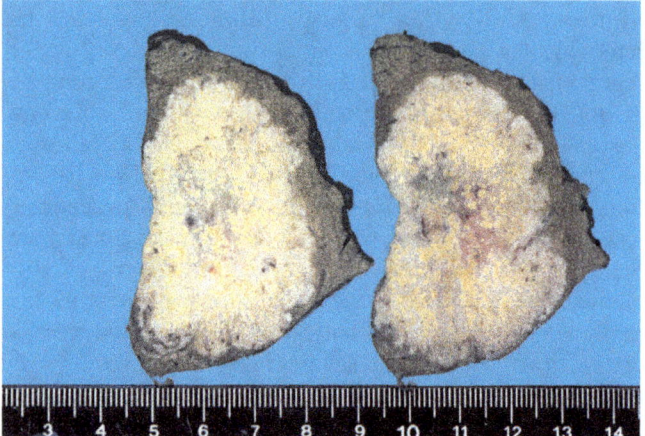

Fig. 40.6: Liver metastasis of a colorectal carcinoma in a liver resection specimen

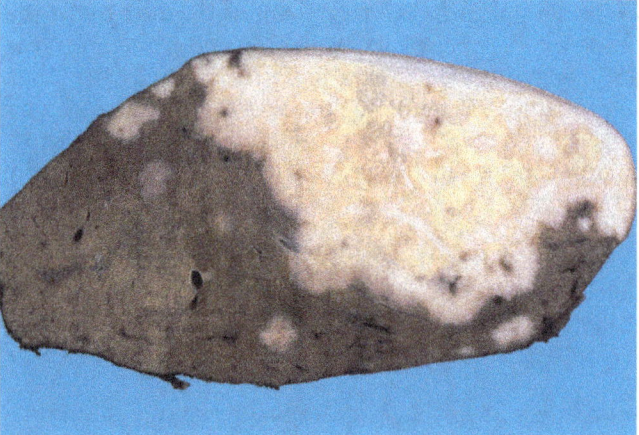

Fig. 40.7: Cholangiocarcinoma (peripheral type) in a liver resection specimen

6.4.3 Regeneration

In 1879 H. TILLMANNS first reported the phenomenon of liver regeneration following a large resection in an animal experiment. This observation was confirmed in 1931 by animal experiments, in which restoration of the liver was demonstrated following two-thirds resection in the rat. (353) • It has meanwhile been shown that liver regeneration begins directly after resection with a cascade of biochemical and molecular mechanisms. It becomes measurable three to four weeks later. Numerous examinations revealed that the remaining liver reaches its initial, normal size again within three to six months. (348) Even in chronic hepatitis or cirrhosis, the liver demonstrates its regenerative capacity after extensive resection, albeit more slowly and to a lesser extent than a liver with healthy parenchyma. • Regeneration appears to depend on (*1.*) regeneration-stimulating factors in the portal blood after resection (e. g. endotoxin), and (*2.*) the quantity (and quality or special characteristics?) of the portal blood flow. • Regulatory factors of growth can be divided into: (*1.*) *mitogens* (which stimulate synthesis of DNA and mitosis of hepatocytes), such as EGF, TGFα, HGF and FGF; (*2.*) *inhibitors*, such as TGFβ, HPI and some interleukins; (*3.*) *co-mitogens* (which enhance the effect of mitogens and reduce the effect of inhibitors), such as insulin and glucagon ("goodies of the liver"), TNFα, IL 1, IL 6 and hormones. The genetically steered interplay of numerous factors in separate phases of development leads to a closely controlled regeneration process. What is important for the result is the relationship between liver mass and body mass. (346, 362, 366) (s. p. 408!) • Regeneration did not occur in a portacaval end-to-side shunt under experimental conditions. Liver cirrhosis induced in animal experiments proved to have regenerative capacity, an observation which was confirmed by clinical findings. It is assumed that in resection-related regeneration, "other" mechanisms (apart from age) are set in motion than in cirrhosis-related regenerative processes. (367) The type and extent of the cirrhosis also seem to be important factors with regard to resection-stimulated regeneration in residual cirrhosis.

Complete regeneration of the right liver lobe occurred in two women following right lobectomy; surprisingly, the regenerated right lobe showed exactly the same external shape as the original one. This led to the well-founded assumption that there is both (*1.*) resection-stimulated hyperplasia of the remaining liver, and (*2.*) regeneration of its resected part. The causes of these two developments are still unclear, as is the varying capacity of a cirrhotic liver to regenerate. Several different methods of elucidating the regenerative processes have been suggested. (346) (s. pp 5!, 408)

6.5 Liver injuries

▶ Liver injuries, particularly caused by weapons and accidents, have been known ever since the dawn of mankind. There are numerous reports dating from antiquity and later centuries of liver injuries and surgical attempts to heal them. • About 1600, F. HILDANUS reported an excision of a prolapsed part of the liver after trauma – the patient survived. In 1716 G. BERTA succeeded in treating a prolapsed and severely injured liver in a madman who had cut open his belly with a knife. • Laparotomy has been used since 1886 to manage liver injuries; mortality rates were 60% (L. EDLER, 1887), 81% (F. TERRIER, 1896) and 44% (B. T. TILTUN, 1905).

The following **classification** is used to assess liver injury (H. BOCKHORN et al., 1982):

> Type Ia: Superficial parenchymal lesions
> Ib: Deep liver ruptures
> Ic: Visible parenchymal destruction, with or without bile-duct injury
> Type II: Additional injuries of the porta hepatis (bile ducts, portal vein, hepatic artery)
> Type III: Injuries of the portal vein hilum
> Type IV: Liver injuries combined with lesions of the vena cava

Whereas penetrating injuries are less common today, the number of blunt injuries has increased, frequently accompanied by liver rupture. A liver injury is involved in up to 40% of patients with blunt abdominal trauma. Conservative treatment is recommended as far as possible in order to avoid unnecessary laparotomy. (379) The overall mortality rates were 11.8% and 16.8% respectively. (371, 373) In many cases, the urgency of the situation does not allow the requisite examinations to be made (e.g. US, CT (376, 378), angiography, laparoscopy). An emergency operation has to be performed. Such an operation must even be done under shock if the patient does not respond directly to conservative methods.

The **surgical treatment** chosen depends on the type of injury, but also on the patient's condition at the time. Some 40–65% of all deaths are due to exsanguination, while 35–60% are caused by postoperative organ failure. Intra-abdominal formation of abscesses is deemed to be the most common complication. (370, 375) Based on the findings available, the following **surgical methods** are used: (1.) drainage, (2.) superficial suture with drainage, (3.) haemostasis by means of transcatheter arterial embolization (372, 374), fibrin glue, infrared coagulator or electrocoagulation, (4.) anastomosis techniques (e.g. intracaval shunt), (5.) hepatorrhaphy, (6.) resection techniques (e.g. debridement, segmentectomy), etc. (369, 370, 375, 377) An overall mortality rate of 10.5% was reported in 1,000 consecutive liver injuries.

7 Liver transplantation

> ▶ The first liver transplantation was carried out on a dog by C.S. WELCH et al. in 1955. (443) • After a five-year period of experimental preparations, T.E. STARZL et al. were able to carry out the first orthotopic liver transplantation for extrahepatic biliary atresia on a three-year-old boy in Denver (USA) on **1st March 1963**; however, the boy bled to death during the operation. Another four transplant recipients lived 6–23 days. (434) • In 1968 R.Y. CALNE et al. began carrying out liver transplantations in Cambridge (England). In Germany, A. GÜTGEMANN et al. started performing liver transplantations in 1968, followed by R. PICHLMAYR et al. in 1979. • While surgical techniques were constantly undergoing improvement, the problem of organ rejection could not be solved in a satisfactory way by the substances used at that time.

It was not until the introduction of cyclosporine A (R.Y. CALNE et al., 1979) and the combination of cyclosporine A + prednisolone (T.E. STARZL et al., 1980) that the ultimate breakthrough was achieved. In 1983, liver transplantation (LTX, LT) was recognized as an important option for patients in the final stage of chronic liver disease. • By 1993, a total of 26,500 liver transplantations had been carried out worldwide (R. BELLE et al., 1993). Due to the rapidly rising number of centres (about 300 worldwide), the *total number of liver transplantations was thought to have reached about 80,000 worldwide by the end of 2000.* • In Germany, the number of liver transplantations rose from 502 in 1992 to 779 in 2004. Currently, the number of LTX performed every year is 4,000 in Europe and 6,000 in the USA. • The 1-, 5- and 10-year survival rates amount to >90%, >80% and >75% respectively. However, the demand for liver transplantation is far greater than the supply of donor organs. This lack has **practical consequences**: (1.) on the indication for LT, (2.) on the development of more sophisticated liver-support devices for bridging a life-threatening situation and for avoiding LT should the diseased liver meanwhile become restored (s. p. 389), (3.) on the search for alternative transplantation techniques (e.g. split-liver, APOLT, LDLT) for optimizing the use of cadaveric livers, and (4.) on the mortality rate among patients waiting for a suitable organ. • The waiting period is currently 6–12 or even 12–18 months. *(see chapter 20. 5.4)*

> **Potential indications** for liver transplantation are given in almost any kind of life-threatening liver disease (1.) which has taken a progressive and irreversible course (e.g. chronic liver disease in the end stage, acute liver failure, hepatic neoplasias) or (2.) in which a period of time has to be bridged between the patient's irresponsiveness to treatment and the probable reversibility of the diseased liver. • The motivation and compliance of the patient are prerequisites for LT.

7.1 Indications

If the indication for LT is given, the case should be registered with a liver transplantation centre. The patient is then checked regarding the indication, and all contraindications should be excluded. Subsequent to phase-1 and phase-2 evaluation, the patient is added to the waiting list. Principally, only those patients will be selected for LT (1.) who have a realistic chance of surviving the perioperative phase and (2.) whose chances of survival are much better following LT. Children under one year of age can also be successfully transplanted. (384, 397, 435)

| 1. **Cirrhosis**
Alcoholic cirrhosis
Autoimmune hepatitis
Cryptogenic cirrhosis
HBV and HDV
HCV
2. **Cholestatic diseases**
Alagille syndrome
Bile-duct atresia
Bile-duct papillomatosis
Biliary cirrhosis after cholangitis
Biliary cirrhosis after PBC
Biliary cirrhosis after PSC
Caroli's disease
Cholangiodysplasia
Cholestatic sarcoidosis
Graft-versus-host disease
3. **Acute liver failure**
Acute episode of a chronic liver disease
Fatty liver of pregnancy
Fulminant viral hepatitis (393)
HELLP syndrome
Intoxications, poisoning (386)
Postoperative, posttraumatic
4. **Mycosis**
Candidiasis
Coccidiodomycosis | 5. **Hepatic tumours**
Benign tumours
Cystic liver (403, 422)
– echinococcosis (402)
– focal nodular hyperplasia
Sarcoidosis

Malignant tumours
– selected biliary carcinomas
– selected gall-bladder carcinomas
– selected hepatic carcinomas
– selected metastases
6. **Vascular diseases**
Budd-Chiari syndrome
Haemangiomatosis
Veno-occlusive disease
7. **Metabolic diseases**
α_1-antitrypsin deficiency
Aminoacidurias
Amyloidosis
Byler's disease
Crigler-Najjar syndrome
Familial cholestasis
Fructose intolerance
Galactosaemia
Gaucher's disease
Glycogenosis I, IV (432)
Haemochromatosis (423) | Haemophilia
Hypercholesterinaemia
Hyperlipoproteinaemia II
Niemann-Pick disease
Oxalosis
Porphyria
Reye's disease
Sanfilippo's syndrome
Sickle cell anaemia
Thalassaemia (β)
Tyrosinaemia
Urea cycle defects
Wilson's disease (436)
Wolman's disease
8. **Complications in cirrhosis**
Ascites unresponsive to treatment
Hepatopulmonary syndrome
Hepatorenal syndrome
Recurrent varix bleeding
Severe hypoalimentation
Spontaneous bacterial peritonitis
9. **Retransplantation**
Acute rejection
Arterial thrombosis
Chronic rejection
Initial dysfunction
Portal vein thrombosis
Recidivism of the underlying disease |

Tab. 40.15: Indications for liver transplantation: *safe, putative* and *limited* indications (as have been published) (with some references)

The spectrum of **indications** for liver transplantation has widened enormously due to more sophisticated presurgical diagnosis, more exact evaluation of risk factors, better management of intraoperative techniques and supplementary measures, improvement in immunosuppressive agents and more qualified aftercare. The indications may be grouped into **eight main categories**, subdivided into *frequent* and *rare*. In addition, differentiation is made between *safe, possible* and *limited* indications for liver transplantation. (s. tab. 40.14)

The indication for LT depends on (*1.*) **type of liver disease**, and (*2.*) **stage of disease**, i.e. at what point LT is carried out during the course of disease. It should be noted that the preparations necessary for LT should commence as from stage Child B. • Eurotransplant assigns the status "high urgent" only to patients suffering from acute liver failure or acute transplant failure following LT. Patients suffering from acute deterioration of an existing liver disease are not included in this category. High urgent registrations undergo meticulous examination by Eurotransplant. In such cases, the waiting period is 6–30 hours. Important parameters regarding an indication for LT in acute liver failure include (*1.*) advancing encephalopathy, (*2.*) atrophy of the liver (daily US!), (*3.*) development of an ascites, (*4.*) decrease in the transaminases and Quick's value, and (*5.*) progressive renal insufficiency. In order to bridge the time until a transplant is available, the use of a liver-support device can be most helpful. (s. p. 389)

Three indication categories are differentiated according to the overall condition of the patient, respective liver function, the effects of the liver disease on other organs, and existing risk factors:

(*1.*) **Elective indication:** The general condition is stable and the nutritional state is still good or can be improved; liver function is decreasing, but still sufficient; bilirubin is constantly rising; there are as yet no severe extrahepatic complications (e. g. encephalopathy, ascites, hepatorenal or hepatopulmonary syndrome).

(*2.*) **Late indication:** The general condition is poor and the nutritional state is considerably reduced; liver function is severely compromised and shows increasing deterioration; there are complications and additional risk factors.

(*3.*) **Emergency indication:** Failure of vital functions; severe complications are observed (HE stages II–IV, kidney insufficiency, respiratory insufficiency). • This situation may develop either (*1.*) as the final phase of a long-standing, preexisting liver disease or in an abrupt manner, or (*2.*) as an urgent indication in acute liver failure (386, 387, 392, 428) or acute liver transplant failure.

Time of indication: Determining the best time for LT is very important, but it is also difficult. Although Child-Pugh classification is used as a standard in liver cirrhosis, it has not turned out to be a valuable tool regarding the timing of LT. • Important **criteria** for determining the best time of indication are (*1.*) *type of liver disease*, including its natural course and risks due to complications, (*2.*) *subjective drop in performance of the patient*, and (*3.*) progressive deterioration of certain *laboratory parameters*. In this context, a slow but steady decrease

I. Liver disease	
1. Type: primary hepatocellular / primary biliary	
2. Natural course	
II. Subjective deterioration in condition	
III. Changes in laboratory values	
1. *Enzymatic activity*	
• GPT, GOT	< 10 U/l
2. *Endogenous function values*	
• Albumins	< 3 g/dl
• Quick's value	< 40%
• Cholinesterase	< 1,000 U/l
• Bilirubin	> 5 mg/dl
3. *Exogenous function values*	
• Indocyanine green	> 5 min.
• Galactose elimination capacity	< 5 mg
• MEGX	
• Aminopyrine ^{14}C	
4. *Biliary function*	
• Alkaline phosphatase	> 1,500 U/l

Tab. 40.16: Important criteria in timing liver transplantation

in GPT and GOT to subnormal values points to severe and irreparable loss of parenchyma. Deterioration of endogenous functional values also suggests that the final phase is imminent. This is likewise confirmed by the fact that the results of exogenous function tests worsen. Such tests are easy to carry out, do not entail side effects, cause little inconvenience and are highly reliable, particularly in combination. (s. tab. 40.15) The ICG and the aminopyrine ^{14}C breath test have proved to be valuable transplant control measures. (391)

It is important not to miss the right moment for LT. A long waiting period with conservative therapy generally leads to an increase in intraoperative risks as well as a decrease in postoperative survival time. Any complications further worsen the prognosis and put LT into the "late indication" category. (380) • In addition to rising bilirubin and AP values, the consequences of impaired bile flow (e.g. undernourishment and malnutrition, catabolism, osteoporosis, malabsorption, hypercholesterolaemia and pruritus) are prognostically relevant in primary biliary diseases – while liver function tests still show good values in most cases.

Liver transplantation has the following aims: (*1.*) improvement in life expectancy, and (*2.*) improvement in the quality of life.

7.2 Contraindications

As the management of liver transplantation has improved, absolute and relative contraindications have been established. Relative contraindications may question the success of LT in some cases. Obesity leads to an increased rate of postoperative complications, but it does not influence the survival rate. (417, 424) (s. tab. 40.16) • Contraindications should also be considered in urgent LT due to acute liver failure – possibly accompanied by necrotizing pancreatitis, septic shock and problems with assisted respiration. • Visceral inversion is not deemed to be a contraindication: a successful LT was indeed carried out under such conditions by G. B. KLINTMALM et al. in 1993.

Absolute contraindications
1. Severe cardiac disease
2. Severe pulmonary disease
3. Extrahepatic metastases
4. Malignant secondary disease
5. Florid sepsis
6. AIDS
7. Severe irreversible brain damage
8. Active alcohol or drug abuse
9. Anatomical or postoperative anomalies
10. Portal vein plus superior mesenteric vein thromboses
11. Severe osteopenia
12. Poor nutritional state

Relative contraindications
1. Portacaval shunts
2. Portal vein thrombosis (with open superior mesenteric vein)
3. Age > 65 – 70 years (biological age is more important!)
4. Condition after complex hepatobiliary surgery
5. Chronic renal insufficiency
6. Muscular atrophy
7. Unstable personality structure
8. Unstable psychosocial environment
9. Obesity (> 100 kg BW)
10. Retransplantation

Tab. 40.17: Absolute and relative contraindications for liver transplantation. (The relative contraindications should be determined for each individual case)

7.3 Preoperative diagnostics

Clinical examination prior to LT comprises (*1.*) meticulous anamnesis including all previous findings, (*2.*) thorough internal examination, (*3.*) psychosocial and psychiatric assessment, and (*4.*) broad spectrum of laboratory parameters. *The medical "work-up" prior to LT takes about 10 – 12 days.*

Specific laboratory parameters comprise (*1.*) blood group and antibodies, (*2.*) HLA typing, (*3.*) hepatitis serology, including HCV RNA (by PCR) and HBV DNA, (*4.*) serology, including HSV I and II, EBV, CMV, HIV and varicella, (*5.*) coagulation status, (*6.*) thyroid function, (*7.*) renal function, and (*8.*) immunology, including ANA, AMA, SMA, anti-LKM and anti-SLA.

Technical examinations comprise (1.) thoracic X-ray, (2.) ECG, (3.) echocardiography, (4.) pulmonary function, (5.) gastroscopy, (6.) EEG, (7.) US and colour-encoded duplex sonography of the abdomen, (8.) radiology (including CT and angiography of the coeliac trunk) and right renal arteriography (to exclude high right kidney) as well as MRI cholangiography. With regard to post-operative osteoporosis, bone densitometry is recommended prior to LT. (390)

This **extensive programme** is, on the one hand, essential for preoperative diagnostics and the documentation of initial findings, while on the other hand, postoperative changes in the findings can be evaluated more easily. • The **indication** for LT is determined by an interdisciplinary team. If possible, both assessment and registration of cirrhosis patients should be carried out during Child B as soon as progressive deterioration is observed. • When preoperative diagnostics have been completed, patients grouped in the elective category may spend the **waiting period** at home. However, even if the findings are constant, there is always a risk of acute and unforeseeable complications.

Previous **shunt operations** and **TIPS** need to be removed in order to guarantee that the transplanted liver is sufficiently supplied with portovenous blood. In these cases, the portal system is checked preoperatively for thromboses by means of colour-encoded duplex sonography and X-ray techniques. In any case, the confluence of superior mesenteric vein and splenic vein must be free. (411) • The main advantage of portacaval end-to-side anastomosis is its low thrombosis rate of <5%; in addition, there is no need for a distal shunt ligature. In shunts distal to the hilus (mesocaval, distal splenorenal), no preparation of the liver hilus is required; however, in 10% of cases, these shunts show portal vein thrombosis (in TIPS, up to 15%). • Usually, all surgical shunts are disconnected or ligated before the liver transplantation is completed in order to avoid a steal effect. • Although portal vein thrombosis, previous operations in the liver hilus and portosystemic shunt surgery are (sometimes considerable) obstacles to liver transplantation, they are not regarded as contraindications. When there is isolated or partial portal vein thrombosis, a connection to the portal vein can often be restored by thrombectomy or bypass techniques; the survival rate is similar to that in patients with a primary open portal vein. Nevertheless, the conditions for a successful LT are more favourable if there is no portal vein thrombosis and the liver hilus does not require special preparatory measures.

7.4 Preparation of patients

(1.) During the waiting period, it is important to maintain or even improve the patient's **nutritional status.** Protein tolerance can be monitored by using simple *psychometric tests*. A protein intake of 1.0–1.5 g/kg BW/day would be ideal. Supplementation by *branched-chain amino acids* may be helpful. The *calorie supply* has to be adjusted to the optimal requirement of the patient. (s. pp 765, 878, 888)

(2.) The daily food intake should be spread over **five meals.** However, it is almost impossible to achieve an optimum supply of water-soluble and fat-soluble **vitamins.** Administration of multivitamin preparations is therefore recommended. **Sodium chloride** intake should not exceed 7–8 g/day. (s. pp 286, 753, 765)

(3.) Depending on the patient's condition, regular **muscle training** should be carried out daily if possible in order to improve anabolism as well as urea and glutamine metabolism in the muscles. (s. pp 683, 755)

(4.) The administration of **lactulose** over an extended period of time (dosage aim = 2–3 stools per day) is recommended. (858) • It is advisable to use a combination with *metronidazole* or with *non-absorbable antibiotics* (e.g. paramomycine) preoperatively in order to suppress the gram-negative intestinal flora and thus also the formation of endotoxins. If necessary, **antimycotics** may be administered in addition.

(5.) *Latent encephalopathy*, detectable by psychometric tests (s. p. 211), is frequent; experience has shown that it can rapidly become manifest. Of the urea-cycle amino acids suitable for therapy, **ornithine aspartate** has proved the most successful — also as an i.v. infusion in the post-operative phase. (s. pp 287, 756)

(6.) The relevant literature additionally recommends **vaccination** against pneumococcus and influenza as well as hepatitis B (unless there is already immunity).

7.5 Surgical aspects

Compatibility of blood groups

Interestingly, compatibility within the **blood group system** has proved to be the decisive factor in liver transplantation to date. • Although the *HLA system* is usually determined (for retrospective evaluation), it seems to be of minor importance. This is also true of so-called *"cross-matching"* between patient serum and donor lymphocytes. No other compatibilities between recipient and donor (apart from body weight, height and thorax size) are known to be required.

Quality of a donor liver

The quality of the donor liver is of crucial importance for successful LT. First of all, careful and proper **organ retrieval** *by a qualified team is an important prerequisite. Most centres now have such a designated multi-organ retrieval team.* • Any information pertaining to the donor (e.g. clinical results, anamnesis, laboratory values, current medication, further findings) is listed in the **donor protocol.** Of equal importance in the evaluation of a donor liver are the circumstances leading to the donor's death (cause of death, intensive care measures, etc.). • Using more suitable **preservation solutions** (Ringer's lactate, University of Wisconsin solution), the conservation time of donor livers could be prolonged to 15—20 hours. Great emphasis is being placed on achieving further improvements in this area. • During removal by the surgeon, the **donor liver** is assessed macroscopically and by palpation. This requires considerable experience, particularly since no other criteria for assessing the quality of the donor organ are available. (442) The **transplant** should be almost identical to the recipient's organ in terms of size, weight and vascular diameter (portal vein, superior/inferior vena cava). • The use of *size-reduced transplants* is being further developed as a possible method for the future.

Zero biopsy: Immediately after reperfusion of the donor liver, a biopsy is taken. This is seen as a starting point and reference value for the detection of pre-existing liver disease and assessment of organ quality (damage during preservation and respective reperfusion).

Types of transplantation

(*1.*) Normally, **orthotopic liver transplantation** (OLT) is used; in this technique, the donor liver is implanted at the site where the recipient's organ has been removed. The average survival rate is >90% after 1 year and >80% after 5 years. (s. p. 391)

(*2.*) A modified procedure, so-called **orthotopic segment liver transplantation** (OSLT), has proved successful (H. BISMUTH et al., 1984); this involves implanting parts of an adult liver, i.e. segments II and III or I—IV depending on the size of the recipient's organ, into a young recipient ("reduced size").

(*3.*) In **split liver transplantation** (SLT) (R. PICHLMAYR et al., 1989), it is possible to transplant segments V—VIII, which are left over in OSLT, into an adult. This means that two recipients can be supplied with one donor organ. The surgical splitting of the donor liver subjects the organ to considerable stress, and therefore its quality has to meet particularly high standards. (389, 444)

(*4.*) In **living donation** (LDLT) (R. W. STRONG et al., 1990), segments II and III are taken from a parent and transplanted into the child. The surgical risk for the living donor, which was quite high at the beginning, has been reduced considerably in the meantime to about 0.24%. The survival chance of the recipient is 27—92%. To date, more than 3000 transplantations of this kind have been carried out worldwide. The technique has now been generally established for children. About 5% of all LT patients are also suitable for an LDLT. Therefore, the possibility of such an LDLT should be discussed in all those cases where the waiting time for a regular LT would prove to be a problem. More than 75% of the donors are free from complications. In LDLT involving adults, the volume of the donor organ should be equivalent to approx. 1% of the body weight of the recipient. The respective size of the transplant, which is usually taken from the right lobe, is determined by means of CT volumetry. • After LDLT, bile leaks (7—10%) and biliary strictures (16—20%) frequently appear. In such suspected complications, ERC is recommended. (387, 403, 412, 413, 416, 430, 433, 445)

(*5.*) In **heterotopic liver transplantation** (HLT), the donor liver is transplanted as an auxiliary (additional) organ into the right upper abdomen, but the recipient retains the diseased liver (K. ABSOLON et al., 1965; J. G. FORTNER et al., 1970). This technique is not easy to carry out in terms of surgical requirements; it involves the so-called *piggyback method* and is used particularly for young patients suffering from acute liver failure. (s. p. 391)

(*6.*) **Auxiliary partial orthotopic liver transplantation** (APOLT) was introduced by G. GUBERNATIS et al. in 1991. In this procedure, segments II and III of the diseased liver are removed, while segments II—IV (or sometimes only segments II and III) of the donor organ are transplanted. The bile duct is reconstructed as a biliodigestive anastomosis. Full reversibility of the existing liver disease is a precondition for the surgical concept of APOLT. (428) (s. p. 391)

▶ The importance of an adequate supply of **zinc** is now accepted. In most cases, however, there is already a deficiency of this important trace element (unless previous medication has remedied the situation). Due to the scale of the operation, there is a considerable loss of zinc, which usually cannot be balanced even by intravenous substitution. Experience has shown that pronounced and extremely detrimental *zincuria* may be kept in check by i.v. application of **potassium canrenoate**. (s. p. 812!)

Venous bypass: Insertion of a combined venovenous and portovenous bypass reduces the negative effects of the anhepatic operative phase (lasting 30—120 minutes) by interrupting the blood flow in the portal vein and inferior vena cava. This measure allows greater haemodynamic stability during the anhepatic phase.

Biliary anastomosis: Reconstruction of the biliary flow is achieved by side-to-side anastomosis of the two choledochal stumps or, when primary bile-duct disease is present in the recipient, by anastomosis using a jejunum sling in the Roux-en-Y technique.

Duration of the operation: The duration of the operation varies greatly owing to the widely differing conditions during surgery. On average, it takes 5—10 hours. • The blood loss also differs considerably: 6—15 units of blood are normally substituted, but this quantity may be much higher in some cases. The number of units of blood can be reduced by administering *aprotinin*, which inhibits fibrinolysis after reperfusion.

Nitric oxide: Ischemia is the main cause of dysfunction in the transplanted liver. Inhalation of NO during the operation helps to reduce the frequency of dysfunction in the initial phase, since the transplanted liver produces insufficient NO at this time.

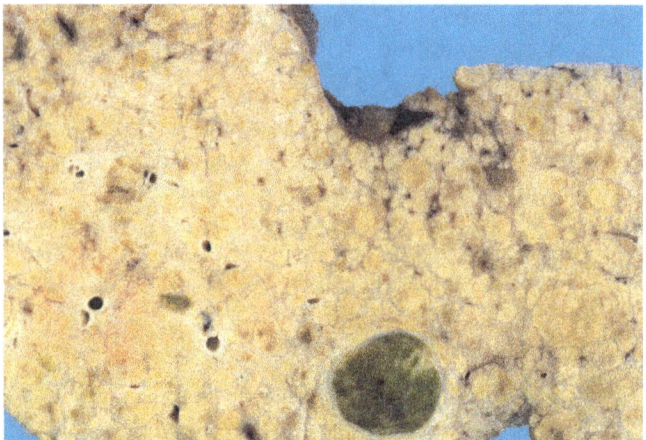

Fig. 40.8: End-stage liver cirrhosis with a small hepatocellular carcinoma in a non-cirrhotic explanted liver

7.6 Postoperative features

The postoperative phase has **three main objectives:** (*1.*) monitoring the functional condition of the transplanted liver, (*2.*) adjustment of immunosuppression, and (*3.*) early detection and treatment of complications.

Early postoperative phase: Extubation is carried out as soon as possible with subsequent regular breathing exercises and optimal infusion therapy. This takes into account all problems arising from such extensive surgery, e.g. lactate-free volume replacement, stability of circulation and coagulation, pain therapy, electrolytes, zinc, vitamins, acid-base balance, energy carriers. Loss of protein is substituted by fresh-frozen plasma and albumin. The onset of bile production and a decrease in lactate values are initial signs that the transplant is functioning well. In addition, factor V and thromboplastin time generally increase. Occasionally, ascites can occur. (388) From the seventh day, the transaminases fall steadily. Antibiotic prophylaxis, which began during surgery, is usually discontinued on the second or third day. Oral and bodily hygiene as well as monitoring of infection are also part of the intensive-care programme. Special surveillance protocols have been carefully designed for this purpose.

Immunosuppression

Induction and adjustment of immunosuppression follow established protocols, which can, however, be executed in various ways. New immunosuppressants are meanwhile in use (tacrolimus, sirolimus, mycophenolate mofetile, brequinar, leflunomide, etc.). Cyclosporine and tacrolimus include a calcineurine inhibitor. Initially, the patients receive *triple therapy*: tacrolimus (or cyclosporine) + prednisolone + mycophenolate, occasionally with interleukin-2 receptor antagonist (e.g. basiliximab, diclizumab). • After three months, the patient is given *dual therapy*, generally with tacrolimus (or cyclosporine) + prednisolone or with tacrolimus + mycophenolate; after a further six months, the patient is put on *monotherapy* with tacrolimus (or cyclosporine). During dual therapy, the dosage of prednisolone is reduced slowly until the drug is ultimately discontinued (except in cases with AIH as an underlying disease). (426) • In patients with HCC, immunosuppression based on rapamycin has often proved more efficacious, and appears to have an antitumourigenic effect. • The monitoring of tacrolimus (or cyclosporine) is carried out at regular intervals using the respective values in the blood. • Long-term follow-up is performed by the family doctor or internal specialist and, at certain intervals, by the outpatient department of the transplantation centre. (394) • The **toxicity** of immunosuppressive agents is the main cause of complications (e.g. hypertension, kidney damage and even kidney failure, severe headaches, altered blood values, nervousness, trembling, peripheral paraesthesia, increase in liver enzymes). Such toxicity-related complications may also be due to **interactions** between cyclosporine and other drugs. Differential diagnosis of transplant rejection may prove difficult.

Tolerance: Donor cells have sometimes been detected in the blood of liver transplant recipients. This chimerism may influence the immune system of the host with development of tolerance to donor tissue. (440) That would mean that a donor liver might, in some cases, be spontaneously accepted. As a result, it is possible to stop the administration of immunosuppressants. • Usually, after five-year survival of a primary graft, one third of all patients are able to cease immunotherapy.

Complications

Major complications after LT include (*1.*) non-function of primary graft (1st–2nd day), (*2.*) infection (3rd–14th day, and longer), and (*3.*) rejection (5th–10th day). The clinical features of these complications are similar:

▶ liver	• fever
– large	• leucocytosis
– firm	• jaundice
– tender on pressure	

Such findings require immediate and extensive examination: US, Doppler sonography, CT, HIDA scintigraphy, and cholangiography. • Further complications are (*1.*) afterbleeding (10–15%), (*2.*) portal vein thrombosis (up to 2.2%) or hepatic vein occlusion, (*3.*) hepatic artery thrombosis or stenosis, (*4.*) pleural effusion, and (*5.*) subcapsular necrosis (due to the disproportionate size of donor and recipient liver). Stenosing of the suprahepatic vena cava is a particularly dangerous condition, which can lead to ALF. • The most frequent complication affects the **biliary system** in the form of leaks or strictures (5—25% of cases). They can be diagnosed with the help of T-drain radiology or ERC. (409)

Infection

One of the major problems following LT and immunosuppression are infections. During the early postoperative phase, the danger of **bacterial** or **fungal infection** is particularly great due to high-dosage immunosuppression and intensive medical care at a time when the patient's physical condition is considerably impaired. Monitoring of infection, accompanied by optimal hygiene and prophylactic measures, is required as well as (possibly) immediate treatment with antibiotics. In order to avoid translocation of gram-negative microorganisms, decontamination of the intestinal tract, already initiated in the preoperative phase, is often continued; in addition, the use of an antimycotic agent is recommended (e.g. against candidiasis or coccidioidomycosis). (399, 401, 425, 438) • **Viral infections** are most frequent two to four months after LT. A particular danger, both in adults and children, may come from new infection with or reactivation of CMV (431, 439), EBV, herpes-6 virus, varicella-zoster or Listeria monocytogenes. (406) CMV infection is associated with a higher rate of rejection. Early diagnosis (by PCR) and early treatment (e.g. intravenous ganciclovir) are required. Of the various viral infections, especially condylomas caused by papilloma viruses are to be feared in the long term, since a high percentage of them can develop into squamous-cell carcinoma. A new form of treatment with *imiquimod* may prove effective.

Transplant rejection

Hyperacute form: Transplant rejection may occur as an antibody-related complication within a short period of time after LT (= humoral rejection). This rare event is caused by donor antigens coming into contact with preformed antibodies in the recipient, which results in damage to the endothelial cells of the arteries with vascular occlusion. The outcome is necrosis of the transplant.

Acute form: This condition appears in the first three postoperative weeks. Some 40—60% of patients have one or even several rejection reactions of varying intensity, accompanied by discomfort, fever, exhaustion and, occasionally, mild jaundice. Early diagnosis is only possible by detecting an increase in liver enzymes, particularly GDH; the diagnosis is confirmed histologically. Percutaneous biopsy should be carried out with antibiotic protection. (405) Histology reveals the presence of large lymphocytes, plasma cells, macrophages and granulocytes in the portal fields in this type of cellular reaction. The interlobular bile ducts are damaged, and there is subsequent cholestasis. It is possible to observe adherence of lymphocytes to the venous and arterial endothelium, resulting in subendothelial inflammation (= **endothelialitis**). (s. fig. 40.9) • *Therapy* is based on prednisolone (500 mg i.v. for 3 days). In cases showing no reaction, the dosage of tacrolimus should be increased, and, occasionally, mycophenolate (2 x 1g/day) or rapamycin can be added. In non-responders, therapy with OKT3 is recommended (after histology has shown persistent rejection). Thus, an acute rejection does not pose a risk for long-term prognosis. In most cases, drug therapy is successful and without morphological residues. (383) • *Retransplantation* is seldom necessary.

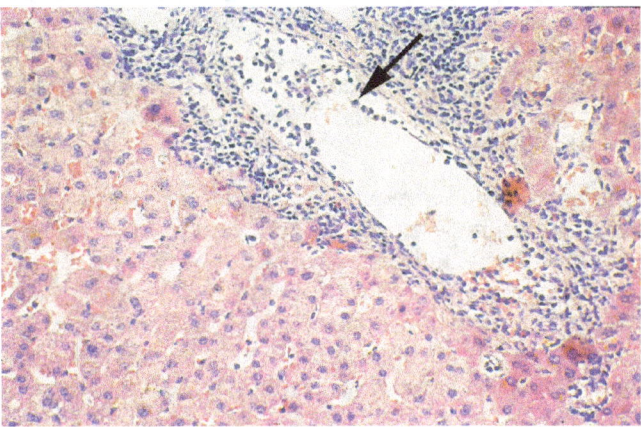

Fig. 40.9: Acute rejection: portal/periportal inflammation and portovenous endothelialitis (↓) (HE)

Chronic form: This condition is no longer observed very often (2—3%). It usually sets in one to nine months after LT and is characterized by progressive cholestasis. This form may develop after repeated acute attacks or develop insidiously from the beginning. There is a ductopenic reaction, whereby the interlobular bile ducts are infiltrated and destroyed by mononuclear cells; ultimately, the bile ducts disappear. Duct loss can be calculated from the ratio of the number of hepatic arteries to the number of bile ducts within a portal field (normal = > 0.7), whereby 20 portal fields should be examined. At the same time, obliterating arteritis develops, with fibrinoid wall necrosis and deposition of foam cells within the intima. (414) The result is portal and periportal fibrosis. (s. fig. 40.10) Differential diagnosis is difficult

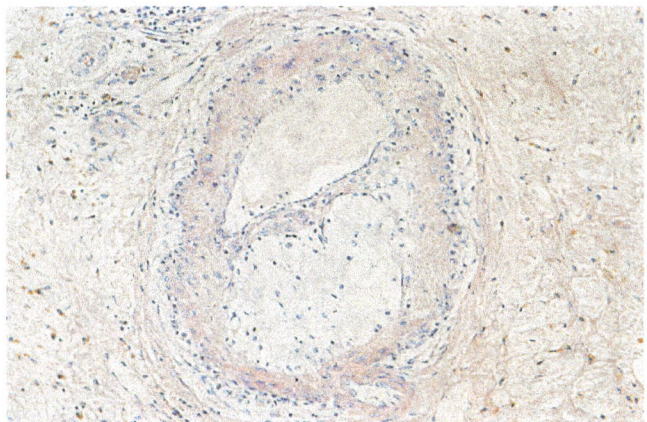

Fig. 40.10: Chronic rejection: stenosing foamy cell arteriopathy (HE)

and may require repeated biopsies. Chronic rejection can be graded histologically in a mild, moderate or severe form. (418) • *Therapy* with tacrolimus halted progression in some cases. Tacrolimus and mycophenolate may generally bring about a reduction in the chronic rejection response. Should the treatment fail, the only alternative is *retransplantation*. In this case, an elective indication for retransplantation is given, since liver functions remain intact for a relatively long time. • In acute and chronic rejection accompanied by an increase in alkaline phosphatase, *ursodeoxycholic acid* should be used as supportive therapy. • With regard to unclarified **complicative situations,** it is essential to determine the level of immunosuppressants in the blood (underdosage? toxicity?). Subsequently, US, colour-encoded duplex sonography, CT and MRI are indicated. Radiology-dependent interventions may be required.

Retransplantation is required in 5–10% of patients. The main indications are primary graft failure, hepatic arterial thrombosis and chronic rejection. • Results of retransplantation are not so satisfactory as with the first LT: the survival rate is shorter and mortality (usually due to sepsis) is mostly within six months. Nevertheless, the prognosis is improving steadily. (427)

Relapse of the underlying disease

Some 25% of hepatocellular and up to 70% of cholangiocellular **carcinomas** are subject to relapse within 12 months. Tumour relapse is caused by the presence of undetected extrahepatic metastases, which find their way back into the transplanted liver, and on the suppressed state of the immune system. According to some observations, the probability of relapse depends on the stage of the primary tumour. For this reason, only (selected) early tumour stages are a possible indication for LT. (s. fig. 40.10) • Reinfection of the transplant occurs in 80–100% of cases due to **hepatitis B** from extrahepatic reservoirs, most likely in the early postoperative (low-defence) stage. Of these cases, about 15% follow a fulminant course, about 15% show persistent hepatitis, 5% reach chronic carrier stage, and 20–25% develop fibrosing cholestatic hepatitis with a high rate of viral replication and an unfavourable course. (385) In some patients with severe reinfection, cirrhosis can develop within a few years. **HDV infection** may lead to a similar outcome. With such a negative outlook, it is important to consider every possibility of avoiding reinfection. The prophylaxis is based on HBIG (10,000 IU intraoperatively and then daily) + lamivudine until HBsAg has disappeared from the serum. In this way, the risk of reinfection can be reduced to 10–20%. (s. p. 725) Should reinfection nevertheless occur (renewed evidence of HBsAg), new nucleoside analogues (e.g. adefovir, entecavir, tenofir) are available under certain conditions. (381) • In **hepatitis C,** the transplant is reinfected in 90–100% of cases, although only about half the patients display HCV antibodies when immunosuppressives are administered. HCV replication occurs already in the first week after LT. The infection follows a mild course both in terms of clinical findings and morphology; fulminant or cholestatic courses are rare. In 10–30% of patients, chronic hepatitis, or even cirrhosis, appears. Nevertheless, in view of the great effort involved in performing an LT, the use of peg IFN-α with ribavirin, and occasionally in combination with amantadine, must be considered. (s. p. 723) (395, 399, 410, 419, 427, 439) • **HGV infection** (generally a result of numerous blood transfusions!) is of no clinical significance. (400) • **Alcoholic liver disease** is followed by relapse within two years in about 20% of cases. (421) • Relapses have been observed following **primary biliary cholangitis** (404, 437) or **primary sclerosing cholangitis** (< 5%) (396, 407), **autoimmune hepatitis** (despite immunosuppression in 10–30%) (382, 413), **BCS** (without anticoagulant in 100%) and **non-alcoholic steatohepatitis.** (415)

7.7 Aftercare and rehabilitation

LT patients need seven to ten days in an intensive care unit and about three weeks in a normal ward of the hospital. The patient is usually fully rehabilitated after six months. Subsequent to inpatient treatment, *follow-up therapy* is carried out at a **rehabilitation clinic** which is specialized in hepatology. Generally, this stationary rehabilitation phase lasts four to six weeks and includes various **tasks** and **objectives**. (s. tab. 40.17)

Risk of infection: Patients are subject to a high risk of infection at public events, when using public transport, and particularly during waves of influenza. Interdigital mycosis also presents an infection risk. A further problem can derive from indoor plants (beware of fungal spores in potting compost!). Domestic animals similarly constitute a risk factor; it is of great importance that no

---

1. Step-by-step reorientation of the individual patient from the clinical atmosphere to the more "normal" daily routine in a rehabilitation centre. Medical follow-ups, including monitoring of the immunosuppressive adjustment.
2. Gradual social and cultural reintegration within the rehabilitation community.
3. Detailed information for the patient regarding personal hygiene, nutrition, lifestyle, significance of aftercare, recognizing complaints or abnormalities, etc.
4. Improvement in the patient's nutritional state.
5. General physiotherapeutic measures; targeted training of the muscle groups atrophied to a varying extent in the individual patient.
6. Psychotherapeutic support (particularly in how to handle the fear of complications), opportunities for psychosocial care, discussion of questions relating to the patient's occupation, etc.

Tab. 40.18: Tasks and objectives of aftercare and rehabilitation in specialized clinics

new pets are introduced. Towels and bed linen must be changed regularly. Shower water, which is usually heated to 60 °C in the boiler, should be run for an extended period two to three times a week in order to prevent legionellosis. Vaccinations with live vaccines should be avoided. Intake of tap water and non-pasteurized milk is forbidden as these liquids have a high bacteria count. Lettuce and vegetables need to be washed several times and with particular care. Fruit that is difficult to clean (raspberries, etc.) should not be eaten; preference is to be given to fruit which can be peeled. Raw steak tartare must not be consumed. • These numerous recommendations and warnings are not designed to create hysteria, but to help minimize the risk of infection at a realistic and, for the patient, comprehensible level.

Nutrition: The patient's diet should comply with the basic principles of physiological nutrition. (429) It is recommended to take three main and two minor meals per day. Foodstuffs causing flatulence and containing poorly digestible fats (e. g. lard) must be avoided. It is important to consider the influence of glucocorticoids on appetite as well as their metabolic side effects (e. g. restriction of sodium chloride, loss of potassium).

Medical aftercare: This comprises adjusting and monitoring *immunosuppressants*, providing the patient with all necessary information as well as recognizing and controlling side effects. • Occasionally, *pleural effusion* has to be monitored and, if necessary, aspirated. *Ascites*, often evident as a local accumulation of fluid in the abdomen, may still be present. • Sometimes, *wound care*, treatment of postoperative wound complications or removal of a T-drainage, generally after six weeks, may still be required. • The *renal function* needs to be monitored carefully, even if there is no obvious progressive renal damage. • The *vascular system* (portal vein, inferior vena cava, hepatic artery) has to be checked by colour-encoded duplex sonography for the occurrence of thromboses, stenoses or aneurysms. Bile leakage or stenoses may appear in the *bile ducts*. • In 60—80% of patients, *hypertension* can be anticipated due to treatment with cyclosporin. In 20—30% of cases (more often with tacrolimus than with cyclosporine), *diabetes mellitus* or *hypercholesterolaemia* develops. • *Fatigue* is indeed a major and often difficult treatable problem. (441)

If this wide spectrum of sophisticated rehabilitation measures is carried out with great care — and with success — fewer problems will arise in the aftercare of outpatients when they return to their normal daily routine. The *length of stay* at a specialized clinic should be tailored to the patient's individual needs; on average, this lasts four to six weeks. In view of the high costs involved in LT and the great inconvenience to which the patient is subjected, the rehabilitation phase assumes an essential role; follow-up therapy is thus both necessary and recommended for achieving long-term survival and improved quality of life with reintegration into the work process.

Inpatient monitoring is succeeded by **outpatient control protocols**. The check-ups are carried out by the family doctor or internist in close cooperation with the transplantation centre. • The one-year survival rate after liver transplantation is 80—95%. The five-year survival rate varies depending on the underlying disease, e. g. 70—80% in cirrhotic patients, 45—50% in acute liver failure, and 35% in malignancies. (408) About two-thirds of the patients begin working again despite a long phase of being unable to work due to chronic liver disease. Most liver transplant recipients are very satisfied with their newly acquired quality of life. (420, 421)

8 Sociomedical aspects

Health awareness on the part of the individual as well as *preventive* and *rehabilitative medicine* in general are exerting more and more influence on developments in the medical world — and thus also on hepatology. These changes in medical practice are an inevitable and characteristic feature of a modern society. • Consequently, physicians will need to devote more attention to *"prevention"* in the healthy person in order to keep the curative phase of an illness as short as possible. And to an increasing degree, they will also have to undertake *"rehabilitation"* in order to reduce to a tolerable minimum any periods in which the individual cannot perform efficiently and is also unfit for work. (s. fig. 40.11)

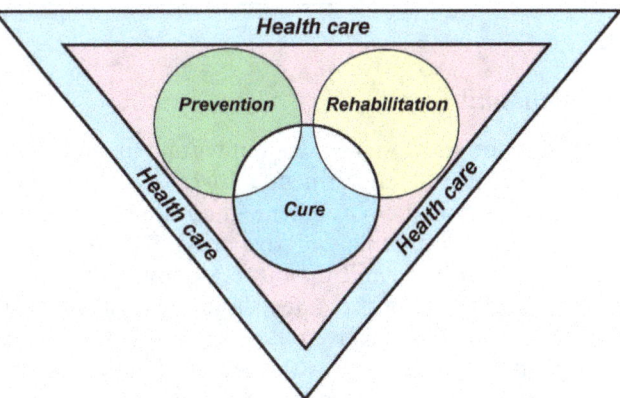

Fig. 40.11: Combination of prevention and rehabilitation in health awareness

8.1 Health awareness

▶ This term subsumes all factors which reduce potential damage to health. These include protective measures promoted by the state, various authorized institutions and associations as well as by industry, science and the medical professions. Above all, however, every individual should assume personal responsibility for maintaining his or her state of health through appropriate behaviour. • *The media must also accept a vital role in this context!*

> **Health awareness with regard to hepatology**
>
> - Healthy diet and normal body weight
> - Hygiene concerning drinking water and food
> - Physical/muscular fitness
> - No alcohol abuse
>   No medication abuse
>   No drugs
> - Avoidance of occupation-related damage
> - Prevention of infections by observing basic hygiene

8.2 Preventive medicine

These are health measures which are carried out by individuals of their own accord, sponsored by the state, accepted by medical insurance companies, and basically feasible; they enable monitoring and preservation of health as well as early recognition of diseases.

> **Prevention with regard to hepatology**
>
> - Prophylactic vaccinations
> - Safe blood transfusions
>   Safe blood products
> - Prevention of infections
>   (antibacterial and antiparasitic measures)
> - Occupation-related measures
> - Regular medical check-ups

8.3 Rehabilitation

Rehabilitation is designed to reintegrate people with physical or mental impairment into both their professional and personal environment. It comprises aftercare with a social component in the sense that society is called upon to help, and thus it is a communal undertaking. Rehabilitative measures should start as early as possible during the curative phase. Once the disease has consolidated and as soon as the prognosis offers a realistic perspective, the physician should address the question of rehabilitation. The necessity for rehabilitation depends on the severity of the symptoms and/or the psychosocial problems involved.

The indications for **medical rehabilitation** are subject to strict legal stipulations. First of all, an expertise including a detailed medical evaluation is required from a physician. In rehabilitation centres specialized in hepatology, all necessary interdisciplinary diagnostic and therapeutic measures are applied. It is important that the rehabilitee cooperates actively.

Measures necessary for **occupational rehabilitation** are initiated at the same time. These include options for vocational retraining and additional qualifications, redesigning the workplace to fit the needs of the handicapped person, reintegration into the work process, personal support, etc. Occupational rehabilitation also depends on the rehabilitee being adequately motivated. Furthermore, it is important to evaluate individual vocational preferences and prospects of success. Job-related psychological and aptitude tests together with measures aimed at finding a suitable job must be carried out before a final decision can be made.

> **Rehabilitation with regard to hepatology**
>
> - Adjustment to disease-dependent changes in lifestyle
>   - special diets (e.g. low iron, low copper, MCT)
>   - administration of medication (e.g. interferon, immunosuppressants, penicillamine, UDCA)
> - Introduction of secondary prevention
>   - elimination of risk factors (alcohol abuse, overweight, faulty nutrition, *etc.*)
>   - vaccination prophylaxis
> - Information about particular risks
>   - hepatic encephalopathy, water retention, variceal bleeding, side effects of medication, *etc.*
> - Muscular/physical exercise
> - Psychological guidance for liver transplantees
> - Assessment of the individual's remaining capacity for everyday life
> - Introduction of occupational rehabilitation measures

▶ Altogether, the measures and objectives of our time do justice to the demands made by RITTER VON BUSS (a German specialist in constitutional law) who coined the term **rehabilitation** in 1844 with the words:

"The diseased who can be cured shall be completely rehabilitated, he shall rise again to the position from which he has descended, he shall regain the feeling of personal dignity and thus a new life."

8.4 Capacity for work

A positive and negative profile of a patient's capacity for performing certain tasks should be compiled on the basis of the respective disease phase. For the rehabilitation process, it is important to assess the remaining capacity of the individual in combination with any personal strengths. In addition, liver function and potential health risks have to be considered. The medical evaluation of the patient's capacity for work forms the basis for the respective sociolegal decision. It should be noted, however, that the medical expertise and the legal decision are independent of each other — such legal terms as *"incapacity for work"* or *"inability to practise the learned profession"* must be avoided in the medical report. • Capacity for work also includes *fitness to drive a vehicle* (e.g. in encephalopathy) or *fitness for public service* (e.g. in the educational or judicial sector). In severe cases of advanced liver disease, evaluation is not difficult. However, this is not so easy in less severe cases (e.g. diffuse fibrosis, no complications) or low-grade to moderate inflammatory processes. Objectivation of the findings is only possible by extensive diagnostic clarification of the function and morphology of the liver — as well as of other affected organs.

The physician's assessment of a patient's capacity for work considers individual factors in a certain type of liver disease and thus forms the basis for determining (*1.*) **unfitness for work**, (*2.*) **inability to practise the learned profession**, and (*3.*) **inability to earn** within the sociolegal framework of the country concerned. This involves reviewing the overall situation in a concrete manner, i.e. if there is a workplace available that is appropriate to the patient's capacity for work. Pension allowances paid due to inability to practise the learned profession are generally lower than those paid due to unfitness for work. Assessment of the inability to earn does not depend on whether the person has recently worked or on current job prospects. It should be noted that clearly defined standards of assessment are required under pension law. For accident insurance, severe disability and social compensation, the principle of abstract damage assessment applies. Inability to practise the learned profession and inability to earn must be permanent. All indications for rehabilitation have to be checked carefully and with regard to the relevant conditions. **Unfitness for public service** is a term generally used for civil servants, but it also applies to soldiers and persons doing community work.

The hepatological diagnosis should be as accurate as possible, so that the physician is able to assess the (positive and negative) capacity profile. In this connection, the insured person is not obliged to tolerate **invasive examinations** (e.g. laparoscopy, percutaneous liver biopsy). However, the risk of underestimating the reduction in earning capacity can be detrimental for the individual. Moreover, the possibility of *further deterioration of a disease* is not included in an assessment; thus a follow-up report may be required after a certain time.

The original International Classification of Impairment, Disability and Handicap (ICIDH) has been revised as the International Classification of Functioning (ICF). This new classification requires a precise description of the disease-related impairments of the individual patient. Subjective complaints should be considered although they cannot, of course, be evaluated objectively. Aggravations must be treated with caution.

> **Objective assessment** can be based on clinical findings (s. fig. 4.21), enzymatic and mesenchymal activity (s. tabs. 5.15; 5.23), serological or immunological findings (s. tabs. 5.17; 5.20), and liver function tests (s. tab. 5.14), (s. fig. 5.2). Ultrasound, colour-encoded Doppler sonography, elastography or even CT give an impression of the morphological structure of the liver, especially in cases where patients refuse to have a biopsy. The assessment programme should also contain psychometric tests. (s. pp 210–214)

The term **reduction in earning capacity** is used in civil law to assess claims payments. It denotes the difference between the income earned before the accident happened and afterwards, i.e. the actual and proven pecuniary loss is determined.

The term (severe) **disability** was defined by the World Health Organisation (WHO) in 1980. It contains guidelines for protecting severely disabled persons by law. The principle of abstract damage assessment applies when determining the degree of disability. A small part of the labour market should be kept open for severely disabled persons.

The above statements only serve as general criteria for a physician's evaluation of patients with liver disease. More detailed information is usually available from the insurance provider. Thus it is desirable that medical practitioners cooperate closely with sociomedical specialists, making it possible to deal directly with any application for compensation, disability pension, etc.

Although there are **guidelines** for evaluating the reduction in earning capacity, the actual degree of disability may be assessed differently depending on the existing disease. In the individual case, the physician can propose percentage values concerning the disability which are higher or lower than the recommended rate. • The assessment of chronic hepatitis B and C is of great importance (H. SELMAIR et al., 1998), and it should be made according to the aetiological-morphological nomenclature. (s. pp 714–716) (s. tab. 40.18)

Altogether, **three criteria** are important in the assessment of a liver disease:

> 1. its effects on the patient's capacity for work
> 2. its connection with a specific damaging event
> 3. its rehabilitation potential

Medical evaluations are simply opinions of an advisory nature; they have to be assessed by administrative and legal experts before a final decision can be made. • The physician, however, is responsible for the medical determination of a disease and the resulting diagnosis of *unfitness for work*.

Functional hyperbilirubinaemia	0–10%
Acute viral hepatitis	100%
Asymptomatic HBsAg carrier status	0%
Chronic active hepatitis	
– low inflammatory activity	20–30%
– moderate inflammatory activity	30–40%
– severe inflammatory activity	50–70%
– fibrosis (low → severe)	20–60%
Scarred liver without complications (depending on the functional reduction)	20–40%
Chronic cholangitis	20–100%
Fatty liver disease	0–10%
– with hepatitis (low → severe)	20–100%
Fatty cirrhosis	40–100%
Cirrhosis, compensated	
– inactive (stable)	40%
– moderately active	50%
– distinctly active	60–100%
with severe functional reduction	80–100%
with shunt surgery	60–100%
Cirrhosis, decompensated	80–100%
Liver lobe resection	> 50%
Tumour resection	100%
Liver transplantation (after consolidation lasting two years with 100% DOD/REC, and later on no less than 60%)	100%
Primary liver cell carcinoma (within the first five years of consolidation, the REC remains at 100%)	100%

Tab. 40.19: Guidelines for assessing reduction in earning capacity (REC) and degree of disability (DOD) in liver diseases. • If the hepatological picture cannot be classified in relation to a diagnosis shown in the above table, it should be described and classified according to its functional disturbances in line with the above diagnoses

8.5 Self-help groups

In most countries, there are numerous self-help groups for liver patients. Participation in such self-help groups is generally beneficial. They are highly valued for their constant availability and their counselling competence. As a rule, the patient can remain anonymous and all counselling is strictly confidential. Moreover, this useful service is offered free of charge. Self-help groups provide the participants with information on all important topics (including the latest developments) by means of printed material, special meetings and reports in the media; in addition, they facilitate a mutual exchange of experience among the patients.

References:

Clinical studies
1. **Brown, R.S.:** Strategies and pitfalls in quality of life research. Hepatology 1999; 29 (Suppl.): 9–12
2. **Bull, J.P.:** The historical development of clinical therapeutic trials. J. Chron. Dis. 1959; 10: 218–248
3. **Burkhardt, R., Kienle, G.:** Controlled trials. A social challenge. Eur. J. Clin. Pharmacol. 1981; 20: 311–319
4. **De Craen, A.J.M., Kaptchuk, T.J., Tijssen, J.G.P., Kleijnen, J.:** Placebos and placebo effects in medicine: historical overview. J. Royal Soc. Med. 1999; 92: 511–515
5. **De Dombal, F.T.:** The controlled, randomized clinical trial – sacred duty or sacred cow? Klin. Wschr. 1980; 58: 649–652
6. **Hill, A.B.:** Principles of medical statistics. The Lancer Lim. London, 1937
7. **Imperiale, T.R.:** Meta-Analysis: when and how. Hepatology 1999; 29 (Suppl. 1): 26–31
8. **Martini, P.:** Methodenlehre der therapeutischen Untersuchung. (in German) Verlag J. Springer, Berlin, 1932, 69 pages, 9 figures
9. **Ohmann, C., Albrecht, J.:** Lessons to be learned for gastroenterology from recent issues in clinical trial methodology. Can. J. Gastroenterol. 2000; 14: 293–298
10. **Rosner, F.:** The ethics of randomized clinical trials. Amer. J. Med. 1987; 82: 283–290
11. **Sackett, D.L., Gent, M.:** Controversy in counting and attributing events in clinical trials. New Engl. J. Med. 1979; 301: 1410–1412
12. **Spiegelhalter, D.J.:** Statistical issues in studies of individual response. Scand. J. Gastroenterol. 1988; 23: 40–45

Principles of liver therapy
13. **Bayliss, M.S.:** Methods in outcomes research in hepatology: definition and domains of quality of life. Hepatology 1999; 29 (Suppl. 1): 3–6
14. **Foster, G.R., Goldin, R.D., Thomas, H.C.:** Chronic hepatitis C virus infection causes a significant reduction in quality of life in the absence of cirrhosis. Hepatology 1998; 27: 209–212
15. **Kamath, P.S., Kim, W.R.:** The model for endstage liver disease (MELD). Hepatology 2007; 45: 797–805
16. **Kuntz, E.:** Fundamental and contemporary views on the therapy of liver diseases. (in German) Med. Welt 1991; 42: 668–673
17. **Malinchoc, M., Kamath, P.S., Gordon, F.D., Peine, C.J., Rank, J., Borg, P.C.:** A model to predict poor survival in patients undergoing transjugular intrahepatic portosystemic shunts. Hepatology 2000; 31: 864–871
18. **Propst, A., Propst, T., Zangerl, G., Öfner, D., Judmaier, G., Vogel, W.:** Prognosis life expectancy in chronic liver disease. Dig. Dis. Sci. 1995; 40: 1805–1815
19. **Younossi, Z.M., Boparai, N., McCormick, M., Price, L.L., Guyatt, G.:** Assessment of utilities and health-related quality of life in patients with chronic liver disease. Amer. J. Gastroenterol. 2001; 96: 579–583

Nutritional therapy of liver diseases
20. **Alpers, D.H.:** Liver complications and failure in patients on home parenteral nutrition. Gastroenterology 2001; 17: 147–149
21. **Baker, A.L., Rosenberg, I.H.:** Hepatic complications of total parenteral nutrition. Amer. J. Med. 1987; 82: 489–497
22. **Bories, P.N., Campillo, B.:** One-month regular oral nutrition in alcoholic cirrhotic patients. Changes of nutritional status, hepatic function and serum lipid pattern. Brit. J. Nutr. 1994; 72: 937–946
23. **Buchman, A.L., Ament, M.E., Sohel, M., Dubin, M., Jenden, D.J., Roch, M., Pownall, H., Farley, W., Awal, M., Ahn, C.:** Choline deficiency causes reversible hepatic abnormalities in patients receiving parenteral nutrition: Proof of a human choline requirement: A placebo-controlled trial. J. Parenter. Enter. Nutr. 2001; 25: 260–268
24. **Campillo, B., Richardet, J.P., Bories, P.N.:** Validation of body mass index for the diagnosis of malnutrition in patients with liver cirrhosis. Gastroenterol. Clin. Biol. 2006; 30: 1137–1143
25. **Crawford, D.H.G., Cuneo, R.C., Shepherd, R.W.:** Pathogenesis and assessment of malnutrition in liver disease. J. Gastroenterol. Hepatol. 1993; 8: 89–94
26. **Fan, S.T.:** Nutritional support for patients with cirrhosis (review). J. Gastroenterol. Hepatol. 1997; 12: 282–286
27. **Gaddipati, K., Yang, P.:** Hepatobiliary complications of parenteral nutrition. Gastroenterologist 1996; 4: 98–106
28. **Guglielmi, F.W., Boggio-Bertinet, D., Federico, A., Forte, G.B., Guglielmi, A., Loguercio, C., Mazzuoli, S., Merli, M., Palmo, A., Panella, C., Pironi, L., Francavilla, A.:** Total parenteral nutrition-related gastroenterological complications (review). Dig. Liver Dis. 2006; 387: 623–642
29. **Hasse, J.M., Blue, L.S., Liepa, G.V., Goldstein, R.M., Jennings, L.W., Mor, E., Husberg, B.S., Levy, M.F., Gonwa, T.A., Klintman, G.B.:** Early enteral nutrition support in patients undergoing liver transplantation. J. Parenter. Enter. Nutr. 1995; 19: 437–443
30. **Henkel, A.S., Buchman, A.L.:** Nutritional support in patients with chronic liver disease. Nat. Clin. Pract. Gastroenterol. Hepatol. 2006; 3: 202–209
31. **Kearns, P.J., Young, H., Garcia, G., Blaschke, T., O'Hanlon, G., Rinki, M., Sucher, K., Gregory, P.:** Accelerated improvement of alcoholic liver disease with enteral nutrition. Gastroenterology 1992; 102: 200–205
32. **Kestell, M.F., Lee, S.P.:** Clinical nutrition in acute and chronic liver disease. Semin. Gastrointest. Dis. 1993; 4: 116–126

33. **Lautz, H.U., Selberg, O., Körber, J., Bürger, M., Müller, M.J.:** Forms of malnutrition in patients with liver cirrhosis. Clin. Invest. 1992; 70: 478–486
34. **Leonard, J.V.:** The nutritional management of urea cycle disorders. J. Pediatr. 2001; 138: 40–44
35. **Marsano, L.S., Martin, A.E., Randall, H.B.:** Current nutrition in liver disease. Curr. Opin. Gastroenterol. 2002; 18: 246–253
36. **McCullough, A.J.:** Malnutrition in liver disease. Liver Transplant. 2000; 6 (Suppl. 1): 85–96
37. **Moriwaki, H.:** Nutritional assessment in liver cirrhosis (editorial). J. Gastroenterol. 2006; 41: 511–512
38. **Müller, M.J., Böttcher, J., Selberg, O.:** Energy expenditure and substrate metabolism in liver cirrhosis. Intern. J. Obes. 1993; 17 (Suppl. 3): 102–106
39. **Nielsen, K., Kondrup, J., Martinsen, L., Dossing, H., Larsson, B., Stilling, B., Jensen, M.G.:** Long-term oral refeeding of patients with cirrhosis of the liver. Brit. J. Nutrit. 1995; 74: 557–567
40. **Sarin, S.K., Dhingra, N., Bansal, A., Malhotra, S., Guptan, R.C.:** Dietary and nutritional abnormalities in alcoholic liver disease: a comparison with chronic alcoholics without liver disease. Amer. J. Gastroenterol. 1997; 92: 777–783
41. **Siriboonkoom, W., Gramlich, L.:** Nutrition and chronic liver disease. Can. J. Gastroenterol. 1998; 12: 201–207
42. **Wang, H., Khaoustov, V.I., Krishnan, B., Cai, W., Stoll, B., Burrin, D.G., Yoffe, B.:** Total parenteral nutrition induces liver steatosis and apoptosis in neonatal piglets. J. Nutrit. 2006; 136: 2547–2552

Interferon
43. **Bruno, R., Sacchi, P., Ciappina, V., Zochetti, C., Patruno, S., Maiocchi, L., Filice, G.:** Viral dynamics and pharmacokinetics of peginterferon alpha-2a and peginterferon alpha-2b in naïve patients with chronic hepatitis C: a randomized, controlled study. Antiviral Ther. 2004; 9: 491–497
44. **Dianzani, F.:** Biological basis for the clinical use of interferon. Gut 1993; 34 (Suppl. 2): 74–76
45. **Foster, G.R.:** Review article: Pegylated interferons: chemical and clinical differences. Aliment. Pharmacol. Ther. 2004; 20: 825–830
46. **Isaacs, A., Lindenmann, J.:** Virus interference: I The interferon. Proc. Royal Soc. (London) 1957; 147: 258–267
47. **Ito, Y., Takeda, N., Ishimori, M., Akai, A., Miura, K., Yasuda, K.:** Effects of long-term interferon-alpha treatment on glucose tolerance in patients with chronic hepatitis C. J. Hepatol. 1999; 31: 215–220
48. **Peters, M.:** Mechanisms of action of interferons. Semin. Liver Dis. 1989; 9: 235–239
49. **Renauld, P.F., Hoofnagle, J.H.:** Side effects of alpha interferon. Semin. Liver Dis. 1989; 9: 273–277
50. **Shakil, A.O., DiBisceglie, A.M., Hoofnagle, J.H.:** Seizures during interferon therapy. J. Hepatol. 1996; 24: 48–51
51. **Thomas, H., Foster, G., Platis, D.:** Mechanisms of action of interferon and nucleoside analogues. J. Hepatol. 2003; 39 (Suppl. 1): 93–09
52. **Zeuzem, S., Welsch, C., Herrmann, E.:** Pharmacokinetics of peginterferons. Semin. Liver Dis. 2003; 23 (Suppl. 1): 23–28

Nucleoside analogues
53. **Bacon, T.H.:** Famciclovir, from the bench to the patient – a comprehensive review of the preclinical data. Int. J. Antimicrobiol. Agents 1996; 7: 119–134
54. **Colledge, D., Locarnini, S., Shaw, T.:** Synergistic inhibition of hepadnaviral replication by lamivudine in combination with penciclovir in vitro. Hepatology 1997; 26: 216–225
55. **Glue, P.:** The clinical pharmacology of ribavirin. Semin. Liver Dis. 1999; 19 (Suppl. 1): 17–24
56. **Korba, M., Gerin, J.L.:** Use of standardized cell culture assay to assess activities of nucleoside analogs against hepatitis B virus replication. Antiviral Res. 1992; 19: 55–75
57. **Pawlothsky, J.-M., Dahari, H., Neumann, A.U., Hezode, C., Germanidis, G., Lonjon, I., Castera, L., Dhumeaux, D.:** Antiviral action of ribavirin in chronic hepatitis C. Gastroenterology 2004; 126: 703–714
58. **Schalm, S.W., de Man, R.A., Heijtink, R.A., Niesters, H.G.M.:** New nucleoside analogues for chronic hepatitis B. J. Hepatol. 1995; 22 (Suppl. 1): 52–56
59. **Tam, R.C., Lau, J.Y.N., Hong, Z.:** Mechanisms of action of ribavirin in antiviral therapies. Antiviral Chem. Chemother. 2002; 12: 261–272
60. **Yuen, G.J., Morris, D.M., Mydlow, P.K., Haidar, S., Hall, S.T., Hussey, E.K.:** Pharmacokinetics, absolute bioavailability, and absorption characteristics of lamivudine. J. Clin. Pharmacol. 1995; 35: 1174–1180
61. **Zoulim, F., Trepo, C.:** Nucleoside analogs in the treatment of chronic viral hepatitis. Efficacy and complications. J. Hepatol. 1994; 21: 142–144

Immunosuppressants
62. **Anstey, A., Lear, J.T.:** Azathioprine. Clinical pharmacology and curent indications in autoimmune disorders. BioDrugs 1998; 9: 33–47
63. **Casanovas Taltavull, T.:** Impact of cyclosporine on the development of immunosuppressive therapy in liver transplantation. Transplant. Proc. 2004; 36 (Suppl. 1): 291–294
64. **Fung, J.J., Eliasziw, M., Todo, S., Jain, A., Demetris, A.J., McMichael, J.P., Starzl, T.E., Meier, P., Donner, A.:** The Pittsburgh randomized trial of tacrolimus compared to cyclosporine for hepatic transplantation. J. Amer. Coll. Surg. 1996; 183: 117–125
65. **Jonas, S., Neuhaus, R., Junge, G., Klu, J., Theruvat, T., Langrehr, J.M., Settmacher, U., Neuhaus, P.:** Primary immunosuppression with tacrolimus after liver transplantation: 12-years follow-up. Internat. Immunopharm. 2005; 5: 125–128
66. **Mackay, I.R., Weiden, S., Ungar, B.:** Treatment of active chronic hepatitis with 6-mercaptopurine and azathioprine. Lancet 1964/I: 899–902
67. **Pratschke, J., Neuhaus, R., Tullius, S.G., Haller, G.W., Jonas, S., Steinmueller, T., Bechstein, W.O., Neuhaus, P.:** Treatment of cyclosporine-related adverse effects by conversion to tacrolimus after liver transplantation. Transplantation 1997; 64: 938–940
68. **Pratt, D.S., Flavin, D.P., Kaplan, M.M.:** The successful treatment of autoimmune hepatitis with 6-mercaptopurine after failure with azathioprine. Gastroenterology 1996; 110: 271–274
69. **Schrem, H., Lück, R., Becker, T., Nashan, B., Klempnauer, J.:** Update on liver transplantation using cyclosporine. Transplant. Proc. 2004; 36: 2525–2531
70. **Sciveres, M., Caprai, S., Palla, G., Uglu, C., Maggiore, G.:** Effectiveness and safety of ciclosporin as therapy for autoimmune diseases of the liver in children and adolescents. Aliment. Pharmacol. Ther. 2004; 19: 209–217
71. **Van Thiel, D.H., Wright, H., Carroll, P., Abu Elmagd, K., Rodriguez-Rilo, H., McMichael, J., Irish, W., Starzl, T.E.:** Tacrolimus: a potential new treatment for autoimmune chronic active hepatitis: results of an open-label preliminary trial. Amer. J. Gastroenterol. 1995; 90: 771–776
72. **Watashi, K., Hijikata, M., Hosaka, M., Yamaji, M., Shimotohno, K.:** Cyclosporin A suppresses replication of hepatitis C virus genome in cultured hepatocytes. Hepatology 2003; 38: 1282–1288

Immunostimulants
73. **Antoniello, S., Auletta, M., Cerini, R., Capasso, A.:** Zinc deficiency and hepatic encephalopathy. Ital. J. Gastroenterol. 1986; 18: 27–29
74. **Baraldi, M., Caselgrandi, E., Borella, P., Zeneroli, M.L.:** Decrease of brain zinc in experimental hepatic encephalopathy. Brain Res. 1983; 258: 170–172
75. **Chien, R.-N., Liaw, Y.-F., Chen, T.-C., Yeh, C.-T., Sheen, I.-S.:** Efficacy of thymosin α_1 in patients with chronic hepatitis B: a randomized, controlled trial. Hepatology 1998; 27: 1383–1387
76. **Kiremidjian-Schumacher, L., Roy, M., Wishe, H.I., Cohen, M.W., Stotzky, G.:** Supplementation with selenium and human immune cell functions. II. Effect on cytotoxic lymphocytes and natural killer cells. Biol. Trace Elem. Res. 1994; 41: 115–127
77. **Köhrle, J.:** Exciting new perspectives and further necessity for selenium research in Europe. (Editorial) J. Trace Elem. Med. Biol. 2004; 17: 275–276
78. **Low, T.L.K., Goldstein, A.L.:** Thymosins: structure, function and therapeutic applications. Thymus 1984; 6: 27–42
79. **McKenzie, R.C., Rafferty, T.S., Beckett, G.J.:** Selenium: an essential element for immune function. Immunol. Today 1998; 19: 342–345
80. **Prasad, A.S.:** Zinc: an overview. Nutrition 1995; 11 (Suppl.) 93–99
81. **Raymond, R.S., Fallon, M.B., Abrams, G.A.:** Oral thymic extract for chronic hepatitis C in patients previously treated with interferon – a randomized, double-blind, placebo-controlled trial. Ann. Int. Med. 1998; 129: 797–800
82. **Sandstead, H.:** Understanding zinc: Recent observations and interpretations. J. Lab. Clin. Med. 1994; 124: 322–327
83. **Sherman, K.E., Sjogren, M., Creager, R.L., Damiano, M.A., Freeman, S., Lewey, S., Davis, D., Root, S., Weber, F.L., Ishak, K.G., Goodman, Z.D.:** Combination therapy with thymosin α_1 and interferon for the treatment of chronic hepatitis C infection: a randomized, placebo-controlled double-blind trial. Hepatology 1998; 27: 1128–1135

Ursodeoxycholic acid
84. **Arslanoglu, S., Moro, G.E., Tauschel, H.D., Boehm, G.:** Ursodeoxycholic acid treatment in preterm infants: a pilot study for the prevention of cholestasis associated with total parenteral nutrition. J. Pediatr. Gastroenterol. Nutr. 2008; 46: 228–231
85. **Barnes, D., Talenti, D., Cammell, G., Goormastic, M., Farquhar, L., Henderson, M., Vogt, D., Mayes, J., Westveer, M.K., Carey, W.:** A randomized clinical trial of ursodeoxycholic acid as adjuvant treatment to prevent liver transplant rejection. Hepatology 1997; 26: 853–857
86. **Bertolotti, M., Morselli-Labate, A.M., Riusticali, A.G., Loria, P., Carulli, N.:** Ursodeoxycholic acid improves liver tests in chronic hepatitis. Results of a randomized controlled trial. Clin. Drug Invest. 1999; 17: 425–434
87. **Beuers, U.:** Drug insight: Mechanisms and sites of action of ursodeoxycholic acid in cholestasis. Nat. Clin. Pract. Gastroenterol Hepatol. 2006; 3: 318–328
88. **Calmus, Y., Weill, B., Ozier, Y., Chéreau, C., Houssin, D., Poupon, R.:** Immunosuppressive properties of chenodeoxycholic and ursodeoxycholic acids in the mouse. Gastroenterology 1992; 103: 617–621
89. **Charatcharoenwitthaya, P., Pimentel, S., Talwalkar, J.A., Enders, F.T., Lindor, K.D., Krom, R.A., Wiesner, R.H.:** Long-term survival and impact of ursodeoxycholic acid treatment for recurrent primary biliary cirrhosis after liver transplantation. Liver Transpl. 2007; 13: 1236–1245
90. **Crosignani, A., Podda, M., Batezzati, P.M., Bertolini, E., Zuin, M., Watson, D., Setchell, K.D.R.:** Changes in bile acid composition in patients with primary biliary cirrhosis induced by ursodeoxycholic acid administration. Hepatology 1991; 14: 1000–1007
91. **Desmond, C.P., Wilson, J., Bailey, M., Clark, D., Roberts, S.K.:** The benign course of liver disease in adults with cystic fibrosis and the effect of ursodeoxycholic acid. Liver Int. 2007; 27: 1402–1408

92. Fedorowski, T., Salen, G., Colallilo, A., Tint, G.S., Mosbach, E.H., Hall, J.C.: Metabolism of ursodeoxycholic acid in man. Gastroenterology 1977; 73: 1131–1137
93. Fischer, S., Neubrand, M., Paumgartner, G.: Biotransformation of orally administered ursodeoxycholic acid in man as observed in gallbladder bile, serum and urine. Eur. J. Clin. Invest. 1993; 23: 28–36
94. Galsky, J., Bansky, G., Holubová, T., König, J.: Effect of ursodeoxycholic acid in acute viral hepatitis. J. Clin. Gastroenterol. 1999; 28: 249–253
95. Glantz, A., Reilly, S.J., Benthin, L., Lammert, F., Mattsson, L.A., Marschall, H.U.: Intrahepatic cholestasis of pregnancy: Amelioration of pruritus by UDCA is associated with decreased progesterone disulphates in urine. Hepatology 2008; 47: 544–541
96. Güldütuna, S., Zimmer, G., Imhof, M., Bhatti, S., You, T., Leuschner, U.: Molecular aspects of membrane stabilization by ursodeoxycholic acid. Gastroenterology 1993; 104: 1736–1744
97. Harnois, D.M., Angulo, P., Jorgensen, R.A., LaRusso, N.F., Lindor, K.D.: High-dose ursodeoxycholic acid as a therapy for patients with primary sclerosing cholangitis. Amer. J. Gastroenterol. 2001; 96: 1558–1562
98. Hempfling, W., Dilger, K., Breuers, U.: Systematic review: Ursodeoxycholic acid − Adverse effects and drug interactions. Aliment. Pharm. Ther. 2003; 18: 963–972
99. Heumann, D.M.: Hepatoprotective properties of ursodeoxycholic acid. Gastroenterology 1993; 104: 1865–1870
100. Hofmann, A.F.: Biliary secretion and excretion in health and disease: current concepts. Ann. Hepatol. 2007; 6: 15–27
101. Ikegami, T., Matsuzaki, Y.: Ursodeoxycholic acid: Mechanism of action and novel clinical applications. Hepatol. Res. 2008; 38: 123–131
102. Lacaille, F., Paradis, K.: The immunosuppressive effect of ursodeoxycholic acid: a comparative in vitro study on human peripheral blood mononuclear cells. Hepatology 1993; 18: 165–172
103. Leuschner, U., Kurtz, W.: Pharmacological aspects and therapeutic effects of ursodeoxycholic acid. Dig. Dis. 1990; 8: 12–22
104. Li, L.J., Xu, X.W., Zao, N.F.: Effects of ursodeoxycholic acid on intrahepatic cholestasis in rats. Chin. Med. J. 2003; 116: 1099–1103
105. Mazzella, G., Rizzo, N., Azzaroli, F., Simoni, P., Bovicelli, L., Miracolo, A., Simonazzi, G., Colecchia, A., Nigro, G., Mwangemi, C., Festi, D., Roda, E.: Ursodeoxycholic acid administration in patients with cholestasis of pregnancy: Effects of primary bile acids in babies and mothers. Hepatology 2001; 33: 504–508
106. Omata, M., Yoshida, H., Toyota, J., Tomita, E., Nishiguchi, S., Hayashi, N., Iino, S., Makino, I., Okita, K., Toda, G., Tanikawa, K., Kumada, H.: Japanese C-Viral Hepatitis Network. A large-scale, multicentre, double-blind trial of ursodeoxycholic acid in patients with chronic hepatitis C. Gut. 2007; 56: 1747–1753
107. Pardi, D.S., Loftus, E.V. Jr., Kremers, W.K., Keach, J., Lindor, K.D.: Ursodeoxycholic acid as a chemopreventive agent in patients with ulcerative colitis and primary sclerosing cholangitis. Gastroenterology 2003; 124: 889–893
108. Paumgartner, G., Pusl, T.: Medical treatment of cholestatic liver disease. Clin. Liver Dis. 2008; 12: 53–80
109. Poo, J.L., Feldmann, G., Erlinger, S., Braillon, A., Gaudin, C., Dumont, M., Lebrec, D.: Ursodeoxycholic acid limits liver histologic alterations and portal hypertension induced by bile duct ligation in the rat. Gastroenterology 1992; 102: 1752–1759
110. Queneau, P.-E., Montet, J.-C.: Hepatoprotection by hydrophilic bile salts. J. Hepatol. 1994; 21: 260–268
111. Rodriguez-Ortigosa, C.M., Cincu, R.N., Sanz, S., Ruiz, F., Quiroga, J., Prieto, J.: Effect of ursodeoxycholic acid on methionine adenosyltransferase activity and hepatic glutathione metabolism in rats. Gut 2002; 50: 701–706
112. Rudolph, G., Kloeters-Plachky, P., Rost, D., Stiehl, A.: The incidence of cholangiocarcinoma in primary sclerosing cholangitis after longtime treatment with ursodeoxycholic acid. Eur. J. Gastroenterol. Hepatol. 2007; 19: 487–491
113. Simko, V., Michael, S., Prego, V.: Ursodeoxycholic therapy in chronic liver disease: A meta-analysis in primary biliary cirrhosis and in chronic hepatitis. Amer. J. Gastroenterol. 1994; 89: 392–398
114. Solá, S., Aranha, M.M., Steer, C.J., Rodrigues, C.M.: Game and players: mitochondrial apoptosis and the therapeutic potential of ursodeoxycholic acid. Curr. Topics Mol. Biol. 2007; 9: 123–138
115. Takano, S., Ito, Y., Yokosuka, M., Ohto, M., Uchiumi, K., Hirota, K., Omata, M.: A multicenter randomized controlled dose study of ursodeoxycholic acid for chronic hepatitis C. Hepatology 1994; 20: 558–564
116. Tay, J., Tinmouth, A., Fergusson, D., Huebsch, L., Allan, D.S.: Systematic review of controlled clinical trials on the use of ursodeoxycholic acid for the prevention of hepatic veno-occlusive disease in hematopoietic stem cell transplantation. Biol. Blood Marrow Transplant. 2007; 13: 206–217
117. Trauner, M., Graziadei, I.W.: Review article: mechanisms of action and therapeutic applications of ursodeoxycholic acid in chronic liver disease. Aliment. Pharm. Ther. 1999; 13: 979–995
118. Tung, B.Y., Emond, M.J., Haggitt, R.C., Bronner, M.P., Kimmey, M.B., Kowdley, K.V., Brentnall, T.A.: Ursodiol use is associated with lower prevalence of colonic neoplasia in patients with ulcerative colitis and primary sclerosing cholangitis. Ann. Intern. Med. 2001; 134: 89–95
119. Weitzel, C., Stark, D., Kullmann, F., Schölmerich, J., Holstege, A., Falk, W.: Ursodeoxycholic acid induced activation of the glucocorticoid receptor in primary rat hepatocytes. Eur. J. Gastroenterol. Hepatol. 2005; 17: 169–177
120. Yoshikawa, M., Tsujii, T., Matsumura, K., Yamao, J., Matsumura, Y., Kubo, R., Fukui, H., Ishizaka, S.: Immunomodulatory effects of ursodeoxycholic acid on immune response. Hepatology 1992; 16: 358–364
121. Yoshikawa, M., Matsumura, K., Matsumura, Y., Yamao, J., Kuriyama, S., Ishizaka, S., Fukui, H., Hozumi, N., Tsujii, T.: Effects of ursodeoxycholic acid on antigen presentation. Int. Hepatol. Commun. 1993; 1: 243–249

Lactulose
122. Conn, H.O.: A clinical hepatologist's predictions about non-absorbed carbohydrates for the early twenty-first century. Scand. J. Gastroenterol. 1997; 32 (Suppl. 222): 88–92
123. Fernandes, J., Morali, G., Wolever, T.M.S., Blendis, L.M., Koo, M., Jenkins, D.J.A., Rao, A.V.: Effect of acute lactulose administration on serum acetate levels in cirrhosis. Clin. Invest. Med. 1994; 17: 218–225
124. Horsmans, Y., Solbreux, P.M., Daenens, J.P., Geubel, A.P.: Lactulose improves psychometric testing in cirrhotic patients with subclinical encephalopathy. Aliment. Pharm. Ther. 1997; 11: 165–170
125. Masini, A., Efrati, C., Merli, M., Attili, A.F., Amodio, P., Ceccanti, M., Riggio, O.: Effect of lactitol on blood ammonia response to oral glutamine challenge in cirrhotic patients: evidence for an effect of non-absorbable disaccharides on small intestine ammonia generation. Amer. J. Gastroenterol. 1999; 94: 3323–3327
126. Özaslan, C., Türkcapar, A.g., Kesenci, M., Karayalcin, K., Yerdel, M.A., Bengisun, S., Törüner, A.: Effect of lactulose on bacterial translocation. Eur. J. Surg. 1997; 163: 463–467
127. Uribe-Esquivel, M., Moran, S., Poo, J.L., Munoz, R.M.: In vitro and in vivo lactose and lactulose effects on colonic fermentation and portal-systemic encephalopathy parameters. Scand. J. Gastroenterol. 1997; 32 (Suppl. 222): 49–52
128. Watanabe, A., Sakai, T., Sato, S., Imai, F., Ohto, M., Arakawa, Y., Toda, G., Kobayashi, K., Muto, Y., Tsujii, T., Kawasaki, H., Okita, K., Tanikawa, K., Fujiyama, S., Shimada, S.: Clinical efficacy of lactulose in cirrhotic patients with and without subclinical hepatic encephalopathy. Hepatology 1997; 26: 1410–1414
129. Weber, F.L.jr.: Effects of lactulose on nitrogen metabolism. Scand. J. Gastroenterol. 1997; 32 (Suppl. 222): 83–87

Branched-chain amino acids
130. Charlton, M.R.: Branched chains revisited. Gastroenterology 1996; 111: 252–255
131. Charlton, M.: Branched-chain amino acid enriched supplements as therapy for liver disease. J. Nutrit. 2006; 136: 295–295
132. Fabbri, A., Magrini, N., Bianchi, G., Zoli, M., Marchesini, G.: Overview of randomized clinical trials of oral branched-chain amino acid treatment in chronic hepatic encephalopathy. J. Parenter. Enter. Nutr. 1996; 20: 159–164
133. Fischer, J.E.: Branched-chain-enriched amino acid solutions in patients with liver failure: an early example of nutritional pharmacology. J. Parenter. Enter. Nutr. 1990; 14 (Suppl. 5): 249–256
134. Ghanta, R.K., Salvino, R.M., Mullen, K.D.: Branched chain amino acid supplements in liver disease (editorial). Clin. Gastroenterol. Hepatol. 2005; 3: 631–632
135. Harris, R.A., Joshi, M., Jeoung, N.H.: Mechanisms responsible for regulation of branched-chain amino acid metabolism. Biochem. Biophys. Res. Com. 2004; 313: 391–396
136. Hayashi, M., Ikezawa, K., Ono, A., Okabayashi, S., Hayashi, Y., Shimizu, S., Mzuno, T., Maeda, K., Akasaka, T., Naito, M., Michida, T., Ueshima, D., Nada, T., Kawaguchi, K., Nakamura, T., Katayama, K.: Evaluation of the effects of combination therapy with branched-chain amino acid and zinc supplements on nitrogen metabolism in liver cirrhosis. Hepatol. Res. 2007; 37: 619–619
137. Higashiguchi, T., Ito, A., Kitagawa, M., Taoka, H., Kawarada, Y.: Administration of branched-chain amino acids prevents bacterial translocation after liver resection in the cirrhotic rat. Hepat. Bil. Pancr. Surg. 1996; 3: 291–296
138. Ichida, T., Shibasaki, K., Muto, Y., Satoh, S., Watanabe, A., Ichida, F.: Clinical study of an enteral branched-chain amino acid solution in decompensated liver cirrhosis with hepatic encephalopathy. Nutrition 1995; 11 (Suppl. 2): 238–244
139. Kajiwara, K., Okuno, M., Kobayashi, T., Honma, N., Maki, T., Kato, M., Ohnishi, H., Muto, Y., Moriwaki, H.: Oral supplementation with branched-chain amino acids improves survival rate of rats with carbon tetrachloride-induced liver cirrhosis. Dig. Dis. Sci. 1998; 43: 1572–1579
140. Kato, M., Miwa, Y., Tajika, M., Hiraoka, T., Muto, Y., Moriwaki, H.: Preferential use of branched-chain amino acids as an energy substrate in patients with liver cirrhosis. Intern. Med. 1998; 37: 429–434
141. Khanna, S., Gopalan, S.: Role of branched-chain amino acids in liver disease: the evidence for and against. Curr. Opin. Clin. Nutr. Metab. Care. 2007; 10: 297–303
142. Kimball, S.R., Jefferson, L.S.: Regulation of global and specific mRNA translation by oral administration of branched-chain amino acids. Biochem. Biophys. Res. Com. 2004; 313: 423–427
143. Marchesini, G., Marzocchi, R., Noia, M., Bianchi, G.: Branched-chain amino acid supplementation in patients with liver diseases. J. Nutr. 2005; 135 (Suppl.): 1596–1601
144. Miwa, Y., Kato, M., Moriwaki, H., Okuno, M., Sugihara, J., Ohnishi, H., Yoshida, T., Muto, Y., Nakayama, M., Morioka, Y., Asagi, K.:

Effects of branched-chain amino acid infusion on protein metabolism in rats with acute hepatic failure. Hepatology 1995; 22: 291–296
145. **Moriwaki, H., Miwa, Y., Tajika, M., Kato, M., Fukushima, H., Shiraki, M.:** Branched-chain amino acids as a protein- and energy-source in liver cirrhosis. Biochem. Biophys. Res. Com. 2004; 313: 405–409
146. **Muto, Y., Sato, S., Watanabe, A., Moriwaki, H., Suzuki, K., Kato, A., Kato, M., Nakamura, T., Higuchi, K., Nishigudu, S., Kumada, H.:** Effects of oral branched-chain amino acids granules on event-free survival in patients with liver cirrhosis. Clin. Gastroenterol. Hepatol. 2005; 3: 705–713
147. **Platell, C., Kong, S.E., McCauley, R., Hall, J.C.:** Branched-chain amino acids. J. Gastroenterol. Hepatol. 2000; 15: 706–717
148. **Tabaru, A., Shirohara, H., Moriyama, A., Otsuki, M.:** Effects of branched-chain-enriched amino acid solution on insulin and glucagons secretion and blood glucose level in liver cirrhosis. Scand. J. Gastroenterol. 1998; 33: 853–859
149. **Tessari, P., Zanetti, M., Barazzoni, R., Biolo, G., Orlando, R., Vettore, M., Inchiostro, S., Perini, P., Tiengo, A.:** Response of phenylalanine and leucine kinetics to branched chain-enriched amino acids and insuline in patients with cirrhosis. Gastroenterology 1996; 111: 127–137
150. **Tomiya, T., Omata, M., Fujiwara, K.:** Significance of branched-chain amino acids as possible stimulators of hepatocyte growth factor. Biochem. Biophys. Res. Com. 2004; 313: 411–416
151. **Urata, Y., Okita, K., Korenaga, K., Uchida, K., Yamasaki, T., Sakaida, I.:** The effect of supplementation with branched-chain amino acids in patients with liver cirrhosis. Hepatol. Res. 2007; 37: 510–516

Amino acids of the urea cycle
152. **Bessmann, S.P.:** The reduction of blood ammonia levels by certain amino acids. J. Clin. Invest. 1956; 35: 690
153. **Cohen, N.S., Cheung, C.-W., Raijman, L.:** The effects of ornithine on mitochondrial carbamylphosphate synthesis. J. Biol. Chem. 1980; 255: 10248–10255
154. **Cynober, L., Vaubourdolle, M., Dore, A., Giboudeau, J.:** Kinetics and metabolic effects of orally administered ornithine α-ketoglutarate in healthy subjects fed with a standardized regimen. Amer. J. Clin. Nutr. 1984; 39: 514–519
155. **Gebhardt, R., Backers, G., Gaunitz, F., Haupt, W., Jonitza, D., Klein, S., Scheja, L.:** Treatment of cirrhotic rats with L-ornithine-L-aspartate enhances urea synthesis and lowers serum ammonia levels. J. Pharmacol. Exper. Ther. 1997; 283: 1–6
156. **Greenstein, J.P., Winitz, M., Gullino, P., Birnbaum, S.M., Otey, M.C.:** Studies on the metabolism of amino acids and related compounds in vivo. III. Prevention of ammonia toxicity by arginine and related compounds. Arch. Biochem. 1956; 64: 342–354
157. **Krebs, H.A., Henseleit, K.:** Untersuchungen über die Harnstoffbildung im Tierkörper. Hoppe-Seyler's Z. Physiol. Chem. 1932; 210: 33–66
158. **Kuntz, E. (Hrsg.):** Die hepatische Enzephalopathie. Aspekte der Diagnose und Behandlung. Univ. Verlag Jena, 1992; 125 Seiten
159. **Lescoat, G., Desvergne, B., Loreal, O., Pasdeloup, N., Deugnier, Y., Bourel, M., Brissot, P.:** Modulation of albumin secretion by ornithine alpha-ketoglutarate in adult rat hepatocyte cultures and a human hepatoma cell line (Hep G$_2$). Ann. Nutrit. Metab. 1989; 33: 252–260
160. **Najarian, J.-S., Harper, H.A.:** A clinical study of the effect of arginine on blood ammonia. Amer. J. Med. 1956; 21: 832–842
161. **O'Sullivan, D., Brosnan, J.T., Brosnan, M.E.:** Hepatic zonation of the catabolism of arginine and ornithine in the perfused rat liver. Biochem. J. 1998; 330: 627–632
162. **Rose, C., Michalak, A., Rama Rao, K.V., Quack, G., Kircheis, G., Butterworth, R.F.:** L-ornithine-L-aspartate lowers plasma and cerebrospinal fluid ammonia and prevents brain edema in rats with acute liver failure. Hepatology 1999; 30: 636–640
163. **Staedt, U., Leweling, H., Gladisch, R., Kortsick, C., Hagmüller, E., Holm, E.:** Effects of ornithine aspartate on plasma ammonia and plasma amino acids in patients with cirrhosis. A double-blind, randomized study using a four-fold crossover design. J. Hepatol. 1993; 19: 424–430
164. **Vogels, B.A.P.M., Karlsen, O.T., Maas, M.A.W., Boveé, W.M.M.J., Chamuleau, R.A.F.M.:** L-Ornithine vs. L-ornithine-L-aspartate as a treatment for hyperammonemia-induced encephalopathy in rats. J. Hepatol. 1997; 26: 174–182
165. **Zieve, L., Lyftogt, C., Raphael, D.:** Ammonia toxicity: comparative protective effect of various arginine and ornithine derivatives, aspartate, benzoate, and carbamyl glutamate. Metab. Brain Dis. 1986; 1: 25–35

D-penicillamine
166. **Bavdekar, A.R., Bhave, S.A., Pradhan, A.M., Pandit, A.N., Tanner, M.S.:** Long term survival in Indian childhood cirrhosis treated with D-penicillamine. Arch. Dis. Childh. 1996; 74: 32–35
167. **Bodenheimer, H.C., Charland, C., Thayer, W.R., Schaffner, F., Staples, P.J.:** Effects of penicillamine on serum immunoglobulins and immune complex-reactive material in primary biliary cirrhosis. Gastroenterology 1985; 88: 412–417
168. **Kukovetz, W.R., Beubler, E., Kreuzig, F., Moritz, A.J., Nirnberger, G., Werner-Breitenecker, L.:** Bioavailability and pharmacokinetics of D-penicillamine. J. Rheumat. 1983; 10: 90–94

Somatostatin
169. **Cicera, I., Feu, F., Luca, A., Garcia-Pagan, J.C., Fernandez, M., Escorsell, A., Bosch, J., Rodes, J.:** Effects of bolus injections and continuous infusions of somatostatin and placebo in patients with cirrhosis: a double-blind hemodynamic investigation. Hepatology 1995; 22: 106–111
170. **Hadengue, A.:** Somatostatin or octreotide in acute variceal bleeding. Digestion 1999; 60 (Suppl. 2): 31–41
171. **Villanueva, C., Ortiz, J., Sabat, M., Gallego, A., Torras, X., Soriano, G., Sainz, S., Boadas, J., Cusso, X., Guarner, C., Balanzo, J.:** Somatostatin alone or combined with emergency sclerotherapy in the treatment of acute esophageal variceal bleeding: A prospective randomized trial. Hepatology 1999; 30: 384–389

Terlipressin
172. **Escorsell, A., Bandi, J.C., Moitinho, E., Feu, F., Garcia-Pagan, J.C., Bosch, J., Rodes, J.:** Time profile of the haemodynamic effects of terlipressin in portal hypertension. J. Hepatol. 1997; 26: 621–627
173. **Halimi, C., Bonnard, P., Bernard, B., Mathurin, P., Mofredj, A., di M, V., Demontis, R., Henry-Blabaud, E., Flevet, P., Opolon, P., Poynard, T., Cadranel, J.F.:** Effect of terlipressin (Glypressin) on hepatorenal syndrome in cirrhotic patients: results of a multicentre pilot study. Eur. J. Gastroenterol. Hepatol. 2002; 14: 153–158
174. **Moller, S., Bendtsen, F., Henriksen, J.H.:** Splanchnic and systemic hemodynamic derangement in decompensated cirrhosis. Can. J. Gastroenterol. 2001; 15: 94–106
175. **Nevens, F., van Steenbergen, W., Yap, S.H., Fevery, J.:** Assessment of variceal pressure by continuous non-invasive endoscopic registration: a placebo controlled evaluation of the effect of terlipressin and octreotide. Gut 1996; 38: 129–134
176. **Walker, S., Kreichgauer, H.-P., Bode, J.C.:** Terlipressin (Glypressin) versus somatostatin in the treatment of bleeding esophageal varices. – Final report of a placebo-controlled, double-blind study. Z. Gastroenterol. 1996; 34: 692–698

S-adenosyl-L-methionine
177. **Alvaro, D., Gigliozzi, A., Piat, C., Carli, L., Bini, A., La Rosa, T., Furfaro, S., Capocaccia, L.:** Effect of S-adenosyl-L-methionine on ethanol cholestasis and hepatotoxicity in isolated perfused rat liver. Dig. Dis. Sci. 1995; 40: 1592–1600
178. **Bontemps, F., van den Berghe, G.:** Metabolism of exogenous S-adenosylmethionine in isolated rat hepatocyte suspensions: methylation of plasma-membrane phospholipids without intracellular uptake. Biochem. J. 1997; 327: 383–389
179. **Bottiglieri, T.:** S-adenosyl-L-methionine (SAMe): from the bench to the bedside. Molecular basis of a pleiotrophic molecule. Amer. J. Clin. Nutr. 2002; 76: 1151–1157
180. **Cincu, F.N., Rodriguez-Ortigosa, C.M., Vesperinas, I., Quiroga, J., Prieto, J.:** S-adenosyl-L-methionine protects the liver against the cholestatic, cytotoxic, and vasoactive effects of leukotriene D-4: a study with isolated and perfused rat liver. Hepatology 1997; 26: 330–335
181. **Friedel, H.A., Goa, K.L., Benfield, P.:** S-adenosyl-L-methionine. A review of its pharmacological properties and therapeutic potential in liver dysfunction and affective disorders in relation to its physiological role in cell metabolism. Drugs 1989; 38: 389–416
182. **Gasso, M., Rubio, M., Varela, G., Cabre, M., Caballeria, J., Alonso, E., Deulofem, R., Camps, J., Gimenez, A., Pajares, M., Pares, A., Mato, J.M., Rodes, J.:** Effects of S-adenosylmethionine on lipid peroxidation and liver fibrogenesis in carbon tetrachloride-induced cirrhosis. J. Hepatol. 1996; 25: 200–205
183. **Gonzalez-Correa, J.A., De la Cruz, J.P., Martin-Aurioles, E., Lopez-Egea, M.A., Ortiz, P., De la Cuesta, F.S.:** Effects of S-adenosyl-L-methionine on hepatic and renal oxidative stress in an experimental model of acute biliary obstruction in rats. Hepatology 1997; 26: 121–127
184. **Horne, D.W., Holloway, R.S., Wagner, C.:** Transport of S-adenosyl-L-methionine in isolated rat liver mitochondria. Arch. Biochem. Biophys. 1997; 343: 201–206
185. **Jeon, B.R., Lee, S.M.:** S-adenosylmethionine protects post-ischemic mitochondrial injury in rat liver. J. Hepatol. 2001; 34: 395–401
186. **Lieber, C.S., Packer, L.:** S-adenosyl-L-methionine: molecular, biological, and clinical aspects – an introduction. Amer. J. Clin. Nutr. 2002; 76: 1148–1150
187. **Lieber, C.S.:** S-adenosyl-L-methionine: Its role in the treatment of liver disorders. Amer. J. Clin. Nutr. 2002; 76: 1183–1187
188. **Martinez-Chantar, M.L., Garcia-Trevijano, E.R., Latasa, M.U., Perez-Mato, I., Sanchez-del-Pino, M.M., Corrales, F.J., Avila, M.A., Mato, J.M.:** Importance of a deficiency in S-adenosyl-L-methionine synthesis in the pathogenesis of liver injury. Amer. J. Nutr. 2002; 76: 1177–1182
189. **Pastor, A., Collado, P.S., Almar, M., Gonzalez-Gallego, J.:** Microsonal function in biliary obstructed rats: effects of S-adenosyl-methionine. J. Hepatol. 1996; 24: 353–359
190. **Roman, I.D., Johnson, G.D., Coleman, R.:** S-adenosyl-L-methionine prevents disruption of canalicular function and pericanalicular cytoskeleton integrity caused by cyclosporine A in isolated rat hepatocyte couplets. Hepatology 1996; 24: 134–140
191. **Simile, M.M., Saviozzi, M., De Miglio, M.R., Muroni, M.R., Nufris, A., Pascale, R.M., Malvaldi, G., Feo, F.:** Persistent chemopreventive effect of S-adenosyl-L-methionine on the development of liver putative preneoplastic lesions induced by thiobenzamide in diethylnitrosamine-initiated rats. Carcinogenesis 1996, 17: 1533–1537
192. **Wu, J., Söderbergh, H., Karlsson, K., Danielsson, A.:** Protective effect of S-adenosyl-L-methionine on bromobenzene- and D-galactosamine-induced toxicity to isolated rat hepatocytes. Hepatology 1996; 23: 359–365

Haemarginate

193. **Herrick, A., McLellan, A., Brodie, M.J., McColl, K.E.L., Moore, M.R., Goldberg, A.:** Effect of haem arginate therapy on porphyrin metabolism and mixed function oxygenase activity in acute hepatic porphyria. Lancet 1987/II: 1178–1179
194. **Mustajoki, P., Nordmann, Y.:** Early administration of haem arginate for acute porphyric attacks. Arch. Intern. Med. 1993; 153: 2004–2008
195. **Tenhunen, R., Tokola, O., Linden, I.B.:** Haem arginate: a new stabl haem compound. J. Pharm. Pharmacol. 1987; 39: 780–786

Phytotherapeutics

196. **Concepcion-Navarro, M., Pilar-Montilla, M., Martin, A., Jimenez, J., Pilar-Utrilla, M.:** Free radical scavenger and antihepatotoxic activity of Rosmarinus tomentosus. Planta Med. 1993; 59: 312–314
197. **Sharma, A., Singh, R.T., Sehgal, V., Handa, S.S.:** Antihepatotoxic activity of some plants used in herbal formulations. Fitoterapia. 1991; 62: 131–138
198. **Thabrew, M.I., Hughes, R.D.:** Phytogenic agents in the therapy of liver disease. Phytother. Res. 1996; 10: 461–467
199. **Wasser, S., Ho, J.M.S., Ang, H.K., Tan, C.E.L.:** Salvia miltorrhiza reduces experimentally-induced hepatic fibrosis in rats. J. Hepatol. 1998; 29: 760–771

Essential phospholipids

200. **Kuntz, E.:** The "essential" phospholipids and their role in liver therapy. Monography (in German) carried out for Nattermann (Cologne) (as per 31.12.1988) with 16 figures, 19 tables, 288 quoted references
201. **Aleynik, S.I., Leo, M.A., Ma, X., Aleynik, M.K., Lieber, C.S.:** Polyenylphosphatidylcholine prevents carbon tetrachloride-induced lipid peroxidation while it attenuates liver fibrosis. J. Hepatol. 1997; 27: 554–561
202. **Aleynik, M.K., Leo, M.A., Aleynik, S.L., Lieber, C.S.:** Polyenylphosphatidylcholine opposes the increase of cytochrome P-4502E1 by ethanol and corrects its iron-induced decrease. Alcohol. Clin. Exp. Res. 1999; 23: 96–100
203. **Aleynik, S.I., Lieber, C.S.:** Polyenylphosphatidylcholine corrects the alcohol-induced hepatic oxidative stress by restoring S-adenosylmethionine. Alcohol Alcoholisms 2003; 38: 208–212
204. **Baraona, E., Zeballos, G.A., Shoichet, L., Mal, K.M., Lieber, C.S.:** Ethanol consumption increases nitric oxide production in rats, and its peroxynitrite-mediated toxicity is attenuated by polyenylphosphatidylcholine. Alcoh. Clin. Exp. Res. 2002; 26: 883–889
205. **Chanussot, F., Benkoel, L.:** Prevention by dietary (n-6) polyunsaturated phosphatidylcholines of intrahepatic cholestasis induced by cyclosporine A in animals. Life Sci. 2003; 73: 381–392
206. **Brady, L.M., Fox, E.S., Fimmel, C.J.:** Polyenylphosphatidylcholine inhibits PDGF-induced proliferation in rat hepatic stellate cells. Biochem. Biophys. Res. Comm. 1998; 248: 174–179
207. **Bruha, R., Mareczek, Z.:** Essential phospholipids in the treatment of hepatic encephalopathy. Vnitr. Lek. 2000; 46: 199–204
208. **Buko, V., Artsukevich, A., Maltsev, A., Nikitin, V., Ignatenko, V., Gundermann, K.-J., Schumacher, R.:** Effect of polyunsaturated phosphatidylcholine on lipid structure and camp-dependent signal transduction in the liver of rats chronically intoxicated with ethanol. Exp. Toxic. Pathol. 1994; 46: 375–382
209. **Cao, Q., Mak, K.M., Lieber, C.S.:** Dilinoleoylphosphatidylcholine prevents transforming growth factor β1-mediated collagen accumulation in cultured rat hepatic stellate cells. J. Lab. Clin. Med. 2002; 139: 202–210
210. **Chirkin, A.A., Konevalova, N.Y., Grebennikov, I.N., Kulikov, V.A., Saraev, Y.V., Buko, V.U., Chirkina, I.A., Danchenko, E.O., Gundermann, K.-J.:** Effect of polyunsaturated phosphatidylcholine on lipid transport system in alcoholic liver injury. Addiction Biol. 1998; 3: 65–70
211. **Demirbilek, S., Karaman, A., Gürünluoglu, K., Tas, E., Akin, M., Aksoy, R.T., Türkmen, E., Edali, M.N., Baykarabulut, A.:** Polyenylphosphatidylcholine pre-treatment protects rat liver from ischemia/reperfusion injury. Hepat. 2006; 34: 84–91
212. **Dinakaran, N.:** Safety and efficacy of Essentiale-L on the treatment of non-alcoholic fatty liver disease. Indian J. Clin. Practice 2003; 14: 512–518
213. **Geetha, J., Manjula, R., Malathi, S., Usha, K.:** Efficacy of essential phospholipid substance of Soya bean oil and Phyllanthus niruri in acute viral hepatitis. J. Gen. Med. (India) 1992; 4: 53–58
214. **Gonciarz, Z., Besser, P., Lelek, E., Gundermann, K.J., Johannes, K.J.:** Randomized placebo-controlled double blind trial on "essential" phospholipids in the treatment of fatty liver associated with diabetes. Med. Chir. Dig. 1988; 17: 61–65
215. **Holecek, M., Mraz, J., Koldova, P., Skopec, F.:** Effect of polyunsaturated phosphatidylcholine on liver regeneration onset after hepatectomy in the rat. Drug. Res. 1992; 42: 337–339
216. **Holoman, J., Glasa, J., Hlavaty, I., Veningerova, M., Prachar, V., Lukacsova, M.:** Favourable effects of essential phospholipids and the arrangement of life routine in patients with toxic damage liver. Bratisl. Lek Listy 1998; 99: 75–81
217. **Hu, G.-P., Liu, N., Wang, S., Tang, H., Zhao, L.-S.:** Polyunsaturated phosphatidylcholine (Essentiale) for chronic hepatitis: a systematic review. Chin. J. Evid. Bas. Med. 2005; 5: 543–548
218. **Ilic, V., Kordac, V., Alvarez, S.Z.:** Clinical experience with long-term administration of "essential" phospholipids in chronic active hepatitis. Review of 3 double-blind studies. (tschech.) Cas. Lek. Ces. 1992; 131: 801–804
219. **Kharbanda, K.K., Mailliard, M.E., Beckenhauer, H.C., Sorrell, M.F., Tuma, D.J.:** Betaine attenuates alcoholic steatosis by restoring phosphatidylcholine generation via the phosphatidylethanolamine methyltransferase pathway. J. Hepatol. 2007; 46: 314–321
220. **Koga, S., Irisa, T., Miyata, Y., Sakai, H., Tsuji, Y., Fujimoto, Y., Masumoto, A., Matsuura, T., Sato, M., Yokota, M., Yamamoto, F., Tokumatso, M.:** Clinical progress of 51 fatty liver cases analyzed by liver function tests and ultrasonic screening and results of EPL administered cases. Prog. Med. 1991; 11: 1891–1899
221. **Kuntz, E.:** Pilotstudie mit Polyenylphosphatidylcholin bei schwerer Leberinsuffizienz. Med. Welt 1989; 40: 1327–1329
222. **Kuntz, E.:** "Essentielle" Porpholipide in der Hepatologie – 50 Jahre experimentelle und klinische Erfahrung. Z. Gastroenterol. 1991; 29 (Suppl. 2): 7–13
223. **Kuntz, E.:** The "essential" phospholipids in hepatology. Experimental and clinical experiences. Progr. Hepatol. Pharmacol. 1995; 1: 156–167
224. **Li, J., Kim, C.-I., Leo, M.A., Mak, K.M., Rojkind, M., Lieber, C.S.:** Polyunsaturated lecithin prevents acetaldehyde-mediated hepatic collagen accumulation by stimulating collagenase activity in cultured lipocytes. Hepatology 1992; 15: 373–381
225. **Lieber, C.S., DeCarli, L.M., Mak, K.M., Kim, C.-I., Leo, M.A.:** Attenuation of alcohol-induced hepatic fibrosis by polyunsaturated lecithin. Hepatology 1990; 12: 1390–1398
226. **Lieber, C.S., Robins, S.J., Li, J., DeCarli, L.M., Mak, K.M., Fasulo, J.M., Leo, M.A.:** Phosphatidylcholine protects against fibrosis and cirrhosis in the baboon. Gastroenterology 1994; 106: 152–159
227. **Lieber, C.S., Robins, S.J., Leo, M.A.:** Hepatic phosphatidyl ethanolamine methyltransferase activity is decreased by ethanol and increased by phosphatidylcholine. Alcohol Clin. Exp. Res. 1994; 18: 592–595
228. **Lieber, C.S., Leo, M.A., Aleynik, S.I., Aleynik, M.K., DeCarli, L.M.:** Polyenylphosphatidylcholine decreases alcohol-induced oxidative stress in the baboon. Alcohol. Clin. Exp. Res. 1997; 21: 375–379
229. **Lieber, C.S.:** Prevention and treatment of liver fibrosis based on pathogenesis. Alcohol. Clin. Exp. Res. 1999; 23: 944–949
230. **Lieber, C.S.:** Alcoholic liver disease: new insights in pathogenesis lead to new treatments. J. Hepatol. 2000; 32 (Suppl. 1): 113–128
231. **Liu, E.:** The curative effect observation of Essentiale on treating severe jaundice type of hepatitis. Modern. J. Integr. Trad. Chin. West. Med. 2003; 12: 402
232. **Ma., X., Zhao, J., Lieber, C.S.:** Polyenylphosphatidylcholine attenuates non-alcoholic hepatic fibrosis and accelerates its regression. J. Hepatol. 1996; 24: 604–613
233. **Machoy-Mokrzynska, A., Put, A., Ceglecka, M., Mysliwie, Z.:** Influence of essential phospholipids (EPL) on selected biochemical parameters of lipid metabolism in rats chronically exposed to ammonium fluoride vapours. Fluoride 1994; 27: 201–204
234. **Mak, K.M., Wen; K., Ren, C., Lieber, C.S.:** Dilinoleoylphosphatidylcholine reproduces the antiapoptotic actions of polyenylphosphatidylcholine against ethanol-induced hepatocyte apoptosis. Alcoh. Clin. Exp. Res. 2003; 27: 997–1005
235. **Mathur, S.N., Simon, I., Lokesh, B.R., Spector, A.A.:** Phospholipid fatty acid modification of rat liver microsomes affects acylcoenzyme A: cholesterol acyltransferase activity. Biochem. Biophys. Acta 1983; 751: 401–411
236. **Mi, L.-J., Mak, K.M., Lieber, C.S.:** Attenuation of alcohol-induced apoptosis of hepatocytes in rat livers by polyenylphosphatidylcholine (PPC). Alcohol. Clin. Exp. Res. 2000; 24: 207–212
237. **Navder, K.P., Baraona, E., Lieber, C.S.:** Polyenylphosphatidylcholine attenuates alcohol-induced fatty liver and hyperlipemia in rats. J. Nutr. 1997; 127: 1800–1806
238. **Navder, K.P., Baraona, E., Leo, M.A., Lieber, C.S.:** Oxidation of LDL in baboons is increased by alcohol and attenuated by polyenylphosphatidylcholine- J. Lipid Res. 1999; 40: 983–987
239. **Niederau, C., Strohmeyer, G., Heintges, T., Peter, K., Göpfert, E.:** Polyunsaturated phosphatidyl-choline and interferon alpha for treatment of chronic hepatitis B and C: a multi-center, randomized, double-blind, placebo-controlled trial. Hepato-Gastroenterol. 1998; 45: 797–804
240. **Nolan, B., Semententes, J., Bankey, P.:** Hepatocyte polyunsaturated fatty acid enrichment increases acute phase protein synthesis. Surgery 1998; 124: 471–476
241. **Oette, K., Kühn, E., Römer, A., Niemann, R., Gundermann, K.-J., Schumacher, R.:** The absorption of dilinoleoyl-phosphatidylcholine after oral administration. Drug. Res. 1995; 45: 875–879
242. **Oneta, C.M., Mak, K.M., Lieber, C.S.:** Dilinoleoylphosphatidylcholine selectively modulates lipopolysaccharide-induced Kupffer cell activation. J. Lab. Clin. Med. 1999; 134: 466–470
243. **Poniachik, J., Baraona, E., Zhao, J., Lieber, C.S.:** Dilinoleoylphosphatidylcholine decreases hepatic stellate cell activation. J. Lab. Clin. Med. 1999; 133: 342–348
244. **Put, A., Samochowiec, L., Ceglecka, M., Tustanowski, S., Birkenfeld, B., Zaborek, B.:** Clinical efficacy of "essential" phospholipids in patients chronically exposed to organic solvents. J. Int. Med. Res. 1993; 21: 185–191
245. **Shinuzu, Y., Kusano, M.:** The efficacy of polyenylphosphatidylcholine for liver disease. (Editorial). Hepatol. Res. 2006; 34: 74–75
246. **Wang, X.D., Andersson, R., Soltesz, V., Wang, W.Q., Ar'Rajab, A., Bengmark, S.:** Pospholipids prevent enteric bacterial translocation in the early stage of experimental acute liver failure in the rat. Scand. J. Gastroenterol. 1994; 29: 1117–1121

Silymarin

247. **Kuntz, E.:** The role of the active agent silymarin in liver disease (in German) with 75 pages, 10 figures, 8 tables, 247 quoted references; 1994. • Addendum 1995, English edition 1998 • Falk-Foundation e.V. Freiburg
248. **Bartholomaeus, A.R., Bolton, R., Ahokas, J.T.:** Inhibition of rat liver cytosolic glutathione S-transferase by silybin. Xenobiotica 1994; 24: 17−24
249. **Basaga, H., Poli, G., Tekkaya, C., Aras, I.:** Free radical scavenging and antioxidative properties of "silibin" complexes on microsomal lipid peroxidation. Cell Biochem. Funct. 1997; 15: 27−33
250. **Beckmann-Knopp, S., Rietbrock, S., Weyhenmeyer, R., Böker, R.H., Beckurts, K.T., Lang, W., Hunz, M., Fuhr, U.:** Inhibitory effects of silibinin on cytochrome P-450 enzymes in human liver microsomes. Pharm. Toxicol. 2000; 86: 250−256
251. **Boigk, G., Stroedter, L., Herbst, H., Waldschmidt, J., Riecken, E.O., Schuppan, D.:** Silymarin retards collagen accumulation in early and advanced biliary fibrosis secondary to complete bile duct obliteration in rats. Hepatology 1997; 26: 643−649
252. **Carducci, R., Armellino, M.F., Volpe, C., Basile, G., Caso, N., Apicella, A., Basile, V.:** Silibinina e intossicazione acuta da Amanita phalloides. Min. Anest. 1996; 62: 187−193
253. **Chrungoo, V.J., Reen, R.K., Singh, K., Singh, J.:** Effects of Silymarin on UDP-glucuronic acid and glucuronidation activity in the rat isolated hepatocytes and liver in relation to D-galactosamine toxicity. Ind. J. Exp. Biol. 1997; 35: 256−263
254. **Chrungoo, V.J., Singh, K., Singh, J.:** Silymarin mediated differential modulation of toxicity induced by carbon tetrachloride, paracetamol and D-galactosamine in freshly isolated rat hepatocytes. Ind. J. Exp. Biol. 1997; 35: 611−617
255. **Crocenci, F.A., Sanchez-Pozzi, E.J., Pellegrino, J.M., Rodriguez-Garay, E.A., Mottino, A.D., Roma, M.G.:** Preventive effect of silymarin against taurolithocholate-induced cholestasis in the rat. Biochem. Pharmacol. 2003; 66: 355−364
256. **Dehmlow, C., Erhard, J., de Groot, H.:** Inhibition of Kupffer cell functions as an explanation for the hepatoprotective properties of silibinin. Hepatology 1996; 23: 749−754
257. **Dehmlow, C., Murawski, N., de Groot, H.:** Scavenging of reactive oxygen species and inhibition of arachidonic acid metabolism by silibinin in human cells. Life Sci. 1996; 58: 1591−1600
258. **Dvorak, Z., Kosina, P., Walterova, D., Simanek, V., Bachteda, P., Ulrichova, J.:** Primary cultures of human hepatocytes as a tool in cytotoxicity studies: Cell protection against model toxins by flavonolignans obtained from Silybum marianum. Toxicol. Letters 2003; 137: 201−212
259. **Farghali, H., Kamenikowa, L., Hynie, S., Kmonickova, E.:** Silymarin effects on intracellular calcium and cytotoxicity: a study in perfused rat hepatocytes after oxidative stress injury. Pharm. Res. 2000; 41: 231−237
260. **Favari, L., Perez-Alvarez, V.:** Comparative effects of colchicine and silymarin on CCl_4-chronic liver damage in rats. Arch. Med. Res. 1997; 28: 11−17
261. **Favari, L., Soto, C., Mourelle, M.:** Effect of portal vein ligation and silymarin treatment on aspirin metabolism and disposition in rats. Biopharm. Drug Dispos. 1997; 18: 53−64
262. **Flora, K., Hahn, M., Rosen, H., Benner, K.:** Milk thistle (Silybum marianum) for the therapy of liver disease. Amer. J. Gastroenterol. 1998; 93: 139−143
263. **Fraschini, F., Demartini, G., Esposti, D.:** Pharmacology of silymarin. Clin. Drug Invest. 2002; 22: 51−65
264. **Fuchs, E.C., Weyhenmeyer, R., Weiner, O.H.:** Effects of silibinin and of a synthetic analogue on isolated rat hepatic stellate cells and myofibroblasts. Drug Res. 1997; 47: 1383−1387
265. **Gonzales-Correa, J.A., de la Cruz, J.P., Cordillo, J., Urena, I., Redondo, L., de la Cuesta, F.S.:** Effects of silymarin MZ-80 on hepatic oxidative stress in rats with biliary obstruction. Pharmacology 2002; 64: 18−27
266. **Gyorgy, I., Antus, S., Blazovics, A., Foldiak, G.:** Substituent effects in the free radical reactions of silybin: radiation-induced oxidation of the flavonoid at neutral pH. Int. J. Radiat. Biol. 1992; 61: 603−609
267. **Ignatowicz, E., Szaefer, H., Zielinska, M., Korczowska, I., Fenrych, W.:** Silybin and silydianin diminish the oxidative metabolism of human polymorphnuclear neutrophils. Acta Biochim. Polon. 1997; 44: 127−130
268. **Jia, J.D., Bauer, M., Cho, J.J., Ruehl, M., Milani, S., Boigk, G., Riecken, E.O., Schuppan, D.:** Antifibrotic effect of silymarin in rat secondary biliary fibrosis is mediated by downregulated of procollagen alpha 1 (I) and TIMP-1. J. Hepatol. 2001; 35: 392−398
269. **Katiyar, S.K., Korman, N.J., Mukhtar, H., Agarwal, R.:** Protective effects of silymarin against photocarcinogenesis in a mouse skin model. J. Natl. Canc. Inst. 1997; 89: 556−566
270. **Kim, D.H., Jin, Y.H., Park, J.B., Kobashi, K.:** Silymarin and its components are inhibitors of beta-glucuronidase. Biol. Pharm. Bull. 1994; 17: 443−445
271. **Lang, I., Deak, G., Muzes, G., Pronai, L., Feher, J.:** Effect of the natural bioflavonoid antioxidant silymarin on superoxide dismutase (SOD) activity and expression in vitro. Biotechnol. Ther. 1993; 4: 263−270
272. **Lieber, C.S., Leo, M.A., Cao, Q., Ren, C.L., deCarli, L.M.:** Silymarin retards the progression of alcohol-induced hepatic fibrosis in baboons. J. Clin. Gastroenterol. 2003; 37: 336−339
273. **Mira, L., Silva, M., Manso, C.F.:** Scavenging of reactive oxygen species by silibinin dihemisuccinate. Biochem. Pharmacol. 1994; 48: 753−759
274. **Muriel, P., Garciapina, T., Perez-Alvarez, V., Mourelle, M.:** Silymarin protects against paracetamol-induced lipid peroxidation and liver damage. J. Appl. Toxicol. 1992; 12: 439−442
275. **Palasciano, G., Portincasa, P., Palmieri, V., Ciani, D., Vendemiale, G., Altomare, E.:** The effect of silymarin on plasma levels of malon-dialdehyde in patients receiving long-term treatment with psychotropic drugs. Curr. Ther. Res. 1994; 55: 537−545
276. **Pares, A., Planas, R., Torres, M., Caballeria, J., Viver, J.M., Acero, D., Panes, J., Rigau, J., Santos, J., Rodes, J.:** Effects of silymarin in alcoholic patients with cirrhosis of the liver: results of a controlled, double-blind, randomized and multicenter trial. J. Hepatol. 1998; 28: 615−621
277. **Pietrangelo, A., Borella, F., Casalgrandi, G., Montosi, G., Ceccarelli, D., Gallesi, D., Giovannini, F., Gasparetto, A., Masini, A.:** Antioxidant activity of silybin in vivo during long-term iron overload in rats. Gastroenterology 1995; 109: 1941−1949
278. **Ramadan, L.A., Roushdy, H.M., Abu-Senna, G.M., Amin, N.E., El-Deshw, O.A.:** Radioprotective effect of silymarin against radiation-induced hepatotoxicity. Pharmacol. Res. 2002; 45: 447−454
279. **Schürmann, J., Prockl, J., Kremer, A.K., Vollmar, A.M., Bang, R., Tiegs, G.:** Silibinin protects mice from T cell-dependent liver injury. J. Hepatol. 2003; 39: 333−340
280. **Takahara, E., Ohta, S., Hirobe, M.:** Stimulatory effects of silibinin on the DNA synthesis in partially hepatectomized rat livers: Nonresponse in hepatoma and other malignant cell lines. Biochem. Pharmacol. 1986; 35: 538−541
281. **Thamsborg, S.M., Jorgensen, R.J., Brummerstedt, E., Bjerregard, J.:** Putative effect of silymarin on Sawfly (Arge pullata) − induced hepatotoxicosis in sheep. Vet. Hum. Toxicol. 1996; 38: 89−91
282. **Valenzuela, A., Garrido, A.:** Biochemical bases of the pharmacological action of the flavonoid silymarin and of its structural isomer silibinin. Biol. Res. 1994; 27: 105−112
283. **Varghese, L., Agarwal, C., Tyagi, A., Singh, R.P., Agarwal, R.:** Silibinin efficacy against human hepatocellular carcinoma. Clin. Canc. Res. 2005; 11: 8441−8448
284. **Velussi, M., Cernigoi, A.M., de Monte, A., Dapas, F., Caffau, C., Zilli, M.:** Long-term (12 month) treatment with an anti-oxidant drug (silymarin) is effective on hyperinsulinemia, exogenous insulin need and malondialdehyde levels in cirrhotic diabetic patients. J. Hepatol. 1997; 26: 871−879
285. **Venkataramanan, R., Ramachandran, V., Komoroski, B.J., Zhang, S.M., Schiff, P.L., Strom, S.C.:** Milk thistle, a herbal supplement decreases the activity of CYP3A4 and uridine diphosphoglucuronosyl transferase in human hepatocyte cultures. Drug Metabol. Dispos. 2000; 28: 1270−1273
286. **Wang, M., La Grange, L., Tao, J., Reyes, E.:** Hepatoprotective properties of Silybum marianum herbal preparation on ethanol-induced liver damage. Fitoterapia 1996; 67: 166−171
287. **Wenzel, S., Stolte, H., Soose, M.:** Effects of silibinin and antioxidants on high glucose-induced alterations of fibronectin turnover in human mesangial cell cultures. J. Pharmacol. Exper. Therap. 1996; 279: 1520−1526
288. **Wu, C.G., Chamuleau, R.A., Bosch, K.S., Frederiks, W.M.:** Protective effect of silymarin on rat liver injury induced by ischemia. Virch. Arch. B. Cell Pathol. Mol. Pathol. 1993; 64: 259−263

EPL and Silymarin combination

289. **Barzaghi, N., Crema, F., Gatti, G., Pifferi, G., Perucca, E.:** Pharmacokinetic studies on IdB 1016, a silybin-phosphatidylcholine complex, in healthy human subjects. Eur. J. Drug Met. Pharmacokinet. 1990: 15: 333−338
290. **Buzzelli, G., Moscarella, S., Giusti, A., Duchini, A., Marena, C., Lampertico, M.:** A pilot study on the liver protective effect of silybin-phosphatidylcholine complex (IdB 1016) in chronic active hepatitis. Int. J. Clin. Pharmacol. Ther. Toxicol. 1993; 31: 456−460
291. **Carini, R., Comoglio, A., Albano, E., Poli, G.:** Lipid peroxidation and irreversible damage in the rat hepatocyte model. Protection by the silybin-phospholipid complex IdB 1016. Biochem. Pharmacol. 1992; 43: 2111−2115
292. **Comoglio, A., Tomasi, A., Malandrino, S., Poli, G., Albano, E.:** Scavenging effect of silipide, a new silybin-phospholipid complex, on ethanol-derived free radicals. Biochem. Pharmacol. 1995; 50: 1313−1316
293. **Di Sario, A., Bendia, E., Taffetani, S., Omenetti, A., Candelaresi, C., Marzioni, M., De Minicis, S., Benedetti, A.:** Hepatoprotective and antifibrotic effect of a new silybinphosphatidylcholine-vitamin E complex in rats. Dig. Liver Dis. 2005; 37: 869−876
294. **Morazzoni, P., Montalbetti, A., Malandrino, S., Pifferi, G.:** Comparative pharmacokinetics of silipide and silymarin in rats. Eur. J. Drug. Metab. Pharmacokinet. 1993; 18: 289−297
295. **Schandalik, R., Perrucca, E.:** Pharmacokinetics of silybin following oral administration of silipide in patients with extrahepatic biliary obstruction. Drugs Exp. Clin. Res. 1994; 20: 37−42

Glycyrrhizin

296. **Acharya, S.K., Dasarathy, S., Tandon, A., Joshi, Y.K., Tandon, B.N.:** A preliminary open trial on interferon stimulator (SNMC) derived from Glycyrrhiza glabra in the treatment of sub-acute hepatic failure. Ind. J. Med. Res. 1993; 98: 69−74
297. **Ismair, M.G., Stanca, C., Ha, H.R., Renner, E.L., Meier, P.J., Kullak-Ublick:** Interactions of glycyrrhizin with organic anion transporting polypeptides of rat and human liver. Hepatol. Res. 2003; 26: 343−347

298. Takahara, T., Watanabe, A., Shiraki, K.: Effects of glycyrrhizin on hepatitis B surface antigen: a biochemical and morphological study. J. Hepatol 1994; 21: 601–609
299. Van Rossum, T.G.J., Vulto, A.G., de Man, R.A., Brouwer, J.T., Schalm, S.W.: Review article: glycyrrhizin as a potential treatment for chronic hepatitis C. Aliment. Pharm. Ther. 1998; 12: 199–205

Colchicine
300. Cedillo, A., Mourelle, M., Muriel, P.: Effect of colchicine and tri-methylcolchicinic acid on CCl_4-induced cirrhosis in the rat. Pharm. Toxicol. 1996; 79: 241–246
301. Dällenbach, A., Renner, E.L.: Colchicine does not inhibit secretin-induced choleresis in rats exhibiting hyperplasia of bile ductules: evidence against a pivotal role of exocytic vesicle insertion. J. Hepatol. 1995; 22: 338–348
302. Ikeda, T., Tozuka, S., Noguchi, O., Kobayashi, F., Sakamoto, S., Marumo, F., Sato, C.: Effects of additional administration of colchicine in ursodeoxycholic acid-treated patients with primary biliary cirrhosis: a prospective randomized study. J. Hepatol. 1996; 24: 88–94
303. Lin, D.-Y., Sheen, I.-S., Chu, C.-M., Liaw, Y.-F.: A prospective randomized trial of colchicine in prevention of liver cirrhosis in chronic hepatitis B patients. Aliment. Pharmacol. Therap. 1996; 10: 961–966
304. Muriel, P., Quintanar, E., Perez-Alvarez, V.: Effect of colchicine on acetaminophen-induced liver damage. Liver 1993; 13: 217–221
305. Nikolaidis, N., Kountouras, J., Gioulome, O., Tzarou, V., Chatzizisi, O., Patsiaoura, K., Papageorgiou, A., Leontsini, M., Eugenidis, N., Zamboulis, C.: Colchicine treatment of liver fibrosis. Hepato-Gastroenterol. 2006; 53: 281–285
306. Olsson, R., Broomé, U., Danielsson, A., Hägerstrand, I., Järnerot, G., Lööf, L., Prytz, H., Ryden, B.-O., Wallerstedt, S.: Colchicine treatment of primary sclerosing cholangitis. Gastroenterology 1995; 108: 1199–1203
307. Poo, J.L., Feldmann, G., Moreau, A., Gaudin, C., Lebrec, D.: Early colchicine administration reduces hepatic fibrosis and portal hypertension in rats with bile duct ligation. J. Hepatol. 1993; 19: 90–94
308. Rao, V.C., Mehendale, H.M.: Effect of antimitotic agent colchicine on carbon tetrachloride toxicity. Arch. Toxicol. 1993; 67: 392–400
309. Rudi, J., Raedsch, R., Gerteis, C., Schlenker, T., Plachky, J., Walter-Sack, I., Sabouraud, A., Scherrmann, J.M., Kommerell, B.: Plasma kinetics and biliary excretion of colchicine in patients with chronic liver disease after oral administration of a single dose and after long-term treatment. Scand. J. Gastroenterol. 1994; 29: 346–351
310. Sabouraud, A., Rochdi, M., Urtizberea, M., Christen, M.O., Achtert, G., Scherrmann, J.M.: Pharmacokinetics of colchicine: a review of experimental and clinical data. Z. Gastroenterol. 1992; 30 (Suppl. 1): 35–39
311. Solis-Herruzo, J.A., De Gando, M., Ferrer, M.P., Hernandez Munoz, I., Fernandez-Boya, B., De La Torre, M.P., Munoz-Yague, M.T.: Reversal of carbon tetrachloride induced changes in microviscosity and lipid composition of liver plasma membrane by colchicine in rats. Gut 1993; 34: 1438–1442
312. Wang, Y.-J., Lee, S.-D., Hsieh, M.-C., Lin, H.-C., Lee, F.-Y., Tsay, S.-H., Tsai, Y.-T., Hu, O.Y.-P., King, M.-L., Lo, K.-J.: A double-blind randomized controlled trial of colchicine in patients with hepatitis B virus-related postnecrotic cirrhosis. J. Hepatol. 1994; 21: 872–877

Bupleurum falcatum
313. Kayano, K., Sakaida, I., Uchida, K., Okita, K.: Inhibitory effects of the herbal medicine Sho-saiko-to (TJ-9) on cell proliferation and procollagen gene expressions in cultured rat hepatic stellate cells. J. Hepatol. 1998; 29: 642–649
314. Sakaida, I., Matsumura, Y., Akiyama, S., Hayashi, K., Ishige, A., Okita, K.: Herbal medicine Sho-saiko-to (TJ-9) prevents liver fibrosis and enzyme-altered lesions in rat liver cirrhosis induced by a choline-deficient L-amino acid-defined diet. J. Hepatol. 1998; 28: 298–306
315. Shimizu, I., Ma, Y.-R., Mizobuchi, Y., Liu, F., Miura, T., Nakai, Y., Yasuda, M., Shiba, M., Horie, T., Amagaya, S., Kawada, N., Hori, H., Ito, S.: Effects of Sho-saiko-to, a Japanese herbal medicine, on hepatic fibrosis in rats. Hepatology 1999; 29: 149–160
316. Tajiri, H., Kozaiwa, K., Ozaki, Y., Miki, K., Shimuzu, K., Okada, S.: Effect of Sho-Saiko to (Xiao-Chai-Hu-Tang) on HBeAg clearance in children with chronic hepatitis B virus infection and with sustained liver disease. Amer. J. Chin. Med. 1991; 19: 121–129

Phyllanthus amarus
317. Doshi, J.C., Vaidya, A.B., Antarkar, D.S., Deolalikar, R., Antani, D.H.: A two-stage clinical trial of Phyllanthus amarus on hepatitis B carriers: Failure to eradicate the surface antigen. Indian J. Gastroenterol. 1994; 13: 7–8
318. Niu, J., Wang, Y., Quiao, M., Gowans, E., Edwards, P., Thyagarajan, S.P., Gust, I., Locarnini, S.: Effect of Phyllanthus amarus on duck hepatitis B virus replication in vivo. J. Med. Virol. 1990; 32: 212–218
319. Ott, M., Thyagarajan, S.P., Gupta, S.: Phyllantus amarus suppresses hepatitis B virus by interrupting interactions between HBV enhancer I and cellular transcription factors. Eur. J. Clin. Invest. 1997; 27: 908–915
320. Thyagarajan, S.P., Jayaram, S., Valliamma, T., Madanagopalan, N.: Phyllanthus amarus and hepatitis B. Lancet 1990; 2: 949–950
321. Venkateswaran, P.S., Millman, I., Blumberg, S.: Effects of an extract from Phyllanthus niruri on hepatitis B and Woodchuck hepatitis viruses: in-vitro and in-vivo studies. Proc. Natl. Acad. Sci. USA 1987; 84: 274–278

Schizandra chinensis
322. Hikino, H., Kiso, Y., Taguchi, H., Ikeya, Y.: Antihepatotoxic actions of lignoids from Schizandra chinensis fruits. Planta Med. 1984; 51: 213–218
323. Kiso, Y., Tohkin, M., Hikino, H., Ikeya, Y., Taguchi, H.: Mechanism of antihepatotoxic activity of Wuweizisu C and Gomisin A1. Planta Med. 1985; 52: 331–334
324. Langmead, L., Rampton, D.S.: Review article: Herbal treatment in gastrointestinal and liver disease: benefits and dangers. Aliment. Pharm. Ther. 2001; 15: 1239–1252
325. Liu, K.T., Lesca, P.: Pharmacological properties of Dibenzo (a,c) cyclooctene derivatives isolated from fructus Schizandra chinensis III. Inhibitory effects on carbon tetrachloride-induced lipid peroxidation, metabolism and covalent binding of carbon tetrachloride to lipids. Chem. Biol. Interact. 1982; 41: 39–47
326. Maeda, S., Takeda, S., Miyamoto, Y., Aburada, M., Harada, M.: Effects of Gomisin A on liver functions in hepatotoxic chemicals-treated rats. Jpn. J. Pharmacol. 1985; 38: 347–353
327. Miyamoto, K., Wakusawa, S., Nomura, M., Sanae, F., Sakai, R., Sudo, K., Ohtaki, Y., Takeda, S., Fujii, Y.: Effects of Gomisin A on hepatocarcinogenesis by 3'-methyl-4-dimethylaminoazobenzene in rats. Japan J. Pharmacol. 1991; 57: 71–77
328. Nagai, H., Yakuo, I., Aoki, M., Teshima, K., Ono, Y., Sengoku, T., Shimazawa, T., Aburada, M., Koda, A.: The effect of Gomisin A on immunologic liver injury in mice. Planta Med. 1989; 55: 13–17
329. Thyagarajan, S.P., Subramanian, S., Thirunalasundari, T., Venkateswaran, P.S., Blumberg, B.S.: Effect of Phyllanthus amarus on chronic carriers of hepatitis B virus. Lancet 1988; 2: 764–766

TIPS
330. Crenshaw, W.B., Gordon, F.D., McEniff, N.J., Perry, L.J., Hartnell, G., Anastopoulos, H., Jenkins, R.L., Lewis, W.D., Wheeler, H.G., Clouse, M.E.: Severe Ascites: efficacy of the transjugular intrahepatic portosystemic shunt in treatment. Radiology 1996; 200: 185–192
331. Kerlan, R.K., LaBerge, J.M., Gordon, R.L., Ring, E.J.: Transjugular intrahepatic portosystemic shunts: current status. Amer. J. Radiol. 1995; 164: 1059–1066
332. Lake, D., Guimaraes, M., Ackerman, S., Hannegan, C., Schonholz, C., Selby, J.B., Uflacker, R.: Comparative results of Doppler sonography after TIPS using covered and bare stents. Amer. J. Roentgenol. 2006; 186: 1138–1143
333. Ochs, A.: Transjugular intrahepatic portosystemic shunt. Dig. Dis. Sci. 2005; 23: 56–64
334. Sanyal, A.J., Freedman, A.M., Luketic, V.A., Purdum, P.P., Shiffman, M.L., Tisnado, J., Cole, P.E.: Transjugular intrahepatic portosystemic shunts for patients with active variceal hemorrhage unresponsive to sclerotherapy. Gastroenterology 1996; 111: 138–146
335. Somberg, K.A., Lake, J.R., Tomlanovich, S.J., LaBerge, J.M., Feldstein, V., Bass, N.M.: Transjugular intrahepatic portosystemic shunts for refractory ascites: assessment of clinical and hormonal response and renal function. Hepatology 1995; 21: 709–716
336. Wachsberg, R.H.: Doppler ultrasound evaluation of transjugular intrahepatic portosystemic shunt function. Pitfalls and artifacts. Ultrasound Quart. 2003; 19: 139–148
337. Wong, F.: The use of TIPS in chronic liver disease. Ann. Hepatol. 2006; 5: 5–15

Shunt
338. Borgonovo, G., Costantini, M., Grange, D., Vons, C., Smadja, C., Franco, D.: Comparison of a modified Sugiura procedure with portal systemic shunt for prevention of recurrent variceal bleeding in cirrhosis. Surgery 1996; 119: 214–221
339. Capussotti, L., Vergara, V., Polastri, R., Bouzari, H., Galatola, G.: Liver function and encephalopathy after partial vs direct side-to-side portacaval shunt: a prospective randomized clinical trial. Surgery 2000; 127: 614–621
340. Hillebrand, D.J., Kojouri, K., Cao, S., Runyon, B.A., Ojogho, O., Conception, U.: Small-diameter portocaval H-graft shunt: a paradigm shift back to surgical shunting in the management of variceal bleeding in patients with preserved liver function. Liver Transplant. 2000; 6: 459–465
341. Mercado, M.A., Morales-Linares, J.C., Granados-Garcia, J., Gomez-Mendez, T.J.M., Chan, C., Orozco, H.: Distal splenorenal shunt versus 10 mm low-diameter mesocaval shunt for variceal hemorrhage. Amer. J. Surg. 1996; 171: 591–595
342. Orug, T., Soonawalla, Z.F., Tekin, K., Olliff, S.P., Buckels, J.A.C., Mayer, A.D.: Role of surgical portosystemic shunts in the era of interventional radiology and liver transplantation. Brit. J. Surg. 2004; 91: 769–773
343. Tajiri, T., Onada, M., Yoshida, H., Mamada, Y., Taniai, N., Umehara, M., Toba, M., Yamashita, K.: Long-term results of modified distal splenorenal shunts for the treatment of esophageal varices. Hepato-Gastroenterol. 2000; 47: 720–723
344. Wolff, M., Hirner, A.: Current state of portosystemic shunt surgery. Langenbecks Arch. Surg. 2003; 388: 141–149

Liver resection
345. Aldrighetti, L., Arru, M., Caterini, R., Finazzi, R., Comotti, L., Torri, G., Ferla, G.: Impact of advanced age on the outcome of liver resection. World J. Surg. 2003; 27: 1149–1154
346. Assy, N., Minuk, G.Y.: Liver regeneration: methods for monitoring and their applications. J. Hepatol. 1997; 26: 945–952

347. Belghiti, J., Hiramatsu, K., Benoist, S., Massault, P.P., Sauvanet, A., Farges, O.: Seven hundred forty-seven hepatectomies in the 1990s: an update to evaluate the actual risk of liver resection. J. Amer. Coll. Surg. 2000; 191: 38−46
348. Boeckl, O., Ortner, W., Galvan, G.: Komplette Regeneration der rechten Leber nach Hemihepatektomie. Dtsch. Med. Wschr. 1984; 109: 581−585
349. Buell, J.F., Rosen, S., Yoshida, A., Labow, D., Limsrichamrern, S., Cronin, D.C., Bruce, D.S., Wen, M., Michelassi, F., Millis, J.M., Posner, M.C.: Hepatic resection: effective treatment for primary and secondary tumors. Surgery 2000; 128: 686−692
350. Chouillard, E., Cherqui, D., Tayar, C., Brunetti, F., Fagniez, P.L.: Anatomical bi- and trisegmentectomies as alternatives to extensive liver resections. Arch. Surg. 2003; 238: 29−34
351. Couinaud, C.: Liver anatomy: portal (and suprahepatic) or biliary segmentation. Dig. Surg. 1999; 16: 459−467
352. Finch, M.D., Crosbie, J.L., Currie, E., Garden, O.J.: An 8-year experience of hepatic resection: indications and outcome. Brit. J. Surg. 1998; 85: 315−319
353. Higgins, G.M., Anderson, R.M.: Experimental pathology of the liver − I. Resection of the liver of the white rat following partial surgical removal. Arch. Pathol. 1931; 12: 186−202
354. Holt, D.R., van Thiel, D., Edelstein, S., Brems, J.J.: Hepatic resections. Arch. Surg. 2000; 135: 1353−1358
355. Imamura, H., Seyama, Y., Kokudo, N., Maema, A., Sugawara, Y., Sano, K., Takayama, T., Makuuchi, M.: One thousand fifty-six hepatectomies without mortality in 8 years. Arch. Surg. 2003; 138: 1198−1206
356. Kogure, K., Kuwano, H., Fujimaki, N., Ishikawa, H., Takada, K.: Reproposal for Hjortjo's segmental anatomy on the anterior segment in human liver. Arch. Surg. 2002; 137: 1118−1124
357. Kooby, D.A., Fong, Y., Suriawinata, A., Gonen, M., Allen, P.J., Klimstra, D.S., DeMatteo, R.P., D'Angelica, M., Blumgart, L.H., Jarnagin, W.R.: Impact of steatosis on perioperative outcome following hepatic resection. J. Gastroenterol. Surg. 2003; 7: 1034−1044
358. Kubo, S., Nishiguchi, S., Hamba, H., Hirohashi, K., Tanaka, H., Shuto, T., Kinoshita, H., Kuroki, T.: Reactivation of viral replication after liver resection in patients infected with hepatitis B virus. Ann. Surg. 2001; 233: 139−145
359. Lam, C.M., Lo, C:M;, LIU; C.L., Fan, S.T.: Biliary complications during liver resection. World J. Surg. 2001; 25: 1273−1276
360. Lamadé, W., Glombitza, G., Demiris, A..M., Cardenas, C., Meinzer, H.P., Richter, G., Lehnert, Th., Herfarth, C.: Virtual operation planning in liver surgery. Chirurg 1999; 70: 239−245
361. Lang, H., Sotiropoulos, G.C., Dömland, M., Frühauf, N.R., Paul, A., Hüsing, J., Malago, M., Broelsch, C.E.: Liver resection for hepatocellular carcinoma in non-cirrhotic liver without unterlying viral hepatitis. Brit. J. Surg. 2005; 92: 198−202
362. Mangnall, D., Bird, N.C., Majeed, A.W.: The molecular physiology of liver regeneration following partial hepatectomy (review). Liver Internat. 2003; 23: 124−138
363. Nanashima, A., Yamaguchi, H., Shibasaki, S., Morino, S., Ide, N., Takeshita, H., Sawai, T., Nakagoe, T., Nagayasu, T., Ogawa, Y.: Relationship between indocyanine green test and technetium-aam galactosyl serum albumin scintigraphy in patients scheduled for hepatectomy: Clinical evaluation and patient outcome. Hepatol. Res. 2004; 28: 184−190
364. Redaelli, C.A., Dufour, J.F., Wagner, M., Schilling, M., Hüsler, J., Krähenbühl, L., Büchler, M.W., Reichen, J.: Preoperative galactose elimination capacity predicts complications and survival after hepatic resection. Ann. Surg. 2002; 235: 77−85
365. Richter, B., Schmandra, T.C., Glling, M., Bechstein, W.O.: Nutritional support after open liver resection: A systematic review. Dig. Surg. 2006; 23: 139−145
366. Shamberger, R.C., Leichtner, A.M., Jonas, M.M., LaQuaglia, M.P.: Long-term hepatic regeneration and function in infants and children following liver resection. Amer. Coll. Surg. 1996; 182: 515−519
367. Shan, Y.S., Hsieh, Y.H., Sy, E.D., Chiu, N.T., Lin, P.W.: The influence of spleen size on liver regeneration after major hepatectomy in normal and early cirrhotic liver. Liver Internat. 2005; 25: 96−100
368. Van Gulik, T., Lang, H.: Isolated resection of segment 1 of the liver. Dig. Surg. 2005; 22: 146−148

Liver injuries
369. Brammer, R.D., Bramhall, S.R., Mirza, D.F., Mayer, A.D., McMaster, P., Buckels, J.A.C.: A 10-year experience of complex liver trauma. Brit. J. Surg. 2002; 89: 1532−1537
370. Cox, E.F., Flancbaum, L., Dauterive, A.H., Paulson, R.L.: Blunt trauma to the liver. Analysis of management and mortality in 323 consecutive patients. Ann. Surg. 1988; 207: 126−134
371. Gao, J.M., Du, D.Y., Zhao, X.Y., Liu, G.L., Yang, J., Zhao, S.H., Lin, X.: Liver trauma: Experience in 348 cases. World J. Surg. 2003; 27: 703−708
372. Greco, L., Francioso, G., Pratichizzo, A., Testini, M., Impedovo, G., Ettorre, G.C.: Arterial embolization in the treatment of severe blunt hepatic trauma. Hepato-Gastroenterol. 2003; 50: 746−749
373. Gür, S., Örsel, A., Atahan, K., Hökmez, A., Tarcan, E.: Surgical treatment of liver trauma (analysis of 244 patients). Hepato-Gastroenterol. 2003; 50: 2109−2111
374. Hagiwara, A., Yukioka, T., Ohta, S., Tokunaga, T., Ohta, S., Matsuda, H., Shimazaki, S.: Nonsurgical management of patients with blunt hepatic injury: efficacy of transcatheter arterial embolization. Amer. J. Roentgenol. 1997; 169: 1151−1156
375. Marr, J.D.F., Krige, J.E.J., Terblanche, J.: Analysis of 153 gunshot wounds of the liver. Brit. J. Surg. 2000; 87: 1030−1034
376. Matthes, G., Stengel, D., Seifert, J., Rademacher, G., Mutze, S., Ekkernkamp, A.: Blunt liver injuries in polytrauma: Results from a cohort study with the regular use of whole-body helical computed tomography. World J. Surg. 2003; 27: 1124−1130
377. Richardson, J.D., Franklin, G.A., Lukan, J.K., Carrillo, E.H., Spain, D.A., Miller, F.B., Wilson, M.A., Polk, H.C., Flint, L.M.: Evolution in the management of hepatic trauma: a 25-year perspective. Ann. Surg. 2000; 232: 324−329
378. Romano, L., Giovine, S., Guidi, G., Tortora, G., Cinque, T., Romano, S.: Hepatic trauma: CT findings and considerations based on our experience in emergency diagnostic imaging. Eur. J. Radiol. 2004; 50: 59−66
379. Velmahos, G.C., Toutouzas, K., Radin, R., Chan, L., Rhee, P., Tillou, A., Demetriades, D.: High success with nonoperative management of blunt hepatic trauma. The liver is a sturdy organ. Arch. Surg. 2003; 138: 475−480

Liver transplantation
380. Adam, R., Cailliez, V., Majno, P., Karam, V., McMaster, P., Caine, R.Y., O'Grady, J., Pichlmayr, R., Neuhaus, P., Ottl, J.-B., Hoeckerstedt, K., Bismuth, H.: Normalised intrinsic mortality risk in liver transplantation: European Liver Transplant Registry study. Lancet 2000; 356: 621−627
381. Angus, P.W., McCaughan, G.W., Gane, E.J., Crawford, D.H.G., Harley, H.: Combination low-dose hepatitis B immune globulin and lamivudine therapy provides effective prophylaxis against posttransplantation hepatitis B. Liver Transplant. 2000; 6: 429−433
382. Ayata, G., Gordon, F.D., Lewis, W.D., Pomfret, E., Pomposelli, J.J., Jenkins, R.L., Khettry, U.: Liver transplantation for autoimmune hepatitis: a long-term pathologic study. Hepatology 2000; 32: 185−192
383. Bartlett, A.S., Ramadas, R., Furness, S., Gane, E., McCall, J.L.: The natural history of acute histologic rejection without biochemical graft dysfunction in orthotopic liver transplantation: A systematic review. Liver Transplant. 2002; 8: 1147−1153
384. Beath, S.V., Brook, G.D., Kelly, D.A., Cash, A.J., McMaster, P., Mayer, A.D., Buckels, J.A.: Successful liver transplantation in babies under 1 year. Brit. Med. J. 1993; 307: 825−828
385. Ben-Ari, Z., Pappo, O., Mor, E.: Intrahepatic cholestasis after liver transplantation (review). Liver Transplant. 2003; 9: 1005−1018
386. Berger, J., Hart, J., Millis, M., Baker, A.L.: Fulminant hepatic failure from heat stroke requiring liver transplantation. J. Clin. Gastroenterol. 2000; 30: 429−431
387. Broelsch, C.E., Malago, M., Testa, G., Gamazo, C.V.: Living donor liver transplantation in adults: outcome in Europe. Liver Transplant. 2000; 6 (Suppl. 2): 64−65
388. Cirera, I., Navasa, M., Rimola, A., Garcia-Pagan, J.C., Grande, L., Garcia-Valdecasas, J.C., Fuster, J., Bosch, J., Rodes, J.: Ascites after liver transplantation. Liver Transplant. 2000; 6: 157−162
389. Colledan, M., Andorno, E., Segalin, A., Lucianetti, A., Spada, M., Corno, V., Valente, U., Antonucci, A., Gridelli, B.: Alternative split liver technique: The equal size split. Transplant. Proc. 2001; 33: 1335−1336
390. Compston, J.E.: Osteoporosis after liver transplantation (review). Liver Transplant. 2003; 9: 321−330
391. Di Campli, C., Angelini, G., Armuzzi, A., Nardo, B., Zocco, M.A., Candelli, M., Santoliquido, A., Cavallari, A., Bernardi, M., Gasbarrini, A.: Quantitative evaluation of liver function by the methionine and aminopyrine breath tests in the early stages of liver transplantation. Eur. J. Gastroenterol. Hepatol. 2003; 15: 727−732
392. Farmer, D.G., Anselmo, D.M., Ghobrial, R.M., Yersiz, H., McDiarmid, S.V., Cao, C., Weaver, J., Figueroa, J., Khan, K., Vargas, J., Saab, S., Han, S., Durazo, F., Goldstein, L., Holt, C., Busuttil, R.W.: Liver transplantation for fulminant hepatic failure. Experience with more than 200 patients over a 17-year period. Ann. Surg. 2003; 237: 666−676
393. Feranchak, A.P., Tyson, R.W., Narkewicz, M.R., Karrer, F.M., Sokol, R.J.: Fulminant Epstein-Barr viral hepatitis: orthotopic liver transplantation and review of the literature. Liver Transplant. Surg. 1998; 4: 469−476
394. Fung, J., Kelly, D., Kadry, Z., Patel-Tom, K., Eghtesad, B.: Immunosuppression in liver transplantation beyond calcineurin inhibitors (review). Liver Transplant. 2005; 11: 267−280
395. Gopal, D.V., Rabkin, J.M., Berk, B.S., Corless, C.L., Chou, S.W., Olyaei, A., Orloff, S.L., Rosen, H.R.: Treatment of progressive hepatitis C recurrence after liver transplantation with combination interferon plus ribavirin. Liver Transplant. 2001; 7: 181−190
396. Goss, J.A., Shackleton, C.R., Farmer, D.G., Arnaout, W.S., Seu, P., Markowitz, J.S., Martin, P., Stribling, R.J., Goldstein, L.I., Busuttil, R.W.: Orthotopic liver transplantation for primary sclerosing cholangitis: a 12-year single center experience. Ann. Surg. 1997; 225: 472−481
397. Grabhorn, E., Schulz, A., Helmke, K., Hinrichs, B., Rogiers, X., Broering, D.C., Burdelski, M., Ganschow, R.: Short- and long-term results of liver transplantation in infants aged less than 6 months. Transplantation 2004; 78: 235−241
398. Hata, S., Sugawara, Y., Kishi, Y., Niiya, T., Kaneko, J., Sano, K., Imamura, H., Kokudo, N., Makuuchi, M.: Volume regeneration after right liver donation. Liver Transplant. 2004; 10: 65−70

399. Holt, C.D., Winston, D.J., Kubak, B., Imagawa, D.K., Martin, P., Goldstein, L., Olthoff, K., Millis, J.M., Shaked, A., Shackleton, C.R., Busuttil, R.W.: Coccidioidomycosis in liver transplant patients. Clin. Infect. Dis. 1997; 24: 216–221
400. Humar, A., Kumar, D., Caliendo, A.M., Moussa, G., Ashi-Sulaiman, A., Levy, G., Mazzulli, T.: Clinical impact of human herpesvirus 6 infection after liver transplantation. Transplantation 2002; 73: 599–604
401. Kaneko, J., Sugawara, Y., Makuuchi, M.: Aspergillus osteomyelitis after liver transplantation. Liver Transplant. 2002; 8: 1073–1075
402. Koch, S., Bresson-Hadni, S., Miguet, J.P., Crumbach, J.P., Gillet, M., Mantion, G.A., Heyd, B., Vuitton, D.A., Minello, A., Kurtz, S.: Experience of liver transplantation for incurable alveolar echinococcosis: A 45-case European collaborative report. Transplantation 2003; 75: 856–863
403. Koyama, I., Fuchinoue, S., Urashima, Y., Kato, Y., Tsuji, K., Kawase, T., Murakami, T., Tojimbara, T., Nakajima, I., Teraoka, S.: Living related liver transplantation for polycystic liver disease. Transplant Internat. 2002; 15: 578–580
404. Kurdow, R., Marks, H.G., Kraemer-Hansen, H., Luttges, J., Kremer, B., Henne-Bruns, D.: Recurrence of primary biliary cirrhosis after orthotopic liver transplantation. Hepato-Gastroenterol. 2003; 50: 322–325
405. Larson, A.M., Chan, G.C., Wartelle, C.F., McVicar, J.P., Carithers, R.L., Hamill, G.M., Kowdley, K.V.: Infection complicating percutaneous liver biopsy in liver transplant recipients. Hepatology 1997; 26: 1406–1409
406. Limaye, A.P., Perkins, J.D., Kowdley, K.V.: Listeria infection after liver transplantation: report of a case and review of the literature. Amer. J. Gastroenterol. 1998; 93: 1942–1944
407. MacLean, A.R., Lilly, L., Cohen, Z., O'Connor, B., McLeod, R.S.: Outcome of patients undergoing liver transplantation for primary sclerosing cholangitis. Dis. Col. Rect. 2003; 46: 1124–1128
408. Markmann, J.F., Markowitz, J.S., Yersiz, H., Morrisey, M., Farmer, D.G., Farmer, D.A., Goss, J., Ghobrial,.R., McDiarmid, S.V., Stribling, R., Martin, P., Goldstein, L.I., Seu, P., Shackleton, C., Busuttil, R.W.: Long-term survival after retransplantation of the liver. Ann. Surg. 1997; 226: 408–418
409. Mata, A., Bordas, J.M., Llach, J., Gines, A., Mondelo, F., Lopez Serrano, A., Valdecasas, J.C.G., Pique, J.M., Arroyo, V.: ERCP in orthotopic liver transplanted patients. Hepato-Gastroenterol. 2004; 51: 1801–1804
410. Mazzaferro, V., Tagger, A., Schiaro, M., Regalia, E., Pulvirenti, A., Ribero, M.L., Coppa, J., Romito, R., Burgoa, L., Zucchini, N., Urbanek, T., Bonino, F.: Prevention of recurrent hepatitis C after liver transplantation with early interferon and ribavirin treatment. Transplant. Proc. 2001; 33: 1355–1357
411. Menegaux, F., Keeffe, E.B., Baker, E., Egawa, H., Concepcion, W., Russell, T.R., Esquivel, C.O.: Comparison of transjugular and surgical portosystemic shunts on the outcome of liver transplantation. Arch. Surg. 1994; 129: 1018–1024
412. Middleton, P.F., Duffield, M., Lynch, S.V., Padbury, R.T.A., House, T., Stanton, P., Verran, D., Maddern, G.: Living donor liver transplantation – Adult donor outcomes: A systematic review. Liver Transplant. 2006; 12: 24–30
413. Miyagawa-Hayashino, A., Haga, H., Egawa, H., Hayashino, Y., Sakurai, T., Minamiguchi, S., Tanaka, K., Manabe, T.: Outcome and risk factors of de novo autoimmune hepatitis in living-donor liver transplantation. Transplantation 2004; 78: 128–135
414. Miyagawa-Hayashino, A., Tsuruyama, T., Haga, H., Oike, F., Il-Deok, K., Egawa, H., Hiai, H., Tanaka, K., Manabe, T.: Arteriopathy in chronic allograft rejection in liver transplantation. Liver Transplant. 2004; 10: 513–519
415. Molloy, R.M., Komorowski, R., Varma, R.R.: Recurrent nonalcoholic steatohepatitis and cirrhosis after liver transplantation. Liver Transplant. Surg. 1997; 3: 177–178
416. Nadalin, S., Testa, G., Malago, M., Beste, M., Frilling, A., Schroeder, T., Jochum, C., Gerken, G., Broelsch, C.E.: Volumetric and functional recovery of the liver after right hepatectomy for living donation. Liver Transplant. 2004; 10: 1024–1029
417. Nair, S., Cohen, D.B., Cohen, C., Tan, H., Maley, W., Thuluvath, P.J.: Postoperative morbidity, mortality, costs, and long-term survival in severely obese patients undergoing orthotopic liver transplantation. Amer. J. Gastroenterol. 2001; 96: 842–845
418. Neil, D.A., Hubscher, S.G.: Histological and biochemical changes during the evolution of chronic rejection of liver allografts. Hepatology 2002; 35: 639–651
419. Neumann, U.P., Berg, T., Bahra, M., Puhl, G., Guckelberger, O., Langrehr, J.M., Neuhaus, P.: Long-term outcome of liver transplants for chronic hepatitis C.: A 10-year follow-up. Transplantation 2004; 77: 226–231
420. Painter, P., Krasnoff, J., Paul, S.M., Aascher, N.L.: Physical activity and health-related quality of life in liver transplant recipients. Liver Transplant. 2001; 7: 213–219
421. Pereira, S.P., Howard, L.M., Muiesan, P., Rela, M., Heaton, N., Williams, R.: Quality of life after liver transplantation for alcoholic liver disease. Liver Transplant. 2000; 6: 762–768
422. Pirenne, J., Aerts, R., Yoong, K., Gunson, B., Koshiba, T., Fourneau, I., Mayer, D., Buckels, J., Mirza, D., Roskams, T., Elias, E., Nevens, F., Fevery, J., McMaster, P.: Liver transplantation for polycystic liver disease. Liver Transplant. 2001; 7: 238–245
423. Poulos, J.E., Bacon, B.R.: Liver transplantation for hereditary hemochromatosis. Dig. Dis. Sci. 1996; 14: 316–322
424. Pruett, T.: Obesity and the liver transplant recipient. Liver Transplant. 2002; 8: 171–173
425. Rabkin, J.M., Oroloff, S.L., Corless, C.L., Benner, K.G., Flora, K.D., Rosen, H.R., Olyaei, A.J.: Association of fungal infection and increased mortality in liver transplant recipients. Amer. J. Surg. 2000; 179: 426–430
426. Ringe, B., Braun, F., Schütz, E., Füzesi, L., Lorf, T., Canelo, R., Oellerich, M., Ramadori, G.: A novel management strategy of steroid-free immunosuppression after liver transplantation: Efficacy and safety of tacrolimus and mycophenolate mofetil. Transplantation 2001; 71: 508–515
427. Roayaie, S., Schiano, T.D., Thung, S.N., Emre, S.H., Fishbein, T.M., Miller, C.M., Schwartz, M.E.: Results of retransplantation for recurrent hepatitis C. Hepatology 2003; 38: 1428–1436
428. Rosenthal, P., Roberts, J.P., Ascher, N.L., Emond, J.C.: Auxiliary liver transplant in fulminant failure. Pediatrics 1997; 100: 101–103
429. Sanchez, A.J., Aranda-Michel, J.: Nutrition for the liver transplant patient. Liver Transplant. 2006; 12: 1310–1316
430. Schiano, T.D., Kim-Schluger, L., Gondolesi, G., Miller, C.: Adult living donor liver transplantation: the hepatologist's perspective. Hepatology 2001; 33: 3–9
431. Seehofer, D., Rayes, N., Tullius, S.G., Schmidt, C.A., Neumann, U.P., Radke, C., Settmacher, U., Müller, A.R., Steinmüller, T., Neuhaus, P.: CMV hepatitis after liver transplantation. Incidence, clinical course, and long-term follow-up. Liver Transplant. 2002; 8: 1138–1146
432. Selby, R., Starzl, T.E., Yunis, E., Brown, B.I., Kendall, R.S., Tzakis, A.: Liver transplantation for type IV glycogen storage disease. New Engl. J. Med. 1991; 324: 39–42
433. Shah, S.A., Levy, G.A., Adcock, L.D., Gallagher, G., Grant, D.R.: Adult-to-adult living donor liver transplantation (review). Can. J. Gastroenterol. 2006; 20: 339–343
434. Starzl, T.E., Marchioro, T.L., v. Kaulla, K.N., Hermann, G., Brittain, R.S., Waddell, W.R.: Homotransplantation of the liver in humans. Surg. Gynec. Obstetr. 1963; 117: 659–676
435. Sundaram, S.S., Alonso, E.M., Whitington, P.E.: Liver transplantation in neonates (review). Liver Transplant. 2003; 9: 783–788
436. Sutcliffe, R.P., Maguire, D.D., Muiesan, P., Dhawan, A., MieliVergani, G., Ogrady, J.G., Rela, M., Heaton, N.D.: Liver transplantation for Wilson's disease: Long-term results and quality-of-life assessment. Transplantation 2003; 75: 1003–1006
437. Sylvestre, P.B., Batts, K.P., Burgart, L.J., Poterucha, J.J., Wiesner, R.H.: Recurrence of primary biliary cirrhosis after liver transplantation: Histologic estimate of incidence and natural history. Liver Transplant. 2003; 9: 1086–1093
438. Tang, T.J., Janssen, H.L.A., van der Vlies, C.H., de Man, R.A., Metselaar, H.J., Tilanus, H.W., de Marie, S.: Aspergillus osteomyelitis after liver transplantation: conservative or surgical treatment. Eur. J. Gastroenterol. Hepatol. 2000; 12: 123–126
439. Teixeira, R., Pastacaldi, S., Davies, S., Dhillon, A.P., Emery, V.C., Rolles, K., Davidson, B., Patch, D., Burroughs, A.K.: The influence of cytomegalovirus viraemia on the outcome of recurrent hepatitis C after liver transplantation. Transplantation 2000; 70: 1454–1458
440. Ten Hove, W.R., van Hoek, B., Bajema, I.M., Ringers, J., van Krieken, J.H.J.M., Lagaaij, E.L.: Extensive chimerism in liver transplants: Vascular endothelium, bile duct epithelium, and hepatocytes. Liver Transplant. 2003; 9: 552–556
441. Van den Berg-Emons, R., van Ginneken, B., Wijffels, M., Tilanus, H., Metselaar, H., Stam, H., Kazemier, G.: Fatigue is a major problem after liver transplantation (review). Can. J. Gastroenterol. 2006; 20: 339–343
442. Verran, D., Kusyk, T., Painter, D., Fisher, J., Koorey, D., Strasser, S., Stewart, G., McCaughan, G.: Clinical experience gained from the use of 120 steatotic donor livers for orthotopic liver transplantation. Liver Transplant. 2003; 9: 500–505
443. Welch, C.S.: A note on transplantation of the whole liver in dogs. Transplant. Bull. 1955; 2: 54–55
444. Yersiz, H., Renz, J.F., Farmer, D.G., Hisatake, G.M., McDiarmid, S.V., Busuttil, R.W.: One hundred in situ split-liver transplantations. A single-center experience. Ann. Surg. 2003; 238: 496–507
445. Yilmaz, F., Aydin, U., Nart, D., Zeytunlu, M., Karasu, Z., Kaya, T., Ozer, I., Yuce, G., Aydogdu, S.: The incidence and management of acute and chronic rejection after living donor liver transplantation. Transplant. Proc. 2006; 38: 1435–1437

> The wish and the hope expressed by a Babylonian haruspex (a diviner whose predictions are based on inspecting the entrails of sacrificed animals) in the following sentence, which he inscribed as a repeating stereotype on a clay model of a sheep's liver (ca. 2000 BC) (s. fig. 1.1), is dedicated to all patients suffering from liver disease and also to all users of *"Hepatology – Textbook and Atlas"*:
>
> **"May your liver be smooth"**

> **"In the heart the physician grows,
> from God he proceeds ...
> The highest ground of all remedies is love."**

**Theophrastus Bombastus von Hohenheim,
known as PARACELSUS (1493–1541)**

Index

A

Aagenaes type 241, 699
Abdominal baldness 84, 90
Abdominal palpation 6, 81
Abdominal wall varices 264
Abdominoscopy 157
Abernethy malformation 860
Abetalipoproteinaemia 616
Acamprosat 550
Acanthosis nigricans 632
Aceruloplasminaemia 637
Accessory lobe 19, 32
Acetaldehyde 69, 75, 410, 534, 535, 538, 553, 918
Acetic acid injection 809
Acholic stool 248, 429, 680
Aciclovir 475, 476, 730, 882, 884
Acid-base disorders 384
Acid-base metabolism 64
Acidophilic bodies 406
Acinus 10, 11, 26, 27, 29, 37, 41, 62, 101, 274, 407, 549, 739, 779
Acrodermatitis papulosa 88
Actin filament 32
Actinomycosis 492
Activity 127
– enzymatic 116, 127, 747
– histological 127, 715
– immunological 127
– mesenchymal 116, 118, 127, 747
Acute fatty liver, pregnancy 606
Acute heart insufficiency 853
Acute intermittent porphyria 624
Acute leukaemia 838
Acute liver failure 91, 225, 256, 273, 279, 330, 380, 471, 519, 564, 588, 839, 847, 903
Acute phase protein 70, 111
Acute viral hepatitis 118, 411, 421
– history 421
– morphology 422
Addiction memory 533
Addictive substances 536
Adefovir 723, 726, 728, 734, 735, 882, 910
Adenocarcinoma 198, 405, 515, 814, 820, 822, 832
Adenoma 142, 181, 188, 202, 563, 569, 773, 776, 794, 900
Adenovirus hepatitis 477
Adhesiolysis 160
Adhesion 159
Adhesive glycoprotein 22
Adjuvant therapy 248, 271, 289, 358, 589, 603, 644, 730, 827, 873
Adrenalectomy 321
Adult polycystic disease 669, 697, 784
Adult Still's disease 846
Aerobilia 143, 186, 674
Aetiocholanolone fever 383, 761
Aflatoxin 57, 519, 581, 587, 591, 605, 799, 815, 828
African iron overload 646
African sleeping sickness 504
Airport malaria 502
Agent orange 585
Alagille's syndrome 649, 666, 687, 699, 710, 904
Alanine transaminase 101, 646
Albumin 53, 111, 228, 304, 314, 324, 335, 765, 858
– gradient 306
– synthesis 109, 112, 116, 266
Albumin dialyse 390
Alcohol 59, 64, 256, 532
– absorption 65
– abstinence 546, 550, 764
– alcoholism 533
– abuse 532, 645
– addiction 533
– biochemical effects 534
– biochemical values 65
– blood concentration 65
– catalase 68
– consumption 532, 542
– degradation 66
– endogenous synthesis 64
– lethal concentration 66
– malate-aspartate cycle 67
– MEOS 67, 534, 536
– uptake 64
– Widmark's formula 65
Alcohol dehydrogenase 66, 68, 75, 100, 534, 536, 553
Alcohol injection, percutaneous 809
Alcoholic fatty liver 118, 531, 534, 539, 543, 550, 593, 646, 918
Alcoholic foamy degeneration 402, 417, 544, 554
Alcoholic hyalin 538, 540
Alcoholic liver disease 533
– clinical features 543
– diagnostic markers 548
– morphology 537
– pathogenesis 541
– steatohepatitis 544
– therapy 550
Alcoholic porphyria 531, 535
Alcoholism 533
– diagnostic markers 548
– physical dependence 533
– psychological dependence 533
– types 533
Aldehyde dehydrogenase 68, 75, 100, 534, 554
Aldolase 96, 100, 613, 649, 803
Aldosterone 298, 299
Aldosteronism 274, 278, 293, 313, 462
Alemtuzumal 844
Algorithmic diagnostics 127
Alkaline phosphatase 107
– elevation 107
– decrease 108
Allgoewer-Burri index 355
Allopurinol, test 611
Alpha-antichymotrypsin 610
Alpha-antitrypsin 307, 607, 699
Alpha-foetoprotein 112, 129, 453, 748, 763, 803, 829, 868
ALT (GPT) 102
Alzheimer glia type II 277
Amanita phalloides 382, 388, 587
Amantadine 444, 730, 884
Amino acids 42, 275
– aromatic 42, 275, 753
– biochemistry 42
– classification 42, 43
– degradation 42
– imbalance 275, 753
– pool 42
Aminopyrine 14C breath test 115
Ammonia 61, 113, 259, 274, 284, 888, 890
– detoxification 42, 61, 62, 63
– formation 61
– glutamine cycle 62
– metabolism 61
– neurotoxicity 61
– tolerance test 113, 747
Amoebiasis 498
– abscess 201, 500
– amoeboma 499
Amyloidosis 88, 487, 609
Anabolism 51
Anabolite 556
Anamnesis 80, 232, 566
Anasarka 295
Anatomia Mundini 8
Anatomy 17
Anaxagoras 6
Andersen's disease 613
Androgens 39, 50, 70, 609, 775, 779, 798, 799
Angiography 186, 260, 373
Angiolipoma 782
Angiomyolipoma 782
Angiosarcoma 818
Angular cheilosis 86, 87
Anorectal varices 251, 259, 260, 264, 378, 737, 760, 770
Antibiogram 310
Antibiotics 288
Antibodies 123, 124, 245, 567, 657
– antihistone 95, 124, 127, 537, 546, 884
– antinuclear 124
– antiribosomal 687
– granulocytes 127
– liver-kidney microsomes 125
– liver membrane 125
– mitochondria 126
– smooth muscle 125
– soluble liver protein 126
– system 124
Antidiuretic hormon 299, 325, 330
Antifibrinogen 410, 894
Anti-GOR 95, 127, 452, 658, 659, 666, 690, 721
Antihistone 95, 124, 127, 537, 546, 884
Antioxidants 68, 71, 72, 603
Antiporter 74
Antipyrine test 115
Antiquity 2
Antithrombin III 111, 351
– concentrate 353
Antral vascular ectasia 354, 760
Apolipoproteins 41, 46, 48, 244, 540, 550, 557
APOLT 392, 395, 903, 907
Apoprotein B 616
Apoptosis 25, 238, 406
APUD cells 25, 819
Arenavirus 478
Aretaios 7, 224
Arginine deiminase 811
Arias syndrome 229
Aristoteles 6, 252
Aromatic amines 58, 579, 585, 586, 799
Aromatic amino acids 42, 273, 275, 276, 278, 286, 753, 890
Arsenic 181, 580, 586
Artefacts 133
Arterial aneurysm 864
Arterial bruit 92
Arterial ligation 322
Arterial occlusion 865
Arteriography 187
Arteriohepatic dysplasia 699
Arterioportal fistula 254, 861
Arteriosclerosis 866
Arthropathy 634, 641, 643, 645, 652, 758, 803
Ascaris lumbricoides 504
Ascites 6, 7, 83, 141, 164, 296, 385, 756, 899
– albumin gradient 306
– bacterial peritonitis 308, 757
– complications 308
– differential diagnosis 306, 308
– formation 297
– hydrothorax 304
– latent 303, 311
– lymph cysts 297, 298
– lymph imbalance theory 300

– overflow theory 300
– portal 302
– refractory 316
– reinfusion 316
– sonography 141, 304
– surgical procedures 321, 322
– transsudate 306
– ultrafiltration 317
– underfill theory 300
– vasodilation theory 300
Asiaglycoprotein receptor 125, 658
Aspartate transaminase 101
Aspergillosis 519
Assessment scale 98
AST (GOT) 102
Asterixis 208, 214, 280, 282, 284, 382
Asteroid bodies 788
Atransferrinaemia 637
Atrial natriuretic factor 299
Atrophic cirrhosis 741
Auscultation, scratch 83
Australian antigen 119, 422
Autoantibodies 123
Autoimmune cholangitis 693
– morphology 694
– therapy 694
Autoimmune hepatitis 655
– classification 658
– morphology 660
– pathogenesis 656
– therapy 663
Autoimmune polyendocrine syndrome 659
Avicenna 8
Azathioprine 664, 683, 684, 685
Azotaemia 278, 314, 332, 333, 335, 586
Azure lunulae 632

B

Babylonian 2, 5
Bacterial cholangitis 671
Bacterial infections 384, 387, 484, 754
Bacterial pathogens 484
Bacterial peliosis hepatis 404
Bacteriocholia 670, 671
Balloon dilatation 693, 858
Balloon tamponade 365
– Linton-Nachlas 365
– Minnesota tube 365
– Sengstaken-Blakemore 365
Ballooned hepatocytes 401, 424, 446, 539, 544, 560
Banti's syndrome 255
BCLC classification 806
Beef-like cells 486
BELS 391
Benfotiamine 551
Bengal rose iodine test 116
Benign recurrent cholestasis 241
Benign tumours 416, 563, 774
– classification 774
Benzpyrene 587
Berlin-blue reaction 54, 621, 638

Beta blocker 366, 762, 767, 772, 860, 877
Beta-hexosaminidase 550
Betaine 897
Bezafibrate 683
Bicarbonate neutralization 35, 57, 63, 64
– acid-base metabolism 64
– metabolic acidosis 63
– metabolic alkalosis 63
Bifidum milk 287
Bile 10, 39, 41
– canalicular 41
– ductular 42
– lipids 42
– salts 40
Bile acids 10, 39, 107, 244
– cholesterol-hydroxylase 39
– functions 41
– function test 101
– pool 40
– primary 39
– pump system 41
– secondary 40
– tertiary 40
– transport 41
Bile drainage 671, 675
Bile droplets 236, 246, 560
Bile-duct adenoma 785
Bile-duct papillomatosis 786
Bile infarct 236, 238, 246
Bile lipids 42
Bile pigments, urine 106
– urinary dipstick 106
Bile thrombi 238, 560
Bilharziosis 509
Biliary atresia 696, 739
Biliary cirrhosis 415, 673, 679, 696, 739, 743, 744
Biliary epithelial cell 15, 17, 26
Biliary hamartoma 787
Biliary leakage 154, 166, 202
Biliary pneumonia 485
Biliary steatorrhoea 248
Biliary system 21
– biliferous ductule 21
– canaliculus 21
– cholangiole 21
– choledochus 6, 21
– common hepatic duct 21
Biliary varices 265
Biliorenal syndrome 674
Bilirubin 12, 37, 38, 105, 106, 225, 244
– bilirubin-albumin complex 37
– conjugation 38, 225
– delta 38, 105, 225, 244
– direct 38, 105
– excretion 38
– indirect 38, 105
– shunt bilirubin 37
– unconjugated 225
Bilirubinostasis 236, 237, 246, 401, 403, 424, 561
Bilirubinuria 106
Bilitranslocase 38
Biliverdin 12, 37
Bioartificial liver systems 391

Biochemical dysfunction 98
Biochemical check list 99
Biopsy needle 151
– Menghini 151, 155, 159, 169
– Trucut 133, 152, 155, 156, 165, 169, 171, 173
– Jamshidi 152, 155, 156, 157
– spring-loaded 152
– Vim-Silverman 152, 155, 165, 169, 173, 750, 751
Biotoxometabolite 57, 59, 68, 377, 556, 565, 581
Biotransformation 56, 68, 244, 556, 581
– enzyme adaptation 58
– enzyme induction 59
– enzyme inhibition 59
– fat-soluble substances 56
– glucuronidation capacity 57
– water-soluble substances 56
Bipolar probe 357
Black liver jaundice 231
Black tea 644, 727, 881
Blastogenesis 16
Blastomycosis 520
Blebbing stage 406
Block surgery 370, 900
Blood circulation 9, 202, 252, 384
Blood sample collection 97
BLSS 391
Body mass index 605
Boiling stage 406
Booster effect 119, 431, 444
Borreliosis 490
Bosentan 344, 759
Boswellinic acids 665, 685, 693
Botkin's disease 421
Boutonneuse fever 491
Bowel purgation 356, 357
Brain 208, 272
– disorders 208
– functions 208, 272
Brain's reward system 533
Branched-chain amino acids 39, 42, 43, 44, 271, 273, 275, 276, 287, 288, 292, 334, 335, 387, 535, 550, 589, 747, 752, 753, 756, 763, 769, 770, 771, 810, 871, 877, 881, 889, 890, 916, 917
– modes of action 890
Breast-milk jaundice 228
Bridging necrosis 407
Bright (white) liver 138
Brimstone fibrosis 413
Brimstone liver 489
Bromocriptine 289
Bromopyruvate 811
Bromsulphthalein test 117
Bronchial varices 265
Bronze diabetes 88, 635, 641
Brown atrophy 604
Brucellosis 490
Bruit de diable 92
B-symptomatology 816
Budd-Chiari syndrome 140, 182, 200, 257, 562, 587, 840, 856

– clinical findings 857
– morphology 857
Budesonide 664, 665, 685, 693, 702, 704
Bull's eye phenomenon 144, 804
Bunyavirus 468, 478
Bupleurum 568, 726, 898
Burkholderia pseudomallei 492
Bush pattern 805
Butterfly sign 88, 680
Byler's disease 242
Byler's syndrome 242

C

Caffeine elimination test 115
CAGE test 548
Calcareous foci 799
Calcium homoeostasis 408, 557, 853
Campylobacter colitis 491
Canaliculus 16, 21
Cancer umbilicus 821
Candidosis 519
Capacity for work 913
– guidelines for evaluation 913
– reduction in earning capacity 913
Capecitabin 827
Capillaria hepatica 506
Capillarization, sinusoidal 413, 540, 541, 567, 586, 592, 742, 743
Capillary permeability 297, 302, 411
Caput Medusae 91, 92, 254, 264, 265, 749, 861
Carbamoyl phosphate 62
Carbohydrate metabolism 11, 35, 36, 44, 45, 52, 595, 737, 746, 752
– glucolysis 35, 45
– gluconeogenesis 35, 45, 50
– glucose paradox 45
– glucose pool 45
– glycogenesis 45
– glycogenolysis 45
Carbohydrate-deficient transferrin 549, 552, 553, 554
Carbon dioxide venography 260
Carbon pigment 403
Carbon tetrachloride 584
Carcinoid 171, 795, 797, 820, 823, 834, 835
Cardiac cirrhosis 18, 739, 852, 855, 859, 867
Cardiovascular diseases 852
– morphology 853
– pathophysiology 852
Caroli's disease 182, 697, 785
Caroli's syndrome 785
Carotene jaundice 224
Carrier, chronic, HBsAg 434
Catabolism 51, 753
Catabolite 556

Catalase 68
Catalase reaction 72
Catechin 898
Catecholamin 50
Cat-scratch fever 404, 492
Caudate lobe 18, 20, 137, 139, 856, 857
Cavernous haemangioma 182, 185, 188, 195, 203, 205, 412, 774, 780, 789, 818, 902
Cavernous transformation 141, 253, 861, 862
Cavography 191
Cell death 406
– programmed 406
– provoked 406
Cell necrosis 407
Cell nucleus 29, 30
Cellular bilirubinostasis 236
Cellular hydrops 246, 401, 539, 560
Cellular infiltration 562
Cellular polarization 25
Cellular transport processess 73
Celsus 7
Central dot sign 697
Central hepatic vein 21, 27
Central hyaline sclerosis 414
Central vein lobule 26
Centrilobular perivenular fibrosis 414, 540
Centrocytic lymphoma 845
Cerebral functions 209, 214, 281, 283, 290, 305, 890
Cerebral oedema 290, 381, 383, 384, 387, 388, 392, 394, 395, 577, 588
Cerebrohepatorenal syndrome 242, 620
Cerebrotendinous xanthomatosis 616
Ceroid 73, 403, 405, 423, 447, 604, 619, 840, 855
Ceruloplasmin 54, 629, 633
Cestodes 510
Chagas' disease 504
Chameleon phenomenon 144
Charcot's triad 672
Check list 74, 79, 81, 92, 99, 128, 282, 567, 768, 747
Chemical lesion 58, 59
Chemical substances 582
– historical review 580
– morphology 582
– pathophysiology 582
Chemoembolization 809, 810
Chemotherapy 808, 809, 811, 826, 827
Chenodeoxycholic acid 39, 40, 242, 616, 623, 649, 699, 886
Cherry red spots 360
Chiari's disease 257
Chiari's triad 856
Chicken-wire fibrosis 413, 414, 540
Chilaiditi syndrome 19, 82
Childhood fibropolycystic disease 697
Child-Pugh criteria 347, 360, 750, 807

Chinese herbs 567
Chinese liver fluke 507
Chlamydia 491
Chlorambucil 570, 585, 683, 703
Chloroquine 500, 503, 570, 598, 624, 628
Cholangiocarcinoma 503, 507, 508, 691, 813
– clinical features 815
– morphology 814
Cholangiodysplasia 255, 696
Cholangiography 191
– direct 191, 674
– indirect 191
– intraoperative 194
– laparoscopic 194
– MRCP 191
– percutaneous 194
– postoperative 194
– transvenous 194
Cholangiolitis lenta 485
Cholangitis 501, 670
– acute 672
– aetiology 670
– ascending 670
– autoimmune 693
– bacterial 671
– chronic 672
– chronic non-suppurative destructive 675, 678
– classification 670
– descending 670
– morphology 672
– obstructive 671
– parasitic 671
– tuberculous 486
Cholate stasis 237, 561, 788
Choledochal cyst 183
Choledocholithiasis 691
Cholehepatic shunt 40, 887
Cholelithiasis 672, 691, 761
– cholesterol-calcium pigment 672
Cholemie simple familiale 229
Cholestasis 107, 123, 236, 402, 539, 547, 560, 690
– bile acids 9, 10, 39, 107, 244, 595
– bile infarct 238
– bile lake 236, 238, 865
– bile thrombi 238
– biliary steatorrhoea 248
– bilirubinostasis 237
– cholate stasis 237, 561, 788
– enzymatic markers 107, 236, 244
– feathery degeneration 238, 246, 424
– histology 246
– intrahepatic 238, 239
– liver cell rosette 237, 407, 424, 660
– malabsorption 248, 765
– network necrosis 238
– obstructive 236, 238
– paralytic 237
– pregnancy 240
– progressive familiale 241
– pruritus 89, 240, 243, 683, 692

– scintigraphy 202
– scratch marks 89, 240, 243
Cholestatic course 419, 424, 426, 430, 431, 441, 445, 452, 458, 544, 604, 910
Cholestatic syndrome 202, 250, 547
Cholesterol 11, 48, 49, 108
Cholesterol ester storage 402, 615
Cholestyramine 229, 233, 241, 249, 250, 431, 445, 623, 683, 755
Cholic acid 39
Cholinesterase 109
Chondroma 782
CHOP 845
Chromium 56
Chronic heart insufficiency 854
Chronic hepatitis 117, 399, 632, 692, 712
– clinical findings 717
– cryptogenic 660, 696, 716
– extrahepatic manifestations 719
– grading 714
– historical review 712
– lobular 712
– minimal 712
– morphology 712, 717
– necrotizing 712
– non-viral 714, 717
– persistent 712
– scoring systems 716
– septal 712
– staging 714
Chronic hepatitis B 719
– classification 720
– immunostimulants 726
– morphology 720
– nucleoside analogues 725
– serology 720
– therapy 722
Chronic hepatitis C 721
– course 721
– morphology 721
– therapy 727
– triple therapy 730
Chronic liver insufficiency 385
– compensated 385
– decompensated 385
– global 385
– partial 385
– therapy 387, 389, 391, 392
Chronic lymphatic leukaemia 843
Chronic myeloid leukaemia 839
Chronic non-suppurative destructive cholangitis 499, 675, 678, 705
Churg-Strauss vasculitis 847
Chvostek's body type 84
Chylomicrons 47
Chylous ascites 306, 318, 323, 822, 868, 900
Cirrhosis 168, 181, 188, 200, 414, 541, 546, 716, 720, 738
– aetiology 743

– atrophic 739, 741
– Child-Pugh 347, 360, 750, 807
– classification 738, 745
– complete 742
– cryptogenic 744
– decompensation 745, 746
– endoscopy 750
– evaluation programme 768
– hypertrophic 739
– incomplete septal 740, 742
– laboratory findings 747
– laparoscopy 168, 169, 749
– macronodular 415, 740
– micronodular 415, 541, 740
– mixed nodular 415, 741
– morphology 742
– pseudolobular 741
– psychological guidance 766
– Nagayo type 740
– postdystrophic 415, 742
– smooth 256, 415, 739
Circulating immune complex 123
Cirrhotic glomerular sclerosis 757
Clay pipe-stem fibrosis 255, 413, 509
Clearance function 70, 105
Clevudine 726
Clinical findings 80, 92
Clinical studies 60, 551, 873, 878
– cohort 873
– comparability 874
– controlled 873
– difficulties 874
– placebo 874
– prospective 873
– retrolective 873
– retrospective 873
– trohoc 873
– types 873
CLIP score 806
Clonidine 207
Clonorchis sinensis 507
Clostridium 491
Cluster sign 525
Coagulation 110, 348
– cascade system 110, 349
– factors 110
Coagulation necrosis 407, 560, 739, 810, 826
Coagulopathy 348, 384, 386
– DIC 350, 384
– fibrinolysis 348
– forms of haemostasis 348
– therapy 352
Cobalt 56
Coccidioidomycosis 520
Coelioscopy 157
Cohort 873
Colchicine 551, 683, 692, 897
Collagen 22, 424, 410
Collateral circulation 262
Collidon 561
Colliquation necrosis 407
Colloidosmotic pressure 296, 297
Colombi index 111, 350, 439

927

Index

Colour-encoded duplex sonography 134, 749
Comet-tail phenomenon 142, 525
Common bile duct 21
Common hepatic artery 20, 187, 864
Complaints 81, 232, 746, 802
Complete responder 724
Computer tomography 178, 804
– contraindications 179
– contrast media 179
– grew liver 180
– Hounsfield unit 178
– indications 180
– principle 178
– volumetry 179
Concomitant virus hepatitis 474
Congenital erythropoietic porphyria 623
Congenital hepatic cyst 141
Congenital liver fibrosis 239, 255, 333, 669, 687, 697, 698, 785
Congestion index 260
Congestive liver 138, 854
Congestive fibrosis 855
Coniothyrium 521
Conjugated bile acids 39
Conjugated bilirubin 38, 225, 232
Conjugation reaction 58
Connective tissue 10, 23
Consensus IFN 723, 730, 882, 883
Constrictive pericarditis 859
Contraceptive 563, 564
Conversion syndrome 696
Copper 54, 108, 245, 629, 633
Coproporphyrin 39
Corbicula portalis 27
Cori's disease 613
Corpus Hippocraticum 6
Cotton wool sign 780
Cough furrow 18
Councilman body 402, 406, 423, 446, 451, 478, 482, 660, 713, 840
Cowdry type 402, 475
Coxsackie hepatitis 477
Crane hepatitis 431
Crigler-Najjar syndrome 229
Critical flicker frequency 211, 281
Cross circulation 389
Cruveilhier-von Baumgarten disease 91, 254, 861
Cruveilhier-von Baumgarten syndrome 91, 140, 163, 254, 359, 861
Cryoglobulinaemia 719
Cryosurgery 807, 808, 826, 831
Cryptococcosis 520
Cryptosporidiosis 501
Crystalloid solution 356
Cupruria 633
Cyanosis 342

Cyclin 409
Cyclophosphamide 665, 885
Cyclosporine 665, 683, 684, 885
Cynara scolymus 898
CYP 2 E1 67, 552
Cyst 141, 182, 698, 783
Cystadenocarcinoma 816
Cystadenoma 784
Cystic fibrosis 620
Cystinosis 611
Cytochrome P-450 58, 456, 584, 585, 896, 918, 919
Cytokine 24, 50, 537
Cytomegalovirus 476
Cytoplasm 29
Cytoplast 32
Cytoskeleton 32
Cytosol 29, 39

D

Dacie's syndrome 221
Dane particle 119, 121, 422
Dark liver 138, 642
Dark liver cell 29, 446
Darlrymple's sign 90
Darrow-Yanett principle 295
DDT 584
Debre' s syndrome 617
Decholine test 189
Decompensation 385
– metabolic 745, 746
– portal 385, 745
Deferoxamine 72, 105, 569, 642, 644, 654, 840, 877
Dehydration 295
Deiodase 55
Delta-aminolaevulinic acid 39
Delta-bilirubin 38, 105, 225, 244
Dengue fever 479
Dentistry, hepatitis 438
Denver shunt 317
Deoxycholic acid 40
DeRitis quotient 101, 429, 439, 566, 601, 602, 822
Des-γ-carboxyprothrombin 748, 763, 803, 804, 829, 830, 831
Desmopressine 152, 353
Desmosome 25
Desmoteric infection 437
Diabetes mellitus 605, 641, 752
Diacytosis 74
Diagnosis 78
– accuracy 80, 98
– complaints 81
– detailed 78, 80, 169
– early 78
– pillars 79
– questions 81
– rational 78
– specificity 80
– targets 79
Diaita 6
Dialysis unit 438
Diaplacental infection 436
Diazo reaction 105, 227, 230, 232

Diazoxide 827
Dicrocoelium dentriciticum 507
Diet 765, 878
Dietary advice 311
Dimethyl sulphoxide 610
Diogenes 6, 411
Dioxin 581, 585
Direct bilirubin 38, 105, 225
Disability 913
Disorientation 272
Disseminated intravascular coagulopathy 350
Disse's space 22, 23
Disulfiram 536
Diuretics 278, 312, 313
– resistance 314
– sequential nephron blockade 314
– side effects 314
Documentation sheet 283, 286, 311, 756, 766, 768, 880, 881
Dolichol 550
Donnan equilibrium 295
Dopamine 276, 335, 388
Doppler sonography 133, 259
Doss porphyria 626
Double-barrelled-gun phenomenon 141, 245
Double-flow principle 19
Double wheel structure 526
Downhill varices 263
Dronabinol 241, 249
Dropsy 6
Drug therapy 881
– efficacy 874
– marketability 874
– metabolism 854
– placebo 874
– quality 874
– safety 874
Drug-induced damage 91, 117, 424, 556, 575, 577, 710
– clinical aspects 565
– idiosyncratic 558
– immunological type 558
– metabolic type 558
– morphological reactions 559
– pathogenesis 557
– re-exposure trial 569
– withdrawal trial 568
Drumstick fingers 90, 342, 343
Dubin-Johnson syndrome 230, 430
Duck hepatitis virus 431
Ductal plate 16
Ductal plate malformation 696
Duct of Arantius 16
Ductopenia 560, 696, 697, 699, 700
Ductular bile 42
Ductular bilirubinostasis 236
Ductus venosus 9, 16
Duodenal varices 364
Duplex sonography 134
Dupuytren's contracture 87
Durio Zibethinus 64
Dwarf threadworm 506

Dyscrasia 6
Dysontogenetic cyst 182
Dysplastic lesions 416, 801
Dyspnoea 342
Dysproteinaemia 111
Dystrophia lenta 586

E

Ebola virus 479
Ecchymosis 90
Echinococcus 510
– alveolaris 144, 182, 188, 510, 512
– cysticus 182, 510
– oligarthus 510
– vogeli 510
Echofree lesions 141
Echogenicity 138
ECHO virus hepatitis 477
Eck's fistula 286
Ecstasy 588
Ectopic varices 262, 760
EEG 208, 280, 283
– endogenous evoked 209, 283
– P-300 wave 209, 283
– spontaneous 208, 284
– visual evoked 209, 284
Effector hormones 50
Effemination 84
Ehrlichiosis 486
Eicosanoid 24, 49, 50, 69, 70, 408
ELAD 391
Elastin 22
Elastrography 135
Electrohydrothermoprobe 358
Electrolyte balance 283, 293, 294, 298, 299, 302, 305, 334, 374, 445, 756, 880, 881, 893
Embryogenesis 16
Embryology 16
Embryonal sarcoma 817
Empedokles 6
Emperipolesis 407, 660
Empirical therapy 872
Emtricitabine 726
Encephalopathy 208, 272, 382, 385, 756
– amino acids 275
– ammonia 274, 284
– asterixis 208, 214, 280, 282, 284, 382
– benzodiazepine 276
– brain oedema 273, 383
– clinical forms 278, 281
– coma check-lists 282
– coma hepaticum 284, 380, 386
– documentation sheet 283, 286, 311, 756, 766, 768, 880, 881
– EEG 280, 283
– flapping tremor 282
– flumazenil 289
– gliopathy 273
– Golytely solution 286
– Helicobacter pylori 61, 66, 274, 545, 756

- hepatic foetor 91, 275, 383
- hyperammoniaemia 274
- lactulose 287
- latent (minimal) 280
- mannitol solution 286
- mercaptan 275
- morphology 277
- neuropsychological test 280
- ornithine aspartate 287
- pathogenesis 273
- portacaval myelopathy 281
- portosystemic 280
- protein intake 277, 286, 765
- proton MR spectroscopy 280
- psychometric test 211, 281, 283, 284, 881
- subclinical 280

Endemic spotted fever 491
Endocrinopathy 754, 641
Endocytosis 74
Endogenous ligands 58
Endoplasmic reticulum 31
- rough 30, 44
- smooth 30, 59, 57, 218, 400, 537, 559

Endosonography 135
Endothelial cells 24
Endothelialitis 909
Endothelin 300, 344
Endotoxin 70, 237, 300, 588, 761
Enemas 285, 357
Energy balance 751
Entamoeba histolytica 498
Entecavir 726
Enteral feeding 879
Enterohepatic circulation 12, 38, 40, 106
Enzymes 99
- adaptation 58
- classification 100
- elevation 100
- enzymatic activity 116
- enzyme code 99
- enzyme distortion 100
- enzyme elimination 100
- enzyme pattern 100, 109
- enzyme ratios 101, 552
- induction 59
- inhibition 59

Eosinophilic granulomatous vasculitis 847
Episodes of acute hepatitis 426
Epithelioid haemangioendothelioma 817
EPL (s. Essent. phospholipids) 388, 551, 569, 589, 603, 605, 647, 727, 894, 895, 896, 918, 919
Epomediol 241
Epoprostenol 344, 345, 346, 759
Epping disease 581, 586
Eppinger 96
Epstein-Barr virus 474
Erasistratos 7
ERC 177, 191, 674, 690
Erdheim-Chester disease 799

Erythema diffusum hepaticum 88
Erythropoietic porphyria 623
Escape phenomenon 299
Escherichia coli 485
Essential phospholipids (s. EPL) 48, 228, 240, 334, 388, 394, 543, 551, 553, 569, 589, 603, 605, 620, 647, 727, 730, 765, 767, 871, 876, 877, 879, 880, 893, 894, 895, 896, 897, 898, 918
- cytoprotective effects 895
- indications 895
- membrane functions 895
- modes of action 895

Ethacrynic acid 313
Ethanol injection 809
Ethylglucuronide 549
Etruscans 3
Eucrasia 6
Euler-Liljestrand reflex 342
Exanthema 88
Exchange transfusion 389
Exocytosis 74
Exotic hepatotropic viruses 478
Explorative laparoscopy 158, 806, 815
Extracellular matrix 22, 410
Extramedullary haemopoiesis 838

F

Fabri's disease 618
Facies cirrhotica 84
Facilitated diffusion 73
Factor II index 804
Factor VIII 95, 110, 351, 383, 393, 413, 428, 748, 818, 862, 868
Factor XIII 348, 350, 351, 353
Facultative hepatotoxins 558
Falciform ligament 9, 16, 18, 20, 22, 26, 136, 137, 144, 146, 153, 163, 164, 179, 194, 298, 824, 899
Famciclovir 725, 883
Familiar quotations 5
Fanconi's syndrome 610, 611, 614
Fasciola hepatica 507
Fasciolopsis buski 508
Fat cysts 540, 597
Fat embolism 548, 602
Fatigue 91, 243, 475, 717, 746, 846
Fat-soluble vitamins 51, 683, 753
Fat storing cells 24
Fatty acid-binding protein 48
Fatty acid degeneration 48
Fatty acid-synthesis 47
Fatty degeneration 596, 598
Fatty infiltration 596
Fatty liver 138, 180, 185, 539, 596
- acute, pregnancy 606
- cryptogenic 599
- fat cysts 540, 597

- fat embolism 548, 602
- fatty infiltration 596
- focal 144, 180, 598, 599, 782
- macrovesicular 560, 597
- microvesicular 560, 598, 606, 607
- morphology 596
- pathogenesis 596
- segmental 598

Faulty nutrition 604
Feathery degeneration 238, 246, 402, 560
Felty's syndrome 846
Fenestra 24
Fenton reaction 71
Ferritin 54, 104, 307, 403, 638, 642
Ferrochelatase 39, 535, 621, 622, 623, 626
Fetogenesis 16
Fever 164, 383, 761
FGF 16
Fibrinogen 110, 348, 353
Fibrinolysis 348
Fibrin-ring granuloma 430
Fibrogenesis 410, 540, 742
Fibrolamellar carcinoma 813
Fibronectin 307
Fibrosarcoma 819
Fibrosis 118, 165, 412, 540, 714
- brushwood-like 413
- centrilobular perivenular 414, 540
- chicken-wire 413, 540
- clay pipe stem 255, 413, 509
- holly leaf 413
- marker 118, 412
- periductular 413
- periportal 413, 540
- perisinusoidal 413, 540
- perivenous 414
- portal 413, 561
- septal 414, 742

Fibrotic cholestatic hepatitis 441
Fibrous histiocytoma 819
Fibrous tumour 783
Filoviruses 478
Filtration pressure 296
Fine-needle biopsy 133, 157, 204, 775, 781, 806, 808, 825
Finger clubbing 90
Fitz-Hugh-Curtis syndrome 92, 477, 485, 491
Five-finger rule 589
Flapping tremor 282
Flare-up 720, 724
Flavin icterus 84, 224
Flaviviridae 478
Flow diagram 79, 145, 184, 186, 199, 204, 205, 232, 247, 372, 674
Fluctuation wave 83
Fluid spaces 294
Flumazenil 289, 756
Fluorouracil 827
Flushing syndrome 66, 70, 536
Fly agaric liver 789

Foam cells 70, 246, 402, 488, 547, 607, 615, 616, 617, 618, 619, 909
Focal fatty infiltration 142, 146, 180, 181, 186, 195, 196, 598, 602, 646, 782
Focal lesions 141, 168, 181, 186, 201
Focal nodular hyperplasia 142, 181, 186, 188, 202, 563, 777
Focal reduction of fat 142
Forbes subtype 613
Forbes-Hers subtype 613
Forceps biopsy 165, 775, 806
Forward flow hypothesis 252
Francisella tularense 491
Free diffusion 73
Free fatty acids 48
Free radicals disease 73
Frerichs 12
Fresh frozen plasma 352, 356
Friction rub 92
Fructose intolerance 614, 615
Ftorafur 827
Fucosidosis 620
Fulminant hepatitis 279
Fulminant liver failure 382, 425, 430, 441, 458, 476, 477, 564, 632
Funnel liver 413, 738
Furosemide 313, 757
Fuzzy coat 24

G

GABA 276
Galactosaemia 614
Galactose 812, 828
- elimination capacity 95, 113, 114, 129, 394, 544, 601, 602, 612, 614, 680, 705, 747, 751, 791, 803, 853, 905, 925
- test 612, 613

Galactosyl-neoglycoalbumin 203
Galenos 7, 252
Gall-bladder carcinoma 167
Gallium 203
Gamma globulin 117
Gamma glutamyl transferase 59, 103, 537, 549
- alcohol marker 104
- physiological elevation 59, 104

Gamna-Gandy nodule 261
Ganciclovir 476, 477, 481, 735, 882, 884, 909
Gangliosidosis 618
Gap junctions 25
Gastric alcohol dehydrogenase 66, 553, 554
Gastrinoma 820
Gastric antral vascular ectasia 760
Gastric varices 363
Gastrin 332
Gastrointestinal haemorrhage 353

929

Index

– lower 372
– upper 353
Gastrolavage 356
Gaucher cells 402, 617
Gaucher's disease 88, 617
GB viruses 459
GDH 102
Gianotti-Crosti syndrome 88, 439
Giant cell arteriitis 846
Giant-cell hepatitis 425, 476, 477, 503
Giant gall-bladder staghorn 800
Giant mitochondria 237, 401, 538, 544, 559
Gierke's disease 612
Gilbert-Meulengracht syndrome 229
Glasgow scale 282
Gliopathy 277
Glisson 10, 252
– Glisson's capsule 9, 23
– Glisson's triangle 9, 22, 24, 27
Glomangioma 783
Glucagon 50, 274
– test 612, 615
Glucocerebroside 617
Glucocorticoids 50, 389, 663, 884
Glucolysis 45
Gluconeogenesis 45, 50
Glucose-alanine cycle 43
Glucose metabolism 46
Glucose paradox 45
Glucose pool 45
Glucose tolerance factor 56
Glucostate 45, 752
GLUT 45
Glutamate dehydrogenase 102
Glutamic oxaloacetic transaminase 101
Glutamic pyruvic transaminase 101
Glutamine 62, 274
Glutamine cycle 62
Glycerol 45
Glyceryl trinitrate 367
Glycogen 45
Glycogen storage disease 612
Glycogen vacuolation of nuclei 120, 402, 540, 597, 600, 605, 613, 630, 639
Glycogenolysis 45, 752
Glycoproteins 44
Glycyrrhiza glabra 897, 726
Goat's milk, raw 765
Golgi complex 30, 31
Golytely solution 286, 357
GOT (AST) 102
– mitochondrial 102
Gout 606
GPT (ALT) 102, 538
– screening enzyme 102
Grading 714
Granular cell swelling 401, 538
Granuloma 405, 499, 500, 501, 502, 503, 509, 561, 787
– eosinophilic 405

– epithelioid 787
– fibrin-ring 430
– foreign-body 405
– immune 405
– lipogranuloma 405
– lipophagic 539
Granulomatosis infantiseptica 490
Granulomatous hepatitis 405, 470, 487
Grey liver 602
Griseofulvin 587
Ground squirrel hepatitis 431
Ground-glass cell 120, 402, 432, 559, 720, 802
Gumma 490
Gynaecomastia 87
Gyromitrin 588

H

Haber-Weiss reaction 71
Haem 37, 38, 621
Haemangioma 143, 203, 779
Haemarginate 625, 893
Haematemesis 354, 361, 760
Haematoma 143, 154, 182, 188
Haematopoiesis 16
Haematopoietic system 838
Haemobilia 154, 167, 171, 172, 187, 188, 193, 194, 227, 239, 354, 369, 505, 508, 787, 865
Haemochezia 373
Haemochromatosis 88, 181, 185, 635, 880
– arthropathy 641
– bronze diabetes 88, 641
– cardiomyopathy 641
– classification 636
– clinical findings 641
– deferoxamine test 105
– endocrinopathy 641
– morphology 639
– neonatal 637
– pathogenesis 637
– therapy 643
Haemoclips 358
Haemocystic spots 360
Haemodiaabsorption 389
Haemofiltration 389
Haemolysis 97, 226, 228, 633, 840
Haemoperfusion 389
Haemopexin 54
Haemorrhage 352, 386, 899
– ecchymosis 90
– lower gastrointestinal 372
– petechia 90
– purpura 90
– suffusion 90
– suggilation 90
– upper gastrointestinal 353
– varices 358
– vibices 90
Haemorrhoides 264
Haemosiderin 54, 88, 104, 226, 403, 638, 639, 839
Haemozoin 502

Hair changes 84
Hairy cell leukaemia 844
Haller 10, 11
Haller's tripod 20
Halo sign 144, 197, 682, 706, 804
Halogenated hydrocarbons 584
Halothane 560
Hamartoma 88, 783
Handwriting-specimen test 211
Harris-Benedict equation 880
Haruspices 3, 5
Head-out water immersion 335
Health awareness 911
Heater technique 357
Helicobacter pylori 61, 66, 274, 290, 291, 292, 545, 553, 554, 756, 760, 771, 772
HELLP 228
Helminthiasis 504
Helvella esculenta 588
Hepadnavirus 431
Hepar 2
Hepar lobatum 19, 490
Hepar succenturiatum 19, 630
Hepatic amoebiasis 499
Hepatic artery 20, 864
– aneurysm 864
– arteriosclerosis 866
– disorders 864
– occlusion 865
Hepatic blood flow 20, 57, 200, 252, 371, 445, 835, 839, 852, 853, 854, 877, 878, 900
Hepatic blood volume 762, 852
Hepatic brucelloma 490
Hepatic coma 284, 380, 386
– check-list 282
– electrolyte coma 285, 386
– endogenous 280, 386
– exogenous 285, 386
– profile 282
Hepatic foetor 77, 91, 92, 275, 280, 383, 425
Hepatic hydrothorax 304, 305, 308, 323, 324, 327, 759, 769, 770, 899
Hepatic porphyria 623
– acute intermittent 624
– cutanea tarda 626
– Doss porphyria 626
– erythropoietic 623
– hereditary coproporphyria 625
– PB-synthase defect 626
– variegate 625
Hepatic resistance 252
Hepatic storage disease 231
Hepatic triglyceride lipase 48
Hepatic vein 21, 856
Hepatic vein pressure 191, 197, 254, 376, 852, 853, 856, 860, 861, 863
Hepatic volume fraction 381
Hepatitis 411, 421
– anicteric 425

– cholestatic 424
– fulminant 425
– histomorphology 423
– history 421
– minimal 424
Hepatitis A virus 118, 119, 426
– clinical findings 429
– detection 427
– epidemiology 427
– immunization 430
– inactivation 427
– pathogen 118, 427
– serology 120, 121, 429
– transmission 427
Hepatitis B virus 119, 431
– chronic carrier 434
– clinical stages 439
– determinant "a" 419, 434
– ground-glass cell 120, 402, 432
– healing 446
– immunization 443
– inactivation 432
– pathogen 119, 431
– serology 120, 122, 431
– specific courses 434, 440
– therapy 445
– transmission 435
– variants 433
Hepatitis C virus 121, 448
– clinical stages 451
– epidemiology 449
– genotypes 121, 448
– morphology 451
– pathogen 448
– serology 121, 449
– transmission 450
Hepatitis D virus 122, 454
– coinfection 122, 455
– pathogen 454
– transmission 454
– serology 122, 455
– superinfection 122, 455
Hepatitis E virus 123, 456, 457
Hepatitis G virus 123, 458
Hepatitis mononucleosa 474
Hepatitis NANE 458
Hepatitis oedematosa 303, 445
Hepatoblast 16
Hepatoblastoma 817
Hepatocellular carcinoma 144, 183, 203, 442, 453, 548, 643, 719, 762, 798
– bull's eye 804
– bush pattern 805
– chemoembolization 809, 810
– consensus conference 807
– metastatic spread 802
– morphology 800, 802
– nodule-in-nodule 804
– risk factors 798
– score/classification 806
– spontaneous regression 807
– sunburst sign 805
– surgical therapy 807
Hepatocytes 11, 23, 25
– cellular polarization 25

– desmosome 25
– gap junctions 25
– tight junctions 25
Hepatocytolysis 432
Hepatoerythropoietic porphyria 628
Hepatogenesis 16
Hepatojugular reflux 855
Hepatolithiasis 674
Hepatomegaly 82, 218, 219, 400
Hepato-ovarian syndrome 754
Hepatopathy 78, 398
Hepatopexy 321, 898
Hepatoportal sclerosis 254, 862
Hepatopulmonary syndrome 340, 758
– clinical aspects 342
– pathogenesis 340
Hepatorenal glycogenosis 612
Hepatorenal syndrome 330, 386, 757
– azotaemia 332
– clinical course 331
– hyponatraemia 332
– oliguria 332
– pseudohepatorenal 333
– resistance index 332
Hepatoscopy 2, 158
– clay model 3, 4
– haruspices 3, 5
– inspection of entrails 2
– predictions 5
– sacrificial priests 2
Hepatosis 397, 404, 411, 412, 478
Hepatotesticular syndrome 754
Hepatotoxic remedies 569–575
Hepatotoxins 556
– facultative 557
– obligate 558
Hepatovenous pressure gradient 261
Herbal remedies 567, 894
Hereditary coproporphyria 625
Hereditary haemorrhagic telangiectasia 866
Hering's canal 22
Heron hepatitis 431
Herophilus 6, 252
Herpes virus hepatitis 475
Hers' disease 613
Herzberg-Potjan-Gebauer syndrome 84
Hexachlorobenzene 581, 626
HGM-CoA reductase 49
High-density lipoproteins 47, 550, 650
High-grade malignant NHL 837, 845
Hippie hepatitis 424
Hippocrates 6, 272
Histiocytosis X 848
Histological activity 127
Histological activity index 716
Histon 2B antibody 127, 537

Histoplasmosis 520
History 2
HIV 478
– cholangiopathy 478, 671
– hepatitis 478
HLA 640, 656, 675, 687
Hodgkin lymphoma 840
Hoesch test 623
Holly leaf fibrosis 413, 639
Homer 5
Homocysteine 748
Homocystinuria 612
Homotaurocholic acid test 202
Hormones 50
– classification 50
– effector hormones 50
Hounsfield unit 177, 178, 179, 602
Hour-glass nails 90, 342, 343, 758
Human albumin 314, 356
Human herpes virus 476
Human parvovirus B19 478
Hunter's syndrome 619
Hyaline bodies 401, 402, 423, 424, 831
Hyaline drops 401
Hyaline inclusion bodies 802
Hyaloplasm 29
Hyaluronan 410, 747, 750, 770
Hybridization test 121
Hydatid cyst 141, 510
Hydatid sand 510
Hydrocarbon derivatives 585
Hydrophylic xenobiotics 56
Hydropic liver cell 29, 218, 401, 539, 560
Hydrostatic pressure 297
Hydroxyethyl starch 757
Hydroxynonenal 73
Hypalbuminaemia 86, 95, 111, 112, 276, 296, 297, 302, 322, 332, 637
Hyperaminoaciduria 631
Hyperammonaemia 113, 274, 611, 753
Hyperbilirubinaemia 106, 225
– conjugated 225
– unconjugated 225
Hypercalciuria 631
Hypercholesterolaemia 109
Hyperdynamic circulation 85, 252, 253, 266, 268, 301, 342, 384, 745, 747, 762, 769, 862
Hyperechoic lesions 143
Hyperfibrinolysis 351
Hyperglycaemia 534
Hyperhydration 295
Hyperlipidaemia 534, 605
Hyperpigmentation 691
Hyperplasia of SER 559
Hypersiderinaemia 104, 642
Hypersplenism 221, 746
Hypertensive colonopathy 265
Hypertensive gastropathy 265, 760
Hypertrichosis 84
Hypertrophic osteoarthropathy 90, 342, 339, 340, 345, 758

Hyperuricaemia 535
Hypoalbuminaemia 86, 95, 111
Hypoalphalipoproteinaemia 617
Hypocoagulability 351
Hypoechoic lesions 142
Hypoglycaemia 384, 534, 752
Hypogonadism 641, 754
Hyponatraemia 314, 332, 334, 625
Hypotrichosis 84
Hypovitaminoses 753
Hypoxaemia 334, 342, 758

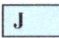

Icterus 6, 7, 8, 84, 106, 140, 224, 244, 383, 560
– carotene 224
– classification 224
– differential diagnosis 232
– flavin 80, 224
– haemolysis 226
– intermittens 229
– intrahepatic 226
– kernicterus 221, 228
– melas 80, 224
– neonatal 227
– posthepatic 227
– postoperative 227
– prehepatic 226
– rubin 80, 224
– scleral 84, 89, 106, 224
– subicterus 224
– verdin 80, 224
Idiopathic ductopenia 700
Idiosyncrasy 558, 559
Imiglucerase 618
Imaging procedures 132, 178, 184, 186, 191, 200, 748, 525, 775
Immune deficiency 533, 731, 754
Immunization 430, 443
Immunocytoma 844
Immunoglobulins 116, 443, 549
Immunogram 117
Immunologic tolerance 656
Immunostimulants 711, 723, 726, 730, 811, 871, 877, 885, 908, 915
Immunosuppressants 884
Inability to earn 913
Inactivation 57
Inclusion cell disease 620
Incomplete responder 724
Indian childhood cirrhosis 635
Indirect bilirubin 38, 105
Indocyanine green test 95, 98, 113, 114, 544, 601, 602, 747, 803, 808, 921
Indol 276
Indometacin 761
Induced cell 402
Industrial toxins 584
Infantile haemangioendothelioma 781
Infantile sclerosis 605

Infectious mononucleosis 474
Inferior vena cava 21
Inflammatory criteria 414, 803, 815, 823, 841, 842, 843, 845, 846, 847
Inflammatory pseudotumour 789
Infrequent blinking 90
Initiation 800
Innsbruck coma scale 282
Inspection 83
Insufficiency 400
– global 400
– partial 400
Insulin 50
Insulin resistance 600, 752
Insulin-glucagon quotient 48
Integrins 22
Intelligence 208
– crystalline 208, 280
– fluid 208, 280
Interdisciplinary conference 807, 825
Interface hepatitis 407, 660, 679, 712, 713, 725
Interferon 453, 723, 728, 882
– consensus 723, 883
– lymphoblastoid 723, 883
– modes of action 883
– pegylated 723, 728, 883
Interleukin 726
Interlobular artery 20
Interlobular vein 21
Intermediate filament 32
Interstitial syphilitic hepatitis 489
Intestinal varices 264, 760
Intestinal vasculopathy 265
Intoxication, chronic 588
Intranuclear inclusions 402
Ionogram 294
Iris-diaphragm phenomenon 143, 182, 780
Iron 54, 104, 637, 638, 727
– binding capacity 642
– body iron content 54
– depletion 637, 644, 727, 764
– index 640, 642
– low-iron diet 644, 727
Iron-copper constellations 108
Ischaemic infarction 865
Isocitrate dehydrogenase 100
Isohydria 295
Isotonicity 295
Isovolaemia 294, 295
Itching s. Pruritus
Ito cells 16, 24

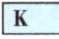

Jamshidi needle 152, 155, 156, 157
Jaundice s. icterus
Juberg-Clayton type 242

K

Kala-azar 501
Kalk's point 162

Index

Kallikrein-kinin system 299
Kaposi sarkoma 476
Karyoplasm 29
Kasabach-Merritt syndrome 781, 782
Kayser-Fleischer corneal ring 90, 245, 631
Kernicterus 37, 228, 229
Ketoacidosis 547, 605
Ketogenesis 46
Ketolithocholic acid 40
Ketone bodies 753
Kirros 738
Klatskin's tumour 814
Koller's test 111, 244
Kupffer cell 16, 24
Kurorinone 726
Kwashiorkor 84, 88, 604

L

Laboratory diagnostics 96, 98, 305, 548, 803
– algorithmic diagnostics 127
– check-list 92, 99, 283, 567, 768
– four epochs 96
– specimen transport 96
– substrat stability 96
Labrea fever 402
Lacquered lips 87
Lactate dehydrogenase 95, 100, 103
Lactitol 287
Lactoferrin 54
Lactulose 287, 887
– chemistry 887
– modes of action 888
– pharmacology 888
Lafora body 403, 620
Lafora's disease 620
Lakeland plain 141
Lambliasis 500
Lamivudine 389, 725, 883
Langhans' giant cell 486, 788
LAP 108
Laparoscopy 138, 157
– adhesiolysis 159
– adiposity 161
– children 161
– cirrhosis/fibrosis 165, 168
– complications 167
– contraindications 159
– diagnostic validity 168
– extrahepatic findings 166
– hernias 161
– history 157
– indications 158
– inspection schedule 162
– mini-laparoscopy 170
– photodocumentation 164
– portal hypertension 260
– serosa syndrome 160
– sonography 170
– technique 161
Large intestinal fluke 508
Large liver fluke 507
Laronidase 619
Lassa fever 480
Late bleeding 154

Latent ascites 311, 768
Latent HE 208, 280, 756
Latent oedema 280, 296, 303, 311
Lattice fibre network 23
LDH 103
– ratio 103, 307
– LDH/GOT ratio 101
L-dopa 289
Lead 586
Lebara 2
Lecithin-cholesterol-acyltransferase 48
Lectin receptor 812
Leiomyoma 783
Leiomyosarcoma 818
Leishmaniasis 501
Lepra granuloma 488
Leptin 605
Leptospirosis 488
Leroy syndrome 620
Lethargy 272
Leucine arylamidase 108
Leukaemia 838
– acute 838
– chronic lymphatic 843
– chronic myeloid 839
– hairy cell 844
– plasma cell 844
Leukotriene 676
LeVeen shunt 317
Li-Fraumeni syndrome 800
Ligand 49, 58
Ligandin 225
Light bulb sign 780
Limiting plate 24, 26, 27
Line-tracing test 213
Linolenic acid 48
Linolic acid 48
Linton-Nachlas tube 365
Lipid accumulation 402
Lipid metabolism 46, 753
Lipid peroxidation 73, 408, 536, 538, 603
Lipid topogenesis 47
Lipiodol 809
Lipoamide dehydrogenase 426
Lipofuscin 401, 403, 423, 559, 604
Lipogenesis 47, 753
Lipogranuloma 405
Lipoma 782
Lipophagic granuloma 539
Lipophilic xenobiotics 56
Lipoprotein X 112, 244
Lipoproteins 46, 48, 70, 244, 753
Liposarcoma 819
Lipotropic substances 603
Liquorice 311, 314
Listeriosis 490
Lithocholic acid 40
LITT 810, 826
Liver abscess 142, 183, 186, 500, 524, 787
– cluster sign 525
– comet-tail phenomenon 525
– double wheel structure 526
– pathogens 524
– target phenomenon 526

Liver atrophy 82, 381
Liver biopsy 18, 150, 165, 602, 805
– children 155
– complications 154
– contraindications 152
– history 150
– indications 151
– outpatient biopsy 156
– postpuncture complaints 153
– technique 152, 153
– transfemoral 156
– transjugular 156
Liver capsule 22
Liver cell rosette 237, 407, 424, 660
Liver clay model 2, 3, 4
Liver decompensation 385
Liver dystrophy 425
Liver collapse fibrosis 414
Liver colour 18
Liver function tests 98, 101, 113, 747
Liver infarction 182
Liver injury 182, 902
Liver in shock 853
Liver insufficiency 380
– acute 380
– compensation 385
– decompensation 385
– global 380, 385
– partial 380, 385
Liver lobule 26, 28, 29
Liver palpation 6, 81
Liver position 18
Liver regeneration 5, 17
Liver resection 516, 807, 825, 900
– dorsocranial 901
– functional reserve 900
– hemihepatectomy 901
– lobectomy 901
– metastasectomy 825
– R-resection 826
– segmentectomy 825, 901
Liver segments 9, 10, 19, 135, 137, 147, 901
Liver shape 18
Liver siderosis 539, 645
Liver size 18, 383
Liver stem cells 17
Liver stroma 22
Liver support system 389
Liver surface 18
– diaphragmatic 18
– visceral 18
Liver therapy 875
– active substances 876
– aims 876
– antidotes 876
– drug 881
Liver tongue 87
Liver topography 18
Liver transplantation 268, 322, 336, 343, 372, 392, 665, 686, 693, 730, 903
– aftercare 910
– APOLT 392, 907
– endothelialitis 909
– heterotopic 392, 907

– immunosuppression 908
– indications 903
– infection 907, 909
– living donation 392, 907
– orthotopic 392, 907
– postoperative features 908
– preoperative diagnostics 905
– rehabilitation 910
– relapse 910
– shunt and TIPS 906
– split liver 392, 907
– transplant rejection 909
– xenotransplantation 393
Liver weeping 297, 298
Liver weight 17
Lobar agenesis 19
Lobar atrophy 19
Lobucavir 725, 855, 882, 884
Looser-Milkman syndrome 755
Losartan 366, 757
Low-density lipoproteins 47
Lower gastrointestinal bleeding 372
Low-grade malignant NHL 843
Low-T3 syndrome 754
Lucey-Driscoll syndrome 228
Lues 489
Lumbar blockade 335
Lunulae 88, 632, 651
Lupoid hepatitis 656, 660
Lupus erythematosus 847
Luteoskyrin 587
Lutzner cell 844
Lycopenaemia 224
Lyme hepatitis 490
Lymphangioma 787
Lymph imbalance theory 300
Lymphadenopathy 143, 662, 718, 721
Lymphatic vessels 7, 10, 12, 22, 149, 164, 193, 224, 231, 241, 297, 679, 759
Lymphcysts 265, 298
Lymphoblastoid IFN 883
Lysosomes 30, 630

M

Machinery murmur 254, 259
Macroenzymes 101
Macrovesicular steatosis 560, 597
Maddrey risk index 545
Magna form 499
Magnetic resonance imaging 184
– basic informations 184
Malabsorption 248
Malaria 501
– pathogen 501
– pigment 403, 502
– prophylaxis 502
– therapy 503
Malate-aspartate cycle 67
Malignant lymphoma 183, 820
Malignant melanoma 164, 819
Malignant tumour 186, 188, 416, 564, 796

– classification 796
– TNM staging 797
Mall's space 22, 23
Mallory-Denk body 237, 403, 404, 451, 538, 544, 598, 602, 612, 630, 679, 720, 802,
Mallory-Weiss syndrome 760
Malnutrition 543, 604, 802, 880
Malondialdehyde 73
MALT 548, 820
Maltrozyne 587
Manganese 55, 277
Mannite solution 286
Mannitol 314, 335
Mannitol test 314
Mannosidosis 620
Marburg virus disease 479
Marchand's cirrhosis 740
Maroteauy-Lamy syndrome 620
MARS 336, 390, 552, 683
MAST 548
Mastocytosis 847
Matrix metalloproteinase 743
Mauriac syndrome 607
McBurney point 305
McCurdy cell 535
MCT 810
Mean corpuscular volume 549
Measles hepatitis 477
Medium-chain fatty acid 241, 683
Melaena 355, 373
Melas icterus 84, 224
MELS 391
Membrane 31
– flip-flop 31
– fluidity 31
– hyperplasia 59, 400, 537, 559
– lateral diffusion 31
Membrofenin 116
Menghini biopsy 151, 157, 165
MEOS 67, 534, 536
Mercaptan 275
Mesenchymal activity 117, 118, 747
Mesenchymal hamartoma 783
Mesenchymal reaction 561
Mesenchymal tumour 797, 817
Mesothelioma 783
Metabolic acidosis 63
Metabolic alkalosis 63
Metabolic detoxification 57
Metabolic disease 595, 881
Metabolic functions 595
Metabolic heterogeneity 27
Metabolism 36
– decompensation 745
– disorders 595
– functions 36, 595
– heterogeneity 27, 36
– periportal zone 37
– perivenous zone 38
Metabolite 556
Metabonate 556
Metallothioneine 55
Metastasis 183, 186, 201, 820
– calcified 823
– morphology 821

– spontaneous regression 821
– surgical therapy 825
Meteorism 83, 304, 385, 747
Methanol 536, 542
Methotrexate 683, 684, 885
Methylene blue 343, 346, 759, 771, 901
Methylene dianiline 581, 585
Methylumbelliferone 57, 98, 113, 854
Metoclopramide 367
Metronidazole 289, 310, 492, 500, 501, 527, 536, 624, 675, 683, 693, 756, 906
Meyenburg complex 698, 787
MgSO$_4$ solution 286
MHC system 656
Micelle formation 41
Microhamartoma 698
Microtrabecula 32
Microtubule 32
Microvesicular steatosis 560
Microvilli 21
MIGET 342
Miliary tuberculosis 486
Mini-laparoscopy 170
Minimal hepatitis 424
Minnesota tube 365
Minuta form 499
Mirizzi syndrome 227, 671
Misoprostol 335, 336, 446, 463
Misty mesentery 305
Mitochondria 30, 31, 39
Mitochondrial GOT 102, 549
Mixed cryoglobulinaemia 719
Mixed tumour 796
Mn-SOD 676
Moist warmth 445
Molecular mimicry 656, 677
Molsidomine 267, 366, 367, 368, 759, 760, 767
Monoethylglycinexylidide test 115
Monopolar probe 357
Morphological lesions 98, 423, 559, 714, 715, 739, 774
Morquio's syndrome 620
Morrison's pouch 141
Morula cells 402
Mount St. Helen's sign 360
Mucoepidermoid carcinoma 814
Mucolipidosis 620
Mucopolysaccharidosis 619
Mucormycosis 520
Mucoviscidosis 620, 699
Muehrke's nail lines 86
Multicentric Castelman disease 476
Multiple myeloma 845
Muralium 16
Muscle cramps 746
Mycobacterium 486
Mycophenolate mofetil 665, 666, 684, 703, 908, 922
Mycoplasma pneumoniae 485
Mycosis 518
Mycosis fungoides 844
Mycotoxin 587
Mycotoxin theory 676

Myelolipoma 782
Myeloproliferative syndrome 839

N

N-acetylcysteine 72, 335, 336, 387, 389, 395, 569, 588, 589, 876
NaCl-tolerance test 300
Nadolol 267, 268, 366, 367, 368, 375, 377, 378, 760, 767, 770
Nagayo type 740
Naloxone 241, 243, 249, 683
Naltrexone 233, 241, 249, 250, 683
Natriuretic factors 299
N-butyl-cyanoacrylate 358, 362, 363
Necrapoptosis 407
Necrosis 406, 539
– bridging 407
– coagulation 407, 560
– colliquation 407
– confluent 407
– piecemeal 407, 649
– single-cell 407, 539, 559
Nectins 22
Needlestick-injury 438, 443, 450, 453, 466
Neisseria gonorrhoeae 485
Nematodes 504
Neodymium YAG laser 358
Neomycin 288
Neonatal haemochromatosis 637
Neonatal jaundice 227
Nervous system 26
Network necrosis 238
Neuroblastoma 825
Neuroendocrine tumour 203, 819
Neuropsychological test 209, 281
– test combinations 209
Neurotensin 813
Neurotransmitter 276
Newcastle infection 437
Nicotine acid test 230
Niemann-Pick disease 619
Nikolsky's phenomenon 627
Nitric oxide 302, 330, 340
Nitrovasodilator 366
Nodular periarteritis 865
Nodular regenerative hyperplasia 144, 779
Nodule-in-nodule 804
Non-alcoholic fatty liver 595
Non-alcoholic steatohepatitis 599
– diagnosis 601
– morphology 600
– pathogenesis 600
– therapy 603
Non-Hodgkin lymphoma 842
Non-Indian childhood cirrhosis 635
Non-responder 444, 445, 655, 665, 730

Non-specific reactive hepatitis 398, 399, 477, 484, 501, 503, 509, 562, 712, 847
Noradrenaline 276, 300
North American Indian cirrhosis 699
Nosocomial infection 309, 427, 437, 450
Notifiable disease 118, 428, 435, 449, 498
Nucleosides 725, 883
Nucleotidase 108
Number-connection test 212
Nutmeg liver 855
Nutrition 550, 765, 878
– arterial 879
– enteral 879
– parenteral 766, 879
– reference values 880
– resting energy expenditure 880
– special diets 880, 881

O

Obesity 550, 593, 599, 605, 646, 647, 828, 905, 922
Obligate hepatotoxins 558
Obligation for notification 428, 435, 474, 478, 484, 498
Obliterative hepatic endophlebitis 257
Obstructive cholestasis 236
Obstructive jaundice 101, 111, 140, 152, 193, 227, 246, 591, 793
Occult blood 259, 355, 373
Occupational disease 438, 583
Ochratoxin 587
Octopamine 276
Octreotide 305, 335, 367, 811, 820
Oedema 295, 311, 386
Oedema disease 296
Oedematization 296
Oesophageal varices 262, 358, 760
– balloon tamponade 365, 366
– endoscopy 359
– endosonography 360
– gastric varices 363
– sclerotherapy 361
– surgical treatment 369
– variceal ligation 364
– varices pressure 262
Oesophagogastroscopy 260, 359
Oestrogens 50
Old Testament 3, 5
Oliguria 332
Omentopexie 321
Omphaloportography 190
Ondansetron 241, 249
Open reading frame 119
Opioid peptides 536
Opisthorchis felineus 508
Opisthorchis viverrini 508
Opsonin 70
Organelle 25, 29, 30, 36

Organoscopy 157
Oriental cholangiohepatitis 672
Ornipressin 314, 335, 336, 337, 770
Ornithine-α-ketoglutarate 287
Ornithine aspartate 287, 288, 319, 334, 351, 388, 589, 743, 764, 767, 880, 891, 906, 917
Ornithine carbamoyl transferase 100
Ornithine cycle 61
Ornithosis 491
Orthodeoxia 342, 345, 346
Osler-Rendu-Weber disease 348, 866
Osmolality 295
Osmolarity 295
Osmotic diuresis 314
Osteoarthropathy 90, 339, 340, 342, 345, 758
Osteomalacia 755
Osteomyelofibrosis 839
Osteopathy 248, 648, 683, 691, 754, 755
Osteoporosis 546, 754
Osteoprotegerin 546
Osteosarcoma 819
Outlier syndromes 695
Overflow theory 300
Overlap syndrome 695
Owl's eyes 476
Oxaliplatin 827
Oxidative energy 48
Oxidation reaction 58
Oxidative stress 73, 381, 408
Oxygen consumption 21, 48, 752, 852
Oyster hepatitis 427

P

P-300 wave 209, 283
Pain on pressure 82
Paints, varnishes 585
PAIR 511
Palmar erythema 85
Palpation 6, 81, 83
– Chauffard 81
– Gilbert 81
– liver 81
– spleen 83
Paltauf-Sternberg cell 840
pANCA 127, 687, 691
Paper money skin 86
Papyrus Ebers 5
Paracelsus XIX, 9, 83, 923
Paracentesis 7, 314, 757
Paracetamol 382, 388
Paralytic cholestasis 237
Paramyxovirus 477
Paraneoplastic symptoms 803
Parasitic cholangitis 671
Parasitic cysts 784
Parasitic infection 498, 815
Parchment skin 86
Parenchyma 6, 10, 26
Parenteral feeding 387, 879
Paromomycin 288

Parotid enlargement 84
Parotitis hepatitis 477
Paroxysmal haemoglobinuria 840
Partial nodular hyperplasia 779
Partial responder 724
Patellar chondromalacia 631
Paucity, bile ducts 697
Paul-Bunnel test 474
Pegylated IFN 453, 727, 882
PEI 826
Pel-Ebstein fever 841
Peliosis hepatis 404, 487, 787
Penicillamine 628, 633, 635, 683, 892
Pentastomum denticulatum 506
Pentoxifylline 544, 552
Pepper's syndrome 825
Percussion 83
– ascites 83
– liver 83
– spleen 83
Periarteritis nodosa 846
Peribiliary plexus 864
Pericanalicular ectoplasm 21
Pericholangitis 688
Perihepatitis gonorrhoica 485
Perinatal infection 436
Peripolesis 407
Periportal inflammation 713
Periportal zone 37
Peritoneoscopy 157
Perisinusoidal functional unit 24
Perisplenitis cartilaginea 839
Peritoneal tuberculosis 167
Peritoneovenous shunt 317, 336, 899
Perivascular connective tissue 23
Perivenous zone 37
Perivenular fibrosis 414, 540
Perna disease 584
Peroxisome 30, 31, 68, 630
PET 203, 805
Petechia 90
Petren's venous plexus 266
Pfaundler-Hurler syndrome 619
Phagocytosis 24, 69
Pharmacogenetics 57
Phenobarbital 249
Phenols 275
Phenylethanolamine 276
Phlebography 190
Phlogogram 307
Phosphaturia 631
Phosphatidylcholine (s. EPL) 48, 228, 240, 388, 394, 543, 551, 553, 647, 767, 893, 894, 895, 896, 898, 918, 919
Phosphohexoisomerase 100
Phospholipidosis 559, 598
Phospholipids 48, 543
Phosphorus 382, 394, 580, 583, 584, 586, 590, 591, 599, 744, 880
Phototherapy 228, 229, 233, 234, 241, 249

Phyllanthus 726, 898
Physical activity 551, 683, 755, 765
Phytotherapeutics 894
Phytotoxin 257, 579, 587, 599, 605, 744, 799, 857
Pi nomenclature 608
Pick cell 619
Picornavirus 118
Piecemeal necrosis 407, 414, 415, 656, 660, 679, 689, 712, 713, 714, 715
Pigment calculus 633, 761, 840
Pigment cirrhosis 639
Pigmentation 88, 618, 632, 635
Pin cells 402
Pinguecula 90, 618
Pinocytosis 24
Piracetam 289
Pit cell 25
Placebo 874
Plantar erythema 85
Plasma cell leukaemia 845
Plasma perfusion 389
Plasmapheresis 228, 233, 234, 241, 389, 395, 450, 466, 628, 635, 644, 707
Plasminogen 319
Plasmocytoma 844
Platon 6
Platypnoea 342
Pleural effusion 304, 759
Pleural spider naevi 341
Plexogenic arteriopathy 344, 758
Plinius 7
Pneumoperitoneum 162
Poems syndrome 302, 316
Poisoning 589
– five-finger rule 589
– information centre 589
Polidocanol 358, 362
Polycystic liver disease, adult 141, 784
Polycythaemia vera 839
Polyendocrine syndrome 659
Polyenylphosphatidylcholine (s. EPL) 388, 394, 894, 918
Polymerase-chain reaction 121
Polymyalgia rheumatica 846
Polymyositis 846
Pompe's disease 613
Porcelain liver 800
Pores 24
Porphobilinogen 39, 627
Porphyria cutanea tarda 84, 88, 166, 626, 645
Porphyria, alcoholic 535
Porphyrias 621
– biochemistry 621
– haem 37, 38
– metabolism 38
– red fluorescence 39
Portacaval anastomosis 113, 290, 321, 330, 370, 761
Portacaval myelopathy 281
Portal biliopathy 266
Portal fibrosis 413, 561
Portal field 24

Portal hepatitis 712, 713
Portal hypertension 139, 163, 252, 509, 547, 548, 641, 681, 745
– intrahepatic 254
– posthepatic 257
– prehepatic 253
– presinusoidal block 255
– postsinusoidal block 256
– segmental 254
– sequelae 261
– shunt operation 267
– sonography 259
– splenic infarction 261
– vasculopathy 265
Portal hypertensive gastropathy 760
Portal tract 24
Portal vein 21, 163, 252, 860
– anomalies 860
– aneurysm 863
– disorders 860
– double-flow principle 19
– inner root 21
– thrombosis 141, 254, 840, 862
Portal vein amputation 140
Portal vein lobule 27
Portal vein pressure 261, 266
Portography 189
Portopulmonary hypertension 266, 758
Portosystemic encephalopathy 280
Posner test 210
Postsinusoidal block 256
Potassium canrenoate 312, 313, 324, 811, 812, 828, 907
Potassium sulphide 635
Potato liver 381, 740
Power Doppler US 134
PPSB 353
Prealbumin 44, 111, 112, 129
Preanalytical phase 97
Prednimustine 685
Prednisolone 605, 612, 613, 683
Pregnancy 436, 442
Pressure gradient 359
Preventive medicine 912
Primary biliary cholangitis 126, 675
– aetiology 675
– clinical courses 679
– complications 680
– morphology 678
– pathogenesis 677
– therapy 683
Primary sclerosing cholangitis 686
– aetiopathogenesis 687
– clinical aspects 689
– diagnosis 689
– morphology 688
– systematics 686
– therapy 692
Probiotics 287
Procalcitonin 384
Procollagen-III-peptide 118, 540, 550, 855
Profibrinogen 410

Progesterone 50
Progressive cholestasis 241
Proliferation 739
Prometheus 5
Prometheus system 390
Promotion 800
Proper hepatic artery 20
Propranolol 267, 367
Prostaglandins 299, 389
Protein 44
− metabolism 44, 64
− tolerance threshold 278, 286
Proteoglycane 22
Prothrombin 111, 348
Proton MR spectroscopy 209, 280
Protoporphyrin 37, 39, 237, 621, 622, 623, 624, 625, 626
− degradation 64
Protothecosis 520
Protozoiasis 498
Pruritus 89, 240, 243, 249, 683, 692
PSE syndrome test 211
Pseudoaldosteronism 897
Pseudo-Bartter syndrome 314
Pseudo-double-barrelled gun 139
Pseudo-Gaucher cells 402
Pseudohepatorenal syndrome 329, 332, 333
Pseudo-Lafora body 403
Pseudo-parallel channel sign 545
Psittacosis 491
Psychometric tests 211, 281, 283, 881
− critical flicker test 211, 281
− graphological identity 211
− handwriting-specimen 211
− line-tracing 213
− multiple choice device 210
− number-connection 212
− Posner test 210
− pychometric test set 211
− serial-subtraction 213
− SIP 210
− star-construction 213
− story-retelling 214
− test programme 210, 880
PTC 193, 674
PTCS 194
Puddle sign 304
Pugh criteria 763
Purpura 90, 386
Push enteroscopy 373
Pylephlebitis 862
Pyridoxin deficiency 635
Pyrrolizidine alkaloids 257, 568, 579, 587, 859

Q

Quality of life 878
Quartan malaria 501
Quick's value 111, 244
Quadrate lobe 18, 20, 137, 139, 187, 749, 770, 901
Questions 81
Q-fever 491

R

RAAS 298, 756
R-classification 808
Radiofrequency thermal ablation 811, 827
Radionuclids 200
Reactive oxygen intermediate 71, 408
− formation 71
− inactivation 71
− radicals 71
Recombinant IFN 882
Recurrent cholestasis, pregnancy 240, 241
Red fluorescence 166, 622
Red wall markings 360
Re-exposure trial 569
Reflex density 138
Reflex distribution 138
Refractory ascites 316
Refsum's syndrome 242
Regeneration 5, 385, 408, 416, 424, 742, 902
Regenerative nodes 139, 256, 416, 610, 689, 739, 742, 774, 779, 855
Regulator protein 409
Rehabilitation 912
Reichenstein disease 580
Renal failure 384
Renal natriuretic factor 299
Rendu-Osler-Weber disease 866
Respiratory insufficiency 384
RES-scintigraphy 200
Resting energy expenditure 880
Reticulin 23, 124, 412, 413, 751, 779, 841
Reticuloendothelial system 69
− functions 69
Retinol ester 24, 25, 44, 51, 55, 535, 753
Retothelial nodule 404, 487
Retraction of the eyelid 90
Retroperitoneal varices 265
Retzius veins 265
Rex-Cantlie's line 19, 20
Reye's syndrome 279, 606
Reynold's pentad 672
RFTA 826, 810
Rhabdomyolysis 632
Rhabdomyosarcoma 819
Rheumatoid arthritis 845
Rheumatoid factor 124, 845
Rhodanine 630
Ribavirin 729, 884
Ribosome 23, 29, 30, 31, 36, 44, 109, 124, 125, 537
Rickettsiosis 491
Riedel's lobe 18, 82, 137
Rifampicin 225, 226, 230, 234, 249, 382, 487, 488, 491, 565, 574, 576, 599, 624, 626, 683, 703, 895
Rift Valley fever 480
Rima coeci Halleri 18
Rituximab 843
RNA polymerases 44
Robbers forceps 165, 169, 170, 453, 563, 776, 806
Rochalimaea 492
Rocky Mountain spotted fever 491
Rotor syndrome 231
Rough endoplasmic reticulum 23, 29, 30, 36, 44, 47, 48, 109, 230, 539, 559, 560, 566, 596
Round ligament 21, 18, 136, 162, 163, 179, 254, 264, 265, 818, 860
Rubella hepatitis 477
Rubin icterus 84, 224
Rufus 7

S

Sacrificial priest 2
S-adenosyl-L-methionine 233, 241, 249, 543, 552, 893
Saint's venous plexus 266
Salad oil 581
Salmonellosis 486
Sanded nuclei 402, 720
Sanfilippo's syndrome 619
Sappey's vein 92, 265
Sarcoidosis 405, 406, 788
Saturnism 586
Scarred liver 381, 412, 738, 751
Scavenger 72, 551, 896
Schaumann bodies 788
Schistosomiasis 255, 509
Schizandra 726, 898
Schoenlein-Henoch disease 348
Schwannoma 783, 819
Scintigraphy 200, 373
Scleral icterus 84, 89, 106, 224
Sclerosing hyaline fibrosis 540
Sclerotherapy 361
Scoring systems 716
Scratch auscultation 83
Scratch mark 89, 240, 243
Screening enzyme 102
Sea-anemone phenomenon 141, 304
Sea-blue histiocytes 619
Secondary aldosteronism 275, 278, 299, 462
Section planes 136
Segmental portal hypertension 254
Segmental subdivisions 19, 20, 135, 137, 899, 901
Selenite 310, 388
Selenium 55, 444, 551, 811, 885
Self-help groups 914
Senecio alkaloids 563
Sengstaken-Blakemore tube 365
Senile atrophy 136
SEN virus 460
Septa 742, 414
Septal fibrosis 397, 413, 414, 541, 553, 661, 678, 720, 722
Sequential nephron blockade 314
Sequential scintigraphy 201

Serial-subtraction test 213
Serological markers 118, 122, 429, 432, 449, 455, 458, 657
Serosa syndrome 160
Serotonin 276
Sertraline 241, 249, 574, 577
Sexually transmitted disease 436, 467
Sezary syndrome 844
Sheep lice 446
Shigella 486
Shock liver 853
Short-chain fatty acid 47, 271, 273, 275, 276, 752, 753
Sho-Saiko-To 898
Shunt operation 267, 370, 899
Shunt-bilirubin 37
Siberian liver fluke 508
Sickle-cell anaemia 840
Sickness impact profile 210
Siderin 423
Sideronecrosis 639
Siderophile hepatitis 639
Siderosis 539
Sieve plate 24
Signal substances 24, 49, 70
Silibinin 587, 896
Silvestrini-Corda syndrome 754
Silymarin 385, 551, 644, 727, 896
Simian cleft 19, 630, 741
Simvastatin 683
Sinusoidal block 255
Sinusoidal cell 24
Sinusoids 13, 16, 21, 24
SIP 210
Sirolimus 908
Sjögren's syndrome 846
Skatol 276
Skin stigmata in liver diseases 84, 747
Skirros 6, 738
Small-duct PSC 688
Smooth cirrhosis 256, 739
Smooth endoplasmic reticulum 23, 28, 29, 30, 51, 57, 59, 68, 105, 125, 218, 229, 237, 400, 401, 432, 537, 542, 559, 560, 606
Smooth red tongue 86
Snowball 143
Sociomedical aspects 911
− capacity for work 912
− disability 913
− guidelines for evaluation 913
− health awareness 911
− inability to earn 913
− preventive medicine 912
− rehabilitation 912
− unfitness for work 913
Sodium benzoate 287
Somatostatin 366, 811, 892
Somnolence 272
Sonography 132, 304, 804, 823
− artefacts 133
− basic information 132
− biopsy 133
− contrast medium 135

935

Index

– echo types 132
– endoscopic 135
– section planes 136
Sopor 272
Sorbitol clearance 116
Sorbitoldehydrogenase 100
SPAD 390
Specimen identification 97
– specimen stability 97
SPECT 196, 200, 201, 202, 203, 205, 206, 756, 763, 792, 805, 842
Speculative therapy 872
Sphingomyelin 619
Spider naevus 84
– incomplete 85
– liver surface 627
Spill-over effect 761
Spiral-CT 179
Spironolactone 87, 267, 299, 311, 312, 366, 767
Spleen 83, 145, 163, 220
– scintigraphy 220
Splendore-Hoeppli syndrome 404, 509
Splenic infarction 261, 747
Splenomegaly 83, 145, 220, 261
Splenoportography 189, 260
– direct 189, 260
– indirect 190, 260
Splenorenal varices 265
Spontaneous bacterial peritonitis 293, 308, 316, 324, 331, 334, 546, 746, 764
Spontaneous Talma 160, 264, 163
Spring-summer encephalitis hepatitis 479
SQUID biosusceptiometer 640, 642
Staghorn calculus 691, 790
Staging 714, 715
Standard test meal 259
Staphylococcus 485
Star-construction test 213
Star-filled sky 585
Starling forces 294, 297
Statutory maternal guideline 436
Steatosis 539, 596, 721
– centroacinar 539, 598
– diffuse 539
– peripheral 539, 597
– zonal 539, 598
Stein-Leventhal syndrome 167
Stellate cell nodule 423, 561
Stellwag's sign 90
Stem cell 17
Stent insertion 693
Stercobilin 12, 38, 106
Steroid hormone 50
Stift cell 407
Still's disease 845
Storage diseases 595
Story-retelling test 214
Streaming liver 28
Streptococcus 485
Stress metabolism 753
Stroma 22
Strongyloides stercoralis 506
Stuart-Bras symdrome 256, 257, 859
Stupor 272, 273, 279, 286, 382
Subacute liver failure 381
Subicterus 224
Sublingual varices 265
Suffusion 90
Sugar-icing spleen 839
Suggillation 90, 386
Sulpholithocholic acid 40
Summerskill-Tygstrup type 241
Sunburst sign 805
Sunflower cataract 90, 631
Superoxide dismutase 54, 55, 56, 59, 70, 72, 603, 676, 705, 886, 897, 919
Surgical therapy 898
Symporter 74
Syphilis 489
Syphiloma 489
Systematization 398

T

Tacrolimus 665, 885
Tangier disease 617
Target phenomenon 144, 526
Tarry stool 6, 355, 373
Tauro-ursodeoxycholic acid 684
Techneticum 200, 202
Telangiectasis 86, 866
Telbivudine 728
Tenofovir 726, 728
Terlipressin 335, 366, 760, 892
Terminal hepatic vein 21, 27
Terracotta model 2
Tertian malaria 501
Testicular atrophy 90, 641
Thalassaemia 840
Thalidomide 845
Therapy 872
– adjuvant measures 248, 271, 289, 358, 589, 603, 644, 730, 811, 817, 827, 828, 873
– drug therapy 881
– empirical 872
– mythological 872
– speculative 872
– statistical 872
Thermotherapy 810
Thesaurismoses 595
Thin spot 360
Thioacetamide 581
Thioredoxin 605
Thorotrast 580, 586
Threefold pattern 566
Thrombocytopenia 349
Thrombocytosis, essential 840
Thromboplastin time 111
Thymosin 726, 886
Thyroid hormone 51
Tight junctions 25
TIPS 267, 320, 336, 343, 368, 899
Tityos 5
TNM staging 163, 798
Togavirus 474
Topography 18
Torasemide 312, 313, 314, 324, 325, 335, 757
Torres bodies 402, 478
Torsade de points 361, 362
Torulopsosis 520
Toxic substances 580
Toxocariasis 506
Toxoplasmosis 503
Trace elements 53
Trail-making test 212
Transaminase 101, 102
Transarterial radiation 810
Transcuprin 629
Transcytosis 74
Transferrin 54, 638
– saturation 642
Transport protein 44
Transthyretin 609
Trematodes 507
Treponema pallidum 489
Tricarboxylic-acid cycle 43
Trichinella spiralis 507
Trichosporosis 520
Triethylene tetramine 635
Triglyceride 48, 595
Trocar 162
Trohoc 873
Tropheryma whippeli 491
Tropical juvenile cirrhosis 605
Tropical malaria 501
Tru-Cut needle 133, 152, 155, 156, 165, 169, 171, 173
Trypanosomiasis 504
Tryptophan 43, 276
TT virus 459
Tuberculoma 486
Tuberculosis 143, 166, 183, 486
Tuberculous pseudocirrhosis 487
Tularaemia 491
Tumour marker 822
Tumour staging 163
Tumour-suppressor gene 442, 800
Turkish non-syndromic paucity 699
TVC 194
Tympanic intestinal resonance 83
Typhoma 486
Tyrosinaemia 610

U

Ubiquitine 404, 538, 600, 647, 702
Ubiquinone 52, 765
Ullrich-Scheie syndrome 619
Ultrastructural heterogeneity 28
Underfill theory 300
Undernourishment 543
Unfit to drive 280
Unfitness for work 913
Uniporter 74
Uphill varices 262
Upper gastrointestinal bleeding 353
Urea cycle 61, 274, 611, 890
– ornithine aspartase 890
Urinary dipstick 106
Urobilin 12, 13, 38
Urobilinogen 38, 106
Urobilinogenuria 106, 226, 429, 747
Uroporphyrin 39
Ursodeoxycholic acid 40, 205, 233, 241, 242, 243, 248, 249, 250, 431, 445, 463, 464, 569, 575, 589, 603, 604, 620, 647, 650, 655, 664, 665, 683, 684, 692 - 697, 699, 700, 702 -710, 727, 730, 735, 764, 770, 785, 871, 876, 886, 887, 897, 910, 912, 915, 916, 920
– modes of action 886
– pharmacology 887
UV fluorescence 39, 153, 166, 622

V

Vaccination 431, 443, 723
Vagus shock 153
Valsalva's manoeuvre 141
Vancomycin 289
Vanishing bile-duct 240, 286, 296, 560, 696, 849
Variceal ligation 364
Varicella-zoster hepatitis 476
Varices 262, 358, 360
Variegate porphyria 625
Vascular reactions 562
Vascular star 778
Vasodilation theory 301
Veins of Retzius 265
Veins of Sappey 265
Venesection 628, 638, 641, 642, 643, 644, 645, 727
Venography 191
Veno-occlusive disease 140, 257, 562, 587, 839, 840, 859
Venous hum 92, 861
Ventroscopy 157
Verdin icterus 84, 224
Veres canula 161
Very low-density lipoprotein 47, 596
Vesalius 9
Vesicular transport 74
Vibices 90
Vim-Silverman needle 152, 155, 165, 169, 173, 750, 751
Vinyl chloride 581, 584, 818
Viral load 723
Virchow cell 488
Virtual liver surgery 807
Virus docking 431
Virustatics 881, 883
Visceropexie 321
Visually evoked potentials 209
Vital hepatocytes 391
Vitamins 51
– classification 51, 52
– fat-soluble 51, 52, 256
– water-soluble 52
Vitiligo 86
Volumen replacement 355, 361

W

Warren shunt 371
Wasting syndrome 752, 753
Water equilibrium 294
Watson-Schwartz test 623
Wegener's granulomatosis 847
Weibel-Palade body 818
Weil's disease 488
Wheels-within-wheels 519
Wheel-spoke phenomenon 141, 143, 778
Whipple disease 492
White liver 601, 642
White nails 86
White nipple sign 360
White spots, skin 86
WHVP 254, 255, 256, 257, 261, 262, 359, 893
Widmark's formula 65
Wieland test 588
Wilm's tumour 825
Wilson's disease 88, 628
Wireless capsule endoscopy 373
Withdrawal syndrome 551, 568
Wolman's disease 615
Woodchuck hepatitis virus 431

X

Xanthelasma 89, 243, 691
Xanthodermia 224
Xanthoma 89, 243, 615, 681
Xanthoma cells 238
Xanthomatous neuropathy 243, 681, 706
Xenobiotics 56, 556
– hydrophilic 56
– lipophilic 56
Xenotransplantation 392
Xipamide 313

Y

Yellow fever virus 478
Yellow spot 598, 782
Yersinia enterocolitica 484, 485, 486, 493, 529, 530, 643, 671, 701

Z

Zahn's furrow 18
Zahn's infarct 821, 862
Zellweger's syndrome 242, 620, 699
Ziehl-Neelsen 788
Zieve's syndrome 109, 239, 531, 536, 539, 547, 550
Zinc 55, 66, 105, 286, 444, 551, 635, 811, 885, 907
– metalloenzyme 55
Zinc deficiency 55, 683
Zonal heterogeneity 37